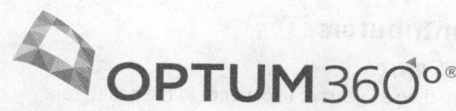

Current Procedural Coding Expert

CPT® codes with Medicare essentials for enhanced accuracy

2022

optum360coding.com

Notice

The *2022 Current Procedural Coding Expert, Professional Edition,* is designed to be an accurate and authoritative source of information about the CPT® coding system. Every effort has been made to verify the accuracy of the listings, and all information is believed reliable at the time of publication. Absolute accuracy cannot be guaranteed, however. This publication is made available with the understanding that the publisher is not engaged in rendering legal or other services that require a professional license.

American Medical Association Notice

Our Commitment to Accuracy

Optum360 is committed to producing accurate and reliable materials.

To report corrections, please email accuracy@optum.com. You can also reach customer service by calling 1.800.464.3649, option 1.

Copyright

Acknowledgments

Gregory A. Kemp, MA, *Product Manager*
Stacy Perry, *Manager, Desktop Publishing*
Elizabeth Leibold, RHIT, *Subject Matter Expert*
Anita Schmidt, BS, RHIA, AHIMA-approved ICD-10-CM/PCS Trainer, *Subject Matter Expert*
LaJuana Green, RHIA, CCS, *Subject Matter Expert*
Tracy Betzler, *Senior Desktop Publishing Specialist*
Hope M. Dunn, *Senior Desktop Publishing Specialist*
Katie Russell, *Desktop Publishing Specialist*
Kate Holden, *Editor*

About the Contributors

Elizabeth Leibold, RHIT

Ms. Leibold has more than 25 years of experience in the health care profession. She has served in a variety of roles, ranging from patient registration to billing and collections, and has an extensive background in both physician and hospital outpatient coding and compliance. She has worked for large health care systems and health information management services companies, and has wide-ranging experience in facility and professional component coding, along with CPT expertise in interventional procedures, infusion services, emergency department, observation, and ambulatory surgery coding. Her areas of expertise include chart-to-claim coding audits and providing staff education to both tenured and new coding staff. She is an active member of the American Health Information Management Association (AHIMA) and West Tennessee Health Information Management Association (WTHIMA).

Anita Schmidt, BS, RHIA, AHIMA-approved ICD-10-CM/PCS Trainer

Ms. Schmidt has expertise in ICD-10-CM/PCS, DRG, and CPT with more than 15 years' experience in coding in multiple settings, including inpatient, observation, and same-day surgery. Her experience includes analysis of medical record documentation, assignment of ICD-10-CM and PCS codes, and DRG validation. She has conducted training for ICD-10-CM/PCS and electronic health record. She has also collaborated with clinical documentation specialists to identify documentation needs and potential areas for physician education. Most recently she has been developing content for resource and educational products related to ICD-10-CM, ICD-10-PCS, DRG, and CPT. Ms. Schmidt is an AHIMA-approved ICD-10-CM/PCS trainer and is an active member of the American Health Information Management Association (AHIMA) and the Minnesota Health Information Management Association.

LaJuana Green, RHIA, CCS

Ms. Green is a Registered Health Information Administrator with over 35 years of experience in multiple areas of information management. She has proven expertise in the analysis of medical record documentation, assignment of ICD-10-CM and PCS codes, DRG validation, and CPT code assignment in ambulatory surgery units and the hospital outpatient setting. Her experience includes serving as a director of a health information management department, clinical technical editing, new technology research and writing, medical record management, utilization review activities, quality assurance, tumor registry, medical library services, and chargemaster maintenance. Ms. Green is an active member of the American Health Information Management Association (AHIMA).

Contents

Introduction

Welcome to Optum360's *Current Procedural Coding Expert, Professional Edition*, an exciting Medicare coding and reimbursement tool and definitive procedure coding source that combines the work of the Centers for Medicare and Medicaid Services (CMS), American Medical Association (AMA), and Optum360 experts with the technical components you need for proper reimbursement and coding accuracy.

This approach to CPT® Medicare coding utilizes innovative and intuitive ways of communicating the information you need to code claims accurately and efficiently. *Includes* and *Excludes* notes, similar to those found in the ICD-10-CM manual, help determine what services are related to the codes you are reporting. Icons help you crosswalk the code you are reporting to laboratory and radiology procedures necessary for proper reimbursement. CMS-mandated icons and relative value units (RVUs) help you determine which codes are most appropriate for the service you are reporting. Add to that additional information identifying age and sex edits, ambulatory surgery center (ASC) and ambulatory payment classification (APC) indicators, and Medicare coverage and payment rule citations, and *Current Procedural Coding Expert, Professional Edition* provides the best in Medicare procedure reporting.

Current Procedural Coding Expert, Professional Edition includes the information needed to submit claims to federal contractors and most commercial payers, and is correct at the time of printing. However, CMS, federal contractors, and commercial payers may change payment rules at any time throughout the year. *Current Procedural Coding Expert, Professional Edition* includes effective codes that will not be published in the AMA's Current Procedural Terminology (CPT) book until the following year. Commercial payers will announce changes through monthly news or information posted on their websites. CMS will post changes in policy on its website at http://www.cms.gov/transmittals. National and local coverage determinations (NCDs and LCDs) provide universal and individual contractor guidelines for specific services. The existence of a procedure code does not imply coverage under any given insurance plan.

Current Procedural Coding Expert, Professional Edition is based on the AMA's Current Procedural Terminology coding system, which is copyrighted and owned by the physician organization. The CPT codes are the nation's official, Health Information Portability and Accountability Act (HIPAA) compliant code set for procedures and services provided by physicians, ambulatory surgery centers (ASCs), and hospital outpatient services, as well as laboratories, imaging centers, physical therapy clinics, urgent care centers, and others.

Getting Started with *Current Procedural Coding Expert, Professional Edition*

Current Procedural Coding Expert, Professional Edition is an exciting tool combining the most current material at the time of our publication from the AMA's CPT 2022, CMS's online manual system, the Correct Coding initiative, CMS fee schedules, official Medicare guidelines for reimbursement and coverage, the Integrated Outpatient Code Editor (I/OCE), and Optum360's own coding expertise.

These coding rules and guidelines are incorporated into more specific section notes and code notes. Section notes are listed under a range of codes and apply to all codes in that range. Code notes are found under individual codes and apply to the single code.

Material is presented in a logical fashion for those billing Medicare, Medicaid, and many private payers. The format, based on customer comments, better addresses what customers tell us they need in a comprehensive Medicare procedure coding guide.

Designed to be easy to use and full of information, this product is an excellent companion to your AMA CPT manual, and other Optum360 and Medicare resources.

In anticipation of severe acute respiratory syndrome coronavirus 2 (SARS-CoV-2) (COVID-19) vaccines receiving Emergency Use Authorization (EUA) and/or FDA approval, and in order to expedite the availability of codes for coding and reimbursement, the AMA released a set of codes (0001A–0104A, 91300–91310) to be utilized upon receipt of EUA or FDA approval. In *Current Procedural Coding Expert, Professional Edition* these codes have been designated as placeholders and **PLACEHOLDER ONLY** appears next to the code. When the AMA releases an official code descriptor, Optum360 will update the corresponding electronic files and will provide updates to customers to allow them to update their *Current Procedural Coding Expert, Professional Edition* book.

For mid-year code updates, official errata changes, correction notices, and any other changes pertinent to the information in *Current Procedural Coding Expert, Professional Edition*, see our product update page at https://www.optum360coding.com/ProductUpdates/. The password for 2022 is PROCEDURE2022.

Note: The AMA releases code changes quarterly as well as errata or corrections to CPT codes and guidelines and posts them on their website. Some of these changes may not appear in the AMA's CPT book until the following year. *Current Procedural Coding Expert, Professional Edition* incorporates the most recent errata or release notes found on the AMA's website at our publication time, including new, revised and deleted codes. *Current Procedural Coding Expert, Professional Edition* identifies these new or revised codes from the AMA website errata or release notes with an icon similar to the AMA's current new ● and revised ▲ icons. For purposes of this publication, new CPT codes and revisions that won't be in the AMA book until the next edition are indicated with a ● and a ▲ icon. CPT codes that are new or revised during 2021 but do not appear in the AMA's CPT code book until 2023 are identified in appendix B as "Web Release New, Revised, and Deleted Codes." For the next year's edition of *Current Procedural Coding Expert, Professional Edition*, these codes will appear with standard black new or revised icons, as appropriate, to correspond with those changes as indicated in the AMA's CPT book.

General Conventions

Many of the sources of information in this book can be determined by color.

- All CPT codes and descriptions and the Evaluation and Management guidelines from the American Medical Association are in **black text**.
- Includes, Excludes, and other notes appear in **blue text**. The resources used for this information are a variety of Medicare policy manuals, the *National Correct Coding Initiative Policy Manual* (NCCI), AMA resources and guidelines, and specialty association resources and our Optum360 clinical experts.

Resequencing of CPT Codes

The American Medical Association (AMA) employs a numbering methodology of resequencing, which is the practice of displaying codes outside of their numerical order according to the description relationship. According to the AMA, there are instances in which a new code is needed within an existing grouping of codes, but an unused code number is not available. In these situations, the AMA will resequence the codes. In other words, it will assign a code that is not in numeric sequence with the related codes.

An example of resequencing from *Current Procedural Coding Expert, Professional Edition* follows:

	21555	Excision, tumor, soft tissue of neck or anterior thorax, subcutaneous; less than 3 cm
#	21552	3 cm or greater
	21556	Excision, tumor, soft tissue of neck or anterior thorax, subfascial (eg, intramuscular); less than 5 cm
#	21554	5 cm or greater

In *Current Procedural Coding Expert, Professional Edition* the resequenced codes are listed twice. They appear in their resequenced position as shown above as well as in their original numeric position with a note indicating that the code is out of numerical sequence and where it can be found. (See example below.)

21554   **Resequenced code. See code following 21556.**

This differs from the AMA CPT book, in which the coder is directed to a code range that contains the resequenced code and description, rather than to a specific location.

Resequenced codes will appear in brackets in the headers, section notes, and code ranges. For example:

> 27327-27339 [27337, 27339] Excision Soft Tissue Tumors Femur/Knee. Codes [27337, 27339] are included in section 27327-27339 in their resequenced positions.

> Code also toxoid/vaccine (90476-90749 [90619, 90620, 90621, 90625, 90630, 90644, 90672, 90673, 90674, 90750, 90756])

> This shows codes 90619, 90620, 90621, 90625, 90630, 90644, 90672, 90673, 90674, 90750, and 90756 are resequenced in this range of codes.

Code Ranges for Medicare Billing

Appendix E identifies all resequenced CPT codes. Optum360 will display the resequenced coding as assigned by the AMA in its CPT products so that the user may understand the code description relationships.

Each particular group of CPT codes in *Current Procedural Coding Expert, Professional Edition* is organized in a more intuitive fashion for Medicare billing, being grouped by the Medicare rules and regulations as found in the official CMS online manuals that govern payment of these particular procedures and services, as in this example:

99221-99233 Inpatient Hospital Visits: Initial and Subsequent
CMS: 100-4,11,40.1.3 Independent Attending Physician Services; 100-4,12,30.6.10 Consultation Services; 100-4,12,30.6.15.1 Prolonged Services With Direct Face-to-Face Patient Contact; 100-4,12,30.6.4 Services Furnished Incident to Physician's Service; 100-4,12,30.6.9 Hospital Visit and Critical Care on Same Day

Icons

● **New Codes**
Codes that have been added since the last edition of the AMA CPT book was printed.

▲ **Revised Codes**
Codes that have been revised since the last edition of the AMA CPT book was printed.

● **New Web Release**
Codes that are new for the current year but will not be in the AMA CPT book until 2023.

▲ **Revised Web Release**
Codes that have been revised for the current year, but will not be in the AMA CPT book until 2023.

Resequenced Codes
Codes that are out of numeric order but apply to the appropriate category.

★ **Telemedicine Services**
Codes that may be reported for telemedicine services. Modifier 95 must be appended to code.

○ **Reinstated Code**
Codes that have been reinstated since the last edition of the book was printed.

Pink Color Bar—Not Covered by Medicare
Services and procedures identified by this color bar are never covered benefits under Medicare. Services and procedures that

are not covered may be billed directly to the patient at the time of the service.

Gray Color Bar—Unlisted Procedure
Unlisted CPT codes report procedures that have not been assigned a specific code number. An unlisted code delays payment due to the extra time necessary for review.

Green Color Bar—Resequenced Codes
Resequenced codes are codes that are out of numeric sequence—they are indicated with a green color bar. They are listed twice, in their resequenced position as well as in their original numeric position with a note that the code is out of numerical sequence and where the resequenced code and description can be found.

INCLUDES   **Includes notes**
Includes notes identify procedures and services that would be bundled in the procedure code. These are derived from AMA, CMS, NCCI, and Optum360 coding guidelines. This is not meant to be an all-inclusive list.

EXCLUDES   **Excludes notes**
Excludes notes may lead the user to other codes. They may identify services that are not bundled and may be separately reported, OR may lead the user to another more appropriate code. These are derived from AMA, CMS, NCCI, and Optum360 coding guidelines. This is not meant to be an all-inclusive list.

Code Also   This note identifies an additional code that should be reported with the service and may relate to another CPT code or an appropriate HCPCS code(s) that should be reported along with the CPT code when appropriate.

Code First   Found under add-on codes, this note identifies codes for primary procedures that should be reported first, with the add-on code reported as a secondary code.

◣   **Laboratory/Pathology Crosswalk**
This icon denotes CPT codes in the laboratory and pathology section of CPT that may be reported separately with the primary CPT code.

✥   **Radiology Crosswalk**
This icon denotes codes in the radiology section that may be used with the primary CPT code being reported.

TC   **Technical Component Only**
Codes with this icon represent only the technical component (staff and equipment costs) of a procedure or service. Do not use either modifier 26 (professional component) or TC (technical component) with these codes.

26   **Professional Component**
Only codes with this icon represent the physician's work or professional component of a procedure or service. Do not use either modifier 26 (professional component) or TC (technical component) with these codes.

50   **Bilateral Procedure**
This icon identifies codes that can be reported bilaterally when the same surgeon provides the service for the same patient on the same date. Medicare allows payment for both procedures at 150 percent of the usual amount for one procedure. The modifier does not apply to bilateral procedures inclusive to one code.

80   **Assist-at-Surgery Allowed**
Services noted by this icon are allowed an assistant at surgery with a Medicare payment equal to 16 percent of the allowed amount for the global surgery for that procedure. No documentation is required.

80   **Assist-at-Surgery Allowed with Documentation**
Services noted by this icon are allowed an assistant at surgery with a Medicare payment equal to 16 percent of the allowed amount for the global surgery for that procedure. Documentation is required.

+ Add-on Codes

This icon identifies procedures reported in addition to the primary procedure. The icon "**+**" denotes add-on codes. An add-on code is neither a stand-alone code nor subject to multiple procedure rules since it describes work in addition to the primary procedure.

According to Medicare guidelines, add-on codes may be identified in the following ways:

- The code is found on Change Request (CR) 7501 or successive CRs as a Type I, Type II, or Type III add-on code.

- The add-on code most often has a global period of "ZZZ" in the Medicare Physician Fee Schedule Database.

- The code is found in the CPT book with the icon "**+**" appended. Add-on code descriptors typically include the phrases "each additional" or "(List separately in addition to primary procedure)."

㊿ Optum Modifier 50 Exempt

Codes identified by this icon indicate that the procedure should not be reported with modifier 50 (Bilateral procedures).

⊘ Modifier 51 Exempt

Codes identified by this icon indicate that the procedure should not be reported with modifier 51 (Multiple procedures).

�51 Optum Modifier 51 Exempt

Codes identified by this Optum360 icon indicate that the procedure should not be reported with modifier 51 (Multiple procedures). Any code with this icon is backed by official AMA guidelines but was not identified by the AMA with their modifier 51 exempt icon.

▣ Correct Coding Initiative (CCI)

Current Procedural Coding Expert, Professional Edition identifies those codes with corresponding CCI edits. The CCI edits define correct coding practices that serve as the basis of the national Medicare policy for paying claims. The code noted is the major service/procedure. The code may represent a column 1 code within the column 1/column 2 correct coding edits table or a code pair that is mutually exclusive of each other.

✖ CLIA Waived Test

This symbol is used to distinguish those laboratory tests that can be performed using test systems that are waived from regulatory oversight established by the Clinical Laboratory Improvement Amendments of 1988 (CLIA). The applicable CPT code for a CLIA waived test may be reported by providers who perform the testing but do not hold a CLIA license.

�63 Modifier 63 Exempt

This icon identifies procedures performed on infants that weigh less than 4 kg. Due to the complexity of performing procedures on infants less than 4 kg, modifier 63 may be added to the surgery codes to inform the payers of the special circumstances involved.

A2 – Z3 ASC Payment Indicators

This icon identifies ASC status payment indicators. They indicate how the ASC payment rate was derived and/or how the procedure, item, or service is treated under the revised ASC payment system. For more information about these indicators and how they affect billing, consult Optum360's *Revenue Cycle Pro*.

A2 Surgical procedure on ASC list in 2007; payment based on OPPS relative payment weight.

B5 Alternative code may be available; no payment made.

D5 Deleted/discontinued code; no payment made.

F4 Corneal tissue acquisition; hepatitis B vaccine; paid at reasonable cost.

G2 Non-office-based surgical procedure added in CY 2008 or later; payment based on OPPS relative payment weight.

H2 Brachytherapy source paid separately when provided integral to a surgical procedure on ASC list; payment based on OPPS rate.

J7 OPPS pass-through device paid separately when provided integral to a surgical procedure on ASC list; payment contractor-priced.

J8 Device-intensive procedure; paid at adjusted rate.

K2 Drugs and biologicals paid separately when provided integral to a surgical procedure on ASC list; payment based on OPPS rate.

K7 Unclassified drugs and biologicals; payment contractor-priced.

L1 Influenza vaccine; pneumococcal vaccine. Packaged item/service; no separate payment made.

L6 New technology intraocular lens (NTIOL); special payment.

N1 Packaged service/item; no separate payment made.

P2 Office-based surgical procedure added to ASC list in CY 2008 or later with MPFS nonfacility practice expense (PE) RVUs; payment based on OPPS relative payment weight.

P3 Office-based surgical procedure added to ASC list in CY 2008 or later with MPFS nonfacility PE RVUs; payment based on MPFS nonfacility PE RVUs.

R2 Office-based surgical procedure added to ASC list in CY 2008 or later without MPFS nonfacility PE RVUs; payment based on OPPS relative payment weight.

Z2 Radiology or diagnostic service paid separately when provided integral to a surgical procedure on ASC list; payment based on OPPS relative payment weight.

Z3 Radiology or diagnostic service paid separately when provided integral to a surgical procedure on ASC list; payment based on MPFS nonfacility PE RVUs.

A Age Edit

This icon denotes codes intended for use with a specific age group, such as neonate, newborn, pediatric, and adult. This edit is based on age specifications in the CPT code descriptors, the product/service represented by the code *may* have age restrictions, and/or updates from the Integrated Outpatient Code Editor (I/OCE). Carefully review the code description to ensure the code you report most appropriately reflects the patient's age.

M Maternity

This icon identifies procedures that by definition should be used only for maternity patients generally between 9 and 64 years of age based on CMS I/OCE designations.

♀ Female Only

This icon identifies procedures designated by CMS for females only based on CMS I/OCE designations.

♂ Male Only

This icon identifies procedures designated by CMS for males only based on CMS I/OCE designations.

🖫 Facility RVU

This icon precedes the facility RVU from CMS's 2018 physician fee schedule (PFS). It can be found under the code description.

New codes include no RVU information.

⚒ Nonfacility RVU

This icon precedes the nonfacility RVU from CMS's 2018 PFS. It can be found under the code description.

New codes include no RVU information.

FUD: Global days are sometimes referred to as "follow-up days" or FUDs. The global period is the time following surgery during which routine care by the physician is considered postoperative and included in the surgical fee. Office visits or other routine care related to the original surgery cannot be separately reported if provided during the global period. The statuses are:

000   No follow-up care included in this procedure

010   Normal postoperative care is included in this procedure for ten days

090   Normal postoperative care is included in the procedure for 90 days

MMM   Maternity codes; usual global period does not apply

XXX   The global concept does not apply to the code

YYY   The carrier is to determine whether the global concept applies and establishes postoperative period, if appropriate, at time of pricing

ZZZ   The code is related to another service and is always included in the global period of the other service

CMS: This notation indicates that there is a specific CMS guideline pertaining to this code in the CMS Online Manual System which includes the internet-only manual (IOM) *National Coverage Determinations Manual* (NCD). These CMS sources present the rules for submitting these services to the federal government or its contractors and a link to the IOMs is included in appendix G of this book.

AMA: This indicates discussion of the code in the American Medical Association's *CPT Assistant* newsletter. Use the citation to find the correct issue. This includes citations for the current year and the preceding six years. In the event no citations can be found during this time period, the most recent citations that can be found are used.

✗   **Drug Not Approved by FDA**
The AMA CPT Editorial Panel is publishing new vaccine product codes prior to Food and Drug Administration approval. This symbol indicates which of these codes are pending FDA approval at press time.

A – Y   **OPPS Status Indicators (OPSI)**
Status indicators identify how individual CPT codes are paid or not paid under the latest available hospital outpatient prospective payment system (OPPS). The same status indicator is assigned to all the codes within an ambulatory payment classification (APC). Consult your payer or other resource to learn which CPT codes fall within various APCs.

A   Services furnished to a hospital outpatient that are paid under a fee schedule or payment system other than OPPS. For example:
- Ambulance services
- Separately payable clinical diagnostic laboratory services
- Separately payable non-implantable prosthetics and orthotics
- Physical, occupational, and speech therapy
- Diagnostic mammography
- Screening mammography

B   Codes that are not recognized by OPPS when submitted on an outpatient hospital Part B bill type (12x and 13x)

C   Inpatient procedures

D   Discontinued codes

E1   Items, codes, and services:
- Not covered by any Medicare outpatient benefit category
- Statutorily excluded by Medicare

- Not reasonable and necessary

E2   Items, codes, and services for which pricing information and claims data are not available

F   Corneal tissue acquisition; certain CRNA services and hepatitis B vaccines

G   Pass-through drugs and biologicals

H   Pass-through device categories

J1   Hospital Part B services paid through a comprehensive APC

J2   Hospital Part B services that may be paid through a comprehensive APC

K   Nonpass-through drugs and nonimplantable biologicals, including therapeutic radiopharmaceuticals

L   Influenza vaccine; pneumococcal pneumonia vaccine

M   Items and services not billable to the MAC

N   Items and services packaged into APC rates

P   Partial hospitalization

Q1   STV-packaged codes

Q2   T-packaged codes

Q3   Codes that may be paid through a composite APC

Q4   Conditionally packaged laboratory tests

R   Blood and blood products

S   Procedure or service, not discounted when multiple

T   Procedure or service, multiple procedure reduction applies

U   Brachytherapy sources

V   Clinic or emergency department visit

Y   Nonimplantable durable medical equipment

Appendixes

Appendix A: Modifiers—This appendix identifies modifiers. A modifier is a two-position alpha or numeric code that is appended to a CPT or HCPCS code to clarify the services being reported. Modifiers provide a means by which a service can be altered without changing the procedure code. They add more information, such as anatomical site, to the code. In addition, they help eliminate the appearance of duplicate billing and unbundling. Modifiers are used to increase the accuracy in reimbursement and coding consistency, ease editing, and capture payment data.

Appendix B: New, Revised, and Deleted Codes—This is a list of new, revised, and deleted CPT codes for the current year. This appendix also includes a list of web release new, revised, and deleted codes, which indicate official code changes in *Current Procedural Coding Expert, Professional Edition* that will not be in the CPT code book until the following year.

Appendix C: Evaluation and Management Extended Guidelines—This appendix presents an overview of evaluation and management (E/M) services that augment the official AMA CPT E/M services. It includes tables that distinguish documentation components of each E/M code and the federal documentation guidelines (1995 and 1997) currently in use by the Centers for Medicare and Medicaid Services (CMS).

Appendix D: Crosswalk of Deleted Codes—This appendix is a cross-reference from a deleted CPT code to an active code when one is available. The deleted code cross-reference will also appear under the deleted code description in the tabular section of the book.

Appendix E: Resequenced Codes—This appendix contains a list of codes that are not in numeric order in the book. AMA resequenced some of the code numbers to relocate codes in the same category but not in numeric sequence. In addition to the list of codes, this appendix provides the page number where the resequenced code may be found.

Appendix F: Add-on, Optum Modifier 50 Exempt, Modifier 51 Exempt, Optum Modifier 51 Exempt, Modifier 63 Exempt, and Modifier 95 Telemedicine Services—This list includes add-on codes that cannot be reported alone, codes that are exempt from modifiers 50 and 51, codes that should not be reported with modifier 63, and codes identified by the ★ icon to which modifier 95 may be appended when the service is provided as a synchronous telemedicine service.

Appendix G: Medicare Internet-only Manual (IOMs)—Previously, this appendix contained a verbatim printout of the Medicare Internet-only Manual references pertaining to specific codes. This appendix now contains a link to the IOMs on the Centers for Medicare and Medicaid Services website. The IOM references applicable to specific codes can still be found at the code level. For example:

93784-93790 Ambulatory Blood Pressure Monitoring
CMS: 100-3,20.19 Ambulatory Blood Pressure Monitoring (20.19); 100-4,32,10.1 Ambulatory Blood Pressure Monitoring Billing Requirements

Appendix H: Quality Payment Program (QPP)—Previously, this appendix contained lists of the numerators and denominators applicable to the Medicare PQRS. However, with the implementation of the Quality Payment Program (QPP) mandated by passage of the Medicare Access and Chip Reauthorization Act (MACRA) of 2015, the PQRS system will be obsolete. This appendix now contains information pertinent to that legislation as well as a brief overview of the proposed changes for the following year, as is available by the date of this publication.

Appendix I: Medically Unlikely Edits—This appendix contains the published medically unlikely edits (MUEs). These edits establish maximum daily allowable units of service. The edits will be applied to the services provided to the same patient, for the same CPT code, on the same date of service when billed by the same provider. Included are the physician and facility edits.

Appendix J: Inpatient-Only Procedures—This appendix identifies services with the status indicator "C." Medicare will not pay an OPPS hospital or ASC when these procedures are performed on a Medicare patient as an outpatient. Physicians should refer to this list when scheduling Medicare patients for surgical procedures. CMS updates this list quarterly.

Appendix K: Place of Service and Type of Service—This appendix contains lists of place-of-service codes that should be used on professional claims and type-of-service codes used by the Medicare Common Working File.

Appendix L: Multianalyte Assays with Algorithmic Analyses—This appendix lists the administrative codes for multianalyte assays with algorithmic analyses. The AMA updates this list three times a year.

Appendix M: Glossary—This appendix contains general terms and definitions that may be helpful for coding and reimbursement.

Appendix N: Listing of Sensory, Motor, and Mixed Nerves—This appendix lists a summary of each sensory, motor, and mixed nerve with its appropriate nerve conduction study code.

Note: All data current as of November 1, 2021.

Anatomical Illustrations

Body Planes and Movements

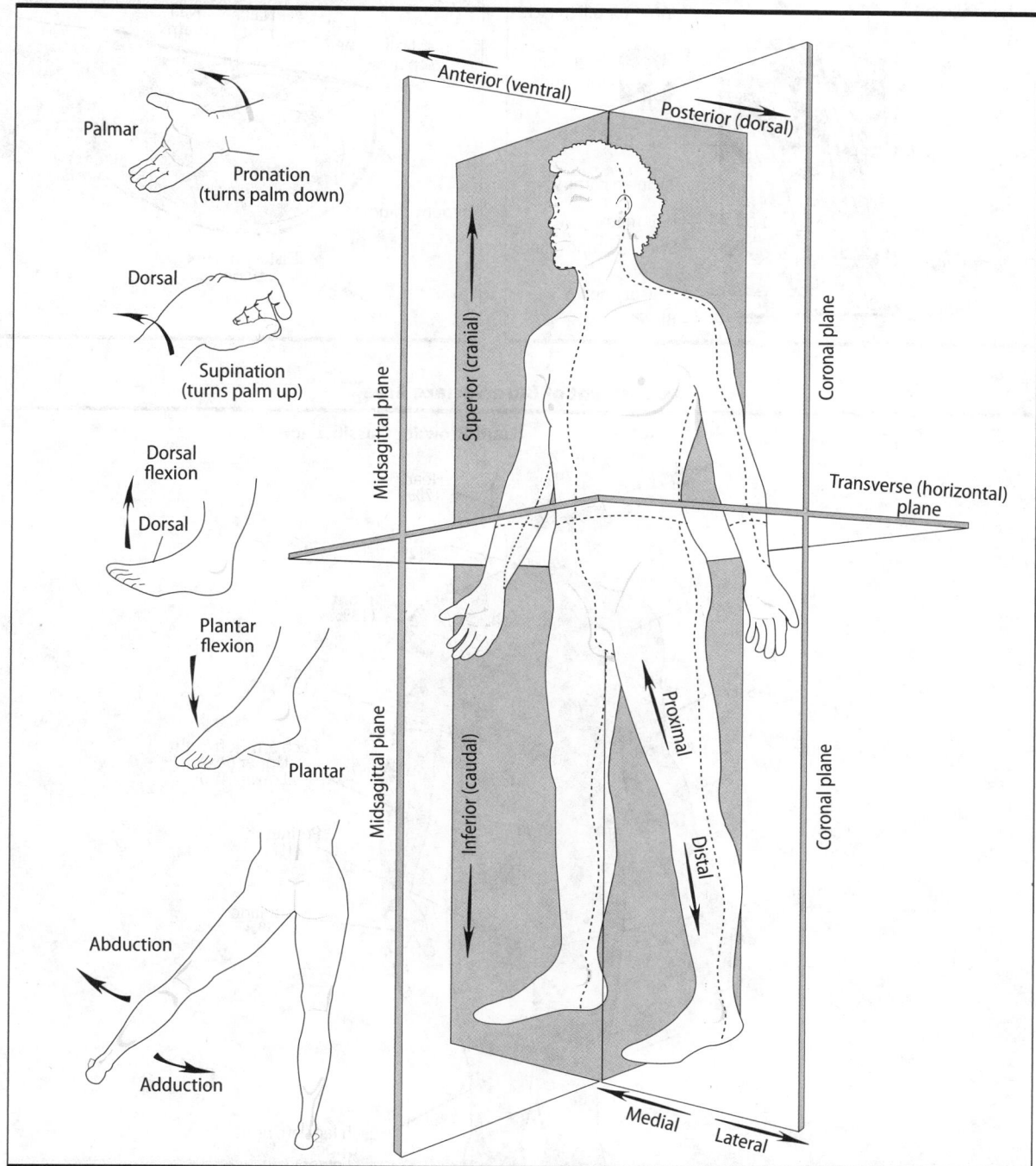

Integumentary System

Skin and Subcutaneous Tissue

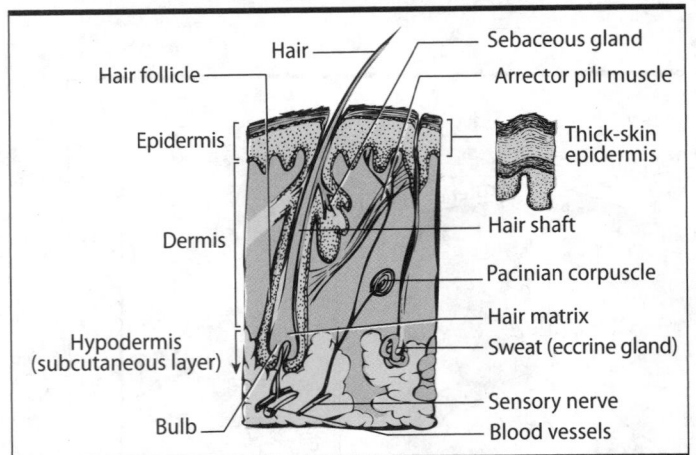

Hair
Hair follicle
Epidermis
Dermis
Hypodermis (subcutaneous layer)
Bulb

Sebaceous gland
Arrector pili muscle
Thick-skin epidermis
Hair shaft
Pacinian corpuscle
Hair matrix
Sweat (eccrine gland)
Sensory nerve
Blood vessels

Nail Anatomy

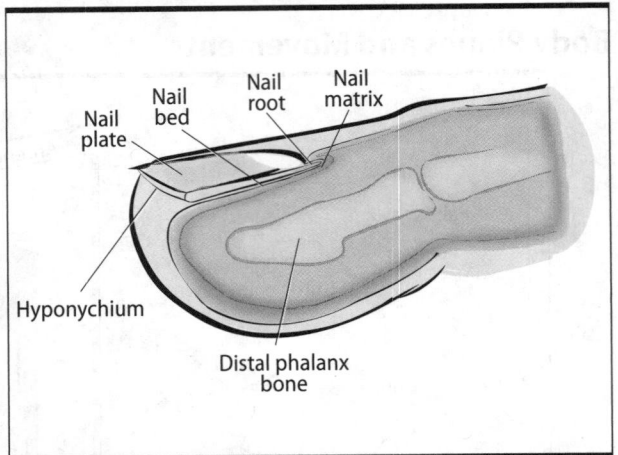

Nail plate
Nail bed
Nail root
Nail matrix
Hyponychium
Distal phalanx bone

Assessment of Burn Surface Area

Rule of Nines **Lund-Browder Classification**

Head and neck (9%)
Front (18%)
Back (18%)
Arm (9%)
Perineum (1%)
Leg (18%)

Head (7%)
Neck (2%)
Front (13%)
Back (13%)
Each arm/left/right Upper (4%) Lower (4%)
Perineum (1%)
Each hand (2.5%)
Each leg/left/right Upper (9.5%) Lower (7%)

Musculoskeletal System

Bones and Joints

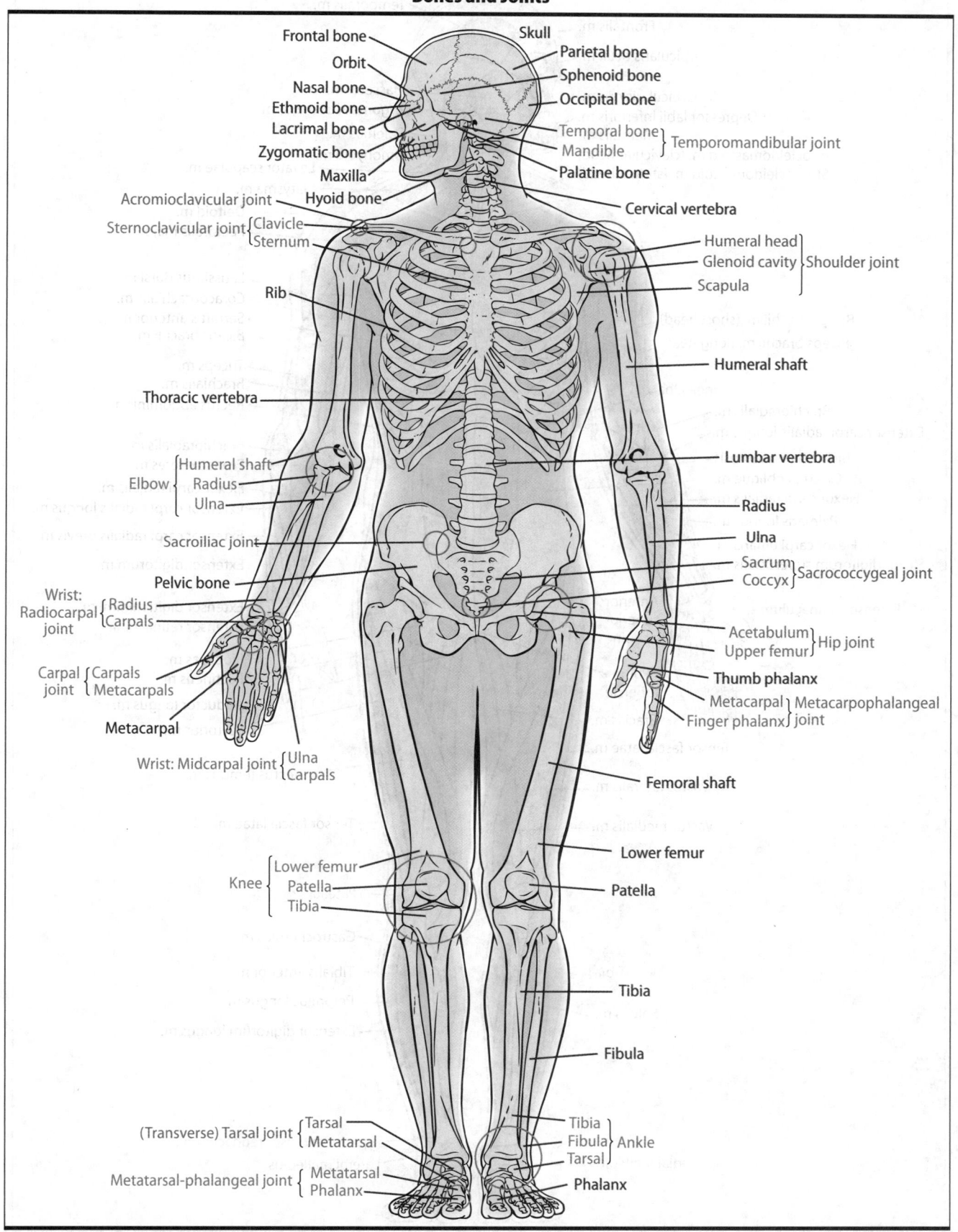

Frontal bone
Orbit
Nasal bone
Ethmoid bone
Lacrimal bone
Zygomatic bone
Maxilla
Hyoid bone
Skull
Parietal bone
Sphenoid bone
Occipital bone
Temporal bone
Mandible
} Temporomandibular joint
Palatine bone

Acromioclavicular joint
Sternoclavicular joint { Clavicle
Sternum
Cervical vertebra
Humeral head
Glenoid cavity } Shoulder joint
Scapula
Rib
Humeral shaft

Thoracic vertebra

Lumbar vertebra

Humeral shaft
Elbow { Radius
Ulna
Radius
Ulna

Sacroiliac joint
Pelvic bone
Sacrum
Coccyx } Sacrococcygeal joint

Wrist:
Radiocarpal
joint { Radius
Carpals
Acetabulum
Upper femur } Hip joint
Thumb phalanx

Carpal
joint { Carpals
Metacarpals
Metacarpal
Finger phalanx } Metacarpophalangeal joint
Metacarpal

Wrist: Midcarpal joint { Ulna
Carpals
Femoral shaft

Lower femur

Knee { Lower femur
Patella
Tibia
Patella

Tibia

Fibula

(Transverse) Tarsal joint { Tarsal
Metatarsal
Tibia
Fibula
Tarsal } Ankle

Metatarsal-phalangeal joint { Metatarsal
Phalanx
Phalanx

Anatomical Illustrations—Musculoskeletal System

Muscles

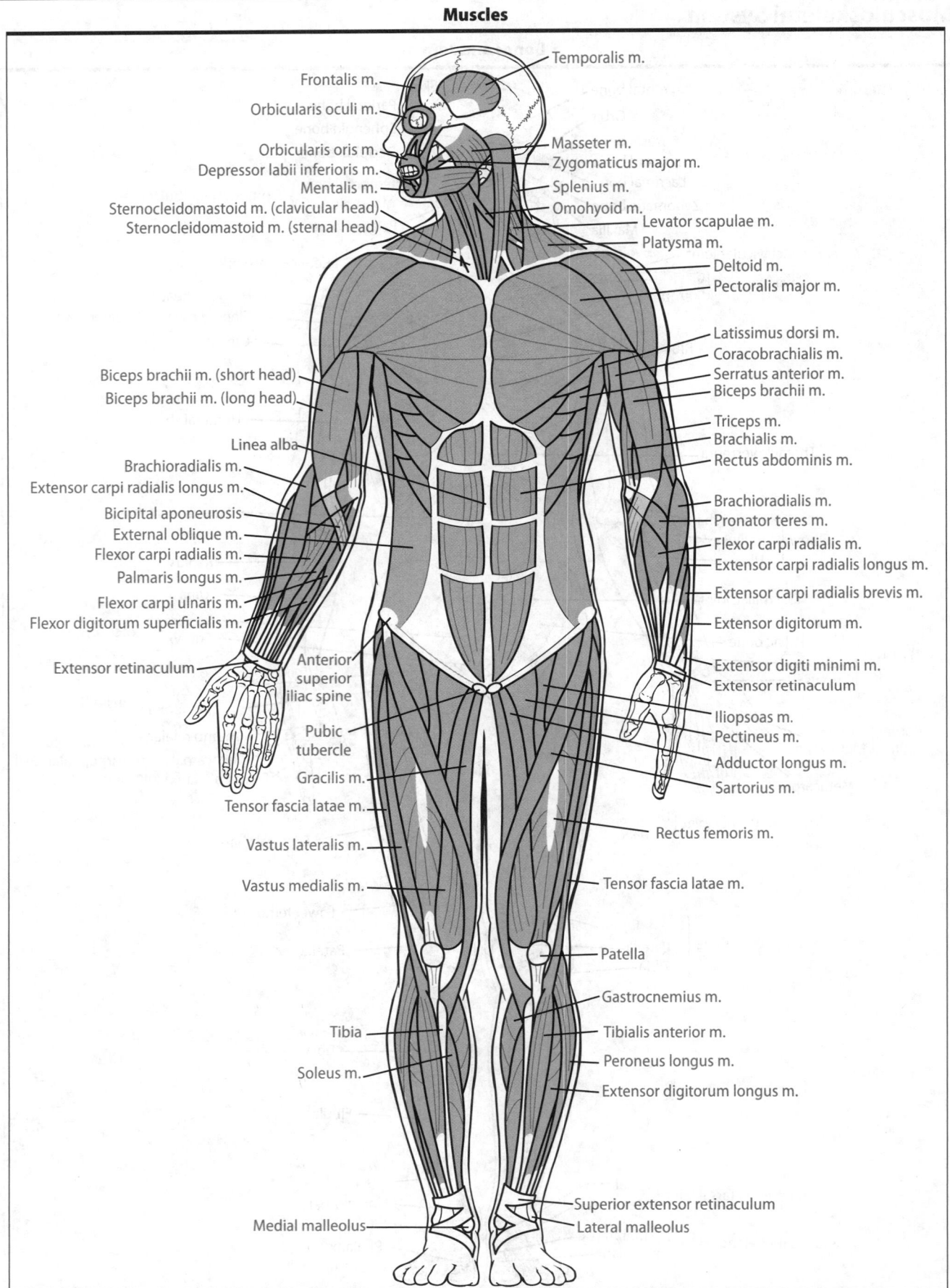

- Temporalis m.
- Frontalis m.
- Orbicularis oculi m.
- Orbicularis oris m.
- Depressor labii inferioris m.
- Mentalis m.
- Masseter m.
- Zygomaticus major m.
- Splenius m.
- Omohyoid m.
- Sternocleidomastoid m. (clavicular head)
- Sternocleidomastoid m. (sternal head)
- Levator scapulae m.
- Platysma m.
- Deltoid m.
- Pectoralis major m.
- Latissimus dorsi m.
- Coracobrachialis m.
- Serratus anterior m.
- Biceps brachii m.
- Biceps brachii m. (short head)
- Biceps brachii m. (long head)
- Triceps m.
- Brachialis m.
- Rectus abdominis m.
- Linea alba
- Brachioradialis m.
- Extensor carpi radialis longus m.
- Bicipital aponeurosis
- External oblique m.
- Flexor carpi radialis m.
- Palmaris longus m.
- Flexor carpi ulnaris m.
- Flexor digitorum superficialis m.
- Brachioradialis m.
- Pronator teres m.
- Flexor carpi radialis m.
- Extensor carpi radialis longus m.
- Extensor carpi radialis brevis m.
- Extensor digitorum m.
- Extensor digiti minimi m.
- Extensor retinaculum
- Extensor retinaculum
- Anterior superior iliac spine
- Iliopsoas m.
- Pectineus m.
- Adductor longus m.
- Sartorius m.
- Pubic tubercle
- Gracilis m.
- Tensor fascia latae m.
- Vastus lateralis m.
- Rectus femoris m.
- Vastus medialis m.
- Tensor fascia latae m.
- Patella
- Gastrocnemius m.
- Tibia
- Tibialis anterior m.
- Soleus m.
- Peroneus longus m.
- Extensor digitorum longus m.
- Superior extensor retinaculum
- Medial malleolus
- Lateral malleolus

Head and Facial Bones

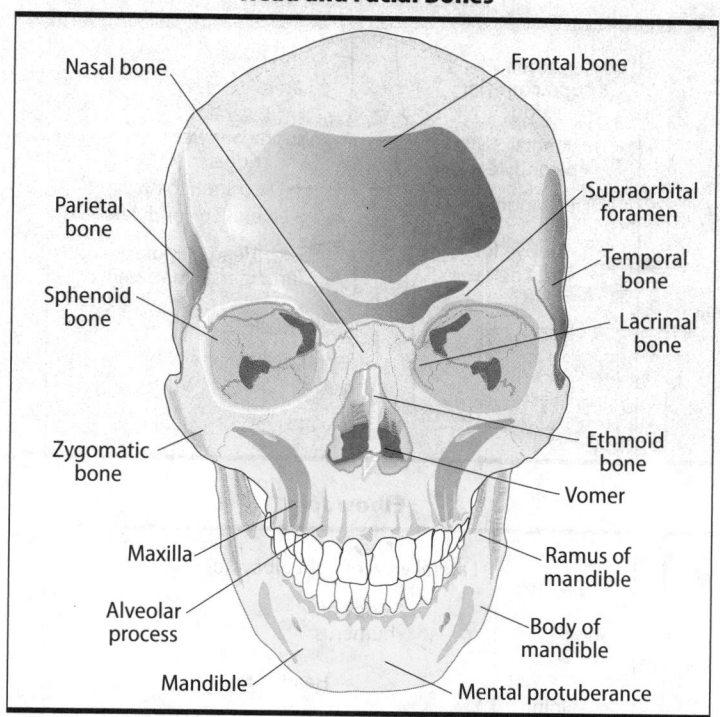

Nasal bone
Frontal bone
Supraorbital foramen
Parietal bone
Temporal bone
Sphenoid bone
Lacrimal bone
Zygomatic bone
Ethmoid bone
Vomer
Maxilla
Ramus of mandible
Alveolar process
Body of mandible
Mandible
Mental protuberance

Nose

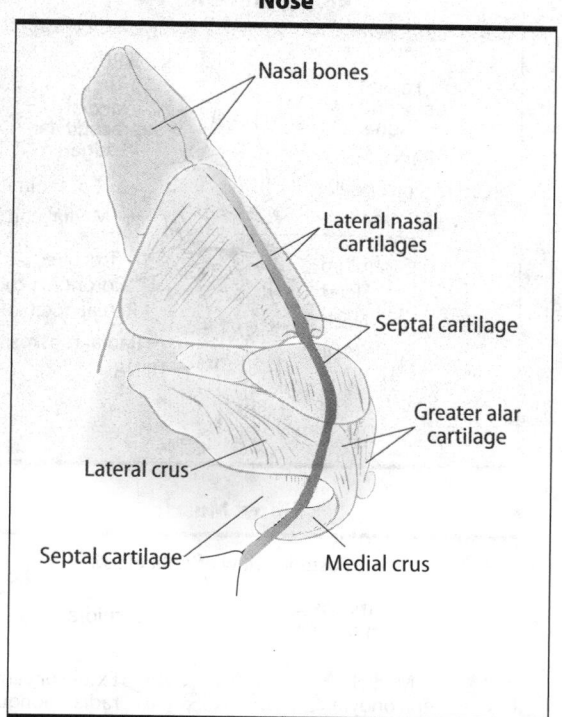

Nasal bones
Lateral nasal cartilages
Septal cartilage
Greater alar cartilage
Lateral crus
Septal cartilage
Medial crus

Shoulder (Anterior View)

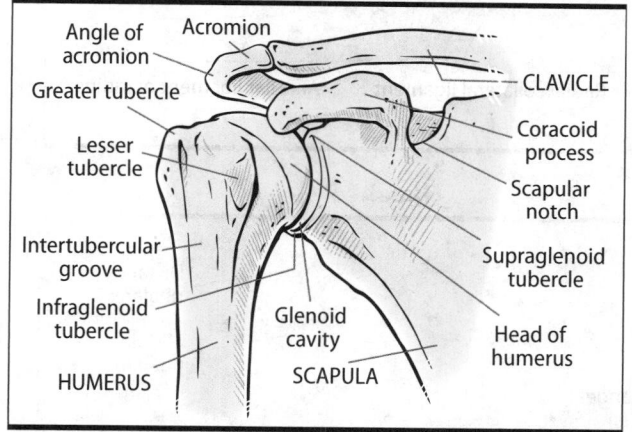

Angle of acromion
Acromion
CLAVICLE
Greater tubercle
Coracoid process
Lesser tubercle
Scapular notch
Intertubercular groove
Supraglenoid tubercle
Infraglenoid tubercle
Glenoid cavity
Head of humerus
HUMERUS
SCAPULA

Shoulder (Posterior View)

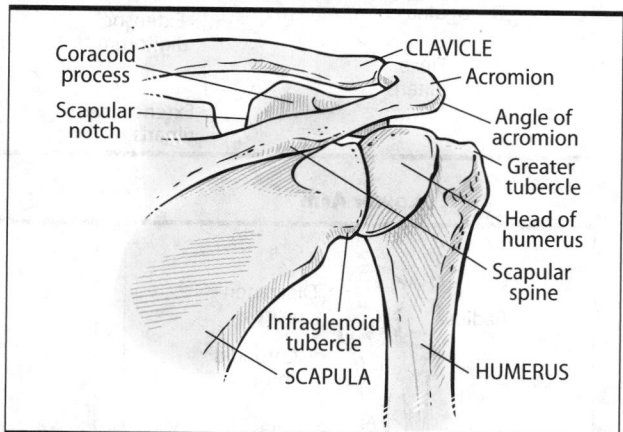

Coracoid process
CLAVICLE
Acromion
Scapular notch
Angle of acromion
Greater tubercle
Head of humerus
Scapular spine
Infraglenoid tubercle
SCAPULA
HUMERUS

Shoulder Muscles

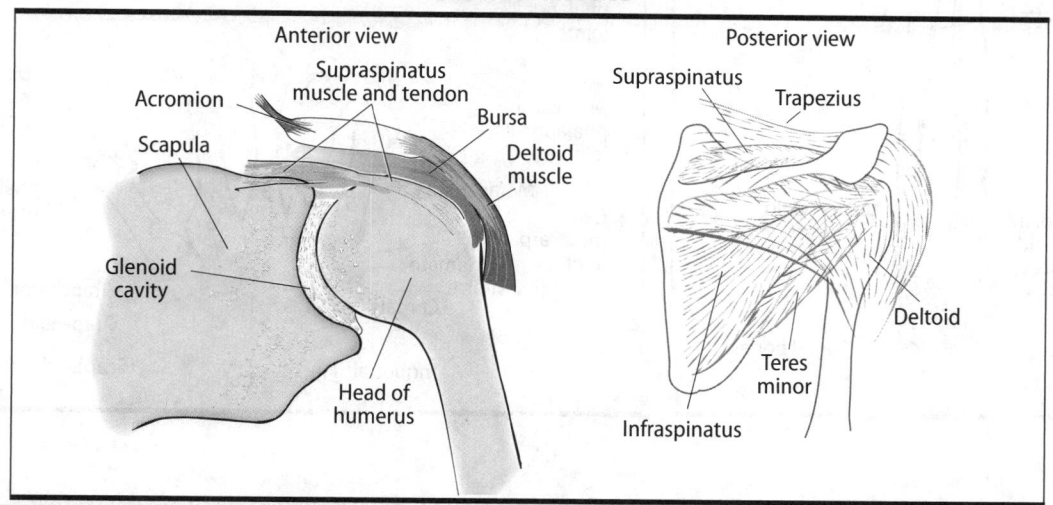

Anterior view
Supraspinatus muscle and tendon
Acromion
Bursa
Scapula
Deltoid muscle
Glenoid cavity
Head of humerus

Posterior view
Supraspinatus
Trapezius
Deltoid
Teres minor
Infraspinatus

Anatomical Illustrations—Musculoskeletal System

Elbow (Anterior View)

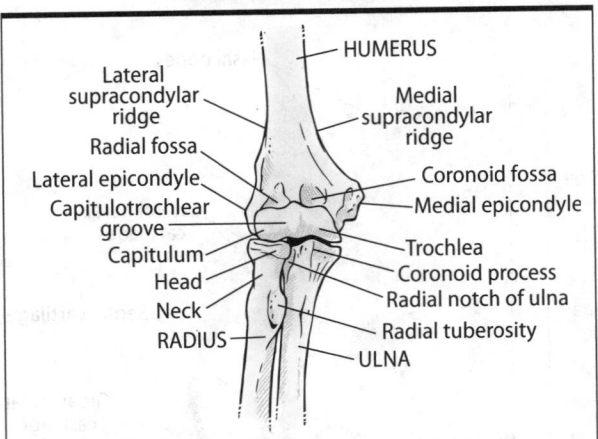

- HUMERUS
- Lateral supracondylar ridge
- Medial supracondylar ridge
- Radial fossa
- Lateral epicondyle
- Coronoid fossa
- Capitulotrochlear groove
- Medial epicondyle
- Capitulum
- Trochlea
- Head
- Coronoid process
- Neck
- Radial notch of ulna
- RADIUS
- Radial tuberosity
- ULNA

Elbow (Posterior View)

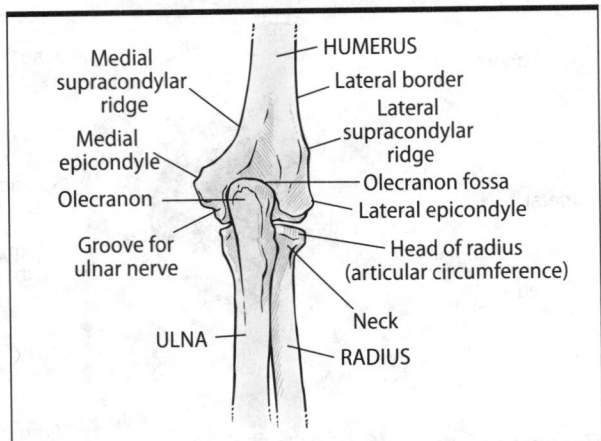

- Medial supracondylar ridge
- HUMERUS
- Lateral border
- Medial epicondyle
- Lateral supracondylar ridge
- Olecranon
- Olecranon fossa
- Lateral epicondyle
- Groove for ulnar nerve
- Head of radius (articular circumference)
- Neck
- ULNA
- RADIUS

Elbow Muscles

Posterior view of right elbow

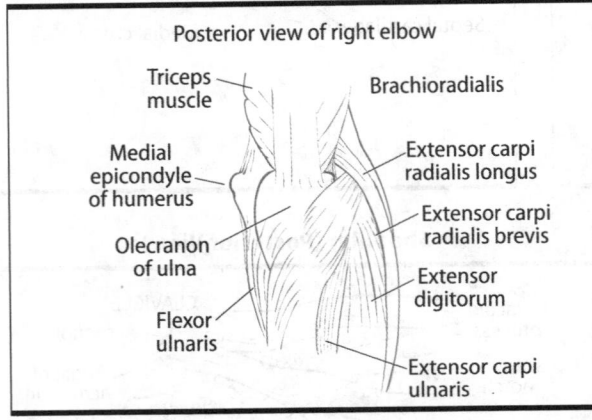

- Triceps muscle
- Brachioradialis
- Medial epicondyle of humerus
- Extensor carpi radialis longus
- Olecranon of ulna
- Extensor carpi radialis brevis
- Extensor digitorum
- Flexor ulnaris
- Extensor carpi ulnaris

Elbow Joint

Lateral view of right elbow joint

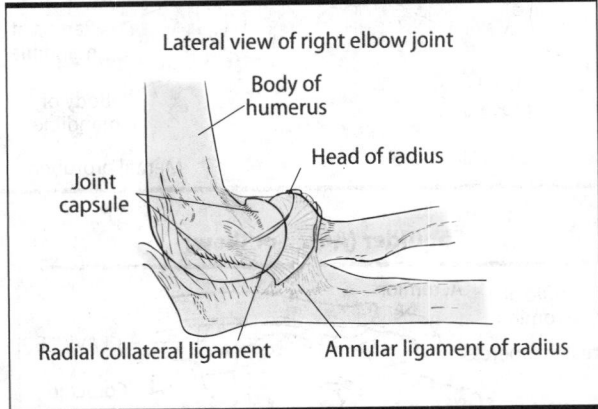

- Body of humerus
- Head of radius
- Joint capsule
- Radial collateral ligament
- Annular ligament of radius

Lower Arm

- Radius
- Olecranon process
- Coronoid process
- Ulna
- Shafts
- Radial styloid process
- Ulnar styloid process
- Carpal bones

Hand

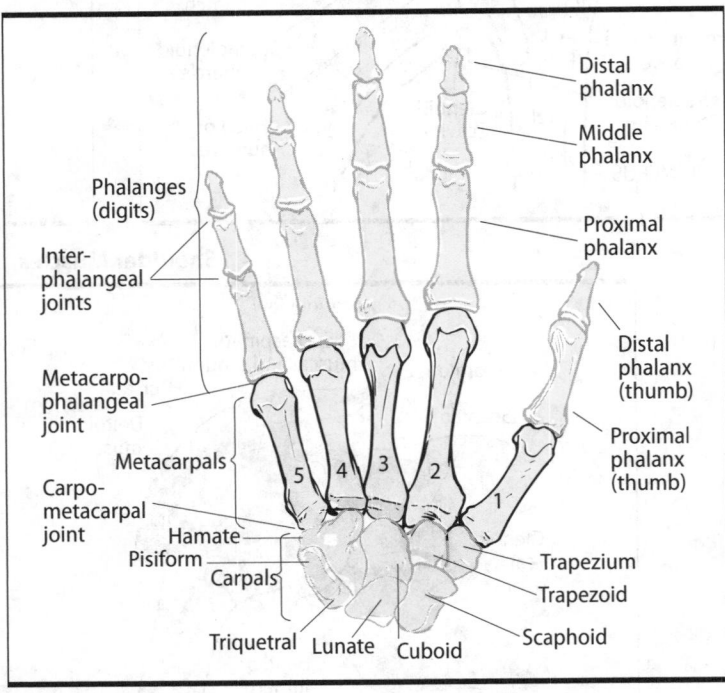

- Distal phalanx
- Middle phalanx
- Phalanges (digits)
- Proximal phalanx
- Interphalangeal joints
- Distal phalanx (thumb)
- Metacarpophalangeal joint
- Proximal phalanx (thumb)
- Metacarpals
- Carpometacarpal joint
- Hamate
- Pisiform
- Carpals
- Trapezium
- Trapezoid
- Scaphoid
- Triquetral
- Lunate
- Cuboid

© 2021 Optum360, LLC

Hip (Anterior View)

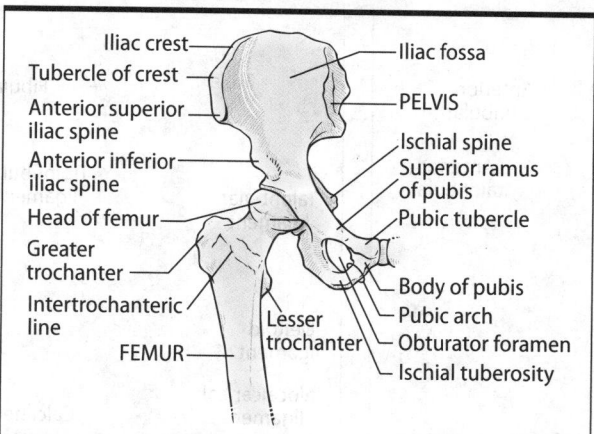

- Iliac crest
- Tubercle of crest
- Anterior superior iliac spine
- Anterior inferior iliac spine
- Head of femur
- Greater trochanter
- Intertrochanteric line
- FEMUR
- Iliac fossa
- PELVIS
- Ischial spine
- Superior ramus of pubis
- Pubic tubercle
- Body of pubis
- Pubic arch
- Lesser trochanter
- Obturator foramen
- Ischial tuberosity

Hip (Posterior View)

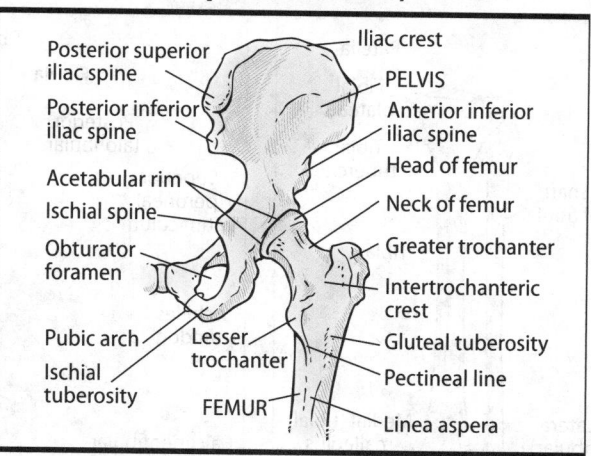

- Posterior superior iliac spine
- Posterior inferior iliac spine
- Acetabular rim
- Ischial spine
- Obturator foramen
- Pubic arch
- Ischial tuberosity
- Lesser trochanter
- FEMUR
- Iliac crest
- PELVIS
- Anterior inferior iliac spine
- Head of femur
- Neck of femur
- Greater trochanter
- Intertrochanteric crest
- Gluteal tuberosity
- Pectineal line
- Linea aspera

Knee (Anterior View)

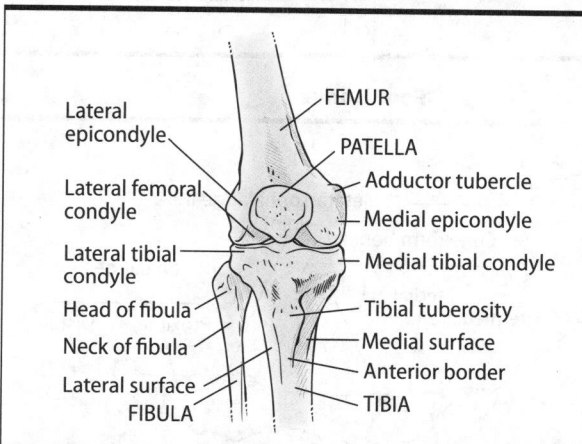

- Lateral epicondyle
- Lateral femoral condyle
- Lateral tibial condyle
- Head of fibula
- Neck of fibula
- Lateral surface
- FIBULA
- FEMUR
- PATELLA
- Adductor tubercle
- Medial epicondyle
- Medial tibial condyle
- Tibial tuberosity
- Medial surface
- Anterior border
- TIBIA

Knee (Posterior View)

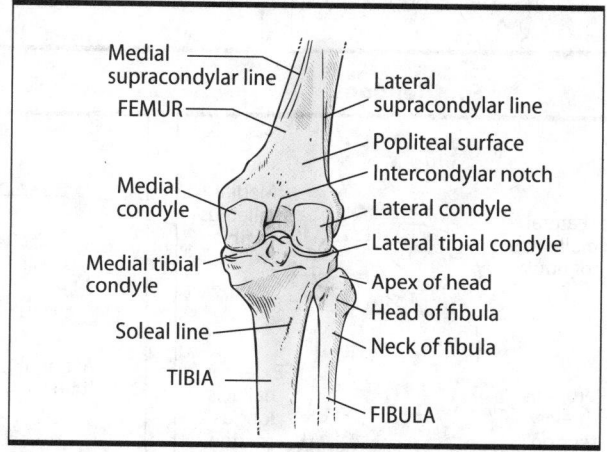

- Medial supracondylar line
- FEMUR
- Medial condyle
- Medial tibial condyle
- Soleal line
- TIBIA
- Lateral supracondylar line
- Popliteal surface
- Intercondylar notch
- Lateral condyle
- Lateral tibial condyle
- Apex of head
- Head of fibula
- Neck of fibula
- FIBULA

Knee Joint (Anterior View)

- Patella
- Medial meniscus cartilage
- Lateral meniscus cartilage

Knee Joint (Lateral View)

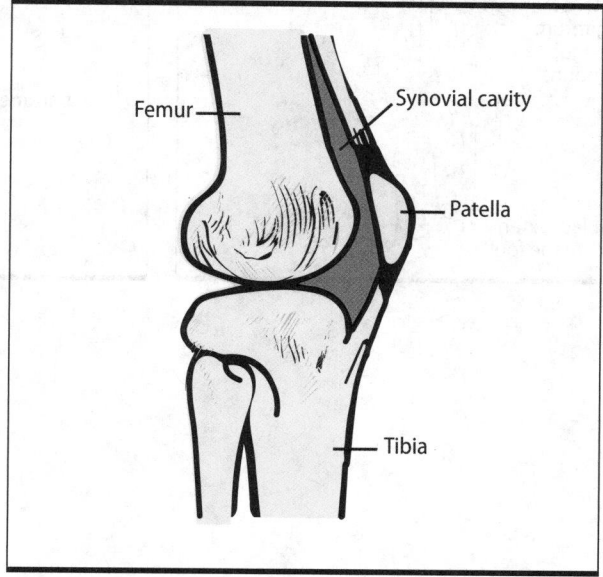

- Femur
- Synovial cavity
- Patella
- Tibia

Anatomical Illustrations—Musculoskeletal System

Lower Leg

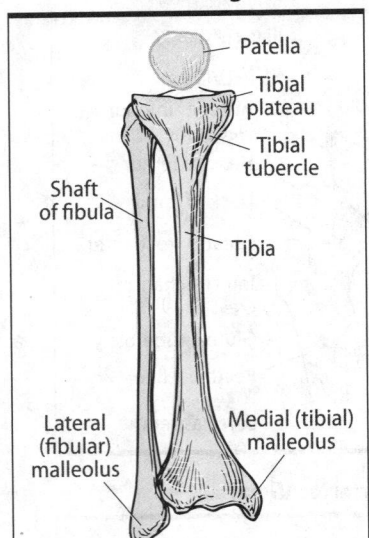

- Patella
- Tibial plateau
- Tibial tubercle
- Shaft of fibula
- Tibia
- Lateral (fibular) malleolus
- Medial (tibial) malleolus

Ankle Ligament (Lateral View)

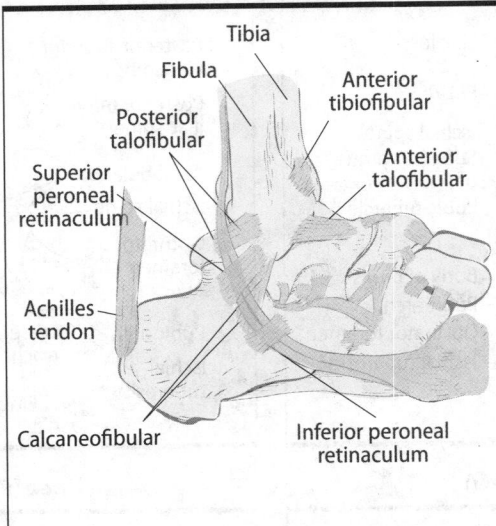

- Tibia
- Fibula
- Anterior tibiofibular
- Posterior talofibular
- Anterior talofibular
- Superior peroneal retinaculum
- Achilles tendon
- Calcaneofibular
- Inferior peroneal retinaculum

Ankle Ligament (Posterior View)

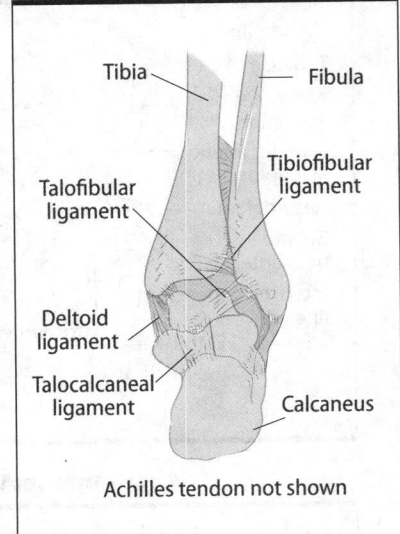

- Tibia
- Fibula
- Talofibular ligament
- Tibiofibular ligament
- Deltoid ligament
- Talocalcaneal ligament
- Calcaneus

Achilles tendon not shown

Foot Tendons

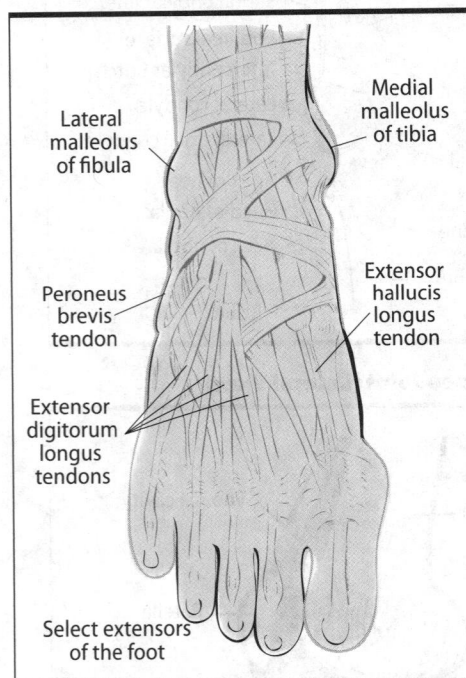

- Lateral malleolus of fibula
- Medial malleolus of tibia
- Peroneus brevis tendon
- Extensor hallucis longus tendon
- Extensor digitorum longus tendons

Select extensors of the foot

Foot Bones

- Tarsals
- Metatarsophalangeal joint
- Cuneiform bones
- Medial
- Lateral
- Phalanges
- Navicular
- Intermediate
- Proximal
- Distal
- Astragalus (talus)
- Calcaneus
- Cuboid
- Metatarsals
- Tarsometatarsal joint
- Medial
- Interphalangeal joints

Respiratory System

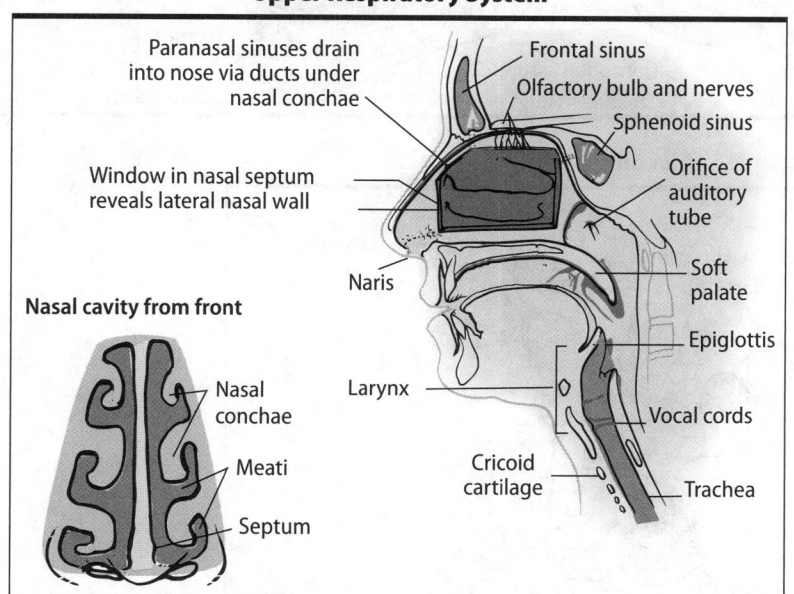

Nasal cavity and paranasal sinuses
Nostril
Oral cavity
Pharynx
Larynx
Trachea
Right lung
Right main / primary bronchus
Diaphragm
Pleura
Left lung
Carina of trachea
Left main/primary bronchus
Secondary (lobar) bronchi
Tertiary (segmental) bronchi
Bronchioles
Alveoli

Upper Respiratory System

Paranasal sinuses drain into nose via ducts under nasal conchae
Window in nasal septum reveals lateral nasal wall
Frontal sinus
Olfactory bulb and nerves
Sphenoid sinus
Orifice of auditory tube
Soft palate
Epiglottis
Vocal cords
Trachea
Naris
Larynx
Cricoid cartilage

Nasal cavity from front
Nasal conchae
Meati
Septum

Nasal Turbinates

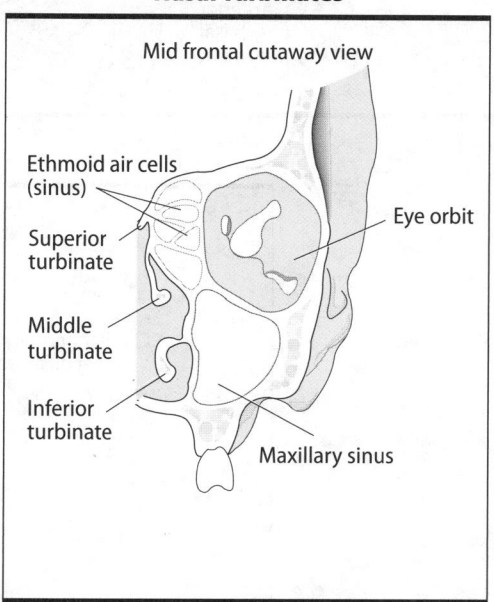

Mid frontal cutaway view
Ethmoid air cells (sinus)
Superior turbinate
Middle turbinate
Inferior turbinate
Eye orbit
Maxillary sinus

Anatomical Illustrations—Respiratory System

Paranasal Sinuses

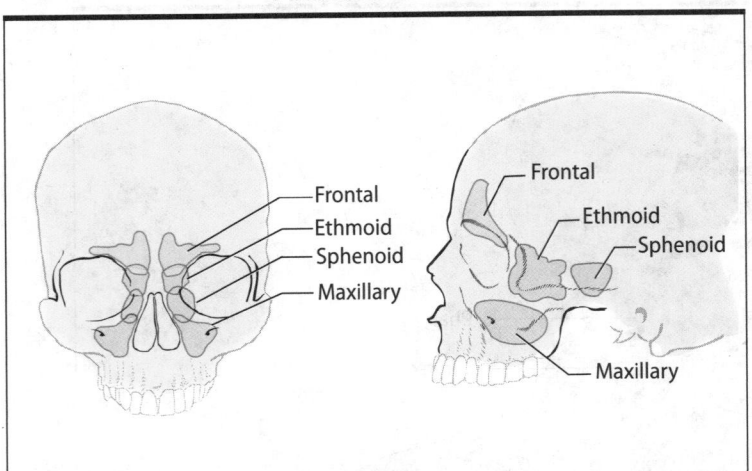

Frontal
Ethmoid
Sphenoid
Maxillary

Frontal
Ethmoid
Sphenoid
Maxillary

Lower Respiratory System

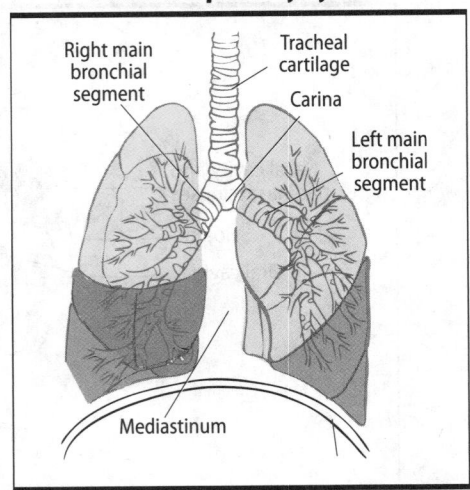

Right main bronchial segment
Tracheal cartilage
Carina
Left main bronchial segment
Mediastinum

Lung Segments

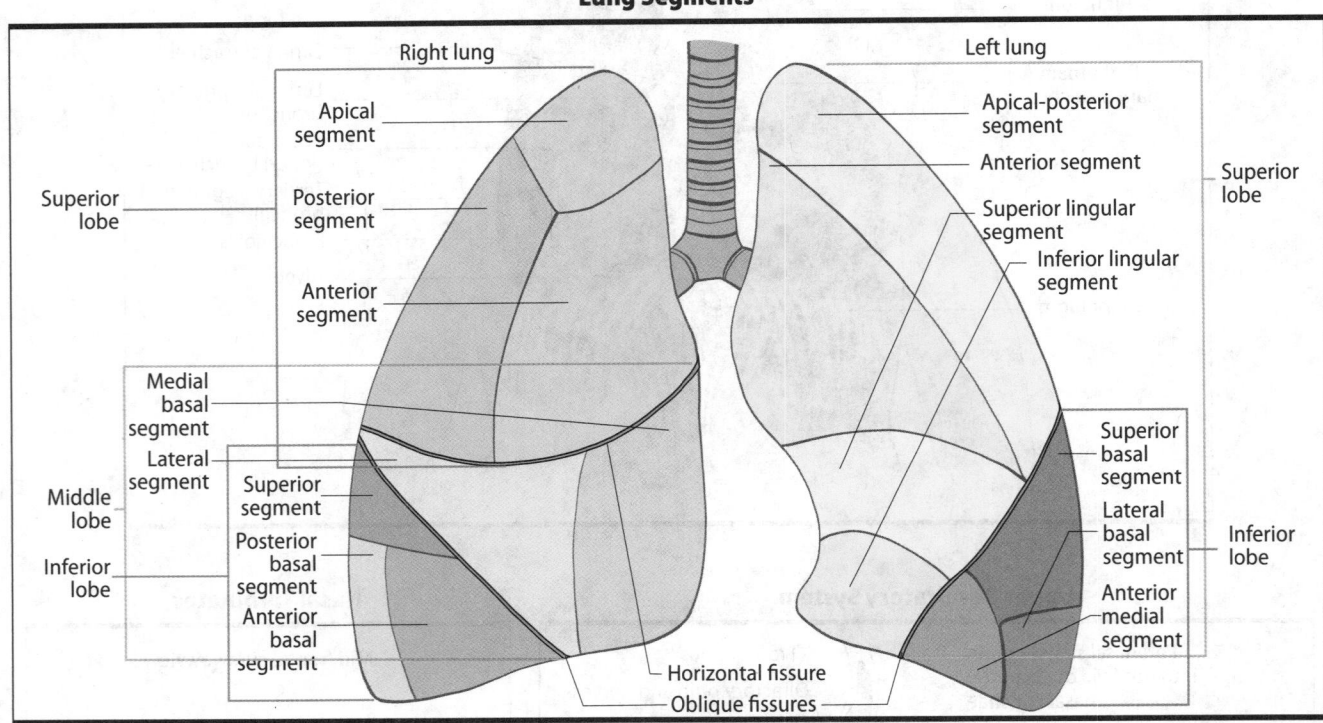

Right lung

Apical segment
Superior lobe
Posterior segment
Anterior segment

Medial basal segment
Lateral segment
Middle lobe
Superior segment
Posterior basal segment
Inferior lobe
Anterior basal segment

Left lung

Apical-posterior segment
Anterior segment
Superior lobe
Superior lingular segment
Inferior lingular segment

Superior basal segment
Lateral basal segment
Inferior lobe
Anterior medial segment

Horizontal fissure
Oblique fissures

Alveoli

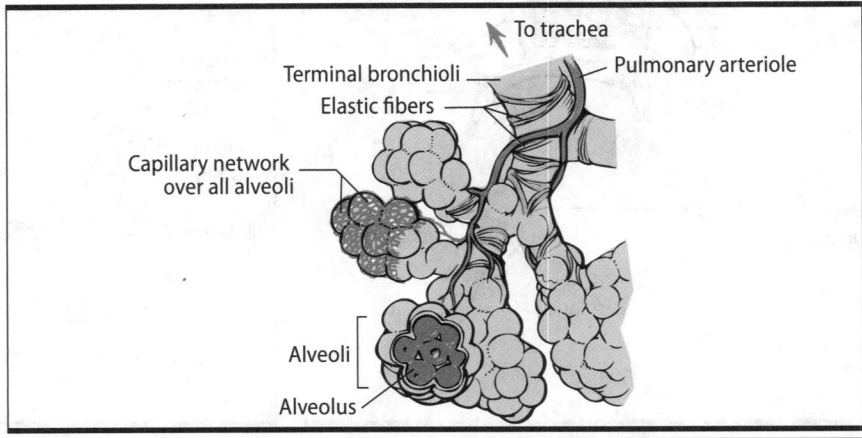

To trachea
Terminal bronchioli
Pulmonary arteriole
Elastic fibers
Capillary network over all alveoli
Alveoli
Alveolus

Arterial System

Upper Arteries:

Middle temporal a.
Transverse facial a.
Superficial temporal a.
External carotid a.
Internal carotid a.
Common carotid a.
Vertebral a.
Subclavian a.
Superior thyroid a.
Inferior thyroid a.
Innominate a.
Ascending aorta
Internal thoracic a. (mammary)
Brachial a.
Common hepatic a.
Celiac trunk (artery)
R. gastric a.
Arch of aorta
Pulmonary a.
Axillary a.
Descending aorta
L. gastric a.
Splenic a.
Renal a.
Superior mesenteric a.
R. colic a.
Abdominal aorta
L. colic a.
Radial a.
Ulnar a.
Inferior mesenteric a.
Common iliac a.
Internal iliac a.
External iliac a.
Uterine a.

Lower Arteries:

Femoral a.
Popliteal a.
Anterior tibial a.
Peroneal a.
Posterior tibial a.

Branches of Abdominal Aorta

Common hepatic
Hepatic
Cystic
Right gastric
Colic
Celiac trunk
Left gastric
Short gastric
Splenic
Gastroepiploic
Superior mesenteric
Ileocolic
Inferior mesenteric
Superior rectal
Left colic

Internal Carotid and Arteries and Branches

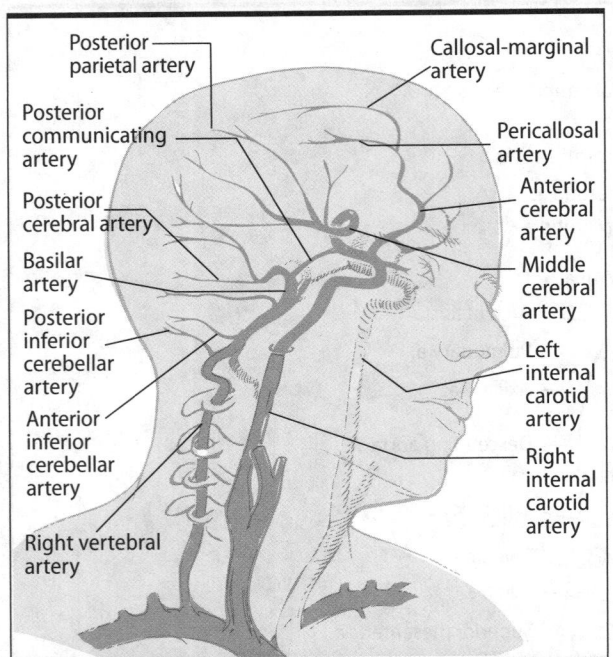

- Posterior parietal artery
- Callosal-marginal artery
- Posterior communicating artery
- Pericallosal artery
- Anterior cerebral artery
- Posterior cerebral artery
- Middle cerebral artery
- Basilar artery
- Left internal carotid artery
- Posterior inferior cerebellar artery
- Anterior inferior cerebellar artery
- Right internal carotid artery
- Right vertebral artery

External Carotid Arteries and Branches

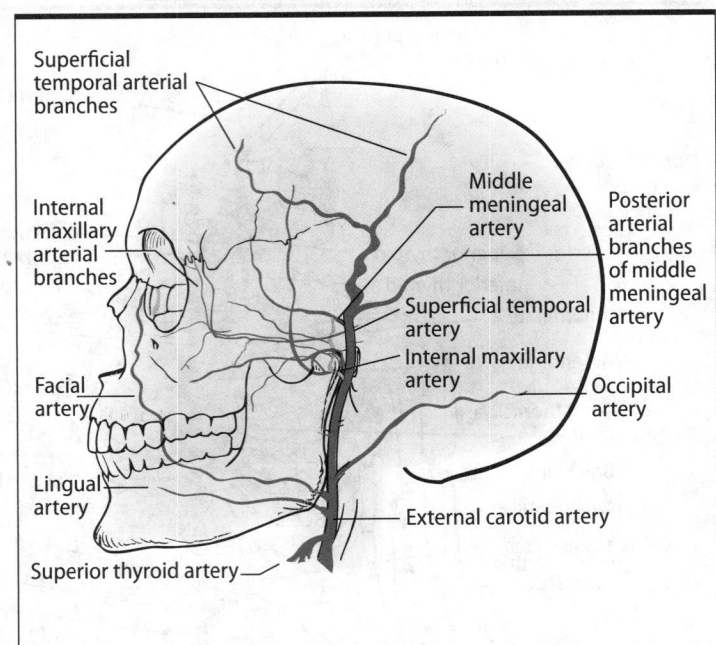

- Superficial temporal arterial branches
- Middle meningeal artery
- Posterior arterial branches of middle meningeal artery
- Internal maxillary arterial branches
- Superficial temporal artery
- Internal maxillary artery
- Facial artery
- Occipital artery
- Lingual artery
- External carotid artery
- Superior thyroid artery

Upper Extremity Arteries

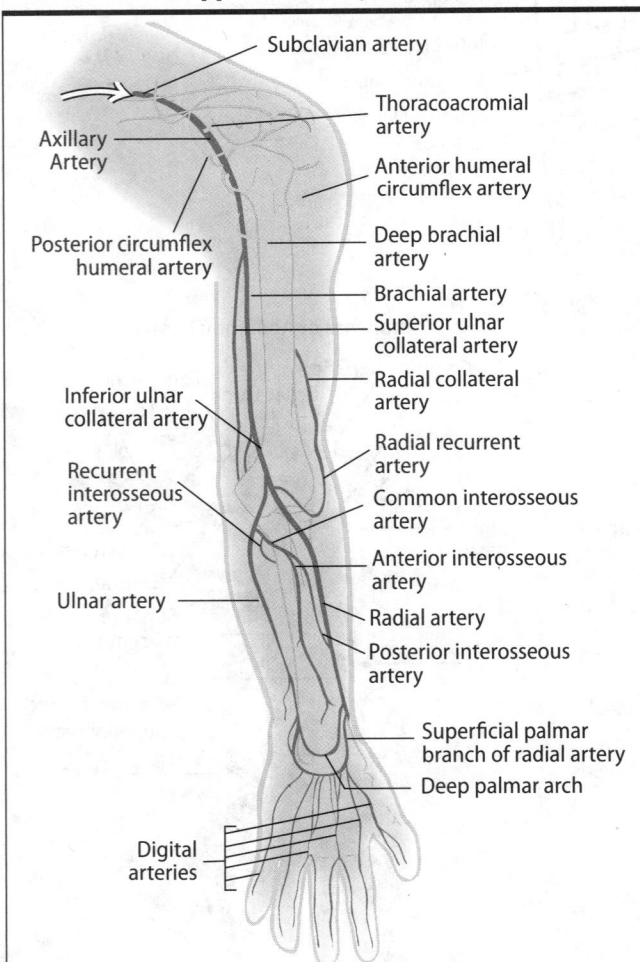

- Subclavian artery
- Thoracoacromial artery
- Axillary Artery
- Anterior humeral circumflex artery
- Deep brachial artery
- Posterior circumflex humeral artery
- Brachial artery
- Superior ulnar collateral artery
- Radial collateral artery
- Inferior ulnar collateral artery
- Radial recurrent artery
- Recurrent interosseous artery
- Common interosseous artery
- Anterior interosseous artery
- Ulnar artery
- Radial artery
- Posterior interosseous artery
- Superficial palmar branch of radial artery
- Deep palmar arch
- Digital arteries

Lower Extremity Arteries

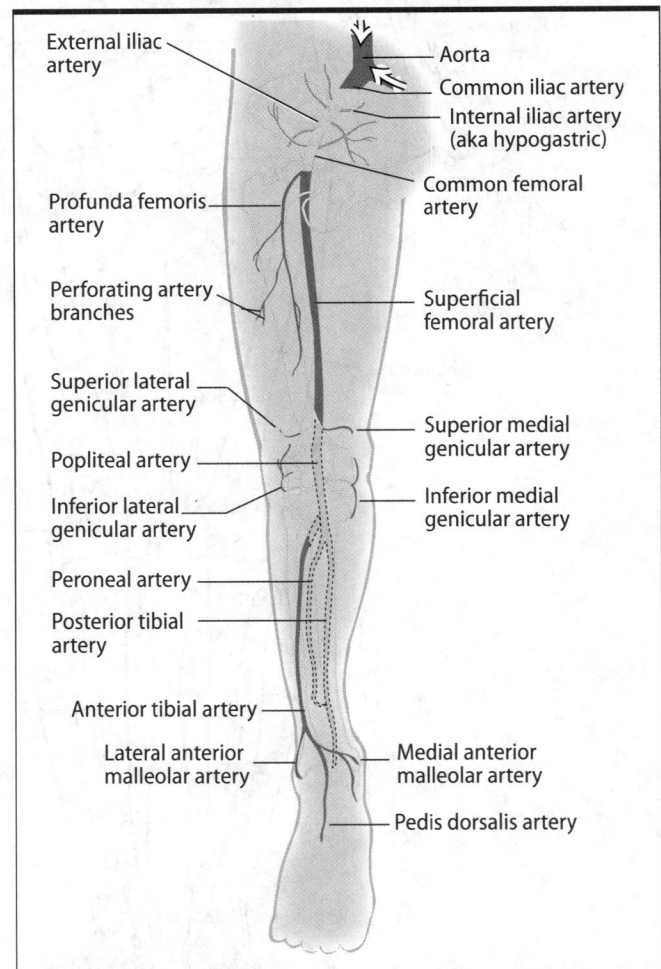

- External iliac artery
- Aorta
- Common iliac artery
- Internal iliac artery (aka hypogastric)
- Profunda femoris artery
- Common femoral artery
- Perforating artery branches
- Superficial femoral artery
- Superior lateral genicular artery
- Popliteal artery
- Superior medial genicular artery
- Inferior lateral genicular artery
- Inferior medial genicular artery
- Peroneal artery
- Posterior tibial artery
- Anterior tibial artery
- Lateral anterior malleolar artery
- Medial anterior malleolar artery
- Pedis dorsalis artery

Venous System

Superficial temporal v.
Vertebral v.
Internal jugular v.
External jugular v.
Subclavian v.
Innominate v.
Azygos v.
Axillary v.
Brachial v.
Hemiazygos v.
Inferior vena cava
Cephalic v.
Common hepatic v.
Basilic v.
Portal v.
Esophageal v.
R. gastric v.
L. gastric v.
R. colic v.
Splenic v.
Radial v.
Renal v.
Ulnar v.
Inferior mesenteric v.
Superior mesenteric v.
L. colic v.
Common iliac v.
Internal iliac v.
(Hypogastric v.)
External iliac v.
Internal pudendal v.
Rectal venous plexus
Femoral v.
Greater saphenous v.
Popliteal v.
Lesser saphenous v.
Anterior tibial v.
Lesser saphenous v.
Posterior tibial v.
Greater saphenous v.

Portal Venous Circulation
Inferior vena cava

Gastric
Portal
Splenic
Superior mesenteric
Right colic
Ileocolic
Inferior mesenteric
Left colic

Head and Neck Veins

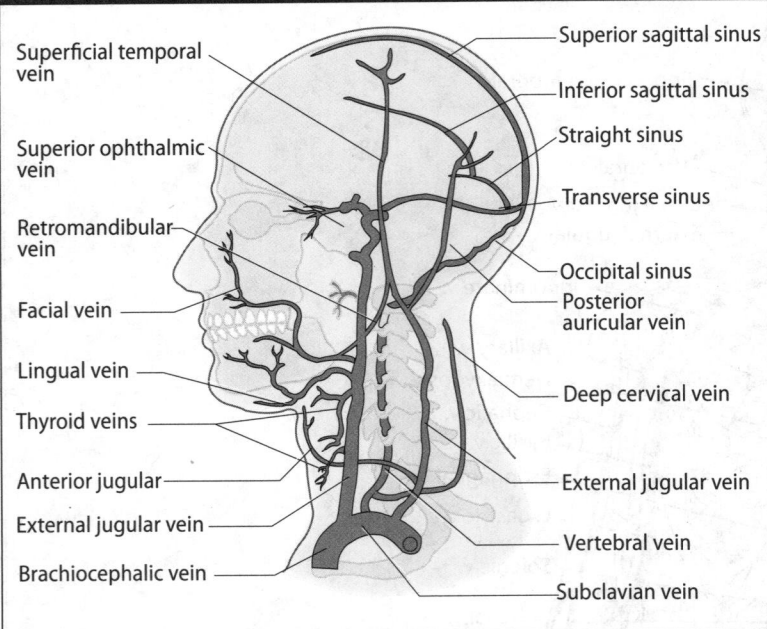

- Superficial temporal vein
- Superior ophthalmic vein
- Retromandibular vein
- Facial vein
- Lingual vein
- Thyroid veins
- Anterior jugular
- External jugular vein
- Brachiocephalic vein
- Superior sagittal sinus
- Inferior sagittal sinus
- Straight sinus
- Transverse sinus
- Occipital sinus
- Posterior auricular vein
- Deep cervical vein
- External jugular vein
- Vertebral vein
- Subclavian vein

Venae Comitantes

- Artery
- Venae comitantes

Upper Extremity Veins

- Axillary
- Cephalic
- Brachial
- Basilic
- Median cubital
- Median forearm

Venous Blood Flow

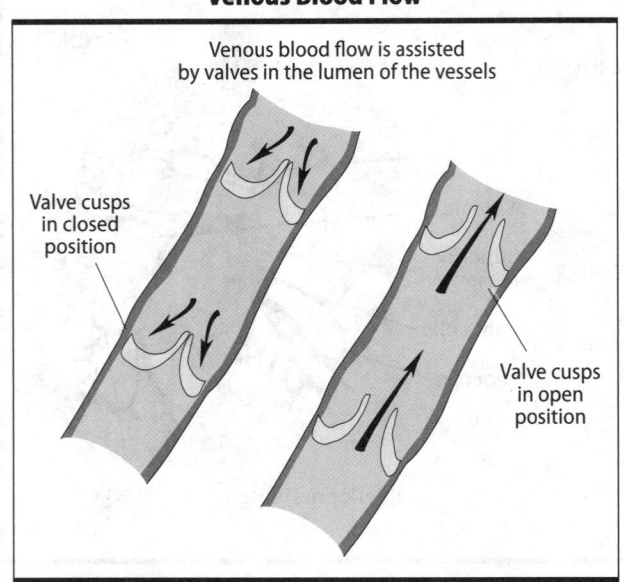

Venous blood flow is assisted by valves in the lumen of the vessels

- Valve cusps in closed position
- Valve cusps in open position

Abdominal Veins

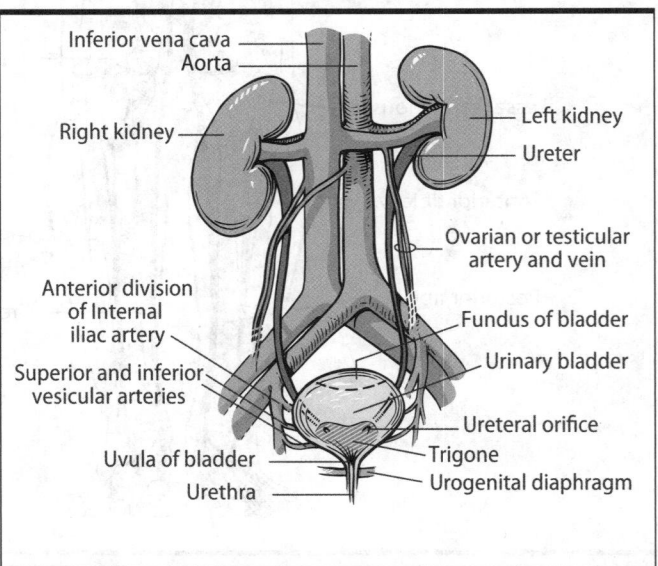

- Inferior vena cava
- Aorta
- Right kidney
- Left kidney
- Ureter
- Ovarian or testicular artery and vein
- Anterior division of Internal iliac artery
- Superior and inferior vesicular arteries
- Uvula of bladder
- Urethra
- Fundus of bladder
- Urinary bladder
- Ureteral orifice
- Trigone
- Urogenital diaphragm

Cardiovascular System

Coronary Veins

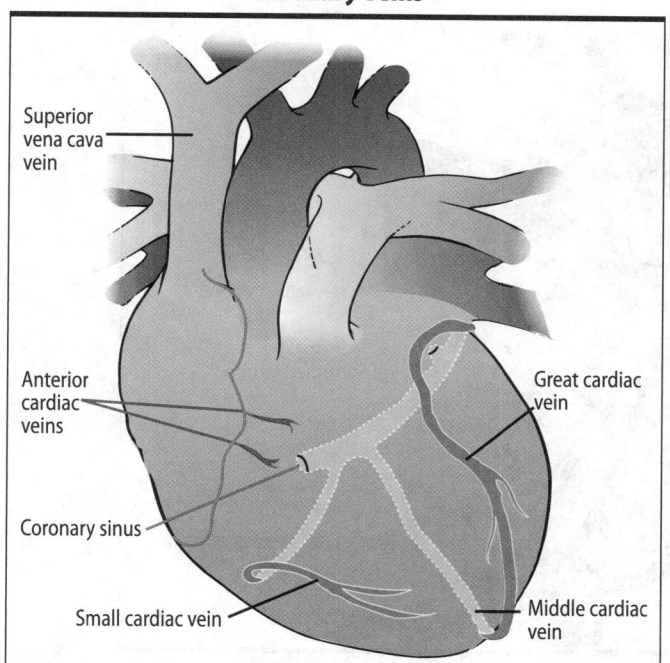

Superior vena cava vein

Anterior cardiac veins

Coronary sinus

Small cardiac vein

Great cardiac vein

Middle cardiac vein

Anatomy of the Heart

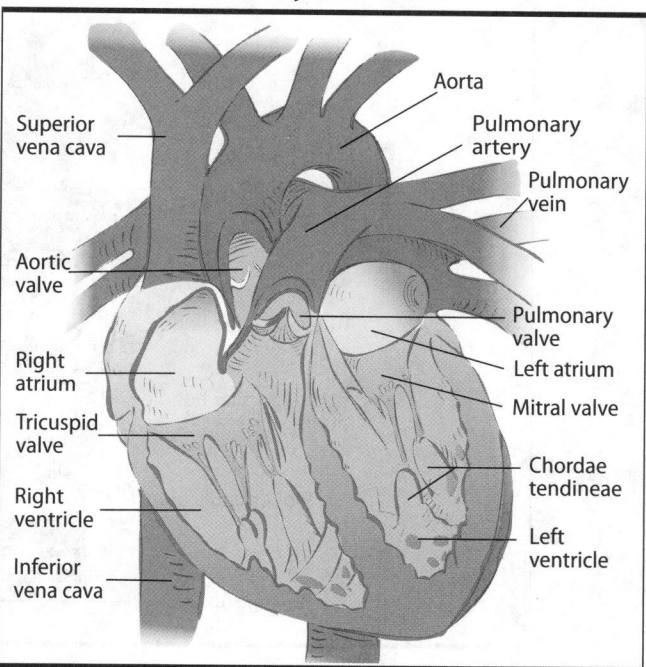

Superior vena cava

Aortic valve

Right atrium

Tricuspid valve

Right ventricle

Inferior vena cava

Aorta

Pulmonary artery

Pulmonary vein

Pulmonary valve

Left atrium

Mitral valve

Chordae tendineae

Left ventricle

Heart Cross Section

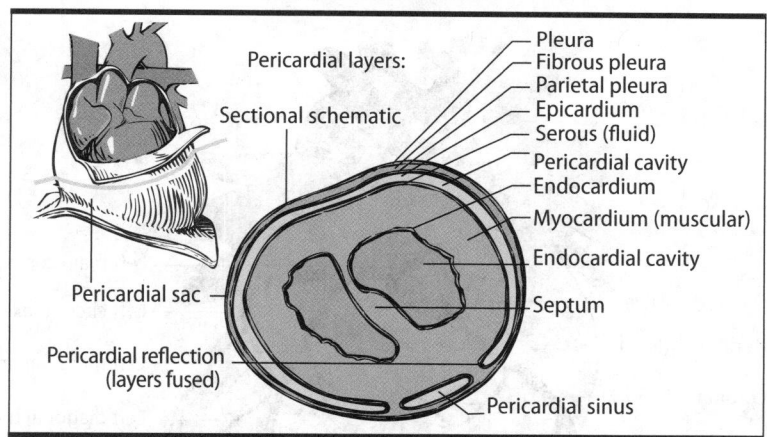

Pericardial layers:

Sectional schematic

Pericardial sac

Pericardial reflection (layers fused)

Pleura
Fibrous pleura
Parietal pleura
Epicardium
Serous (fluid)
Pericardial cavity
Endocardium
Myocardium (muscular)
Endocardial cavity
Septum

Pericardial sinus

Heart Valves

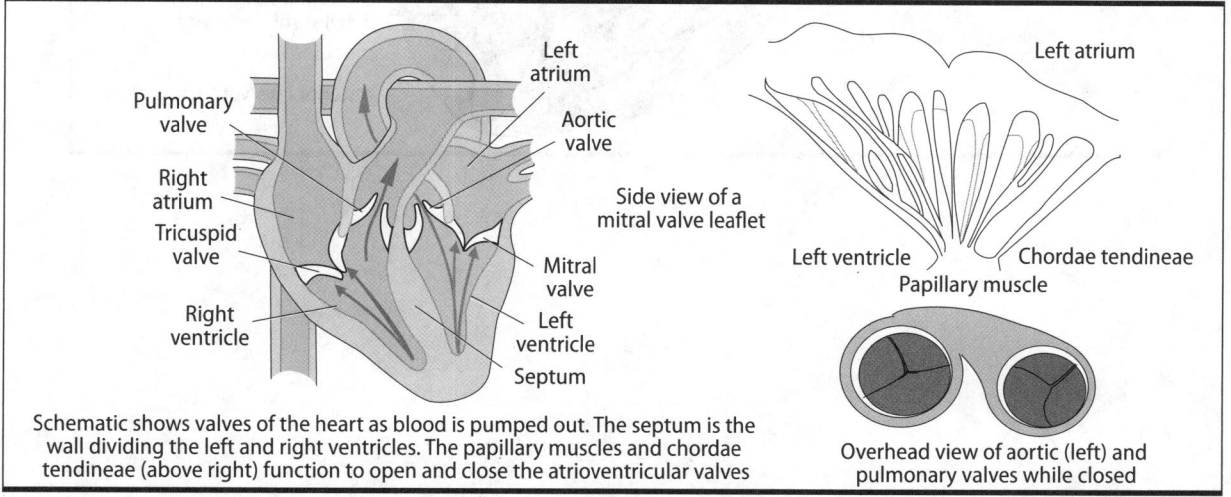

Pulmonary valve

Right atrium

Tricuspid valve

Right ventricle

Left atrium

Aortic valve

Mitral valve

Left ventricle

Septum

Left atrium

Side view of a mitral valve leaflet

Left ventricle

Chordae tendineae

Papillary muscle

Schematic shows valves of the heart as blood is pumped out. The septum is the wall dividing the left and right ventricles. The papillary muscles and chordae tendineae (above right) function to open and close the atrioventricular valves

Overhead view of aortic (left) and pulmonary valves while closed

Anatomical Illustrations—Cardiovascular System

Heart Conduction System

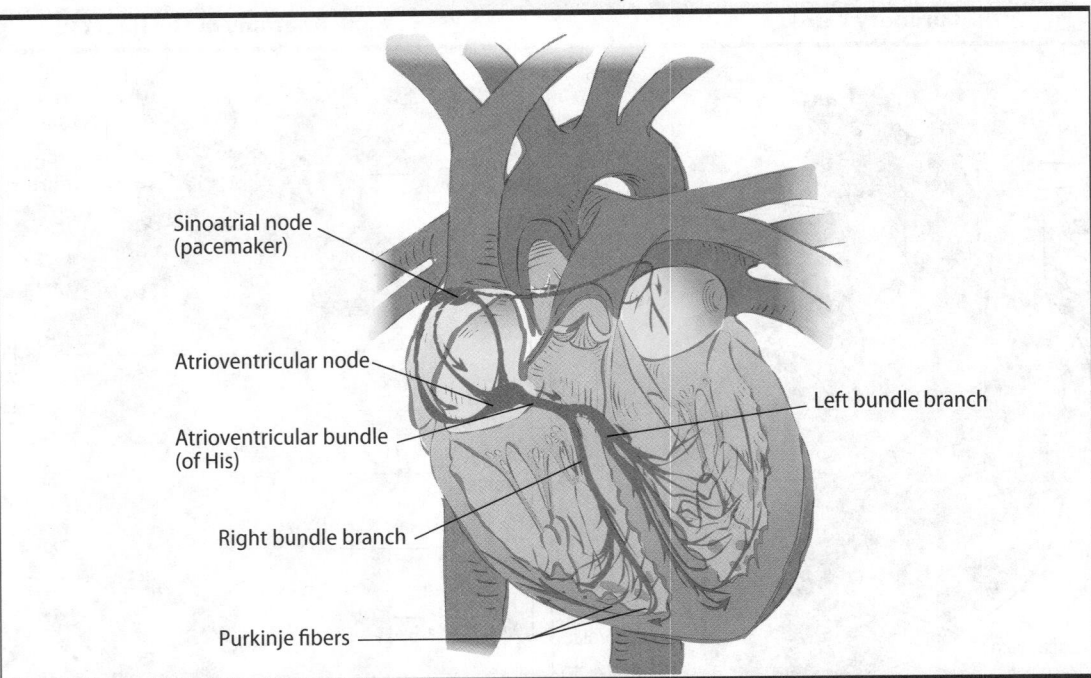

Sinoatrial node (pacemaker)

Atrioventricular node

Atrioventricular bundle (of His)

Right bundle branch

Purkinje fibers

Left bundle branch

Coronary Arteries

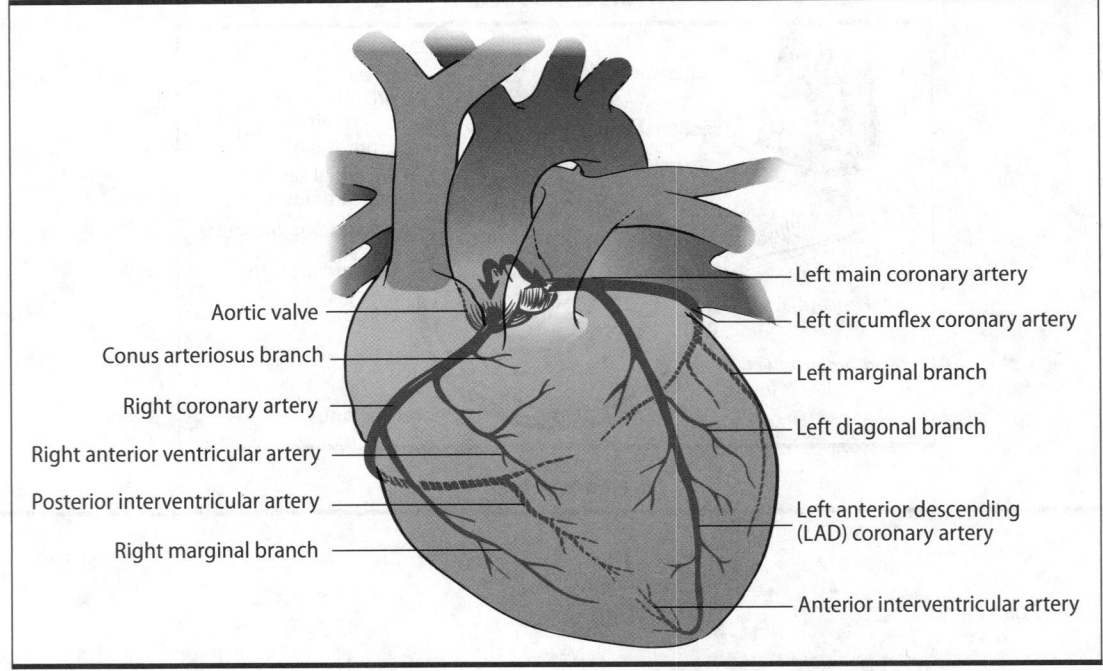

Aortic valve

Conus arteriosus branch

Right coronary artery

Right anterior ventricular artery

Posterior interventricular artery

Right marginal branch

Left main coronary artery

Left circumflex coronary artery

Left marginal branch

Left diagonal branch

Left anterior descending (LAD) coronary artery

Anterior interventricular artery

Lymphatic System

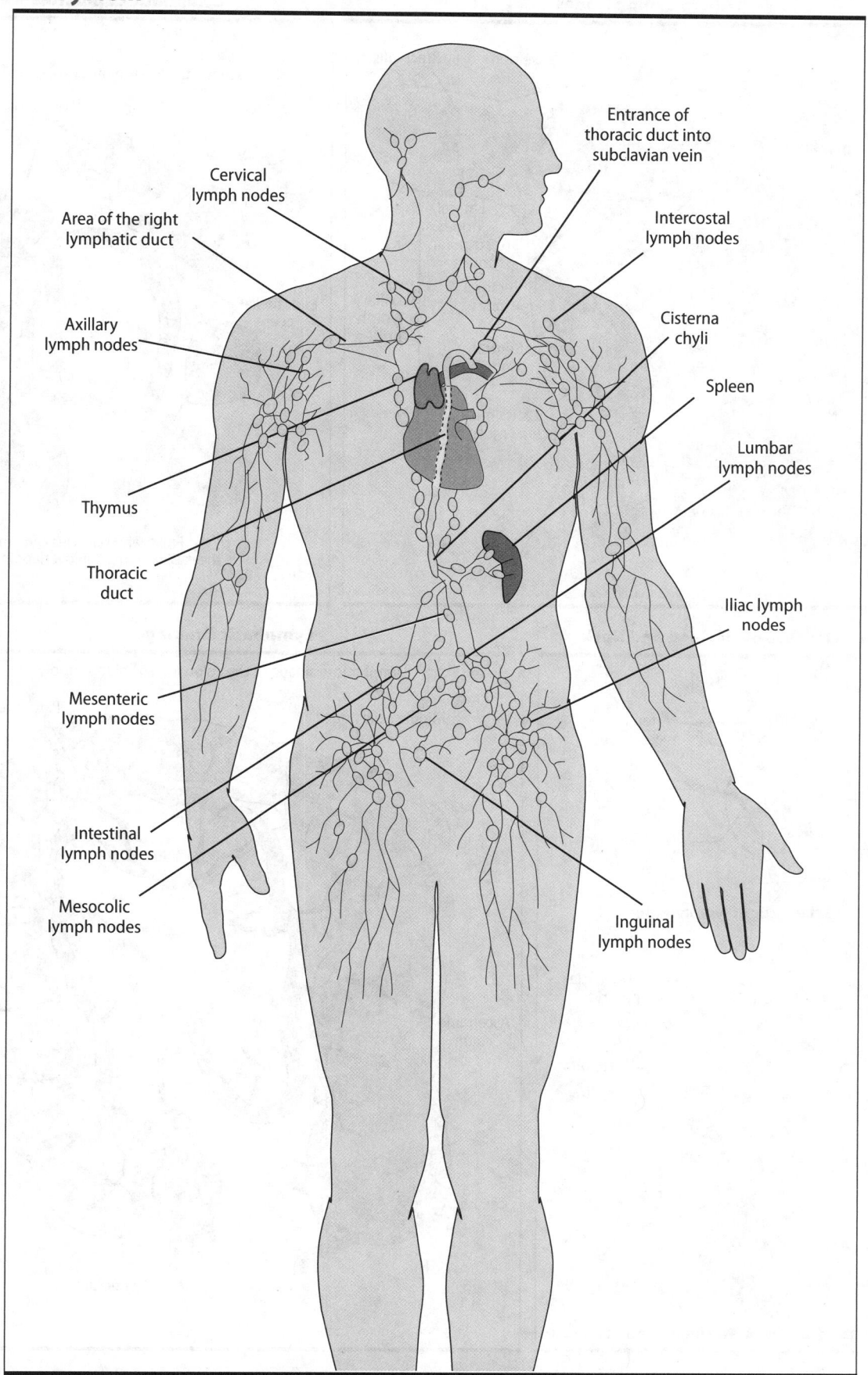

Cervical lymph nodes

Area of the right lymphatic duct

Axillary lymph nodes

Thymus

Thoracic duct

Mesenteric lymph nodes

Intestinal lymph nodes

Mesocolic lymph nodes

Entrance of thoracic duct into subclavian vein

Intercostal lymph nodes

Cisterna chyli

Spleen

Lumbar lymph nodes

Iliac lymph nodes

Inguinal lymph nodes

Anatomical Illustrations—Lymphatic System

Axillary Lymph Nodes

Lymphatic Capillaries

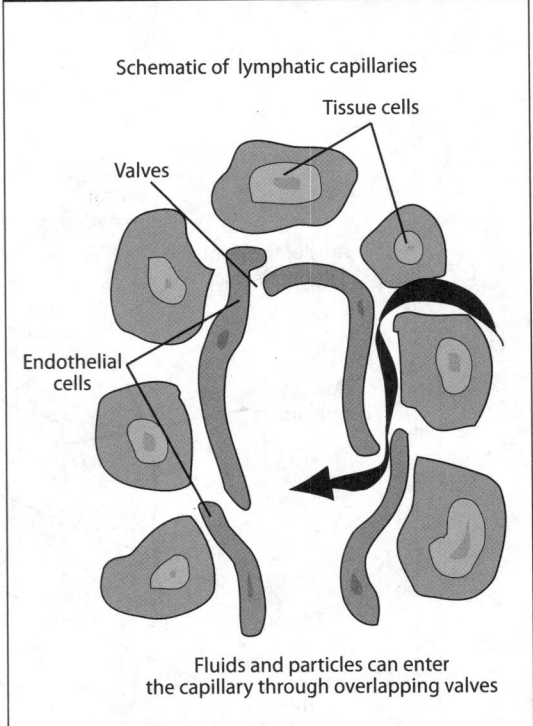

Schematic of lymphatic capillaries

Fluids and particles can enter
the capillary through overlapping valves

Lymphatic System of Head and Neck

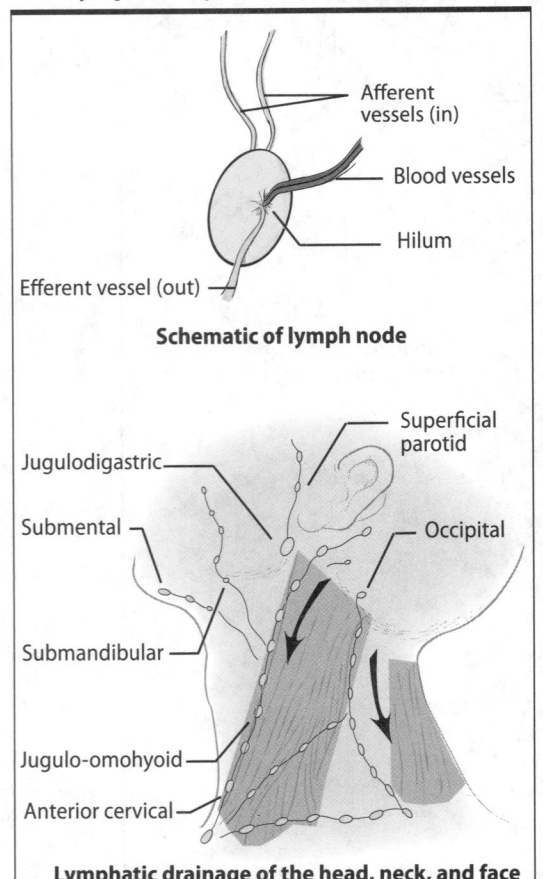

Schematic of lymph node

Lymphatic drainage of the head, neck, and face

Lymphatic Drainage

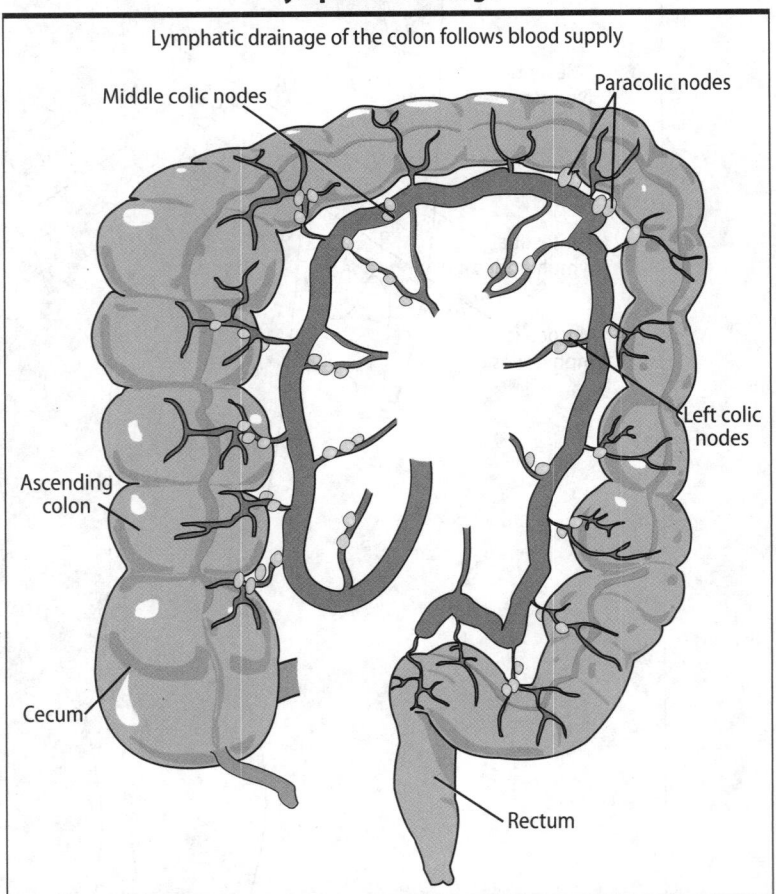

Lymphatic drainage of the colon follows blood supply

Spleen Internal Structures

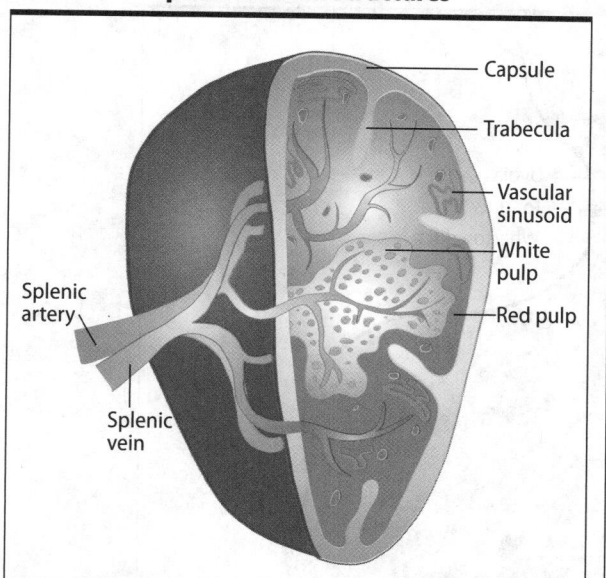

- Capsule
- Trabecula
- Vascular sinusoid
- White pulp
- Red pulp
- Splenic artery
- Splenic vein

Spleen External Structures

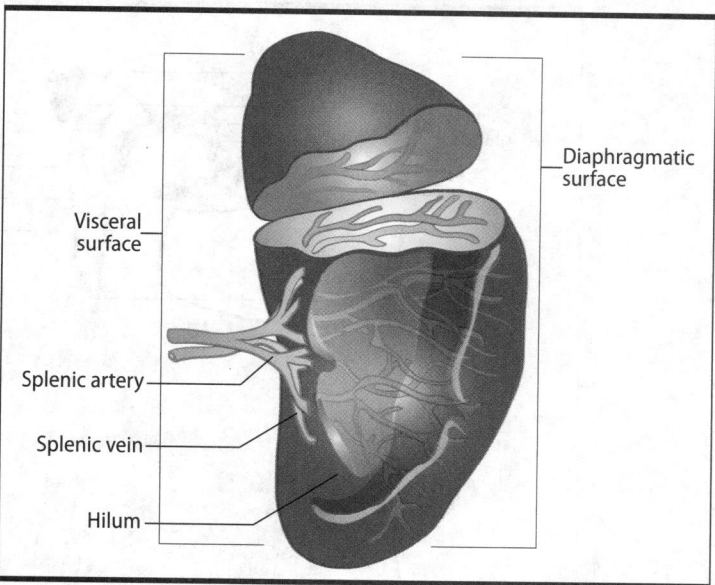

- Diaphragmatic surface
- Visceral surface
- Splenic artery
- Splenic vein
- Hilum

Digestive System

Pharynx

Salivary glands
Parotid
Sublingual
Submandibular
Oral cavity

Uvula
Tongue
Wharton duct

Esophagus

Stomach

Splenic flexure

Liver
Pancreas
Gallbladder
Common bile duct
Hepatic flexure

Duodenum
Jejunum — Small intestine
Ileum

Mesentery

Transverse colon
Ascending colon
Ileocecal valve
Cecum
Appendix
Rectum

Anus

Descending colon

Sigmoid colon

Gallbladder

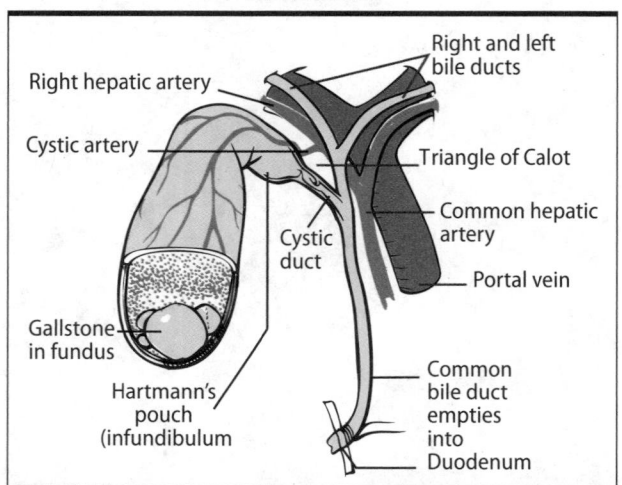

Right hepatic artery
Cystic artery
Gallstone in fundus
Hartmann's pouch (infundibulum

Right and left bile ducts
Triangle of Calot
Common hepatic artery
Portal vein
Cystic duct
Common bile duct empties into Duodenum

Stomach

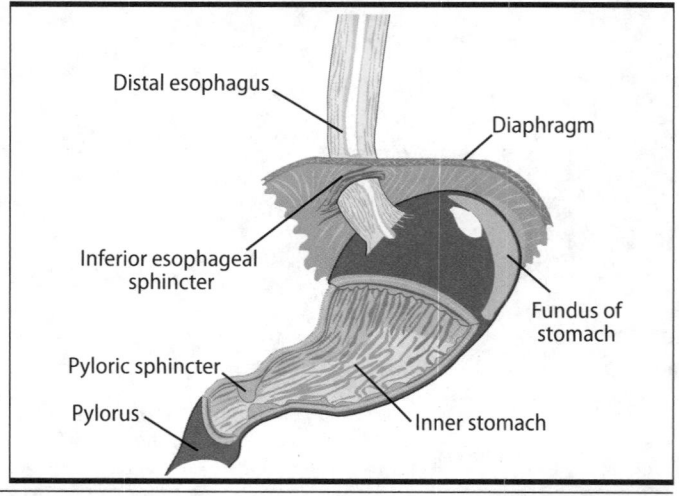

Distal esophagus
Inferior esophageal sphincter
Pyloric sphincter
Pylorus

Diaphragm
Fundus of stomach
Inner stomach

Mouth (Upper)

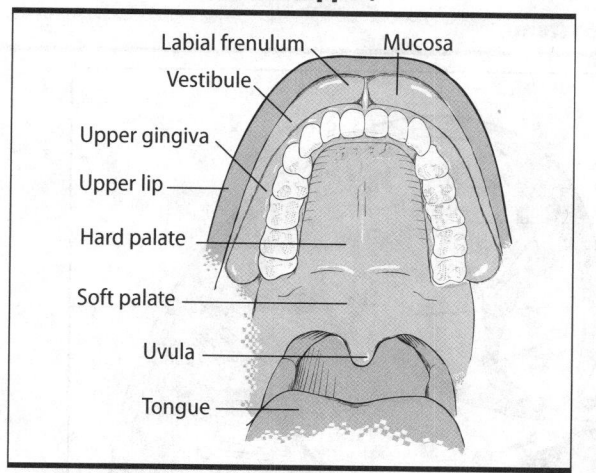

Labial frenulum
Mucosa
Vestibule
Upper gingiva
Upper lip
Hard palate
Soft palate
Uvula
Tongue

Mouth (Lower)

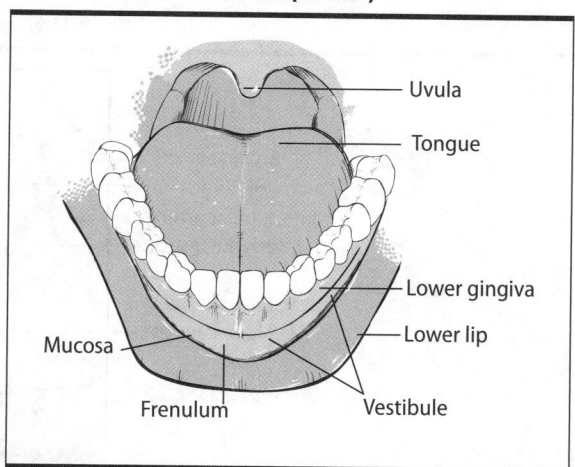

Uvula
Tongue
Lower gingiva
Lower lip
Mucosa
Vestibule
Frenulum

Pancreas

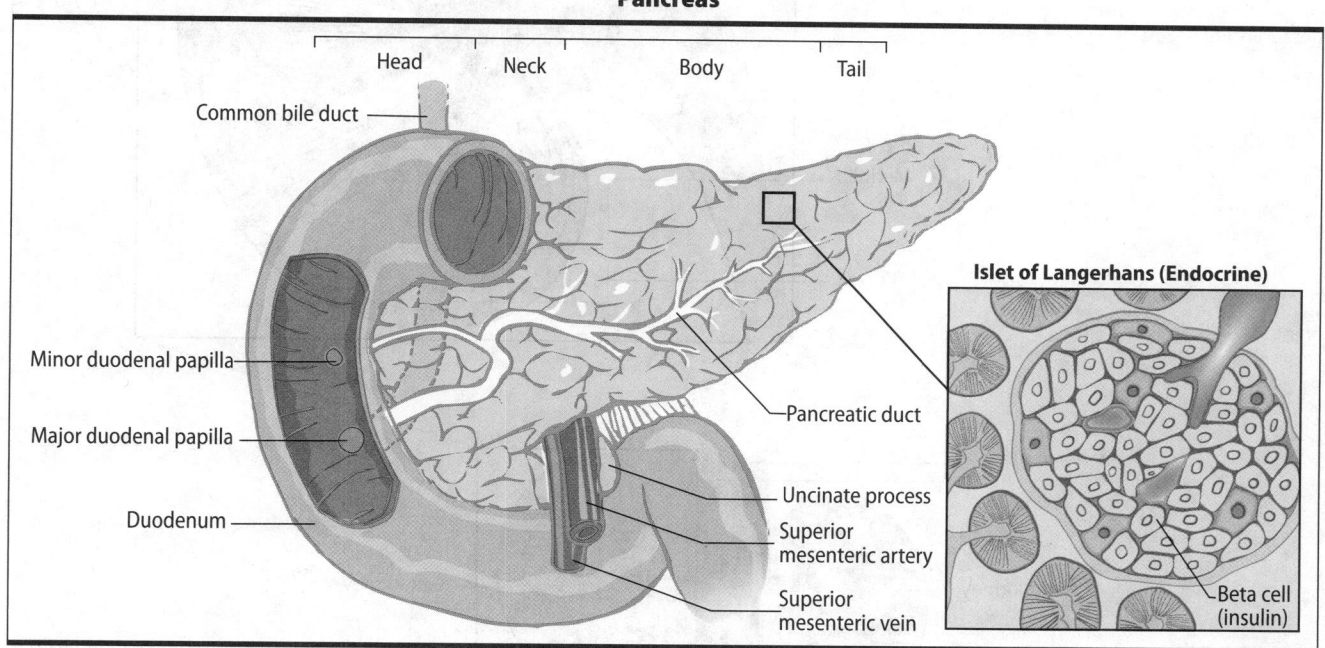

Head   Neck   Body   Tail

Common bile duct
Minor duodenal papilla
Major duodenal papilla
Duodenum
Pancreatic duct
Uncinate process
Superior mesenteric artery
Superior mesenteric vein

Islet of Langerhans (Endocrine)

Beta cell (insulin)

Liver

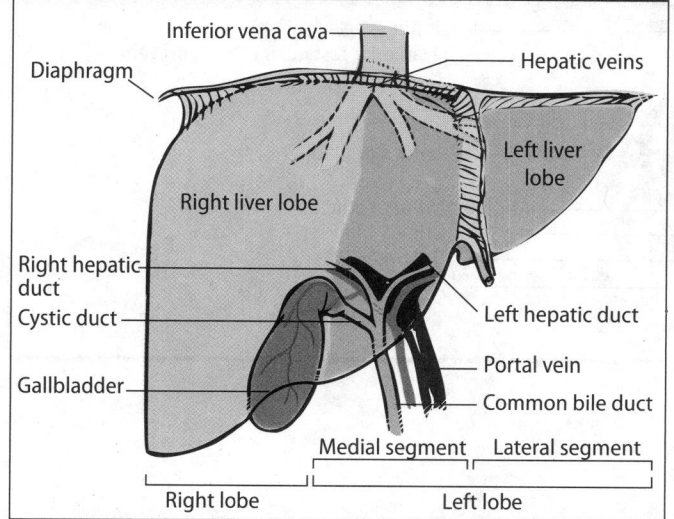

Inferior vena cava
Diaphragm
Hepatic veins
Left liver lobe
Right liver lobe
Right hepatic duct
Cystic duct
Gallbladder
Left hepatic duct
Portal vein
Common bile duct
Medial segment
Lateral segment
Right lobe
Left lobe

Anus

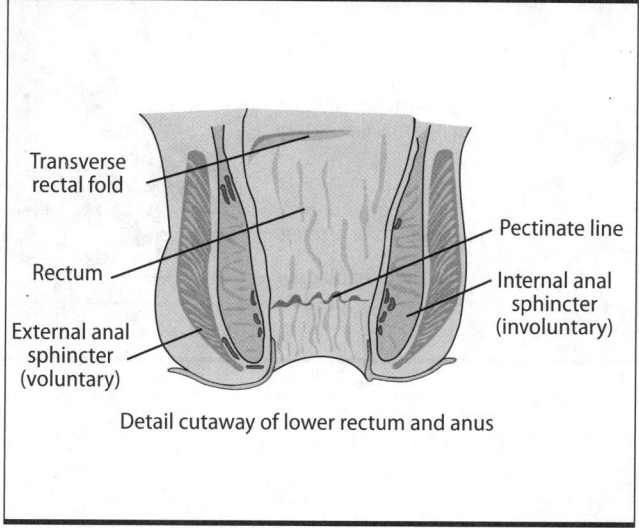

Transverse rectal fold
Rectum
External anal sphincter (voluntary)
Pectinate line
Internal anal sphincter (involuntary)

Detail cutaway of lower rectum and anus

Genitourinary System

Urinary System

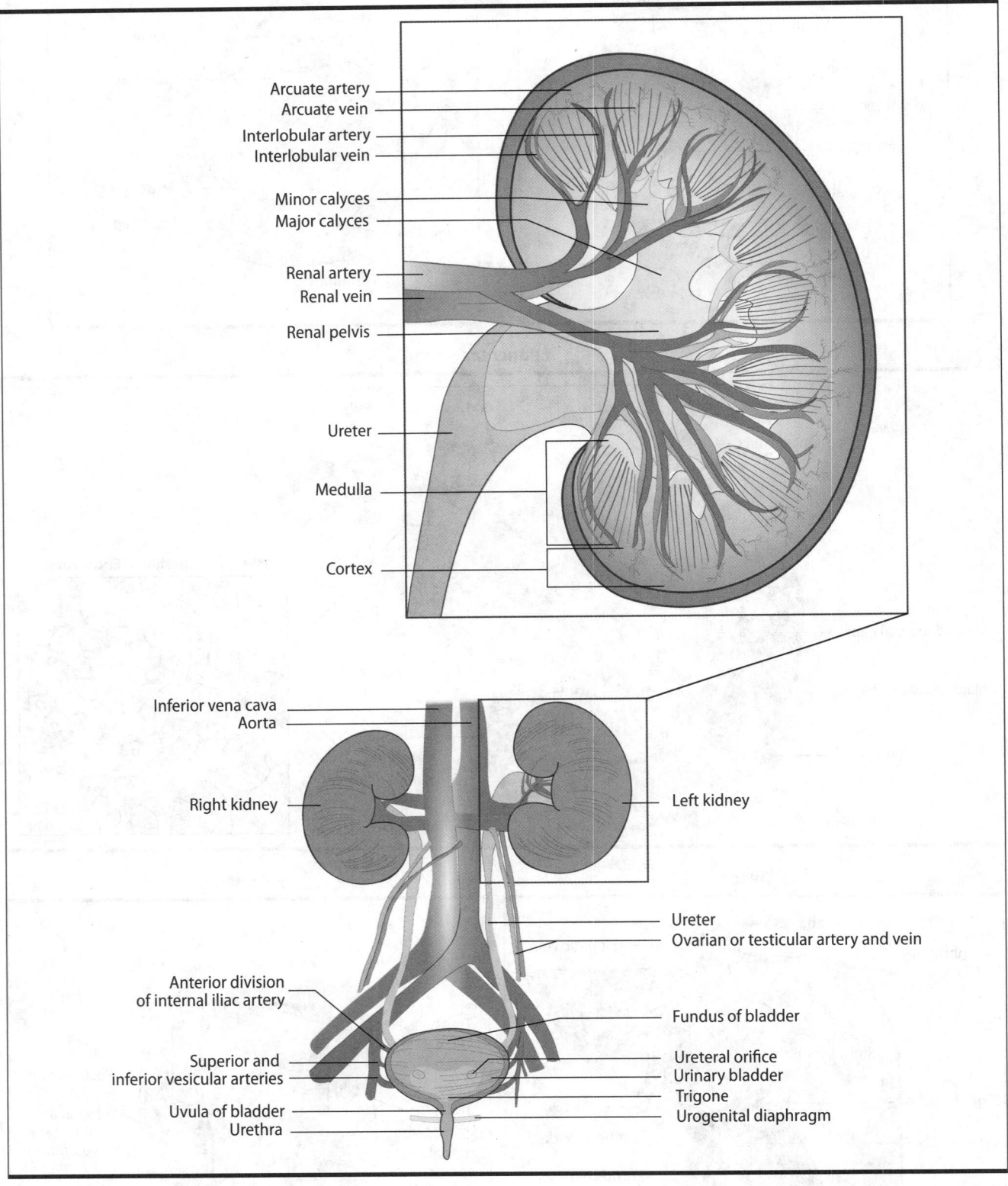

- Arcuate artery
- Arcuate vein
- Interlobular artery
- Interlobular vein
- Minor calyces
- Major calyces
- Renal artery
- Renal vein
- Renal pelvis
- Ureter
- Medulla
- Cortex

- Inferior vena cava
- Aorta
- Right kidney
- Left kidney
- Ureter
- Ovarian or testicular artery and vein
- Anterior division of internal iliac artery
- Fundus of bladder
- Superior and inferior vesicular arteries
- Ureteral orifice
- Urinary bladder
- Trigone
- Uvula of bladder
- Urogenital diaphragm
- Urethra

© 2021 Optum360, LLC

Nephron

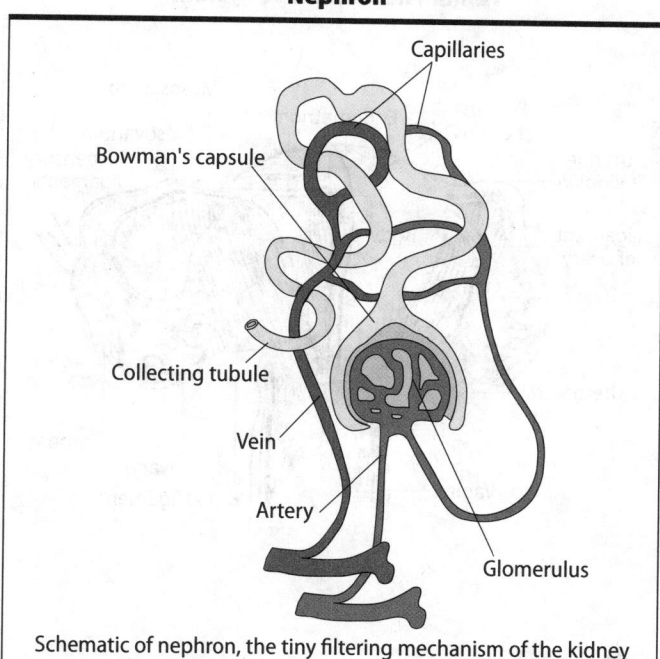

Schematic of nephron, the tiny filtering mechanism of the kidney

Male Genitourinary

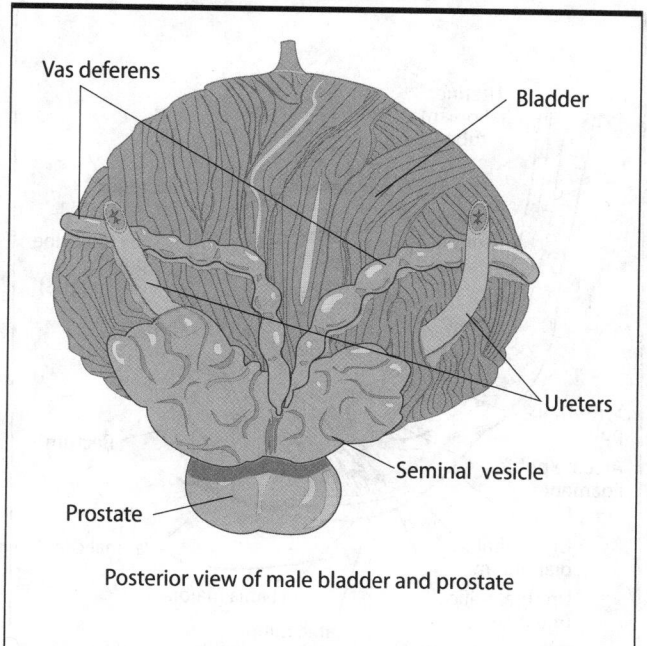

Posterior view of male bladder and prostate

Testis and Associate Structures

Male Genitourinary System

Female Genitourinary

Female Reproductive System

Female Bladder

Female Breast

Endocrine System

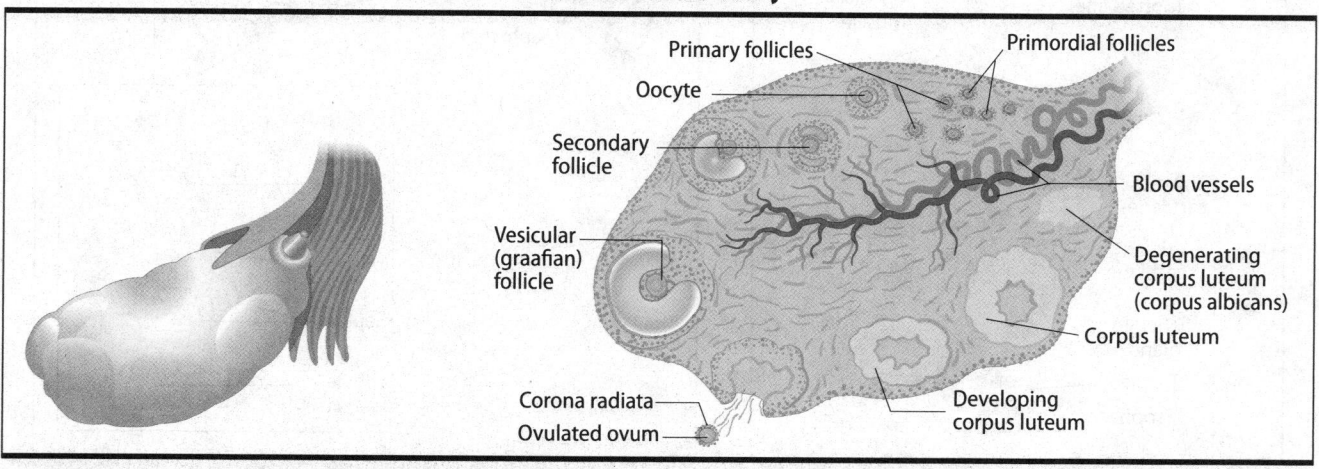

Pineal gland

Hypothalamus

Pituitary gland

Thyroid

Parathyroid gland

Adrenal gland

Pancreas

Ovaries

Structure of an Ovary

Primary follicles

Primordial follicles

Oocyte

Secondary follicle

Blood vessels

Vesicular (graafian) follicle

Degenerating corpus luteum (corpus albicans)

Corpus luteum

Developing corpus luteum

Corona radiata

Ovulated ovum

Anatomical Illustrations—Endocrine System

Thyroid and Parathyroid Glands

Posterior view

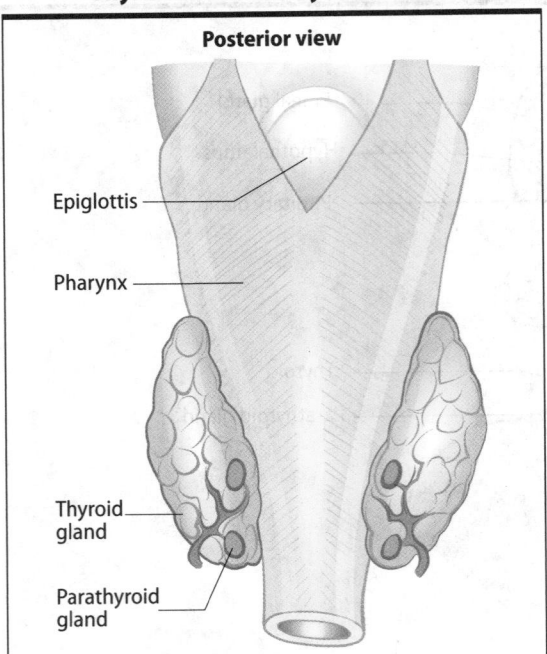

Epiglottis

Pharynx

Thyroid gland

Parathyroid gland

Adrenal Gland

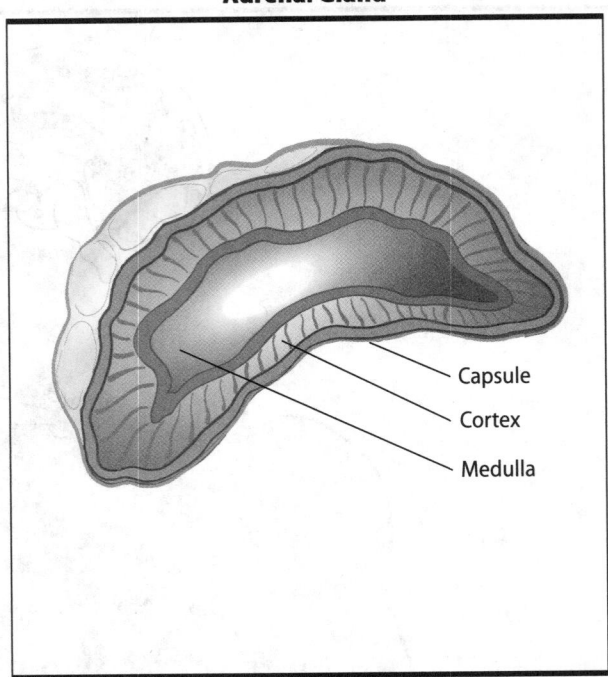

Capsule

Cortex

Medulla

Thyroid

Anterior view

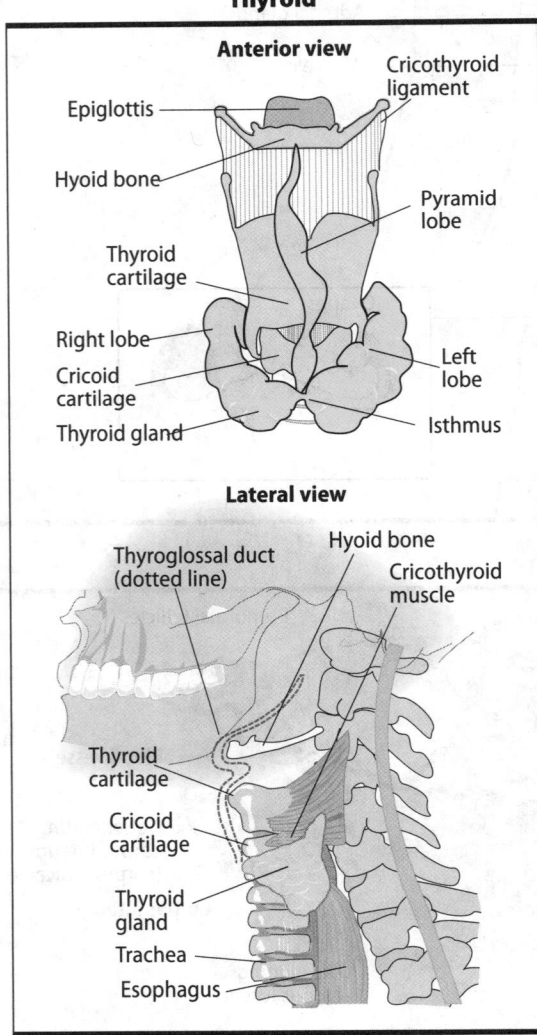

Cricothyroid ligament

Epiglottis

Hyoid bone

Pyramid lobe

Thyroid cartilage

Right lobe

Cricoid cartilage

Thyroid gland

Left lobe

Isthmus

Lateral view

Thyroglossal duct (dotted line)

Hyoid bone

Cricothyroid muscle

Thyroid cartilage

Cricoid cartilage

Thyroid gland

Trachea

Esophagus

Thymus

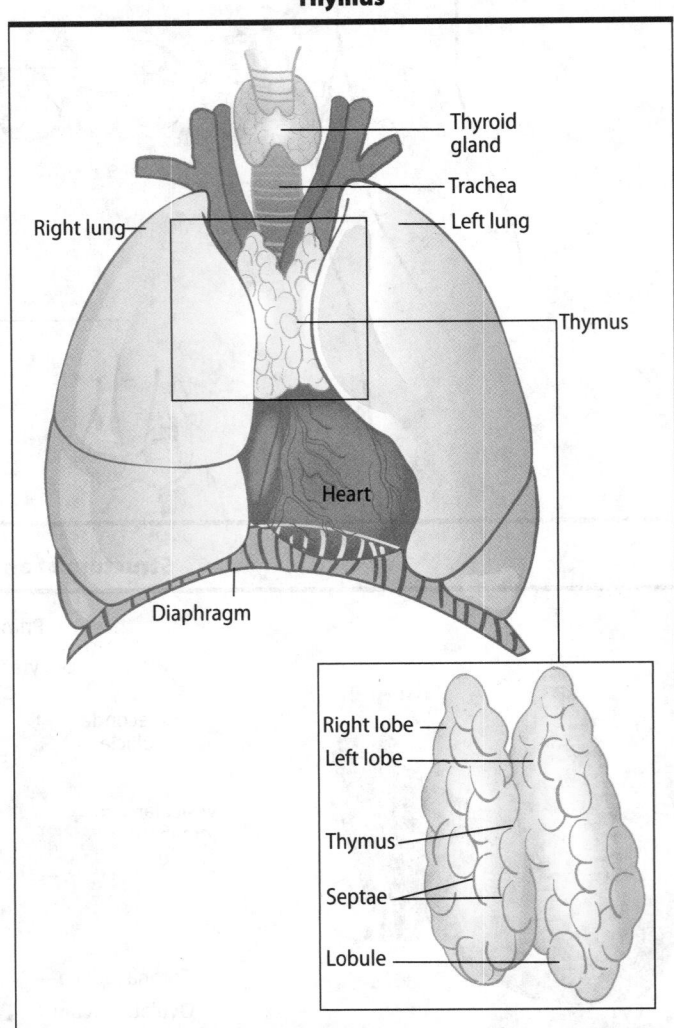

Thyroid gland

Trachea

Right lung

Left lung

Thymus

Heart

Diaphragm

Right lobe

Left lobe

Thymus

Septae

Lobule

Nervous System

Brain

Cranial Nerves

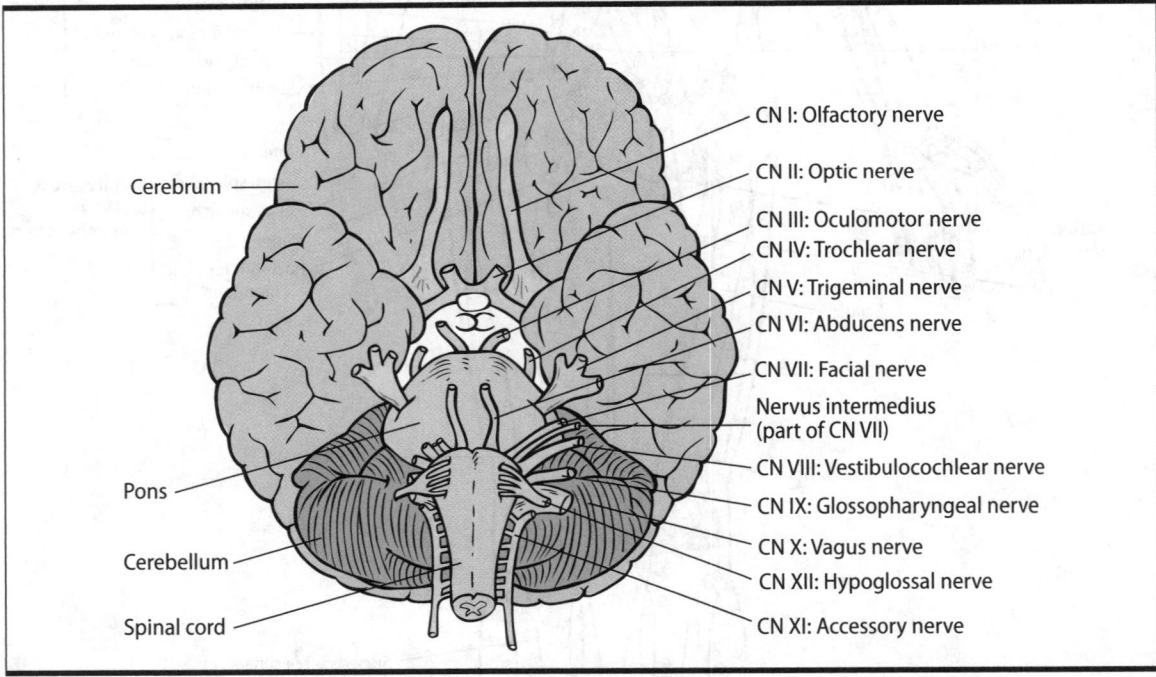

Spinal Cord and Spinal Nerves

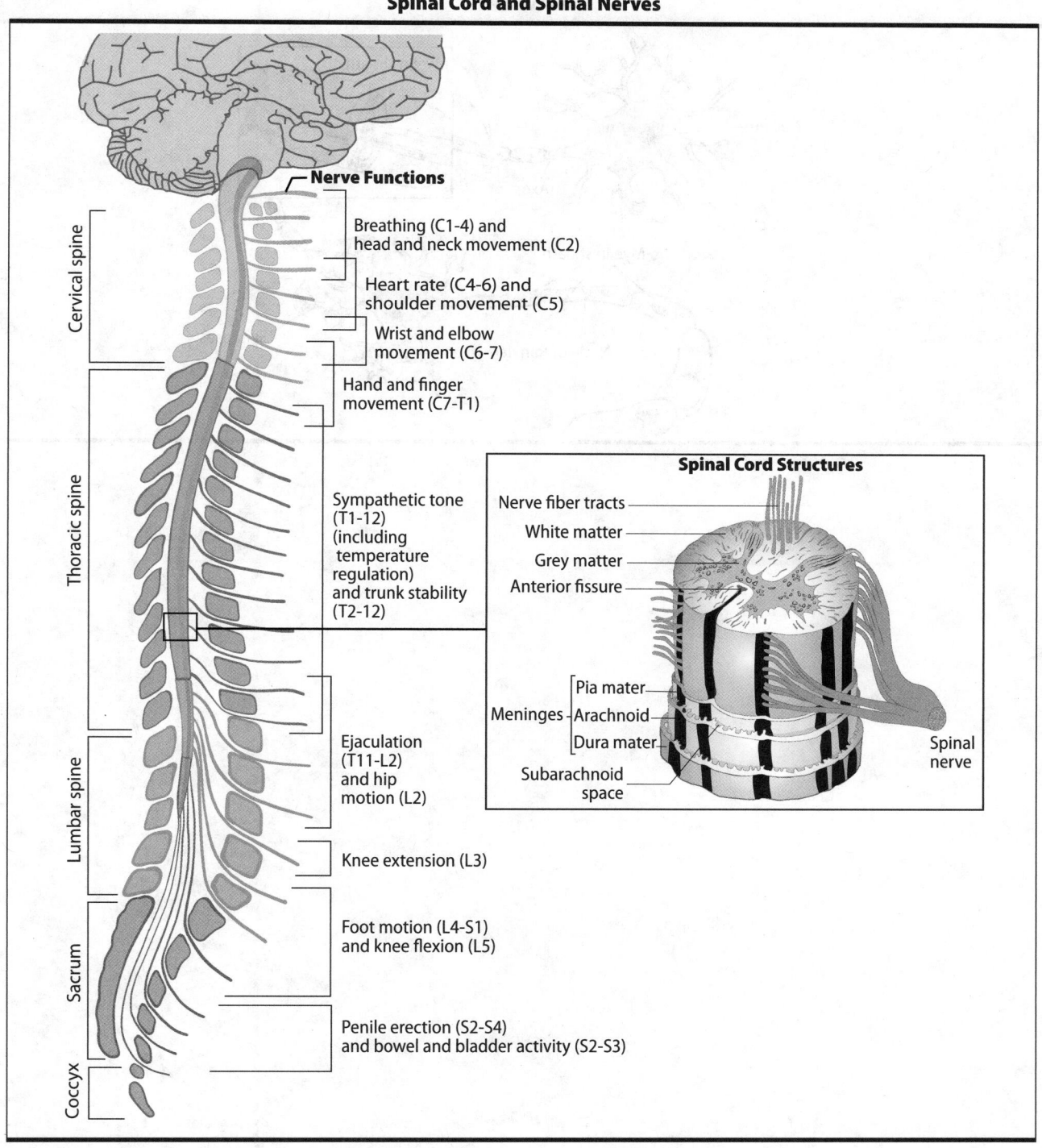

Nerve Functions

Cervical spine

Breathing (C1-4) and head and neck movement (C2)

Heart rate (C4-6) and shoulder movement (C5)

Wrist and elbow movement (C6-7)

Hand and finger movement (C7-T1)

Thoracic spine

Sympathetic tone (T1-12) (including temperature regulation) and trunk stability (T2-12)

Lumbar spine

Ejaculation (T11-L2) and hip motion (L2)

Knee extension (L3)

Sacrum

Foot motion (L4-S1) and knee flexion (L5)

Coccyx

Penile erection (S2-S4) and bowel and bladder activity (S2-S3)

Spinal Cord Structures

Nerve fiber tracts

White matter

Grey matter

Anterior fissure

Meninges — Pia mater, Arachnoid, Dura mater

Subarachnoid space

Spinal nerve

Anatomical Illustrations—Nervous System

Nerve Cell

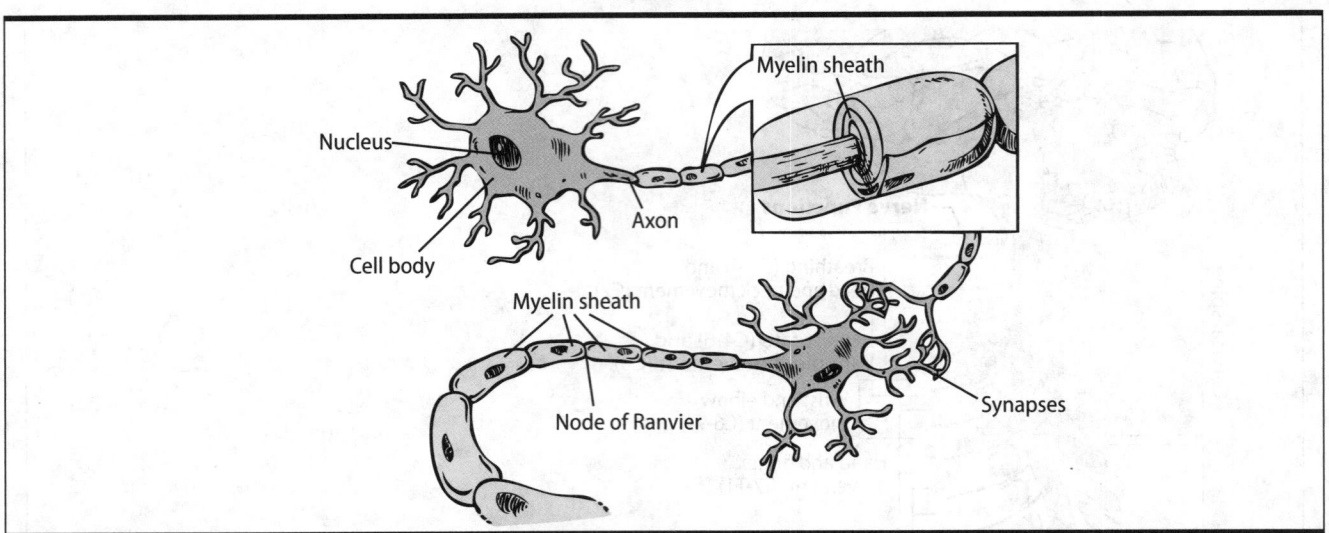

Eye

Eye Structure

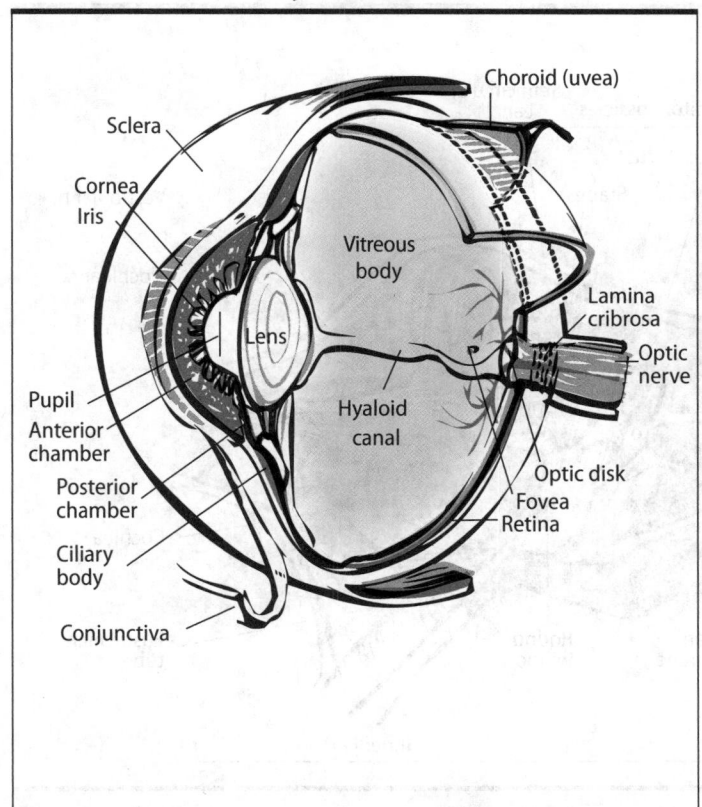

- Sclera
- Cornea
- Iris
- Choroid (uvea)
- Vitreous body
- Lamina cribrosa
- Optic nerve
- Lens
- Pupil
- Anterior chamber
- Posterior chamber
- Hyaloid canal
- Ciliary body
- Optic disk
- Fovea
- Retina
- Conjunctiva

Posterior Pole of Globe/Flow of Aqueous Humor

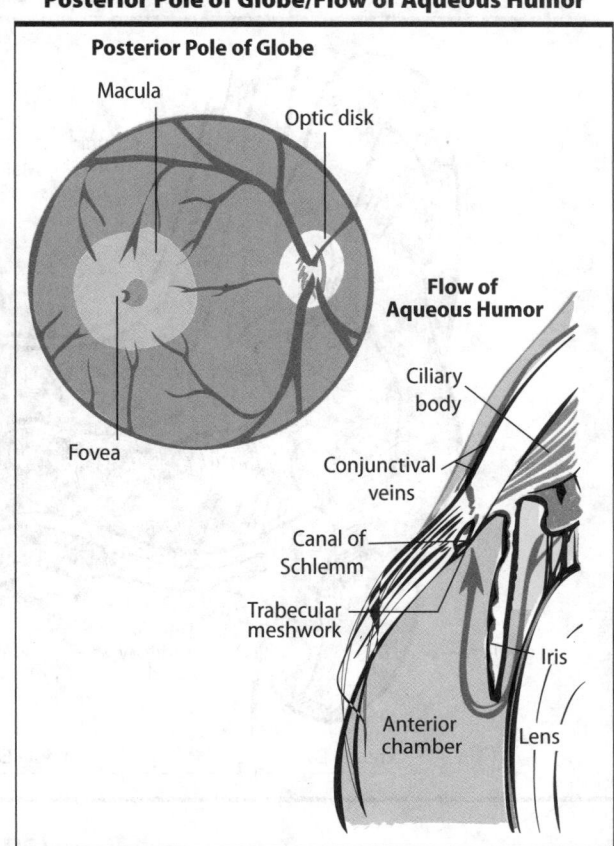

Posterior Pole of Globe
- Macula
- Optic disk
- Fovea

Flow of Aqueous Humor
- Ciliary body
- Conjunctival veins
- Canal of Schlemm
- Trabecular meshwork
- Iris
- Lens
- Anterior chamber

Eye Musculature

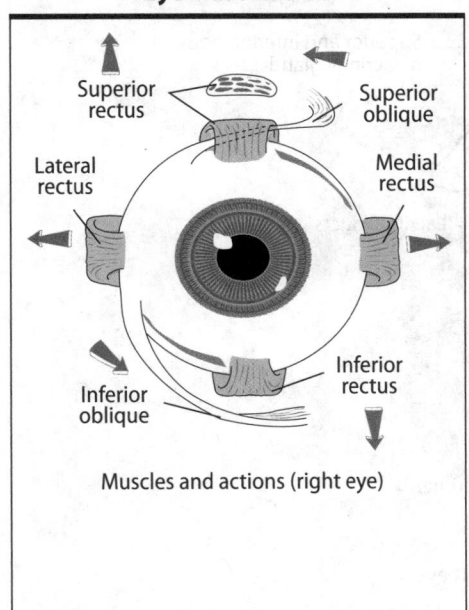

- Superior rectus
- Superior oblique
- Lateral rectus
- Medial rectus
- Inferior oblique
- Inferior rectus

Muscles and actions (right eye)

Eyelid Structures

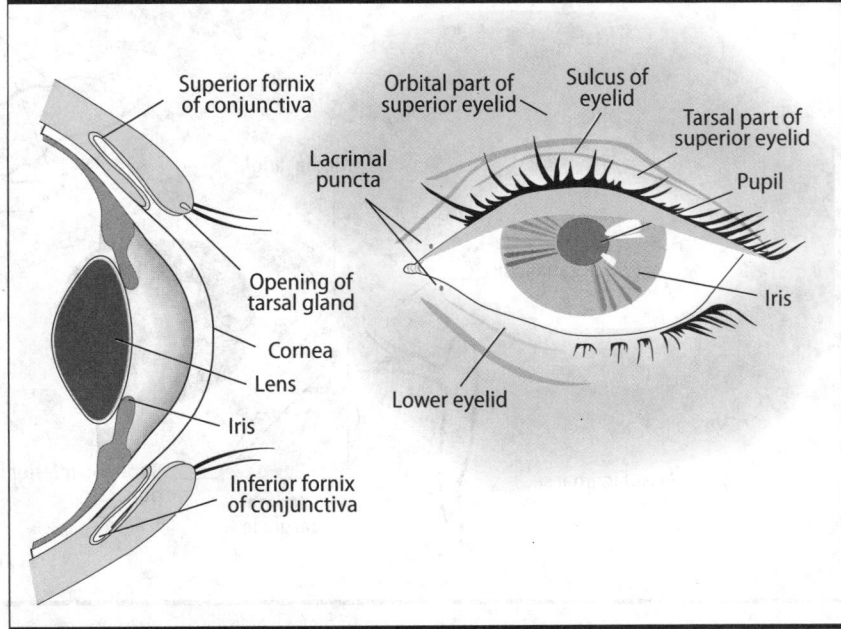

- Superior fornix of conjunctiva
- Orbital part of superior eyelid
- Sulcus of eyelid
- Tarsal part of superior eyelid
- Lacrimal puncta
- Pupil
- Opening of tarsal gland
- Cornea
- Lens
- Iris
- Iris
- Lower eyelid
- Inferior fornix of conjunctiva

Ear and Lacrimal System

Ear Anatomy

Lacrimal System

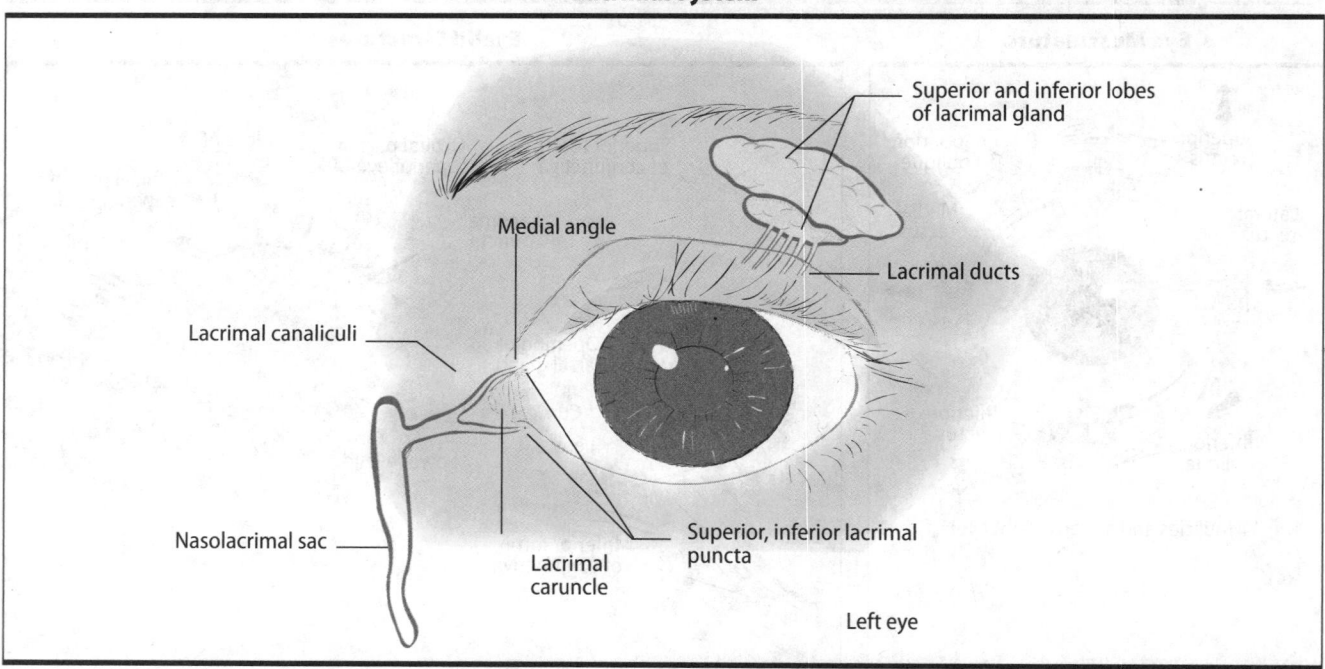

　　　　　　CPT © 2021 American Medical Association. All Rights Reserved.　　　　　　© 2021 Optum360, LLC

[Resequenced]

Adalimumab
Assay, 80145
Adamantinoma, Pituitary
See Craniopharyngioma
ADAMTS-13, 85397
Adaptive Behavior
Assessments, 0362T, [97151], [97152]
Treatment, 0373T, [97153], [97154], [97155], [97156], [97157], [97158]
Addam Operation, 26040-26045
Adductor Tenotomy of Hip
See Tenotomy, Hip, Adductor
Adelson
Crosby Immersion Method, 85999
Adenoidectomy
Primary
Age 12 or Over, 42831
Younger Than Age 12, 42830
Secondary
Age 12 or Over, 42836
Younger Than Age 12, 42835
with Tonsillectomy, 42820, 42821
Adenoids
Excision, 42830-42836
with Tonsillectomy, 42820, 42821
Unlisted Services and Procedures, 42999
Adenoma
Pancreas
Excision, 48120
Parathyroid
Injection for Localization, 78808
Thyroid Gland
Excision, 60200
Adenosine 3', 5' Monophosphate, 82030
Adenosine Diphosphate
Blood, 82030
Adenosine Monophosphate (AMP)
Blood, 82030
Adenovirus
Antibody, 86603
Antigen Detection
Enzyme Immunoassay, 87301-87451
Immunofluorescence, 87260
Adenovirus Vaccine, 90476-90477
ADH (Antidiuretic Hormone), 84588
ADHD Emotional/Behavioral Assessment, [96127]
Adhesion, Adhesions
Epidural, 62263, 62264
Eye
Corneovitreal, 65880
Incision
Anterior Segment, 65860-65870
Posterior Segment, 65875
Intermarginal
Construction, 67880
Transposition of Tarsal Plate, 67882
Intestinal
Enterolysis, 44005
Laparoscopic, 44180
Intracranial
Lysis, 62161
Intranasal Synechia, 30560
Intrauterine
Lysis, 58559
Labial
Lysis, 56441
Lungs
Pneumolysis, 32124, 32940
Pelvic
Lysis, 58660, 58662, 58740
Penile
Lysis
Post–Circumcision, 54162
Preputial
Lysis, 54450
Urethral
Lysis, 53500
Adipectomy, 15830-15839, 15876-15879
Adjustment
External Fixation, 20693, 20696
Transperineal Periurethral Balloon Continence Device, 53454
ADL
Activities of Daily Living, 97535, 97537
Administration
Health Risk Assessment, 96160-96161

Administration — *continued*
Immunization
Severe Acute Respiratory Syndrome Coronavirus (SARS-CoV, SARS-CoV-2 [COVID-19]), [0001A, 0002A, 0003A, 0004A], [0011A, 0012A, 0013A], [0021A, 0022A], [0031A], [0034A], [0041A, 0042A], [0051A, 0052A, 0053A, 0054A], [0064A], [0071A, 0072A]
with Counseling, 90460-90461
without Counseling, 90471-90474
Injection
Intramuscular Antibiotic, 96372
Therapeutic, Diagnostic, Prophylactic
Intra–arterial, 96373
Intramuscular, 96372
Intravenous, 96374-96376
Subcutaneous, 96372
Occlusive Substance During Bronchoscopy, 31634
Pharmacologic Agent w/Monitoring
Endovascular Intracranial for Other Than Thrombolysis, 61650-61651
with Monitoring, 93463
Administrative Codes for Multianalyte Assays with Algorithmic Analyses, 0002M-0004M, 0006M-0007M, 0011M, 0012M, 0013M, 0014M, 0015M, 0016M, 0017M, 0018M
ADP (Adenosine Diphosphate), 82030
ADRB2, 81401
Adrenal Cortex Hormone, 83491
Adrenal Gland
Biopsy, 60540, 60545
Excision
Laparoscopy, 60650
Retroperitoneal, 60545
Exploration, 60540, 60545
Nuclear Medicine
Imaging, 78075
Adrenal Medulla
See Medulla
Adrenalectomy, 60540
Anesthesia, 00866
Laparoscopic, 60650
with Excision Retroperitoneal Tumor, 60545
Adrenalin
Blood, 82383, 82384
Fractionated, 82384
Urine, 82382, 82384
Adrenaline or Noradrenaline
Testing, 82382-82384
Adrenocorticotropic Hormone (ACTH), 80400-80406, 80412, 80418, 82024
Blood or Urine, 82024
Stimulation Panel, 80400-80406
Adrenogenital Syndrome, 56805, 57335
Adson Test, 95870
Adult T Cell Leukemia Lymphoma Virus I, 86687, 86689
Advance Care Planning, 99497-99498
Advance Directives, 99497-99498
Advanced Life Support
Emergency Department Services, 99281-99288
Physician Direction, 99288
Advancement
Genioglossus, 21199
Tendon
Foot, 28238
Genioglossus, 21199
Advancement Flap
Skin, Adjacent Tissue Transfer, 14000-14350
AEP, [92650], [92651], [92652], [92653]
Aerosol Inhalation
Inhalation Treatment, 94640, 94664
Pentamidine, 94642
AF4/FMR2, 81171-81172
AFB (Acid Fast Bacilli), 87116
AFBG, 35539, 35540, 35646
AFF2, 81171-81172
Afferent Nerve
See Sensory Nerve
AFG3L2, 81406
AFGE, 66020
AFI, 76815

Afluria, 90655-90658
AFP, 82105, 82106
After Hours Medical Services, 99050-99060
Afterloading Brachytherapy, 77767-77768, 77770-77772
Agents, Anticoagulant
See Clotting Inhibitors
Agglutinin
Cold, 86156, 86157
Febrile, 86000
Aggregation
Platelet, 85576
AGL, 81407
AGTR1, 81400
AGTT, 82951, 82952
AHG (Antihemophilic Globulin), 85240
AHI1, 81407
Ahmed Glaucoma Valve
Insertion, 66180
Removal, 67120
Revision, 66185
AICD (Pacing Cardioverter–Defibrillator), 0571T-0580T, 33223, 93282, 93289, 93292, 93295
Heart
Defibrillator, 33240-33249 [33230, 33231, 33262, 33263, 33264], 93282, 93292, 93295
Pacemaker, 33212-33214 [33221], 33233-33237 [33227, 33228, 33229]
Aid, Hearing
Bone Conduction, 69710-69711
Check, 92590-92595
AIDS
Antibodies, 86687-86689, 86701-86703
Virus, 86701, 86703
A–II (Angiotensin II), 82163
Air Contrast Barium Enema (ACBE), 74280
AIRE, 81406
Airway
Integrity Testing Car Seat/Bed Neonate, 94780-94781
Resistance by Oscillometry, 94728
ALA (Aminolevulinic Acid), 82135
Alanine 2 Oxoglutarate Aminotransferase
See Transaminase, Glutamic Pyruvic
Alanine Amino (ALT), 84460
Alanine Transaminase
See Transaminase, Glutamic Pyruvic
Albumin
Cobalt Binding (ACB), 82045
Ischemia Modified, 82045
Other Source, [82042]
Serum Plasma, 82040
Urine, 82043-82044
Whole Blood, 82040
Alcohol, [80320]
Abuse Screening and Intervention, 99408-99409
Biomarkers, [80321, 80322]
Breath, 82075
Ethylene Glycol, 82693
Other Source, 82077
Alcohol Dehydrogenase
See Antidiuretic Hormone
Alcohol, Isopropyl
See Isopropyl Alcohol
Alcohol, Methyl
See Methanol
ALDH7A1, 81406, [81419]
Aldolase
Blood, 82085
Aldosterone
Blood, 82088
Suppression Evaluation, 80408
Urine, 82088
Alexander's Operation, 58400-58410
ALIF (Anterior Lumbar Interbody Fusion), 22558-22585
Alimentary Canal
See Gastrointestinal Tract
ALK (Automated Lamellar Keratoplasty), 65710
Alkaline Phosphatase, 84075-84080
Leukocyte, 85540
WBC, 85540
Alkaloids, [80323]
See Also Specific Drug

Allergen Bronchial Provocation Tests, 95070
Allergen Challenge, Endobronchial, 95070
Allergen Immunotherapy
Allergen
Allergenic Extracts
Extract Supply with Injection, 95120-95134
Injection, 95115, 95117
with Extract Supply, 95120-95134
Injection Only, 95115-95117
Antigens, 95144-95165
IgE, 86003, 86005, 86008
IgG, 86001
Injection
with Extract Supply, 95120, 95125
without Extract Supply, 95115, 95117
Insect Venom
Prescription
Supply, 95145-95149
Injection, 95130-95134
Prescription
Supply, 95165
Insect, Whole Body, 95170
Rapid Desensitization, 95180
Unlisted Services and Procedures, 95199
Allergy Services/Procedures
See Allergen Immunotherapy
Allergy Tests
Challenge Test
Bronchial, 95070
Ingestion, 95076, 95079
Eye Allergy, 95060
Food Allergy, 95076, 95079
Intradermal
Allergen Extract, 95024, 95028
Biologicals or Drugs, 95018
Incremental, 95027
Venoms, 95017
Nasal Mucous Membrane Test, 95065
Nose Allergy, 95065
Patch
Application Tests, 95044
Photo Patch, 95052
Photosensitivity, 95056
Skin Tests
Allergen Extract, 95004, 95024, 95027
Biologicals or Drugs, 95018
End Point Titration, 95027
Venoms, 95017
Allogeneic Donor
Backbench Preparation
Intestine, 44715-44721
Kidney, 50323-50329
Liver, 47143-47147
Pancreas, 48551-48552
Lymphocyte Infusion, 38242
Allogeneic Transplantation
See Homograft
Backbench Preparation, 44715-44721
Intestine, 44715-44721
Kidney, 50323-50329
Liver, 47143-47147
Pancreas, 48551-48552
Hematopoietic Progenitor Cells, 38240
Allograft
Aortic Valve, 33406, 33413
Bone, Structural, 20931-20932
Cartilage
Knee, 27415
Elbow, 24370-24371
Lung Transplant, 32850
Osteoarticular, 20932
Sacroiliac Joint (Stabilization), 27279
Shoulder, 23473-23474
Skin Substitute Graft, 15271-15278
Spine Surgery
Morselized, 20930
Osteopromotive Material, 20930
Structural, 20931
Uterus
Backbench Reconstruction, 0669T-0670T
Standard Preparation, 0668T
Allograft Preparation
Cornea, 65757
Heart, 33933, 33944
Intestines, 44715-44721

[Resequenced]   CPT © 2021 American Medical Association. All Rights Reserved.   © 2021 Optum360, LLC

Index — Analysis
Analysis — Analysis

Analysis — continued

Multianalyte Assays with Algorithmic Analysis — continued
  Probability Predicted Main Cancer Type/Subtype, [81540]
  Recurrence Score, 81519, 81525
  Rejection Risk Score, [81595]
  Risk Score, 81493, 81506-81512, 81539-81551 [81503, 81504, 81546], [81500]
  Tissue Similarity, [81504]
  Unlisted Assay, 81599
Pacemaker, 93279-93281, 93288, 93293-93294
Patient Specific Findings, 99199
Physiologic Data, Remote, [99091], [99453, 99454], [99457]
Prostate Tissue Fluorescence Spectroscopy, 0443T
Protein
  Tissue
    Western Blot, 88372
Semen, 89320-89322
  Sperm Isolation, 89260, 89261
Spectrum, 82190
Tear Osmolarity, 83861
Tissue Composition
  Quantitative Magnetic Resonance, 0648T, 0649T
  Mulitple Organs, [0697T], [0698T]
Translocation
  PML/RARalpha, 81315-81316
  t(9;22) (BCF/ABL1), [81206, 81207, 81208, 81209]
  t(15;17), 81315-81316
X Chromosome Inactivation, [81204]

Anaspadias
See Epispadias

Anastomosis
Arteriovenous Fistula
  Direct, 36821
  Revision, 36832, 36833
    with Thrombectomy, 36833
    without Thrombectomy, 36832
  with Bypass Graft, 35686
  with Graft, 36825, 36830, 36832
  with Thrombectomy, 36831
Artery
  to Aorta, 33606
  to Artery
    Cranial, 61711
Bile Duct
  to Bile Duct, 47800
  to Intestines, 47760, 47780
Bile Duct to Gastrointestinal, 47760, 47780, 47785
Broncho–Bronchial, 32486
Caval to Mesenteric, 37160
Cavopulmonary, 33622, 33768
Colorectal, 44620, 44626
Epididymis
  to Vas Deferens
    Bilateral, 54901
    Unilateral, 54900
Excision
  Trachea, 31780, 31781
    Cervical, 31780
Fallopian Tube, 58750
Gallbladder to Intestine, 47720-47740
Gallbladder to Pancreas, 47999
Hepatic Duct to Intestine, 47765, 47802
Ileo–Anal, 45113
Intestine to Intestine, 44130
Intestines
  Colo–anal, 45119
  Cystectomy, 51590
  Enterocystoplasty, 51960
  Enterostomy, 44620-44626
  Ileoanal, 44157-44158
  Resection
    Laparoscopic, 44202-44205
Intrahepatic Portosystemic, 37182, 37183
Jejunum, 43820-43825
Microvascular
  Free Transfer Jejunum, 43496
Nerve
  Facial to Hypoglossal, 64868

Anastomosis — continued
Nerve — continued
  Facial to Spinal Accessory, 64864, 64865
Oviduct, 58750
Pancreas to Intestines, 48520, 48540, 48548
Polya, 43632
Portocaval, 37140
Pulmonary, 33606
Renoportal, 37145
Splenorenal, 37180, 37181
Stomach, 43825
  to Duodenum, 43810
  to Jejunum, 43820, 43825, 43860, 43865
Tubotubal, 58750
Ureter
  to Bladder, 50780-50785
  to Colon, 50810, 50815
    Removal, 50830
  to Intestine, 50800, 50820, 50825
    Removal, 50830
  to Kidney, 50727-50750
  to Ureter, 50725-50728, 50760, 50770
Vein
  Saphenopopliteal, 34530
Vein to Vein, 37140-37183

Anastomosis, Aorta–Pulmonary Artery
See Aorta, Anastomosis, to Pulmonary Artery

Anastomosis, Bladder, to Intestine
See Enterocystoplasty

Anastomosis, Hepatic Duct
See Hepatic Duct, Anastomosis

Anastomosis of Lacrimal Sac to Conjunctival Sac
See Conjunctivorhinostomy

Anastomosis of Pancreas
See Pancreas, Anastomosis

Anatomic
Guide, 3D Printed, 0561T-0562T
Model, 3D Printed, 0559T-0560T

ANC, 85048
Anderson Tibial Lengthening, 27715
Androstanediol Glucuronide, 82154
Androstanolone
See Dihydrotestosterone

Androstenedione
Blood or Urine, 82157

Androstenolone
See Dehydroepiandrosterone

Androsterone
Blood or Urine, 82160

Anesthesia
See Also Analgesia
Abbe–Estlander Procedure, 00102
Abdomen
  Abdominal Wall, 00700-00730, 00800, 00802, 00820-00836
    Halsted Repair, 00750-00756
  Blood Vessels, 00770, 00880-00882, 01930, 01931
    Inferior Vena Cava Ligation, 00882
    Transvenous Umbrella Insertion, 01930
  Endoscopy, 00731-00732, 00811-00813
  Extraperitoneal, 00860, 00862, 00866-00868, 00870
  Hernia Repair, 00830-00836
    Diaphragmatic, 00756
    Halsted Repair, 00750-00756
    Omphalocele, 00754
  Intraperitoneal, 00790-00797, 00840-00851
  Laparoscopy, 00790
  Liver Transplant, 00796
  Pancreatectomy, 00794
  Renal Transplant, 00868
Abdominoperineal Resection, 00844
Abortion
  Incomplete, 01965
  Induced, 01966
Achilles Tendon Repair, 01472
Acromioclavicular Joint, 01620
Adrenalectomy, 00866
Amniocentesis, 00842
Amputation
  Femur, 01232
  Forequarter, 01636
  Interthoracoscapular, 01636

Anesthesia — continued
Amputation — continued
  Penis
    Complete, 00932
    Radical with Bilateral Inguinal and Iliac Lymphadenectomy, 00936
    Radical with Bilateral Inguinal Lymphadenectomy, 00934
Aneurysm
  Axillary–Brachial, 01652
  Knee, 01444
  Popliteal Artery, 01444
Angiography, 01920
Angioplasty, 01924-01926
Ankle, 00400, 01462-01522
  Achilles Tendon, 01472
  Nerves, Muscles, Tendons, 01470
  Skin, 00400
Anorectal Procedure, 00902
Anus, 00902
Arm
  Lower, 00400, 01810-01860
    Arteries, 01842
    Bones, Closed, 01820
    Bones, Open, 01830
    Cast Application, 01860
    Cast Removal, 01860
    Embolectomy, 01842
    Nerves, Muscle, Tendons, 01810
    Phleborrhaphy, 01852
    Shunt Revision, 01844
    Skin, 00400
    Total Wrist, 01832
    Veins, 01850
  Upper Arm, and Elbow, 00400, 01710-01782
    Nerves, Muscles, Tendons, 01710
      Tenodesis, 01716
      Tenoplasty, 01714
      Tenotomy, 01712
    Skin, 00400
Arrhythmias, 00410
Arteriograms, 01916
Arteriography, 01916
Arteriovenous (AV) Fistula, 01432
Arthroplasty
  Hip, 01214, 01215
  Knee, 01402
Arthroscopic Procedures
  Ankle, 01464
  Elbow, 01732-01740
  Foot, 01464
  Hip, 01202
  Knee, 01382, 01400, 01464
  Shoulder, 01610-01638
  Wrist, 01829-01830
Auditory Canal, External
  Removal Foreign Body, 69205
Axilla, 00400, 01610-01670
Back Skin, 00300
Batch–Spittler–McFaddin Operation, 01404
Biopsy, 00100
  Anorectal, 00902
  Clavicle, 00454
  External Ear, 00120
  Inner Ear, 00120
  Intraoral, 00170
  Liver, 00702
  Middle Ear, 00120
  Nose, 00164
  Parotid Gland, 00100
  Salivary Gland, 00100
  Sinuses, Accessory, 00164
  Sublingual Gland, 00100
  Submandibular Gland, 00100
Bladder, 00870, 00912
Blepharoplasty, 00103
Brain, 00210-00218, 00220-00222
Breast, 00402-00406
  Augmentation Mammoplasty, 00402
  Breast Reduction, 00402
  Muscle Flaps, 00402
Bronchi, 00542
  Intrathoracic Repair of Trauma, 00548
  Reconstruction, 00539

Anesthesia — continued
Bronchoscopy, 00520
Burns
  Debridement and/or Excision, 01951-01953
  Dressings and/or Debridement, 16020-16030
Burr Hole, 00214
Bypass Graft
  Coronary Artery without Pump Oxygenator, 00566
  Leg
    Lower, 01500
    Upper, 01270
  Shoulder, Axillary, 01654, 01656
  with Pump Oxygenator, Younger Than One Year of Age, 00561
Cardiac Catheterization, 01920
Cardioverter, 00534, 00560
Cast
  Application
    Body Cast, 01130
    Forearm, 01860
    Hand, 01860
    Knee Joint, 01420
    Lower Leg, 01490
    Pelvis, 01130
    Shoulder, 01680
    Wrist, 01860
  Removal
    Forearm, 01860
    Hand, 01860
    Knee Joint, 01420
    Lower Leg, 01490
    Shoulder, 01680
  Repair
    Forearm, 01860
    Hand, 01860
    Knee Joint, 01420
    Lower Leg, 01490
    Shoulder, 01680
Central Venous Circulation, 00532
Cervical Cerclage, 00948
Cervix, 00948
Cesarean Section, 01961, 01963, 01968, 01969
Chest, 00400-00410, 00470-00474, 00522, 00530-00539, 00542, 00546-00550
Chest Skin, 00400
Childbirth
  Cesarean Delivery, 01961, 01963, 01968, 01969
  External Cephalic Version, 01958
  Vaginal Delivery, 01960, 01967
Clavicle, 00450, 00454
Cleft Lip Repair, 00102
Cleft Palate Repair, 00172
Colpectomy, 00942
Colporrhaphy, 00942
Colpotomy, 00942
Conscious Sedation, 99151-99157
Corneal Transplant, 00144
Coronary Procedures, 00560-00580
Craniectomy, 00211
Cranioplasty, 00215
Craniotomy, 00211
Culdoscopy, 00950
Cystectomy, 00864
Cystolithotomy, 00870
Cystourethroscopy
  Local, 52265
  Spinal, 52260
Decortication, 00542
Defibrillator, 00534, 00560
Diaphragm, 00540-00541
Disarticulation
  Hip, 01212
  Knee, 01404
  Shoulder, 01634
Discography, 01937-01938
Donor
  Nephrectomy, 00862
Dressing Change, 15852
Drug Administration
  Epidural or Subarachnoid, 01996
Ear, 00120-00126
ECT, 00104

Bladder — *continued*
 Radiotracer, 51020, 52250
 Reconstruction
  Radiofrequency Micro-Remodeling, 53860
  with Intestines, 51960
  with Urethra, 51800, 51820
 Removal
  Calculus, 51050, 51065, 52310, 52315, 52352
  Foreign Body, 52310, 52315
  Litholapaxy, 52317-52318
  Lithotripsy, 51065, 52353
  Urethral Stent, 52310, 52315
 Repair
  Diverticulum, 52305
  Exstrophy, 51940
  Fistula, 44660, 44661, 45800, 45805, 51880-51925
  Neck, 51845
  Wound, 51860, 51865
 Resection, 52500
 Residual Study, 78730
 Sphincter Surgery, 52277
 Suspension, 51990
 Suture
  Fistula, 44660, 44661, 45800, 45805, 51880-51925
  Wound, 51860, 51865
 Tumor
  Excision, 51530
  Fulguration, 52234-52240
  Resection, 52234-52240
 Unlisted Services and Procedures, 53899
 Ureterocele, 51535
 Urethrocystography, 74450, 74455
 Urethrotomy, 52270-52276
 Urinary Incontinence Procedures
  Laparoscopy, 51990, 51992
  Plan of Care Documented, 0509F
  Radiofrequency Micro-Remodeling, 53860
  Sling Operation, 51992
  Urethral Suspension, 51990
 Uroflowmetry, 51736-51741
 Voiding Pressure Studies, 51727-51729 [51797]
 X-ray, 74430
  with Contrast, 74450, 74455
Blair Arthrodesis, 27870
Blalock–Hanlon Procedure, 33735-33737
Blalock–Taussig Procedure, 33750
Blast Transformation
 See Blastogenesis
Blastocyst Transfer
 See Embryo Transfer
Blastogenesis, 86353
Blastomyces
 Antibody, 86612
Blastomycosis, European
 See Cryptococcus
Blatt Capsulodesis, 25320
Bleeding
 See Hemorrhage
Bleeding, Anal
 See Anus, Hemorrhage
Bleeding Disorder
 See Coagulopathy
Bleeding Time, 85002
Bleeding, Uterine
 See Hemorrhage, Uterus
Bleeding, Vaginal
 See Hemorrhage, Vagina
Blepharoplasty, 15820-15823
 See Canthoplasty
 Anesthesia, 00103
 Ectropion
  Excision Tarsal Wedge, 67916
  Extensive, 67917
 Entropion
  Excision Tarsal Wedge, 67923
  Extensive, 67924
Blepharoptosis
 Repair, 67901-67909
  Frontalis Muscle Technique, 67901
   with Fascial Sling, 67902

Blepharoptosis — *continued*
 Repair — *continued*
  Superior Rectus Technique with Fascial Sling, 67906
  Tarso Levator Resection Advancement
   External Approach, 67904
   Internal Approach, 67903
Blepharorrhaphy
 See Tarsorrhaphy
Blepharospasm
 Chemodenervation, 64612
Blepharotomy, 67700
Blister
 See Bulla
BLM, 81412, [81209]
Blom–Singer Prosthesis, 31611
Blood
 Banking
  Frozen Blood Preparation, 86930-86932, 88240
  Frozen Plasma Preparation, 86927
  Physician Services, 86077-86079
 Bleeding Time, 85002
 Blood Clot
  Assay, 85396
  Clotting
   Factor, 85250-85293
   Factor Test, 85210
   Inhibitors, 85300-85301
  Coagulation Time, 85345-85348
  Lysis Time, 85175
  Retraction, 85170
  Thrombolytic Agents
   Tissue Plasminogen Activator (tPA), 4077F
 Cell
  CD4 and CD8
   Including Ratio, 86360
  Enzyme Activity, 82657
  Exchange, 36511-36513
  Sedimentation Rate
   Automated, 85652
   Manual, 85651
 Cell Count
  Automated, 85049
  B–Cells, 86355
  Blood Smear, 85007, 85008
  Complete Blood Count (CBC), 85025, 85027
  Differential WBC Count, 85004-85007, 85009
  Hematocrit, 85014
  Hemoglobin, 85018
  Hemogram
   Added Indices, 85025-85027
   Automated, 85025-85027
   Manual, 85032
  Microhematocrit, 85013
  Natural Killer (NK) Cells, 86357
  Red
   See Red Blood Cell (RBC), Count
  Red Blood Cells, 85032-85041
  Reticulocyte, 85044-85046
  Stem Cells, 86367
  T Cell, 86359-86361
  White
   See White Blood Cell, Count
  White Blood Cell, 85032, 85048, 89055
 Clot
  Assay, 85396
   Activity, 85397
    ADAMTS-13, 85397
  Clot Lysis Time, 85175
  Clot Retraction, 85170
  Clotting Factor, 85250-85293
  Clotting Factor Test, 85210-85244
  Clotting Inhibitors, 85300-85303, 85305-85307, 85335, 85337
  Coagulation Time, 85345-85348
  Factor Inhibitor Test, 85335
 Coagulation
  Factor I, 85384, 85385
  Factor II, 85210
  Factor III, 85730, 85732
  Factor IV, 82310

Blood — *continued*
 Coagulation — *continued*
  Factor IX, 85250
  Factor V, 85220
  Factor VII, 85230
  Factor VIII, 85244, 85247
  Factor X, 85260
  Factor XI, 85270
  Factor XIII, 85290, 85291
 Collection, for Autotransfusion
  Intraoperative, 86891
  Preoperative, 86890
 Feces, 82270, 82272
  by Hemoglobin Immunoassay, 82274
 Flow Check
  Graft, 15860, 90940
 Gases
  by Pulse Oximetry, 94760
  CO2, 82803
  HCO3, 82803
  Hemoglobin–Oxygen Affinity, 82820
  O2, 82803-82810
  O2 Saturation, 82805, 82810
  pCO2, 82803
  pH, 82800, 82803
  pO2, 82803, 82820
 Gastric Contents, 82271
 Hemoglobin
  Concentration, 85046
  Quantitative, 88740
  Transcutaneous
   Carboxyhemoglobin, 88740
   Methemoglobin, 88741
 Hemoglobin A1c (HbA1c) Level, 3044F-3046F
 Injection
  Plasma, 0232T
 Nuclear Medicine
  Flow Imaging, 78445
  Red Cell, 78140
  Red Cell Survival, 78130
 Occult, 82270
 Osmolality, 83930
 Other Sources, 82271
 Patch, 62273
 Plasma
  Exchange, 36514-36516
  Frozen Preparation, 86927
  Injection, 0232T
  Volume, 78110-78111
 Platelet
  Aggregation, 85576
  Automated Count, 85049
  Count, 85008
  Manual Count, 85032
  Phospholipid Neutralization, 85597-85598
 Pool Imaging, 78472, 78473, 78481, 78483, 78494, 78496
 Products
  Irradiation, 86945
  Pooling, 86965
  Splitting, 86985
  Volume Reduction, 86960
 Reticulocyte, 85046
 Sample
  Fetal, 59030
 Smear, 85060
  Microorganism Identification, 87205-87207
  Microscopic Examination, 85007-85008
  Peripheral, 85060
  Sex Chromatin, 88140
  Surgical Pathology, 88312-88313, 88319
 Stem Cell
  Count, 86367
  Donor Search, 38204
  Erythropoietin Therapy, 3160F, 4090F-4095F
  Harvesting, 38205-38206
  Preparation, 38207-38209
  Transplantation, 38240-38242
   Cell Concentration, 38215
   Cryopreservation, 38207, 88240
   Plasma Depletion, 38214
   Platelet Depletion, 38213

Blood — *continued*
 Stem Cell — *continued*
  Transplantation — *continued*
   Red Blood Cell Depletion, 38212
   T–Cell Depletion, 38210
   Thawing, 38208-38209, 88241
   Tumor Cell Depletion, 38211
   Washing, 38209
 Test(s)
  Iron Stores, 3160F
  Kt/V, 3082F-3084F
  Nuclear Medicine
   Plasma Volume, 78110, 78111
   Platelet Survival, 78191
   Red Cell Survival, 78130
   Red Cell Volume, 78120, 78121
   Whole Blood Volume, 78122
  Panels
   Electrolyte, 80051
   General Health Panel, 80050
   Hepatic Function, 80076
   Hepatitis, Acute, 80074
   Lipid Panel, 80061
   Metabolic Panel, Basic
    Basic, 80047-80048
    Comprehensive, 80053
    Ionized Calcium, 80047
    Total Calcium, 80048
   Obstetric Panel, 80055, [80081]
   Renal Function, 80069
  Volume Determination, 78122
 Transcutaneous
  Carboxyhemoglobin, 88740
  Methemoglobin, 88741
 Transfusion, 36430, 36440
  Exchange, 36455
   Newborn, 36450
   Partial, 36456
  Fetal, 36460
  Push
   Infant, 36440
 Typing
  ABO Only, 86900
  Antigen Testing, 86902, 86904
  Crossmatch, 86920-86923
  Other RBC Antigens, 86905
  Paternity Testing, 86910, 86911
  Rh(D), 86901
  Rh Phenotype, 86906
 Unlisted Services and Procedures, 85999
 Urea Nitrogen, 84520, 84525
 Urine, 83491
 Viscosity, 85810
 Volume
  Plasma, 78110-78111
  Red Blood Cells, 78120-78121
  Whole Blood, 78122
Blood Coagulation Defect
 See Coagulopathy
Blood Coagulation Disorders
 See Clot
Blood Coagulation Test
 See Coagulation
Blood Component Removal
 See Apheresis
Blood Count, Complete
 See Complete Blood Count (CBC)
Blood Letting
 See Phlebotomy
Blood Lipoprotein
 See Lipoprotein
Blood, Occult
 See Occult Blood
Blood Pressure
 Baroactivation Device, 0266T-0273T
 Central Arterial Analysis, Non-invasive, 93050
 Diastolic, 3078F-3080F
 Monitoring, 24 hour, 93784-93990
 Systolic, 3074F-3075F
 Venous, 93770
Blood Serum
 See Serum
Blood Transfusion, Autologous
 See Autotransfusion
Blood Vessel(s)
 See Artery; Vein

Burr Hole — *continued*
Skull — *continued*
Drainage
Abscess, 61150, 61151
Cyst, 61150, 61151
Hematoma, 61154, 61156
Exploration
Infratentorial, 61253
Supratentorial, 61250
Implant
Catheter, 61210
Cerebral Monitoring Device, 61210
Cerebral Thermal Perfusion Probe, 61107, 61210
Device for Pressure Recording, 61210
EEG Electrode, 61210
Neurostimulator Array, 61850, 61863-61868
Strip Electrodes, 61531
Injection, Contrast Media, 61120
Insertion
Catheter, 61210
Pump, 61210
Reservoir, 61210
Lesion Creation, 61720
Stereotactic
Laser Interstitial Thermal Therapy (LITT), 61736-61737
Localization, 61770
Ventricular Puncture, 61020
Contrast Media Injection, 61120
Diagnostic or Therapeutic Injection, 61026
with Injection, 61120
Burrow's Operation, 14000-14350
Bursa
Ankle, 27604
Aspiration or Injection, 20605-20606
Arm
Lower, 25031
Aspiration or Injection, 20605-20606
Upper, 23031, 23931
Aspiration or Injection, 20610-20611
Elbow, 23931
Aspiration or Injection, 20605-20606
Excision, 24105
Femur, 27062
Finger, 20600-20604
Foot, 28001
Hand, 26025-26030
Hip, 26991
Aspiration or Injection, 20610-20611
Injection, 20600-20611
Ischial, 27060
Joint, 20600-20611
Knee
Aspiration or Injection, 20610-20611
Excision, 27340
Incision and Drainage, 27301
Leg
Lower, 27604
Aspiration or Injection, 20605-20606
Upper, 27301
Aspiration or Injection, 20610-20611
Palm, 26025, 26030
Pelvis, 26991
Shoulder
Aspiration or Injection, 20610-20611
Drainage, 23031
Toe, 20600-20604
Trochanteric Bursa, 27062
Wrist
Aspiration or Injection, 20605-20606
Excision, 25115, 25116
Incision and Drainage, 25031
Bursectomy
of Hand, 26989
Bursitis, Radiohumeral
See Tennis Elbow
Bursocentesis
See Aspiration, Bursa

Buttock
Excision
Excess Skin, 15835
Button
Bone Graft, 20900
Nasal Septal Prosthesis, 30220
Voice Prosthesis, 31611
Butyrylcholine Esterase
See Cholinesterase
Bypass
Cardiopulmonary, 33510-33516
Bypass Graft
Aortobifemoral, 35540, 35646
Aortobi-iliac, 35538, 35638
Aortocarotid, 35526, 35626
Aortoceliac, 35531, 35631
Aortofemoral, 35539, 35647
Aortoiliac, 35537, 35637
Aortoinnominate, 35526, 35626
Aortomesenteric, 35531, 35631
Aortorenal, 35560, 35631
Aortosubclavian, 35526, 35626
Axillary Artery, 35516-35522, 35533, 35616-35623, 35650, 35654
Brachial Artery, 35510, 35512, 35522-35525
Brachial-Ulnar or -Radial, 35523
Carotid Artery, 33891, 35501-35510, 35601, 35606, 35642
Celiac Artery, 35341, 35631-35632
Coronary Artery
Arterial, 33533-33536
Arterial-Venous, 33517-33519, 33521-33523, 33530
Venous Graft, 33510-33516
Excision
Abdomen, 35907
Extremity, 35903
Neck, 35901
Thorax, 35905
Femoral Artery, 35521, 35533, 35539, 35540, 35556, 35558, 35566, 35621, 35646, 35647, 35654-35661, 35666, 35700
Harvest
Endoscopic
Artery, 33509
Vein, 33508
Open
Lower Extremity Vein, 35572
Upper Extremity Artery, 35600
Upper Extremity Vein, 35500
Hepatorenal, 35535
Iliac Artery, 35537, 35538, 35563, 35637, 35638, 35663
Ilio-Celiac, 35632
Iliofemoral, 35565, 35665
Ilioiliac, 35563, 35663
Ilio-Mesenteric, 35633
Iliorenal, 35634
Mesenteric Artery, 35531, 35631
Peroneal Artery, 35566, 35570-35571, 35585, 35587, 35666, 35671
Peroneal-Tibial Vein, 35570
Placement
Vein Patch, 35685
Popliteal Artery, 35556, 35571, 35583, 35623, 35656, 35671, 35700
Renal Artery, 35536, 35560, 35631, 35636
Reoperation, 35700
Repair
Abdomen, 35907
Extremity, 35903
Lower Extremity
with Composite Graft, 35681-35683
Neck, 35901
Thorax, 35905
Revascularization
Extremity, 35903
Neck, 35901
Thorax, 35905
Revision
Lower Extremity
Femoral Artery, 35883-35884
with Angioplasty, 35879
with Vein Interposition, 35881
Secondary Repair, 35870

Bypass Graft — *continued*
Splenic Artery, 35536, 35636
Subclavian Artery, 35506, 35511-35516, 35526, 35606-35616, 35626, 35645, 35693-35694
Thrombectomy, 35875, 35876, 37184-37186
Other Than Hemodialysis Graft or Fistula, 35875-35876
Tibial Artery, 35566, 35571, 35623, 35666, 35671
Tibial-Tibial Vein, 35570
Vertebral Artery, 35508, 35515, 35642, 35645
with Composite Graft, 35681-35683
Autogenous
Three or More Segments
Two Locations, 35683
Two Segments
Two Locations, 35682
Bypass In Situ
Femoral Artery, 35583-35585
Peroneal Artery, 35585, 35587
Popliteal Artery, 35583, 35587
Tibial Artery, 35585, 35587
Ventricular Restoration, 33548

C

C10orf2, 81404
C-13
Urea Breath Test, 83013, 83014
Urease Activity, 83013, 83014
C-14
Urea Breath Test, 78267, 78268
Urease Activity, 83013, 83014
C481F/C481R/C481S, *[81233]*
CA, 82310-82340
CABG, 33503-33505, 33510-33536
CACNA1A, *[81184, 81185, 81186], [81419]*
CACNB2, 81406
Cadaver Donor
Organ Perfusion System
Lung(s)
Initiation and Monitoring, 0495T-0496T
Surgical Preparation and Cannulation, 0494T
Cadmium
Urine, 82300
Caffeine
Assay, 80155
Caffeine Halothane Contracture Test (CHCT), 89049
Calcaneus
Bone Graft, 28420
Craterization, 28120
Cyst
Excision, 28100-28103
Diaphysectomy, 28120
Excision, 28118-28120
Fracture
Closed Treatment, 28400, 28405
Open Treatment, 28415, 28420
Percutaneous Fixation, 28406
with Bone Graft, 28420
with Manipulation, 28405, 28406
without Manipulation, 28400
Repair
Osteotomy, 28300
Saucerization, 28120
Sequestrectomy, 28120
Spur, 28119
Tumor
Excision, 28100-28103
Radical Resection, 27647
X-ray, 73650
Calcareous Deposits
Subdeltoid
Removal, 23000
Calcifediol
Blood Serum Level 25 Hydroxy, 82306
I, 25 Dihydroxy, *[82652]*
Calciferol
Blood Serum Level 25 Hydroxy, 82306
I, 25 Dihydroxy, *[82652]*
Calcification
See Calcium, Deposits

Calciol
See Calcifediol
Calcitonin
Blood or Urine, 82308
Stimulation Panel, 80410
Calcium
Blood
Infusion Test, 82331
Deposits
Removal, Calculi–Stone
Bile Duct, 43264, 47420, 47425, 47554
Bladder, 51050, 52310-52318
Gallbladder, 47480
Hepatic Duct, 47400
Kidney, 50060-50081, 50130, 50561, 50580
Pancreas, 48020
Pancreatic Duct, 43264
Salivary Gland, 42330-42340
Ureter, 50610-50630, 50961, 50980, 51060, 51065, 52320-52330
Urethra, 52310, 52315
Ionized, 82330
Panel, 80047
Total, 82310
Panel, 80048
Urine, 82340
Calcium Voltage-gated Channel Subunit Alpha 1A, *[81184]*
Calcium–Binding Protein, Vitamin K–Dependent
See Osteocalcin
Calcium–Pentagastrin Stimulation, 80410
Calculus
Analysis, 82355-82370
Destruction
Bile Duct, 43265
Kidney
Extracorporeal Shock Wave Lithotripsy, 50590
Pancreatic Duct, 43265
Ureter
Lithotripsy, 52353, *[52356]*
Removal
Bile Duct, 43264, 47554
Biliary Tract, 47400, 47420, 47425, 47480
Bladder, 51050, 52310-52318, 52352
Kidney, 50060-50081, 50130, 50561, 50580, 52352
Liver, 47400
Pancreatic Duct, 43264, 48020
Ureter, 50610-50630, 50945, 50961, 50980, 51060, 51065, 52310-52315, 52320, 52325, 52352
Urethra, 52310, 52315, 52352
Calculus of Kidney
See Calculus, Removal, Kidney
Caldwell–Luc Procedure(s), 21385, 31030, 31032
Orbital Floor Blowout Fracture, 21385
Sinusotomy, 31030, 31032
Caliper
Application
Removal, 20660
Callander Knee Disarticulation, 27598
Callosum, Corpus
See Corpus Callosum
Calmette Guerin Bacillus Vaccine
See BCG Vaccine
Caloric Vestibular Test, 92533, 92537-92538
Calprotectin
Fecal, 83993
Calycoplasty, 50405
Camey Enterocystoplasty, 50825
CAMP
See Cyclic AMP
Campbell Arthrodesis, 27870
Campbell Procedure, 27422
Campylobacter
Antibody, 86625
Antigen, 86628
Skin Test, 86485
Campylobacter Pylori
Antibody, 86677
Antigen Detection Enzyme Immunoassay, 87338-87339
Blood Test, 83009

[Resequenced]   CPT © 2021 American Medical Association. All Rights Reserved.   © 2021 Optum360, LLC

Chromosome Analysis — *continued*
  Tissue Culture — *continued*
    Unlisted Cytogenic Study, 88299
    Unlisted Services and Procedures, 88299
Chromotubation
  Oviduct, 58350
Chronic Erection
  See Priapism
Chronic Interstitial Cystitides
  See Cystitis, Interstitial
Chronic Lymphocytic Leukemia, *[81233]*
Ciliary Body
  Cyst
    Destruction
      Cryotherapy, 66720
      Cyclodialysis, 66740
      Cyclophotocoagulation, 66710-
        66711
      Diathermy, 66700
      Nonexcisional, 66770
    Destruction
      Cyclophotocoagulation, 66710, 66711
      Cyst or Lesion, 66770
      Endoscopic, 66711
    Lesion
      Destruction, 66770
    Repair, 66680
Cimino Type Procedure, 36821
Cinefluorographies
  See Cineradiography
Cineplasty
  Arm, Lower, 24940
  Arm, Upper, 24940
Cineradiography
  Esophagus, 74230
  Pharynx, 70371, 74230
  Speech Evaluation, 70371
  Swallowing Evaluation, 74230
  Unlisted Services and Procedures, 76120,
    76125
Circulation Assist
  Aortic, 33967, 33970
  Balloon Counterpulsation, 33967, 33970
    Removal, 33971
  Cardioassist Method
    External, 92971
    Internal, 92970
  External, 33946-33949
Circulation, Extracorporeal
  See Extracorporeal Circulation
Circumcision
  Adhesions, 54162
  Incomplete, 54163
  Repair, 54163
  Surgical Excision
    28 Days or Less, 54160
    Older Than 28 Days, 54161
    with Clamp or Other Device, 54150
Cisternal Puncture, 61050, 61055
Cisternography, 70015
  Nuclear, 78630
Citrate
  Blood or Urine, 82507
CK, 82550-82554
  Total, 82550
Cl, 82435-82438
Clagett Procedure
  Chest Wall, Repair, Closure, 32810
Clavicle
  Arthrocentesis, 20605
  Arthrotomy
    Acromioclavicular Joint, 23044, 23101
    Sternoclavicular Joint, 23044, 23101,
      23106
  Claviculectomy
    Arthroscopic, 29824
    Partial, 23120
    Total, 23125
  Craterization, 23180
  Cyst
    Excision, 23140
      with Allograft, 23146
      with Autograft, 23145
  Diaphysectomy, 23180

Clavicle — *continued*
  Dislocation
    Acromioclavicular Joint
      Closed Treatment, 23540, 23545
      Open Treatment, 23550, 23552
    Sternoclavicular Joint
      Closed Treatment, 23520, 23525
      Open Treatment, 23530, 23532
    without Manipulation, 23540
  Excision, 23170
    Partial, 23120, 23180
    Total, 23125
  Fracture
    Closed Treatment
      with Manipulation, 23505
      without Manipulation, 23500
    Open Treatment, 23515
  Osteotomy, 23480
    with Bone Graft, 23485
  Pinning, Wiring, Etc., 23490
  Prophylactic Treatment, 23490
  Repair Osteotomy, 23480, 23485
  Saucerization, 23180
  Sequestrectomy, 23170
  Tumor
    Excision, 23140, 23146, 23200
      with Allograft, 23146
      with Autograft, 23145
    Radical Resection, 23200
  X–ray, 73000
Clavicula
  See Clavicle
Claviculectomy
  Arthroscopic, 29824
  Partial, 23120
  Total, 23125
Claw Finger Repair, 26499
Clayton Procedure, 28114
CLCN1, 81406
CLCNKB, 81406
Cleft, Branchial
  See Branchial Cleft
Cleft Cyst, Branchial
  See Branchial Cleft, Cyst
Cleft Foot
  Reconstruction, 28360
Cleft Hand
  Repair, 26580
Cleft Lip
  Repair, 40700-40761
  Rhinoplasty, 30460, 30462
Cleft Palate
  Repair, 42200-42225
  Rhinoplasty, 30460, 30462
Clinical Act of Insertion
  See Insertion
Clitoroplasty
  for Intersex State, 56805
Closed [Transurethral] Biopsy of Bladder
  See Biopsy, Bladder , Cystourethroscopy
Clostridial Tetanus
  See Tetanus
Clostridium Botulinum Toxin
  See Chemodenervation
Clostridium Difficile Toxin
  Amplified Probe Technique, 87493
  Antigen Detection
    Enzyme Immunoassay, 87324
    by Immunoassay
      with Direct Optical Observation, 87803
  Tissue Culture, 87230
Clostridium Tetani ab
  See Antibody, Tetanus
Closure
  Anal Fistula, 46288
  Appendiceal Fistula, 44799
  Atrial Appendage
    with Implant, 33340
  Atrial Septal Defect, 33641, 33647
  Atrioventricular Valve, 33600
  Cardiac Valve, 33600, 33602
  Cystostomy, 51880
  Diaphragm
    Fistula, 39599
  Enterostomy, 44620-44626
    Laparoscopic, 44227

Closure — *continued*
  Esophagostomy, 43420-43425
  Fistula
    Anal, 46288, 46706
    Anorectal, 46707
    Bronchi, 32815
    Carotid-Cavernous, 61710
    Chest Wall, 32906
    Enterovesical, 44660-44661
    Ileoanal Pouch, 46710-46712
    Kidney, 50520-50526
    Lacrimal, 68770
    Nose, 30580-30600
    Oval Window, 69666
    Rectovaginal, 57305-57308
    Tracheoesophageal, 43305, 43312,
      43314
    Ureter, 50920-50930
    Urethra, 53400-53405
    Urethrovaginal, 57310-57311
    Vesicouterine, 51920-51925
    Vesicovaginal, 51900, 57320, 57330
  Gastrostomy, 43870
  Lacrimal Fistula, 68770
  Lacrimal Punctum
    Plug, 68761
    Thermocauterization, Ligation, or Laser
      Surgery, 68760
  Meningocele, 63700-63702
  Patent Ductus Arteriosus, 93582
  Rectovaginal Fistula, 57300-57308
  Semilunar Valve, 33602
  Septal Defect, 33615
    Ventricular, 33675-33677, 33681-33688,
      93581
  Skin
    Abdomen
      Complex, 13100-13102
      Intermediate, 12031-12037
      Layered, 12031-12037
      Simple, 12001-12007
      Superficial, 12001-12007
    Arm, Arms
      Complex, 13120-13122
      Intermediate, 12031-12037
      Layered, 12031-12037
      Simple, 12001-12007
      Superficial, 12001-12007
    Axilla, Axillae
      Complex, 13131-13133
      Intermediate, 12031-12037
      Layered, 12031-12037
      Simple, 12001-12007
      Superficial, 12001-12007
    Back
      Complex, 13100-13102
      Intermediate, 12031-12037
      Layered, 12031-12037
      Simple, 12001-12007
      Superficial, 12001-12007
    Breast
      Complex, 13100-13102
      Intermediate, 12031-12037
      Layered, 12031-12037
      Simple, 12001-12007
      Superficial, 12001-12007
    Buttock
      Complex, 13100-13102
      Intermediate, 12031-12037
      Layered, 12031-12037
      Simple, 12001-12007
      Superficial, 12001-12007
    Cheek, Cheeks
      Complex, 13131-13133
      Intermediate, 12051-12057
      Layered, 12051-12057
      Simple, 12011-12018
      Superficial, 12011-12018
    Chest
      Complex, 13100-13102
      Intermediate, 12031-12037
      Layered, 12031-12037
      Simple, 12001-12007
      Superficial, 12001-12007
    Chin
      Complex, 13131-13133

Closure — *continued*
  Skin — *continued*
    Chin — *continued*
      Intermediate, 12051-12057
      Layered, 12051-12057
      Simple, 12011-12018
      Superficial, 12011-12018
    Ear, Ears
      Complex, 13151-13153
      Intermediate, 12051-12057
      Layered, 12051-12057
      2.5 cm or Less, 12051
      Simple, 12011-12018
      Superficial, 12011-12018
    External
      Genitalia
        Intermediate, 12041-12047
        Layered, 12041-12047
        Simple, 12001-12007
        Superficial, 12001-12007
    Extremity, Extremities
      Intermediate, 12031-12037
      Layered, 12031-12037
      Simple, 12001-12007
      Superficial, 12001-12007
    Eyelid, Eyelids
      Complex, 13151-13153
      Intermediate, 12051-12057
      Layered, 12051-12057
      Simple, 12011-12018
      Superficial, 12011-12018
    Face
      Complex, 13131-13133
      Intermediate, 12051-12057
      Layered, 12051-12057
      Simple, 12011-12018
      Superficial, 12011-12018
    Feet
      Complex, 13131-13133
      Intermediate, 12041-12047
      Layered, 12041-12047
      Simple, 12001-12007
      Superficial, 12001-12007
    Finger, Fingers
      Complex, 13131-13133
      Intermediate, 12041-12047
      Layered, 12041-12047
      Simple, 12001-12007
      Superficial, 12001-12007
    Foot
      Complex, 13131-13133
      Intermediate, 12041-12047
      Layered, 12041-12047
      Simple, 12001-12007
      Superficial, 12001-12007
    Forearm, Forearms
      Complex, 13120-13122
      Intermediate, 12031-12037
      Layered, 12031-12037
      Simple, 12001-12007
      Superficial, 12001-12007
    Forehead
      Complex, 13131-13133
      Intermediate, 12051-12057
      Layered, 12051-12057
      Simple, 12011-12018
      Superficial, 12011-12018
    Genitalia
      Complex, 13131-13133
      External
        Intermediate, 12041-12047
        Layered, 12041-12047
        Simple, 12001-12007
        Superficial, 12001-12007
    Hand, Hands
      Complex, 13131-13133
      Intermediate, 12041-12047
      Layered, 12041-12047
      Simple, 12001-12007
      Superficial, 12001-12007
    Leg, Legs
      Complex, 13120-13122
      Intermediate, 12031-12037
      Layered, 12031-12037
      Simple, 12001-12007
      Superficial, 12001-12007

Closure — *continued*
Skin — *continued*
Lip, Lips
Complex, 13151-13153
Intermediate, 12051-12057
Layered, 12051-12057
Simple, 12011-12018
Superficial, 12011-12018
Lower
Arm, Arms
Complex, 13120-13122
Intermediate, 12031-12037
Layered, 12031-12037
Simple, 12001-12007
Superficial, 12001-12007
Extremity, Extremities
Intermediate, 12031-12037
Layered, 12031-12037
Simple, 12001-12007
Superficial, 12001-12007
Leg, Legs
Complex, 13120-13122
Intermediate, 12031-12037
Layered, 12031-12037
Simple, 12001-12007
Superficial, 12001-12007
Mouth
Complex, 13131-13133
Mucous Membrane, Mucous Membranes
Intermediate, 12051-12057
Layered, 12051-12057
Simple, 12011-12018
Superficial, 12011-12018
Neck
Complex, 13131-13133
Intermediate, 12041-12047
Layered, 12041-12047
Simple, 12001-12007
Superficial, 12001-12007
Nose
Complex, 13151-13153
Intermediate, 12051-12057
Layered, 12051-12057
Simple, 12011-12018
Superficial, 12011-12018
Palm, Palms
Complex, 13131-13133
Intermediate, 12041-12047
Layered, 12041-12047
Simple, 12001-12007
Superficial, 12001-12007
Scalp
Complex, 13120-13122
Intermediate, 12031-12037
Layered, 12031-12037
Simple, 12001-12007
Superficial, 12001-12007
Toe, Toes
Complex, 13131-13133
Intermediate, 12041-12047
Layered, 12041-12047
Simple, 12001-12007
Superficial, 12001-12007
Trunk
Complex, 13100-13102
Intermediate, 12031-12037
Layered, 12031-12037
Simple, 12001-12007
Superficial, 12001-12007
Upper
Arm, Arms
Complex, 13120-13122
Intermediate, 12031-12037
Layered, 12031-12037
Simple, 12001-12007
Superficial, 12001-12007
Extremity
Intermediate, 12031-12037
Layered, 12031-12037
Simple, 12001-12007
Superficial, 12001-12007
Leg, Legs
Complex, 13120-13122
Intermediate, 12031-12037
Layered, 12031-12037
Simple, 12001-12007

Closure — *continued*
Skin — *continued*
Upper — *continued*
Leg, Legs — *continued*
Superficial, 12001-12007
Sternotomy, 21750
Vagina, 57120
Ventricular Septal Defect, 33675-33677, 33681-33688, 93581
Clot, 34001-34490, 35875, 35876, 50230
Lysis Time, 85175
Retraction, 85170
Clot Lysis Time
Euglobin Lysis, 85360
Whole Blood Dilution, 85175
Clotting, 85210-85293
Disorder, 85390
Factor, 85210-85293
Factor II (Prothrombin), 85210
Factor III (Thromboplastin) Inhibition, 85705
Factor IX (Christmas Factor), 85250
Factor VII, 85230
Factor VIII
AHG, 85240
Related Antigen, 85244
von Willebrand Factor, 85247
VW Factor, 85245-85246
Factor X (Stuart-Prower), 85260
Factor X (Thrombokinase), 85260
Factor XI, 85270
Factor XII (Hageman Factor), 85280
Factor XIII (Fibrin Stabilizing), 85290-85291
Fitzgerald Factor Assay, 85293
Fletcher Factor Assay, 85292
High Molecular Weight Kininogen Assay, 85293
Inhibition Test, 85347
Partial Time, 85730-85732
Plasma Thromboplastin Antecedent (TPA), 85270
Prekallikrein Assay, 85292
Inhibitors, 85300-85305, 85307
Test
Antithrombin III, 85300-85301
Factor Inhibitor, 85335
Mixed Screen, 85611, 85732
Protein C, 85302-85303, 85307
Protein S, 85305-85306
Thrombomodulin, 85337
Thromboplastin Inhibition, 85705
Time, 85345-85348
Cloverleaf Skull
Suture of, 61558
Clozapine
Assay, 80159
CLRN1, 81400, 81404, 81430
Clubfoot Cast, 29450
Wedging, 29750
CMG (Cystometrogram), 51725-51729
CMRI (Cardiac Magnetic Resonance Imaging)
for Morphology and Function, 75557-75563
Velocity Flow Mapping, 75565
with Contrast, 75561-75563
without Contrast, 75557-75559
CMV (Cytomegalovirus)
Antibody, 86644, 86645
Antigen Detection
Enzyme Immunoassay, 87332
Nucleic Acid, 87495-87497
CNBP, *[81187]*
CNP, 94662
CNPB (Continuous Negative Pressure Breathing), 94662
CNTNAP2, 81406
CO₂
CO_2
See Carbon Dioxide
Coaching
Well-being, 0591T-0593T
Coagulation
Defect, 85390
Assay, 85130
Factor I, 85384, 85385
Factor II, 85210
Factor II, Prothrombin Gene Analysis, 81240

Coagulation — *continued*
Factor III, 85730, 85732
Factor IV, 82310
Factor IX, 85250
Factor V, 85220
Factor V Gene Analysis, 81241
Factor VII, 85230
Factor VIII, 85244, 85247
Factor X, 85260
Factor XI, 85270
Factor XII, 85280
Factor XIII, 85290, 85291
Fibrinolysis, 85396-85397
Time, 85345-85348
Unlisted Services and Procedures, 85999
Coagulin
See Thromboplastin
Coagulopathy, 85390
Assay, 85130
Cocaine, *[80305, 80306, 80307]*, *[80353]*
Coccidioides
Antibody, 86635
Coccidioidin Test
Streptokinase, Antibody, 86590
Coccidioidomycosis
Skin Test, 86490
Coccygeal Spine Fracture
See Coccyx, Fracture
Coccygectomy, 15920, 15922, 27080
Coccyx
Excision, 27080
Fracture
Closed Treatment, 27200
Open Treatment, 27202
Pressure Ulcer, 15920, 15922
Tumor
Excision, 49215
X-ray, 72220
Cochlear Device
Analysis, 92601-92604
Insertion, 69930
Osseointegrated Implant
Implantation, *[69714]*, *[69716]*
Removal, *[69726]*, *[69727]*
Revision or Replacement, *[69717]*, *[69719]*
Programming, 92601-92604
Codeine Screen, *[80305, 80306, 80307]*, *[80361, 80362]*
Co-Factor I, Heparin
See Antithrombin III
Cofactor Protein S
See Protein S
Coffey Operation
Uterus, Repair, Suspension, 58400
with Presacral Sympathectomy, 58410
Cognitive Behavioral Therapy
Online, Digital, 0702T-0703T
Cognitive Function Tests, 96116, 96121, *[96125]*
See Neurology, Diagnostic
Cognitive Skills Development, 97129-97130
See Physical Medicine/Therapy/Occupational Therapy
COHB, 82375-82376
COL1A1, 81408
COL1A1/PDGFB, 81402
COL1A2, 81408
COL3A1, 81410-81411
COL4A1, 81408
COL4A3, 81408
COL4A4, 81407
COL4A5, 81408
COL6A2, 81406-81407
COL6A3, 81407
Cold Agglutinin, 86156, 86157
Cold Pack Treatment, 97010
Cold Preservation
See Cryopreservation
Cold Therapies
See Cryotherapy
Colectomy
Miles', 44155
Partial, 44140
Transanal Approach, 44147
with
Anastomosis, 44140

Colectomy — *continued*
Partial — *continued*
with — *continued*
Anastomosis — *continued*
Laparoscopic, 44213
Coloproctostomy, 44145-44146
Colostomy, 44141-44144
Laparoscopic, 44205
Ileocolostomy, Laparoscopic, 44205
Ileostomy, 44144
Mobilization Splenic Flexure, 44139
Laparoscopic, 44213
Removal Ileum, 44160
Total
Laparoscopic
with
Ileoproctostomy, 44210
Ileostomy, 44210-44212
Proctectomy, 44211-44212
Proctectomy and Ileoanal Anastomosis, 44211
Proctectomy and Ileostomy, 44212
Rectal Mucosectomy, 44211
without Proctectomy, 44210
Open
with
Complete Proctectomy, 45121
Ileal Reservoir, 44158
Ileoanal Anastomosis, 44157
Ileoproctostomy, 44150
Ileostomy, 44150-44151
Proctectomy, 44155-44158
Collagen Cross Links, 82523
Collagen Injection, 11950-11954
Collapse
Nasal Valve, Repair, 30468
Collar Bone
Craterization, 23180
Cyst
Excision, 23140
with
Allograft, 23146
Autograft, 23145
Diaphysectomy, 23180
Dislocation
Acromioclavicular Joint
Closed Treatment, 23540, 23545
Open Treatment, 23550, 23552
Sternoclavicular Joint
Closed Treatment, 23520, 23525
Open Treatment, 23530, 23532
with Manipulation, 23540
Excision
Partial, 23120, 23180
Total, 23125
Fracture
Closed Treatment
with Manipulation, 23505
without Manipulation, 23500
Open Treatment, 23515
Osteotomy, 23480, 23485
Pinning, Wiring, Etc., 23490
Prophylactic Treatment, 23490
Repair Osteotomy, 23480, 23485
Saucerization, 23180
Sequestrectomy, 23170
Tumor
Excision, 23140
with Allograft, 23146
with Autograft, 23145
Radical Resection, 23200
X-ray, 73000
Collateral Ligament
Ankle
Repair, 27695-27698
Interphalangeal Joint, 26545
Knee Joint
Repair, 27409
Knee Repair, 27405, 27409
Metacarpophalangeal Joint Repair, 26540-26542
Reconstruction
Elbow, 24346
Interphalangeal Joint, 26545

 [Resequenced]   CPT © 2021 American Medical Association. All Rights Reserved.   © 2021 Optum360, LLC

Culture — *continued*
  Oocyte/Embryo — *continued*
    for In Vitro Fertilization — *continued*
      with Co–Culture of Embryo, 89251
  Pathogen
    by Kit, 87084
    Screening Only, 87081
  Skin
    Chromosome Analysis, 88233
  Stool, 87045-87046
  Tissue
    Drug Resistance, 87903-87904
    Homogenization, 87176
    Toxin
      Antitoxin, 87230
      Toxin Virus, 87252, 87253
    Tubercle Bacilli, 87116
  Tumor Tissue
    Chromosome Analysis, 88239
  Typing, 87140-87158
    Culture, 87140-87158
  Unlisted Services and Procedures, 87999
  Yeast, 87106
Curettage
  See Dilation and Curettage
  Anal Fissure, 46940
  Cervix
    Endocervical, 57454, 57456, 57505
  Cornea, 65435, 65436
    Chelating Agent, 65436
  Dentoalveolar, 41830
  Hydatidiform Mole, 59870
  Postpartum, 59160
  Uterus
    Endometrial, 58356
    Postpartum, 59160
Curettage and Dilatation
  See Dilation and Curettage
Curettage, Uterus
  See Uterus, Curettage
Curettement
  Skin Lesion, 11055-11057, 17004, 17110,
    17270, 17280
    Benign Hyperkeratotic Lesion, 11055-
      11057
    Malignant, 17260-17264, 17266, 17270-
      17274, 17280-17284, 17286
    Premalignant, 17000, 17003-17004,
      17110-17111
Curietherapy
  See Brachytherapy
Custodial Care
  See Domiciliary Services; Nursing Facility Ser-
    vices
Cutaneolipectomy
  See Lipectomy
Cutaneous Electrostimulation, Analgesic
  See Application, Neurostimulation
Cutaneous Tag
  See Skin, Tags
Cutaneous Tissue
  See Integumentary System
Cutaneous–Vesicostomy
  See Vesicostomy, Cutaneous
CVAD (Central Venous Access Device)
  Insertion
    Central, 36555-36558, 36560-36561,
      36563, 36565-36566, 36578,
      36580-36583
    Peripheral, 36568-36569, 36570-36571,
      36584-36585, [36572, 36573]
  Removal, 36589
  Repair, 36575
  Replacement, 36580-36585
  Repositioning, 36597
CVS, 59015
CXL, Collagen Cross-Linking, Cornea, 0402T
CXR, 71045-71048
Cyanide
  Blood, 82600
  Tissue, 82600
Cyanocobalamin, 82607, 82608
Cyclic AMP, 82030
Cyclic Citrullinated Peptide (CCP), Antibody,
  86200

Cyclic Somatostatin
  See Somatostatin
Cyclocryotherapy
  See Cryotherapy, Destruction, Ciliary Body
Cyclodialysis
  Destruction
    Ciliary Body, 66740
Cyclophotocoagulation
  Destruction
    Ciliary Body, 66710, 66711
Cyclosporine
  Assay, 80158
CYP11B1, 81405
CYP17A1, 81405
CYP1B1, 81404
CYP21A2, 81402, 81405
CYP2C19, 81225
CYP2C9, [81227]
CYP2D6, 81226
CYP3A4, [81230]
CYP3A5, [81231]
Cyst
  Abdomen
    Destruction, 49203-49205
    Excision, 49203-49205
    Laparoscopy with Aspiration, 49322
  Ankle
    Capsule, 27630
    Tendon Sheath, 27630
  Bartholin's Gland
    Excision, 56740
    Marsupialization, 56440
    Puncture Aspiration, 10160
    Repair, 56440
  Bile Duct
    Excision, 47715
  Bladder
    Excision, 51500
  Bone
    Drainage, 20615
    Injection, 20615
  Brain
    Drainage, 61150, 61151, 61156, 62161,
      62162
    Excision, 61516, 61524, 62162
  Branchial Cleft
    Excision, 42810, 42815
  Breast
    Excision, 19020
    Puncture Aspiration, 19000, 19001
  Calcaneus, 28100-28103
  Carpal, 25130-25136
  Choledochal
    Excision, 47715
  Ciliary Body
    Destruction, 66770
  Clavicle
    Excision, 23140-23146
  Conjunctiva, 68020
  Dermoid
    Nose
      Excision, 30124, 30125
  Drainage
    Contrast Injection, 49424
      with X–ray, 76080
    Image-guided by catheter, 10030
  Enucleation
    Mandible, 21040
    Maxilla, 21030
    Zygoma, 21030
  Excision
    Cheekbone, 21030
    Clavicle, 23140
      with Allograft, 23146
      with Autograft, 23145
    Femur, 27065-27067, 27355-27358
    Foot, 28090
    Ganglion
      See Ganglion
    Hand
      Capsule, 26160
      Tendon Sheath, 26160
    Humerus, 24120-24126
      Proximal, 23150-23156
    Hydatid
      See Echinococcosis

Cyst — *continued*
  Excision — *continued*
    Lymphatic
      See Lymphocele
    Maxilla, 21030
    Mediastinum, 32662
    Mouth
      Dentoalveolar, 41800
      Lingual, 41000
      Masticator Space, 41009, 41018
      Sublingual, 41005-41006, 41015
      Submandibular, 41008, 41017
      Submental, 41007, 41016
      Vestibular, 40800-40801
    Olecranon Process, 24120
      with Allograft, 24126
      with Autograft, 24125
    Ovarian, 58925
    Pancreas
      Anastomosis, 48520, 48540
      Excision, 48120
      Marsupialization, 48500
    Pericardial, 32661
      Resection, 33050
    Pilonidal, 11770-11772
    Radius, 24120
      with Allograft, 24126
      with Autograft, 24125
    Scapula, 23140
      with Allograft, 23146
      with Autograft, 23145
    Symphysis Pubis, 27065-27067
    Ulna, 24120, 25120
      with Allograft, 24126, 25125
      with Autograft, 24125, 25126
    Wrist, 25111-25112, 25130, 25135-25136
    Zygoma, 21030
  Facial Bones
    Excision, 21030
  Femur
    Excision, 27065-27067, 27355-27358
  Fibula, 27635-27638
  Finger, 26210, 26215
  Ganglion
    Aspiration/Injection, 20612
  Gums
    Incision and Drainage, 41800
  Hand
    Capsule, 26160
    Tendon Sheath, 26160
  Hip, 27065-27067
  Humerus
    Excision, 23150-23156, 24110
      with Allograft, 24116
      with Autograft, 24115
  Ilium, 27065-27067
  Incision and Drainage, 10060, 10061
    Mouth, 41800
      Dentoalveolar, 41800
      Lingual, 41000
      Masticator Space, 41009, 41018
      Sublingual, 41005-41006
      Submandibular, 41008, 41017
      Submental, 41007, 41016
      Vestibular, 40800-40801
    Pilonidal, 10080, 10081
    Puncture Aspiration, 10160
  Iris
    Destruction, 66770
  Kidney
    Ablation, 50541
    Aspiration, 50390
    Excision, 50280, 50290
    Injection, 50390
    X–ray, 74470
  Knee
    Baker's, 27345
    Excision, 27347
  Leg, Lower
    Capsule, 27630
    Tendon Sheath, 27630
  Liver
    Aspiration, 47015
    Incision and Drainage
      Open, 47010
    Marsupialization, 47300

Cyst — *continued*
  Liver — *continued*
    Repair, 47300
  Lung
    Incision and Drainage, 32200
    Removal, 32140
  Lymph Node
    Axillary
      Cervical
        Excision, 38550, 38555
  Mandible
    Excision, 21040, 21046, 21047
  Maxilla, 21030, 21048-21049
  Mediastinal
    Excision, 32662
    Resection, 39200
  Metacarpal, 26200, 26205
  Metatarsal, 28104-28107
  Mouth
    Dentoalveolar, 41800
    Lingual, 41000
    Masticator Space, 41009, 41018
    Sublingual, 41005-41006
    Submandibular, 41008, 41017
    Submental, 41007, 41016
    Vestibular, 40800-40801
  Mullerian Duct
    Excision, 55680
  Nose
    Excision, 30124, 30125
  Olecranon, 24120, 24125-24126
  Opening or Removal of (Incision and Drainage)
    Acne Surgery, 10040
  Ovarian
    Excision, 58925
    Incision and Drainage, 58800, 58805
  Pancreas
    Anastomosis, 48520, 48540
    Excision, 48120
    Marsupialization, 48500
  Pelvis
    Aspiration, 50390
    Injection, 50390
  Pericardial
    Excision, 33050
  Phalanges
    Finger, 26210, 26215
    Toe, 28092, 28108
  Pilonidal
    Excision, 11770-11772
    Incision and Drainage, 10080, 10081
  Pubis, 27065-27067
  Radius
    Excision, 24120, 25120-25126
  Rathke's Pouch
    See Craniopharyngioma
  Removal
    Skin, 10040
  Retroperitoneum
    Destruction, 49203-49205
    Excision, 49203-49205
  Salivary Gland
    Drainage, 42409
    Excision, 42408
    Marsupialization, 42409
  Scapula
    Excision, 23140-23146
  Seminal Vesicles
    Excision, 55680
  Skene's Gland
    Destruction, 53270
    Drainage, 53060
  Skin
    Incision and Drainage, 10060-10061
    Puncture Aspiration, 10160
    Removal, 10040
  Spinal Cord
    Aspiration, 62268
    Incision and Drainage, 63172, 63173
  Sublingual Gland
    Drainage, 42409
    Excision, 42408
  Symphysis Pubis, 27065-27067
  Talus, 28100-28103
  Tarsal, 28104-28107

[Resequenced]

[Resequenced]

Dislocation — continued
Interphalangeal Joint
Finger(s)/Hand
Closed Treatment, 26770, 26775
Open Treatment, 26785
Percutaneous Fixation, 26776
Toe(s)/Foot, 28660-28675
Closed Treatment, 28660, 28665
Open Treatment, 28675
Percutaneous Fixation, 28666
Knee
Closed Treatment, 27550, 27552
Open Treatment, 27556-27558, 27566, 27730
Patella, 27560-27562
Recurrent, 27420-27424
Lunate
Closed Treatment, 25690
Open Treatment, 25695
with Manipulation, 25690, 26670-26676, 26700-26706
Metacarpophalangeal Joint
Closed Treatment, 26700-26706
Open Treatment, 26715
Metatarsophalangeal Joint
Closed Treatment, 28630, 28635
Open Treatment, 28645
Percutaneous Fixation, 28636
Patella
Closed Treatment, 27560, 27562
Open Treatment, 27566
Recurrent, 27420-27424
Pelvic Ring
Closed Treatment, 27197-27198
Open Treatment, 27217, 27218
Percutaneous Fixation, 27216
Percutaneous Fixation
Metacarpophalangeal, 26705
Peroneal Tendons, 27675, 27676
Radiocarpal Joint
Closed Treatment, 25660
Open Treatment, 25670
Radioulnar Joint
Closed Treatment, 25675
with Radial Fracture, 25520
Galeazzi, 25520, 25525-25526
Open Treatment, 25676
with Radial Fracture, 25525, 25526
Radius
Closed Treatment, 24640
with Fracture, 24620, 24635
Closed Treatment, 24620
Open Treatment, 24635
Shoulder
Closed Treatment
with Manipulation, 23650, 23655
with Fracture of Greater
Humeral Tuberosity, 23665
Open Treatment, 23670
with Surgical or Anatomical
Neck Fracture, 23675
Open Treatment, 25680
Open Treatment, 23660
Recurrent, 23450-23466
Sternoclavicular Joint
Closed Treatment
with Manipulation, 23525
without Manipulation, 23520
Open Treatment, 23530, 23532
Talotarsal Joint
Closed Treatment, 28570, 28575
Open Treatment, 28546
Percutaneous Fixation, 28576
Tarsal
Closed Treatment, 28540, 28545
Open Treatment, 28555
Percutaneous Fixation, 28545, 28546
Tarsometatarsal Joint
Closed Treatment, 28600, 28605
Open Treatment, 28615
Percutaneous Fixation, 28606
Temporomandibular Joint
Closed Treatment, 21480, 21485
Open Treatment, 21490

Dislocation — continued
Thumb
Closed Treatment, 26641, 26645
Open Treatment, 26665
Percutaneous Fixation, 26650
with Fracture, 26645
Open Treatment, 26665
Percutaneous Fixation, 26650, 26665
with Manipulation, 26641-26650
Tibiofibular Joint
Closed Treatment, 27830, 27831
Open Treatment, 27832
Toe
Closed Treatment, 26770, 26775, 28630-28635
Open Treatment, 28645
Percutaneous Fixation, 26776, 28636
Trans-scaphoperilunar, 25680
Closed Treatment, 25680
Open Treatment, 25685
Vertebrae
Additional Segment, Any Level
Open Treatment, 22328
Cervical
Open Treatment, 22318-22319, 22326
Closed Treatment
with Manipulation, Casting and/or
Bracing, 22315
without Manipulation, 22310
Lumbar
Open Treatment, 22325
Thoracic
Open Treatment, 22327
with Debridement, 11010-11012
Wrist
Intercarpal
Closed Treatment, 25660
Open Treatment, 25670
Percutaneous, 25671
Radiocarpal
Closed Treatment, 25660
Open Treatment, 25670
Radioulnar
Closed Treatment, 25675
Open Treatment, 25676
Percutaneous Fixation, 25671
with Fracture
Closed Treatment, 25680
Open Treatment, 25685

Disorder
Blood Coagulation
See Coagulopathy
Penis
See Penis
Retinal
See Retina

Displacement Therapy
Nose, 30210

Dissection
Axial Vessel for Island Pedicle Flap, 15740
Cavernous Sinus, 61613
Cranial Adhesions, 62161
Donor Organs
Heart, 33944
Heart/Lung, 33933
Kidney, 50323, 50325
Liver, 47143
Lung, 32855
Pancreas, 48551
for Debulking Malignancy, 58952-58954
Hygroma, Cystic
Axillary, 38550, 38555
Cervical, 38550, 38555
Infrarenal Aneurysm, 34701-34712, 34830-34832
Lymph Nodes, 38542
Mediastinal, 60521-60522
Neurovascular, 32503
Sclera, 67107
Urethra, 54328, 54332, 54336, 54348, 54352

Dissection, Neck, Radical
See Radical Neck Dissection

Distention
See Dilation

Diverticulectomy, 44800
Esophagus, 43130, 43135

Diverticulectomy, Meckel's
See Meckel's Diverticulum, Excision

Diverticulopexy
Esophagus, 43499
Pharynx, 43499

Diverticulum
Bladder
See Bladder, Diverticulum
Meckel's
Excision, 44800
Unlisted Procedure, 44899
Repair
Excision, 53230, 53235
Large Intestine, 44604-44605
Marsupialization, 53240
Small Intestine, 44602-44603
Urethroplasty, 53400, 53405

Division
Anal Sphincter, 46080
Flap, 15600, 15610, 15620, 15630
Intrauterine Septum, 58560
Muscle
Foot, 28250
Neck
Scalenus Anticus, 21700, 21705
Sternocleidomastoid, 21720, 21725
Plantar Fascia
Foot, 28250
Rectal Stricture, 45150
Saphenous Vein, 37700, 37718, 37722, 37735

Division, Isthmus, Horseshoe Kidney
See Symphysiotomy, Horseshoe Kidney

Division, Scalenus Anticus Muscle
See Muscle Division, Scalenus Anticus

DLAT, 81406
DLD, 81406
DM1 Protein Kinase, *[81234]*
DMD (Dystrophin), 81408, *[81161]*
DMO
See Dimethadione
DMPK, *[81234]*, *[81239]*
DNA Antibody, 86225, 86226
DNA Endonuclease
See DNAse
DNA Probe
See Cytogenetics Studies; Nucleic Acid Probe
DNAse, 86215
DNAse Antibody, 86215
DNMT3A, 81403
Domiciliary Services
See Nursing Facility Services
Assisted Living, 99339-99340
Care Plan Oversight, 99339-99340
Discharge Services, 99315, 99316
Established Patient, 99334-99337
New Patient, 99324-99328
Supervision, 99374-99375

Donor Procedures
Backbench Preparation Prior to Transplantation
Intestine, 44715-44721
Kidney, 50323-50329
Liver, 47143-47147
Pancreas, 48551-48552
Uterus, 0668T, 0669T, 0670T
Bone Harvesting, 20900-20902
Bone Marrow Harvesting, 38230, 38232
Conjunctival Graft, 68371
Heart Excision, 33940
Heart–Lung Excision, 33930
Hysterectomy, 0664T, 0665T, 0666T, 0667T
Intestine, 44132-44133
Kidney, 50300, 50320
Liver, 47133, 47140-47142
Lung, 32850
Mucosa of Vestibule of Mouth, 40818
Pancreas, 48550
Preparation Fecal Microbiota, 44705
Stem Cells
Donor Search, 38204
Transplantation Rejection Risk Score, 81560

Dopamine
See Catecholamines
Blood, 82383, 82384

Dopamine — continued
Urine, 82382, 82384

Doppler Echocardiography, 76827, 76828, 93320-93350
3D Imaging During Procedure for Congenital
Anomalies, *[93319]*
Hemodialysis Access, 93990
Prior to Access Creation, 93985-93986
Intracardiac, 93662
Strain Imaging, *[93356]*
Transesophageal, 93318
Transthoracic, 93303-93317
with Myocardial Contrast Perfusion, 0439T

Doppler Scan
Arterial Studies
Coronary Flow Reserve, 93571-93572
Extracranial, 93880-93882
Extremities, 93922-93924
Fetal
Middle Cerebral Artery, 76821
Umbilical Artery, 76820
Intracranial, 93886-93893
Saline Infusion Sonohysterography (SIS), 76881
Transplanted Kidney, 76776

Dor Procedure, 33548
Dorsal Vertebra
See Vertebra, Thoracic
Dose Plan
Radiation Therapy, 77300, 77331, 77399
Brachytherapy, 77316-77318
Teletherapy, 77306-77307, 77321

Dosimetry
Radiation Therapy, 77300, 77331, 77399
Brachytherapy, 77316-77318
Dose Limits Established Before Therapy, 0520F
Intensity Modulation, 77301, 77338
Special, 77331
Teletherapy, 77306-77307, 77321
Unlisted Dosimetry Procedure, 77399

Double–J Stent, 52332
Cystourethroscopy, 52000, 52601, 52647, 52648

Double–Stranded DNA
See Deoxyribonucleic Acid
Douglas–Type Procedure, 41510
Doxepin
Assay, *[80335, 80336, 80337]*
DPH
See Phenytoin
DPYD, 81232
Drainage
See Excision; Incision; Incision and Drainage
Abdomen
Abdominal Fluid, 49082-49083
Paracentesis, 49082-49083
Peritoneal, 49020
Peritoneal Lavage, 49084
Peritonitis, Localized, 49020
Retroperitoneal, 49060
Subdiaphragmatic, 49040
Subphrenic, 49040
Wall
Skin and Subcutaneous Tissue, 10060, 10061
Complicated, 10061
Multiple, 10061
Simple, 10060
Single, 10060
Abscess
Abdomen, 49040
Peritoneal
Open, 49020
Peritonitis, localized, 49020
Retroperitoneal
Open, 49060
Skin and Subcutaneous Tissue
Complicated, 10061
Multiple, 10061
Simple, 10060
Single, 10060
Subdiaphragmatic, 49040
Subphrenic, 49040

Drainage

Drainage — *continued*
Abscess — *continued*
Anal
Incision and Drainage, 46045, 46050, 46060
Ankle
Incision and Drainage, 27603
Appendix
Incision and Drainage, 44900
Arm, Lower, 25028
Incision and Drainage, 25035
Arm, Upper
Incision and Drainage, 23930-23935
Auditory Canal, External, 69020
Bartholin's Gland
Incision and Drainage, 56420
Puncture Aspiration, 10160
Biliary Tract, 47400, 47420, 47425, 47480, 47533-47536
Bladder
Cystotomy or Cystostomy, 51040
Incision and Drainage, 51080
Brain
by
Burrhole, 61150, 61151
Craniotomy/Craniectomy, 61320, 61321
Neuroendoscopy, 62160, 62162, 62164
Breast
Incision and Drainage, 19020
Carpals
Incision, Deep, 25035
Clavicle
Sequestrectomy, 23170
Contrast Injection, 49424
with X–ray, 75989, 76080
Dentoalveolar Structures, 41800
Ear, External
Complicated, 69005
Simple, 69000
Elbow
Incision and Drainage, 23930-23935
Epididymis
Incision and Drainage, 54700
Eyelid
Incision and Drainage, 67700
Facial Bone(s)
Excision, 21026
Finger
Incision and Drainage, 26010, 26011, 26034
Tendon Sheath, 26020
Foot
Incision, 28005
Ganglion Cyst, 20600-20605
Gums
Incision and Drainage, 41800
Hand
Incision and Drainage, 26034
Hematoma
Brain, 61154-61156
Incision and Drainage, 27603
Vagina, 57022, 57023
Hip
Incision and Drainage, 26990-26992
Humeral Head, 23174
Humerus
Incision and Drainage, 23935
Kidney
Incision and Drainage
Open, 50020
Knee, 27301
Leg, Lower, 27603
Incision and Drainage, 27603
Liver
Incision and Drainage
Open, 47010
Injection, 47015
Repair, 47300
Localization
Nuclear Medicine, 78300, 78305, 78306, 78315

Drainage — *continued*
Abscess — *continued*
Lung
Bronchoscopy, 31645-31646
Open Drainage, 32200, 32201
Lymph Node, 38300, 38305
Lymphocele, 49062, 49185
Mandible
Excision, 21025
Mouth
Lingual, 41000
Masticator Space, 41009, 41018
Sublingual, 41005-41006, 41015, 42310
Submandibular Space, 41008, 41017
Submaxillary, 42310, 42320
Submental Space, 41007, 41016
Nasal Septum
Incision and Drainage, 30020
Neck
Incision and Drainage, 21501, 21502
Nose
Incision and Drainage, 30000, 30020
Ovary
Incision and Drainage
Abdominal Approach, 58822
Vaginal Approach, 58820
Palate
Incision and Drainage, 42000
Paraurethral Gland
Incision and Drainage, 53060
Parotid Gland, 42300, 42305
Pelvic
Percutaneous, 49406
Supralevator, 45020
Transrectal, 49407
Transvaginal, 49407
Pelvis, 26990
Incision and Drainage, 26990-26992, 45000
Perineum
Incision and Drainage, 56405
Perirenal or Renal
Open, 50020
Peritoneum
Open, 49020
Peritonsillar, 42700
Pharyngeal, 42720, 42725
Prostate
Incision and Drainage
Prostatotomy, 55720, 55725
Transurethral, 52700
Radius
Incision, Deep, 25035
Rectum
Incision and Drainage, 45005, 45020, 46040, 46060
Renal, 50020
Retroperitoneal
Laparoscopic, 49323
Open, 49060
Salivary Gland, 42300-42320
Scapula
Sequestrectomy, 23172
Scrotum
Incision and Drainage, 54700, 55100
Shoulder
Incision and Drainage, 23030
Skene's Gland
Incision and Drainage, 53060
Skin
Incision and Drainage
Complicated, 10061
Multiple, 10061
Simple, 10060
Single, 10060
Puncture Aspiration, 10160
Soft Tissue
Image-Guided by Catheter, 10030
Percutaneous, 10030
Subfascial, 22010, 22015
Spine, Subfascial, 22010, 22015

Drainage — *continued*
Abscess — *continued*
Subdiaphragmatic
Incision and Drainage, 49040
Sublingual Gland, 42310, 42320
Submaxillary Gland, 42310, 42320
Subphrenic, 49040
Testis
Incision and Drainage, 54700
Thigh, 27301
Thoracostomy, 32551
Thorax
Incision and Drainage, 21501, 21502
Throat
Incision and Drainage, 42700-42725
Tongue
Incision and Drainage, 41000-41006, 41015-41018
Tonsil
Incision and Drainage, 42700
Ulna
Incision, Deep, 25035
Urethra
Incision and Drainage, 53040
Uvula
Incision and Drainage, 42000
Vagina
Incision and Drainage, 57010
Vestibule of Mouth, 40800-40801
Visceral, 49405
Vulva
Incision and Drainage, 56405
Wrist
Incision and Drainage, 25028, 25035
X-ray, 75989, 76080
Amniotic Fluid
Diagnostic Aspiration, 59000
Therapeutic Aspiration, 59001
Aqueous, 0449T-0450T, 0474T, 66179-66180, 66183, [0253T], [0671T]
Bile Duct
Transhepatic, 47533-47534
Brain Fluid, 61070
Bursa
Arm, Lower, 25031
Arm, Upper, 23931
Arthrocentesis, 20600-20615
Elbow, 23931
Foot, 28001-28003
Hip, 26991
Knee, 27301
Leg, 27604
Palm, 26025, 26030
Pelvis, 26991
Shoulder, 23031
Thigh, 27301
Wrist, 25031
Cerebrospinal Fluid, 61000-61020, 61050, 61070, 62272
Cervical Fluid, 61050
Cisternal Fluid, 61050
Cyst
Bone, 20615
Brain, 61150, 61151, 62161, 62162
Breast, 19000, 19001
Conjunctiva, 68020
Dentoalveolar Structures, 41800
Ganglion, 20612
Intramedullary, 63172-63173
Liver, 47010
Lung, 32200
Mouth
Lingual, 41000
Masticator Space, 41009, 41018
Sublingual, 41005-41006, 41015
Submandibular Space, 41008, 41017
Submental Space, 41007, 41016
Vestibule, 40800-40801
Ovary, 58800, 58805
Pilonidal, 10080-10081
Salivary Gland, 42409
Skene's Gland, 53060

Drainage — *continued*
Cyst — *continued*
Sublingual Gland, 42409
Elbow, 23930
Empyema, 32036, 32810
Extraperitoneal Lymphocele
Laparoscopic, 49323
Open, 49062
Percutaneous, Sclerotherapy, 49185
Eye
Anterior Chamber
Aqueous Drainage Device, 66183
into Subconjunctival Space, 0449T-0450T
into Suprachoroidal Space, [0253T]
into Supraciliary Space, 0474T
Paracentesis
with Diagnostic Aspiration of Aqueous, 65800
Removal Blood, 65815
Removal Vitreous and/or Discission Anterior Hyaloid Membrane, 65810
Lacrimal Gland, 68400
Lacrimal Sac, 68420
Fetal Fluid, 59074
Fluid
Abdominal, 49082-49083
Amniotic Fluid, 59001
Cerebrospinal, 62272
Fetal, 59074
Peritoneal
Percutaneous, 49406
Transrectal, 49407
Transvaginal, 49407
Retinal, 67108, 67113
Retroperitoneal
Percutaneous, 49406
Transrectal, 49407
Transvaginal, 49407
Tendon Sheath Hand, 26020
Visceral, 49405
Ganglion Cyst, 20612
Hematoma
Ankle, 27603
Arm, Lower, 25028
Brain, 61108, 61154, 61156
Dentoalveolar Structures, 41800
Ear, External, 69000, 69005
Joint, 20600-20610
Mouth
Lingual, 41000
Masticator Space, 41009, 41018
Sublingual, 41005-41006, 41015
Submandibular Space, 41008, 41017
Submental Space, 41007, 41016
Vestibule, 40800-40801
Subungual, 11740
Superficial, 10140
Vagina, 57022, 57023
Wrist, 25028
Joint
Acromioclavicular, 23044
Ankle, 27610
Carpometacarpal, 26070
Glenohumeral, 23040
Hip, 26990, 27030
Interphalangeal, 26080, 28024
Intertarsal, 28020
Knee, 27301, 29871
Metacarpophalangeal, 26075
Metatarsophalangeal, 28022
Midcarpal, 25040
Pelvis, 26990
Radiocarpal, 25040
Sternoclavicular, 23044
Thigh, 27301
Wrist, 29843
Kidney, 50040
Liver
Abscess or Cyst, 47010
Lymph Node, 38300-38305
Lymphocele, 49062
Laparoscopic, 49323
Percutaneous, Sclerotherapy, 49185

E1, 82679
E2, 82670
E2A/PBX1 (t(1;19)), 81401
E3, 82677
Ear
　Collection of Blood From, 36416
　Drum, 69420, 69421, 69424, 69433, 69436,
　　69450, 69610, 69620
　　See Tympanic Membrane
　External
　　Abscess
　　　Incision and Drainage
　　　　Complicated, 69005
　　　　Simple, 69000
　　Biopsy, 69100, 69105
　　Customized Prosthesis, 21086
　　Debridement Mastoidectomy Cavity,
　　　69220-69222
　　Excision
　　　Exostosis, 69140
　　　Partial, 69110
　　　Soft Tissue, 69145
　　　　with Neck Dissection, 69155
　　　　without Neck Dissection,
　　　　　69150
　　　Total, 69120
　　Hematoma
　　　Incision and Drainage, 69000,
　　　　69005
　　Reconstruction
　　　External Auditory Canal, 69310,
　　　　69320
　　　Protruding Ear(s), 69300
　　　with Graft, 21230, 21235
　　　with Tissue Transfer, 14060-14061
　　Removal
　　　Cerumen, 69209-69210
　　　Foreign Body, 69200, 69205
　　Repair
　　　Complex, 13151-13153
　　　Intermediate, 12051-12057
　　　Simple, 12011-12018
　　　Superficial, 12011-12018
　　Unlisted Services and Procedures, 69399
　Inner
　　CT Scan, 70480-70482
　　Excision
　　　Labyrinth, 61596, 69905, 69910
　　Exploration
　　　Endolymphatic Sac, 69805, 69806
　　Incision
　　　Labyrinth, 69801
　　Insertion
　　　Cochlear Device, 69930
　　Labyrinthectomy, 61596, 69905, 69910
　　Labyrinthotomy, 69801
　　Unlisted Services and Procedures, 69949
　　Vestibular Evoked Myogenic Potential
　　　(VEMP) Testing, [92517], [92518],
　　　[92519]
　　Vestibular Nerve Section, 69915
　Meatoplasty, 69310
　　for Congenital Atresia, 69320
　Middle
　　CT Scan, 70480-70482
　　Excision
　　　Aural Polyp, 69540
　　　Glomus Tumor, 69550, 69552,
　　　　69554
　　　Polyp, 69540
　　Exploration, 69440
　　Facial Nerve
　　　Decompression, 69720, 69725
　　　Suture, 69740, 69745
　　Lesion
　　　Excision, 69540
　　Reconstruction
　　　Tympanoplasty with Antrotomy or
　　　　Mastoidectomy, 69635-
　　　　69637
　　　Tympanoplasty with Mastoidecto-
　　　　my, 69641-69646
　　　Tympanoplasty without Mastoidec-
　　　　tomy, 69631-69633
　　Removal
　　　Ventilating Tube, 69424

Ear — *continued*
　Middle — *continued*
　　Repair
　　　Fistula, 69666-69667
　　　Oval Window, 69666
　　　Round Window, 69667
　　Revision
　　　Stapes, 69662
　　Stapes
　　　Mobilization, 69650
　　　Stapedectomy, 69660-69662
　　　Stapedotomy, 69660-69662
　　Tumor
　　　Excision, 69550-69554
　　Unlisted Services and Procedures, 69799
　Outer
　　CT Scan, 70480-70482
　　Skin Graft
　　　Delay of Flap, 15630
　　　Full Thickness, 15260, 15261
　　　Pedicle Flap, 15576
　　　Split, 15120, 15121
　　Tissue Transfer, Adjacent, 14060-14061
　　Removal Skin Lesions
　　　Excision
　　　　Benign, 11440-11446
　　　　Malignant, 11640-11646
　　　Shaving, 11310-11313
　　Temporal Bone
　　　Bone Conduction Hearing Device
　　　　Implantation, 69710
　　　　Removal, 69711
　　　　Repair, 69711
　　　Osseointegrated Implant
　　　　Implantation, [69714], [69716]
　　　　Removal, [69726, 69727]
　　　　Replacement, [69717], [69719]
　　　Resection, 69535
　　　Unlisted Service or Procedure, 69799
Ear Canal
　See Auditory Canal
Ear Cartilage
　Graft
　　to Face, 21230
　　to Nose or Ear, 21230, 21235
Ear Lobes
　Pierce, 69090
Ear, Nose, and Throat
　Acoustic, 92568
　Audiometry
　　Conditioning Play, 92582
　　Evoked Response, [92650], [92651],
　　　[92652], [92653]
　　Picture, 92583
　　Pure Tone, 92552-92553, 0208T-0209T
　　Select Picture, 92583
　　Speech, 92555-92557, 0210T-0212T
　　Tympanometry and Reflex, 92550
　　Visual Reinforcement, 92579
　Binocular Microscopy, 92504
　Brainstem Evoked Response, [92650], [92651],
　　[92652], [92653]
　Central Auditory Function Evaluation, 92620-
　　92621
　Comprehensive Audiometry Threshold Evalu-
　　ation, 92557
　Diagnostic Analysis
　　Auditory Brainstem Implant, 92640
　　Cochlear Implant, 92601-92604
　Ear Protector Evaluation, 92596
　Electrocochleography, 92584
　Evaluation
　　Auditory Rehabilitation Status, 92626-
　　　92627, 92630, 92633
　　Communication Device
　　　Non-speech Generating, 92605,
　　　　[92618]
　　　Speech Generating, 92607-92608
　　Language Comprehensive and Expres-
　　　sion, 92523
　　Laryngeal Sensory Testing, 92614-92617
　　Speech Fluency, 92521
　　Speech Sound Production, 92522
　　Swallowing, 92610-92613, 92616
　　Voice and Resonance Analysis, 92524
　Examination Under Anesthesia, 92502

Ear, Nose, and Throat — *continued*
　Facial Nerve Function Study, 92516
　Filtered Speech, 92571
　Hearing Aid Evaluation, 92590-92595
　Hearing, Language, and Speech Evaluation,
　　92521-92524
　Immittance Testing, 92570
　Impedance Testing, 92567
　Laryngeal Function Study, 92520
　Lombard Test, 92700
　Loudness Balance, 92562
　Nasal Function Study, 92512
　Nasopharyngoscopy, 92511
　Reflex, 92568
　Screening Test, 92551
　Treatment
　　Hearing, Language, Speech Disorder,
　　　92507-92508
　　Oral Function for Feeding, 92526
　　Swallowing Dysfunction, 92526
Ear Protector Attenuation, 92596
　See Hearing Aid Services
Ear Wax
　See Cerumen
Ebstein Anomaly Repair, 33468
EBV, 86663-86665
ECCE, 66840-66852, 66940
Eccrine Glands
　Chemodenervation
　　Axillae, 64650
　　Feet, 64999
　　Hands, 64999
　　Other Areas, 64653
ECG, 93000-93024, 93040-93278 *[93241, 93242,*
　93243, 93244, 93245, 93246, 93247, 93248]
　External, 93224-93272 *[93241, 93242, 93243,*
　93244, 93245, 93246, 93247, 93248]
　Signal-Averaged, 93278
Echinococcosis, 86171, 86280
ECHO, 76825, 93303-93312, 93314, 93315, 93317-
　93321, 93350, *[93356]*
Echocardiography
　Cardiac, 93320-93350
　　Intracardiac, 93662
　　Strain Imaging, *[93356]*
　　Transesophageal, 93318
　　Transthoracic, 93303-93317
　　　with Myocardial Contrast Perfu-
　　　　sion, 0439T
　　　with Stress Test, 93350-93352
　Doppler, 93303-93321, 93350, 93662
　Fetal Heart, 76825-76828
　　Doppler
　　　Complete, 76827
　　　Follow–up or Repeat Study, 76828
　　for Assessment of Myocardial Ischemia/Viabil-
　　　ity, 0439T
　　for Congenital Anomalies
　　　3D Imaging During Procedure, *[93319]*
　　　Transesophageal, 93315-93317
　　　Transthoracic, 93303, 93304
　　Intracardiac, 93662
　　M Mode and Real Time, 93306
　　Myocardial Contrast Perfusion, 0439T
　　Strain Imaging, *[93356]*
　　Stress Test, 93350-93351
　　　with Contrast, 93352
　　　with Myocardial Contrast Perfusion,
　　　　0439T
　　Transesophageal, 93312-93318
　　　for Congenital Anomalies, 93315-93317
　　　　3D Imaging During Procedure,
　　　　　[93319]
　　　for Guidance Intracardiac or Great Vessel
　　　　Intervention, 93355
　　　for Monitoring Purposes, 93318
　　Transthoracic, 93303-93308, 93350-93352
　　　for Congenital Anomalies, 93303, 93304
　　　　3D Imaging During Procedure,
　　　　　[93319]
　　　with Myocardial Contrast Perfusion,
　　　　0439T
　　　with Stress Test, 93350-93352
Echoencephalography, 76506
Echography
　Abdomen, 76700-76705

Echography — *continued*
　Arm
　　Complete, 76881
　　Limited, 76882
　Cardiac, 0439T, 93303-93317, 93320-93321,
　　93350-93352, 93662
　　Guidance for Biopsy, 76932
　Chest, 76604
　Extracranial Arteries, 93880, 93882
　Eyes, 76510-76529
　Head, 76536
　Heart, 0439T, 93303-93317, 93320-93321,
　　93350-93352, 93662
　　Guidance for Biopsy, 76932
　Hip
　　Infant, 76885, 76886
　Intracranial Arteries, 93886-93893
　Intraoperative, 76998
　Kidney
　　Transplant, 76776
　Leg
　　Complete, 76881
　　Limited, 76882
　Neck, 76536
　Pelvis, 76856, 76857
　Pregnant Uterus, 76801-76828
　Prostate, 76872-76873
　Retroperitoneal, 76770, 76775
　Scrotum, 76870
　Spine, 76800
　Transrectal, 76872, 76873
　Transvaginal, 76817, 76830
　Unlisted Ultrasound, 76999
　Vagina, 76817, 76830
Echotomography
　See Echography
ECLS (Extracorporeal Life Support Services)
　Cannulization
　　Insertion, 33951-33956
　　Removal, *[33965, 33966, 33969, 33984,*
　　　33985, 33986]
　　Repositioning, 33957-33959 *[33962,*
　　　33963, 33964]
　Creation Graft Conduit, *[33987]*
　Daily Management, 33948-33949
　Initiation, 33946-33947
　Left Heart Vent Insertion, *[33988]*
　Left Heart Vent Removal, *[33989]*
ECMO (Extracorporeal Membrane Oxygenation)
　Cannulization
　　Insertion, 33951-33956
　　Isolated with Chemotherapy Perfusion,
　　　36823
　　Removal, *[33965, 33966, 33969, 33984,*
　　　33985, 33986]
　　Repositioning, 33957-33959 *[33962,*
　　　33963, 33964]
　Creation Graft Conduit, *[33987]*
　Daily Management, 33948-33949
　Initiation, 33946-33947
　Left Heart Vent Insertion, *[33988]*
　Left Heart Vent Removal, *[33989]*
ECS
　See Emission Computerized Tomography
ECSF (Erythrocyte Colony Stimulating Factor)
　See Erythropoietin
ECT (Emission Computerized Tomography), 78803
ECT (Electroconvulsive Therapy), 90870
Ectasia
　See Dilation
Ectopic Pregnancy
　See Obstetrical Care
　Abdominal, 59130
　Cervix, 59140
　Interstitial
　　Partial Resection Uterus, 59136
　Laparoscopy, 59150
　　with Salpingectomy and/or Oophorecto-
　　　my, 59151
　Ovarian
　　with Salpingectomy and/or Oophorecto-
　　　my, 59120
　　without Salpingectomy and/or
　　　Oophorectomy, 59121

Electron Microscopy — Endoscopy

Electron Microscopy, 88348
Electronic Analysis
  Cardiac Rhythm Monitor System, 93285,
    93290-93291, 93297-93298
    Data Analysis, 93291, 93297-93298
    Evaluation of Programming, 0650T,
      93285, 93291, 93297-93298
  Cardioverter–Defibrillator
    Evaluation
      in Person, 0575T-0576T, 93289,
        93640, 93642
      Remote, 0578T-0579T, 93295-
        93296
      with Reprogramming, 0577T, 93282-
        93284, 93287, 93642, 93644
      without Reprogramming, 93289, 93292,
        93295, 93640-93641
  Data Analysis, 93289
  Defibrillator, 93282, 93289, 93292, 93295
  Drug Infusion Pump, 62367-62370, 95990-
    95991
  Neurostimulator Pulse Generator, 0589T-
    0590T, 95970-95982 *[95983, 95984]*
  Pulse Generator, 0589T-0590T, 95970-95982
    [95983, 95984]
    Field Stimulation, 64999
    Gastric Neurostimulator, 95980-95982
Electro–Oculography, 92270
Electrophoresis
  Hemoglobin, 83020
  High Resolution, 83701
  Immuno–, 86320-86327
  Immunofixation, 86334-86335
  Protein, 84165-84166
  Unlisted Services and Procedures, 82664
Electrophysiology Procedure, 93600-93660
Electroporation, Irreversible
  Ablation, Tumor, 0600T, 0601T
Electroretinography, 0509T, 92273-92274
Electrostimulation, Analgesic Cutaneous
  See Application, Neurostimulation
Electrosurgery
  Anal, 46924
  Penile, 54065
  Rectal Tumor, 45190
  Skin Lesion, 17000-17111, 17260-17286
  Skin Tags, 11200-11201
  Trichiasis
    Correction, 67825
  Vaginal, 57061, 57065
  Vulva, 56501, 56515
Electroversion, Cardiac
  See Cardioversion
Elevation, Scapula, Congenital
  See Sprengel's Deformity
Elliot Operation, 66130
  Excision, Lesion, Sclera, 66130
Eloesser Procedure, 32035, 32036
Eloesser Thoracoplasty, 32905
Embolectomy
  Aortoiliac Artery, 34151, 34201
  Axillary Artery, 34101
  Brachial Artery, 34101
  Carotid Artery, 34001
  Celiac Artery, 34151
  Femoral, 34201
  Iliac, 34151, 34201
  Innominate Artery, 34001-34101
  Mesentery Artery, 34151
  Peroneal Artery, 34203
  Popliteal Artery, 34201, 34203
  Pulmonary Artery, 33910-33916
  Radial Artery, 34111
  Renal Artery, 34151
  Subclavian Artery, 34001-34101
  Tibial Artery, 34203
  Ulnar Artery, 34111
Embolic Protection Device
  Insertion
    Cerebral, 33370
Embolization
  Arterial (Not Hemorrhage or Tumor), 37242
  Hemorrhage
    Arterial, 37244
    Venous, 37244
  Infarction, 37243

Embolization — *continued*
  Leiomyomata, 37243
  Lymphatic Extravasation, 37244
  Organ Ischemia, 37243
  Tumors, 37243
  Ureter, 50705
  Venous Malformations, 37241
Embryo
  Biopsy, 89290, 89291
  Carcinoembryonic Antigen, 82378
  Cryopreservation, 89258
  Cryopreserved
    Preparation/Thawing, 89352
  Culture, 89250
    Extended Culture, 89272
    with Co–Culture Oocyte, 89251
  Hatching
    Assisted Microtechnique, 89253
  Preparation for Transfer, 89255
  Storage, 89342
Embryo Implantation
  See Implantation
Embryo Transfer
  In Vitro Fertilization, 58970, 58974, 58976
    Intrafallopian Transfer, 58976
    Intrauterine Transfer, 58974
    Preparation for Transfer, 89255
Embryo/Fetus Monitoring
  See Monitoring, Fetal
Embryonated Eggs
  Inoculation, 87250
EMD, 81404-81405
Emergency Department Services, 99281-99288
  See Critical Care; Emergency Department
  Anesthesia, 99140
    in Office, 99058
  Physician Direction of Advanced Life Support,
    99288
Emesis Induction, 99175
EMG (Electromyography, Needle), 51784, 51785,
  92265, 95860-95872 *[95885, 95886, 95887]*
EMI Scan
  See CT Scan
Emission Computerized Tomography, 78803
Emission Computerized Tomography, Single–Photon
  See Also SPECT
EML4/ALK, 81401
Emmet Operation, 57720
Empyema
  Closure
    Chest Wall, 32810
  Empyemectomy, 32540
  Enucleation, 32540
  Thoracostomy, 32035, 32036, 32551
Empyemectomy, 32540
EMS, 99288
Encephalitis
  Antibody, 86651-86654
Encephalitis Virus Vaccine, 90738
Encephalocele
  Repair, 62120
    Craniotomy, 62121
Encephalography, A–Mode, 76506
Encephalon
  See Brain
Endarterectomy
  Coronary Artery, 33572
    Anomaly, 33500-33507
  Pulmonary, 33916
Endemic Flea–Borne Typhus
  See Murine Typhus
End–Expiratory Pressure, Positive
  See Pressure Breathing, Positive
Endobronchial Challenge Tests
  See Bronchial Challenge Test
Endocavitary Fulguration
  See Electrocautery
Endocrine, Pancreas
  See Islet Cell
Endocrine System
  Unlisted Services and Procedures, 60699,
    78099
Endocrinology (Type 2 Diabetes) Biochemical
  Assays, 81506

Endograft
  Aorta, 34701-34706
  Iliac Artery, 34707-34711
  Infrarenal Artery, 34701-34706
Endolaser Photocoagulation
  Focal, 67039
  Panretinal, 67040
Endoluminal Imaging, *[92978, 92979]*
Endolymphatic Sac
  Exploration
    with Shunt, 69806
    without Shunt, 69805
Endometrial Ablation, 0404T, 58353, 58356, 58563
  Curettage, 58356
  Exploration via Hysteroscopy, 58563
Endometrioma
  Abdomen
    Destruction, 49203-49205
    Excision, 49203-49205
  Mesenteric
    Destruction, 49203-49205
    Excision, 49203-49205
  Peritoneal
    Destruction, 49203-49205
    Excision, 49203-49205
  Retroperitoneal
    Destruction, 49203-49205
    Excision, 49203-49205
Endometriosis, Adhesive
  See Adhesions, Intrauterine
Endometrium
  Ablation, 0404T, 58353, 58356, 58563
  Biopsy, 58100, 58110, 58558
  Curettage, 58356
Endomyocardial
  Biopsy, 93505
Endomysial Antibody (EMA), 86231
Endonuclease, DNA
  See DNAse
Endopyelotomy, 50575
Endorectal Pull–Through
  Proctectomy, Total, 45110, 45112, 45120,
    45121
Endoscopic Retrograde Cannulation of Pancreatic
  Duct (ERCP)
  See Cholangiopancreatography
Endoscopic Retrograde Cholangiopancreatography
  Ablation Lesion/Polyp/Tumor, *[43278]*
  Balloon Dilation, *[43277]*
  Destruction of Calculi, 43265
  Diagnostic, 43260
  Measure Pressure Sphincter of Oddi, 43263
  Placement
    Stent, *[43274]*
      with Removal and Replacement,
        [43276]
  Removal
    Calculi or Debris, 43264
    Foreign Body, *[43275]*
    Stent, *[43275]*
      with Stent Exchange, *[43276]*
    Removal Calculi or Debris, 43264
  with Optical Endomicroscopy, 0397T
Endoscopies, Pleural
  See Thoracoscopy
Endoscopy
  See Arthroscopy; Thoracoscopy
  Adrenal Gland
    Biopsy, 60650
    Excision, 60650
  Anal
    Ablation
      Polyp, 46615
      Tumor, 46615
    Biopsy, 46606, 46607
    Collection of Specimen, 46600-46601
    Diagnostic, 46600-46601
    Dilation, 46604
    Exploration, 46600
    Hemorrhage, 46614
    High Resolution, 46601, 46607
    Removal
      Foreign Body, 46608
      Polyp, 46610, 46612
      Tumor, 46610, 46612

Endoscopy — *continued*
  Atria, 33265-33266
  Bile Duct
    Biopsy, 47553
    Cannulation, 43273
    Catheterization, 74328, 74330
    Destruction
      Calculi (Stone), 43265
      Tumor, *[43278]*
    Diagnostic, 47552
    Dilation, 47555, 47556, *[43277]*
    Exchange
      Stent, *[43276]*
    Exploration, 47552
    Intraoperative, 47550
    Percutaneous, 47552-47556
    Removal
      Calculi (Stone), 43264, 47554
      Foreign Body, *[43275]*
      Stent, *[43275]*
    Specimen Collection, 43260
    Sphincter Pressure, 43263
    Sphincterotomy, 43262, *[43274]*
    Stent Placement, *[43274]*
  Bladder
    Biopsy, 52204, 52250, 52354
    Catheterization, 52005, 52010
    Destruction, 52354
      Lesion, 52400
      Polyps, 52285
      with Fulguration, 52214
    Diagnostic, 52000
    Dilation, 52260, 52265
    Evacuation
      Clot, 52001
    Excision
      Tumor, 52355
    Exploration, 52351
    Insertion
      Radioactive Substance, 52250
      Stent, 52282, 53855
    Instillation, 52010
    Irrigation, 52010
    Lesion, 52224, 52234-52235, 52240,
      52400
    Litholapaxy, 52317-52318
    Lithotripsy, 52353
    Neck, 51715
    Removal
      Calculus, 52310, 52315, 52352
      Urethral Stent, 52310, 52315
  Bladder Neck
    Injection of Implant Material, 51715
  Brain
    Catheterization, 62160
    Dissection
      Adhesions, 62161
      Cyst, 62162
    Drainage, 62162
    Excision
      Brain Tumor, 62164
      Cyst, 62162
      Pituitary Tumor, 62165
    Shunt Creation, 62201
  Bronchi
    Aspiration, 31645-31646
    Biopsy, 31625, 31632, 31633
    Computer-Assisted Image Guidance,
      31627
    Destruction
      Lesion, 31641, 96570-96571
      Tumor, 31641, 96570-96571
    Dilation, 31630-31631, 31636-31638
    Excision Tumor, 31640
    Exploration, 31622
    Lavage, 31624
    Lesion, 31641
      Destruction, 31641, 96570-96571
    Needle Biopsy, 31629, 31633
    Occlusion, 31634
    Placement
      Fiducial Marker, 31626
      Radioelement Catheter, 31643
      Stent, 31631, 31636-31637
    Removal
      Foreign Body, 31635

[Resequenced] © 2021 Optum360, LLC

Index

Endoscopy — Epiphyseal Separation

Epiphyseal Separation — *continued*
Femur — *continued*
Open Treatment, 27519
Percutaneous Treatment, 27509
Radius
Closed Treatment, 25600, 25605
Open Treatment, 25607, 25608-25609
Percutaneous Treatment, 25606
Epiphysiodesis
See Epiphyseal Arrest
Epiphysis
See Bone; Specific Bone
Epiploectomy, 49255
EPIS, 59300, 95925-95930 *[95938, 95939]*, *[92650]*, *[92651]*, *[92652]*, *[92653]*
Episiotomy, 59300, 59610, 59612
Epispadias
Penis
Reconstruction, 54385
Repair, 54380-54390
with Exstrophy of Bladder, 54390
with Incontinence, 54385
Epistaxis
Control, 30901-30906
with Nasal
Sinus Endoscopy, 31238
Epley Maneuver, 95992
EPM2A, 81404
EPO, 82668
EPS, 93600-93660
Epstein–Barr Virus
Antibody, 86663-86665
Equina, Cauda
Decompression, 63005, 63011, 63017, 63047-63048, 63055
Exploration, 63005, 63011, 63017
ER, 99281-99288
ERCP (Cholangiopancreatography), 43260-43270 *[43274, 43275, 43276, 43277, 43278]*
ERG (Electroretinography), 0509T, 92273-92274
Ergocalciferol
See Calciferol
Ergocalciferols
See Calciferol
Ergonovine Provocation Test, 93024
ERMAP, 81403
Erythrocyte
See Red Blood Bell (RBC)
Erythrocyte ab
See Antibody, Red Blood Cell
Erythrocyte Count
See Red Blood Cell (RBC), Count
Erythropoietin, 82668
Escharotomy
Burns, 16035, 16036
Graft Site, 15002-15005
Escherichia Coli O157
Antigen Detection
Enzyme Immunoassay, 87335
ESD
See Endoscopy, Gastrointestinal, Upper
Esophageal Acid Infusion Test, 91030
Esophageal Myotomy
Cricopharyngeal, 43030
Lower Esophageal, 43497
Esophageal Polyp
See Polyp, Esophagus
Esophageal Tumor
See Tumor, Esophagus
Esophageal Varices
Decompression, 37181
Injection Sclerosis, 43204, 43243
Ligation, 43205, 43244, 43400
Esophagectomy
McKeown, 43112
Partial, 43116-43124
Total, 43107-43113, 43124, 43286-43288
Tri-incisional, *[43211]*
Esophagoenterostomy
with Total Gastrectomy, 43260
Esophagogastroduodenoscopy
Ablation Lesions/Polyps/Tumors, *[43270]*
Band Ligation of Varices, 43244
Biopsy (Single or Multiple), 0653T, 43239
Collection of Specimen, 43235
Control of Bleeding, 43255

Esophagogastroduodenoscopy — *continued*
Delivery of Thermal Energy, 43257
Diagnostic, 0652T, 43235
Dilation, 43245, 43248-43249, *[43233]*
Directed Submucosal Injection(s), 43236
Drainage of Pseudocyst, 43240
Endoscopic Ultrasound Examination, 43237, 43259
Fine Needle Aspiration/Biopsy(s), 43238, 43242
Guide Wire Insertion, 43248
Injection
Anesthetic Agent, 43253
Diagnostic Substance(s), 43253
Fiducial Marker(s), 43253
Neurolytic Agent, 43253
Sclerosis Agent, 43243
Submucosal, 43236
Therapeutic Substance(s), 43253
Injection Varices, 43243
Insertion Intraluminal Tube or Catheter, 0654T, 43241
Mucosal Resection, 43254
Optical Endomicroscopy, 43252
Placement
Endoscopic Stent, *[43266]*
Gastrostomy Tube, 43246
Removal
Foreign Body, 43247
Lesion/Polyp/Tumor, 43250-43251
Transnasal, 0652T-0655T
Ultrasound Guided, 43237-43238, 43253, 43259
Esophagogastrostomy, 43112, 43320
Esophagojejunostomy, 43340, 43341
Esophagomyotomy, 32665, 43330, 43331
Abdominal, 43330
Heller Type, 32665, 43279, 43330
Laparoscopic, 43279
Thoracic Approach, 43331
Thoracoscopic, 32665
With Fundoplasty, 43279
Esophagoplasty, 43300-43312
Congenital Defect, 43313-43314
Esophagorrphaphy
See Esophagus, Suture
Esophagoscopies
See Endoscopy, Esophagus
Esophagoscopy
Dilation Over Guidewire, 43196
Operative By Incision, 43499
Through Artificial Stoma, 43499
Transnasal
Biopsy, 43198
Collection of Specimen, 43197
Transoral
Ablation of Lesion, 43229
Collection of Specimen, 43191, 43200
Dilation, 43195-43196, 43220 *[43212, 43213, 43214]*, 43226, 43229
Exploration, 43200
Guide Wire Insertion, 43196, 43226, 43229, *[43212]*
Hemorrhage, 43227
Injection, 43192, 43201, 43204
Ligation of Varices, 43205
Mucosal Resection, *[43211]*
Needle Biopsy, 43232
Removal
Foreign Body, 43194, 43215
Polyp, 43216-43217, 43229
Tumor, 43216-43217, 43229
Stent Placement, *[43212]*
With Diverticulectomy, 43180
With Optical Endomicroscopy, 43206
With Ultrasound Examination, 43231-43232
Ultrasound, 43231-43232
Vein Ligation, 43205
With Optical Endomicroscopy, 43206
Esophagostomy
Closure, 43420, 43425
External Fistulization, 43351-43352
With Esophagectomy, 43124
Esophagotomy, 43020, 43045
Esophagotracheal Fistula
See Fistula, Tracheoesophageal

Esophagus
Ablation
Lesion, 43229
Polyp, 43229
Tumor, 43229
Acid Perfusion Test, 91030
Acid Reflux Tests, 91034-91035, 91037-91038
Balloon Distension, 43249, *[43233]*
Provocation Study, 91040
Biopsy
Endoscopy, 43198, 43202
Forceps, 3150F
Cineradiography, 74230
Cricopharyngeal Myotomy, 43030
Dilation, 43450, 43453
Endoscopic, 43195-43196, 43220 *[43212, 43213, 43214]*, 43226, 43229, 43248-43249, *[43233]*
Strictures
Duodenal, 43245
Gastric, 43245
Surgical, 43510
Endoscopy
Biopsy, 43193, 43198, 43202
Diagnostic, 43191, 43197, 43200
Dilation, 43220, 43226
Balloon, 43195, *[43214]*, *[43233]*
Dilator Over Guide Wire, 43196, 43226, 43248
Retrograde by Balloon or Dilator, *[43213]*
Transendoscopic with Balloon, 43220, 43249
Exploration, 43200
Hemorrhage, 43227
Injection, 43192, 43201, 43204, 43243, 43253
Insertion Stent, *[43212]*
Mucosal Resection, *[43211]*
Needle Biopsy, 43232
Removal
Foreign Body, 43194, 43215
Polyp, 43216-43217
Tumor, 43216-43217
Specimen Collection, 43191, 43197, 43200
Ultrasound, 43231, 43232
Vein Ligation, 43205
Excision
Diverticula, 43130, 43135
Partial, 43116-43124
Total, 43107-43113, 43124
Exploration
Endoscopy, 43200
Hemorrhage, 43227
Imaging Studies
Motility, 78258
Obstructions, 74360
Reflux, 78262
Removal Foreign Body, 74235
Strictures, 74360
Swallowing Function Cineradiography, 74230
X-ray, 74210, 74220
Incision, 43020, 43045
Muscle, 43030
Injection
Sclerosis Agent, 43204
Submucosal, 43192, 43201
Insertion
Sengstaken Tamponade, 43460
Stent, *[43212]*
Tamponade, 43460
Tube, 43510
Intraluminal Imaging, 91110-91111
Intubation with Specimen Collection, 43753-43755
Lengthening, 43283, 43338
Lesion
Excision, 43100, 43101
Ligation, 43405
Motility Study, 78258, 91010-91013
Mucosal Resection, *[43211]*
Myotomy
Cricopharyngeal, 43030
Lower Esophageal, 43497

Esophagus — *continued*
Needle Biopsy
Endoscopy, 43232
Nuclear Medicine
Imaging (motility), 78258
Reflux Study, 78262
Reconstruction, 43300, 43310, 43313
Creation
Stoma, 43351-43352
Esophagostomy, 43351-43352
Fistula, 43305, 43312, 43314
Gastrointestinal, 43360, 43361
Removal
Foreign Bodies, 43020, 43045, 43194, 43215, 74235
Lesion, 43216-43217
Polyp, 43216-43217
Repair, 43300, 43310, 43313
Esophagogastric Fundoplasty, 43325-43328
Laparoscopic, 43280
Esophagogastrostomy, 43112, 43320
Esophagojejunostomy, 43340, 43341
Esophagomyotomy, 43279
Esophagoplasty, 43300, 43305, 43310, 43312
Fistula, 43305, 43312, 43314, 43420, 43425
Heller Esophagomyotomy, 32665
Muscle, 43330, 43331
Nissan Procedure, 43280
Paraesophageal Hernia
Laparoscopic, 43281-43282
Laparotomy, 43332-43333
Thoracoabdominal Incision, 43336-43337
Thoracotomy, 43334-43335
Pre–existing Perforation, 43405
Thal-Nissen Procedure, 43325
Toupet Procedure, 43280
Wound, 43410, 43415
Stapling Gastroesophageal Junction, 43405
Suture
Gastroesophageal Junction, 43405
Wound, 43410, 43415
Ultrasound, 43231, 43232
Unlisted Services and Procedures, 43289, 43499
Vein
Ligation, 43205, 43400
Video, 74230
X-ray, 74220
Esophagus Neoplasm
See Tumor, Esophagus
Esophagus, Varix
See Esophageal Varices
ESR, 85651, 85652
ESR1/PGR, 81402
ESRD, 90951-90961, 90967-90970
Home, 90963-90966
EST, 90870
Established Patient
Critical Care, 99291-99292
Domiciliary or Rest Home Visit, 99334-99337, 99339-99340
Emergency Department Services, 99281-99285
Evaluation Services
Basic Life and/or Disability, 99450
Work-related or Medical Disability, 99455
Home Services, 99347-99350, 99601-99602
Hospital Inpatient Services, 99221-99239
Hospital Observation Services, 99217-99220, 99234-99236, *[99224, 99225, 99226]*
Initial Inpatient Consultation, 99251-99255
Nursing Facility, 99304-99310, 99315-99316, 99318
Office and/or Other Outpatient Consultations, 99241-99245
Office Visit, 99211-99215
Online Evaluation and Management Services
Nonphysician, 98970-98973
Physician, *[99421, 99422, 99423]*
Ophthalmological Services, 92012, 92014
Outpatient Visit, 99211-99215
Preventive Services, 99391-99397

Excision — continued

Breast
- Biopsy, 19100-19101
- Chest Wall Tumor, 21601-21603
- Cyst, 19120-19126
- Lactiferous Duct Fistula, 19112
- Lesion, 19120-19126
  - by Needle Localization, 19125, 19126
- Mastectomy, 19300-19307
- Nipple Exploration, 19110

Bulbourethral Gland, 53250

Bullae
- Lung, 32141
  - Endoscopic, 32655

Burns, 15002-15003, 15004-15005

Bursa
- Elbow, 24105
- Excision, 27060
- Femur, 27062
- Ischial, 27060
- Knee, 27340
- Wrist, 25115, 25116

Bypass Graft, 35901-35907

Calcaneus, 28118-28120

Calculi (Stone)
- Parotid Gland, 42330, 42340
- Salivary Gland, 42330-42340
- Sublingual Gland, 42330, 42335
- Submandibular Gland, 42330, 42335

Carotid Artery, 60605

Carpal, 25145, 25210, 25215

Cartilage
- Knee Joint, 27332, 27333
- Shoulder Joint, 23101
- Temporomandibular Joint, 21060
- Wrist, 25107

Caruncle, Urethra, 53265

Cataract
- Secondary, 66830

Cervix
- Electrode, 57460
- Radical, 57531
- Stump
  - Abdominal Approach, 57540, 57545
  - Vaginal Approach, 57550-57556
- Total, 57530

Chalazion
- Multiple
  - Different Lids, 67805
  - Same Lid, 67801
- Single, 67800
  - with Anesthesia, 67808

Chest Wall Tumor, 21601-21603

Choroid Plexus, 61544

Clavicle
- Partial, 23120, 23180
- Sequestrectomy, 23170
- Total, 23125
- Tumor
  - Radical Resection, 23200

Coccyx, 27080

Colon
- Excision
  - Partial, 44140-44147, 44160
    - with Anastomosis, 44140
  - Total, 44150-44156
- Laparoscopic
  - with Anastomosis, 44204, 44207-44208
  - with Colostomy, 44206, 44208
  - with Ileocolostomy, 44205

Condyle
- Temporomandibular Joint, 21050

Condylectomy, 21050

Constricting Ring
- Finger, 26596

Cornea
- Epithelium, 65435
  - with Chelating Agent, 65436
- Scraping, 65430

Coronoidectomy, 21070

Cowper's gland, 53250

Cranial Bone
- Tumor, 61563, 61564

Excision — continued

Cyst
- *See* Ganglion Cyst
- Bile Duct, 47715
- Bladder, 51500
- Brain, 61516, 61524, 62162
- Branchial, 42810, 42815
- Breast, 19120
- Calcaneus, 28100-28103
- Carpal, 25130-25136
- Cheekbone, 21030
- Clavicle, 23140
  - with Allograft, 23146
  - with Autograft, 23145
- Facial Bone, 21030
- Femur, 27065-27067, 27355-27358
- Fibula, 27635-27638
- Finger, 26034, 26160
- Foot, 28090
- Hand, 26160
- Hip, 27065-27067
- Humerus, 23150, 24110
  - with Allograft, 23156, 24116
  - with Autograft, 23155, 24115
- Ilium, 27065-27067, 27070-27071, 27075-27076
- Intra-abdominal, 49203-49205
- Kidney, 50280, 50290
- Knee, 27345, 27347
- Lung, 32140
- Mandible, 21040, 21046-21047
- Maxilla, 21030, 21048-21049
- Mediastinum, 32662
- Metacarpal, 26200, 26205
- Metatarsal, 28104-28107
- Mullerian Duct, 55680
- Nose, 30124-30125
- Olecranon (Process), 24120
  - with Allograft, 24126
  - with Autograft, 24125
- Ovarian, 58925
  - *See* Cystectomy, Ovarian
- Pericardial, 33050
  - Endoscopic, 32661
- Phalanges
  - Finger, 26210, 26215
  - Toe, 28108
- Pilonidal, 11770-11772
- Pubis, 27066, 27067
- Radius, 24120, 25120-25126
  - with Allograft, 24126
  - with Autograft, 24125
- Salivary Gland, 42408
- Scapula, 23140
  - with Allograft, 23146
  - with Autograft, 23145
- Seminal Vesicle, 55680
- Sublingual Gland, 42408
- Talus, 28100-28103
- Tarsal, 28104-28107
- Thyroglossal Duct, 60280, 60281
- Thyroid Gland, 60200
- Tibia, 27635-27638
- Toe, 28092
- Ulna, 24120, 25120
  - with Allograft, 24126
  - with Autograft, 24125
- Urachal
  - Bladder, 51500
- Vaginal, 57135

Destruction of the Vestibule of the Mouth
- *See* Mouth, Vestibule of, Excision, Destruction

Diverticulum, Meckel's
- *See* Meckel's Diverticulum, Excision

Ear, External
- Partial, 69110
- Total, 69120

Ear, Inner
- Labyrinthectomy, 61596, 69905, 69910

Elbow Joint, 24155

Electrode, 57522

Embolectomy/Thrombectomy
- Aortoiliac Artery, 34151, 34201
- Axillary Artery, 34101
- Brachial Artery, 34101

Excision — continued

Embolectomy/Thrombectomy — *continued*
- Carotid Artery, 34001
- Celiac Artery, 34151
- Femoral Artery, 34201
- Heart, 33310-33315
- Iliac Artery, 34151, 34201
- Innominate Artery, 34001-34101
- Mesentery Artery, 34151
- Peroneal Artery, 34203
- Popliteal Artery, 34203
- Radial Artery, 34111
- Renal Artery, 34151
- Subclavian Artery, 34001-34101
- Tibial Artery, 34203
- Ulnar Artery, 34111

Embolism
- Pulmonary Artery, 33910-33916

Empyema
- Lung, 32540
- Pleural, 32540

Endometriomas
- Intra-abdominal, 49203-49205

Epididymis
- Bilateral, 54861
- Unilateral, 54860

Epiglottis, 31420

Epikeratoplasty, 65767

Epiphyseal Bar, 20150

Esophagus
- Diverticulum, 43130, 43135
- Partial, 43116-43124
- Total, 43107-43113, 43124

Excess Skin
- Abdomen, 15830

Eye
- *See* Enucleation, Eye

Fallopian Tubes
- Salpingectomy, 58700
- Salpingo–Oophorectomy, 58720

Fascia
- *See* Fasciectomy
- Femur, 27360
  - Partial, 27070, 27071
- Fibula, 27360, 27455, 27457, 27641

Fistula
- Anal, 46270-46285

Foot
- Fasciectomy, 28060
  - Radical, 28062

Gallbladder
- Open, 47600-47620
- via Laparoscopy
  - Cholecystectomy, 47562
    - with Cholangiography, 47563
    - with Exploration Common Duct, 47564

Ganglion Cyst
- Knee, 27347
- Wrist, 25111, 25112

Gingiva, 41820

Gums, 41820
- Alveolus, 41830
- Operculum, 41821

Heart
- Donor, 33940
- Lung
  - Donor, 33930

Hemangioma, 11400-11446

Hemorrhoids, 46221, 46250
- Clot, [46320]
- Complex, 46260-46262
- Simple, 46255
- with Fissurectomy, 46257, 46258

Hip
- Partial, 27070, 27071

Hippocampus, 61566

Humeral Head
- Resection, 23195
- Sequestrectomy, 23174

Humerus, 23184, 23220, 24134, 24140, 24150

Hydrocele
- Spermatic Cord, 55500
- Tunica Vaginalis, 55040, 55041
  - Bilateral, 55041

Excision — continued

Hydrocele — *continued*
- Tunica Vaginalis — *continued*
  - Unilateral, 55040

Hygroma, Cystic
- Axillary
  - Cervical, 38550, 38555

Hymenotomy, 56700
- *See* Hymen, Excision

Ileum
- Ileoanal Reservoir, 45136
- Partial, 27070, 27071

Inner Ear
- *See* Ear, Inner, Excision

Interphalangeal Joint
- Toe, 28160

Intervertebral Disc
- Decompression, 62380, 63075-63078
- Hemilaminectomy, 63040, 63043, 63044
- Herniated, 62380, 63020-63044, 63055-63066

Intestine
- Laparoscopic
  - with Anastomosis, 44202, 44203

Intestines
- Donor, 44132, 44133

Intestines, Small, 44120-44128
- Transplanted Allograft, 44137

Iris
- Iridectomy
  - Optical, 66635
  - Peripheral, 66625
  - Sector, 66630
  - with Corneoscleral or Corneal Section, 66600
  - with Cyclectomy, 66605

Kidney
- Donor, 50300, 50320, 50547
- Partial, 50240
- Recipient, 50340
- Transplantation, 50370
- with Ureters, 50220-50236

Kneecap, 27350

Labyrinth
- Transcanal, 69905
- with Mastoidectomy, 69910

Lacrimal Gland
- Partial, 68505
- Total, 68500

Lacrimal Sac, 68520

Laparoscopy
- Adrenalectomy, 60650

Larynx
- Endoscopic, 31545-31546
- Partial, 31367-31382
- Total, 31360-31365
- with Pharynx, 31390, 31395

Leg, 27630

Leg, Lower, 27630

Lesion
- Anal, 45108, 46922
- Ankle, 27630
  - Arthroscopic, 29891
- Arm, 25110
- Arthroscopic
  - Ankle, 29891
  - Talus, 29891
  - Tibia, 29891
- Auditory Canal, External
  - Exostosis, 69140
  - Radical with Neck Dissection, 69155
  - Radical without Neck Dissection, 69150
  - Soft Tissue, 69145
- Bladder, 52224
- Brain, 61534, 61536-61540
- Brainstem, 61575, 61576
- Carotid Body, 60600, 60605
- Colon, 44110, 44111
- Conjunctiva, 68110-68130
  - Over One Centimeter, 68115
  - with Adjacent Sclera, 68130
- Cornea, 65400
  - without Graft, 65420
- Ear, Middle, 69540

Excision — *continued*
- Synovium — *continued*
  - Tarsometatarsal Joint, 28070
  - Wrist, 25105, 25115-25119
- Tag
  - Anus, 46230 *[46220]*
  - Skin, 11200-11201
- Talus, 28120, 28130
  - Arthroscopic, 29891
- Tarsal, 28116, 28122
- Temporal Bone, 69535
- Temporal, Petrous
  - Apex, 69530
- Tendon
  - Finger, 26180, 26390, 26415
  - Forearm, 25109
  - Hand, 26390, 26415
  - Palm, 26170
  - Wrist, 25109
- Tendon Sheath
  - Finger, 26145
  - Foot, 28086, 28088
  - Forearm, 25110
  - Palm, 26145
  - Wrist, 25115, 25116
- Testis
  - Extraparenchymal Lesion, 54512
  - Laparoscopic, 54690
  - Partial, 54522
  - Radical, 54530, 54535
  - Simple, 54520
  - Tumor, 54530, 54535
- Thrombectomy
  - Axillary Vein, 34490
  - Bypass Graft, 35875, 35876
  - Femoropopliteal Vein, 34401-34451
  - Iliac Vein, 34401-34451
  - Subclavian Vein, 34471, 34490
  - Vena Cava, 34401-34451
- Thromboendarterectomy
  - Aorta, Abdominal, 35331
  - Aortoiliac, 35361
  - Aortoiliofemoral, 35363
  - Axillary Artery, 35321
  - Brachial Artery, 35321
  - Carotid Artery, 35301, 35390
  - Celiac Artery, 35341
  - Femoral Artery, 35302, 35371, 35372
  - Iliac, 35361, 35363
  - Iliac Artery, 35351
  - Iliofemoral Artery, 35355, 35363
  - Innominate Artery, 35311
  - Mesenteric Artery, 35341
  - Peroneal Artery, 35305-35306
  - Popliteal Artery, 35303
  - Renal Artery, 35341
  - Subclavian Artery, 35301, 35311, 35331, 35390
  - Superficial Femoral Artery, 35302
  - Tibial Artery, 35305-35306
  - Tibioperoneal Trunk, 35304
  - Vertebral Artery, 35301, 35390
- Thymus Gland, 60521
- Thyroid Gland
  - for Malignancy, 60252, 60254
    - Limited Neck Dissection, 60252
    - Radical Neck Dissection, 60254
  - Partial, 60210-60225
  - Removal All Thyroid Tissue, 60260
  - Secondary, 60260
  - Total, 60240
    - Cervical Approach, 60271
    - Sternal Split
      - Transthoracic, 60270
- Tibia, 27360, 27640
  - Arthroscopic, 29891
- Toe, 28092
- Tongue
  - Complete, 41140-41155
  - Frenum, 41115
  - Partial, 41120-41135
  - with Mouth Resection, 41150, 41153
  - with Radical Neck Dissection, 41135, 41145-41155
- Tonsils
  - Lingual, 42870

Excision — *continued*
- Tonsils — *continued*
  - Radical, 42842-42845
    - Closure Local Flap, 42844, 42845
  - Tag, 42860
  - Tonsillectomy and Adenoidectomy
    - Age 12 or Over, 42821
    - Younger Than Age 12, 42820
  - Tonsillectomy, Primary or Secondary
    - Age 12 or Over, 42826
    - Younger Than Age 12, 42825
- Torus Mandibularis, 21031
- Total, 31360, 31365
- Trachea
  - Stenosis, 31780, 31781
- Transcervical Approach, 60520
- Tricuspid Valve, 33460-33465
- Tumor
  - Abdomen, 49203-49205
  - Abdominal Wall, 22900-22905
  - Acetabulum, 27076
  - Ankle, 27615-27619 *[27632, 27634]*, 27647
  - Arm, Lower, 25075-25078 *[25071, 25073]*, 25120-25126, 25170
  - Arm, Upper, 23220, 24075-24079 *[24071, 24073]*, 24110-24126, 24150-24152
  - Back
    - Flank, 21930, 21935
  - Bile Duct, 47711, 47712
  - Bladder, 51530, 52234-52240, 52355
  - Brain, 61510, 61518, 61520, 61521, 61526, 61530, 61545, 62164
  - Bronchi, 31640, 31641
  - Calcaneus, 27647, 28100-28103
    - with Allograft, 28103
    - with Autograft, 28102
  - Carpal, 25075-25078 *[25071, 25073]*, 25130-25136
  - Cheekbone, 21030, 21034, 21048-21049
  - Clavicle, 23075-23078 *[23071, 23073]*, 23140, 23200
    - with Allograft, 23146
    - with Autograft, 23145
  - Ear, Middle
    - Extended, 69554
    - Transcanal, 69550
    - Transmastoid, 69552
  - Elbow, 24075-24079 *[24071, 24073]*, 24120-24126, 24152
  - Esophagus
    - Endoscopic, 43216-43217
  - Face or Scalp, 21011-21016
  - Facial
    - Bones, 21029, 21030, 21034, 21040, 21046-21049
    - Tissue, 21011-21016
  - Femur, 27327-27328 *[27337, 27339]*, 27355-27358, 27364-27365 *[27329]*
  - Fibula, 27615-27619 *[27632, 27634]*, 27635-27638, 27646
  - Finger, 26115-26118 *[26111, 26113]*, 26210-26215, 26260-26262
  - Foot, 28043-28047 *[28039, 28041]*, 28100-28107, 28171-28175
  - Gums, 41825-41827
  - Hand, 26115-26118 *[26111, 26113]*, 26200-26205, 26250
  - Heart, 33120, 33130
  - Hip, 27047-27049 *[27043, 27045, 27059]*, 27065-27067, 27076-27078
  - Humerus, 23150-23156, 23220, 24075-24079 *[24071, 24073]*, 24110, 24150
    - Radial Head or Neck, 24152
    - with Allograft, 23156, 24116
    - with Autograft, 23155, 24115
  - Ilium, 27065-27067, 27070-27071, 27075-27076
  - Innominate, 27047-27049 *[27043, 27045, 27059]*, 27077
  - Intestines
    - Small, 43250

Excision — *continued*
- Tumor — *continued*
  - Ischial, 27047-27049 *[27043, 27045, 27059]*, 27078
  - Kidney, 52355
  - Knee, 27327-27328 *[27337, 27339]*, 27364-27365 *[27329]*
  - Lacrimal Gland
    - Frontal Approach, 68540
    - Involving Osteotomy, 68550
  - Larynx, 31300
    - Endoscopic, 31540, 31541, 31578
  - Leg, Lower, 27615-27619 *[27632, 27634]*, 27635-27638, 27645-27647
  - Leg, Upper, 27327-27328 *[27337, 27339]*, 27355-27358, 27364-27365 *[27329]*
  - Mandible, 21040-21047
  - Maxilla, 21030, 21034, 21048, 21049
  - Mediastinum, 32662
  - Metacarpal, 26115-26118 *[26111, 26113]*, 26200-26205
  - Metatarsal, 28043-28047 *[28039, 28041]*, 28100-28107, 28173
  - Neck, 21555-21558 *[21552, 21554]*
  - Olecranon Process, 24075-24079 *[24071, 24073]*, 24120
    - with Allograft, 24126
    - with Autograft, 24125
  - Parotid Gland, 42410-42426
  - Pelvis, 27047-27049 *[27043, 27045, 27059]*, 27065-27067
  - Pericardium, 32661
  - Phalanges
    - Finger, 26115-26118 *[26111, 26113]*, 26210, 26215, 26260-26262
    - Toe, 28043-28047 *[28039, 28041]*, 28108, 28175
  - Pituitary Gland, 61546, 61548, 62165
  - Presacral, 49215
  - Pubis, 27065-27067
  - Radius, 24152
  - Rectum, 0184T, 45160, 45171-45172
    - Transanal Endoscopic, 0184T
  - Retropharyngeal
    - Anesthesia, 00174
  - Sacrococcygeal, 49215
  - Scalp or Face, 21011-21014
  - Scapula, 23140
    - with Allograft, 23146
    - with Autograft, 23145
  - Shoulder, 23075-23078 *[23071, 23073]*
  - Skull, 61500
  - Spermatocele
    - *See* Spermatocele, Excision
  - Spinal Cord, 63275-63290
  - Spleen, Total
    - *See* Splenectomy, Total
  - Sternum, 21630
  - Stomach, 43610
  - Talus, 27647
  - Tarsal
    - Benign, 28104
      - with Allograft, 28107
      - with Autograft, 28106
    - Radical, 28171
  - Thigh, 27327-27328 *[27337, 27339]*, 27355-27358, 27364-27365 *[27329]*
  - Thorax, 21555-21558 *[21552, 21554]*
  - Thyroid, 60200
  - Tibia, 27615-27619 *[27632, 27634]*, 27635-27638, 27645
  - Toe, 28043-28047 *[28039, 28041]*, 28108, 28175
  - Trachea
    - Cervical, 31785
    - Thoracic, 31786
  - Ulna, 25075-25078 *[25071, 25073]*, 25120-25126, 25170
  - Ureter, 52355
  - Urethra, 52234, 52235, 52240, 52355, 53220
  - Uterus
    - Abdominal, 58140, 58146

Excision — *continued*
- Tumor — *continued*
  - Uterus — *continued*
    - Laparoscopic, 58545-58546
    - Vaginal, 58145, 58561
  - Uvula, 42120
  - Vagina, 57135
  - Vertebra
    - Lumbar, 22102
    - Thoracic, 22101
  - Wrist, 25075-25078 *[25071, 25073]*, 25120-25126
  - Zygoma, 21030, 21034
- Turbinate, 30130, 30140
- Tympanic Nerve, 69676
- Ulcer
  - Stomach, 43610
- Ulna, 24147, 25145
  - Complete, 25240
  - Partial, 24147, 25150, 25240
  - Radical, 25170
- Umbilicus, 49250
- Ureter
  - *See* Ureterectomy
- Ureterocele, 51535
- Urethra
  - Diverticulum, 53230, 53235
  - Prolapse, 53275
  - Total
    - Female, 53210
    - Male, 53215
- Uterus
  - Abdominal
    - Myomectomy, 58140, 58146
    - Partial, 58180
    - Radical, 58210
    - Total, 58150, 58152, 58200
  - Laparoscopic, 58541-58544, 58548-58554
    - Adhesions, 58559
    - Leiomyomata, 58561
    - Myomas, 58545-58546
  - Vaginal, 58260-58294
    - Myomectomy, 58145
    - Removal Tube(s) and/or Ovary(ies), 58262-58263, 58291-58292
    - with Colpectomy, 58275-58280
    - with Colpo–Urethrocystopexy, 58267
    - with Repair of Enterocele, 58270, 58280, 58292, 58294
- Uvula, 42104-42107, 42140, 42145
- Vagina
  - Closure, 57120
  - Complete
    - with Removal of Paravaginal Tissue, 57111
    - with Removal of Vaginal Wall, 57110
  - Partial
    - with Removal of Paravaginal Tissue, 57107
    - with Removal of Paravaginal Tissue with Lymphadenectomy, 57109
    - with Removal of Vaginal Wall, 57106
  - Septum, 57130
  - Total, 57110
    - with Hysterectomy, 58275, 58280
    - Repair of Enterocele, 58280
    - with Colpectomy, 58275
- Varicocele
  - Spermatic Cord, 55530-55540
    - Abdominal Approach, 55535
    - with Hernia Repair, 55540
- Vas Deferens, 55250
- Vascular Malformation
  - Finger, 26115
  - Hand, 26115
- Vein
  - Varicose, 37765, 37766
- Vertebra
  - Additional Segment, 22103, 22116
  - Cervical, 22110
    - for Tumor, 22100, 22110

Eye — *continued*
Analysis, Movement, 0615T
Biometry, 76516, 76519, 92136
Blood Flow Measurement, 0198T
Computerized Corneal Topography, 92025
Dilation
Aqueous Outflow Canal, 66174-66175
Discission of Secondary Membranous Cataract, 66821
Drainage
Anterior Chamber, 65800-65815
Diagnostic Aspiration of Aqueous, 65800
Removal of Blood, 65815
Therapeutic Drainage of Aqueous, 66183
Aqueous, 65800
Anterior Segment Device, 66183
Aqueous Shunt, 66179-66180
Insertion, Subconjunctival Space, 0449T-0450T
Insertion, Supraciliary Space, 0474T
Revision of Aqueous Shunt, 66184-66185
Aspiration, 65800
Removal
Blood, 65815
Vitreous, 65810
Vitreous and/or Discission of Anterior Hyaloid Membrane, 65810
Drug Delivery
Suprachoroidal, 67299
Endoscopy, 66990
Enucleation, 65101-65105
Evisceration, 65091, 65093
Exam
Dilated Fundus, 2021F
Established Patient, 92012, 92014
New Patient, 92002, 92004
Radiologic, 70030
with Anesthesia, 92018, 92019
Exenteration
Ocular Contents
with Implant, 65093
without Implant, 65091
with Muscle or Myocutaneous Flap, 65114
Muscles Attached, 65105
Exercises
Training, 92065
Goniotomy, 65820
Implantation
Anterior Segment Drainage Device, 66183
Aqueous Shunt, 0449T-0450T, 0474T, 66179-66180
Corneal Ring Segment, 65785
Drainage Device, 66183, *[0253T], [0671T]*
Drug Delivery System, 67027
Electrode Array, 0100T
Foreign Material for Reinforcement, 65155
Pharmacologic Agent, 68399
Incision
Adhesions
Anterior Synechiae, 65860, 65870
Corneovitreal Adhesions, 65880
Goniosynechiae, 65865
Posterior Synechiae, 65875
Anterior Chamber, 65820
Trabecula, 65850
Injection
Air, 66020
Medication, 66030
Posterior Chamber, 0699T
Suprachoroidal, 0465T
Insertion
Corneal Ring Segment, 65785
Drainage Device, 66183, *[0253T], [0671T]*
Drug Delivery System, 67027
Lacrimal Canaliculus, 68841
Electrode Array, 0100T
Foreign Material for Reinforcement, 65155

Eye — *continued*
Insertion — *continued*
Ocular Implant
After
Enucleation
Muscles Attached to Implant, 65140
Muscles Not Attached to Implant, 65135
Evisceration, 65130
Pharmacologic Agent, 68399
Reinsertion, 65150
Scleral Shell, 65130
Interferometry
Biometry, 92136
Intraocular Drug-Eluting System
Implant, 0660T
Removal or Reimplantation, 0661T
Intraocular Pressure
Measurement Blood Flow, 0198T
Monitoring, 0329T
Laser
Anterior Segment Adhesions, 65860
Corneovitreal Adhesions, 66821
Iridectomy, 66761
Iridotomy, 66761
Lacrimal Punctum, 68760
Posterior Lens, 66821
Secondary Cataract, 66821
Vitreous Strands/Adhesions, 67031
Lesion
Excision, 65900
Muscles
Biopsy, 67346
Extraocular Muscle, 67346
Repair
Strabismus
Adjustable Sutures, 67335
Exploration and/or Repair Detached Extraocular Muscle, 67340
on Patient with Previous Surgery, 67331
One Vertical Muscle, 67314
Posterior Fixation Suture, 67334
Recession or Resection, 67311, 67312
Release of Scar Tissue without Detaching Extraocular Muscle, 67343
Two or More Vertical Muscles, 67316
with Scarring Extraocular Muscles, 67332
with Superior Oblique Muscle, 67318
Transposition, 67320
Unlisted Procedure, Ocular Muscle, 67399
Nerve
Destruction, 67345
Paracentesis
Anterior Chamber
with Diagnostic Aspiration of Aqueous, 65800
with Removal of Blood, 65815
Removal of Vitreous and/or Discission Anterior Hyaloid Membrane, 65810
Photocoagulation
Iridoplasty, 66762
Lesion
Choroid, 67220
Cornea, 65450
Retina, 67210, 67227-67228
Retinal Detachment, 67105, 67107-67108, 67113, 67145
Retinopathy, 67228-67229
Vitrectomy, 67039-67040, 67043
Photodynamic Therapy Choroidal Lesions, 67221, 67225
Placement
Pharmacologic Agent, 68399
Prosthesis, 21077, 65770, 66982-66985
Loan, 92358

Eye — *continued*
Pupillometry, Quantitative, 92499
Radial Keratotomy, 65771
Reconstruction
Amniotic Membrane, 65780
Conjunctiva, 65782
Removal
Blood Clot, 65930
Bone, 65112
Foreign Body
Conjunctival Embedded, 65210
Conjunctival Superficial, 65205
Corneal with Slit Lamp, 65222
Corneal without Slit Lamp, 65220
Intraocular, 65235-65265
Implant, 65175
Anterior Segment, 65920
Muscles Not Attached, 65103
Posterior Segment, 67120, 67121
Repair
Conjunctiva
by Mobilization and Rearrangement with Hospitalization, 65273
by Mobilization and Rearrangement without Hospitalization, 65272
Direct Closure, 65270
Cornea
Nonperforating, 65275
Perforating, 65280, 65285
Muscles, 65290
Sclera
Anterior Segment, 66250
with Graft, 66225
with Tissue Glue, 65286
Trabecular Meshwork, 65855
Wound
by Mobilization and Rearrangement, 65272, 65273
Direct Closure, 65270
Shunt, Aqueous
into Subconjunctival Space, 0449T-0450T
into Supraciliary Space, 0474T
to Extraocular Reservoir, 66179-66180
Stem Cell Transplantation, 65781
Tear Film Imaging, 0330T
Tear Osmolarity, 83861
Transluminal Dilation
Aqueous Outflow Canal, 66174-66175
Ultrasound, 76510-76514
Biometry, 76516, 76519
Foreign Body, 76529
Unlisted Services and Procedures
Anterior Segment, 66999
Posterior Segment, 67299
X-ray, 70030

Eye Socket
See Orbit; Orbital Contents; Orbital Floor; Periorbital Region

Eyebrow
Repair
Ptosis, 67900

Eyeglasses
See Spectacle Services

Eyelashes
Repair Trichiasis
Epilation
by Forceps Only, 67820
by Other Than Forceps, 67825
Incision of Lid Margin, 67830
with Free Mucous Membrane Graft, 67835

Eyelid
Abscess
Incision and Drainage, 67700
Biopsy, *[67810]*
Blepharoplasty, 15820-15823
Chalazion
Excision
Multiple, 67801, 67805
Single, 67800
with Anesthesia, 67808
Closure by Suture, 67875
Drug-Eluting Ocular Insert Placement, 0444T-0445T, 68841

Eyelid — *continued*
Evacuation
Meibomian Glands, 0207T, *[0563T]*
Incision
Canthus, 67715
Injection
Subconjunctival, 68200
Sutures, 67710
Lesion
Destruction, 67850
Excision
Multiple, 67801, 67805
Single, 67800
with Anesthesia, 67808
without Closure, 67840
Meibomian Glands Evacuation, 0207T, *[0563T]*
Placement, Drug-Eluting Ocular Insert, 0444T-0445T, 68841
Ptosis, 67901-67908
Reconstruction
Canthus, 67950
Total Eyelid
Conjunctivo–Tarso–Muller's Muscle–Levator Resection, 67908
Lower, 67973
Second Stage, 67975
Upper, 67974
Second Stage, 67975
Full Thickness, 67973-67975
Transfer of Tarsoconjunctival Flap from Opposing Eyelid, 67971
Removal
Foreign Body, 67938
Repair, 21280, 21282
Blepharoptosis
Conjunctivo-Tarso-Muller's Muscle-Levator Resection, 67908
Frontalis Muscle Technique, 67901-67904
Reduction Overcorrection of Ptosis, 67909
Superior Rectus Technique with Fascial Sling, 67906
Ectropion
Excision Tarsal Wedge, 67916
Extensive, 67917
Suture, 67914
Thermocauterization, 67915
Entropion
Excision Tarsal Wedge, 67923
Extensive, 67924
Suture, 67921
Thermocauterization, 67922
Excisional, 67961
Over One–Fourth of Lid Margin, 67966
Lagophthalmos, 67912
Lashes
Epilation, by Forceps Only, 67820
Epilation by Other Than Forceps, 67825
Lid Margin, 67830, 67835
Wound
Full Thickness, 67935
Partial Thickness, 67930
Skin Graft
Delay of Flap, 15630
Full Thickness, 15260, 15261, 67961
Pedicle Flap, 15576
Split, 15120, 15121, 67961
Suture, 67880
with Transposition of Tarsal Plate, 67882
Tissue Transfer, Adjacent, 14060, 14061, 67961
Unlisted Services and Procedures, 67999
EYS, 81434
EZH2, 81236-81237

F

F11, 81401
F12, 81403
F13B, 81400
F2, 81240, 81400
F5, 81241, 81400
F7, 81400
F8, 81403, 81406-81407

Fertility Control
See Contraception

Fertility Test
Semen Analysis, 89300-89322
Sperm Evaluation
Cervical Mucus Penetration Test, 89330
Hamster Penetration, 89329

Fertilization
Oocytes (Eggs)
In Vitro, 89250-89251
Assisted (Microtechnique), 89280, 89281
with Co–Culture of Embryo, 89251

Fertilization in Vitro
See In Vitro Fertilization

Fetal Aneuploidy, 81507

Fetal Biophysical Profile, 76818, 76819

Fetal Congenital Abnormalities Biochemical Assays, 81508-81512

Fetal Contraction Stress Test, 59020

Fetal Hemoglobin, 83030, 83033, 85460, 85461

Fetal Lung Maturity Assessment, Lecithin Sphingomyelin Ratio, 83661

Fetal Monitoring
See Monitoring, Fetal

Fetal Non–stress Test, 59025
Ultrasound, 76818

Fetal Procedure
Amnioinfusion, 59070
Cord Occlusion, 59072
Fluid Drainage, 59074
Shunt Placement, 59076
Unlisted Fetal Invasive Procedure, 59897
Unlisted Laparoscopy Procedure Maternity and Delivery, 59898
Unlisted Procedure Maternity and Delivery, 59899

Fetal Testing
Amniotic Fluid Lung Maturity, 83661, 83663-83664
Biophysical Profile, 76818-76819
Lung Maturity, 83661, 83663, 83664
Heart, 76825, 76826
Doppler
Complete, 76827
Follow–up or Repeat Study, 76828
Magnetic Cardiac Signal, 0475T-0478T
Hemoglobin, 83030, 83033, 85460, 85461
Magnetic Cardiac Signal Recording, 0475T-0478T
Scalp Blood Sampling, 59020
Ultrasound, 76801-76828
Heart, 76825
Middle Cerebral Artery, 76821
Umbilical Artery, 76820

Fetuin
See Alpha–Fetoprotein

Fever, Australian Q
See Q Fever

Fever, Japanese River
See Scrub Typhus

FFR (Fractional Flow Reserve), 0501T-0504T, [0523T]

FGB, 81400

FGF23, 81404

FGFR1, 81400, 81405

FGFR2, 81404

FGFR3, 81400-81401, 81403-81404

FH, 81405

FHL1, 81404

Fibrillation
Atrial, 33254-33256
Documentation, 1060F-1061F

Fibrillation, Heart
See Heart, Fibrillation

Fibrin Degradation Products, 85362-85380

Fibrin Deposit
Removal, 32150

Fibrin Stabilizing Factor, 85290, 85291

Fibrinase
See Plasmin

Fibrinogen, 85384, 85385

Fibrinolysin
See Plasmin

Fibrinolysins, 85390

Fibrinolysis
ADAMTS-13, 85397
Alpha–2 Antiplasmin, 85410
Assay, 85396
Functional Activity, 85397
Plasmin, 85400
Plasminogen, 85420, 85421
Plasminogen Activator, 85415
Pleural Cavity
Instillation of Agent, 32561-32562

Fibroadenoma
Ablation
Cryosurgical, 19105
Radiofrequency, 0404T
Excision, 19120-19126

Fibroblastoma, Arachnoidal
See Meningioma

Fibrocutaneous Tags
Destruction, 11200, 11201

Fibroid Tumor of Uterus
Ablation
Radiofrequency, 0404T, [58674]
Ultrasound, 0071T-0072T
Excision
Abdominal Approach, 58140
Vaginal Approach, 58145

Fibromatosis, Dupuytrens's
See Dupuytren's Contracture

Fibromatosis, Penile
See Peyronie Disease

Fibromyoma
See Leiomyomata

Fibronectin, Fetal, 82731

Fibrosis, Penile
See Peyronie Disease

Fibrosis, Retroperitoneal
See Retroperitoneal Fibrosis

Fibrous Cavernitides
See Peyronie Disease

Fibrous Dysplasia, 21029, 21181-21184
Reconstruction
Cranial, 21181
Facial, 21029
Orbital Walls, 21182
40 cm to 80 cm, 21183
80 cm or More, 21184

Fibula
See Ankle; Knee; Tibia
Bone Graft with Microvascular Anastomosis, 20955
Craterization, 27360, 27641
Cyst
Excision, 27635-27638
Diaphysectomy, 27360, 27641
Excision, 27360, 27641
Epiphyseal Bar, 20150
Fracture
Malleolus
Bimalleolar
Closed Treatment, 27808
with Manipulation, 27810
Open Treatment, 27814
Lateral
Closed Treatment, 27786
with Manipulation, 27788
Open Treatment, 27792
Medial
Closed Treatment, 27760
with Manipulation, 27762
Open Treatment, 27766
Trimalleolar
Closed Treatment, 27816
with Manipulation, 27818
Open Treatment, 27822
with Fixation, 27823
Nonunion or Malunion, 27726
Shaft
Closed Treatment, 27780
with Manipulation, 27781
Open Treatment, 27784
Incision, 27607

Fibula — continued
Osteoplasty
Lengthening, 27715
Repair
Epiphysis, 27477-27485, 27730-27742
Nonunion or Malunion, 27726
Osteotomy, 27707-27712
Saucerization, 27360, 27641
Tumor
Excision, 27635-27638
Radical Resection, 27615-27616, 27646
X–ray, 73590

FIG4, 81406

Figure of Eight Cast, 29049

Filariasis, 86280

Filtering Operation
Incision, Sclera, Fistulization
Sclerectomy with Punch or Scissors with Iridectomy, 66160
Thermocauterization with Iridectomy, 66155
Trabeculectomy ab Externo in Absence Previous Surgery, 66170
Trephination with Iridectomy, 66150
with Iridectomy, 66160

Filtration Implant, Glaucoma
See Aqueous Shunt

Fimbrioplasty, 58760
Laparoscopic, 58672

Fine Needle Aspiration, 10021, [10004, 10005, 10006, 10007, 10008, 10009, 10010, 10011, 10012]
Evaluation
Abdominal Mass, 49180
Bone, 20220, 20225
Breast, 19081-19086
Epididymis, 54800
Evaluation, 88172-88173, [88177]
General, 10021, [10004, 10005, 10006, 10007, 10008, 10009, 10010, 10011, 10012]
Intervertebral Disc, 62267
Kidney, 50200
Lung, 32408
Mediastinum, 32408
Muscle, 20206
Nucleus Pulposus, 62267
Orbital Contents, 67415
Pancreas, 48102
Paravertebral Tissue, 62267
Pleura, 32400
Prostate, 55700, 55706
with Fluorescence Spectroscopy, 0443T
Retroperitoneal Mass, 49180
Salivary Gland, 42400
Soft Tissue Drainage, 10030
Spinal Cord, 62269
Testis, 54500
Thyroid, 60100
Transendoscopic
Colon, 45392
Esophagogastroduodenoscopy, 43238, 43242
Esophagus, 43238
Surgically Altered Stomach, 43242
with Fluorescence Spectroscopy, 0443T

Finger
See Phalanx, Finger
Abscess
Bone
Incision and Drainage, 26034
Incision and Drainage, 26010, 26011
Amputation, 26951
with Exploration or Removal, 26910
Arthrocentesis, 20600-20604
Arthrodesis
Interphalangeal Joint, 26860-26863
Metacarpophalangeal Joint, 26850, 26852
Bone
Incision and Drainage, 26034
Cast, 29086
Collection of Blood, 36415, 36416
Decompression, 26035
Excision, 26235-26236

Finger — continued
Excision — continued
Constricting Ring, 26596
Tendon, 26180, 26390, 26415
Flap
Tissue Transfer, 14350
Insertion
Tendon Graft, 26392
Magnetic Resonance Imaging (MRI), 73221
Reconstruction
Extra Digit, 26587
Toe to Hand Transfer, 26551-26554, 26556
Removal
Implantation, 26320
Tube, 26392, 26416
Repair
Blood Vessel, 35207
Claw Finger, 26499
Extra Digit, 26587
Macrodactylia, 26590
Tendon
Dorsum, 26418, 26420
Extensor, 26415-26434, 26445, 26449, 26460
Central Slip, 26426, 26428
Distal Insertion, 26432, 26433
Excision with Implantation, 26415
Hand, 26410
with Graft, 26412
Realignment, Hand, 26437
Flexor, 26356-26358, 26440, 26442, 26455
Flexor Excision with Implantation, 26390
Lengthening, 26476, 26478
Opponensplasty, 26490-26496
Profundus, 26370-26373
Removal Tube or Rod
Extensor, 26416
Flexor, 26392
Shortening, 26477, 26479
Tenodesis, 26471, 26474
Tenolysis, 26440-26449
Tenotomy, 26450-26460
Transfer or Transplant, 26485, 26489, 26497, 26498
Volar Plate, 26548
Web Finger, 26560-26562
Replantation, 20816, 20822
Reposition, 26555
Sesamoidectomy, 26185
Splint, 29130, 29131
Strapping, 29280
Tendon Sheath
Excision, 26145
Incision, 26055
Incision and Drainage, 26020
Tenotomy, 26060, 26460
Flexor, 26455
Tumor
Excision, 26115-26116 [26111] [26113]
Radical Resection, 26117-26118
Unlisted Services and Procedures/Hands or Fingers, 26989
X–ray, 73140

Finger Joint
See Intercarpal Joint

FIP1L1/PDGFRA, 81401

FISH, 88365

Fissure in Ano
See Anus, Fissure

Fissurectomy, 46200, 46261-46262

Fistula
Anal
Repair, 46262-46288, 46706
Anorectal
Repair, 46707
Arteriovenous, 36831-36833
Injection, 36901-36903
Revision
with Thrombectomy, 36831
without Thrombectomy, 36832
Thrombectomy without revision, 36831
Autogenous Graft, 36825

Fistula — *continued*
Bronchi
Repair, 32815
Carotid–Cavernous Repair, 61710
Chest Wall
Repair, 32906
Conjunctiva
with Tube or Stent, 68750
without Tube, 68745
Enterovesical
Closure, 44660, 44661
Ileoanal Pouch
Repair, 46710-46712
Kidney, 50520-50526
Lacrimal Gland
Closure, 68770
Dacryocystorhinostomy, 68720
Nose
Repair, 30580, 30600
Window, 69666
Oval Window, 69666
Postauricular, 69700
Rectovaginal
Abdominal Approach, 57305
Transperineal Approach, 57308
with Concomitant Colostomy, 57307
Round Window, 69667
Sclera
Sclerectomy with Punch or Scissors with
Iridectomy, 66160
Thermocauterization with Iridectomy,
66155
Trabeculectomy ab Externo in Absence
Previous Surgery, 66170
Trabeculectomy ab Externo with Scar-
ring, 66172
Trephination with Iridectomy, 66150
Suture
Kidney, 50520-50526
Ureter, 50920, 50930
Trachea, 31755
Tracheoesophageal
Repair, 43305, 43312, 43314
Speech Prosthesis, 31611
Transperineal Approach, 57308
Ureter, 50920, 50930
Urethra, 53400, 53405
Urethrovaginal, 57310
with Bulbocavernosus Transplant, 57311
Vesicouterine
Closure, 51920, 51925
Vesicovaginal
Closure, 51900
Transvesical and Vaginal Approach,
57330
Vaginal Approach, 57320
X–ray, 76080
Fistula Arteriovenous
See Arteriovenous Fistula
Fistulectomy
Anal, 46060, 46262-46285
Fistulization
Conjunction to Nasal Cavity, 68745
Esophagus, 43351-43352
Intestines, 44300-44346
Laparoscopic, 44187-44188
Mucofistula, 44144
Lacrimal Sac to Nasal Cavity, 68720
Penis, 54435
Pharynx, 42955
Tracheopharyngeal, 31755
Fistulization, Interatrial
See Septostomy, Atrial
Fistulotomy
Anal, 46270-46280
Fitting
Cervical Cap, 57170
Contact Lens, 92071-92072, 92310-92313
Diaphragm, 57170
Low Vision Aid, 92354, 92355
See Spectacle Services
Spectacle Prosthesis, 92352, 92353
Spectacles, 92340-92342
Fitzgerald Factor, 85293

Fixation (Device)
See Application; Bone; Fixation; Spinal Instru-
mentation
Application, External, 20690-20697
Insertion, 20690-20697, 22841-22844, 22853-
22854, 22867-22870, *[22859]*
Reinsertion, 22849
Interdental without Fracture, 21497
Pelvic
Insertion, 22848
Removal
External, 20694
Internal, 20670, 20680
Sacrospinous Ligament
Vaginal Prolapse, 57282
Shoulder, 23700
Skeletal
Humeral Epicondyle
Percutaneous, 24566
Spinal
Insertion, 22841-22847, 22853-22854,
22867-22870, *[22859]*
Reinsertion, 22849
Fixation, External
See External Fixation
Fixation, Kidney
See Nephropexy
Fixation, Rectum
See Proctopexy
Fixation Test Complement
See Complement, Fixation Test
Fixation, Tongue
See Tongue, Fixation
FKRP, 81404
FKTN, 81400, 81405
Flank
See Back/Flank
Flap
See Skin Graft and Flap
Delay of Flap at Trunk, 15600
at Eyelids, Nose Ears, or Lips, 15630
at Forehead, Cheeks, Chin, Neck, Axillae,
Genitalia, Hands, Feet, 15620
at Scalp, Arms, or Legs, 15610
Section Pedicle of Cross Finger, 15620
Fasciocutaneous, 15733-15738
Free
Breast Reconstruction (fTRAM, DIEP,
SIEA, GAP), 19364
Closure Following Pharyngeal Wall Re-
section (Muscle, Skin, Fascia),
42894
Microvascular Transfer, 15756-15758,
20969-20973, 42894, 49906
Muscle for Facial Nerve Paralysis, 15842
Omental, 49906
Osteocutaneous
Great Toe, 20973
Iliac Crest, 20970
Metatarsal, 20972
Other Than Iliac Crest, Metatarsal,
Great Toe, 20969
Grafts, 15574-15650, 15842
Composite, 15760
Derma–Fat–Fascia, 15770
Cross Finger Flap, 15574
Punch for Hair Transplant
Less Than 15, 15775
More Than 15, 15776
Island Pedicle, 15740
Neurovascular Pedicle, 15750
Latissimus Dorsi
Breast Reconstruction, 19361
Midface, 15730
Muscle, 15733-15738
Myocutaneous, 15733-15738
Omentum
Free
with Microvascular Anastomosis,
49906
Transfer
Intermediate of Any Pedicle, 15650
Transverse Rectus Abdominis Myocutaneous
(TRAM)
Breast Reconstruction, 19367-19369
Zygomaticofacial, 15730

Flatfoot Correction, 28735
Flea Typhus
See Murine Typhus
Flecainide Assay, *[80181]*
Fletcher Factor, 85292
FLG, 81401
Flick Method Testing, 93598
Flow Cytometry, 3170F, 86356, 88182-88189
Flow Volume Loop/Pulmonary, 94375
See Pulmonology, Diagnostic
FLT3, *[81245, 81246]*
Flu Vaccines, 90647-90648, 90653-90668 *[90630,
90672, 90673, 90674, 90756]*
FLUARIX, 90656
Flublok, *[90673]*
Flucelvax, 90661
Fluid, Amniotic
See Amniotic Fluid
Fluid, Body
See Body Fluid
Fluid, Cerebrospinal
See Cerebrospinal Fluid
Fluid Collection
Incision and Drainage
Skin, 10140
Fluid Drainage
Abdomen, 49082-49084
Flulaval, 90658, 90688
FluMist, 90660
Fluorescein
Angiography, Ocular, 92242, 92287
Intravenous Injection
Vascular Flow Check, Graft, 15860
Fluorescein, Angiography
See Angiography, Fluorescein
Fluorescence Wound Imaging
Noncontact, 0598T, 0599T
Fluorescent Antibody, 86255, 86256
Fluorescent In Situ Hybridization, 88365
Cytopathology, 88120-88121
Fluoride
Blood, 82735
Urine, 82735
Fluoride Varnish Application, 99188
Fluoroscopy
Bile Duct
Guide for Catheter, 74328, 74330
Chest
Bronchoscopy, 31622-31646
Complete (Four views), 71048, 76000
Partial (Two views), 71046, 76000
Drain Abscess, 75989
GI Tract
Guidance Intubation, 74340
Hourly, 76000
Introduction
GI Tube, 74340
Larynx, 70370
Nasogastric, 43752
Needle Biopsy, 77002
Orogastric, 43752
Pancreatic Duct
Catheter, 74329, 74330
Pharynx, 70370
Sacroiliac Joint
Injection Guidance, 27096
Spine/Paraspinous
Guide Catheter
Needle, 77003
Unlisted Procedure, 76496
Venous Access Device, 36598, 77001
Flurazepam, *[80346, 80347]*
Fluvirin, 90656, 90658
Fluzone, 90655-90658
Fluzone High Dose, 90662
FMR1, 81243-81244
FMRI (Functional MRI), 70554-70555
Fms-Related Tyrosine Kinase 3 Gene Analysis,
[81245]
FNA (Fine Needle Aspiration), 10021, *[10004, 10005,
10006, 10007, 10008, 10009, 10010, 10011,
10012]*
Foam Stability Test, 83662
FOBT (Fecal Occult Blood Test), 82270, 82272,
82274

Focal Laser Ablation
Prostate
Transperineal, 0655T
Fold, Vocal
See Vocal Cords
Foley Operation Pyeloplasty
See Pyeloplasty
Foley Y–Pyeloplasty, 50400, 50405
Folic Acid, 82746
RBC, 82747
Follicle Stimulating Hormone (FSH), 80418, 80426,
83001
Follicular Lymphoma, 81401, *[81278]*
Folliculin
See Estrone
Follitropin
See Follicle Stimulating Hormone (FSH)
Follow–up Services
See Hospital Services; Office and/or Other
Outpatient Services
Post–op, 99024
Fontan Procedure, 33615, 33617
Foot
See Metatarsal; Tarsal
Amputation, 28800, 28805
Bursa
Incision and Drainage, 28001
Capsulotomy, 28260-28264
Cast, 29450
Cock Up Fifth Toe, 28286
Fasciectomy, 28060
Radical, 28060, 28062
Fasciotomy, 28008
Endoscopic, 29893
Hammertoe Operation, 28285
Incision, 28002-28005
Joint
See Talotarsal Joint; Tarsometatarsal
Joint
Magnetic Resonance Imaging (MRI),
73721-73723
Lesion
Excision, 28080, 28090
Magnetic Resonance Imaging (MRI), 73718-
73720
Morton's
Destruction, 64632
Excision, 28080
Injection, 64455
Nerve
Destruction, 64632
Excision, 28055
Incision, 28035
Neurectomy, 28055
Neuroma
Destruction, 64632
Excision, 28080, 64782-64783
Injection, 64455
Ostectomy, Metatarsal Head, 28288
Reconstruction
Cleft Foot, 28360
Removal
Foreign Body, 28190-28193
Repair
Muscle, 28250
Tendon
Advancement Posterior Tibial,
28238
Capsulotomy; Metatarsopha-
langeal, 28270
Interphalangeal, 28272
Capsulotomy, Midfoot; Medial Re-
lease, 28260
Capsulotomy, Midtarsal (Heyman
Type), 28264
Extensor, Single, 28208
Secondary with Free Graft,
28210
Flexor, Single, with Free Graft,
28200
Secondary with Free Graft,
28202
Tenolysis, Extensor
Multiple Through Same Inci-
sion, 28226

Fracture Treatment — *continued*
  Ulna — *continued*
    Open Treatment — *continued*
      Proximal End, 24685
      Radial AND Ulnar Shaft, 25574,
        25575
      Shaft, 25545
    Shaft
      Closed Treatment, 25530, 25535
      Open Treatment, 25545, 25574
    Styloid Process
      Closed Treatment, 25650
      Open Treatment, 25652
      Percutaneous Fixation, 25651
    with Dislocation, 24620, 24635
      Closed Treatment, 24620
      Monteggia, 24620, 24635
      Open Treatment, 24635
    with Manipulation, 25535, 25565
    with Radius, 25560, 25565
      Open Treatment, 25574-25575
    without Manipulation, 25530
  Vertebra
    Additional Segment
      Open Treatment, 22328
    Cervical
      Open Treatment, 22326
    Closed Treatment
      with Manipulation, Casting and/or
        Bracing, 22315
      without Manipulation, 22310
    Lumbar
      Open Treatment, 22325
    Posterior
      Open Treatment, 22325-22327
    Thoracic
      Open Treatment, 22327
  Vertebral Process
    Closed Treatment
      See Evaluation and Management
        Codes
  Wrist
    with Dislocation, 25680, 25685
      Closed Treatment, 25680
      Open Treatment, 25685
  Zygomatic Arch
    Open Treatment, 21356, 21360-21366
    with Manipulation, 21355
Fragile–X
  Chromosome Analysis, 88248
  Mental Retardation 1 Gene Analysis, 81243-
    81244
Fragility
  Red Blood Cell
    Mechanical, 85547
    Osmotic, 85555, 85557
Frames, Stereotactic
  See Stereotactic Frame
Francisella, 86000
  Antibody, 86668
Frataxin, *[81284, 81285, 81286]*
FRAXE, 81171-81172
Frazier-Spiller Procedure, 61450
Fredet–Ramstedt Procedure, 43520
Free E3
  See Estriol
Free Skin Graft
  See Skin, Grafts, Free
Free T4
  See Thyroxine, Free
Frei Disease
  See Lymphogranuloma Venereum
Frenectomy, 40819, 41115
Frenoplasty, 41520
Frenotomy, 40806, 41010
Frenulectomy, 40819
Frenuloplasty, 41520
Frenum
  See Lip
  Lip
    Incision, 40806
Frenumectomy, 40819
Frickman Operation, 45550
Friederich Ataxia, *[81284, 81285, 81286]*
Frontal Craniotomy, 61556

Frontal Sinus
  See Sinus, Frontal
Frontal Sinusotomy
  See Exploration, Sinus, Frontal
Frost Suture
  Eyelid
    Closure by Suture, 67875
Frozen Blood Preparation, 86930-86932
Fructose, 84375
  Semen, 82757
Fructose Intolerance Breath Test, 91065
Fruit Sugar
  See Fructose
FSF, 85290, 85291
FSH, 83001
  with Additional Tests, 80418, 80426
FSHMD1A, 81404
FSP, 85362-85380
FT–4, 84439
FTG, 15200-15261
FTI, 84439
fTRAM Flap
  Breast Reconstruction, 19364
FTSG, 15200-15261
FTSJ1, 81405-81406
Fulguration
  See Destruction
  Bladder, 51020
  Cystourethroscopy with, 52214
    Lesion, 52224
    Tumor, 52234-52240
  Ureter, 50957, 50976
  Ureterocele
    Ectopic, 52301
    Orthotopic, 52300
Fulguration, Endocavitary
  See Electrocautery
Full Thickness Graft, 15200-15261
Function, Study, Nasal
  See Nasal Function Study
Function Test, Lung
  See Pulmonology, Diagnostic
Function Test, Vestibular
  See Vestibular Function Tests
Functional Ability
  See Activities of Daily Living
Functional MRI, 70554-70555
Fundoplasty
  Esophagogastric
    Endoscopic, *[43210]*
    Laparoscopic, 43279-43280, 43283
    Laparotomy, 43327
    Thoracotomy, 43328
    with Gastroplasty, 43842-43843
  Esophagomyotomy
    Laparoscopic, 43279
    with Fundic Patch, 43325
    with Paraesophageal Hernia
      Laparoscopic, 43281-43282
      with Fundoplication
        Laparotomy, 43332-43333
        Thoracoabdominal Incisional,
          43336-43337
      Thoracotomy, 43334-43335
Fundoplication
  See Fundoplasty, Esophagogastric
Fungal Wet Prep, 87220
Fungus
  Antibody, 86671
  Culture
    Blood, 87103
    Hair, 87101
    Identification, 87106
    Nail, 87101
    Other, 87102
    Skin, 87101
  Tissue Exam, 87220
Funnel Chest
  See Pectus Excavatum
Furuncle
  Incision and Drainage, 10060, 10061
Furuncle, Vulva
  See Abscess, Vulva
FUS/DDIT3, 81401, 81406
Fusion
  See Arthrodesis

Fusion — *continued*
  Pleural Cavity, 32560
  Thumb
    in Opposition, 26820
Fusion, Epiphyseal–Diaphyseal
  See Epiphyseal Arrest
Fusion, Joint
  See Arthrodesis
Fusion, Joint, Ankle
  See Ankle, Arthrodesis
Fusion, Joint, Interphalangeal, Finger
  See Arthrodesis, Finger Joint, Interphalangeal
FXN, *[81284, 81285, 81286], [81289]*

G

G6PC, *[81250]*
G6PD, 81247-81249
  Common Variants, 81247
  Full Gene Sequence, 81249
  Known Familial Variants, 81248
GAA, 81406
Gabapentin
  Assay, *[80171]*
GABRG2, 81405, *[81419]*
Gago Procedure
  Repair, Tricuspid Valve, 33463-33465
Gait Training, 97116
Galactogram, 77053, 77054
  Injection, 19030
Galactokinase
  Blood, 82759
Galactose
  Blood, 82760
  Urine, 82760
Galactose–1–Phosphate
  Uridyl Transferase, 82775-82776
Galactosemia, 81401, 81406, *[81419], [81443]*
GALC, 81401, 81406
Galeazzi Dislocation
  Fracture
    Closed Treatment, 25520
    Open Treatment, 25525, 25526
Galectin-3, 82777
Gallbladder
  See Bile Duct
  Anastomosis
    with Intestines, 47720-47741
  Cholecystectomy, 47600
    Laparoscopic, 47562
      with Cholangiogram, 47564
    Open, 47600
      with Cholangiogram, 47605
      with Choledochoenterostomy,
        47612
      with Exploration Common Duct,
        47610
      with Transduodenal Sphincterotomy or Sphincteroplasty,
        47620
  Cholecystostomy
    for Drainage, 47480
    for Exploration, 47480
    for Removal of Stone, 47480
    Percutaneous, 47490
  Excision, 47562-47564, 47600-47620
  Exploration, 47480
  Incision, 47490
  Incision and Drainage, 47480
  Nuclear Medicine
    Imaging, 78226-78227
  Removal Calculi, 47480
  Repair
    with Gastroenterostomy, 47741
    with Intestines, 47720-47740
  Unlisted Services and Procedures, 47999
  X–ray with Contrast, 74290
GALT, 81401, 81406
Galvanocautery
  See Electrocautery
Galvanoionization
  See Iontophoresis
Gamete Intrafallopian Transfer (GIFT), 58976
Gamete Transfer
  In Vitro Fertilization, 58976
Gamma Camera Imaging
  See Nuclear Medicine

Gamma Glutamyl Transferase, 82977
Gamma Seminoprotein
  See Antigen, Prostate Specific
Gammacorten
  See Dexamethasone
Gammaglobulin
  Blood, 82784-82787
Gamulin Rh
  See Immune Globulins, Rho (D)
Ganglia, Trigeminal
  See Gasserian Ganglion
Ganglion
  See Gasserian Ganglion
  Cyst
    Aspiration/Injection, 20612
    Drainage, 20612
    Wrist
      Excision, 25111, 25112
  Injection
    Anesthetic, 64505, 64510
Ganglion Cervicothoracicum
  See Stellate Ganglion
Ganglion, Gasser's
  See Gasserian Ganglion
Ganglion Pterygopalatinum
  See Sphenopalatine Ganglion
GAP Flap
  Breast Reconstruction, 19364
GARDASIL, 90649
Gardner Operation, 63700, 63702
Gardnerella Vaginalis Detection, 87510-87512
GARS, 81406
Gasser Ganglion
  See Gasserian Ganglion
Gasserian Ganglion
  Sensory Root
    Decompression, 61450
    Section, 61450
    Stereotactic, 61790
Gastrectomy
  Longitudinal, 43775
  Partial, 43631
    Distal with Vagotomy, 43635
    with Gastroduodenostomy, 43631
      with Roux–en–Y Reconstruction,
        43633
    with Gastrojejunostomy, 43632
    with Intestinal Pouch, 43634
  Sleeve, 43775
  Total, 43621, 43622
    with Esophagoenterostomy, 43620
    with Intestinal Pouch, 43622
Gastric, 82930
  Acid, 82930
  Analysis Test, 43755-43757
  Electrodes
    Neurostimulator
      Implantation
        Laparoscopic, 43647
        Open, 43881
      Removal
        Laparoscopic, 43648
        Open, 43882
      Replacement
        Laparoscopic, 43647
        Open, 43881
      Revision
        Laparoscopic, 43648
        Open, 43882
  Intubation, 43753-43755
    Diagnostic, 43754-43757
    Therapeutic, 43753
  Lavage
    Therapeutic, 43753
  Restrictive Procedure
    Laparoscopy, 43770-43774
    Open, 43886-43888
  Tests
    Manometry, 91020
Gastric Ulcer Disease
  See Stomach, Ulcer
Gastrin, 82938, 82941
Gastrocnemius Recession
  Leg, Lower, 27687
Gastroduodenostomy, 43810

Gastroduodenostomy — *continued*
  Revision of Anastomosis with Reconstruction, 43850
    with Vagotomy, 43855
    with Gastrectomy, 43631, 43632
Gastroenterology, Diagnostic
  Breath Hydrogen Test, 91065
  Colon Motility Study, 91117
  Duodenal Intubation and Aspiration, 43756-43757
  Esophagus Tests
    Acid Perfusion, 91030
    Acid Reflux Test, 91034-91038
    Balloon Distension Provocation Study, 91040
    Intubation with Specimen Collection, 43754-43755
    Manometry, 91020
    Motility Study, 91010-91013
  Gastric Tests
    Manometry, 91020
  Gastroesophageal Reflux Test
    See Acid Reflux, 91034-91038
  Manometry, 91020
  Rectum
    Manometry, 91122
    Sensation, Tone, and Compliance Test, 91120
  Stomach
    Intubation with Specimen Collection, 43754-43755
    Manometry, 91020
    Stimulation of Secretion, 43755
  Unlisted Services and Procedures, 91299
Gastroenterostomy
  for Obesity, 43644-43645, 43842-43848
Gastroesophageal Reflux Test, 91034-91038
Gastrointestinal Endoscopies
  See Endoscopy, Gastrointestinal
Gastrointestinal Exam
  Nuclear Medicine
    Blood Loss Study, 78278
    Protein Loss Study, 78282
    Shunt Testing, 78291
    Unlisted Services and Procedures, 78299
Gastrointestinal Prophylaxis for NSAID Use Prescribed, 4017F
Gastrointestinal Tract
  Imaging Intraluminal
    Colon, *[91113]*
    Distal Ileum, *[91113]*
    Esophagus, 91111
    Esophagus Through Ileum, 91110
    Reconstruction, 43360, 43361
    Transit and Pressure Measurements, 91112
  Upper
    Dilation, 43249
    X–ray, 74240, 74248
      Guide Dilator, 74360
      Guide Intubation, 49440, 74340
      with Contrast, 74246, 74248
Gastrointestinal, Upper
  Biopsy
    Endoscopy, 43239
  Dilation
    Endoscopy, 43245
    Esophagus, 43248
  Endoscopy
    Catheterization, 43241
    Destruction
      Lesion, *[43270]*
    Dilation, 43245
    Drainage
      Pseudocyst, 43240
    Exploration, 43235
    Hemorrhage, 43255
    Inject Varices, 43243
    Needle Biopsy, 43238, 43242
    Removal
      Foreign Body, 43247
      Lesion, 43250-43251
      Polyp, 43250-43251
      Tumor, 43250-43251
    Resection, Mucosa, 43254
    Stent Placement, *[43266]*
    Thermal Radiation, 43257

Gastrointestinal, Upper — *continued*
  Endoscopy — *continued*
    Tube Placement, 43246
    Ultrasound, 43237, 43238, 43242, 43253, 76975
  Exploration
    Endoscopy, 43235
  Hemorrhage
    Endoscopic Control, 43255
  Injection
    Submucosal, 43236
    Varices, 43243
  Lesion
    Destruction, *[43270]*
  Ligation of Vein, 43244
  Needle Biopsy
    Endoscopy, 43238, 43242
  Removal
    Foreign Body, 43247
    Lesion, 43250-43251
    Polyp, 43250-43251
    Tumor, 43250-43251
  Stent Placement, *[43266]*
  Tube Placement
    Endoscopy, 43237, 43238, 43246
  Ultrasound
    Endoscopy, 43237, 43238, 43242, 43259, 76975
Gastrojejunostomy, 43860, 43865
  Contrast Injection, 49465
  Conversion from Gastrostomy Tube, 49446
  Removal
    Obstructive Material, 49460
  Replacement
    Tube, 49452
  Revision, 43860
    with Vagotomy, 43865
  with Duodenal Exclusion, 48547
  with Partial Gastrectomy, 43632
  with Vagotomy, 43825
  without Vagotomy, 43820
Gastropexy
  with Insertion Gastrostomy Tube, 0647T
Gastroplasty
  Collis, 43283, 43338
  Esophageal Lengthening Procedure, 43283, 43338
  Laparoscopic, 43283, 43644-43645
  Restrictive for Morbid Obesity, 43842-43843, 43845-43848
    Other Than Vertical Banded, 43843
  Wedge, 43283, 43338
Gastrorrhaphy, 43840
Gastroschisis, 49605-49606
Gastrostomy
  Closure, 43870
  Laparoscopic
    Permanent, 43832
    Temporary, 43653
  Temporary, 43830
    Laparoscopic, 43653
    Neonatal, 43831
  Tube
    Change of, 43762-43763
    Conversion to Gastro-jejunostomy Tube, 49446
    Directed Placement
      Endoscopic, 43246
      Percutaneous, 49440
    Insertion
      Endoscopic, 43246
      Percutaneous, 49440
        with Magnetic Gastropexy, 0647T
    Percutaneous, 49440
    Removal
      Obstructive Material, 49460
    Replacement, 49450
    Repositioning, 43761
  with Pancreatic Drain, 48001
  with Pyloroplasty, 43640
  with Vagotomy, 43640
Gastrotomy, 43500, 43501, 43510
Gaucher Disease Genomic Sequence Analysis, 81412, *[81443]*
GBA, 81251, 81412

GCDH, 81406
GCH1, 81405
GCK, 81406
GDAP1, 81405
GDH, 82965
GE
  Reflux, 78262
Gel Diffusion, 86331
Gene Analysis
  See Analysis, Gene
Genioplasty, 21120-21123
  Augmentation, 21120, 21123
  Osteotomy, 21121-21123
Genitalia
  Female
    Anesthesia, 00940-00952
  Male
    Anesthesia, 00920-00938
  Skin Graft
    Delay of Flap, 15620
    Full Thickness, 15240, 15241
    Pedicle Flap, 15574
    Split, 15120, 15121
    Tissue Transfer, Adjacent, 14040, 14041
Genitourinary Sphincter, Artificial
  See Prosthesis, Urethral Sphincter
Genotype Analysis
  See Analysis, Gene
Gentamicin, 80170
  Assay, 80170
Gentiobiase, 82963
Genus: Human Cytomegalovirus Group
  See Cytomegalovirus
GERD
  See Gastroesophageal Reflux Test
German Measles
  See Rubella
Gestational Trophoblastic Tumor
  See Hydatidiform Mole
GFAP, 81405
GFR
  See Glomerular Filtration Rate
GGT, 82977
GH, 83003
GH1, 81404
GHb, 83036
GHR, 81405
GHRHR, 81405
GI Tract
  See Gastrointestinal Tract
  X-rays, 74240, 74248, 74250-74251, 74340, 74360
Giardia
  Antigen Detection
    Enzyme Immunoassay, 87329
    Immunofluorescence, 87269
Giardia Lamblia
  Antibody, 86674
Gibbons Stent, 52332
GIF, 84307
GIFT, 58976
Gill Operation, 63012
Gillies Approach
  Fracture
    Zygomatic Arch, 21356
Gingiva
  See Gums
Gingiva, Abscess
  See Abscess
  Fracture
    See Abscess, Gums; Gums
    Zygomatic Arch
      See Abscess, Gums; Gums, Abscess
Gingivectomy, 41820
Gingivoplasty, 41872
Girdlestone Laminectomy
  See Laminectomy
Girdlestone Procedure
  Acetabulum, Reconstruction, 27120, 27122
GJB1, 81403, *[81448]*
GJB2, 81252-81253, 81430
GJB6, 81254
GLA, 81405
Gla Protein (Bone)
  See Osteocalcin

Glabellar Frown Lines
  Rhytidectomy, 15826
Gland
  See Specific Gland
Gland, Adrenal
  See Adrenal Gland
Gland, Bartholin's
  See Bartholin's Gland
Gland, Bulbourethral
  See Bulbourethral Gland
Gland, Lacrimal
  See Lacrimal Gland
Gland, Mammary
  See Breast
Gland, Parathyroid
  See Parathyroid Gland
Gland, Parotid
  See Parotid Gland
Gland, Pituitary
  See Pituitary Gland
Gland, Salivary
  See Salivary Glands
Gland, Sublingual
  See Sublingual Gland
Gland, Sweat
  See Sweat Glands
Gland, Thymus
  See Thymus Gland
Gland, Thyroid
  See Thyroid Gland
Glasses
  See Spectacle Services
Glaucoma
  Cryotherapy, 66720
  Cyclophotocoagulation, 66710, 66711
  Diathermy, 66700
  Fistulization of Sclera, 66150
Glaucoma Drainage Implant
  See Aqueous Shunt
Glenn Procedure, 33622, 33766-33767
Glenohumeral Joint
  Arthrotomy, 23040
    with Biopsy, 23100
    with Synovectomy, 23105
  Exploration, 23107
  Removal
    Foreign or Loose Body, 23107
Glenoid Fossa
  Reconstruction, 21255
Gliadin Deamidated Antibody (DGP), 86258
Glioblastoma Multiforme, *[81287]*, *[81345]*
GLN, 82127-82131
Globulin
  Antihuman, 86880-86886
  Immune, 90281-90399
  Sex Hormone Binding, 84270
Globulin, Corticosteroid–Binding, 84449
Globulin, Rh Immune, 90384-90386
Globulin, Thyroxine–Binding, 84442
Glomerular Filtration Rate (GFR)
  Measurement, 0602T
  Monitoring, 0603T
Glomerular Procoagulant Activity
  See Thromboplastin
Glomus Caroticum
  See Carotid Body
Glossectomies, 41120-41155
Glossectomy, 41120-41155
Glossorrhaphy
  See Suture, Tongue
Glucagon, 82943
  Tolerance Panel, 80422, 80424
  Tolerance Test, 82946
Glucose, 80422, 80424, 80430-80435, 95251 *[95249]*
  Blood Test, 82947-82950, 82962
  Body Fluid, 82945
  Hormone Panel, 80430
  Interstitial Fluid
    Continuous Monitoring, 95250-95251 *[95249]*
  Interstitial Sensor (Implantable), 0446T-0448T
  Tolerance Test, 82951, 82952
Glucose Phosphate Isomerase, 84087
Glucose Phosphate Isomerase Measurement, 84087

© 2021 Optum360, LLC

Glucose-6-Phosphatase, Catalytic Subunit Gene Analysis, [81250]
Glucose-6-Phosphate
  Dehydrogenase, 82955, 82960
Glucosidase, 82963
  Beta Acid Gene Analysis, 81251
Glucuronide Androstanediol, 82154
GLUD1, 81406
Glue
  Cornea Wound, 65286
  Sclera Wound, 65286
Glukagon
  See Glucagon
Glutamate Dehydrogenase, 82965
Glutamate Pyruvate Transaminase, 84460
Glutamic Alanine Transaminase, 84460
Glutamic Aspartic Transaminase, 84450
Glutamic Dehydrogenase, 82965
Glutamine, 82127-82131
Glutamyltransferase, Gamma, 82977
Glutathione, 82978
  Glutathione Reductase, 82979
Glycanhydrolase, N-Acetylmuramide
  See Lysozyme
Glycated Hemoglobins
  See Glycohemoglobin
Glycated Protein, 82985
Glycerol, Phosphatidyl
  See Phosphatidylglycerol
Glycerol Phosphoglycerides
  See Phosphatidylglycerol
Glycerophosphatase
  See Alkaline Phosphatase
Glycinate, Theophylline Sodium
  See Theophylline
Glycocholic Acid
  See Cholylglycine
Glycohemoglobin, 83036-83037
Glycol, Ethylene
  See Ethylene Glycol
Glycols, Ethylene
  See Ethylene Glycol
Glycosaminoglycan
  See Mucopolysaccharides
GNAQ, 81403
GNE, 81400, 81406
Goeckerman Treatment
  Photochemotherapy, 96910-96913
Gold
  Assay, [80375]
Goldwaite Procedure
  Reconstruction, Patella, for Instability, 27422
Golfer's Elbow, 24357-24359
Gol-Vernet Operation, 50120
Gonadectomy, Female
  See Oophorectomy
Gonadectomy, Male
  See Excision, Testis
Gonadotropin
  Chorionic, 84702, 84703
  FSH, 83001
  ICSH, 83002
  LH, 83002
Gonadotropin Panel, 80426
Goniophotography, 92285
Gonioscopy, 92020
Goniotomy, 65820
Gonococcus
  See Neisseria Gonorrhoeae
Goodenough Harris Drawing Test, 96112-96116
GOTT
  See Transaminase, Glutamic Oxaloacetic
GP1BA, [81106]
GP1BB, 81404
GPUT, 82775-82776
Graefe's Operation, 66830
Graft
  Anal, 46753
  Aorta, 33845, 33852, 33858-33859, 33863-33864, 33866, 33871-33877
  Artery
    Coronary, 33503-33505
  Bone
    See Bone Marrow, Transplantation
    Anastomosis, 20969-20973
    Harvesting, 20900, 20902

Graft — *continued*
  Bone — *continued*
    Microvascular Anastomosis, 20955-20962
    Osteocutaneous Flap with Microvascular Anastomosis, 20969-20973
    Vascular Pedicle, 25430
    Vertebra, 0222T
      Cervical, 0219T
      Lumbar, 0221T
      Thoracic, 0220T
  Bone and Skin, 20969-20973
  Cartilage
    Costochondral, 20910
    Ear to Face, 21235
    Harvesting, 20910, 20912
      See Cartilage Graft
    Rib to Face, 21230
      Three or More Segments
        Two Locations, 35682, 35683
  Composite, 35681-35683
  Conjunctiva, 65782
    Harvesting, 68371
  Cornea
    with Lesion Excision, 65426
    Corneal Transplant
      Allograft Preparation, 65757
      Endothelial, 65756
      in Aphakia, 65750
      in Pseudophakia, 65755
      Lamellar, 65710
      Penetrating, 65730
  Dura
    Spinal Cord, 63710
  Eye
    Amniotic Membrane, 65780
    Conjunctiva, 65782
      Harvesting, 68371
    Stem Cell, 65781
  Facial Nerve Paralysis, 15840-15845
  Fascia Graft
    Cheek, 15840
  Fascia Lata
    Harvesting, 20920, 20922
  Gum Mucosa, 41870
  Heart
    See Heart, Transplantation
  Heart Lung
    See Transplantation, Heart-Lung
  Hepatorenal, 35535
  Kidney
    See Kidney, Transplantation
  Liver
    See Liver, Transplantation
  Lung
    See Lung, Transplantation
  Muscle
    Cheek, 15841-15845
  Nail Bed Reconstruction, 11762
  Nerve, 64885-64907
  Oral Mucosa, 40818
  Organ
    See Transplantation
  Osteochondral
    Knee, 27415-27416
    Talus, 28446
  Pancreas
    See Pancreas, Transplantation
  Peroneal-Tibial, 35570
  Skin
    Autograft, 15150-15152, 15155-15157
    Biological, 15271-15278
    Blood Flow Check, Graft, 15860
      See Skin Graft and Flap
    Check Vascular Flow Injection, 15860
    Composite, 15760, 15770
    Delayed Flap, 15600-15630
    Free Flap, 15757
    Full Thickness, Free
      Axillae, 15240, 15241
      Cheeks, Chin, 15240, 15241
      Ears, Eyelids, 15260, 15261
      Extremities (Excluding Hands/Feet), 15240, 15241
      Feet, Hands, 15240, 15241
      Forehead, 15240, 15241

Graft — *continued*
  Skin — *continued*
    Full Thickness, Free — *continued*
      Genitalia, 15240, 15241
      Lips, Nose, 15260, 15261
      Mouth, Neck, 15240, 15241
      Scalp, 15220, 15221
      Trunk, 15200, 15201
    Harvesting
      for Tissue Culture, 15040
    Pedicle
      Direct, 15570, 15576
      Transfer, 15650
    Pinch Graft, 15050
    Preparation Recipient Site, 15002, 15004-15005
    Split Graft, 15100, 15101, 15120, 15121
    Substitute, 15271-15278
    Vascular Flow Check, Graft, 15860
  Tendon
    Finger, 26392
    Hand, 26392
    Harvesting, 20924
  Tibial/Peroneal Trunk-Tibial, 35570
  Tibial-Tibial, 35570
  Tissue
    Harvesting, 15771-15774, [15769]
  Vein
    Cross-over, 34520
  Vertebra, 0222T
    Cervical, 0219T
    Lumbar, 0221T
    Thoracic, 0220T
Grain Alcohol
  See Alcohol, Ethyl
Granulation Tissue
  Cauterization, Chemical, 17250
Gravis, Myasthenia
  See Myasthenia Gravis
Gravities, Specific
  See Specific Gravity
Great Toe
  Free Osteocutaneous Flap with Microvascular Anastomosis, 20973
Great Vessel(s)
  Shunt
    Aorta to Pulmonary Artery
      Ascending, 33755
      Descending, 33762
    Central, 33764
    Subclavian to Pulmonary Artery, 33750
    Vena Cava to Pulmonary Artery, 33766, 33767
  Unlisted Services and Procedures, 33999
Great Vessels Transposition
  See Transposition, Great Arteries
Greater Tuberosity Fracture
  with Shoulder Dislocation
    Closed Treatment, 23665
    Open Treatment, 23670
Greater Vestibular Gland
  See Bartholin's Gland
Green Operation
  See Scapulopexy
Greenfield Filter Insertion, 37191
Grice Arthrodesis, 28725
GRIN2A, [81419]
Grippe, Balkan
  See Q Fever
Gritti Operation, 27590-27592
  See Amputation, Leg, Upper; Radical Resection; Replantation
GRN, 81406
Groin Area
  Repair
    Hernia, 49550-49557
Gross Type Procedure, 49610, 49611
Group Health Education, 99078
Grouping, Blood
  See Blood Typing
Growth Factors, Insulin-Like
  See Somatomedin
Growth Hormone, 83003
  Human, 80418, 80428, 80430, 86277
  with Arginine Tolerance Test, 80428

Growth Hormone Release Inhibiting Factor
  See Somatostatin
Growth Stimulation Expressed Gene, 83006
GTT, 82951, 82952
Guaiac Test
  Blood in Feces, 82270
Guanylic Acids
  See Guanosine Monophosphate
Guard Stain, 88313
Guide
  3D Printed, Anatomic, 0561T-0562T
Gullet
  See Esophagus
Gums
  Abscess
    Incision and Drainage, 41800
  Alveolus
    Excision, 41830
  Cyst
    Incision and Drainage, 41800
  Excision
    Gingiva, 41820
    Operculum, 41821
  Graft
    Mucosa, 41870
  Hematoma
    Incision and Drainage, 41800
  Lesion
    Destruction, 41850
    Excision, 41822-41828
  Mucosa
    Excision, 41828
  Reconstruction
    Alveolus, 41874
    Gingiva, 41872
  Removal
    Foreign Body, 41805
  Tumor
    Excision, 41825-41827
  Unlisted Services and Procedures, 41899
Gunning-Lieben Test, 82009, 82010
Gunther Tulip Filter Insertion, 37191
Guthrie Test, 84030
GYPA, 81403
GYPB, 81403
GYPE, 81403

H

H Flu
  See Hemophilus Influenza
H19, 81401
HAA (Hepatitis Associated Antigen), 87340-87380, 87516-87527
  See Hepatitis Antigen, B Surface
HAAb (Antibody, Hepatitis), 86708, 86709
HADHA, 81406
HADHB, 81406
Haemoglobin F
  See Fetal Hemoglobin
Haemorrhage
  See Hemorrhage
Haemorrhage Rectum
  See Hemorrhage, Rectum
Hageman Factor, 85280
  Clotting Factor, 85210-85293
Haglund's Deformity Repair, 28119
HAI (Hemagglutination Inhibition Test), 86280
Hair
  Electrolysis, 17380
  KOH Examination, 87220
  Microscopic Evaluation, 96902
  Transplant
    Punch Graft, 15775, 15776
    Strip Graft, 15220, 15221
Hair Removal
  See Removal, Hair
Hallux
  See Great Toe
Hallux Rigidus
  Correction with Cheilectomy, 28289, 28291
Hallux Valgus, 28292-28299
Halo
  Body Cast, 29000
  Cranial, 20661
    for Thin Skull Osteology, 20664
  Femur, 20663

Halo — *continued*
  Maxillofacial, 21100
  Pelvic, 20662
  Removal, 20665
Haloperidol
  Assay, 80173
Halstead-Reitan Neuropsychological Battery, 96132-96133, 96136-96139, 96146
Halsted Mastectomy, 19305
Halsted Repair
  Hernia, 49495
Ham Test
  Hemolysins, 85475
    with Agglutinins, 86940, 86941
Hammertoe Repair, 28285, 28286
Hamster Penetration Test, 89329
Hand
  See Carpometacarpal Joint; Intercarpal Joint
  Abscess, 26034
  Amputation
    at Metacarpal, 25927
    at Wrist, 25920
      Revision, 25922
    Revision, 25924, 25929, 25931
  Arthrodesis
    Carpometacarpal Joint, 26843, 26844
    Intercarpal Joint, 25820, 25825
  Bone
    Incision and Drainage, 26034
  Cast, 29085
  Decompression, 26035, 26037
  Dislocation
    Carpal
      Closed, 25690
      Open, 25695
    Carpometacarpal
      Closed, 26670, 26675
      Open, 26685-26686
      Percutaneous, 26676
    Interphalangeal
      Closed, 26770, 26775
      Open, 26785
      Percutaneous, 26776
    Lunate
      Closed, 25690
      Open, 25695
    Metacarpophalangeal
      Closed, 26700-26705
      Open, 26715
      Percutaneous, 26706
    Radiocarpal
      Closed, 25660
      Open, 25670
    Thumb
      See Dislocation Thumb
    Wrist
      See Dislocation, Wrist
  Dupuytren's Contracture(s)
    Fasciotomy
      Open Partial, 26045
      Percutaneous, 26040
    Injection
      Enzyme, 20527
      Manipulation, 26341
    Palmar Fascial Cord
      Injection
        Enzyme, 20527
        Manipulation, 26341
  Excision
    Excess Skin, 15837
  Fracture
    Carpometacarpal, 26641-26650
    Interphalangeal, 26740-26746
    Metacarpal, 26600
    Metacarpophalangeal, 26740-26746
    Phalangeal, 26720-26735, 26750-26765
  Implantation
    Removal, 26320
      Tube/Rod, 26392, 26416
    Tube/Rod, 26390
  Insertion
    Tendon Graft, 26392
  Magnetic Resonance Imaging (MRI), 73218-73223
  Reconstruction
    Tendon Pulley, 26500-26502

Hand — *continued*
  Removal
    Implant, 26320
  Repair
    Blood Vessel, 35207
    Cleft Hand, 26580
    Muscle, 26591, 26593
      Release, 26593
    Tendon
      Extensor, 26410-26416, 26426, 26428, 26433-26437
      Flexor, 26350-26358, 26440
      Profundus, 26370-26373
  Replantation, 20808
  Skin Graft
    Delay of Flap, 15620
    Full Thickness, 15240, 15241
    Pedicle Flap, 15574
    Split, 15100, 15101
  Strapping, 29280
  Tendon
    Excision, 26390
      Extensor, 26415
    Tenotomy, 26450, 26460
  Tissue Transfer, Adjacent, 14040, 14041
  Tumor
    Excision, 26115 *[26111]*
    Radical Resection, 26116-26118 *[26113]*, 26250
  Unlisted Services and Procedures, 26989
  X–ray, 73120, 73130
Hand Phalange
  See Finger, Bone
Handling
  Device, 99002
  Radioelement, 77790
  Specimen, 99000, 99001
Hanganutziu Deicher Antibodies
  See Antibody, Heterophile
Haptoglobin, 83010, 83012
Hard Palate
  See Palate
Harelip Operation
  See Cleft Lip, Repair
Harrington Rod
  Insertion, 22840
  Removal, 22850
Hartley-Krause, 61450
Hartmann Procedure, 44143
  Closure of, 44227, 44626
  Laparoscopy
    Partial Colectomy with Colostomy, 44206
  Open, 44143
Harvesting
  Bone Graft, 20900, 20902
  Bone Marrow
    Allogeneic, 38230
    Autologous, 38232
  Cartilage, 20910, 20912
  Conjunctival Graft, 68371
  Eggs for In Vitro Fertilization, 58970
  Endoscopic
    Artery for Bypass Graft, 33509
    Vein for Bypass Graft, 33508
  Fascia Lata Graft, 20920, 20922
  Intestines, 44132, 44133
  Kidney, 50300, 50320, 50547
  Liver, 47133, 47140-47142
  Lower Extremity Vein for Vascular Reconstruction, 35572
  Skin, 15040
  Stem Cell, 38205, 38206
  Tendon Graft, 20924
  Tissue Grafts, 15771-15774, *[15769]*
  Upper Extremity Artery
    for Coronary Artery Bypass Graft, 35600
  Upper Extremity Vein
    for Bypass Graft, 35500
Hauser Procedure
  Reconstruction, Patella, for Instability, 27420
HAVRIX, 90632-90634
Hayem's Elementary Corpuscle
  See Blood, Platelet
Haygroves Procedure, 27120, 27122
Hb Bart Hydrops Fetalis Syndrome, *[81257]*
HBA1/HBA2, *[81257, 81258, 81259], [81269]*

HBA1/HBA2 — *continued*
  Duplication/Deletion Variant(s), *[81269]*
  Full Gene Sequence, *[81259]*
  Known Familial Variant(s), *[81258]*
HBB, *[81361, 81362, 81363, 81364]*
  Duplication/Deletion Variant(s), *[81363]*
  Full Gene Sequence, *[81364]*
  Known Familial Variant(s), *[81362]*
HBcAb, 86704, 86705
HBeAb, 86707
HBeAg, 87350
HbH Disease, *[81257]*
HBsAb, 86706
HBsAg (Hepatitis B Surface Antigen), 87340
HCG, 84702-84704
HCO3
  See Bicarbonate
Hct, 85013, 85014
HCV Antibodies
  See Antibody, Hepatitis C
  Biochemical Assay, *[81596]*
HD, 27295
HDL (High Density Lipoprotein), 83718
Head
  Angiography, 70496, 70544-70546
  CT Scan, 70450-70470, 70496
  Excision, 21015-21070
  Fracture and/or Dislocation, 21315-21497
  Incision, 21010, 61316, 62148
  Introduction, 21076-21116
  Lipectomy, Suction Assisted, 15876
  Magnetic Resonance Angiography (MRA), 70544-70546
  Nerve
    Graft, 64885, 64886
  Other Procedures, 21299, 21499
  Repair
    Revision and/or Reconstruction, 21120-21296
  Ultrasound Examination, 76506, 76536
  Unlisted Services and Procedures, 21499
  X–ray, 70350
Head Brace
  Application, 21100
  Removal, 20661
Head Rings, Stereotactic
  See Stereotactic Frame
Heaf Test
  TB Test, 86580
Health and Well-being
  Assessment, Individual, 0591T
  Follow-up Session, 0592T
  Group Session, 0593T
Health Behavior
  Alcohol and/or Substance Abuse, 99408-99409
  Assessment, 96156
  Family Intervention, *[96167, 96168, 96170, 96171]*
  Group Intervention, 0403T, *[96164, 96165]*
  Individual Intervention, 96158-96159
  Re-assessment, 96156
  Smoking and Tobacco Cessation, 99406-99407
Health Risk Assessment Instrument, 96160-96161
Hearing Aid
  Bone Conduction
    Implant, 69710
    Removal, 69711
    Repair, 69711
    Replace, 69710
  Check, 92592, 92593
Hearing Aid Services
  Electroacoustic Test, 92594, 92595
  Examination, 92590, 92591
Hearing Tests
  See Audiologic Function Tests; Hearing Evaluation
Hearing Therapy, 92507, 92601-92604
Heart
  Ablation
    Arrhythmogenic Focus
      Intracardiac Catheter, 93650-93657
      Open, 33250-33261
    Ventricular Septum
      Transcatheter Alcohol Septal Ablation, 93583

Heart — *continued*
  Acoustic Cardiography with Computer Analysis, 93799
  Allograft Preparation, 33933, 33944
  Angiography, 93454-93461
    Injection, 93563-93568
  Aortic Arch
    with Cardiopulmonary Bypass, 33853
    without Cardiopulmonary Bypass, 33852
  Aortic Valve
    Implantation, 33361-33369, 33405-33413
    Repair
      Left Ventricle, 33414
      Transcatheter Closure, 93591-93592
    Replacement, 33405-33413
      Transcatheter, 33361-33369
      with Cardiopulmonary Bypass, 33405-33406, 33410
  Arrhythmogenic Focus
    Destruction, 33250, 33251, 33261
  Atria
    See Atria
  Biopsy, 93505
    Radiologic Guidance, 76932
  Blood Vessel
    Repair, 33320-33322
  Cardiac Output Measurements
    by Indicator Dilution, 93598
  Cardiac Rehabilitation, 93797, 93798
  Cardiac Rhythm Monitor System
    Insertion, 93290-93291
    Interrogation, 93297-93298
    Programming, 0650T, 93285
  Cardioassist, 92970, 92971
  Cardiopulmonary Bypass
    Lung Transplant, 32852, 32854
    Replacement Ventricular Assist Device, 33983
  Cardioverter–Defibrillator
    Evaluation and Testing, 0575T-0579T, 93640, 93641, 93642
  Catheterization, 93451-93453, 93456-93462
    Combined Left and Right Heart, 93596-93597
    Flow–Directed, 93503
    Left Heart, 93595
    Right Heart, 93593-93594
  Closure
    Patent Ductus Arteriosus, 93582
    Septal Defect, 33615
      Ventricular, 33675-33677, 33681-33688, 33776, 33780, 93581
    Valve
      Atrioventricular, 33600
      Semilunar, 33602
  Commissurotomy, Right Ventricle, 33476, 33478
  CT Scan, 75571-75573
    Angiography, 75574
  Defibrillator
    Body Surface-activation Mapping, 0695T-0696T
    Removal, 33243, 33244
      Pulse Generator Only, 33241
    Repair, 33218, 33220
    Replacement, Leads, 33216, 33217, 33249
    Wearable Device, 93745
  Destruction
    Arrhythmogenic Focus, 33250, 33261
  Electrical Recording
    3D Mapping, 93613
    Acoustic Cardiography, 93799
    Atria, 93602
    Atrial Electrogram, Esophageal (or Transesophageal), 93615, 93616
    Bundle of His, 93600
    Comprehensive, 93619-93622
    Right Ventricle, 93603
    Tachycardia Sites, 93609
  Electroconversion, 92960, 92961
  Electrode
    Insertion, 33202-33203

   [Resequenced]

Heart — *continued*
Electrophysiologic Follow–up Study, 93624
Electrophysiology Procedures, 93600-93660
Endoscopy
Atrial, 33265-33266
Evaluation of Device, 93640
Excision
Donor, 33930, 33940
Tricuspid Valve, 33460, 33465
Exploration, 33310, 33315
Fibrillation
Atrial, 33254, 33255-33256
Great Vessels
See Great Vessels
Heart–Lung Bypass
See Cardiopulmonary Bypass
Heart–Lung Transplantation
See Transplantation, Heart–Lung
Hemodynamic Monitoring
with Pharmacologic Agent, 93463
with Physiologic Exercise Study, 93464
Implantable Defibrillator
Data Analysis, 93289, 93295-93296
Evaluation
In Person, 93282-93284, 93287,
93289
Remote, 93295-93296
Initial Setup and Programming, 93745
Insertion Electrodes, 33216, 33217,
33224-33225, 33249
Pulse Generator, 33240
Insertion, 33240 *[33230, 33231]*
Removal, 33241
Replacement, *[33262, 33263,
33264]*
System, 33249, *[33270]*
Reposition Electrodes, 33215, 33226
Implantation
Artificial Heart, Intracorporeal, 33927
Intracorporeal, 33979
Total Replacement Heart System, Intra-
corporeal, 33927
Ventricular Assist Device
Extracorporeal, 33975-33976,
33981
Intracorporeal, 33979, 33982-
33983
Percutaneous, 33990-33991,
[33995]
Incision
Atrial, 33254, 33255-33256
Exploration, 33310, 33315
Injection
Radiologic, 93565-93566
Insertion
Balloon Device, 33973
Defibrillator, 33212-33213
Electrode, 33210, 33211, 33214-33217,
33224-33225
Pacemaker, 33206-33208, 33212, 33213
Catheter, 33210
Pulse Generator, 33212-33214
[33221]
Ventricular Assist Device
Extracorporeal, 33975-33976,
33981
Intracorporeal, 33979, 33982-
33983
Percutaneous, 33990-33991,
[33995]
Intraoperative Pacing and Mapping, 93631
Ligation
Fistula, 37607
Magnetic Resonance Imaging (MRI), 75557-
75565
with Contrast Material, 75561-75563
with Velocity Flow Mapping, 75565
without Contrast Material, 75557-75559
without Contrast Material, Followed by
Contrast Material, 75561-75563
Mitral Valve
See Mitral Valve
Muscle
See Myocardium
Myocardial Contrast Perfusion, 0439T

Heart — *continued*
Myocardial Infarction tPA Administration
Documented, 4077F
Myocardial Strain Imaging, *[93356]*
Myocardial Sympathetic Innervation Imaging,
0331T-0332T
Myocardium
Imaging, Nuclear, 78466-78469
Perfusion Study, 78451-78454
Sympathetic Innervation Imaging,
0331T-0332T
Nuclear Medicine
Blood Flow Study, 78414
Blood Pool Imaging, 78472, 78473,
78481, 78483, 78494, 78496
Myocardial Imaging, 78466-78469
Myocardial Perfusion, 0439T, 78451-
78454
Shunt Detection (Test), 78428
Unlisted Services and Procedures, 78499
Open Chest Massage, 32160
Output, 93598
Pacemaker
Body Surface-activation Mapping,
0695T-0696T
Conversion, 33214
Evaluation
In Person, 93279-93281, 93286,
93288
Remote, 93293-93294, 93296
Insertion, 33206-33208
Pulse Generator, 33212, 33213
Leadless, Ventricular
Insertion, *[33274]*
Removal, *[33275]*
Replacement, *[33274]*
Removal, 33233-33237 *[33227, 33228,
33229]*
Replacement, 33206-33208
Catheter, 33210
Upgrade, 33214
Pacing
Arrhythmia Induction, 93618
Atria, 93610
Transcutaneous
Temporary, 92953
Ventricular, 93612
Positron Emission Tomography (PET), 78459,
[78429], *[78434]*
Perfusion Study, 78491, 78492 *[78430,
78431, 78432, 78433]*
Pulmonary Valve
See Pulmonary Valve
Rate Increase
See Tachycardia
Reconstruction
Atrial Septum, 33735-33737
Vena Cava, 34502
Recording
Left Ventricle, 93622
Right Ventricle, 93603
Tachycardia Sites, 93609
Reduction
Ventricular Septum
Non–surgical, 93799
Removal
Balloon Device, 33974
Electrode, 33238
Ventricular Assist Device, 33977, 33978
Intracorporeal, 33980, 33999
Removal Single/Dual Chamber
Electrodes, 33243, 33244
Pulse Generator, 33241
Repair, 33218, 33220
Repair
Anomaly, 33615, 33617
Aortic Sinus, 33702-33720
Aortic Valve, 93591-93592
Atrial Septum, 33254, 33255-33256,
33641, 33647, 93580
Atrioventricular Canal, 33660, 33665
Complete, 33670
Prosthetic Valve, 33670
Atrioventricular Valve, 33660, 33665
Cor Triatriatum, 33732
Electrode, 33218

Heart — *continued*
Repair — *continued*
Fenestration, 93580
Prosthetic Valve, 33670
Infundibular, 33476, 33478
Mitral Valve, 33420-33430, 93590-93592
Myocardium, 33542
Outflow Tract, 33476, 33478
Patent Ductus Arteriosus, 93582
Postinfarction, 33542, 33545
Prosthetic Valve Dysfunction, 33496
Septal Defect, 33608, 33610, 33660,
33813, 33814, 93581
Sinus of Valsalva, 33702-33720
Sinus Venosus, 33645
Tetralogy of Fallot, 33692-33697, 33924
Tricuspid Valve, 0569T-0570T, 33460-
33468
Ventricle, 33611, 33612
Obstruction, 33619
Ventricular Septum, 33545, 33647,
33681-33688, 33692-33697,
93581
Wound, 33300, 33305
Replacement
Artificial Heart, Intracorporeal, 33928
Electrode, 33210, 33211, 33217
Mitral Valve, 33430
Total Replacement Heart System, Intra-
corporeal, 33928
Tricuspid Valve, 33465
Ventricular Assist Device, 0459T, 33981-
33983
Repositioning
Electrode, 33215, 33217, 33226
Tricuspid Valve, 33468
Resuscitation, 92950
Septal Defect
Repair, 33782-33783, 33813-33814
Ventricular
Closure, 33675-33688
Open, 33675-33688
Percutaneous, 93581
Stimulation and Pacing, 93623
Thrombectomy, 33310-33315
Ventricular Assist Device, 33976
Intracorporeal, 33979
Transplantation, 33935, 33945
Allograft Preparation, 33933, 33944
Anesthesia, 00580
Tricuspid Valve
See Tricuspid Valve
Tumor
Excision, 33120, 33130
Ultrasound
Myocardial Strain Imaging, *[93356]*
Radiologic Guidance, 76932
Unlisted Services and Procedures, 33999
Ventriculography
See Ventriculography
Ventriculomyectomy, 33416
Ventriculomyotomy, 33416
Wound
Repair, 33300, 33305
Heart Biopsy
Ultrasound, Radiologic Guidance, 76932
Heart Vessels
Angiography, 93454-93461, 93563-93566
Angioplasty, *[92920, 92921]*, *[92928, 92929]*,
[92937, 92938], *[92941]*, *[92943, 92944]*
Injection, 93452-93461, 93563-93568
Insertion
Graft, 33330-33335
Thrombolysis, *[92975, 92977]*
Valvuloplasty
See Valvuloplasty
Percutaneous, 92986-92990
Heat Unstable Haemoglobin
See Hemoglobin, Thermolabile
Heavy Lipoproteins
See Lipoprotein
Heavy Metal, 83015, 83018
Heel
See Calcaneus
Collection of Blood, 36415, 36416
X–ray, 73650

Heel Bone
See Calcaneus
Heel Fracture
See Calcaneus, Fracture
Heel Spur
Excision, 28119
Heine Operation
See Cyclodialysis
Heine–Medin Disease
See Polio
Heinz Bodies, 85441, 85445
Helicobacter Pylori
Antibody, 86677
Antigen Detection
Enzyme Immunoassay, 87338, 87339
Breath Test, 78267, 78268, 83013
Stool, 87338
Urease Activity, 83009, 83013, 83014
Heller Procedure, 32665, 43279, 43330-43331
Helminth
Antibody, 86682
Hemagglutination Inhibition Test, 86280
Hemangioma, 17106-17108
Hemapheresis, 36511-36516
Hematochezia, 82270, 82274
Hematologic Test
See Blood Tests
Hematology
Unlisted Services and Procedures, 85999
Hematolymphoid Neoplasm or Disorder, 81450,
81455
Hematoma
Ankle, 27603
Arm, Lower, 25028
Arm, Upper
Incision and Drainage, 23930
Brain
Drainage, 61154, 61156
Evacuation, 61312-61315
Incision and Drainage, 61312-61315
Drain, 61108
Ear, External
Complicated, 69005
Simple, 69000
Elbow
Incision and Drainage, 23930
Epididymis
Incision and Drainage, 54700
Gums
Incision and Drainage, 41800
Hip, 26990
Incision and Drainage
Neck, 21501, 21502
Skin, 10140
Thorax, 21501, 21502
Knee, 27301
Leg, Lower, 27603
Leg, Upper, 27301
Mouth, 41005-41009, 41015-41018
Incision and Drainage, 40800, 40801
Nasal Septum
Incision and Drainage, 30020
Nose
Incision and Drainage, 30000, 30020
Pelvis, 26990
Puncture Aspiration, 10160
Scrotum
Incision and Drainage, 54700
Shoulder
Drainage, 23030
Skin
Incision and Drainage, 10140
Puncture Aspiration, 10160
Subdural, 61108
Subungual
Evacuation, 11740
Testis
Incision and Drainage, 54700
Tongue, 41000-41006, 41015
Vagina
Incision and Drainage, 57022, 57023
Wrist, 25028
Hematopoietic Stem Cell Transplantation
See Stem Cell, Transplantation
Hematopoietin
See Erythropoietin

© 2021 Optum360, LLC

Insertion — *continued*
Radioactive Material — *continued*
Remote Afterloading Brachytherapy,
77767-77768, 77770-77772
Receiver
Brain, 61885, 61886
Spinal Cord, 63685
Reservoir
Brain, 61210, 61215
Spinal Cord, 62360
Shunt, 36835
Abdomen
Vein, 49425
Venous, 49426
Interatrial Septal Shunt
Percutaneous, Transcatheter,
0613T
Intrahepatic Portosystemic, 37182
Spinal Instrument, 22849
Spinous Process, 22841, 22867-22870
Spinal Instrumentation
Anterior, 22845-22847
Internal Spinal Fixation, 22841, 22853-
22854, 22867-22870, [22859]
Pelvic Fixation, 22848
Posterior Non–segmental
Harrington Rod Technique, 22840
Posterior Segmental, 22842-22844
Stent
Bile Duct, 47801, [43274]
Bladder, 51045
Conjunctiva, 68750
Esophagus, [43212]
Gastrointestinal, Upper, [43266]
Indwelling, 50605
Lacrimal Canaliculus, Drug-Eluting,
68841
Lacrimal Duct, 68810-68815
Pancreatic Duct, [43274]
Small Intestines, 44370, 44379
Ureteral, 50688, 50693-50695, 50947,
52332
Urethral, 52282, 53855
Tamponade
Esophagus, 43460
Tandem
Uterus
for Brachytherapy, 57155
Tendon Graft
Finger, 26392
Hand, 26392
Testicular Prosthesis
See Prosthesis, Testicular, Insertion
Tissue Expanders, Skin, 11960-11971
Tube
Cecostomy, 49442
Duodenostomy or Jejunostomy, 49441
Esophagus, 43510
Gastrointestinal, Upper, 43241
Gastrostomy, 49440
Small Intestines, 44379
Trachea, 31730
Ureter, 50688, 50693-50695
Urethral
Catheter, 51701-51703
Guide Wire, 52344
Implant Material, 51715
Intraurethral Valve Pump, 0596T, 0597T
Suppository, 53660-53661
Vascular Pedicle
Carpal Bone, 25430
Venous Access Device
Central, 36560-36566
Peripheral, 36570, 36571
Venous Shunt
Abdomen, 49425
Ventilating Tube, 69433
Ventricular Assist Device
Extracorporeal, 33975-33976, 33981
Intracorporeal, 33979, 33982-33983
Percutaneous, 33990-33991, [33995]
Wire
Skeletal Traction, 20650
Wireless Cardiac Stimulator, 0515T-0517T

Inspiratory Positive Pressure Breathing
See Intermittent Positive Pressure Breathing
(IPPB)
Instillation
Agent for Pleurodesis, 32560-32562
Drugs
Bladder, 51720
Kidney, 50391
Ureter, 50391
Instillation, Bladder
See Bladder, Instillation
Instrumentation
See Application; Bone; Fixation; Spinal Instru-
mentation
Spinal
Insertion, 22840-22848, 22853-22854,
22867-22870, [22859]
Reinsertion, 22849
Removal, 22850, 22852, 22855
Insufflation, Eustachian Tube
See Eustachian Tube, Inflation
Insulin, 80422, 80432-80435
Antibody, 86337
Blood, 83525
Free, 83527
Insulin C–Peptide Measurement
See C–Peptide
Insulin Like Growth Factors
See Somatomedin
Insurance
Basic Life and/or Disability Evaluation Services,
99450
Examination, 99450-99456
Integumentary System
Ablation
Breast, 19105
Biopsy, 11102-11107
Breast
Ablation, 19105
Excision, 19100-19126, 21601-21603
Incision, 19000-19030
Localization Device, 19281-19288
with Biopsy, 19081-19086
Reconstruction, 19316-19396
Repair, 19316-19396
Unlisted Services and Procedures, 19499
Burns, 15002-15003, 15005, 16000-16036
Debridement, 11000-11006, 11010-11044
[11045, 11046], 96574
Destruction
See Dermatology
Actinotherapy, 96900
Benign Lesion, 17000-17004
by Photodynamic Therapy, 96567
Chemical Exfoliation, 17360
Cryotherapy, 17340
Electrolysis Epilation, 17380
Malignant Lesion, 17260-17286
Mohs Micrographic Surgery, 17311-
17315
Photodynamic Therapy, 96567, 96570,
96571, 96573-96574
Premalignant Lesion, 17000-17004
Unlisted Services and Procedures, 17999
Drainage, 10040-10180
Excision
Benign Lesion, 11400-11471
Debridement, 11000-11006, 11010-
11044 [11045, 11046]
Malignant Lesion, 11600-11646
Graft, 14000-14350, 15002-15278
Autograft, 15040-15157
Skin Substitute, 15271-15278
Surgical Preparation, 15002-15005
Tissue Transfer or Rearrangement,
14000-14350
Implantation Biologic Implant, 15777
Incision, 10040-10180
Introduction
Drug Delivery Implant, 11981, 11983
Nails, 11719-11765
Paring, 11055-11057
Photography, 96904
Pressure Ulcers, 15920-15999
Removal
Drug Delivery Implant, 11982, 11983

Integumentary System — *continued*
Repair
Adjacent Tissue Transfer
Rearrangement, 14000-14350
Complex, 13100-13160
Flaps, 15740-15776
Free Skin Grafts, 15002-15005, 15050-
15136, 15200-15261
Implantation Acellular Dermal Matrix,
15777
Intermediate, 12031-12057
Other Procedures, 15780-15879
Simple, 12001-12021
Skin and/or Deep Tissue, 15570-15738
Skin Substitute, 15271-15278
Shaving of Epidermal or Dermal Lesion, 11300-
11313
Skin Tags
Removal, 11200, 11201
Integumentum Commune
See Integumentary System
Intelligence Test
Computer-Assisted, 96130-96131, 96136-
96139, 96146
Psychiatric Diagnosis, Psychological Testing,
96112-96113, 96116, 96121, 96130-
96146
Intensity Modulated Radiation Therapy (IMRT)
Complex, [77386]
Plan, 77301
Simple, [77385]
Intensive Care
Low Birth Weight Infant, 99478-99479
Neonatal
Initial Care, 99479
Subsequent Care, 99478
Intercarpal Joint
Arthrodesis, 25820, 25825
Dislocation
Closed Treatment, 25660
Repair, 25447
Intercostal Nerve
Destruction, 64620
Injection
Anesthetic or Steroid, 64420, 64421
Neurolytic Agent, 64620
Intercranial Arterial Perfusion
Thrombolysis, 61624
Interdental Fixation
Device
Application, 21110
Mandibular Fracture
Closed Treatment, 21453
Open Treatment, 21462
without Fracture, 21497
Interdental Papilla
See Gums
Interdental Wire Fixation
Closed Treatment
Craniofacial Separation, 21431
Interferometry
Eye
Biometry, 92136
Interleukin-6 (IL-6), [83529]
Intermediate Care Facility (ICF) Visits, 99304-
99318
Intermittent Positive Pressure Breathing (IPPB)
See Continuous Negative Pressure Breathing
(CNPB); Continuous Positive Airway
Pressure (CPAP)
Internal Breast Prostheses
See Breast, Implants
Internal Ear
See Ear, Inner
Internal Rigid Fixation
Reconstruction
Mandibular Rami, 21196
International Normalized Ratio
Test Review, 93792-93793
Internet E/M Service
Nonphysician, 98970-98972
Physician, [99421, 99422, 99423]
Interphalangeal Joint
Arthrodesis, 26860-26863
Arthroplasty, 26535, 26536
Arthrotomy, 26080, 28054

Interphalangeal Joint — *continued*
Biopsy
Synovium, 26110
Capsule
Excision, 26525
Incision, 26525
Dislocation
Closed Treatment, 26770
Fingers/Hand
Closed Treatment, 26770, 26775
Open Treatment, 26785
Percutaneous Fixation, 26776
with Manipulation, 26340
Open Treatment, 26785
Percutaneous Fixation, 26776
Toes/Foot
Closed Treatment, 28660, 28665
Open Treatment, 28675
Percutaneous Fixation, 28666
with Manipulation, 26340
Excision, 28160
Exploration, 26080, 28024
Fracture
Closed Treatment, 26740
Open Treatment, 26746
with Manipulation, 26742
Fusion, 26860-26863
Great Toe
Arthrodesis, 28755
with Tendon Transfer, 28760
Fusion, 28755
with Tendon Transfer, 28760
Removal
Foreign Body, 26080
Loose Body, 28024
Repair
Collateral Ligament, 26545
Volar Plate, 26548
Synovectomy, 26140
Synovial
Biopsy, 28054
Toe, 28272
Arthrotomy, 28024
Biopsy
Synovial, 28054
Dislocation, 28660-28665, 28675
Percutaneous Fixation, 28666
Excision, 28160
Exploration, 28024
Removal
Foreign Body, 28024
Loose Body, 28024
Synovial
Biopsy, 28054
Interrogation
Cardiac Rhythm Monitor System, 0650T, 93285,
93291, 93297-93298
Cardiac Stimulator, 0521T
Cardio-Defibrillator, 93289, 93292, 93295
Cardiovascular Physiologic Monitoring System,
93290, 93297-93298
Carotid Sinus Baroreflex Activation Device,
0272T-0273T
Pacemaker, 93288, 93294, 93296
Ventricular Assist Device, 33999, 93750
Interruption
Vein
Femoral, 37650
Iliac, 37660
Intersex State
Clitoroplasty, 56805
Vaginoplasty, 57335
Intersex Surgery
Female to Male, 55980
Male to Female, 55970
Interstitial Cell Stimulating Hormone
See Luteinizing Hormone (LH)
Cystitides, Chronic
See Cystitis, Interstitial
Cystitis
See Cystitis, Interstitial
Fluid Pressure
Monitoring, 20950
Interstitial Glucose Sensor
Insertion, 0446T, 0448T
Removal, 0447T-0448T

Kidney

Abscess
  Incision and Drainage
    Open, 50020
Allograft Preparation, 50323-50329
  Donor Nephrectomy, 50300, 50320, 50547
  Implantation of Graft, 50360
  Recipient Nephrectomy, 50340, 50365
  Reimplantation Kidney, 50380
  Removal Transplant Renal Autograft, 50370
Anesthesia
  Donor, 00862
  Recipient, 00868
Biopsy, 50200, 50205
  Endoscopic, 50555-50557, 52354
  Renal Pelvis, 50606
Catheterization
  Endoscopic, 50572
Cyst
  Ablation, 50541
  Aspiration, 50390
  Excision, 50280, 50290
  Injection, 50390
  X-ray, 74470
Destruction
  Calculus, 50590
  Endoscopic, 50557, 50576, 52354
Dilation, [50436, 50437]
Endoscopy
  Biopsy, 50555, 50574-50576, 52354
  Catheterization, 50553, 50572
  Destruction, 50557, 50576, 52354
  Dilation
    Intrarenal Stricture, 52343, 52346
    Ureter, 50553
  Excision
    Tumor, 52355
  Exploration, 52351
  Lithotripsy, 52353
  Removal
    Calculus, 50561, 50580, 52352
    Foreign Body, 50561, 50580
  via Incision, 50570-50580
  via Stoma, 50551-50561
  with Endopyelotomy, 50575
Excision
  Donor, 50300, 50320, 50547
  Partial, 50240
  Recipient, 50340
  Transplantation, 50370
  with Ureters, 50220-50236
Exploration, 50010, 50045, 50120
Incision, 50010, 50045, 50120, 50130, 50135
Incision and Drainage, 50040, 50125
Injection
  Drugs, 50391
Insertion
  Guide, [50436, 50437]
Instillation
  Drugs, 50391
Lithotripsy, 50590
Manometry
  Pressure, 50396
Mass
  Ablation, 50542
    Cryosurgical, 50250
    Radiofrequency, 50592
Mass Ablation, 50542
Needle Biopsy, 50200
Nuclear Medicine
  Blood Flow, 78701-78709
  Function Study, 78725
  Imaging, 78700-78707, 78803
  Unlisted Services and Procedures, 78799
Removal
  Calculus, 50060-50081, 50130, 50561
  Foreign Body, 50561, 50580
  Tube
    Nephrostomy, 50389
Renal Pelvis, 50405
Repair
  Blood Vessels, 50100
  Fistula, 50520-50526
  Horseshoe Kidney, 50540

Kidney — continued

Repair — continued
  Renal Pelvis, 50400, 50405
  Wound, 50500
Solitary, 50405
Suture
  Fistula, 50520-50526
  Horseshoe Kidney, 50540
Transplantation
  Allograft Preparation, 50323-50329
  Anesthesia
    Donor, 00862
    Recipient, 00868
  Donor Nephrectomy, 50300-50320, 50547
  Graft Implantation, 50360-50365
  Implantation of Graft, 50360
  Recipient Nephrectomy, 50340, 50365
  Reimplantation Kidney, 50380
  Removal Transplant Allograft, 50370
Tumor
  Ablation
    Cryotherapy, 50250, 50593
  Ultrasound, 76770-76775, 76776

Kidney Stone

Removal, Calculi, 50060-50081, 50130, 50561, 50580

Killer Cell Immunoglobulin-like Receptor (KIR) Gene Family, 81403

Killian Operation, 31020
  Sinusotomy, Frontal, 31070-31087

Kinase Creatine
  Blood, 82550-82552

Kinematic and Kinetic Motion Analysis, 0693T

Kineplasty
  Arm, Lower or Upper, 24940

Kinetic Therapy, 97530

Kininase A, 82164

Kininogen, 85293

Kininogen, High Molecular Weight, 85293

Kirsten Rat Sarcoma Viral Oncogene Homolog Gene Analysis, 81275

KIT, 81272
  D816 Variant, 81273

Kleihauer–Betke Test, 85460

Kloramfenikol, 82415

Knee

See Femur; Fibula; Patella; Tibia
Abscess, 27301
Arthrocentesis, 20610-20611
Arthrodesis, 27580
Arthroplasty, 27440-27445, 27447
  Revision, 27486, 27487
Arthroscopy
  Diagnostic, 29870
  Surgical, 29866-29868, 29871-29889
Arthrotomy, 27310, 27330-27335, 27403
Autograft, Osteochondral, Open, 27416
Biopsy, 27323, 27324, 27330, 27331
  Synovium, 27330-27331
Bone
  Drainage, 27303
Bursa, 27301
  Excision, 27340
Cyst
  Excision, 27345, 27347
Disarticulation, 27598
Dislocation
  Closed Treatment, 27550, 27552, 27560, 27562
  Open Treatment, 27556-27558, 27566
Drainage, 27310
Excision
  Cartilage, 27332, 27333
  Ganglion, 27347
  Lesion, 27347
  Synovial Lining, 27334, 27335
Exploration, 27310, 27331
Fasciotomy, 27305, 27496-27499
Fracture, 27520, 27524
  Arthroscopic Treatment, 29850, 29851
Fusion, 27580
Hematoma, 27301
Incision
  Capsule, 27435

Knee — continued

Injection
  X-ray, 27369
Magnetic Resonance Imaging (MRI), 73721-73723
Manipulation, 27570
Meniscectomy, 27332, 27333
Osteochondral Graft, 27415-27416
Reconstruction, 27437, 27438
  Ligament, 27427-27429
    with Implantation, 27445
    with Prosthesis, 27445
Removal
  Foreign Body, 27310, 27331, 27372
  Loose Body, 27331
  Prosthesis, 27488
Repair
  Ligament, 27405-27409
    Collateral, 27405
    Collateral and Cruciate, 27409
    Cruciate, 27407, 27409
  Meniscus, 27403
  Tendon, 27380, 27381
Replacement, 27447
Retinacular
  Release, 27425
Strapping, 29530
Suture
  Tendon, 27380, 27381
Transplantation
  Chondrocytes, 27412
  Meniscus, 29868
  Osteochondral
    Allograft, 27415, 29867
    Autograft, 27412, 29866
Tumor, 27327-27328 [27337, 27339], 27355-27358, 27364-27365 [27329]
Unlisted Services and Procedures, 27599
X-ray, 73560-73564
  Arthrography, 73580
  Bilateral, 73565
X-ray with Contrast
  Angiography, 73706
  Arthrography, 73580

Knee Prosthesis
  See Prosthesis, Knee

Kneecap
  Excision, 27350
  Repair
    Instability, 27420-27424

Knock–Knee Repair, 27455, 27457

Kocher Operation, 23650-23680
  See Clavicle; Scapula; Shoulder, Dislocation, Closed Treatment

Kocher Pylorectomy
  Gastrectomy, Partial, 43631

Kock Pouch, 44316
  Formation, 50825

Kock Procedure, 44316

KOH
  Hair, Nails, Tissue, Examination for Fungi, 87220

Konno Procedure, 33412

Koop Inguinal Orchiopexy, 54640

KRAS, 81275-81276, 81405

Kraske Procedure, 45116

Krause Operation
  Gasserian Ganglion, Sensory Root, Decompression, 61450

Kroenlein Procedure, 67420

Krukenberg Procedure, 25915

Krupin-Denver Valve
  Implant, 66180
  Removal, 67120
  Revision, 66185

KS, 83586, 83593

KUB, 74420

Kuhlmann Test, 96112-96116

Kuhnt–Szymanowski Procedure, 67917

Kyphectomy
  More Than Two Segments, 22819
  Up to Two Segments, 22818

Kyphoplasty, 22513-22515

L

L Ascorbic Acid
  See Ascorbic Acid

L Aspartate 2 Oxoglutarate Aminotransferase
  See Transaminase, Glutamic Oxaloacetic

L Glutamine
  See Glutamine

L1CAM, 81407

Labial Adhesions
  Lysis, 56441

Labyrinth
  See Ear, Inner

Labyrinthectomy
  Transcanal, 69905
  with Mastoidectomy, 69910
  with Skull Base Surgery, 61596

Labyrinthotomy
  Transcanal, 69801

Laceration Repair
  See Repair, Laceration, Skin

Lacrimal Duct
  Balloon, 68816
  Canaliculi
    Incision, 68899
    Repair, 68700
  Dilation, 68816
  Exploration, 68810
    Canaliculi, 68840
    Stent, 68815
    with Anesthesia, 68811
  Insertion
    Stent, 68815
  Nasolacrimal Duct Probing, 68816
  Removal
    Dacryolith, 68530
    Foreign Body, 68530
  X-ray with Contrast, 70170

Lacrimal Gland
  Biopsy, 68510
  Close Fistula, 68770
  Excision
    Partial, 68505
    Total, 68500
  Fistulization, 68720
  Incision and Drainage, 68400
  Injection
    X-ray, 68850
  Nuclear Medicine
    Tear Flow, 78660
  Removal
    Dacryolith, 68530
    Foreign Body, 68530
  Repair
    Fistula, 68770
  Tumor
    Excision
      with Osteotomy, 68550
      without Closure, 68540
  X-ray, 70170

Lacrimal Punctum
  Closure
    by Plug, 68761
    by Thermocauterization, Ligation or Laser Surgery, 68760
  Dilation, 68801
  Incision, 68440
  Repair, 68705

Lacrimal Sac
  Biopsy, 68525
  Excision, 68520
  Incision and Drainage, 68420

Lacrimal System
  Unlisted Services and Procedures, 68899

Lacryoaptography
  Nuclear, 78660

Lactase Deficiency Breath Test, 91065

Lactate, 83605

Lactic Acid, 83605

Lactic Acid Measurement
  See Lactate

Lactic Cytochrome Reductase
  See Lactic Dehydrogenase

Lactic Dehydrogenase, 83615, 83625

Lactiferous Duct
  Excision, 19112
  Exploration, 19110

Microvascular Anastomosis — *continued*
  Osteocutaneous Flap with, 20969-20973
  Skin Flap, Free, 15757
Microvite A, 84590
Microvolt T-Wave Alternans, 93025
Microwave Therapy, 97024
  See Physical Medicine/Therapy/Occupational Therapy
Midbrain
  See Brain; Brainstem; Mesencephalon; Skull Base Surgery
Midcarpal Medioccipital Joint
  Arthrotomy, 25040
Middle Cerebral Artery Velocimetry, 76821
Middle Ear
  See Ear, Middle
Midface
  Reconstruction
    Forehead Advancement, 21159, 21160
    with Bone Graft, 21145-21159, 21188
    without Bone Graft, 21141-21143
Mile Operation, 44155, 44156
Milia, Multiple
  Removal, 10040
Miller Procedure, 28737
Miller–Abbott Intubation, 44500, 74340
Millin-Read Operation, 57288
Minerva Cast, 29040
  Removal, 29710
Minimum Inhibitory Concentration, 87186
Minimum Lethal Concentration, 87187
Minnesota Multiple Personality Inventory, 96112-96116
Miscarriage
  Incomplete Abortion, 59812
  Missed Abortion
    First Trimester, 59820
    Second Trimester, 59821
  Septic Abortion, 59830
Missed Abortion
  First Trimester, 59820
  Second Trimester, 59821
Mitochondrial Antibody, 86255, 86256, 86381
Mitochondrial Genome Deletions, 81405
Mitogen Blastogenesis, 86353
Mitral Valve
  Implantation or Replacement
    Percutaneous, 0483T
    Transthoracic, 0484T
  Incision, 33420, 33422
  Repair, 33420-33427
    Incision, 33420, 33422
    Transcatheter, 0345T, 33418-33419, 93590, 93592
  Replacement, 33430
Mitrofanoff Operation, 50845
Miyagawanella
  See Chlamydia
  Antibody, 86631-86632
  Antigen Detection
    Direct Fluorescence, 87270
    Enzyme Immunoassay, 87320
  Culture, 87110
MLB Test, 92562
MLC, 86821
MLH1, 81432-81433, 81435-81436, *[81288, 81292, 81293, 81294]*
MLL/AFF1 (t(4;11)), 81401
MLL/MLLT3 (t(9;11)), 81401
MMAA, 81405
MMAB, 81405
MMACHC, 81404
MMK, 51841
MMPI, 96112-96116
  Computer Assisted, 96130-96131, 96136-96139, 96146
MMR Vaccine, 90707
MMRV, 90710
Mobilization
  Splenic Flexure, 44139
    Laparoscopic, 44213
  Stapes, 69650
Model
  3D Printed, Anatomic, 0559T-0560T
Moderate Sedation, 99151-99157
Modified Radical Mastectomy, 19307

Modulation System, Cardiac, 0408T-0418T
Mohs Micrographic Surgery, 17311-17315
Molar Pregnancy
  Evacuation and Curettage, 59870
  Excision, 59100
Mold
  Culture, 87107
Mole, Carneous
  See Abortion
Mole, Hydatid
  Evacuation and Curettage, 59870
  Excision, 59100
Molecular
  Cytogenetics, 88271-88275
    Interpretation and Report, 88291
  Fluorescent Imaging
    Nevus, 0700T-0701T
  MAAA
    Administrative, 0002M-0004M, 0006M-0007M, 0011M-0018M
    Category I, 81490-81599 *[81500, 81503, 81504, 81522, 81540, 81546, 81595, 81596]*
  Oxygen Saturation, 82803-82810
  Pathology
    Tier 1 Procedures, 81170-81383 *[81105, 81106, 81107, 81108, 81109, 81110, 81111, 81112, 81120, 81121, 81161, 81162, 81163, 81164, 81165, 81166, 81167, 81168, 81173, 81174, 81184, 81185, 81186, 81187, 81188, 81189, 81190, 81191, 81192, 81193, 81194, 81200, 81201, 81202, 81203, 81204, 81205, 81206, 81207, 81208, 81209, 81210, 81219, 81227, 81230, 81231, 81233, 81234, 81238, 81239, 81245, 81246, 81250, 81257, 81258, 81259, 81261, 81262, 81263, 81264, 81265, 81266, 81267, 81268, 81269, 81271, 81274, 81277, 81278, 81279, 81283, 81284, 81285, 81286, 81287, 81288, 81289, 81291, 81292, 81293, 81294, 81295, 81301, 81302, 81303, 81304, 81306, 81307, 81308, 81309, 81312, 81320, 81324, 81325, 81326, 81332, 81334, 81336, 81337, 81338, 81339, 81343, 81344, 81345, 81347, 81348, 81351, 81352, 81353, 81357, 81361, 81362, 81363, 81364]*
    Tier 2 Procedures, 81400-81408, *[81479]*
Molluscum Contagiosum Destruction
  Anus, 46900-46924
  Penis, 54050-54065
  Skin, 17110-17111
  Vulva, 56501-56515
Molteno Procedure, 66180
Molteno Valve
  Insertion, 66180
  Removal, 67120
  Revision, 66185
Monilia
  Antibody, 86628
  Skin Test, 86485
Monitoring
  Blood Pressure, 24 hour, 93784-93790
  Cardiac Rhythm, 33285-33286
  Electrocardiogram
    External, 93224-93272
  Electroencephalogram, 95812, 95813
    Long Term Set Up, *[95700, 95705, 95706, 95707, 95708, 95709, 95710, 95711, 95712, 95713, 95714, 95715, 95716, 95717, 95718, 95719, 95720, 95721, 95722, 95723, 95724, 95725, 95726]*
    with Drug Activation, 95954
    with Physical Activation, 95954
    with WADA Activation, 95958
  Fetal
    During Labor, 59050, 59051, 99500

Monitoring — *continued*
  Fetal — *continued*
    During Labor — *continued*
      Interpretation Only, 59051
  Glomerular Filtration Rate (GFR), 0603T
  Glucose
    Interstitial Fluid, 95250-95251, *[95249]*
  INR, 93792-93793
  Interstitial Fluid Pressure, 20950
  Intracardiac Ischemic Monitoring
    Insertion
      Electrode Only, 0526T
      Implantable Monitor Only, 0527T
      Monitoring System, 0525T
    Interrogation, 0529T
    Programming, 0528T
    Removal
      Complete System, 0530T
      Electrode Only, 0531T
      Implantable Monitor Only, 0532T
    Replacement, 0525T
  Intraocular Pressure, 0329T
  Pediatric Apnea, 94774-94777
  Prolonged, with Physician Attendance, 99354-99360
  Pulmonary Fluid System, 0607T, 0608T
  Seizure, 61531, 61760
  Therapeutic, Remote, 98975-98977
    Treatment Management Services, 98980-98981
Monitoring, Sleep, 95808-95811
Monoethylene Glycol, 82693
Mononuclear Cell Antigen
  Quantitative, 86356
Mononucleosis Virus, Infectious, 86663-86665
Monophosphate, Adenosine, 82030
Monophosphate, Adenosine Cyclic, 82030
Monospot Test, 86308
Monteggia Fracture, 24620, 24635
Monticelli Procedure, 20690, 20692
Morbilli
  See Rubeola
Morcellation Operation
  Hysterectomy, Vaginal, 58260-58270, 58550
Morphine Methyl Ether
  See Codeine
Morphometric Analysis
  Nerve, 88356
  Skeletal Muscle, 88355
  Tumor, 88358-88361
Morton's Neuroma
  Excision, 28080
Mosaicplasty, 27416, 29866-29867
Moschcowitz Operation
  Repair, Hernia, Femoral, 49550-49557
Mosenthal Test, 81002
Mother Cell
  See Stem Cell
Motility Study
  Colon, 91117
  Duodenal, 91022
  Esophagus, 91010, 91013
    Imaging, 78258
  Sperm, 89300
Motion Analysis
  by Video and 3D Kinematics, 96000, 96004
  Computer–Based, 96000, 96004
Motor Function Mapping Using nTMS, 64999
Mousseaux–Barbin Procedure, 43510
Mouth
  Abscess
    Incision and Drainage, 40800, 40801, 41005-41009, 41015-41018
  Biopsy, 40808, 41108
  Cyst
    Incision and Drainage, 40800, 40801, 41005-41009, 41015-41018
  Excision
    Frenum, 40819
  Hematoma
    Incision and Drainage, 40800, 40801, 41005-41009, 41015-41018
  Lesion
    Destruction, 40820
    Excision, 40810-40816, 41116

Mouth — *continued*
  Lesion — *continued*
    Vestibule of
      Destruction, 40820
      Repair, 40830
  Mucosa
    Excision, 40818
  Reconstruction, 40840-40845
  Removal
    Foreign Body, 40804, 40805
  Repair
    Laceration, 40830, 40831
  Skin Graft
    Full Thickness, 15240, 15241
    Pedicle Flap, 15574
    Split, 15120, 15121
  Tissue Transfer, Adjacent, 14040, 14041
  Unlisted Services and Procedures, 40899, 41599
  Vestibule
    Excision
      Destruction, 40808-40820
      Incision, 40800-40806
      Other Procedures, 40899
    Removal
      Foreign Body, 40804
    Repair, 40830-40845
Move
  See Transfer
  Finger, 26555
  Toe Joint, 26556
  Toe to Hand, 26551-26554
Movement Disorder Symptom Recording
  Complete Procedure, 0533T
  Data Upload, Analysis, Initial Report, 0535T
  Download Review, Interpretation, Report, 0536T
  Set-up, Training, Monitor Configuration, 0534T
MPI, 81405
MPL, *[81338], [81339]*
MPO, 83876
MPR (Multifetal Pregnancy Reduction), 59866
MPV17, 81404-81405
MPZ, 81405, *[81448]*
MR Spectroscopy
  See Magnetic Resonance Spectroscopy
MRA (Magnetic Resonance Angiography), 71555, 72159, 72198, 73225, 73725, 74185
MRCP (Magnetic Resonance Cholangiopancreatography), 74181
MRI (Magnetic Resonance Imaging)
  3D Rendering, 76376-76377
  Abdomen, 74181-74183
  Ankle, 73721-73723
  Arm, 73218-73220, 73223
  Bone Marrow Study, 77084
  Brain, 70551-70553
    Functional, 70554-70555
    Intraoperative, 0398T, 70557-70559
  Breast, 77046-77049
  Chest, 71550-71552
  Elbow, 73221
  Face, 70540-70543
  Fetal, 74712-74713
  Finger Joint, 73221
  Foot, 73718, 73719
  Foot Joints, 73721-73723
  Guidance
    Intracranial Stereotactic Ablation Lesion, 0398T
    Needle Placement, 77021
    Parenchymal Tissue Ablation, 77022
    Tissue Ablation, 77022
  Hand, 73218-73220, 73223
  Heart, 75557-75563
    Complete Study, 75557-75563, 75565
    Flow Mapping, 75565
    Morphology, 75557-75563
  Joint
    Lower Extremity, 73721-73723
    Upper Extremity, 73221-73223
  Knee, 73721-73723
  Leg, 73718-73720
  Neck, 70540-70543
  Orbit, 70540-70543
  Pelvis, 72195-72197

Nasal — *continued*
- Smear
  - Eosinophils, 89190
- Turbinate
  - Fracture
    - Therapeutic, 30930

Nasoethmoid Complex
- Fracture
  - Open Treatment, 21338, 21339
  - Percutaneous Treatment, 21340
- Reconstruction, 21182-21184

Nasogastric Tube
- Placement, 43752

Nasolacrimal Duct
- Exploration, 68810
  - with Anesthesia, 68811
- Insertion
  - Stent, 68815
- Probing, 68816
- X–ray
  - with Contrast, 70170

Nasomaxillary
- Fracture
  - Closed Treatment, 21345
  - Open Treatment, 21346-21348
    - with Bone Grafting, 21348

Nasopharynges
- *See* Nasopharynx

Nasopharyngoscopy, 92511
- Surgical
  - Dilation Eustachian Tube, 69705, 69706

Nasopharynx
- *See* Pharynx
- Biopsy, 42804, 42806
- Hemorrhage, 42970-42972
- Unlisted Services and Procedures, 42999

Natriuretic Peptide, 83880

Natural Killer Cells (NK)
- Total Count, 86357

Natural Ostium
- Sinus
  - Maxillary, 31000
  - Sphenoid, 31002

Navicular
- Arthroplasty
  - with Implant, 25443
- Fracture
  - Closed Treatment, 25622
  - Open Treatment, 25628
    - with Manipulation, 25624
- Repair, 25440

Navigation
- Computer Assisted, 20985, 61781-61783

NDP, 81403-81404
NDUFA1, 81404
NDUFAF2, 81404
NDUFS1, 81406
NDUFS4, 81404
NDUFS7, 81405
NDUFS8, 81405
NDUFV1, 81405

Near-Infrared
- Dual Imaging of Meibomian Glands, 0507T
- Spectroscopy Studies
  - Contact, 0493T
  - Noncontact, [0640T, 0641T, 0642T]

NEB, 81400, 81408

Neck
- Angiography, 70498, 70547-70549
- Artery
  - Ligation, 37615
- Biopsy, 21550
- Bypass Graft, 35901
- CT Scan, 70490-70492, 70498
- Dissection, Radical
  - *See* Radical Neck Dissection
- Exploration
  - Blood Vessels, 35800
  - Lymph Nodes, 38542
- Incision and Drainage
  - Abscess, 21501, 21502
  - Hematoma, 21501, 21502
- Lipectomy, Suction Assisted, 15876
- Magnetic Resonance Angiography (MRA), 70547-70549

Neck — *continued*
- Magnetic Resonance Imaging (MRI), 70540-70543
- Nerve
  - Graft, 64885, 64886
- Repair
  - Blood Vessel, 35201
    - with Other Graft, 35261
    - with Vein Graft, 35231
  - Rhytidectomy, 15825, 15828
- Skin
  - Revision, 15819
- Skin Graft
  - Delay of Flap, 15620
  - Full Thickness, 15240, 15241
  - Pedicle Flap, 15574
  - Split, 15120, 15121
- Surgery, Unlisted, 21899
- Tissue Transfer, Adjacent, 14040, 14041
- Tumor, 21555-21558 [21552, 21554]
- Ultrasound Exam, 76536
- Unlisted Services and Procedures, 21899
- Urinary Bladder
  - *See* Bladder, Neck
- Wound Exploration
  - Penetrating, 20100
- X–ray, 70360

Neck, Humerus
- Fracture
  - with Shoulder Dislocation
    - Closed Treatment, 23680
    - Open Treatment, 23675

Neck Muscle
- Division, Scalenus Anticus, 21700, 21705
- Sternocleidomastoid, 21720-21725

Necropsy
- Coroner Examination, 88045
- Forensic Examination, 88040
- Gross and Microscopic Examination, 88020-88029
- Gross Examination, 88000-88016
- Organ, 88037
- Regional, 88036
- Unlisted Services and Procedures, 88099

Needle Biopsy
- *See* Biopsy
- Abdomen Mass, 49180
- Bone, 20220, 20225
- Bone Marrow, 38221
- Breast, 19100
- Colon
  - Endoscopy, 45392
- Colon Sigmoid
  - Endoscopy, 45342
- CT Scan Guidance, 77012
- Epididymis, 54800
- Esophagus
  - Endoscopy, 43232, 43238
- Fluoroscopic Guidance, 77002
- Gastrointestinal, Upper
  - Endoscopy, 43238, 43242
- Kidney, 50200
- Liver, 47000, 47001
- Lung, 32408
- Lymph Node, 38505
- Mediastinum, 32408
- Muscle, 20206
- Pancreas, 48102
- Pleura, 32400
- Prostate, 55700
  - with Fluorescence Spectroscopy, 0443T
- Retroperitoneal Mass, 49180
- Salivary Gland, 42400
- Spinal Cord, 62269
- Testis, 54500
- Thyroid Gland, 60100
- Transbronchial, 31629, 31633

Needle Insertion, Dry, [20560, 20561]

Needle Localization
- Breast
  - Placement, 19281-19288
    - with Biopsy, 19081-19086
    - with Lesion Excision, 19125, 19126
  - Magnetic Resonance Guidance, 77021

Needle Manometer Technique, 20950

Needle Wire
- Introduction
  - Trachea, 31730
- Placement
  - Breast, 19281-19288

Neer Procedure, 23470

NEFL, 81405

Negative Pressure Wound Therapy (NPWT), 97605-97608

Neisseria Gonorrhoeae, 87590-87592, 87850

Neisseria Meningitidis
- Antibody, 86741

Neoblader
- Construction, 51596

Neonatal Alloimmune Thrombocytopenia [NAIT], [81105, 81106, 81107, 81108, 81109, 81110, 81111, 81112]

Neonatal Critical Care, 99468-99469

Neonatal Intensive Care
- *See* Newborn Care
- Initial, 99477-99480
- Subsequent, 99478-99480

Neoplasm
- See Tumor

Neoplastic Growth
- *See* Tumor

Nephelometry, 83883

Nephrectomy
- Donor, 50300, 50320, 50547
- Laparoscopic, 50545-50548
- Partial, 50240
  - Laparoscopic, 50543
- Recipient, 50340
- with Ureters, 50220-50236, 50546, 50548

Nephrolith
- *See* Calculus, Removal, Kidney

Nephrolithotomy, 50060-50075

Nephropexy, 50400, 50405

Nephroplasty
- *See* Kidney, Repair

Nephropyeloplasty, 50400-50405, 50544

Nephrorrhaphy, 50500

Nephroscopy
- *See* Endoscopy, Kidney

Nephrostogram, [50430, 50431]

Nephrostolithotomy
- Percutaneous, 50080, 50081

Nephrostomy
- Change Tube, [50435]
  - with Drainage, 50400
- Closure, 53899
- Endoscopic, 50562-50570
  - with Exploration, 50045
- Percutaneous, 52334

Nephrostomy Tract
- Establishment, [50436, 50437]

Nephrotomogram
- *See* Nephrotomography

Nephrotomography, 74415

Nephrotomy, 50040, 50045
- with Exploration, 50045

Nerve
- Cranial
  - *See* Cranial Nerve
- Facial
  - *See* Facial Nerve
- Foot
  - Incision, 28035
- Intercostal
  - *See* Intercostal Nerve
- Median
  - *See* Median Nerve
- Obturator
  - *See* Obturator Nerve
- Peripheral
  - *See* Peripheral Nerve
- Phrenic
  - *See* Phrenic Nerve
- Sciatic
  - *See* Sciatic Nerve
- Spinal
  - *See* Spinal Nerve
- Tibial
  - *See* Tibial Nerve
- Ulnar
  - *See* Ulnar Nerve

Nerve — *continued*
- Vestibular
  - *See* Vestibular Nerve

Nerve Conduction
- Motor and/or Sensory, 95905-95913

Nerve II, Cranial
- *See* Optic Nerve

Nerve Root
- *See* Cauda Equina; Spinal Cord
- Decompression, 62380, 63020-63048, 63055-63103
- Incision, 63185, 63190
- Section, 63185, 63190

Nerve Stimulation, Transcutaneous
- *See* Application, Neurostimulation

Nerve Teasing, 88362

Nerve V, Cranial
- *See* Trigeminal Nerve

Nerve VII, Cranial
- *See* Facial Nerve

Nerve X, Cranial
- *See* Vagus Nerve

Nerve XI, Cranial
- *See* Accessory Nerve

Nerve XII, Cranial
- *See* Hypoglossal Nerve

Nerves
- Anastomosis
  - Facial to Hypoglossal, 64868
  - Facial to Spinal Accessory, 64866
- Avulsion, 64732-64772
- Biopsy, 64795
- Cryoablation, Percutaneous, 0440T-0442T
- Decompression, 62380, 64702-64727
- Destruction, 64600-64681 [64633, 64634, 64635, 64636]
  - Intraosseous Basivertebral, [64628], [64629]
  - Paravertebral Facet Joint, [64633, 64634, 64635, 64636]
- Foot
  - Excision, 28055
  - Incision, 28035
- Graft, 64885-64907
- Implantation
  - Electrode, 64553-64581
  - to Bone, 64787
  - to Muscle, 64787
- Incision, 43640, 43641, 64732-64772
- Injection
  - Anesthetic or Steroid, 01991-01992, 64400-64530
  - Neurolytic Agent, 64600-64681 [64633, 64634, 64635, 64636]
- Insertion
  - Electrode, 64553-64581
- Lesion
  - Excision, 64774-64792
- Neurofibroma
  - Excision, 64788-64792
- Neurolemmoma
  - Excision, 64788-64792
- Neurolytic
  - Internal, 64727
- Neuroma
  - Excision, 64774-64786
- Neuroplasty, 64702-64721
- Nuclear Medicine
  - Unlisted Services and Procedures, 78699
- Removal
  - Electrode, 64585
- Repair
  - Graft, 64885-64911
  - Microdissection
    - with Surgical Microscope, 69990
  - Suture, 64831-64876
- Spinal Accessory
  - Incision, 63191
  - Section, 63191
- Suture, 64831-64876
- Sympathectomy
  - Excision, 64802-64818
- Transection, 43640, 43641, 64732-64772
- Transposition, 64718-64721
- Unlisted Services and Procedures, 64999

ORIF — *continued*
Fracture — *continued*
Ulna, Ulnar — *continued*
Shaft — *continued*
or Radial, Radius, 25574
Vertebral, 22325-22328
Zygomatic Arch, 21365-21366

Ormond Disease
Ureterolysis, 50715

Orogastric Tube
Placement, 43752

Oropharynx
Biopsy, 42800

Orthodontic Cephalogram, 70350

Orthomyxoviridae
Antibody, 86710
by Immunoassay with Direct Optical Observation, 87804

Orthomyxovirus, 86710, 87804

Orthopantogram, 70355

Orthopedic Cast
See Cast

Orthopedic Surgery
Computer Assisted Navigation, 20985
Stereotaxis
Computer Assisted, 20985

Orthoptic Training, 92065

Orthoroentgenogram, 77073

Orthosis/Orthotics
Management/Training, 97760, 97763

Os Calcis Fracture
Open Treatment, 28415-28420
Percutaneous Fixation, 28406
with Manipulation, 28405-28406
without Manipulation, 28400

Oscillometry, 94728

Osmolality
Blood, 83930
Urine, 83935

Osseous Survey, 77074-77076

Osseous Tissue
See Bone

Ossicles
Excision
Stapes
with Footplate Drill Out, 69661
without Foreign Material, 69660-69661
Reconstruction
Ossicular Chain
Tympanoplasty with Antrotomy or Mastoidotomy, 69636-69637
Tympanoplasty with Mastoidectomy, 69642, 69644, 69646
Tympanoplasty without Mastoidectomy, 69632-69633
Release
Stapes, 69650
Replacement
with Prosthesis, 69633, 69637

OST, 59020

Ostectomy
Carpal, 25215
Femur, 27365
Humerus, 24999
Metacarpal, 26250
Metatarsal, 28288
Phalanges
Fingers, 26260-26262
Pressure Ulcer
Ischial, 15941, 15945
Sacral, 15933, 15935, 15937
Trochanteric, 15951, 15953, 15958
Radius, 25999
Scapula, 23190
Sternum, 21620
Ulna, 25999

Osteocalcin, 83937

Osteocartilaginous Exostosis
Auditory Canal
Excision, 69140

Osteochondroma
Auditory Canal
Excision, 69140

Osteoclasis
Carpal, 26989
Clavicle, 23929
Femur, 27599
Humerus, 24999
Metacarpal, 26989
Metatarsal, 28899
Patella, 27599
Radius, 26989
Scapula, 23929
Tarsal, 28899
Thorax, 23929
Ulna, 26989

Osteocutaneous Flap
with Microvascular Anastomosis, 20969-20973

Osteoma
Sinusotomy
Frontal, 31075

Osteomyelitis
Excision
Clavicle, 23180
Facial, 21026
Femur, 27360
Fibula
Distal, 27641
Proximal, 27360
Humerus, 24140
Proximal, 23184
Mandible, 21025
Metacarpal, 26230
Olecranon Process, 24147
Pelvis/Hip Joint
Deep, 27071
Superficial, 27070
Phalanx (Finger)
Phalanx (Toe), 28124
Distal, 26236
Proximal or Middle, 26235
Radial Head/Neck, 24145
Scapula, 23182
Talus/Calcaneus, 28120
Tarsal/Metatarsal, 28122
Tibia
Distal, 27640
Proximal, 27360
Ulna, 25150
Incision
Elbow, 23935
Femur, 27303
Foot, 28005
Forearm, 25035
Hand/Finger, 26034
Hip Joint, 26992
Humerus, 23935
Knee, 27303
Leg/Ankle, 27607
Pelvis, 26992
Shoulder, 23035
Thorax, 21510
Wrist, 25035
Sequestrectomy
Clavicle, 23170
Forearm, 25145
Humeral Head, 23174
Humerus, Shaft or Distal, 24134
Olecranon Process, 24138
Radial Head/Neck, 24136
Scapula, 23172
Skull, 61501
Wrist, 25145

Osteopathic Manipulation, 98925-98929

Osteophytectomy, 63075-63078

Osteoplasty
Carpal Bone, 25394
Facial Bones
Augmentation, 21208
Reduction, 21209
Femoral Neck, 27179
Femur, 27179
Lengthening, 27466-27468
Shortening, 27465, 27468
Fibula
Lengthening, 27715
Humerus, 24420
Metacarpal, 26568

Osteoplasty — *continued*
Phalanges
Finger, 26568
Toe, 28299, 28310-28312
Radius, 25390-25393
Tibia
Lengthening, 27715
Ulna, 25390-25393
Vertebra
Cervicothoracic, 22510, 22512
Lumbosacral, 22511-22512

Osteotomy
Blount, 27455, 27475-27485
Calcaneus, 28300
Chin, 21121-21123
Clavicle, 23480-23485
Femur
Femoral Neck, 27161
for Slipped Epiphysis, 27181
Greater Trochanter, 27140
with Fixation, 27165
with Open Reduction of Hip, 27156
with Realignment, 27454
without Fixation, 27448-27450
Fibula, 27707-27712
Hip, 27146-27156
Femoral
with Open Reduction, 27156
Femur, 27151
Humerus, 24400-24410
with Intramedullary Lengthening, 0594T
Mandible, 21198-21199
Extraoral, 21047
Intraoral, 21046
Maxilla, 21206
Extraoral, 21049
Intraoral, 21048
Metacarpal, 26565
Metatarsal, 28306-28309
Orbit Reconstruction, 21256
Patella
Wedge, 27448
Pelvis, 27158
Pemberton, 27147
Periorbital
Orbital Hypertelorism, 21260-21263
Osteotomy with Graft, 21267-21268
Phalanges
Finger, 26567
Toe, 28299, 28310-28312
Radius
and Ulna, 25365, 25375
Distal Third, 25350
Middle or Proximal Third, 25355
Multiple, 25370
Salter, 27146
Skull Base, 61582-61585, 61592
Spine
Anterior, 22220-22226
Posterior/Posterolateral, 22210-22214
Cervical, 22210
Each Additional Vertebral Segment, 22208, 22216
Lumbar, 22207, 22214
Thoracic, 22206, 22212
Three-Column, 22206-22208
Talus, 28302
Tarsal, 28304-28305
Tibia, 27455-27457, 27705, 27709-27712
Ulna, 25360
and Radius, 25365, 25375
Multiple, 25370
Vertebra
Additional Segment
Anterior Approach, 22226
Posterior/Posterolateral Approach, 22208, 22216
Cervical
Anterior Approach, 22220
Posterior/Posterolateral Approach, 22210
Lumbar
Anterior Approach, 22224
Posterior/Posterolateral Approach, 22214

Osteotomy — *continued*
Vertebra — *continued*
Thoracic
Anterior Approach, 22222
Posterior/Posterolateral Approach, 22212
with Graft
Reconstruction
Periorbital Region, 21267-21268

OTC, 81405

Other Nonoperative Measurements and Examinations
Acid Perfusion
Esophagus, 91013, 91030
Acid Reflux
Esophagus, 91034-91035, 91037-91038
Attenuation Measurements
Ear Protector, 92596
Bernstein Test, 91030
Breath Hydrogen, 91065
Bronchial Challenge Testing, 95070
Gastric Motility (Manometric) Studies, 91020
Iontophoresis, 97033
Laryngeal Function Studies, 92520
Manometry
Anorectal, 91122
Esophageal, 91010
Photography
Anterior Segment, 92286
External Ocular, 92285

Otoacoustic Emission Evaluation, 92587-92588

Otolaryngology
Diagnostic
Exam Under Anesthesia, 92502

Otomy
See Incision

Otoplasty, 69300

Otorhinolaryngology
Diagnostic
Otolaryngology Exam, 92502
Unlisted Services and Procedures, 92700

Ouchterlony Immunodiffusion, 86331

Outer Ear
CT Scan, 70480-70482

Outpatient Visit, 99202-99215

Output, Cardiac
by Indicator Dilution, 93598

Ova
Smear, 87177

Oval Window
Repair Fistula, 69666

Oval Window Fistula
Repair, 69666

Ovarian Cyst
Excision, 58925
Incision and Drainage, 58800-58805

Ovarian Vein Syndrome
Ureterolysis, 50722

Ovariectomies, 58940-58943
for Ectopic Pregnancy, 59120, 59151
with Hysterectomy, 58262-58263, 58291-58292, 58542, 58544, 58552, 58554, 58571, 58573

Ovariolysis, 58740

Ovary
Abscess
Incision and Drainage, 58820-58822
Abdominal Approach, 58822
Vaginal Approach, 58820
Biopsy, 58900
Cryopreservation, 88240
Cyst
Incision and Drainage, 58800-58805
Ovarian, 58805
Excision, 58662, 58720
Cyst, 58925
Partial
Oophorectomy, 58661, 58940
Ovarian Malignancy, 58943
Peritoneal Malignancy, 58943
Tubal Malignancy, 58943
Wedge Resection, 58920
Total, 58940-58943
Laparoscopy, 58660-58662, 58679
Lysis
Adhesions, 58660, 58740

Penis — continued
Replacement — continued
Prosthesis — continued
Semi–Rigid, 54416-54417
Replantation, 54438
Revascularization, 37788
Rigidity Test, 54250
Test Erection, 54250
Unlisted Services and Procedures, 54699, 55899
Venous Studies, 93980-93981

Penis Adhesions
Lysis
Post–circumcision, 54162

Penis Prostheses
See Penile Prosthesis

Pentagastrin Test, 43755-43757

Pentamidine
Inhalation Treatment, 94640-94644

Peptidase P
Angiotensin Converting Enzyme (ACE), 82164

Peptidase S
Leucine Aminopeptidase, 83670

Peptide, Connecting, 80432, 84681

Peptide, Vasoactive Intestinal, 84586

Peptidyl Dipeptidase A
Angiotensin Converting Enzyme (ACE), 82164

Percutaneous
Access, Biliary, 47541
Aspiration
Bartholin's Gland, 10160
Gallbladder, 47999
Seminal Vesicle, 54699, 55899
Atherectomies, 0234T-0238T, 37225, 37227, 37229, 37231, 37233, 37235
Biopsy, Gallbladder/Bile Ducts, 47553
Cardiopulmonary Bypass, 33999
Cystostomy, 51100-51102, 53899
Discectomies, 62287
Electric Nerve Stimulation
Electrode Insertion, 64553-64566
Injection
Intervertebral Disc, Lumbar, 0627T, 0628T, 0629T, 0630T
Laminotomy/Laminectomy for Decompression
Neural Elements, 0274T-0275T
Lumbar Discectomy, 62287
Lysis of Adhesions
Epidural, 62263-62264
Nephrostomies, 52334, [50436, 50437]
Transcatheter
Interatrial Septal Shunt, 0613T
Ultrasound Ablation, 0632T
Transluminal Angioplasty
Aortic, 33897, [37246, 37247]
Brachiocephalic, [37246, 37247]
Coronary Artery, [92920, 92921]
with Atherectomy, [92924, 92925], [92933, 92934, 92937, 92938, 92941, 92943, 92944]
with Stent, [92928, 92929, 92933, 92934, 92937, 92938, 92941, 92943, 92944]
Femoral, Popliteal, 37224-37227
Iliac, 37220-37223
Pulmonary, 92997, 92998
Renal, [37246, 37247]
Tibioperoneal, 37228-37235
Vein, [37248, 37249]
Visceral, [37246, 37247]
Vertebral Augmentation, 22513-22515
Vertebroplasty, 22510-22512

Pereyra Procedure, 51845, 57289, 58267

Performance Measures
See Also Physician Quality Reporting System (PQRS)
ACE Inhibitor Therapy, 4010F
Acute Otitis
Examination
Membrane Mobility, 2035F
History
Auricular Pain, 1116F
Intervention
Antimicrobial Therapy, 4131F-4132F

Performance Measures — continued
Acute Otitis — continued
Intervention — continued
Effusion Antihistamines, 4133F-4134F
Systemic Antimicrobials, 4131F-4132F
Systemic Steroids, 4135F-4136F
Topical Therapy, 4130F
Anginal Symptom Assessment, 1002F
Antiplatelet Therapy, 4011F
Aortic Aneurysm, 9001F-9004F
Beta–Blocker Therapy, 4008F
Blood Pressure, 2000F
Postpartum Care Visit, 0503F
Prenatal Care Visit Initial, 0500F
Prenatal Care Visit Subsequent, 0502F
Prenatal Flow Sheet, 0501F
Carotid Stenosis, 9005F-9007F
Statin Therapy, 4013F
Tobacco Use
Assessment, 1000F, 1034F-1036F
Counseling, 4000F
Pharmacologic Therapy, 4001F

Performance Test
See Also Physical Medicine/Therapy/Occupational Therapy
Cognitive, 96112-96116 [96127], 96121, [96125]
Performance Test Physical Therapy, 97750
Psychological Test, 96112-96146

Perfusion
Brain
Imaging, 0042T
Myocardial, 78451-78454
Imaging, 0439T, 78466-78469
Positron Emission Tomography (PET)
Myocardial Imaging, 78491-78492
Pulmonary, 78580, 78582, 78597-78598

Perfusion, Intracranial Arterial
Percutaneous, 61645
Thrombolysis, 61624

Perfusion Pump
See Infusion Pump

Pericardectomies, 33030-33031
Endoscopic, 32659

Pericardial Cyst
See Cyst, Pericardial
Excision, 33050
Thoracoscopic, 32661

Pericardial Sac
Biopsy, 32604
Drainage, 32659

Pericardial Window
for Drainage, 33025
Thoracoscopic, 32659

Pericardiectomy
Complete, 33030-33031
Subtotal, 33030-33031

Pericardiocentesis, 33016-33019

Pericardiostomy
Tube, 33017-33019

Pericardiotomy
Removal
Clot/Foreign Body, 33020
via Thoracoscopy, 32658

Pericardium
Cyst
Excision, 32661, 33050
Excision, 32659, 33030-33031
Incision, 33030-33031
Removal
Clot, 33020
Foreign Body, 33020
with Tube, 33017-33019
Incision and Drainage, 33025
Puncture Aspiration, 33016-33019
Removal
Clot
Endoscopic, 32658
Foreign Body
Endoscopic, 32658
Tumor
Excision, 32661, 33050

Peridural Anesthesia
See Anesthesia, Epidural

Peridural Injection, 62281-62282, 62320-62327, 64479-64484

Perineal Prostatectomy
Partial, 55801
Radical, 55810-55815

Perineoplasty, 56810

Perineorrhaphy
Repair
Rectocele, 57250

Perineum
Abscess
Incision and Drainage, 56405
Biopsy, 56605-56606
Colposcopy, 99170
Debridement
Infected, 11004, 11006
Removal
Prosthesis, 53442
Repair, 56810
X–ray with Contrast, 74775

Perionychia, 10060-10061

Periorbital Region
Reconstruction–Osteotomy
with Graft, 21267-21268
Repair–Osteotomy, 21260-21263

Peripheral Artery Disease (PAD) Rehabilitation, 93668

Peripheral Blood Stem Cell Transplant, 38240-38242

Peripheral Nerve
Repair/Suture
Major, 64856, 64859

Periprostatic Placement Biodegradable Material
Transperineal, 55874

Periprosthetic Capsulotomy
Breast, 19371

Peristaltic Pumps
See Infusion Pump

Peritoneal Dialysis, 4055F, 90945-90947
Kt/V Level, 3082F-3084F
Training
Counseling, 90989, 90993

Peritoneal Free Air, 49400

Peritoneal Lavage, 49084

Peritoneoscopy
Biopsy, 49321
Exploration, 49320

Peritoneum
Abscess
Incision and Drainage, 49020
Chemotherapy Administration, 96446
Exchange
Drainage Catheter, 49423
Injection
Contrast
Via Catheter, 49424
Laparoscopic
Drainage
Lymphocele, 49323
Ligation
Shunt, 49428
Removal
Cannula
Catheter, 49422
Foreign Body, 49402
Shunt, 49429
Tumor
Resection, 58950-58954
Unlisted Services and Procedures, 49999
Venous Shunt, 49427
X–ray, 74190

Persistent, Omphalomesenteric Duct
Excision, 44800

Persistent Truncus Arteriosus
See Truncus Arteriosus
Repair, 33786

Personal Care
See Self Care

Personality Test, 96112-96121

Pertussis Immunization, 90715, 90723

Pessary
Insertion, 57160

Pesticides
Chlorinated Hydrocarbons, 82441

PET Scan
See Also Specific Site; Nuclear Medicine

PET Scan — continued
Brain, 78608-78609
Heart, 78414
Absolute Quantitation, [78434]
Blood Pool Imaging, 78472-78473, 78481, 78483, 78494, 78496
Myocardial Imaging, 78459, 78466-78469, [78429]
Myocardial Perfusion, 0439T, 78451-78454, 78491-78492 [78430, 78431, 78432, 78433, 78434]
Limited Area, 78811
Skull Base to Mid-thigh, 78812
Whole Body, 78813
with Computed Tomography (CT)
Limited Area, 78814
Skull Base to Mid-thigh, 78815
Whole Body, 78816

Petrous Temporal
Excision
Apex, 69530

Peyronie Disease
Injection, 54200
Surgical Exposure, 54205
with Graft, 54110-54112

PFG (Percutaneous Fluoroscopic Gastrostomy), 49440

PFT (Pulmonary Function Test), 94010-94799

PG, 84081, 84150

pH
Blood Gases, 82800-82805
Body Fluid, Not Otherwise Specified, 83986
Exhaled Breath Condensate, 83987

Phacoemulsification
Removal
Extracapsular Cataract, 66982, 66983, 66984, [66987], [66988]
Secondary Membranous Cataract, 66850

Phagocytosis
White Blood Cells, 86344

Phalangectomy
Toe, 28150
Partial, 28160

Phalanges (Hand)
See Also Finger, Bone
Incision, Bone Cortex, 26034

Phalanx, Finger
Craterization, 26235, 26236
Cyst
Excision, 26210, 26215
Diaphysectomy, 26235, 26236
Excision, 26235, 26236
Radical
for Tumor, 26260-26262
Fracture
Articular
Closed Treatment, 26740
Open Treatment, 26746
with Manipulation, 26742
Distal, 26755, 26756
Closed Treatment, 26750
Open Treatment, 26765
Percutaneous, 26756
Open Treatment, 26735
Distal, 26765
Percutaneous Fixation, 26756
Shaft, 26720-26727
Open Treatment, 26735
Incision and Drainage, 26034
Ostectomy
Radical
for Tumor, 26260-26262
Repair
Lengthening, 26568
Nonunion, 26546
Osteotomy, 26567
Saucerization, 26235, 26236
Thumb
Fracture
Shaft, 26720-26727
Tumor, 26115-26118 [26111, 26113], 26210-26215, 26260-26262

Phalanx, Great Toe
See Also Phalanx, Toe
Fracture
Closed Treatment, 28490

Phalanx, Great Toe — *continued*
  Fracture — *continued*
    Closed Treatment — *continued*
      with Manipulation, 28495
      Open Treatment, 28505
      Percutaneous Skeletal Fixation, 28496
Phalanx, Toe
  Condyle
    Excision, 28126
  Craterization, 28124
  Cyst
    Excision, 28108
  Diaphysectomy, 28124
  Excision, 28124, 28150-28160
  Fracture
    Open Treatment, 28525
    with Manipulation, 28515
    without Manipulation, 28510
  Repair
    Osteotomy, 28310, 28312
  Saucerization, 28124
  Tumor
    Excision, 28108, 28175
Pharmaceutic Preparations
  See Drug
Pharmacotherapies
  See Chemotherapy
Pharyngeal Tonsil
  Excision, 42830-42836
    with Tonsils, 42820-42821
  Unlisted Services/Procedures, 42999
Pharyngectomy
  Partial, 42890
Pharyngolaryngectomy, 31390, 31395
Pharyngoplasty, 42950
Pharyngorrhaphy, 42900
Pharyngostomy, 42955
Pharyngotomy
  See Incision, Pharynx
Pharyngotympanic Tube
  Inflation
    with Myringotomy, 69420-69421
Pharynx
  See Also Nasopharynx; Throat
  Biopsy, 42800-42806
  Cineradiography, 70371, 74230
  Creation
    Stoma, 42955
  Excision, 42145
    Partial, 42890
    Resection, 42892, 42894
    with Larynx, 31390, 31395
  Hemorrhage, 42960-42962
  Lesion
    Destruction, 42808
    Excision, 42808
  Reconstruction, 42950
  Removal, Foreign Body, 42809
  Repair
    with Esophagus, 42953
  Unlisted Services and Procedures, 42999
  Video, 70371, 74230
  X-ray, 70370, 74210
Phencyclidine, *[83992]*
Phenobarbital, *[80345]*
  Assay, 80184
Phenothiazine, *[80342, 80343, 80344]*
Phenotype Analysis
  by Nucleic Acid
    Infectious Agent
      HIV-1 Drug Resistance, 87903, 87904
Phenotype Prediction
  by Generic Database
    HIV-1
      Drug Susceptibility, 87900
  Using Regularly Updated Genotypic Bioinformatics, 87900
Phenylalanine, 84030
Phenylalanine-Tyrosine Ratio, 84030
Phenylketones, 84035
Phenylketonuria, 84030
  Genomic Sequence Analysis, *[81443]*
Phenytoin
  Assay, 80185, 80186
Pheochromocytoma, 80424

Pheresis, 36511-36516
PHEX, 81406
Phlebectasia
  Ablation, 36473-36479
  Removal, 37718-37735, 37765-37785
    with Tissue Excision, 37735-37760
Phlebectomy
  Stab, 37765-37766
Phlebographies, 75820-75880, 75885, 75893, 78445, 78457-78458
  Injection, 36005
Phleborrhaphy
  Femoral, 37650
  Iliac, 37660
Phlebotomy
  Therapeutic, 99195
Phonocardiogram
  Evaluation, 93799
  Intracardiac, 93799
  Tracing, 93799
Phoria
  See Strabismus
Phosphatase
  Alkaline, 84075, 84080
    Blood, 84078
Phosphatase, Acid, 84060
  Blood, 84066
Phosphate, Pyridoxal, 84207
Phosphatidyl Glycerol, 84081
Phosphatidylcholine Cholinephosphohydrolase
  See Tissue Typing
Phosphatidylglycerol, 84081
Phosphocreatine Phosphotransferase, ADP, 82550-82552
Phosphogluconate-6
  Dehydrogenase, 84085
Phosphoglycerides, Glycerol, 84081
Phosphohexose Isomerase, 84087
Phosphohydrolases
  Alkaline, 84075-84080
Phosphokinase, Creatine, 82550-82552
Phospholipase C
  See Tissue Typing
  C Gamma 2, *[81320]*
Phospholipid
  Antibody, 86147-86148
  Neutralization, 85598
Phosphomonoesterase, 84075-84080
Phosphoric Monoester Hydrolases, 84075-84080
Phosphorous, 84100
  Urine, 84105
Phosphotransferase, ADP Phosphocreatine, 82550-82552
Photo Patch
  Allergy Test, 95052
    See Also Allergy Tests
Photochemotherapies, Extracorporeal, 36522
Photochemotherapy, 96910-96913
  See Also Dermatology
  Endoscopic Light, 96570-96571
Photocoagulation
  Endolaser Panretinal
    Vitrectomy, 67040
  Focal Endolaser
    Vitrectomy, 67040
  Iridoplasty, 66762
  Lesion
    Choroid, 67220
    Cornea, 65450
    Retina, 67210, 67228, 67229
  Retinal Detachment
    Prophylaxis, 67145
    Repair, 67105, 67107, 67108, 67113
  Retinopathy, 67228-67229
Photodynamic Therapy
  Choroidal Lesions Eye, 67221, 67225
  External, 96567, 96573-96574
Photography
  Ocular
    Anterior Segment, 92286, 92287
    External, 92285
    Fundus, 92250
  Skin, Diagnostic, 96904
Photopheresis
  Extracorporeal, 36522

Photophoresis
  See Actinotherapy; Photochemotherapy
Photoradiation Therapies
  See Actinotherapy
Photoscreen
  Ocular, 99174
Photosensitivity Testing, 95056
  See Also Allergy Tests
Phototherapies
  See Actinotherapy
Phototherapy, Ultraviolet, 96900
PHOX2B, 81403-81404
Phrenic Nerve
  Avulsion, 64746
  Incision, 64746
  Injection
    Anesthetic or Steroid, 64999
  Transection, 64746
Physical Examination
  Office and/or Other Outpatient Services, 99202-99215
Physical Medicine/Therapy/Occupational Therapy
  See Also Neurology, Diagnostic
  Activities of Daily Living, 97535, 99509
  Aquatic Therapy
    with Exercises, 97113
  Athletic Training
    Evaluation, *[97169, 97170, 97171]*
    Re-evaluation, *[97172]*
  Cognitive Skills Development, 97129-97130
  Community/Work Reintegration, 97537
  Evaluation, *[97161, 97162, 97163, 97164, 97165, 97166, 97167, 97168, 97169, 97170, 97171, 97172]*
  Hydrotherapy
    Hubbard Tank, 97036
    Pool with Exercises, 97036, 97113
  Joint Mobilization, 97140
  Kinetic Therapy, 97530
  Manipulation, 97140
  Manual Therapy, 97140
  Modalities
    Contrast Baths, 97034
    Diathermy Treatment, 97024
    Electric Stimulation
      Attended, Manual, 97032
      Unattended, 97014
    Hot or Cold Pack, 97010
    Hydrotherapy (Hubbard Tank), 97036
    Infrared Light Treatment, 97026
    Iontophoresis, 97033
    Microwave Therapy, 97024
    Paraffin Bath, 97018
    Traction, 97012
    Ultrasound, 97035
    Ultraviolet Light, 97028
    Unlisted Services and Procedures, 97039
    Vasopneumatic Device, 97016
    Whirlpool Therapy, 97022
  Orthotics Training, 97760, 97763
  Osteopathic Manipulation, 98925-98929
  Procedures
    Aquatic Therapy, 97113
    Direct, 97032
    Gait Training, 97116
    Group Therapeutic, 97150
    Massage Therapy, 97124
    Neuromuscular Reeducation, 97112
    Physical Performance Test, 97750
    Supervised, 97010-97028
    Therapeutic Exercises, 4018F, 97110
    Traction Therapy, 97140
    Work Hardening, 97545, 97546
  Prosthetic Training, 97761
  Sensory Integration, 97533
  Therapeutic Activities, 97530
  Unlisted Services and Procedures, 97139, 97799
  Wheelchair Management, 97542
  Work Reintegration, 97537
Physical Therapy
  See Physical Medicine/Therapy/Occupational Therapy
Physician Services
  Care Plan Oversight Services, 99339-99340, 99374-99380

Physician Services — *continued*
  Care Plan Oversight Services — *continued*
    Domiciliary Facility, 99339-99340
    Home Health Agency Care, 99374
    Home/Rest Home Care, 99339-99340
    Hospice, 99377, 99378
    Nursing Facility, 99379, 99380
  Case Management Services, 99366-99368
  Direction, Advanced Life Support, 99288
  Online, *[99421, 99422, 99423]*
  Prolonged, *[99417]*
    with Direct Patient Contact, 99354-99357
      Outpatient Office, 99354, 99355
    with Direct Patient Services
      Inpatient, 99356, 99357
    without Direct Patient Contact, 99358, 99359
  Standby, 99360
  Supervision, Care Plan Oversight Services, 99339-99340, 99374-99380
  Team Conference, 99367
  Telephone, 99441-99443
Physiologic Recording of Tremor, 95999
PICC Line Insertion, 36568-36569, 36584, *[36572, 36573]*
Pierce Ears, 69090
Piercing of Ear Lobe, 69090
PIK3CA, *[81309]*
Piles
  See Hemorrhoids
Pilon Fracture Treatment, 27824
Pilonidal Cyst
  Excision, 11770-11772
  Incision and Drainage, 10080, 10081
Pin
  See Also Wire
  Insertion
    Removal
      Skeletal Traction, 20650
  Prophylactic Treatment
    Femur, 27187
    Humerus, 24498
    Shoulder, 23490, 23491
Pinch Graft, 15050
Pineal Gland
  Excision
    Partial, 60699
    Total, 60699
  Incision, 60699
PINK1, 81405
Pinna
  See Ear, External
Pinworms
  Examination, 87172
Pirogoff Procedure, 27888
Pituitary Epidermoid Tumor
  See Craniopharyngioma
Pituitary Fossa
  Exploration, 60699
Pituitary Gland
  Excision, 61546, 61548
  Incision, 60699
  Tumor
    Excision, 61546, 61548, 62165
Pituitary Growth Hormone
  See Growth Hormone
Pituitary Lactogenic Hormone
  See Prolactin
Pituitectomy
  See Excision, Pituitary Gland
PKD1, 81407
PKD2, 81406
PKHD1, 81408
PKLR, 81405
PKP, 65730-65755
PKP2, 81406, 81439
PKU, 84030
PL, 80418, 84146
PLA Codes
  See Proprietary Laboratory Analyses (PLA)
Placement
  Adjustable Gastric Restrictive Device, 43770
  Amniotic Membrane
    Ocular Surface, 65778-65779
  Aqueous Drainage Device, 0449T-0450T, 0474T, 66179-66185, *[0253T]*, *[0671T]*

Index

Proctosigmoidoscopy — Proprietary Laboratory Analysis (PLA)

Psoriasis Treatment — QSART

Radical Neck Dissection
- Laryngectomy, 31365-31368
- Pharyngolaryngectomy, 31390, 31395
- with Auditory Canal Surgery, 69155
- with Thyroidectomy, 60254
- with Tongue Excision, 41135, 41145, 41153, 41155

Radical Vaginal Hysterectomy, 58285
Radical Vulvectomy, 56630-56640
Radioactive Colloid Therapy, 79300
Radioactive Substance
- Insertion
  - Prostate, 55860

Radiocarpal Joint
- Arthrotomy, 25040
- Dislocation
  - Closed Treatment, 25660
  - Open Treatment, 25670

Radiocinematographies
- Esophagus, 74230
- Pharynx, 70371, 74230
- Speech Evaluation, 70371
- Swallowing Evaluation, 74230
- Unlisted Services and Procedures, 76120-76125

Radioelement
- Application, 77761-77772
  - Surface, 77789
    - with Ultrasound, 76965
  - Handling, 77790
  - Infusion, 77750
  - Placement
    - *See* Radioelement Substance

Radioelement Substance
- Catheter Placement
  - Breast, 19296-19298
  - Bronchus, 31643
  - Head and/or Neck, 41019
  - Muscle and/or Soft Tissue, 20555
  - Pelvic Organs or Genitalia, 55920
  - Prostate, 55875
- Catheterization, 55875
- Needle Placement
  - Head and/or Neck, 41019
  - Muscle and/or Soft Tissue, 20555
  - Pelvic Organs and Genitalia, 55920
  - Prostate, 55875

Radiofrequency Remodeling for Incontinence, 53860
- Endovaginal
  - Bladder Neck and Proximal Urethra, 0672T

Radiofrequency Spectroscopy
- Partial Mastectomy, 0546T

Radiography
- *See* Radiology, Diagnostic; X–ray

Radioimmunosorbent Test
- Gammaglobulin, Blood, 82784-82785

Radioisotope Brachytherapy
- *See* Brachytherapy

Radioisotope Scan
- *See* Nuclear Medicine

Radiological Marker
- Preoperative Placement
  - Excision of Breast Lesion, 19125, 19126

Radiology
- *See Also* Nuclear Medicine, Radiation Therapy, X–ray, Ultrasound
- Diagnostic
  - Unlisted Services and Procedures, 76499
  - Examination, 70030
    - Stress Views, 77071
  - Joint Survey, 77077
- Therapeutic
  - Field Set–up, 77280-77290
  - Planning, 77261-77263, 77299
  - Port Film, 77417

Radionuclide Therapy
- Heart, 79440
- Interstitial, 79300
- Intra–arterial, 79445
- Intra–articular, 79440
- Intracavitary, 79200
- Intravascular, 79101
- Intravenous, 79101, 79403
- Intravenous Infusion, 79101, 79403
- Oral, 79005

Radionuclide Therapy — *continued*
- Remote Afterloading, 77767-77768, 77770-77772
- Unlisted Services and Procedures, 79999

Radionuclide Tomography, Single–Photon Emission–Computed
- *See* Specific Site; Nuclear Medicine

Radiopharmaceutical Localization of Tumor, 78800-78803 *[78804, 78830, 78831, 78832]*, *[78835]*

Radiopharmaceutical Therapy
- Heart, 79440
- Interstitial, 79300
  - Colloid Administration, 79300
- Intra-arterial Particulate, 79445
- Intra–articular, 79440
- Intracavitary, 79200
- Intravascular, 79101
- Intravenous, 78808, 79101, 79403
- Oral, 79005
- Unlisted Services and Procedures, 79999

Radiostereometric Analysis
- Lower Extremity, 0350T
- Placement Interstitial Device, 0347T
- Spine, 0348T
- Upper Extremity, 0349T

Radiosurgery
- Cranial Lesion, 61796-61799
- Spinal Lesion, 63620-63621

Radiotherapeutic
- *See* Radiation Therapy

Radiotherapies
- *See* Irradiation

Radiotherapy
- Afterloading, 77767-77768, 77770-77772
  - Catheter Insertion, 19296-19298
  - Planning, 77316-77318

Radiotherapy, Surface, 77789

Radioulnar Joint
- Arthrodesis
  - with Ulnar Resection, 25830
- Dislocation
  - Closed Treatment, 25525, 25675
  - Open Treatment, 25676
  - Percutaneous Fixation, 25671

Radius
- *See Also* Arm, Lower; Elbow; Ulna
- Arthroplasty, 24365
  - with Implant, 24366, 25441
- Craterization, 24145, 25151
- Cyst
  - Excision, 24125, 24126, 25120-25126
- Diaphysectomy, 24145, 25151
- Dislocation
  - Partial, 24640
  - Subluxate, 24640
  - with Fracture
    - Closed Treatment, 24620
    - Open Treatment, 24635
- Excision, 24130, 24136, 24145, 24152
  - Epiphyseal Bar, 20150
  - Partial, 25145
  - Styloid Process, 25230
- Fracture, 25605
  - Closed Treatment, 25500, 25505, 25520, 25600, 25605
    - with Manipulation, 25605
    - without Manipulation, 25600
  - Colles, 25600, 25605
  - Distal, 25600-25609
    - Closed Treatment, 25600-25605
    - Open Treatment, 25607-25609
  - Head/Neck
    - Closed Treatment, 24650, 24655
    - Open Treatment, 24665, 24666
  - Open Treatment, 25515, 25525, 25526, 25574
  - Percutaneous Fixation, 25606
  - Shaft, 25500-25526
    - Open Treatment, 25515, 25574-25575
    - with Ulna, 25560, 25565
      - Open Treatment, 25575
- Implant
  - Removal, 24164
- Incision and Drainage, 25035

Radius — *continued*
- Osteomyelitis, 24136, 24145
- Osteoplasty, 25390-25393
- Prophylactic Treatment, 25490, 25492
- Repair
  - Epiphyseal Arrest, 25450, 25455
  - Epiphyseal Separation
    - Closed, 25600
    - Closed with Manipulation, 25605
    - Open Treatment, 25607, 25608-25609
    - Percutaneous Fixation, 25606
  - Malunion or Nonunion, 25400, 25415
  - Osteotomy, 25350, 25355, 25370, 25375 and Ulna, 25365
    - with Graft, 25405, 25420-25426
- Saucerization, 24145, 25151
- Sequestrectomy, 24136, 25145
- Subluxation, 24640
- Tumor
  - Cyst, 24120
  - Excision, 24125, 24126, 25120-25126, 25170

RAF1, 81404, 81406
RAI1, 81405
Ramstedt Operation
- Pyloromyotomy, 43520

Ramus Anterior, Nervus Thoracicus
- Destruction, 64620
- Injection
  - Anesthetic or Steroid, 64420-64421
  - Neurolytic, 64620

Range of Motion Test
- Extremities, 95851
- Eye, 92018, 92019
- Hand, 95852
- Rectum
  - Biofeedback, 90912-90913
- Trunk, 97530

Ranula
- Treatment of, 42408

Rapid Heart Rate
- Heart
  - Recording, 93609

Rapid Plasma Reagin Test, 86592, 86593
Rapid Test for Infection, 86308, 86403, 86406
- Monospot Test, 86308

Rapoport Test, 52005
Raskind Procedure, 33735-33737
Rastelli Procedure, 33786
Rat Typhus, 86000
Rathke Pouch Tumor
- Excision, 61545

Rays, Roentgen
- *See* X–ray

Raz Procedure, 51845
RBC, 78120, 78121, 78130-78140, 85007, 85014, 85041, 85547, 85555, 85557, 85651-85660, 86850-86870, 86970-86978
RBC ab, 86850-86870
RBL (Rubber Band Ligation)
- Hemorrhoids, 46221
- Skin Tags, 11200-11201
RCM, 96931-96936
RDH12,, 81434
Reaction
- Lip
  - without Reconstruction, 40530
Realignment
- Femur, with Osteotomy, 27454
- Knee, Extensor, 27422
- Muscle, 20999
  - Hand, 26989
- Tendon, Extensor, 26437
Reattachment
- Muscle, 20999
- Thigh, 27599
Receptor
- CD4, 86360
- Estrogen, 84233
- Progesterone, 84234
- Progestin, 84234
Receptor Assay
- Endocrine, 84235
- Estrogen, 84233
- Non–hormone, 84238

Receptor Assay — *continued*
- Progesterone, 84234
Recession
- Gastrocnemius
  - Leg, Lower, 27687
- Tendon
  - Hand, 26989
RECOMBIVAX HB, 90740, 90743-90744, 90746
Reconstruction
- *See Also* Revision
- Abdominal Wall
  - Omental Flap, 49905
- Acetabulum, 27120, 27122
- Anal
  - Congenital Absence, 46730-46740
  - Fistula, 46742
  - Graft, 46753
  - Sphincter, 46750, 46751, 46760-46761
- Ankle, 27700-27703
- Apical–Aortic Conduit, 33404
- Atrial, 33254-33259
  - Endoscopic, 33265-33266
  - Open, 33254-33259
- Auditory Canal, External, 69310, 69320
- Bile Duct
  - Anastomosis, 47800
- Bladder
  - from Colon, 50810
  - from Intestines, 50820, 51960
  - with Urethra, 51800, 51820
- Breast
  - Augmentation, 19325
  - Mammoplasty, 19318-19325
    - Biesenberger, 19318
  - Nipple, 19350, 19355
  - Reduction, 19318
  - Revision, 19380
  - Transverse Rectus Abdominis Myocutaneous (TRAM) Flap, 19367-19369
  - with Free Flap (fTRAM, DIEP, SIEA, GAP), 19364
  - with Latissimus Dorsi Flap, 19361
  - with Tissue Expander, 19357
- Bronchi
  - Graft Repair, 31770
  - Stenosis, 31775
  - with Lobectomy, 32501
  - with Segmentectomy, 32501
- Canthus, 67950
- Cardiac Anomaly, 33622
- Carpal, 25443
- Carpal Bone, 25394, 25430
- Cheekbone, 21270
- Chest Wall
  - Omental Flap, 49905
  - Trauma, 32820
- Cleft Palate, 42200-42225
- Conduit
  - Apical–Aortic, 33404
- Conjunctiva, 68320-68335
  - with Flap
    - Bridge or Partial, 68360
    - Total, 68362
- Cranial Bone
  - Extracranial, 21181-21184
- Ear, Middle
  - Tympanoplasty with Antrotomy or Mastoidotomy, 69635
    - with Ossicular Chain Reconstruction, 69636, 69637
  - Tympanoplasty with Mastoidectomy, 69641
    - Radical or Complete, 69644, 69645
    - with Intact or Reconstructed Wall, 69643, 69644
    - with Ossicular Chain Reconstruction, 69642
  - Tympanoplasty without Mastoidectomy, 69631
    - with Ossicular Chain Reconstruction, 69632, 69633
- Elbow, 24360
  - Total Replacement, 24363
  - with Implant, 24361, 24362
- Esophagus, 43300, 43310, 43313

Removal — *continued*

Cataract
  Dilated Fundus Evaluation, 2021F
  with Replacement
    Extracapsular, 66982, 66984, *[66987]*, *[66988]*
    Intracapsular, 66983
    Not Associated with Concurrent, 66983
Catheter
  Central Venous, 36589
  Peritoneum, 49422
  Pleural, 32552
  Spinal Cord, 62355
Cerclage
  Cervix, 59871
Cerumen
  Auditory Canal, External, 69209-69210
Chest Wall Respiratory Sensor Electrode/Electrode Array
Clot
  Pericardium, 33020
  Endoscopic, 32658
Comedones, 10040
Contraceptive Capsules, 11976
Cranial Tongs, 20665
Cyst, 10040
Dacryolith
  Lacrimal Duct, 68530
  Lacrimal Gland, 68530
Defibrillator
  Heart, 33244
    Pulse Generator Only, 33241
      via Thoracotomy, 33243
    Subcutaneous Defibrillator Electrode Removal, *[33272]*
    Subcutaneous Pulse Generator, 33241, *[0614T]*, *[33262, 33263, 33264]*
Drug Delivery Implant, 11982, 11983
Ear Wax
  Auditory Canal, External, 69210
Electrode
  Brain, 61535, 61880
  Cranial Nerve, 64570
  Heart, 0573T, 0580T, 33234-33238
  Nerve, 64585
  Neurostimulator, 64584, 64999
  Spinal Cord, 63661-63664
  Stomach, 43648, 43882
Embolus, Artery
  Aortoiliac, 34151-34201
  Axillary, 34101
  Brachial, 34101
  Carotid, 34001
  Celiac, 34151
  Femoropopliteal, 34201
  Iliac, 34151, 34201
  Innominate, 34001-34101
  Mesentery, 34151
  Peroneal, 34203
  Popliteal, 34203
  Pulmonary, 33910-33916
  Radial, 34111
  Renal, 34151
  Subclavian, 34001-34101
  Tibial, 34203
  Ulnar, 34111
External Fixation System, 20694, 20697
Eye
  Bone, 67414, 67445
  Ocular Contents
    with Implant, 65093
    without Implant, 65091
  Orbital Contents Only, 65110
  with Bone, 65112
  with Implant
    Muscles Attached, 65105
    Muscles Not Attached, 65103
  with Muscle or Myocutaneous Flap, 65114
  without Implant, 65101
Fallopian Tube
  Laparoscopy, 58661
    with Hysterectomy, 58542, 58544, 58548

Removal — *continued*

Fat
  Lipectomy, 15876-15879
Fecal Impaction
  Rectum, 45915
Fibrin Deposit, 32150
Fixation Device, 20670, 20680
Foreign Bodies
  Adenoid, 42999
  Anal, 46608
  Ankle Joint, 27610, 27620
  Arm
    Lower, 25248
    Upper, 24200, 24201
  Auditory Canal, External, 69200
    with Anesthesia, 69205
  Bile Duct, *[43275]*
  Bladder, 52310, 52315
  Brain, 61570
  Bronchi, 31635
  Colon, 44025, 44390, 45379
  Colon–Sigmoid, 45332
  Conjunctival Embedded, 65210
  Cornea
    with Slit Lamp, 65222
    without Slit Lamp, 65220
  Duodenum, 44010
  Elbow, 24000, 24101, 24200, 24201
  Esophagus, 43020, 43045, 43194, 43215, 74235
  External Eye, 65205
  Eyelid, 67938
  Finger, 26075, 26080
  Foot, 28190-28193
  Gastrointestinal, Upper, 43247
  Gum, 41805
  Hand, 26070
  Hip, 27033, 27086, 27087
  Hysteroscopy, 58562
  Interphalangeal Joint
    Toe, 28024
  Intertarsal Joint, 28020
  Intestines, Small, 44020, 44363
  Intraocular, 65235
  Kidney, 50561, 50580
  Knee Joint, 27310, 27331, 27372
  Lacrimal Duct, 68530
  Lacrimal Gland, 68530
  Larynx, 31511, 31530, 31531, 31577
  Leg, Upper, 27372
  Lung, 32151
  Mandible, 41806
  Maxillary Sinus, 31299
  Mediastinum, 39000, 39010
  Metatarsophalangeal Joint, 28022
  Mouth, 40804, 40805
  Muscle, 20520, 20525
    Stimulator
      Skeletal, 20999
  Nose, 30300
    Anesthesia, Under, 30310
    Lateral Rhinotomy, 30320
  Orbit, 67413, 67430
    with Bone Flap, 67430
    without Bone Flap, 67413
  Pancreatic Duct, *[43275]*
  Patella
    See Patellectomy
  Pelvis, 27086, 27087
  Penile Tissue, 54115
  Penis, 54115
  Pericardium, 33020
    Endoscopic, 32658
  Peritoneum, 49402
  Pharynx, 42809
  Pleura, 32150, 32151
    Endoscopic, 32653
  Posterior Segment
    Magnetic Extraction, 65260
    Nonmagnetic Extraction, 65265
  Rectum, 45307, 45915
  Scrotum, 55120
  Shoulder, 23040, 23044
    Deep, 23333
    Subcutaneous, 23330

Removal — *continued*

Foreign Bodies — *continued*
  Skin
    with Debridement, 11010-11012
  Stomach, 43500
  Subcutaneous, 10120, 10121
    with Debridement, 11010-11012
  Tarsometatarsal Joint, 28020
  Tendon Sheath, 20520, 20525
  Toe, 28022
  Ureter, 50961, 50980
  Urethra, 52310, 52315
  Uterus, 58562
  Vagina, 57415
  Wrist, 25040, 25101, 25248
Hair
  by Electrolysis, 17380
Halo, 20665
Harrington Rod, 22850
Hearing Aid
  Bone Conduction, 69711
Hematoma
  Brain, 61312-61315
Implant, 20670, 20680
  Ankle, 27704, *[0510T, 0511T]*
  Contraceptive Capsules, 11976
  Disc, 0164T, 22865
  Elbow, 24160
  Eye, 67120, 67121
  Finger, 26320
  Hand, 26320
  Pin, 20670, 20680
  Radius, 24164
  Rod, 20670, 20680
  Screw, 20670, 20680
  Wrist, 25449
Implantable Defibrillator, 33241
Infusion Pump
  Intra–arterial, 36262
  Intravenous, 36590
  Spinal Cord, 62365
Interstitial Glucose Sensor, 0447T-0448T
Intra–aortic Balloon, 33974
  Assist Device, 33968, 33971
Intracardiac Mass, 0644T
Intraocular Drug-Eluting Implant, 0661T
Intrauterine Device (IUD), 58301
Intravascular Vena Cava (IVC) Filter, 37193
Keel
  Laryngoplasty, 31580
Kidney
  Mechanical, 53899
Lacrimal Gland
  Partial, 68505
  Total, 68500
Lacrimal Sac
  Excision, 68520
Laryngocele, 31300
Leiomyomata, 58545, 58546, 58561
Lens, 66920-66940
Lens Material, 66840-66852
Lesion
  Conjunctiva, 68040
  Larynx
    Endoscopic, 31512, 31545-31546, 31578
Loose Body
  Ankle, 27620
  Carpometacarpal Joint, 26070
  Elbow, 24101
  Foot, 28020
  Interphalangeal Joint, Toe, 28024
  Intertarsal Joint, 28020
  Knee Joint, 27331
  Metatarsophalangeal Joint, 28022
  Tarsometatarsal Joint, 28020
  Toe, 28022
  Wrist, 25101
Lung
  Apical Tumor, 32503-32504
  Bronchoplasty, 32501
  Completion Pneumonectomy, 32488
  Cyst, 32140
  Emphysematous, 32491
  Extrapleural, 32445
  Pneumonectomy, 32440-32445

Removal — *continued*

Lung — *continued*
  Single Lobe, 32480
  Single Segment, 32484
  Sleeve Lobectomy, 32486
  Sleeve Pneumonectomy, 32442
  Two Lobes, 32482
  Volume Reduction, 32491
Lymph Nodes
  Abdominal, 38747
  Inguinofemoral, 38760, 38765
  Pelvic, 38770
  Retroperitoneal Transabdominal, 38780
  Thoracic, 38746
Mammary Implant, 19328, 19330
Mass, Intracardiac, 0644T
Mastoid
  Air Cells, 69670
Mesh
  Abdominal Wall, 11008
Milia, Multiple, 10040
Nail, 11730, 11732, 11750
  Finger, 26236
  Toe, 28124, 28160
Nephrostomy Tube, 50389
Neurostimulator
  Electrode, 63661-63662, 64999
  Pulse Generator, 64595, 64999
  Receiver, 64595
Obstructive Material
  Gastrostomy, Duodenostomy, Jejunostomy, Gastro-jejunostomy, or Cecostomy Tube, 49460
Ocular Implant, 65175, 65920
Orbital Implant, 67560
Ovaries
  Laparoscopy, 58661
    with Hysterectomy, 58542, 58544, 58548
Pacemaker
  Heart, 33233-33237 *[33227, 33228, 33229]*
Patella, Complete, 27424
Plate
  Skull, 62142
Polyp
  Anal, 46610, 46612
  Antrochoanal, 31032
  Colon, 44392, 45385
  Colon–Sigmoid, 45333
  Endoscopy, 44364, 44365, 44394
  Esophagus, 43217, 43250
  Gastrointestinal, Upper, 43250, 43251
  Rectum, 45315
  Sphenoid Sinus, 31051
Prosthesis
  Abdomen, 49606
  Abdominal Wall, 11008
  Elbow, 24160
  Hip, 27090, 27091
  Knee, 27488
  Penis, 54406, 54410-54417
  Perineum, 53442
  Radius, 24164
  Shoulder, 23334-23335
  Skull, 62142
  Urethral Sphincter, 53446, 53447
  Wrist, 25250, 25251
Pulse Generator
  Brain, 61888
  Neurostimulator, 64999
  Spinal Cord, 63688
  Substernal Implantable Defibrillator, *[0614T]*
  Vagus Nerve Blocking Therapy, 0314T-0315T
Pustules, 10040
Receiver
  Brain, 61888
  Spinal Cord, 63688
    Reservoir, 62365
Seton
  Anal, 46030
Shoulder Joint
  Foreign or Loose Body, 23107

Removal — *continued*
Shunt
Brain, 62256, 62258
Heart, 33924
Peritoneum, 49429
Spinal Cord, 63746
Skin Tags, 11200, 11201
Sling
Urethra, 53442
Vagina, 57287
Spinal Instrumentation
Anterior, 22855
Posterior Nonsegmental
Harrington Rod, 22850
Posterior Segmental, 22852
Stent
Bile Duct, [43275, 43276]
Pancreatic Duct, [43275, 43276]
Ureteral, 50382-50386
Stone (Calculi)
Bile Duct, 43264, 47420, 47425
Percutaneous, 47554
Bladder, 51050, 52310-52318, 52352
Gallbladder, 47480
Hepatic Duct, 47400
Kidney, 50060-50081, 50130, 50561,
50580, 52352
Pancreas, 48020
Pancreatic Duct, 43264
Salivary Gland, 42330-42340
Ureter, 50610-50630, 50961, 50980,
51060, 51065, 52320-52330,
52352
Urethra, 52310, 52315
Subcutaneous Port for Gastric Restrictive Pro-
cedure, 43887-43888
Suture
Anal, 46754
Anesthesia, 15850, 15851
Thrombus
See Thrombectomy
Tissue
Vaginal, Partial, 57107
Tissue Expanders, 11971
Transperineal Periurethral Balloon Device,
0550T
Continence Device, 53453
Transplant Intestines, 44137
Transplant Kidney, 50370
Tube
Ear, Middle, 69424
Finger, 26392, 26416
Hand, 26392, 26416
Nephrostomy, 50389
Tumor
Temporal Bone, 69970
Ureter
Ligature, 50940
Stent, 50382-50386
Urethral Stent
Bladder, 52310, 52315
Urethra, 52310, 52315
Vagina
Partial
Tissue, 57106
Wall, 57107, 57110, 57111
with Nodes, 57109
Vein
Clusters, 37785
Perforation, 37760
Saphenous, 37718-37735, 37780
Secondary, 37785
Varicose, 37765, 37766
Venous Access Device
Obstruction, 75901-75902
Ventilating Tube
Ear, Middle, 69424
Ventricular Assist Device, 33977, 33978
Intracorporeal, 33980, 33999
Vitreous
Partial, 67005, 67010
Wire
Anal, 46754
Wireless Cardiac Stimulator, 0518T-0520T
Renal Abscess
Incision and Drainage, 50020

Renal Arteries
Aneurysm, 35121-35122
Angiography, 36251-36253
Angioplasty, [37246, 37247]
Atherectomy, 0234T
Bypass Graft, 35536, 35560, 35631-35636
Embolectomy, 34151
Thrombectomy, 34151
Thromboendarterectomy, 35341
Renal Autotransplantation, 50380
Renal Calculus
Removal, 50060-50081, 50130, 50561, 50580,
52352
Renal Cyst
Ablation, 50541
Aspiration, 50390
Excision, 50280, 50290
Injection, 50390
X-ray, 74470
Renal Dialysis
Blood Flow Study, 90940
Documented Plan of Care, 0505F
Duplex Scan of Access, 93990
Prior to Access Creation, 93985-93986
Kt/V Level, 3082F-3084F
via Catheter, 4054F
via Functioning Arteriovenous Fistula, 4052F
via Functioning Arteriovenous Graft, 4053F
Renal Disease Services
Arteriovenous Fistula
Revision, 36832, 36833
Thrombectomy, 36831
Arteriovenous Shunt
Revision, 36832, 36833
Thrombectomy, 36831
End Stage Renal Disease, 90951-90956, 90964,
90968
Hemodialysis, 90935, 90937
Blood Flow Study, 90940
Hemoperfusion, 90997
Patient Training, 90989, 90993
Peritoneal Dialysis, 90945-90947
Renal Pelvis Biopsy, 50606
Renal Transplantation
Allograft Preparation, 50323-50329
Anesthesia
Donor, 00862
Recipient, 00868
Donor Nephrectomy, 50300-50320, 50547
Graft Implantation, 50360-50365
Recipient Nephrectomy, 50340, 50365
Reimplantation Kidney, 50380
Removal Transplanted Allograft, 50370
Rendezvous Procedure
Biliary Tree Access, 47541
Renin, 80408, 80416, 84244
Peripheral Vein, 80417
Renin–Converting Enzyme, 82164
Reoperation
Carotid
Thromboendarterectomy, 35390
Coronary Artery Bypass
Valve Procedure, 33530
Distal Vessel Bypass, 35700
Repair
See Also Revision
Abdomen, 49900
Hernia, 49491-49525, 49565, 49570,
49582-49590
Omphalocele, 49600-49611
Suture, 49900
Abdominal Wall, 15830, 15847, 17999
Anal
Anomaly, 46744-46748
Fistula, 46288, 46706-46716
High Imperforate, 46730, 46735, 46740,
46742
Low Imperforate, 46715-46716
Park Posterior, 46761
Stricture, 46700, 46705
Aneurysm
Aorta
Abdominal, 34701-34706, 34830-
34832, 34841-34848,
35081-35103

Repair — *continued*
Aneurysm — *continued*
Aorta — *continued*
Abdominal — *continued*
Iliac Vessels, 34707-34711
[34717, 34718], 35102-
35103, 37220-37223
Visceral Vessels, 35091-35092
Infrarenal, 34701-34706, 34830-
34832
Thoracic, 33877-33886
Arteriovenous, 36832
Axillary-Brachial Artery, 35011, 35013
Carotid Artery, 35001-35002
Endovascular
Abdominal Aorta, 34701-34712
[34717, 34718]
Iliac Artery, 34707-34711 [34717,
34718], 35102-35103,
37220-37223
Infrarenal Artery, 34701-34706
Thoracic Aorta, 33880-33891
Visceral Artery, 34841-34848
Femoral, 35141-35142
Hepatic, Celiac, Renal, or Mesenteric
Artery, 35121-35122
Iliac Artery, 34701-34706, 35131-35132
Innominate, Subclavian Artery, 35021-
35022
Intracranial Artery, 61697-61708
Popliteal Artery, 35151-35152
Radial or Ulnar Artery, 35045
Sinus of Valsalva, 33720
Subclavian Artery, 35001-35002, 35021-
35022
Vertebral Artery, 35005
Ankle
Ligament, 27695-27698
Tendon, 27612, 27650-27654, 27680-
27687
Anomaly
Artery Arborization, 33925-33926
Cardiac, 33608, 33610, 33615, 33617
Coronary Artery, 33502-33507
Pulmonary Venous Return, 33730
Aorta, 33320-33322, 33802, 33803
Coarctation, 33840-33851, 33894-33895
Graft, 33858-33859, 33863-33877
Sinus of Valsalva, 33702-33720
Thoracic
Endovascular, 33880-33891,
33894-33895
Prosthesis Placement, 33886
Radiological Supervision and Inter-
pretation, 75956-75959
Visceral
Endovascular, 34841-34848
Aortic Arch
with Cardiopulmonary Bypass, 33853
without Cardiopulmonary Bypass, 33852
Aortic Valve, 93591-93592
Obstruction
Outflow Tract, 33414
Septal Hypertrophy, 33416
Stenosis, 33415
Valvuloplasty, 93591-93592
Arm
Lower, 25260, 25263, 25270
Fasciotomy, 24495
Secondary, 25265, 25272, 25274
Tendon, 25290
Tendon Sheath, 25275
Muscle, 24341
Tendon, 24332, 24341, 25280, 25295,
25310-25316
Upper
Muscle Revision, 24330, 24331
Muscle Transfer, 24301, 24320
Tendon Lengthening, 24305
Tendon Revision, 24320
Tendon Transfer, 24301
Tenotomy, 24310
Arteriovenous Aneurysm, 36832
Arteriovenous Fistula
Abdomen, 35182
Acquired or Traumatic, 35189

Repair — *continued*
Arteriovenous Fistula — *continued*
Extremities, 35184
Acquired or Traumatic, 35190
Head, 35180
Acquired or Traumatic, 35188
Neck, 35180
Acquired or Traumatic, 35188
Thorax, 35182
Acquired or Traumatic, 35189
Arteriovenous Malformation
Intracranial, 61680-61692
Intracranial Artery, 61705, 61708
Spinal Artery, 62294
Spinal Cord, 63250-63252
Artery
Angioplasty, 36902-36903, 36905-36908
Aorta, 33897, [37246, 37247]
Axillary, [37246, 37247]
Brachiocephalic, [37246, 37247]
Bypass Graft, 35501-35571, 35601-
35683, 35691-35700
Bypass In–Situ, 35583-35587
Bypass Venous Graft, 33510-33516,
35510-35525
Coronary
Anomalous, 33502-33507
Dialysis Circuit, 36902-36903, 36905-
36908
Iliac, 34707-34711 [34717, 34718], 35102-
35103, 37220-37223
Occlusive Disease, 35001, 35005-35021,
35045, 35081, 35091, 35102,
35111, 35121, 35131, 35141,
35151
Pulmonary, 33690, 33925-33926
Renal, [37246, 37247]
Renal or Visceral, [37246, 37247]
Subclavian, [37246, 37247]
Thromboendarterectomy, 35301-35321,
35341-35390
Venous Graft, 33510-33516, 35510-
35525
Visceral, [37246, 37247]
Arytenoid Cartilage, 31400
Atria
Laparoscopic, 33265-33266
Open, 33254-33256
Atrial Fibrillation, 33254, 33255-33256
Atrioventricular Canal, 33660-33670
Bile Duct, 47701
with Intestines, 47760, 47780, 47785
Wound, 47900
Bladder
Exstrophy, 51940
Fistula, 44660, 44661, 45800, 45805,
51880-51925
Neck, 51845
Resection, 52500
Wound, 51860, 51865
Blepharoptosis
Conjunctivo-Tarso-Muller's Muscle Resec-
tion, 67908
Frontalis Muscle Technique
with Fascial Sling, 67902
Superior Rectus Technique with Fascial
Sling, 67906
Tarso Levator Resection or Advance-
ment, 67903-67904
Blood Vessel(s)
Abdomen, 35221, 35251, 35281
with Other Graft, 35281
with Vein Graft, 35251
Chest, 35211, 35216
with Other Graft, 35271, 35276
with Vein Graft, 35241, 35246
Finger, 35207
Graft Defect, 35870
Hand, 35207
Intrathoracic, 35211, 35216, 35241,
35246, 35271, 35276
Kidney, 50100
Lower Extremity, 35226, 35256, 35286
with Other Graft, 35286
with Vein Graft, 35256
Neck, 35201, 35231, 35261

Repair — continued

Laceration, Skin — continued
Scalp — continued
Intermediate, 12031-12037
Layered, 12031-12037
Simple, 12001-12007
Superficial, 12001-12007
Toe, Toes
Complex, 13131-13133
Intermediate, 12041-12047
Layered, 12041-12047
Simple, 12001-12007
Superficial, 12001-12007
Trunk
Complex, 13100-13102
Intermediate, 12031-12037
Layered, 12031-12037
Simple, 12001-12007
Superficial, 12001-12007
Upper
Arm, Arms
Complex, 13120-13122
Intermediate, 12031-12037
Layered, 12031-12037
Simple, 12001-12007
Superficial, 12001-12007
Extremity
Complex, 13120-13122
Intermediate, 12031-12037
Layered, 12031-12037
Simple, 12001-12007
Superficial, 12001-12007
Leg, Legs
Complex, 13120-13122
Intermediate, 12031-12037
Layered, 12031-12037
Simple, 12001-12007
Superficial, 12001-12007
Larynx
Fracture, 31584
Reinnervation
Neuromuscular Pedicle, 31590
Leak
Cerebrospinal Fluid, 31290-31291
Leg
Lower
Fascia, 27656
Tendon, 27658-27692
Upper
Muscles, 27385, 27386, 27400, 27430
Tendon, 27393-27400
Ligament
Ankle, 27695-27696, 27698
Anterior Cruciate, 29888
Collateral
Elbow, 24343, 24345
Metacarpophalangeal or Interpha-
langeal Joint, 26540
Knee, 27405, 27407, 27409
Posterior Cruciate Ligament, 29889
Lip, 40650-40654
Cleft Lip, 40700-40761
Fistula, 42260
Liver
Abscess, 47300
Cyst, 47300
Wound, 47350-47361
Lung
Hernia, 32800
Pneumolysis, 32940
Tear, 32110
Macrodactylia, 26590
Malunion
Femur, 27470, 27472
Fibula, 27726
Humerus, 24430
Metatarsal, 28322
Radius, 25400, 25405, 25415, 25420
Tarsal Bones, 28320
Tibia, 27720, 27722, 27724-27725
Ulna, 25400, 25405, 25415, 25420
Mastoidectomy
Complete, 69601
Modified Radical, 69602
Radical, 69603

Repair — continued

Mastoidectomy — continued
with Tympanoplasty, 69604
Maxilla
Osteotomy, 21206
Meningocele, 63700, 63702
Meniscus
Knee, 27403, 29882-29883
Mesentery, 44850
Metacarpal
Lengthen, 26568
Nonunion, 26546
Osteotomy, 26565
Metacarpophalangeal Joint
Capsulodesis, 26516-26518
Collateral Ligament, 26540-26542
Fusion, 26516-26518
Metatarsal, 28322
Osteotomy, 28306-28309
Microsurgery, 69990
Mitral Valve, 0543T-0544T, 33420-33427, 93590, 93592
Mouth
Floor, 41250
Laceration, 40830, 40831
Vestibule of, 40830-40845
Muscle
Hand, 26591
Upper Arm or Elbow, 24341
Musculotendinous Cuff, 23410, 23412
Myelomeningocele, 63704, 63706
Nail Bed, 11760
Nasal Deformity
Cleft Lip, 40700-40761
Nasal Septum, 30630
Navicular, 25440
Neck Muscles
Scalenus Anticus, 21700, 21705
Sternocleidomastoid, 21720, 21725
Nerve, 64876
Facial, 69955
Graft, 64885-64907
Microrepair
with Surgical Microscope, 69990
Suture, 64831-64876
Nonunion
Carpal Bone, 25431
Femur, 27470, 27472
Fibula, 27726
Humerus, 24430
Metacarpal, 26546
Metatarsal, 28322
Navicular, 25440
Phalanx, 26546
Radius, 25400, 25405, 25415, 25420
Scaphoid, 25440
Tarsal Bones, 28320
Tibia, 27720, 27722, 27724-27725
Ulna, 25400, 25405, 25415, 25420
Nose
Adhesions, 30560
Fistula, 30580, 30600, 42260
Nasal Valve Collapse, 30468
Rhinophyma, 30120
Septum, 30540, 30545, 30630
Synechia, 30560
Vestibular Stenosis, 30465
Obstruction
Ventricular Outflow, 33414, 33619
Omentum, 49999
Omphalocele, 49600-49611
Osteochondritis Dissecans Lesion, 29892
Osteotomy
Femoral Neck, 27161
Radius and Ulna, 25365
Ulna and Radius, 25365
Vertebra
Additional Segment, 22216, 22226
Cervical, 22210, 22220
Lumbar, 22214, 22224
Thoracic, 22212, 22222
Oval Window
Fistula, 69666-69667
Oviduct, 58752
Create Stoma, 58770

Repair — continued

Pacemaker
Heart
Electrode(s), 33218, 33220
Palate
Laceration, 42180, 42182
Vomer Flap, 42235
Pancreas
Cyst, 48500
Pseudocyst, 48510
Paravaginal Defect, 57284-57285, 57423
Pectus Carinatum, 21740-21742
with Thoracoscopy, 21743
Pectus Excavatum, 21740-21742
with Thoracoscopy, 21743
Pectus Excavatum or Carinatum, 21740, 21742-21743
Pelvic Floor
with Prosthesis, 57267
Pelvis
Osteotomy, 27158
Tendon, 27098
Penis
Corporeal Tear, 54437
Fistulization, 54435
Injury, 54440
Priapism, 54420-54435
Prosthesis, 54408
Replantation, 54438
Shunt, 54420, 54430
Perforation
Septal, 30630
Perineum, 56810
Periorbital Region
Osteotomy, 21260-21263
Peritoneum, 49999
Phalanges
Finger
Lengthening, 26568
Osteotomy, 26567
Nonunion, 26546
Toe
Osteotomy, 28310, 28312
Pharynx
with Esophagus, 42953
Pleura, 32215
Prosthesis
Penis, 54408
Pseudarthrosis
Tibia, 27727
Pulmonary Artery, 33917, 33920, 33925-33926
Reimplantation, 33788
Pulmonary Valve, 33471-33474
Pulmonary Venous
Anomaly, 33724
Stenosis, 33726
Quadriceps, 27430
Radius
Epiphyseal, 25450, 25455
Malunion or Nonunion, 25400-25420
Osteotomy, 25350, 25355, 25370, 25375
with Graft, 25405, 25420-25426
Rectocele, 45560, 57250
Rectovaginal Fistula, 57308
Rectum
Fistula, 45800-45825, 46706-46707, 46715-46716, 46740, 46742
Injury, 45562-45563
Prolapse, 45505-45541, 45900
Rectocele, 45560, 57250
Stenosis, 45500
with Sigmoid Excision, 45550
Retinal Detachment, 67101-67113
Rotator Cuff, 23410-23412, 23420, 29827
Salivary Duct, 42500, 42505
Fistula, 42600
Scalenus Anticus, 21700, 21705
Scapula
Fixation, 23400
Scapulopexy, 23400
Sclera
Reinforcement
with Graft, 67255
without Graft, 67250
Staphyloma
with Graft, 66225

Repair — continued

Sclera — continued
with Glue, 65286
Wound
Operative, 66250
Tissue Glue, 65286
Scrotum, 55175, 55180
Septal Defect, 33813-33814
Septum, Nasal, 30420
Shoulder
Capsule, 23450-23466
Cuff, 23410, 23412
Ligament Release, 23415
Muscle Transfer, 23395, 23397
Musculotendinous (Rotator) Cuff, 23410, 23412
Rotator Cuff, 23415, 23420
Tendon, 23410, 23412, 23430, 23440
Tenomyotomy, 23405, 23406
Simple, Integumentary System, 12001-12021
Sinus
Ethmoid
Cerebrospinal Fluid Leak, 31290
Meningocele, 63700, 63702
Myelomeningocele, 63704, 63706
Sphenoid
Cerebrospinal Fluid Leak, 31291
Sinus of Valsalva, 33702-33720
Skin
See Also Repair, Laceration
Wound
Complex, 13100-13160
Intermediate, 12031-12057
Simple, 12020, 12021
Skull
Cerebrospinal Fluid Leak, 62100
Encephalocele, 62120
SLAP Lesion, 29807
Spectacles, 92370, 92371
Prosthesis, 92371
Sphincter, 53449
Spica Cast, 29720
Spinal Cord, 63700
Cerebrospinal Fluid Leak, 63707, 63709
Meningocele, 63700, 63702
Myelomeningocele, 63704, 63706
Spinal Meningocele, 63700-63702
Spine
Cervical Vertebra, 22510, 22512
Lumbar Vertebra, 22511-22512, 22514-22515
Osteotomy, 22210-22226
Sacral Vertebra, 22511-22512
Thoracic Vertebra, 22510, 22512, 22513, 22515
Spleen, 38115
Stenosis
Nasal Vestibular, 30465
Pulmonary, 33782-33783
Sternocleidomastoid, 21720, 21725
Stomach
Esophagogastrostomy, 43112, 43320
Fistula, 43880
Fundoplasty, 43325-43328
Laceration, 43501, 43502
Stoma, 43870
Ulcer, 43501
Symblepharon, 68330, 68335, 68340
Syndactyly, 26560-26562
Talus
Osteotomy, 28302
Tarsal, 28320
Osteotomy, 28304, 28305
Tear
Lung, 32110
Tendon
Achilles, 27650, 27652, 27654
Extensor, 26410, 26412, 26418, 26420, 26426, 26428, 26433-26434, 27664-27665
Foot, 28208, 28210
Flexor, 26350, 26352, 26356-26358, 27658-27659
Leg, 28200, 28202
Foot, 28200, 28202, 28208, 28210
Leg, 27658-27659, 27664-27665

[Resequenced]   CPT © 2021 American Medical Association. All Rights Reserved.   © 2021 Optum360, LLC

Rhinectomy — *continued*
  Total, 30160
Rhinomanometry, 92512
Rhinopharynx
  Biopsy, 42804-42806
  Hemorrhage, 42970-42972
  Unlisted Services/Procedures, 42999
Rhinophyma
  Repair, 30120
Rhinoplasty
  Cleft Lip
    Cleft Palate, 30460-30462
    Primary, 30400-30420
    Secondary, 30430-30450
Rhinoscopy
  Diagnostic, 31231-31235
  Surgical, 31237-31294 *[31253, 31257, 31259]*
  Unlisted Services/Procedures, 31299
Rhinotomy
  Lateral, 30118, 30320
Rhizotomy, 63185, 63190
RHO, 81404, 81434
Rho(D) Vaccine, 90384-90386
Rho Variant Du, 86905
Rhythm Monitor, Cardiac, 33285-33286
Rhytidectomy, 15824-15829
  Cheek, 15828
  Chin, 15828
  Forehead, 15824
  Glabellar Frown Lines, 15826
  Neck, 15825, 15828
  Superficial Musculoaponeurotic System, 15829
Rhytidoplasties, 15824-15829
Rib
  Antibody, 86756
  Antigen Detection by Immunoassay with Direct Optical Observation
    Direct Fluorescence, 87280
    Enzyme Immunoassay, 87420
  Bone Graft
    with Microvascular Anastomosis, 20962
  Excision, 21600-21616, 32900
  Fracture
    Closed Treatment
      See E&M codes
    External Fixation, 21899
    Open Treatment, 21811-21813
  Free Osteocutaneous Flap with Microvascular Anastomosis, 20969
  Graft
    to Face, 21230
  Resection, 21601-21603, 32900
  X-ray, 71100-71111
Riboflavin, 84252
Richardson Operation Hysterectomy, 58150
  See Also Hysterectomy, Abdominal, Total
Richardson Procedure, 53460
Rickettsia
  Antibody, 86757
Ridell Operation
  Sinusotomy, Frontal, 31075-31087
Ridge, Alveolar
  Fracture Treatment
    Closed, 21440
    Open, 21445
RIG (Rabies Immune Globulin), 90375, 90376, 90377
Right Atrioventricular Valve, 33460-33468
Right Heart Cardiac Catheterization, 93456-93457
  for Congenital Anomalies, 93593-93594
Ripstein Operation
  Laparoscopic, 45400
    with Sigmoid Resection, 45402
  Open, 45540-45541
    with Sigmoid Excision, 45550
Risk Factor Reduction Intervention
  Behavior Change Interventions, 99406-99409
  Group Counseling, 0403T, 99411-99412
  Individual Counseling, 99401-99404
Risk Score Cancer, mRNA
  Prostate, 0011M
  Urothelial, 0012M-0013M
Risser Jacket, 29010-29015
  Removal, 29710
RK, 65771

Robotic Assistance
  Prostatectomy, 55866
Rocky Mountain Spotted Fever, 86000
Roentgen Rays
  See X-ray
Roentgenographic
  See X-ray
Roentgenography
  See Radiology, Diagnostic
ROM, 95851-95852, 97110, 97530
Ropes Test, 83872
Rorschach Test, 96112-96116
Ross Information Processing Assessment, *[96125]*
Ross Procedure, 33413
Ross-Konno Procedure, *[33440]*
Rotarix, 90681
RotaTeq, 90680
Rotation Flap, 14000-14350
Rotator Cuff
  Repair, 23410-23420
Rotavirus
  Antibody, 86759
  Antigen Detection
    Enzyme Immunoassay, 87425
Rotavirus Vaccine, 90680-90681
Round Window
  Repair Fistula, 69667
Round Window Fistula, 69667
Roux-en-Y Procedures
  Biliary Tract, 47740-47741, 47780-47785
  Pancreas, 48540
  Stomach, 43621, 43633, 43644, 43846
    Laparoscopic, 43644
RP1, 81404, 81434
RP2, 81434
RPE65, 81406, 81434
RPGR, 81434
RPP (Radical Perineal Prostatectomy), 55810-55815
RPR, 86592-86593
RPS19, 81405
RRM2B, 81405
RRP (Radical Retropubic Prostatectomy), 55840-55845
RSV
  Antibody, 86756
  Antigen Detection
    Direct Fluorescent Antibody, 87280
    Enzyme Immunoassay, 87420
  Recombinant, 90378
RT3, 84482
Rubber Band Ligation
  Hemorrhoids, 46221
  Skin Tags, 11200-11201
Rubella
  Antibody, 86762
  Vaccine, 90707-90710
Rubella HI Test
  Hemagglutination Inhibition Test, 86280
Rubella Immunization
  MMR, 90707
  MMRV, 90710
Rubeola
  Antibody, 86765
  Antigen Detection
    Immunofluorescence, 87283
Rufinamide Assay, *[80210]*
Ruiz-Mora Procedure, 28286
RUNX1/RUNX1T1, 81401, *[81334]*
Russell Viper Venom Time, 85612-85613
RYR1, 81406, 81408
RYR2, 81408

S

Sac, Endolymphatic
  Exploration, 69805-69806
Saccomanno Technique, 88108
Sacral Nerve
  Implantation
    Electrode, 64561, 64581
  Insertion
    Electrode, 64561, 64581
Sacroiliac Joint
  Arthrodesis, 27280
  Arthrotomy, 27050
  Biopsy, 27050

Sacroiliac Joint — *continued*
  Dislocation
    Open Treatment, 27218
  Fusion, 27280
  Injection for Arthrography, 27096
  Stabilization for Arthrodesis, 27279
  X-ray, 72200-72202, 73525
Sacroplasty, 0200T-0201T
Sacrum
  Augmentation, 0200T-0201T
  Pressure Ulcer, 15931-15937
  Tumor
    Excision, 49215
    X-ray, 72220
SAECG, 93278
SAH, 61566
Salabrasion, 15780-15787
Salicylate
  Assay, *[80179]*, *[80329, 80330, 80331]*
Saline-Solution Abortion, 59850-59851
Salivary Duct
  Catheterization, 42660
  Dilation, 42650-42660
  Ligation, 42665
  Repair, 42500-42505
    Fistula, 42600
Salivary Gland Virus
  Antibody, 86644-86645
  Antigen Detection
    Direct Fluorescence, 87271
    Enzyme Immunoassay, 87332
    Nucleic Acid, 87495-87497
Salivary Glands
  Abscess
    Incision and Drainage, 42310-42320
  Biopsy, 42405
  Calculi (Stone)
    Excision, 42330-42340
  Cyst
    Drainage, 42409
    Excision, 42408
  Injection
    X-ray, 42550
  Needle Biopsy, 42400
  Nuclear Medicine
    Function Study, 78232
    Imaging, 78230-78231
  Parotid
    Abscess, 42300-42305
  Unlisted Services and Procedures, 42699
  X-ray, 70380-70390
    with Contrast, 70390
Salmonella
  Antibody, 86768
Salpingectomy, 58262-58263, 58291-58292, 58552, 58554, 58661, 58700
  Ectopic Pregnancy
    Laparoscopic Treatment, 59151
    Surgical Treatment, 59120
  Oophorectomy, 58943
Salpingography, 0568T
Salpingohysterostomy, 58752
Salpingolysis, 58660, 58740
Salpingoneostomy, 58673, 58770
Salpingo-Oophorectomy, 58720
  Resection Ovarian Malignancy, 58950-58956
  Resection Peritoneal Malignancy, 58950-58956
  Resection Tubal Malignancy, 58950-58956
Salpingostomy, 58673, 58770
  Laparoscopic, 58673
SALT, 84460
Salter Osteotomy of the Pelvis, 27146
Sampling
  See Biopsy; Brush Biopsy; Needle Biopsy
Sang-Park Procedure
  Septectomy, Atrial, 33735-33737, 33741
Sao Paulo Typhus, 86000
SAST, 84450
Saucerization
  Calcaneus, 28120
  Clavicle, 23180
  Femur, 27070, 27360
  Fibula, 27360, 27641
  Hip, 27070
  Humerus, 23184, 24140
  Ileum, 27070

Saucerization — *continued*
  Metacarpal, 26230
  Metatarsal, 28122
  Olecranon Process, 24147
  Phalanges
    Finger, 26235-26236
    Toe, 28124
  Pubis, 27070
  Radius, 24145, 25151
  Scapula, 23182
  Talus, 28120
  Tarsal, 28122
  Tibia, 27360, 27640
  Ulna, 24147, 25150
Saundby Test, 82270, 82272
Sauve-Kapandji Procedure
  Arthrodesis, Distal Radioulnar Joint, 25830
SAVER (Surgical Anterior Ventricular Endocardial Restoration), 33548
SBFT, 74246, 74248
SBRT (Stereotactic Body Radiation Therapy), 77373
Scabies, 87220
Scalenotomy, 21700-21705
Scalenus Anticus
  Division, 21700-21705
Scaling
  Chemical for Acne, 17360
Scalp
  Cooling, 0662T, 0663T
  Skin Graft
    Delay of Flap, 15610
    Full Thickness, 15220-15221
    Pedicle Flap, 15572
    Split, 15100-15101
  Tissue Transfer, Adjacent, 14020-14021
  Tumor Excision, 21011-21016
Scalp Blood Sampling, 59030
Scan
  See Also Specific Site; Nuclear Medicine
  Abdomen
    Computed Tomography, 74150-74175, 75635
  Computerized
    Ophthalmic, 92132-92134
  CT
    See CT Scan
  MRI
    See Magnetic Resonance Imaging
  PET
    See Specific Site; Nuclear Medicine
  Radionuclide, Brain, 78803
  Retinal Polarization, 0469T
Scanning Radioisotope
  See Nuclear Medicine
Scanogram, 77073
Scaphoid
  Fracture
    Closed Treatment, 25622
    Open Treatment, 25628
    with Manipulation, 25624
Scapula
  Craterization, 23182
  Cyst
    Excision, 23140
      with Allograft, 23146
      with Autograft, 23145
  Diaphysectomy, 23182
  Excision, 23172, 23190
    Partial, 23182
  Fracture
    Closed Treatment
      with Manipulation, 23575
      without Manipulation, 23570
    Open Treatment, 23585
  Ostectomy, 23190
  Repair
    Fixation, 23400
    Scapulopexy, 23400
  Saucerization, 23182
  Sequestrectomy, 23172
  Tumor
    Excision, 23140, 23210
      with Allograft, 23146
      with Autograft, 23145
    Radical Resection, 23210

© 2021 Optum360, LLC

CPT © 2021 American Medical Association. All Rights Reserved.

[Resequenced]

Index — 119

Rhinectomy — Scapula

Index

Scapula — *continued*
X–ray, 73010
Scapulopexy, 23400
Scarification
Pleural, 32215
Scarification of Pleura
Agent for Pleurodesis, 32560
Endoscopic, 32650
SCBE (Single Contrast Barium Enema), 74270
Schanz Operation, 27448
Schauta Operation, 58285
Schede Procedure, 32905-32906
Scheie Procedure, 66155
Schlatter Operation, 43620
Schlemm's Canal Dilation, 66174-66175
Schlichter Test, 87197
Schocket Procedure, 66180
Schuchardt Procedure
Osteotomy
Maxilla, 21206
Schwannoma, Acoustic
See Brain, Tumor, Excision
Sciatic Nerve
Decompression, 64712
Injection
Anesthetic or Steroid, 64445-64446
Lesion
Excision, 64786
Neuroma
Excision, 64786
Neuroplasty, 64712
Release, 64712
Repair
Suture, 64858
Scintigraphy
See Emission Computerized Tomography
See Nuclear Medicine
Scissoring
Skin Tags, 11200-11201
Sclera
Excision, 66130
Sclerectomy with Punch or Scissors, 66160
Fistulization
Sclerectomy with Punch or Scissors with Iridectomy, 66160
Thermocauterization with Iridectomy, 66155
Trabeculectomy ab Externo in Absence of Previous Surgery, 66170
Trephination with Iridectomy, 66150
Incision (Fistulization)
Sclerectomy with Punch or Scissors with Iridectomy, 66160
Thermocauterization with Iridectomy, 66155
Trabeculectomy ab Externo in Absence of Previous Surgery, 66170
Trephination with Iridectomy, 66150
Lesion
Excision, 66130
Repair
Reinforcement
with Graft, 67255
without Graft, 67250
Staphyloma
with Graft, 66225
with Glue, 65286
Wound (Operative), 66250
Tissue Glue, 65286
Trabeculostomy Ab Interno
by Laser, 0621T
with Ophthalmic Endoscope, 0622T
Scleral Buckling Operation
Retina, Repair, Detachment, 67107-67108, 67113
Scleral Ectasia
Repair with Graft, 66225
Sclerectomy, 66160
Sclerotherapy
Percutaneous (Cyst, Lymphocele, Seroma), 49185
Venous, 36468-36471
Sclerotomy, 66150-66170
SCN1A, 81407, *[81419]*
SCN1B, 81404, *[81419]*

SCN2A, *[81419]*
SCN4A, 81406
SCN5A, 81407
SCN8A, *[81419]*
SCNN1A, 81406
SCNN1B, 81406
SCNN1G, 81406
SCO1, 81405
SCO2, 81404
Scoliosis Evaluation, Radiologic, 72081-72084
Scrambler Therapy, 0278T
Screening
Abdominal Aortic Aneurysm (AAA), 76706
Developmental, 96110, 96112-96113
Drug
Alcohol and/or Substance Abuse, 99408-99409
Evoked Otoacoustic Emissions, *[92558]*
Mammography, 77067
Scribner Cannulization, 36810
Scrotal Varices
Excision, 55530-55540
Scrotoplasty, 55175-55180
Scrotum
Abscess
Incision and Drainage, 54700, 55100
Excision, 55150
Exploration, 55110
Hematoma
Incision and Drainage, 54700
Removal
Foreign Body, 55120
Repair, 55175-55180
Ultrasound, 76870
Unlisted Services and Procedures, 55899
Scrub Typhus, 86000
SDHA, 81406
SDHB, 81405, 81437-81438
SDHC, 81404-81405, 81437-81438
SDHD, 81404, 81437-81438
Second Look Surgery
Carotid Thromboendarterectomy, 35390
Coronary Artery Bypass, 33530
Distal Vessel Bypass, 35700
Valve Procedure, 33530
Section
See Also Decompression
Cesarean
See Cesarean Delivery
Cranial Nerve, 61460
Spinal Access, 63191
Gasserian Ganglion
Sensory Root, 61450
Nerve Root, 63185-63190
Spinal Accessory Nerve, 63191
Spinal Cord Tract, 63197
Vestibular Nerve
Transcranial Approach, 69950
Translabyrinthine Approach, 69915
Sedation
Moderate, 99155-99157
with Independent Observation, 99151-99153
Seddon–Brookes Procedure, 24320
Sedimentation Rate
Blood Cell
Automated, 85652
Manual, 85651
Segmentectomy
Breast, 19301-19302
Lung, 32484, 32669
Selective Cellular Enhancement Technique, 88112
Selenium, 84255
Self Care
See Also Physical Medicine/ Therapy/Occupational Therapy
Training, 97535, 98960-98962, 99509
Sella Turcica
CT Scan, 70480-70482
X–ray, 70240
Semen
Cryopreservation
Storage (Per Year), 89343
Thawing, Each Aliquot, 89353
Semen Analysis, 89300-89322
Sperm Analysis, 89329-89331

Semen Analysis — *continued*
Sperm Analysis — *continued*
Antibodies, 89325
with Sperm Isolation, 89260-89261
Semenogelase, 84152-84154
Semilunar
Bone
See Lunate
Seminal Vesicle
Cyst
Excision, 55680
Excision, 55650
Incision, 55600, 55605
Mullerian Duct
Excision, 55680
Unlisted Services and Procedures, 55899
Seminal Vesicles
Vesiculography, 74440
X–ray with Contrast, 74440
Seminin, 84152-84154
Semiquantitative, 81005
Semont Maneuver, 95992
Sengstaken Tamponade
Esophagus, 43460
Senning Procedure
Repair, Great Arteries, 33774-33777
Senning Type, 33774-33777
Sensitivity Study
Antibiotic
Agar, 87181
Disc, 87184
Enzyme Detection, 87185
Macrobroth, 87188
MIC, 87186
Microtiter, 87186
MLC, 87187
Mycobacteria, 87190
Antiviral Drugs
HIV–1
Tissue Culture, 87904
Sensor, Interstitial Glucose, 0446T-0448T
Sensor, Transcatheter Placement, 34701-34708
Sensorimotor Exam, 92060
Sensory Nerve
Common
Repair/Suture, 64834
Sensory Testing
Quantitative (QST), Per Extremity
Cooling Stimuli, 0108T
Heat–Pain Stimuli, 0109T
Touch Pressure Stimuli, 0106T
Using Other Stimuli, 0110T
Vibration Stimuli, 0107T
Sentinel Node
Injection Procedure, 38792
SEP (Somatosensory Evoked Potentials), 95925-95927 *[95938]*
Separation
Craniofacial
Closed Treatment, 21431
Open Treatment, 21432-21436
SEPT9, 81327
Septal Defect
Repair, 33813-33814
Ventricular
Closure
Open, 33675-33688
Percutaneous, 93581
Septectomy
Atrial, 33735-33737, 33741
Closed, 33735
Noncongenital Anomaly(ies), 93799
Submucous Nasal, 30520
Septic Abortion, 59830
Septin9, 81327
Septoplasty, 30520
Septostomy
Atrial, 33735-33737, 33741
Noncongenital Anomaly(ies), 93799
Septum, Nasal
See Nasal Septum
Sequestrectomy
Calcaneus, 28120
Carpal, 25145
Clavicle, 23170
Forearm, 25145

Sequestrectomy — *continued*
Humeral Head, 23174
Humerus, 24134
Olecranon Process, 24138
Radius, 24136, 25145
Scapula, 23172
Skull, 61501
Talus, 28120
Ulna, 24138, 25145
with Alveolectomy, 41830
Wrist, 25145
Serialography
Aorta, 75625
Serodiagnosis, Syphilis, 86592-86593
Serologic Test for Syphilis, 86592-86593
Seroma
Incision and Drainage
Skin, 10140
Sclerotherapy, Percutaneous, 49185
Serotonin, 84260
Serpin Peptidase Inhibitor, Clade A, Alpha-1 Antiproteinase, Antitrypsin, Member 1 Gene Analysis, *[81332]*
SERPINA1, *[81332]*
SERPINE1, 81400
Serum
Albumin, 82040
Antibody Identification
Pretreatment, 86975-86978
CPK, 82550
Serum Immune Globulin, 90281-90284
Serum Globulin Immunization, 90281-90284
Sesamoid Bone
Excision, 28315
Finger
Excision, 26185
Foot
Fracture, 28530-28531
Thumb
Excision, 26185
Sesamoidectomy
Toe, 28315
SETX, 81406
Sever Procedure, 23020
Severing of Blepharorrhaphy, 67710
Sex Change Operation
Female to Male, 55980
Male to Female, 55970
Sex Chromatin, 88130
Sex Chromatin Identification, 88130-88140
Sex Hormone Binding Globulin, 84270
Sex–Linked Ichthyoses, 86592-86593
SF3B1, *[81347]*
SG, 84315, 93503
SGCA, 81405
SGCB, 81405
SGCD, 81405
SGCE, 81405-81406
SGCG, 81404-81405
SGOT, 84450
SGPT, 84460
SH2D1A, 81403-81404
SH3TC2, 81406
Shaving
Skin Lesion, 11300-11313
SHBG, 84270
Shelf Procedure
Osteotomy, Hip, 27146-27151
Femoral with Open Reduction, 27156
Shiga–Like Toxin
Antigen Detection
Enzyme Immunoassay, 87427
Shigella
Antibody, 86771
Shirodkar Operation, 57700
SHOC2, 81400, 81405
Shock Wave Lithotripsy, 50590
Shock Wave (Extracorporeal) Therapy, 0101T-0102T, 20999, 28890, 28899, 43265, 50590, 52353, *[0512T, 0513T]*
Shock Wave, Ultrasonic
See Ultrasound
Shop Typhus of Malaya, 86000
Shoulder
See Also Clavicle; Scapula

[Resequenced]
CPT © 2021 American Medical Association. All Rights Reserved.
© 2021 Optum360, LLC

Speech — *continued*
  Evaluation — *continued*
    for Prosthesis, 92607, 92608, *[92597]*
    Video, 70371
  Prosthesis
    Creation, 31611
    Evaluation for Speech, 92567, 92607, 92608
    Insertion, 31611
    Preparation of, 21084
  Therapy, 92507, 92508
Speech Evaluation, 92521-92524
Sperm
  Antibodies, 89325
  Cryopreservation, 89259
  Evaluation, 89329-89331
  Identification
    from Aspiration, 89257
    from Testis Tissue, 89264
    Medicolegal, 88125
  Isolation, 89260-89261
  Storage (per year), 89343
  Thawing, 89353
Sperm Analysis
  Antibodies, 89325
  Cervical Mucus Penetration Test, 89330
  Cryopreservation, 89259
  Hamster Penetration Test, 89329
  Identification
    from Aspiration, 89257
    from Testis Tissue, 89264
  Isolation and Preparation, 89260-89261
Sperm Evaluation, Cervical Mucus Penetration Test, 89330
Sperm Washing, 58323
Spermatic Cord
  Hydrocele
    Excision, 55500
    Laparoscopy, 55559
  Lesion
    Excision, 55520
  Repair
    Veins, 55530
      Abdominal Approach, 55535
      with Hernia Repair, 55540
  Varicocele
    Excision, 55530-55540
Spermatic Veins
  Excision, 55530-55540
  Laparoscopic, 55550
Spermatocele
  Excision, 54840
Spermatocystectomy, 54840
SPG11, *[81448]*
SPG7, 81405-81406
Sphenoid Sinus
  See Sinuses, Sphenoid
Sphenoidotomy
  with Nasal
    Sinus Endoscopy, 31287, 31288, *[31257]*, *[31259]*
Sphenopalatine Ganglion
  Injection
    Anesthetic, 64505
Sphenopalatine Ganglionectomy, 64999
Sphincter
  See Also Specific Sphincter
  Anal
    Dilation, 45905
    Incision, 46080
  Artificial Genitourinary, 53444-53449
  Esophageal Augmentation, 43284-43285
  Pyloric
    Incision, 43520
    Reconstruction, 43800
Sphincter of Oddi
  Pressure Measurement
    Endoscopy, 43263
Sphincteroplasty
  Anal, 46750-46751, 46760-46761
  Bile Duct, 47460, 47542
  Bladder Neck, 51800, 51845
  Pancreatic, 48999
Sphincterotomy
  Anal, 46080
  Bile Duct, 47460

Sphincterotomy — *continued*
  Bladder, 52277
Sphingomyelin Phosphodiesterase 1, Acid Lysosomal Gene Analysis, 81330
Spica Cast
  Hip, 29305, 29325
  Repair, 29720
  Shoulder, 29055
Spinal Accessory Nerve
  Anastomosis
    to Facial Nerve, 64866
  Incision, 63191
  Section, 63191
Spinal Column
  See Spine
Spinal Cord
  Biopsy, 63275-63290
  Cyst
    Aspiration, 62268
    Incision and Drainage, 63172, 63173
  Decompression, 62380, 63001-63103
    with Cervical Laminoplasty, 63050-63051
  Drain Fluid, 62272
  Exploration, 63001-63044
  Graft
    Dura, 63710
  Implantation
    Electrode, 63650, 63655
    Pulse Generator, 63685
    Receiver, 63685
  Incision, 63200
    Nerve Root, 63185-63190
    Tract, 63170, 63197
  Injection
    Anesthesia, 62320-62327
    Blood, 62273
    CT Scan, 62284
    Neurolytic Agent, 62280-62282
    Other, 62320-62327
    X-ray, 62284
  Insertion
    Electrode, 63650, 63655
    Pulse Generator, 63685
    Receiver, 63685
  Lesion
    Destruction, 62280-62282
    Excision, 63265-63273, 63300-63308
  Needle Biopsy, 62269
  Neoplasm
    Excision, 63275-63290
  Puncture (Tap)
    Diagnostic, 62270
    Drainage of Fluid, 62272
    Lumbar, 62270
  Reconstruction
    Dorsal Spine Elements, 63295
  Release, 63200
  Removal
    Catheter, 62355
    Electrode, 63661-63662
    Pulse Generator, 63688
    Pump, 62365
    Receiver, 63688
    Reservoir, 62365
  Repair
    Cerebrospinal Fluid Leak, 63707-63709
    Meningocele, 63700-63702
    Myelomeningocele, 63704-63706
  Revision
    Electrode, 63663-63664
    Neurostimulator, 63688
  Section
    Nerve Root, 63185-63190
    Tract, 63170, 63197
  Shunt
    Create, 63740, 63741
    Irrigation, 63744
    Removal, 63746
    Replacement, 63744
  Stereotaxis
    Creation Lesion, 63600
    Stimulation, 63610
  Syrinx
    Aspiration, 62268
  Tumor
    Excision, 63275-63290

Spinal Cord Neoplasms
  Excision, 63275-63290
Spinal Fluid
  Immunoelectrophoresis, 86325
  Nuclear Imagine, 78630-78650
Spinal Fracture
  See Fracture, Vertebra
Spinal Instrumentation
  Anterior, 22845-22847
    Removal, 22855
  Internal Fixation, 22841
  Pelvic Fixation, 22848
  Posterior Nonsegmental
    Harrington Rod Technique, 22840
    Harrington Rod Technique Removal, 22850
  Posterior Segmental, 22842-22844
  Posterior Segmental Removal, 22852
  Prosthetic Device, 22853-22854, 22867-22870, *[22859]*
  Reinsertion of Spinal Fixation Device, 22849
Spinal Manipulation, 98940-98942
Spinal Muscular Atrophy, 81329
Spinal Nerve
  Avulsion, 64772
  Transection, 64772
Spinal Tap
  Cervical Puncture, 61050-61055
  Cisternal Puncture, 61050-61055
  Drainage of Fluid, 62272
  Lumbar, 62270
  Subdural Tap, 61000-61001
  Ventricular Puncture, 61020-61026, 61105-61120
Spine
  See Also Intervertebral Disc; Spinal Cord; Vertebra; Vertebral Body; Vertebral Process
  Allograft
    Morselized, 20930
    Structural, 20931
  Arthroplasty
    Cervical, 0098T, 22856, 22861, 22864, *[22858]*
    Lumbar, 0163T-0165T, 22857, 22862, 22865
  Augmentation
    Lumbar Vertebra, 22514-22515
    Thoracic Vertebra, 22513, 22515
  Autograft
    Local, 20936
    Morselized, 20937
    Structural, 20938
  Biopsy, 20250, 20251
  CT Scan
    Cervical, 72125-72127
    Lumbar, 72131-72133
    Thoracic, 72128-72130
  Fixation, 22842
  Fusion
    Anterior, 22808-22812
    Anterior Approach, 22548-22585, 22812
    Exploration, 22830
    Lateral Extracavitary, 22532-22534
    Posterior Approach, 22590-22802
  Incision and Drainage
    Abscess, 22010-22015
  Insertion
    Instrumentation, 22840-22848, 22853-22854, 22867-22870, *[22859]*
  Kyphectomy, 22818, 22819
  Magnetic Resonance Angiography, 72159
  Magnetic Resonance Imaging
    Cervical, 72141, 72142, 72156-72158
    Lumbar, 72148-72158
    Thoracic, 72146, 72147, 72156-72158
  Manipulation
    Anesthesia, 22505
  Myelography
    Cervical
      Radiological Supervision and Interpretation Only, 72240
      with Radiological Supervision and Interpretation, 62302
    Lumbosacral
      Radiological Supervision and Interpretation Only, 72265

Spine — *continued*
  Myelography — *continued*
    Lumbosacral — *continued*
      with Radiological Supervision and Interpretation, 62304
    Thoracic
      Radiological Supervision and Interpretation Only, 72255
      with Radiological Supervision and Interpretation, 62303
    Two or More Regions
      Radiological Supervision and Interpretation Only, 72270
      with Radiological Supervision and Interpretation, 62305
  Percutaneous Vertebral Augmentation, 22513-22515
  Percutaneous Vertebroplasty, 22510-22512
  Reconstruction
    Dorsal Spine Elements, 63295
  Reinsertion Instrumentation, 22849
  Removal Instrumentation, 22850, 22852-22855
  Repair, Osteotomy
    Anterior, 22220-22226
    Posterior, 22210-22214
      Cervical Laminoplasty, 63050-63051
      Posterolateral, 22216
  Spinocerebellar Ataxia, 81178, 81179, 81180, 81181, 81182, 81183, 81321-81332 *[81332, 81334, 81336, 81337, 81343, 81344, 81347, 81348]*, *[81184]*, *[81185]*, *[81186]*
  Surgery, NOS, 22899
  Ultrasound, 76800
  Unlisted Services and Procedures, 22899
  X-ray, 72020
    Absorptiometry, 77080
    Cervical, 72040-72052
    Lumbosacral, 72100-72120
    Thoracic, 72070-72074
    Thoracolumbar, 72080, 72084
    Thoracolumbar Junction, 72080
    with Contrast
      Cervical, 72240
      Lumbosacral, 72265
      Thoracic, 72255
      Total, 72270
Spine Chemotherapy
  Administration, 96450
  See Also Chemotherapy
Spirometry, 94010-94070
  Patient Initiated, 94014-94016
Splanchnicectomy, 64802-64818
Spleen
  Excision, 38100-38102
    Laparoscopic, 38120
  Injection
    Radiologic, 38200
  Nuclear Medicine
    Imaging, 78185, 78215, 78216
  Repair, 38115
Splenectomy
  Laparoscopic, 38120
  Partial, 38101
  Partial with Repair, Ruptured Spleen, 38115
  Total, 38100
    En Bloc, 38102
Splenoplasty, 38115
Splenoportography, 75810
  Injection Procedures, 38200
Splenorrhaphy, 38115
Splenotomy, 38999
Splint
  See Also Casting; Strapping
  Arm
    Long, 29105
    Short, 29125-29126
  Finger, 29130-29131
  Leg
    Long, 29505
    Short, 29515
  Oral Surgical, 21085
  Ureteral, 50400-50405
Split Grafts, 15100-15101, 15120-15121
Split Renal Function Test, 52005

Surgical — *continued*
 Preparation
  Cadaver Donor Lung(s), 0494T
 Removal, Eye
  with Implant, 65103-65105
  without Implant, 65101
 Revision
  Cardiac Valve Procedure, 33530
  Carotid Thromboendarterectomy, 35390
  Coronary Artery Bypass, 33530
  Distal Vessel Bypass, 35700
 Services
  Postoperative Visit, 99024
 Ventricular Restoration, 33548
Surgical Correction
 Uterus
  Inverted, 59899
Surgical Services
 Postoperative Visit, 99024
Surveillance
 See Monitoring
 Survival of Motor Neuron1, Telomeric, 81329
Survival of Motor Neurons, Telomeric, 81329,
  [81336, 81337]
Suspension
 Aorta, 33800
 Hyoid, 21685
 Kidney, 50400-50405
 Tongue Base, 41512
 Urethra, 51990, 57289
 Uterine, 58400-58410
 Vagina, 57280-57283, 57425
 Vesical Neck, 51845
Suture
 See Also Repair
 Abdomen, 49900
 Anus, 46999
 Aorta, 33320, 33321
 Bile Duct
  Wound, 47900
 Bladder
  Fistulization, 44660-44661, 45800-45805,
    51880-51925
   Vesicouterine, 51920-51925
   Vesicovaginal, 51900
  Wound, 51860-51865
 Cervix, 57720
 Colon
  Diverticula, 44604-44605
  Fistula, 44650-44661
  Plication, 44680
  Stoma, 44620-44625
  Ulcer, 44604-44605
  Wound, 44604-44605
 Esophagus
  Wound, 43410, 43415
 Eyelid, 67880
  Closure of, 67875
  with Transposition of Tarsal Plate, 67882
  Wound
   Full Thickness, 67935
   Partial Thickness, 67930
 Facial Nerve
  Intratemporal
   Lateral to Geniculate Ganglion,
     69740
   Medial to Geniculate Ganglion,
     69745
 Fallopian Tube
  Simple, 58999
 Foot
  Tendon, 28200-28210
 Gastroesophageal, 43405
 Great Vessel, 33320-33322
 Hemorrhoids, [46945], [46946]
 Hepatic Duct, 47765, 47802
 Intestines
  Large, 44604-44605
  Small, 44602-44603
   Fistula, 44640-44661
   Plication, 44680
   Stoma, 44620-44625
 Iris
  with Ciliary Body, 66682
 Kidney
  Fistula, 50520-50526

Suture — *continued*
 Kidney — *continued*
  Horseshoe, 50540
  Wound, 50500
 Leg, Lower
  Tendon, 27658-27665
 Leg, Upper
  Muscles, 27385, 27386
 Liver
  Wound, 47350-47361
 Mesentery, 44850
 Nerve, 64831-64876
 Pancreas, 48545
 Pharynx
  Wound, 42900
 Rectum
  Fistula, 45800-45825
  Prolapse, 45540, 45541
 Removal
  Anesthesia, 15850, 15851
 Spleen, 38115
 Stomach
  Fistula, 43880
  Laceration, 43501, 43502
  Stoma, 43870
  Ulcer, 43501, 43840
  Wound, 43840
 Tendon
  Foot, 28200-28210
  Knee, 27380, 27381
 Testis
  Injury, 54670
  Suspension, 54620, 54640
 Thoracic Duct
  Abdominal Approach, 38382
  Cervical Approach, 38380
  Thoracic Approach, 38381
 Throat
  Wound, 42900
 Tongue
  to Lip, 41510
 Trachea
  Fistula, 31825
   with Plastic Repair, 31825
   without Plastic Repair, 31820
  Stoma, 31825
   with Plastic Repair, 31825
   without Plastic Repair, 31820
  Wound
   Cervical, 31800
   Intrathoracic, 31805
 Ulcer, 44604-44605
 Ureter, 50900, 50940
  Deligation, 50940
  Fistula, 50920-50930
 Urethra
  Fistula, 45820-45825, 53520
  Stoma, 53520
  to Bladder, 51840-51841
  Wound, 53502-53515
 Uterus
  Fistula, 51920-51925
  Rupture, 58520, 59350
  Suspension, 58400-58410
 Vagina
  Cystocele, 57240, 57260
  Enterocele, 57265
  Fistula
   Rectovaginal, 57300-57307
   Transvesical and Vaginal Approach,
     57330
   Urethrovaginal, 57310-57311
   Vesicovaginal, 51900, 57320-57330
  Rectocele, 57250-57260
  Suspension, 57280-57283
  Wound, 57200-57210
 Vas Deferens, 55400
 Vein
  Femoral, 37650
  Iliac, 37660
  Vena Cava, 37619
 Wound, 44604-44605
  Skin
   Complex, 13100-13160
   Intermediate, 12031-12057
   Simple, 12020-12021

SUZI (Sub-Zonal Insemination), 89280
SVR (Surgical Ventricular Restoration), 33548
Swallowing
 Cine, 74230
 Evaluation, 92610-92613, 92616-92617
 Therapy, 92526
 Video, 74230
Swan-Ganz Catheter Insertion, 93503
Swanson Procedure
 Repair, Metatarsal, 28322
  Osteotomy, 28306-28309
Sweat Collection
 Iontophoresis, 89230
Sweat Glands
 Excision
  Axillary, 11450, 11451
  Inguinal, 11462, 11463
  Perianal, 11470, 11471
  Perineal, 11470, 11471
  Umbilical, 11470, 11471
Sweat Test
 Chloride, Blood, 82435
Swenson Procedure, 45120
Syme Procedure, 27888
Sympathectomy
 Artery
  Digital, 64820
  Radial, 64821
   Superficial Palmar Arch, 64823
   Ulnar, 64822
 Cervical, 64802
 Cervicothoracic, 64804
 Digital Artery with Magnification, 64820
 Lumbar, 64818
 Presacral, 58410
 Renal, 0338T-0339T
 Thoracic, 32664
 Thoracolumbar, 64809
  with Rib Excision, 21616
Sympathetic Nerve
 Excision, 64802-64818
 Injection
  Anesthetic, 64520-64530
Sympathins, 80424, 82382-82384
Symphysiotomy
 Horseshoe Kidney, 50540
Symphysis, Pubic, 27282
Synagis, 90378
Syncytial Virus, Respiratory
 Antibody, 86756
 Antigen Detection
  Direct Fluorescence, 87280
  Direct Optical Observation, 87807
  Enzyme Immunoassay, 87420
Syndactylism, Toes, 28280
Syndactyly
 Repair, 26560-26562
Syndesmotomy
 Coracoacromial
  Arthroscopic, 29826
  Open, 23130, 23415
 Lateral Retinacular
  Endoscopic, 29873
  Open, 27425
 Transverse Carpal, 29848
Syndrome
 Adrenogenital, 56805, 57335
 Ataxia–Telangiectasia
  Chromosome Analysis, 88248
 Bloom
  Chromosome Analysis, 88245
  Genomic Sequence Analysis, 81412
 Carpal Tunnel
  Decompression, 64721
 Costen's
  See Temporomandibular Joint (TMJ)
 Crigler-Najjar, 81404
 Erb–Goldflam, 95857
 Gilbert, 81350
 Ovarian Vein
  Ureterolysis, 50722
 Synechiae, Intrauterine
  Lysis, 58559
 Treacher Collins
  Midface Reconstruction, 21150-21151

Syndrome — *continued*
 Urethral
  Cystourethroscopy, 52285
SYNGAP1, [81419]
Syngesterone, 84144
Synostosis (Cranial)
 Bifrontal Craniotomy, 61557
 Extensive Craniectomy, 61558-61559
 Frontal Craniotomy, 61556
 Parietal Craniotomy, 61556
Synovectomy
 Arthrotomy with
  Glenohumeral Joint, 23105
  Sternoclavicular Joint, 23106
 Elbow, 24102
 Excision
  Carpometacarpal Joint, 26130
  Finger Joint, 26135-26140
  Hip Joint, 27054
  Interphalangeal Joint, 26140
  Knee Joint, 27334-27335
  Metacarpophalangeal Joint, 26135
  Palm, 26145
 Wrist, 25105, 25115-25119
  Radical, 25115-25116
Synovial
 Bursa
  See Also Bursa
  Joint Aspiration, 20600-20611
 Cyst
  See Also Ganglion
  Aspiration, 20612
 Membrane
  See Synovium
  Popliteal Space, 27345
Synovium
 Biopsy
  Carpometacarpal Joint, 26100
  Interphalangeal Joint, 26110
  Knee Joint, 27330-27331
  Metacarpophalangeal Joint
   with Synovial Biopsy, 26105
 Excision
  Carpometacarpal Joint, 26130
  Finger Joint, 26135-26140
  Hip Joint, 27054
  Interphalangeal Joint, 26140
  Knee Joint, 27334-27335
Syphilis Nontreponemal Antibody, 86592-86593
Syphilis Test, 86592, 86593
Syrinx
 Pulmonary Fluid Monitoring, 0607T, 0608T
 Spinal Cord
  Aspiration, 62268
System
 Cardiac Contractility Modulation, 0408T-0418T
 Diaphragmatic Stimulation
  Evaluation/Interrogation, 0684T-0685T
  Insertion or Replacement, 0674T-0676T
   Pulse Generator Only, 0680T
  Programming, 0683T
  Removal, 0679T
   Pulse Generator Only, 0682T
  Repositioning, 0677T-0678T
   Pulse Generator Only, 0681T
 Neurostimulator
  Central Sleep Apnea, 0424T-0436T
 Pulmonary Fluid Monitoring, 0607T-0608T
 Tympanostomy
  Automated Tube Delivery, 0583T
System, Body
 Auditory, 69000-69979
 Cardiovascular, 33016-37799 [33221, 33227,
   33228, 33229, 33230, 33231, 33262,
   33263, 33264, 33270, 33271, 33272,
   33273, 33274, 33275, 33440, 33962,
   33963, 33964, 33965, 33966, 33969,
   33984, 33985, 33986, 33987, 33988,
   33989, 34717, 34718, 34812, 34820,
   34833, 34834, 36465, 36466, 36482,
   36483, 36572, 36573, 37246, 37247,
   37248, 37249]

Thoracoscopy — *continued*
Surgical — *continued*
Wedge Resection, 32666-32668
Thoracostomy
Empyema, 32035, 32036
Tube, 32551
Thoracotomy
Biopsy, 32096-32098
Cardiac Massage, 32160
Cyst Removal, 32140
Esophagogastric Fundoplasty, 43328
Exploration, 32100
for Postoperative Complications, 32120
Hemorrhage, 32110
Hiatal Hernia Repair, 43334-43335
Neonatal, 39503
Lung Repair, 32110
Open Intrapleural Pneumolysis, 32124
Removal
Bullae, 32141
Cyst, 32140
Defibrillator, 33243
Electrodes, 33238
Foreign Body
Intrapleural, 32150
Intrapulmonary, 32151
Pacemaker, 33236, 33237
Resection-Plication of Bullae, 32141
Transmyocardial Laser Revascularization, 33140, 33141
Wedge Resection, 32505-32507
Thorax
See Also Chest; Chest Cavity; Mediastinum
Angiography, 71275
Biopsy, 21550
CT Scan, 71250-71275
Incision
Empyema, 32035, 32036
Pneumothorax, 32551
Incision and Drainage
Abscess, 21501, 21502
Deep, 21510
Hematoma, 21501, 21502
Strapping, 29200
Tumor, 21555-21558 *[21552, 21554]*
Unlisted Services and Procedures, 21899
THRB, 81405
Three Glass Test
Urinalysis, Glass Test, 81020
Three–Day Measles
Antibody, 86762
Vaccine, 90707-90710
Throat
See Also Pharynx
Abscess
Incision and Drainage, 42700-42725
Biopsy, 42800-42806
Hemorrhage, 42960-42962
Reconstruction, 42950
Removal
Foreign Body, 42809
Repair
Pharyngoesophageal, 42953
Wound, 42900
Suture
Wound, 42900
Unlisted Services and Procedures, 42999
Thrombectomy
Aortoiliac Artery, 34151, 34201
Arterial, Mechanical, 37184-37185
Arteriovenous Fistula
Graft, 36904-36906
Axillary Artery, 34101
Axillary Vein, 34490
Brachial Artery, 34101
Bypass Graft, 35875, 35876
Noncoronary/Nonintracranial, 37184-37186
Carotid Artery, 34001
Celiac Artery, 34151
Dialysis Circuit, 36904-36906
Dialysis Graft
without Revision, 36831
Femoral, 34201
Femoropopliteal Vein, 34421, 34451
Iliac Artery, 34151, 34201

Thrombectomy — *continued*
Iliac Vein, 34401-34451
Innominate Artery, 34001-34101
Intracranial, Percutaneous, 61645
Mesenteric Artery, 34151
Percutaneous
Coronary Artery, *[92973]*
Noncoronary, Nonintracranial, 37184-37186
Vein, 37187-37188
Peroneal Artery, 34203
Popliteal Artery, 34203
Radial Artery, 34111
Renal Artery, 34151
Subclavian Artery, 34001-34101
Subclavian Vein, 34471, 34490
Tibial Artery, 34203
Ulnar Artery, 34111
Vena Cava, 34401-34451
Vena Caval, 50230
Venous, Mechanical, 37187-37188
Thrombin Inhibitor I, 85300-85301
Thrombin Time, 85670, 85675
Thrombocyte (Platelet)
Aggregation, 85576
Automated Count, 85049
Count, 85008
Manual Count, 85032
Thrombocyte ab, 86022-86023
Thromboendarterectomy
See Also Thrombectomy
Aorta, Abdominal, 35331
Aortoiliofemoral Artery, 35363
Axillary Artery, 35321
Brachial Artery, 35321
Carotid Artery, 35301, 35390
Celiac Artery, 35341
Femoral Artery, 35302, 35371-35372
Iliac Artery, 35351, 35361, 35363
Iliofemoral Artery, 35355, 35363
Innominate Artery, 35311
Mesenteric Artery, 35341
Peroneal Artery, 35305-35306
Popliteal Artery, 35303
Renal Artery, 35341
Subclavian Artery, 35301, 35311
Tibial Artery, 35305-35306
Vertebral Artery, 35301
Thrombokinase, 85260
Thrombolysin, 85400
Thrombolysis
Cerebral
Intravenous Infusion, 37195
Coronary Vessels, *[92975, 92977]*
Cranial Vessels, 37195
Intracranial, 61645
Other Than Coronary or Intracranial, *[37211, 37212, 37213, 37214]*
Thrombolysis Biopsy Intracranial
Arterial Perfusion, 61624
Thrombolysis Intracranial, 61645, 65205
See Also Ciliary Body; Cornea; Eye, Removal, Foreign Body; Iris; Lens; Retina; Sclera; Vitreous
Thrombomodulin, 85337
Thromboplastin
Inhibition, 85705
Inhibition Test, 85347
Partial Time, 85730, 85732
Thromboplastin Antecedent, Plasma, 85270
Thromboplastinogen, 85210-85293
Thromboplastinogen B, 85250
Thromboxane Metabolite(s), 84431
Thumb
Amputation, 26910-26952
Arthrodesis
Carpometacarpal Joint, 26841, 26842
Dislocation
with Fracture, 26645, 26650
Open Treatment, 26665
with Manipulation, 26641
Fracture
with Dislocation, 26645, 26650
Open Treatment, 26665
Fusion
in Opposition, 26820

Thumb — *continued*
Reconstruction
from Finger, 26550
Opponensplasty, 26490-26496
Repair
Muscle, 26508
Muscle Transfer, 26494
Tendon Transfer, 26510
Replantation, 20824, 20827
Sesamoidectomy, 26185
Unlisted Services and Procedures, 26989
Thymectomy, 60520, 60521
Sternal Split
Transthoracic Approach, 60521, 60522
Transcervical Approach, 60520
Thymotaxin, 82232
Thymus Gland, 60520
Excision, 60520, 60521
Exploration
Thymus Field, 60699
Incision, 60699
Other Operations, 60699
Repair, 60699
Transplantation, 60699
Thyrocalcitonin, 80410, 82308
Thyroglobulin, 84432
Antibody, 86800
Thyroglossal Duct
Cyst
Excision, 60280, 60281
Thyroid Carcinoma, 81346
Thyroid Gland
Ablation
Nodule, 0673T
Biopsy
Open, 60699
Cyst
Aspiration, 60300
Excision, 60200
Incision and Drainage, 60000
Injection, 60300
Excision
for Malignancy
Limited Neck Dissection, 60252
Radical Neck Dissection, 60254
Partial, 60210-60225
Secondary, 60260
Total, 60240, 60271
Cervical Approach, 60271
Removal All Thyroid Tissue, 60260
Sternal Split
Transthoracic Approach, 60270
Transcervical Approach, 60520
Metastatic Cancer
Nuclear Imaging, 78015-78018
Needle Biopsy, 60100
Nuclear Medicine
Imaging for Metastases, 78015-78018
Metastases Uptake, 78020
Suture, 60699
Tissue
Reimplantation, 60699
Tumor
Excision, 60200
Thyroid Hormone Binding Ratio, 84479
Thyroid Hormone Uptake, 84479
Thyroid Isthmus
Transection, 60200
Thyroid Simulator, Long Acting, 80438-80439
Thyroid Stimulating Hormone (TSH), 80418, 80438, 84443
Thyroid Stimulating Hormone Receptor ab, 80438-80439
Thyroid Stimulating Immune Globulins (TSI), 84445
Thyroid Suppression Test
Nuclear Medicine Thyroid Uptake, 78012, 78014
Thyroidectomy
Partial, 60210-60225
Secondary, 60260
Total, 60240, 60271
Cervical Approach, 60271

Thyroidectomy — *continued*
Total — *continued*
Cervical Approach — *continued*
for Malignancy
Limited Neck Dissection, 60252
Radical Neck Dissection, 60254
Removal All Thyroid Tissue, 60260
Sternal Split
Transthoracic Approach, 60270
Thyrolingual Cyst
Incision and Drainage, 60000
Thyrotomy, 31300
Thyrotropin Receptor ab, 80438-80439
Thyrotropin Releasing Hormone (TRH), 80438, 80439
Thyrotropin Stimulating Immunoglobulins, 84445
Thyroxine
Free, 84439
Neonatal, 84437
Total, 84436
True, 84436
Thyroxine Binding Globulin, 84442
Tiagabine
Assay, 80199
TIBC, 83550
Tibia
See Also Ankle
Arthroscopy Surgical, 29891, 29892
Craterization, 27360, 27640
Cyst
Excision, 27635-27638
Diaphysectomy, 27360, 27640
Excision, 27360, 27640
Epiphyseal Bar, 20150
Fracture
Arthroscopic Treatment, 29855, 29856
Plafond, 29892
Closed Treatment, 27824, 27825
with Manipulation, 27825
without Manipulation, 27824
Distal, 27824-27828
Intercondylar, 27538, 27540
Malleolus, 27760-27766, 27808-27814
Open Treatment, 27535, 27536, 27758, 27759, 27826-27828
Plateau, 29855, 29856
Closed Treatment, 27530, 27532
Shaft, 27752-27759
with Manipulation, 27825
without Manipulation, 27824
Incision, 27607
Osteoplasty
Lengthening, 27715
Prophylactic Treatment, 27745
Reconstruction, 27418
at Knee, 27440-27443, 27446
Repair, 27720-27725
Epiphysis, 27477-27485, 27730-27742
Osteochondritis Dissecans Arthroscopy, 29892
Osteotomy, 27455, 27457, 27705, 27709, 27712
Pseudoarthrosis, 27727
Saucerization, 27360, 27640
Tumor
Excision, 27635-27638, 27645
X-ray, 73590
Tibial
Arteries
Bypass Graft, 35566-35571, 35666-35671
Bypass In-Situ, 35585-35587
Embolectomy, 34203
Thrombectomy, 34203
Thromboendarterectomy, 35305-35306
Nerve
Repair/Suture
Posterior, 64840
Tibiofibular Joint
Arthrodesis, 27871
Dislocation, 27830-27832
Disruption
Open Treatment, 27829
Fusion, 27871
TIG, 90389

[Resequenced]

[Resequenced]

Index

Trachea — Transplantation

[Resequenced]

[Resequenced]

CPT © 2021 American Medical Association. All Rights Reserved.

© 2021 Optum360, LLC

Index

Unlisted Services or Procedures — Urethra

Index

Vaccines — Varicocele

Vulva — *continued*
Excision — *continued*
Partial, 56620, 56630-56632
Radical, 56630, 56631, 56633-56640
Complete, 56633-56640
Partial, 56630-56632
Simple
Complete, 56625
Partial, 56620
Lesion
Destruction, 56501, 56515
Perineum
Biopsy, 56605, 56606
Incision and Drainage, 56405
Repair
Obstetric, 59300
Vulvectomy
Complete, 56625, 56633-56640
Partial, 56620, 56630-56632
Radical, 56630-56640
Complete
with Bilateral Inguinofemoral
Lymphadenectomy, 56637
with Inguinofemoral, Iliac, and
Pelvic Lymphadenectomy,
56640
with Unilateral Inguinofemoral
Lymphadenectomy, 56634
Partial, 56630-56632
Simple
Complete, 56625
Partial, 56620
Tricuspid Valve, 33460-33465
VWF, 81401, 81403-81406, 81408
V–Y Operation, Bladder, Neck, 51845
V–Y Plasty
Skin, Adjacent Tissue Transfer, 14000-14350
VZIG, 90396

W

WADA Activation Test, 95958
WAIS
Psychiatric Diagnosis, Psychological Testing,
96112-96116
Waldenstrom's Macroglobulinemia, 81305
Wall, Abdominal
See Abdominal Wall
Walldius Procedure, 27445
Walsh Modified Radical Prostatectomy, 55810
Warfarin Therapy, 4012F
Warts
Flat
Destruction, 17110, 17111
WAS, 81406
Washing
Sperm, 58323
Wasserman Test
Syphilis Test, 86592-86593
Wassmund Procedure
Osteotomy
Maxilla, 21206
Water Wart
Destruction
Penis, 54050-54060
Skin, 17110-17111
Vulva, 56501-56515
Waterjet Ablation
Prostate, 0421T
Waterston Procedure, 33755
Watson–Jones Procedure
Repair, Ankle, Ligament, 27695-27698
Wave, Ultrasonic Shock
See Ultrasound
WBC, 85007, 85009, 85025, 85048, 85540
WDR62, 81407
Webbed
Toe
Repair, 28280
Wechsler Memory Scales, 96132-96146
Wedge Excision
Osteotomy, 21122
Wedge Resection
Chest, 32505-32507, 32666-32668
Ovary, 58920
Weight Recorded, 2001F

Well Child Care, 99381-99384, 99391-99394, 99460-
99463
Well-being Coaching, 0591T-0593T
Wellness Behavior
Alcohol and/or Substance Abuse, 99408-99409
Assessment, 96156
Family Intervention, [96167, 96168, 96170,
96171]
Group Intervention, 0403T, [96164, 96165]
Individual Intervention, 96158-96159
Re-assessment, 96156
Smoking and Tobacco Cessation Counseling,
99406-99407
Wernicke–Posadas Disease, 86490
Wertheim Hysterectomy, 58210
Wertheim Operation, 58210
West Nile Virus
Antibody, 86788-86789
Westergren Test
Sedimentation Rate, Blood Cell, 85651, 85652
Western Blot
HIV, 86689
Protein, 84181, 84182
Tissue Analysis, 88371, 88372
Wharton Ducts
Ligation of, 42510
Wheelchair Management
Propulsion
Training, 97542
Wheeler Knife Procedure, 66820
Wheeler Procedure
Blepharoplasty, 67924
Discission Secondary Membranous Cataract,
66820
Whipple Procedure, 48150
without Pancreatojejunostomy, 48152
Whirlpool Therapy, 97022
White Blood Cell
Alkaline Phosphatase, 85540
Antibody, 86021
Count, 85032, 85048, 89055
Differential, 85004-85007, 85009
Histamine Release Test, 86343
Phagocytosis, 86344
Transfusion, 86950
Whitehead Hemorrhoidectomy, 46260
Whitehead Operation, 46260
Whitman Astragalectomy, 28120, 28130
Whitman Procedure (Hip), 27120
Wick Catheter Technique, 20950
Widal Serum Test
Agglutinin, Febrile, 86000
Wilke Type Procedure, 42507
Window
Oval
Fistula Repair, 69666
Round
Fistula Repair, 69667
Window, Pericardial, 33017-33019
Windpipe
See Trachea
Winiwarter Operation, 47720-47740
Winter Procedure, 54435
Wintrobe Test
Sedimentation Rate, Blood Cell, 85651, 85652
Wire
Insertion
Removal
Skeletal Traction, 20650
Intradental
without Fracture, 21497
Wireless Cardiac Stimulator
Insertion
Battery and Transmitter, 0517T
Battery Only, 0517T
Complete System, 0515T
Electrode Only, 0516T
Transmitter Only, 0517T
Interrogation, 0521T
Programming, 0522T
Removal Only
Battery, 0520T
Battery and Transmitter, 0520T
Transmitter, 0520T
Removal with Replacement
Battery, 0519T

Wireless Cardiac Stimulator — *continued*
Removal with Replacement — *continued*
Battery and Transmitter, 0519T
Battery and/or Transmitter and Elec-
trode, 0520T
Transmitter, 0519T
Wiring
Prophylactic Treatment
Humerus, 24498
Wirsung Duct
See Pancreatic Duct
Wisconsin Card Sorting Test, 96132-96146
Witzel Operation, 43500, 43520, 43830-43832
Wolff–Parkinson–White Procedure, 33250
Womb
See Uterus
Work Hardening, 97545-97546
Work Reintegration, 97545, 97546
Work Related Evaluation Services, 99455, 99456
Worm
Helminth Antibody, 86682
Wound
Abdominal Wall, 49900
Debridement
Non–selective, 97602
Selective, 97597-97598
Dehiscence
Repair
Abdominal Wall, 49900
Secondary
Abdominal Wall, 49900
Skin and Subcutaneous Tissue
Complex, 13160
Complicated, 13160
Extensive, 13160
Skin and Subcutaneous Tissue
Simple, 12020
with Packing, 12021
Superficial, 12020
with Packing, 12021
Suture
Secondary
Abdominal Wall, 49900
Skin and Subcutaneous Tissue
Complex, 13160
Complicated, 13160
Extensive, 13160
Skin and Subcutaneous Tissue
Simple, 12020
with Packing, 12021
Superficial, 12020
with Packing, 12021
Exploration
Parathyroidectomy, 60502
Penetrating
Abdomen/Flank/Back, 20102
Chest, 20101
Extremity, 20103
Neck, 20100
Penetrating Trauma, 20100-20103
Imaging
Noncontact, Fluorescence, 0598T, 0599T
Infection
Incision and Drainage
Postoperative, 10180
Negative Pressure Therapy, 97605-97608
Repair
Skin
Complex, 13100-13160
Intermediate, 12031-12057
Simple, 12001-12021
Urethra, 53502-53515
Secondary
Abdominal Wall, 49900
Skin and Subcutaneous Tissue
Complex, 13160
Complicated, 13160
Extensive, 13160
Simple, 12020
Simple with Packing, 12021
Superficial, 12020
with Packing, 12021
Suture
Bladder, 51860, 51865
Kidney, 50500

Wound — *continued*
Suture — *continued*
Trachea
Cervical, 31800
Intrathoracic, 31805
Urethra, 53502-53515
Vagina
Repair, 57200, 57210
W–Plasty
Skin Surgery, Adjacent Tissue Transfer, 14000-
14350
Wrist
See Also Arm, Lower; Carpal Bone
Abscess, 25028
Arthrocentesis, 20605-20606
Arthrodesis, 25800
with Graft, 25810
with Sliding Graft, 25805
Arthrography, 73115
Arthroplasty, 25332, 25443, 25447
Revision, 25449
Total Replacement, 25446
with Implant, 25441, 25442, 25444,
25445
Arthroscopy
Diagnostic, 29840
Surgical, 29843-29848
Arthrotomy, 25040, 25100-25105
for Repair, 25107
Biopsy, 25065, 25066, 25100, 25101
Bursa
Excision, 25115, 25116
Incision and Drainage, 25031
Capsule
Incision, 25085
Cast, 29085
Cyst, 25130-25136
Decompression, 25020, 25023
Disarticulation, 25920
Reamputation, 25924
Revision, 25922
Dislocation
Closed Treatment, 25660
Intercarpal, 25660
Open Treatment, 25670
Open Treatment, 25660, 25670, 25676
Percutaneous Fixation, 25671
Radiocarpal, 25660
Open Treatment, 25670
Radioulnar
Closed Treatment, 25675
Percutaneous Fixation, 25671
with Fracture
Closed Treatment, 25680
Open Treatment, 25685
with Manipulation, 25259, 25660, 25675
Excision
Carpal, 25210, 25215
Cartilage, 25107
Tendon Sheath, 25115, 25116
Tumor, 25075-25078 [25071, 25073]
Exploration, 25040, 25101
Fasciotomy, 25020-25025
Fracture, 25645
Closed Treatment, 25622, 25630
Open Treatment, 25628
with Dislocation, 25680, 25685
with Manipulation, 25259, 25624, 25635
Ganglion Cyst
Excision, 25111, 25112
Hematoma, 25028
Incision, 25040, 25100-25105
Tendon Sheath, 25000, 25001
Injection
Carpal Tunnel
Therapeutic, 20526
X–ray, 25246
Joint
See Radiocarpal Joint
Lesion
Excision, 25110
Tendon Sheath, 25000
Magnetic Resonance Imaging, 73221
Reconstruction
Capsulectomy, 25320
Capsulorrhaphy, 25320

X

Y

Z

00100-00126 Anesthesia for Cleft Lip, Ear, ECT, Eyelid, and Salivary Gland Procedures

CMS: 100-04,12,140.1 Qualified Nonphysician Anesthetists; 100-04,12,140.3 Payment for Qualified Nonphysician Anesthetists; 100-04,12,140.3.3 Billing Modifiers; 100-04,12,140.3.4 General Billing Instructions; 100-04,12,140.4.1 An Anesthesiologist and Qualified Nonphysician Anesthetist Work Together; 100-04,12,140.4.2 Anesthetist and Anesthesiologist in a Single Procedure; 100-04,12,140.4.3 Payment for Medical /Surgical Services by CRNAs; 100-04,12,140.4.4 Conversion Factors for Anesthesia Services; 100-04,12,140.5 Payment for Anesthesia Services Furnished by a Teaching CRNA; 100-04,4,250.3.2 Anesthesia in a Hospital Outpatient Setting

00100 **Anesthesia for procedures on salivary glands, including biopsy**
0.00   0.00   **FUD** XXX
AMA: 2019,Oct,10; 2018,Jan,8; 2017,Dec,8; 2017,Jan,8; 2016,Jan,13

00102 **Anesthesia for procedures involving plastic repair of cleft lip**
0.00   0.00   **FUD** XXX
AMA: 2019,Oct,10; 2018,Jan,8; 2017,Dec,8; 2017,Jan,8; 2016,Jan,13

00103 **Anesthesia for reconstructive procedures of eyelid (eg, blepharoplasty, ptosis surgery)**
0.00   0.00   **FUD** XXX
AMA: 2019,Oct,10; 2018,Jan,8; 2017,Dec,8; 2017,Jan,8; 2016,Jan,13

00104 **Anesthesia for electroconvulsive therapy**
0.00   0.00   **FUD** XXX
AMA: 2019,Oct,10; 2018,Jan,8; 2017,Dec,8; 2017,Jan,8; 2016,Jan,13

00120 **Anesthesia for procedures on external, middle, and inner ear including biopsy; not otherwise specified**
0.00   0.00   **FUD** XXX
AMA: 2019,Oct,10; 2018,Jan,8; 2017,Dec,8; 2017,Jan,8; 2016,Jan,13

00124 **otoscopy**
0.00   0.00   **FUD** XXX
AMA: 2019,Oct,10; 2018,Jan,8; 2017,Dec,8; 2017,Jan,8; 2016,Jan,13

00126 **tympanotomy**
0.00   0.00   **FUD** XXX
AMA: 2019,Oct,10; 2018,Jan,8; 2017,Dec,8; 2017,Jan,8; 2016,Jan,13

00140-00148 Anesthesia for Eye Procedures

CMS: 100-04,12,140.1 Qualified Nonphysician Anesthetists; 100-04,12,140.3 Payment for Qualified Nonphysician Anesthetists; 100-04,12,140.3.3 Billing Modifiers; 100-04,12,140.3.4 General Billing Instructions; 100-04,12,140.4.1 An Anesthesiologist and Qualified Nonphysician Anesthetist Work Together; 100-04,12,140.4.2 Anesthetist and Anesthesiologist in a Single Procedure; 100-04,12,140.4.3 Payment for Medical /Surgical Services by CRNAs; 100-04,12,140.4.4 Conversion Factors for Anesthesia Services; 100-04,12,140.5 Payment for Anesthesia Services Furnished by a Teaching CRNA; 100-04,4,250.3.2 Anesthesia in a Hospital Outpatient Setting

00140 **Anesthesia for procedures on eye; not otherwise specified**
0.00   0.00   **FUD** XXX
AMA: 2019,Oct,10; 2018,Jan,8; 2017,Dec,8; 2017,Jan,8; 2016,Jan,13

00142 **lens surgery**
0.00   0.00   **FUD** XXX
AMA: 2019,Oct,10; 2018,Jan,8; 2017,Dec,8; 2017,Jan,8; 2016,Jan,13

00144 **corneal transplant**
0.00   0.00   **FUD** XXX
AMA: 2019,Oct,10; 2018,Jan,8; 2017,Dec,8; 2017,Jan,8; 2016,Jan,13

00145 **vitreoretinal surgery**
0.00   0.00   **FUD** XXX
AMA: 2019,Oct,10; 2018,Jan,8; 2017,Dec,8; 2017,Jan,8; 2016,Jan,13

00147 **iridectomy**
0.00   0.00   **FUD** XXX
AMA: 2019,Oct,10; 2018,Jan,8; 2017,Dec,8; 2017,Jan,8; 2016,Jan,13

00148 **ophthalmoscopy**
0.00   0.00   **FUD** XXX
AMA: 2019,Oct,10; 2018,Jan,8; 2017,Dec,8; 2017,Jan,8; 2016,Jan,13

00160-00326 Anesthesia for Face and Head Procedures

CMS: 100-04,12,140.1 Qualified Nonphysician Anesthetists; 100-04,12,140.3 Payment for Qualified Nonphysician Anesthetists; 100-04,12,140.3.3 Billing Modifiers; 100-04,12,140.3.4 General Billing Instructions; 100-04,12,140.4.1 An Anesthesiologist and Qualified Nonphysician Anesthetist Work Together; 100-04,12,140.4.2 Anesthetist and Anesthesiologist in a Single Procedure; 100-04,12,140.4.4 Conversion Factors for Anesthesia Services; 100-04,12,140.5 Payment for Anesthesia Services Furnished by a Teaching CRNA; 100-04,4,250.3.2 Anesthesia in a Hospital Outpatient Setting

00160 **Anesthesia for procedures on nose and accessory sinuses; not otherwise specified**
0.00   0.00   **FUD** XXX
AMA: 2019,Oct,10; 2018,Jan,8; 2017,Dec,8; 2017,Jan,8; 2016,Jan,13

00162 **radical surgery**
0.00   0.00   **FUD** XXX
AMA: 2019,Oct,10; 2018,Jan,8; 2017,Dec,8; 2017,Jan,8; 2016,Jan,13

00164 **biopsy, soft tissue**
0.00   0.00   **FUD** XXX
AMA: 2019,Oct,10; 2018,Jan,8; 2017,Dec,8; 2017,Jan,8; 2016,Jan,13

00170 **Anesthesia for intraoral procedures, including biopsy; not otherwise specified**
0.00   0.00   **FUD** XXX
AMA: 2019,Oct,10; 2018,Jan,8; 2017,Dec,8; 2017,Jan,8; 2016,Jan,13

00172 **repair of cleft palate**
0.00   0.00   **FUD** XXX
AMA: 2019,Oct,10; 2018,Jan,8; 2017,Dec,8; 2017,Jan,8; 2016,Jan,13

00174 **excision of retropharyngeal tumor**
0.00   0.00   **FUD** XXX
AMA: 2019,Oct,10; 2018,Jan,8; 2017,Dec,8; 2017,Jan,8; 2016,Jan,13

00176 **radical surgery**
0.00   0.00   **FUD** XXX
AMA: 2019,Oct,10; 2018,Jan,8; 2017,Dec,8; 2017,Jan,8; 2016,Jan,13

00190 **Anesthesia for procedures on facial bones or skull; not otherwise specified**
0.00   0.00   **FUD** XXX
AMA: 2019,Oct,10; 2018,Jan,8; 2017,Dec,8; 2017,Jan,8; 2016,Jan,13

00192 **radical surgery (including prognathism)**
0.00   0.00   **FUD** XXX
AMA: 2019,Oct,10; 2018,Jan,8; 2017,Dec,8; 2017,Jan,8; 2016,Jan,13

00210 **Anesthesia for intracranial procedures; not otherwise specified**
0.00   0.00   **FUD** XXX
AMA: 2019,Oct,10; 2018,Jan,8; 2017,Dec,8; 2017,Jan,8; 2016,Jan,13

00211 **craniotomy or craniectomy for evacuation of hematoma**
0.00   0.00   **FUD** XXX
AMA: 2019,Oct,10; 2018,Jan,8; 2017,Dec,8; 2017,Jan,8; 2016,Jan,13

00212 **subdural taps**
0.00   0.00   **FUD** XXX
AMA: 2019,Oct,10; 2018,Jan,8; 2017,Dec,8; 2017,Jan,8; 2016,Jan,13

00214 **burr holes, including ventriculography**
0.00   0.00   **FUD** XXX
AMA: 2019,Oct,10; 2018,Jan,8; 2017,Dec,8; 2017,Jan,8; 2016,Jan,13

00215 cranioplasty or elevation of depressed skull fracture, extradural (simple or compound)
🚑 0.00   ⅋ 0.00   **FUD** XXX   C 🔲
AMA: 2019,Oct,10; 2018,Jan,8; 2017,Dec,8; 2017,Jan,8; 2016,Jan,13

00216 vascular procedures
🚑 0.00   ⅋ 0.00   **FUD** XXX   N 🔲
AMA: 2019,Oct,10; 2018,Jan,8; 2017,Dec,8; 2017,Jan,8; 2016,Jan,13

00218 procedures in sitting position
🚑 0.00   ⅋ 0.00   **FUD** XXX   N 🔲
AMA: 2019,Oct,10; 2018,Jan,8; 2017,Dec,8; 2017,Jan,8; 2016,Jan,13

00220 cerebrospinal fluid shunting procedures
🚑 0.00   ⅋ 0.00   **FUD** XXX   N 🔲
AMA: 2019,Oct,10; 2018,Jan,8; 2017,Dec,8; 2017,Jan,8; 2016,Jan,13

00222 electrocoagulation of intracranial nerve
🚑 0.00   ⅋ 0.00   **FUD** XXX   N 🔲
AMA: 2019,Oct,10; 2018,Jan,8; 2017,Dec,8; 2017,Jan,8; 2016,Jan,13

00300 Anesthesia for all procedures on the integumentary system, muscles and nerves of head, neck, and posterior trunk, not otherwise specified
🚑 0.00   ⅋ 0.00   **FUD** XXX   N 🔲
AMA: 2019,Oct,10; 2018,Jan,8; 2017,Dec,8; 2017,Jan,8; 2016,Jan,13

00320 Anesthesia for all procedures on esophagus, thyroid, larynx, trachea and lymphatic system of neck; not otherwise specified, age 1 year or older
🚑 0.00   ⅋ 0.00   **FUD** XXX   N 🔲
AMA: 2019,Oct,10; 2018,Jan,8; 2017,Dec,8; 2017,Jan,8; 2016,Jan,13

00322 needle biopsy of thyroid
EXCLUDES *Cervical spine and spinal cord procedures (00600, 00604, 00670)*
🚑 0.00   ⅋ 0.00   **FUD** XXX   N 🔲
AMA: 2019,Oct,10; 2018,Jan,8; 2017,Dec,8; 2017,Jan,8; 2016,Jan,13

00326 Anesthesia for all procedures on the larynx and trachea in children younger than 1 year of age   A
INCLUDES *Anesthesia for patient of extreme age, younger than 1 year and older than 70 (99100)*
🚑 0.00   ⅋ 0.00   **FUD** XXX   N 🔲
AMA: 2019,Oct,10; 2018,Jan,8; 2017,Dec,8; 2017,Jan,8; 2016,Jan,13

00350-00352 Anesthesia for Neck Vessel Procedures

CMS: 100-04,12,140.1 Qualified Nonphysician Anesthetists; 100-04,12,140.3 Payment for Qualified Nonphysician Anesthetists; 100-04,12,140.3.3 Billing Modifiers; 100-04,12,140.3.4 General Billing Instructions; 100-04,12,140.4.1 An Anesthesiologist and Qualified Nonphysician Anesthetist Work Together; 100-04,12,140.4.2 Anesthetist and Anesthesiologist in a Single Procedure; 100-04,12,140.4.3 Payment for Medical /Surgical Services by CRNAs; 100-04,12,140.4.4 Conversion Factors for Anesthesia Services; 100-04,12,140.5 Payment for Anesthesia Services Furnished by a Teaching CRNA; 100-04,4,250.3.2 Anesthesia in a Hospital Outpatient Setting
EXCLUDES *Arteriography (01916)*

00350 Anesthesia for procedures on major vessels of neck; not otherwise specified
🚑 0.00   ⅋ 0.00   **FUD** XXX   N 🔲
AMA: 2019,Oct,10; 2018,Jan,8; 2017,Dec,8; 2017,Jan,8; 2016,Jan,13

00352 simple ligation
🚑 0.00   ⅋ 0.00   **FUD** XXX   N 🔲
AMA: 2019,Oct,10; 2018,Jan,8; 2017,Dec,8; 2017,Jan,8; 2016,Jan,13

00400-00529 Anesthesia for Chest/Pectoral Girdle Procedures

CMS: 100-04,12,140.1 Qualified Nonphysician Anesthetists; 100-04,12,140.3 Payment for Qualified Nonphysician Anesthetists; 100-04,12,140.3.3 Billing Modifiers; 100-04,12,140.3.4 General Billing Instructions; 100-04,12,140.4.1 An Anesthesiologist and Qualified Nonphysician Anesthetist Work Together; 100-04,12,140.4.2 Anesthetist and Anesthesiologist in a Single Procedure; 100-04,12,140.4.3 Payment for Medical /Surgical Services by CRNAs; 100-04,12,140.4.4 Conversion Factors for Anesthesia Services; 100-04,12,140.5 Payment for Anesthesia Services Furnished by a Teaching CRNA; 100-04,4,250.3.2 Anesthesia in a Hospital Outpatient Setting

00400 Anesthesia for procedures on the integumentary system on the extremities, anterior trunk and perineum; not otherwise specified
🚑 0.00   ⅋ 0.00   **FUD** XXX   N 🔲
AMA: 2019,Oct,10; 2018,Jan,8; 2017,Dec,8; 2017,Jan,8; 2016,Jan,13

00402 reconstructive procedures on breast (eg, reduction or augmentation mammoplasty, muscle flaps)
🚑 0.00   ⅋ 0.00   **FUD** XXX   N 🔲
AMA: 2019,Oct,10; 2018,Jan,8; 2017,Dec,8; 2017,Jan,8; 2016,Jan,13

00404 radical or modified radical procedures on breast
🚑 0.00   ⅋ 0.00   **FUD** XXX   N 🔲
AMA: 2019,Oct,10; 2018,Jan,8; 2017,Dec,8; 2017,Jan,8; 2016,Jan,13

00406 radical or modified radical procedures on breast with internal mammary node dissection
🚑 0.00   ⅋ 0.00   **FUD** XXX   N 🔲
AMA: 2019,Oct,10; 2018,Jan,8; 2017,Dec,8; 2017,Jan,8; 2016,Jan,13

00410 electrical conversion of arrhythmias
🚑 0.00   ⅋ 0.00   **FUD** XXX   N 🔲
AMA: 2019,Oct,10; 2018,Jan,8; 2017,Dec,8; 2017,Jan,8; 2016,Jan,13

00450 Anesthesia for procedures on clavicle and scapula; not otherwise specified
🚑 0.00   ⅋ 0.00   **FUD** XXX   N 🔲
AMA: 2019,Oct,10; 2018,Jan,8; 2017,Dec,8; 2017,Jan,8; 2016,Jan,13

00454 biopsy of clavicle
🚑 0.00   ⅋ 0.00   **FUD** XXX   N 🔲
AMA: 2019,Oct,10; 2018,Jan,8; 2017,Dec,8; 2017,Jan,8; 2016,Jan,13

00470 Anesthesia for partial rib resection; not otherwise specified
🚑 0.00   ⅋ 0.00   **FUD** XXX   N 🔲
AMA: 2019,Oct,10; 2018,Jan,8; 2017,Dec,8; 2017,Jan,8; 2016,Jan,13

00472 thoracoplasty (any type)
🚑 0.00   ⅋ 0.00   **FUD** XXX   N 🔲
AMA: 2019,Oct,10; 2018,Jan,8; 2017,Dec,8; 2017,Jan,8; 2016,Jan,13

00474 radical procedures (eg, pectus excavatum)
🚑 0.00   ⅋ 0.00   **FUD** XXX   C 🔲
AMA: 2019,Oct,10; 2018,Jan,8; 2017,Dec,8; 2017,Jan,8; 2016,Jan,13

00500 Anesthesia for all procedures on esophagus
🚑 0.00   ⅋ 0.00   **FUD** XXX   N 🔲
AMA: 2019,Oct,10; 2018,Jan,8; 2017,Dec,8; 2017,Jan,8; 2016,Jan,13

00520 Anesthesia for closed chest procedures; (including bronchoscopy) not otherwise specified
🚑 0.00   ⅋ 0.00   **FUD** XXX   N 🔲
AMA: 2019,Oct,10; 2018,Jan,8; 2017,Dec,8; 2017,Jan,8; 2016,Jan,13

00522 needle biopsy of pleura
🚑 0.00   ⅋ 0.00   **FUD** XXX   N 🔲
AMA: 2019,Oct,10; 2018,Jan,8; 2017,Dec,8; 2017,Jan,8; 2016,Jan,13

| 26/TC PC/TC Only | A2-Z3 ASC Payment | 50 Bilateral | ♂ Male Only | ♀ Female Only | 🚑 Facility RVU | ⅋ Non-Facility RVU | CCI | ✖ CLIA |
| **FUD** Follow-up Days | **CMS:** IOM | **AMA:** CPT Asst | A-Y OPPSI | 80/80 Surg Assist Allowed / w/Doc | Lab Crosswalk | | Radiology Crosswalk | |

© 2021 Optum360, LLC

00524	**pneumocentesis**

🚑 0.00   ⚕ 0.00   **FUD** XXX   C 🔲

AMA: 2019,Oct,10; 2018,Jan,8; 2017,Dec,8; 2017,Jan,8; 2016,Jan,13

00528	**mediastinoscopy and diagnostic thoracoscopy not utilizing 1 lung ventilation**

EXCLUDES   *Tracheobronchial reconstruction (00539)*

🚑 0.00   ⚕ 0.00   **FUD** XXX   N 🔲

AMA: 2019,Oct,10; 2018,Jan,8; 2017,Dec,8; 2017,Jan,8; 2016,Jan,13

00529	**mediastinoscopy and diagnostic thoracoscopy utilizing 1 lung ventilation**

🚑 0.00   ⚕ 0.00   **FUD** XXX   N 🔲

AMA: 2019,Oct,10; 2018,Jan,8; 2017,Dec,8; 2017,Jan,8; 2016,Jan,13

00530 Anesthesia for Cardiac Pacemaker Procedure

CMS: 100-03,10.6 Anesthesia in Cardiac Pacemaker Surgery; 100-04,12,140.1 Qualified Nonphysician Anesthetists; 100-04,12,140.3 Payment for Qualified Nonphysician Anesthetists; 100-04,12,140.3.3 Billing Modifiers; 100-04,12,140.3.4 General Billing Instructions; 100-04,12,140.4.1 An Anesthesiologist and Qualified Nonphysician Anesthetist Work Together; 100-04,12,140.4.2 Anesthetist and Anesthesiologist in a Single Procedure; 100-04,12,140.4.3 Payment for Medical /Surgical Services by CRNAs; 100-04,12,140.4.4 Conversion Factors for Anesthesia Services; 100-04,12,140.5 Payment for Anesthesia Services Furnished by a Teaching CRNA; 100-04,4,250.3.2 Anesthesia in a Hospital Outpatient Setting

00530	**Anesthesia for permanent transvenous pacemaker insertion**

🚑 0.00   ⚕ 0.00   **FUD** XXX   N 🔲

AMA: 2019,Oct,10; 2018,Jan,8; 2017,Dec,8; 2017,Jan,8; 2016,Jan,13

00532-00550 Anesthesia for Heart and Lung Procedures

CMS: 100-04,12,140.1 Qualified Nonphysician Anesthetists; 100-04,12,140.3 Payment for Qualified Nonphysician Anesthetists; 100-04,12,140.3.3 Billing Modifiers; 100-04,12,140.3.4 General Billing Instructions; 100-04,12,140.4.1 An Anesthesiologist and Qualified Nonphysician Anesthetist Work Together; 100-04,12,140.4.2 Anesthetist and Anesthesiologist in a Single Procedure; 100-04,12,140.4.3 Payment for Medical /Surgical Services by CRNAs; 100-04,12,140.4.4 Conversion Factors for Anesthesia Services; 100-04,12,140.5 Payment for Anesthesia Services Furnished by a Teaching CRNA; 100-04,4,250.3.2 Anesthesia in a Hospital Outpatient Setting

00532	**Anesthesia for access to central venous circulation**

🚑 0.00   ⚕ 0.00   **FUD** XXX   N 🔲

AMA: 2019,Oct,10; 2018,Jan,8; 2017,Dec,8; 2017,Jan,8; 2016,Jan,13

00534	**Anesthesia for transvenous insertion or replacement of pacing cardioverter-defibrillator**

EXCLUDES   *Transthoracic approach (00560)*

🚑 0.00   ⚕ 0.00   **FUD** XXX   N 🔲

AMA: 2019,Oct,10; 2018,Jan,8; 2017,Dec,8; 2017,Jan,8; 2016,Jan,13

00537	**Anesthesia for cardiac electrophysiologic procedures including radiofrequency ablation**

🚑 0.00   ⚕ 0.00   **FUD** XXX   N 🔲

AMA: 2019,Oct,10; 2018,Jan,8; 2017,Dec,8; 2017,Jan,8; 2016,Jan,13

00539	**Anesthesia for tracheobronchial reconstruction**

🚑 0.00   ⚕ 0.00   **FUD** XXX   N 🔲

AMA: 2019,Oct,10; 2018,Jan,8; 2017,Dec,8; 2017,Jan,8; 2016,Jan,13

00540	**Anesthesia for thoracotomy procedures involving lungs, pleura, diaphragm, and mediastinum (including surgical thoracoscopy); not otherwise specified**

EXCLUDES   *Thoracic spine and spinal cord procedures via anterior transthoracic approach (00625-00626)*

🚑 0.00   ⚕ 0.00   **FUD** XXX   C 🔲

AMA: 2019,Oct,10; 2018,Jan,8; 2017,Dec,8; 2017,Jan,8; 2016,Jan,13

00541	**utilizing 1 lung ventilation**

EXCLUDES   *Thoracic spine and spinal cord procedures via anterior transthoracic approach (00625-00626)*

🚑 0.00   ⚕ 0.00   **FUD** XXX   N 🔲

AMA: 2019,Oct,10; 2018,Jan,8; 2017,Dec,8; 2017,Jan,8; 2016,Jan,13

00542	**decortication**

🚑 0.00   ⚕ 0.00   **FUD** XXX   C 🔲

AMA: 2019,Oct,10; 2018,Jan,8; 2017,Dec,8; 2017,Jan,8; 2016,Jan,13

00546	**pulmonary resection with thoracoplasty**

🚑 0.00   ⚕ 0.00   **FUD** XXX   C 🔲

AMA: 2019,Oct,10; 2018,Jan,8; 2017,Dec,8; 2017,Jan,8; 2016,Jan,13

00548	**intrathoracic procedures on the trachea and bronchi**

🚑 0.00   ⚕ 0.00   **FUD** XXX   N 🔲

AMA: 2019,Oct,10; 2018,Jan,8; 2017,Dec,8; 2017,Jan,8; 2016,Jan,13

00550	**Anesthesia for sternal debridement**

🚑 0.00   ⚕ 0.00   **FUD** XXX   N 🔲

AMA: 2019,Oct,10; 2018,Jan,8; 2017,Dec,8; 2017,Jan,8; 2016,Jan,13

00560-00580 Anesthesia for Open Heart Procedures

CMS: 100-04,12,140.1 Qualified Nonphysician Anesthetists; 100-04,12,140.3 Payment for Qualified Nonphysician Anesthetists; 100-04,12,140.3.3 Billing Modifiers; 100-04,12,140.3.4 General Billing Instructions; 100-04,12,140.4.1 An Anesthesiologist and Qualified Nonphysician Anesthetist Work Together; 100-04,12,140.4.2 Anesthetist and Anesthesiologist in a Single Procedure; 100-04,12,140.4.3 Payment for Medical /Surgical Services by CRNAs; 100-04,12,140.4.4 Conversion Factors for Anesthesia Services; 100-04,12,140.5 Payment for Anesthesia Services Furnished by a Teaching CRNA; 100-04,4,250.3.2 Anesthesia in a Hospital Outpatient Setting

00560	**Anesthesia for procedures on heart, pericardial sac, and great vessels of chest; without pump oxygenator**

🚑 0.00   ⚕ 0.00   **FUD** XXX   C 🔲

AMA: 2019,Oct,10; 2018,Jan,8; 2017,Dec,8; 2017,Jan,8; 2016,Jan,13

00561	**with pump oxygenator, younger than 1 year of age** A

INCLUDES   Anesthesia complicated by utilization of controlled hypotension (99135)
Anesthesia complicated by utilization of total body hypothermia (99116)
Anesthesia for patient of extreme age, younger than 1 year and older than 70 (99100)

🚑 0.00   ⚕ 0.00   **FUD** XXX   C 🔲

AMA: 2019,Oct,10; 2018,Jan,8; 2017,Dec,8; 2017,Jan,8; 2016,Jan,13

00562	**with pump oxygenator, age 1 year or older, for all noncoronary bypass procedures (eg, valve procedures) or for re-operation for coronary bypass more than 1 month after original operation** A

🚑 0.00   ⚕ 0.00   **FUD** XXX   C 🔲

AMA: 2019,Oct,10; 2018,Jan,8; 2017,Dec,8; 2017,Jan,8; 2016,Jan,13

00563	**with pump oxygenator with hypothermic circulatory arrest**

🚑 0.00   ⚕ 0.00   **FUD** XXX   N 🔲

AMA: 2019,Oct,10; 2018,Jan,8; 2017,Dec,8; 2017,Jan,8; 2016,Jan,13

00566	**Anesthesia for direct coronary artery bypass grafting; without pump oxygenator**

🚑 0.00   ⚕ 0.00   **FUD** XXX   N 🔲

AMA: 2019,Oct,10; 2018,Jan,8; 2017,Dec,8; 2017,Jan,8; 2016,Jan,13

00567	**with pump oxygenator**

🚑 0.00   ⚕ 0.00   **FUD** XXX   C 🔲

AMA: 2019,Oct,10; 2018,Jan,8; 2017,Dec,8; 2017,Jan,8; 2016,Jan,13

00580	**Anesthesia for heart transplant or heart/lung transplant**

🚑 0.00   ⚕ 0.00   **FUD** XXX   C 🔲

AMA: 2019,Oct,10; 2018,Jan,8; 2017,Dec,8; 2017,Jan,8; 2016,Jan,13

Anesthesia

00600 — 00792

00600-00670 Anesthesia for Spinal Procedures

CMS: 100-04,12,140.1 Qualified Nonphysician Anesthetists; 100-04,12,140.3 Payment for Qualified Nonphysician Anesthetists; 100-04,12,140.3.3 Billing Modifiers; 100-04,12,140.3.4 General Billing Instructions; 100-04,12,140.4.1 An Anesthesiologist and Qualified Nonphysician Anesthetist Work Together; 100-04,12,140.4.2 Anesthetist and Anesthesiologist in a Single Procedure; 100-04,12,140.4.3 Payment for Medical /Surgical Services by CRNAs; 100-04,12,140.4.4 Conversion Factors for Anesthesia Services; 100-04,12,140.5 Payment for Anesthesia Services Furnished by a Teaching CRNA; 100-04,4,250.3.2 Anesthesia in a Hospital Outpatient Setting

00600 **Anesthesia for procedures on cervical spine and cord; not otherwise specified**

EXCLUDES Percutaneous image-guided spine and spinal cord anesthesia services (01937-01942)

🖅 0.00 ⚖ 0.00 **FUD** XXX N▣

AMA: 2019,Oct,10; 2018,Jan,8; 2017,Dec,8; 2017,Jan,8; 2016,Jan,13

00604 **procedures with patient in the sitting position**

🖅 0.00 ⚖ 0.00 **FUD** XXX C▣

AMA: 2019,Oct,10; 2018,Jan,8; 2017,Dec,8; 2017,Jan,8; 2016,Jan,13

00620 **Anesthesia for procedures on thoracic spine and cord, not otherwise specified**

🖅 0.00 ⚖ 0.00 **FUD** XXX N▣

AMA: 2019,Oct,10; 2018,Jan,8; 2017,Dec,8; 2017,Jan,8; 2016,Jan,13

00625 **Anesthesia for procedures on the thoracic spine and cord, via an anterior transthoracic approach; not utilizing 1 lung ventilation**

EXCLUDES Anesthesia services for thoracotomy procedures other than spine (00540-00541)

🖅 0.00 ⚖ 0.00 **FUD** XXX N▣

AMA: 2019,Oct,10; 2018,Jan,8; 2017,Dec,8; 2017,Jan,8; 2016,Jan,13

00626 **utilizing 1 lung ventilation**

EXCLUDES Anesthesia services for thoracotomy procedures other than spine (00540-00541)

🖅 0.00 ⚖ 0.00 **FUD** XXX N▣

AMA: 2019,Oct,10; 2018,Jan,8; 2017,Dec,8; 2017,Jan,8; 2016,Jan,13

00630 **Anesthesia for procedures in lumbar region; not otherwise specified**

🖅 0.00 ⚖ 0.00 **FUD** XXX N▣

AMA: 2019,Oct,10; 2018,Jan,8; 2017,Dec,8; 2017,Jan,8; 2016,Jan,13

00632 **lumbar sympathectomy**

🖅 0.00 ⚖ 0.00 **FUD** XXX C▣

AMA: 2019,Oct,10; 2018,Jan,8; 2017,Dec,8; 2017,Jan,8; 2016,Jan,13

00635 **diagnostic or therapeutic lumbar puncture**

🖅 0.00 ⚖ 0.00 **FUD** XXX N▣

AMA: 2019,Oct,10; 2018,Jan,8; 2017,Dec,8; 2017,Jan,8; 2016,Jan,13

00640 **Anesthesia for manipulation of the spine or for closed procedures on the cervical, thoracic or lumbar spine**

🖅 0.00 ⚖ 0.00 **FUD** XXX N▣

AMA: 2019,Oct,10; 2018,Jan,8; 2017,Dec,8; 2017,Jan,8; 2016,Jan,13

00670 **Anesthesia for extensive spine and spinal cord procedures (eg, spinal instrumentation or vascular procedures)**

🖅 0.00 ⚖ 0.00 **FUD** XXX C▣

AMA: 2019,Oct,10; 2018,Jan,8; 2017,Dec,8; 2017,Jan,8; 2016,Jan,13

00700-00882 Anesthesia for Abdominal Procedures

CMS: 100-04,12,140.1 Qualified Nonphysician Anesthetists; 100-04,12,140.3 Payment for Qualified Nonphysician Anesthetists; 100-04,12,140.3.3 Billing Modifiers; 100-04,12,140.3.4 General Billing Instructions; 100-04,12,140.4.1 An Anesthesiologist and Qualified Nonphysician Anesthetist Work Together; 100-04,12,140.4.2 Anesthetist and Anesthesiologist in a Single Procedure; 100-04,12,140.4.3 Payment for Medical /Surgical Services by CRNAs; 100-04,12,140.4.4 Conversion Factors for Anesthesia Services; 100-04,12,140.5 Payment for Anesthesia Services Furnished by a Teaching CRNA; 100-04,4,250.3.2 Anesthesia in a Hospital Outpatient Setting

00700 **Anesthesia for procedures on upper anterior abdominal wall; not otherwise specified**

🖅 0.00 ⚖ 0.00 **FUD** XXX N▣

AMA: 2019,Oct,10; 2018,Jan,8; 2017,Dec,8; 2017,Jan,8; 2016,Jan,13

00702 **percutaneous liver biopsy**

🖅 0.00 ⚖ 0.00 **FUD** XXX N▣

AMA: 2019,Oct,10; 2018,Jan,8; 2017,Dec,8; 2017,Jan,8; 2016,Jan,13

00730 **Anesthesia for procedures on upper posterior abdominal wall**

🖅 0.00 ⚖ 0.00 **FUD** XXX N▣

AMA: 2019,Oct,10; 2018,Jan,8; 2017,Dec,8; 2017,Jan,8; 2016,Jan,13

00731 **Anesthesia for upper gastrointestinal endoscopic procedures, endoscope introduced proximal to duodenum; not otherwise specified**

EXCLUDES Combination upper and lower endoscopic gastrointestinal procedures (00813)

🖅 0.00 ⚖ 0.00 **FUD** XXX N▣

AMA: 2019,Oct,10; 2018,Jan,8; 2017,Dec,8

00732 **endoscopic retrograde cholangiopancreatography (ERCP)**

EXCLUDES Combination upper and lower endoscopic gastrointestinal procedures (00813)

🖅 0.00 ⚖ 0.00 **FUD** XXX N▣

AMA: 2019,Oct,10; 2018,Jan,8; 2017,Dec,8

00750 **Anesthesia for hernia repairs in upper abdomen; not otherwise specified**

🖅 0.00 ⚖ 0.00 **FUD** XXX N▣

AMA: 2019,Oct,10; 2018,Jan,8; 2017,Dec,8; 2017,Jan,8; 2016,Jan,13

00752 **lumbar and ventral (incisional) hernias and/or wound dehiscence**

🖅 0.00 ⚖ 0.00 **FUD** XXX N▣

AMA: 2019,Oct,10; 2018,Jan,8; 2017,Dec,8; 2017,Jan,8; 2016,Jan,13

00754 **omphalocele**

🖅 0.00 ⚖ 0.00 **FUD** XXX N▣

AMA: 2019,Oct,10; 2018,Jan,8; 2017,Dec,8; 2017,Jan,8; 2016,Jan,13

00756 **transabdominal repair of diaphragmatic hernia**

🖅 0.00 ⚖ 0.00 **FUD** XXX N▣

AMA: 2019,Oct,10; 2018,Jan,8; 2017,Dec,8; 2017,Jan,8; 2016,Jan,13

00770 **Anesthesia for all procedures on major abdominal blood vessels**

🖅 0.00 ⚖ 0.00 **FUD** XXX N▣

AMA: 2019,Oct,10; 2018,Jan,8; 2017,Dec,8; 2017,Jan,8; 2016,Jan,13

00790 **Anesthesia for intraperitoneal procedures in upper abdomen including laparoscopy; not otherwise specified**

🖅 0.00 ⚖ 0.00 **FUD** XXX N▣

AMA: 2019,Oct,10; 2018,Jan,8; 2017,Dec,8; 2017,Jan,8; 2016,Jan,13

00792 **partial hepatectomy or management of liver hemorrhage (excluding liver biopsy)**

🖅 0.00 ⚖ 0.00 **FUD** XXX C▣

AMA: 2019,Oct,10; 2018,Jan,8; 2017,Dec,8; 2017,Jan,8; 2016,Jan,13

26/TC PC/TC Only | A2-Z3 ASC Payment | 50 Bilateral | ♂ Male Only | ♀ Female Only | 🖅 Facility RVU | ⚖ Non-Facility RVU | ▣ CCI | ✖ CLIA
FUD Follow-up Days | **CMS:** IOM | **AMA:** CPT Asst | A-Y OPPSI | 80/80 Surg Assist Allowed / w/Doc | Lab Crosswalk | Radiology Crosswalk

4

00794 pancreatectomy, partial or total (eg, Whipple procedure)
🔲 0.00 ⚕ 0.00 **FUD** XXX   C 🖵
AMA: 2019,Oct,10; 2018,Jan,8; 2017,Dec,8; 2017,Jan,8; 2016,Jan,13

00796 liver transplant (recipient)
EXCLUDES *Physiological support during liver harvest (01990)*
🔲 0.00 ⚕ 0.00 **FUD** XXX   C 🖵
AMA: 2019,Oct,10; 2018,Jan,8; 2017,Dec,8; 2017,Jan,8; 2016,Jan,13

00797 gastric restrictive procedure for morbid obesity
🔲 0.00 ⚕ 0.00 **FUD** XXX   N 🖵
AMA: 2019,Oct,10; 2018,Jan,8; 2017,Dec,8; 2017,Jan,8; 2016,Jan,13

00800 Anesthesia for procedures on lower anterior abdominal wall; not otherwise specified
🔲 0.00 ⚕ 0.00 **FUD** XXX   N 🖵
AMA: 2019,Oct,10; 2018,Jan,8; 2017,Dec,8; 2017,Jan,8; 2016,Jan,13

00802 panniculectomy
🔲 0.00 ⚕ 0.00 **FUD** XXX   C 🖵
AMA: 2019,Oct,10; 2018,Jan,8; 2017,Dec,8; 2017,Jan,8; 2016,Jan,13

00811 Anesthesia for lower intestinal endoscopic procedures, endoscope introduced distal to duodenum; not otherwise specified
🔲 0.00 ⚕ 0.00 **FUD** XXX   N 🖵
AMA: 2019,Oct,10; 2018,Jan,8; 2017,Dec,8

00812 screening colonoscopy
INCLUDES *Anesthesia services for all screening colonoscopy irrespective of findings*
🔲 0.00 ⚕ 0.00 **FUD** XXX   N 🖵
AMA: 2019,Oct,10; 2018,Jan,8; 2017,Dec,8

00813 Anesthesia for combined upper and lower gastrointestinal endoscopic procedures, endoscope introduced both proximal to and distal to the duodenum
🔲 0.00 ⚕ 0.00 **FUD** XXX   N 🖵
AMA: 2019,Oct,10; 2018,Jan,8; 2017,Dec,8

00820 Anesthesia for procedures on lower posterior abdominal wall
🔲 0.00 ⚕ 0.00 **FUD** XXX   N 🖵
AMA: 2019,Oct,10; 2018,Jan,8; 2017,Dec,8; 2017,Jan,8; 2016,Jan,13

00830 Anesthesia for hernia repairs in lower abdomen; not otherwise specified
EXCLUDES *Anesthesia for hernia repairs on infants one year old or less (00834, 00836)*
🔲 0.00 ⚕ 0.00 **FUD** XXX   N 🖵
AMA: 2019,Oct,10; 2018,Jan,8; 2017,Dec,8; 2017,Jan,8; 2016,Jan,13

00832 ventral and incisional hernias
EXCLUDES *Anesthesia for hernia repairs on infants one year old or less (00834, 00836)*
🔲 0.00 ⚕ 0.00 **FUD** XXX   N 🖵
AMA: 2019,Oct,10; 2018,Jan,8; 2017,Dec,8; 2017,Jan,8; 2016,Jan,13

00834 Anesthesia for hernia repairs in the lower abdomen not otherwise specified, younger than 1 year of age   A
INCLUDES *Anesthesia for patient of extreme age, younger than 1 year and older than 70 (99100)*
🔲 0.00 ⚕ 0.00 **FUD** XXX   N 🖵
AMA: 2019,Oct,10; 2018,Jan,8; 2017,Dec,8; 2017,Jan,8; 2016,Jan,13

00836 Anesthesia for hernia repairs in the lower abdomen not otherwise specified, infants younger than 37 weeks gestational age at birth and younger than 50 weeks gestational age at time of surgery   A
INCLUDES *Anesthesia for patient of extreme age, younger than 1 year and older than 70 (99100)*
🔲 0.00 ⚕ 0.00 **FUD** XXX   N 🖵
AMA: 2019,Oct,10; 2018,Jan,8; 2017,Dec,8; 2017,Jan,8; 2016,Jan,13

00840 Anesthesia for intraperitoneal procedures in lower abdomen including laparoscopy; not otherwise specified
🔲 0.00 ⚕ 0.00 **FUD** XXX   N 🖵
AMA: 2019,Oct,10; 2018,Jan,8; 2017,Dec,8; 2017,Jan,8; 2016,Jan,13

00842 amniocentesis   M ♀
🔲 0.00 ⚕ 0.00 **FUD** XXX   N 🖵
AMA: 2019,Oct,10; 2018,Jan,8; 2017,Dec,8; 2017,Jan,8; 2016,Jan,13

00844 abdominoperineal resection
🔲 0.00 ⚕ 0.00 **FUD** XXX   C 🖵
AMA: 2019,Oct,10; 2018,Jan,8; 2017,Dec,8; 2017,Jan,8; 2016,Jan,13

00846 radical hysterectomy   ♀
🔲 0.00 ⚕ 0.00 **FUD** XXX   C 🖵
AMA: 2019,Oct,10; 2018,Jan,8; 2017,Dec,8; 2017,Jan,8; 2016,Jan,13

00848 pelvic exenteration
🔲 0.00 ⚕ 0.00 **FUD** XXX   C 🖵
AMA: 2019,Oct,10; 2018,Jan,8; 2017,Dec,8; 2017,Jan,8; 2016,Jan,13

00851 tubal ligation/transection   ♀
🔲 0.00 ⚕ 0.00 **FUD** XXX   N 🖵
AMA: 2019,Oct,10; 2018,Jan,8; 2017,Dec,8; 2017,Jan,8; 2016,Jan,13

00860 Anesthesia for extraperitoneal procedures in lower abdomen, including urinary tract; not otherwise specified
🔲 0.00 ⚕ 0.00 **FUD** XXX   N 🖵
AMA: 2019,Oct,10; 2018,Jan,8; 2017,Dec,8; 2017,Jan,8; 2016,Jan,13

00862 renal procedures, including upper one-third of ureter, or donor nephrectomy
🔲 0.00 ⚕ 0.00 **FUD** XXX   N 🖵
AMA: 2019,Oct,10; 2018,Jan,8; 2017,Dec,8; 2017,Jan,8; 2016,Jan,13

00864 total cystectomy
🔲 0.00 ⚕ 0.00 **FUD** XXX   C 🖵
AMA: 2019,Oct,10; 2018,Jan,8; 2017,Dec,8; 2017,Jan,8; 2016,Jan,13

00865 radical prostatectomy (suprapubic, retropubic)   ♂
🔲 0.00 ⚕ 0.00 **FUD** XXX   C 🖵
AMA: 2019,Oct,10; 2018,Jan,8; 2017,Dec,8; 2017,Jan,8; 2016,Jan,13

00866 adrenalectomy
🔲 0.00 ⚕ 0.00 **FUD** XXX   C 🖵
AMA: 2019,Oct,10; 2018,Jan,8; 2017,Dec,8; 2017,Jan,8; 2016,Jan,13

00868 renal transplant (recipient)
EXCLUDES *Anesthesia for donor nephrectomy (00862)*
          Physiological support during kidney harvest (01990)
🔲 0.00 ⚕ 0.00 **FUD** XXX   C 🖵
AMA: 2019,Oct,10; 2018,Jan,8; 2017,Dec,8; 2017,Jan,8; 2016,Jan,13

00870 cystolithotomy
🔲 0.00 ⚕ 0.00 **FUD** XXX   N 🖵
AMA: 2019,Oct,10; 2018,Jan,8; 2017,Dec,8; 2017,Jan,8; 2016,Jan,13

● New Code ▲ Revised Code ○ Reinstated ● New Web Release ▲ Revised Web Release + Add-on Unlisted Not Covered # Resequenced
㊿ Optum Mod 50 Exempt ⚕ AMA Mod 51 Exempt ⑤ Optum Mod 51 Exempt ⑥ Mod 63 Exempt ⚡ Non-FDA Drug ★ Telemedicine M Maternity A Age Edit

00872 **Anesthesia for lithotripsy, extracorporeal shock wave; with water bath**
 🔲 0.00 🔲 0.00 **FUD** XXX   N 🔲
 AMA: 2019,Oct,10; 2018,Jan,8; 2017,Dec,8; 2017,Jan,8; 2016,Jan,13

00873 **without water bath**
 🔲 0.00 🔲 0.00 **FUD** XXX   N 🔲
 AMA: 2019,Oct,10; 2018,Jan,8; 2017,Dec,8; 2017,Jan,8; 2016,Jan,13

00880 **Anesthesia for procedures on major lower abdominal vessels; not otherwise specified**
 🔲 0.00 🔲 0.00 **FUD** XXX   N 🔲
 AMA: 2019,Oct,10; 2018,Jan,8; 2017,Dec,8; 2017,Jan,8; 2016,Jan,13

00882 **inferior vena cava ligation**
 🔲 0.00 🔲 0.00 **FUD** XXX   C 🔲
 AMA: 2019,Oct,10; 2018,Jan,8; 2017,Dec,8; 2017,Jan,8; 2016,Jan,13

00902-00952 Anesthesia for Genitourinary Procedures

CMS: 100-04,12,140.1 Qualified Nonphysician Anesthetists; 100-04,12,140.3 Payment for Qualified Nonphysician Anesthetists; 100-04,12,140.3.3 Billing Modifiers; 100-04,12,140.3.4 General Billing Instructions; 100-04,12,140.4.1 An Anesthesiologist and Qualified Nonphysician Anesthetist Work Together; 100-04,12,140.4.2 Anesthetist and Anesthesiologist in a Single Procedure; 100-04,12,140.4.3 Payment for Medical /Surgical Services by CRNAs; 100-04,12,140.4.4 Conversion Factors for Anesthesia Services; 100-04,12,140.5 Payment for Anesthesia Services Furnished by a Teaching CRNA; 100-04,4,250.3.2 Anesthesia in a Hospital Outpatient Setting

EXCLUDES Procedures on perineal skin, muscles, and nerves (00300, 00400)

00902 **Anesthesia for; anorectal procedure**
 🔲 0.00 🔲 0.00 **FUD** XXX   N 🔲
 AMA: 2019,Oct,10; 2018,Jan,8; 2017,Dec,8; 2017,Jan,8; 2016,Jan,13

00904 **radical perineal procedure**
 🔲 0.00 🔲 0.00 **FUD** XXX   C 🔲
 AMA: 2019,Oct,10; 2018,Jan,8; 2017,Dec,8; 2017,Jan,8; 2016,Jan,13

00906 **vulvectomy** ♀
 🔲 0.00 🔲 0.00 **FUD** XXX   N 🔲
 AMA: 2019,Oct,10; 2018,Jan,8; 2017,Dec,8; 2017,Jan,8; 2016,Jan,13

00908 **perineal prostatectomy** ♂
 🔲 0.00 🔲 0.00 **FUD** XXX   C 🔲
 AMA: 2019,Oct,10; 2018,Jan,8; 2017,Dec,8; 2017,Jan,8; 2016,Jan,13

00910 **Anesthesia for transurethral procedures (including urethrocystoscopy); not otherwise specified**
 🔲 0.00 🔲 0.00 **FUD** XXX   N 🔲
 AMA: 2019,Oct,10; 2018,Jan,8; 2017,Dec,8; 2017,Jan,8; 2016,Jan,13

00912 **transurethral resection of bladder tumor(s)**
 🔲 0.00 🔲 0.00 **FUD** XXX   N 🔲
 AMA: 2019,Oct,10; 2018,Jan,8; 2017,Dec,8; 2017,Jan,8; 2016,Jan,13

00914 **transurethral resection of prostate** ♂
 🔲 0.00 🔲 0.00 **FUD** XXX   N 🔲
 AMA: 2019,Oct,10; 2018,Jan,8; 2017,Dec,8; 2017,Jan,8; 2016,Jan,13

00916 **post-transurethral resection bleeding**
 🔲 0.00 🔲 0.00 **FUD** XXX   N 🔲
 AMA: 2019,Oct,10; 2018,Jan,8; 2017,Dec,8; 2017,Jan,8; 2016,Jan,13

00918 **with fragmentation, manipulation and/or removal of ureteral calculus**
 🔲 0.00 🔲 0.00 **FUD** XXX   N 🔲
 AMA: 2019,Oct,10; 2018,Jan,8; 2017,Dec,8; 2017,Jan,8; 2016,Jan,13

00920 **Anesthesia for procedures on male genitalia (including open urethral procedures); not otherwise specified** ♂
 🔲 0.00 🔲 0.00 **FUD** XXX   N 🔲
 AMA: 2019,Oct,10; 2018,Jan,8; 2017,Dec,8; 2017,Jan,8; 2016,Jan,13

00921 **vasectomy, unilateral or bilateral** ♂
 🔲 0.00 🔲 0.00 **FUD** XXX   N 🔲
 AMA: 2019,Oct,10; 2018,Jan,8; 2017,Dec,8; 2017,Jan,8; 2016,Jan,13

00922 **seminal vesicles** ♂
 🔲 0.00 🔲 0.00 **FUD** XXX   N 🔲
 AMA: 2019,Oct,10; 2018,Jan,8; 2017,Dec,8; 2017,Jan,8; 2016,Jan,13

00924 **undescended testis, unilateral or bilateral** ♂
 🔲 0.00 🔲 0.00 **FUD** XXX   N 🔲
 AMA: 2019,Oct,10; 2018,Jan,8; 2017,Dec,8; 2017,Jan,8; 2016,Jan,13

00926 **radical orchiectomy, inguinal** ♂
 🔲 0.00 🔲 0.00 **FUD** XXX   N 🔲
 AMA: 2019,Oct,10; 2018,Jan,8; 2017,Dec,8; 2017,Jan,8; 2016,Jan,13

00928 **radical orchiectomy, abdominal** ♂
 🔲 0.00 🔲 0.00 **FUD** XXX   N 🔲
 AMA: 2019,Oct,10; 2018,Jan,8; 2017,Dec,8; 2017,Jan,8; 2016,Jan,13

00930 **orchiopexy, unilateral or bilateral** ♂
 🔲 0.00 🔲 0.00 **FUD** XXX   N 🔲
 AMA: 2019,Oct,10; 2018,Jan,8; 2017,Dec,8; 2017,Jan,8; 2016,Jan,13

00932 **complete amputation of penis** ♂
 🔲 0.00 🔲 0.00 **FUD** XXX   C 🔲
 AMA: 2019,Oct,10; 2018,Jan,8; 2017,Dec,8; 2017,Jan,8; 2016,Jan,13

00934 **radical amputation of penis with bilateral inguinal lymphadenectomy** ♂
 🔲 0.00 🔲 0.00 **FUD** XXX   C 🔲
 AMA: 2019,Oct,10; 2018,Jan,8; 2017,Dec,8; 2017,Jan,8; 2016,Jan,13

00936 **radical amputation of penis with bilateral inguinal and iliac lymphadenectomy** ♂
 🔲 0.00 🔲 0.00 **FUD** XXX   C 🔲
 AMA: 2019,Oct,10; 2018,Jan,8; 2017,Dec,8; 2017,Jan,8; 2016,Jan,13

00938 **insertion of penile prosthesis (perineal approach)** ♂
 🔲 0.00 🔲 0.00 **FUD** XXX   N 🔲
 AMA: 2019,Oct,10; 2018,Jan,8; 2017,Dec,8; 2017,Jan,8; 2016,Jan,13

00940 **Anesthesia for vaginal procedures (including biopsy of labia, vagina, cervix or endometrium); not otherwise specified** ♀
 🔲 0.00 🔲 0.00 **FUD** XXX   N 🔲
 AMA: 2019,Oct,10; 2018,Jan,8; 2017,Dec,8; 2017,Jan,8; 2016,Jan,13

00942 **colpotomy, vaginectomy, colporrhaphy, and open urethral procedures** ♀
 🔲 0.00 🔲 0.00 **FUD** XXX   N 🔲
 AMA: 2019,Oct,10; 2018,Jan,8; 2017,Dec,8; 2017,Jan,8; 2016,Jan,13

00944 **vaginal hysterectomy** ♀
 🔲 0.00 🔲 0.00 **FUD** XXX   C 🔲
 AMA: 2019,Oct,10; 2018,Jan,8; 2017,Dec,8; 2017,Jan,8; 2016,Jan,13

00948 **cervical cerclage** ♀
 🔲 0.00 🔲 0.00 **FUD** XXX   N 🔲
 AMA: 2019,Oct,10; 2018,Jan,8; 2017,Dec,8; 2017,Jan,8; 2016,Jan,13

00950	**culdoscopy** ♀
	⚕ 0.00 ⚗ 0.00 **FUD** XXX N 🖵
	AMA: 2019,Oct,10; 2018,Jan,8; 2017,Dec,8; 2017,Jan,8; 2016,Jan,13

00952	**hysteroscopy and/or hysterosalpingography** ♀
	⚕ 0.00 ⚗ 0.00 **FUD** XXX N 🖵
	AMA: 2019,Oct,10; 2018,Jan,8; 2017,Dec,8; 2017,Jan,8; 2016,Jan,13

01112-01522 Anesthesia for Lower Extremity Procedures

CMS: 100-04,12,140.1 Qualified Nonphysician Anesthetists; 100-04,12,140.3 Payment for Qualified Nonphysician Anesthetists; 100-04,12,140.3.3 Billing Modifiers; 100-04,12,140.3.4 General Billing Instructions; 100-04,12,140.4.1 An Anesthesiologist and Qualified Nonphysician Anesthetist Work Together; 100-04,12,140.4.2 Anesthetist and Anesthesiologist in a Single Procedure; 100-04,12,140.4.3 Payment for Medical /Surgical Services by CRNAs; 100-04,12,140.4.4 Conversion Factors for Anesthesia Services; 100-04,12,140.5 Payment for Anesthesia Services Furnished by a Teaching CRNA; 100-04,4,250.3.2 Anesthesia in a Hospital Outpatient Setting

01112	**Anesthesia for bone marrow aspiration and/or biopsy, anterior or posterior iliac crest**
	⚕ 0.00 ⚗ 0.00 **FUD** XXX N 🖵
	AMA: 2019,Oct,10; 2018,Jan,8; 2017,Dec,8; 2017,Jan,8; 2016,Jan,13

01120	**Anesthesia for procedures on bony pelvis**
	⚕ 0.00 ⚗ 0.00 **FUD** XXX N 🖵
	AMA: 2019,Oct,10; 2018,Jan,8; 2017,Dec,8; 2017,Jan,8; 2016,Jan,13

01130	**Anesthesia for body cast application or revision**
	⚕ 0.00 ⚗ 0.00 **FUD** XXX N 🖵
	AMA: 2019,Oct,10; 2018,Jan,8; 2017,Dec,8; 2017,Jan,8; 2016,Jan,13

01140	**Anesthesia for interpelviabdominal (hindquarter) amputation**
	⚕ 0.00 ⚗ 0.00 **FUD** XXX C 🖵
	AMA: 2019,Oct,10; 2018,Jan,8; 2017,Dec,8; 2017,Jan,8; 2016,Jan,13

01150	**Anesthesia for radical procedures for tumor of pelvis, except hindquarter amputation**
	⚕ 0.00 ⚗ 0.00 **FUD** XXX C 🖵
	AMA: 2019,Oct,10; 2018,Jan,8; 2017,Dec,8; 2017,Jan,8; 2016,Jan,13

01160	**Anesthesia for closed procedures involving symphysis pubis or sacroiliac joint**
	⚕ 0.00 ⚗ 0.00 **FUD** XXX N 🖵
	AMA: 2019,Oct,10; 2018,Jan,8; 2017,Dec,8; 2017,Jan,8; 2016,Jan,13

01170	**Anesthesia for open procedures involving symphysis pubis or sacroiliac joint**
	⚕ 0.00 ⚗ 0.00 **FUD** XXX N 🖵
	AMA: 2019,Oct,10; 2018,Jan,8; 2017,Dec,8; 2017,Jan,8; 2016,Jan,13

01173	**Anesthesia for open repair of fracture disruption of pelvis or column fracture involving acetabulum**
	⚕ 0.00 ⚗ 0.00 **FUD** XXX N 🖵
	AMA: 2019,Oct,10; 2018,Jan,8; 2017,Dec,8; 2017,Jan,8; 2016,Jan,13

01200	**Anesthesia for all closed procedures involving hip joint**
	⚕ 0.00 ⚗ 0.00 **FUD** XXX N 🖵
	AMA: 2019,Oct,10; 2018,Jan,8; 2017,Dec,8; 2017,Jan,8; 2016,Jan,13

01202	**Anesthesia for arthroscopic procedures of hip joint**
	⚕ 0.00 ⚗ 0.00 **FUD** XXX N 🖵
	AMA: 2019,Oct,10; 2018,Jan,8; 2017,Dec,8; 2017,Jan,8; 2016,Jan,13

01210	**Anesthesia for open procedures involving hip joint; not otherwise specified**
	⚕ 0.00 ⚗ 0.00 **FUD** XXX N 🖵
	AMA: 2019,Oct,10; 2018,Jan,8; 2017,Dec,8; 2017,Jan,8; 2016,Jan,13

01212	**hip disarticulation**
	⚕ 0.00 ⚗ 0.00 **FUD** XXX C 🖵
	AMA: 2019,Oct,10; 2018,Jan,8; 2017,Dec,8; 2017,Jan,8; 2016,Jan,13

01214	**total hip arthroplasty**
	⚕ 0.00 ⚗ 0.00 **FUD** XXX C 🖵
	AMA: 2019,Oct,10; 2018,Jan,8; 2017,Dec,8; 2017,Jan,8; 2016,Jan,13

01215	**revision of total hip arthroplasty**
	⚕ 0.00 ⚗ 0.00 **FUD** XXX N 🖵
	AMA: 2019,Oct,10; 2018,Jan,8; 2017,Dec,8; 2017,Jan,8; 2016,Jan,13

01220	**Anesthesia for all closed procedures involving upper two-thirds of femur**
	⚕ 0.00 ⚗ 0.00 **FUD** XXX N 🖵
	AMA: 2019,Oct,10; 2018,Jan,8; 2017,Dec,8; 2017,Jan,8; 2016,Jan,13

01230	**Anesthesia for open procedures involving upper two-thirds of femur; not otherwise specified**
	⚕ 0.00 ⚗ 0.00 **FUD** XXX N 🖵
	AMA: 2019,Oct,10; 2018,Jan,8; 2017,Dec,8; 2017,Jan,8; 2016,Jan,13

01232	**amputation**
	⚕ 0.00 ⚗ 0.00 **FUD** XXX C 🖵
	AMA: 2019,Oct,10; 2018,Jan,8; 2017,Dec,8; 2017,Jan,8; 2016,Jan,13

01234	**radical resection**
	⚕ 0.00 ⚗ 0.00 **FUD** XXX C 🖵
	AMA: 2019,Oct,10; 2018,Jan,8; 2017,Dec,8; 2017,Jan,8; 2016,Jan,13

01250	**Anesthesia for all procedures on nerves, muscles, tendons, fascia, and bursae of upper leg**
	⚕ 0.00 ⚗ 0.00 **FUD** XXX N 🖵
	AMA: 2019,Oct,10; 2018,Jan,8; 2017,Dec,8; 2017,Jan,8; 2016,Jan,13

01260	**Anesthesia for all procedures involving veins of upper leg, including exploration**
	⚕ 0.00 ⚗ 0.00 **FUD** XXX N 🖵
	AMA: 2019,Oct,10; 2018,Jan,8; 2017,Dec,8; 2017,Jan,8; 2016,Jan,13

01270	**Anesthesia for procedures involving arteries of upper leg, including bypass graft; not otherwise specified**
	⚕ 0.00 ⚗ 0.00 **FUD** XXX N 🖵
	AMA: 2019,Oct,10; 2018,Jan,8; 2017,Dec,8; 2017,Jan,8; 2016,Jan,13

01272	**femoral artery ligation**
	⚕ 0.00 ⚗ 0.00 **FUD** XXX C 🖵
	AMA: 2019,Oct,10; 2018,Jan,8; 2017,Dec,8; 2017,Jan,8; 2016,Jan,13

01274	**femoral artery embolectomy**
	⚕ 0.00 ⚗ 0.00 **FUD** XXX C 🖵
	AMA: 2019,Oct,10; 2018,Jan,8; 2017,Dec,8; 2017,Jan,8; 2016,Jan,13

01320	**Anesthesia for all procedures on nerves, muscles, tendons, fascia, and bursae of knee and/or popliteal area**
	⚕ 0.00 ⚗ 0.00 **FUD** XXX N 🖵
	AMA: 2019,Oct,10; 2018,Jan,8; 2017,Dec,8; 2017,Jan,8; 2016,Jan,13

01340	**Anesthesia for all closed procedures on lower one-third of femur**
	⚕ 0.00 ⚗ 0.00 **FUD** XXX N 🖵
	AMA: 2019,Oct,10; 2018,Jan,8; 2017,Dec,8; 2017,Jan,8; 2016,Jan,13

01360	**Anesthesia for all open procedures on lower one-third of femur**
	⚕ 0.00 ⚗ 0.00 **FUD** XXX N 🖵
	AMA: 2019,Oct,10; 2018,Jan,8; 2017,Dec,8; 2017,Jan,8; 2016,Jan,13

● New Code ▲ Revised Code ○ Reinstated ● New Web Release ▲ Revised Web Release + Add-on Unlisted Not Covered # Resequenced
50 Optum Mod 50 Exempt ⚗ AMA Mod 51 Exempt 51 Optum Mod 51 Exempt 63 Mod 63 Exempt ✔ Non-FDA Drug ★ Telemedicine M Maternity A Age Edit

01380 Anesthesia for all closed procedures on knee joint

🛏 0.00 ⚕ 0.00 **FUD** XXX N 🖬

AMA: 2019,Oct,10; 2018,Jan,8; 2017,Dec,8; 2017,Jan,8; 2016,Jan,13

01382 Anesthesia for diagnostic arthroscopic procedures of knee joint

🛏 0.00 ⚕ 0.00 **FUD** XXX N 🖬

AMA: 2019,Oct,10; 2018,Jan,8; 2017,Dec,8; 2017,Jan,8; 2016,Jan,13

01390 Anesthesia for all closed procedures on upper ends of tibia, fibula, and/or patella

🛏 0.00 ⚕ 0.00 **FUD** XXX N 🖬

AMA: 2019,Oct,10; 2018,Jan,8; 2017,Dec,8; 2017,Jan,8; 2016,Jan,13

01392 Anesthesia for all open procedures on upper ends of tibia, fibula, and/or patella

🛏 0.00 ⚕ 0.00 **FUD** XXX N 🖬

AMA: 2019,Oct,10; 2018,Jan,8; 2017,Dec,8; 2017,Jan,8; 2016,Jan,13

01400 Anesthesia for open or surgical arthroscopic procedures on knee joint; not otherwise specified

🛏 0.00 ⚕ 0.00 **FUD** XXX N 🖬

AMA: 2019,Oct,10; 2018,Jan,8; 2017,Dec,8; 2017,Jan,8; 2016,Jan,13

01402 total knee arthroplasty

🛏 0.00 ⚕ 0.00 **FUD** XXX C 🖬

AMA: 2019,Oct,10; 2018,Jan,8; 2017,Dec,8; 2017,Jan,8; 2016,Jan,13

01404 disarticulation at knee

🛏 0.00 ⚕ 0.00 **FUD** XXX C 🖬

AMA: 2019,Oct,10; 2018,Jan,8; 2017,Dec,8; 2017,Jan,8; 2016,Jan,13

01420 Anesthesia for all cast applications, removal, or repair involving knee joint

🛏 0.00 ⚕ 0.00 **FUD** XXX N 🖬

AMA: 2019,Oct,10; 2018,Jan,8; 2017,Dec,8; 2017,Jan,8; 2016,Jan,13

01430 Anesthesia for procedures on veins of knee and popliteal area; not otherwise specified

🛏 0.00 ⚕ 0.00 **FUD** XXX N 🖬

AMA: 2019,Oct,10; 2018,Jan,8; 2017,Dec,8; 2017,Jan,8; 2016,Jan,13

01432 arteriovenous fistula

🛏 0.00 ⚕ 0.00 **FUD** XXX N 🖬

AMA: 2019,Oct,10; 2018,Jan,8; 2017,Dec,8; 2017,Jan,8; 2016,Jan,13

01440 Anesthesia for procedures on arteries of knee and popliteal area; not otherwise specified

🛏 0.00 ⚕ 0.00 **FUD** XXX N 🖬

AMA: 2019,Oct,10; 2018,Jan,8; 2017,Dec,8; 2017,Jan,8; 2016,Jan,13

01442 popliteal thromboendarterectomy, with or without patch graft

🛏 0.00 ⚕ 0.00 **FUD** XXX C 🖬

AMA: 2019,Oct,10; 2018,Jan,8; 2017,Dec,8; 2017,Jan,8; 2016,Jan,13

01444 popliteal excision and graft or repair for occlusion or aneurysm

🛏 0.00 ⚕ 0.00 **FUD** XXX C 🖬

AMA: 2019,Oct,10; 2018,Jan,8; 2017,Dec,8; 2017,Jan,8; 2016,Jan,13

01462 Anesthesia for all closed procedures on lower leg, ankle, and foot

🛏 0.00 ⚕ 0.00 **FUD** XXX N 🖬

AMA: 2019,Oct,10; 2018,Jan,8; 2017,Dec,8; 2017,Jan,8; 2016,Jan,13

01464 Anesthesia for arthroscopic procedures of ankle and/or foot

🛏 0.00 ⚕ 0.00 **FUD** XXX N 🖬

AMA: 2019,Oct,10; 2018,Jan,8; 2017,Dec,8; 2017,Jan,8; 2016,Jan,13

01470 Anesthesia for procedures on nerves, muscles, tendons, and fascia of lower leg, ankle, and foot; not otherwise specified

🛏 0.00 ⚕ 0.00 **FUD** XXX N 🖬

AMA: 2019,Oct,10; 2018,Jan,8; 2017,Dec,8; 2017,Jan,8; 2016,Jan,13

01472 repair of ruptured Achilles tendon, with or without graft

🛏 0.00 ⚕ 0.00 **FUD** XXX N 🖬

AMA: 2019,Oct,10; 2018,Jan,8; 2017,Dec,8; 2017,Jan,8; 2016,Jan,13

01474 gastrocnemius recession (eg, Strayer procedure)

🛏 0.00 ⚕ 0.00 **FUD** XXX N 🖬

AMA: 2019,Oct,10; 2018,Jan,8; 2017,Dec,8; 2017,Jan,8; 2016,Jan,13

01480 Anesthesia for open procedures on bones of lower leg, ankle, and foot; not otherwise specified

🛏 0.00 ⚕ 0.00 **FUD** XXX N 🖬

AMA: 2019,Oct,10; 2018,Jan,8; 2017,Dec,8; 2017,Jan,8; 2016,Jan,13

01482 radical resection (including below knee amputation)

🛏 0.00 ⚕ 0.00 **FUD** XXX N 🖬

AMA: 2019,Oct,10; 2018,Jan,8; 2017,Dec,8; 2017,Jan,8; 2016,Jan,13

01484 osteotomy or osteoplasty of tibia and/or fibula

🛏 0.00 ⚕ 0.00 **FUD** XXX N 🖬

AMA: 2019,Oct,10; 2018,Jan,8; 2017,Dec,8; 2017,Jan,8; 2016,Jan,13

01486 total ankle replacement

🛏 0.00 ⚕ 0.00 **FUD** XXX C 🖬

AMA: 2019,Oct,10; 2018,Jan,8; 2017,Dec,8; 2017,Jan,8; 2016,Jan,13

01490 Anesthesia for lower leg cast application, removal, or repair

🛏 0.00 ⚕ 0.00 **FUD** XXX N 🖬

AMA: 2019,Oct,10; 2018,Jan,8; 2017,Dec,8; 2017,Jan,8; 2016,Jan,13

01500 Anesthesia for procedures on arteries of lower leg, including bypass graft; not otherwise specified

🛏 0.00 ⚕ 0.00 **FUD** XXX N 🖬

AMA: 2019,Oct,10; 2018,Jan,8; 2017,Dec,8; 2017,Jan,8; 2016,Jan,13

01502 embolectomy, direct or with catheter

🛏 0.00 ⚕ 0.00 **FUD** XXX C 🖬

AMA: 2019,Oct,10; 2018,Jan,8; 2017,Dec,8; 2017,Jan,8; 2016,Jan,13

01520 Anesthesia for procedures on veins of lower leg; not otherwise specified

🛏 0.00 ⚕ 0.00 **FUD** XXX N 🖬

AMA: 2019,Oct,10; 2018,Jan,8; 2017,Dec,8; 2017,Jan,8; 2016,Jan,13

01522 venous thrombectomy, direct or with catheter

🛏 0.00 ⚕ 0.00 **FUD** XXX N 🖬

AMA: 2019,Oct,10; 2018,Jan,8; 2017,Dec,8; 2017,Jan,8; 2016,Jan,13

26/TC PC/TC Only   A2-Z3 ASC Payment   50 Bilateral   ♂ Male Only   ♀ Female Only   🛏 Facility RVU   ⚕ Non-Facility RVU   🖬 CCI   ❌ CLIA
FUD Follow-up Days   CMS: IOM   AMA: CPT Asst   A-Y OPPSI   80/80 Surg Assist Allowed / w/Doc   ⚕ Lab Crosswalk   Radiology Crosswalk

8   CPT © 2021 American Medical Association. All Rights Reserved.   © 2021 Optum360, LLC

01610-01680 Anesthesia for Shoulder Procedures

CMS: 100-04,12,140.1 Qualified Nonphysician Anesthetists; 100-04,12,140.3 Payment for Qualified Nonphysician Anesthetists; 100-04,12,140.3.3 Billing Modifiers; 100-04,12,140.3.4 General Billing Instructions; 100-04,12,140.4.1 An Anesthesiologist and Qualified Nonphysician Anesthetist Work Together; 100-04,12,140.4.2 Anesthetist and Anesthesiologist in a Single Procedure; 100-04,12,140.4.3 Payment for Medical /Surgical Services by CRNAs; 100-04,12,140.4.4 Conversion Factors for Anesthesia Services; 100-04,12,140.5 Payment for Anesthesia Services Furnished by a Teaching CRNA; 100-04,4,250.3.2 Anesthesia in a Hospital Outpatient Setting

INCLUDES   Acromioclavicular joint
            Humeral head and neck
            Shoulder joint
            Sternoclavicular joint

01610   **Anesthesia for all procedures on nerves, muscles, tendons, fascia, and bursae of shoulder and axilla**
            ⏚ 0.00   ⚕ 0.00   **FUD** XXX   N ▢
            AMA: 2019,Oct,10; 2018,Jan,8; 2017,Dec,8; 2017,Jan,8; 2016,Jan,13

01620   **Anesthesia for all closed procedures on humeral head and neck, sternoclavicular joint, acromioclavicular joint, and shoulder joint**
            ⏚ 0.00   ⚕ 0.00   **FUD** XXX   N ▢
            AMA: 2019,Oct,10; 2018,Jan,8; 2017,Dec,8; 2017,Jan,8; 2016,Jan,13

01622   **Anesthesia for diagnostic arthroscopic procedures of shoulder joint**
            ⏚ 0.00   ⚕ 0.00   **FUD** XXX   N ▢
            AMA: 2019,Oct,10; 2018,Jan,8; 2017,Dec,8; 2017,Jan,8; 2016,Jan,13

01630   **Anesthesia for open or surgical arthroscopic procedures on humeral head and neck, sternoclavicular joint, acromioclavicular joint, and shoulder joint; not otherwise specified**
            ⏚ 0.00   ⚕ 0.00   **FUD** XXX   N ▢
            AMA: 2019,Oct,10; 2018,Jan,8; 2017,Dec,8; 2017,Jan,8; 2016,Jan,13

01634   **shoulder disarticulation**
            ⏚ 0.00   ⚕ 0.00   **FUD** XXX   C ▢
            AMA: 2019,Oct,10; 2018,Jan,8; 2017,Dec,8; 2017,Jan,8; 2016,Jan,13

01636   **interthoracoscapular (forequarter) amputation**
            ⏚ 0.00   ⚕ 0.00   **FUD** XXX   C ▢
            AMA: 2019,Oct,10; 2018,Jan,8; 2017,Dec,8; 2017,Jan,8; 2016,Jan,13

01638   **total shoulder replacement**
            ⏚ 0.00   ⚕ 0.00   **FUD** XXX   C ▢
            AMA: 2019,Oct,10; 2018,Jan,8; 2017,Dec,8; 2017,Jan,8; 2016,Jan,13

01650   **Anesthesia for procedures on arteries of shoulder and axilla; not otherwise specified**
            ⏚ 0.00   ⚕ 0.00   **FUD** XXX   N ▢
            AMA: 2019,Oct,10; 2018,Jan,8; 2017,Dec,8; 2017,Jan,8; 2016,Jan,13

01652   **axillary-brachial aneurysm**
            ⏚ 0.00   ⚕ 0.00   **FUD** XXX   C ▢
            AMA: 2019,Oct,10; 2018,Jan,8; 2017,Dec,8; 2017,Jan,8; 2016,Jan,13

01654   **bypass graft**
            ⏚ 0.00   ⚕ 0.00   **FUD** XXX   C ▢
            AMA: 2019,Oct,10; 2018,Jan,8; 2017,Dec,8; 2017,Jan,8; 2016,Jan,13

01656   **axillary-femoral bypass graft**
            ⏚ 0.00   ⚕ 0.00   **FUD** XXX   C ▢
            AMA: 2019,Oct,10; 2018,Jan,8; 2017,Dec,8; 2017,Jan,8; 2016,Jan,13

01670   **Anesthesia for all procedures on veins of shoulder and axilla**
            ⏚ 0.00   ⚕ 0.00   **FUD** XXX   N ▢
            AMA: 2019,Oct,10; 2018,Jan,8; 2017,Dec,8; 2017,Jan,8; 2016,Jan,13

01680   **Anesthesia for shoulder cast application, removal or repair, not otherwise specified**
            ⏚ 0.00   ⚕ 0.00   **FUD** XXX   N ▢
            AMA: 2019,Oct,10; 2018,Jan,8; 2017,Dec,8; 2017,Jan,8; 2016,Jan,13

01710-01860 Anesthesia for Upper Extremity Procedures

CMS: 100-04,12,140.1 Qualified Nonphysician Anesthetists; 100-04,12,140.3 Payment for Qualified Nonphysician Anesthetists; 100-04,12,140.3.3 Billing Modifiers; 100-04,12,140.3.4 General Billing Instructions; 100-04,12,140.4.1 An Anesthesiologist and Qualified Nonphysician Anesthetist Work Together; 100-04,12,140.4.2 Anesthetist and Anesthesiologist in a Single Procedure; 100-04,12,140.4.3 Payment for Medical /Surgical Services by CRNAs; 100-04,12,140.4.4 Conversion Factors for Anesthesia Services; 100-04,12,140.5 Payment for Anesthesia Services Furnished by a Teaching CRNA; 100-04,4,250.3.2 Anesthesia in a Hospital Outpatient Setting

01710   **Anesthesia for procedures on nerves, muscles, tendons, fascia, and bursae of upper arm and elbow; not otherwise specified**
            ⏚ 0.00   ⚕ 0.00   **FUD** XXX   N ▢
            AMA: 2019,Oct,10; 2018,Jan,8; 2017,Dec,8; 2017,Jan,8; 2016,Jan,13

01712   **tenotomy, elbow to shoulder, open**
            ⏚ 0.00   ⚕ 0.00   **FUD** XXX   N ▢
            AMA: 2019,Oct,10; 2018,Jan,8; 2017,Dec,8; 2017,Jan,8; 2016,Jan,13

01714   **tenoplasty, elbow to shoulder**
            ⏚ 0.00   ⚕ 0.00   **FUD** XXX   N ▢
            AMA: 2019,Oct,10; 2018,Jan,8; 2017,Dec,8; 2017,Jan,8; 2016,Jan,13

01716   **tenodesis, rupture of long tendon of biceps**
            ⏚ 0.00   ⚕ 0.00   **FUD** XXX   N ▢
            AMA: 2019,Oct,10; 2018,Jan,8; 2017,Dec,8; 2017,Jan,8; 2016,Jan,13

01730   **Anesthesia for all closed procedures on humerus and elbow**
            ⏚ 0.00   ⚕ 0.00   **FUD** XXX   N ▢
            AMA: 2019,Oct,10; 2018,Jan,8; 2017,Dec,8; 2017,Jan,8; 2016,Jan,13

01732   **Anesthesia for diagnostic arthroscopic procedures of elbow joint**
            ⏚ 0.00   ⚕ 0.00   **FUD** XXX   N ▢
            AMA: 2019,Oct,10; 2018,Jan,8; 2017,Dec,8; 2017,Jan,8; 2016,Jan,13

01740   **Anesthesia for open or surgical arthroscopic procedures of the elbow; not otherwise specified**
            ⏚ 0.00   ⚕ 0.00   **FUD** XXX   N ▢
            AMA: 2019,Oct,10; 2018,Jan,8; 2017,Dec,8; 2017,Jan,8; 2016,Jan,13

01742   **osteotomy of humerus**
            ⏚ 0.00   ⚕ 0.00   **FUD** XXX   N ▢
            AMA: 2019,Oct,10; 2018,Jan,8; 2017,Dec,8; 2017,Jan,8; 2016,Jan,13

01744   **repair of nonunion or malunion of humerus**
            ⏚ 0.00   ⚕ 0.00   **FUD** XXX   N ▢
            AMA: 2019,Oct,10; 2018,Jan,8; 2017,Dec,8; 2017,Jan,8; 2016,Jan,13

01756   **radical procedures**
            ⏚ 0.00   ⚕ 0.00   **FUD** XXX   C ▢
            AMA: 2019,Oct,10; 2018,Jan,8; 2017,Dec,8; 2017,Jan,8; 2016,Jan,13

01758   **excision of cyst or tumor of humerus**
            ⏚ 0.00   ⚕ 0.00   **FUD** XXX   N ▢
            AMA: 2019,Oct,10; 2018,Jan,8; 2017,Dec,8; 2017,Jan,8; 2016,Jan,13

01760   **total elbow replacement**
            ⏚ 0.00   ⚕ 0.00   **FUD** XXX   N ▢
            AMA: 2019,Oct,10; 2018,Jan,8; 2017,Dec,8; 2017,Jan,8; 2016,Jan,13

01770	**Anesthesia for procedures on arteries of upper arm and elbow; not otherwise specified**
	🔧 0.00 ⚕ 0.00 **FUD** XXX N ▣
	AMA: 2019,Oct,10; 2018,Jan,8; 2017,Dec,8; 2017,Jan,8; 2016,Jan,13

01772	**embolectomy**
	🔧 0.00 ⚕ 0.00 **FUD** XXX N ▣
	AMA: 2019,Oct,10; 2018,Jan,8; 2017,Dec,8; 2017,Jan,8; 2016,Jan,13

01780	**Anesthesia for procedures on veins of upper arm and elbow; not otherwise specified**
	🔧 0.00 ⚕ 0.00 **FUD** XXX N ▣
	AMA: 2019,Oct,10; 2018,Jan,8; 2017,Dec,8; 2017,Jan,8; 2016,Jan,13

01782	**phleborrhaphy**
	🔧 0.00 ⚕ 0.00 **FUD** XXX N ▣
	AMA: 2019,Oct,10; 2018,Jan,8; 2017,Dec,8; 2017,Jan,8; 2016,Jan,13

01810	**Anesthesia for all procedures on nerves, muscles, tendons, fascia, and bursae of forearm, wrist, and hand**
	🔧 0.00 ⚕ 0.00 **FUD** XXX N ▣
	AMA: 2019,Oct,10; 2018,Jan,8; 2017,Dec,8; 2017,Jan,8; 2016,Jan,13

01820	**Anesthesia for all closed procedures on radius, ulna, wrist, or hand bones**
	🔧 0.00 ⚕ 0.00 **FUD** XXX N ▣
	AMA: 2019,Oct,10; 2018,Jan,8; 2017,Dec,8; 2017,Jan,8; 2016,Jan,13

01829	**Anesthesia for diagnostic arthroscopic procedures on the wrist**
	🔧 0.00 ⚕ 0.00 **FUD** XXX N ▣
	AMA: 2019,Oct,10; 2018,Jan,8; 2017,Dec,8; 2017,Jan,8; 2016,Jan,13

01830	**Anesthesia for open or surgical arthroscopic/endoscopic procedures on distal radius, distal ulna, wrist, or hand joints; not otherwise specified**
	🔧 0.00 ⚕ 0.00 **FUD** XXX N ▣
	AMA: 2019,Oct,10; 2018,Jan,8; 2017,Dec,8; 2017,Jan,8; 2016,Jan,13

01832	**total wrist replacement**
	🔧 0.00 ⚕ 0.00 **FUD** XXX N ▣
	AMA: 2019,Oct,10; 2018,Jan,8; 2017,Dec,8; 2017,Jan,8; 2016,Jan,13

01840	**Anesthesia for procedures on arteries of forearm, wrist, and hand; not otherwise specified**
	🔧 0.00 ⚕ 0.00 **FUD** XXX N ▣
	AMA: 2019,Oct,10; 2018,Jan,8; 2017,Dec,8; 2017,Jan,8; 2016,Jan,13

01842	**embolectomy**
	🔧 0.00 ⚕ 0.00 **FUD** XXX N ▣
	AMA: 2019,Oct,10; 2018,Jan,8; 2017,Dec,8; 2017,Jan,8; 2016,Jan,13

01844	**Anesthesia for vascular shunt, or shunt revision, any type (eg, dialysis)**
	🔧 0.00 ⚕ 0.00 **FUD** XXX N ▣
	AMA: 2019,Oct,10; 2018,Jan,8; 2017,Dec,8; 2017,Jan,8; 2016,Jan,13

01850	**Anesthesia for procedures on veins of forearm, wrist, and hand; not otherwise specified**
	🔧 0.00 ⚕ 0.00 **FUD** XXX N ▣
	AMA: 2019,Oct,10; 2018,Jan,8; 2017,Dec,8; 2017,Jan,8; 2016,Jan,13

01852	**phleborrhaphy**
	🔧 0.00 ⚕ 0.00 **FUD** XXX N ▣
	AMA: 2019,Oct,10; 2018,Jan,8; 2017,Dec,8; 2017,Jan,8; 2016,Jan,13

01860	**Anesthesia for forearm, wrist, or hand cast application, removal, or repair**
	🔧 0.00 ⚕ 0.00 **FUD** XXX N ▣
	AMA: 2019,Oct,10; 2018,Jan,8; 2017,Dec,8; 2017,Jan,8; 2016,Jan,13

01916-01942 Anesthesia for Interventional Radiology Procedures

01916	**Anesthesia for diagnostic arteriography/venography**
	EXCLUDES *Anesthesia for therapeutic interventional radiological procedures involving arterial system (01924-01926)*
	Anesthesia for therapeutic interventional radiological procedures involving venous/lymphatic system (01930-01933)
	🔧 0.00 ⚕ 0.00 **FUD** XXX N ▣
	AMA: 2019,Oct,10; 2018,Jan,8; 2017,Dec,8; 2017,Jan,8; 2016,Jan,13

01920	**Anesthesia for cardiac catheterization including coronary angiography and ventriculography (not to include Swan-Ganz catheter)**
	🔧 0.00 ⚕ 0.00 **FUD** XXX N ▣
	AMA: 2019,Oct,10; 2018,Jan,8; 2017,Dec,8; 2017,Jan,8; 2016,Jan,13

01922	**Anesthesia for non-invasive imaging or radiation therapy**
	🔧 0.00 ⚕ 0.00 **FUD** XXX N ▣
	AMA: 2019,Oct,10; 2018,Jan,8; 2017,Dec,8; 2017,Jan,8; 2016,Jan,13

01924	**Anesthesia for therapeutic interventional radiological procedures involving the arterial system; not otherwise specified**
	🔧 0.00 ⚕ 0.00 **FUD** XXX N ▣
	AMA: 2019,Oct,10; 2018,Jan,8; 2017,Dec,8; 2017,Jan,8; 2016,Jan,13

01925	**carotid or coronary**
	🔧 0.00 ⚕ 0.00 **FUD** XXX N ▣
	AMA: 2019,Oct,10; 2018,Jan,8; 2017,Dec,8; 2017,Jan,8; 2016,Jan,13

01926	**intracranial, intracardiac, or aortic**
	🔧 0.00 ⚕ 0.00 **FUD** XXX N ▣
	AMA: 2019,Oct,10; 2018,Jan,8; 2017,Dec,8; 2017,Jan,8; 2016,Jan,13

01930	**Anesthesia for therapeutic interventional radiological procedures involving the venous/lymphatic system (not to include access to the central circulation); not otherwise specified**
	🔧 0.00 ⚕ 0.00 **FUD** XXX N ▣
	AMA: 2019,Oct,10; 2018,Jan,8; 2017,Dec,8; 2017,Jan,8; 2016,Jan,13

01931	**intrahepatic or portal circulation (eg, transvenous intrahepatic portosystemic shunt[s] [TIPS])**
	🔧 0.00 ⚕ 0.00 **FUD** XXX N ▣
	AMA: 2019,Oct,10; 2018,Jan,8; 2017,Dec,8; 2017,Jan,8; 2016,Jan,13

01932	**intrathoracic or jugular**
	🔧 0.00 ⚕ 0.00 **FUD** XXX N ▣
	AMA: 2019,Oct,10; 2018,Jan,8; 2017,Dec,8; 2017,Jan,8; 2016,Jan,13

01933	**intracranial**
	🔧 0.00 ⚕ 0.00 **FUD** XXX N ▣
	AMA: 2019,Oct,10; 2018,Jan,8; 2017,Dec,8; 2017,Jan,8; 2016,Jan,13

~~01935~~	~~**Anesthesia for percutaneous image-guided procedures on the spine and spinal cord; diagnostic**~~
	To report, see (01937-01942)

~~01936~~	~~**therapeutic**~~
	To report, see (01937-01942)

| 26/TC PC/TC Only | A2-Z3 ASC Payment | 50 Bilateral | ♂ Male Only | ♀ Female Only | 🔧 Facility RVU | ⚕ Non-Facility RVU | ▣ CCI | ✖ CLIA |
| **FUD** Follow-up Days | **CMS:** IOM | **AMA:** CPT Asst | A-Y OPPSI | 80/80 Surg Assist Allowed / w/Doc | ◼ Lab Crosswalk | ◼ Radiology Crosswalk |

10   CPT © 2021 American Medical Association. All Rights Reserved.   © 2021 Optum360, LLC

● 01937 Anesthesia for percutaneous image-guided injection, drainage or aspiration procedures on the spine or spinal cord; cervical or thoracic

EXCLUDES Anesthesia for percutaneous image-guided destruction (01939)

● 01938 lumbar or sacral

EXCLUDES Anesthesia for percutaneous image-guided destruction (01940)

● 01939 Anesthesia for percutaneous image-guided destruction procedures by neurolytic agent on the spine or spinal cord; cervical or thoracic

EXCLUDES Anesthesia for percutaneous injection, drainage or aspiration (01937)

● 01940 lumbar or sacral

EXCLUDES Anesthesia for percutaneous injection, drainage or aspiration (01938)

● 01941 Anesthesia for percutaneous image-guided neuromodulation or intravertebral procedures (eg, kyphoplasty, vertebroplasty) on the spine or spinal cord; cervical or thoracic

● 01942 lumbar or sacral

01951-01953 Anesthesia for Burn Procedures

CMS: 100-04,12,140.1 Qualified Nonphysician Anesthetists; 100-04,12,140.3 Payment for Qualified Nonphysician Anesthetists; 100-04,12,140.3.3 Billing Modifiers; 100-04,12,140.3.4 General Billing Instructions; 100-04,12,140.4.1 An Anesthesiologist and Qualified Nonphysician Anesthetist Work Together; 100-04,12,140.4.2 Anesthetist and Anesthesiologist in a Single Procedure; 100-04,12,140.4.3 Payment for Medical /Surgical Services by CRNAs; 100-04,12,140.4.4 Conversion Factors for Anesthesia Services; 100-04,12,140.5 Payment for Anesthesia Services Furnished by a Teaching CRNA; 100-04,4,250.3.2 Anesthesia in a Hospital Outpatient Setting

01951 Anesthesia for second- and third-degree burn excision or debridement with or without skin grafting, any site, for total body surface area (TBSA) treated during anesthesia and surgery; less than 4% total body surface area

🗂 0.00 ⚖ 0.00 FUD XXX N 🖵

AMA: 2019,Oct,10; 2018,Jan,8; 2017,Dec,8; 2017,Jan,8; 2016,Jan,13

01952 between 4% and 9% of total body surface area

🗂 0.00 ⚖ 0.00 FUD XXX N 🖵

AMA: 2019,Oct,10; 2018,Jan,8; 2017,Dec,8; 2017,Jan,8; 2016,Jan,13

+ 01953 each additional 9% total body surface area or part thereof (List separately in addition to code for primary procedure)

Code first (01952)

🗂 0.00 ⚖ 0.00 FUD XXX N 🖵

AMA: 2019,Oct,10; 2018,Jan,8; 2017,Dec,8; 2017,Jan,8; 2016,Jan,13

01958-01969 Anesthesia for Obstetric Procedures

CMS: 100-04,12,140.1 Qualified Nonphysician Anesthetists; 100-04,12,140.3 Payment for Qualified Nonphysician Anesthetists; 100-04,12,140.3.3 Billing Modifiers; 100-04,12,140.3.4 General Billing Instructions; 100-04,12,140.4.1 An Anesthesiologist and Qualified Nonphysician Anesthetist Work Together; 100-04,12,140.4.2 Anesthetist and Anesthesiologist in a Single Procedure; 100-04,12,140.4.3 Payment for Medical /Surgical Services by CRNAs; 100-04,12,140.4.4 Conversion Factors for Anesthesia Services; 100-04,12,140.5 Payment for Anesthesia Services Furnished by a Teaching CRNA; 100-04,4,250.3.2 Anesthesia in a Hospital Outpatient Setting

01958 Anesthesia for external cephalic version procedure M

🗂 0.00 ⚖ 0.00 FUD XXX N 🖵

AMA: 2019,Oct,10; 2018,Jan,8; 2017,Dec,8; 2017,Jan,8; 2016,Jan,13

01960 Anesthesia for vaginal delivery only M ♀

🗂 0.00 ⚖ 0.00 FUD XXX N 🖵

AMA: 2019,Oct,10; 2018,Jan,8; 2017,Dec,8; 2017,Jan,8; 2016,Jan,13

01961 Anesthesia for cesarean delivery only M ♀

🗂 0.00 ⚖ 0.00 FUD XXX N 🖵

AMA: 2019,Oct,10; 2018,Jan,8; 2017,Dec,8; 2017,Jan,8; 2016,Jan,13

01962 Anesthesia for urgent hysterectomy following delivery M ♀

🗂 0.00 ⚖ 0.00 FUD XXX N 🖵

AMA: 2019,Oct,10; 2018,Jan,8; 2017,Dec,8; 2017,Jan,8; 2016,Jan,13

01963 Anesthesia for cesarean hysterectomy without any labor analgesia/anesthesia care M ♀

🗂 0.00 ⚖ 0.00 FUD XXX N 🖵

AMA: 2019,Oct,10; 2018,Jan,8; 2017,Dec,8; 2017,Jan,8; 2016,Jan,13

01965 Anesthesia for incomplete or missed abortion procedures M ♀

🗂 0.00 ⚖ 0.00 FUD XXX N 🖵

AMA: 2019,Oct,10; 2018,Jan,8; 2017,Dec,8; 2017,Jan,8; 2016,Jan,13

01966 Anesthesia for induced abortion procedures M ♀

🗂 0.00 ⚖ 0.00 FUD XXX N 🖵

AMA: 2019,Oct,10; 2018,Jan,8; 2017,Dec,8; 2017,Jan,8; 2016,Jan,13

01967 Neuraxial labor analgesia/anesthesia for planned vaginal delivery (this includes any repeat subarachnoid needle placement and drug injection and/or any necessary replacement of an epidural catheter during labor) M ♀

🗂 0.00 ⚖ 0.00 FUD XXX N 🖵

AMA: 2019,Oct,10; 2018,Jan,8; 2017,Dec,8; 2017,Jan,8; 2016,Jan,13

+ 01968 Anesthesia for cesarean delivery following neuraxial labor analgesia/anesthesia (List separately in addition to code for primary procedure performed) M ♀

Code first (01967)

🗂 0.00 ⚖ 0.00 FUD XXX N 🖵

AMA: 2019,Oct,10; 2018,Jan,8; 2017,Dec,8; 2017,Jan,8; 2016,Jan,13

+ 01969 Anesthesia for cesarean hysterectomy following neuraxial labor analgesia/anesthesia (List separately in addition to code for primary procedure performed) M ♀

Code first (01967)

🗂 0.00 ⚖ 0.00 FUD XXX N 🖵

AMA: 2019,Oct,10; 2018,Jan,8; 2017,Dec,8; 2017,Jan,8; 2016,Jan,13

01990-01999 Anesthesia Miscellaneous

CMS: 100-04,12,140.1 Qualified Nonphysician Anesthetists; 100-04,12,140.3 Payment for Qualified Nonphysician Anesthetists; 100-04,12,140.3.3 Billing Modifiers; 100-04,12,140.3.4 General Billing Instructions; 100-04,12,140.4.1 An Anesthesiologist and Qualified Nonphysician Anesthetist Work Together; 100-04,12,140.4.2 Anesthetist and Anesthesiologist in a Single Procedure; 100-04,12,140.4.3 Payment for Medical /Surgical Services by CRNAs; 100-04,12,140.4.4 Conversion Factors for Anesthesia Services; 100-04,12,140.5 Payment for Anesthesia Services Furnished by a Teaching CRNA; 100-04,4,250.3.2 Anesthesia in a Hospital Outpatient Setting

01990 Physiological support for harvesting of organ(s) from brain-dead patient

🗂 0.00 ⚖ 0.00 FUD XXX C 🖵

AMA: 2019,Oct,10; 2018,Jan,8; 2017,Dec,8; 2017,Jan,8; 2016,Jan,13

01991 Anesthesia for diagnostic or therapeutic nerve blocks and injections (when block or injection is performed by a different physician or other qualified health care professional); other than the prone position

EXCLUDES Bier block for pain management (64999)
Moderate Sedation (99151-99153, 99155-99157)
Pain management via intra-arterial or IV therapy (96373-96374)
Regional or local anesthesia arms or legs for surgical procedure

🗂 0.00 ⚖ 0.00 FUD XXX N 🖵

AMA: 2019,Oct,10; 2018,Jan,8; 2017,Dec,8; 2017,Jan,8; 2016,Jan,13

● New Code ▲ Revised Code ○ Reinstated ● New Web Release ▲ Revised Web Release + Add-on Unlisted Not Covered # Resequenced
🔟 Optum Mod 50 Exempt ⊘ AMA Mod 51 Exempt �51 Optum Mod 51 Exempt 63 Mod 63 Exempt ✀ Non-FDA Drug ★ Telemedicine M Maternity A Age Edit

01992   **prone position**

> EXCLUDES   *Bier block for pain management (64999)*
> *Moderate sedation (99151-99153, 99155-99157)*
> *Pain management via intra-arterial or IV therapy (96373-96374)*
> *Regional or local anesthesia arms or legs for surgical procedure*
>
> 🖙 0.00   ⅀ 0.00   **FUD** XXX   N 🔲
>
> **AMA:** 2019,Oct,10; 2018,Jan,8; 2017,Dec,8; 2017,Jan,8; 2016,Jan,13

01996   **Daily hospital management of epidural or subarachnoid continuous drug administration**

> INCLUDES   Continuous epidural or subarachnoid drug services performed after insertion epidural or subarachnoid catheter
>
> 🖙 0.00   ⅀ 0.00   **FUD** XXX   N 🔲
>
> **AMA:** 2019,Oct,10; 2018,Jan,8; 2017,Dec,8; 2017,Sep,6; 2017,Jan,8; 2016,Jan,13

01999   **Unlisted anesthesia procedure(s)**

> 🖙 0.00   ⅀ 0.00   **FUD** XXX   N 🔲
>
> **AMA:** 2019,Oct,10; 2018,Jan,8; 2017,Dec,8; 2017,Jan,8; 2016,Jan,13

26/TC PC/TC Only   A2-Z3 ASC Payment   50 Bilateral   ♂ Male Only   ♀ Female Only   🖙 Facility RVU   ⅀ Non-Facility RVU   🔲 CCI   ❌ CLIA
FUD Follow-up Days   CMS: IOM   AMA: CPT Asst   A-Y OPPSI   80/80 Surg Assist Allowed / w/Doc   🔲 Lab Crosswalk   🔲 Radiology Crosswalk

12   CPT © 2021 American Medical Association. All Rights Reserved.   © 2021 Optum360, LLC

10004-10012 [10004, 10005, 10006, 10007, 10008, 10009, 10010, 10011, 10012] Fine Needle Aspiration

EXCLUDES
Core needle biopsy, lung or mediastinum (32408)
Percutaneous localization clip placement during breast biopsy (19081-19086)
Percutaneous needle biopsy:
  Abdominal or retroperitoneal mass (49180)
  Epididymis (54800)
  Kidney (50200)
  Liver (47000-47001)
  Lymph node (38505)
  Muscle (20206)
  Nucleus pulposus, paravertebral tissue, intervertebral disc (62267)
  Pancreas (48102)
  Pleura (32400)
  Prostate (55700, 55706)
  Salivary gland (42400)
  Spinal cord (62269)
  Testis (54500)
  Thyroid (60100)
Soft tissue percutaneous fluid drainage by catheter using image guidance (10030)
Thyroid cyst (60300)

Code also multiple biopsies on same service date:
  FNA biopsies using same imaging guidance: report imaging add-on code for second and successive procedures
  FNA biopsies separate lesions, different imaging guidance: append modifier 59 to codes for additional imaging modality used
  FNA and core needle biopsy same lesion, same imaging guidance, procedure includes imaging guidance for core needle procedure
  FNA and core needle biopsies separate lesions, same or different imaging guidance, append modifier 59 to code for core needle biopsy and imaging guidance

10004 Resequenced code. See code following 10021.

10005 Resequenced code. See code following 10021.

10006 Resequenced code. See code following 10021.

10007 Resequenced code. See code following 10021.

10008 Resequenced code. See code following 10021.

10009 Resequenced code. See code following 10021.

10010 Resequenced code. See code following 10021.

10011 Resequenced code. See code following 10021.

10012 Resequenced code. See code following 10021.

10021 Fine needle aspiration biopsy, without imaging guidance; first lesion
- (88172-88173, [88177])
- 1.60 2.80 **FUD** XXX T P3 80
- **AMA:** 2019,May,10; 2019,Apr,4; 2019,Feb,8; 2018,Jan,8; 2017,Jan,8; 2016,Jan,13

+ # **10004** each additional lesion (List separately in addition to code for primary procedure)
- EXCLUDES *Fine needle biopsy using other imaging methods for same lesion ([10005, 10006, 10007, 10008, 10009, 10010, 10011, 10012])*
- *Imaging guidance (76942)*
- Code first (10021)
- (88172-88173, [88177])
- 1.25 1.48 **FUD** ZZZ N1 80
- **AMA:** 2019,Apr,4; 2019,Feb,8

10005 Fine needle aspiration biopsy, including ultrasound guidance; first lesion
- INCLUDES Imaging guidance (76942)
- (88172-88173, [88177])
- 2.10 3.59 **FUD** XXX G2 80
- **AMA:** 2019,May,10; 2019,Feb,8; 2019,Apr,4

+ # **10006** each additional lesion (List separately in addition to code for primary procedure)
- INCLUDES Imaging guidance (76942)
- Code first ([10005])
- (88172-88173, [88177])
- 1.42 1.70 **FUD** ZZZ N1 80
- **AMA:** 2019,Apr,4; 2019,Feb,8

10007 Fine needle aspiration biopsy, including fluoroscopic guidance; first lesion
- INCLUDES Imaging guidance (77002)
- (88172-88173, [88177])
- 2.70 8.09 **FUD** XXX P3 80
- **AMA:** 2019,Apr,4; 2019,Feb,8

+ # **10008** each additional lesion (List separately in addition to code for primary procedure)
- INCLUDES Imaging guidance (77002)
- Code first ([10007])
- (88172-88173, [88177])
- 1.76 4.79 **FUD** ZZZ N1 80
- **AMA:** 2019,Apr,4; 2019,Feb,8

10009 Fine needle aspiration biopsy, including CT guidance; first lesion
- INCLUDES Imaging guidance (77012)
- (88172-88173, [88177])
- 3.28 13.3 **FUD** XXX G2 80
- **AMA:** 2019,Apr,4; 2019,Feb,8

+ # **10010** each additional lesion (List separately in addition to code for primary procedure)
- INCLUDES Imaging guidance (77012)
- Code first ([10009])
- (88172-88173, [88177])
- 2.38 8.02 **FUD** ZZZ N1 80
- **AMA:** 2019,Apr,4; 2019,Feb,8

10011 Fine needle aspiration biopsy, including MR guidance; first lesion
- INCLUDES Imaging guidance (77021)
- (88172-88173, [88177])
- 0.00 0.00 **FUD** XXX R2 80
- **AMA:** 2019,Apr,4; 2019,Feb,8

+ # **10012** each additional lesion (List separately in addition to code for primary procedure)
- INCLUDES Imaging guidance (77021)
- Code first ([10011])
- (88172-88173, [88177])
- 0.00 0.00 **FUD** ZZZ N1 80
- **AMA:** 2019,Apr,4; 2019,Feb,8

10030-10180 Treatment of Lesions: Skin and Subcutaneous Tissues

EXCLUDES *Excision benign lesion (11400-11471)*

10030 Image-guided fluid collection drainage by catheter (eg, abscess, hematoma, seroma, lymphocele, cyst), soft tissue (eg, extremity, abdominal wall, neck), percutaneous
- INCLUDES Radiologic guidance (75989, 76942, 77002-77003, 77012, 77021)
- EXCLUDES *Percutaneous drainage with imaging guidance:*
  Peritoneal or retroperitoneal collections (49406)
  Visceral collections (49405)
  Transvaginal or transrectal drainage with imaging guidance peritoneal or retroperitoneal collections (49407)
- Code also every instance of fluid collection drained using a separate catheter (10030)
- 3.98 17.5 **FUD** 000 T G2 80
- **AMA:** 2019,Apr,4; 2018,Jan,8; 2017,Aug,9; 2017,Jan,8; 2016,Jan,13

10035 **Placement of soft tissue localization device(s) (eg, clip, metallic pellet, wire/needle, radioactive seeds), percutaneous, including imaging guidance; first lesion**

INCLUDES Radiologic guidance (76942, 77002, 77012, 77021)

EXCLUDES *Sites with more specific code descriptor, such as breast*
Reporting code more than one time per site, regardless number markers used

Code also each additional target on same or opposite side (10036)

🏥 2.46 ⚕ 12.8 **FUD** 000 T N1 80 50 ▢

AMA: 2018,Jan,8; 2017,Jan,8; 2016,Jun,3

+ **10036** **each additional lesion (List separately in addition to code for primary procedure)**

INCLUDES Radiologic guidance (76942, 77002, 77012, 77021)

EXCLUDES *Sites with more specific code descriptor, such as breast*
Reporting code more than one time per site, regardless number markers used

Code first (10035)

🏥 1.25 ⚕ 11.7 **FUD** ZZZ N N1 80 ▢

AMA: 2018,Jan,8; 2017,Jan,8; 2016,Jun,3

10040 **Acne surgery (eg, marsupialization, opening or removal of multiple milia, comedones, cysts, pustules)**

🏥 1.53 ⚕ 3.11 **FUD** 010 Q1 N1 ▢

AMA: 2018,Jan,8; 2017,Jan,8; 2016,Jan,13

10060 **Incision and drainage of abscess (eg, carbuncle, suppurative hidradenitis, cutaneous or subcutaneous abscess, cyst, furuncle, or paronychia); simple or single**

🏥 2.87 ⚕ 3.44 **FUD** 010 T P3 ▢

AMA: 2018,Jan,8; 2017,Jan,8; 2016,Jan,13

10061 **complicated or multiple**

🏥 5.16 ⚕ 5.87 **FUD** 010 T P3 ▢

AMA: 2018,Jan,8; 2017,Jan,8; 2016,Jan,13

10080 **Incision and drainage of pilonidal cyst; simple**

🏥 2.95 ⚕ 5.99 **FUD** 010 T P3 ▢

AMA: 2018,Jan,8; 2017,Jan,8; 2016,Jan,13

10081 **complicated**

EXCLUDES *Excision pilonidal cyst (11770-11772)*

🏥 4.93 ⚕ 8.67 **FUD** 010 T P3 ▢

AMA: 2018,Jan,8; 2017,Jan,8; 2016,Jan,13

10120 **Incision and removal of foreign body, subcutaneous tissues; simple**

🏥 2.94 ⚕ 4.31 **FUD** 010 T P3 ▢

AMA: 2018,Jan,8; 2017,Jan,8; 2016,Jan,13

10121 **complicated**

EXCLUDES *Debridement associated with fracture or dislocation (11010-11012)*
Exploration penetrating wound (20100-20103)

🏥 5.33 ⚕ 7.76 **FUD** 010 J A2 ▢

AMA: 2018,Jan,8; 2017,Jan,8; 2016,Jan,13

10140 **Incision and drainage of hematoma, seroma or fluid collection**

📷 (76942, 77002, 77012, 77021)

🏥 3.40 ⚕ 4.77 **FUD** 010 J P3 ▢

AMA: 2018,Jan,8; 2017,Jan,8; 2016,Jan,13

Hematoma may be decompressed with a hemostat

Drain may be placed to allow further drainage

10160 **Puncture aspiration of abscess, hematoma, bulla, or cyst**

📷 (76942, 77002, 77012, 77021)

🏥 2.71 ⚕ 3.71 **FUD** 010 T P3 ▢

AMA: 2018,Jan,8; 2017,Aug,9; 2017,Jan,8; 2016,Jan,13

10180 **Incision and drainage, complex, postoperative wound infection**

EXCLUDES *Wound dehiscence (12020-12021, 13160)*

🏥 5.10 ⚕ 7.12 **FUD** 010 J A2 ▢

AMA: 2018,Jan,8; 2017,Jan,8; 2016,Jan,13

11000-11012 Removal of Foreign Substances and Infected/Devitalized Tissue

EXCLUDES *Debridement:*
Burns (16000-16030)
Deeper tissue (11042-11047 [11045, 11046])
Nails (11720-11721)
Nonelective debridement/active care management (97597-97598)
Wounds (11042-11047 [11045, 11046])
Dermabrasions (15780-15783)
Pressure ulcer excision (15920-15999)

11000 **Debridement of extensive eczematous or infected skin; up to 10% of body surface**

EXCLUDES *Necrotizing soft tissue infection:*
Abdominal wall (11005-11006)
External genitalia and perineum (11004, 11006)

🏥 0.82 ⚕ 1.61 **FUD** 000 T P3 ▢

AMA: 2018,Feb,10; 2018,Jan,8; 2017,Jan,8; 2016,Jan,13

+ **11001** **each additional 10% of the body surface, or part thereof (List separately in addition to code for primary procedure)**

EXCLUDES *Necrotizing soft tissue infection:*
Abdominal wall (11005-11006)
External genitalia and perineum (11004, 11006)

Code first (11000)

🏥 0.41 ⚕ 0.62 **FUD** ZZZ N N1 ▢

AMA: 2018,Feb,10; 2018,Jan,8; 2017,Jan,8; 2016,Jan,13

11004 **Debridement of skin, subcutaneous tissue, muscle and fascia for necrotizing soft tissue infection; external genitalia and perineum**

Code also skin grafts or flaps, when performed (14000-14350, 15040-15770 [15769], 15771-15776)

🏥 16.6 ⚕ 16.6 **FUD** 000 C ▢

AMA: 2019,Nov,14; 2018,Feb,10; 2018,Jan,8; 2017,Jan,8; 2016,Jan,13

| 26/TC PC/TC Only | A2-Z3 ASC Payment | 50 Bilateral | ♂ Male Only | ♀ Female Only | 🏥 Facility RVU | ⚕ Non-Facility RVU | ▢ CCI | ✖ CLIA |
| **FUD** Follow-up Days | **CMS:** IOM | **AMA:** CPT Asst | A-Y OPPSI | 80/80 Surg Assist Allowed / w/Doc | ▢ Lab Crosswalk | ▢ Radiology Crosswalk | | |

14

CPT © 2021 American Medical Association. All Rights Reserved.

© 2021 Optum360, LLC

11005   **abdominal wall, with or without fascial closure**
Code also skin grafts or flaps, when performed (14000-14350, 15040-15770 [15769], 15771-15776)
🔪 22.6   ⚕ 22.6   **FUD** 000   Ⓒ 80 ▦
AMA: 2019,Nov,14; 2018,Feb,10; 2018,Jan,8; 2017,Jan,8; 2016,Jan,13

11006   **external genitalia, perineum and abdominal wall, with or without fascial closure**
EXCLUDES Orchiectomy (54520)
Testicular transplant (54680)
Code also skin grafts or flaps, when performed (14000-14350, 15040-15770 [15769], 15771-15776)
🔪 20.4   ⚕ 20.4   **FUD** 000   Ⓒ ▦
AMA: 2019,Nov,14; 2018,Jan,8; 2017,Jan,8; 2016,Jan,13

+ **11008**   **Removal of prosthetic material or mesh, abdominal wall for infection (eg, for chronic or recurrent mesh infection or necrotizing soft tissue infection) (List separately in addition to code for primary procedure)**
EXCLUDES Debridement (11000-11001, 11010-11044 [11045, 11046])
Insertion mesh (49568)
Code also skin grafts or flaps, when performed (14000-14350, 15040-15770 [15769], 15771-15776)
Code first (10180, 11004-11006)
🔪 7.99   ⚕ 7.99   **FUD** ZZZ   Ⓒ 80 ▦
AMA: 2019,Jan,14; 2018,Jan,8; 2017,Jan,8; 2016,Jan,13

11010   **Debridement including removal of foreign material at the site of an open fracture and/or an open dislocation (eg, excisional debridement); skin and subcutaneous tissues**
🔪 7.96   ⚕ 13.5   **FUD** 010   Ⓣ A2 ▦
AMA: 2018,Jan,8; 2017,Jan,8; 2016,Jan,13

11011   **skin, subcutaneous tissue, muscle fascia, and muscle**
🔪 8.68   ⚕ 15.4   **FUD** 000   Ⓣ A2 ▦
AMA: 2018,Jan,8; 2017,Jan,8; 2016,Jan,13

11012   **skin, subcutaneous tissue, muscle fascia, muscle, and bone**
🔪 12.0   ⚕ 19.3   **FUD** 000   Ⓙ A2 ▦
AMA: 2018,Jan,8; 2017,Jan,8; 2016,Jan,13

11042-11047 [11045, 11046] Removal of Infected/Devitalized Tissue

INCLUDES Debridement reported by size and depth
Debridement reported for multiple wounds by adding total surface area wounds with same depth
Injuries, wounds, chronic ulcers, infections
EXCLUDES Debridement:
Burn (16020-16030)
Eczematous or infected skin (11000-11001)
Nails (11720-11721)
Necrotizing soft tissue infection external genitalia, perineum, or abdominal wall (11004-11006)
Non-elective debridement/active care management same wound (97597-97602)
Dermabrasions (15780-15783)
Excision pressure ulcers (15920-15999)
Code also each additional single wound with different depths
Code also modifier 59 for additional wound debridement
Code also multiple wound groups with different depths

11042   **Debridement, subcutaneous tissue (includes epidermis and dermis, if performed); first 20 sq cm or less**
🔪 1.75   ⚕ 3.57   **FUD** 000   Ⓣ A2 ▦
AMA: 2018,Jan,8; 2017,Jan,8; 2016,Oct,3; 2016,Aug,9; 2016,Feb,13; 2016,Jan,13

+ # **11045**   **each additional 20 sq cm, or part thereof (List separately in addition to code for primary procedure)**
Code first (11042)
🔪 0.77   ⚕ 1.19   **FUD** ZZZ   Ⓝ N1 80 ▦
AMA: 2018,Jan,8; 2017,Jan,8; 2016,Oct,3; 2016,Aug,9; 2016,Jan,13

11043   **Debridement, muscle and/or fascia (includes epidermis, dermis, and subcutaneous tissue, if performed); first 20 sq cm or less**
🔪 4.47   ⚕ 6.64   **FUD** 000   Ⓣ A2 ▦
AMA: 2020,Apr,8; 2018,Jan,8; 2017,Jan,8; 2016,Oct,3; 2016,Aug,9; 2016,Jan,13

+ # **11046**   **each additional 20 sq cm, or part thereof (List separately in addition to code for primary procedure)**
Code first (11043)
🔪 1.62   ⚕ 2.12   **FUD** ZZZ   Ⓝ N1 80 ▦
AMA: 2018,Jan,8; 2017,Jan,8; 2016,Oct,3; 2016,Aug,9; 2016,Jan,13

11044   **Debridement, bone (includes epidermis, dermis, subcutaneous tissue, muscle and/or fascia, if performed); first 20 sq cm or less**
🔪 6.58   ⚕ 8.93   **FUD** 000   Ⓙ A2 ▦
AMA: 2018,Jan,8; 2017,Jan,8; 2016,Oct,3; 2016,Aug,9; 2016,Jan,13

11045   **Resequenced code. See code following 11042.**

11046   **Resequenced code. See code following 11043.**

+ **11047**   **each additional 20 sq cm, or part thereof (List separately in addition to code for primary procedure)**
Code first (11044)
🔪 2.86   ⚕ 3.53   **FUD** ZZZ   Ⓝ N1 80 ▦
AMA: 2018,Jan,8; 2017,Jan,8; 2016,Oct,3; 2016,Aug,9; 2016,Jan,13

11055-11057 Excision Benign Hypertrophic Skin Lesions

CMS: 100-04,32,80.8 CSF Edits: Routine Foot Care
EXCLUDES Destruction benign lesions other than cutaneous vascular proliferative lesions or skin tags (17110-17111)

11055   **Paring or cutting of benign hyperkeratotic lesion (eg, corn or callus); single lesion**
🔪 0.46   ⚕ 1.78   **FUD** 000   01 N1 ▦
AMA: 2018,Jan,8; 2017,Jan,8; 2016,Jan,13

11056   **2 to 4 lesions**
🔪 0.65   ⚕ 1.90   **FUD** 000   01 N1 ▦
AMA: 2018,Jan,8; 2017,Jan,8; 2016,Jan,13

11057   **more than 4 lesions**
🔪 0.85   ⚕ 2.31   **FUD** 000   Ⓣ P3 ▦
AMA: 2018,Jan,8; 2017,Jan,8; 2016,Jan,13

11102-11107 Surgical Biopsy Skin and Mucous Membranes

INCLUDES Attaining tissue for pathologic exam
EXCLUDES Biopsies performed during related procedures
Biopsy:
Anterior 2/3 tongue (41100)
Conjunctiva (68100)
Ear (69100)
Eyelid ([67810])
Floor of mouth (41108)
Intranasal (30100)
Lip (40490)
Nail (11755)
Penis (54100)
Perineum/vulva (56605-56606)
Vestibule of mouth (40808)

11102   **Tangential biopsy of skin (eg, shave, scoop, saucerize, curette); single lesion**
🔪 1.12   ⚕ 2.84   **FUD** 000   P3 ▦
AMA: 2020,May,13; 2019,Dec,9; 2019,Jan,9

+ **11103**   **each separate/additional lesion (List separately in addition to code for primary procedure)**
Code first different biopsy techniques used for additional separate lesions, when performed (11102, 11104, 11106)
🔪 0.66   ⚕ 1.51   **FUD** ZZZ   N1 ▦
AMA: 2020,May,13; 2019,Dec,9; 2019,Jan,9

11104   **Punch biopsy of skin (including simple closure, when performed); single lesion**
🔪 1.40   ⚕ 3.57   **FUD** 000   P3 ▦
AMA: 2019,Dec,9; 2019,Jan,9

+　　11105　　**each separate/additional lesion (List separately in addition to code for primary procedure)**
　　　　　　　　Code first different biopsy techniques used for additional separate lesions, when performed (11104, 11106)
　　　　　　　　📋 0.76　　✂ 1.72　　**FUD** ZZZ　　　　　　　N1 ⌷
　　　　　　　　AMA: 2019,Dec,9; 2019,Jan,9

　　11106　　**Incisional biopsy of skin (eg, wedge) (including simple closure, when performed); single lesion**
　　　　　　　　📋 1.74　　✂ 4.26　　**FUD** 000　　　　　　　P3 ⌷
　　　　　　　　AMA: 2019,Dec,9; 2019,Jan,9

+　　11107　　**each separate/additional lesion (List separately in addition to code for primary procedure)**
　　　　　　　　Code first (11106)
　　　　　　　　📋 0.93　　✂ 2.04　　**FUD** ZZZ　　　　　　　N1 ⌷
　　　　　　　　AMA: 2019,Dec,9; 2019,Jan,9

11200-11201 Skin Tag Removal - All Techniques

INCLUDES	Chemical destruction
	Electrocauterization
	Electrosurgical destruction
	Ligature strangulation
	Removal with or without local anesthesia
	Sharp excision or scissoring

　　11200　　**Removal of skin tags, multiple fibrocutaneous tags, any area; up to and including 15 lesions**
　　　　　　　　📋 2.10　　✂ 2.52　　**FUD** 010　　　　　　　01 N1 ⌷
　　　　　　　　AMA: 2018,Jan,8; 2017,Jan,8; 2016,Jan,13

+　　11201　　**each additional 10 lesions, or part thereof (List separately in addition to code for primary procedure)**
　　　　　　　　Code first (11200)
　　　　　　　　📋 0.48　　✂ 0.54　　**FUD** ZZZ　　　　　　　N N1 ⌷
　　　　　　　　AMA: 2018,Jan,8; 2017,Jan,8; 2016,Jan,13

11300-11313 Skin Lesion Removal: Shaving

INCLUDES	Local anesthesia
	Partial thickness excision by horizontal slicing
	Wound cauterization

　　11300　　**Shaving of epidermal or dermal lesion, single lesion, trunk, arms or legs; lesion diameter 0.5 cm or less**
　　　　　　　　📋 0.99　　✂ 2.84　　**FUD** 000　　　　　　　01 N1 80 ⌷
　　　　　　　　AMA: 2019,Jan,9; 2018,Feb,10; 2018,Jan,8; 2017,Dec,14; 2017,Jan,8; 2016,Jan,13

Shave excision of an elevated lesion; technique also used to biopsy

Elliptical excision is often used when tissue removal is larger than 4 mm or when deep pathology is suspected

A punch biopsy cuts a core of tissue as the tool is twisted downward

　　11301　　**lesion diameter 0.6 to 1.0 cm**
　　　　　　　　📋 1.50　　✂ 3.45　　**FUD** 000　　　　　　　01 N1 80 ⌷
　　　　　　　　AMA: 2019,Jan,9; 2018,Feb,10; 2018,Jan,8; 2017,Dec,14; 2017,Jan,8; 2016,Jan,13

　　11302　　**lesion diameter 1.1 to 2.0 cm**
　　　　　　　　📋 1.76　　✂ 3.99　　**FUD** 000　　　　　　　01 N1 80 ⌷
　　　　　　　　AMA: 2019,Jan,9; 2018,Feb,10; 2018,Jan,8; 2017,Dec,14; 2017,Jan,8; 2016,Jan,13

　　11303　　**lesion diameter over 2.0 cm**
　　　　　　　　📋 2.07　　✂ 4.39　　**FUD** 000　　　　　　　01 N1 80 ⌷
　　　　　　　　AMA: 2019,Jan,9; 2018,Feb,10; 2018,Jan,8; 2017,Dec,14; 2017,Jan,8; 2016,Jan,13

　　11305　　**Shaving of epidermal or dermal lesion, single lesion, scalp, neck, hands, feet, genitalia; lesion diameter 0.5 cm or less**
　　　　　　　　📋 1.12　　✂ 2.90　　**FUD** 000　　　　　　　01 N1 80 ⌷
　　　　　　　　AMA: 2019,Jan,9; 2018,Feb,10; 2018,Jan,8; 2017,Dec,14; 2017,Jan,8; 2016,Jan,13

　　11306　　**lesion diameter 0.6 to 1.0 cm**
　　　　　　　　📋 1.45　　✂ 3.50　　**FUD** 000　　　　　　　01 N1 80 ⌷
　　　　　　　　AMA: 2019,Jan,9; 2018,Feb,10; 2018,Jan,8; 2017,Dec,14; 2017,Jan,8; 2016,Jan,13

　　11307　　**lesion diameter 1.1 to 2.0 cm**
　　　　　　　　📋 1.87　　✂ 4.09　　**FUD** 000　　　　　　　T P2 80 ⌷
　　　　　　　　AMA: 2019,Jan,9; 2018,Feb,10; 2018,Jan,8; 2017,Dec,14; 2017,Jan,8; 2016,Jan,13

　　11308　　**lesion diameter over 2.0 cm**
　　　　　　　　📋 2.11　　✂ 4.37　　**FUD** 000　　　　　　　01 N1 80 ⌷
　　　　　　　　AMA: 2019,Jan,9; 2018,Feb,10; 2018,Jan,8; 2017,Dec,14; 2017,Jan,8; 2016,Jan,13

　　11310　　**Shaving of epidermal or dermal lesion, single lesion, face, ears, eyelids, nose, lips, mucous membrane; lesion diameter 0.5 cm or less**
　　　　　　　　📋 1.34　　✂ 3.29　　**FUD** 000　　　　　　　T P3 80 ⌷
　　　　　　　　AMA: 2019,Jan,9; 2018,Feb,10; 2018,Jan,8; 2017,Dec,14; 2017,Jan,8; 2016,Jan,13

　　11311　　**lesion diameter 0.6 to 1.0 cm**
　　　　　　　　📋 1.88　　✂ 3.86　　**FUD** 000　　　　　　　T P2 80 ⌷
　　　　　　　　AMA: 2019,Jan,9; 2018,Feb,10; 2018,Jan,8; 2017,Dec,14; 2017,Jan,8; 2016,Jan,13

　　11312　　**lesion diameter 1.1 to 2.0 cm**
　　　　　　　　📋 2.17　　✂ 4.51　　**FUD** 000　　　　　　　T P3 80 ⌷
　　　　　　　　AMA: 2019,Jan,9; 2018,Feb,10; 2018,Jan,8; 2017,Dec,14; 2017,Jan,8; 2016,Jan,13

　　11313　　**lesion diameter over 2.0 cm**
　　　　　　　　📋 2.82　　✂ 5.27　　**FUD** 000　　　　　　　T P3 80 ⌷
　　　　　　　　AMA: 2019,Jan,9; 2018,Feb,10; 2018,Jan,8; 2017,Dec,14; 2017,Jan,8; 2016,Jan,13

11400-11446 Skin Lesion Removal: Benign

INCLUDES	Biopsy on same lesion
	Cicatricial lesion excision
	Full thickness removal including margins
	Lesion measurement before excision at largest diameter plus margin
	Local anesthesia
	Simple, nonlayered closure
EXCLUDES	*Adjacent tissue transfer: report only adjacent tissue transfer (14000-14302)*
	Biopsy eyelid ([67810])
	Destruction:
	Benign lesions, any method (17110-17111)
	Cutaneous vascular proliferative lesions (17106-17108)
	Destruction of eyelid lesion (67850)
	Malignant lesions (17260-17286)
	Premalignant lesions (17000, 17003-17004)
	Escharotomy (16035-16036)
	Excision and reconstruction eyelid (67961-67975)
	Excision chalazion (67800-67808)
	Eyelid procedures involving more than skin (67800 and subsequent codes)
	Laser fenestration for scars (0479T-0480T)
	Shave removal (11300-11313)

Code also:
　Complex closure (13100-13153)
　Each separate lesion
　Intermediate closure (12031-12057)
　Modifier 22 when excision complicated or unusual
　Reconstruction (15002-15261, 15570-15770)

　　11400　　**Excision, benign lesion including margins, except skin tag (unless listed elsewhere), trunk, arms or legs; excised diameter 0.5 cm or less**
　　　　　　　　📋 2.33　　✂ 3.57　　**FUD** 010　　　　　　　T P3 ⌷
　　　　　　　　AMA: 2019,Nov,3; 2018,Sep,7; 2018,Feb,10; 2018,Jan,8; 2017,Jan,8; 2016,Apr,3; 2016,Jan,13

　　11401　　**excised diameter 0.6 to 1.0 cm**
　　　　　　　　📋 2.96　　✂ 4.35　　**FUD** 010　　　　　　　T P3 ⌷
　　　　　　　　AMA: 2019,Nov,3; 2018,Sep,7; 2018,Feb,10; 2018,Jan,8; 2017,Jan,8; 2016,Apr,3; 2016,Jan,13

　　11402　　**excised diameter 1.1 to 2.0 cm**
　　　　　　　　📋 3.29　　✂ 4.78　　**FUD** 010　　　　　　　T P3 ⌷
　　　　　　　　AMA: 2019,Nov,3; 2018,Sep,7; 2018,Feb,10; 2018,Jan,8; 2017,Jan,8; 2016,Apr,3; 2016,Jan,13

26/TC PC/TC Only　　**A2-Z3** ASC Payment　　**50** Bilateral　　♂ Male Only　　♀ Female Only　　📋 Facility RVU　　✂ Non-Facility RVU　　⌷ CCI　　✗ CLIA
FUD Follow-up Days　　**CMS:** IOM　　**AMA:** CPT Asst　　**A-Y** OPPSI　　**80/80** Surg Assist Allowed / w/Doc　　Lab Crosswalk　　Radiology Crosswalk

16　　　　　　　　　　　　　　　CPT © 2021 American Medical Association. All Rights Reserved.　　　　　　　　　　　　　© 2021 Optum360, LLC

11403   excised diameter 2.1 to 3.0 cm
    4.23   5.58   **FUD** 010   T P3
    AMA: 2019,Nov,3; 2018,Sep,7; 2018,Feb,10; 2018,Jan,8; 2017,Jan,8; 2016,Apr,3; 2016,Jan,13

11404   excised diameter 3.1 to 4.0 cm
    4.66   6.34   **FUD** 010   J A2
    AMA: 2019,Nov,3; 2018,Sep,7; 2018,Feb,10; 2018,Jan,8; 2017,Jan,8; 2016,Apr,3; 2016,Jan,13

11406   excised diameter over 4.0 cm
    7.09   9.07   **FUD** 010   J A2
    AMA: 2019,Nov,3; 2018,Sep,7; 2018,Feb,10; 2018,Jan,8; 2017,Jan,8; 2016,Apr,3; 2016,Jan,13

11420   **Excision, benign lesion including margins, except skin tag (unless listed elsewhere), scalp, neck, hands, feet, genitalia; excised diameter 0.5 cm or less**
    2.34   3.60   **FUD** 010   J P3
    AMA: 2019,Nov,3; 2018,Sep,7; 2018,Feb,10; 2018,Jan,8; 2017,Jan,8; 2016,Apr,3; 2016,Jan,13

11421   excised diameter 0.6 to 1.0 cm
    3.15   4.49   **FUD** 010   T P3
    AMA: 2019,Nov,3; 2018,Sep,7; 2018,Feb,10; 2018,Jan,8; 2017,Jan,8; 2016,Apr,3; 2016,Jan,13

11422   excised diameter 1.1 to 2.0 cm
    3.88   5.11   **FUD** 010   J P3
    AMA: 2019,Nov,3; 2018,Sep,7; 2018,Feb,10; 2018,Jan,8; 2017,Jan,8; 2016,Apr,3; 2016,Jan,13

11423   excised diameter 2.1 to 3.0 cm
    4.45   5.81   **FUD** 010   J P3
    AMA: 2019,Nov,3; 2018,Sep,7; 2018,Feb,10; 2018,Jan,8; 2017,Jan,8; 2016,Apr,3; 2016,Jan,13

11424   excised diameter 3.1 to 4.0 cm
    5.11   6.71   **FUD** 010   J A2
    AMA: 2019,Nov,3; 2018,Sep,7; 2018,Feb,10; 2018,Jan,8; 2017,Jan,8; 2016,Apr,3; 2016,Jan,13

11426   excised diameter over 4.0 cm
    7.89   9.63   **FUD** 010   J A2
    AMA: 2019,Nov,3; 2018,Sep,7; 2018,Feb,10; 2018,Jan,8; 2017,Jan,8; 2016,Apr,3; 2016,Jan,13

11440   **Excision, other benign lesion including margins, except skin tag (unless listed elsewhere), face, ears, eyelids, nose, lips, mucous membrane; excised diameter 0.5 cm or less**
    2.96   3.91   **FUD** 010   T P3
    AMA: 2019,Nov,3; 2019,Jan,14; 2018,Sep,7; 2018,Feb,10; 2018,Jan,8; 2017,Jan,8; 2016,Apr,3; 2016,Jan,13

The physician removes a benign lesion from the external ear, nose, or mucous membranes

11441   excised diameter 0.6 to 1.0 cm
    3.73   4.88   **FUD** 010   T P3
    AMA: 2019,Nov,3; 2019,Jan,14; 2018,Sep,7; 2018,Feb,10; 2018,Jan,8; 2017,Jan,8; 2016,Apr,3; 2016,Jan,13

11442   excised diameter 1.1 to 2.0 cm
    4.14   5.43   **FUD** 010   T P3
    AMA: 2019,Nov,3; 2019,Jan,14; 2018,Sep,7; 2018,Feb,10; 2018,Jan,8; 2017,Jan,8; 2016,Apr,3; 2016,Jan,13

11443   excised diameter 2.1 to 3.0 cm
    5.08   6.45   **FUD** 010   J P3
    AMA: 2019,Nov,3; 2019,Jan,14; 2018,Sep,7; 2018,Feb,10; 2018,Jan,8; 2017,Jan,8; 2016,Apr,3; 2016,Jan,13

11444   excised diameter 3.1 to 4.0 cm
    6.49   8.09   **FUD** 010   J A2
    AMA: 2019,Nov,3; 2019,Jan,14; 2018,Sep,7; 2018,Feb,10; 2018,Jan,8; 2017,Jan,8; 2016,Apr,3; 2016,Jan,13

11446   excised diameter over 4.0 cm
    9.33   11.1   **FUD** 010   J A2
    AMA: 2019,Nov,3; 2019,Jan,14; 2018,Sep,7; 2018,Feb,10; 2018,Jan,8; 2017,Jan,8; 2016,Apr,3; 2016,Jan,13

11450-11471 Treatment of Hidradenitis: Excision and Repair

Code also closure by skin graft or flap (14000-14350, 15040-15770 [15769], 15771-15776)

11450   **Excision of skin and subcutaneous tissue for hidradenitis, axillary; with simple or intermediate repair**
    7.36   11.6   **FUD** 090   J A2 50
    AMA: 2019,Nov,3; 2018,Sep,7; 2018,Feb,10; 2018,Jan,8; 2017,Jan,8; 2016,Aug,9; 2016,Jan,13

Hidradenitis is a disease process stemming from clogged specialized sweat glands, principally located in the axilla and groin areas

Hair shaft

Hidradenitis of the axilla

Hair matrix

Sweat (eccrine gland)

11451   with complex repair
    9.41   14.5   **FUD** 090   J A2 80 50
    AMA: 2019,Nov,3; 2018,Sep,7; 2018,Feb,10; 2018,Jan,8; 2017,Jan,8; 2016,Aug,9; 2016,Jan,13

11462   **Excision of skin and subcutaneous tissue for hidradenitis, inguinal; with simple or intermediate repair**
    7.01   11.3   **FUD** 090   J A2 80 50
    AMA: 2019,Nov,3; 2018,Sep,7; 2018,Feb,10; 2018,Jan,8; 2017,Jan,8; 2016,Aug,9; 2016,Jan,13

11463   with complex repair
    9.42   14.3   **FUD** 090   J A2 80 50
    AMA: 2019,Nov,3; 2018,Sep,7; 2018,Feb,10; 2018,Jan,8; 2017,Jan,8; 2016,Aug,9; 2016,Jan,13

11470   **Excision of skin and subcutaneous tissue for hidradenitis, perianal, perineal, or umbilical; with simple or intermediate repair**
    8.08   12.0   **FUD** 090   J A2
    AMA: 2019,Nov,3; 2018,Sep,7; 2018,Feb,10; 2018,Jan,8; 2017,Jan,8; 2016,Aug,9; 2016,Jan,13

11471   with complex repair
    10.0   15.0   **FUD** 090   J A2 80
    AMA: 2019,Nov,3; 2018,Sep,7; 2018,Feb,10; 2018,Jan,8; 2017,Jan,8; 2016,Aug,9; 2016,Jan,13

11600-11646 Skin Lesion Removal: Malignant

INCLUDES Biopsy on same lesion
Excision additional margin at same operative session
Full thickness removal including margins
Lesion measurement before excision at largest diameter plus margin
Local anesthesia
Simple, nonlayered closure

EXCLUDES *Adjacent tissue transfer. Report only adjacent tissue transfer (14000-14302)*
Destruction (17260-17286)
Excision additional margin at subsequent operative session (11600-11646)

Code also:
Complex closure (13100-13153)
Each separate lesion
Intermediate closure (12031-12057)
Modifier 22 when excision complicated or unusual
Reconstruction (15002-15261, 15570-15770)

11600 **Excision, malignant lesion including margins, trunk, arms, or legs; excised diameter 0.5 cm or less**
🗗 3.46   ⚕ 5.61   **FUD** 010   T P3 ▢
AMA: 2019,Nov,3; 2018,Sep,7; 2018,Jan,8; 2017,Jan,8; 2016,Jan,13

11601 **excised diameter 0.6 to 1.0 cm**
🗗 4.29   ⚕ 6.52   **FUD** 010   T P3 ▢
AMA: 2019,Nov,3; 2018,Sep,7; 2018,Jan,8; 2017,Jan,8; 2016,Jan,13

11602 **excised diameter 1.1 to 2.0 cm**
🗗 4.63   ⚕ 7.02   **FUD** 010   T P3 ▢
AMA: 2019,Nov,3; 2018,Sep,7; 2018,Jan,8; 2017,Jan,8; 2016,Jan,13

11603 **excised diameter 2.1 to 3.0 cm**
🗗 5.54   ⚕ 8.00   **FUD** 010   T P3 ▢
AMA: 2019,Nov,3; 2018,Sep,7; 2018,Jan,8; 2017,Jan,8; 2016,Jan,13

11604 **excised diameter 3.1 to 4.0 cm**
🗗 6.12   ⚕ 8.93   **FUD** 010   T A2 ▢
AMA: 2019,Nov,3; 2018,Sep,7; 2018,Jan,8; 2017,Jan,8; 2016,Jan,13

11606 **excised diameter over 4.0 cm**
🗗 9.24   ⚕ 12.8   **FUD** 010   J A2 ▢
AMA: 2019,Nov,3; 2018,Sep,7; 2018,Jan,8; 2017,Jan,8; 2016,Jan,13

11620 **Excision, malignant lesion including margins, scalp, neck, hands, feet, genitalia; excised diameter 0.5 cm or less**
🗗 3.50   ⚕ 5.64   **FUD** 010   J P3 ▢
AMA: 2019,Nov,3; 2018,Sep,7; 2018,Jan,8; 2017,Jan,8; 2016,Jan,13

11621 **excised diameter 0.6 to 1.0 cm**
🗗 4.27   ⚕ 6.55   **FUD** 010   T P3 ▢
AMA: 2019,Nov,3; 2018,Sep,7; 2018,Jan,8; 2017,Jan,8; 2016,Jan,13

11622 **excised diameter 1.1 to 2.0 cm**
🗗 4.93   ⚕ 7.30   **FUD** 010   T P3 ▢
AMA: 2019,Nov,3; 2018,Sep,7; 2018,Jan,8; 2017,Jan,8; 2016,Jan,13

11623 **excised diameter 2.1 to 3.0 cm**
🗗 6.03   ⚕ 8.52   **FUD** 010   J P3 ▢
AMA: 2019,Nov,3; 2018,Sep,7; 2018,Jan,8; 2017,Jan,8; 2016,Jan,13

11624 **excised diameter 3.1 to 4.0 cm**
🗗 6.85   ⚕ 9.65   **FUD** 010   J A2 ▢
AMA: 2019,Nov,3; 2018,Sep,7; 2018,Jan,8; 2017,Jan,8; 2016,Jan,13

11626 **excised diameter over 4.0 cm**
🗗 8.44   ⚕ 11.6   **FUD** 010   J A2 ▢
AMA: 2019,Nov,3; 2018,Sep,7; 2018,Jan,8; 2017,Jan,8; 2016,Jan,13

11640 **Excision, malignant lesion including margins, face, ears, eyelids, nose, lips; excised diameter 0.5 cm or less**
EXCLUDES *Eyelid excision involving more than skin (67800-67808, 67840-67850, 67961-67966)*
🗗 3.59   ⚕ 5.77   **FUD** 010   T P3 ▢
AMA: 2019,Nov,3; 2018,Sep,7; 2018,Jan,8; 2017,Jan,8; 2016,Jan,13

11641 **excised diameter 0.6 to 1.0 cm**
EXCLUDES *Eyelid excision involving more than skin (67800-67808, 67840-67850, 67961-67966)*
🗗 4.45   ⚕ 6.78   **FUD** 010   T P3 ▢
AMA: 2019,Nov,3; 2018,Sep,7; 2018,Jan,8; 2017,Jan,8; 2016,Jan,13

11642 **excised diameter 1.1 to 2.0 cm**
EXCLUDES *Eyelid excision involving more than skin (67800-67808, 67840-67850, 67961-67966)*
🗗 5.30   ⚕ 7.73   **FUD** 010   T P3 ▢
AMA: 2019,Nov,3; 2018,Sep,7; 2018,Jan,8; 2017,Jan,8; 2016,Jan,13

11643 **excised diameter 2.1 to 3.0 cm**
EXCLUDES *Eyelid excision involving more than skin (67800-67808, 67840-67850, 67961-67966)*
🗗 6.55   ⚕ 9.06   **FUD** 010   J P3 ▢
AMA: 2019,Nov,3; 2018,Sep,7; 2018,Jan,8; 2017,Jan,8; 2016,Jan,13

11644 **excised diameter 3.1 to 4.0 cm**
EXCLUDES *Eyelid excision involving more than skin (67800-67808, 67840-67850, 67961-67966)*
🗗 8.14   ⚕ 11.1   **FUD** 010   J A2 ▢
AMA: 2019,Nov,3; 2018,Sep,7; 2018,Jan,8; 2017,Jan,8; 2016,Jan,13

11646 **excised diameter over 4.0 cm**
EXCLUDES *Eyelid excision involving more than skin (67800-67808, 67840-67850, 67961-67966)*
🗗 11.2   ⚕ 14.5   **FUD** 010   J A2 ▢
AMA: 2019,Nov,3; 2018,Sep,7; 2018,Jan,8; 2017,Jan,8; 2016,Jan,13

11719-11765 Nails and Supporting Structures

CMS: 100-02,15,290 Foot Care
EXCLUDES *Drainage paronychia or onychia (10060-10061)*

11719 **Trimming of nondystrophic nails, any number**
🗗 0.22   ⚕ 0.41   **FUD** 000   Q1 N1 ▢
AMA: 2018,Jan,8; 2017,Jan,8; 2016,Jan,13

11720 **Debridement of nail(s) by any method(s); 1 to 5**
🗗 0.42   ⚕ 0.93   **FUD** 000   Q1 N1 ▢
AMA: 2018,Jan,8; 2017,Jan,8; 2016,Jan,13

11721 **6 or more**
🗗 0.72   ⚕ 1.29   **FUD** 000   Q1 N1 ▢
AMA: 2018,Jan,8; 2017,Jan,8; 2016,Jan,13

11730 **Avulsion of nail plate, partial or complete, simple; single**
🗗 1.57   ⚕ 3.14   **FUD** 000   Q1 N1 ▢
AMA: 2018,Jan,8; 2017,Jan,8; 2016,Jan,13

+ 11732 **each additional nail plate (List separately in addition to code for primary procedure)**
Code first (11730)
🗗 0.50   ⚕ 0.95   **FUD** ZZZ   N N1 ▢
AMA: 2018,Jan,8; 2017,Jan,8; 2016,Jan,13

11740 **Evacuation of subungual hematoma**
🗗 0.90   ⚕ 1.52   **FUD** 000   Q1 N1 ▢
AMA: 2018,Jan,8; 2017,Jan,8; 2016,Jan,13

11750 **Excision of nail and nail matrix, partial or complete (eg, ingrown or deformed nail), for permanent removal;**
EXCLUDES *Pinch graft (15050)*
🗗 2.92   ⚕ 4.41   **FUD** 010   T P3 ▢
AMA: 2018,Jan,8; 2017,Jan,8; 2016,Jan,13

CPT © 2021 American Medical Association. All Rights Reserved.   © 2021 Optum360, LLC

11755–11983 (left column)

11755 Biopsy of nail unit (eg, plate, bed, matrix, hyponychium, proximal and lateral nail folds) (separate procedure)
🚑 1.79   ⚕ 3.47   **FUD** 000   T P3 80 ▣
AMA: 2019,Jan,9; 2018,Jan,8; 2017,Jan,8; 2016,Jan,13

11760 Repair of nail bed
🚑 3.27   ⚕ 5.46   **FUD** 010   T P3 ▣
AMA: 2018,Jan,8; 2017,Jan,8; 2016,Jan,13

11762 Reconstruction of nail bed with graft
🚑 5.33   ⚕ 8.15   **FUD** 010   T P3 ▣
AMA: 2018,Jan,8; 2017,Jan,8; 2016,Jan,13

11765 Wedge excision of skin of nail fold (eg, for ingrown toenail)
INCLUDES Cotting's operation
🚑 2.64   ⚕ 4.80   **FUD** 010   Q1 N1 ▣
AMA: 2018,Jan,8; 2017,Jan,8; 2016,Jan,13

11770-11772 Treatment Pilonidal Cyst: Excision
EXCLUDES Incision of pilonidal cyst (10080-10081)

11770 Excision of pilonidal cyst or sinus; simple
🚑 5.34   ⚕ 8.92   **FUD** 010   J A2 ▣

11771 extensive
🚑 12.7   ⚕ 17.2   **FUD** 090   J A2 ▣

11772 complicated
🚑 16.6   ⚕ 20.9   **FUD** 090   J A2 ▣
AMA: 2018,Jan,8; 2017,Jan,8; 2016,Jan,13

11900-11901 Treatment of Lesions: Injection
EXCLUDES Injection local anesthesia performed preoperatively
Injection veins (36470-36471)
Intralesional chemotherapy (96405-96406)

11900 Injection, intralesional; up to and including 7 lesions
🚑 0.90   ⚕ 1.54   **FUD** 000   Q1 N1 ▣
AMA: 2018,Jan,8; 2017,Jan,8; 2016,Jan,13

11901 more than 7 lesions
🚑 1.36   ⚕ 1.97   **FUD** 000   Q1 N1 ▣
AMA: 2018,Jan,8; 2017,Jan,8; 2016,Jan,13

11920-11971 Tattoos, Tissue Expanders, and Dermal Fillers
CMS: 100-02,16,10 Exclusions from Coverage; 100-02,16,120 Cosmetic Procedures; 100-02,16,180 Services Related to Noncovered Procedures

11920 Tattooing, intradermal introduction of insoluble opaque pigments to correct color defects of skin, including micropigmentation; 6.0 sq cm or less
🚑 3.23   ⚕ 5.33   **FUD** 000   T P3 80 ▣
AMA: 2018,Jan,8; 2017,Jan,8; 2016,Aug,9

11921 6.1 to 20.0 sq cm
🚑 3.81   ⚕ 6.08   **FUD** 000   T P3 80 ▣
AMA: 2018,Jan,8; 2017,Jan,8; 2016,Aug,9

+ 11922 each additional 20.0 sq cm, or part thereof (List separately in addition to code for primary procedure)
Code first (11921)
🚑 0.86   ⚕ 1.71   **FUD** ZZZ   N N1 80 ▣

11950 Subcutaneous injection of filling material (eg, collagen); 1 cc or less
🚑 1.51   ⚕ 2.26   **FUD** 000   T P3 80 ▣
AMA: 2019,Aug,10; 2018,Jan,8; 2017,Jan,8; 2016,Jan,13

11951 1.1 to 5.0 cc
🚑 1.98   ⚕ 2.80   **FUD** 000   T P3 80 ▣
AMA: 2019,Aug,10; 2018,Jan,8; 2017,Jan,8; 2016,Jan,13

11952 5.1 to 10.0 cc
🚑 3.03   ⚕ 4.13   **FUD** 000   T P3 80 ▣
AMA: 2019,Aug,10; 2018,Jan,8; 2017,Jan,8; 2016,Jan,13

11954 over 10.0 cc
🚑 3.21   ⚕ 4.41   **FUD** 000   T P3 80 ▣
AMA: 2019,Aug,10; 2018,Jan,8; 2017,Jan,8; 2016,Jan,13

(right column)

11960 Insertion of tissue expander(s) for other than breast, including subsequent expansion
EXCLUDES Breast reconstruction with tissue expander(s) (19357)
Decompression, nerve (64722-64726)
Endoscopic release transverse carpal ligament (29848)
Neuroplasty (64702-64721)
Removal tissue expander without implant insertion (11971)
Secondary closure, surgical wound or dehiscence (13160)
🚑 28.1   ⚕ 28.1   **FUD** 090   T A2 ▣
AMA: 1991,Win,1

11970 Replacement of tissue expander with permanent implant
🚑 17.6   ⚕ 17.6   **FUD** 090   J J8 50 ▣
AMA: 2018,Jan,8; 2017,Jan,8; 2016,Jan,13

11971 Removal of tissue expander without insertion of implant
EXCLUDES Insertion/replacement tissue expander (11960, 11970)
🚑 9.31   ⚕ 13.7   **FUD** 090   Q2 A2 80 50 ▣
AMA: 2018,Jan,8; 2017,Jan,8; 2016,Jan,13

11976-11983 Drug Implantation

11976 Removal, implantable contraceptive capsules   ♀
🚑 2.73   ⚕ 4.15   **FUD** 000   Q2 P3 80 ▣
AMA: 1992,Win,1; 1991,Win,1

11980 Subcutaneous hormone pellet implantation (implantation of estradiol and/or testosterone pellets beneath the skin)
🚑 1.61   ⚕ 2.69   **FUD** 000   Q1 N1 ▣
AMA: 2018,Jan,8; 2017,Jan,8; 2016,Jan,13

▲ 11981 Insertion, drug-delivery implant (ie, bioresorbable, biodegradable, non-biodegradable)
EXCLUDES Removal bioresorbable/biodegradable drug-delivery implant (17999)
Insertion deep drug-delivery device:
Intra-articular (20704)
Intramedullary (20702)
Subfascial (20700)
🚑 1.86   ⚕ 2.96   **FUD** 000   Q1 N1 80 ▣
AMA: 2018,Jan,8; 2017,Jan,8; 2016,Jan,13

11982 Removal, non-biodegradable drug delivery implant
EXCLUDES Removal deep drug-delivery device:
Intra-articular (20705)
Intramedullary (20703)
Subfascial (20701)
🚑 2.87   ⚕ 4.49   **FUD** XXX   Q1 N1 80 ▣

11983 Removal with reinsertion, non-biodegradable drug delivery implant
🚑 3.01   ⚕ 4.15   **FUD** 000   Q1 N1 80 ▣

● New Code   ▲ Revised Code   ○ Reinstated   ● New Web Release   ▲ Revised Web Release   + Add-on   Unlisted   Not Covered   # Resequenced
50 Optum Mod 50 Exempt   Ⓢ AMA Mod 51 Exempt   51 Optum Mod 51 Exempt   63 Mod 63 Exempt   ✕ Non-FDA Drug   ★ Telemedicine   Ⓜ Maternity   Ⓐ Age Edit

Integumentary System

12001 — 12041

12001-12021 Suturing of Superficial Wounds

INCLUDES   Administration local or topical anesthesia
        Hemostasis
        Repair that involves:
            Routine debridement and decontamination
            Simple one layer closure
            Superficial tissues
            Sutures, staples, tissue adhesives
            Total length several repairs in same code category
        Simple:
            Exploration nerves, blood vessels, tendons
            Vessel ligation, in wound

EXCLUDES   *Complex repair nerves, blood vessels, tendons (see appropriate anatomical section)*
        Debridement requiring:
            Comprehensive cleaning
            Removal significant tissue
            Removal soft tissue and/or bone, no fracture/dislocation, performed separately (11042-11047 [11045, 11046])
            Removal soft tissue and/or bone with open fracture/dislocation (11010-11012)
        Deep tissue repair (12031-13153)
        Major exploration (20100-20103)
        Repair/closure limited to:
            Adhesive strips only, see appropriate E/M service
            Chemical cauterization, see appropriate E/M service
            Electrocauterization, see appropriate E/M service
        Secondary closure/dehiscence (13160)
        Repair nerves, blood vessels, tendons (See appropriate anatomical section. These repairs include simple and intermediate closure. Report complex closure with modifier 59.)

Code also modifier 59 added to less complicated procedure code when reporting more than one wound repair classification

12001   **Simple repair of superficial wounds of scalp, neck, axillae, external genitalia, trunk and/or extremities (including hands and feet); 2.5 cm or less**
       🔧 1.27   ✂ 2.53   **FUD** 000   01 N1 ▭
       AMA: 2018,Sep,7; 2018,Jan,8; 2017,Dec,14; 2017,Jan,8; 2016,Jan,13

12002   **2.6 cm to 7.5 cm**
       🔧 1.67   ✂ 3.08   **FUD** 000   01 N1 ▭
       AMA: 2018,Sep,7; 2018,Jan,8; 2017,Jan,8; 2016,Jan,13

12004   **7.6 cm to 12.5 cm**
       🔧 2.15   ✂ 3.69   **FUD** 000   01 N1 ▭
       AMA: 2018,Sep,7; 2018,Jan,8; 2017,Jan,8; 2016,Jan,13

12005   **12.6 cm to 20.0 cm**
       🔧 2.71   ✂ 4.69   **FUD** 000   01 A2 ▭
       AMA: 2018,Sep,7; 2018,Jan,8; 2017,Jan,8; 2016,Jan,13

12006   **20.1 cm to 30.0 cm**
       🔧 3.33   ✂ 5.54   **FUD** 000   02 A2 ▭
       AMA: 2018,Sep,7; 2018,Jan,8; 2017,Jan,8; 2016,Jan,13

12007   **over 30.0 cm**
       🔧 4.15   ✂ 6.37   **FUD** 000   T A2 ▭
       AMA: 2018,Sep,7; 2018,Jan,8; 2017,Jan,8; 2016,Jan,13

12011   **Simple repair of superficial wounds of face, ears, eyelids, nose, lips and/or mucous membranes; 2.5 cm or less**
       🔧 1.57   ✂ 3.09   **FUD** 000   01 N1 ▭
       AMA: 2018,Sep,7; 2018,Jan,8; 2017,Jan,8; 2016,Nov,7; 2016,Jan,13

12013   **2.6 cm to 5.0 cm**
       🔧 1.72   ✂ 3.29   **FUD** 000   01 N1 ▭
       AMA: 2018,Sep,7; 2018,Jan,8; 2017,Jan,8; 2016,Jan,13

12014   **5.1 cm to 7.5 cm**
       🔧 2.14   ✂ 3.88   **FUD** 000   01 N1 ▭
       AMA: 2018,Sep,7; 2018,Jan,8; 2017,Jan,8; 2016,Jan,13

12015   **7.6 cm to 12.5 cm**
       🔧 2.78   ✂ 4.84   **FUD** 000   01 G2 ▭
       AMA: 2018,Sep,7; 2018,Jan,8; 2017,Jan,8; 2016,Jan,13

12016   **12.6 cm to 20.0 cm**
       🔧 3.77   ✂ 6.16   **FUD** 000   01 A2 ▭
       AMA: 2018,Sep,7; 2018,Jan,8; 2017,Jan,8; 2016,Jan,13

12017   **20.1 cm to 30.0 cm**
       🔧 4.48   ✂ 4.48   **FUD** 000   01 A2 80 ▭
       AMA: 2018,Sep,7; 2018,Jan,8; 2017,Jan,8; 2016,Jan,13

12018   **over 30.0 cm**
       🔧 5.08   ✂ 5.08   **FUD** 000   01 A2 80 ▭
       AMA: 2018,Sep,7; 2018,Jan,8; 2017,Jan,8; 2016,Jan,13

12020   **Treatment of superficial wound dehiscence; simple closure**
       EXCLUDES   *Secondary closure major/complex wound or dehiscence (13160)*
       🔧 5.43   ✂ 8.41   **FUD** 010   T A2 ▭
       AMA: 2019,Nov,3; 2018,Jan,8; 2017,Jan,8; 2016,Jan,13

12021   **with packing**
       EXCLUDES   *Secondary closure major/complex wound or dehiscence (13160)*
       🔧 4.01   ✂ 4.90   **FUD** 010   T A2 ▭
       AMA: 2019,Nov,3; 2018,Jan,8; 2017,Jan,8; 2016,Jan,13

12031-12057 Suturing of Intermediate Wounds

INCLUDES   Administration local anesthesia
        Repair that involves:
            Closure contaminated single layer wound
            Layered closure (e.g., subcutaneous tissue, superficial fascia)
            Limited undermining
            Removal foreign material (e.g., gravel, glass)
            Routine debridement and decontamination
        Simple:
            Exploration nerves, blood vessels, tendons in wound
            Vessel ligation, in wound
        Total length several repairs in same code category

EXCLUDES   *Debridement requiring:*
            Removal soft tissue and/or bone, no fracture/dislocation, performed separately (11042-11047 [11045, 11046])
            Removal soft tissue/bone due to open fracture/dislocation (11010-11012)
        Major exploration (20100-20103)
        Repair nerves, blood vessels, tendons (See appropriate anatomical section. These repairs include simple and intermediate closure. Report complex closure with modifier 59.)
        Secondary closure major/complex wound or dehiscence (13160)
        Wound repair involving more than layered closure

Code also modifier 59 added to less complicated procedure code when reporting more than one wound repair classification

12031   **Repair, intermediate, wounds of scalp, axillae, trunk and/or extremities (excluding hands and feet); 2.5 cm or less**
       🔧 4.36   ✂ 7.17   **FUD** 010   T P2 ▭
       AMA: 2019,Nov,3; 2018,Sep,7; 2018,Jan,8; 2017,Jan,8; 2016,Jan,13

12032   **2.6 cm to 7.5 cm**
       🔧 5.58   ✂ 8.65   **FUD** 010   T P2 ▭
       AMA: 2019,Nov,3; 2018,Sep,7; 2018,Jan,8; 2017,Jan,8; 2016,Jan,13

12034   **7.6 cm to 12.5 cm**
       🔧 5.99   ✂ 8.92   **FUD** 010   T A2 ▭
       AMA: 2019,Nov,3; 2018,Sep,7; 2018,Jan,8; 2017,Jan,8; 2016,Jan,13

12035   **12.6 cm to 20.0 cm**
       🔧 6.94   ✂ 11.0   **FUD** 010   T A2 ▭
       AMA: 2019,Nov,3; 2018,Sep,7; 2018,Jan,8; 2017,Jan,8; 2016,Jan,13

12036   **20.1 cm to 30.0 cm**
       🔧 8.05   ✂ 12.1   **FUD** 010   T A2 ▭
       AMA: 2019,Nov,3; 2018,Sep,7; 2018,Jan,8; 2017,Jan,8; 2016,Jan,13

12037   **over 30.0 cm**
       🔧 9.53   ✂ 14.0   **FUD** 010   T A2 80 ▭
       AMA: 2019,Nov,3; 2018,Sep,7; 2018,Jan,8; 2017,Jan,8; 2016,Jan,13

12041   **Repair, intermediate, wounds of neck, hands, feet and/or external genitalia; 2.5 cm or less**
       🔧 4.22   ✂ 7.19   **FUD** 010   02 P2 ▭
       AMA: 2019,Nov,3; 2018,Sep,7; 2018,Jan,8; 2017,Jan,8; 2016,Jan,13

26/TC PC/TC Only   A2-Z3 ASC Payment   50 Bilateral   ♂ Male Only   ♀ Female Only   🔧 Facility RVU   ✂ Non-Facility RVU   ▭ CCI   ✖ CLIA
FUD Follow-up Days   **CMS:** IOM   **AMA:** CPT Asst   A-Y OPPSI   80/80 Surg Assist Allowed / w/Doc   Lab Crosswalk   Radiology Crosswalk

20   CPT © 2021 American Medical Association. All Rights Reserved.   © 2021 Optum360, LLC

12042	**2.6 cm to 7.5 cm**

🚑 5.64   ⚕ 8.54   **FUD** 010   T P2 ▭

AMA: 2019,Nov,3; 2018,Sep,7; 2018,Jan,8; 2017,Jan,8; 2016,Jan,13

12044	**7.6 cm to 12.5 cm**

🚑 6.16   ⚕ 10.6   **FUD** 010   T A2 ▭

AMA: 2019,Nov,3; 2018,Sep,7; 2018,Jan,8; 2017,Jan,8; 2016,Jan,13

12045	**12.6 cm to 20.0 cm**

🚑 7.71   ⚕ 11.4   **FUD** 010   T A2 ▭

AMA: 2019,Nov,3; 2018,Sep,7; 2018,Jan,8; 2017,Jan,8; 2016,Jan,13

12046	**20.1 cm to 30.0 cm**

🚑 9.01   ⚕ 13.8   **FUD** 010   T A2 80 ▭

AMA: 2019,Nov,3; 2018,Sep,7; 2018,Jan,8; 2017,Jan,8; 2016,Jan,13

12047	**over 30.0 cm**

🚑 10.1   ⚕ 15.4   **FUD** 010   T A2 80 ▭

AMA: 2019,Nov,3; 2018,Sep,7; 2018,Jan,8; 2017,Jan,8; 2016,Jan,13

12051	**Repair, intermediate, wounds of face, ears, eyelids, nose, lips and/or mucous membranes; 2.5 cm or less**

🚑 4.85   ⚕ 7.73   **FUD** 010   T P2 ▭

AMA: 2019,Nov,3; 2018,Sep,7; 2018,Jan,8; 2017,Jan,8; 2016,Jan,13

12052	**2.6 cm to 5.0 cm**

🚑 5.85   ⚕ 8.55   **FUD** 010   T P2 ▭

AMA: 2019,Nov,3; 2018,Sep,7; 2018,Jan,8; 2017,Jan,8; 2016,Jan,13

12053	**5.1 cm to 7.5 cm**

🚑 6.20   ⚕ 10.1   **FUD** 010   T P2 ▭

AMA: 2019,Nov,3; 2018,Sep,7; 2018,Jan,8; 2017,Jan,8; 2016,Jan,13

12054	**7.6 cm to 12.5 cm**

🚑 6.35   ⚕ 10.7   **FUD** 010   02 A2 ▭

AMA: 2019,Nov,3; 2018,Sep,7; 2018,Jan,8; 2017,Jan,8; 2016,Jan,13

12055	**12.6 cm to 20.0 cm**

🚑 8.66   ⚕ 13.9   **FUD** 010   T A2 ▭

AMA: 2019,Nov,3; 2018,Sep,7; 2018,Jan,8; 2017,Jan,8; 2016,Jan,13

12056	**20.1 cm to 30.0 cm**

🚑 11.0   ⚕ 16.0   **FUD** 010   02 A2 80 ▭

AMA: 2019,Nov,3; 2018,Sep,7; 2018,Jan,8; 2017,Jan,8; 2016,Jan,13

12057	**over 30.0 cm**

🚑 12.3   ⚕ 17.0   **FUD** 010   T A2 80 ▭

AMA: 2019,Nov,3; 2018,Sep,7; 2018,Jan,8; 2017,Jan,8; 2016,Jan,13

13100-13160 Suturing of Complicated Wounds

INCLUDES Creation limited defect for repair
Debridement complicated wounds/avulsions
Repair with layered closure that involves at least one of the following:
  Debridement wound edges
  Exposure underlying structures, such as bone, cartilage, tendon, or named neovascular structure
  Extensive undermining
  Free margin involvement helical or nostril rim or vermillion border
  Retention suture placement
Simple:-
  Exploration nerves, vessels, tendons in wound
  Vessel ligation in wound
Total length several repairs in same code category

EXCLUDES *Excision:*
  Benign lesions (11400-11446)
  Extensive debridement open fracture/dislocation (11010-11012)
  Extensive debridement penetrating or blunt trauma not associated with open fracture/dislocation (11042-11047 [11045, 11046])
  Malignant lesions (11600-11646)
  Surgical preparation wound bed (15002-15005)
Extensive exploration (20100-20103)
Repair nerves, blood vessel, tendons (See appropriate anatomical section. These repairs include simple and intermediate closure. Report complex closure with modifier 59.)
Code also modifier 59 added to less complicated procedure code when reporting more than one wound repair classification

13100	**Repair, complex, trunk; 1.1 cm to 2.5 cm**

EXCLUDES *Complex repair 1.0 cm or less (12001, 12031)*

🚑 5.81   ⚕ 9.72   **FUD** 010   T A2 ▭

AMA: 2019,Nov,14; 2019,Nov,3; 2018,Sep,7; 2018,Jan,8; 2017,Apr,9; 2017,Jan,8; 2016,Jan,13

13101	**2.6 cm to 7.5 cm**

🚑 7.14   ⚕ 11.4   **FUD** 010   T A2 ▭

AMA: 2019,Dec,14; 2019,Nov,3; 2018,Sep,7; 2018,Jan,8; 2017,Apr,9; 2017,Jan,8; 2016,Jan,13

+	13102	**each additional 5 cm or less (List separately in addition to code for primary procedure)**

Code first (13101)

🚑 2.14   ⚕ 3.46   **FUD** ZZZ   N N1 ▭

AMA: 2019,Nov,14; 2019,Nov,3; 2018,Sep,7; 2018,Jan,8; 2017,Apr,9; 2017,Jan,8; 2016,Jan,13

13120	**Repair, complex, scalp, arms, and/or legs; 1.1 cm to 2.5 cm**

EXCLUDES *Complex repair 1.0 cm or less (12001, 12031)*

🚑 6.68   ⚕ 10.1   **FUD** 010   T A2 ▭

AMA: 2019,Nov,3; 2018,Sep,7; 2018,Jan,8; 2017,Jan,8; 2016,Jan,13

13121	**2.6 cm to 7.5 cm**

🚑 7.67   ⚕ 12.2   **FUD** 010   T A2 ▭

AMA: 2019,Nov,3; 2018,Sep,7; 2018,Jan,8; 2017,Jan,8; 2016,Jan,13

+	13122	**each additional 5 cm or less (List separately in addition to code for primary procedure)**

Code first (13121)

🚑 2.42   ⚕ 3.74   **FUD** ZZZ   N N1 ▭

AMA: 2019,Nov,3; 2018,Sep,7; 2018,Jan,8; 2017,Jan,8; 2016,Jan,13

13131	**Repair, complex, forehead, cheeks, chin, mouth, neck, axillae, genitalia, hands and/or feet; 1.1 cm to 2.5 cm**

EXCLUDES *Complex repair 1.0 cm or less (12001, 12011, 12031, 12041, 12051)*

🚑 7.04   ⚕ 11.1   **FUD** 010   T A2 ▭

AMA: 2019,Nov,3; 2018,Sep,7; 2018,Jan,8; 2017,Apr,9; 2017,Jan,8; 2016,Jan,13

13132	**2.6 cm to 7.5 cm**

🚑 8.81   ⚕ 13.5   **FUD** 010   T A2 ▭

AMA: 2019,Nov,3; 2018,Sep,7; 2018,Jan,8; 2017,Apr,9; 2017,Jan,8; 2016,Jan,13

Integumentary System

13133 — 14350

+ **13133** each additional 5 cm or less (List separately in addition to code for primary procedure)

Code first (13132)

🔾 3.77   ⚕ 5.06   **FUD** ZZZ   N N1 ▢

AMA: 2019,Nov,3; 2018,Sep,7; 2018,Jan,8; 2017,Apr,9; 2017,Jan,8; 2016,Jan,13

13151 Repair, complex, eyelids, nose, ears and/or lips; 1.1 cm to 2.5 cm

EXCLUDES   *Complex repair 1.0 cm or less (12011, 12051)*

🔾 8.25   ⚕ 12.1   **FUD** 010   T A2 ▢

AMA: 2019,Nov,3; 2018,Sep,7; 2018,Jan,8; 2017,Jan,8; 2016,Jan,13

13152 2.6 cm to 7.5 cm

🔾 9.74   ⚕ 14.3   **FUD** 010   T A2 ▢

AMA: 2019,Nov,3; 2018,Sep,7; 2018,Jan,8; 2017,Jan,8; 2016,Jan,13

+ **13153** each additional 5 cm or less (List separately in addition to code for primary procedure)

Code first (13152)

🔾 4.02   ⚕ 5.45   **FUD** ZZZ   N N1 ▢

AMA: 2019,Nov,3; 2018,Sep,7; 2018,Jan,8; 2017,Jan,8; 2016,Jan,13

13160 Secondary closure of surgical wound or dehiscence, extensive or complicated

EXCLUDES   *Insertion tissue expander, other than breast (11960)*
Packing or simple secondary wound closure (12020-12021)

🔾 22.9   ⚕ 22.9   **FUD** 090   T A2 ▢

AMA: 2019,Nov,3; 2018,Jan,8; 2017,Jan,8; 2016,Jan,13

14000-14350 Reposition Contiguous Tissue

INCLUDES   Excision (with or without lesion) with repair by adjacent tissue transfer or tissue rearrangement
Size includes primary (due to excision) and secondary (due to flap design)
Z-plasty, W-plasty, VY-plasty, rotation flap, advancement flap, double pedicle flap, random island flap

EXCLUDES   *Closure wounds by undermining surrounding tissue without additional incisions (13100-13160)*
Full thickness closure:
Eyelid (67930-67935, 67961-67975)
Lip (40650-40654)

Code also skin graft necessary to repair secondary defect (15040-15731)

14000 Adjacent tissue transfer or rearrangement, trunk; defect 10 sq cm or less

INCLUDES   Burrow's operation

EXCLUDES   *Excision lesion with repair by adjacent tissue transfer or tissue rearrangement (11400-11446, 11600-11646)*

🔾 14.3   ⚕ 17.8   **FUD** 090   T A2 ▢

AMA: 2018,Jan,8; 2017,Oct,9; 2017,Jan,8; 2016,Jan,13

Example of common Z-plasty. Lesion is removed with oval-shaped incision

Two additional incisions (a. and b.) intersect the area

Skin of each incision is reflected back

The flaps are then transposed and the repair is closed

An adjacent flap, or other rearrangement flap, is performed to repair a defect

14001 defect 10.1 sq cm to 30.0 sq cm

EXCLUDES   *Excision lesion with repair by adjacent tissue transfer or tissue rearrangement (11400-11446, 11600-11646)*

🔾 18.7   ⚕ 22.8   **FUD** 090   T A2 ▢

AMA: 2018,Jan,8; 2017,Oct,9; 2017,Jan,8; 2016,Jan,13

14020 Adjacent tissue transfer or rearrangement, scalp, arms and/or legs; defect 10 sq cm or less

EXCLUDES   *Excision lesion with repair by adjacent tissue transfer or tissue rearrangement (11400-11446, 11600-11646)*

🔾 16.0   ⚕ 19.8   **FUD** 090   T A2 ▢

AMA: 2018,Jan,8; 2017,Jan,8; 2016,Jan,13

14021 defect 10.1 sq cm to 30.0 sq cm

EXCLUDES   *Excision lesion with repair by adjacent tissue transfer or tissue rearrangement (11400-11446, 11600-11646)*

🔾 20.5   ⚕ 24.7   **FUD** 090   T A2 ▢

AMA: 2018,Jan,8; 2017,Jan,8; 2016,Jan,13

14040 Adjacent tissue transfer or rearrangement, forehead, cheeks, chin, mouth, neck, axillae, genitalia, hands and/or feet; defect 10 sq cm or less

INCLUDES   Krimer's palatoplasty

EXCLUDES   *Excision lesion with repair by adjacent tissue transfer or tissue rearrangement (11400-11446, 11600-11646)*

🔾 18.1   ⚕ 21.7   **FUD** 090   T A2 ▢

AMA: 2018,Jan,8; 2017,Nov,6; 2017,Jan,8; 2016,Jan,13

14041 defect 10.1 sq cm to 30.0 sq cm

EXCLUDES   *Excision lesion with repair by adjacent tissue transfer or tissue rearrangement (11400-11446, 11600-11646)*

🔾 22.3   ⚕ 26.7   **FUD** 090   T A2 ▢

AMA: 2018,Jan,8; 2017,Nov,6; 2017,Jan,8; 2016,Jan,13

14060 Adjacent tissue transfer or rearrangement, eyelids, nose, ears and/or lips; defect 10 sq cm or less

INCLUDES   Denonvillier's operation

EXCLUDES   *Excision lesion with repair by adjacent tissue transfer or tissue rearrangement (11400-11446, 11600-11646)*
Eyelid, full thickness (67961-67966)

🔾 19.0   ⚕ 21.9   **FUD** 090   T A2 ▢

AMA: 2018,Jan,8; 2017,Nov,6; 2017,Jan,8; 2016,Jan,13

14061 defect 10.1 sq cm to 30.0 sq cm

EXCLUDES   *Excision lesion with repair by adjacent tissue transfer or tissue rearrangement (11400-11446, 11600-11646)*
Eyelid, full thickness (67961 and subsequent codes)

🔾 23.4   ⚕ 28.3   **FUD** 090   T A2 ▢

AMA: 2018,Jan,8; 2017,Nov,6; 2017,Jan,8; 2016,Jan,13

14301 Adjacent tissue transfer or rearrangement, any area; defect 30.1 sq cm to 60.0 sq cm

EXCLUDES   *Excision lesion with repair by adjacent tissue transfer or tissue rearrangement (11400-11446, 11600-11646)*

🔾 25.0   ⚕ 30.8   **FUD** 090   T 62 80 ▢

AMA: 2018,Jan,8; 2017,Nov,6; 2017,Apr,9; 2017,Jan,8; 2016,Jan,13

+ **14302** each additional 30.0 sq cm, or part thereof (List separately in addition to code for primary procedure)

EXCLUDES   *Excision lesion with repair by adjacent tissue transfer or tissue rearrangement (11400-11446, 11600-11646)*

Code first (14301)

🔾 6.31   ⚕ 6.31   **FUD** ZZZ   N N1 80 ▢

AMA: 2018,Jan,8; 2017,Nov,6; 2017,Jan,8; 2016,Jan,13

14350 Filleted finger or toe flap, including preparation of recipient site

🔾 19.6   ⚕ 19.6   **FUD** 090   T A2 80 ▢

AMA: 2018,Jan,8; 2017,Jan,8; 2016,Jan,13

26/TC PC/TC Only   A2-Z3 ASC Payment   50 Bilateral   ♂ Male Only   ♀ Female Only   🔾 Facility RVU   ⚕ Non-Facility RVU   ▢ CCI   ☒ CLIA
FUD Follow-up Days   CMS: IOM   AMA: CPT Asst   A-Y OPPSI   80/80 Surg Assist Allowed / w/Doc   Lab Crosswalk   Radiology Crosswalk

22   CPT © 2021 American Medical Association. All Rights Reserved.   © 2021 Optum360, LLC

15002-15005 Development of Base for Tissue Grafting

INCLUDES Add together surface area multiple wounds in same anatomical locations as indicated in code descriptor groups, such as face and scalp. Do not add together multiple wounds at different anatomical site groups such as trunk and face
Ankle or wrist when code description describes leg or arm
Cleaning and preparing viable wound surface for grafting or negative pressure wound therapy used to heal wound primarily
Code selection based on defect size and location
Percentage applies to children younger than age 10
Removal nonviable tissue in nonchronic wounds for primary healing
Square centimeters applies to children and adults age 10 or older

EXCLUDES Chronic wound management on wounds left to heal by secondary intention (11042-11047 [11045, 11046], 97597-97598)
Necrotizing soft tissue infections for specific anatomical locations (11004-11008)

15002 Surgical preparation or creation of recipient site by excision of open wounds, burn eschar, or scar (including subcutaneous tissues), or incisional release of scar contracture, trunk, arms, legs; first 100 sq cm or 1% of body area of infants and children

EXCLUDES Linear scar revision (13100-13153)
6.45   10.0   FUD 000   T A2 80
AMA: 2019,Nov,3; 2018,Jan,8; 2017,Jan,8; 2016,Jan,13

+ **15003** each additional 100 sq cm, or part thereof, or each additional 1% of body area of infants and children (List separately in addition to code for primary procedure)
Code first (15002)
1.32   2.11   FUD ZZZ   N N1 80
AMA: 2019,Nov,3; 2018,Jan,8; 2017,Jan,8; 2016,Jan,13

15004 Surgical preparation or creation of recipient site by excision of open wounds, burn eschar, or scar (including subcutaneous tissues), or incisional release of scar contracture, face, scalp, eyelids, mouth, neck, ears, orbits, genitalia, hands, feet and/or multiple digits; first 100 sq cm or 1% of body area of infants and children
7.65   11.4   FUD 000   T A2 80
AMA: 2019,Nov,3; 2018,Jan,8; 2017,Jan,8; 2016,Jan,13

+ **15005** each additional 100 sq cm, or part thereof, or each additional 1% of body area of infants and children (List separately in addition to code for primary procedure)
Code first (15004)
2.66   3.50   FUD ZZZ   N N1 80
AMA: 2019,Nov,3; 2018,Jan,8; 2017,Jan,8; 2016,Jan,13

15040 Obtain Autograft

INCLUDES Ankle or wrist when code description describes leg or arm
Percentage applies to children younger than age 10
Square centimeters applies to children and adults age 10 or older

15040 Harvest of skin for tissue cultured skin autograft, 100 sq cm or less
3.60   7.47   FUD 000   T A2
AMA: 2018,Jan,8; 2017,Jan,8; 2016,Jan,13

15050 Pinch Graft

INCLUDES Autologous skin graft harvest and application
Current graft removal
Fixation and anchoring skin graft
Simple cleaning

EXCLUDES Removal devitalized tissue from wound(s), non-selective debridement, without anesthesia (97602)
Code also graft or flap necessary to repair donor site

15050 Pinch graft, single or multiple, to cover small ulcer, tip of digit, or other minimal open area (except on face), up to defect size 2 cm diameter
13.0   16.7   FUD 090   T A2
AMA: 2018,Jan,8; 2017,Jan,8; 2016,Jun,8; 2016,Jan,13

15100-15261 Skin Grafts and Replacements

INCLUDES Add together surface area multiple wounds in same anatomical locations as indicated in code descriptor groups, such as face and scalp. Do not add together multiple wounds at different anatomical site groups such as trunk and face
Ankle or wrist when code description describes leg or arm
Autologous skin graft harvest and application
Code selection based on recipient site location and graft size and type
Current graft removal
Fixation and anchoring skin graft
Percentage applies to children younger than age 10
Simple cleaning
Simple tissue debridement
Square centimeters applies to children and adults age 10 or older

EXCLUDES Debridement without immediate primary closure, when wound grossly contaminated and extensive cleaning needed, or when necrotic or contaminated tissue removed (11042-11047 [11045, 11046], 97597-97598)
Removal devitalized tissue from wound(s), non-selective debridement, without anesthesia (97602)
Code also:
Graft or flap necessary to repair donor site
Primary procedure requiring skin graft for definitive closure

15100 Split-thickness autograft, trunk, arms, legs; first 100 sq cm or less, or 1% of body area of infants and children (except 15050)
20.5   24.5   FUD 090   T A2
AMA: 2018,Jan,8; 2017,Jan,8; 2016,Jun,8; 2016,Jan,13

+ **15101** each additional 100 sq cm, or each additional 1% of body area of infants and children, or part thereof (List separately in addition to code for primary procedure)
Code first (15100)
3.24   5.40   FUD ZZZ   N N1
AMA: 2018,Jan,8; 2017,Jan,8; 2016,Jun,8; 2016,Jan,13

15110 Epidermal autograft, trunk, arms, legs; first 100 sq cm or less, or 1% of body area of infants and children
19.9   23.1   FUD 090   T A2
AMA: 2018,Jan,8; 2017,Jan,8; 2016,Jan,13

+ **15111** each additional 100 sq cm, or each additional 1% of body area of infants and children, or part thereof (List separately in addition to code for primary procedure)
Code first (15110)
3.02   3.33   FUD ZZZ   N N1
AMA: 2018,Jan,8; 2017,Jan,8; 2016,Jan,13

15115 Epidermal autograft, face, scalp, eyelids, mouth, neck, ears, orbits, genitalia, hands, feet, and/or multiple digits; first 100 sq cm or less, or 1% of body area of infants and children
19.6   22.8   FUD 090   T A2
AMA: 2018,Jan,8; 2017,Jan,8; 2016,Jan,13

+ **15116** each additional 100 sq cm, or each additional 1% of body area of infants and children, or part thereof (List separately in addition to code for primary procedure)
Code first (15115)
4.39   4.81   FUD ZZZ   N N1
AMA: 2018,Jan,8; 2017,Jan,8; 2016,Jan,13

15120 Split-thickness autograft, face, scalp, eyelids, mouth, neck, ears, orbits, genitalia, hands, feet, and/or multiple digits; first 100 sq cm or less, or 1% of body area of infants and children (except 15050)
EXCLUDES Other eyelid repair (67961-67975)
19.9   24.3   FUD 090   T A2
AMA: 2018,Jan,8; 2017,Jan,8; 2016,Jun,8; 2016,Jan,13

+ **15121** each additional 100 sq cm, or each additional 1% of body area of infants and children, or part thereof (List separately in addition to code for primary procedure)
EXCLUDES Other eyelid repair (67961-67975)
Code first (15120)
3.90   6.05   FUD ZZZ   N N1
AMA: 2018,Jan,8; 2017,Jan,8; 2016,Jun,8; 2016,Jan,13

15130 Dermal autograft, trunk, arms, legs; first 100 sq cm or less, or 1% of body area of infants and children
🚗 17.1 ⚖ 20.6 **FUD** 090   T A2 ▣
AMA: 2018,Jan,8; 2017,Jan,8; 2016,Jan,13

+ 15131 each additional 100 sq cm, or each additional 1% of body area of infants and children, or part thereof (List separately in addition to code for primary procedure)
Code first (15130)
🚗 2.65 ⚖ 2.86 **FUD** ZZZ   N N1 ▣
AMA: 2018,Jan,8; 2017,Jan,8; 2016,Jan,13

15135 Dermal autograft, face, scalp, eyelids, mouth, neck, ears, orbits, genitalia, hands, feet, and/or multiple digits; first 100 sq cm or less, or 1% of body area of infants and children
🚗 21.7 ⚖ 25.0 **FUD** 090   T A2 ▣
AMA: 2018,Jan,8; 2017,Jan,8; 2016,Jan,13

+ 15136 each additional 100 sq cm, or each additional 1% of body area of infants and children, or part thereof (List separately in addition to code for primary procedure)
Code first (15135)
🚗 2.65 ⚖ 2.83 **FUD** ZZZ   N N1 ▣
AMA: 2018,Jan,8; 2017,Jan,8; 2016,Jan,13

15150 Tissue cultured skin autograft, trunk, arms, legs; first 25 sq cm or less
🚗 18.4 ⚖ 20.3 **FUD** 090   T A2 ▣
AMA: 2018,Jan,8; 2017,Jan,8; 2016,Jan,13

+ 15151 additional 1 sq cm to 75 sq cm (List separately in addition to code for primary procedure)
EXCLUDES Grafts over 75 sq cm (15152)
Reporting code more than one time per session
Code first (15150)
🚗 3.19 ⚖ 3.45 **FUD** ZZZ   N N1 ▣
AMA: 2018,Jan,8; 2017,Jan,8; 2016,Jan,13

+ 15152 each additional 100 sq cm, or each additional 1% of body area of infants and children, or part thereof (List separately in addition to code for primary procedure)
Code first (15151)
🚗 4.22 ⚖ 4.47 **FUD** ZZZ   N N1 ▣
AMA: 2018,Jan,8; 2017,Jan,8; 2016,Jan,13

15155 Tissue cultured skin autograft, face, scalp, eyelids, mouth, neck, ears, orbits, genitalia, hands, feet, and/or multiple digits; first 25 sq cm or less
🚗 21.1 ⚖ 23.0 **FUD** 090   T A2 ▣
AMA: 2018,Jan,8; 2017,Jan,8; 2016,Jan,13

+ 15156 additional 1 sq cm to 75 sq cm (List separately in addition to code for primary procedure)
EXCLUDES Grafts over 75 sq cm (15157)
Reporting code more than one time per session
Code first (15155)
🚗 4.39 ⚖ 4.64 **FUD** ZZZ   N N1 ▣
AMA: 2018,Jan,8; 2017,Jan,8; 2016,Jan,13

+ 15157 each additional 100 sq cm, or each additional 1% of body area of infants and children, or part thereof (List separately in addition to code for primary procedure)
Code first (15156)
🚗 4.82 ⚖ 5.19 **FUD** ZZZ   N N1 ▣
AMA: 2018,Jan,8; 2017,Jan,8; 2016,Jan,13

15200 Full thickness graft, free, including direct closure of donor site, trunk; 20 sq cm or less
🚗 19.2 ⚖ 23.9 **FUD** 090   T A2 ▣
AMA: 2018,Jan,8; 2017,Jan,8; 2016,Jun,8; 2016,Jan,13

+ 15201 each additional 20 sq cm, or part thereof (List separately in addition to code for primary procedure)
Code first (15200)
🚗 2.26 ⚖ 4.20 **FUD** ZZZ   N N1 ▣
AMA: 2018,Jan,8; 2017,Jan,8; 2016,Jun,8; 2016,Jan,13

15220 Full thickness graft, free, including direct closure of donor site, scalp, arms, and/or legs; 20 sq cm or less
🚗 17.4 ⚖ 21.9 **FUD** 090   T A2 ▣
AMA: 2018,Jan,8; 2017,Jan,8; 2016,Jun,8; 2016,Jan,13

+ 15221 each additional 20 sq cm, or part thereof (List separately in addition to code for primary procedure)
Code first (15220)
🚗 2.03 ⚖ 3.86 **FUD** ZZZ   N N1 ▣
AMA: 2018,Jan,8; 2017,Jan,8; 2016,Jun,8; 2016,Jan,13

15240 Full thickness graft, free, including direct closure of donor site, forehead, cheeks, chin, mouth, neck, axillae, genitalia, hands, and/or feet; 20 sq cm or less
EXCLUDES Fingertip graft (15050)
Syndactyly repair fingers (26560-26562)
🚗 23.0 ⚖ 26.6 **FUD** 090   T A2 ▣
AMA: 2018,Jan,8; 2017,Jan,8; 2016,Jun,8; 2016,Jan,13

+ 15241 each additional 20 sq cm, or part thereof (List separately in addition to code for primary procedure)
Code first (15240)
🚗 3.18 ⚖ 5.22 **FUD** ZZZ   N N1 ▣
AMA: 2018,Jan,8; 2017,Jan,8; 2016,Jun,8; 2016,Jan,13

15260 Full thickness graft, free, including direct closure of donor site, nose, ears, eyelids, and/or lips; 20 sq cm or less
EXCLUDES Other eyelid repair (67961-67975)
🚗 24.1 ⚖ 28.5 **FUD** 090   T A2 ▣
AMA: 2018,Jan,8; 2017,Jan,8; 2016,Jun,8; 2016,Jan,13

+ 15261 each additional 20 sq cm, or part thereof (List separately in addition to code for primary procedure)
EXCLUDES Other eyelid repair (67961-67975)
Code first (15260)
🚗 3.96 ⚖ 5.99 **FUD** ZZZ   N N1 ▣
AMA: 2018,Jan,8; 2017,Jan,8; 2016,Jun,8; 2016,Jan,13

15271-15278 Skin Substitute Graft Application

INCLUDES Add together surface area multiple wounds in same anatomical locations as indicated in code descriptor groups, such as face and scalp. Do not add together multiple wounds at different anatomical site groups such as trunk and face

Ankle or wrist when code description describes leg or arm

Code selection based on defect site location and size

Fixation and anchoring skin graft

Graft types include:

Biological material used for tissue engineering (e.g., scaffold) for growing skin

Nonautologous human skin such as:

Acellular

Allograft

Cellular

Dermal

Epidermal

Homograft

Nonhuman grafts

Percentage applies to children younger than age 10

Removing current graft

Simple cleaning

Simple tissue debridement

Square centimeters applies to children and adults age 10 or older

EXCLUDES Application nongraft dressing

Injected skin substitutes

Removal devitalized tissue from wound(s), non-selective debridement, without anesthesia (97602)

Skin application procedures, low cost (C5271-C5278)

Code also:

Biologic implant for soft tissue reinforcement (15777)

Primary procedure requiring skin graft for definitive closure

Supply high-cost skin substitute product (C1849, C9363, Q4101, Q4103-Q4110, Q4116, Q4121-Q4123, Q4126-Q4128, Q4132-Q4133, Q4137-Q4138, Q4140-Q4141, Q4143, Q4146-Q4148, Q4150-Q4161, Q4163-Q4164, Q4167, Q4169, Q4173, Q4175, Q4176, Q4178-Q4184, Q4186-Q4188, Q4190, Q4193-Q4198, Q4200-Q4201, Q4203, Q4205, Q4208-Q4209, Q4211, Q4219, Q4222, Q4226, Q4227, Q4232, Q4234, Q4237-Q4239, Q4249)

15271 **Application of skin substitute graft to trunk, arms, legs, total wound surface area up to 100 sq cm; first 25 sq cm or less wound surface area**

EXCLUDES *Total wound area greater than or equal to 100 sq cm (15273-15274)*

2.45   4.29   **FUD** 000   T G2 ▭

AMA: 2018,Jan,8; 2017,Oct,9; 2017,Jan,8; 2016,Jan,13

+ 15272 **each additional 25 sq cm wound surface area, or part thereof (List separately in addition to code for primary procedure)**

EXCLUDES *Total wound area greater than or equal to 100 sq cm (15273-15274)*

Code first (15271)

0.51   0.75   **FUD** ZZZ   N M1 ▭

AMA: 2018,Jan,8; 2017,Jan,8; 2016,Jan,13

15273 **Application of skin substitute graft to trunk, arms, legs, total wound surface area greater than or equal to 100 sq cm; first 100 sq cm wound surface area, or 1% of body area of infants and children**

EXCLUDES *Total wound surface area up to 100 cm (15271-15272)*

5.84   8.73   **FUD** 000   T G2 ▭

AMA: 2018,Jan,8; 2017,Jan,8; 2016,Jan,13

+ 15274 **each additional 100 sq cm wound surface area, or part thereof, or each additional 1% of body area of infants and children, or part thereof (List separately in addition to code for primary procedure)**

EXCLUDES *Total wound surface area up to 100 cm (15271-15272)*

Code first (15273)

1.32   2.26   **FUD** ZZZ   N M1 ▭

AMA: 2018,Jan,8; 2017,Jan,8; 2016,Jan,13

15275 **Application of skin substitute graft to face, scalp, eyelids, mouth, neck, ears, orbits, genitalia, hands, feet, and/or multiple digits, total wound surface area up to 100 sq cm; first 25 sq cm or less wound surface area**

EXCLUDES *Total wound area greater than or equal to 100 sq cm (15277-15278)*

2.75   4.48   **FUD** 000   T G2 ▭

AMA: 2018,Jan,8; 2017,Jan,8; 2016,Jan,13

+ 15276 **each additional 25 sq cm wound surface area, or part thereof (List separately in addition to code for primary procedure)**

EXCLUDES *Total wound area greater than or equal to 100 sq cm (15277-15278)*

Code first (15275)

0.75   0.98   **FUD** ZZZ   N M1 ▭

AMA: 2018,Jan,8; 2017,Jan,8; 2016,Jan,13

15277 **Application of skin substitute graft to face, scalp, eyelids, mouth, neck, ears, orbits, genitalia, hands, feet, and/or multiple digits, total wound surface area greater than or equal to 100 sq cm; first 100 sq cm wound surface area, or 1% of body area of infants and children**

EXCLUDES *Total surface area up to 100 sq cm (15275-15276)*

6.60   9.55   **FUD** 000   T G2 ▭

AMA: 2018,Jan,8; 2017,Jan,8; 2016,Jan,13

+ 15278 **each additional 100 sq cm wound surface area, or part thereof, or each additional 1% of body area of infants and children, or part thereof (List separately in addition to code for primary procedure)**

EXCLUDES *Total surface area up to 100 sq cm (15275-15276)*

Code first (15277)

1.66   2.54   **FUD** ZZZ   N M1 ▭

AMA: 2018,Jan,8; 2017,Jan,8; 2016,Jan,13

15570-15731 Wound Reconstruction: Skin Flaps

INCLUDES   Ankle or wrist when code description describes leg or arm
Code selection based on recipient site when flap attached in transfer or to final site and based on donor site when tube created for transfer later or when flap delayed prior to transfer
Fixation and anchoring skin graft
Simple tissue debridement
Tube formation for later transfer

EXCLUDES   *Contiguous tissue transfer flaps (14040-14041, 14060-14061, 14301-14302)*
Debridement without immediate primary closure (11042-11047 [11045, 11046], 97597-97598)
Excision:
  Benign lesion (11400-11471)
  Burn eschar or scar (15002-15005)
  Malignant lesion (11600-11646)
Microvascular repair (15756-15758)
Primary procedure--see appropriate anatomical site
Code also:
  Application extensive immobilization apparatus
  Repair donor site with skin grafts or flaps

15570   **Formation of direct or tubed pedicle, with or without transfer; trunk**
  INCLUDES   Flaps without vascular pedicle
  🔪 21.1   ⚕ 26.2   **FUD** 090   T A2 ▥
  AMA: 2018,Jan,8; 2017,Jan,8; 2016,Jan,13

Pedicle flap

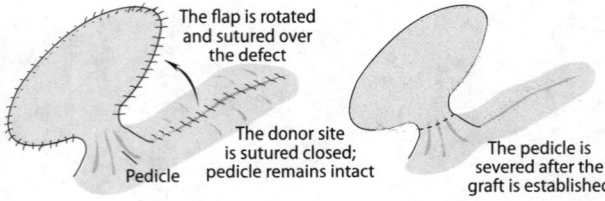

Defective tissue is identified   And removed   A nearby flap is lifted; a pedicle remains attached to provide an intact blood supply

The flap is rotated and sutured over the defect

Pedicle   The donor site is sutured closed; pedicle remains intact   The pedicle is severed after the graft is established

15572   **scalp, arms, or legs**
  INCLUDES   Flaps without vascular pedicle
  🔪 21.2   ⚕ 25.3   **FUD** 090   T A2 ▥
  AMA: 2018,Jan,8; 2017,Jan,8; 2016,Jan,13

15574   **forehead, cheeks, chin, mouth, neck, axillae, genitalia, hands or feet**
  INCLUDES   Flaps without vascular pedicle
  🔪 21.6   ⚕ 25.7   **FUD** 090   T A2 ▥
  AMA: 2018,Jan,8; 2017,Jan,8; 2016,Jan,13

15576   **eyelids, nose, ears, lips, or intraoral**
  INCLUDES   Flaps without vascular pedicle
  🔪 19.1   ⚕ 22.9   **FUD** 090   T A2 ▥
  AMA: 2018,Jan,8; 2017,Jan,8; 2016,Jan,13

15600   **Delay of flap or sectioning of flap (division and inset); at trunk**
  🔪 5.96   ⚕ 9.47   **FUD** 090   T A2 80 ▥
  AMA: 2019,Jun,14; 2018,Jan,8; 2017,Jan,8; 2016,Jan,13

15610   **at scalp, arms, or legs**
  🔪 6.89   ⚕ 10.2   **FUD** 090   T A2 80 ▥
  AMA: 2018,Jan,8; 2017,Jan,8; 2016,Jan,13

15620   **at forehead, cheeks, chin, neck, axillae, genitalia, hands, or feet**
  🔪 9.26   ⚕ 12.6   **FUD** 090   T A2 ▥
  AMA: 2018,Jan,8; 2017,Jan,8; 2016,Jan,13

15630   **at eyelids, nose, ears, or lips**
  🔪 9.77   ⚕ 13.0   **FUD** 090   T A2 ▥
  AMA: 2018,Jan,8; 2017,Jan,8; 2016,Jan,13

15650   **Transfer, intermediate, of any pedicle flap (eg, abdomen to wrist, Walking tube), any location**
  EXCLUDES   *Defatting, revision, or rearranging transferred pedicle flap or skin graft (13100-14302)*
  Eyelids, ears, lips, and nose - refer to anatomical area
  🔪 10.9   ⚕ 14.5   **FUD** 090   T A2 80 ▥
  AMA: 2018,Jan,8; 2017,Jan,8; 2016,Jan,13

15730   **Midface flap (ie, zygomaticofacial flap) with preservation of vascular pedicle(s)**
  🔪 26.3   ⚕ 42.9   **FUD** 090   T G2 ▥
  AMA: 2018,Apr,10; 2018,Jan,8; 2017,Nov,6

15731   **Forehead flap with preservation of vascular pedicle (eg, axial pattern flap, paramedian forehead flap)**
  EXCLUDES   *Muscle, myocutaneous, or fasciocutaneous flap head or neck (15733)*
  🔪 28.6   ⚕ 32.0   **FUD** 090   T A2 80 ▥
  AMA: 2018,Jan,8; 2017,Nov,6; 2017,Jan,8; 2016,Jan,13

15733-15738 Wound Reconstruction: Muscle Flaps

INCLUDES   Code based on donor site
EXCLUDES   *Contiguous tissue transfer flaps (14040-14041, 14060-14061, 14301-14302)*
Microvascular repair (15756-15758)
Code also:
  Application extensive immobilization apparatus
  Repair donor site with skin grafts or flaps

15733   **Muscle, myocutaneous, or fasciocutaneous flap; head and neck with named vascular pedicle (ie, buccinators, genioglossus, temporalis, masseter, sternocleidomastoid, levator scapulae)**
  INCLUDES   Repair extracranial defect by anterior pericranial flap on vascular pedicle (15731)
  🔪 29.9   ⚕ 29.9   **FUD** 090   T A2 ▥
  AMA: 2018,Apr,10; 2018,Jan,8; 2017,Nov,6

15734   **trunk**
  🔪 43.6   ⚕ 43.6   **FUD** 090   T A2 80 ▥
  AMA: 2018,Aug,10; 2018,Jan,8; 2017,Nov,6; 2017,Jan,8; 2016,Jan,13

15736   **upper extremity**
  🔪 35.3   ⚕ 35.3   **FUD** 090   T A2 ▥
  AMA: 2018,Jan,8; 2017,Nov,6; 2017,Jan,8; 2016,Jan,13

15738   **lower extremity**
  🔪 37.4   ⚕ 37.4   **FUD** 090   T A2 80 ▥
  AMA: 2018,Jan,8; 2017,Nov,6; 2017,Jan,8; 2016,Jan,13

15740-15758 Wound Reconstruction: Other

INCLUDES   Fixation and anchoring skin graft
Routine dressing
Simple tissue debridement
EXCLUDES   *Adjacent tissue transfer (14000-14302)*
Excision:
  Benign lesion (11400-11471)
  Burn eschar or scar (15002-15005)
  Malignant lesion (11600-11646)
Flaps without vascular pedicle addition (15570-15576)
Primary procedure--see appropriate anatomical section
Skin graft for repair donor site (15050-15278)
Code also repair donor site with skin grafts or flaps (14000-14350, 15050-15278)

15740   **Flap; island pedicle requiring identification and dissection of an anatomically named axial vessel**
  EXCLUDES   *V-Y subcutaneous flaps, random island flaps, and other flaps from adjacent areas (14000-14302)*
  🔪 24.2   ⚕ 28.8   **FUD** 090   T A2 ▥
  AMA: 2018,Jan,8; 2017,Dec,14; 2017,Jan,8; 2016,Jan,13

15750 **neurovascular pedicle**

EXCLUDES *V-Y subcutaneous flaps, random island flaps, and other flaps from adjacent areas (14000-14302)*

26.4   26.4   **FUD** 090   T A2 80

AMA: 2018,Jan,8; 2017,Dec,14

15756 **Free muscle or myocutaneous flap with microvascular anastomosis**

INCLUDES Operating microscope (69990)

66.0   66.0   **FUD** 090   C 80

AMA: 2019,Dec,5; 2018,Jan,8; 2017,Jan,8; 2016,Feb,12; 2016,Jan,13

15757 **Free skin flap with microvascular anastomosis**

INCLUDES Operating microscope (69990)

65.5   65.5   **FUD** 090   C 80

AMA: 2019,Dec,5; 2018,Jan,8; 2017,Jan,8; 2016,Apr,8; 2016,Feb,12; 2016,Jan,13

15758 **Free fascial flap with microvascular anastomosis**

INCLUDES Operating microscope (69990)

66.0   66.0   **FUD** 090   C 80

AMA: 2019,Dec,5; 2018,Jan,8; 2017,Jan,8; 2016,Feb,12; 2016,Jan,13

15760-15774 [15769] Other Grafts

EXCLUDES *Adjacent tissue transfer (14000-14302)*
Excision:
  Benign lesion (11400-11471)
  Burn eschar or scar (15002-15005)
  Malignant lesion (11600-11646)
Flaps without vascular pedicle addition (15570-15576)
Microvascular repair (15756-15758)
Primary procedure (see appropriate anatomical site)
Repair donor site with skin grafts or flaps (14000-14350, 15050-15278)

15760 **Graft; composite (eg, full thickness of external ear or nasal ala), including primary closure, donor area**

INCLUDES Fixation and anchoring skin graft
Routine dressing
Simple tissue debridement

20.0   24.1   **FUD** 090   T A2

AMA: 2018,Jan,8; 2017,Jan,8; 2016,Jan,13

15769   **Resequenced code. See code following 15770.**

15770 **derma-fat-fascia**

INCLUDES Fixation and anchoring skin graft
Routine dressing
Simple tissue debridement

19.0   19.0   **FUD** 090   T A2 80

AMA: 2019,Oct,5; 2018,Jan,8; 2017,Jan,8; 2016,Jan,13

\# **15769** **Grafting of autologous soft tissue, other, harvested by direct excision (eg, fat, dermis, fascia)**

INCLUDES Excisional graft harvest and recipient site placement

EXCLUDES *Autologous grafts specific tissue types, such as skin, bone, nerve, tendon, fascia lata, or vessels*
Autologous white blood cell concentrate injection (0481T)
Harvesting adipose tissue for adipose-derived regenerative cell therapy (0489T-0490T)
Platelet-rich plasma injection (0232T)
Suction assisted lipectomy (15876-15879)

13.8   13.8   **FUD** 090   G2

15771 **Grafting of autologous fat harvested by liposuction technique to trunk, breasts, scalp, arms, and/or legs; 50 cc or less injectate**

INCLUDES Add together injectate volume harvested from each anatomical area indicated in code description, such as face and neck, to report total volume. Do not add together injectate harvested from different anatomical site groups, such as trunk and face
Code based on recipient site

EXCLUDES *Autologous white blood cell concentrate injection (0481T)*
Liposuction not for grafting purposes (15876-15879)
Obtaining tissue for adipose-derived regenerative cell therapy (0489T-0490T)
Platelet-rich plasma injection (0232T)
Subcutaneous injection filling material, at same anatomical site (11950-11954)
Reporting code more than one time per session

13.7   16.5   **FUD** 090   G2

AMA: 2020,Apr,10

\+ **15772** **each additional 50 cc injectate, or part thereof (List separately in addition to code for primary procedure)**

Code first (15771)

4.07   5.22   **FUD** ZZZ

AMA: 2020,Apr,10

15773 **Grafting of autologous fat harvested by liposuction technique to face, eyelids, mouth, neck, ears, orbits, genitalia, hands, and/or feet; 25 cc or less injectate**

INCLUDES Add together injectate volume harvested from each anatomical area indicated in code description, such as face and neck, to report total volume. Do not add together injectate harvested from different anatomical site groups, such as trunk and face
Code based on recipient site

EXCLUDES *Autologous white blood cell concentrate injection (0481T)*
Liposuction not for grafting purposes (15876-15879)
Obtaining tissue for adipose-derived regenerative cell therapy (0489T-0490T)
Platelet-rich plasma injection (0232T)
Reporting code more than one time per session
Subcutaneous injection filling material, at same anatomical site (11950-11954)

13.9   16.7   **FUD** 090   G2

\+ **15774** **each additional 25 cc injectate, or part thereof (List separately in addition to code for primary procedure)**

Code first (15773)

3.91   5.06   **FUD** ZZZ

Integumentary System

15775 — 15829

15775-15839 Plastic, Reconstructive, and Aesthetic Surgery

CMS: 100-02,16,10 Exclusions from Coverage; 100-02,16,120 Cosmetic Procedures; 100-02,16,180 Services Related to Noncovered Procedures

15775 Punch graft for hair transplant; 1 to 15 punch grafts

EXCLUDES Strip transplant (15220)

🔧 6.42   ⚕ 8.74   **FUD** 000   T A2 80 ▢

AMA: 2018,Jan,8; 2017,Jan,8; 2016,Jan,13

Hair shaft within follicle
Epidermis
Sebaceous gland attached to hair follicle
Eccrine sweat gland with duct open directly to surface
Apocrine sweat gland connected by duct to a hair follicle
Typical male pattern hair loss

15776 more than 15 punch grafts

EXCLUDES Strip transplant (15220)

🔧 10.2   ⚕ 14.5   **FUD** 000   T A2 80 ▢

AMA: 2018,Jan,8; 2017,Jan,8; 2016,Jan,13

+ 15777 Implantation of biologic implant (eg, acellular dermal matrix) for soft tissue reinforcement (ie, breast, trunk) (List separately in addition to code for primary procedure)

EXCLUDES Application high cost skin substitute to external wound (15271-15278)
Application low cost skin substitute to external wound (C5271–C5278)
Mesh implantation for:
  Open repair ventral or incisional hernia (49560–49566) and (49568)
  Repair devitalized soft tissue infection (11004-11006) and (49568)
  Repair pelvic floor (57267)
Repair anorectal fistula with plug (46707)
Reporting modifier 50 for bilateral breast procedure. Report once for each side when performed bilaterally
Soft tissue reinforcement with biologic implants other than in the breast or trunk (17999)

Code also:
  Supply biologic implant
  Synthetic or nonbiological implant to reinforce abdominal wall (0437T)
Code first primary procedure

🔧 6.25   ⚕ 6.25   **FUD** ZZZ   N N1 ▢

AMA: 2019,Nov,14; 2019,Jan,14; 2018,Jan,8; 2017,Jan,8; 2016,Jan,13

15780 Dermabrasion; total face (eg, for acne scarring, fine wrinkling, rhytids, general keratosis)

🔧 19.3   ⚕ 25.2   **FUD** 090   J P3 80 ▢

AMA: 2018,Jan,8; 2017,Jan,8; 2016,Jan,13

15781 segmental, face

🔧 12.3   ⚕ 15.6   **FUD** 090   T P2 ▢

AMA: 1997,Nov,1

15782 regional, other than face

🔧 11.2   ⚕ 15.3   **FUD** 090   J P3 80 ▢

AMA: 1997,Nov,1

15783 superficial, any site (eg, tattoo removal)

🔧 10.6   ⚕ 13.6   **FUD** 090   T P2 80 ▢

AMA: 2018,Jan,8; 2017,Jan,8; 2016,Jan,13

15786 Abrasion; single lesion (eg, keratosis, scar)

🔧 3.85   ⚕ 6.87   **FUD** 010   Q1 N1 ▢

AMA: 1997,Nov,1

+ 15787 each additional 4 lesions or less (List separately in addition to code for primary procedure)

Code first (15786)

🔧 0.50   ⚕ 1.27   **FUD** ZZZ   N N1 ▢

AMA: 1997,Nov,1

15788 Chemical peel, facial; epidermal

🔧 6.55   ⚕ 12.2   **FUD** 090   Q1 N1 ▢

AMA: 1997,Nov,1; 1993,Win,1

15789 dermal

🔧 11.6   ⚕ 15.3   **FUD** 090   T P2 ▢

AMA: 1997,Nov,1; 1993,Win,1

15792 Chemical peel, nonfacial; epidermal

🔧 6.61   ⚕ 10.9   **FUD** 090   Q1 N1 80 ▢

AMA: 1997,Nov,1; 1993,Win,1

15793 dermal

🔧 10.0   ⚕ 13.6   **FUD** 090   Q1 N1 ▢

AMA: 1997,Nov,1; 1993,Win,1

15819 Cervicoplasty

🔧 22.7   ⚕ 22.7   **FUD** 090   T G2 80 ▢

AMA: 1997,Nov,1

15820 Blepharoplasty, lower eyelid;

🔧 14.5   ⚕ 16.2   **FUD** 090   T A2 80 50 ▢

AMA: 2018,Jan,8; 2017,Jan,8; 2016,Jan,13

15821 with extensive herniated fat pad

🔧 15.5   ⚕ 17.4   **FUD** 090   T A2 80 50 ▢

AMA: 2018,Jan,8; 2017,Jan,8; 2016,Jan,13

15822 Blepharoplasty, upper eyelid;

🔧 11.2   ⚕ 12.9   **FUD** 090   T A2 50 ▢

AMA: 2018,Jan,8; 2017,Jan,8; 2016,Jan,13

15823 with excessive skin weighting down lid

🔧 15.5   ⚕ 17.4   **FUD** 090   T A2 50 ▢

AMA: 2018,Jan,8; 2017,Jan,8; 2016,Jan,13

15824 Rhytidectomy; forehead

EXCLUDES Repair brow ptosis (67900)

🔧 0.00   ⚕ 0.00   **FUD** 000   T A2 80 50 ▢

AMA: 2018,Jan,8; 2017,Apr,9

Frontalis (elevates brow)
Forehead rhytidectomy incision
Procerus (wrinkles nose)
Corrugators (move brows medially)
A rhytidectomy is an excision to eliminate wrinkles. This procedure in the forehead region typically involves an incision just inside the scalp line. Skin and underlying tissues are then manipulated to eliminate wrinkles in the forehead

15825 neck with platysmal tightening (platysmal flap, P-flap)

🔧 0.00   ⚕ 0.00   **FUD** 000   T A2 80 50 ▢

AMA: 2018,Jan,8; 2017,Apr,9

15826 glabellar frown lines

🔧 0.00   ⚕ 0.00   **FUD** 000   T A2 80 50 ▢

AMA: 1997,Nov,1

15828 cheek, chin, and neck

🔧 0.00   ⚕ 0.00   **FUD** 000   T A2 80 50 ▢

AMA: 1997,Nov,1

15829 superficial musculoaponeurotic system (SMAS) flap

🔧 0.00   ⚕ 0.00   **FUD** 000   T A2 80 50 ▢

AMA: 1997,Nov,1

15830   Excision, excessive skin and subcutaneous tissue (includes lipectomy); abdomen, infraumbilical panniculectomy

EXCLUDES   For same wound:
Adjacent tissue transfer, trunk (14000-14001, 14302)
Complex wound repair, trunk (13100-13102)
Intermediate wound repair, trunk (12031-12032, 12034-12037)
Other abdominoplasty (17999)
Code also, when performed (15847)
33.9   33.9   FUD 090   J A2 80

15832   thigh
26.5   26.5   FUD 090   J A2 80 50
AMA: 1997,Nov,1

15833   leg
25.2   25.2   FUD 090   J A2 80 50
AMA: 1997,Nov,1

15834   hip
25.7   25.7   FUD 090   J A2 80 50
AMA: 1997,Nov,1

15835   buttock
26.9   26.9   FUD 090   J A2 80
AMA: 1997,Nov,1

15836   arm
22.6   22.6   FUD 090   J A2 80 50
AMA: 1997,Nov,1

15837   forearm or hand
20.6   24.7   FUD 090   J G2 80
AMA: 1997,Nov,1

15838   submental fat pad
18.5   18.5   FUD 090   J G2 80
AMA: 1998,Feb,1; 1997,Nov,1

15839   other area
21.2   25.4   FUD 090   J A2 80
AMA: 1997,Nov,1

15840-15845 Reanimation of the Paralyzed Face

INCLUDES   Routine dressing and supplies
EXCLUDES   Intravenous fluorescein evaluation blood flow in graft or flap (15860)
Nerve:
Decompression (69720, 69725, 69955)
Pedicle transfer (64905, 64907)
Suture (64831-64876, 69740, 69745)
Code also repair donor site with skin grafts or flaps

15840   Graft for facial nerve paralysis; free fascia graft (including obtaining fascia)
28.9   28.9   FUD 090   T A2
AMA: 1997,Nov,1

15841   free muscle graft (including obtaining graft)
51.2   51.2   FUD 090   T A2 80
AMA: 1997,Nov,1

15842   free muscle flap by microsurgical technique
INCLUDES   Operating microscope (69990)
78.5   78.5   FUD 090   T G2 80
AMA: 2016,Feb,12

15845   regional muscle transfer
28.8   28.8   FUD 090   T A2 80
AMA: 1998,Feb,1; 1997,Nov,1

15847 Removal of Excess Abdominal Tissue Add-on

CMS: 100-02,16,10 Exclusions from Coverage; 100-02,16,120 Cosmetic Procedures; 100-02,16,180 Services Related to Noncovered Procedures

+   15847   Excision, excessive skin and subcutaneous tissue (includes lipectomy), abdomen (eg, abdominoplasty) (includes umbilical transposition and fascial plication) (List separately in addition to code for primary procedure)
EXCLUDES   Abdominal wall hernia repair (49491-49587)
Other abdominoplasty (17999)
Code first (15830)
0.00   0.00   FUD YYY   N N1 80

15850-15852 Suture Removal/Dressing Change: Anesthesia Required

15850   Removal of sutures under anesthesia (other than local), same surgeon
1.14   2.57   FUD XXX   T G2
AMA: 2018,Jan,8; 2017,Jan,8; 2016,Jan,13

15851   Removal of sutures under anesthesia (other than local), other surgeon
1.31   2.85   FUD 000   T P3
AMA: 2018,Jan,8; 2017,Jan,8; 2016,Jan,13

15852   Dressing change (for other than burns) under anesthesia (other than local)
EXCLUDES   Dressing change for burns (16020-16030)
1.34   1.34   FUD 000   Q1 N1
AMA: 1997,Nov,1

15860 Injection for Vascular Flow Determination

15860   Intravenous injection of agent (eg, fluorescein) to test vascular flow in flap or graft
3.13   3.13   FUD 000   Q1 N1 80
AMA: 2002,May,7; 1997,Nov,1

15876-15879 Liposuction

CMS: 100-02,16,10 Exclusions from Coverage; 100-02,16,120 Cosmetic Procedures; 100-02,16,180 Services Related to Noncovered Procedures
EXCLUDES   Liposuction for autologous fat grafting (15771-15774)
Obtaining tissue for adipose-derived regenerative cell therapy (0489T-0490T)

15876   Suction assisted lipectomy; head and neck
0.00   0.00   FUD 000   T A2 80
AMA: 2019,Oct,5; 2019,Aug,10; 2018,Sep,12

Cannula typically inserted through incision in front of ear

15877   trunk
0.00   0.00   FUD 000   T A2 80
AMA: 2019,Oct,5; 2019,Aug,10; 2018,Sep,12; 2018,Jan,8; 2017,Jan,8; 2016,Jan,13

15878   upper extremity
0.00   0.00   FUD 000   T A2 80 50
AMA: 2019,Oct,5; 2019,Aug,10; 2018,Sep,12

15879   lower extremity
0.00   0.00   FUD 000   T A2 80 50
AMA: 2019,Oct,5; 2019,Aug,10; 2018,Sep,12

15920-15999 Treatment of Decubitus Ulcers

Code also free skin graft to repair ulcer or donor site

15920   Excision, coccygeal pressure ulcer, with coccygectomy; with primary suture
17.8   17.8   FUD 090   J A2 80
AMA: 2011,May,3-5; 1997,Nov,1

15922   with flap closure
22.8   22.8   FUD 090   T A2 80
AMA: 2011,May,3-5; 1997,Nov,1

15931   **Excision, sacral pressure ulcer, with primary suture;**
🚗 20.1   ⚕ 20.1   **FUD** 090   J A2 ▭
AMA: 2011,May,3-5; 1997,Nov,1

15933   **with ostectomy**
🚗 24.5   ⚕ 24.5   **FUD** 090   J A2 80 ▭
AMA: 2011,May,3-5; 1997,Nov,1

15934   **Excision, sacral pressure ulcer, with skin flap closure;**
🚗 27.3   ⚕ 27.3   **FUD** 090   T A2 ▭
AMA: 2011,May,3-5; 1997,Nov,1

15935   **with ostectomy**
🚗 31.6   ⚕ 31.6   **FUD** 090   T A2 80 ▭
AMA: 2011,May,3-5; 1997,Nov,1

15936   **Excision, sacral pressure ulcer, in preparation for muscle or myocutaneous flap or skin graft closure;**
Code also any defect repair with:
Muscle or myocutaneous flap (15734, 15738)
Split skin graft (15100-15101)
🚗 26.0   ⚕ 26.0   **FUD** 090   T A2 ▭
AMA: 2011,May,3-5; 1998,Nov,1

15937   **with ostectomy**
Code also any defect repair with:
Muscle or myocutaneous flap (15734, 15738)
Split skin graft (15100-15101)
🚗 29.8   ⚕ 29.8   **FUD** 090   T A2 ▭
AMA: 2011,May,3-5; 1998,Nov,1

15940   **Excision, ischial pressure ulcer, with primary suture;**
🚗 20.1   ⚕ 20.1   **FUD** 090   J A2 ▭
AMA: 2011,May,3-5; 1997,Nov,1

15941   **with ostectomy (ischiectomy)**
🚗 26.4   ⚕ 26.4   **FUD** 090   J A2 80 ▭
AMA: 2011,May,3-5; 1997,Nov,1

15944   **Excision, ischial pressure ulcer, with skin flap closure;**
🚗 26.2   ⚕ 26.2   **FUD** 090   T A2 80 ▭
AMA: 2011,May,3-5; 1997,Nov,1

15945   **with ostectomy**
🚗 29.3   ⚕ 29.3   **FUD** 090   T A2 80 ▭
AMA: 2011,May,3-5; 1997,Nov,1

15946   **Excision, ischial pressure ulcer, with ostectomy, in preparation for muscle or myocutaneous flap or skin graft closure**
Code also any defect repair with:
Muscle or myocutaneous flap (15734, 15738)
Split skin graft (15100-15101)
🚗 47.0   ⚕ 47.0   **FUD** 090   T A2 ▭
AMA: 2018,Jan,8; 2017,Jan,8; 2016,Jan,13

15950   **Excision, trochanteric pressure ulcer, with primary suture;**
🚗 17.6   ⚕ 17.6   **FUD** 090   J A2 ▭
AMA: 2011,May,3-5; 1997,Nov,1

15951   **with ostectomy**
🚗 25.3   ⚕ 25.3   **FUD** 090   J A2 80 ▭
AMA: 2011,May,3-5; 1997,Nov,1

15952   **Excision, trochanteric pressure ulcer, with skin flap closure;**
🚗 26.3   ⚕ 26.3   **FUD** 090   T A2 80 ▭
AMA: 2011,May,3-5; 1997,Nov,1

15953   **with ostectomy**
🚗 28.9   ⚕ 28.9   **FUD** 090   T A2 ▭
AMA: 2011,May,3-5; 1997,Nov,1

15956   **Excision, trochanteric pressure ulcer, in preparation for muscle or myocutaneous flap or skin graft closure;**
Code also any defect repair with:
Muscle or myocutaneous flap (15734, 15738)
Split skin graft (15100-15101)
🚗 33.3   ⚕ 33.3   **FUD** 090   T A2 ▭
AMA: 2011,May,3-5; 1998,Nov,1

15958   **with ostectomy**
Code also any defect repair with:
Muscle or myocutaneous flap (15734-15738)
Split skin graft (15100-15101)
🚗 34.0   ⚕ 34.0   **FUD** 090   T A2 ▭
AMA: 2011,May,3-5; 1998,Nov,1

15999   **Unlisted procedure, excision pressure ulcer**
🚗 0.00   ⚕ 0.00   **FUD** YYY   T 80 ▭
AMA: 2011,May,3-5; 1997,Nov,1

16000-16036 Burn Care

INCLUDES   Local care burn surface only
EXCLUDES   Application skin grafts and flaps including all services described in:
(15100-15777)
E/M services
Laser fenestration for scars (0479T-0480T)

16000   **Initial treatment, first degree burn, when no more than local treatment is required**
🚗 1.33   ⚕ 2.09   **FUD** 000   Q1 N1 ▭
AMA: 2018,Jan,8; 2017,Jan,8; 2016,Jan,13

16020   **Dressings and/or debridement of partial-thickness burns, initial or subsequent; small (less than 5% total body surface area)**
INCLUDES   Wound coverage other than skin graft
🚗 1.56   ⚕ 2.35   **FUD** 000   Q1 N1 ▭
AMA: 2018,Jan,8; 2017,Jan,8; 2016,Jan,13

16025   **medium (eg, whole face or whole extremity, or 5% to 10% total body surface area)**
INCLUDES   Wound coverage other than skin graft
🚗 3.16   ⚕ 4.26   **FUD** 000   T A2 ▭
AMA: 2018,Jan,8; 2017,Jan,8; 2016,Jan,13

16030   **large (eg, more than 1 extremity, or greater than 10% total body surface area)**
INCLUDES   Wound coverage other than skin graft
🚗 3.82   ⚕ 5.40   **FUD** 000   T A2 ▭
AMA: 2018,Jan,8; 2017,Jan,8; 2016,Jan,13

16035   **Escharotomy; initial incision**
EXCLUDES   Debridement scraping of burn (16020-16030)
🚗 5.71   ⚕ 5.71   **FUD** 000   T G2 ▭
AMA: 2018,Jan,8; 2017,Jan,8; 2016,Jan,13

+ **16036**   **each additional incision (List separately in addition to code for primary procedure)**
EXCLUDES   Debridement or scraping burn (16020-16030)
Code first (16035)
🚗 2.37   ⚕ 2.37   **FUD** ZZZ   C ▭
AMA: 2018,Jan,8; 2017,Jan,8; 2016,Jan,13

17000-17004 Destruction Any Method: Premalignant Lesion

CMS: 100-03,140.5 Laser Procedures

EXCLUDES *Cryotherapy acne (17340)*
Destruction, skin:
  Benign lesions other than cutaneous vascular proliferative lesions
    (17110-17111)
  Cutaneous vascular proliferative lesions (17106-17108)
  Malignant lesions (17260-17286)
Destruction lesion:
  Anus (46900-46917, 46924)
  Conjunctiva (68135)
  Eyelid (67850)
  Penis (54050-54057, 54065)
  Vagina (57061, 57065)
  Vestibule of mouth (40820)
  Vulva (56501, 56515)
Destruction or excision skin tags (11200-11201)
Escharotomy (16035-16036)
Excision benign lesion (11400-11446)
Laser fenestration for scars (0479T-0480T)
Localized chemotherapy treatment see appropriate office visit service code
Paring or excision benign hyperkeratotic lesion (11055-11057)
Shaving skin lesions (11300-11313)
Treatment inflammatory skin disease via laser (96920-96922)

17000 **Destruction (eg, laser surgery, electrosurgery, cryosurgery, chemosurgery, surgical curettement), premalignant lesions (eg, actinic keratoses); first lesion**
    🔲 1.53   ⚖ 1.85   **FUD** 010   [Q1][N1][▭]
    AMA: 2018,Jan,8; 2017,Dec,14; 2017,Jan,8; 2016,Apr,3; 2016,Jan,13

+ 17003 **second through 14 lesions, each (List separately in addition to code for first lesion)**
    Code first (17000)
    🔲 0.06   ⚖ 0.17   **FUD** ZZZ   [N][N1][▭]
    AMA: 2018,Jan,8; 2017,Dec,14; 2017,Jan,8; 2016,Apr,3; 2016,Jan,13

17004 **Destruction (eg, laser surgery, electrosurgery, cryosurgery, chemosurgery, surgical curettement), premalignant lesions (eg, actinic keratoses), 15 or more lesions**
    EXCLUDES *Reporting code for destruction less than 15 lesions (17000-17003)*
    🔲 2.85   ⚖ 4.31   **FUD** 010   [T][P3][▭]
    AMA: 2018,Jan,8; 2017,Dec,14; 2017,Jan,8; 2016,Apr,3; 2016,Jan,13

17106-17250 Destruction Any Method: Vascular Proliferative Lesion

CMS: 100-02,16,10 Exclusions from Coverage; 100-02,16,120 Cosmetic Procedures

EXCLUDES *Cryotherapy acne (17340)*
Destruction, skin:
  Malignant lesions (17260-17286)
  Premalignant lesions (17000-17004)
Destruction lesion:
  Anus (46900-46917, 46924)
  Conjunctiva (68135)
  Eyelid (67850)
  Penis (54050-54057, 54065)
  Vagina (57061, 57065)
  Vestibule of mouth (40820)
  Vulva (56501, 56515)
Destruction or excision skin tags (11200-11201)
Escharotomy (16035-16036)
Excision benign lesion (11400-11446)
Laser fenestration for scars (0479T-0480T)
Localized chemotherapy treatment see appropriate office visit service code
Paring or excision benign hyperkeratotic lesion (11055-11057)
Shaving skin lesions (11300-11313)
Treatment inflammatory skin disease via laser (96920-96922)

17106 **Destruction of cutaneous vascular proliferative lesions (eg, laser technique); less than 10 sq cm**
    🔲 7.84   ⚖ 9.72   **FUD** 090   [T][P2][▭]
    AMA: 2019,Sep,10; 2018,Jan,8; 2017,Dec,14; 2017,Jan,8; 2016,Apr,3; 2016,Jan,13

17107 **10.0 to 50.0 sq cm**
    🔲 10.1   ⚖ 12.7   **FUD** 090   [T][P2][▭]
    AMA: 2018,Jan,8; 2017,Dec,14; 2017,Jan,8; 2016,Apr,3; 2016,Jan,13

17108 **over 50.0 sq cm**
    🔲 15.0   ⚖ 18.1   **FUD** 090   [T][P3][80][▭]
    AMA: 2018,Jan,8; 2017,Dec,14; 2017,Jan,8; 2016,Apr,3; 2016,Jan,13

17110 **Destruction (eg, laser surgery, electrosurgery, cryosurgery, chemosurgery, surgical curettement), of benign lesions other than skin tags or cutaneous vascular proliferative lesions; up to 14 lesions**
    🔲 1.91   ⚖ 3.17   **FUD** 010   [Q1][N1][▭]
    AMA: 2020,Apr,10; 2018,Jan,8; 2017,Dec,14; 2017,Jan,8; 2016,Apr,3; 2016,Jan,13

17111 **15 or more lesions**
    EXCLUDES *Destruction neurofibromas, 50-100 lesions (0419T-0420T)*
    🔲 2.34   ⚖ 3.72   **FUD** 010   [Q1][N1][▭]
    AMA: 2018,Jan,8; 2017,Dec,14; 2017,Jan,8; 2016,Apr,3; 2016,Jan,13

17250 **Chemical cauterization of granulation tissue (ie, proud flesh)**
    EXCLUDES *Chemical cauterization when applied for wound hemostasis*
      Excision/removal codes for same lesion
      Wound care management (97597-97598, 97602)
    🔲 1.05   ⚖ 2.31   **FUD** 000   [Q1][N1][▭]
    AMA: 2018,Jan,8; 2017,Dec,14; 2017,Jan,8; 2016,Jan,13

17260-17286 Destruction, Any Method: Malignant Lesion

CMS: 100-03,140.5 Laser Procedures

EXCLUDES *Cryotherapy acne (17340)*
Destruction, skin:
  Benign lesions other than cutaneous vascular proliferative lesions
    (17110-17111)
  Cutaneous vascular proliferative lesions (17106-17108)
  Premalignant lesions (17000-17004)
Destruction lesion:
  Anus (46900-46917, 46924)
  Conjunctiva (68135)
  Eyelid (67850)
  Penis (54050-54057, 54065)
  Vestibule of mouth (40820)
  Vulva (56501-56515)
Destruction or excision skin tags (11200-11201)
Escharotomy (16035-16036)
Excision benign lesion (11400-11446)
Laser fenestration for scars (0479T-0480T)
Localized chemotherapy treatment see appropriate office visit service code
Paring or excision benign hyperkeratotic lesion (11055-11057)
Shaving skin lesion (11300-11313)
Treatment inflammatory skin disease via laser (96920-96922)

17260 **Destruction, malignant lesion (eg, laser surgery, electrosurgery, cryosurgery, chemosurgery, surgical curettement), trunk, arms or legs; lesion diameter 0.5 cm or less**
    🔲 2.03   ⚖ 2.71   **FUD** 010   [Q1][N1][▭]
    AMA: 2018,Jan,8; 2017,Dec,14; 2017,Jan,8; 2016,Jan,13

17261 **lesion diameter 0.6 to 1.0 cm**
    🔲 2.58   ⚖ 4.11   **FUD** 010   [Q1][N1][▭]
    AMA: 2018,Jan,8; 2017,Dec,14; 2017,Jan,8; 2016,Jan,13

17262 **lesion diameter 1.1 to 2.0 cm**
    🔲 3.30   ⚖ 5.01   **FUD** 010   [Q1][N1][▭]
    AMA: 2018,Jan,8; 2017,Dec,14; 2017,Jan,8; 2016,Jan,13

17263 **lesion diameter 2.1 to 3.0 cm**
    🔲 3.55   ⚖ 5.45   **FUD** 010   [Q1][N1][▭]
    AMA: 2018,Jan,8; 2017,Dec,14; 2017,Jan,8; 2016,Jan,13

17264 **lesion diameter 3.1 to 4.0 cm**
    🔲 3.79   ⚖ 5.84   **FUD** 010   [T][P3][▭]
    AMA: 2018,Jan,8; 2017,Dec,14; 2017,Jan,8; 2016,Jan,13

Integumentary System

17266 — 17360

17266   lesion diameter over 4.0 cm
🔲 4.47   ⚕ 6.66   **FUD** 010   T P3 🖿
AMA: 2018,Jan,8; 2017,Dec,14; 2017,Jan,8; 2016,Jan,13

17270   Destruction, malignant lesion (eg, laser surgery, electrosurgery, cryosurgery, chemosurgery, surgical curettement), scalp, neck, hands, feet, genitalia; lesion diameter 0.5 cm or less
🔲 2.74   ⚕ 4.22   **FUD** 010   T P2 🖿
AMA: 2018,Jan,8; 2017,Dec,14; 2017,Jan,8; 2016,Jan,13

17271   lesion diameter 0.6 to 1.0 cm
🔲 3.14   ⚕ 4.67   **FUD** 010   T P2 🖿
AMA: 2018,Jan,8; 2017,Dec,14; 2017,Jan,8; 2016,Jan,13

17272   lesion diameter 1.1 to 2.0 cm
🔲 3.63   ⚕ 5.33   **FUD** 010   Q1 N1 🖿
AMA: 2018,Jan,8; 2017,Dec,14; 2017,Jan,8; 2016,Jan,13

17273   lesion diameter 2.1 to 3.0 cm
🔲 4.11   ⚕ 5.94   **FUD** 010   T P3 🖿
AMA: 2018,Jan,8; 2017,Dec,14; 2017,Jan,8; 2016,Jan,13

17274   lesion diameter 3.1 to 4.0 cm
🔲 5.04   ⚕ 7.01   **FUD** 010   T P3 🖿
AMA: 2018,Jan,8; 2017,Dec,14; 2017,Jan,8; 2016,Jan,13

17276   lesion diameter over 4.0 cm
🔲 5.86   ⚕ 8.07   **FUD** 010   T P3 🖿
AMA: 2018,Jan,8; 2017,Dec,14; 2017,Jan,8; 2016,Jan,13

17280   Destruction, malignant lesion (eg, laser surgery, electrosurgery, cryosurgery, chemosurgery, surgical curettement), face, ears, eyelids, nose, lips, mucous membrane; lesion diameter 0.5 cm or less
🔲 2.48   ⚕ 3.94   **FUD** 010   Q1 N1 🖿
AMA: 2018,Jan,8; 2017,Dec,14; 2017,Jan,8; 2016,Jan,13

17281   lesion diameter 0.6 to 1.0 cm
🔲 3.54   ⚕ 5.09   **FUD** 010   T P3 🖿
AMA: 2018,Jan,8; 2017,Dec,14; 2017,Jan,8; 2016,Jan,13

17282   lesion diameter 1.1 to 2.0 cm
🔲 3.97   ⚕ 5.82   **FUD** 010   T P3 🖿
AMA: 2018,Jan,8; 2017,Dec,14; 2017,Jan,8; 2016,Jan,13

17283   lesion diameter 2.1 to 3.0 cm
🔲 4.97   ⚕ 6.94   **FUD** 010   T P3 🖿
AMA: 2018,Jan,8; 2017,Dec,14; 2017,Jan,8; 2016,Jan,13

17284   lesion diameter 3.1 to 4.0 cm
🔲 5.80   ⚕ 7.90   **FUD** 010   T P3 🖿
AMA: 2018,Jan,8; 2017,Dec,14; 2017,Jan,8; 2016,Jan,13

17286   lesion diameter over 4.0 cm
🔲 7.86   ⚕ 10.1   **FUD** 010   T P3 🖿
AMA: 2018,Jan,8; 2017,Dec,14; 2017,Jan,8; 2016,Jan,13

17311-17315 Mohs Surgery

INCLUDES   Surgical/pathology services performed by same physician or other qualified health care provider:
Evaluation skin margins by surgeon
Pathology exam on Mohs surgery specimen (by Mohs surgeon) (88302-88309)
Routine frozen section stain (88314)
Tumor removal, mapping, preparation, and examination lesion

EXCLUDES   *Frozen section if no prior diagnosis determination has been performed (88331)*
Code also:
Any special histochemical stain on frozen section, nonroutine and append modifier 59 (88311-88314, 88342)
Biopsy when no prior diagnosis determination has been performed, biopsy indeterminate, or performed more than 90 days preoperatively and append modifier 59 (11102, 11104, 11106)
Complex repair (13100-13160)
Flaps or grafts (14000-14350, 15050-15770)
Intermediate repair (12031-12057)
Simple repair (12001-12021)

17311   Mohs micrographic technique, including removal of all gross tumor, surgical excision of tissue specimens, mapping, color coding of specimens, microscopic examination of specimens by the surgeon, and histopathologic preparation including routine stain(s) (eg, hematoxylin and eosin, toluidine blue), head, neck, hands, feet, genitalia, or any location with surgery directly involving muscle, cartilage, bone, tendon, major nerves, or vessels; first stage, up to 5 tissue blocks
🔲 10.4   ⚕ 18.8   **FUD** 000   T P2 🖿
AMA: 2018,Jan,8; 2017,Jan,8; 2016,Jan,13

+ 17312   each additional stage after the first stage, up to 5 tissue blocks (List separately in addition to code for primary procedure)
Code first (17311)
🔲 5.55   ⚕ 11.3   **FUD** ZZZ   N N1 🖿
AMA: 2018,Jan,8; 2017,Jan,8; 2016,Jan,13

17313   Mohs micrographic technique, including removal of all gross tumor, surgical excision of tissue specimens, mapping, color coding of specimens, microscopic examination of specimens by the surgeon, and histopathologic preparation including routine stain(s) (eg, hematoxylin and eosin, toluidine blue), of the trunk, arms, or legs; first stage, up to 5 tissue blocks
🔲 9.34   ⚕ 17.6   **FUD** 000   T P2 🖿
AMA: 2018,Jan,8; 2017,Jan,8; 2016,Jan,13

+ 17314   each additional stage after the first stage, up to 5 tissue blocks (List separately in addition to code for primary procedure)
Code first (17313)
🔲 5.14   ⚕ 10.8   **FUD** ZZZ   N N1 🖿
AMA: 2018,Jan,8; 2017,Jan,8; 2016,Jan,13

+ 17315   Mohs micrographic technique, including removal of all gross tumor, surgical excision of tissue specimens, mapping, color coding of specimens, microscopic examination of specimens by the surgeon, and histopathologic preparation including routine stain(s) (eg, hematoxylin and eosin, toluidine blue), each additional block after the first 5 tissue blocks, any stage (List separately in addition to code for primary procedure)
Code first (17311-17314)
🔲 1.47   ⚕ 2.22   **FUD** ZZZ   N N1 🖿
AMA: 2018,Jan,8; 2017,Jan,8; 2016,Jan,13

17340-17999 Treatment for Active Acne and Permanent Hair Removal

CMS: 100-02,16,10 Exclusions from Coverage; 100-02,16,120 Cosmetic Procedures

17340   Cryotherapy (CO2 slush, liquid N2) for acne
🔲 1.40   ⚕ 1.49   **FUD** 010   Q1 N1 🖿
AMA: 2018,Jan,8; 2017,Jan,8; 2016,Jan,13

17360   Chemical exfoliation for acne (eg, acne paste, acid)
🔲 2.77   ⚕ 3.61   **FUD** 010   Q1 N1 🖿
AMA: 2018,Jan,8; 2017,Jan,8; 2016,Jan,13

17380-19101

17380 Electrolysis epilation, each 30 minutes

> EXCLUDES *Actinotherapy (96900)*
> 🔲 0.00 ⚕ 0.00 **FUD** 000 T R2 80 🔲
> **AMA:** 2018,Jan,8; 2017,Jan,8; 2016,Jan,13

17999 Unlisted procedure, skin, mucous membrane and subcutaneous tissue

> 🔲 0.00 ⚕ 0.00 **FUD** YYY Q1 80 🔲
> **AMA:** 2019,Sep,10; 2019,Mar,10; 2019,Jan,14; 2018,Jan,8; 2017,Dec,13; 2017,Jan,8; 2016,May,13; 2016,Jan,13

19000-19030 Treatment of Breast Abscess and Cyst with Injection, Aspiration, Incision

19000 Puncture aspiration of cyst of breast;

> 🔁 (76942, 77021)
> 🔲 1.26 ⚕ 3.12 **FUD** 000 T P3 🔲
> **AMA:** 2018,Jan,8; 2017,Jan,8; 2016,Jan,13

+ 19001 each additional cyst (List separately in addition to code for primary procedure)

> Code first (19000)
> 🔁 (76942, 77021)
> 🔲 0.62 ⚕ 0.77 **FUD** ZZZ N N1 🔲
> **AMA:** 2018,Jan,8; 2017,Jan,8; 2016,Jan,13

19020 Mastotomy with exploration or drainage of abscess, deep

> 🔲 8.93 ⚕ 13.5 **FUD** 090 J A2 50 🔲
> **AMA:** 2018,Jan,8; 2017,Jan,8; 2016,Jan,13

19030 Injection procedure only for mammary ductogram or galactogram

> 🔁 (77053-77054)
> 🔲 2.23 ⚕ 4.74 **FUD** 000 N N1 50 🔲
> **AMA:** 2018,Jan,8; 2017,Jan,8; 2016,Jan,13

19081-19086 Breast Biopsy with Imaging Guidance

CMS: 100-03,220.13 Percutaneous Image-guided Breast Biopsy; 100-04,12,40.7 Bilateral Procedures; 100-04,13,80.1 Physician Presence; 100-04,13,80.2 S&I Multiple Procedure Reduction

> INCLUDES Breast biopsy with placement localization devices
> Fluoroscopic guidance for needle placement (77002)
> Magnetic resonance guidance for needle placement (77021)
> Radiological examination, surgical specimen (76098)
> Ultrasonic guidance for needle placement (76942)
>
> EXCLUDES *Biopsy breast without imaging guidance (19100-19101)*
> *Lesion removal without concentration on surgical margins (19110-19126)*
> *Open biopsy after placement localization device (19101)*
> *Partial mastectomy (19301-19302)*
> *Placement localization devices only (19281-19288)*
> *Total mastectomy (19303-19307)*
> Code also additional biopsies performed with different imaging modalities

19081 Biopsy, breast, with placement of breast localization device(s) (eg, clip, metallic pellet), when performed, and imaging of the biopsy specimen, when performed, percutaneous; first lesion, including stereotactic guidance

> 🔲 4.82 ⚕ 17.3 **FUD** 000 J G2 80 50 🔲
> **AMA:** 2019,Apr,4; 2018,Jan,8; 2017,Jan,8; 2016,Jun,3; 2016,Jan,13

+ 19082 each additional lesion, including stereotactic guidance (List separately in addition to code for primary procedure)

> Code first (19081)
> 🔲 2.42 ⚕ 13.9 **FUD** ZZZ N N1 80 🔲
> **AMA:** 2019,Apr,4; 2018,Jan,8; 2017,Jan,8; 2016,Jun,3; 2016,Jan,13

19083 Biopsy, breast, with placement of breast localization device(s) (eg, clip, metallic pellet), when performed, and imaging of the biopsy specimen, when performed, percutaneous; first lesion, including ultrasound guidance

> 🔲 4.56 ⚕ 17.1 **FUD** 000 J G2 80 50 🔲
> **AMA:** 2019,Apr,4; 2018,Jan,8; 2017,Jan,8; 2016,Jun,3; 2016,Jan,13

+ 19084 each additional lesion, including ultrasound guidance (List separately in addition to code for primary procedure)

> Code first (19083)
> 🔲 2.25 ⚕ 13.6 **FUD** ZZZ N N1 80 🔲
> **AMA:** 2019,Apr,4; 2018,Jan,8; 2017,Jan,8; 2016,Jun,3; 2016,Jan,13

19085 Biopsy, breast, with placement of breast localization device(s) (eg, clip, metallic pellet), when performed, and imaging of the biopsy specimen, when performed, percutaneous; first lesion, including magnetic resonance guidance

> 🔲 5.28 ⚕ 26.1 **FUD** 000 J G2 80 50 🔲
> **AMA:** 2019,Apr,4; 2018,Jan,8; 2017,Jan,8; 2016,Jun,3; 2016,Jan,13

+ 19086 each additional lesion, including magnetic resonance guidance (List separately in addition to code for primary procedure)

> Code first (19085)
> 🔲 2.65 ⚕ 21.9 **FUD** ZZZ N N1 80 🔲
> **AMA:** 2019,Apr,4; 2018,Jan,8; 2017,Jan,8; 2016,Jun,3; 2016,Jan,13

19100-19101 Breast Biopsy Without Imaging Guidance

> EXCLUDES *Biopsy breast with imaging guidance (19081-19086)*
> *Lesion removal without concentration on surgical margins (19110-19126)*
> *Partial mastectomy (19301-19302)*
> *Total mastectomy (19303-19307)*

19100 Biopsy of breast; percutaneous, needle core, not using imaging guidance (separate procedure)

> EXCLUDES *Fine needle aspiration:*
> *With imaging guidance ([10005, 10006, 10007, 10008, 10009, 10010, 10011, 10012])*
> *Without imaging guidance (10021, [10004])*
> 🔲 2.03 ⚕ 4.32 **FUD** 000 J A2 50 🔲
> **AMA:** 2018,Jan,8; 2017,Jan,8; 2016,Jan,13

Clavicle — Tail of Spence area — Deltoid — Brachialis — Parasternal nodes — Lateral nodes — Subscapular nodes — Pectoral nodes — Axillary lymph nodes — Central nodes — Lactiferous ducts and gland lobules — Latissimus dorsi muscle — Areola — Nipple

19101 open, incisional

> Code also placement localization device with imaging guidance (19281-19288)
> 🔲 6.45 ⚕ 9.62 **FUD** 010 . J A2 50 🔲
> **AMA:** 2018,Jan,8; 2017,Jan,8; 2016,Jan,13

19105 Treatment of Fibroadenoma: Cryoablation

CMS: 100-04,13,80.1 Physician Presence; 100-04,13,80.2 S&I Multiple Procedure Reduction

INCLUDES Adjacent lesions treated with one cryoprobe
Ultrasound guidance (76940, 76942)

EXCLUDES *Cryoablation malignant breast tumors (0581T)*

19105 **Ablation, cryosurgical, of fibroadenoma, including ultrasound guidance, each fibroadenoma**

🗖 6.14 ⚕ 77.6 **FUD** 000 J J8 50 ▭

AMA: 2007,Mar,7-8

19110-19126 Excisional Procedures: Breast

INCLUDES Open removal breast mass without concentration on surgical margins
Code also placement localization device with imaging guidance (19281-19288)

19110 **Nipple exploration, with or without excision of a solitary lactiferous duct or a papilloma lactiferous duct**

🗖 9.94 ⚕ 13.9 **FUD** 090 J A2 50 ▭

AMA: 2018,Jan,8; 2017,Jan,8; 2016,Jan,13

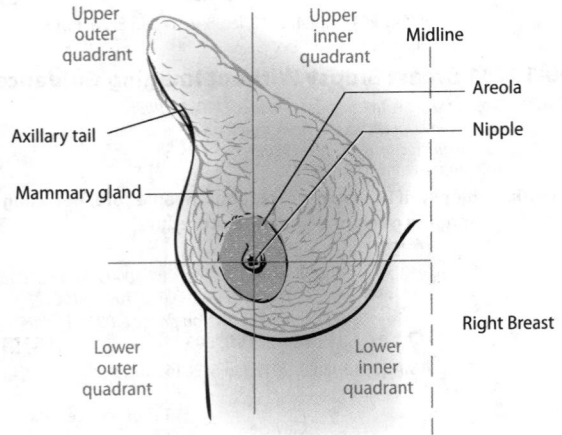

Upper outer quadrant — Upper inner quadrant — Midline — Areola — Nipple — Axillary tail — Mammary gland — Lower outer quadrant — Lower inner quadrant — Right Breast

19112 **Excision of lactiferous duct fistula**

🗖 9.12 ⚕ 13.2 **FUD** 090 J A2 80 50 ▭

AMA: 2018,Jan,8; 2017,Jan,8; 2016,Jan,13

19120 **Excision of cyst, fibroadenoma, or other benign or malignant tumor, aberrant breast tissue, duct lesion, nipple or areolar lesion (except 19300), open, male or female, 1 or more lesions**

🗖 12.0 ⚕ 14.5 **FUD** 090 J A2 50 ▭

AMA: 2018,Jan,8; 2017,Jan,8; 2016,Jan,13

19125 **Excision of breast lesion identified by preoperative placement of radiological marker, open; single lesion**

INCLUDES Intraoperative clip placement

🗖 13.2 ⚕ 15.8 **FUD** 090 J A2 50 ▭

AMA: 2018,Jan,8; 2017,Jan,8; 2016,Jan,13

+ **19126** **each additional lesion separately identified by a preoperative radiological marker (List separately in addition to code for primary procedure)**

INCLUDES Intraoperative clip placement

Code first (19125)

🗖 4.68 ⚕ 4.68 **FUD** ZZZ N N1 ▭

AMA: 2018,Jan,8; 2017,Jan,8; 2016,Jan,13

19281-19288 Placement of Localization Markers

INCLUDES Placement localization devices only

EXCLUDES *Biopsy breast without imaging guidance (19100-19101)*
When performed on same lesion:
Fluoroscopic guidance for needle placement (77002)
Localization device placement with biopsy breast (19081-19086)
Magnetic resonance guidance for needle placement (77021)
Ultrasonic guidance for needle placement (76942)

Code also:
Open excision of breast lesion when performed after localization device placement (19110-19126)
Open incisional breast biopsy when performed after localization device placement (19101)
Radiography surgical specimen (76098)

19281 **Placement of breast localization device(s) (eg, clip, metallic pellet, wire/needle, radioactive seeds), percutaneous; first lesion, including mammographic guidance**

🗖 2.91 ⚕ 6.90 **FUD** 000 Q1 N1 80 50 ▭

AMA: 2018,Jan,8; 2017,Jan,8; 2016,Jun,3; 2016,Jan,13

+ **19282** **each additional lesion, including mammographic guidance (List separately in addition to code for primary procedure)**

Code first (19281)

🗖 1.46 ⚕ 4.92 **FUD** ZZZ N N1 80 ▭

AMA: 2018,Jan,8; 2017,Jan,8; 2016,Jun,3; 2016,Jan,13

19283 **Placement of breast localization device(s) (eg, clip, metallic pellet, wire/needle, radioactive seeds), percutaneous; first lesion, including stereotactic guidance**

🗖 2.93 ⚕ 7.74 **FUD** 000 Q1 N1 80 50 ▭

AMA: 2018,Jan,8; 2017,Jan,8; 2016,Jun,3; 2016,May,13; 2016,Jan,13

+ **19284** **each additional lesion, including stereotactic guidance (List separately in addition to code for primary procedure)**

Code first (19283)

🗖 1.49 ⚕ 5.90 **FUD** ZZZ N N1 80 ▭

AMA: 2018,Jan,8; 2017,Jan,8; 2016,Jun,3; 2016,May,13; 2016,Jan,13

19285 **Placement of breast localization device(s) (eg, clip, metallic pellet, wire/needle, radioactive seeds), percutaneous; first lesion, including ultrasound guidance**

🗖 2.49 ⚕ 12.9 **FUD** 000 Q1 N1 80 50 ▭

AMA: 2018,Jan,8; 2017,Jan,8; 2016,Jun,3; 2016,May,13; 2016,Jan,13

+ **19286** **each additional lesion, including ultrasound guidance (List separately in addition to code for primary procedure)**

Code first (19285)

🗖 1.25 ⚕ 11.9 **FUD** ZZZ N N1 80 ▭

AMA: 2018,Jan,8; 2017,Jan,8; 2016,Jun,3; 2016,May,13; 2016,Jan,13

19287 **Placement of breast localization device(s) (eg clip, metallic pellet, wire/needle, radioactive seeds), percutaneous; first lesion, including magnetic resonance guidance**

🗖 3.72 ⚕ 22.1 **FUD** 000 Q1 N1 80 50 ▭

AMA: 2018,Jan,8; 2017,Jan,8; 2016,Jun,3; 2016,May,13; 2016,Jan,13

+ **19288** **each additional lesion, including magnetic resonance guidance (List separately in addition to code for primary procedure)**

Code first (19287)

🗖 1.87 ⚕ 19.7 **FUD** ZZZ N N1 80 ▭

AMA: 2018,Jan,8; 2017,Jan,8; 2016,Jun,3; 2016,May,13; 2016,Jan,13

26/TC PC/TC Only A2-Z3 ASC Payment 50 Bilateral ♂ Male Only ♀ Female Only 🗖 Facility RVU ⚕ Non-Facility RVU ▭ CCI ☒ CLIA
FUD Follow-up Days **CMS:** IOM **AMA:** CPT Asst A-Y OPPSI 80/80 Surg Assist Allowed / w/Doc ▭ Lab Crosswalk ▭ Radiology Crosswalk

34

19294-19298 Radioelement Application

+ 19294 Preparation of tumor cavity, with placement of a radiation therapy applicator for intraoperative radiation therapy (IORT) concurrent with partial mastectomy (List separately in addition to code for primary procedure)
Code first (19301-19302)
🔧 4.71 ⚕ 4.71 **FUD** ZZZ Ⓝ N1 80 ▭
AMA: 2020,May,9

19296 Placement of radiotherapy afterloading expandable catheter (single or multichannel) into the breast for interstitial radioelement application following partial mastectomy, includes imaging guidance; on date separate from partial mastectomy
🔧 6.11 ⚕ 114. **FUD** 000 Ⓙ J8 80 50 ▭
AMA: 2020,May,9; 2018,Jan,8; 2017,Jan,8; 2016,Jan,13

+ 19297 concurrent with partial mastectomy (List separately in addition to code for primary procedure)
Code first (19301-19302)
🔧 2.75 ⚕ 2.75 **FUD** ZZZ Ⓝ N1 80 ▭
AMA: 2020,May,9; 2019,Apr,10; 2018,Jan,8; 2017,Jan,8; 2016,Jan,13

19298 Placement of radiotherapy after loading brachytherapy catheters (multiple tube and button type) into the breast for interstitial radioelement application following (at the time of or subsequent to) partial mastectomy, includes imaging guidance
🔧 9.22 ⚕ 28.4 **FUD** 000 Ⓙ G2 80 50 ▭
AMA: 2020,May,9; 2018,Jan,8; 2017,Jan,8; 2016,Jan,13

19300-19307 Mastectomies: Partial, Simple, Radical

CMS: 100-04,12,40.7 Bilateral Procedures
INCLUDES Intraoperative clip placement
EXCLUDES Insertion prosthesis (19340, 19342)

19300 Mastectomy for gynecomastia ♂
EXCLUDES Removal breast tissue for:
  Other than gynecomastia (19318)
  Treatment or prevention breast cancer (19301-19307)
🔧 12.1 ⚕ 15.8 **FUD** 090 Ⓙ A2 50 ▭
AMA: 2020,May,9; 2018,Jan,8; 2017,Jan,8; 2016,Jan,13

19301 Mastectomy, partial (eg, lumpectomy, tylectomy, quadrantectomy, segmentectomy);
EXCLUDES Insertion radiotherapy afterloading balloon during separate encounter (19296)
Code also:
  3D volumetric specimen imaging, when performed (0694T)
  Insertion radiotherapy afterloading balloon catheter, when performed at same time (19297)
  Insertion radiotherapy afterloading brachytherapy catheter, when performed at same time (19298)
  Intraoperative radiofrequency spectroscopy margin assessment and report (0546T)
  Tumor cavity preparation with intraoperative radiation therapy applicator, when performed (19294)
🔧 19.0 ⚕ 19.0 **FUD** 090 Ⓙ A2 80 50 ▭
AMA: 2020,May,9; 2018,Jan,8; 2017,Oct,9; 2017,Jan,8; 2016,Jan,13

19302 with axillary lymphadenectomy
EXCLUDES Insertion radiotherapy afterloading balloon during separate encounter (19296)
Code also:
  3D volumetric specimen imaging, when performed (0694T)
  Insertion radiotherapy afterloading balloon catheter, when performed at same time (19297)
  Insertion radiotherapy afterloading brachytherapy catheter, when performed at same time (19298)
  Intraoperative radiofrequency spectroscopy margin assessment and report (0546T)
  Tumor cavity preparation with intraoperative radiation therapy applicator, when performed (19294)
🔧 25.9 ⚕ 25.9 **FUD** 090 Ⓙ A2 80 50 ▭
AMA: 2020,Nov,12; 2020,May,9; 2019,Feb,8; 2018,Jan,8; 2017,Jan,8; 2016,Jan,13

19303 Mastectomy, simple, complete
EXCLUDES Excision pectoral muscles and axillary or internal mammary lymph nodes
  Removal breast tissue for:
    Gynecomastia (19300)
    Other than gynecomastia (19318)
🔧 27.8 ⚕ 27.8 **FUD** 090 Ⓙ A2 80 50 ▭
AMA: 2020,May,9; 2019,Dec,4; 2018,Jan,8; 2017,Jan,8; 2016,Jan,13

19305 Mastectomy, radical, including pectoral muscles, axillary lymph nodes
🔧 33.0 ⚕ 33.0 **FUD** 090 Ⓒ 80 50 ▭
AMA: 2020,May,9; 2018,Jan,8; 2017,Jan,8; 2016,Jan,13

19306 Mastectomy, radical, including pectoral muscles, axillary and internal mammary lymph nodes (Urban type operation)
🔧 34.6 ⚕ 34.6 **FUD** 090 Ⓒ 80 50 ▭
AMA: 2020,May,9; 2018,Jan,8; 2017,Jan,8; 2016,Jan,13

19307 Mastectomy, modified radical, including axillary lymph nodes, with or without pectoralis minor muscle, but excluding pectoralis major muscle
🔧 34.6 ⚕ 34.6 **FUD** 090 Ⓙ G2 80 50 ▭
AMA: 2020,May,9; 2019,Feb,8; 2018,Jan,8; 2017,Jan,8; 2016,Jan,13

19316-19499 Plastic, Reconstructive, and Aesthetic Breast Procedures

CMS: 100-03,140.2 Breast Reconstruction Following Mastectomy; 100-04,12,40.7 Bilateral Procedures
Code also biologic implant for tissue reinforcement (15777)

19316 Mastopexy
🔧 22.3 ⚕ 22.3 **FUD** 090 Ⓙ A2 80 50 ▭
AMA: 2018,Jan,8; 2017,Jan,8; 2016,Jan,13

19318 Breast reduction
INCLUDES Aries-Pitanguy mammaplasty
  Biesenberger mammaplasty
🔧 31.5 ⚕ 31.5 **FUD** 090 Ⓙ A2 80 50 ▭
AMA: 2020,May,9; 2018,Jan,8; 2017,Jan,8; 2016,Jan,13

19325 Breast augmentation with implant
EXCLUDES Flap or graft (15100-15650)
Code also fat grafting, when performed (15771-15772)
🔧 18.6 ⚕ 18.6 **FUD** 090 Ⓙ G2 80 50 ▭
AMA: 2018,Jan,8; 2017,Jan,8; 2016,Jan,13

19328 Removal of intact breast implant
EXCLUDES Removal tissue expander (11970-11971)
  Revision peri-implant capsule, breast (19370)
🔧 14.4 ⚕ 14.4 **FUD** 090 02 A2 50 ▭
AMA: 2018,Jan,8; 2017,Jan,8; 2016,Jan,13

19330 Removal of ruptured breast implant, including implant contents (eg, saline, silicone gel)
EXCLUDES Insertion new breast implant during same operative session (19342)
  Removal ruptured tissue expander (11970-11971)
🔧 18.1 ⚕ 18.1 **FUD** 090 02 A2 50 ▭
AMA: 2018,Jan,8; 2017,Jan,8; 2016,Jan,13

19340   **Insertion of breast implant on same day of mastectomy (ie, immediate)**

    EXCLUDES *Preparation moulage for custom breast implant (19396)*
          Supply prosthetic implant (99070, C1789, L8600)

    🚑 28.6   ✂ 28.6   **FUD** 090   J A2 50 📄

    AMA: 2020,May,9; 2018,Jan,8; 2017,Jan,8; 2016,Jan,13

19342   **Insertion or replacement of breast implant on separate day from mastectomy**

    EXCLUDES *Preparation moulage for custom breast implant (19396)*
          Removal intact breast implant (19328)
          Removal tissue expander with insertion breast implant (11970)
          Supply prosthetic implant (99070, C1789, L8600)

    🚑 26.7   ✂ 26.7   **FUD** 090   J A2 80 50 📄

    AMA: 2020,May,9; 2018,Jan,8; 2017,Jan,8; 2016,Jan,13

19350   **Nipple/areola reconstruction**

    INCLUDES Adjacent tissue transfer, trunk (14000-14001)
          Full-thickness graft, trunk (15200-15201)
          Split-thickness autograft, trunk, arms, legs (15100)
          Tattooing to correct skin color defects (11920-11922)

    🚑 19.4   ✂ 23.8   **FUD** 090   J A2 50 📄

    AMA: 2018,Jan,8; 2017,Jan,8; 2016,Aug,9; 2016,Jan,13

19355   **Correction of inverted nipples**

    🚑 17.7   ✂ 21.5   **FUD** 090   J A2 80 50 📄

    AMA: 2018,Jan,8; 2017,Jan,8; 2016,Jan,13

19357   **Tissue expander placement in breast reconstruction, including subsequent expansion(s)**

    🚑 43.1   ✂ 43.1   **FUD** 090   J J8 80 50 📄

    AMA: 2018,Jan,8; 2017,Jan,8; 2016,Jan,13

19361   **Breast reconstruction; with latissimus dorsi flap**

    INCLUDES Closure donor site
          Harvesting skin graft
          Inset shaping flap into breast

    EXCLUDES *Implant prosthesis with latissimus dorsi implant:*
          performed different day than mastectomy (19342)
          performed same day as mastectomy (19340)
          Insertion tissue expander with latissimus dorsi flap (19357)

    🚑 45.4   ✂ 45.4   **FUD** 090   C 80 50 📄

    AMA: 2019,Nov,14; 2018,Jan,8; 2017,Jan,8; 2016,Jan,13

19364   **with free flap (eg, fTRAM, DIEP, SIEA, GAP flap)**

    INCLUDES Closure donor site
          Harvesting skin graft
          Inset shaping flap into breast
          Microvascular repair
          Operating microscope (69990)

    🚑 79.7   ✂ 79.7   **FUD** 090   C 80 50 📄

    AMA: 2020,Dec,11; 2019,Nov,14; 2018,Jan,8; 2017,Jan,8; 2016,Feb,12; 2016,Jan,13

19367   **with single-pedicled transverse rectus abdominis myocutaneous (TRAM) flap**

    INCLUDES Closure donor site
          Harvesting skin graft
          Inset shaping flap into breast

    🚑 51.5   ✂ 51.5   **FUD** 090   C 80 50 📄

    AMA: 2019,Nov,14; 2018,Jan,8; 2017,Jan,8; 2016,Jan,13

19368   **with single-pedicled transverse rectus abdominis myocutaneous (TRAM) flap, requiring separate microvascular anastomosis (supercharging)**

    INCLUDES Closure donor site
          Harvesting skin graft
          Inset shaping flap into breast
          Operating microscope (69990)

    🚑 63.2   ✂ 63.2   **FUD** 090   C 80 50 📄

    AMA: 2019,Nov,14; 2018,Jan,8; 2017,Jan,8; 2016,Feb,12; 2016,Jan,13

19369   **with bipedicled transverse rectus abdominis myocutaneous (TRAM) flap**

    INCLUDES Closure donor site
          Harvesting skin graft
          Inset shaping flap into breast

    🚑 59.0   ✂ 59.0   **FUD** 090   C 80 50 📄

    AMA: 2019,Nov,14; 2018,Jan,8; 2017,Jan,8; 2016,Jan,13

19370   **Revision of peri-implant capsule, breast, including capsulotomy, capsulorrhaphy, and/or partial capsulectomy**

    EXCLUDES *Removal and replacement with new implant (19342)*
          Removal intact breast implant (19328)

    🚑 19.9   ✂ 19.9   **FUD** 090   J A2 50 📄

    AMA: 2018,Jan,8; 2017,Jan,8; 2016,Jan,13

19371   **Peri-implant capsulectomy, breast, complete, including removal of all intracapsular contents**

    EXCLUDES *Removal and replacement with new implant (19342)*
          Removal intact breast implant (19328)
          Removal ruptured breast implant (19330)
          Revision peri-implant capsule on same breast (19370)

    🚑 22.5   ✂ 22.5   **FUD** 090   J A2 50 📄

    AMA: 2018,Jan,8; 2017,Jan,8; 2016,Jan,13

19380   **Revision of reconstructed breast (eg, significant removal of tissue, re-advancement and/or re-inset of flaps in autologous reconstruction or significant capsular revision combined with soft tissue excision in implant-based reconstruction)**

    INCLUDES Removal portion or reshaping flap
          Revision flap position on chest wall
          Revision scar(s)
          When performed on same breast:
              Breast reduction (19318)
              Mastopexy (19316)
              Repair complex, trunk (13100-13102)
              Repair intermediate, trunk (12031-12037)
              Revision peri-implant capsule, breast (19370)
              Suction assisted lipectomy; trunk (15877)

    EXCLUDES *Autologuous fat graft (15771-15772)*
          Implant replacement (19342)

    🚑 22.4   ✂ 22.4   **FUD** 090   J A2 50 📄

    AMA: 2019,Nov,14; 2018,Jan,8; 2017,Dec,13; 2017,Jan,8; 2016,Jan,13

19396   **Preparation of moulage for custom breast implant**

    🚑 4.17   ✂ 8.23   **FUD** 000   J G2 80 50 📄

    AMA: 2018,Jan,8; 2017,Jan,8; 2016,Jan,13

19499   **Unlisted procedure, breast**

    🚑 0.00   ✂ 0.00   **FUD** YYY   J 80 50 📄

    AMA: 2019,Aug,10; 2019,Apr,10; 2018,Jan,8; 2017,Jan,8; 2016,Dec,16; 2016,Jan,13

26/TC PC/TC Only   A2-Z3 ASC Payment   50 Bilateral   ♂ Male Only   ♀ Female Only   🚑 Facility RVU   ✂ Non-Facility RVU   CCI   CLIA
FUD Follow-up Days   CMS: IOM   AMA: CPT Asst   A-Y OPPSI   80/80 Surg Assist Allowed / w/Doc   Lab Crosswalk   Radiology Crosswalk

36   CPT © 2021 American Medical Association. All Rights Reserved.   © 2021 Optum360, LLC

20100-20103 Exploratory Surgery of Traumatic Wound

INCLUDES Debridement
Expanded dissection wound for exploration
Extraction foreign material
Open examination
Tying or coagulation small vessels

EXCLUDES Cutaneous/subcutaneous incision and drainage procedures (10060-10061)
Laparotomy (49000-49010)
Repair major vessels:
  Abdomen (35221, 35251, 35281)
  Chest (35211, 35216, 35241, 35246, 35271, 35276)
  Extremity (35206-35207, 35226, 35236, 35256, 35266, 35286)
  Neck (35201, 35231, 35261)
Thoracotomy (32100-32160)

20100 **Exploration of penetrating wound (separate procedure); neck**
17.4 17.4 **FUD** 010   T G2 80 50
AMA: 2018,Jan,8; 2017,Jan,8; 2016,Jan,13

20101 **chest**
6.10 13.7 **FUD** 010   T G2
AMA: 2018,Jan,8; 2017,Jan,8; 2016,Jan,13

20102 **abdomen/flank/back**
7.43 14.7 **FUD** 010   T G2
AMA: 2020,Jan,6; 2018,Jan,8; 2017,Jan,8; 2016,Jan,13

20103 **extremity**
9.99 16.6 **FUD** 010   T G2 80
AMA: 2018,Jan,8; 2017,Jan,8; 2016,Jan,13

20150 Epiphyseal Bar Resection

20150 **Excision of epiphyseal bar, with or without autogenous soft tissue graft obtained through same fascial incision**
29.0 29.0 **FUD** 090   J G2 80 50
AMA: 1996,Nov,1

20200-20206 Muscle Biopsy

EXCLUDES Removal of muscle tumor (see appropriate anatomic section)

20200 **Biopsy, muscle; superficial**
2.73 5.95 **FUD** 000   J A2
AMA: 2020,NovBULL,1

20205 **deep**
4.48 8.35 **FUD** 000   J A2

20206 **Biopsy, muscle, percutaneous needle**
EXCLUDES Fine needle aspiration (10021, [10004, 10005, 10006, 10007, 10008, 10009, 10010, 10011, 10012])
(76942, 77002, 77012, 77021)
(88172-88173)
1.67 6.76 **FUD** 000   J A2
AMA: 2019,Apr,4

20220-20225 Percutaneous Bone Biopsy

EXCLUDES Bone marrow aspiration(s) or biopsy(ies) (38220-38222)

20220 **Biopsy, bone, trocar, or needle; superficial (eg, ilium, sternum, spinous process, ribs)**
(77002, 77012, 77021)
2.06 4.79 **FUD** 000   J A2
AMA: 2018,Jan,8; 2017,Jan,8; 2016,Jan,13

20225 **deep (eg, vertebral body, femur)**
EXCLUDES When performed at same level:
  Percutaneous sacral augmentation (sacroplasty) (0200T-0201T)
  Percutaneous vertebroplasty (22510-22515)
(77002, 77012, 77021)
3.07 14.7 **FUD** 000   J A2
AMA: 2018,Jan,8; 2017,Jan,8; 2016,Jan,13

20240-20251 Open Bone Biopsy

EXCLUDES Sequestrectomy or incision and drainage of bone abscess of:
  Calcaneus (28120)
  Carpal bone (25145)
  Clavicle (23170)
  Humeral head (23174)
  Humerus (24134)
  Olecranon process (24138)
  Radius (24136, 25145)
  Scapula (23172)
  Skull (61501)
  Talus (28120)
  Ulna (24138, 24145)

20240 **Biopsy, bone, open; superficial (eg, sternum, spinous process, rib, patella, olecranon process, calcaneus, tarsal, metatarsal, carpal, metacarpal, phalanx)**
4.21 4.21 **FUD** 000   J A2
AMA: 2018,Jan,8; 2017,Jan,8; 2016,Jan,13

20245 **deep (eg, humeral shaft, ischium, femoral shaft)**
10.1 10.1 **FUD** 000   J A2
AMA: 2018,Jan,8; 2017,Jan,8; 2016,Jan,13

20250 **Biopsy, vertebral body, open; thoracic**
11.3 11.3 **FUD** 010   J A2
AMA: 2018,Jan,8; 2017,Jan,8; 2016,Jan,13

20251 **lumbar or cervical**
12.4 12.4 **FUD** 010   J A2 80
AMA: 2018,Jan,8; 2017,Jan,8; 2016,Jan,13

20500-20501 Injection Fistula/Sinus Tract

EXCLUDES Arthrography injection of:
  Ankle (27648)
  Elbow (24220)
  Hip (27093, 27095)
  Sacroiliac joint (27096)
  Shoulder (23350)
  Temporomandibular joint (TMJ) (21116)
  Wrist (25246)
Autologous adipose-derived regenerative cells injection (0489T-0490T)

20500 **Injection of sinus tract; therapeutic (separate procedure)**
(76080)
2.49 3.25 **FUD** 010   T P3

20501 **diagnostic (sinogram)**
EXCLUDES Contrast injection or injections for radiological evaluation existing gastrostomy, duodenostomy, jejunostomy, gastro-jejunostomy, or cecostomy (or other colonic) tube from percutaneous approach (49465)
(76080)
1.09 3.62 **FUD** 000   N M1

20520-20525 Foreign Body Removal

20520 **Removal of foreign body in muscle or tendon sheath; simple**
4.22 6.03 **FUD** 010   J P3

20525 **deep or complicated**
7.11 13.6 **FUD** 010   J A2

20526-20561 [20560, 20561] Therapeutic Injections: Tendons, Trigger Points

20526 **Injection, therapeutic (eg, local anesthetic, corticosteroid), carpal tunnel**
1.66 2.20 **FUD** 000   T P3 50
AMA: 2018,Jan,8; 2017,Jan,8; 2016,Jan,13

20527 **Injection, enzyme (eg, collagenase), palmar fascial cord (ie, Dupuytren's contracture)**
EXCLUDES Post injection palmar fascial cord manipulation (26341)
1.90 2.43 **FUD** 000   T P3 50
AMA: 2018,Jan,8; 2017,Jan,8; 2016,Jan,13

● New Code   ▲ Revised Code   ○ Reinstated   ● New Web Release   ▲ Revised Web Release   + Add-on   Unlisted   Not Covered   # Resequenced
50 Optum Mod 50 Exempt   ⊘ AMA Mod 51 Exempt   51 Optum Mod 51 Exempt   63 Mod 63 Exempt   ✎ Non-FDA Drug   ★ Telemedicine   M Maternity   A Age Edit

Musculoskeletal System

20550 — 20650

20550   Injection(s); single tendon sheath, or ligament, aponeurosis (eg, plantar "fascia")
- EXCLUDES   Autologous WBC injection (0481T)
  Morton's neuroma (64455, 64632)
  Platelet rich plasma injection (0232T)
- (76942, 77002, 77021)
- 1.13   1.51   **FUD** 000   [T] [P3] [50]
- AMA: 2018,Jan,8; 2017,Jan,8; 2016,Jan,13

20551   single tendon origin/insertion
- EXCLUDES   Autologous WBC injection (0481T)
  Platelet rich plasma injection (0232T)
- (76942, 77002, 77021)
- 1.15   1.53   **FUD** 000   [T] [P3]
- AMA: 2018,Jan,8; 2017,Dec,13; 2017,Jan,8; 2016,Jan,13

20552   Injection(s); single or multiple trigger point(s), 1 or 2 muscle(s)
- EXCLUDES   Autologous WBC injection (0481T)
  Needle insertion(s) without injection(s) for same muscle(s) ([20560, 20561])
  Platelet rich plasma injection (0232T)
- (76942, 77002, 77021)
- 1.11   1.59   **FUD** 000   [T] [P3]
- AMA: 2020,Feb,9; 2018,Jan,8; 2017,Dec,13; 2017,Jun,10; 2017,Jan,8; 2016,Jan,13

20553   single or multiple trigger point(s), 3 or more muscles
- EXCLUDES   Needle insertion(s) without injection(s) for same muscle(s) ([20560, 20561])
- (76942, 77002, 77021)
- 1.25   1.82   **FUD** 000   [T] [P3]
- AMA: 2020,Feb,9; 2018,Dec,8; 2018,Dec,8; 2018,Jan,8; 2017,Jun,10; 2017,Jan,8; 2016,Jan,13

\# **20560**   **Needle insertion(s) without injection(s); 1 or 2 muscle(s)**
- INCLUDES   Dry needling and trigger-point acupuncture
- 0.47   0.74   **FUD** XXX
- AMA: 2020,Feb,9

\# **20561**   **3 or more muscles**
- INCLUDES   Dry needling and trigger-point acupuncture
- 0.71   1.10   **FUD** XXX
- AMA: 2020,Feb,9

20555-20561 [20560, 20561] Placement of Catheters/Needles for Brachytherapy

Code also interstitial radioelement application (77770-77772, 77778)

20555   Placement of needles or catheters into muscle and/or soft tissue for subsequent interstitial radioelement application (at the time of or subsequent to the procedure)
- EXCLUDES   Interstitial radioelement:
  Devices placed into breast (19296-19298)
  Placement needle, catheters, or devices into muscle or soft tissue head and neck (41019)
  Placement needles or catheters into pelvic organs or genitalia (55920)
  Placement needles or catheters into prostate (55875)
- (76942, 77002, 77012, 77021)
- 9.48   9.48   **FUD** 000   [J] [R2] [80]
- AMA: 2018,Jan,8; 2017,Jan,8; 2016,Jan,13

20560   Resequenced code. See code following 20553.

20561   Resequenced code. See code before 20555.

20600-20611 Aspiration and/or Injection of Joint

CMS: 100-03,150.7 Prolotherapy, Joint Sclerotherapy, and Ligamentous Injections with Sclerosing Agents

20600   Arthrocentesis, aspiration and/or injection, small joint or bursa (eg, fingers, toes); without ultrasound guidance
- EXCLUDES   Autologous adipose-derived regenerative cells injection (0489T-0490T)
  Platelet rich plasma (PRP) injections (0232T)
  Ultrasound guidance (76942)
- (77002, 77012, 77021)
- 1.04   1.44   **FUD** 000   [T] [P3] [50]
- AMA: 2018,Sep,12; 2018,Jan,8; 2017,Aug,9; 2017,Jan,8; 2016,Jan,13

20604   with ultrasound guidance, with permanent recording and reporting
- INCLUDES   Ultrasound guidance (76942)
- EXCLUDES   Autologous adipose-derived regenerative cells injection (0489T-0490T)
  Platelet rich plasma (PRP) injections (0232T)
- (77002, 77012, 77021)
- 1.32   2.17   **FUD** 000   [T] [P3] [50]
- AMA: 2018,Sep,12; 2018,Jan,8; 2017,Jan,8; 2016,Jan,13

20605   Arthrocentesis, aspiration and/or injection, intermediate joint or bursa (eg, temporomandibular, acromioclavicular, wrist, elbow or ankle, olecranon bursa); without ultrasound guidance
- EXCLUDES   Ultrasound guidance (76942)
- (77002, 77012, 77021)
- 1.08   1.49   **FUD** 000   [T] [P3] [50]
- AMA: 2018,Jan,8; 2017,Aug,9; 2017,Jan,8; 2016,Jan,13

20606   with ultrasound guidance, with permanent recording and reporting
- INCLUDES   Ultrasound guidance (76942)
- EXCLUDES   Platelet rich plasma (PRP) injections (0232T)
- (77002, 77012, 77021)
- 1.53   2.28   **FUD** 000   [T] [P3] [50]
- AMA: 2018,Jan,8; 2017,Jan,8; 2016,Jan,13

20610   Arthrocentesis, aspiration and/or injection, major joint or bursa (eg, shoulder, hip, knee, subacromial bursa); without ultrasound guidance
- EXCLUDES   Injection contrast for knee arthrography (27369)
  Platelet rich plasma (PRP) injections (0232T)
  Ultrasound guidance (76942)
- (77002, 77012, 77021)
- 1.32   1.77   **FUD** 000   [T] [P3] [50]
- AMA: 2019,Aug,7; 2018,Jan,8; 2017,Apr,9; 2017,Jan,8; 2016,Jan,13

20611   with ultrasound guidance, with permanent recording and reporting
- INCLUDES   Ultrasound guidance (76942)
- EXCLUDES   Injection contrast for knee arthrography (27369)
  Platelet rich plasma (PRP) injections (0232T)
- (77002, 77012, 77021)
- 1.76   2.58   **FUD** 000   [T] [P3] [50]
- AMA: 2019,Aug,7; 2018,Jan,8; 2017,Jan,8; 2016,Jan,13

20612-20615 Aspiration and/or Injection of Cyst

20612   Aspiration and/or injection of ganglion cyst(s) any location
Code also modifier 59 for multiple ganglion aspirations or injections
- 1.19   1.76   **FUD** 000   [T] [P3]

20615   Aspiration and injection for treatment of bone cyst
- EXCLUDES   Bone marrow lesions bone-substitute material injection (0707T)
- 4.60   7.10   **FUD** 010   [T] [P3]

20650-20697 Procedures Related to Bony Fixation

20650   Insertion of wire or pin with application of skeletal traction, including removal (separate procedure)
- 4.54   6.08   **FUD** 010   [J] [A2]

26/TC PC/TC Only   A2-Z3 ASC Payment   50 Bilateral   ♂ Male Only   ♀ Female Only   🗲 Facility RVU   Non-Facility RVU   CCI   CLIA
FUD Follow-up Days   CMS: IOM   AMA: CPT Asst   A-Y OPPSI   80/80 Surg Assist Allowed / w/Doc   Lab Crosswalk   Radiology Crosswalk

38   CPT © 2021 American Medical Association. All Rights Reserved.   © 2021 Optum360, LLC

20660   Application of cranial tongs, caliper, or stereotactic frame, including removal (separate procedure)
 🚗 7.00 ✂ 7.00 **FUD** 000 [Q2] [G2] ▣
 AMA: 2018,Jan,8; 2017,Jan,8; 2016,Jan,13

20661   Application of halo, including removal; cranial
 🚗 14.4 ✂ 14.4 **FUD** 090 [C] ▣
 AMA: 2018,Jan,8; 2017,Jan,8; 2016,Jan,13

20662 pelvic
 🚗 14.8 ✂ 14.8 **FUD** 090 [J] [R2] [80] ▣

20663 femoral
 🚗 13.6 ✂ 13.6 **FUD** 090 [J] [R2] [80] [50] ▣

20664   Application of halo, including removal, cranial, 6 or more pins placed, for thin skull osteology (eg, pediatric patients, hydrocephalus, osteogenesis imperfecta)
 🚗 25.0 ✂ 25.0 **FUD** 090 [C] ▣
 AMA: 2018,Jan,8; 2017,Jan,8; 2016,Jan,13

20665   Removal of tongs or halo applied by another individual
 🚗 2.68 ✂ 3.19 **FUD** 010 [Q1] [G2] [80] ▣
 AMA: 2018,Jan,8; 2017,Jan,8; 2016,Jan,13

20670   Removal of implant; superficial (eg, buried wire, pin or rod) (separate procedure)
 🚗 4.18 ✂ 10.5 **FUD** 010 [Q2] [A2] ▣
 AMA: 2018,Jan,3; 2018,Jan,8; 2017,Jan,8; 2016,Jan,13

20680 deep (eg, buried wire, pin, screw, metal band, nail, rod or plate)
  EXCLUDES *Removal and reinsertion sinus tarsi implant ([0511T])*
   Removal sinus tarsi implant ([0510T])
 🚗 12.1 ✂ 17.6 **FUD** 090 [Q2] [A2] [80] ▣
 AMA: 2018,Jan,3; 2018,Jan,8; 2017,Jan,8; 2016,Nov,9; 2016,Jan,13

20690   Application of a uniplane (pins or wires in 1 plane), unilateral, external fixation system
  Code also:
   For replacement traction device during or after global period
   Traction device supplies
 🚗 17.2 ✂ 17.2 **FUD** 090 [J] [J8] ▣
 AMA: 2018,Jan,3; 2018,Jan,8; 2017,Jan,8; 2016,Jan,13

20692   Application of a multiplane (pins or wires in more than 1 plane), unilateral, external fixation system (eg, Ilizarov, Monticelli type)
  Code also:
   For replacement traction device during or after global period
   Traction device supplies
 🚗 32.2 ✂ 32.2 **FUD** 090 [J] [J8] [80] ▣
 AMA: 2019,May,10; 2018,Jan,8; 2018,Jan,3; 2017,Jan,8; 2016,Jan,13

20693   Adjustment or revision of external fixation system requiring anesthesia (eg, new pin[s] or wire[s] and/or new ring[s] or bar[s])
 🚗 12.7 ✂ 12.7 **FUD** 090 [J] [A2] ▣
 AMA: 2018,Jan,3; 2018,Jan,8; 2017,Jan,8; 2016,Jan,13

20694   Removal, under anesthesia, of external fixation system
 🚗 9.72 ✂ 12.2 **FUD** 090 [Q2] [A2] ▣
 AMA: 2018,Jan,3; 2018,Jan,8; 2017,Jan,8; 2016,Jan,13

20696   Application of multiplane (pins or wires in more than 1 plane), unilateral, external fixation with stereotactic computer-assisted adjustment (eg, spatial frame), including imaging; initial and subsequent alignment(s), assessment(s), and computation(s) of adjustment schedule(s)
  EXCLUDES *Application multiplane external fixation system (20692)*
   Osteotomy with insertion intramedullary lengthening device, humerus (0594T)
   Removal and replacement each strut (20697)
 🚗 34.4 ✂ 34.4 **FUD** 090 [J] [J8] [80] ▣
 AMA: 2018,Jan,3; 2018,Jan,8; 2017,Jan,8; 2016,Jan,13

20697 exchange (ie, removal and replacement) of strut, each
  EXCLUDES *Application multiplane external fixation system (20692)*
   Exchange strut for multiplane external fixation system (20697)
 🚗 58.9 ✂ 58.9 **FUD** 000 ⊘ [J] [P2] [80] [TC]
 AMA: 2018,Jan,3; 2018,Jan,8; 2017,Jan,8; 2016,Jan,13

20700-20705 Drug Delivery Device

+ **20700**   Manual preparation and insertion of drug-delivery device(s), deep (eg, subfascial) (List separately in addition to code for primary procedure)
  INCLUDES Combining therapeutic agents, including antibiotics, with carrier substance during operative episode
   Forming resulting mixture into drug delivery devices (beads, nails, spacers)
   Insertion therapeutic device/agent once per anatomic location
  EXCLUDES *Insertion drug delivery implant, non-biodegradable (11981)*
   Insertion prefabricated drug device
  Code first (11010-11012, 11043, [11046], 11044, 11047, 20240-20251, 21010, 21025-21026, 21501-21510, 21627-21630, 22010-22015, 23030-23044, 23170-23184, 23334-23335, 23930-24000, 24134-24140, 24147, 24160, 25031-25040, 25145-25151, 26070, 26230-26236, 26990-26992, 27030, 27070-27071, 27090, 27301-27303, 27310, 27360, 27603-27604, 27610, 27640-27641, 28001-28003, 28020, 28120-28122)
 🚗 2.44 ✂ 2.44 **FUD** ZZZ [80] ▣

+ **20701**   Removal of drug-delivery device(s), deep (eg, subfascial) (List separately in addition to code for primary procedure)
  INCLUDES Removal therapeutic device/agent once per anatomic location from subfascial tissues
  EXCLUDES *Removal drug delivery device, performed alone (20680)*
   Removal drug delivery implant, non-biodegradable (11982)
  Code first (11010-11012, 11043, [11046], 11044, 11047, 20240-20251, 21010, 21025-21026, 21501-21510, 21627-21630, 22010-22015, 23030-23044, 23170-23184, 23334-23335, 23930-24000, 24134-24140, 24147, 24160, 25031-25040, 25145-25151, 26070, 26230-26236, 26990-26992, 27030, 27070-27071, 27090, 27301-27303, 27310, 27360, 27603-27604, 27610, 27640-27641, 28001-28003, 28020, 28120-28122)
 🚗 1.82 ✂ 1.82 **FUD** ZZZ [80] ▣

+ **20702**   Manual preparation and insertion of drug-delivery device(s), intramedullary (List separately in addition to code for primary procedure)
  INCLUDES Combining therapeutic agents, including antibiotics, with carrier substance during operative episode
   Forming resulting mixture into drug delivery devices (beads, nails, spacers)
   Insertion therapeutic device/agent once per anatomic location into intramedullary spaces
  EXCLUDES *Insertion drug delivery implant, non-biodegradable (11981)*
   Insertion prefabricated drug device
  Code first (20680-20692, 20694, 20802-20805, 20838, 21510, 23035, 23170, 23180, 23184, 23515, 23615, 23935, 24134, 24138-24140, 24147, 24430, 24516, 25035, 25145-25151, 25400, 25515, 25525-25526, 25545, 25574-25575, 27245, 27259, 27360, 27470, 27506, 27640, 27720)
 🚗 4.06 ✂ 4.06 **FUD** ZZZ [80] ▣

+ **20703**   Removal of drug-delivery device(s), intramedullary (List separately in addition to code for primary procedure)
  INCLUDES Removal therapeutic device/agent once per anatomic location from intramedullary spaces
  EXCLUDES *Removal drug delivery device, performed alone (20680)*
   Removal drug delivery implant, non-biodegradable (11982)
  Code first (20690-20692, 20694, 20802-20805, 20838, 21510, 23035, 23170, 23180, 23184, 23515, 23615, 23935, 24134, 24138-24140, 24147, 24430, 24516, 25035, 25145-25151, 25400, 25515, 25525-25526, 25545, 25574-25575, 27245, 27259, 27360, 27470, 27506, 27640, 27720)
 🚗 2.91 ✂ 2.91 **FUD** ZZZ [80] ▣

● New Code ▲ Revised Code ○ Reinstated ● New Web Release ▲ Revised Web Release + Add-on Unlisted Not Covered # Resequenced
⑤⓪ Optum Mod 50 Exempt ⊘ AMA Mod 51 Exempt ⑤ Optum Mod 51 Exempt ⑥ Mod 63 Exempt ✗ Non-FDA Drug ★ Telemedicine Ⓜ Maternity Ⓐ Age Edit

+ **20704** **Manual preparation and insertion of drug-delivery device(s), intra-articular (List separately in addition to code for primary procedure)**

INCLUDES Combining therapeutic agents, including antibiotics, with carrier substance during operative episode
Forming resulting mixture into drug delivery devices (beads, nails, spacers)
Insertion therapeutic device/agent once per anatomic location into intra-articular spaces

EXCLUDES Insertion drug delivery implant, non-biodegradable (11981)
Insertion prefabricated drug device
Removal hip prosthesis (27091)
Removal knee prosthesis (27488)

Code first (22864-22865, 23040-23044, 23334, 24000, 24160, 25040, 25250-25251, 26070-26080, 26990, 27030, 27090, 27301, 27310, 27603, 27610, 28020)

⏱ 4.23 ⚕ 4.23 **FUD** ZZZ `80` `□`

+ **20705** **Removal of drug-delivery device(s), intra-articular (List separately in addition to code for primary procedure)**

INCLUDES Removal therapeutic device/agent once per anatomic location from intra-articular space(s)

EXCLUDES Open treatment femoral neck fracture/internal fixation or prosthetic replacement (27236)
Partial knee replacement (27446)
Partial or total hip replacement (27125-27130)
Patella arthroplasty with prosthesis (27438)
Removal drug delivery device, performed alone (20680)
Removal drug delivery implant, non-biodegradable (11982)
Removal hip prosthesis (27091)
Removal knee prosthesis (27488)
Removal shoulder prosthesis (23335)
Revision hip arthroplasty (27134-27138)
Revision knee arthroplasty (27486-27487)

Code first (22864-22865, 23040-23044, 23334, 24000, 24160, 25040, 25250-25251, 26070-26080, 26990, 27030, 27090, 27301, 27310, 27603, 27610, 28020)

⏱ 3.48 ⚕ 3.48 **FUD** ZZZ `80` `□`

20802-20838 Reimplantation Procedures

EXCLUDES Repair incomplete amputation (see individual repair codes for bone(s), ligament(s), tendon(s), nerve(s), or blood vessel(s) and append modifier 52)

20802 **Replantation, arm (includes surgical neck of humerus through elbow joint), complete amputation**

⏱ 79.5 ⚕ 79.5 **FUD** 090 `C` `80` `50` `□`
AMA: 1997,Apr,4

20805 **Replantation, forearm (includes radius and ulna to radial carpal joint), complete amputation**

⏱ 94.7 ⚕ 94.7 **FUD** 090 `C` `80` `50` `□`
AMA: 1997,Apr,4

20808 **Replantation, hand (includes hand through metacarpophalangeal joints), complete amputation**

⏱ 114. ⚕ 114. **FUD** 090 `C` `80` `50` `□`
AMA: 1997,Apr,4

20816 **Replantation, digit, excluding thumb (includes metacarpophalangeal joint to insertion of flexor sublimis tendon), complete amputation**

⏱ 59.5 ⚕ 59.5 **FUD** 090 `C` `80` `□`
AMA: 2018,Jan,8; 2017,Jan,8; 2016,Jan,13

20822 **Replantation, digit, excluding thumb (includes distal tip to sublimis tendon insertion), complete amputation**

⏱ 51.2 ⚕ 51.2 **FUD** 090 `J` `62` `80` `□`
AMA: 1997,Apr,4

20824 **Replantation, thumb (includes carpometacarpal joint to MP joint), complete amputation**

⏱ 59.7 ⚕ 59.7 **FUD** 090 `C` `80` `50` `□`
AMA: 1997,Apr,4

20827 **Replantation, thumb (includes distal tip to MP joint), complete amputation**

⏱ 52.6 ⚕ 52.6 **FUD** 090 `C` `80` `50` `□`
AMA: 1997,Apr,4

20838 **Replantation, foot, complete amputation**

⏱ 80.6 ⚕ 80.6 **FUD** 090 `C` `80` `50` `□`
AMA: 1997,Apr,4

20900-20924 Bone and Tissue Autografts

EXCLUDES Acquisition autogenous bone, bone marrow, cartilage, tendon, fascia lata or other grafts through distinct incision unless included in code description
Autologous fat graft obtained by liposuction (15771-15774)
Bone graft procedures on spine (20930-20938)
Other autologous soft tissue grafts (fat, dermis, fascia) harvested by direct excision ([15769])

20900 **Bone graft, any donor area; minor or small (eg, dowel or button)**

⏱ 5.33 ⚕ 11.6 **FUD** 000 `J` `A2` `80` `□`
AMA: 2020,May,13; 2018,Jul,14; 2018,Jan,8; 2017,Jan,8; 2016,Jan,13

20902 **major or large**

⏱ 8.20 ⚕ 8.20 **FUD** 000 `J` `A2` `80` `□`
AMA: 2020,May,13; 2018,Jul,14; 2018,Jan,8; 2017,Jan,8; 2016,Jan,13

20910 **Cartilage graft; costochondral**

EXCLUDES Graft with ear cartilage (21235)

⏱ 13.5 ⚕ 13.5 **FUD** 090 `T` `A2` `80` `□`
AMA: 2020,May,13; 2018,Jul,14; 2018,Jan,8; 2017,Jan,8; 2016,Jan,13

20912 **nasal septum**

EXCLUDES Graft with ear cartilage (21235)

⏱ 13.6 ⚕ 13.6 **FUD** 090 `T` `A2` `80` `□`
AMA: 2020,May,13; 2018,Jul,14

20920 **Fascia lata graft; by stripper**

⏱ 11.5 ⚕ 11.5 **FUD** 090 `T` `A2`
AMA: 2020,May,13; 2018,Jul,14; 2018,Jan,8; 2017,Jan,8; 2016,Jan,13

20922 **by incision and area exposure, complex or sheet**

⏱ 13.9 ⚕ 17.0 **FUD** 090 `T` `A2` `80` `□`
AMA: 2020,May,13; 2018,Jul,14; 2018,Jan,8; 2017,Jan,8; 2016,Jan,13

20924 **Tendon graft, from a distance (eg, palmaris, toe extensor, plantaris)**

⏱ 14.6 ⚕ 14.6 **FUD** 090 `J` `A2` `80` `□`
AMA: 2020,May,13; 2018,Jul,14

20930-20939 Bone Allograft and Autograft of Spine

EXCLUDES Acquisition autogenous bone, bone marrow, cartilage, tendon, fascia lata, or other grafts through distinct incision unless included in code description
Autologous fat graft obtained by liposuction (15771-15774)
Other autologous soft tissue grafts (fat, dermis, fascia) harvested by direct excision ([15769])

+ **20930** **Allograft, morselized, or placement of osteopromotive material, for spine surgery only (List separately in addition to code for primary procedure)**

Code first (22319, 22532-22533, 22548-22558, 22590-22612, 22630, 22633-22634, 22800-22812)

⏱ 0.00 ⚕ 0.00 **FUD** XXX `N` `M1` `□`
AMA: 2020,May,13; 2019,May,7; 2018,Jul,14; 2018,Jan,8; 2017,Mar,7; 2017,Jan,8; 2016,Jan,13

+ **20931** **Allograft, structural, for spine surgery only (List separately in addition to code for primary procedure)**

Code first (22319, 22532-22533, 22548-22558, 22590-22612, 22630, 22633-22634, 22800-22812)

⏱ 3.22 ⚕ 3.22 **FUD** ZZZ `N` `M1` `□`
AMA: 2020,May,13; 2019,May,7; 2018,Jul,14; 2018,Jan,8; 2017,Mar,7; 2017,Jan,8; 2016,Jan,13

`26`/`TC` PC/TC Only `A2`-`Z3` ASC Payment `50` Bilateral ♂ Male Only ♀ Female Only ⏱ Facility RVU ⚕ Non-Facility RVU `□` CCI `✕` CLIA
FUD Follow-up Days **CMS:** IOM **AMA:** CPT Asst `A`-`Y` OPPSI `80`/`80` Surg Assist Allowed / w/Doc `▣` Lab Crosswalk `▣` Radiology Crosswalk

40 CPT © 2021 American Medical Association. All Rights Reserved. © 2021 Optum360, LLC

+ **20932** **Allograft, includes templating, cutting, placement and internal fixation, when performed; osteoarticular, including articular surface and contiguous bone (List separately in addition to code for primary procedure)**

> EXCLUDES *Allograft, intercalary (20933-20934)*
> *Injection contrast for ankle arthrography (27648)*
> *Osteotomy, femur (27448)*
> *Radical resection tumor:*
> > *Clavicle (23200)*
> > *Fibula (27646)*
> > *Ischial tuberosity/greater trochanter femur (27078)*
> > *Radial head or neck (24152)*
> > *Talus or calcaneus (27647)*
> > *Removal hip prosthesis (27090-27091)*
>
> Code also insertion joint prosthesis
> Code first (23210, 23220, 24150, 25170, 27075-27077, 27365, 27645, 27704)
>
> 20.6 20.6 **FUD** ZZZ   N1 80

> **AMA:** 2020,May,13; 2019,May,7

+ **20933** **hemicortical intercalary, partial (ie, hemicylindrical) (List separately in addition to code for primary procedure)**

> EXCLUDES *Allograft, intercalary, complete (20934)*
> *Allograft, osteoarticular (20932)*
> *Arthroplasty procedures, hip (27130, 27132, 27134, 27138)*
> *Bone graft (20955-20957, 20962)*
> *Excision cyst with allograft (23146, 23156, 24116, 24126, 25126, 25136, 27356, 27638, 28103, 28107)*
> *Injection contrast for ankle arthrography (27648)*
> *Open treatment femoral fractures (27236, 27244)*
> *Osteotomy, femur (27448)*
> *Radical resection tumor:*
> > *Clavicle (23200)*
> > *Fibula (27646)*
> > *Ischial tuberosity/greater trochanter femur (27078)*
> > *Radial head or neck (24152)*
> > *Talus or calcaneus (27647)*
> > *Removal hip prosthesis (27090-27091)*
>
> Code also insertion joint prosthesis
> Code first (23210, 23220, 24150, 25170, 27075-27077, 27365, 27645, 27704)
>
> 18.9 18.9 **FUD** ZZZ   N1 80

> **AMA:** 2020,May,13; 2019,May,7

+ **20934** **intercalary, complete (ie, cylindrical) (List separately in addition to code for primary procedure)**

> EXCLUDES *Allograft, intercalary, partial (20933)*
> *Allograft, osteoarticular (20932)*
> *Excision cyst with allograft (23146, 23156)*
> *Injection contrast for ankle arthrography (27648)*
> *Osteotomy, femur (27448)*
> *Radical resection tumor:*
> > *Clavicle (23200)*
> > *Fibula (27646)*
> > *Ischial tuberosity/greater trochanter femur (27078)*
> > *Radial head or neck (24152)*
> > *Talus or calcaneus (27647)*
> > *Removal hip prosthesis (27090-27091)*
>
> Code also insertion joint prosthesis
> Code first (23210, 23220, 24150, 25170, 27075-27077, 27365, 27645, 27704)
>
> 20.6 20.6 **FUD** ZZZ   N1 80

> **AMA:** 2020,May,13; 2019,May,7

+ **20936** **Autograft for spine surgery only (includes harvesting the graft); local (eg, ribs, spinous process, or laminar fragments) obtained from same incision (List separately in addition to code for primary procedure)**

> Code first (22319, 22532-22533, 22548-22558, 22590-22612, 22630, 22633-22634, 22800-22812)
>
> 0.00 0.00 **FUD** XXX   N N1

> **AMA:** 2020,May,13; 2018,Jul,14; 2018,Jan,8; 2017,Mar,7; 2017,Jan,8; 2016,Jan,13

+ **20937** **morselized (through separate skin or fascial incision) (List separately in addition to code for primary procedure)**

> Code first (22319, 22532-22533, 22548-22558, 22590-22612, 22630, 22633-22634, 22800-22812)
>
> 4.85 4.85 **FUD** ZZZ   N N1 80

> **AMA:** 2020,May,13; 2018,Jul,14; 2018,Jan,8; 2017,Mar,7; 2017,Jan,8; 2016,Jan,13

+ **20938** **structural, bicortical or tricortical (through separate skin or fascial incision) (List separately in addition to code for primary procedure)**

> EXCLUDES *Bone marrow for bone grafting in spinal surgery (20939)*
> Code first (22319, 22532-22533, 22548-22558, 22590-22612, 22630, 22633-22634, 22800-22812)
>
> 5.34 5.34 **FUD** ZZZ   N N1 80

> **AMA:** 2020,May,13; 2018,Jul,14; 2018,Jan,8; 2017,Mar,7; 2017,Jan,8; 2016,Jan,13

+ **20939** **Bone marrow aspiration for bone grafting, spine surgery only, through separate skin or fascial incision (List separately in addition to code for primary procedure)**

> EXCLUDES *Bone marrow aspiration for other than bone grafting in spinal surgery (20999)*
> *Diagnostic bone marrow aspiration (38220, 38222)*
> *Platelet rich plasma injection (0232T)*
> *Reporting with modifier 50. Report once for each side when performed bilaterally*
> Code first (22319, 22532-22534, 22548, 22551-22552, 22554, 22556, 22558, 22590, 22595, 22600, 22610, 22612, 22630, 22633-22634, 22800, 22802, 22804, 22808, 22810, 22812)
>
> 2.03 2.03 **FUD** ZZZ   N N1 80

> **AMA:** 2018,May,3

20950 Measurement of Intracompartmental Pressure

20950 **Monitoring of interstitial fluid pressure (includes insertion of device, eg, wick catheter technique, needle manometer technique) in detection of muscle compartment syndrome**

> 2.56 7.43 **FUD** 000   T 62 80

> **AMA:** 2018,Jan,8; 2017,Jan,8; 2016,Jan,13

20955-20973 Bone and Osteocutaneous Grafts

> INCLUDES Operating microscope (69990)

20955 **Bone graft with microvascular anastomosis; fibula**

> 70.9 70.9 **FUD** 090   C 80

> **AMA:** 2019,Dec,5; 2019,May,7; 2018,Jan,8; 2017,Jan,8; 2016,Feb,12; 2016,Jan,13

20956 **iliac crest**

> 76.5 76.5 **FUD** 090   C 80

> **AMA:** 2019,Dec,5; 2019,May,7; 2018,Jan,8; 2017,Jan,8; 2016,Feb,12; 2016,Jan,13

20957 **metatarsal**

> 79.6 79.6 **FUD** 090   C 80

> **AMA:** 2019,Dec,5; 2019,May,7; 2018,Jan,8; 2017,Jan,8; 2016,Feb,12; 2016,Jan,13

20962 **other than fibula, iliac crest, or metatarsal**

> 76.9 76.9 **FUD** 090   C 80

> **AMA:** 2019,Dec,5; 2019,May,7; 2016,Feb,12

20969 **Free osteocutaneous flap with microvascular anastomosis; other than iliac crest, metatarsal, or great toe**

> 78.6 78.6 **FUD** 090   C 80

> **AMA:** 2019,Dec,5; 2019,Oct,10; 2018,Jan,8; 2017,Jan,8; 2016,Feb,12; 2016,Jan,13

20970 **iliac crest**

> 82.6 82.6 **FUD** 090   C 80

> **AMA:** 2019,Dec,5; 2018,Jan,8; 2017,Jan,8; 2016,Feb,12; 2016,Jan,13

20972 **metatarsal**

> 82.4 82.4 **FUD** 090   J 62 80

> **AMA:** 2019,Dec,5; 2018,Jan,8; 2017,Jan,8; 2016,Feb,12; 2016,Jan,13

Musculoskeletal System

20973 — 21026

20973   **great toe with web space**

> *EXCLUDES*   *Great toe wrap-around with bone graft (26551)*
> 🚑 87.0   ⚕ 87.0   **FUD** 090   J R2 80 50 ▢
>
> **AMA:** 2019,Dec,5; 2018,Jan,8; 2017,Jan,8; 2016,Feb,12; 2016,Jan,13

20974-20979 Osteogenic Stimulation

CMS: 100-03,150.2 Osteogenic Stimulation

20974   **Electrical stimulation to aid bone healing; noninvasive (nonoperative)**

> 🚑 1.45   ⚕ 2.26   **FUD** 000   ⊘ A ▢
>
> **AMA:** 2018,Jan,8; 2017,Jan,8; 2016,Jan,13

20975   **invasive (operative)**

> 🚑 5.18   ⚕ 5.18   **FUD** 000   ⊘ N N1 80 ▢
>
> **AMA:** 2002,Apr,13; 2000,Nov,8

20979   **Low intensity ultrasound stimulation to aid bone healing, noninvasive (nonoperative)**

> 🚑 0.93   ⚕ 1.53   **FUD** 000   01 N1 ▢
>
> **AMA:** 2018,Jan,8; 2017,Jan,8; 2016,Jan,13

20982-20999 General Musculoskeletal Procedures

20982   **Ablation therapy for reduction or eradication of 1 or more bone tumors (eg, metastasis) including adjacent soft tissue when involved by tumor extension, percutaneous, including imaging guidance when performed; radiofrequency**

> *EXCLUDES*   *Radiologic guidance (76940, 77002, 77013, 77022)*
> 🚑 10.5   ⚕ 110.   **FUD** 000   J G2 50 ▢
>
> **AMA:** 2018,Jan,8; 2017,Jan,8; 2016,Jan,13

20983   **cryoablation**

> *EXCLUDES*   *Radiologic guidance (76940, 77002, 77013, 77022)*
> 🚑 10.3   ⚕ 170.   **FUD** 000   J G2 50 ▢
>
> **AMA:** 2018,Jan,8; 2017,Jan,8; 2016,Jan,13

+   **20985**   **Computer-assisted surgical navigational procedure for musculoskeletal procedures, image-less (List separately in addition to code for primary procedure)**

> *EXCLUDES*   *Image guidance derived from intraoperative and preoperative obtained images (0054T-0055T)*
>   *Stereotactic computer-assisted navigational procedure; cranial or intradural (61781-61783)*
> Code first primary procedure
> 🚑 4.24   ⚕ 4.24   **FUD** ZZZ   N N1 80 ▢
>
> **AMA:** 2018,Jan,8; 2017,Jan,8; 2016,Jan,13

20999   **Unlisted procedure, musculoskeletal system, general**

> 🚑 0.00   ⚕ 0.00   **FUD** YYY   T 80 ▢
>
> **AMA:** 2018,May,3; 2018,Jan,8; 2017,Jan,8; 2016,Jan,13

21010 Temporomandibular Joint Arthrotomy

21010   **Arthrotomy, temporomandibular joint**

> *EXCLUDES*   *Cutaneous/subcutaneous abscess and hematoma drainage (10060-10061)*
>   *Excision foreign body from dentoalveolar site (41805-41806)*
> 🚑 22.0   ⚕ 22.0   **FUD** 090   J A2 80 50 ▢
>
> **AMA:** 2002,Apr,13

21011-21016 Excision Soft Tissue Tumors Face and Scalp

INCLUDES   Any necessary elevation tissue planes or dissection
          Measurement tumor and necessary margin at greatest diameter prior to excision
          Simple and intermediate repairs
          Excision types:
            Fascial or subfascial soft tissue tumors: simple and marginal resection tumors found either in or below deep fascia, not including bone or excision substantial amount normal tissue; primarily benign and intramuscular tumors
            Radical resection soft tissue tumor: wide resection tumor involving substantial margins normal tissue and may include tissue removal from one or more layers; most often malignant or aggressive benign
            Subcutaneous: simple and marginal resection tumors in subcutaneous tissue above deep fascia; most often benign

EXCLUDES   *Complex repair*
          Excision benign cutaneous lesions (eg, sebaceous cyst) (11420-11426)
          Radical resection cutaneous tumors (eg, melanoma) (11620-11646)
          Significant vessel exploration or neuroplasty

21011   **Excision, tumor, soft tissue of face or scalp, subcutaneous; less than 2 cm**

> 🚑 7.38   ⚕ 10.3   **FUD** 090   J P3 80 ▢
>
> **AMA:** 2018,Sep,7; 2018,Jan,8; 2017,Jan,8; 2016,Jan,13

21012   **2 cm or greater**

> 🚑 9.72   ⚕ 9.72   **FUD** 090   J R2 80 ▢
>
> **AMA:** 2018,Sep,7; 2018,Jan,8; 2017,Jan,8; 2016,Jan,13

21013   **Excision, tumor, soft tissue of face and scalp, subfascial (eg, subgaleal, intramuscular); less than 2 cm**

> 🚑 11.5   ⚕ 15.1   **FUD** 090   J P3 80 ▢
>
> **AMA:** 2018,Sep,7; 2018,Jan,8; 2017,Jan,8; 2016,Jan,13

21014   **2 cm or greater**

> 🚑 15.0   ⚕ 15.0   **FUD** 090   J R2 80 ▢
>
> **AMA:** 2018,Sep,7; 2018,Jan,8; 2017,Jan,8; 2016,Jan,13

21015   **Radical resection of tumor (eg, sarcoma), soft tissue of face or scalp; less than 2 cm**

> *EXCLUDES*   *Removal of cranial tumor for osteomyelitis (61501)*
> 🚑 20.3   ⚕ 20.3   **FUD** 090   J G2 ▢
>
> **AMA:** 2018,Sep,7; 2018,Jan,8; 2017,Jan,8; 2016,Jan,13

21016   **2 cm or greater**

> 🚑 29.0   ⚕ 29.0   **FUD** 090   J G2 80 ▢
>
> **AMA:** 2018,Sep,7; 2018,Jan,8; 2017,Jan,8; 2016,Jan,13

21025-21070 Procedures of Cranial and Facial Bones

INCLUDES   Any necessary elevation tissue planes or dissection
          Measurement tumor and necessary margins prior to excision
          Radical resection bone tumor involves resection tumor (may include entire bone) and wide margins normal tissue primarily for malignant or aggressive benign tumors
          Simple and intermediate repairs

EXCLUDES   *Complex repair*
          Excision soft tissue tumors, face and scalp (21011-21016)
          Radical resection cutaneous tumors (e.g., melanoma) (11620-11646)
          Significant vessel exploration, neuroplasty, reconstruction, or complex bone repair

21025   **Excision of bone (eg, for osteomyelitis or bone abscess); mandible**

> 🚑 19.9   ⚕ 23.6   **FUD** 090   J A2 ▢
>
> **AMA:** 2018,Sep,7; 2018,Jan,8; 2017,Jan,8; 2016,Jan,13

21026   **facial bone(s)**

> 🚑 12.9   ⚕ 16.0   **FUD** 090   J A2 ▢
>
> **AMA:** 2018,Sep,7

26/TC PC/TC Only   A2-Z3 ASC Payment   50 Bilateral   ♂ Male Only   ♀ Female Only   🚑 Facility RVU   ⚕ Non-Facility RVU   ▢ CCI   ✖ CLIA
FUD Follow-up Days   CMS: IOM   AMA: CPT Asst   A-Y OPPSI   80/80 Surg Assist Allowed / w/Doc   Lab Crosswalk   Radiology Crosswalk

42   CPT © 2021 American Medical Association. All Rights Reserved.   © 2021 Optum360, LLC

21029 **Removal by contouring of benign tumor of facial bone (eg, fibrous dysplasia)**
17.9 21.8 **FUD** 090
J A2 80
AMA: 2018,Sep,7

Vestibular incision

Area of benign bone growth

Burrs, files, and osteotomes used to remove bone

21030 **Excision of benign tumor or cyst of maxilla or zygoma by enucleation and curettage**
11.1 14.0 **FUD** 090
J P3 50
AMA: 2018,Sep,7; 2018,Jan,8; 2017,Jan,8; 2016,Jan,13

21031 **Excision of torus mandibularis**
8.03 11.1 **FUD** 090
J P3 50
AMA: 2018,Sep,7

21032 **Excision of maxillary torus palatinus**
8.21 11.3 **FUD** 090
J P3
AMA: 2018,Sep,7

21034 **Excision of malignant tumor of maxilla or zygoma**
33.0 37.5 **FUD** 090
J A2 80
AMA: 2018,Sep,7; 2018,Jan,8; 2017,Jan,8; 2016,Jan,13

21040 **Excision of benign tumor or cyst of mandible, by enucleation and/or curettage**
INCLUDES Removal benign tumor or cyst without osteotomy
EXCLUDES *Removal benign tumor or cyst with osteotomy (21046-21047)*
11.1 14.1 **FUD** 090
J A2
AMA: 2018,Sep,7; 2018,Jan,8; 2017,Jan,8; 2016,Jan,13

21044 **Excision of malignant tumor of mandible;**
25.0 25.0 **FUD** 090
J A2 80
AMA: 2018,Sep,7

21045 **radical resection**
Code also bone graft procedure (21215)
34.6 34.6 **FUD** 090
C 80
AMA: 2018,Sep,7

21046 **Excision of benign tumor or cyst of mandible; requiring intra-oral osteotomy (eg, locally aggressive or destructive lesion[s])**
30.0 30.0 **FUD** 090
J A2 80
AMA: 2018,Sep,7; 2018,Jan,8; 2017,Jan,8; 2016,Jan,13

21047 **requiring extra-oral osteotomy and partial mandibulectomy (eg, locally aggressive or destructive lesion[s])**
36.7 36.7 **FUD** 090
J A2 80
AMA: 2018,Sep,7; 2018,Jan,8; 2017,Jan,8; 2016,Jan,13

21048 **Excision of benign tumor or cyst of maxilla; requiring intra-oral osteotomy (eg, locally aggressive or destructive lesion[s])**
30.5 30.5 **FUD** 090
J R2 80
AMA: 2018,Sep,7; 2018,Jan,8; 2017,Jan,8; 2016,Jan,13

21049 **requiring extra-oral osteotomy and partial maxillectomy (eg, locally aggressive or destructive lesion[s])**
34.7 34.7 **FUD** 090
J 62 80
AMA: 2018,Sep,7; 2018,Jan,8; 2017,Jan,8; 2016,Jan,13

21050 **Condylectomy, temporomandibular joint (separate procedure)**
25.2 25.2 **FUD** 090
J A2 80 50
AMA: 2018,Sep,7

21060 **Meniscectomy, partial or complete, temporomandibular joint (separate procedure)**
22.9 22.9 **FUD** 090
J A2 80 50
AMA: 2018,Sep,7

21070 **Coronoidectomy (separate procedure)**
18.3 18.3 **FUD** 090
J A2 80 50
AMA: 2018,Sep,7

21073 Temporomandibular Joint Manipulation with Anesthesia

21073 **Manipulation of temporomandibular joint(s) (TMJ), therapeutic, requiring an anesthesia service (ie, general or monitored anesthesia care)**
EXCLUDES *Closed treatment TMJ dislocation (21480, 21485)*
Manipulation TMJ without general or MAC anesthesia (97140, 98925-98929, 98943)
7.19 10.9 **FUD** 090
T P3 80 50
AMA: 2018,Sep,7; 2018,Jan,8; 2018,Jan,3; 2017,Jan,8; 2016,Jan,13

21076-21089 Medical Impressions for Fabrication Maxillofacial Prosthesis

INCLUDES Design, preparation, and professional services rendered by physician or other qualified health care professional
EXCLUDES *Application or removal caliper or tongs (20660, 20665)*
Professional services rendered for outside laboratory designed and prepared prosthesis

21076 **Impression and custom preparation; surgical obturator prosthesis**
23.1 27.6 **FUD** 010
T P3 80
AMA: 2018,Sep,7; 2018,Jan,8; 2017,Jan,8; 2016,Jan,13

21077 **orbital prosthesis**
53.4 64.0 **FUD** 090
J P3 80 50
AMA: 2018,Sep,7; 2018,Jan,8; 2017,Jan,8; 2016,Jan,13

21079 **interim obturator prosthesis**
38.8 46.6 **FUD** 090
J P3
AMA: 2018,Sep,7; 2018,Jan,8; 2017,Jan,8; 2016,Jan,13

21080 **definitive obturator prosthesis**
40.4 49.8 **FUD** 090
J P3
AMA: 2018,Sep,7; 2018,Jan,8; 2017,Jan,8; 2016,Jan,13

21081 **mandibular resection prosthesis**
37.0 45.7 **FUD** 090
J P3 80
AMA: 2018,Sep,7; 2018,Jan,8; 2017,Jan,8; 2016,Jan,13

21082 **palatal augmentation prosthesis**
34.0 42.4 **FUD** 090
J P3 80
AMA: 2018,Sep,7; 2018,Jan,8; 2017,Jan,8; 2016,Jan,13

21083 **palatal lift prosthesis**
31.6 40.4 **FUD** 090
J P3 80
AMA: 2018,Sep,7; 2018,Jan,8; 2017,Jan,8; 2016,Jan,13

21084 **speech aid prosthesis**
36.5 46.2 **FUD** 090
J P3 80
AMA: 2018,Sep,7; 2018,Jan,8; 2017,Jan,8; 2016,Jan,13

21085 **oral surgical splint**
15.7 21.0 **FUD** 010
T P2
AMA: 2018,Sep,7; 2018,Jan,8; 2017,Sep,14; 2017,Jan,8; 2016,Jan,13

21086 **auricular prosthesis**
39.4 47.6 **FUD** 090
J P3 80 50
AMA: 2018,Sep,7; 2018,Jan,8; 2017,Jan,8; 2016,Jan,13

21087 nasal prosthesis
🔲 42.7 ⚕ 51.1 **FUD** 090   J P3 80 ▭
AMA: 2018,Sep,7; 2018,Jan,8; 2017,Jan,8; 2016,Jan,13

21088 facial prosthesis
🔲 0.00 ⚕ 0.00 **FUD** 090   J R2 80 ▭
AMA: 2018,Sep,7; 2018,Jan,8; 2017,Jan,8; 2016,Jan,13

21089 Unlisted maxillofacial prosthetic procedure
🔲 0.00 ⚕ 0.00 **FUD** YYY   T ▭
AMA: 2018,Sep,7; 2018,Jan,8; 2017,Jan,8; 2016,Jan,13

21100-21110 Application Fixation Device

21100 Application of halo type appliance for maxillofacial fixation, includes removal (separate procedure)
🔲 10.6 ⚕ 18.9 **FUD** 090   J A2 80 ▭
AMA: 2018,Sep,7

21110 Application of interdental fixation device for conditions other than fracture or dislocation, includes removal
> EXCLUDES   *Interdental fixation device removal by different provider (20670-20680)*
🔲 19.5 ⚕ 23.3 **FUD** 090   Q2 P2 ▭
AMA: 2018,Sep,7; 2018,Jan,8; 2017,Jan,8; 2016,Jan,13

21116 Injection for TMJ Arthrogram

CMS: 100-02,15,150.1 Treatment of Temporomandibular Joint (TMJ) Syndrome; 100-04,13,80.1 Physician Presence; 100-04,13,80.2 S&I Multiple Procedure Reduction

21116 Injection procedure for temporomandibular joint arthrography
🔲 (70332)
🔲 1.34 ⚕ 5.62 **FUD** 000   N M1 50 ▭
AMA: 2018,Sep,7; 2018,Jan,8; 2017,Jan,8; 2016,May,13; 2016,Jan,13

21120-21299 Repair/Reconstruction Craniofacial Bones

> EXCLUDES   *Cranioplasty (21179-21180, 62120, 62140-62147)*

21120 Genioplasty; augmentation (autograft, allograft, prosthetic material)
🔲 15.0 ⚕ 19.2 **FUD** 090   J G2 ▭
AMA: 2018,Sep,7

Nasal bone
Frontal bone
Supraorbital margin
Frontonsal suture
Parietal bone
Zygomatic process
Zygomatic bone
Frontomaxillary suture
Nasal septum
Internasal suture
Zygomaxillary suture
Nasomaxillary suture
Maxilla
Ramus
Alveolar process of maxilla
Body of mandible
Mental foramen

21121 sliding osteotomy, single piece
🔲 17.8 ⚕ 20.9 **FUD** 090   J A2 80 ▭
AMA: 2018,Sep,7

21122 sliding osteotomies, 2 or more osteotomies (eg, wedge excision or bone wedge reversal for asymmetrical chin)
🔲 22.1 ⚕ 22.1 **FUD** 090   J A2 80 ▭
AMA: 2018,Sep,7

21123 sliding, augmentation with interpositional bone grafts (includes obtaining autografts)
🔲 26.1 ⚕ 26.1 **FUD** 090   J A2 80 ▭
AMA: 2018,Sep,7

21125 Augmentation, mandibular body or angle; prosthetic material
🔲 19.8 ⚕ 80.8 **FUD** 090   J A2 80 ▭
AMA: 2018,Sep,7

21127 with bone graft, onlay or interpositional (includes obtaining autograft)
🔲 24.6 ⚕ 112. **FUD** 090   J A2 80 ▭
AMA: 2018,Sep,7

21137 Reduction forehead; contouring only
🔲 21.7 ⚕ 21.7 **FUD** 090   J G2 80 ▭
AMA: 2018,Sep,7

21138 contouring and application of prosthetic material or bone graft (includes obtaining autograft)
🔲 26.5 ⚕ 26.5 **FUD** 090   J G2 80 ▭
AMA: 2018,Sep,7

21139 contouring and setback of anterior frontal sinus wall
🔲 32.1 ⚕ 32.1 **FUD** 090   J G2 80 ▭
AMA: 2018,Sep,7

21141 Reconstruction midface, LeFort I; single piece, segment movement in any direction (eg, for Long Face Syndrome), without bone graft
🔲 39.4 ⚕ 39.4 **FUD** 090   C 80 ▭
AMA: 2018,Sep,7

21142 2 pieces, segment movement in any direction, without bone graft
🔲 40.5 ⚕ 40.5 **FUD** 090   C 80 ▭
AMA: 2018,Sep,7

21143 3 or more pieces, segment movement in any direction, without bone graft
🔲 41.0 ⚕ 41.0 **FUD** 090   C 80 ▭
AMA: 2018,Sep,7

21145 single piece, segment movement in any direction, requiring bone grafts (includes obtaining autografts)
🔲 46.2 ⚕ 46.2 **FUD** 090   C 80 ▭
AMA: 2018,Sep,7

21146 2 pieces, segment movement in any direction, requiring bone grafts (includes obtaining autografts) (eg, ungrafted unilateral alveolar cleft)
🔲 48.2 ⚕ 48.2 **FUD** 090   C 80 ▭
AMA: 2018,Sep,7

21147 3 or more pieces, segment movement in any direction, requiring bone grafts (includes obtaining autografts) (eg, ungrafted bilateral alveolar cleft or multiple osteotomies)
🔲 50.8 ⚕ 50.8 **FUD** 090   C 80 ▭
AMA: 2018,Sep,7

21150 Reconstruction midface, LeFort II; anterior intrusion (eg, Treacher-Collins Syndrome)
🔲 47.3 ⚕ 47.3 **FUD** 090   J G2 80 ▭
AMA: 2018,Sep,7

21151 any direction, requiring bone grafts (includes obtaining autografts)
🔲 52.0 ⚕ 52.0 **FUD** 090   C 80 ▭
AMA: 2018,Sep,7

21154 Reconstruction midface, LeFort III (extracranial), any type, requiring bone grafts (includes obtaining autografts); without LeFort I
🔲 56.4 ⚕ 56.4 **FUD** 090   C 80 ▭
AMA: 2018,Sep,7

26/TC PC/TC Only   A2-Z3 ASC Payment   50 Bilateral   ♂ Male Only   ♀ Female Only   🔲 Facility RVU   ⚕ Non-Facility RVU   ▭ CCI   ✖ CLIA
FUD Follow-up Days   **CMS:** IOM   **AMA:** CPT Asst   A-Y OPPSI   80/80 Surg Assist Allowed / w/Doc   Lab Crosswalk   Radiology Crosswalk

44   CPT © 2021 American Medical Association. All Rights Reserved.   © 2021 Optum360, LLC

21155 **with LeFort I**
🔧 62.2 ✂ 62.2 **FUD** 090 Ⓒ 80 ▭
AMA: 2018,Sep,7

Bicoronal scalp flap
Lower eyelid
Circum-vestibular

Typical transcutaneous and transoral incisions

LeFort III with LeFort I down-fracture

21159 **Reconstruction midface, LeFort III (extra and intracranial) with forehead advancement (eg, mono bloc), requiring bone grafts (includes obtaining autografts); without LeFort I**
🔧 75.0 ✂ 75.0 **FUD** 090 Ⓒ 80 ▭
AMA: 2018,Sep,7

21160 **with LeFort I**
🔧 81.4 ✂ 81.4 **FUD** 090 Ⓒ 80 ▭
AMA: 2018,Sep,7

21172 **Reconstruction superior-lateral orbital rim and lower forehead, advancement or alteration, with or without grafts (includes obtaining autografts)**
EXCLUDES *Frontal or parietal craniotomy for craniosynostosis (61556)*
🔧 60.2 ✂ 60.2 **FUD** 090 J G2 80 ▭
AMA: 2018,Sep,7

21175 **Reconstruction, bifrontal, superior-lateral orbital rims and lower forehead, advancement or alteration (eg, plagiocephaly, trigonocephaly, brachycephaly), with or without grafts (includes obtaining autografts)**
EXCLUDES *Bifrontal craniotomy for craniosynostosis (61557)*
🔧 64.3 ✂ 64.3 **FUD** 090 J G2 80 ▭
AMA: 2018,Sep,7

21179 **Reconstruction, entire or majority of forehead and/or supraorbital rims; with grafts (allograft or prosthetic material)**
EXCLUDES *Extensive craniotomy for numerous suture craniosynostosis (61558-61559)*
🔧 44.2 ✂ 44.2 **FUD** 090 Ⓒ 80 ▭
AMA: 2018,Sep,7

21180 **with autograft (includes obtaining grafts)**
EXCLUDES *Extensive craniotomy for numerous suture craniosynostosis (61558-61559)*
🔧 49.0 ✂ 49.0 **FUD** 090 Ⓒ 80 ▭
AMA: 2018,Sep,7

21181 **Reconstruction by contouring of benign tumor of cranial bones (eg, fibrous dysplasia), extracranial**
🔧 21.4 ✂ 21.4 **FUD** 090 J A2 80 ▭
AMA: 2018,Sep,7

21182 **Reconstruction of orbital walls, rims, forehead, nasoethmoid complex following intra- and extracranial excision of benign tumor of cranial bone (eg, fibrous dysplasia), with multiple autografts (includes obtaining grafts); total area of bone grafting less than 40 sq cm**
EXCLUDES *Removal obenign tumor of the skull (61563-61564)*
🔧 61.6 ✂ 61.6 **FUD** 090 Ⓒ 80 ▭
AMA: 2018,Sep,7

21183 **total area of bone grafting greater than 40 sq cm but less than 80 sq cm**
EXCLUDES *Removal benign tumor of the skull (61563-61564)*
🔧 66.7 ✂ 66.7 **FUD** 090 Ⓒ 80 ▭
AMA: 2018,Sep,7

21184 **total area of bone grafting greater than 80 sq cm**
EXCLUDES *Removal benign tumor of the skull (61563-61564)*
🔧 72.3 ✂ 72.3 **FUD** 090 Ⓒ 80 ▭
AMA: 2018,Sep,7

21188 **Reconstruction midface, osteotomies (other than LeFort type) and bone grafts (includes obtaining autografts)**
🔧 48.2 ✂ 48.2 **FUD** 090 Ⓒ 80 ▭
AMA: 2018,Sep,7

21193 **Reconstruction of mandibular rami, horizontal, vertical, C, or L osteotomy; without bone graft**
🔧 36.8 ✂ 36.8 **FUD** 090 J G2 80 ▭
AMA: 2018,Sep,7; 2018,Jan,8; 2017,Jan,8; 2016,Jan,13

21194 **with bone graft (includes obtaining graft)**
🔧 42.3 ✂ 42.3 **FUD** 090 Ⓒ 80 ▭
AMA: 2018,Sep,7; 2018,Jan,8; 2017,Jan,8; 2016,Jan,13

21195 **Reconstruction of mandibular rami and/or body, sagittal split; without internal rigid fixation**
🔧 39.5 ✂ 39.5 **FUD** 090 J J8 80 ▭
AMA: 2018,Sep,7; 2018,Jan,8; 2017,Jan,8; 2016,Jan,13

21196 **with internal rigid fixation**
🔧 40.9 ✂ 40.9 **FUD** 090 Ⓒ 80 ▭
AMA: 2018,Sep,7; 2018,Jan,8; 2017,Jan,8; 2016,Jan,13

21198 **Osteotomy, mandible, segmental;**
EXCLUDES *Total maxillary osteotomy (21141-21160)*
🔧 33.0 ✂ 33.0 **FUD** 090 J G2 80 ▭
AMA: 2018,Sep,7; 2018,Jan,8; 2017,Jan,8; 2016,Jan,13

21199 **with genioglossus advancement**
EXCLUDES *Total maxillary osteotomy (21141-21160)*
🔧 31.0 ✂ 31.0 **FUD** 090 J G2 80 ▭
AMA: 2018,Sep,7; 2018,Jan,8; 2017,Jan,8; 2016,Jan,13

21206 **Osteotomy, maxilla, segmental (eg, Wassmund or Schuchard)**
🔧 34.1 ✂ 34.1 **FUD** 090 J A2 80 ▭
AMA: 2018,Sep,7

21208 **Osteoplasty, facial bones; augmentation (autograft, allograft, or prosthetic implant)**
🔧 23.2 ✂ 49.9 **FUD** 090 J P3 80 ▭
AMA: 2018,Sep,7

21209 **reduction**
🔧 17.4 ✂ 22.9 **FUD** 090 J A2 80 ▭
AMA: 2018,Sep,7

21210 **Graft, bone; nasal, maxillary or malar areas (includes obtaining graft)**
EXCLUDES *Cleft palate procedures (42200-42225)*
🔧 23.9 ✂ 60.2 **FUD** 090 J A2 ▭
AMA: 2018,Sep,7

21215 **mandible (includes obtaining graft)**
🔧 24.9 ✂ 114. **FUD** 090 J A2 ▭
AMA: 2018,Sep,7

21230 Graft; rib cartilage, autogenous, to face, chin, nose or ear (includes obtaining graft)

EXCLUDES Augmentation facial bones (21208)

📷 21.3 ✂ 21.3 **FUD** 090 J A2 80 ▱

AMA: 2018,Sep,7

21235 ear cartilage, autogenous, to nose or ear (includes obtaining graft)

EXCLUDES Augmentation facial bones (21208)

📷 16.2 ✂ 20.7 **FUD** 090 J A2 ▱

AMA: 2018,Sep,7; 2018,Jan,8; 2017,Jan,8; 2016,Jan,13

21240 Arthroplasty, temporomandibular joint, with or without autograft (includes obtaining graft)

📷 30.8 ✂ 30.8 **FUD** 090 J A2 80 50 ▱

AMA: 2018,Sep,7

TMJ syndrome is often related to stress and tooth-grinding; in other cases, arthritis, injury, poorly aligned teeth, or ill-fitting dentures may be the cause

Upper joint space
Lower joint space
Articular disc (meniscus)
Cutaway detail
Condyle
Mandible

Cutaway view of temporomandibular joint (TMJ)

Symptoms include facial pain and chewing problems; TMJ syndrome occurs more frequently in women

21242 Arthroplasty, temporomandibular joint, with allograft

📷 30.0 ✂ 30.0 **FUD** 090 J A2 80 50 ▱

AMA: 2018,Sep,7

21243 Arthroplasty, temporomandibular joint, with prosthetic joint replacement

📷 48.9 ✂ 48.9 **FUD** 090 J J8 80 50 ▱

AMA: 2018,Sep,7

21244 Reconstruction of mandible, extraoral, with transosteal bone plate (eg, mandibular staple bone plate)

📷 29.3 ✂ 29.3 **FUD** 090 J J8 80 ▱

AMA: 2018,Sep,7

21245 Reconstruction of mandible or maxilla, subperiosteal implant; partial

📷 26.8 ✂ 34.5 **FUD** 090 J A2 80 ▱

AMA: 2018,Sep,7

21246 complete

📷 25.4 ✂ 25.4 **FUD** 090 J A2 80 ▱

AMA: 2018,Sep,7

21247 Reconstruction of mandibular condyle with bone and cartilage autografts (includes obtaining grafts) (eg, for hemifacial microsomia)

📷 45.9 ✂ 45.9 **FUD** 090 C 80 50 ▱

AMA: 2018,Sep,7

21248 Reconstruction of mandible or maxilla, endosteal implant (eg, blade, cylinder); partial

EXCLUDES Midface reconstruction (21141-21160)

📷 25.3 ✂ 31.1 **FUD** 090 J A2 ▱

AMA: 2018,Sep,7

21249 complete

EXCLUDES Midface reconstruction (21141-21160)

📷 33.4 ✂ 40.1 **FUD** 090 J A2 80 ▱

AMA: 2018,Sep,7

21255 Reconstruction of zygomatic arch and glenoid fossa with bone and cartilage (includes obtaining autografts)

📷 40.6 ✂ 40.6 **FUD** 090 C 80 50 ▱

AMA: 2018,Sep,7

21256 Reconstruction of orbit with osteotomies (extracranial) and with bone grafts (includes obtaining autografts) (eg, micro-ophthalmia)

📷 35.7 ✂ 35.7 **FUD** 090 J 62 80 50 ▱

AMA: 2018,Sep,7

21260 Periorbital osteotomies for orbital hypertelorism, with bone grafts; extracranial approach

📷 40.1 ✂ 40.1 **FUD** 090 J 62 80 ▱

AMA: 2018,Sep,7

21261 combined intra- and extracranial approach

📷 71.1 ✂ 71.1 **FUD** 090 J 62 80 ▱

AMA: 2018,Sep,7

21263 with forehead advancement

📷 65.7 ✂ 65.7 **FUD** 090 J 62 80 ▱

AMA: 2018,Sep,7

A frontal craniotomy is performed, the brain retracted, and the orbit approached from inside the skull; frontal bone is advanced and secured

Grafts

Osteotomies are cut 360 degrees around the orbit; portions of nasal and ethmoid bones are removed

Grafts are placed and the bony orbits realigned

21267 Orbital repositioning, periorbital osteotomies, unilateral, with bone grafts; extracranial approach

📷 46.8 ✂ 46.8 **FUD** 090 J J8 80 50 ▱

AMA: 2018,Sep,7

21268 combined intra- and extracranial approach

📷 58.8 ✂ 58.8 **FUD** 090 C 80 50 ▱

AMA: 2018,Sep,7

21270 Malar augmentation, prosthetic material

EXCLUDES Augmentation procedure with bone graft (21210)

📷 21.7 ✂ 29.1 **FUD** 090 J A2 80 50 ▱

AMA: 2018,Sep,7

21275 Secondary revision of orbitocraniofacial reconstruction

📷 24.1 ✂ 24.1 **FUD** 090 J 62 80 ▱

AMA: 2018,Sep,7

21280 Medial canthopexy (separate procedure)

EXCLUDES Reconstruction canthus (67950)

📷 16.4 ✂ 16.4 **FUD** 090 J A2 80 50 ▱

AMA: 2018,Sep,7

21282 Lateral canthopexy

📷 11.0 ✂ 11.0 **FUD** 090 J A2 50 ▱

AMA: 2018,Sep,7

21295 Reduction of masseter muscle and bone (eg, for treatment of benign masseteric hypertrophy); extraoral approach

📷 5.39 ✂ 5.39 **FUD** 090 T A2 80 50 ▱

AMA: 2018,Sep,7

26/TC PC/TC Only   A2-Z3 ASC Payment   50 Bilateral   ♂ Male Only   ♀ Female Only   📷 Facility RVU   ✂ Non-Facility RVU   ▱ CCI   ✖ CLIA
FUD Follow-up Days   CMS: IOM   AMA: CPT Asst   A-Y OPPSI   80/80 Surg Assist Allowed / w/Doc   ▱ Lab Crosswalk   ▱ Radiology Crosswalk

46   CPT © 2021 American Medical Association. All Rights Reserved.   © 2021 Optum360, LLC

21296	**intraoral approach**

🚑 11.6   ⚕ 11.6   **FUD** 090   [J] [A2] [80] [50] 🖵

AMA: 2018,Sep,7

21299	**Unlisted craniofacial and maxillofacial procedure**

🚑 0.00   ⚕ 0.00   **FUD** YYY   [T] [80] 🖵

AMA: 2018,Sep,7

21310-21499 Care of Fractures/Dislocations of the Cranial and Facial Bones

EXCLUDES Closed treatment skull fracture, report with appropriate E/M service
Open treatment skull fracture (62000-62010)

21310	~~Closed treatment of nasal bone fracture without manipulation~~

▲	21315	**Closed treatment of nasal bone fracture with manipulation; without stabilization**

EXCLUDES Closed treatment without manipulation or stabilization, report appropriate E/M service

🚑 4.31   ⚕ 7.80   **FUD** 010   [T] [A2] 🖵

AMA: 2019,Nov,12; 2019,Sep,3; 2018,Sep,7; 2018,Jan,3

▲	21320	**with stabilization**

EXCLUDES Closed treatment without maniputaion or stabilization, report appropriate E/M service

🚑 3.83   ⚕ 7.23   **FUD** 010   [J] [A2] 🖵

AMA: 2019,Sep,3; 2018,Sep,7

21325	**Open treatment of nasal fracture; uncomplicated**

🚑 12.4   ⚕ 12.4   **FUD** 090   [J] [A2] [80] 🖵

AMA: 2018,Sep,7

21330	**complicated, with internal and/or external skeletal fixation**

🚑 16.0   ⚕ 16.0   **FUD** 090   [J] [A2] [80] 🖵

AMA: 2018,Sep,7

21335	**with concomitant open treatment of fractured septum**

🚑 20.3   ⚕ 20.3   **FUD** 090   [J] [A2] 🖵

AMA: 2018,Sep,7

21336	**Open treatment of nasal septal fracture, with or without stabilization**

🚑 18.2   ⚕ 18.2   **FUD** 090   [J] [A2] [80] 🖵

AMA: 2018,Sep,7

21337	**Closed treatment of nasal septal fracture, with or without stabilization**

🚑 8.41   ⚕ 11.7   **FUD** 090   [J] [A2] [80] 🖵

AMA: 2019,Sep,3; 2018,Sep,7

21338	**Open treatment of nasoethmoid fracture; without external fixation**

🚑 18.8   ⚕ 18.8   **FUD** 090   [J] [J8] [80] 🖵

AMA: 2018,Sep,7

21339	**with external fixation**

🚑 21.3   ⚕ 21.3   **FUD** 090   [J] [A2] [80] 🖵

AMA: 2018,Sep,7

21340	**Percutaneous treatment of nasoethmoid complex fracture, with splint, wire or headcap fixation, including repair of canthal ligaments and/or the nasolacrimal apparatus**

🚑 21.3   ⚕ 21.3   **FUD** 090   [J] [A2] [80] 🖵

AMA: 2018,Sep,7

21343	**Open treatment of depressed frontal sinus fracture**

🚑 30.7   ⚕ 30.7   **FUD** 090   [C] [80] 🖵

AMA: 2018,Sep,7

21344	**Open treatment of complicated (eg, comminuted or involving posterior wall) frontal sinus fracture, via coronal or multiple approaches**

🚑 39.7   ⚕ 39.7   **FUD** 090   [C] [80] 🖵

AMA: 2018,Sep,7

21345	**Closed treatment of nasomaxillary complex fracture (LeFort II type), with interdental wire fixation or fixation of denture or splint**

🚑 17.9   ⚕ 22.2   **FUD** 090   [T] [A2] [80] 🖵

AMA: 2018,Sep,7

21346	**Open treatment of nasomaxillary complex fracture (LeFort II type); with wiring and/or local fixation**

🚑 27.4   ⚕ 27.4   **FUD** 090   [J] [62] 🖵

AMA: 2018,Sep,7

21347	**requiring multiple open approaches**

🚑 29.0   ⚕ 29.0   **FUD** 090   [C] [80] 🖵

AMA: 2018,Sep,7

21348	**with bone grafting (includes obtaining graft)**

🚑 31.0   ⚕ 31.0   **FUD** 090   [C] [80] 🖵

AMA: 2018,Sep,7

21355	**Percutaneous treatment of fracture of malar area, including zygomatic arch and malar tripod, with manipulation**

🚑 9.18   ⚕ 12.2   **FUD** 010   [J] [A2] [80] [50] 🖵

AMA: 2018,Sep,7

21356	**Open treatment of depressed zygomatic arch fracture (eg, Gillies approach)**

🚑 10.7   ⚕ 14.2   **FUD** 010   [J] [A2] [80] [50] 🖵

AMA: 2018,Sep,7

21360	**Open treatment of depressed malar fracture, including zygomatic arch and malar tripod**

🚑 14.6   ⚕ 14.6   **FUD** 090   [J] [62] [80] [50] 🖵

AMA: 2018,Sep,7

21365	**Open treatment of complicated (eg, comminuted or involving cranial nerve foramina) fracture(s) of malar area, including zygomatic arch and malar tripod; with internal fixation and multiple surgical approaches**

🚑 31.6   ⚕ 31.6   **FUD** 090   [J] [62] [80] [50] 🖵

AMA: 2018,Sep,7

21366	**with bone grafting (includes obtaining graft)**

🚑 36.5   ⚕ 36.5   **FUD** 090   [C] [80] [50] 🖵

AMA: 2018,Sep,7

21385	**Open treatment of orbital floor blowout fracture; transantral approach (Caldwell-Luc type operation)**

🚑 21.5   ⚕ 21.5   **FUD** 090   [J] [62] [80] [50] 🖵

AMA: 2018,Sep,7

21386	**periorbital approach**

🚑 18.7   ⚕ 18.7   **FUD** 090   [J] [62] [80] [50] 🖵

AMA: 2018,Sep,7

21387	**combined approach**

🚑 22.5   ⚕ 22.5   **FUD** 090   [J] [62] [80] [50] 🖵

AMA: 2018,Sep,7

21390	**periorbital approach, with alloplastic or other implant**

🚑 22.9   ⚕ 22.9   **FUD** 090   [J] [62] [80] [50] 🖵

AMA: 2020,Dec,11; 2018,Sep,7

21395	**periorbital approach with bone graft (includes obtaining graft)**

🚑 29.0   ⚕ 29.0   **FUD** 090   [J] [62] [80] [50] 🖵

AMA: 2018,Sep,7

21400	**Closed treatment of fracture of orbit, except blowout; without manipulation**

🚑 4.59   ⚕ 5.77   **FUD** 090   [T] [A2] [80] [50] 🖵

AMA: 2018,Sep,7

21401	**with manipulation**

🚑 9.23   ⚕ 14.7   **FUD** 090   [T] [A2] [80] [50] 🖵

AMA: 2018,Sep,7

21406	**Open treatment of fracture of orbit, except blowout; without implant**

🚑 16.5   ⚕ 16.5   **FUD** 090   [J] [62] [80] [50] 🖵

AMA: 2020,Dec,11; 2018,Sep,7

21407	**with implant**

🚑 18.4   ⚕ 18.4   **FUD** 090   [J] [62] [80] [50] 🖵

AMA: 2020,Dec,11; 2018,Sep,7

21408	**with bone grafting (includes obtaining graft)**

🚑 26.1   ⚕ 26.1   **FUD** 090   [J] [62] [80] [50] 🖵

AMA: 2018,Sep,7

● New Code   ▲ Revised Code   ○ Reinstated   ⬤ New Web Release   ▲ Revised Web Release   + Add-on   Unlisted   Not Covered   # Resequenced
⑤⓪ Optum Mod 50 Exempt   Ⓢ AMA Mod 51 Exempt   ⑤① Optum Mod 51 Exempt   ⑥③ Mod 63 Exempt   ✗ Non-FDA Drug   ★ Telemedicine   Ⓜ Maternity   Ⓐ Age Edit

21421 Closed treatment of palatal or maxillary fracture (LeFort I type), with interdental wire fixation or fixation of denture or splint
　　🚗 16.1　⚕ 19.1　**FUD** 090　　　　　J A2 80 ▭
AMA: 2018,Sep,7

21422 Open treatment of palatal or maxillary fracture (LeFort I type);
　　🚗 18.4　⚕ 18.4　**FUD** 090　　　　　C 80 ▭
AMA: 2018,Sep,7

21423 complicated (comminuted or involving cranial nerve foramina), multiple approaches
　　🚗 22.0　⚕ 22.0　**FUD** 090　　　　　C 80 ▭
AMA: 2018,Sep,7

21431 Closed treatment of craniofacial separation (LeFort III type) using interdental wire fixation of denture or splint
　　🚗 19.9　⚕ 19.9　**FUD** 090　　　　　C 80 ▭
AMA: 2018,Sep,7

21432 Open treatment of craniofacial separation (LeFort III type); with wiring and/or internal fixation
　　🚗 20.7　⚕ 20.7　**FUD** 090　　　　　C 80 ▭
AMA: 2018,Sep,7

21433 complicated (eg, comminuted or involving cranial nerve foramina), multiple surgical approaches
　　🚗 50.5　⚕ 50.5　**FUD** 090　　　　　C 80 ▭
AMA: 2018,Sep,7

21435 complicated, utilizing internal and/or external fixation techniques (eg, head cap, halo device, and/or intermaxillary fixation)
　　EXCLUDES Removal internal or external fixation (20670)
　　🚗 40.7　⚕ 40.7　**FUD** 090　　　　　C 80 ▭
AMA: 2018,Sep,7

21436 complicated, multiple surgical approaches, internal fixation, with bone grafting (includes obtaining graft)
　　🚗 59.2　⚕ 59.2　**FUD** 090　　　　. C 80 ▭
AMA: 2018,Sep,7

21440 Closed treatment of mandibular or maxillary alveolar ridge fracture (separate procedure)
　　🚗 14.0　⚕ 17.3　**FUD** 090　　　　　J P3 80 ▭
AMA: 2018,Sep,7

21445 Open treatment of mandibular or maxillary alveolar ridge fracture (separate procedure)
　　🚗 17.9　⚕ 22.2　**FUD** 090　　　　　J A2 80 ▭
AMA: 2018,Sep,7

21450 Closed treatment of mandibular fracture; without manipulation
　　🚗 13.4　⚕ 16.4　**FUD** 090　　　　　T J8 80 ▭
AMA: 2018,Sep,7

21451 with manipulation
　　🚗 18.0　⚕ 21.5　**FUD** 090　　　　　T A2 80 ▭
AMA: 2018,Sep,7

21452 Percutaneous treatment of mandibular fracture, with external fixation
　　🚗 12.0　⚕ 20.1　**FUD** 090　　　　　J J8 80 ▭
AMA: 2018,Sep,7

Comminuted fractures

Metal or acrylic bar

Rods and pins placed in drilled holes

21453 Closed treatment of mandibular fracture with interdental fixation
　　🚗 23.6　⚕ 27.6　**FUD** 090　　　　　J A2 80 ▭
AMA: 2018,Sep,7; 2018,Jan,8; 2017,Jan,8; 2016,Jan,13

21454 Open treatment of mandibular fracture with external fixation
　　🚗 15.6　⚕ 15.6　**FUD** 090　　　　　J J8 80 ▭
AMA: 2018,Sep,7

21461 Open treatment of mandibular fracture; without interdental fixation
　　🚗 28.8　⚕ 57.4　**FUD** 090　　　　　J J8 ▭
AMA: 2018,Sep,7

21462 with interdental fixation
　　🚗 31.9　⚕ 61.4　**FUD** 090　　　　　J J8 80 ▭
AMA: 2018,Sep,7

21465 Open treatment of mandibular condylar fracture
　　🚗 24.1　⚕ 24.1　**FUD** 090　　　　　J J8 80 50 ▭
AMA: 2018,Sep,7

21470 Open treatment of complicated mandibular fracture by multiple surgical approaches including internal fixation, interdental fixation, and/or wiring of dentures or splints
　　🚗 34.5　⚕ 34.5　**FUD** 090　　　　　J J8 80 ▭
AMA: 2018,Sep,7; 2018,Jan,8; 2017,Jan,8; 2016,Jan,13

21480 Closed treatment of temporomandibular dislocation; initial or subsequent
　　🚗 0.91　⚕ 3.07　**FUD** 000　　　　　T A2 50 ▭
AMA: 2018,Sep,7

21485 complicated (eg, recurrent requiring intermaxillary fixation or splinting), initial or subsequent
　　🚗 20.6　⚕ 25.2　**FUD** 090　　　　　T A2 80 50 ▭
AMA: 2018,Sep,7

21490 Open treatment of temporomandibular dislocation
　　EXCLUDES Closed treatment larynx fracture, report with appropriate E/M service
　　　　　　Interdental wiring (21497)
　　🚗 23.7　⚕ 23.7　**FUD** 090　　　　　J A2 80 50 ▭
AMA: 2018,Sep,7

21497 Interdental wiring, for condition other than fracture
　　🚗 16.4　⚕ 19.6　**FUD** 090　　　　　T A2 80 ▭
AMA: 2018,Sep,7; 2018,Jan,8; 2017,Jan,8; 2016,Jan,13

21499 Unlisted musculoskeletal procedure, head
　　EXCLUDES Unlisted procedures craniofacial or maxillofacial areas (21299)
　　🚗 0.00　⚕ 0.00　**FUD** YYY　　　　　T 80 ▭
AMA: 2018,Sep,7

21501-21510 Surgical Incision for Drainage: Chest and Soft Tissues of Neck

> EXCLUDES
> *Biopsy flank or back (21920-21925)*
> *Simple incision and drainage abscess or hematoma (10060, 10140)*
> *Tumor removal flank or back (21930-21936)*

21501 **Incision and drainage, deep abscess or hematoma, soft tissues of neck or thorax;**

> EXCLUDES
> *Deep incision and drainage posterior spine (22010-22015)*

🔪 9.37 ☘ 13.4 **FUD** 090   J A2 🔲

AMA: 2018,Sep,7; 2018,Jan,8; 2017,Jan,8; 2016,Jan,13

21502 **with partial rib ostectomy**

🔪 14.5 ☘ 14.5 **FUD** 090   J A2 80 🔲

AMA: 2018,Sep,7

21510 **Incision, deep, with opening of bone cortex (eg, for osteomyelitis or bone abscess), thorax**

🔪 12.9 ☘ 12.9 **FUD** 090   C 80 🔲

AMA: 2018,Sep,7

21550 Soft Tissue Biopsy of Chest or Neck

> EXCLUDES
> *Biopsy bone (20220-20251)*
> *Soft tissue needle biopsy (20206)*

21550 **Biopsy, soft tissue of neck or thorax**

🔪 4.47 ☘ 7.50 **FUD** 010   J G2 🔲

AMA: 2018,Sep,7

21552-21558 [21552, 21554] Excision Soft Tissue Tumors Chest and Neck

> INCLUDES
> Any necessary elevation tissue planes or dissection
> Measurement tumor and necessary margin at greatest diameter prior to excision
> Resection without removal significant normal tissue
> Simple and intermediate repairs
> Excision types:
>   Fascial or subfascial soft tissue tumors: simple and marginal resection tumors found either in or below deep fascia, not involving bone or excision substantial amount normal tissue; primarily benign and intramuscular tumors
>   Radical resection soft tissue tumor: wide resection tumor, involving substantial margins normal tissue and may involve tissue removal from one or more layers; most often malignant or aggressive benign
>   Subcutaneous: simple and marginal resection tumors in subcutaneous tissue above deep fascia; most often benign

> EXCLUDES
> *Complex repair*
> *Excision benign cutaneous lesions (eg, sebaceous cyst) (11400-11426)*
> *Radical resection cutaneous tumors (eg, melanoma) (11600-11626)*
> *Significant vessel exploration or neuroplasty*

21552 **Resequenced code. See code following 21555.**

21554 **Resequenced code. See code following 21556.**

21555 **Excision, tumor, soft tissue of neck or anterior thorax, subcutaneous; less than 3 cm**

🔪 8.79 ☘ 12.2 **FUD** 090   J G2 🔲

AMA: 2018,Sep,7; 2018,Jan,8; 2017,Jan,8; 2016,Jan,13

\# **21552** **3 cm or greater**

🔪 12.8 ☘ 12.8 **FUD** 090   J G2 80 🔲

AMA: 2018,Sep,7

21556 **Excision, tumor, soft tissue of neck or anterior thorax, subfascial (eg, intramuscular); less than 5 cm**

🔪 15.2 ☘ 15.2 **FUD** 090   J G2 🔲

AMA: 2018,Sep,7

\# **21554** **5 cm or greater**

🔪 21.0 ☘ 21.0 **FUD** 090   J G2 80 🔲

AMA: 2018,Sep,7

21557 **Radical resection of tumor (eg, sarcoma), soft tissue of neck or anterior thorax; less than 5 cm**

🔪 27.4 ☘ 27.4 **FUD** 090   J G2 80 🔲

AMA: 2020,Apr,10; 2018,Sep,7; 2018,Jan,8; 2017,Jan,8; 2016,Jan,13

21558 **5 cm or greater**

🔪 38.7 ☘ 38.7 **FUD** 090   J G2 80 🔲

AMA: 2020,Apr,10; 2018,Sep,7

21600-21632 Bony Resection Chest and Neck

21600 **Excision of rib, partial**

> EXCLUDES
> *Extensive debridement (11044, 11047)*
> *Radical resection, chest wall/rib cage for tumor (21601)*

🔪 15.9 ☘ 15.9 **FUD** 090   J A2 80 🔲

AMA: 2018,Sep,7; 2018,Jan,8; 2017,Jan,8; 2016,Jan,13

21601 **Excision of chest wall tumor including rib(s)**

> EXCLUDES
> *Exploratory thoracotomy (32100)*
> *Resection apical lung tumor (32503-32504)*
> *Thoracentesis (32554-32555)*
> *Tube thoracostomy (32551)*

🔪 34.1 ☘ 34.1 **FUD** 090   G2 80 🔲

AMA: 2019,Dec,4

21602 **Excision of chest wall tumor involving rib(s), with plastic reconstruction; without mediastinal lymphadenectomy**

> EXCLUDES
> *Exploratory thoracotomy (32100)*
> *Resection apical lung tumor (32503-32504)*
> *Thoracentesis (32554-32555)*
> *Tube thoracostomy (32551)*

🔪 45.8 ☘ 45.8 **FUD** 090   80 🔲

AMA: 2019,Dec,4

21603 **with mediastinal lymphadenectomy**

> EXCLUDES
> *Exploratory thoracotomy (32100)*
> *Resection apical lung tumor (32503-32504)*
> *Thoracentesis (32554-32555)*
> *Tube thoracostomy (32551)*

🔪 50.7 ☘ 50.7 **FUD** 090   80 🔲

AMA: 2019,Dec,4

21610 **Costotransversectomy (separate procedure)**

🔪 34.5 ☘ 34.5 **FUD** 090   J A2 80 🔲

AMA: 2018,Sep,7

21615 **Excision first and/or cervical rib;**

🔪 17.8 ☘ 17.8 **FUD** 090   C 80 50 🔲

AMA: 2018,Sep,7; 2018,Jan,8; 2017,Jan,8; 2016,Jan,13

21616 **with sympathectomy**

🔪 20.7 ☘ 20.7 **FUD** 090   C 80 50 🔲

AMA: 2018,Sep,7

21620 **Ostectomy of sternum, partial**

🔪 14.5 ☘ 14.5 **FUD** 090   C 80 🔲

AMA: 2018,Sep,7

21627 **Sternal debridement**

> EXCLUDES
> *Debridement with sternotomy closure (21750)*

🔪 15.4 ☘ 15.4 **FUD** 090   C 80 🔲

AMA: 2018,Sep,7; 2018,Jan,8; 2017,Jan,8; 2016,Jan,13

21630 **Radical resection of sternum;**

🔪 35.1 ☘ 35.1 **FUD** 090   C 80 🔲

AMA: 2018,Sep,7

21632 **with mediastinal lymphadenectomy**

🔪 34.9 ☘ 34.9 **FUD** 090   C 80 🔲

AMA: 2018,Sep,7

21685-21750 Repair/Reconstruction Chest and Soft Tissues Neck

> EXCLUDES
> *Repair simple wounds (12001-12007)*

21685 **Hyoid myotomy and suspension**

🔪 28.2 ☘ 28.2 **FUD** 090   J G2 80 🔲

AMA: 2018,Sep,7; 2018,Jan,8; 2017,Jan,8; 2016,Jan,13

21700 **Division of scalenus anticus; without resection of cervical rib**

🔪 10.3 ☘ 10.3 **FUD** 090   J A2 80 50 🔲

AMA: 2018,Sep,7

21705 **with resection of cervical rib**

🔪 15.5 ☘ 15.5 **FUD** 090   C 80 50 🔲

AMA: 2018,Sep,7; 2018,Jan,8; 2017,Jan,8; 2016,Jan,13

● New Code   ▲ Revised Code   ○ Reinstated   ● New Web Release   ▲ Revised Web Release   + Add-on   Unlisted   Not Covered   # Resequenced
50 Optum Mod 50 Exempt   Ⓢ AMA Mod 51 Exempt   51 Optum Mod 51 Exempt   63 Mod 63 Exempt   ✏ Non-FDA Drug   ★ Telemedicine   M Maternity   A Age Edit

21720 Division of sternocleidomastoid for torticollis, open operation; without cast application

> EXCLUDES *Transection spinal accessory and cervical nerves (63191, 64722)*

> 📷 15.0   ✂ 15.0   **FUD** 090   J A2 80 📋

> **AMA:** 2018,Sep,7

21725 with cast application

> EXCLUDES *Transection spinal accessory and cervical nerves (63191, 64722)*

> 📷 15.5   ✂ 15.5   **FUD** 090   T A2 80 📋

> **AMA:** 2018,Sep,7

21740 Reconstructive repair of pectus excavatum or carinatum; open

> 📷 29.7   ✂ 29.7   **FUD** 090   C 80 📋

> **AMA:** 2018,Sep,7

21742 minimally invasive approach (Nuss procedure), without thoracoscopy

> 📷 0.00   ✂ 0.00   **FUD** 090   J 62 80 📋

> **AMA:** 2018,Sep,7

21743 minimally invasive approach (Nuss procedure), with thoracoscopy

> 📷 0.00   ✂ 0.00   **FUD** 090   J 62 80 📋

> **AMA:** 2019,Nov,14; 2018,Sep,7

21750 Closure of median sternotomy separation with or without debridement (separate procedure)

> 📷 19.7   ✂ 19.7   **FUD** 090   C 80 📋

> **AMA:** 2018,Sep,7; 2018,Jan,8; 2017,Jan,8; 2016,Jan,13

21811-21825 Fracture Care: Ribs and Sternum

> EXCLUDES *Closed treatment uncomplicated rib fractures, report appropriate E/M services*

21811 Open treatment of rib fracture(s) with internal fixation, includes thoracoscopic visualization when performed, unilateral; 1-3 ribs

> 📷 17.2   ✂ 17.2   **FUD** 000   J 80 50 📋

> **AMA:** 2018,Sep,7; 2018,Jan,8; 2017,Jan,8; 2016,Jan,13

21812 4-6 ribs

> 📷 21.0   ✂ 21.0   **FUD** 000   J 80 50 📋

> **AMA:** 2018,Sep,7; 2018,Jan,8; 2017,Jan,8; 2016,Jan,13

21813 7 or more ribs

> 📷 28.7   ✂ 28.7   **FUD** 000   J 80 50 📋

> **AMA:** 2018,Sep,7; 2018,Jan,8; 2017,Jan,8; 2016,Jan,13

21820 Closed treatment of sternum fracture

> 📷 4.10   ✂ 4.08   **FUD** 090   T A2 📋

> **AMA:** 2018,Sep,7

21825 Open treatment of sternum fracture with or without skeletal fixation

> EXCLUDES *Treatment sternoclavicular dislocation (23520-23532)*

> 📷 15.6   ✂ 15.6   **FUD** 090   C 80 📋

> **AMA:** 2018,Sep,7

21899 Unlisted Procedures of Chest or Neck

CMS: 100-04,4,180.3 Unlisted Service or Procedure

21899 Unlisted procedure, neck or thorax

> 📷 0.00   ✂ 0.00   **FUD** YYY   T 80 📋

> **AMA:** 2018,Sep,7; 2018,Jan,8; 2017,Jan,8; 2016,Jan,13

21920-21925 Biopsy Soft Tissue of Back and Flank

> EXCLUDES *Soft tissue needle biopsy (20206)*

21920 Biopsy, soft tissue of back or flank; superficial

> 📷 4.55   ✂ 7.30   **FUD** 010   J P3 📋

> **AMA:** 2018,Sep,7

21925 deep

> 📷 10.4   ✂ 13.4   **FUD** 090   J A2 📋

> **AMA:** 2018,Sep,7

21930-21936 Excision Soft Tissue Tumors Back or Flank

> INCLUDES Any necessary elevation tissue planes or dissection
> Measurement tumor and necessary margin at greatest diameter prior to excision
> Simple and intermediate repairs
> Excision types:
> Fascial or subfascial soft tissue tumors: simple and marginal resection tumors found either in or below deep fascia, not involving bone or excision substantial amount normal tissue; most often benign and intramuscular tumors
> Radical resection soft tissue tumor: wide resection of tumor, involving substantial margins normal tissue and may include tissue removal from one or more layers; most often malignant or aggressive benign
> Subcutaneous: simple and marginal resection tumors in subcutaneous tissue above deep fascia; most often benign

> EXCLUDES *Complex repair*
> *Excision benign cutaneous lesions (eg, sebaceous cyst) (11400-11406)*
> *Radical resection cutaneous tumors (eg, melanoma) (11600-11606)*
> *Significant vessel exploration or neuroplasty*

21930 Excision, tumor, soft tissue of back or flank, subcutaneous; less than 3 cm

> 📷 10.4   ✂ 13.8   **FUD** 090   J 62 📋

> **AMA:** 2018,Sep,7; 2018,Jan,8; 2017,Jan,8; 2016,Jan,13

21931 3 cm or greater

> 📷 13.6   ✂ 13.6   **FUD** 090   J 62 80 📋

> **AMA:** 2018,Sep,7

21932 Excision, tumor, soft tissue of back or flank, subfascial (eg, intramuscular); less than 5 cm

> 📷 19.0   ✂ 19.0   **FUD** 090   J 62 80 📋

> **AMA:** 2018,Sep,7

21933 5 cm or greater

> 📷 21.3   ✂ 21.3   **FUD** 090   J 62 80 📋

> **AMA:** 2018,Sep,7

21935 Radical resection of tumor (eg, sarcoma), soft tissue of back or flank; less than 5 cm

> 📷 29.7   ✂ 29.7   **FUD** 090   J 62 📋

> **AMA:** 2018,Sep,7

21936 5 cm or greater

> 📷 40.9   ✂ 40.9   **FUD** 090   J 62 80 📋

> **AMA:** 2018,Sep,7

22010-22015 Incision for Drainage of Deep Spinal Abscess

> EXCLUDES *Incision and drainage hematoma (10060, 10140)*
> *Injection:*
> *Chemonucleolysis (62292)*
> *Discography (62290-62291)*
> *Facet joint (64490-64495, [64633, 64634, 64635, 64636])*
> *Myelography (62284)*
> *Needle/trocar biopsy (20220-20225)*

22010 Incision and drainage, open, of deep abscess (subfascial), posterior spine; cervical, thoracic, or cervicothoracic

> 📷 27.7   ✂ 27.7   **FUD** 090   C 80 📋

> **AMA:** 2018,Sep,7

22015 lumbar, sacral, or lumbosacral

> EXCLUDES *Incision and drainage, complex, postoperative wound infection (10180)*
> *Incision and drainage, open, deep abscess (subfascial), posterior spine; cervical, thoracic, or cervicothoracic (22010)*
> *Removal posterior nonsegmental instrumentation (eg, Harrington rod) (22850)*
> *Removal posterior segmental instrumentation (22852)*

> 📷 27.2   ✂ 27.2   **FUD** 090   C 📋

> **AMA:** 2018,Sep,7

| 26/TC PC/TC Only | A2-Z3 ASC Payment | 50 Bilateral | ♂ Male Only | ♀ Female Only | 📷 Facility RVU | ✂ Non-Facility RVU | 📋 CCI | CLIA |
| **FUD** Follow-up Days | **CMS:** IOM | **AMA:** CPT Asst | A-Y OPPSI | 80/80 Surg Assist Allowed / w/Doc | Lab Crosswalk | Radiology Crosswalk | | |

50

CPT © 2021 American Medical Association. All Rights Reserved.

© 2021 Optum360, LLC

22100-22103 Partial Resection Vertebral Component

EXCLUDES Back or flank biopsy (21920-21925)
Bone biopsy (20220-20251)
Bone grafting procedures (20930-20938)
Harvest bone graft (20931, 20938)
Injection:
 Chemonucleolysis (62292)
 Discography (62290-62291)
 Facet joint (64490-64495, [64633, 64634, 64635, 64636])
 Myelography (62284)
Osteotomy (22210-22226)
Reconstruction after vertebral body resection (22585, 63082, 63086, 63088, 63091)
Removal tumor flank or back (21930)
Soft tissue needle biopsy (20206)
Spinal reconstruction with bone graft or vertebral body prosthesis:
 Cervical (20931, 20938, 22554, 63081)
 Lumbar (20931, 20938, 22558, 63087, 63090)
 Thoracic (20931, 20938, 22556, 63085, 63087)
Vertebral corpectomy (63081-63091)

22100 **Partial excision of posterior vertebral component (eg, spinous process, lamina or facet) for intrinsic bony lesion, single vertebral segment; cervical**
24.8   24.8   **FUD** 090   `J` `62` `80`
AMA: 2018,Sep,7; 2018,Jan,8; 2017,Mar,7; 2017,Jan,8; 2016,Jan,13

22101 **thoracic**
25.1   25.1   **FUD** 090   `J` `62` `80`
AMA: 2018,Sep,7; 2018,Jan,8; 2017,Mar,7; 2017,Jan,8; 2016,Jan,13

22102 **lumbar**
Code also posterior spinous process distraction device insertion, when applicable (22867-22870)
23.4   23.4   **FUD** 090   `J` `62` `80`
AMA: 2018,Sep,7; 2018,Jan,8; 2017,Mar,7; 2017,Jan,8; 2016,Jan,13

+ **22103** **each additional segment (List separately in addition to code for primary procedure)**
Code first (22100-22102)
4.09   4.09   **FUD** ZZZ   `N` `N1` `80`
AMA: 2018,Sep,7

22110-22116 Partial Resection Vertebral Component without Decompression

EXCLUDES Back or flank biopsy (21920-21925)
Bone biopsy (20220-20251)
Bone grafting procedures (20930-20938)
Harvest bone graft (20931, 20938)
Injection:
 Chemonucleolysis (62292)
 Discography (62290-62291)
 Facet joint (64490-64495, [64633, 64634, 64635, 64636])
 Myelography (62284)
Osteotomy (22210-22226)
Reconstruction after vertebral body resection (22585, 63082, 63086, 63088, 63091)
Removal tumor flank or back (21930)
Soft tissue needle biopsy (20206)
Spinal reconstruction with bone graft or vertebral body prosthesis:
 Cervical (20931, 20938, 22554, 22853-22854 [22859], 63081)
 Lumbar (20931, 20938, 22558, 22853-22854 [22859], 63087, 63090)
 Thoracic (20931, 20938, 22556, 22853-22854 [22859], 63085, 63087)
Vertebral corpectomy (63081-63091)

22110 **Partial excision of vertebral body, for intrinsic bony lesion, without decompression of spinal cord or nerve root(s), single vertebral segment; cervical**
30.1   30.1   **FUD** 090   `C` `80`
AMA: 2018,Sep,7; 2018,Jan,8; 2017,Mar,7; 2017,Jan,8; 2016,Jan,13

22112 **thoracic**
32.7   32.7   **FUD** 090   `C` `80`
AMA: 2018,Sep,7; 2018,Jan,8; 2017,Mar,7; 2017,Jan,8; 2016,Jan,13

22114 **lumbar**
32.4   32.4   **FUD** 090   `C` `80`
AMA: 2018,Sep,7; 2018,Jan,8; 2017,Mar,7; 2017,Jan,8; 2016,Jan,13

+ **22116** **each additional vertebral segment (List separately in addition to code for primary procedure)**
Code first (22110-22114)
4.12   4.12   **FUD** ZZZ   `C` `80`
AMA: 2018,Sep,7

22206-22216 Spinal Osteotomy: Posterior/Posterolateral Approach

EXCLUDES Decompression spinal cord and/or nerve roots (63001-63308)
Injection:
 Chemonucleolysis (62292)
 Discography (62290-62292)
 Facet joint (64490-64495, [64633, 64634, 64635, 64636])
 Myelography (62284)
Vertebral corpectomy (63081-63091)
Code also:
 Arthrodesis (22590-22632)
 Bone grafting procedures (20930-20938)
 Spinal instrumentation (22840-22855 [22859])

22206 **Osteotomy of spine, posterior or posterolateral approach, 3 columns, 1 vertebral segment (eg, pedicle/vertebral body subtraction); thoracic**
EXCLUDES Osteotomy spine, posterior or posterolateral approach, lumbar (22207)
Procedures performed at same level (22210-22226, 22830, 63001-63048, 63055-63066, 63075-63091, 63101-63103)
71.3   71.3   **FUD** 090   `C` `80`
AMA: 2018,Sep,7; 2018,Jan,8; 2017,Mar,7; 2017,Jan,8; 2016,Jan,13

22207 **lumbar**
EXCLUDES Osteotomy spine, posterior or posterolateral approach, thoracic (22206)
Procedures performed at same level (22210-22226, 22830, 63001-63048, 63055-63066, 63075-63091, 63101-63103)
69.8   69.8   **FUD** 090   `C` `80`
AMA: 2018,Sep,7; 2018,Jan,8; 2017,Mar,7; 2017,Jan,8; 2016,Jan,13

+ **22208** **each additional vertebral segment (List separately in addition to code for primary procedure)**
EXCLUDES Procedures performed at same level (22210-22226, 22830, 63001-63048, 63055-63066, 63075-63091, 63101-63103)
Code first (22206, 22207)
17.1   17.1   **FUD** ZZZ   `C` `80`
AMA: 2018,Sep,7; 2018,Jan,8; 2017,Jan,8; 2016,Jan,13

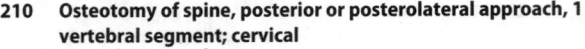

22210   **Osteotomy of spine, posterior or posterolateral approach, 1 vertebral segment; cervical**

🛏 51.7   ⚕ 51.7   **FUD** 090   C 80 ▣

AMA: 2018,Sep,7; 2018,Jan,8; 2017,Mar,7; 2017,Jan,8; 2016,Jan,13

Patient is stabilized by halo and traction to correct cervical problem

Several sections may be removed

C-6
C-7
T-1

Physician removes spinous processes, lamina

22212   **thoracic**

🛏 43.2   ⚕ 43.2   **FUD** 090   C 80 ▣

AMA: 2018,Sep,7; 2018,Jan,8; 2017,Mar,7; 2017,Jan,8; 2016,Jan,13

22214   **lumbar**

🛏 43.4   ⚕ 43.4   **FUD** 090   C 80 ▣

AMA: 2018,Sep,7; 2018,Jan,8; 2017,Mar,7; 2017,Jan,8; 2016,Jan,13

+ 22216   **each additional vertebral segment (List separately in addition to primary procedure)**

Code first (22210-22214)

🛏 10.5   ⚕ 10.5   **FUD** ZZZ   C 80 ▣

AMA: 2018,Sep,7; 2018,Jan,8; 2017,Jan,8; 2016,Jan,13

22220-22226 Spinal Osteotomy: Anterior Approach

EXCLUDES Decompression spinal cord and/or nerve roots (63001-63308)

Injection:
     Chemonucleolysis (62292)
     Discography (62290-62291)
     Facet joint (64490-64495, [64633, 64634, 64636])
     Myelography (62284)
     Needle/trocar biopsy (20220-20225)
     Verterbral corpectomy (63081-63091)

Code also:
   Arthrodesis (22590-22632)
   Bone grafting procedures (20930-20938)
   Spinal instrumentation (22840-22855 [22859])

22220   **Osteotomy of spine, including discectomy, anterior approach, single vertebral segment; cervical**

🛏 47.0   ⚕ 47.0   **FUD** 090   C 80 ▣

AMA: 2018,Sep,7; 2018,Jan,8; 2017,Mar,7; 2017,Jan,8; 2016,Jan,13

22222   **thoracic**

🛏 51.1   ⚕ 51.1   **FUD** 090   C 80 ▣

AMA: 2018,Sep,7; 2018,Jan,8; 2017,Mar,7; 2017,Jan,8; 2016,Jan,13

22224   **lumbar**

🛏 46.1   ⚕ 46.1   **FUD** 090   C 80 ▣

AMA: 2018,Sep,7; 2018,Jan,8; 2017,Mar,7; 2017,Jan,8; 2016,Jan,13

+ 22226   **each additional vertebral segment (List separately in addition to code for primary procedure)**

Code first (22220-22224)

🛏 10.5   ⚕ 10.5   **FUD** ZZZ   C 80 ▣

AMA: 2018,Sep,7

22310-22315 Closed Treatment Vertebral Fractures

EXCLUDES Injection:
     Chemonucleolysis (62292)
     Discography (62290-62291)
     Facet joint (64490-64495, [64633, 64634, 64635, 64636])
     Myelography (62284)
     Percutaneous vertebroplasty at same level (22510-22515)
     Vertebral fracture care by arthrodesis (22590-22632)

Code also:
   Arthrodesis (22590-22632)
   Bone grafting procedures (20930-20938)
   Spinal instrumentation (22840-22855 [22859])

22310   **Closed treatment of vertebral body fracture(s), without manipulation, requiring and including casting or bracing**

🛏 8.38   ⚕ 8.70   **FUD** 090   T A2 ▣

AMA: 2018,Sep,7; 2018,Jan,8; 2017,Mar,7; 2017,Jan,8; 2016,Jan,13

22315   **Closed treatment of vertebral fracture(s) and/or dislocation(s) requiring casting or bracing, with and including casting and/or bracing by manipulation or traction**

EXCLUDES Spinal manipulation (97140)

🛏 22.2   ⚕ 25.3   **FUD** 090   J A2 ▣

AMA: 2018,Sep,7; 2018,Jan,8; 2017,Mar,7; 2017,Jan,8; 2016,Jan,13

22318-22319 Open Treatment Odontoid Fracture: Anterior Approach

EXCLUDES Injection:
     Chemonucleolysis (62292)
     Discography (62290-62291)
     Facet joint (64490-64495, [64633, 64634, 64635, 64636])
     Myelography (62284)
     Needle/trocar biopsy (20220-20225)

Code also:
   Arthrodesis for fracture care (22590-22632)
   Bone grafting procedures (20930-20938)
   Spinal instrumentation (22840-22855 [22859])

22318   **Open treatment and/or reduction of odontoid fracture(s) and or dislocation(s) (including os odontoideum), anterior approach, including placement of internal fixation; without grafting**

🛏 47.6   ⚕ 47.6   **FUD** 090   C 80 ▣

AMA: 2018,Sep,7; 2018,Jan,8; 2017,Mar,7; 2017,Jan,8; 2016,Jan,13

22319   **with grafting**

🛏 53.6   ⚕ 53.6   **FUD** 090   C 80 ▣

AMA: 2018,Sep,7; 2018,May,3; 2018,Jan,8; 2017,Mar,7; 2017,Jan,8; 2016,Jan,13

22325-22328 Open Treatment Vertebral Fractures: Posterior Approach

EXCLUDES Injection:
     Chemonucleolysis (62292)
     Discography (62290-62291)
     Facet joint (64490-64495, [64633, 64634, 64635, 64636])
     Myelography (62284)
     Needle/trocar biopsy (20220-20225)
     Spine decompression (63001-63091)
     Vertebral corpectomy (63081-63091)

Code also:
   Arthrodesis (22590-22632)
   Bone grafting procedures (20930-20938)
   Spinal instrumentation (22840-22855 [22859])

22325   **Open treatment and/or reduction of vertebral fracture(s) and/or dislocation(s), posterior approach, 1 fractured vertebra or dislocated segment; lumbar**

EXCLUDES Percutaneous vertebral augmentation performed at same level (22514-22515)
     Percutaneous vertebroplasty performed at same level (22511-22512)

🛏 41.9   ⚕ 41.9   **FUD** 090   C 80 ▣

AMA: 2018,Sep,7; 2018,Jan,8; 2017,Aug,9; 2017,Mar,7; 2017,Jan,8; 2016,Jan,13

26/TC PC/TC Only   A2-Z3 ASC Payment   50 Bilateral   ♂ Male Only   ♀ Female Only   🛏 Facility RVU   ⚕ Non-Facility RVU   ▣ CCI   ☒ CLIA

FUD Follow-up Days   **CMS:** IOM   **AMA:** CPT Asst   A-Y OPPSI   80/80 Surg Assist Allowed / w/Doc   ▣ Lab Crosswalk   ▣ Radiology Crosswalk

52   CPT © 2021 American Medical Association. All Rights Reserved.   © 2021 Optum360, LLC

22326 cervical

> EXCLUDES Percutaneous vertebroplasty performed at same level (22510, 22512)

43.4   43.4   **FUD** 090   C 80

AMA: 2018,Sep,7; 2018,Jan,8; 2017,Mar,7; 2017,Jan,8; 2016,Jan,13

22327 thoracic

> EXCLUDES Percutaneous vertebral augmentation performed at same level (22515)
> Percutaneous vertebroplasty performed at same level (22510, 22512-22513)

43.7   43.7   **FUD** 090   C 80

AMA: 2018,Sep,7; 2018,Jan,8; 2017,Mar,7; 2017,Jan,8; 2016,Jan,13

+ 22328 each additional fractured vertebra or dislocated segment (List separately in addition to code for primary procedure)

Code first (22325-22327)

8.25   8.25   **FUD** ZZZ   C 80

AMA: 2018,Sep,7

22505 Spinal Manipulation with Anesthesia

> EXCLUDES Manipulation not requiring anesthesia (97140)

22505 Manipulation of spine requiring anesthesia, any region

3.76   3.76   **FUD** 010   J A2

AMA: 2018,Sep,7; 2018,Jan,8; 2017,Jan,8; 2016,Jan,13

22510-22515 Percutaneous Vertebroplasty/Kyphoplasty

> INCLUDES Radiological guidance
> When performed at same level:
>   Bone biopsy (20225)
>   Closed treatment vertebral fractures (22310, 22315)
>   Open treatment/reduction vertebral fractures (22325, 22327)

> EXCLUDES Sacroplasty/augmentation (0200T-0201T)
> Thermal destruction lumbar or sacral intraosseous basivertebral nerve ([64628, 64629])

22510 Percutaneous vertebroplasty (bone biopsy included when performed), 1 vertebral body, unilateral or bilateral injection, inclusive of all imaging guidance; cervicothoracic

12.5   47.9   **FUD** 010   J G2

AMA: 2018,Sep,7; 2018,Jan,8; 2017,Jan,8; 2016,Jan,13

22511 lumbosacral

11.7   47.3   **FUD** 010   J G2

AMA: 2018,Sep,7; 2018,Jan,8; 2017,Jan,8; 2016,Jan,13

+ 22512 each additional cervicothoracic or lumbosacral vertebral body (List separately in addition to code for primary procedure)

Code first (22510-22511)

5.96   24.4   **FUD** ZZZ   N N1

AMA: 2018,Sep,7; 2018,Jan,8; 2017,Jan,8; 2016,Jan,13

22513 Percutaneous vertebral augmentation, including cavity creation (fracture reduction and bone biopsy included when performed) using mechanical device (eg, kyphoplasty), 1 vertebral body, unilateral or bilateral cannulation, inclusive of all imaging guidance; thoracic

15.0   203.   **FUD** 010   J G2

AMA: 2018,Sep,7; 2018,Jan,8; 2017,Jan,8; 2016,Jan,13

22514 lumbar

14.0   202.   **FUD** 010   J G2

AMA: 2018,Sep,7; 2018,Jan,8; 2017,Jan,8; 2016,Jan,13

+ 22515 each additional thoracic or lumbar vertebral body (List separately in addition to code for primary procedure)

Code first (22513-22514)

6.39   105.   **FUD** ZZZ   N N1

AMA: 2018,Sep,7; 2018,Jan,8; 2017,Jan,8; 2016,Jan,13

22526-22527 Percutaneous Annuloplasty

CMS: 100-04,32,220.1 Thermal Intradiscal Procedures (TIPS)

> INCLUDES Fluoroscopic guidance (77002, 77003)

> EXCLUDES Injection:
>   Chemonucleolysis (62292)
>   Discography (62290-62291)
>   Facet joint (64490-64495, [64633, 64634, 64635, 64636])
>   Myelography (62284)
> Needle/trocar biopsy (20220-20225)
> Procedure performed by other methods (22899)

22526 Percutaneous intradiscal electrothermal annuloplasty, unilateral or bilateral including fluoroscopic guidance; single level

9.76   65.0   **FUD** 010   E

AMA: 2018,Sep,7; 2018,Jan,8; 2017,Jan,8; 2016,Jan,13

+ 22527 1 or more additional levels (List separately in addition to code for primary procedure)

Code first (22526)

4.44   53.1   **FUD** ZZZ   E

AMA: 2018,Sep,7; 2018,Jan,8; 2017,Jan,8; 2016,Jan,13

22532-22534 Spinal Fusion: Lateral Extracavitary Approach

> EXCLUDES Corpectomy (63101-63103)
> Exploration spinal fusion (22830)
> Fracture care (22310-22328)
> Injection:
>   Chemonucleolysis (62292)
>   Discography (62290-62291)
>   Facet joint (64490-64495, [64633, 64634, 64635, 64636])
>   Myelography (62284)
> Laminectomy (63001-63017)
> Needle/trocar biopsy (20220-20225)
> Osteotomy (22206-22226)

Code also:
  Bone grafting procedures (20930-20938)
  Spinal instrumentation (22840-22855 [22859])

22532 Arthrodesis, lateral extracavitary technique, including minimal discectomy to prepare interspace (other than for decompression); thoracic

52.1   52.1   **FUD** 090   C 80

AMA: 2020,May,13; 2018,Sep,7; 2018,May,3; 2018,Jan,8; 2017,Mar,7; 2017,Feb,9; 2017,Jan,8; 2016,Jan,13

22533 lumbar

48.0   48.0   **FUD** 090   C 80

AMA: 2020,May,13; 2018,Sep,7; 2018,May,3; 2018,Jan,8; 2017,Mar,7; 2017,Feb,9; 2017,Jan,8; 2016,Jan,13

+ 22534 thoracic or lumbar, each additional vertebral segment (List separately in addition to code for primary procedure)

Code first (22532-22533)

10.5   10.5   **FUD** ZZZ   C 80

AMA: 2020,May,13; 2018,Sep,7; 2018,May,3; 2017,Feb,9

22548-22634 Spinal Fusion: Anterior and Posterior Approach

EXCLUDES
Corpectomy (63081-63091)
Exploration spinal fusion (22830)
Fracture care (22310-22328)
Injection:
  Chemonucleolysis (62292)
  Discography (62290-62291)
  Facet joint (64490-64495, [64633, 64634, 64635, 64636])
  Myelography (62284)
Laminectomy (63001-63017)
Needle/trocar biopsy (20220-20225)
Osteotomy (22206-22226)
Code also:
  Bone grafting procedures (20930-20938)
  Spinal instrumentation (22840-22855 [22859])

22548   **Arthrodesis, anterior transoral or extraoral technique, clivus-C1-C2 (atlas-axis), with or without excision of odontoid process**

EXCLUDES   *Laminectomy or laminotomy with disc removal (63020-63042)*

🖥 56.4   ⚕ 56.4   **FUD** 090   C 80 ▣

AMA: 2020,May,13; 2018,Sep,7; 2018,May,3; 2018,Jan,8; 2017,Mar,7; 2017,Jan,8; 2016,Jan,13

22551   **Arthrodesis, anterior interbody, including disc space preparation, discectomy, osteophytectomy and decompression of spinal cord and/or nerve roots; cervical below C2**

INCLUDES   Operating microscope (69990)

🖥 49.3   ⚕ 49.3   **FUD** 090   J J8 80 ▣

AMA: 2020,May,13; 2018,Sep,7; 2018,Aug,10; 2018,May,3; 2018,Jan,8; 2017,Mar,7; 2017,Jan,8; 2016,May,13; 2016,Feb,12; 2016,Jan,13

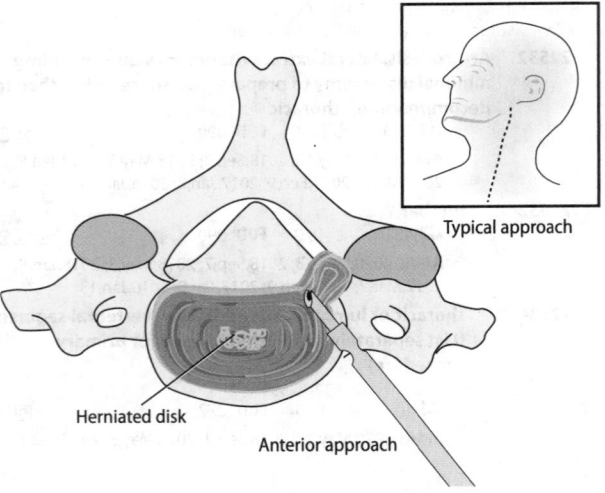

Typical approach

Herniated disk

Anterior approach

+ 22552   **cervical below C2, each additional interspace (List separately in addition to code for separate procedure)**

INCLUDES   Operating microscope (69990)
Code first (22551)

🖥 11.5   ⚕ 11.5   **FUD** ZZZ   N N1 80 ▣

AMA: 2020,May,13; 2018,Sep,7; 2018,Aug,10; 2018,May,3; 2018,Jan,8; 2017,Mar,7; 2017,Jan,8; 2016,Feb,12; 2016,Jan,13

22554   **Arthrodesis, anterior interbody technique, including minimal discectomy to prepare interspace (other than for decompression); cervical below C2**

EXCLUDES   *Anterior discectomy and interbody fusion during same operative session (regardless if performed by multiple surgeons) (22551)*
Discectomy, anterior, with decompression spinal cord and/or nerve root(s), cervical (even by separate individual) (63075-63076)

🖥 36.3   ⚕ 36.3   **FUD** 090   J J8 80 ▣

AMA: 2020,May,13; 2018,Sep,7; 2018,May,3; 2018,Jan,8; 2017,Mar,7; 2017,Jan,8; 2016,Jan,13

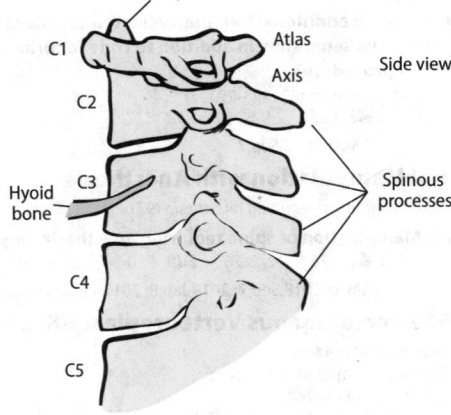

Odontoid process
C1   Atlas
         Axis   Side view
C2
Hyoid
bone   C3   Spinous
               processes
C4
C5

22556   **thoracic**

🖥 48.1   ⚕ 48.1   **FUD** 090   C 80 ▣

AMA: 2020,May,13; 2018,Sep,7; 2018,May,3; 2018,Jan,8; 2017,Mar,7; 2017,Jan,8; 2016,Jan,13

22558   **lumbar**

EXCLUDES   *Arthrodesis using pre-sacral interbody technique (22586)*

🖥 44.3   ⚕ 44.3   **FUD** 090   C 80 ▣

AMA: 2020,May,13; 2018,Sep,7; 2018,May,3; 2018,Jan,8; 2017,Mar,7; 2017,Feb,9; 2017,Jan,8; 2016,Jan,13

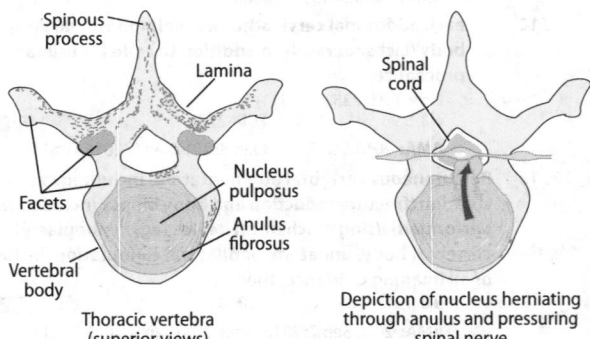

Spinous
process
         Lamina   Spinal
                        cord
Facets
         Nucleus
         pulposus
         Anulus
         fibrosus
Vertebral
body
Thoracic vertebra   Depiction of nucleus herniating
(superior views)   through anulus and pressuring
                        spinal nerve

+ 22585   **each additional interspace (List separately in addition to code for primary procedure)**

EXCLUDES   *Anterior discectomy and interbody fusion during same operative session (regardless if performed by multiple surgeons) (22552)*
Discectomy, anterior, with decompression spinal cord and/or nerve root(s), cervical (even by separate individual) (63075)
Code first (22554-22558)

🖥 9.51   ⚕ 9.51   **FUD** ZZZ   N N1 80 ▣

AMA: 2020,May,13; 2018,Sep,7; 2018,Jan,8; 2017,Jan,8; 2016,Jan,13

2G/TC PC/TC Only   A2-Z3 ASC Payment   50 Bilateral   ♂ Male Only   ♀ Female Only   🖥 Facility RVU   ⚕ Non-Facility RVU   ▣ CCI   ✖ CLIA
FUD Follow-up Days   CMS: IOM   AMA: CPT Asst   A-Y OPPSI   80/80 Surg Assist Allowed / w/Doc   ▣ Lab Crosswalk   ▣ Radiology Crosswalk

54   CPT © 2021 American Medical Association. All Rights Reserved.   © 2021 Optum360, LLC

22586 Arthrodesis, pre-sacral interbody technique, including disc space preparation, discectomy, with posterior instrumentation, with image guidance, includes bone graft when performed, L5-S1 interspace

> *INCLUDES* Radiologic guidance (77002-77003, 77011-77012)
> *EXCLUDES* Allograft and autograft spinal bone (20930-20938)
> Pelvic fixation, other than sacrum (22848)
> Posterior non-segmental instrumentation (22840)

🚑 59.6 ⚕ 59.6 **FUD** 090 [C] [80] ▣

AMA: 2020,May,13; 2018,Sep,7

22590 Arthrodesis, posterior technique, craniocervical (occiput-C2)

> *EXCLUDES* Posterior intrafacet implant insertion (0219T-0222T)

🚑 45.6 ⚕ 45.6 **FUD** 090 [C] [80] ▣

AMA: 2020,May,13; 2018,Sep,7; 2018,May,3; 2018,Jan,8; 2017,Mar,7; 2017,Jan,8; 2016,Jan,13

Skull and cervical vertebrae; posterior view

Occiput

C2 (axis)

Wires and bone graft

The physician fuses skull to C2 (axis) to stabilize cervical vertebrae; anchor holes are drilled in the occiput of the skull

22595 Arthrodesis, posterior technique, atlas-axis (C1-C2)

> *EXCLUDES* Posterior intrafacet implant insertion (0219T-0222T)

🚑 43.5 ⚕ 43.5 **FUD** 090 [C] [80] ▣

AMA: 2020,May,13; 2018,Sep,7; 2018,May,3; 2018,Jan,8; 2017,Mar,7; 2017,Jan,8; 2016,Jan,13

▲ **22600** Arthrodesis, posterior or posterolateral technique, single interspace; cervical below C2 segment

> *EXCLUDES* Posterior intrafacet implant insertion (0219T-0222T)

🚑 37.4 ⚕ 37.4 **FUD** 090 [C] [80] ▣

AMA: 2020,May,13; 2018,Sep,7; 2018,May,3; 2018,Jan,8; 2017,Mar,7; 2017,Jan,8; 2016,Jan,13

▲ **22610** thoracic (with lateral transverse technique, when performed)

> *EXCLUDES* Posterior intrafacet implant insertion (0219T-0222T)

🚑 36.7 ⚕ 36.7 **FUD** 090 [C] [80] ▣

AMA: 2020,May,13; 2018,Sep,7; 2018,May,3; 2018,Jan,8; 2017,Mar,7; 2017,Jan,8; 2016,Jan,13

▲ **22612** lumbar (with lateral transverse technique, when performed)

> *EXCLUDES* Arthrodesis at same interspace using:
> Posterior interbody technique in combination with posterior/posterolateral technique (22633)
> Posterior interbody technique only (22630)
> Posterior intrafacet implant insertion (0219T-0222T)

🚑 46.0 ⚕ 46.0 **FUD** 090 [J] [J8] [80] ▣

AMA: 2020,May,13; 2018,Sep,7; 2018,May,3; 2018,Jan,8; 2017,Mar,7; 2017,Feb,9; 2017,Jan,8; 2016,Jan,13

▲ **+ 22614** each additional interspace (List separately in addition to code for primary procedure)

> *EXCLUDES* Additional interspace athrodesis using:
> Posterior interbody technique in combination with posterior/posterolateral technique (22634)
> Posterior interbody technique only (22632)
> Posterior intrafacet implant insertion (0219T-0222T)
> Code first initial interspace arthrodesis using posterior/posterolateral technique (22600, 22610, 22612)
> Code first initial interspace arthrodesis using posterior interbody technique in combination with posterior/posterolateral technique (22633)
> Code first initial interspace arthrodesis using posterior interbody technique (22630)

🚑 11.4 ⚕ 11.4 **FUD** ZZZ [N] [N1] [80] ▣

AMA: 2020,May,13; 2018,Sep,7; 2018,Jan,8; 2017,Feb,9; 2017,Jan,8; 2016,Jan,13

22630 Arthrodesis, posterior interbody technique, including laminectomy and/or discectomy to prepare interspace (other than for decompression), single interspace; lumbar

> *EXCLUDES* Athrodesis at same interspace using:
> Posterior/posterolateral technique in combination with posterior interbody technique (22633)
> Posterior/posterolateral technique only (22612)
> Code also decompression nerves or spinal components on same vertebral segment or interspace, when performed ([63052])

🚑 45.5 ⚕ 45.5 **FUD** 090 [C] [80] ▣

AMA: 2020,May,13; 2018,Sep,7; 2018,May,3; 2018,Jan,8; 2017,Mar,7; 2017,Feb,9; 2017,Jan,8; 2016,Jan,13

+ **22632** each additional interspace (List separately in addition to code for primary procedure)

> *EXCLUDES* Additional interspace arthrodesis using:
> Posterior/posterolateral technique in combination with posterior interbody technique (22634)
> Posterior/posterolateral technique only (22614)
> Code also decompression nerves or spinal components on same vertebral segment or interspace, when performed ([63053])
> Code first initial interspace arthrodesis using posterior interbody technique (22630)
> Code first initial interspace arthrodesis using posterior/posterolateral technique (22612)
> Code first initial interspace arthrodesis using posterior/posterolateral technique in combination with posterior interbody technique (22633)

🚑 9.36 ⚕ 9.36 **FUD** ZZZ [C] [80] ▣

AMA: 2020,May,13; 2018,Sep,7; 2018,Jan,8; 2017,Feb,9; 2017,Jan,8; 2016,Jan,13

▲ **22633** **Arthrodesis, combined posterior or posterolateral technique with posterior interbody technique including laminectomy and/or discectomy sufficient to prepare interspace (other than for decompression), single interspace; lumbar**

> EXCLUDES *Arthrodesis at same interspace using:*
> *Posterior/posterolateral technique only (22612)*
> *Posterior interbody technique only (22630)*
> Code also decompression nerves or spinal components on same vertebral segment or interspace, when performed ([63052])

🚑 53.8   ⚖ 53.8   **FUD** 090   C 80 ▣

AMA: 2020,May,13; 2018,Sep,7; 2018,Jul,14; 2018,May,9; 2018,May,3; 2018,Jan,8; 2017,Mar,7; 2017,Feb,9; 2017,Jan,8; 2016,Oct,11; 2016,Jan,13

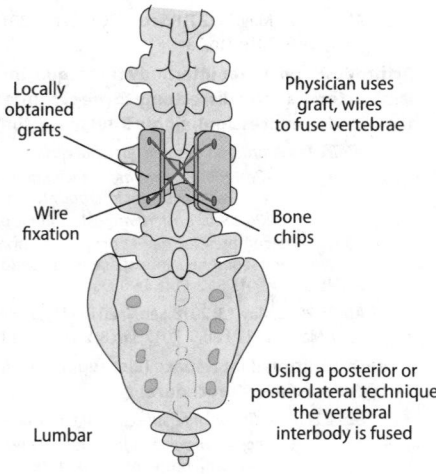

Locally obtained grafts

Physician uses graft, wires to fuse vertebrae

Wire fixation

Bone chips

Using a posterior or posterolateral technique the vertebral interbody is fused

Lumbar

▲ + **22634** **each additional interspace and segment (List separately in addition to code for primary procedure)**

> EXCLUDES *Additional interspace arthrodesis using:*
> *Posterior/posterolateral technique only (22614)*
> *Posterior interbody technique only (22632)*
> Code also decompression nerves or spinal components on same vertebral segment or interspace, when performed ([63053])
> Code first (22633)

🚑 14.4   ⚖ 14.4   **FUD** ZZZ   C 80 ▣

AMA: 2020,May,13; 2018,Sep,7; 2018,Jul,14; 2018,May,3; 2018,Jan,8; 2017,Mar,7; 2017,Feb,9; 2017,Jan,8; 2016,Jan,13

22800-22819 Procedures to Correct Anomalous Spinal Vertebrae

CMS: 100-03,150.2 Osteogenic Stimulation

> EXCLUDES *Facet injection (64490-64495, [64633, 64634, 64635, 64636])*
> *Vertebral body tethering (0656T-0657T)*
> Code also:
> Bone grafting procedures (20930-20938)
> Modifier 62 when two surgeons perform distinct arthrodesis portion
> Spinal instrumentation (22840-22855 [22859])

22800 **Arthrodesis, posterior, for spinal deformity, with or without cast; up to 6 vertebral segments**

🚑 39.3   ⚖ 39.3   **FUD** 090   C 80 ▣

AMA: 2020,May,13; 2018,Sep,7; 2018,May,3; 2018,Jan,8; 2017,Sep,14; 2017,Mar,7; 2017,Feb,9; 2017,Jan,8; 2016,Jan,13

22802 **7 to 12 vertebral segments**

🚑 61.0   ⚖ 61.0   **FUD** 090   C 80 ▣

AMA: 2020,May,13; 2018,Sep,7; 2018,Jul,14; 2018,May,3; 2018,Jan,8; 2017,Sep,14; 2017,Mar,7; 2017,Feb,9; 2017,Jan,8; 2016,Jan,13

22804 **13 or more vertebral segments**

🚑 70.3   ⚖ 70.3   **FUD** 090   C 80 ▣

AMA: 2020,May,13; 2018,Sep,7; 2018,May,3; 2018,Jan,8; 2017,Sep,14; 2017,Mar,7; 2017,Feb,9; 2017,Jan,8; 2016,Jan,13

22808 **Arthrodesis, anterior, for spinal deformity, with or without cast; 2 to 3 vertebral segments**

> INCLUDES Smith-Robinson arthrodesis

🚑 53.1   ⚖ 53.1   **FUD** 090   C 80 ▣

AMA: 2020,May,13; 2018,Sep,7; 2018,May,3; 2018,Jan,8; 2017,Sep,14; 2017,Mar,7; 2017,Jan,8; 2016,Jan,13

22810 **4 to 7 vertebral segments**

🚑 60.2   ⚖ 60.2   **FUD** 090   C 80 ▣

AMA: 2020,May,13; 2018,Sep,7; 2018,May,3; 2018,Jan,8; 2017,Sep,14; 2017,Mar,7; 2017,Jan,8; 2016,Jan,13

22812 **8 or more vertebral segments**

🚑 63.9   ⚖ 63.9   **FUD** 090   C 80 ▣

AMA: 2020,May,13; 2018,Sep,7; 2018,May,3; 2018,Jan,8; 2017,Sep,14; 2017,Mar,7; 2017,Jan,8; 2016,Jan,13

22818 **Kyphectomy, circumferential exposure of spine and resection of vertebral segment(s) (including body and posterior elements); single or 2 segments**

> EXCLUDES *Arthrodesis (22800-22804)*

🚑 62.6   ⚖ 62.6   **FUD** 090   C 80 ▣

AMA: 2020,May,13; 2018,Sep,7; 2018,Jan,8; 2017,Sep,14

22819 **3 or more segments**

> EXCLUDES *Arthrodesis (22800-22804)*

🚑 72.2   ⚖ 72.2   **FUD** 090   C 80 ▣

AMA: 2020,May,13; 2018,Sep,7; 2018,Jan,8; 2017,Sep,14

Excessively kyphotic thoracic spine may be caused by Scheuermann's disease or juvenile kyphosis

Excessive convexity in the thoracic region is known as kyphosis

Excessive concavity in the lumbar region is known as lordosis

Scoliosis is the lateral curvature of the spine; most commonly diagnosed during adolescence; occurrence is higher among females

22830 Surgical Exploration Previous Spinal Fusion

CMS: 100-03,150.2 Osteogenic Stimulation

> EXCLUDES *Arthrodesis (22532-22819)*
> *Bone grafting procedures (20930-20938)*
> *Instrumentation removal (22850, 22852, 22855)*
> *Spinal decompression (63001-63103)*
> Code also spinal instrumentation (22840-22855 [22859])

22830 **Exploration of spinal fusion**

🚑 23.6   ⚖ 23.6   **FUD** 090   C 80 ▣

AMA: 2018,Sep,7; 2018,Jan,8; 2017,Jan,8; 2016,Jan,13

26/TC PC/TC Only   A2-Z3 ASC Payment   50 Bilateral   ♂ Male Only   ♀ Female Only   🚑 Facility RVU   ⚖ Non-Facility RVU   ▣ CCI   ✖ CLIA
FUD Follow-up Days   CMS: IOM   AMA: CPT Asst   A-Y OPPSI   80/80 Surg Assist Allowed / w/Doc   Lab Crosswalk   Radiology Crosswalk

56   CPT © 2021 American Medical Association. All Rights Reserved.   © 2021 Optum360, LLC

22840-22848 Posterior, Anterior, Pelvic Spinal Instrumentation

INCLUDES Removal or revision previously placed spinal instrumentation during same session as insertion new instrumentation at levels including all or part of previously instrumented segments (22849, 22850, 22852, 22855)

EXCLUDES Arthrodesis (22532-22534, 22548-22812)
Bone grafting procedures (20930-20938)
Exploration spinal fusion (22830)
Fracture treatment (22325-22328)
Reporting more than one instrumentation code per incision

+ **22840** **Posterior non-segmental instrumentation (eg, Harrington rod technique, pedicle fixation across 1 interspace, atlantoaxial transarticular screw fixation, sublaminar wiring at C1, facet screw fixation) (List separately in addition to code for primary procedure)**

Code first (22100-22102, 22110-22114, 22206-22207, 22210-22214, 22220-22224, 22310-22327, 22532-22533, 22548-22558, 22590-22612, 22630, 22633-22634, 22800-22812, 63001-63030, 63040-63042, 63045-63047, 63050-63056, 63064, 63075, 63077, 63081, 63085, 63087, 63090, 63101-63102, 63170-63290, 63300-63307)

🚗 22.2 ✂ 22.2 **FUD** ZZZ Ⓝ N1 80 ▭

AMA: 2020,May,13; 2018,Sep,7; 2018,Jan,8; 2017,Jun,10; 2017,Feb,9; 2017,Jan,8; 2016,Jan,13

+ **22841** **Internal spinal fixation by wiring of spinous processes (List separately in addition to code for primary procedure)**

Code first (22100-22102, 22110-22114, 22206-22207, 22210-22214, 22220-22224, 22310-22327, 22532-22533, 22548-22558, 22590-22612, 22630, 22633-22634, 22800-22812, 63001-63030, 63040-63042, 63045-63047, 63050-63056, 63064, 63075, 63077, 63081, 63085, 63087, 63090, 63101-63102, 63170-63290, 63300-63307)

🚗 0.00 ✂ 0.00 **FUD** XXX Ⓒ ▭

AMA: 2020,May,13; 2018,Sep,7; 2018,Jan,8; 2017,Feb,9; 2017,Jan,8; 2016,Jan,13

+ **22842** **Posterior segmental instrumentation (eg, pedicle fixation, dual rods with multiple hooks and sublaminar wires); 3 to 6 vertebral segments (List separately in addition to code for primary procedure)**

Code first (22100-22102, 22110-22114, 22206-22207, 22210-22214, 22220-22224, 22310-22327, 22532-22533, 22548-22558, 22590-22612, 22630, 22633-22634, 22800-22812, 63001-63030, 63040-63042, 63045-63047, 63050-63056, 63064, 63075, 63077, 63081, 63085, 63087, 63090, 63101-63102, 63170-63290, 63300-63307)

🚗 22.1 ✂ 22.1 **FUD** ZZZ Ⓝ N1 80 ▭

AMA: 2020,May,13; 2018,Sep,7; 2018,Jan,8; 2017,Feb,9; 2017,Jan,8; 2016,Jan,13

Example of rod hook; may be attached at top and bottom only, or also at segments

Rod

Segment

+ **22843** **7 to 12 vertebral segments (List separately in addition to code for primary procedure)**

Code first (22100-22102, 22110-22114, 22206-22207, 22210-22214, 22220-22224, 22310-22327, 22532-22533, 22548-22558, 22590-22612, 22630, 22633-22634, 22800-22812, 63001-63030, 63040-63042, 63045-63047, 63050-63056, 63064, 63075, 63077, 63081, 63085, 63087, 63090, 63101-63102, 63170-63290, 63300-63307)

🚗 23.8 ✂ 23.8 **FUD** ZZZ Ⓒ 80 ▭

AMA: 2020,May,13; 2018,Sep,7; 2018,Jul,14; 2018,Jan,8; 2017,Jan,8; 2016,Jan,13

+ **22844** **13 or more vertebral segments (List separately in addition to code for primary procedure)**

Code first (22100-22102, 22110-22114, 22206-22207, 22210-22214, 22220-22224, 22310-22327, 22532-22533, 22548-22558, 22590-22612, 22630, 22633-22634, 22800-22812, 63001-63030, 63040-63042, 63045-63047, 63050-63056, 63064, 63075, 63077, 63081, 63085, 63087, 63090, 63101-63102, 63170-63290, 63300-63307)

🚗 28.6 ✂ 28.6 **FUD** ZZZ Ⓒ 80 ▭

AMA: 2020,May,13; 2018,Sep,7; 2018,Jan,8; 2017,Jan,8; 2016,Jan,13

+ **22845** **Anterior instrumentation; 2 to 3 vertebral segments (List separately in addition to code for primary procedure)**

INCLUDES Dwyer instrumentation technique

EXCLUDES Vertebral body tethering (0656T)

Code first (22100-22102, 22110-22114, 22206-22207, 22210-22214, 22220-22224, 22310-22327, 22532-22533, 22548-22558, 22590-22612, 22630, 22633-22634, 22800-22812, 63001-63030, 63040-63042, 63045-63047, 63050-63056, 63064, 63075, 63077, 63081, 63085, 63087, 63090, 63101-63102, 63170-63290, 63300-63307)

🚗 21.1 ✂ 21.1 **FUD** ZZZ Ⓝ N1 80 ▭

AMA: 2020,May,13; 2018,Sep,7; 2018,Jan,8; 2017,Mar,7; 2017,Jan,8; 2016,May,13; 2016,Jan,13

+ **22846** **4 to 7 vertebral segments (List separately in addition to code for primary procedure)**

INCLUDES Dwyer instrumentation technique

EXCLUDES Vertebral body tethering (0656T)

Code first (22100-22102, 22110-22114, 22206-22207, 22210-22214, 22220-22224, 22310-22327, 22532-22533, 22548-22558, 22590-22612, 22630, 22633-22634, 22800-22812, 63001-63030, 63040-63042, 63045-63047, 63050-63056, 63064, 63075, 63077, 63081, 63085, 63087, 63090, 63101-63102, 63170-63290, 63300-63307)

🚗 22.0 ✂ 22.0 **FUD** ZZZ Ⓒ 80 ▭

AMA: 2020,May,13; 2018,Sep,7; 2018,Jan,8; 2017,Jan,8; 2016,May,13; 2016,Jan,13

+ **22847** **8 or more vertebral segments (List separately in addition to code for primary procedure)**

INCLUDES Dwyer instrumentation technique

EXCLUDES Vertebral body tethering (0657T)

Code first (22100-22102, 22110-22114, 22206-22207, 22210-22214, 22220-22224, 22310-22327, 22532-22533, 22548-22558, 22590-22612, 22630, 22633-22634, 22800-22812, 63001-63030, 63040-63042, 63045-63047, 63050-63056, 63064, 63075, 63077, 63081, 63085, 63087, 63090, 63101-63102, 63170-63290, 63300-63307)

🚗 23.4 ✂ 23.4 **FUD** ZZZ Ⓒ 80 ▭

AMA: 2020,May,13; 2018,Sep,7; 2018,Jan,8; 2017,Jan,8; 2016,May,13; 2016,Jan,13

+ **22848** **Pelvic fixation (attachment of caudal end of instrumentation to pelvic bony structures) other than sacrum (List separately in addition to code for primary procedure)**

Code first (22100-22102, 22110-22114, 22206-22207, 22210-22214, 22220-22224, 22310-22327, 22532-22533, 22548-22558, 22590-22612, 22630, 22633-22634, 22800-22812, 63001-63030, 63040-63042, 63045-63047, 63050-63056, 63064, 63075, 63077, 63081, 63085, 63087, 63090, 63101-63102, 63170-63290, 63300-63307)

🚗 10.4 ✂ 10.4 **FUD** ZZZ Ⓒ 80 ▭

AMA: 2020,May,13; 2018,Sep,7; 2018,Jan,8; 2017,Jan,8; 2016,Jan,13

Musculoskeletal System

22849 — 22861

22849-22855 [22859] Miscellaneous Spinal Instrumentation

EXCLUDES
Arthrodesis (22532-22534, 22548-22812)
Bone grafting procedures (20930-20938)
Exploration spinal fusion (22830)
Facet injection (64490-64495, [64633, 64634, 64635, 64636])
Fracture treatment (22325-22328)

22849 Reinsertion of spinal fixation device
INCLUDES Removal of instrumentation at the same level (22850, 22852, 22855)
37.7   37.7   **FUD** 090   C 80
AMA: 2020,May,13; 2018,Sep,7; 2018,Jan,8; 2017,Jun,10; 2017,Jan,8; 2016,May,13; 2016,Jan,13

22850 Removal of posterior nonsegmental instrumentation (eg, Harrington rod)
21.0   21.0   **FUD** 090   C 80
AMA: 2020,May,13; 2018,Sep,7; 2018,Jan,8; 2017,Jun,10; 2017,Jan,8; 2016,May,13; 2016,Jan,13

22852 Removal of posterior segmental instrumentation
20.2   20.2   **FUD** 090   C 80
AMA: 2020,May,13; 2018,Sep,7; 2018,Jan,8; 2017,Jun,10; 2017,Jan,8; 2016,Jan,13

+ 22853 Insertion of interbody biomechanical device(s) (eg, synthetic cage, mesh) with integral anterior instrumentation for device anchoring (eg, screws, flanges), when performed, to intervertebral disc space in conjunction with interbody arthrodesis, each interspace (List separately in addition to code for primary procedure)
Code also:
Intervertebral bone device/graft application (20930-20931, 20936-20938)
Subsequent disc spaces undergoing device insertion when disc spaces are not connected (22853-22854, [22859])
Code first (22100-22102, 22110-22114, 22206-22207, 22210-22214, 22220-22224, 22310-22327, 22532-22533, 22548-22558, 22590-22612, 22630, 22633-22634, 22800-22812, 63001-63030, 63040, 63042, 63045-63047, 63050-63056, 63064, 63075, 63077, 63081, 63085, 63087, 63090, 63101-63102, 63170-63290, 63300-63307)
7.52   7.52   **FUD** ZZZ   N N1 80
AMA: 2020,May,13; 2018,Sep,7; 2018,Jul,14; 2018,Jan,8; 2017,Aug,9; 2017,Mar,7

+ 22854 Insertion of intervertebral biomechanical device(s) (eg, synthetic cage, mesh) with integral anterior instrumentation for device anchoring (eg, screws, flanges), when performed, to vertebral corpectomy(ies) (vertebral body resection, partial or complete) defect, in conjunction with interbody arthrodesis, each contiguous defect (List separately in addition to code for primary procedure)
Code also:
Intervertebral bone device/graft application (20930-20931, 20936-20938)
Subsequent disc spaces undergoing device insertion when disc spaces are not connected (22853-22854, [22859])
Code first (22100-22102, 22110-22114, 22206-22207, 22210-22214, 22220-22224, 22310-22327, 22532-22533, 22548-22558, 22590-22612, 22630, 22633-22634, 22800-22812, 63001-63030, 63040, 63042, 63045-63047, 63050-63056, 63064, 63075, 63077, 63081, 63085, 63087, 63090, 63101-63102, 63170-63290, 63300-63307)
9.74   9.74   **FUD** ZZZ   N N1 80
AMA: 2020,May,13; 2018,Sep,7; 2018,Jan,8; 2017,Mar,7

+ # 22859 Insertion of intervertebral biomechanical device(s) (eg, synthetic cage, mesh, methylmethacrylate) to intervertebral disc space or vertebral body defect without interbody arthrodesis, each contiguous defect (List separately in addition to code for primary procedure)
Code also:
Intervertebral bone device/graft application (20930-20931, 20936-20938)
Subsequent disc spaces undergoing device insertion when disc spaces are not connected (22853-22854, [22859])
Code first (22100-22102, 22110-22114, 22206-22207, 22210-22214, 22220-22224, 22310-22327, 22532-22533, 22548-22558, 22590-22612, 22630, 22633-22634, 22800-22812, 63001-63030, 63040-63042, 63045-63047, 63050-63056, 63064, 63075, 63077, 63081, 63085, 63087, 63090, 63101-63102, 63170-63290, 63300-63307)
9.74   9.74   **FUD** ZZZ   N N1 80
AMA: 2020,May,13; 2018,Sep,7; 2018,Jan,8; 2017,Mar,7

22855 Removal of anterior instrumentation
32.1   32.1   **FUD** 090   C 80
AMA: 2020,May,13; 2018,Sep,7; 2018,Jan,8; 2017,Jun,10; 2017,Jan,8; 2016,Jan,13

22856-22865 [22858, 22859] Artificial Disc Replacement

EXCLUDES
Fluoroscopy
Spinal decompression (63001-63048)

22856 Total disc arthroplasty (artificial disc), anterior approach, including discectomy with end plate preparation (includes osteophytectomy for nerve root or spinal cord decompression and microdissection); single interspace, cervical
INCLUDES Operating microscope (69990)
EXCLUDES Application intervertebral biomechanical device(s) at same level (22853-22854, [22859])
Arthrodesis at same level (22554)
Discectomy at same level (63075)
Insertion instrumentation at same level (22845)
Code also arthroplasty more than one interspace, when performed ([22858])
47.3   47.3   **FUD** 090   J J8 80
AMA: 2020,May,13; 2018,Sep,7; 2018,Jan,8; 2017,Jan,8; 2016,Feb,12; 2016,Jan,13

+ # 22858 second level, cervical (List separately in addition to code for primary procedure)
Code first (22856)
14.8   14.8   **FUD** ZZZ   N N1 80
AMA: 2020,May,13; 2018,Sep,7; 2018,Jan,8; 2017,Jan,8; 2016,Feb,12; 2016,Jan,13

22857 Total disc arthroplasty (artificial disc), anterior approach, including discectomy to prepare interspace (other than for decompression), single interspace, lumbar
INCLUDES Operating microscope (69990)
EXCLUDES Application intervertebral biomechanical device(s) at same level (22853-22854, [22859])
Arthrodesis at same level (22558)
Insertion instrumentation at same level (22845)
Retroperitoneal exploration (49010)
Code also arthroplasty more than one interspace, when performed (0163T)
51.4   51.4   **FUD** 090   C 80
AMA: 2020,May,13; 2018,Sep,7; 2016,Feb,12

22858 Resequenced code. See code following 22856.

22859 Resequenced code. See code following 22854.

22861 Revision including replacement of total disc arthroplasty (artificial disc), anterior approach, single interspace; cervical
INCLUDES Operating microscope (69990)
EXCLUDES Procedures performed at same level (22845, 22853-22854, [22859], 22864, 63075)
Revision additional cervical arthroplasty (0098T)
66.9   66.9   **FUD** 090   C 80
AMA: 2020,May,13; 2018,Sep,7; 2016,Feb,12

22862 lumbar

> EXCLUDES Arthroplasty revision more than one interspace (0165T)
> Procedures performed at same level (22558, 22845, 22853-22854, [22859], 22865, 49010)

📋 66.8 ⚕ 66.8 **FUD** 090 C 80 ▢

AMA: 2020,May,13; 2018,Sep,7; 2018,Jan,8; 2017,Jan,8; 2016,Jan,13

22864 Removal of total disc arthroplasty (artificial disc), anterior approach, single interspace; cervical

> INCLUDES Operating microscope (69990)
> EXCLUDES Cervical total disc arthroplasty with additional interspace removal (0095T)
> Revision total disc arthroplasty (22861)

📋 59.7 ⚕ 59.7 **FUD** 090 C 80 ▢

AMA: 2020,May,13; 2018,Sep,7

22865 lumbar

> EXCLUDES Arthroplasty more than one level (0164T)
> Exploration, retroperitoneal area with or without biopsy(s) (49010)

📋 65.1 ⚕ 65.1 **FUD** 090 C 80 ▢

AMA: 2020,May,13; 2018,Sep,7; 2018,Jan,8; 2017,Jan,8; 2016,Jan,13

22867-22899 Spinal Distraction/Stabilization Device

22867 Insertion of interlaminar/interspinous process stabilization/distraction device, without fusion, including image guidance when performed, with open decompression, lumbar; single level

> EXCLUDES Interlaminar/interspinous stabilization/distraction device insertion (22869, 22870)
> Procedures at same level (22532-22534, 22558, 22612, 22614, 22630, 22632-22634, 22800, 22802, 22804, 22840-22842, 22869-22870, 63005, 63012, 63017, 63030, 63035, 63042, 63044, 63047-63048, 77003)

📋 28.2 ⚕ 28.2 **FUD** 090 J J8 80 ▢

AMA: 2020,May,13; 2018,Sep,7; 2018,Jan,8; 2017,Feb,9

+ **22868** second level (List separately in addition to code for primary procedure)

> EXCLUDES Interlaminar/interspinous stabilization/distraction device insertion (22869-22870)
> Procedures at same level (22532-22534, 22558, 22612, 22614, 22630, 22632-22634, 22800, 22802, 22804, 22840-22842, 22869-22870, 63005, 63012, 63017, 63030, 63035, 63042, 63044, 63047-63048, 77003)

Code first (22867)

📋 7.08 ⚕ 7.08 **FUD** ZZZ N N1 80 ▢

AMA: 2020,May,13; 2018,Sep,7; 2018,Jan,8; 2017,Feb,9

22869 Insertion of interlaminar/interspinous process stabilization/distraction device, without open decompression or fusion, including image guidance when performed, lumbar; single level

> EXCLUDES Procedures at the same level (22532-22534, 22558, 22612, 22614, 22630, 22632-22634, 22800, 22802, 22804, 22840-22842, 63005, 63012, 63017, 63030, 63035, 63042, 63044, 63047-63048, 77003)

📋 12.8 ⚕ 12.8 **FUD** 090 J J8 80 ▢

AMA: 2020,May,13; 2018,Sep,7; 2018,Jan,8; 2017,Feb,9

+ **22870** second level (List separately in addition to code for primary procedure)

> EXCLUDES Procedures at the same level (22532-22534, 22558, 22612, 22614, 22630, 22632-22634, 22800, 22802, 22804, 22840-22842, 63005, 63012, 63017, 63030, 63035, 63042, 63044, 63047-63048, 77003)

Code first (22869)

📋 3.62 ⚕ 3.62 **FUD** ZZZ N N1 80 ▢

AMA: 2020,May,13; 2018,Sep,7; 2018,Jan,8; 2017,Feb,9

22899 Unlisted procedure, spine

📋 0.00 ⚕ 0.00 **FUD** YYY T 80 ▢

AMA: 2020,Jun,14; 2018,Sep,7; 2018,May,10; 2018,Jan,8; 2017,Feb,9; 2017,Jan,8; 2016,Jan,13

22900-22999 Musculoskeletal Procedures of Abdomen

> INCLUDES Any necessary elevation tissue planes or dissection
> Measurement tumor and necessary margin at greatest diameter prior to excision
> Simple and intermediate repairs
> Excision types:
> Fascial or subfascial soft tissue tumors: simple and marginal resection tumors found either in or below deep fascia, not involving bone or excision substantial amount normal tissue; primarily benign and intramuscular tumors
> Radical resection soft tissue tumor: wide resection tumor involving substantial margins normal tissue and may include tissue removal from one or more layers; most often malignant or aggressive benign
> Subcutaneous: simple and marginal resection tumors in subcutaneous tissue above deep fascia; most often benign

> EXCLUDES Complex repair
> Excision benign cutaneous lesions (eg, sebaceous cyst) (11400-11406)
> Radical resection cutaneous tumors (eg, melanoma) (11600-11606)
> Significant vessel exploration or neuroplasty

22900 Excision, tumor, soft tissue of abdominal wall, subfascial (eg, intramuscular); less than 5 cm

📋 16.3 ⚕ 16.3 **FUD** 090 J 62 80 ▢

AMA: 2018,Sep,7

22901 5 cm or greater

📋 19.3 ⚕ 19.3 **FUD** 090 J 62 80 ▢

AMA: 2018,Sep,7

22902 Excision, tumor, soft tissue of abdominal wall, subcutaneous; less than 3 cm

📋 9.57 ⚕ 13.1 **FUD** 090 J 62 80 ▢

AMA: 2018,Sep,7

22903 3 cm or greater

📋 12.6 ⚕ 12.6 **FUD** 090 J 62 80 ▢

AMA: 2018,Sep,7

22904 Radical resection of tumor (eg, sarcoma), soft tissue of abdominal wall; less than 5 cm

📋 30.5 ⚕ 30.5 **FUD** 090 J 62 80 ▢

AMA: 2018,Sep,7

22905 5 cm or greater

📋 38.5 ⚕ 38.5 **FUD** 090 J 62 80 ▢

AMA: 2018,Sep,7

22999 Unlisted procedure, abdomen, musculoskeletal system

📋 0.00 ⚕ 0.00 **FUD** YYY T 80 ▢

AMA: 2018,Sep,7

23000-23044 Surgical Incision Shoulder: Drainage, Foreign Body Removal, Contracture Release

23000 Removal of subdeltoid calcareous deposits, open

> EXCLUDES Arthroscopic removal calcium deposits bursa (29999)

📋 10.5 ⚕ 16.4 **FUD** 090 J A2 80 50 ▢

AMA: 2018,Sep,7

23020 Capsular contracture release (eg, Sever type procedure)

> EXCLUDES Simple incision and drainage (10040-10160)

📋 19.9 ⚕ 19.9 **FUD** 090 J A2 80 50 ▢

AMA: 2018,Sep,7

23030 Incision and drainage, shoulder area; deep abscess or hematoma

📋 7.20 ⚕ 12.4 **FUD** 010 J A2 ▢

AMA: 2018,Sep,7

Musculoskeletal System

23031 — 23145

23031   **infected bursa**
     6.01   11.5   **FUD** 010   J A2 50
    AMA: 2018,Sep,7

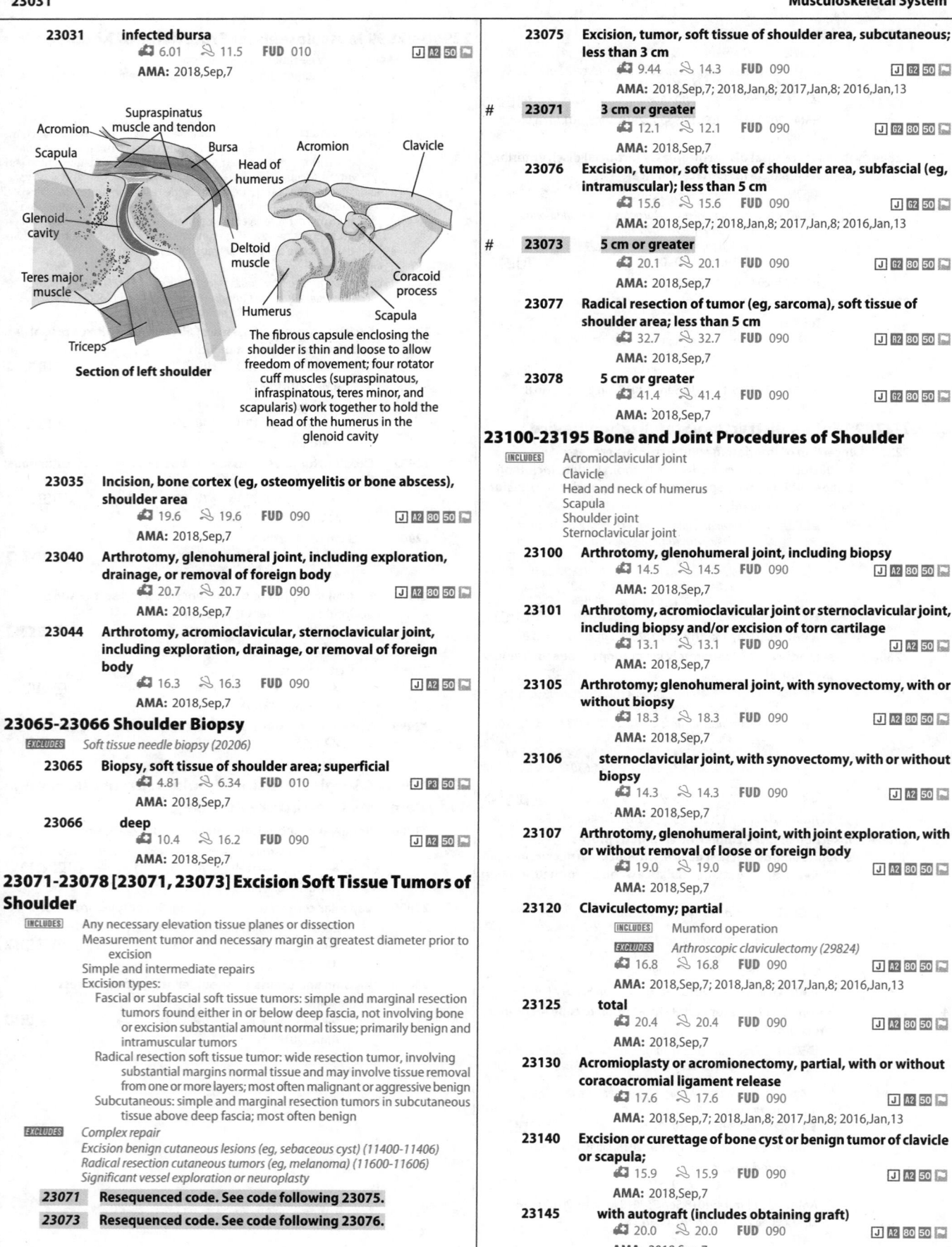

Labels: Supraspinatus muscle and tendon; Acromion; Scapula; Bursa; Acromion; Clavicle; Head of humerus; Glenoid cavity; Deltoid muscle; Teres major muscle; Coracoid process; Humerus; Scapula; Triceps

Section of left shoulder

The fibrous capsule enclosing the shoulder is thin and loose to allow freedom of movement; four rotator cuff muscles (supraspinatous, infraspinatous, teres minor, and scapularis) work together to hold the head of the humerus in the glenoid cavity

23035   **Incision, bone cortex (eg, osteomyelitis or bone abscess), shoulder area**
     19.6   19.6   **FUD** 090   J A2 80 50
    AMA: 2018,Sep,7

23040   **Arthrotomy, glenohumeral joint, including exploration, drainage, or removal of foreign body**
     20.7   20.7   **FUD** 090   J A2 80 50
    AMA: 2018,Sep,7

23044   **Arthrotomy, acromioclavicular, sternoclavicular joint, including exploration, drainage, or removal of foreign body**
     16.3   16.3   **FUD** 090   J A2 50
    AMA: 2018,Sep,7

23065-23066 Shoulder Biopsy

EXCLUDES   *Soft tissue needle biopsy (20206)*

23065   **Biopsy, soft tissue of shoulder area; superficial**
     4.81   6.34   **FUD** 010   J P3 50
    AMA: 2018,Sep,7

23066   **deep**
     10.4   16.2   **FUD** 090   J A2 50
    AMA: 2018,Sep,7

23071-23078 [23071, 23073] Excision Soft Tissue Tumors of Shoulder

INCLUDES   Any necessary elevation tissue planes or dissection
    Measurement tumor and necessary margin at greatest diameter prior to excision
    Simple and intermediate repairs
    Excision types:
      Fascial or subfascial soft tissue tumors: simple and marginal resection tumors found either in or below deep fascia, not involving bone or excision substantial amount normal tissue; primarily benign and intramuscular tumors
      Radical resection soft tissue tumor: wide resection tumor, involving substantial margins normal tissue and may involve tissue removal from one or more layers; most often malignant or aggressive benign
      Subcutaneous: simple and marginal resection tumors in subcutaneous tissue above deep fascia; most often benign

EXCLUDES   *Complex repair*
    Excision benign cutaneous lesions (eg, sebaceous cyst) (11400-11406)
    Radical resection cutaneous tumors (eg, melanoma) (11600-11606)
    Significant vessel exploration or neuroplasty

23071   **Resequenced code. See code following 23075.**

23073   **Resequenced code. See code following 23076.**

23075   **Excision, tumor, soft tissue of shoulder area, subcutaneous; less than 3 cm**
     9.44   14.3   **FUD** 090   J 62 50
    AMA: 2018,Sep,7; 2018,Jan,8; 2017,Jan,8; 2016,Jan,13

\#   **23071**   **3 cm or greater**
     12.1   12.1   **FUD** 090   J 62 80 50
    AMA: 2018,Sep,7

23076   **Excision, tumor, soft tissue of shoulder area, subfascial (eg, intramuscular); less than 5 cm**
     15.6   15.6   **FUD** 090   J 62 50
    AMA: 2018,Sep,7; 2018,Jan,8; 2017,Jan,8; 2016,Jan,13

\#   **23073**   **5 cm or greater**
     20.1   20.1   **FUD** 090   J 62 80 50
    AMA: 2018,Sep,7

23077   **Radical resection of tumor (eg, sarcoma), soft tissue of shoulder area; less than 5 cm**
     32.7   32.7   **FUD** 090   J R2 80 50
    AMA: 2018,Sep,7

23078   **5 cm or greater**
     41.4   41.4   **FUD** 090   J 62 80 50
    AMA: 2018,Sep,7

23100-23195 Bone and Joint Procedures of Shoulder

INCLUDES   Acromioclavicular joint
    Clavicle
    Head and neck of humerus
    Scapula
    Shoulder joint
    Sternoclavicular joint

23100   **Arthrotomy, glenohumeral joint, including biopsy**
     14.5   14.5   **FUD** 090   J A2 80 50
    AMA: 2018,Sep,7

23101   **Arthrotomy, acromioclavicular joint or sternoclavicular joint, including biopsy and/or excision of torn cartilage**
     13.1   13.1   **FUD** 090   J A2 50
    AMA: 2018,Sep,7

23105   **Arthrotomy; glenohumeral joint, with synovectomy, with or without biopsy**
     18.3   18.3   **FUD** 090   J A2 80 50
    AMA: 2018,Sep,7

23106   **sternoclavicular joint, with synovectomy, with or without biopsy**
     14.3   14.3   **FUD** 090   J A2 50
    AMA: 2018,Sep,7

23107   **Arthrotomy, glenohumeral joint, with joint exploration, with or without removal of loose or foreign body**
     19.0   19.0   **FUD** 090   J A2 80 50
    AMA: 2018,Sep,7

23120   **Claviculectomy; partial**
    INCLUDES   Mumford operation
    EXCLUDES   *Arthroscopic claviculectomy (29824)*
     16.8   16.8   **FUD** 090   J A2 80 50
    AMA: 2018,Sep,7; 2018,Jan,8; 2017,Jan,8; 2016,Jan,13

23125   **total**
     20.4   20.4   **FUD** 090   J A2 80 50
    AMA: 2018,Sep,7

23130   **Acromioplasty or acromionectomy, partial, with or without coracoacromial ligament release**
     17.6   17.6   **FUD** 090   J A2 50
    AMA: 2018,Sep,7; 2018,Jan,8; 2017,Jan,8; 2016,Jan,13

23140   **Excision or curettage of bone cyst or benign tumor of clavicle or scapula;**
     15.9   15.9   **FUD** 090   J A2 50
    AMA: 2018,Sep,7

23145   **with autograft (includes obtaining graft)**
     20.0   20.0   **FUD** 090   J A2 80 50
    AMA: 2018,Sep,7

26/TC PC/TC Only   A2-Z3 ASC Payment   50 Bilateral   ♂ Male Only   ♀ Female Only   Facility RVU   Non-Facility RVU   CCI   CLIA
FUD Follow-up Days   CMS: IOM   AMA: CPT Asst   A-Y OPPSI   80/80 Surg Assist Allowed / w/Doc   Lab Crosswalk   Radiology Crosswalk

60   CPT © 2021 American Medical Association. All Rights Reserved.   © 2021 Optum360, LLC

23146   **with allograft**
🔧 17.9   ✂ 17.9   **FUD** 090   J A2 80 50 ▣
AMA: 2019,May,7; 2018,Sep,7

23150   **Excision or curettage of bone cyst or benign tumor of proximal humerus;**
🔧 19.2   ✂ 19.2   **FUD** 090   J A2 80 50 ▣
AMA: 2018,Sep,7

23155   **with autograft (includes obtaining graft)**
🔧 22.7   ✂ 22.7   **FUD** 090   J A2 80 50 ▣
AMA: 2018,Sep,7

23156   **with allograft**
🔧 19.4   ✂ 19.4   **FUD** 090   J A2 80 50 ▣
AMA: 2019,May,7; 2018,Sep,7

23170   **Sequestrectomy (eg, for osteomyelitis or bone abscess), clavicle**
🔧 16.2   ✂ 16.2   **FUD** 090   J A2 50 ▣
AMA: 2018,Sep,7

23172   **Sequestrectomy (eg, for osteomyelitis or bone abscess), scapula**
🔧 16.3   ✂ 16.3   **FUD** 090   J A2 80 50 ▣
AMA: 2018,Sep,7

23174   **Sequestrectomy (eg, for osteomyelitis or bone abscess), humeral head to surgical neck**
🔧 21.9   ✂ 21.9   **FUD** 090   J A2 80 50 ▣
AMA: 2018,Sep,7

23180   **Partial excision (craterization, saucerization, or diaphysectomy) bone (eg, osteomyelitis), clavicle**
🔧 19.1   ✂ 19.1   **FUD** 090   J A2 50 ▣
AMA: 2018,Sep,7

23182   **Partial excision (craterization, saucerization, or diaphysectomy) bone (eg, osteomyelitis), scapula**
🔧 19.0   ✂ 19.0   **FUD** 090   J A2 80 50 ▣
AMA: 2018,Sep,7

23184   **Partial excision (craterization, saucerization, or diaphysectomy) bone (eg, osteomyelitis), proximal humerus**
🔧 21.1   ✂ 21.1   **FUD** 090   J A2 80 50 ▣
AMA: 2018,Sep,7

23190   **Ostectomy of scapula, partial (eg, superior medial angle)**
🔧 16.5   ✂ 16.5   **FUD** 090   J A2 80 50 ▣
AMA: 2018,Sep,7

23195   **Resection, humeral head**
EXCLUDES *Arthroplasty with replacement with implant (23470)*
🔧 21.5   ✂ 21.5   **FUD** 090   J A2 80 50 ▣
AMA: 2018,Sep,7

23200-23220 Radical Resection of Bone Tumors of Shoulder

INCLUDES Any necessary elevation tissue planes or dissection
Excision adjacent soft tissue during bone tumor resection (23071-23078 [23071, 23073])
Measurement tumor and necessary margin at greatest diameter prior to excision
Radical resection cutaneous tumors (e.g., melanoma)
Resection tumor (may include entire bone) and wide margins normal tissues primarily for malignant or aggressive benign tumors
Simple and intermediate repairs
EXCLUDES Complex repair
Significant vessel exploration, neuroplasty, reconstruction, or complex bone repair

23200   **Radical resection of tumor; clavicle**
🔧 43.6   ✂ 43.6   **FUD** 090   C 80 50 ▣
AMA: 2019,May,7; 2018,Sep,7

23210   **scapula**
🔧 51.2   ✂ 51.2   **FUD** 090   C 80 50 ▣
AMA: 2019,May,7; 2018,Sep,7

23220   **Radical resection of tumor, proximal humerus**
🔧 56.3   ✂ 56.3   **FUD** 090   C 80 50 ▣
AMA: 2019,May,7; 2018,Sep,7

23330-23335 Removal Implant/Foreign Body from Shoulder

EXCLUDES *Bursal arthrocentesis or needling (20610)*
K-wire or pin insertion (20650)
K-wire or pin removal (20670, 20680)

23330   **Removal of foreign body, shoulder; subcutaneous**
🔧 4.76   ✂ 8.00   **FUD** 010   T A2 80 50 ▣
AMA: 2018,Sep,7; 2018,Jan,8; 2017,Jan,8; 2016,Jan,13

23333   **deep (subfascial or intramuscular)**
🔧 13.2   ✂ 13.2   **FUD** 090   J G2 80 50 ▣
AMA: 2018,Sep,7; 2018,Jan,8; 2017,Jan,8; 2016,Jan,13

23334   **Removal of prosthesis, includes debridement and synovectomy when performed; humeral or glenoid component**
EXCLUDES *Foreign body removal (23330, 23333)*
Prosthesis removal and replacement in same shoulder (eg, glenoid and/or humeral components) (23473-23474)
🔧 30.8   ✂ 30.8   **FUD** 090   J G2 50 ▣
AMA: 2018,Sep,7; 2018,Jan,8; 2017,Jan,8; 2016,Jan,13

23335   **humeral and glenoid components (eg, total shoulder)**
EXCLUDES *Foreign body removal (23330, 23333)*
Prosthesis removal and replacement in same shoulder (eg, glenoid and/or humeral components) (23473-23474)
🔧 36.7   ✂ 36.7   **FUD** 090   C 50 ▣
AMA: 2018,Sep,7; 2018,Jan,8; 2017,Jan,8; 2016,Jan,13

23350 Injection for Shoulder Arthrogram

23350   **Injection procedure for shoulder arthrography or enhanced CT/MRI shoulder arthrography**
EXCLUDES *Shoulder biopsy (29805-29826)*
📷 (73040, 73201-73202, 73222-73223, 77002)
🔧 1.47   ✂ 3.97   **FUD** 000   N N1 50 ▣
AMA: 2018,Sep,7; 2018,Jan,8; 2017,Jan,8; 2016,May,13; 2016,Jan,13

23395-23491 Repair/Reconstruction of Shoulder

23395   **Muscle transfer, any type, shoulder or upper arm; single**
🔧 37.0   ✂ 37.0   **FUD** 090   J A2 80 ▣
AMA: 2018,Sep,7

23397   **multiple**
🔧 32.9   ✂ 32.9   **FUD** 090   J A2 80 ▣
AMA: 2018,Sep,7

23400   **Scapulopexy (eg, Sprengels deformity or for paralysis)**
🔧 28.0   ✂ 28.0   **FUD** 090   J A2 80 50 ▣
AMA: 2018,Sep,7

23405   **Tenotomy, shoulder area; single tendon**
🔧 17.8   ✂ 17.8   **FUD** 090   J A2 80 ▣
AMA: 2018,Sep,7

23406   **multiple tendons through same incision**
🔧 22.2   ✂ 22.2   **FUD** 090   T A2 80 ▣
AMA: 2018,Sep,7

23410   **Repair of ruptured musculotendinous cuff (eg, rotator cuff) open; acute**
EXCLUDES *Arthroscopic repair (29827)*
🔧 23.6   ✂ 23.6   **FUD** 090   J A2 80 50 ▣
AMA: 2018,Sep,7; 2018,Jan,8; 2017,Jan,8; 2016,Jan,13

23412   **chronic**
EXCLUDES *Arthroscopic repair (29827)*
🔧 24.5   ✂ 24.5   **FUD** 090   J A2 80 50 ▣
AMA: 2018,Sep,7; 2018,Jan,8; 2017,Jan,8; 2016,Jan,13

23415   **Coracoacromial ligament release, with or without acromioplasty**
EXCLUDES *Arthroscopic repair (29826)*
🔧 20.1   ✂ 20.1   **FUD** 090   J A2 50 ▣
AMA: 2018,Sep,7; 2018,Jan,8; 2017,Jan,8; 2016,Jan,13

23420 **Reconstruction of complete shoulder (rotator) cuff avulsion, chronic (includes acromioplasty)**
🔧 28.0　⚕ 28.0　**FUD** 090　　　J A2 80 50 ▭
AMA: 2018,Sep,7; 2018,Jan,8; 2017,Jan,8; 2016,Jan,13

23430 **Tenodesis of long tendon of biceps**
EXCLUDES　*Arthroscopic biceps tenodesis (29828)*
🔧 21.4　⚕ 21.4　**FUD** 090　　　J A2 80 50 ▭
AMA: 2018,Sep,7

23440 **Resection or transplantation of long tendon of biceps**
🔧 21.7　⚕ 21.7　**FUD** 090　　　J A2 80 50 ▭
AMA: 2018,Sep,7

23450 **Capsulorrhaphy, anterior; Putti-Platt procedure or Magnuson type operation**
EXCLUDES　*Arthroscopic thermal capsulorrhaphy (29999)*
🔧 27.3　⚕ 27.3　**FUD** 090　　　J J8 80 50 ▭
AMA: 2018,Sep,7

23455 **with labral repair (eg, Bankart procedure)**
EXCLUDES　*Arthroscopic repair (29806)*
🔧 28.7　⚕ 28.7　**FUD** 090　　　J J8 80 50 ▭
AMA: 2018,Sep,7

23460 **Capsulorrhaphy, anterior, any type; with bone block**
INCLUDES　Bristow procedure
🔧 31.5　⚕ 31.5　**FUD** 090　　　J A2 80 50 ▭
AMA: 2018,Sep,7

23462 **with coracoid process transfer**
EXCLUDES　*Open thermal capsulorrhaphy (23929)*
🔧 30.9　⚕ 30.9　**FUD** 090　　　J A2 80 50 ▭
AMA: 2018,Sep,7

23465 **Capsulorrhaphy, glenohumeral joint, posterior, with or without bone block**
EXCLUDES　*Sternoclavicular and acromioclavicular joint repair (23530, 23550)*
🔧 32.3　⚕ 32.3　**FUD** 090　　　J 62 80 50 ▭
AMA: 2018,Sep,7

23466 **Capsulorrhaphy, glenohumeral joint, any type multi-directional instability**
🔧 32.0　⚕ 32.0　**FUD** 090　　　J A2 80 50 ▭
AMA: 2018,Sep,7

23470 **Arthroplasty, glenohumeral joint; hemiarthroplasty**
🔧 34.7　⚕ 34.7　**FUD** 090　　　J J8 80 50 ▭
AMA: 2018,Sep,7; 2018,Jan,8; 2017,Jan,8; 2016,Jan,13

23472 **total shoulder (glenoid and proximal humeral replacement (eg, total shoulder))**
EXCLUDES　*Proximal humerus osteotomy (24400)*
　　　　　Removal total shoulder components (23334-23335)
🔧 41.9　⚕ 41.9　**FUD** 090　　　C 80 50 ▭
AMA: 2018,Sep,7; 2018,Jan,8; 2017,Jan,8; 2016,Jan,13

23473 **Revision of total shoulder arthroplasty, including allograft when performed; humeral or glenoid component**
EXCLUDES　*Removal prosthesis only (glenoid and/or humeral component) same shoulder/same operative sessions (23334-23335)*
🔧 46.7　⚕ 46.7　**FUD** 090　　　J J8 80 50 ▭
AMA: 2018,Sep,7; 2018,Jan,8; 2017,Jan,8; 2016,Jan,13

23474 **humeral and glenoid component**
EXCLUDES　*Removal prosthesis only (glenoid and/or humeral component) same shoulder/same operative sessions (23334-23335)*
🔧 50.5　⚕ 50.5　**FUD** 090　　　C 80 50 ▭
AMA: 2018,Sep,7; 2018,Jan,8; 2017,Jan,8; 2016,Jan,13

23480 **Osteotomy, clavicle, with or without internal fixation;**
🔧 23.7　⚕ 23.7　**FUD** 090　　　J A2 50 ▭
AMA: 2018,Sep,7

23485 **with bone graft for nonunion or malunion (includes obtaining graft and/or necessary fixation)**
🔧 27.6　⚕ 27.6　**FUD** 090　　　J J8 80 50 ▭
AMA: 2018,Sep,7

23490 **Prophylactic treatment (nailing, pinning, plating or wiring) with or without methylmethacrylate; clavicle**
🔧 24.6　⚕ 24.6　**FUD** 090　　　J A2 80 50 ▭
AMA: 2018,Sep,7

23491 **proximal humerus**
🔧 29.3　⚕ 29.3　**FUD** 090　　　J J8 80 50 ▭
AMA: 2018,Sep,7

23500-23680 Treatment of Shoulder Fracture/Dislocation

23500 **Closed treatment of clavicular fracture; without manipulation**
🔧 6.37　⚕ 6.24　**FUD** 090　　　T A2 50 ▭
AMA: 2018,Sep,7

23505 **with manipulation**
🔧 9.61　⚕ 10.2　**FUD** 090　　　J A2 50 ▭
AMA: 2018,Sep,7

23515 **Open treatment of clavicular fracture, includes internal fixation, when performed**
🔧 20.7　⚕ 20.7　**FUD** 090　　　J J8 80 50 ▭
AMA: 2018,Sep,7; 2018,Jan,8; 2017,Jan,8; 2016,Jan,13

23520 **Closed treatment of sternoclavicular dislocation; without manipulation**
🔧 6.73　⚕ 6.72　**FUD** 090　　　J A2 80 50 ▭
AMA: 2018,Sep,7

23525 **with manipulation**
🔧 10.2　⚕ 11.1　**FUD** 090　　　T A2 80 50 ▭
AMA: 2018,Sep,7

23530 **Open treatment of sternoclavicular dislocation, acute or chronic;**
🔧 16.5　⚕ 16.5　**FUD** 090　　　J A2 80 50 ▭
AMA: 2018,Sep,7

23532 **with fascial graft (includes obtaining graft)**
🔧 17.7　⚕ 17.7　**FUD** 090　　　J J8 80 50 ▭
AMA: 2018,Sep,7

23540 **Closed treatment of acromioclavicular dislocation; without manipulation**
🔧 6.64　⚕ 6.67　**FUD** 090　　　T A2 50 ▭
AMA: 2018,Sep,7

23545 **with manipulation**
🔧 8.93　⚕ 9.91　**FUD** 090　　　T A2 80 50 ▭
AMA: 2018,Sep,7

23550 **Open treatment of acromioclavicular dislocation, acute or chronic;**
🔧 16.3　⚕ 16.3　**FUD** 090　　　J A2 80 50 ▭
AMA: 2018,Sep,7

23552 **with fascial graft (includes obtaining graft)**
🔧 18.8　⚕ 18.8　**FUD** 090　　　J J8 80 50 ▭
AMA: 2019,Nov,14; 2018,Sep,7

23570 **Closed treatment of scapular fracture; without manipulation**
🔧 6.89　⚕ 6.69　**FUD** 090　　　T A2 50 ▭
AMA: 2018,Sep,7

23575 **with manipulation, with or without skeletal traction (with or without shoulder joint involvement)**
🔧 10.8　⚕ 11.6　**FUD** 090　　　J A2 80 50 ▭
AMA: 2018,Sep,7

23585 **Open treatment of scapular fracture (body, glenoid or acromion) includes internal fixation, when performed**
🔧 28.2　⚕ 28.2　**FUD** 090　　　J A2 80 50 ▭
AMA: 2018,Sep,7; 2018,Jan,8; 2017,Jan,8; 2016,Jan,13

23600 **Closed treatment of proximal humeral (surgical or anatomical neck) fracture; without manipulation**
🔧 8.92　⚕ 9.45　**FUD** 090　　　T P2 50 ▭
AMA: 2018,Sep,7

23605   with manipulation, with or without skeletal traction
📋 12.2   ⚖ 13.4   **FUD** 090   J A2 50 ▣
AMA: 2018,Sep,7

23615   Open treatment of proximal humeral (surgical or anatomical neck) fracture, includes internal fixation, when performed, includes repair of tuberosity(s), when performed;
📋 25.5   ⚖ 25.5   **FUD** 090   J J8 80 50 ▣
AMA: 2018,Sep,7; 2018,Jan,8; 2017,Jan,8; 2016,Jan,13

23616   with proximal humeral prosthetic replacement
📋 35.7   ⚖ 35.7   **FUD** 090   J J8 80 50 ▣
AMA: 2018,Sep,7

23620   Closed treatment of greater humeral tuberosity fracture; without manipulation
📋 7.32   ⚖ 7.65   **FUD** 090   T P2 50 ▣
AMA: 2018,Sep,7

23625   with manipulation
📋 10.1   ⚖ 10.9   **FUD** 090   J A2 50 ▣
AMA: 2018,Sep,7

23630   Open treatment of greater humeral tuberosity fracture, includes internal fixation, when performed
📋 22.4   ⚖ 22.4   **FUD** 090   J A2 80 50 ▣
AMA: 2018,Sep,7

23650   Closed treatment of shoulder dislocation, with manipulation; without anesthesia
📋 8.36   ⚖ 9.18   **FUD** 090   T A2 50 ▣
AMA: 2018,Sep,7

23655   requiring anesthesia
📋 11.5   ⚖ 11.5   **FUD** 090   J A2 50 ▣
AMA: 2018,Sep,7

23660   Open treatment of acute shoulder dislocation
EXCLUDES   Chronic dislocation repair (23450-23466)
📋 16.8   ⚖ 16.8   **FUD** 090   A2 80 50 ▣
AMA: 2018,Sep,7; 2018,Jan,8; 2017,Jan,8; 2016,Jan,13

23665   Closed treatment of shoulder dislocation, with fracture of greater humeral tuberosity, with manipulation
📋 11.4   ⚖ 12.3   **FUD** 090   J A2 50 ▣
AMA: 2019,Feb,10; 2018,Sep,7

23670   Open treatment of shoulder dislocation, with fracture of greater humeral tuberosity, includes internal fixation, when performed
📋 25.2   ⚖ 25.2   **FUD** 090   J A2 80 50 ▣
AMA: 2018,Sep,7

23675   Closed treatment of shoulder dislocation, with surgical or anatomical neck fracture, with manipulation
📋 14.4   ⚖ 15.9   **FUD** 090   J A2 50 ▣
AMA: 2018,Sep,7

23680   Open treatment of shoulder dislocation, with surgical or anatomical neck fracture, includes internal fixation, when performed
📋 26.7   ⚖ 26.7   **FUD** 090   J J8 80 50 ▣
AMA: 2018,Sep,7

23700-23929 Other/Unlisted Shoulder Procedures

23700   Manipulation under anesthesia, shoulder joint, including application of fixation apparatus (dislocation excluded)
📋 5.63   ⚖ 5.63   **FUD** 010   J A2 50 ▣
AMA: 2018,Sep,7; 2018,Jan,8; 2017,Jan,8; 2016,Jan,13

23800   Arthrodesis, glenohumeral joint;
📋 29.6   ⚖ 29.6   **FUD** 090   J G2 80 50 ▣
AMA: 2020,May,13; 2018,Sep,7

23802   with autogenous graft (includes obtaining graft)
📋 37.0   ⚖ 37.0   **FUD** 090   J G2 80 50 ▣
AMA: 2020,May,13; 2018,Sep,7

23900   Interthoracoscapular amputation (forequarter)
📋 40.0   ⚖ 40.0   **FUD** 090   C 80 ▣
AMA: 2018,Sep,7

23920   Disarticulation of shoulder;
📋 32.4   ⚖ 32.4   **FUD** 090   C 80 50 ▣
AMA: 2018,Sep,7

23921   secondary closure or scar revision
📋 13.5   ⚖ 13.5   **FUD** 090   T A2 50 ▣
AMA: 2018,Sep,7

23929   Unlisted procedure, shoulder
📋 0.00   ⚖ 0.00   **FUD** YYY   T 80 ▣
AMA: 2018,Sep,7

23930-24006 Surgical Incision Elbow/Upper Arm
EXCLUDES   Simple incision and drainage procedures (10040-10160)

23930   Incision and drainage, upper arm or elbow area; deep abscess or hematoma
📋 6.12   ⚖ 10.2   **FUD** 010   J A2 50 ▣
AMA: 2018,Sep,7

23931   bursa
📋 4.48   ⚖ 8.19   **FUD** 010   J A2 50 ▣
AMA: 2018,Sep,7

23935   Incision, deep, with opening of bone cortex (eg, for osteomyelitis or bone abscess), humerus or elbow
📋 14.7   ⚖ 14.7   **FUD** 090   J A2 80 50 ▣
AMA: 2018,Sep,7

24000   Arthrotomy, elbow, including exploration, drainage, or removal of foreign body
📋 13.7   ⚖ 13.7   **FUD** 090   J A2 80 50 ▣
AMA: 2018,Sep,7

24006   Arthrotomy of the elbow, with capsular excision for capsular release (separate procedure)
📋 20.5   ⚖ 20.5   **FUD** 090   J A2 80 50 ▣
AMA: 2018,Sep,7

24065-24066 Biopsy of Elbow/Upper Arm
EXCLUDES   Soft tissue needle biopsy (20206)

24065   Biopsy, soft tissue of upper arm or elbow area; superficial
📋 4.71   ⚖ 7.41   **FUD** 010   J P3 50 ▣
AMA: 2018,Sep,7

24066   deep (subfascial or intramuscular)
📋 12.0   ⚖ 18.0   **FUD** 090   J A2 50 ▣
AMA: 2018,Sep,7

24071-24079 [24071, 24073] Excision Soft Tissue Tumors Elbow/Upper Arm

INCLUDES   Any necessary elevation tissue planes or dissection
Measurement tumor and necessary margin at greatest diameter prior to excision
Excision types:
Fascial or subfascial soft tissue tumors: simple and marginal resection tumors found either in or below deep fascia, not involving bone or excision substantial amount normal tissue; primarily benign and intramuscular tumors
Radical resection soft tissue tumor: wide resection tumor involving substantial margins normal tissue and may involve tissue removal from one or more layers; most often malignant or aggressive benign
Subcutaneous: simple and marginal resection tumors found in subcutaneous tissue above deep fascia; most often benign
EXCLUDES   Complex repair
Excision benign cutaneous lesion (eg, sebaceous cyst) (11400-11406)
Radical resection cutaneous tumors (eg, melanoma) (11600-11606)
Significant vessel exploration or neuroplasty

24071   Resequenced code. See code following 24075.

24073   Resequenced code. See code following 24076.

24075   Excision, tumor, soft tissue of upper arm or elbow area, subcutaneous; less than 3 cm
📋 9.47   ⚖ 14.8   **FUD** 090   J G2 50 ▣
AMA: 2018,Sep,7

\#   **24071**   **3 cm or greater**
📋 11.7   ⚖ 11.7   **FUD** 090   J G2 80 50 ▣
AMA: 2018,Sep,7

Musculoskeletal System

24076 — 24201

24076 Excision, tumor, soft tissue of upper arm or elbow area, subfascial (eg, intramuscular); less than 5 cm
🔲 15.6 ⚕ 15.6 **FUD** 090 [J] [62] [50] [▣]
AMA: 2018,Sep,7

\# **24073** **5 cm or greater**
🔲 19.9 ⚕ 19.9 **FUD** 090 [J] [62] [80] [50] [▣]
AMA: 2018,Sep,7

24077 Radical resection of tumor (eg, sarcoma), soft tissue of upper arm or elbow area; less than 5 cm
🔲 29.9 ⚕ 29.9 **FUD** 090 [J] [62] [50] [▣]
AMA: 2018,Sep,7

24079 **5 cm or greater**
🔲 38.3 ⚕ 38.3 **FUD** 090 [J] [62] [80] [50] [▣]
AMA: 2018,Sep,7

24100-24149 Bone/Joint Procedures Upper Arm/Elbow

24100 Arthrotomy, elbow; with synovial biopsy only
🔲 12.0 ⚕ 12.0 **FUD** 090 [J] [A2] [80] [50] [▣]
AMA: 2018,Sep,7

24101 with joint exploration, with or without biopsy, with or without removal of loose or foreign body
🔲 14.4 ⚕ 14.4 **FUD** 090 [J] [A2] [80] [50] [▣]
AMA: 2018,Sep,7

24102 with synovectomy
🔲 17.7 ⚕ 17.7 **FUD** 090 [J] [A2] [80] [50] [▣]
AMA: 2018,Sep,7

24105 Excision, olecranon bursa
🔲 10.1 ⚕ 10.1 **FUD** 090 [J] [A2] [50] [▣]
AMA: 2018,Sep,7

24110 Excision or curettage of bone cyst or benign tumor, humerus;
🔲 16.8 ⚕ 16.8 **FUD** 090 [J] [A2] [50] [▣]
AMA: 2018,Sep,7

24115 with autograft (includes obtaining graft)
🔲 21.2 ⚕ 21.2 **FUD** 090 [J] [A2] [80] [50] [▣]
AMA: 2018,Sep,7

24116 with allograft
🔲 24.8 ⚕ 24.8 **FUD** 090 [J] [A2] [80] [50] [▣]
AMA: 2019,May,7; 2018,Sep,7

24120 Excision or curettage of bone cyst or benign tumor of head or neck of radius or olecranon process;
🔲 15.3 ⚕ 15.3 **FUD** 090 [J] [A2] [80] [50] [▣]
AMA: 2018,Sep,7

24125 with autograft (includes obtaining graft)
🔲 17.9 ⚕ 17.9 **FUD** 090 [J] [A2] [80] [50] [▣]
AMA: 2018,Sep,7

24126 with allograft
🔲 18.7 ⚕ 18.7 **FUD** 090 [J] [J8] [80] [50] [▣]
AMA: 2019,May,7; 2018,Sep,7

24130 Excision, radial head
EXCLUDES Radial head arthroplasty with implant (24366)
🔲 14.6 ⚕ 14.6 **FUD** 090 [J] [A2] [50] [▣]
AMA: 2018,Sep,7

24134 Sequestrectomy (eg, for osteomyelitis or bone abscess), shaft or distal humerus
🔲 21.4 ⚕ 21.4 **FUD** 090 [J] [A2] [80] [50] [▣]
AMA: 2018,Sep,7

24136 Sequestrectomy (eg, for osteomyelitis or bone abscess), radial head or neck
🔲 18.2 ⚕ 18.2 **FUD** 090 [J] [A2] [50] [▣]
AMA: 2018,Sep,7

24138 Sequestrectomy (eg, for osteomyelitis or bone abscess), olecranon process
🔲 19.6 ⚕ 19.6 **FUD** 090 [J] [A2] [80] [50] [▣]
AMA: 2018,Sep,7

24140 Partial excision (craterization, saucerization, or diaphysectomy) bone (eg, osteomyelitis), humerus
🔲 20.2 ⚕ 20.2 **FUD** 090 [J] [A2] [80] [50] [▣]
AMA: 2018,Sep,7

24145 Partial excision (craterization, saucerization, or diaphysectomy) bone (eg, osteomyelitis), radial head or neck
🔲 17.1 ⚕ 17.1 **FUD** 090 [J] [A2] [50] [▣]
AMA: 2018,Sep,7

24147 Partial excision (craterization, saucerization, or diaphysectomy) bone (eg, osteomyelitis), olecranon process
🔲 17.9 ⚕ 17.9 **FUD** 090 [J] [A2] [50] [▣]
AMA: 2018,Sep,7

24149 Radical resection of capsule, soft tissue, and heterotopic bone, elbow, with contracture release (separate procedure)
EXCLUDES Capsular and soft tissue release (24006)
🔲 33.8 ⚕ 33.8 **FUD** 090 [J] [62] [80] [50] [▣]
AMA: 2018,Sep,7

24150-24152 Radical Resection Bone Tumor Upper Arm

INCLUDES Any necessary elevation tissue planes or dissection
Excision adjacent soft tissue during bone tumor resection (24071-24079 [24071, 24073])
Measurement tumor and necessary margin at greatest diameter prior to excision
Resection tumor (may include entire bone) and wide margins normal tissue primarily for malignant or aggressive benign tumors
Simple and intermediate repairs
EXCLUDES Complex repair
Significant vessel exploration, neuroplasty, reconstruction, or complex bone repair

24150 Radical resection of tumor, shaft or distal humerus
🔲 44.8 ⚕ 44.8 **FUD** 090 [J] [62] [80] [50] [▣]
AMA: 2019,May,7; 2018,Sep,7

24152 Radical resection of tumor, radial head or neck
🔲 38.9 ⚕ 38.9 **FUD** 090 [J] [62] [80] [50] [▣]
AMA: 2019,May,7; 2018,Sep,7

24155 Elbow Arthrectomy

24155 Resection of elbow joint (arthrectomy)
🔲 24.6 ⚕ 24.6 **FUD** 090 [J] [A2] [80] [50] [▣]
AMA: 2018,Sep,7

24160-24201 Removal Implant/Foreign Body from Elbow/Upper Arm

EXCLUDES Bursal or joint arthrocentesis or needling (20605)
K-wire or pin insertion (20650)
K-wire or pin removal (20670, 20680)

24160 Removal of prosthesis, includes debridement and synovectomy when performed; humeral and ulnar components
INCLUDES Prosthesis removal and replacement in same elbow (eg, humeral and/or ulnar component(s)) (24370-24371)
EXCLUDES Foreign body removal (24200-24201)
Hardware removal other than prosthesis (20680)
🔲 36.3 ⚕ 36.3 **FUD** 090 [02] [A2] [50] [▣]
AMA: 2018,Sep,7; 2018,Jan,8; 2017,Jan,8; 2016,Jan,13

24164 radial head
EXCLUDES Foreign body removal (24200-24201)
Hardware removal other than prosthesis (20680)
🔲 20.8 ⚕ 20.8 **FUD** 090 [02] [A2] [50] [▣]
AMA: 2018,Sep,7; 2018,Jan,8; 2017,Jan,8; 2016,Jan,13

24200 Removal of foreign body, upper arm or elbow area; subcutaneous
🔲 4.05 ⚕ 6.20 **FUD** 010 [J] [P3] [80] [50] [▣]
AMA: 2018,Sep,7; 2018,Jan,8; 2017,Jan,8; 2016,Jan,13

24201 deep (subfascial or intramuscular)
🔲 10.4 ⚕ 15.8 **FUD** 090 [J] [A2] [50] [▣]
AMA: 2018,Sep,7; 2018,Jan,8; 2017,Jan,8; 2016,Jan,13

[26]/[TC] PC/TC Only   [A2]-[Z3] ASC Payment   [50] Bilateral   ♂ Male Only   ♀ Female Only   🔲 Facility RVU   ⚕ Non-Facility RVU   [▣] CCI   ✖ CLIA
FUD Follow-up Days   **CMS:** IOM   **AMA:** CPT Asst   [A]-[Y] OPPSI   [80]/[80] Surg Assist Allowed / w/Doc   Lab Crosswalk   Radiology Crosswalk

64

CPT © 2021 American Medical Association. All Rights Reserved.

© 2021 Optum360, LLC

24220 Injection for Elbow Arthrogram

24220 **Injection procedure for elbow arthrography**
EXCLUDES *Injection tennis elbow (20550)*
(73085)
1.95 4.71 **FUD** 000   N N1 80 50
AMA: 2018,Sep,7; 2018,Jan,8; 2017,Jan,8; 2016,May,13; 2016,Jan,13

24300-24498 Repair/Reconstruction of Elbow/Upper Arm

24300 **Manipulation, elbow, under anesthesia**
EXCLUDES *External fixation (20690, 20692)*
12.0 12.0 **FUD** 090   J G2 50
AMA: 2018,Sep,7

24301 **Muscle or tendon transfer, any type, upper arm or elbow, single (excluding 24320-24331)**
21.6 21.6 **FUD** 090   J A2 80
AMA: 2018,Sep,7

24305 **Tendon lengthening, upper arm or elbow, each tendon**
16.7 16.7 **FUD** 090   J A2 80
AMA: 2018,Sep,7

24310 **Tenotomy, open, elbow to shoulder, each tendon**
13.4 13.4 **FUD** 090   J A2 80
AMA: 2018,Sep,7

24320 **Tenoplasty, with muscle transfer, with or without free graft, elbow to shoulder, single (Seddon-Brookes type procedure)**
22.5 22.5 **FUD** 090   J A2 80
AMA: 2018,Sep,7

24330 **Flexor-plasty, elbow (eg, Steindler type advancement);**
20.7 20.7 **FUD** 090   J A2 80 50
AMA: 2018,Sep,7

24331 **with extensor advancement**
22.7 22.7 **FUD** 090   J A2 80 50
AMA: 2018,Sep,7

24332 **Tenolysis, triceps**
17.6 17.6 **FUD** 090   J G2 50
AMA: 2018,Sep,7

24340 **Tenodesis of biceps tendon at elbow (separate procedure)**
17.7 17.7 **FUD** 090   J A2 80 50
AMA: 2018,Sep,7

24341 **Repair, tendon or muscle, upper arm or elbow, each tendon or muscle, primary or secondary (excludes rotator cuff)**
21.4 21.4 **FUD** 090   J A2 80 50
AMA: 2018,Sep,7

24342 **Reinsertion of ruptured biceps or triceps tendon, distal, with or without tendon graft**
22.3 22.3 **FUD** 090   J A2 80 50
AMA: 2018,Sep,7; 2018,Jan,8; 2017,Apr,9

24343 **Repair lateral collateral ligament, elbow, with local tissue**
20.4 20.4 **FUD** 090   J G2 80 50
AMA: 2018,Sep,7

24344 **Reconstruction lateral collateral ligament, elbow, with tendon graft (includes harvesting of graft)**
31.5 31.5 **FUD** 090   J J8 80 50
AMA: 2018,Sep,7

24345 **Repair medial collateral ligament, elbow, with local tissue**
20.2 20.2 **FUD** 090   J A2 80 50
AMA: 2018,Sep,7

24346 **Reconstruction medial collateral ligament, elbow, with tendon graft (includes harvesting of graft)**
31.7 31.7 **FUD** 090   J G2 80 50
AMA: 2018,Sep,7

24357 **Tenotomy, elbow, lateral or medial (eg, epicondylitis, tennis elbow, golfer's elbow); percutaneous**
EXCLUDES *Arthroscopy, elbow, surgical; debridement (29837-29838)*
11.9 11.9 **FUD** 090   J G2 80 50
AMA: 2018,Sep,7; 2018,Jan,8; 2017,Jan,8; 2016,Jan,13

24358 **debridement, soft tissue and/or bone, open**
EXCLUDES *Arthroscopy, elbow, surgical; debridement (29837-29838)*
15.1 15.1 **FUD** 090   J G2 80 50
AMA: 2018,Sep,7; 2018,Jan,8; 2017,Jan,8; 2016,Jan,13

24359 **debridement, soft tissue and/or bone, open with tendon repair or reattachment**
EXCLUDES *Arthroscopy, elbow, surgical; debridement (29837-29838)*
19.0 19.0 **FUD** 090   J G2 80 50
AMA: 2018,Sep,7; 2018,Jan,8; 2017,Jan,8; 2016,Jan,13

24360 **Arthroplasty, elbow; with membrane (eg, fascial)**
26.0 26.0 **FUD** 090   J J8 80 50
AMA: 2018,Sep,7

24361 **with distal humeral prosthetic replacement**
29.1 29.1 **FUD** 090   J J8 80 50
AMA: 2018,Sep,7

24362 **with implant and fascia lata ligament reconstruction**
30.6 30.6 **FUD** 090   J J8 80 50
AMA: 2018,Sep,7

24363 **with distal humerus and proximal ulnar prosthetic replacement (eg, total elbow)**
EXCLUDES *Total elbow implant revision (24370-24371)*
41.9 41.9 **FUD** 090   J J8 80 50
AMA: 2018,Sep,7; 2018,Jan,8; 2017,Jan,8; 2016,Jan,13

24365 **Arthroplasty, radial head;**
18.4 18.4 **FUD** 090   J J8 80 50
AMA: 2018,Sep,7

24366 **with implant**
19.6 19.6 **FUD** 090   J J8 80 50
AMA: 2018,Sep,7

24370 **Revision of total elbow arthroplasty, including allograft when performed; humeral or ulnar component**
EXCLUDES *Prosthesis removal without replacement in same elbow (eg, humeral and/or ulnar component/s) (24160)*
44.7 44.7 **FUD** 090   J J8 80 50
AMA: 2018,Sep,7; 2018,Jan,8; 2017,Jan,8; 2016,Jan,13

24371 **humeral and ulnar component**
EXCLUDES *Prosthesis removal without replacement in same elbow (eg, humeral and/or ulnar component/s) (24160)*
51.3 51.3 **FUD** 090   J J8 80 50
AMA: 2018,Sep,7; 2018,Jan,8; 2017,Jan,8; 2016,Jan,13

24400 **Osteotomy, humerus, with or without internal fixation**
EXCLUDES *Osteotomy with insertion intramedullary lengthening device, humerus (0594T)*
23.7 23.7 **FUD** 090   J A2 80 50
AMA: 2018,Sep,7; 2018,Jan,8; 2017,Jan,8; 2016,Jan,13

24410 **Multiple osteotomies with realignment on intramedullary rod, humeral shaft (Sofield type procedure)**
EXCLUDES *Osteotomy with insertion intramedullary lengthening device, humerus (0594T)*
30.5 30.5 **FUD** 090   J G2 80 50
AMA: 2018,Sep,7

24420 **Osteoplasty, humerus (eg, shortening or lengthening) (excluding 64876)**
EXCLUDES *Osteotomy with insertion intramedullary lengthening device, humerus (0594T)*
29.5 29.5 **FUD** 090   J A2 80 50
AMA: 2018,Sep,7

24430   **Repair of nonunion or malunion, humerus; without graft (eg, compression technique)**
EXCLUDES   *Repair proximal radius and/or ulna (25400-25420)*
🔲 30.4   ⚖ 30.4   **FUD** 090   J J8 80 50 ▢
AMA: 2018,Sep,7

24435   **with iliac or other autograft (includes obtaining graft)**
EXCLUDES   *Repair proximal radius and/or ulna (25400-25420)*
🔲 31.0   ⚖ 31.0   **FUD** 090   J J8 80 50 ▢
AMA: 2018,Sep,7

24470   **Hemiepiphyseal arrest (eg, cubitus varus or valgus, distal humerus)**
🔲 19.3   ⚖ 19.3   **FUD** 090   J A2 80 50 ▢
AMA: 2018,Sep,7

24495   **Decompression fasciotomy, forearm, with brachial artery exploration**
🔲 21.3   ⚖ 21.3   **FUD** 090   J A2 80 50 ▢
AMA: 2018,Sep,7

24498   **Prophylactic treatment (nailing, pinning, plating or wiring), with or without methylmethacrylate, humeral shaft**
🔲 24.9   ⚖ 24.9   **FUD** 090   J J8 80 50 ▢
AMA: 2018,Sep,7

24500-24685 Treatment of Fracture/Dislocation of Elbow/Upper Arm
INCLUDES   Treatment for either closed or open fractures or dislocations

24500   **Closed treatment of humeral shaft fracture; without manipulation**
🔲 9.35   ⚖ 10.2   **FUD** 090   T A2 50 ▢
AMA: 2018,Sep,7

24505   **with manipulation, with or without skeletal traction**
🔲 12.9   ⚖ 14.3   **FUD** 090   J A2 50 ▢
AMA: 2018,Sep,7

24515   **Open treatment of humeral shaft fracture with plate/screws, with or without cerclage**
🔲 25.3   ⚖ 25.3   **FUD** 090   J J8 80 50 ▢
AMA: 2018,Sep,7

24516   **Treatment of humeral shaft fracture, with insertion of intramedullary implant, with or without cerclage and/or locking screws**
EXCLUDES   *Osteotomy with insertion intramedullary lengthening device, humerus (0594T)*
🔲 24.7   ⚖ 24.7   **FUD** 090   J J8 80 50 ▢
AMA: 2018,Sep,7; 2018,Jan,8; 2018,Jan,3; 2017,Jan,8; 2016,Jan,13

24530   **Closed treatment of supracondylar or transcondylar humeral fracture, with or without intercondylar extension; without manipulation**
🔲 9.96   ⚖ 10.9   **FUD** 090   T A2 50 ▢
AMA: 2018,Sep,7

24535   **with manipulation, with or without skin or skeletal traction**
🔲 16.3   ⚖ 17.6   **FUD** 090   J A2 50 ▢
AMA: 2018,Sep,7

24538   **Percutaneous skeletal fixation of supracondylar or transcondylar humeral fracture, with or without intercondylar extension**
🔲 21.5   ⚖ 21.5   **FUD** 090   J A2 50 ▢
AMA: 2018,Sep,7; 2018,Jan,8; 2017,Jan,8; 2016,Jan,13

24545   **Open treatment of humeral supracondylar or transcondylar fracture, includes internal fixation, when performed; without intercondylar extension**
🔲 26.7   ⚖ 26.7   **FUD** 090   J J8 80 50 ▢
AMA: 2018,Sep,7

24546   **with intercondylar extension**
🔲 29.9   ⚖ 29.9   **FUD** 090   J J8 80 50 ▢
AMA: 2018,Sep,7

24560   **Closed treatment of humeral epicondylar fracture, medial or lateral; without manipulation**
🔲 8.41   ⚖ 9.43   **FUD** 090   T A2 50 ▢
AMA: 2018,Sep,7

24565   **with manipulation**
🔲 14.1   ⚖ 15.3   **FUD** 090   J A2 50 ▢
AMA: 2018,Sep,7

24566   **Percutaneous skeletal fixation of humeral epicondylar fracture, medial or lateral, with manipulation**
🔲 20.6   ⚖ 20.6   **FUD** 090   J A2 50 ▢
AMA: 2018,Sep,7

24575   **Open treatment of humeral epicondylar fracture, medial or lateral, includes internal fixation, when performed**
🔲 21.0   ⚖ 21.0   **FUD** 090   J J8 80 50 ▢
AMA: 2018,Sep,7

24576   **Closed treatment of humeral condylar fracture, medial or lateral; without manipulation**
🔲 8.75   ⚖ 9.80   **FUD** 090   T A2 50 ▢
AMA: 2018,Sep,7

24577   **with manipulation**
🔲 14.4   ⚖ 15.8   **FUD** 090   J A2 50 ▢
AMA: 2018,Sep,7

24579   **Open treatment of humeral condylar fracture, medial or lateral, includes internal fixation, when performed**
EXCLUDES   *Closed treatment without manipulation (24530, 24560, 24576, 24650, 24670)*
Repair with manipulation (24535, 24565, 24577, 24675)
🔲 24.0   ⚖ 24.0   **FUD** 090   J J8 80 50 ▢
AMA: 2018,Sep,7

24582   **Percutaneous skeletal fixation of humeral condylar fracture, medial or lateral, with manipulation**
🔲 23.3   ⚖ 23.3   **FUD** 090   J A2 50 ▢
AMA: 2018,Sep,7

24586   **Open treatment of periarticular fracture and/or dislocation of the elbow (fracture distal humerus and proximal ulna and/or proximal radius);**
🔲 31.2   ⚖ 31.2   **FUD** 090   J 62 80 50 ▢
AMA: 2018,Sep,7

24587   **with implant arthroplasty**
EXCLUDES   *Distal humerus arthroplasty with implant (24361)*
🔲 31.4   ⚖ 31.4   **FUD** 090   J J8 80 50 ▢
AMA: 2018,Sep,7

24600   **Treatment of closed elbow dislocation; without anesthesia**
🔲 9.71   ⚖ 10.6   **FUD** 090   T A2 50 ▢
AMA: 2018,Sep,7

24605   **requiring anesthesia**
🔲 13.5   ⚖ 13.5   **FUD** 090   J A2 50 ▢
AMA: 2018,Sep,7

24615   **Open treatment of acute or chronic elbow dislocation**
🔲 20.6   ⚖ 20.6   **FUD** 090   J A2 80 50 ▢
AMA: 2018,Sep,7

24620   **Closed treatment of Monteggia type of fracture dislocation at elbow (fracture proximal end of ulna with dislocation of radial head), with manipulation**
🔲 15.8   ⚖ 15.8   **FUD** 090   J A2 80 50 ▢
AMA: 2018,Sep,7

24635   **Open treatment of Monteggia type of fracture dislocation at elbow (fracture proximal end of ulna with dislocation of radial head), includes internal fixation, when performed**
🔲 19.3   ⚖ 19.3   **FUD** 090   J J8 80 50 ▢
AMA: 2018,Sep,7

24640   **Closed treatment of radial head subluxation in child, nursemaid elbow, with manipulation**   A
🔲 2.26   ⚖ 2.89   **FUD** 010   T P3 80 50 ▢
AMA: 2018,Sep,7

24650 Closed treatment of radial head or neck fracture; without manipulation
🚗 6.96 ⚕ 7.51 **FUD** 090   T P2 50 📋
AMA: 2018,Sep,7

24655 with manipulation
🚗 11.4 ⚕ 12.6 **FUD** 090   J A2 50 📋
AMA: 2018,Sep,7

24665 Open treatment of radial head or neck fracture, includes internal fixation or radial head excision, when performed;
🚗 18.8 ⚕ 18.8 **FUD** 090   J A2 80 50 📋
AMA: 2018,Sep,7

24666 with radial head prosthetic replacement
🚗 21.1 ⚕ 21.1 **FUD** 090   J J8 80 50 📋
AMA: 2018,Sep,7

24670 Closed treatment of ulnar fracture, proximal end (eg, olecranon or coronoid process[es]); without manipulation
🚗 7.53 ⚕ 8.28 **FUD** 090   T A2 50 📋
AMA: 2018,Sep,7

24675 with manipulation
🚗 11.9 ⚕ 13.1 **FUD** 090   J A2 50 📋
AMA: 2018,Sep,7

24685 Open treatment of ulnar fracture, proximal end (eg, olecranon or coronoid process[es]), includes internal fixation, when performed
EXCLUDES *Arthrotomy, elbow (24100-24102)*
🚗 18.8 ⚕ 18.8 **FUD** 090   J J8 80 50 📋
AMA: 2018,Sep,7; 2018,Jan,3

24800-24999 Other/Unlisted Elbow/Upper Arm Procedures

24800 Arthrodesis, elbow joint; local
🚗 23.9 ⚕ 23.9 **FUD** 090   J A2 80 50 📋
AMA: 2020,May,13; 2018,Sep,7

24802 with autogenous graft (includes obtaining graft)
🚗 28.9 ⚕ 28.9 **FUD** 090   J G2 80 50 📋
AMA: 2020,May,13; 2018,Sep,7

24900 Amputation, arm through humerus; with primary closure
🚗 21.3 ⚕ 21.3 **FUD** 090   C 80 50 📋
AMA: 2018,Sep,7

24920 open, circular (guillotine)
🚗 21.1 ⚕ 21.1 **FUD** 090   C 80 50 📋
AMA: 2018,Sep,7

24925 secondary closure or scar revision
🚗 16.3 ⚕ 16.3 **FUD** 090   J A2 80 50 📋
AMA: 2018,Sep,7

24930 re-amputation
🚗 22.3 ⚕ 22.3 **FUD** 090   C 80 50 📋
AMA: 2018,Sep,7

24931 with implant
🚗 26.9 ⚕ 26.9 **FUD** 090   C 80 50 📋
AMA: 2020,NovBULL,2; 2018,Sep,7

24935 Stump elongation, upper extremity
🚗 33.6 ⚕ 33.6 **FUD** 090   J G2 80 50 📋
AMA: 2018,Sep,7

24940 Cineplasty, upper extremity, complete procedure
🚗 0.00 ⚕ 0.00 **FUD** 090   C 80 50 📋
AMA: 2018,Sep,7

24999 Unlisted procedure, humerus or elbow
🚗 0.00 ⚕ 0.00 **FUD** YYY   T 80 50 📋
AMA: 2018,Sep,7

25000-25001 Incision Tendon Sheath of Wrist

25000 Incision, extensor tendon sheath, wrist (eg, deQuervains disease)
EXCLUDES *Carpal tunnel release (64721)*
🚗 9.70 ⚕ 9.70 **FUD** 090   J A2 50 📋
AMA: 2018,Sep,7

25001 Incision, flexor tendon sheath, wrist (eg, flexor carpi radialis)
🚗 9.88 ⚕ 9.88 **FUD** 090   J G2 50 📋
AMA: 2018,Sep,7

25020-25025 Decompression Fasciotomy Forearm/Wrist

25020 Decompression fasciotomy, forearm and/or wrist, flexor OR extensor compartment; without debridement of nonviable muscle and/or nerve
EXCLUDES *Brachial artery exploration (24495)*
Superficial incision and drainage (10060-10160)
🚗 16.4 ⚕ 16.4 **FUD** 090   J A2 50 📋
AMA: 2018,Sep,7

25023 with debridement of nonviable muscle and/or nerve
EXCLUDES *Debridement (11000-11044 [11045, 11046])*
Decompression fasciotomy with exploration brachial artery exploration (24495)
Superficial incision and drainage (10060-10160)
🚗 34.4 ⚕ 34.4 **FUD** 090   J A2 80 50 📋
AMA: 2018,Sep,7

25024 Decompression fasciotomy, forearm and/or wrist, flexor AND extensor compartment; without debridement of nonviable muscle and/or nerve
🚗 22.5 ⚕ 22.5 **FUD** 090   J A2 50 📋
AMA: 2018,Sep,7

25025 with debridement of nonviable muscle and/or nerve
🚗 34.8 ⚕ 34.8 **FUD** 090   J A2 80 50 📋
AMA: 2018,Sep,7

25028-25040 Incision for Drainage/Foreign Body Removal

25028 Incision and drainage, forearm and/or wrist; deep abscess or hematoma
🚗 17.0 ⚕ 17.0 **FUD** 090   J A2 50 📋
AMA: 2018,Sep,7

25031 bursa
🚗 10.0 ⚕ 10.0 **FUD** 090   J A2 80 50 📋
AMA: 2018,Sep,7

25035 Incision, deep, bone cortex, forearm and/or wrist (eg, osteomyelitis or bone abscess)
🚗 16.8 ⚕ 16.8 **FUD** 090   J A2 80 50 📋
AMA: 2018,Sep,7

25040 Arthrotomy, radiocarpal or midcarpal joint, with exploration, drainage, or removal of foreign body
🚗 16.1 ⚕ 16.1 **FUD** 090   J A2 80 50 📋
AMA: 2018,Sep,7

25065-25066 Biopsy Forearm/Wrist

EXCLUDES *Soft tissue needle biopsy (20206)*

25065 Biopsy, soft tissue of forearm and/or wrist; superficial
🚗 4.59 ⚕ 7.37 **FUD** 010   J P3 50 📋
AMA: 2018,Sep,7

25066 deep (subfascial or intramuscular)
🚗 10.3 ⚕ 10.3 **FUD** 090   J A2 50 📋
AMA: 2018,Sep,7

25071-25078 [25071, 25073] Excision Soft Tissue Tumors Forearm/Wrist

INCLUDES
Any necessary elevation tissue planes or dissection
Measurement tumor and necessary margin at greatest diameter prior to excision
Simple and intermediate repairs
Excision types:
Fascial or subfascial soft tissue tumors: simple and marginal resection tumors found either in or below deep fascia, not involving bone or excision substantial amount normal tissue; primarily benign and intramuscular tumors
Radical resection soft tissue tumor: wide resection tumor involving substantial margins normal tissue and may include tissue removal from one or more layers; most often malignant or aggressive benign
Subcutaneous: simple and marginal resection tumors in subcutaneous tissue above deep fascia; most often benign

EXCLUDES
Complex repair
Excision benign cutaneous lesions (eg, sebaceous cyst) (11400-11406)
Radical resection cutaneous tumors (eg, melanoma) (11600-11606)
Significant vessel exploration or neuroplasty

25071 Resequenced code. See code following 25075.

25073 Resequenced code. See code following 25076.

25075 Excision, tumor, soft tissue of forearm and/or wrist area, subcutaneous; less than 3 cm
🔲 9.09   ⚕ 14.5   **FUD** 090   J G2 50 ▣
AMA: 2018,Sep,7

\# **25071**   3 cm or greater
🔲 12.2   ⚕ 12.2   **FUD** 090   J G2 80 50 ▣
AMA: 2018,Sep,7

25076 Excision, tumor, soft tissue of forearm and/or wrist area, subfascial (eg, intramuscular); less than 3 cm
🔲 14.9   ⚕ 14.9   **FUD** 090   J G2 50 ▣
AMA: 2018,Sep,7

\# **25073**   3 cm or greater
🔲 15.4   ⚕ 15.4   **FUD** 090   J G2 80 50 ▣
AMA: 2018,Sep,7

25077 Radical resection of tumor (eg, sarcoma), soft tissue of forearm and/or wrist area; less than 3 cm
🔲 25.6   ⚕ 25.6   **FUD** 090   J G2 50 ▣
AMA: 2018,Sep,7

25078   3 cm or greater
🔲 33.6   ⚕ 33.6   **FUD** 090   J G2 80 50 ▣
AMA: 2018,Sep,7

25085-25240 Procedures of Bones/Joints Lower Arm/Wrist

25085 Capsulotomy, wrist (eg, contracture)
🔲 12.9   ⚕ 12.9   **FUD** 090   J A2 80 50 ▣
AMA: 2018,Sep,7

25100 Arthrotomy, wrist joint; with biopsy
🔲 10.0   ⚕ 10.0   **FUD** 090   J A2 80 50 ▣
AMA: 2018,Sep,7

25101   with joint exploration, with or without biopsy, with or without removal of loose or foreign body
🔲 11.6   ⚕ 11.6   **FUD** 090   J A2 80 50 ▣
AMA: 2018,Sep,7

25105   with synovectomy
🔲 13.9   ⚕ 13.9   **FUD** 090   J A2 80 50 ▣
AMA: 2018,Sep,7

25107 Arthrotomy, distal radioulnar joint including repair of triangular cartilage, complex
🔲 17.7   ⚕ 17.7   **FUD** 090   J A2 80 50 ▣
AMA: 2018,Sep,7

25109 Excision of tendon, forearm and/or wrist, flexor or extensor, each
🔲 15.4   ⚕ 15.4   **FUD** 090   J G2 50 ▣
AMA: 2018,Sep,7

25110 Excision, lesion of tendon sheath, forearm and/or wrist
🔲 9.84   ⚕ 9.84   **FUD** 090   J A2 50 ▣
AMA: 2018,Sep,7

25111 Excision of ganglion, wrist (dorsal or volar); primary
EXCLUDES   Excision ganglion hand or finger (26160)
🔲 9.24   ⚕ 9.24   **FUD** 090   J A2 50 ▣
AMA: 2018,Sep,7

Synovial sheaths (blue) of the dorsum of right wrist, containing extensor tendons

Ganglion

Anatomical "snuffbox"

Anatomical "snuffbox"

Typical location of ganglion

Ganglions are round cystic swellings usually appearing on the dorsum of the wrist or hand; these swellings often communicate with the synovial sheath

25112   recurrent
EXCLUDES   Excision ganglion hand or finger (26160)
🔲 11.1   ⚕ 11.1   **FUD** 090   J A2 50 ▣
AMA: 2018,Sep,7

25115 Radical excision of bursa, synovia of wrist, or forearm tendon sheaths (eg, tenosynovitis, fungus, Tbc, or other granulomas, rheumatoid arthritis); flexors
EXCLUDES   Finger synovectomy (26145)
🔲 21.8   ⚕ 21.8   **FUD** 090   J A2 50 ▣
AMA: 2018,Sep,7; 2018,Jan,8; 2017,Jan,8; 2016,Jan,13

25116   extensors, with or without transposition of dorsal retinaculum
EXCLUDES   Finger synovectomy (26145)
🔲 17.3   ⚕ 17.3   **FUD** 090   J A2 50 ▣
AMA: 2018,Sep,7

25118 Synovectomy, extensor tendon sheath, wrist, single compartment;
EXCLUDES   Finger synovectomy (26145)
🔲 10.9   ⚕ 10.9   **FUD** 090   J A2 50 ▣
AMA: 2018,Sep,7; 2018,Jan,8; 2017,Jan,8; 2016,Jan,13

25119   with resection of distal ulna
EXCLUDES   Finger synovectomy (26145)
🔲 14.2   ⚕ 14.2   **FUD** 090   J A2 80 50 ▣
AMA: 2018,Sep,7

25120 Excision or curettage of bone cyst or benign tumor of radius or ulna (excluding head or neck of radius and olecranon process);
EXCLUDES   Removal bone cyst or tumor radial head, neck, or olecranon process (24120-24126)
🔲 14.4   ⚕ 14.4   **FUD** 090   J A2 80 50 ▣
AMA: 2018,Sep,7

25125   with autograft (includes obtaining graft)
🔲 16.9   ⚕ 16.9   **FUD** 090   J A2 80 50 ▣
AMA: 2018,Sep,7

25126   with allograft
🔲 17.2   ⚕ 17.2   **FUD** 090   J A2 80 50 ▣
AMA: 2019,May,7; 2018,Sep,7

25130 Excision or curettage of bone cyst or benign tumor of carpal bones;
🔲 12.9   ⚕ 12.9   **FUD** 090   J A2 80 50 ▣
AMA: 2018,Sep,7

28/TC PC/TC Only   A2-Z3 ASC Payment   50 Bilateral   ♂ Male Only   ♀ Female Only   🔲 Facility RVU   ⚕ Non-Facility RVU   ▣ CCI   ✖ CLIA
FUD Follow-up Days   CMS: IOM   AMA: CPT Asst   A-Y OPPSI   80/80 Surg Assist Allowed / w/Doc   Lab Crosswalk   Radiology Crosswalk

68   CPT © 2021 American Medical Association. All Rights Reserved.   © 2021 Optum360, LLC

25135 with autograft (includes obtaining graft)
16.0 16.0 **FUD** 090 J A2 80 50
AMA: 2018,Sep,7

25136 with allograft
14.2 14.2 **FUD** 090 J A2 80 50
AMA: 2019,May,7; 2018,Sep,7

25145 Sequestrectomy (eg, for osteomyelitis or bone abscess), forearm and/or wrist
14.9 14.9 **FUD** 090 A2 80 50
AMA: 2018,Sep,7

25150 Partial excision (craterization, saucerization, or diaphysectomy) of bone (eg, for osteomyelitis); ulna
16.2 16.2 **FUD** 090 J A2 50
AMA: 2018,Sep,7

25151 radius
EXCLUDES *Partial removal radial head, neck, or olecranon process (24145, 24147)*
16.8 16.8 **FUD** 090 A2 80 50
AMA: 2018,Sep,7

25170 Radical resection of tumor, radius or ulna
INCLUDES Any necessary elevation tissue planes or dissection
Excision adjacent soft tissue during bone tumor resection (25071-25078 [25071, 25073])
Measurement tumor and necessary margin at greatest diameter prior to excision
Resection tumor (may include entire bone) and wide margins normal tissues primarily for malignant or aggressive benign tumors
Resection without removal significant normal tissue
Simple and intermediate repairs
EXCLUDES *Complex repair*
Radical resection cutaneous tumors (e.g., melanoma) (11600-11646)
Significant vessel exploration, neuroplasty, reconstruction, or complex bone repair
42.5 42.5 **FUD** 090 J G2 80 50
AMA: 2019,May,7; 2018,Sep,7

25210 Carpectomy; 1 bone
EXCLUDES *Carpectomy with insertion implant (25441-25445)*
14.0 14.0 **FUD** 090 J A2 80
AMA: 2018,Sep,7

25215 all bones of proximal row
17.8 17.8 **FUD** 090 J A2 80 50
AMA: 2019,Dec,14; 2019,Feb,10; 2018,Sep,7

25230 Radial styloidectomy (separate procedure)
12.4 12.4 **FUD** 090 J A2 50
AMA: 2018,Sep,7

25240 Excision distal ulna partial or complete (eg, Darrach type or matched resection)
EXCLUDES *Acquisition fascia for interposition (20920, 20922)*
Implant replacement (25442)
12.3 12.3 **FUD** 090 J A2 80 50
AMA: 2018,Sep,7

25246 Injection for Wrist Arthrogram

25246 Injection procedure for wrist arthrography
EXCLUDES *Excision superficial foreign body (20520)*
(73115)
2.14 5.25 **FUD** 000 N N1 50
AMA: 2018,Sep,7; 2018,Jan,8; 2017,Jan,8; 2016,Jan,13

25248-25251 Removal Foreign Body of Wrist
EXCLUDES *Excision superficial foreign body (20520)*
K-wire, pin, or rod insertion (20650)
K-wire, pin, or rod removal (20670, 20680)

25248 Exploration with removal of deep foreign body, forearm or wrist
11.8 11.8 **FUD** 090 J A2 50
AMA: 2018,Sep,7

25250 Removal of wrist prosthesis; (separate procedure)
15.2 15.2 **FUD** 090 Q2 A2 80 50
AMA: 2018,Sep,7

25251 complicated, including total wrist
20.7 20.7 **FUD** 090 Q2 A2 80 50
AMA: 2018,Sep,7

25259 Manipulation of Wrist with Anesthesia

25259 Manipulation, wrist, under anesthesia
EXCLUDES *Application external fixation (20690, 20692)*
12.1 12.1 **FUD** 090 J G2 50
AMA: 2018,Sep,7; 2018,Jan,8; 2017,Jan,8; 2016,Jan,13

25260-25492 Repair/Reconstruction of Forearm/Wrist

25260 Repair, tendon or muscle, flexor, forearm and/or wrist; primary, single, each tendon or muscle
18.1 18.1 **FUD** 090 J A2
AMA: 2018,Sep,7

25263 secondary, single, each tendon or muscle
18.1 18.1 **FUD** 090 J A2 80
AMA: 2018,Sep,7

25265 secondary, with free graft (includes obtaining graft), each tendon or muscle
21.4 21.4 **FUD** 090 J A2 80
AMA: 2018,Sep,7

25270 Repair, tendon or muscle, extensor, forearm and/or wrist; primary, single, each tendon or muscle
14.1 14.1 **FUD** 090 J A2 80
AMA: 2018,Sep,7

25272 secondary, single, each tendon or muscle
15.9 15.9 **FUD** 090 J A2 80
AMA: 2018,Sep,7

25274 secondary, with free graft (includes obtaining graft), each tendon or muscle
19.1 19.1 **FUD** 090 J A2 80
AMA: 2018,Sep,7

25275 Repair, tendon sheath, extensor, forearm and/or wrist, with free graft (includes obtaining graft) (eg, for extensor carpi ulnaris subluxation)
19.3 19.3 **FUD** 090 J A2 80 50
AMA: 2018,Sep,7

25280 Lengthening or shortening of flexor or extensor tendon, forearm and/or wrist, single, each tendon
16.3 16.3 **FUD** 090 J A2 80
AMA: 2018,Sep,7

25290 Tenotomy, open, flexor or extensor tendon, forearm and/or wrist, single, each tendon
12.5 12.5 **FUD** 090 J A2
AMA: 2018,Sep,7

25295 Tenolysis, flexor or extensor tendon, forearm and/or wrist, single, each tendon
15.1 15.1 **FUD** 090 J A2
AMA: 2018,Sep,7; 2018,Jan,8; 2017,Jan,8; 2016,Jan,13

25300 Tenodesis at wrist; flexors of fingers
19.7 19.7 **FUD** 090 J A2 80 50
AMA: 2018,Sep,7

25301 extensors of fingers
18.5 18.5 **FUD** 090 J A2 80 50
AMA: 2018,Sep,7

25310 Tendon transplantation or transfer, flexor or extensor, forearm and/or wrist, single; each tendon
17.8 17.8 **FUD** 090 J A2 80
AMA: 2018,Sep,7; 2018,Jan,8; 2017,Jan,8; 2016,Jan,13

25312 with tendon graft(s) (includes obtaining graft), each tendon
20.7 20.7 **FUD** 090 J A2 80
AMA: 2018,Sep,7

Musculoskeletal System

25315 — 25449

25315 Flexor origin slide (eg, for cerebral palsy, Volkmann contracture), forearm and/or wrist;
    🦴 22.2   � 22.2   **FUD** 090   J A2 80 50 ▣
    AMA: 2018,Sep,7

25316 with tendon(s) transfer
    🦴 26.4   � 26.4   **FUD** 090   J A2 80 50 ▣
    AMA: 2018,Sep,7

25320 Capsulorrhaphy or reconstruction, wrist, open (eg, capsulodesis, ligament repair, tendon transfer or graft) (includes synovectomy, capsulotomy and open reduction) for carpal instability
    🦴 28.3   � 28.3   **FUD** 090   J A2 80 50 ▣
    AMA: 2018,Sep,7

25332 Arthroplasty, wrist, with or without interposition, with or without external or internal fixation
    EXCLUDES *Acquiring fascia for interposition (20920, 20922)*
    Arthroplasty with prosthesis (25441-25446)
    🦴 24.3   � 24.3   **FUD** 090   J A2 80 50 ▣
    AMA: 2019,Feb,10; 2018,Sep,7; 2018,Jan,8; 2017,Jan,8; 2016,Jan,13

25335 Centralization of wrist on ulna (eg, radial club hand)
    🦴 27.2   � 27.2   **FUD** 090   J A2 80 50 ▣
    AMA: 2018,Sep,7; 2018,May,10

25337 Reconstruction for stabilization of unstable distal ulna or distal radioulnar joint, secondary by soft tissue stabilization (eg, tendon transfer, tendon graft or weave, or tenodesis) with or without open reduction of distal radioulnar joint
    EXCLUDES *Acquiring fascia lata graft (20920, 20922)*
    🦴 25.5   � 25.5   **FUD** 090   J A2 50 ▣
    AMA: 2018,Sep,7

25350 Osteotomy, radius; distal third
    🦴 19.4   � 19.4   **FUD** 090   J J8 80 50 ▣
    AMA: 2018,Sep,7

25355 middle or proximal third
    🦴 22.0   � 22.0   **FUD** 090   J A2 80 50 ▣
    AMA: 2018,Sep,7

25360 Osteotomy; ulna
    🦴 18.8   � 18.8   **FUD** 090   J A2 80 50 ▣
    AMA: 2018,Sep,7

25365 radius AND ulna
    🦴 26.4   � 26.4   **FUD** 090   J A2 80 50 ▣
    AMA: 2018,Sep,7

25370 Multiple osteotomies, with realignment on intramedullary rod (Sofield type procedure); radius OR ulna
    🦴 29.0   � 29.0   **FUD** 090   J A2 80 50 ▣
    AMA: 2018,Sep,7

25375 radius AND ulna
    🦴 27.5   � 27.5   **FUD** 090   J A2 80 50 ▣
    AMA: 2018,Sep,7

25390 Osteoplasty, radius OR ulna; shortening
    🦴 22.1   � 22.1   **FUD** 090   J J8 80 50 ▣
    AMA: 2018,Sep,7

25391 lengthening with autograft
    🦴 28.7   � 28.7   **FUD** 090   J J8 80 50 ▣
    AMA: 2018,Sep,7

25392 Osteoplasty, radius AND ulna; shortening (excluding 64876)
    🦴 29.3   � 29.3   **FUD** 090   J A2 80 50 ▣
    AMA: 2018,Sep,7

25393 lengthening with autograft
    🦴 32.6   � 32.6   **FUD** 090   J A2 80 50 ▣
    AMA: 2018,Sep,7

25394 Osteoplasty, carpal bone, shortening
    🦴 22.6   � 22.6   **FUD** 090   J G2 80 50 ▣
    AMA: 2018,Sep,7

25400 Repair of nonunion or malunion, radius OR ulna; without graft (eg, compression technique)
    🦴 23.1   � 23.1   **FUD** 090   J J8 80 50 ▣
    AMA: 2018,Sep,7

25405 with autograft (includes obtaining graft)
    🦴 29.9   � 29.9   **FUD** 090   J J8 80 50 ▣
    AMA: 2018,Sep,7

25415 Repair of nonunion or malunion, radius AND ulna; without graft (eg, compression technique)
    🦴 27.9   � 27.9   **FUD** 090   J J8 80 50 ▣
    AMA: 2018,Sep,7

25420 with autograft (includes obtaining graft)
    🦴 33.7   � 33.7   **FUD** 090   J J8 80 50 ▣
    AMA: 2018,Sep,7

25425 Repair of defect with autograft; radius OR ulna
    🦴 27.8   � 27.8   **FUD** 090   J A2 80 50 ▣
    AMA: 2018,Sep,7

25426 radius AND ulna
    🦴 32.4   � 32.4   **FUD** 090   J J8 80 50 ▣
    AMA: 2018,Sep,7

25430 Insertion of vascular pedicle into carpal bone (eg, Hori procedure)
    🦴 21.0   � 21.0   **FUD** 090   J G2 50 ▣
    AMA: 2018,Sep,7

25431 Repair of nonunion of carpal bone (excluding carpal scaphoid (navicular)) (includes obtaining graft and necessary fixation), each bone
    🦴 22.7   � 22.7   **FUD** 090   J G2 80 50 ▣
    AMA: 2018,Sep,7

25440 Repair of nonunion, scaphoid carpal (navicular) bone, with or without radial styloidectomy (includes obtaining graft and necessary fixation)
    🦴 22.1   � 22.1   **FUD** 090   J A2 80 50 ▣
    AMA: 2018,Sep,7

25441 Arthroplasty with prosthetic replacement; distal radius
    🦴 27.0   � 27.0   **FUD** 090   J J8 80 50 ▣
    AMA: 2018,Sep,7; 2018,Jan,8; 2017,Aug,9; 2017,Jan,8; 2016,Jan,13

25442 distal ulna
    🦴 23.2   � 23.2   **FUD** 090   J J8 80 50 ▣
    AMA: 2018,Sep,7; 2018,Jan,8; 2017,Aug,9; 2017,Jan,8; 2016,Jan,13

25443 scaphoid carpal (navicular)
    🦴 22.6   � 22.6   **FUD** 090   J J8 80 50 ▣
    AMA: 2018,Sep,7; 2018,Jan,8; 2017,Jan,8; 2016,Jan,13

25444 lunate
    🦴 23.7   � 23.7   **FUD** 090   J J8 80 50 ▣
    AMA: 2018,Sep,7; 2018,Jan,8; 2017,Jan,8; 2016,Jan,13

25445 trapezium
    🦴 20.8   � 20.8   **FUD** 090   J J8 50 ▣
    AMA: 2018,Sep,7; 2018,Jan,8; 2017,Jan,8; 2016,Jan,13

25446 distal radius and partial or entire carpus (total wrist)
    🦴 33.8   � 33.8   **FUD** 090   J J8 80 50 ▣
    AMA: 2018,Sep,7; 2018,Jan,8; 2017,Jan,8; 2016,Jan,13

25447 Arthroplasty, interposition, intercarpal or carpometacarpal joints
    EXCLUDES *Wrist arthroplasty (25332)*
    🦴 23.8   � 23.8   **FUD** 090   J A2 80 50 ▣
    AMA: 2018,Sep,7; 2018,Jan,8; 2017,Jan,8; 2016,Jan,13

25449 Revision of arthroplasty, including removal of implant, wrist joint
    🦴 29.8   � 29.8   **FUD** 090   J A2 80 50 ▣
    AMA: 2018,Sep,7

26/TC PC/TC Only   A2-Z3 ASC Payment   50 Bilateral   ♂ Male Only   ♀ Female Only   🦴 Facility RVU   � Non-Facility RVU   ▣ CCI   ✖ CLIA
FUD Follow-up Days   **CMS:** IOM   **AMA:** CPT Asst   A-Y OPPSI   80/80 Surg Assist Allowed / w/Doc   Lab Crosswalk   Radiology Crosswalk

25450 Epiphyseal arrest by epiphysiodesis or stapling; distal radius OR ulna
🔧 17.7   ✂ 17.7   **FUD** 090   [J] [A2] [50] ▭
AMA: 2018,Sep,7

25455 distal radius AND ulna
🔧 20.9   ✂ 20.9   **FUD** 090   [J] [A2] [50] ▭
AMA: 2018,Sep,7

25490 Prophylactic treatment (nailing, pinning, plating or wiring) with or without methylmethacrylate; radius
🔧 20.7   ✂ 20.7   **FUD** 090   [J] [A2] [80] [50] ▭
AMA: 2018,Sep,7

25491 ulna
🔧 21.3   ✂ 21.3   **FUD** 090   [J] [A2] [80] [50] ▭
AMA: 2018,Sep,7

25492 radius AND ulna
🔧 26.1   ✂ 26.1   **FUD** 090   [J] [A2] [80] [50] ▭
AMA: 2018,Sep,7

25500-25695 Treatment of Fracture/Dislocation of Forearm/Wrist

Code also external fixation, when performed (20690, 20692)

25500 Closed treatment of radial shaft fracture; without manipulation
🔧 7.25   ✂ 7.98   **FUD** 090   [T] [P2] [50] ▭
AMA: 2018,Sep,7

25505 with manipulation
🔧 13.2   ✂ 14.4   **FUD** 090   [J] [A2] [50] ▭
AMA: 2018,Sep,7

25515 Open treatment of radial shaft fracture, includes internal fixation, when performed
🔧 19.2   ✂ 19.2   **FUD** 090   [J] [J8] [80] [50] ▭
AMA: 2018,Sep,7

25520 Closed treatment of radial shaft fracture and closed treatment of dislocation of distal radioulnar joint (Galeazzi fracture/dislocation)
🔧 15.5   ✂ 16.4   **FUD** 090   [J] [A2] [50] ▭
AMA: 2018,Sep,7

25525 Open treatment of radial shaft fracture, includes internal fixation, when performed, and closed treatment of distal radioulnar joint dislocation (Galeazzi fracture/ dislocation), includes percutaneous skeletal fixation, when performed
🔧 22.6   ✂ 22.6   **FUD** 090   [J] [J8] [80] [50] ▭
AMA: 2018,Sep,7

25526 Open treatment of radial shaft fracture, includes internal fixation, when performed, and open treatment of distal radioulnar joint dislocation (Galeazzi fracture/ dislocation), when performed, includes repair of triangular fibrocartilage complex
🔧 27.5   ✂ 27.5   **FUD** 090   [J] [A2] [80] [50] ▭
AMA: 2018,Sep,7

25530 Closed treatment of ulnar shaft fracture; without manipulation
🔧 6.88   ✂ 7.52   **FUD** 090   [T] [P2] [50] ▭
AMA: 2018,Sep,7

25535 with manipulation
🔧 13.0   ✂ 14.0   **FUD** 090   [T] [A2] [50] ▭
AMA: 2018,Sep,7

25545 Open treatment of ulnar shaft fracture, includes internal fixation, when performed
🔧 17.9   ✂ 17.9   **FUD** 090   [J] [J8] [80] [50] ▭
AMA: 2018,Sep,7; 2018,Jan,8; 2017,Jan,8; 2016,Jan,13

25560 Closed treatment of radial and ulnar shaft fractures; without manipulation
🔧 7.31   ✂ 8.15   **FUD** 090   [T] [P2] [50] ▭
AMA: 2018,Sep,7

25565 with manipulation
🔧 13.2   ✂ 14.7   **FUD** 090   [J] [A2] [50] ▭
AMA: 2018,Sep,7

25574 Open treatment of radial AND ulnar shaft fractures, with internal fixation, when performed; of radius OR ulna
🔧 19.4   ✂ 19.4   **FUD** 090   [J] [J8] [80] [50] ▭
AMA: 2018,Sep,7; 2018,Jan,8; 2017,Jan,8; 2016,Jan,13

25575 of radius AND ulna
🔧 25.9   ✂ 25.9   **FUD** 090   [J] [J8] [80] [50] ▭
AMA: 2018,Sep,7

25600 Closed treatment of distal radial fracture (eg, Colles or Smith type) or epiphyseal separation, includes closed treatment of fracture of ulnar styloid, when performed; without manipulation
[INCLUDES]   Closed treatment ulnar styloid fracture (25650)
🔧 9.06   ✂ 9.51   **FUD** 090   [T] [P2] [50] ▭
AMA: 2018,Sep,7; 2018,Jan,8; 2017,Jan,8; 2016,Jan,13

25605 with manipulation
[INCLUDES]   Closed treatment ulnar styloid fracture (25650)
🔧 14.7   ✂ 15.5   **FUD** 090   [J] [A2] [50] ▭
AMA: 2018,Sep,7; 2018,Jan,8; 2017,Jan,8; 2016,Jan,13

25606 Percutaneous skeletal fixation of distal radial fracture or epiphyseal separation
[EXCLUDES]   Closed treatment ulnar styloid fracture (25650)
Open repair ulnar styloid fracture (25652)
Percutaneous repair ulnar styloid fracture (25651)
🔧 19.1   ✂ 19.1   **FUD** 090   [J] [A2] [50] ▭
AMA: 2018,Sep,7

25607 Open treatment of distal radial extra-articular fracture or epiphyseal separation, with internal fixation
[EXCLUDES]   Closed treatment ulnar styloid fracture (25650)
Open repair ulnar styloid fracture (25652)
Percutaneous repair ulnar styloid fracture (25651)
🔧 21.1   ✂ 21.1   **FUD** 090   [J] [J8] [80] [50] ▭
AMA: 2018,Sep,7; 2018,Jan,8; 2017,Jan,8; 2016,Jan,13

25608 Open treatment of distal radial intra-articular fracture or epiphyseal separation; with internal fixation of 2 fragments
[EXCLUDES]   Closed treatment ulnar styloid fracture (25650)
Open repair ulnar styloid fracture (25652)
Open treatment distal radial intra-articular fracture or epiphyseal separation; with internal fixation of 3 or more fragments (25609)
Percutaneous repair ulnar styloid fracture (25651)
🔧 23.7   ✂ 23.7   **FUD** 090   [J] [J8] [80] [50] ▭
AMA: 2018,Sep,7; 2018,Jan,8; 2017,Jan,8; 2016,Jan,13

25609 with internal fixation of 3 or more fragments
[EXCLUDES]   Closed treatment ulnar styloid fracture (25650)
Open repair ulnar styloid fracture (25652)
Percutaneous repair ulnar styloid fracture (25651)
🔧 30.2   ✂ 30.2   **FUD** 090   [J] [J8] [80] [50] ▭
AMA: 2018,Sep,7; 2018,Jan,8; 2017,Jan,8; 2016,Jan,13

25622 Closed treatment of carpal scaphoid (navicular) fracture; without manipulation
🔧 8.07   ✂ 8.76   **FUD** 090   [T] [P2] [50] ▭
AMA: 2018,Sep,7

25624 with manipulation
🔧 12.6   ✂ 13.8   **FUD** 090   [J] [A2] [80] [50] ▭
AMA: 2018,Sep,7

25628 Open treatment of carpal scaphoid (navicular) fracture, includes internal fixation, when performed
🔧 20.7   ✂ 20.7   **FUD** 090   [J] [A2] [80] [50] ▭
AMA: 2018,Sep,7

25630 Closed treatment of carpal bone fracture (excluding carpal scaphoid [navicular]); without manipulation, each bone
🔧 8.13   ✂ 8.77   **FUD** 090   [T] [P2] [50] ▭
AMA: 2018,Sep,7

25635 **with manipulation, each bone**
🛏 11.9   🖐 13.1   **FUD** 090   J A2 80 50 ▭
AMA: 2018,Sep,7

25645 **Open treatment of carpal bone fracture (other than carpal scaphoid [navicular]), each bone**
🛏 16.4   🖐 16.4   **FUD** 090   J A2 80 50 ▭
AMA: 2018,Sep,7

25650 **Closed treatment of ulnar styloid fracture**
EXCLUDES Closed treatment distal radial fracture (25600, 25605)
Open treatment distal radial extra-articular fracture or epiphyseal separation, with internal fixation (25607-25609)
🛏 8.70   🖐 9.35   **FUD** 090   T P2 50 ▭
AMA: 2018,Sep,7; 2018,Jan,8; 2017,Jan,8; 2016,Jan,13

25651 **Percutaneous skeletal fixation of ulnar styloid fracture**
🛏 14.0   🖐 14.0   **FUD** 090   J G2 80 50 ▭
AMA: 2018,Sep,7

25652 **Open treatment of ulnar styloid fracture**
🛏 17.9   🖐 17.9   **FUD** 090   J J8 50 ▭
AMA: 2018,Sep,7; 2018,Jan,8; 2017,Jan,8; 2016,Jan,13

25660 **Closed treatment of radiocarpal or intercarpal dislocation, 1 or more bones, with manipulation**
🛏 11.9   🖐 11.9   **FUD** 090   T A2 80 50 ▭
AMA: 2018,Sep,7

25670 **Open treatment of radiocarpal or intercarpal dislocation, 1 or more bones**
🛏 17.5   🖐 17.5   **FUD** 090   J J8 80 50 ▭
AMA: 2018,Sep,7

25671 **Percutaneous skeletal fixation of distal radioulnar dislocation**
🛏 15.3   🖐 15.3   **FUD** 090   J A2 50 ▭
AMA: 2018,Sep,7

25675 **Closed treatment of distal radioulnar dislocation with manipulation**
🛏 11.3   🖐 12.5   **FUD** 090   T A2 80 50 ▭
AMA: 2018,Sep,7

25676 **Open treatment of distal radioulnar dislocation, acute or chronic**
🛏 18.2   🖐 18.2   **FUD** 090   J A2 80 50 ▭
AMA: 2018,Sep,7

25680 **Closed treatment of trans-scaphoperilunar type of fracture dislocation, with manipulation**
🛏 15.0   🖐 15.0   **FUD** 090   T A2 80 50 ▭
AMA: 2018,Sep,7

25685 **Open treatment of trans-scaphoperilunar type of fracture dislocation**
🛏 21.2   🖐 21.2   **FUD** 090   J A2 80 50 ▭
AMA: 2018,Sep,7

25690 **Closed treatment of lunate dislocation, with manipulation**
🛏 13.9   🖐 13.9   **FUD** 090   J A2 80 50 ▭
AMA: 2018,Sep,7

25695 **Open treatment of lunate dislocation**
🛏 18.2   🖐 18.2   **FUD** 090   J A2 80 50 ▭
AMA: 2018,Sep,7

25800-25830 Wrist Fusion

25800 **Arthrodesis, wrist; complete, without bone graft (includes radiocarpal and/or intercarpal and/or carpometacarpal joints)**
🛏 21.1   🖐 21.1   **FUD** 090   J J8 80 50 ▭
AMA: 2020,May,13; 2018,Sep,7

25805 **with sliding graft**
🛏 24.4   🖐 24.4   **FUD** 090   J J8 80 50 ▭
AMA: 2020,May,13; 2018,Sep,7

25810 **with iliac or other autograft (includes obtaining graft)**
🛏 24.9   🖐 24.9   **FUD** 090   J J8 80 50 ▭
AMA: 2020,May,13; 2018,Sep,7

25820 **Arthrodesis, wrist; limited, without bone graft (eg, intercarpal or radiocarpal)**
🛏 18.1   🖐 18.1   **FUD** 090   J J8 80 50 ▭
AMA: 2020,May,13; 2018,Sep,7

25825 **with autograft (includes obtaining graft)**
🛏 21.9   🖐 21.9   **FUD** 090   J J8 80 50 ▭
AMA: 2020,May,13; 2018,Sep,7; 2018,Jan,8; 2017,Jan,8; 2016,Jan,13

25830 **Arthrodesis, distal radioulnar joint with segmental resection of ulna, with or without bone graft (eg, Sauve-Kapandji procedure)**
🛏 28.1   🖐 28.1   **FUD** 090   J A2 80 50 ▭
AMA: 2020,May,13; 2018,Sep,7

25900-25999 Amputation Through Forearm/Wrist

25900 **Amputation, forearm, through radius and ulna;**
🛏 20.5   🖐 20.5   **FUD** 090   C 80 50 ▭
AMA: 2018,Sep,7

25905 **open, circular (guillotine)**
🛏 20.2   🖐 20.2   **FUD** 090   C 80 50 ▭
AMA: 2018,Sep,7

25907 **secondary closure or scar revision**
🛏 17.6   🖐 17.6   **FUD** 090   J A2 80 50 ▭
AMA: 2018,Sep,7

25909 **re-amputation**
🛏 19.7   🖐 19.7   **FUD** 090   J G2 80 50 ▭
AMA: 2018,Sep,7

25915 **Krukenberg procedure**
🛏 33.7   🖐 33.7   **FUD** 090   C 80 50 ▭
AMA: 2018,Sep,7

25920 **Disarticulation through wrist;**
🛏 20.5   🖐 20.5   **FUD** 090   C 80 50 ▭
AMA: 2018,Sep,7

25922 **secondary closure or scar revision**
🛏 17.7   🖐 17.7   **FUD** 090   J A2 80 50 ▭
AMA: 2018,Sep,7

25924 **re-amputation**
🛏 20.0   🖐 20.0   **FUD** 090   C 80 50 ▭
AMA: 2018,Sep,7

25927 **Transmetacarpal amputation;**
🛏 24.0   🖐 24.0   **FUD** 090   C 80 50 ▭
AMA: 2018,Sep,7

25929 **secondary closure or scar revision**
🛏 17.2   🖐 17.2   **FUD** 090   T A2 80 50 ▭
AMA: 2018,Sep,7

25931 **re-amputation**
🛏 22.1   🖐 22.1   **FUD** 090   J G2 50 ▭
AMA: 2018,Sep,7

25999 **Unlisted procedure, forearm or wrist**
🛏 0.00   🖐 0.00   **FUD** YYY   T 80 50 ▭
AMA: 2019,Feb,10; 2018,Sep,7

26010-26037 Incision Hand/Fingers

26010 Drainage of finger abscess; simple
  🔧 3.97 ✂ 8.62 **FUD** 010   T P2 ▣
  AMA: 2018,Sep,7

The six synovial sheaths (blue) of the dorsum of the wrist branch into nine extensor tendons

Extensor pollicis longus

Anatomical "snuffbox"

Extensor digitorum (five tendons)

Extensor retinaculum

Head of ulna

Fibrous sheaths

Synovium

Flexor tendons

Tendons typically join in a common synovial sheath

26011 complicated (eg, felon)
  🔧 5.32 ✂ 12.4 **FUD** 010   J A2 ▣
  AMA: 2018,Sep,7

26020 Drainage of tendon sheath, digit and/or palm, each
  🔧 15.9 ✂ 15.9 **FUD** 090   J A2 ▣
  AMA: 2018,Sep,7

26025 Drainage of palmar bursa; single, bursa
  🔧 12.1 ✂ 12.1 **FUD** 090   J A2 80 50 ▣
  AMA: 2018,Sep,7

26030 multiple bursa
  🔧 14.0 ✂ 14.0 **FUD** 090   J A2 80 50 ▣
  AMA: 2018,Sep,7

26034 Incision, bone cortex, hand or finger (eg, osteomyelitis or bone abscess)
  🔧 15.6 ✂ 15.6 **FUD** 090   J A2 ▣
  AMA: 2018,Sep,7

26035 Decompression fingers and/or hand, injection injury (eg, grease gun)
  🔧 24.7 ✂ 24.7 **FUD** 090   J G2 80 ▣
  AMA: 2018,Sep,7

26037 Decompressive fasciotomy, hand (excludes 26035)
  EXCLUDES Injection injury (26035)
  🔧 16.3 ✂ 16.3 **FUD** 090   J G2 80 50 ▣
  AMA: 2018,Sep,7

26040-26045 Incision Palmar Fascia

EXCLUDES Enzyme injection fasciotomy (20527, 26341)
  Fasciectomy (26121, 26123, 26125)

26040 Fasciotomy, palmar (eg, Dupuytren's contracture); percutaneous
  🔧 9.00 ✂ 9.00 **FUD** 090   J A2 50 ▣
  AMA: 2018,Sep,7; 2018,Jan,8; 2017,Jan,8; 2016,Jan,13

26045 open, partial
  🔧 13.5 ✂ 13.5 **FUD** 090   J A2 50 ▣
  AMA: 2018,Sep,7; 2018,Jan,8; 2017,Jan,8; 2016,Jan,13

26055-26080 Incision Tendon/Joint of Fingers/Hand

26055 Tendon sheath incision (eg, for trigger finger)
  🔧 8.31 ✂ 15.6 **FUD** 090   J A2 ▣
  AMA: 2018,Sep,7

26060 Tenotomy, percutaneous, single, each digit
  🔧 7.41 ✂ 7.41 **FUD** 090   J A2 80 ▣
  AMA: 2018,Sep,7

26070 Arthrotomy, with exploration, drainage, or removal of loose or foreign body; carpometacarpal joint
  🔧 9.23 ✂ 9.23 **FUD** 090   J A2 50 ▣
  AMA: 2018,Sep,7

26075 metacarpophalangeal joint, each
  🔧 9.64 ✂ 9.64 **FUD** 090   J A2 50 ▣
  AMA: 2018,Sep,7; 2018,Jan,8; 2017,Jan,8; 2016,Jan,13

26080 interphalangeal joint, each
  🔧 11.3 ✂ 11.3 **FUD** 090   J A2 ▣
  AMA: 2018,Sep,7; 2018,Jan,8; 2017,Jan,8; 2016,Jan,13

26100-26110 Arthrotomy with Biopsy of Joint Hand/Fingers

26100 Arthrotomy with biopsy; carpometacarpal joint, each
  🔧 9.64 ✂ 9.64 **FUD** 090   J A2 80 50 ▣
  AMA: 2018,Sep,7

26105 metacarpophalangeal joint, each
  🔧 9.71 ✂ 9.71 **FUD** 090   J A2 80 50 ▣
  AMA: 2018,Sep,7

26110 interphalangeal joint, each
  🔧 9.28 ✂ 9.28 **FUD** 090   J A2 ▣
  AMA: 2018,Sep,7

26111-26118 [26111, 26113] Excision Soft Tissue Tumors Fingers and Hand

INCLUDES Any necessary elevation tissue planes or dissection
  Measurement tumor and necessary margin at greatest diameter prior to excision
  Simple and intermediate repairs
  Excision types:
    Fascial or subfascial soft tissue tumors: simple and marginal resection tumors found either in or below deep fascia, not involving bone or excision substantial amount normal tissue; primarily benign and intramuscular tumors
    Tumors fingers and toes involving joint capsules, tendons and tendon sheaths
    Radical resection soft tissue tumor: wide resection tumor, involving substantial margins normal tissue and may include tissue removal from one or more layers; most often malignant or aggressive benign
    Tumors fingers and toes adjacent to joints, tendons and tendon sheaths
    Subcutaneous: simple and marginal resection tumors found in subcutaneous tissue above deep fascia; most often benign
EXCLUDES Complex repair
  Excision benign cutaneous lesions (eg, sebaceous cyst) (11420-11426)
  Radical resection cutaneous tumors (eg, melanoma) (11620-11626)
  Significant vessel exploration or neuroplasty

26111 Resequenced code. See code following 26115.

26113 Resequenced code. See code following 26116.

26115 Excision, tumor or vascular malformation, soft tissue of hand or finger, subcutaneous; less than 1.5 cm
  🔧 9.51 ✂ 15.2 **FUD** 090   J G2 ▣
  AMA: 2018,Sep,7

\# **26111** 1.5 cm or greater
  🔧 11.9 ✂ 11.9 **FUD** 090   J G2 80 ▣
  AMA: 2018,Sep,7

26116 Excision, tumor, soft tissue, or vascular malformation, of hand or finger, subfascial (eg, intramuscular); less than 1.5 cm
  🔧 15.1 ✂ 15.1 **FUD** 090   J G2 ▣
  AMA: 2018,Sep,7; 2018,Jan,8; 2017,Jan,8; 2016,Jan,13

\# **26113** 1.5 cm or greater
  🔧 15.7 ✂ 15.7 **FUD** 090   J G2 80 ▣
  AMA: 2018,Sep,7

26117 Radical resection of tumor (eg, sarcoma), soft tissue of hand or finger; less than 3 cm
  🔧 21.4 ✂ 21.4 **FUD** 090   J G2 ▣
  AMA: 2018,Sep,7

26118 3 cm or greater
  🔧 30.3 ✂ 30.3 **FUD** 090   J G2 80 ▣
  AMA: 2018,Sep,7

26121-26236 Procedures of Bones, Fascia, Joints and Tendons Hands and Fingers

26121 **Fasciectomy, palm only, with or without Z-plasty, other local tissue rearrangement, or skin grafting (includes obtaining graft)**

> EXCLUDES Enzyme injection fasciotomy (20527, 26341)
> Fasciotomy (26040, 26045)

🔧 17.2 ⚕ 17.2 **FUD** 090 J A2 50 ▭

AMA: 2018,Sep,7; 2018,Jan,8; 2017,Jan,8; 2016,Jan,13

26123 **Fasciectomy, partial palmar with release of single digit including proximal interphalangeal joint, with or without Z-plasty, other local tissue rearrangement, or skin grafting (includes obtaining graft);**

> EXCLUDES Enzyme injection fasciotomy (20527, 26341)
> Fasciotomy (26040, 26045)

🔧 24.0 ⚕ 24.0 **FUD** 090 J A2 50 ▭

AMA: 2018,Sep,7; 2018,Jan,8; 2017,Jan,8; 2016,Jan,13

+ 26125 **each additional digit (List separately in addition to code for primary procedure)**

> EXCLUDES Enzyme injection fasciotomy (20527, 26341)
> Fasciotomy (26040, 26045)
> Code first (26123)

🔧 7.89 ⚕ 7.89 **FUD** ZZZ N N1 ▭

AMA: 2018,Sep,7; 2018,Jan,8; 2017,Jan,8; 2016,Jan,13

26130 **Synovectomy, carpometacarpal joint**

🔧 13.4 ⚕ 13.4 **FUD** 090 J A2 50 ▭

AMA: 2018,Sep,7

26135 **Synovectomy, metacarpophalangeal joint including intrinsic release and extensor hood reconstruction, each digit**

🔧 15.9 ⚕ 15.9 **FUD** 090 J A2 80 ▭

AMA: 2018,Sep,7

26140 **Synovectomy, proximal interphalangeal joint, including extensor reconstruction, each interphalangeal joint**

🔧 14.5 ⚕ 14.5 **FUD** 090 J A2 ▭

AMA: 2018,Sep,7

26145 **Synovectomy, tendon sheath, radical (tenosynovectomy), flexor tendon, palm and/or finger, each tendon**

> EXCLUDES Wrist synovectomy (25115-25116)

🔧 14.7 ⚕ 14.7 **FUD** 090 J A2 ▭

AMA: 2018,Sep,7

26160 **Excision of lesion of tendon sheath or joint capsule (eg, cyst, mucous cyst, or ganglion), hand or finger**

> EXCLUDES Trigger finger (26055)
> Wrist ganglion removal (25111-25112)

🔧 9.04 ⚕ 16.3 **FUD** 090 J A2 ▭

AMA: 2019,Jul,10; 2018,Sep,7

26170 **Excision of tendon, palm, flexor or extensor, single, each tendon**

> EXCLUDES Excision extensor tendon, with implantation synthetic rod for delayed tendon graft, hand or finger, each rod (26415)
> Excision flexor tendon, with implantation synthetic rod for delayed tendon graft, hand or finger, each rod (26390)

🔧 11.6 ⚕ 11.6 **FUD** 090 J A2 80 ▭

AMA: 2018,Sep,7; 2018,Jan,8; 2017,Jan,8; 2016,Jan,13

26180 **Excision of tendon, finger, flexor or extensor, each tendon**

> EXCLUDES Excision extensor tendon, with implantation synthetic rod for delayed tendon graft, hand or finger, each rod (26415)
> Excision flexor tendon, with implantation synthetic rod for delayed tendon graft, hand or finger, each rod (26390)

🔧 12.7 ⚕ 12.7 **FUD** 090 J A2 80 ▭

AMA: 2018,Sep,7

26185 **Sesamoidectomy, thumb or finger (separate procedure)**

🔧 15.8 ⚕ 15.8 **FUD** 090 J A2 80 50 ▭

AMA: 2018,Sep,7

26200 **Excision or curettage of bone cyst or benign tumor of metacarpal;**

🔧 13.0 ⚕ 13.0 **FUD** 090 J A2 80 ▭

AMA: 2018,Sep,7

26205 **with autograft (includes obtaining graft)**

🔧 17.3 ⚕ 17.3 **FUD** 090 J A2 ▭

AMA: 2018,Sep,7

26210 **Excision or curettage of bone cyst or benign tumor of proximal, middle, or distal phalanx of finger;**

🔧 12.7 ⚕ 12.7 **FUD** 090 J A2 ▭

AMA: 2018,Sep,7

26215 **with autograft (includes obtaining graft)**

🔧 16.2 ⚕ 16.2 **FUD** 090 J A2 ▭

AMA: 2018,Sep,7

26230 **Partial excision (craterization, saucerization, or diaphysectomy) bone (eg, osteomyelitis); metacarpal**

🔧 14.4 ⚕ 14.4 **FUD** 090 J A2 80 ▭

AMA: 2018,Sep,7

26235 **proximal or middle phalanx of finger**

🔧 14.1 ⚕ 14.1 **FUD** 090 J A2 80 ▭

AMA: 2019,Jul,10; 2018,Sep,7

26236 **distal phalanx of finger**

🔧 12.6 ⚕ 12.6 **FUD** 090 J A2 ▭

AMA: 2019,Jul,10; 2018,Sep,7

26250-26262 Radical Resection Bone Tumor of Hand/Finger

> INCLUDES Any necessary elevation tissue planes or dissection
> Excision adjacent soft tissue during bone tumor resection (26111-26118 [26111, 26113])
> Measurement tumor and necessary margin at greatest diameter prior to excision
> Resection tumor (may include entire bone) and wide margins normal tissue primarily for malignant or aggressive benign tumors
> Simple and intermediate repairs
>
> EXCLUDES Complex repair
> Significant vessel exploration, neuroplasty, reconstruction, or complex bone repair

26250 **Radical resection of tumor, metacarpal**

🔧 30.8 ⚕ 30.8 **FUD** 090 J A2 80 ▭

AMA: 2018,Sep,7

26260 **Radical resection of tumor, proximal or middle phalanx of finger**

🔧 23.0 ⚕ 23.0 **FUD** 090 J A2 80 ▭

AMA: 2018,Sep,7

26262 **Radical resection of tumor, distal phalanx of finger**

🔧 18.1 ⚕ 18.1 **FUD** 090 J A2 80 ▭

AMA: 2018,Sep,7

26320 Implant Removal Hand/Finger

26320 **Removal of implant from finger or hand**

> EXCLUDES Excision foreign body (20520, 20525)

🔧 9.98 ⚕ 9.98 **FUD** 090 Q2 A2 ▭

AMA: 2018,Sep,7

26340-26548 Repair/Reconstruction of Fingers and Hand

26340 **Manipulation, finger joint, under anesthesia, each joint**

> EXCLUDES Application external fixation (20690, 20692)

🔧 9.67 ⚕ 9.67 **FUD** 090 J G2 50 ▭

AMA: 2018,Sep,7; 2018,Jan,8; 2017,Jan,8; 2016,Jan,13

26341 **Manipulation, palmar fascial cord (ie, Dupuytren's cord), post enzyme injection (eg, collagenase), single cord**

> EXCLUDES Enzyme injection fasciotomy (20527)
> Code also custom orthotic fabrication and/or fitting

🔧 2.17 ⚕ 2.90 **FUD** 010 T P3 50 ▭

AMA: 2018,Sep,7; 2018,Jan,8; 2017,Jan,8; 2016,Jan,13

26350 **Repair or advancement, flexor tendon, not in zone 2 digital flexor tendon sheath (eg, no man's land); primary or secondary without free graft, each tendon**

🔧 20.8 ⚕ 20.8 **FUD** 090 J A2 ▭

AMA: 2018,Sep,7

26/TC PC/TC Only   A2-Z3 ASC Payment   50 Bilateral   ♂ Male Only   ♀ Female Only   🔧 Facility RVU   ⚕ Non-Facility RVU   ▭ CCI   ✖ CLIA
FUD Follow-up Days   CMS: IOM   AMA: CPT Asst   A-Y OPPSI   80/80 Surg Assist Allowed / w/Doc   ▨ Lab Crosswalk   ▧ Radiology Crosswalk

74   CPT © 2021 American Medical Association. All Rights Reserved.   © 2021 Optum360, LLC

26352 secondary with free graft (includes obtaining graft), each tendon
🔧 23.3   ⚕ 23.3   **FUD** 090   J A2 80 ▣
AMA: 2018,Sep,7

26356 Repair or advancement, flexor tendon, in zone 2 digital flexor tendon sheath (eg, no man's land); primary, without free graft, each tendon
🔧 22.8   ⚕ 22.8   **FUD** 090   J A2
AMA: 2018,Sep,7; 2018,Jan,8; 2017,Dec,14; 2017,Jan,8; 2016,Jan,13

26357 secondary, without free graft, each tendon
🔧 25.6   ⚕ 25.6   **FUD** 090   J A2 80 ▣
AMA: 2018,Sep,7

26358 secondary, with free graft (includes obtaining graft), each tendon
🔧 28.3   ⚕ 28.3   **FUD** 090   J A2 80 ▣
AMA: 2018,Sep,7

26370 Repair or advancement of profundus tendon, with intact superficialis tendon; primary, each tendon
🔧 21.9   ⚕ 21.9   **FUD** 090   J A2 80 ▣
AMA: 2018,Sep,7; 2018,Jan,8; 2017,Jan,8; 2016,Jan,13

26372 secondary with free graft (includes obtaining graft), each tendon
🔧 25.7   ⚕ 25.7   **FUD** 090   J A2 80 ▣
AMA: 2018,Sep,7

26373 secondary without free graft, each tendon
🔧 24.7   ⚕ 24.7   **FUD** 090   J A2 80 ▣
AMA: 2018,Sep,7

26390 Excision flexor tendon, with implantation of synthetic rod for delayed tendon graft, hand or finger, each rod
🔧 23.6   ⚕ 23.6   **FUD** 090   J J8 80 ▣
AMA: 2018,Sep,7

26392 Removal of synthetic rod and insertion of flexor tendon graft, hand or finger (includes obtaining graft), each rod
🔧 27.5   ⚕ 27.5   **FUD** 090   J A2 80 ▣
AMA: 2018,Sep,7

26410 Repair, extensor tendon, hand, primary or secondary; without free graft, each tendon
🔧 16.5   ⚕ 16.5   **FUD** 090   J A2 ▣
AMA: 2018,Sep,7

26412 with free graft (includes obtaining graft), each tendon
🔧 19.7   ⚕ 19.7   **FUD** 090   J A2 80 ▣
AMA: 2018,Sep,7

26415 Excision of extensor tendon, with implantation of synthetic rod for delayed tendon graft, hand or finger, each rod
🔧 23.7   ⚕ 23.7   **FUD** 090   J A2 80 ▣
AMA: 2018,Sep,7

26416 Removal of synthetic rod and insertion of extensor tendon graft (includes obtaining graft), hand or finger, each rod
🔧 25.7   ⚕ 25.7   **FUD** 090   J A2 ▣
AMA: 2018,Sep,7; 2018,Jan,8; 2017,Jan,8; 2016,Jan,13

26418 Repair, extensor tendon, finger, primary or secondary; without free graft, each tendon
🔧 16.2   ⚕ 16.2   **FUD** 090   J A2 ▣
AMA: 2018,Sep,7; 2018,Jan,8; 2017,Jan,8; 2016,Jan,13

26420 with free graft (includes obtaining graft) each tendon
🔧 20.6   ⚕ 20.6   **FUD** 090   J A2 80 ▣
AMA: 2018,Sep,7

26426 Repair of extensor tendon, central slip, secondary (eg, boutonniere deformity); using local tissue(s), including lateral band(s), each finger
🔧 14.4   ⚕ 14.4   **FUD** 090   J A2 ▣
AMA: 2018,Sep,7

26428 with free graft (includes obtaining graft), each finger
🔧 21.3   ⚕ 21.3   **FUD** 090   J A2 80 ▣
AMA: 2018,Sep,7

26432 Closed treatment of distal extensor tendon insertion, with or without percutaneous pinning (eg, mallet finger)
🔧 14.7   ⚕ 14.7   **FUD** 090   J A2 ▣
AMA: 2018,Sep,7

26433 Repair of extensor tendon, distal insertion, primary or secondary; without graft (eg, mallet finger)
EXCLUDES   *Trigger finger (26055)*
🔧 15.6   ⚕ 15.6   **FUD** 090   J A2 ▣
AMA: 2018,Sep,7

26434 with free graft (includes obtaining graft)
EXCLUDES   *Trigger finger (26055)*
🔧 18.2   ⚕ 18.2   **FUD** 090   J A2 80 ▣
AMA: 2018,Sep,7

26437 Realignment of extensor tendon, hand, each tendon
🔧 17.5   ⚕ 17.5   **FUD** 090   J A2 ▣
AMA: 2018,Sep,7

26440 Tenolysis, flexor tendon; palm OR finger, each tendon
🔧 17.4   ⚕ 17.4   **FUD** 090   J A2 ▣
AMA: 2018,Sep,7; 2018,Jan,8; 2017,Jan,8; 2016,Jan,13

26442 palm AND finger, each tendon
🔧 27.1   ⚕ 27.1   **FUD** 090   J A2 ▣
AMA: 2018,Sep,7

26445 Tenolysis, extensor tendon, hand OR finger, each tendon
🔧 16.1   ⚕ 16.1   **FUD** 090   J A2 ▣
AMA: 2018,Sep,7; 2018,Jan,8; 2017,Jan,8; 2016,Jan,13

26449 Tenolysis, complex, extensor tendon, finger, including forearm, each tendon
🔧 19.9   ⚕ 19.9   **FUD** 090   J A2 80 ▣
AMA: 2018,Sep,7

26450 Tenotomy, flexor, palm, open, each tendon
🔧 11.4   ⚕ 11.4   **FUD** 090   J A2 80 ▣
AMA: 2018,Sep,7

26455 Tenotomy, flexor, finger, open, each tendon
🔧 12.1   ⚕ 12.1   **FUD** 090   J A2 80 ▣
AMA: 2018,Sep,7

26460 Tenotomy, extensor, hand or finger, open, each tendon
🔧 11.1   ⚕ 11.1   **FUD** 090   J A2 ▣
AMA: 2018,Sep,7

26471 Tenodesis; of proximal interphalangeal joint, each joint
🔧 18.0   ⚕ 18.0   **FUD** 090   J A2 80 ▣
AMA: 2018,Sep,7

26474 of distal joint, each joint
🔧 17.7   ⚕ 17.7   **FUD** 090   J A2 80 ▣
AMA: 2018,Sep,7

26476 Lengthening of tendon, extensor, hand or finger, each tendon
🔧 16.7   ⚕ 16.7   **FUD** 090   J A2 ▣
AMA: 2018,Sep,7

26477 Shortening of tendon, extensor, hand or finger, each tendon
🔧 16.3   ⚕ 16.3   **FUD** 090   J A2 ▣
AMA: 2018,Sep,7

26478 Lengthening of tendon, flexor, hand or finger, each tendon
🔧 18.2   ⚕ 18.2   **FUD** 090   J A2 80 ▣
AMA: 2018,Sep,7; 2018,Jan,8; 2017,Jan,8; 2016,Jan,13

26479 Shortening of tendon, flexor, hand or finger, each tendon
🔧 17.6   ⚕ 17.6   **FUD** 090   J A2 80 ▣
AMA: 2018,Sep,7

26480 Transfer or transplant of tendon, carpometacarpal area or dorsum of hand; without free graft, each tendon
🔧 21.1   ⚕ 21.1   **FUD** 090   J A2 80 ▣
AMA: 2018,Sep,7; 2018,Jan,8; 2017,Jan,8; 2016,Jan,13

26483 with free tendon graft (includes obtaining graft), each tendon
🗁 24.4 ⬠ 24.4 **FUD** 090 J A2 80 ▭
AMA: 2018,Sep,7

26485 Transfer or transplant of tendon, palmar; without free tendon graft, each tendon
🗁 22.7 ⬠ 22.7 **FUD** 090 J A2 80 ▭
AMA: 2018,Sep,7

26489 with free tendon graft (includes obtaining graft), each tendon
🗁 27.1 ⬠ 27.1 **FUD** 090 J A2 80 ▭
AMA: 2018,Sep,7

26490 Opponensplasty; superficialis tendon transfer type, each tendon
EXCLUDES *Thumb fusion (26820)*
🗁 22.5 ⬠ 22.5 **FUD** 090 J A2 80 ▭
AMA: 2018,Sep,7

26492 tendon transfer with graft (includes obtaining graft), each tendon
EXCLUDES *Thumb fusion (26820)*
🗁 25.0 ⬠ 25.0 **FUD** 090 J A2 80 ▭
AMA: 2018,Sep,7

26494 hypothenar muscle transfer
EXCLUDES *Thumb fusion (26820)*
🗁 23.3 ⬠ 23.3 **FUD** 090 J A2 80 ▭
AMA: 2018,Sep,7

26496 other methods
EXCLUDES *Thumb fusion (26820)*
🗁 24.9 ⬠ 24.9 **FUD** 090 J A2 80 ▭
AMA: 2018,Sep,7

26497 Transfer of tendon to restore intrinsic function; ring and small finger
🗁 25.2 ⬠ 25.2 **FUD** 090 J A2 80 ▭
AMA: 2018,Sep,7

26498 all 4 fingers
🗁 33.2 ⬠ 33.2 **FUD** 090 J A2 80 ▭
AMA: 2018,Sep,7

26499 Correction claw finger, other methods
🗁 24.2 ⬠ 24.2 **FUD** 090 J A2 80 ▭
AMA: 2018,Sep,7

26500 Reconstruction of tendon pulley, each tendon; with local tissues (separate procedure)
🗁 18.2 ⬠ 18.2 **FUD** 090 J A2 80 ▭
AMA: 2018,Sep,7

26502 with tendon or fascial graft (includes obtaining graft) (separate procedure)
🗁 20.8 ⬠ 20.8 **FUD** 090 J A2 80 ▭
AMA: 2018,Sep,7

26508 Release of thenar muscle(s) (eg, thumb contracture)
🗁 18.6 ⬠ 18.6 **FUD** 090 J A2 80 50 ▭
AMA: 2018,Sep,7

26510 Cross intrinsic transfer, each tendon
🗁 16.7 ⬠ 16.7 **FUD** 090 J A2 80 ▭
AMA: 2018,Sep,7

26516 Capsulodesis, metacarpophalangeal joint; single digit
🗁 20.5 ⬠ 20.5 **FUD** 090 J A2 80 50 ▭
AMA: 2018,Sep,7

26517 2 digits
🗁 24.1 ⬠ 24.1 **FUD** 090 J A2 80 50 ▭
AMA: 2018,Sep,7

26518 3 or 4 digits
🗁 24.4 ⬠ 24.4 **FUD** 090 J A2 80 50 ▭
AMA: 2018,Sep,7

26520 Capsulectomy or capsulotomy; metacarpophalangeal joint, each joint
EXCLUDES *Carpometacarpal joint arthroplasty (25447)*
🗁 18.2 ⬠ 18.2 **FUD** 090 J A2 ▭
AMA: 2018,Sep,7

26525 interphalangeal joint, each joint
EXCLUDES *Carpometacarpal joint arthroplasty (25447)*
🗁 18.9 ⬠ 18.9 **FUD** 090 J A2 ▭
AMA: 2018,Sep,7; 2018,Jan,8; 2017,Jan,8; 2016,Jan,13

26530 Arthroplasty, metacarpophalangeal joint; each joint
EXCLUDES *Carpometacarpal joint arthroplasty (25447)*
🗁 15.4 ⬠ 15.4 **FUD** 090 J J8 80 ▭
AMA: 2018,Sep,7

26531 with prosthetic implant, each joint
EXCLUDES *Carpometacarpal joint arthroplasty (25447)*
🗁 18.0 ⬠ 18.0 **FUD** 090 J J8 80 ▭
AMA: 2018,Sep,7; 2018,Jan,8; 2017,Jan,8; 2016,Jan,13

26535 Arthroplasty, interphalangeal joint; each joint
EXCLUDES *Carpometacarpal joint arthroplasty (25447)*
🗁 12.4 ⬠ 12.4 **FUD** 090 J A2 ▭
AMA: 2018,Sep,7

26536 with prosthetic implant, each joint
EXCLUDES *Carpometacarpal joint arthroplasty (25447)*
🗁 20.8 ⬠ 20.8 **FUD** 090 J J8 80 ▭
AMA: 2018,Sep,7

26540 Repair of collateral ligament, metacarpophalangeal or interphalangeal joint
🗁 19.3 ⬠ 19.3 **FUD** 090 J A2 80 ▭
AMA: 2018,Sep,7

26541 Reconstruction, collateral ligament, metacarpophalangeal joint, single; with tendon or fascial graft (includes obtaining graft)
🗁 22.5 ⬠ 22.5 **FUD** 090 J A2 80 ▭
AMA: 2018,Sep,7; 2018,Jan,8; 2017,Jan,8; 2016,Jan,13

26542 with local tissue (eg, adductor advancement)
🗁 19.9 ⬠ 19.9 **FUD** 090 J A2 80 ▭
AMA: 2018,Sep,7; 2018,Jan,8; 2017,Jan,8; 2016,Jan,13

26545 Reconstruction, collateral ligament, interphalangeal joint, single, including graft, each joint
🗁 19.9 ⬠ 19.9 **FUD** 090 J A2 80 ▭
AMA: 2018,Sep,7

26546 Repair non-union, metacarpal or phalanx (includes obtaining bone graft with or without external or internal fixation)
🗁 28.9 ⬠ 28.9 **FUD** 090 J A2 80 50 ▭
AMA: 2018,Sep,7

26548 Repair and reconstruction, finger, volar plate, interphalangeal joint
🗁 22.2 ⬠ 22.2 **FUD** 090 J A2 80 ▭
AMA: 2018,Sep,7

26550-26556 Reconstruction Procedures with Finger and Toe Transplants

26550 Pollicization of a digit
🗁 46.8 ⬠ 46.8 **FUD** 090 J A2 80 50 ▭
AMA: 2018,Sep,7

26551 Transfer, toe-to-hand with microvascular anastomosis; great toe wrap-around with bone graft
INCLUDES Operating microscope (69990)
EXCLUDES *Big toe with web space (20973)*
🗁 95.1 ⬠ 95.1 **FUD** 090 C 80 50 ▭
AMA: 2018,Sep,7; 2018,Jan,8; 2017,Jan,8; 2016,Feb,12; 2016,Jan,13

26/TC PC/TC Only	A2-Z3 ASC Payment	50 Bilateral	♂ Male Only	♀ Female Only	🗁 Facility RVU	⬠ Non-Facility RVU	▭ CCI	✖ CLIA
FUD Follow-up Days	CMS: IOM	AMA: CPT Asst	A-Y OPPSI	80/80 Surg Assist Allowed / w/Doc		Lab Crosswalk	Radiology Crosswalk	

76 CPT © 2021 American Medical Association. All Rights Reserved. © 2021 Optum360, LLC

26553   other than great toe, single

   INCLUDES   Operating microscope (69990)
   💪 94.5   ⚥ 94.5   **FUD** 090   C 80 50 ▣

   AMA: 2018,Sep,7; 2018,Jan,8; 2017,Jan,8; 2016,Feb,12; 2016,Jan,13

26554   other than great toe, double

   INCLUDES   Operating microscope (69990)
   💪 109.   ⚥ 109.   **FUD** 090   C 80 50 ▣

   AMA: 2018,Sep,7; 2018,Jan,8; 2017,Jan,8; 2016,Feb,12; 2016,Jan,13

26555   Transfer, finger to another position without microvascular anastomosis

   💪 39.6   ⚥ 39.6   **FUD** 090   J A2 80 ▣

   AMA: 2018,Sep,7

26556   Transfer, free toe joint, with microvascular anastomosis

   INCLUDES   Operating microscope (69990)
   EXCLUDES   Big toe to hand transfer (20973)
   💪 98.2   ⚥ 98.2   **FUD** 090   C 80 ▣

   AMA: 2018,Sep,7; 2018,Jan,8; 2017,Jan,8; 2016,Feb,12; 2016,Jan,13

26560-26596 Repair of Other Deformities of the Fingers/Hand

26560   Repair of syndactyly (web finger) each web space; with skin flaps

   💪 16.5   ⚥ 16.5   **FUD** 090   J A2 80 ▣

   AMA: 2018,Sep,7

26561   with skin flaps and grafts

   💪 27.5   ⚥ 27.5   **FUD** 090   J A2 80 ▣

   AMA: 2018,Sep,7

26562   complex (eg, involving bone, nails)

   💪 38.8   ⚥ 38.8   **FUD** 090   J A2 80 ▣

   AMA: 2018,Sep,7

26565   Osteotomy; metacarpal, each

   💪 19.0   ⚥ 19.0   **FUD** 090   J A2 80 ▣

   AMA: 2018,Sep,7

26567   phalanx of finger, each

   💪 19.9   ⚥ 19.9   **FUD** 090   J A2 80 ▣

   AMA: 2018,Sep,7; 2018,Jan,8; 2017,Jan,8; 2016,Jan,13

26568   Osteoplasty, lengthening, metacarpal or phalanx

   💪 26.1   ⚥ 26.1   **FUD** 090   J A2 80 ▣

   AMA: 2018,Sep,7

26580   Repair cleft hand

   INCLUDES   Barsky's procedure
   💪 43.7   ⚥ 43.7   **FUD** 090   J A2 80 50 ▣

   AMA: 2018,Sep,7

26587   Reconstruction of polydactylous digit, soft tissue and bone

   EXCLUDES   Soft tissue removal only (11200)
   💪 30.0   ⚥ 30.0   **FUD** 090   J A2 80 ▣

   AMA: 2018,Sep,7; 2018,Jan,8; 2017,Jan,8; 2016,Jan,13

26590   Repair macrodactylia, each digit

   💪 40.7   ⚥ 40.7   **FUD** 090   J A2 80 ▣

   AMA: 2018,Sep,7; 2018,Jan,8; 2017,Jan,8; 2016,Jan,13

26591   Repair, intrinsic muscles of hand, each muscle

   💪 13.0   ⚥ 13.0   **FUD** 090   J A2 80 ▣

   AMA: 2018,Sep,7; 2018,Jan,8; 2017,Jan,8; 2016,Jan,13

26593   Release, intrinsic muscles of hand, each muscle

   💪 17.6   ⚥ 17.6   **FUD** 090   J A2 ▣

   AMA: 2018,Sep,7

26596   Excision of constricting ring of finger, with multiple Z-plasties

   EXCLUDES   Graft repair or scar contracture release (11042, 14040-14041, 15120, 15240)
   💪 21.6   ⚥ 21.6   **FUD** 090   J A2 80 ▣

   AMA: 2018,Sep,7

26600-26785 Treatment of Fracture/Dislocation of Fingers and Hand

   INCLUDES   Closed, percutaneous, and open treatment fractures or dislocations

26600   Closed treatment of metacarpal fracture, single; without manipulation, each bone

   💪 7.94   ⚥ 8.39   **FUD** 090   T P2 ▣

   AMA: 2018,Sep,7

26605   with manipulation, each bone

   💪 8.45   ⚥ 9.33   **FUD** 090   T A2 ▣

   AMA: 2018,Sep,7

26607   Closed treatment of metacarpal fracture, with manipulation, with external fixation, each bone

   💪 13.9   ⚥ 13.9   **FUD** 090   J A2 80 ▣

   AMA: 2018,Sep,7

26608   Percutaneous skeletal fixation of metacarpal fracture, each bone

   💪 13.8   ⚥ 13.8   **FUD** 090   J A2 80 ▣

   AMA: 2018,Sep,7

26615   Open treatment of metacarpal fracture, single, includes internal fixation, when performed, each bone

   💪 16.5   ⚥ 16.5   **FUD** 090   J A2 ▣

   AMA: 2018,Sep,7

26641   Closed treatment of carpometacarpal dislocation, thumb, with manipulation

   💪 9.97   ⚥ 11.0   **FUD** 090   T P2 80 50 ▣

   AMA: 2018,Sep,7

26645   Closed treatment of carpometacarpal fracture dislocation, thumb (Bennett fracture), with manipulation

   💪 11.3   ⚥ 12.3   **FUD** 090   J A2 80 50 ▣

   AMA: 2018,Sep,7

26650   Percutaneous skeletal fixation of carpometacarpal fracture dislocation, thumb (Bennett fracture), with manipulation

   💪 13.7   ⚥ 13.7   **FUD** 090   J A2 50 ▣

   AMA: 2018,Sep,7

26665   Open treatment of carpometacarpal fracture dislocation, thumb (Bennett fracture), includes internal fixation, when performed

   💪 18.0   ⚥ 18.0   **FUD** 090   J A2 50 ▣

   AMA: 2018,Sep,7

26670   Closed treatment of carpometacarpal dislocation, other than thumb, with manipulation, each joint; without anesthesia

   💪 8.87   ⚥ 9.86   **FUD** 090   T P2 80 ▣

   AMA: 2018,Sep,7

26675   requiring anesthesia

   💪 12.0   ⚥ 13.1   **FUD** 090   J A2 80 ▣

   AMA: 2018,Sep,7

26676   Percutaneous skeletal fixation of carpometacarpal dislocation, other than thumb, with manipulation, each joint

   💪 14.5   ⚥ 14.5   **FUD** 090   J A2 ▣

   AMA: 2018,Sep,7

26685   Open treatment of carpometacarpal dislocation, other than thumb; includes internal fixation, when performed, each joint

   💪 16.5   ⚥ 16.5   **FUD** 090   J A2 ▣

   AMA: 2018,Sep,7

26686   complex, multiple, or delayed reduction

   💪 18.0   ⚥ 18.0   **FUD** 090   J A2 80 ▣

   AMA: 2018,Sep,7

26700   Closed treatment of metacarpophalangeal dislocation, single, with manipulation; without anesthesia

   💪 8.86   ⚥ 9.55   **FUD** 090   T P2 ▣

   AMA: 2018,Sep,7

26705   requiring anesthesia

   💪 10.9   ⚥ 11.9   **FUD** 090   J A2 80 ▣

   AMA: 2018,Sep,7

26706 Percutaneous skeletal fixation of metacarpophalangeal dislocation, single, with manipulation
 ⚕ 12.6 ⚕ 12.6 **FUD** 090 [J] [A2] 🖾
AMA: 2018,Sep,7

26715 Open treatment of metacarpophalangeal dislocation, single, includes internal fixation, when performed
 ⚕ 16.4 ⚕ 16.4 **FUD** 090 [J] [A2] [80] 🖾
AMA: 2018,Sep,7

26720 Closed treatment of phalangeal shaft fracture, proximal or middle phalanx, finger or thumb; without manipulation, each
 ⚕ 5.26 ⚕ 5.62 **FUD** 090 [T] [P2] 🖾
AMA: 2018,Sep,7

26725 with manipulation, with or without skin or skeletal traction, each
 ⚕ 8.73 ⚕ 9.75 **FUD** 090 [T] [P2] 🖾
AMA: 2018,Sep,7

26727 Percutaneous skeletal fixation of unstable phalangeal shaft fracture, proximal or middle phalanx, finger or thumb, with manipulation, each
 ⚕ 13.5 ⚕ 13.5 **FUD** 090 [J] [A2] 🖾
AMA: 2018,Sep,7

26735 Open treatment of phalangeal shaft fracture, proximal or middle phalanx, finger or thumb, includes internal fixation, when performed, each
 ⚕ 17.1 ⚕ 17.1 **FUD** 090 [J] [A2] 🖾
AMA: 2018,Sep,7

26740 Closed treatment of articular fracture, involving metacarpophalangeal or interphalangeal joint; without manipulation, each
 ⚕ 6.25 ⚕ 6.60 **FUD** 090 [T] [P2] 🖾
AMA: 2018,Sep,7

26742 with manipulation, each
 ⚕ 9.64 ⚕ 10.6 **FUD** 090 [J] [A2] 🖾
AMA: 2018,Sep,7

26746 Open treatment of articular fracture, involving metacarpophalangeal or interphalangeal joint, includes internal fixation, when performed, each
 ⚕ 21.3 ⚕ 21.3 **FUD** 090 [J] [A2] 🖾
AMA: 2018,Sep,7

26750 Closed treatment of distal phalangeal fracture, finger or thumb; without manipulation, each
 ⚕ 5.35 ⚕ 5.32 **FUD** 090 [T] [P2] 🖾
AMA: 2018,Sep,7

26755 with manipulation, each
 ⚕ 7.77 ⚕ 8.99 **FUD** 090 [T] [G2] 🖾
AMA: 2018,Sep,7

26756 Percutaneous skeletal fixation of distal phalangeal fracture, finger or thumb, each
 ⚕ 12.1 ⚕ 12.1 **FUD** 090 [J] [A2] [80] 🖾
AMA: 2018,Sep,7

26765 Open treatment of distal phalangeal fracture, finger or thumb, includes internal fixation, when performed, each
 ⚕ 14.3 ⚕ 14.3 **FUD** 090 [J] [A2] 🖾
AMA: 2018,Sep,7

26770 Closed treatment of interphalangeal joint dislocation, single, with manipulation; without anesthesia
 ⚕ 7.41 ⚕ 8.08 **FUD** 090 [T] [G2] 🖾
AMA: 2018,Sep,7

26775 requiring anesthesia
 ⚕ 9.96 ⚕ 11.0 **FUD** 090 [T] [P2] 🖾
AMA: 2018,Sep,7

26776 Percutaneous skeletal fixation of interphalangeal joint dislocation, single, with manipulation
 ⚕ 12.8 ⚕ 12.8 **FUD** 090 [J] [A2] 🖾
AMA: 2018,Sep,7

26785 Open treatment of interphalangeal joint dislocation, includes internal fixation, when performed, single
 ⚕ 15.7 ⚕ 15.7 **FUD** 090 [J] [A2] 🖾
AMA: 2018,Sep,7

26820-26863 Fusion of Joint(s) of Fingers or Hand

26820 Fusion in opposition, thumb, with autogenous graft (includes obtaining graft)
 ⚕ 22.2 ⚕ 22.2 **FUD** 090 [J] [J8] [80] [50] 🖾
AMA: 2020,May,13; 2018,Sep,7

26841 Arthrodesis, carpometacarpal joint, thumb, with or without internal fixation;
 ⚕ 21.2 ⚕ 21.2 **FUD** 090 [J] [A2] [80] [50] 🖾
AMA: 2020,May,13; 2018,Sep,7

26842 with autograft (includes obtaining graft)
 ⚕ 22.8 ⚕ 22.8 **FUD** 090 [J] [A2] [80] [50] 🖾
AMA: 2020,May,13; 2018,Sep,7

26843 Arthrodesis, carpometacarpal joint, digit, other than thumb, each;
 ⚕ 21.6 ⚕ 21.6 **FUD** 090 [J] [J8] [80] 🖾
AMA: 2020,May,13; 2018,Sep,7; 2018,Jan,8; 2017,Jan,8; 2016,Jan,13

26844 with autograft (includes obtaining graft)
 ⚕ 23.9 ⚕ 23.9 **FUD** 090 [J] [J8] [80] 🖾
AMA: 2020,May,13; 2018,Sep,7

26850 Arthrodesis, metacarpophalangeal joint, with or without internal fixation;
 ⚕ 20.2 ⚕ 20.2 **FUD** 090 [J] [A2] [80] 🖾
AMA: 2020,May,13; 2018,Sep,7

26852 with autograft (includes obtaining graft)
 ⚕ 23.2 ⚕ 23.2 **FUD** 090 [J] [A2] [80] 🖾
AMA: 2020,May,13; 2018,Sep,7

26860 Arthrodesis, interphalangeal joint, with or without internal fixation;
 ⚕ 15.9 ⚕ 15.9 **FUD** 090 [J] [A2] 🖾
AMA: 2020,May,13; 2018,Sep,7; 2018,Jan,8; 2017,Jan,8; 2016,Jan,13

+ 26861 each additional interphalangeal joint (List separately in addition to code for primary procedure)
Code first (26860)
 ⚕ 2.98 ⚕ 2.98 **FUD** ZZZ [N] [N1] 🖾
AMA: 2020,May,13; 2018,Sep,7; 2018,Jan,8; 2017,Jan,8; 2016,Jan,13

26862 with autograft (includes obtaining graft)
 ⚕ 21.1 ⚕ 21.1 **FUD** 090 [J] [A2] [80] 🖾
AMA: 2020,May,13; 2018,Sep,7

+ 26863 with autograft (includes obtaining graft), each additional joint (List separately in addition to code for primary procedure)
Code first (26862)
 ⚕ 6.62 ⚕ 6.62 **FUD** ZZZ [N] [N1] [80] 🖾
AMA: 2020,May,13; 2018,Sep,7

26910-26989 Amputations and Unlisted Procedures Finger/Hand

26910 Amputation, metacarpal, with finger or thumb (ray amputation), single, with or without interosseous transfer
EXCLUDES Repositioning (26550, 26555)
Transmetacarpal amputation hand (25927)
 ⚕ 21.1 ⚕ 21.1 **FUD** 090 [J] [A2] 🖾
AMA: 2018,Sep,7

26951 Amputation, finger or thumb, primary or secondary, any joint or phalanx, single, including neurectomies; with direct closure
EXCLUDES Repair necessitating flaps or grafts (15050-15758)
Transmetacarpal amputation hand (25927)
 ⚕ 19.1 ⚕ 19.1 **FUD** 090 [J] [A2] 🖾
AMA: 2018,Sep,7

26/TC PC/TC Only A2-Z3 ASC Payment 50 Bilateral ♂ Male Only ♀ Female Only ⚕ Facility RVU ⚕ Non-Facility RVU 🖾 CCI ☒ CLIA
FUD Follow-up Days CMS: IOM AMA: CPT Asst A-Y OPPSI 80/80 Surg Assist Allowed / w/Doc 🖾 Lab Crosswalk 🖾 Radiology Crosswalk

78 CPT © 2021 American Medical Association. All Rights Reserved. © 2021 Optum360, LLC

26952   with local advancement flaps (V-Y, hood)

EXCLUDES   *Repair necessitating flaps or grafts (15050-15758)*
Transmetacarpal amputation hand (25927)

🔧 18.9   ⚙ 18.9   **FUD** 090   J A2 ▭

AMA: 2018,Sep,7

26989   Unlisted procedure, hands or fingers

🔧 0.00   ⚙ 0.00   **FUD** YYY   T ▭

AMA: 2018,Sep,7

26990-26992 Incision for Drainage of Pelvis or Hip

EXCLUDES   *Simple incision and drainage procedures (10040-10160)*

26990   Incision and drainage, pelvis or hip joint area; deep abscess or hematoma

🔧 18.8   ⚙ 18.8   **FUD** 090   J A2 ▭

AMA: 2018,Sep,7

26991   infected bursa

🔧 15.1   ⚙ 20.4   **FUD** 090   J A2 80 ▭

AMA: 2018,Sep,7

26992   Incision, bone cortex, pelvis and/or hip joint (eg, osteomyelitis or bone abscess)

🔧 28.5   ⚙ 28.5   **FUD** 090   C 80 ▭

AMA: 2018,Sep,7; 2018,Jan,8; 2017,Jan,8; 2016,Jan,13

27000-27006 Tenotomy Procedures of Hip

27000   Tenotomy, adductor of hip, percutaneous (separate procedure)

🔧 11.6   ⚙ 11.6   **FUD** 090   J A2 50 ▭

AMA: 2018,Sep,7

27001   Tenotomy, adductor of hip, open

🔧 15.6   ⚙ 15.6   **FUD** 090   J A2 80 50 ▭

AMA: 2018,Sep,7

27003   Tenotomy, adductor, subcutaneous, open, with obturator neurectomy

🔧 17.0   ⚙ 17.0   **FUD** 090   J A2 80 50 ▭

AMA: 2018,Sep,7

27005   Tenotomy, hip flexor(s), open (separate procedure)

🔧 20.8   ⚙ 20.8   **FUD** 090   C 80 50 ▭

AMA: 2018,Sep,7

27006   Tenotomy, abductors and/or extensor(s) of hip, open (separate procedure)

🔧 20.7   ⚙ 20.7   **FUD** 090   J 62 80 50 ▭

AMA: 2018,Sep,7

27025-27036 Surgical Incision of Hip

27025   Fasciotomy, hip or thigh, any type

🔧 26.5   ⚙ 26.5   **FUD** 090   C 80 50 ▭

AMA: 2018,Sep,7

27027   Decompression fasciotomy(ies), pelvic (buttock) compartment(s) (eg, gluteus medius-minimus, gluteus maximus, iliopsoas, and/or tensor fascia lata muscle), unilateral

🔧 25.8   ⚙ 25.8   **FUD** 090   J 62 80 50 ▭

AMA: 2018,Sep,7

27030   Arthrotomy, hip, with drainage (eg, infection)

🔧 27.0   ⚙ 27.0   **FUD** 090   C 80 50 ▭

AMA: 2018,Sep,7

27033   Arthrotomy, hip, including exploration or removal of loose or foreign body

🔧 28.1   ⚙ 28.1   **FUD** 090   J A2 80 50 ▭

AMA: 2018,Sep,7; 2018,Jan,8; 2017,Jan,8; 2016,Jan,13

27035   Denervation, hip joint, intrapelvic or extrapelvic intra-articular branches of sciatic, femoral, or obturator nerves

EXCLUDES   *Transection obturator nerve (64763, 64766)*

🔧 32.8   ⚙ 32.8   **FUD** 090   J A2 80 50 ▭

AMA: 2018,Sep,7; 2018,Jan,8; 2017,Jan,8; 2016,Jan,13

27036   Capsulectomy or capsulotomy, hip, with or without excision of heterotopic bone, with release of hip flexor muscles (ie, gluteus medius, gluteus minimus, tensor fascia latae, rectus femoris, sartorius, iliopsoas)

🔧 29.1   ⚙ 29.1   **FUD** 090   C 80 50 ▭

AMA: 2018,Sep,7

27040-27041 Biopsy of Hip/Pelvis

EXCLUDES   *Soft tissue needle biopsy (20206)*

27040   Biopsy, soft tissue of pelvis and hip area; superficial

🔧 5.70   ⚙ 9.83   **FUD** 010   J A2 50 ▭

AMA: 2018,Sep,7

27041   deep, subfascial or intramuscular

🔧 20.1   ⚙ 20.1   **FUD** 090   J A2 50 ▭

AMA: 2018,Sep,7

27043-27059 [27043, 27045, 27059] Excision Soft Tissue Tumors Hip/ Pelvis

INCLUDES   Any necessary elevation tissue planes or dissection
Measurement tumor and necessary margin at greatest diameter prior to excision
Simple and intermediate repairs
Excision types:
    Fascial or subfascial soft tissue tumors: simple and marginal resection tumors found either in or below deep fascia, not involving bone or excision substantial amount normal tissue; primarily benign and intramuscular tumors
    Radical resection soft tissue tumor: wide resection tumor involving substantial margins normal tissue and may involve tissue removal from one or more layers; mostly malignant or aggressive benign,
    Subcutaneous: simple and marginal resection tumors found in subcutaneous tissue above deep fascia; most often benign

EXCLUDES   *Complex repair*
Excision benign cutaneous lesions (eg, sebaceous cyst) (11400-11406)
Radical resection cutaneous tumors (eg, melanoma) (11600-11606)
Significant vessel exploration, neuroplasty, reconstruction, or complex bone repair

27043   Resequenced code. See code following 27047.

27045   Resequenced code. See code following 27048.

27047   Excision, tumor, soft tissue of pelvis and hip area, subcutaneous; less than 3 cm

🔧 10.4   ⚙ 13.6   **FUD** 090   J 62 50 ▭

AMA: 2018,Sep,7

\# **27043**   3 cm or greater

🔧 13.5   ⚙ 13.5   **FUD** 090   J 62 50 ▭

AMA: 2018,Sep,7

27048   Excision, tumor, soft tissue of pelvis and hip area, subfascial (eg, intramuscular); less than 5 cm

🔧 17.6   ⚙ 17.6   **FUD** 090   J 62 80 50 ▭

AMA: 2018,Sep,7

\# **27045**   5 cm or greater

🔧 21.3   ⚙ 21.3   **FUD** 090   J 62 80 50 ▭

AMA: 2018,Sep,7

27049   Radical resection of tumor (eg, sarcoma), soft tissue of pelvis and hip area; less than 5 cm

🔧 38.6   ⚙ 38.6   **FUD** 090   J 62 80 50 ▭

AMA: 2018,Sep,7

\# **27059**   5 cm or greater

🔧 52.6   ⚙ 52.6   **FUD** 090   J 62 80 50 ▭

AMA: 2018,Sep,7

27050-27071 [27059] Procedures of Bones and Joints of Hip and Pelvis

27050   Arthrotomy, with biopsy; sacroiliac joint

🔧 11.5   ⚙ 11.5   **FUD** 090   J A2 80 50 ▭

AMA: 2018,Sep,7

27052   hip joint

🔧 16.6   ⚙ 16.6   **FUD** 090   J A2 80 50 ▭

AMA: 2018,Sep,7

27054 Arthrotomy with synovectomy, hip joint
🔹 19.8 ⚖ 19.8 **FUD** 090 C 80 50 ▢
AMA: 2018,Sep,7

27057 Decompression fasciotomy(ies), pelvic (buttock) compartment(s) (eg, gluteus medius-minimus, gluteus maximus, iliopsoas, and/or tensor fascia lata muscle) with debridement of nonviable muscle, unilateral
🔹 29.2 ⚖ 29.2 **FUD** 090 J G2 80 50 ▢
AMA: 2018,Sep,7

27059 Resequenced code. See code following 27049.

27060 Excision; ischial bursa
🔹 13.4 ⚖ 13.4 **FUD** 090 J A2 50 ▢
AMA: 2018,Sep,7

27062 trochanteric bursa or calcification
EXCLUDES *Arthrocentesis (20610)*
🔹 13.0 ⚖ 13.0 **FUD** 090 J A2 50 ▢
AMA: 2018,Sep,7

27065 Excision of bone cyst or benign tumor, wing of ilium, symphysis pubis, or greater trochanter of femur; superficial, includes autograft, when performed
🔹 15.0 ⚖ 15.0 **FUD** 090 J A2 80 50 ▢
AMA: 2018,Sep,7

27066 deep (subfascial), includes autograft, when performed
🔹 23.1 ⚖ 23.1 **FUD** 090 J A2 80 50 ▢
AMA: 2018,Sep,7

27067 with autograft requiring separate incision
🔹 29.8 ⚖ 29.8 **FUD** 090 J A2 80 50 ▢
AMA: 2018,Sep,7

27070 Partial excision, wing of ilium, symphysis pubis, or greater trochanter of femur, (craterization, saucerization) (eg, osteomyelitis or bone abscess); superficial
🔹 25.3 ⚖ 25.3 **FUD** 090 C 80 50 ▢
AMA: 2018,Sep,7

27071 deep (subfascial or intramuscular)
🔹 27.2 ⚖ 27.2 **FUD** 090 C 80 50 ▢
AMA: 2018,Sep,7

27075-27078 Radical Resection Bone Tumor of Hip/Pelvis

INCLUDES Any necessary elevation tissue planes or dissection
Excision adjacent soft tissue during bone tumor resection (27043-27049 [27043, 27045, 27059])
Measurement tumor and necessary margin at greatest diameter prior to excision
Resection tumor (may include entire bone) and wide margins normal tissue primarily for malignant or aggressive benign tumors
Simple and intermediate repairs
EXCLUDES *Complex repair*
Significant vessel exploration, neuroplasty, reconstruction, or complex bone repair

27075 Radical resection of tumor; wing of ilium, 1 pubic or ischial ramus or symphysis pubis
🔹 60.5 ⚖ 60.5 **FUD** 090 C 80 ▢
AMA: 2019,May,7; 2018,Sep,7

27076 ilium, including acetabulum, both pubic rami, or ischium and acetabulum
🔹 73.3 ⚖ 73.3 **FUD** 090 C 80 ▢
AMA: 2019,May,7; 2018,Sep,7

27077 innominate bone, total
🔹 81.8 ⚖ 81.8 **FUD** 090 C 80 ▢
AMA: 2019,May,7; 2018,Sep,7

27078 ischial tuberosity and greater trochanter of femur
🔹 59.6 ⚖ 59.6 **FUD** 090 C 80 50 ▢
AMA: 2019,May,7; 2018,Sep,7

27080 Excision of Coccyx

EXCLUDES *Surgical excision decubitus ulcers (15920, 15922, 15931-15958)*

27080 Coccygectomy, primary
🔹 14.7 ⚖ 14.7 **FUD** 090 J A2 80 ▢
AMA: 2018,Sep,7

27086-27091 Removal Foreign Body or Hip Prosthesis

27086 Removal of foreign body, pelvis or hip; subcutaneous tissue
🔹 4.82 ⚖ 8.78 **FUD** 010 J A2 80 50 ▢
AMA: 2018,Sep,7; 2018,Jan,8; 2017,Jan,8; 2016,Jan,13

27087 deep (subfascial or intramuscular)
🔹 17.7 ⚖ 17.7 **FUD** 090 J A2 80 50 ▢
AMA: 2018,Sep,7

A foreign body is removed from the pelvis or hip

27090 Removal of hip prosthesis; (separate procedure)
🔹 24.0 ⚖ 24.0 **FUD** 090 C 80 50 ▢
AMA: 2019,May,7; 2018,Sep,7

27091 complicated, including total hip prosthesis, methylmethacrylate with or without insertion of spacer
🔹 46.0 ⚖ 46.0 **FUD** 090 C 80 50 ▢
AMA: 2019,May,7; 2018,Sep,7; 2018,Jan,8; 2017,Jan,8; 2016,Jan,13

27093-27096 Injection for Arthrogram Hip/Sacroiliac Joint

27093 Injection procedure for hip arthrography; without anesthesia
▦ (73525)
🔹 2.01 ⚖ 5.72 **FUD** 000 N N1 50 ▢
AMA: 2018,Sep,7; 2018,Jan,8; 2017,Jan,8; 2016,Jan,13

27095 with anesthesia
▦ (73525)
🔹 2.43 ⚖ 8.36 **FUD** 000 N N1 50 ▢
AMA: 2018,Sep,7; 2018,Jan,8; 2017,Jan,8; 2016,Jan,13; 2016,Jan,11

27096 Injection procedure for sacroiliac joint, anesthetic/steroid, with image guidance (fluoroscopy or CT) including arthrography when performed
INCLUDES Confirmation intra-articular needle placement with CT or fluoroscopy
Fluoroscopic guidance (77002-77003)
EXCLUDES *Procedure performed without fluoroscopy or CT guidance (20552)*
🔹 2.39 ⚖ 4.61 **FUD** 000 B 50 ▢
AMA: 2018,Sep,7; 2018,Jan,8; 2017,Jan,8; 2016,Jan,13

27097-27187 Revision/Reconstruction Hip and Pelvis

INCLUDES Closed, open and percutaneous treatment fractures and dislocations

27097 Release or recession, hamstring, proximal
🔹 19.7 ⚖ 19.7 **FUD** 090 J A2 80 50 ▢
AMA: 2018,Sep,7

27098 Transfer, adductor to ischium
🔹 20.0 ⚖ 20.0 **FUD** 090 J A2 80 50 ▢
AMA: 2018,Sep,7

27100 **Transfer external oblique muscle to greater trochanter including fascial or tendon extension (graft)**
INCLUDES Eggers procedure
🔪 23.6 ⚕ 23.6 **FUD** 090 J A2 80 50 ▣
AMA: 2018,Sep,7

27105 **Transfer paraspinal muscle to hip (includes fascial or tendon extension graft)**
🔪 25.0 ⚕ 25.0 **FUD** 090 J A2 80 50 ▣
AMA: 2018,Sep,7

27110 **Transfer iliopsoas; to greater trochanter of femur**
🔪 28.0 ⚕ 28.0 **FUD** 090 J J8 80 50 ▣
AMA: 2018,Sep,7

27111 **to femoral neck**
🔪 26.0 ⚕ 26.0 **FUD** 090 J A2 80 50 ▣
AMA: 2018,Sep,7

27120 **Acetabuloplasty; (eg, Whitman, Colonna, Haygroves, or cup type)**
🔪 37.5 ⚕ 37.5 **FUD** 090 C 80 50 ▣
AMA: 2018,Sep,7

27122 **resection, femoral head (eg, Girdlestone procedure)**
🔪 31.7 ⚕ 31.7 **FUD** 090 C 80 50 ▣
AMA: 2018,Sep,7

27125 **Hemiarthroplasty, hip, partial (eg, femoral stem prosthesis, bipolar arthroplasty)**
EXCLUDES *Hip replacement following hip fracture (27236)*
🔪 32.7 ⚕ 32.7 **FUD** 090 C 80 50 ▣
AMA: 2018,Sep,7; 2018,Jan,8; 2017,Jan,8; 2016,Jan,13

Acetabulum remains intact

Prosthesis

27130 **Arthroplasty, acetabular and proximal femoral prosthetic replacement (total hip arthroplasty), with or without autograft or allograft**
🔪 39.2 ⚕ 39.2 **FUD** 090 C J8 80 50 ▣
AMA: 2019,May,7; 2018,Sep,7; 2018,Jan,8; 2017,Jan,8; 2016,Jan,13

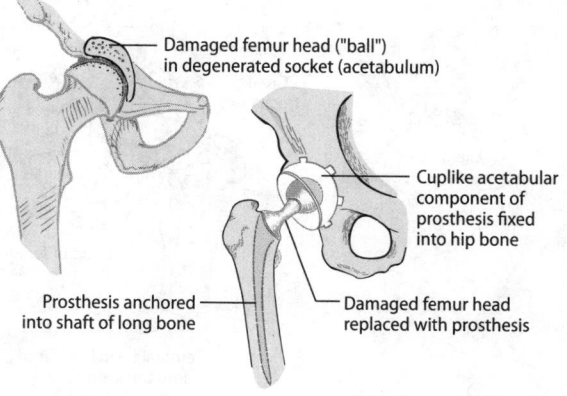

Damaged femur head ("ball") in degenerated socket (acetabulum)

Cuplike acetabular component of prosthesis fixed into hip bone

Prosthesis anchored into shaft of long bone

Damaged femur head replaced with prosthesis

27132 **Conversion of previous hip surgery to total hip arthroplasty, with or without autograft or allograft**
🔪 48.3 ⚕ 48.3 **FUD** 090 C 80 50 ▣
AMA: 2019,May,7; 2018,Sep,7; 2018,Jan,8; 2017,Sep,14; 2017,Jan,8; 2016,Jan,13

27134 **Revision of total hip arthroplasty; both components, with or without autograft or allograft**
🔪 55.3 ⚕ 55.3 **FUD** 090 C 80 50 ▣
AMA: 2019,May,7; 2018,Sep,7; 2018,Jan,8; 2017,Jan,8; 2016,Jan,13

27137 **acetabular component only, with or without autograft or allograft**
🔪 42.5 ⚕ 42.5 **FUD** 090 C 80 50 ▣
AMA: 2018,Sep,7; 2018,Jan,8; 2017,Jan,8; 2016,Jan,13

27138 **femoral component only, with or without allograft**
🔪 44.1 ⚕ 44.1 **FUD** 090 C 80 50 ▣
AMA: 2019,May,7; 2018,Sep,7; 2018,Jan,8; 2017,Jan,8; 2016,Jan,13

27140 **Osteotomy and transfer of greater trochanter of femur (separate procedure)**
🔪 25.8 ⚕ 25.8 **FUD** 090 C 80 50 ▣
AMA: 2018,Sep,7

27146 **Osteotomy, iliac, acetabular or innominate bone;**
INCLUDES Salter osteotomy
🔪 36.9 ⚕ 36.9 **FUD** 090 C 80 50 ▣
AMA: 2018,Sep,7; 2018,Jan,8; 2017,Jan,8; 2016,Jan,13

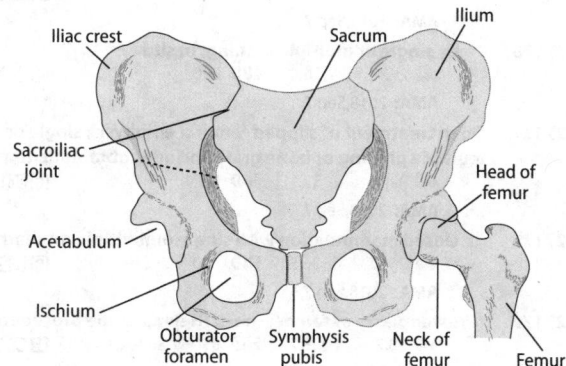

Iliac crest
Sacrum
Ilium
Sacroiliac joint
Head of femur
Acetabulum
Ischium
Obturator foramen
Symphysis pubis
Neck of femur
Femur

27147 **with open reduction of hip**

INCLUDES Pemberton osteotomy

🖥 41.9   ✂ 41.9   **FUD** 090   C 80 50 ▭

AMA: 2018,Sep,7

Ilium

Example of innominate osteotomy

Greater trochanter

Acetabulum

Head of femur

Femoral head is reduced into the acetabulum

Kirschner wires are drilled through the ilium and into lower fragment

27151 **with femoral osteotomy**

🖥 45.9   ✂ 45.9   **FUD** 090   C 80 50 ▭

AMA: 2018,Sep,7

27156 **with femoral osteotomy and with open reduction of hip**

INCLUDES Chiari osteotomy

🖥 48.9   ✂ 48.9   **FUD** 090   C 80 50 ▭

AMA: 2018,Sep,7

27158 **Osteotomy, pelvis, bilateral (eg, congenital malformation)**

🖥 40.5   ✂ 40.5   **FUD** 090   C 80 ▭

AMA: 2018,Sep,7

27161 **Osteotomy, femoral neck (separate procedure)**

🖥 35.2   ✂ 35.2   **FUD** 090   C 80 50 ▭

AMA: 2018,Sep,7

27165 **Osteotomy, intertrochanteric or subtrochanteric including internal or external fixation and/or cast**

🖥 39.6   ✂ 39.6   **FUD** 090   C 80 50 ▭

AMA: 2018,Sep,7; 2018,Jan,8; 2017,Jan,8; 2016,Jan,13

27170 **Bone graft, femoral head, neck, intertrochanteric or subtrochanteric area (includes obtaining bone graft)**

🖥 33.9   ✂ 33.9   **FUD** 090   C 80 50 ▭

AMA: 2018,Sep,7; 2018,Jan,8; 2017,Jan,8; 2016,Jan,13

27175 **Treatment of slipped femoral epiphysis; by traction, without reduction**

🖥 19.2   ✂ 19.2   **FUD** 090   C 80 50 ▭

AMA: 2018,Sep,7

27176 **by single or multiple pinning, in situ**

🖥 26.4   ✂ 26.4   **FUD** 090   C 80 50 ▭

AMA: 2018,Sep,7

27177 **Open treatment of slipped femoral epiphysis; single or multiple pinning or bone graft (includes obtaining graft)**

🖥 32.1   ✂ 32.1   **FUD** 090   C 80 50 ▭

AMA: 2018,Sep,7

27178 **closed manipulation with single or multiple pinning**

🖥 26.5   ✂ 26.5   **FUD** 090   C 80 50 ▭

AMA: 2018,Sep,7

27179 **osteoplasty of femoral neck (Heyman type procedure)**

🖥 28.2   ✂ 28.2   **FUD** 090   J 62 80 50 ▭

AMA: 2018,Sep,7

27181 **osteotomy and internal fixation**

🖥 32.3   ✂ 32.3   **FUD** 090   C 80 50 ▭

AMA: 2018,Sep,7

27185 **Epiphyseal arrest by epiphysiodesis or stapling, greater trochanter of femur**

🖥 20.7   ✂ 20.7   **FUD** 090   C 50 ▭

AMA: 2018,Sep,7

27187 **Prophylactic treatment (nailing, pinning, plating or wiring) with or without methylmethacrylate, femoral neck and proximal femur**

🖥 28.7   ✂ 28.7   **FUD** 090   C 80 50 ▭

AMA: 2018,Sep,7; 2018,Jan,8; 2017,Jan,8; 2016,Jan,13

27197-27269 Treatment of Fracture/Dislocation Hip/Pelvis

27197 **Closed treatment of posterior pelvic ring fracture(s), dislocation(s), diastasis or subluxation of the ilium, sacroiliac joint, and/or sacrum, with or without anterior pelvic ring fracture(s) and/or dislocation(s) of the pubic symphysis and/or superior/inferior rami, unilateral or bilateral; without manipulation**

🖥 3.68   ✂ 3.68   **FUD** 000   T 62 ▭

AMA: 2018,Sep,7; 2018,Jan,8; 2017,Jun,9

27198 **with manipulation, requiring more than local anesthesia (ie, general anesthesia, moderate sedation, spinal/epidural)**

EXCLUDES *Closed treatment anterior pelvic ring, pubic symphysis, inferior rami fracture/dislocation--see appropriate E/M codes*

🖥 8.84   ✂ 8.84   **FUD** 000   T 62 80 ▭

AMA: 2018,Sep,7; 2018,Jan,3; 2018,Jan,8; 2017,Jun,9

27200 **Closed treatment of coccygeal fracture**

🖥 5.40   ✂ 5.32   **FUD** 090   T P2 ▭

AMA: 2018,Sep,7

27202 **Open treatment of coccygeal fracture**

🖥 15.2   ✂ 15.2   **FUD** 090   J A2 80 ▭

AMA: 2018,Sep,7

27215 **Open treatment of iliac spine(s), tuberosity avulsion, or iliac wing fracture(s), unilateral, for pelvic bone fracture patterns that do not disrupt the pelvic ring, includes internal fixation, when performed**

🖥 17.4   ✂ 17.4   **FUD** 090   E ▭

AMA: 2018,Sep,7

27216 **Percutaneous skeletal fixation of posterior pelvic bone fracture and/or dislocation, for fracture patterns that disrupt the pelvic ring, unilateral (includes ipsilateral ilium, sacroiliac joint and/or sacrum)**

EXCLUDES *Sacroiliac joint arthrodesis without fracture and/or dislocation, percutaneous or minimally invasive (27279)*

🖥 25.8   ✂ 25.8   **FUD** 090   E ▭

AMA: 2018,Sep,7; 2018,Jan,8; 2017,Jan,8; 2016,Jan,13

27217 **Open treatment of anterior pelvic bone fracture and/or dislocation for fracture patterns that disrupt the pelvic ring, unilateral, includes internal fixation, when performed (includes pubic symphysis and/or ipsilateral superior/inferior rami)**

🖥 25.0   ✂ 25.0   **FUD** 090   E ▭

AMA: 2018,Sep,7

27218 **Open treatment of posterior pelvic bone fracture and/or dislocation, for fracture patterns that disrupt the pelvic ring, unilateral, includes internal fixation, when performed (includes ipsilateral ilium, sacroiliac joint and/or sacrum)**

EXCLUDES *Sacroiliac joint arthrodesis without fracture and/or dislocation, percutaneous or minimally invasive (27279)*

🖥 34.6   ✂ 34.6   **FUD** 090   E ▭

AMA: 2018,Sep,7; 2018,Jan,8; 2017,Jan,8; 2016,Jan,13

27220 **Closed treatment of acetabulum (hip socket) fracture(s); without manipulation**

🖥 12.2   ✂ 12.4   **FUD** 090   T 62 50 ▭

AMA: 2018,Sep,7

26/TC PC/TC Only   A2-Z3 ASC Payment   50 Bilateral   ♂ Male Only   ♀ Female Only   🖥 Facility RVU   ✂ Non-Facility RVU   ▭ CCI   ✖ CLIA
FUD Follow-up Days   **CMS:** IOM   **AMA:** CPT Asst   A-Y OPPSI   80/80 Surg Assist Allowed / w/Doc   🔲 Lab Crosswalk   🔲 Radiology Crosswalk

82   CPT © 2021 American Medical Association. All Rights Reserved.   © 2021 Optum360, LLC

27222 with manipulation, with or without skeletal traction
🚗 28.1 ⚕ 28.1 **FUD** 090 C 50 ▢
AMA: 2018,Sep,7

27226 Open treatment of posterior or anterior acetabular wall fracture, with internal fixation
🚗 30.4 ⚕ 30.4 **FUD** 090 C 80 50 ▢
AMA: 2018,Sep,7

27227 Open treatment of acetabular fracture(s) involving anterior or posterior (one) column, or a fracture running transversely across the acetabulum, with internal fixation
🚗 47.9 ⚕ 47.9 **FUD** 090 C 80 50 ▢
AMA: 2018,Sep,7

27228 Open treatment of acetabular fracture(s) involving anterior and posterior (two) columns, includes T-fracture and both column fracture with complete articular detachment, or single column or transverse fracture with associated acetabular wall fracture, with internal fixation
🚗 54.3 ⚕ 54.3 **FUD** 090 C 80 50 ▢
AMA: 2018,Sep,7

27230 Closed treatment of femoral fracture, proximal end, neck; without manipulation
🚗 13.6 ⚕ 13.8 **FUD** 090 T A2 50 ▢
AMA: 2018,Sep,7

27232 with manipulation, with or without skeletal traction
🚗 21.6 ⚕ 21.6 **FUD** 090 C 50 ▢
AMA: 2018,Sep,7

27235 Percutaneous skeletal fixation of femoral fracture, proximal end, neck
🚗 26.2 ⚕ 26.2 **FUD** 090 J 62 50 ▢
AMA: 2018,Sep,7; 2018,Jan,8; 2017,Jan,8; 2016,Jan,13

27236 Open treatment of femoral fracture, proximal end, neck, internal fixation or prosthetic replacement
🚗 34.4 ⚕ 34.4 **FUD** 090 C 80 50 ▢
AMA: 2019,May,7; 2018,Sep,7; 2018,Jan,8; 2017,Jan,8; 2016,Nov,9; 2016,Jan,13

27238 Closed treatment of intertrochanteric, peritrochanteric, or subtrochanteric femoral fracture; without manipulation
🚗 13.3 ⚕ 13.3 **FUD** 090 J A2 50 ▢
AMA: 2018,Sep,7; 2018,Jan,8; 2017,Jan,8; 2016,Jan,13

27240 with manipulation, with or without skin or skeletal traction
🚗 27.5 ⚕ 27.5 **FUD** 090 C 50 ▢
AMA: 2018,Sep,7; 2018,Jan,8; 2017,Jan,8; 2016,Jan,13

27244 Treatment of intertrochanteric, peritrochanteric, or subtrochanteric femoral fracture; with plate/screw type implant, with or without cerclage
🚗 35.5 ⚕ 35.5 **FUD** 090 C 80 50 ▢
AMA: 2019,May,7; 2018,Sep,7; 2018,Jan,8; 2017,Jan,8; 2016,Jan,13

27245 with intramedullary implant, with or without interlocking screws and/or cerclage
🚗 35.5 ⚕ 35.5 **FUD** 090 C 80 50 ▢
AMA: 2018,Sep,7; 2018,Jan,8; 2017,Jan,8; 2016,Jan,13

27246 Closed treatment of greater trochanteric fracture, without manipulation
🚗 11.1 ⚕ 11.1 **FUD** 090 T A2 50 ▢
AMA: 2018,Sep,7

27248 Open treatment of greater trochanteric fracture, includes internal fixation, when performed
🚗 21.5 ⚕ 21.5 **FUD** 090 C 80 50 ▢
AMA: 2018,Sep,7

27250 Closed treatment of hip dislocation, traumatic; without anesthesia
🚗 5.33 ⚕ 5.33 **FUD** 000 T A2 50 ▢
AMA: 2018,Sep,7

27252 requiring anesthesia
🚗 21.8 ⚕ 21.8 **FUD** 090 . J A2 50 ▢
AMA: 2018,Sep,7

27253 Open treatment of hip dislocation, traumatic, without internal fixation
🚗 27.2 ⚕ 27.2 **FUD** 090 C 80 50 ▢
AMA: 2018,Sep,7

27254 Open treatment of hip dislocation, traumatic, with acetabular wall and femoral head fracture, with or without internal or external fixation
EXCLUDES *Acetabular fracture treatment (27226-27227)*
🚗 36.4 ⚕ 36.4 **FUD** 090 C 80 50 ▢
AMA: 2018,Sep,7

27256 Treatment of spontaneous hip dislocation (developmental, including congenital or pathological), by abduction, splint or traction; without anesthesia, without manipulation
🚗 6.78 ⚕ 8.73 **FUD** 010 T 62 80 50 ▢
AMA: 2018,Sep,7

27257 with manipulation, requiring anesthesia
🚗 10.4 ⚕ 10.4 **FUD** 010 J A2 80 50 ▢
AMA: 2018,Sep,7

27258 Open treatment of spontaneous hip dislocation (developmental, including congenital or pathological), replacement of femoral head in acetabulum (including tenotomy, etc);
INCLUDES Lorenz's operation
🚗 32.1 ⚕ 32.1 **FUD** 090 C 80 50 ▢
AMA: 2018,Sep,7

27259 with femoral shaft shortening
🚗 44.7 ⚕ 44.7 **FUD** 090 C 80 50 ▢
AMA: 2018,Sep,7

27265 Closed treatment of post hip arthroplasty dislocation; without anesthesia
🚗 11.5 ⚕ 11.5 **FUD** 090 T A2 50 ▢
AMA: 2018,Sep,7

27266 requiring regional or general anesthesia
🚗 16.8 ⚕ 16.8 **FUD** 090 J A2 50 ▢
AMA: 2018,Sep,7

27267 Closed treatment of femoral fracture, proximal end, head; without manipulation
🚗 12.5 ⚕ 12.5 **FUD** 090 J 62 80 50 ▢
AMA: 2018,Sep,7; 2018,Jan,8; 2017,Jan,8; 2016,Jan,13

27268 with manipulation
🚗 15.6 ⚕ 15.6 **FUD** 090 C 80 50 ▢
AMA: 2018,Sep,7; 2018,Jan,8; 2017,Jan,8; 2016,Jan,13

27269 Open treatment of femoral fracture, proximal end, head, includes internal fixation, when performed
EXCLUDES *Arthrotomy, hip (27033)*
Open treatment hip dislocation, traumatic, without internal fixation (27253)
🚗 35.8 ⚕ 35.8 **FUD** 090 C 80 50 ▢
AMA: 2018,Sep,7; 2018,Jan,8; 2017,Jan,8; 2016,Jan,13

27275 Hip Manipulation with Anesthesia

27275 Manipulation, hip joint, requiring general anesthesia
🚗 5.26 ⚕ 5.26 **FUD** 010 J A2
AMA: 2018,Sep,7; 2018,Jan,8; 2017,Jan,8; 2016,May,13; 2016,Jan,11; 2016,Jan,13

27279-27286 Arthrodesis of Hip and Pelvis

27279 Arthrodesis, sacroiliac joint, percutaneous or minimally invasive (indirect visualization), with image guidance, includes obtaining bone graft when performed, and placement of transfixing device
🚗 25.3 ⚕ 25.3 **FUD** 090 J J8 80 50 ▢
AMA: 2020,May,13; 2018,Sep,7

● New Code ▲ Revised Code ○ Reinstated ● New Web Release ▲ Revised Web Release + Add-on Unlisted Not Covered # Resequenced
50 Optum Mod 50 Exempt ⊘ AMA Mod 51 Exempt 51 Optum Mod 51 Exempt 63 Mod 63 Exempt ✗ Non-FDA Drug ★ Telemedicine M Maternity A Age Edit

27280   Arthrodesis, open, sacroiliac joint, including obtaining bone graft, including instrumentation, when performed

> *EXCLUDES*   *Sacroiliac joint arthrodesis without fracture and/or dislocation, percutaneous or minimally invasive (27279)*

   39.2   39.2   **FUD** 090   C 80 50 ⬜

AMA: 2020,May,13; 2018,Sep,7; 2018,Jan,8; 2017,Jan,8; 2016,Jan,13

27282   Arthrodesis, symphysis pubis (including obtaining graft)

   24.7   24.7   **FUD** 090   C 80

AMA: 2020,May,13; 2018,Sep,7

27284   Arthrodesis, hip joint (including obtaining graft);

   46.6   46.6   **FUD** 090   C 80 50 ⬜

AMA: 2020,May,13; 2018,Sep,7

27286   with subtrochanteric osteotomy

   47.6   47.6   **FUD** 090   C 80 50 ⬜

AMA: 2020,May,13; 2018,Sep,7; 2018,Jan,8; 2017,Jan,8; 2016,Jan,13

27290-27299 Amputations and Unlisted Procedures of Hip and Pelvis

27290   Interpelviabdominal amputation (hindquarter amputation)

   46.9   46.9   **FUD** 090   C 80 ⬜

AMA: 2018,Sep,7; 2018,Jan,8; 2017,Jan,8; 2016,Jan,13

27295   Disarticulation of hip

   36.4   36.4   **FUD** 090   C 80 50 ⬜

AMA: 2018,Sep,7; 2018,Jan,8; 2017,Jan,8; 2016,Jan,13

27299   Unlisted procedure, pelvis or hip joint

   0.00   0.00   **FUD** YYY   T 80 50 ⬜

AMA: 2018,Sep,7; 2018,Jan,8; 2017,Jan,8; 2016,Jun,8; 2016,Jan,13

27301-27310 Incisional Procedures Femur or Knee

> *EXCLUDES*   *Superficial incision and drainage (10040-10160)*

27301   Incision and drainage, deep abscess, bursa, or hematoma, thigh or knee region

   14.5   19.4   **FUD** 090   J A2 50 ⬜

AMA: 2018,Sep,7; 2018,Jan,8; 2017,Jan,8; 2016,Jan,13

27303   Incision, deep, with opening of bone cortex, femur or knee (eg, osteomyelitis or bone abscess)

   18.5   18.5   **FUD** 090   C 80 50 ⬜

AMA: 2018,Sep,7

27305   Fasciotomy, iliotibial (tenotomy), open

> *EXCLUDES*   *Ober-Yount (gluteal-iliotibial) fasciotomy (27025)*

   13.8   13.8   **FUD** 090   J A2 80 50 ⬜

AMA: 2018,Sep,7

27306   Tenotomy, percutaneous, adductor or hamstring; single tendon (separate procedure)

   9.87   9.87   **FUD** 090   J A2 80 50 ⬜

AMA: 2018,Sep,7; 2018,Jan,8; 2017,Aug,9

27307   multiple tendons

   13.8   13.8   **FUD** 090   J A2 80 50 ⬜

AMA: 2018,Sep,7; 2018,Jan,8; 2017,Aug,9

27310   Arthrotomy, knee, with exploration, drainage, or removal of foreign body (eg, infection)

   21.1   21.1   **FUD** 090   J A2 80 50 ⬜

AMA: 2018,Sep,7; 2018,Jan,8; 2017,Jan,8; 2016,Jan,13

27323-27324 Biopsy Femur or Knee

> *EXCLUDES*   *Soft tissue needle biopsy (20206)*

27323   Biopsy, soft tissue of thigh or knee area; superficial

   5.08   7.91   **FUD** 010   J A2 50 ⬜

AMA: 2018,Sep,7; 2018,Jan,8; 2017,Jan,8; 2016,Jan,13

27324   deep (subfascial or intramuscular)

   11.6   11.6   **FUD** 090   J A2 50 ⬜

AMA: 2018,Sep,7; 2018,Jan,8; 2017,Jan,8; 2016,Jan,13

27325-27326 Neurectomy

27325   Neurectomy, hamstring muscle

   16.1   16.1   **FUD** 090   J A2 80 50 ⬜

AMA: 2018,Sep,7

27326   Neurectomy, popliteal (gastrocnemius)

   14.9   14.9   **FUD** 090   J A2 80 50 ⬜

AMA: 2018,Sep,7

27327-27339 [27329, 27337, 27339] Excision Soft Tissue Tumors Femur/ Knee

> *INCLUDES*   Any necessary elevation tissue planes or dissection
> Measurement tumor and necessary margin at greatest diameter prior to excision
> Simple and intermediate repairs
> Excision types:
>   Fascial or subfascial soft tissue tumors: simple and marginal resection tumors found either in or below deep fascia, not including bone or excision substantial amount normal tissue; primarily benign and intramuscular tumors
>   Radical resection soft tissue tumor: wide resection tumor involving substantial margins normal tissue and may involve tissue removal from one or more layers; most often malignant or aggressive benign
>   Subcutaneous: simple and marginal resection tumors in subcutaneous tissue above deep fascia; most often benign

> *EXCLUDES*   *Complex repair*
> *Excision benign cutaneous lesions (eg, sebaceous cyst) (11400-11406)*
> *Radical resection cutaneous tumors (eg, melanoma) (11600-11606)*
> *Significant vessel exploration or neuroplasty*

27327   Excision, tumor, soft tissue of thigh or knee area, subcutaneous; less than 3 cm

   9.00   13.5   **FUD** 090   J G2 50 ⬜

AMA: 2018,Sep,7

\#   **27337**   3 cm or greater

   12.1   12.1   **FUD** 090   J G2 80 50 ⬜

AMA: 2018,Sep,7

27328   Excision, tumor, soft tissue of thigh or knee area, subfascial (eg, intramuscular); less than 5 cm

   18.0   18.0   **FUD** 090   J G2 50 ⬜

AMA: 2018,Sep,7; 2018,Jan,8; 2017,Jan,8; 2016,Nov,9

27329   Resequenced code. See code following 27360.

\#   **27339**   5 cm or greater

   21.7   21.7   **FUD** 090   J G2 80 50 ⬜

AMA: 2018,Sep,7

27330-27360 [27337, 27339] Resection Procedures Thigh/Knee

27330   Arthrotomy, knee; with synovial biopsy only

   11.8   11.8   **FUD** 090   J A2 50 ⬜

AMA: 2018,Sep,7; 2018,Jan,8; 2017,Jan,8; 2016,Jan,13

27331   including joint exploration, biopsy, or removal of loose or foreign bodies

   13.6   13.6   **FUD** 090   J A2 80 50 ⬜

AMA: 2018,Sep,7; 2018,Jan,8; 2017,Jan,8; 2016,Jan,13

26/TC PC/TC Only   A2-Z3 ASC Payment   50 Bilateral   ♂ Male Only   ♀ Female Only   🔧 Facility RVU   🔪 Non-Facility RVU   ⬜ CCI   ✖ CLIA

FUD Follow-up Days   **CMS:** IOM   **AMA:** CPT Asst   A-Y OPPSI   80/80 Surg Assist Allowed / w/Doc   Lab Crosswalk   Radiology Crosswalk

84   CPT © 2021 American Medical Association. All Rights Reserved.   © 2021 Optum360, LLC

27332   **Arthrotomy, with excision of semilunar cartilage (meniscectomy) knee; medial OR lateral**
🚑 18.5   ⚕ 18.5   **FUD** 090   J A2 80 50 ▣
AMA: 2018,Sep,7

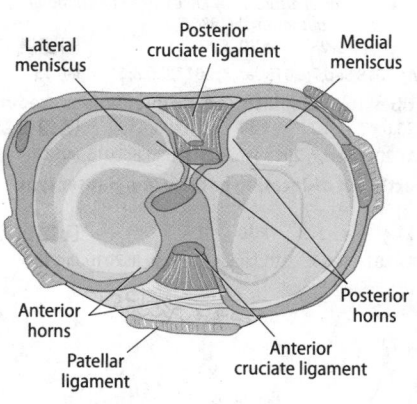

Lateral meniscus — Posterior cruciate ligament — Medial meniscus
Anterior horns
Patellar ligament — Anterior cruciate ligament — Posterior horns

Overhead view of right knee

Bucket handle tear

Radial tear

Meniscus

27333   **medial AND lateral**
🚑 16.9   ⚕ 16.9   **FUD** 090   J A2 80 50 ▣
AMA: 2018,Sep,7; 2018,Jan,8; 2017,Jan,8; 2016,Jan,13

27334   **Arthrotomy, with synovectomy, knee; anterior OR posterior**
🚑 19.7   ⚕ 19.7   **FUD** 090   J A2 80 50 ▣
AMA: 2018,Sep,7

27335   **anterior AND posterior including popliteal area**
🚑 22.0   ⚕ 22.0   **FUD** 090   J A2 80 50 ▣
AMA: 2018,Sep,7

27337   **Resequenced code. See code following 27327.**

27339   **Resequenced code. See code before 27330.**

27340   **Excision, prepatellar bursa**
🚑 10.6   ⚕ 10.6   **FUD** 090   J A2 50 ▣
AMA: 2018,Sep,7

27345   **Excision of synovial cyst of popliteal space (eg, Baker's cyst)**
🚑 13.9   ⚕ 13.9   **FUD** 090   J A2 80 50 ▣
AMA: 2018,Sep,7

27347   **Excision of lesion of meniscus or capsule (eg, cyst, ganglion), knee**
🚑 15.1   ⚕ 15.1   **FUD** 090   J A2 80 50 ▣
AMA: 2018,Sep,7

27350   **Patellectomy or hemipatellectomy**
🚑 18.8   ⚕ 18.8   **FUD** 090   J A2 80 50 ▣
AMA: 2018,Sep,7

27355   **Excision or curettage of bone cyst or benign tumor of femur;**
🚑 17.4   ⚕ 17.4   **FUD** 090   J A2 80 50 ▣
AMA: 2018,Sep,7

27356   **with allograft**
🚑 21.3   ⚕ 21.3   **FUD** 090   J G2 80 50 ▣
AMA: 2019,May,7; 2018,Sep,7

27357   **with autograft (includes obtaining graft)**
🚑 23.5   ⚕ 23.5   **FUD** 090   J A2 80 50 ▣
AMA: 2018,Sep,7; 2018,Jan,8; 2017,Jan,8; 2016,Jan,13

+ 27358   **with internal fixation (List in addition to code for primary procedure)**
Code first (27355-27357)
🚑 8.03   ⚕ 8.03   **FUD** ZZZ   N N1 80 ▣
AMA: 2018,Sep,7

27360   **Partial excision (craterization, saucerization, or diaphysectomy) bone, femur, proximal tibia and/or fibula (eg, osteomyelitis or bone abscess)**
🚑 24.7   ⚕ 24.7   **FUD** 090   J A2 80 50 ▣
AMA: 2018,Sep,7

27329-27365 [27329] Radical Resection Tumor Knee/Thigh

INCLUDES   Any necessary elevation tissue planes or dissection
Excision adjacent soft tissue during bone tumor resection
Measurement tumor and necessary margin at greatest diameter prior to excision
Radical resection bone tumor: resection tumor (may include entire bone) and wide margins normal tissue primarily for malignant or aggressive benign tumors
Radical resection soft tissue tumor: wide resection tumor involving substantial margins normal tissue that may include tissue removal from one or more layers; most often malignant or aggressive benign
Simple and intermediate repairs

EXCLUDES   Complex repair
Radical resection cutaneous tumors (eg, melanoma) (11600-11606)
Significant vessel exploration, neuroplasty, reconstruction, or complex bone repair

 # 27329   **Radical resection of tumor (eg, sarcoma), soft tissue of thigh or knee area; less than 5 cm**
🚑 30.1   ⚕ 30.1   **FUD** 090   J G2 80 50 ▣
AMA: 2018,Sep,7

27364   **5 cm or greater**
🚑 45.2   ⚕ 45.2   **FUD** 090   J G2 80 50 ▣
AMA: 2018,Sep,7

27365   **Radical resection of tumor, femur or knee**
EXCLUDES   Soft tissue tumor excision thigh or knee area (27329, 27364)
🚑 59.6   ⚕ 59.6   **FUD** 090   C 80 50 ▣
AMA: 2019,May,7; 2018,Sep,7

27369 Injection for Arthrogram of Knee

EXCLUDES   Arthrocentesis, aspiration and/or injection, knee (20610-20611)
Arthroscopy, knee (29871)

27369   **Injection procedure for contrast knee arthrography or contrast enhanced CT/MRI knee arthrography**
Code also fluoroscopic guidance, when performed for CT/MRI arthrography (73701-73702, 73722-73723, 77002)
🔀 (73580, 73701-73702, 73722-73723)
🚑 1.17   ⚕ 4.06   **FUD** 000   N1 50 ▣
AMA: 2019,Aug,7

27372 Foreign Body Removal Femur or Knee

EXCLUDES   Arthroscopic procedures (29870-29887)
Removal knee prosthesis (27488)

27372   **Removal of foreign body, deep, thigh region or knee area**
🚑 11.4   ⚕ 17.0   **FUD** 090   J A2 80 50 ▣
AMA: 2018,Sep,7

27380-27499 Repair/Reconstruction of Femur or Knee

27380   **Suture of infrapatellar tendon; primary**
🚑 17.5   ⚕ 17.5   **FUD** 090   J A2 80 50 ▣
AMA: 2018,Sep,7

27381   **secondary reconstruction, including fascial or tendon graft**
🚑 23.0   ⚕ 23.0   **FUD** 090   J J8 80 50 ▣
AMA: 2018,Sep,7

27385   **Suture of quadriceps or hamstring muscle rupture; primary**
🚑 16.9   ⚕ 16.9   **FUD** 090   J A2 80 50 ▣
AMA: 2018,Sep,7; 2018,Jan,8; 2017,Aug,9

27386   secondary reconstruction, including fascial or tendon graft
  🔧 24.3   ✂ 24.3   **FUD** 090   [J] [A2] [80] [50] [🔲]
  AMA: 2020,Apr,10; 2018,Sep,7

27390   Tenotomy, open, hamstring, knee to hip; single tendon
  🔧 12.9   ✂ 12.9   **FUD** 090   [J] [A2] [80] [50] [🔲]
  AMA: 2018,Sep,7

27391   multiple tendons, 1 leg
  🔧 16.2   ✂ 16.2   **FUD** 090   [J] [A2] [80] [🔲]
  AMA: 2018,Sep,7

27392   multiple tendons, bilateral
  🔧 20.5   ✂ 20.5   **FUD** 090   [J] [A2] [80] [🔲]
  AMA: 2018,Sep,7

27393   Lengthening of hamstring tendon; single tendon
  🔧 14.6   ✂ 14.6   **FUD** 090   [J] [A2] [80] [50] [🔲]
  AMA: 2018,Sep,7

27394   multiple tendons, 1 leg
  🔧 18.8   ✂ 18.8   **FUD** 090   [J] [A2] [80] [🔲]
  AMA: 2018,Sep,7

27395   multiple tendons, bilateral
  🔧 25.4   ✂ 25.4   **FUD** 090   [J] [A2] [80] [🔲]
  AMA: 2018,Sep,7

27396   Transplant or transfer (with muscle redirection or rerouting), thigh (eg, extensor to flexor); single tendon
  🔧 17.6   ✂ 17.6   **FUD** 090   [J] [A2] [80] [50] [🔲]
  AMA: 2018,Sep,7

27397   multiple tendons
  🔧 26.4   ✂ 26.4   **FUD** 090   [J] [62] [80] [50] [🔲]
  AMA: 2018,Sep,7

27400   Transfer, tendon or muscle, hamstrings to femur (eg, Egger's type procedure)
  🔧 20.0   ✂ 20.0   **FUD** 090   [J] [A2] [80] [50] [🔲]
  AMA: 2018,Sep,7

27403   Arthrotomy with meniscus repair, knee
  EXCLUDES   Arthroscopic treatment (29882)
  🔧 18.5   ✂ 18.5   **FUD** 090   [J] [A2] [80] [50] [🔲]
  AMA: 2019,May,10; 2018,Sep,7

27405   Repair, primary, torn ligament and/or capsule, knee; collateral
  🔧 19.5   ✂ 19.5   **FUD** 090   [J] [A2] [80] [50] [🔲]
  AMA: 2018,Sep,7; 2018,Jan,8; 2017,Jan,8; 2016,Jan,13

27407   cruciate
  EXCLUDES   Reconstruction (27427)
  🔧 22.9   ✂ 22.9   **FUD** 090   [J] [A2] [80] [50] [🔲]
  AMA: 2018,Sep,7

27409   collateral and cruciate ligaments
  EXCLUDES   Reconstruction (27427-27429)
  🔧 27.9   ✂ 27.9   **FUD** 090   [J] [A2] [80] [50] [🔲]
  AMA: 2018,Sep,7

27412   Autologous chondrocyte implantation, knee
  EXCLUDES   Arthrotomy, knee (27331)
        Autologous fat graft obtained by liposuction (15771-15774)
        Manipulation knee joint under general anesthesia (27570)
        Obtaining chondrocytes (29870)
        Other autologous soft tissue grafts (fat, dermis, fascia) harvested by direct excision ([15769])
  🔧 47.8   ✂ 47.8   **FUD** 090   [J] [62] [80] [50] [🔲]
  AMA: 2018,Sep,7

27415   Osteochondral allograft, knee, open
  EXCLUDES   Arthroscopic procedure (29867)
        Osteochondral autograft knee (27416)
  🔧 39.6   ✂ 39.6   **FUD** 090   [J] [J8] [80] [50] [🔲]
  AMA: 2019,Apr,10; 2018,Sep,7; 2018,Jan,8; 2017,Jan,8; 2016,Jan,13

27416   Osteochondral autograft(s), knee, open (eg, mosaicplasty) (includes harvesting of autograft[s])
  EXCLUDES   Procedures in same compartment (29874, 29877, 29879, 29885-29887)
        Procedures performed at same surgical session (27415, 29870-29871, 29875, 29884)
        Surgical arthroscopy knee with osteochondral autograft(s) (29866)
  🔧 28.3   ✂ 28.3   **FUD** 090   [J] [62] [80] [50] [🔲]
  AMA: 2018,Sep,7; 2018,Jan,8; 2017,Jan,8; 2016,Jan,13

27418   Anterior tibial tubercleplasty (eg, Maquet type procedure)
  🔧 23.8   ✂ 23.8   **FUD** 090   [J] [A2] [80] [50] [🔲]
  AMA: 2018,Sep,7; 2018,Jan,8; 2017,Jan,8; 2016,Jan,13

27420   Reconstruction of dislocating patella; (eg, Hauser type procedure)
  🔧 21.4   ✂ 21.4   **FUD** 090   [J] [A2] [80] [50] [🔲]
  AMA: 2018,Sep,7; 2018,Jan,8; 2017,Jan,8; 2016,Jan,13

Patellar tendon insertion point is resected and shifted

27422   with extensor realignment and/or muscle advancement or release (eg, Campbell, Goldwaite type procedure)
  🔧 21.4   ✂ 21.4   **FUD** 090   [J] [A2] [80] [50] [🔲]
  AMA: 2018,Sep,7; 2018,Jan,8; 2017,Jan,8; 2016,Jan,13

27424   with patellectomy
  🔧 21.5   ✂ 21.5   **FUD** 090   [J] [A2] [80] [50] [🔲]
  AMA: 2018,Sep,7

27425   Lateral retinacular release, open
  EXCLUDES   Arthroscopic release (29873)
  🔧 12.9   ✂ 12.9   **FUD** 090   [J] [A2] [50] [🔲]
  AMA: 2018,Sep,7; 2018,Jan,8; 2017,Jan,8; 2016,Jan,13

27427   Ligamentous reconstruction (augmentation), knee; extra-articular
  EXCLUDES   Primary repair ligament(s) (27405, 27407, 27409)
  🔧 20.5   ✂ 20.5   **FUD** 090   [J] [J8] [80] [50] [🔲]
  AMA: 2018,Sep,7; 2018,Jan,8; 2017,Jan,8; 2016,Jan,13

[26]/[TC] PC/TC Only   [A2]-[Z3] ASC Payment   [50] Bilateral   ♂ Male Only   ♀ Female Only   🔧 Facility RVU   ✂ Non-Facility RVU   [🔲] CCI   [✖] CLIA
FUD Follow-up Days   **CMS:** IOM   **AMA:** CPT Asst   [A]-[Y] OPPSI   [80]/[80] Surg Assist Allowed / w/Doc   [🔲] Lab Crosswalk   [🔲] Radiology Crosswalk

86   CPT © 2021 American Medical Association. All Rights Reserved.   © 2021 Optum360, LLC

27428   intra-articular (open)
EXCLUDES Primary repair ligament(s) (27405, 27407, 27409)
32.2   32.2   **FUD** 090   J A2 80 50
AMA: 2018,Sep,7; 2018,Jan,8; 2017,Jan,8; 2016,Jan,13

27429   intra-articular (open) and extra-articular
EXCLUDES Primary repair ligament(s) (27405, 27407, 27409)
36.2   36.2   **FUD** 090   J J8 80 50
AMA: 2018,Sep,7; 2018,Jan,8; 2017,Jan,8; 2016,Jan,13

27430   Quadricepsplasty (eg, Bennett or Thompson type)
21.2   21.2   **FUD** 090   J A2 80 50
AMA: 2018,Sep,7

27435   Capsulotomy, posterior capsular release, knee
23.2   23.2   **FUD** 090   J A2 80 50
AMA: 2018,Sep,7

27437   Arthroplasty, patella; without prosthesis
19.0   19.0   **FUD** 090   J A2 50
AMA: 2018,Sep,7

27438   with prosthesis
24.3   24.3   **FUD** 090   J J8 80 50
AMA: 2018,Sep,7

27440   Arthroplasty, knee, tibial plateau;
23.0   23.0   **FUD** 090   J J8 80 50
AMA: 2018,Sep,7

27441   with debridement and partial synovectomy
23.8   23.8   **FUD** 090   J 62 80 50
AMA: 2018,Sep,7

27442   Arthroplasty, femoral condyles or tibial plateau(s), knee;
25.2   25.2   **FUD** 090   J J8 80 50
AMA: 2018,Sep,7; 2018,Jan,8; 2017,Jan,8; 2016,Jun,8

27443   with debridement and partial synovectomy
23.4   23.4   **FUD** 090   J J8 80 50
AMA: 2018,Sep,7

27445   Arthroplasty, knee, hinge prosthesis (eg, Walldius type)
EXCLUDES Removal knee prosthesis (27488)
Revision knee arthroplasty (27487)
36.1   36.1   **FUD** 090   C 80 50
AMA: 2018,Sep,7

27446   Arthroplasty, knee, condyle and plateau; medial OR lateral compartment
EXCLUDES Removal knee prosthesis (27488)
Revision knee arthroplasty (27487)
33.4   33.4   **FUD** 090   J J8 80 50
AMA: 2018,Sep,7; 2018,Jan,8; 2017,Dec,13

27447   medial AND lateral compartments with or without patella resurfacing (total knee arthroplasty)
EXCLUDES Removal knee prosthesis (27488)
Revision knee arthroplasty (27487)
39.1   39.1   **FUD** 090   J J8 80 50
AMA: 2018,Sep,7; 2018,Jan,8; 2017,Jan,8; 2016,Jan,13

27448   Osteotomy, femur, shaft or supracondylar; without fixation
23.7   23.7   **FUD** 090   C 80 50
AMA: 2019,May,7; 2018,Sep,7

27450   with fixation
29.3   29.3   **FUD** 090   C 80 50
AMA: 2018,Sep,7

27454   Osteotomy, multiple, with realignment on intramedullary rod, femoral shaft (eg, Sofield type procedure)
37.4   37.4   **FUD** 090   C 80 50
AMA: 2018,Sep,7

27455   Osteotomy, proximal tibia, including fibular excision or osteotomy (includes correction of genu varus [bowleg] or genu valgus [knock-knee]); before epiphyseal closure
27.5   27.5   **FUD** 090   C 80 50
AMA: 2018,Sep,7

27457   after epiphyseal closure
27.8   27.8   **FUD** 090   C 80 50
AMA: 2018,Sep,7

27465   Osteoplasty, femur; shortening (excluding 64876)
36.1   36.1   **FUD** 090   C 80 50
AMA: 2018,Sep,7

27466   lengthening
34.0   34.0   **FUD** 090   C 80 50
AMA: 2018,Sep,7

27468   combined, lengthening and shortening with femoral segment transfer
38.8   38.8   **FUD** 090   C 80 50
AMA: 2018,Sep,7

27470   Repair, nonunion or malunion, femur, distal to head and neck; without graft (eg, compression technique)
33.9   33.9   **FUD** 090   C 80 50
AMA: 2018,Sep,7

27472   with iliac or other autogenous bone graft (includes obtaining graft)
36.4   36.4   **FUD** 090   C 80 50
AMA: 2018,Sep,7

27475   Arrest, epiphyseal, any method (eg, epiphysiodesis); distal femur
19.1   19.1   **FUD** 090   J 62 50
AMA: 2018,Sep,7

27477   tibia and fibula, proximal
21.1   21.1   **FUD** 090   J J8 50
AMA: 2018,Sep,7

27479   combined distal femur, proximal tibia and fibula
26.5   26.5   **FUD** 090   J 62 80 50
AMA: 2018,Sep,7

27485   Arrest, hemiepiphyseal, distal femur or proximal tibia or fibula (eg, genu varus or valgus)
19.3   19.3   **FUD** 090   J 62 50
AMA: 2018,Sep,7

27486   Revision of total knee arthroplasty, with or without allograft; 1 component
40.5   40.5   **FUD** 090   C 80 50
AMA: 2018,Sep,7; 2018,Apr,10; 2018,Jan,8; 2017,Jan,8; 2016,Jan,13

27487   femoral and entire tibial component
50.7   50.7   **FUD** 090   C 80 50
AMA: 2018,Sep,7; 2018,Jan,8; 2017,Jan,8; 2016,Jan,13

27488   Removal of prosthesis, including total knee prosthesis, methylmethacrylate with or without insertion of spacer, knee
34.6   34.6   **FUD** 090   C 80 50
AMA: 2018,Sep,7; 2018,Jan,8; 2017,Jan,8; 2016,Jan,13

27495   Prophylactic treatment (nailing, pinning, plating, or wiring) with or without methylmethacrylate, femur
32.5   32.5   **FUD** 090   C 80 50
AMA: 2018,Sep,7

27496   Decompression fasciotomy, thigh and/or knee, 1 compartment (flexor or extensor or adductor);
15.7   15.7   **FUD** 090   J A2 50
AMA: 2018,Sep,7

27497   with debridement of nonviable muscle and/or nerve
16.7   16.7   **FUD** 090   J A2 80 50
AMA: 2018,Sep,7

27498   Decompression fasciotomy, thigh and/or knee, multiple compartments;
18.8   18.8   **FUD** 090   J A2 80 50
AMA: 2018,Sep,7

27499   with debridement of nonviable muscle and/or nerve
20.2   20.2   **FUD** 090   J A2 80 50
AMA: 2018,Sep,7

● New Code   ▲ Revised Code   ○ Reinstated   ● New Web Release   ▲ Revised Web Release   + Add-on   Unlisted   Not Covered   # Resequenced
50 Optum Mod 50 Exempt   AMA Mod 51 Exempt   51 Optum Mod 51 Exempt   63 Mod 63 Exempt   Non-FDA Drug   ★ Telemedicine   M Maternity   A Age Edit

27500-27566 Treatment of Fracture/Dislocation of Femur/Knee

INCLUDES Closed, percutaneous, and open treatment fractures and dislocations

27500 Closed treatment of femoral shaft fracture, without manipulation
🦴 13.8 ⚕ 15.0 **FUD** 090 T A2 50 ▭
AMA: 2018,Sep,7

27501 Closed treatment of supracondylar or transcondylar femoral fracture with or without intercondylar extension, without manipulation
🦴 14.3 ⚕ 14.5 **FUD** 090 T A2 80 50 ▭
AMA: 2018,Sep,7

27502 Closed treatment of femoral shaft fracture, with manipulation, with or without skin or skeletal traction
🦴 21.9 ⚕ 21.9 **FUD** 090 J A2 50 ▭
AMA: 2018,Sep,7; 2018,Jan,8; 2017,Jan,8; 2016,Jan,13

27503 Closed treatment of supracondylar or transcondylar femoral fracture with or without intercondylar extension, with manipulation, with or without skin or skeletal traction
🦴 23.1 ⚕ 23.1 **FUD** 090 J A2 80 50 ▭
AMA: 2018,Sep,7

27506 Open treatment of femoral shaft fracture, with or without external fixation, with insertion of intramedullary implant, with or without cerclage and/or locking screws
🦴 38.6 ⚕ 38.6 **FUD** 090 C 80 50 ▭
AMA: 2018,Sep,7; 2018,Jan,8; 2017,Jan,8; 2016,Jan,13

27507 Open treatment of femoral shaft fracture with plate/screws, with or without cerclage
🦴 28.0 ⚕ 28.0 **FUD** 090 C 80 50 ▭
AMA: 2018,Sep,7

27508 Closed treatment of femoral fracture, distal end, medial or lateral condyle, without manipulation
🦴 14.3 ⚕ 15.0 **FUD** 090 T A2 50 ▭
AMA: 2018,Sep,7

27509 Percutaneous skeletal fixation of femoral fracture, distal end, medial or lateral condyle, or supracondylar or transcondylar, with or without intercondylar extension, or distal femoral epiphyseal separation
🦴 18.6 ⚕ 18.6 **FUD** 090 J J8 80 50 ▭
AMA: 2018,Dec,10; 2018,Dec,10; 2018,Sep,7

Pins are placed percutaneously

27510 Closed treatment of femoral fracture, distal end, medial or lateral condyle, with manipulation
🦴 19.6 ⚕ 19.6 **FUD** 090 J A2 50 ▭
AMA: 2018,Sep,7

27511 Open treatment of femoral supracondylar or transcondylar fracture without intercondylar extension, includes internal fixation, when performed
🦴 28.8 ⚕ 28.8 **FUD** 090 C 80 50 ▭
AMA: 2018,Sep,7

27513 Open treatment of femoral supracondylar or transcondylar fracture with intercondylar extension, includes internal fixation, when performed
🦴 35.9 ⚕ 35.9 **FUD** 090 C 80 50 ▭
AMA: 2018,Sep,7

27514 Open treatment of femoral fracture, distal end, medial or lateral condyle, includes internal fixation, when performed
🦴 27.9 ⚕ 27.9 **FUD** 090 C 80 50 ▭
AMA: 2018,Sep,7

27516 Closed treatment of distal femoral epiphyseal separation; without manipulation
🦴 13.8 ⚕ 14.7 **FUD** 090 T A2 50 ▭
AMA: 2018,Sep,7

27517 with manipulation, with or without skin or skeletal traction
🦴 19.6 ⚕ 19.6 **FUD** 090 J A2 80 50 ▭
AMA: 2018,Sep,7

27519 Open treatment of distal femoral epiphyseal separation, includes internal fixation, when performed
🦴 25.8 ⚕ 25.8 **FUD** 090 C 80 50 ▭
AMA: 2018,Sep,7

27520 Closed treatment of patellar fracture, without manipulation
🦴 8.46 ⚕ 9.21 **FUD** 090 T A2 50 ▭
AMA: 2018,Sep,7

27524 Open treatment of patellar fracture, with internal fixation and/or partial or complete patellectomy and soft tissue repair
🦴 21.6 ⚕ 21.6 **FUD** 090 J 62 80 50 ▭
AMA: 2018,Sep,7

27530 Closed treatment of tibial fracture, proximal (plateau); without manipulation
EXCLUDES Arthroscopic repair (29855-29856)
🦴 8.05 ⚕ 8.63 **FUD** 090 T A2 50 ▭
AMA: 2018,Sep,7

27532 with or without manipulation, with skeletal traction
EXCLUDES Arthroscopic repair (29855-29856)
🦴 16.5 ⚕ 17.7 **FUD** 090 J A2 50 ▭
AMA: 2018,Sep,7

27535 Open treatment of tibial fracture, proximal (plateau); unicondylar, includes internal fixation, when performed
EXCLUDES Arthroscopic repair (29855-29856)
🦴 25.9 ⚕ 25.9 **FUD** 090 C 80 50 ▭
AMA: 2018,Sep,7

27536 bicondylar, with or without internal fixation
EXCLUDES Arthroscopic repair (29855-29856)
🦴 34.2 ⚕ 34.2 **FUD** 090 C 80 50 ▭
AMA: 2018,Sep,7

27538 Closed treatment of intercondylar spine(s) and/or tuberosity fracture(s) of knee, with or without manipulation
EXCLUDES Arthroscopic repair (29850-29851)
🦴 12.7 ⚕ 13.6 **FUD** 090 T A2 80 50 ▭
AMA: 2018,Sep,7

27540 Open treatment of intercondylar spine(s) and/or tuberosity fracture(s) of the knee, includes internal fixation, when performed
🦴 23.4 ⚕ 23.4 **FUD** 090 C 80 50 ▭
AMA: 2018,Sep,7

26/TC PC/TC Only **A2-Z3** ASC Payment **50** Bilateral ♂ Male Only ♀ Female Only 🦴 Facility RVU ⚕ Non-Facility RVU ▭ CCI ✖ CLIA
FUD Follow-up Days **CMS:** IOM **AMA:** CPT Asst **A-Y** OPPSI **80/80** Surg Assist Allowed / w/Doc Lab Crosswalk Radiology Crosswalk

88 CPT © 2021 American Medical Association. All Rights Reserved. © 2021 Optum360, LLC

27550 Closed treatment of knee dislocation; without anesthesia
13.8   14.9   **FUD** 090   T A2 80 50
AMA: 2018,Sep,7

27552 requiring anesthesia
18.1   18.1   **FUD** 090   J A2 80 50
AMA: 2018,Sep,7

27556 Open treatment of knee dislocation, includes internal fixation, when performed; without primary ligamentous repair or augmentation/reconstruction
25.3   25.3   **FUD** 090   C 80 50
AMA: 2018,Sep,7

27557 with primary ligamentous repair
30.2   30.2   **FUD** 090   C 80 50
AMA: 2018,Sep,7

27558 with primary ligamentous repair, with augmentation/reconstruction
34.5   34.5   **FUD** 090   C 80 50
AMA: 2018,Sep,7

27560 Closed treatment of patellar dislocation; without anesthesia
EXCLUDES Recurrent dislocation (27420-27424)
9.66   10.5   **FUD** 090   T A2 50
AMA: 2018,Sep,7

27562 requiring anesthesia
EXCLUDES Recurrent dislocation (27420-27424)
13.9   13.9   **FUD** 090   T A2 80 50
AMA: 2018,Sep,7

27566 Open treatment of patellar dislocation, with or without partial or total patellectomy
EXCLUDES Recurrent dislocation (27420-27424)
25.8   25.8   **FUD** 090   J A2 80 50
AMA: 2018,Sep,7

27570 Knee Manipulation with Anesthesia

27570 Manipulation of knee joint under general anesthesia (includes application of traction or other fixation devices)
4.34   4.34   **FUD** 010   J A2 50
AMA: 2018,Sep,7; 2018,Jan,8; 2017,Jan,8; 2016,Jan,13

27580 Knee Arthrodesis

27580 Arthrodesis, knee, any technique
42.1   42.1   **FUD** 090   C 80 50
AMA: 2020,May,13; 2018,Sep,7

27590-27599 Amputations and Unlisted Procedures at Femur or Knee

27590 Amputation, thigh, through femur, any level;
23.0   23.0   **FUD** 090   C 80 50
AMA: 2018,Sep,7; 2018,Jan,8; 2017,Dec,13

27591 immediate fitting technique including first cast
27.9   27.9   **FUD** 090   C 80 50
AMA: 2018,Sep,7

27592 open, circular (guillotine)
19.5   19.5   **FUD** 090   C 80 50
AMA: 2018,Sep,7

27594 secondary closure or scar revision
14.6   14.6   **FUD** 090   J A2 50
AMA: 2018,Sep,7

27596 re-amputation
20.6   20.6   **FUD** 090   C 50
AMA: 2018,Sep,7

27598 Disarticulation at knee
INCLUDES Batch-Spittler-McFaddin operation
Callander knee disarticulation
Gritti amputation
20.6   20.6   **FUD** 090   C 80 50
AMA: 2018,Sep,7

27599 Unlisted procedure, femur or knee
0.00   0.00   **FUD** YYY   T 80 50
AMA: 2019,Apr,10; 2018,Dec,10; 2018,Dec,10; 2018,Sep,7; 2018,Apr,10; 2018,Jan,8; 2017,Aug,9; 2017,Mar,10; 2017,Jan,8; 2016,Nov,9; 2016,Jun,8; 2016,Jan,13

27600-27602 Decompression Fasciotomy of Leg
EXCLUDES Fasciotomy with debridement (27892-27894)
Simple incision and drainage (10140-10160)

27600 Decompression fasciotomy, leg; anterior and/or lateral compartments only
11.7   11.7   **FUD** 090   J A2 50
AMA: 2018,Sep,7

27601 posterior compartment(s) only
12.8   12.8   **FUD** 090   J A2 50
AMA: 2018,Sep,7

27602 anterior and/or lateral, and posterior compartment(s)
13.9   13.9   **FUD** 090   J A2 80 50
AMA: 2018,Sep,7

27603-27612 Incisional Procedures Lower Leg and Ankle

27603 Incision and drainage, leg or ankle; deep abscess or hematoma
11.2   15.3   **FUD** 090   J A2 50
AMA: 2018,Sep,7

27604 infected bursa
9.61   13.6   **FUD** 090   J A2 80 50
AMA: 2018,Sep,7

27605 Tenotomy, percutaneous, Achilles tendon (separate procedure); local anesthesia
5.34   9.83   **FUD** 010   J A2 80 50
AMA: 2018,Sep,14; 2018,Sep,7

27606 general anesthesia
7.99   7.99   **FUD** 010   J A2 50
AMA: 2018,Sep,7; 2018,Sep,14

27607 Incision (eg, osteomyelitis or bone abscess), leg or ankle
17.5   17.5   **FUD** 090   J A2 50
AMA: 2018,Sep,7

27610 Arthrotomy, ankle, including exploration, drainage, or removal of foreign body
18.7   18.7   **FUD** 090   J A2 50
AMA: 2018,Sep,7

27612 Arthrotomy, posterior capsular release, ankle, with or without Achilles tendon lengthening
EXCLUDES Lengthening or shortening tendon (27685)
16.0   16.0   **FUD** 090   J A2 80 50
AMA: 2018,Sep,7

27613-27614 Biopsy Lower Leg and Ankle
EXCLUDES Needle biopsy (20206)

27613 Biopsy, soft tissue of leg or ankle area; superficial
4.60   7.22   **FUD** 010   J P3 50
AMA: 2018,Sep,7

27614 deep (subfascial or intramuscular)
11.7   16.6   **FUD** 090   J A2 50
AMA: 2018,Sep,7

27615-27634 [27632, 27634] Excision Soft Tissue Tumors Lower Leg/Ankle

INCLUDES   Any necessary elevation tissue planes or dissection
Measurement tumor and necessary margin at greatest diameter prior to excision
Resection without removal significant normal tissue
Simple and intermediate repairs
Excision types:
  Fascial or subfascial soft tissue tumors: simple and marginal resection most often benign and intramuscular tumors found either in or below deep fascia, not involving bone
  Resection tumor (may include entire bone) and wide margins normal tissue primarily for malignant or aggressive benign tumors
  Subcutaneous: simple and marginal resection most often benign tumors found in subcutaneous tissue above deep fascia

EXCLUDES   Complex repair
Excision benign cutaneous lesions (eg, sebaceous cyst) (11400-11406)
Radical resection cutaneous tumors (eg, melanoma) (11600-11606)
Significant vessel exploration or neuroplasty

27615   **Radical resection of tumor (eg, sarcoma), soft tissue of leg or ankle area; less than 5 cm**
  🔨 29.6   ⚖ 29.6   **FUD** 090   J G2 80 50 ▣
  AMA: 2018,Sep,7

27616   **5 cm or greater**
  🔨 36.6   ⚖ 36.6   **FUD** 090   J G2 80 50 ▣
  AMA: 2018,Sep,7

27618   **Excision, tumor, soft tissue of leg or ankle area, subcutaneous; less than 3 cm**
  🔨 8.83   ⚖ 13.2   **FUD** 090   J G2 50 ▣
  AMA: 2018,Sep,7; 2018,Jan,8; 2017,Jan,8; 2016,Jan,13

\# **27632**   **3 cm or greater**
  🔨 11.9   ⚖ 11.9   **FUD** 090   J G2 80 50 ▣
  AMA: 2018,Sep,7

27619   **Excision, tumor, soft tissue of leg or ankle area, subfascial (eg, intramuscular); less than 5 cm**
  🔨 13.3   ⚖ 13.3   **FUD** 090   J G2 50 ▣
  AMA: 2018,Sep,7

\# **27634**   **5 cm or greater**
  🔨 19.7   ⚖ 19.7   **FUD** 090   J G2 80 50 ▣
  AMA: 2018,Sep,7

27620-27641 [27632, 27634] Bone and Joint Procedures Ankle/Leg

27620   **Arthrotomy, ankle, with joint exploration, with or without biopsy, with or without removal of loose or foreign body**
  🔨 12.9   ⚖ 12.9   **FUD** 090   J A2 80 50 ▣
  AMA: 2018,Sep,7

27625   **Arthrotomy, with synovectomy, ankle;**
  🔨 16.4   ⚖ 16.4   **FUD** 090   J A2 80 50 ▣
  AMA: 2018,Sep,7

27626   **including tenosynovectomy**
  🔨 17.4   ⚖ 17.4   **FUD** 090   J A2 80 50 ▣
  AMA: 2018,Sep,7

27630   **Excision of lesion of tendon sheath or capsule (eg, cyst or ganglion), leg and/or ankle**
  🔨 10.4   ⚖ 15.9   **FUD** 090   J A2 50 ▣
  AMA: 2018,Sep,7

27632   Resequenced code. See code following 27618.

27634   Resequenced code. See code following 27619.

27635   **Excision or curettage of bone cyst or benign tumor, tibia or fibula;**
  🔨 16.7   ⚖ 16.7   **FUD** 090   J A2 50 ▣
  AMA: 2018,Sep,7; 2018,Jan,8; 2017,Jan,8; 2016,Jan,13

27637   **with autograft (includes obtaining graft)**
  🔨 21.5   ⚖ 21.5   **FUD** 090   J A2 80 50 ▣
  AMA: 2018,Sep,7

27638   **with allograft**
  🔨 22.0   ⚖ 22.0   **FUD** 090   J A2 80 50 ▣
  AMA: 2019,May,7; 2018,Sep,7

27640   **Partial excision (craterization, saucerization, or diaphysectomy), bone (eg, osteomyelitis); tibia**
  EXCLUDES   Excision exostosis (27635)
  🔨 23.9   ⚖ 23.9   **FUD** 090   J A2 50 ▣
  AMA: 2018,Sep,7; 2018,Jan,8; 2017,Jan,8; 2016,Jan,13

27641   **fibula**
  EXCLUDES   Excision exostosis (27635)
  🔨 19.0   ⚖ 19.0   **FUD** 090   J A2 50 ▣
  AMA: 2018,Sep,7

27645-27647 Radical Resection Bone Tumor Ankle/Leg

INCLUDES   Any necessary elevation tissue planes or dissection
Excision adjacent soft tissue during bone tumor resection (27615-27619 [27632, 27634])
Measurement tumor and necessary margin at greatest diameter prior to excision
Resection tumor (may include entire bone) and wide margins normal tissue primarily for malignant or aggressive benign tumors
Simple and intermediate repairs

EXCLUDES   Complex repair
Significant vessel exploration, neuroplasty, reconstruction, or complex bone repair

27645   **Radical resection of tumor; tibia**
  🔨 51.2   ⚖ 51.2   **FUD** 090   C 80 50 ▣
  AMA: 2019,May,7; 2018,Sep,7

27646   **fibula**
  🔨 44.6   ⚖ 44.6   **FUD** 090   C 80 50 ▣
  AMA: 2019,May,7; 2018,Sep,7

27647   **talus or calcaneus**
  🔨 29.3   ⚖ 29.3   **FUD** 090   J A2 80 50 ▣
  AMA: 2019,May,7; 2018,Sep,7

27648 Injection for Ankle Arthrogram

EXCLUDES   Arthroscopy (29894-29898)

27648   **Injection procedure for ankle arthrography**
  📷 (73615)
  🔨 1.52   ⚖ 5.22   **FUD** 000   N N1 80 50 ▣
  AMA: 2019,May,7; 2018,Sep,7; 2018,Jan,8; 2017,Jan,8; 2016,Jan,13

27650-27745 Repair/Reconstruction Lower Leg/Ankle

27650   **Repair, primary, open or percutaneous, ruptured Achilles tendon;**
  🔨 18.9   ⚖ 18.9   **FUD** 090   J A2 80 50 ▣
  AMA: 2020,Jun,14; 2018,Sep,7; 2018,Jan,8; 2017,Jan,8; 2016,Jan,13

27652   **with graft (includes obtaining graft)**
  🔨 19.1   ⚖ 19.1   **FUD** 090   J J8 50 ▣
  AMA: 2018,Sep,7; 2018,Jan,8; 2017,Jan,8; 2016,Jan,13

27654   **Repair, secondary, Achilles tendon, with or without graft**
  🔨 20.4   ⚖ 20.4   **FUD** 090   J A2 80 50 ▣
  AMA: 2020,Jun,14; 2020,Apr,8; 2018,Sep,7; 2018,Jan,8; 2017,Jan,8; 2016,Dec,16; 2016,Jan,13

27656   **Repair, fascial defect of leg**
  🔨 11.4   ⚖ 18.2   **FUD** 090   J A2 80 50 ▣
  AMA: 2018,Sep,7

27658   **Repair, flexor tendon, leg; primary, without graft, each tendon**
  🔨 10.6   ⚖ 10.6   **FUD** 090   J A2 80 ▣
  AMA: 2018,Sep,7

27659   **secondary, with or without graft, each tendon**
  🔨 13.5   ⚖ 13.5   **FUD** 090   J A2 80 ▣
  AMA: 2018,Sep,7; 2018,Jan,8; 2017,Jan,8; 2016,Jan,13

27664   **Repair, extensor tendon, leg; primary, without graft, each tendon**
  🔨 10.3   ⚖ 10.3   **FUD** 090   J A2 80 ▣
  AMA: 2018,Sep,7; 2018,Jan,8; 2017,Jan,8; 2016,Jan,13

27665   secondary, with or without graft, each tendon
🔧 11.9   ⚕ 11.9   **FUD** 090   J A2 80 ▣
AMA: 2018,Sep,7

27675   Repair, dislocating peroneal tendons; without fibular osteotomy
🔧 14.1   ⚕ 14.1   **FUD** 090   J A2 80 50 ▣
AMA: 2018,Sep,7

27676   with fibular osteotomy
🔧 17.2   ⚕ 17.2   **FUD** 090   J A2 80 50 ▣
AMA: 2018,Sep,7

27680   Tenolysis, flexor or extensor tendon, leg and/or ankle; single, each tendon
🔧 12.2   ⚕ 12.2   **FUD** 090   J A2
AMA: 2018,Sep,7; 2018,Jan,8; 2017,Jan,8; 2016,Jan,13

27681   multiple tendons (through separate incision[s])
🔧 15.7   ⚕ 15.7   **FUD** 090   J A2 50 ▣
AMA: 2018,Sep,7

27685   Lengthening or shortening of tendon, leg or ankle; single tendon (separate procedure)
🔧 13.3   ⚕ 19.0   **FUD** 090   J A2 80 50 ▣
AMA: 2018,Sep,7; 2018,Sep,14; 2018,Jan,8; 2017,Jan,8; 2016,Jan,13

27686   multiple tendons (through same incision), each
🔧 15.6   ⚕ 15.6   **FUD** 090   J A2 50 ▣
AMA: 2018,Sep,7; 2018,Jan,8; 2017,Jan,8; 2016,Jan,13

27687   Gastrocnemius recession (eg, Strayer procedure)
🔧 13.0   ⚕ 13.0   **FUD** 090   J A2 80 50 ▣
AMA: 2018,Sep,7

27690   Transfer or transplant of single tendon (with muscle redirection or rerouting); superficial (eg, anterior tibial extensors into midfoot)
INCLUDES Toe extensors considered single tendon with transplant into midfoot
🔧 18.4   ⚕ 18.4   **FUD** 090   J A2 80 50 ▣
AMA: 2018,Sep,7

27691   deep (eg, anterior tibial or posterior tibial through interosseous space, flexor digitorum longus, flexor hallucis longus, or peroneal tendon to midfoot or hindfoot)
INCLUDES Barr procedure
Toe extensors considered single tendon with transplant into midfoot
🔧 21.4   ⚕ 21.4   **FUD** 090   J A2 80 50 ▣
AMA: 2018,Sep,7

+ **27692**   each additional tendon (List separately in addition to code for primary procedure)
INCLUDES Toe extensors considered single tendon with transplant into midfoot
Code first (27690-27691)
🔧 3.01   ⚕ 3.01   **FUD** ZZZ   N N1 80 ▣
AMA: 2018,Sep,7

27695   Repair, primary, disrupted ligament, ankle; collateral
🔧 13.6   ⚕ 13.6   **FUD** 090   J A2 50 ▣
AMA: 2018,Nov,11; 2018,Sep,7; 2018,Jan,8; 2017,Jan,8; 2016,Jan,13

Lateral view of right ankle showing components of the collateral ligament

Fibula — Tibia — Posterior talofibular — Anterior talofibular — Calcaneus — Calcaneofibular

27696   both collateral ligaments
🔧 16.0   ⚕ 16.0   **FUD** 090   J A2 50 ▣
AMA: 2018,Nov,11; 2018,Sep,7; 2018,Jan,8; 2017,Jan,8; 2016,Jan,13

27698   Repair, secondary, disrupted ligament, ankle, collateral (eg, Watson-Jones procedure)
🔧 18.3   ⚕ 18.3   **FUD** 090   J A2 80 50 ▣
AMA: 2018,Sep,7; 2018,Jan,8; 2017,Jan,8; 2016,Jan,13

27700   Arthroplasty, ankle;
🔧 17.6   ⚕ 17.6   **FUD** 090   J J8 80 50 ▣
AMA: 2018,Sep,7

27702   with implant (total ankle)
🔧 27.7   ⚕ 27.7   **FUD** 090   C 80 50 ▣
AMA: 2018,Sep,7

27703   revision, total ankle
🔧 32.2   ⚕ 32.2   **FUD** 090   C 80 50 ▣
AMA: 2018,Sep,7

27704   Removal of ankle implant
🔧 16.5   ⚕ 16.5   **FUD** 090   02 A2 50 ▣
AMA: 2019,May,7; 2018,Sep,7

27705   Osteotomy; tibia
EXCLUDES Genu varus or genu valgus repair (27455-27457)
🔧 21.8   ⚕ 21.8   **FUD** 090   J J8 80 50 ▣
AMA: 2018,Sep,7

27707   fibula
EXCLUDES Genu varus or genu valgus repair (27455-27457)
🔧 11.4   ⚕ 11.4   **FUD** 090   J A2 50 ▣
AMA: 2018,Sep,7

27709   tibia and fibula
EXCLUDES Genu varus or genu valgus repair (27455-27457)
🔧 33.6   ⚕ 33.6   **FUD** 090   J J8 80 50 ▣
AMA: 2018,Sep,7

27712   multiple, with realignment on intramedullary rod (eg, Sofield type procedure)
EXCLUDES Genu varus or genu valgus repair (27455-27457)
🔧 31.8   ⚕ 31.8   **FUD** 090   C 80 50 ▣
AMA: 2018,Sep,7

27715   Osteoplasty, tibia and fibula, lengthening or shortening
INCLUDES Anderson tibial lengthening
🔧 30.9   ⚕ 30.9   **FUD** 090   C 80 50 ▣
AMA: 2018,Sep,7

27720 Repair of nonunion or malunion, tibia; without graft, (eg, compression technique)
🔹 25.1 ⚕ 25.1 **FUD** 090   J J8 80 50 ▣
AMA: 2018,Sep,7

27722 with sliding graft
🔹 25.7 ⚕ 25.7 **FUD** 090   J J8 80 50 ▣
AMA: 2018,Sep,7

27724 with iliac or other autograft (includes obtaining graft)
🔹 36.4 ⚕ 36.4 **FUD** 090   C 80 50 ▣
AMA: 2018,Sep,7; 2018,Jan,8; 2017,Jan,8; 2016,Jan,13

27725 by synostosis, with fibula, any method
🔹 35.1 ⚕ 35.1 **FUD** 090   C 80 50 ▣
AMA: 2018,Sep,7

27726 Repair of fibula nonunion and/or malunion with internal fixation
INCLUDES Osteotomy; fibula (27707)
🔹 27.6 ⚕ 27.6 **FUD** 090   J J8 50 ▣
AMA: 2018,Sep,7; 2018,Jan,8; 2017,Jan,8; 2016,Jan,13

27727 Repair of congenital pseudarthrosis, tibia
🔹 29.9 ⚕ 29.9 **FUD** 090   C 80 50 ▣
AMA: 2018,Sep,7

27730 Arrest, epiphyseal (epiphysiodesis), open; distal tibia
🔹 16.9 ⚕ 16.9 **FUD** 090   J A2 50 ▣
AMA: 2018,Sep,7

27732 distal fibula
🔹 12.9 ⚕ 12.9 **FUD** 090   J A2 50 ▣
AMA: 2018,Sep,7

27734 distal tibia and fibula
🔹 18.9 ⚕ 18.9 **FUD** 090   J A2 50 ▣
AMA: 2018,Sep,7

27740 Arrest, epiphyseal (epiphysiodesis), any method, combined, proximal and distal tibia and fibula;
EXCLUDES Epiphyseal arrest proximal tibia and fibula (27477)
🔹 20.4 ⚕ 20.4 **FUD** 090   J G2 80 50 ▣
AMA: 2018,Sep,7

27742 and distal femur
EXCLUDES Epiphyseal arrest proximal tibia and fibula (27477)
🔹 22.4 ⚕ 22.4 **FUD** 090   J A2 80 50 ▣
AMA: 2018,Sep,7

27745 Prophylactic treatment (nailing, pinning, plating or wiring) with or without methylmethacrylate, tibia
🔹 21.7 ⚕ 21.7 **FUD** 090   J J8 80 50 ▣
AMA: 2018,Sep,7

27750-27848 Treatment of Fracture/Dislocation Lower Leg/Ankle

INCLUDES Treatment open or closed fracture or dislocation

27750 Closed treatment of tibial shaft fracture (with or without fibular fracture); without manipulation
🔹 9.18 ⚕ 9.91 **FUD** 090   T A2 50 ▣
AMA: 2018,Sep,7; 2018,Jan,8; 2017,Jan,8; 2016,Jan,13

27752 with manipulation, with or without skeletal traction
🔹 14.1 ⚕ 15.4 **FUD** 090   J A2 50 ▣
AMA: 2018,Sep,7; 2018,Jan,8; 2018,Jan,3; 2017,Jan,8; 2016,Jan,13

27756 Percutaneous skeletal fixation of tibial shaft fracture (with or without fibular fracture) (eg, pins or screws)
🔹 16.6 ⚕ 16.6 **FUD** 090   J A2 80 50 ▣
AMA: 2018,Sep,7; 2018,Jan,8; 2017,Jan,8; 2016,Jan,13

27758 Open treatment of tibial shaft fracture (with or without fibular fracture), with plate/screws, with or without cerclage
🔹 25.8 ⚕ 25.8 **FUD** 090   J J8 80 50 ▣
AMA: 2018,Sep,7; 2018,Jan,8; 2017,Jan,8; 2016,Jan,13

27759 Treatment of tibial shaft fracture (with or without fibular fracture) by intramedullary implant, with or without interlocking screws and/or cerclage
🔹 28.8 ⚕ 28.8 **FUD** 090   J J8 80 50 ▣
AMA: 2018,Sep,7; 2018,Jan,8; 2017,Jan,8; 2016,Jan,13

27760 Closed treatment of medial malleolus fracture; without manipulation
🔹 8.81 ⚕ 9.56 **FUD** 090   T A2 50 ▣
AMA: 2018,Sep,7

27762 with manipulation, with or without skin or skeletal traction
🔹 12.4 ⚕ 13.7 **FUD** 090   J A2 50 ▣
AMA: 2018,Sep,7

27766 Open treatment of medial malleolus fracture, includes internal fixation, when performed
🔹 17.4 ⚕ 17.4 **FUD** 090   J A2 50 ▣
AMA: 2018,Sep,7

27767 Closed treatment of posterior malleolus fracture; without manipulation
EXCLUDES Treatment bimalleolar ankle fracture (27808-27814)
Treatment trimalleolar ankle fracture (27816-27823)
🔹 8.20 ⚕ 8.24 **FUD** 090   T P2 50 ▣
AMA: 2018,Sep,7

27768 with manipulation
EXCLUDES Treatment bimalleolar ankle fracture (27808-27814)
Treatment trimalleolar ankle fracture (27816-27823)
🔹 12.7 ⚕ 12.7 **FUD** 090   J G2 50 ▣
AMA: 2018,Sep,7

27769 Open treatment of posterior malleolus fracture, includes internal fixation, when performed
EXCLUDES Treatment bimalleolar ankle fracture (27808-27814)
Treatment trimalleolar ankle fracture (27816-27823)
🔹 21.0 ⚕ 21.0 **FUD** 090   J G2 50 ▣
AMA: 2018,Sep,7

27780 Closed treatment of proximal fibula or shaft fracture; without manipulation
🔹 8.08 ⚕ 8.80 **FUD** 090   T A2 50 ▣
AMA: 2018,Sep,7; 2018,Jan,8; 2017,Jan,8; 2016,Jan,13

27781 with manipulation
🔹 11.3 ⚕ 12.3 **FUD** 090   J A2 50 ▣
AMA: 2018,Sep,7

27784 Open treatment of proximal fibula or shaft fracture, includes internal fixation, when performed
🔹 20.5 ⚕ 20.5 **FUD** 090   J A2 50 ▣
AMA: 2018,Sep,7; 2018,Jan,8; 2017,Jan,8; 2016,Jan,13

27786 Closed treatment of distal fibular fracture (lateral malleolus); without manipulation
🔹 8.25 ⚕ 9.01 **FUD** 090   T A2 50 ▣
AMA: 2018,Sep,7

27788 with manipulation
🔹 11.1 ⚕ 12.2 **FUD** 090   T A2 50 ▣
AMA: 2018,Sep,7

27792 Open treatment of distal fibular fracture (lateral malleolus), includes internal fixation, when performed
EXCLUDES Repair tibia and fibula shaft fracture (27750-27759)
🔹 18.6 ⚕ 18.6 **FUD** 090   J J8 50 ▣
AMA: 2018,Sep,7; 2018,Jan,8; 2017,Jan,8; 2016,Jan,13

27808 Closed treatment of bimalleolar ankle fracture (eg, lateral and medial malleoli, or lateral and posterior malleoli or medial and posterior malleoli); without manipulation
🔹 8.70 ⚕ 9.57 **FUD** 090   T A2 50 ▣
AMA: 2018,Sep,7

27810 with manipulation
🔹 12.1 ⚕ 13.3 **FUD** 090   J A2 50 ▣
AMA: 2018,Sep,7

27814   Open treatment of bimalleolar ankle fracture (eg, lateral and medial malleoli, or lateral and posterior malleoli, or medial and posterior malleoli), includes internal fixation, when performed
🔧 22.1   ⚕ 22.1   **FUD** 090   J J8 80 50 ▣
AMA: 2018,Sep,7; 2018,Jan,8; 2017,Jan,8; 2016,Feb,13

27816   Closed treatment of trimalleolar ankle fracture; without manipulation
🔧 8.28   ⚕ 9.27   **FUD** 090   T A2 50 ▣
AMA: 2018,Sep,7

27818   with manipulation
🔧 12.4   ⚕ 13.9   **FUD** 090   J A2 50 ▣
AMA: 2018,Sep,7

27822   Open treatment of trimalleolar ankle fracture, includes internal fixation, when performed, medial and/or lateral malleolus; without fixation of posterior lip
🔧 24.9   ⚕ 24.9   **FUD** 090   J J8 80 50 ▣
AMA: 2018,Sep,7

27823   with fixation of posterior lip
🔧 28.0   ⚕ 28.0   **FUD** 090   J J8 80 50 ▣
AMA: 2018,Sep,7

27824   Closed treatment of fracture of weight bearing articular portion of distal tibia (eg, pilon or tibial plafond), with or without anesthesia; without manipulation
🔧 8.71   ⚕ 9.02   **FUD** 090   T A2 50 ▣
AMA: 2018,Sep,7

27825   with skeletal traction and/or requiring manipulation
🔧 14.2   ⚕ 15.7   **FUD** 090   J A2 80 50 ▣
AMA: 2018,Sep,7

27826   Open treatment of fracture of weight bearing articular surface/portion of distal tibia (eg, pilon or tibial plafond), with internal fixation, when performed; of fibula only
🔧 24.2   ⚕ 24.2   **FUD** 090   J J8 80 50 ▣
AMA: 2018,Sep,7

27827   of tibia only
🔧 32.0   ⚕ 32.0   **FUD** 090   J J8 80 50 ▣
AMA: 2018,Sep,7

27828   of both tibia and fibula
🔧 38.1   ⚕ 38.1   **FUD** 090   J J8 80 50 ▣
AMA: 2018,Sep,7; 2018,Jan,8; 2017,Jan,8; 2016,Jan,13

27829   Open treatment of distal tibiofibular joint (syndesmosis) disruption, includes internal fixation, when performed
🔧 20.0   ⚕ 20.0   **FUD** 090   J J8 80 50 ▣
AMA: 2018,Sep,7; 2018,Jan,8; 2017,Jan,8; 2016,Feb,13; 2016,Jan,13

27830   Closed treatment of proximal tibiofibular joint dislocation; without anesthesia
🔧 10.2   ⚕ 11.1   **FUD** 090   T A2 80 50 ▣
AMA: 2018,Sep,7

27831   requiring anesthesia
🔧 11.6   ⚕ 11.6   **FUD** 090   J A2 80 50 ▣
AMA: 2018,Sep,7

27832   Open treatment of proximal tibiofibular joint dislocation, includes internal fixation, when performed, or with excision of proximal fibula
🔧 21.8   ⚕ 21.8   **FUD** 090   J J8 80 50 ▣
AMA: 2018,Sep,7

27840   Closed treatment of ankle dislocation; without anesthesia
🔧 10.7   ⚕ 10.7   **FUD** 090   T A2 50 ▣
AMA: 2018,Sep,7

27842   requiring anesthesia, with or without percutaneous skeletal fixation
🔧 14.2   ⚕ 14.2   **FUD** 090   J A2 50 ▣
AMA: 2018,Sep,7

27846   Open treatment of ankle dislocation, with or without percutaneous skeletal fixation; without repair or internal fixation
EXCLUDES   Arthroscopy (29894-29898)
🔧 20.6   ⚕ 20.6   **FUD** 090   J A2 80 50 ▣
AMA: 2018,Sep,7

27848   with repair or internal or external fixation
EXCLUDES   Arthroscopy (29894-29898)
🔧 23.0   ⚕ 23.0   **FUD** 090   J J8 80 50 ▣
AMA: 2018,Sep,7

27860 Ankle Manipulation with Anesthesia

27860   Manipulation of ankle under general anesthesia (includes application of traction or other fixation apparatus)
🔧 4.91   ⚕ 4.91   **FUD** 010   J A2 80 50 ▣
AMA: 2018,Sep,7

27870-27871 Arthrodesis Lower Leg/Ankle

27870   Arthrodesis, ankle, open
EXCLUDES   Arthroscopic arthrodesis ankle (29899)
🔧 29.5   ⚕ 29.5   **FUD** 090   J J8 80 50 ▣
AMA: 2020,May,13; 2018,Sep,7

27871   Arthrodesis, tibiofibular joint, proximal or distal
🔧 19.8   ⚕ 19.8   **FUD** 090   J J8 80 50 ▣
AMA: 2020,May,13; 2018,Sep,7

27880-27889 Amputations of Lower Leg/Ankle

27880   Amputation, leg, through tibia and fibula;
INCLUDES   Burgess amputation
🔧 26.3   ⚕ 26.3   **FUD** 090   C 80 50 ▣
AMA: 2018,Sep,7

27881   with immediate fitting technique including application of first cast
🔧 24.8   ⚕ 24.8   **FUD** 090   C 80 50 ▣
AMA: 2018,Sep,7

27882   open, circular (guillotine)
🔧 17.2   ⚕ 17.2   **FUD** 090   C 80 50 ▣
AMA: 2018,Sep,7

27884   secondary closure or scar revision
🔧 16.5   ⚕ 16.5   **FUD** 090   J A2 50 ▣
AMA: 2018,Sep,7

27886   re-amputation
🔧 18.9   ⚕ 18.9   **FUD** 090   C 50 ▣
AMA: 2018,Sep,7

27888   Amputation, ankle, through malleoli of tibia and fibula (eg, Syme, Pirogoff type procedures), with plastic closure and resection of nerves
🔧 18.9   ⚕ 18.9   **FUD** 090   C 80 50 ▣
AMA: 2018,Sep,7

27889   Ankle disarticulation
🔧 18.6   ⚕ 18.6   **FUD** 090   J A2 50 ▣
AMA: 2018,Sep,7

27892-27899 Decompression Fasciotomy Lower Leg
EXCLUDES   Decompression fasciotomy without debridement (27600-27602)

27892   Decompression fasciotomy, leg; anterior and/or lateral compartments only, with debridement of nonviable muscle and/or nerve
🔧 15.8   ⚕ 15.8   **FUD** 090   J A2 80 50 ▣
AMA: 2018,Sep,7

27893   posterior compartment(s) only, with debridement of nonviable muscle and/or nerve
🔧 17.5   ⚕ 17.5   **FUD** 090   J A2 80 50 ▣
AMA: 2018,Sep,7

27894   anterior and/or lateral, and posterior compartment(s), with debridement of nonviable muscle and/or nerve
🔧 24.3   ⚕ 24.3   **FUD** 090   J A2 80 50 ▣
AMA: 2018,Sep,7

27899 Unlisted procedure, leg or ankle
🚗 0.00 ⚗ 0.00 **FUD** YYY ⬚ T 80 50 ▢

AMA: 2020,Apr,8; 2018,Sep,7; 2018,Jan,8; 2017,Jan,8; 2016,Dec,16; 2016,Jan,13

28001-28008 Surgical Incision Foot/Toe
EXCLUDES Simple incision and drainage (10060-10160)

28001 Incision and drainage, bursa, foot
🚗 4.90 ⚗ 8.03 **FUD** 010 ⬚ J P3 ▢

AMA: 2018,Sep,7

28002 Incision and drainage below fascia, with or without tendon sheath involvement, foot; single bursal space
🚗 9.20 ⚗ 12.7 **FUD** 010 ⬚ J A2 ▢

AMA: 2018,Sep,7

28003 multiple areas
🚗 16.0 ⚗ 20.1 **FUD** 090 ⬚ J A2 ▢

AMA: 2018,Sep,7

28005 Incision, bone cortex (eg, osteomyelitis or bone abscess), foot
🚗 16.6 ⚗ 16.6 **FUD** 090 ⬚ J A2 ▢

AMA: 2018,Sep,7

28008 Fasciotomy, foot and/or toe
EXCLUDES Plantar fascia division (28250)
  Plantar fasciectomy (28060, 28062)
🚗 8.46 ⚗ 12.5 **FUD** 090 ⬚ J A2 50 ▢

AMA: 2018,Sep,7

28010-28011 Tenotomy/Toe
EXCLUDES Open tenotomy (28230-28234)
  Simple incision and drainage (10140-10160)

28010 Tenotomy, percutaneous, toe; single tendon
🚗 5.99 ⚗ 6.69 **FUD** 090 ⬚ J P3 ▢

AMA: 2018,Sep,7

28011 multiple tendons
🚗 8.10 ⚗ 9.09 **FUD** 090 ⬚ J A2 ▢

AMA: 2018,Sep,7

28020-28024 Arthrotomy Foot/Toe
EXCLUDES Simple incision and drainage (10140-10160)

28020 Arthrotomy, including exploration, drainage, or removal of loose or foreign body; intertarsal or tarsometatarsal joint
🚗 10.4 ⚗ 15.5 **FUD** 090 ⬚ J A2 ▢

AMA: 2018,Sep,7

28022 metatarsophalangeal joint
🚗 9.36 ⚗ 14.0 **FUD** 090 ⬚ J A2 ▢

AMA: 2018,Sep,7

28024 interphalangeal joint
🚗 8.67 ⚗ 13.1 **FUD** 090 ⬚ J A2 ▢

AMA: 2018,Sep,7

28035 Tarsal Tunnel Release
EXCLUDES Other nerve decompression (64722)
  Other neuroplasty (64704)

28035 Release, tarsal tunnel (posterior tibial nerve decompression)
🚗 10.2 ⚗ 15.2 **FUD** 090 ⬚ J A2 50 ▢

AMA: 2018,Sep,7

28039-28047 [28039, 28041] Excision Soft Tissue Tumors Foot/Toe
INCLUDES Any necessary elevation tissue planes or dissection
  Measurement tumor and necessary margin at greatest diameter prior to excision
  Simple and intermediate repairs
  Excision types:
    Fascial or subfascial soft tissue tumors: simple and marginal resection tumors found either in or below deep fascia, not involving bone or excision substantial amount normal tissue; primarily benign and intramuscular tumors
    Tumors fingers and toes involving joint capsules, tendons and tendon sheaths
    Radical resection soft tissue tumor: wide resection tumor, involving substantial margins normal tissue and may involve tissue removal from one or more layers; most often malignant or aggressive benign
    Tumors fingers and toes adjacent to joints, tendons and tendon sheaths
    Subcutaneous: simple and marginal resection tumors in subcutaneous tissue above deep fascia; most often benign
EXCLUDES Complex repair
  Excision benign cutaneous lesions (eg, sebaceous cyst) (11420-11426)
  Radical resection cutaneous tumors (eg, melanoma) (11620-11626)
  Significant vessel exploration, neuroplasty, or reconstruction

28039 Resequenced code. See code following 28043.

28041 Resequenced code. See code following 28045.

28043 Excision, tumor, soft tissue of foot or toe, subcutaneous; less than 1.5 cm
🚗 7.52 ⚗ 11.3 **FUD** 090 ⬚ J 62 50 ▢

AMA: 2018,Sep,7

28039 1.5 cm or greater
🚗 9.94 ⚗ 14.3 **FUD** 090 ⬚ J 62 80 50 ▢

AMA: 2018,Sep,7

28045 Excision, tumor, soft tissue of foot or toe, subfascial (eg, intramuscular); less than 1.5 cm
🚗 9.97 ⚗ 14.0 **FUD** 090 ⬚ J 62 80 50 ▢

AMA: 2018,Sep,7

28041 1.5 cm or greater
🚗 13.0 ⚗ 13.0 **FUD** 090 ⬚ J 62 80 50 ▢

AMA: 2018,Sep,7

28046 Radical resection of tumor (eg, sarcoma), soft tissue of foot or toe; less than 3 cm
🚗 20.6 ⚗ 20.6 **FUD** 090 ⬚ J 62 50 ▢

AMA: 2018,Sep,7

28047 3 cm or greater
🚗 30.1 ⚗ 30.1 **FUD** 090 ⬚ J 62 80 50 ▢

AMA: 2018,Sep,7

28050-28160 Resection Procedures Foot/Toes

28050 Arthrotomy with biopsy; intertarsal or tarsometatarsal joint
🚗 8.03 ⚗ 12.1 **FUD** 090 ⬚ J A2 50 ▢

AMA: 2002,Apr,13; 1998,Nov,1

28052 metatarsophalangeal joint
🚗 8.15 ⚗ 12.8 **FUD** 090 ⬚ J A2 50 ▢

AMA: 2002,Apr,13

28054 interphalangeal joint
🚗 6.77 ⚗ 10.8 **FUD** 090 ⬚ J A2 80 50 ▢

AMA: 2002,Apr,13

28055 Neurectomy, intrinsic musculature of foot
🚗 11.0 ⚗ 11.0 **FUD** 090 ⬚ J A2 80 50 ▢

28060 Fasciectomy, plantar fascia; partial (separate procedure)
EXCLUDES Plantar fasciotomy (28008, 28250)
🚗 10.3 ⚗ 15.0 **FUD** 090 ⬚ J A2 50 ▢

AMA: 2018,Jan,8; 2017,Jan,8; 2016,Jan,13

28062 radical (separate procedure)
EXCLUDES Plantar fasciotomy (28008, 28250)
🚗 11.7 ⚗ 16.7 **FUD** 090 ⬚ J A2 50 ▢

AMA: 2002,Apr,13

26/TC PC/TC Only   A2-Z3 ASC Payment   50 Bilateral   ♂ Male Only   ♀ Female Only   🚗 Facility RVU   ⚗ Non-Facility RVU   CCI   CLIA
FUD Follow-up Days   CMS: IOM   AMA: CPT Asst   A-Y OPPSI   80/80 Surg Assist Allowed / w/Doc   Lab Crosswalk   Radiology Crosswalk

94   CPT © 2021 American Medical Association. All Rights Reserved.   © 2021 Optum360, LLC

28070   Synovectomy; intertarsal or tarsometatarsal joint, each
🖥 10.1   ⚕ 15.2   **FUD** 090   J A2 🖼
AMA: 2002,Apr,13

28072   metatarsophalangeal joint, each
🖥 9.26   ⚕ 14.1   **FUD** 090   J A2 🖼
AMA: 2002,Apr,13

28080   Excision, interdigital (Morton) neuroma, single, each
🖥 10.6   ⚕ 15.1   **FUD** 090   J A2 80 🖼
AMA: 2018,Jan,8; 2017,Jan,8; 2016,Jan,13

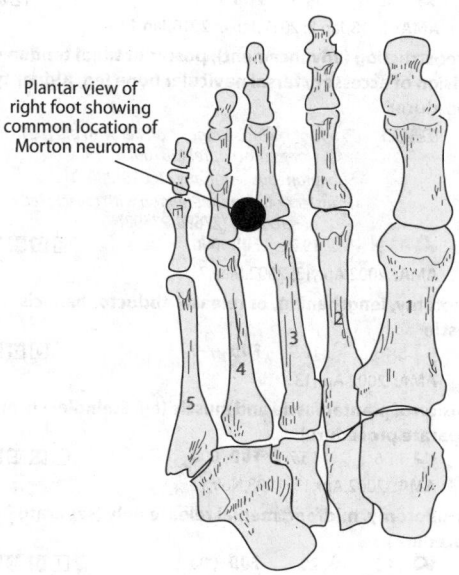

Plantar view of right foot showing common location of Morton neuroma

Morton neuroma is a chronic inflammation or irritation of the nerves in the web space between the heads of the metatarsals and phalanges

28086   Synovectomy, tendon sheath, foot; flexor
🖥 10.2   ⚕ 15.4   **FUD** 090   J A2 80 50 🖼
AMA: 2002,Apr,13

28088   extensor
🖥 7.92   ⚕ 12.5   **FUD** 090   J A2 80 50 🖼
AMA: 2002,Apr,13

28090   Excision of lesion, tendon, tendon sheath, or capsule (including synovectomy) (eg, cyst or ganglion); foot
🖥 8.86   ⚕ 13.5   **FUD** 090   J A2 50 🖼
AMA: 2002,Apr,13; 1998,Nov,1

28092   toe(s), each
🖥 7.75   ⚕ 12.2   **FUD** 090   J A2 🖼
AMA: 2002,Apr,13; 1998,Nov,1

28100   Excision or curettage of bone cyst or benign tumor, talus or calcaneus;
🖥 11.9   ⚕ 17.6   **FUD** 090   J A2 80 50 🖼
AMA: 2002,Apr,13

28102   with iliac or other autograft (includes obtaining graft)
🖥 17.5   ⚕ 17.5   **FUD** 090   J A2 80 50 🖼
AMA: 2002,Apr,13

28103   with allograft
🖥 11.2   ⚕ 11.2   **FUD** 090   J J8 80 50 🖼
AMA: 2019,May,7

28104   Excision or curettage of bone cyst or benign tumor, tarsal or metatarsal, except talus or calcaneus;
🖥 10.2   ⚕ 15.2   **FUD** 090   J A2 80 🖼
AMA: 2002,May,7; 2002,Apr,13

28106   with iliac or other autograft (includes obtaining graft)
🖥 12.3   ⚕ 12.3   **FUD** 090   J A2 80 🖼
AMA: 2002,May,7; 2002,Apr,13

28107   with allograft
🖥 10.0   ⚕ 14.8   **FUD** 090   J J8 80 🖼
AMA: 2019,May,7

28108   Excision or curettage of bone cyst or benign tumor, phalanges of foot
EXCLUDES   Partial excision bone, toe (28124)
🖥 8.30   ⚕ 12.7   **FUD** 090   J A2 🖼
AMA: 2002,Apr,13

28110   Ostectomy, partial excision, fifth metatarsal head (bunionette) (separate procedure)
🖥 8.35   ⚕ 13.3   **FUD** 090   J A2 50 🖼
AMA: 2018,Jan,8; 2017,Jan,8; 2016,Jan,13

28111   Ostectomy, complete excision; first metatarsal head
🖥 9.33   ⚕ 14.0   **FUD** 090   J A2 50 🖼
AMA: 2002,Apr,13

28112   other metatarsal head (second, third or fourth)
🖥 9.00   ⚕ 14.0   **FUD** 090   J A2 50 🖼
AMA: 2002,Apr,13

28113   fifth metatarsal head
🖥 12.1   ⚕ 16.9   **FUD** 090   J A2 80 50 🖼
AMA: 2002,Apr,13

28114   all metatarsal heads, with partial proximal phalangectomy, excluding first metatarsal (eg, Clayton type procedure)
🖥 23.9   ⚕ 30.7   **FUD** 090   J A2 80 50 🖼
AMA: 2002,Apr,13; 1998,Nov,1

28116   Ostectomy, excision of tarsal coalition
🖥 16.6   ⚕ 22.0   **FUD** 090   J A2 50 🖼
AMA: 2002,Apr,13

28118   Ostectomy, calcaneus;
🖥 11.9   ⚕ 17.2   **FUD** 090   J A2 80 50 🖼
AMA: 2018,Jan,8; 2017,Jan,8; 2016,Jan,13

28119   for spur, with or without plantar fascial release
🖥 10.3   ⚕ 15.1   **FUD** 090   J A2 50 🖼
AMA: 2018,Jan,8; 2017,Jan,8; 2016,Jan,13

28120   Partial excision (craterization, saucerization, sequestrectomy, or diaphysectomy) bone (eg, osteomyelitis or bossing); talus or calcaneus
INCLUDES   Barker operation
🖥 14.3   ⚕ 19.5   **FUD** 090   J A2 50 🖼
AMA: 2020,Oct,14; 2018,Jan,8; 2017,Jan,8; 2016,Jan,13

28122   tarsal or metatarsal bone, except talus or calcaneus
EXCLUDES   Hallux rigidus cheilectomy (28289)
            Partial removal talus or calcaneus (28120)
🖥 12.6   ⚕ 17.2   **FUD** 090   J A2 80 50 🖼
AMA: 2020,Aug,14

28124   phalanx of toe
🖥 9.54   ⚕ 13.8   **FUD** 090   J P3 50 🖼
AMA: 2002,Apr,13

28126   Resection, partial or complete, phalangeal base, each toe
🖥 7.11   ⚕ 11.3   **FUD** 090   J A2 🖼
AMA: 2018,Jan,8; 2017,Jan,8; 2016,Jan,13

28130   Talectomy (astragalectomy)
INCLUDES   Whitman astragalectomy
EXCLUDES   Calcanectomy (28118)
🖥 18.2   ⚕ 18.2   **FUD** 090   J A2 80 50 🖼
AMA: 2002,Apr,13

28140   Metatarsectomy
🖥 12.5   ⚕ 16.9   **FUD** 090   J A2 🖼
AMA: 2002,Apr,13

28150   Phalangectomy, toe, each toe
🖥 8.04   ⚕ 12.2   **FUD** 090   J A2 🖼
AMA: 2002,Apr,13; 1998,Nov,1

28153   Resection, condyle(s), distal end of phalanx, each toe
🖥 7.63   ⚕ 11.9   **FUD** 090   J A2 🖼
AMA: 2018,Jan,8; 2017,Jan,8; 2016,Jan,13

Musculoskeletal System

28160 — 28264

28160 **Hemiphalangectomy or interphalangeal joint excision, toe, proximal end of phalanx, each**
🔧 7.69   ✂ 11.9   **FUD** 090   J A2 ▢
AMA: 2002,Apr,13; 1998,Nov,1

28171-28175 Radical Resection Bone Tumor Foot/Toes

INCLUDES   Any necessary elevation tissue planes or dissection
Excision adjacent soft tissue during bone tumor resection (28039-28047 [28039, 28041])
Measurement tumor and necessary margin at greatest diameter prior to excision
Resection tumor (may include entire bone) and wide margins normal tissue primarily for malignant or aggressive benign tumors
Simple and intermediate repairs

EXCLUDES   Complex repair
Radical tumor resection calcaneus or talus (27647)
Significant vessel exploration, neuroplasty, reconstruction, or complex bone repair

28171 **Radical resection of tumor; tarsal (except talus or calcaneus)**
🔧 32.2   ✂ 32.2   **FUD** 090   J A2 80 ▢
AMA: 2002,Apr,13; 1994,Win,1

28173 **metatarsal**
🔧 21.3   ✂ 21.3   **FUD** 090   J A2 ▢
AMA: 2002,Apr,13; 1994,Win,1

28175 **phalanx of toe**
🔧 13.6   ✂ 13.6   **FUD** 090   J A2 ▢
AMA: 2002,Apr,13

28190-28193 Foreign Body Removal: Foot

28190 **Removal of foreign body, foot; subcutaneous**
🔧 3.85   ✂ 7.35   **FUD** 010   T P3 50 ▢
AMA: 2018,Jan,8; 2017,Jan,8; 2016,Jan,13

28192 **deep**
🔧 9.01   ✂ 13.5   **FUD** 090   J A2 50 ▢
AMA: 2018,Jan,8; 2017,Jan,8; 2016,Jan,13

28193 **complicated**
🔧 10.6   ✂ 15.2   **FUD** 090   J A2 50 ▢
AMA: 2002,Apr,13

28200-28360 [28295] Repair/Reconstruction of Foot/Toe

INCLUDES   Closed, open, and percutaneous treatment fractures and dislocations

28200 **Repair, tendon, flexor, foot; primary or secondary, without free graft, each tendon**
🔧 9.33   ✂ 14.2   **FUD** 090   J A2 ▢
AMA: 2018,Jan,8; 2017,Jan,8; 2016,Feb,15; 2016,Jan,13

28202 **secondary with free graft, each tendon (includes obtaining graft)**
🔧 12.4   ✂ 17.4   **FUD** 090   J A2 80 ▢
AMA: 2002,Apr,13

28208 **Repair, tendon, extensor, foot; primary or secondary, each tendon**
🔧 9.11   ✂ 13.9   **FUD** 090   J A2 ▢
AMA: 2002,Apr,13; 1998,Nov,1

28210 **secondary with free graft, each tendon (includes obtaining graft)**
🔧 12.0   ✂ 16.9   **FUD** 090   J A2 80 ▢
AMA: 2002,Apr,13

28220 **Tenolysis, flexor, foot; single tendon**
🔧 8.72   ✂ 13.0   **FUD** 090   J P3 50 ▢
AMA: 2002,Apr,13; 1998,Nov,1

28222 **multiple tendons**
🔧 10.2   ✂ 14.9   **FUD** 090   J A2 50 ▢
AMA: 2002,Apr,13; 1998,Nov,1

28225 **Tenolysis, extensor, foot; single tendon**
🔧 7.59   ✂ 12.0   **FUD** 090   J A2 50 ▢
AMA: 2002,Apr,13; 1998,Nov,1

28226 **multiple tendons**
🔧 11.3   ✂ 17.6   **FUD** 090   J A2 50 ▢
AMA: 2002,Apr,13; 1998,Nov,1

28230 **Tenotomy, open, tendon flexor; foot, single or multiple tendon(s) (separate procedure)**
🔧 8.16   ✂ 12.5   **FUD** 090   J P3 50 ▢
AMA: 2002,Apr,13; 1998,Nov,1

28232 **toe, single tendon (separate procedure)**
🔧 6.95   ✂ 11.1   **FUD** 090   J P3 ▢
AMA: 2020,Apr,10; 2018,Jan,8; 2017,Jan,8; 2016,Jan,13

28234 **Tenotomy, open, extensor, foot or toe, each tendon**
EXCLUDES   Tendon transfer (27690-27691)
🔧 7.59   ✂ 11.8   **FUD** 090   J A2 ▢
AMA: 2018,Jan,8; 2017,Jan,8; 2016,Jan,13

28238 **Reconstruction (advancement), posterior tibial tendon with excision of accessory tarsal navicular bone (eg, Kidner type procedure)**
EXCLUDES   Extensor hallucis longus transfer with big toe fusion (Jones procedure) (28760)
Subcutaneous tenotomy (28010-28011)
Transfer or transplant tendon with muscle redirection or rerouting (27690-27692)
🔧 13.9   ✂ 19.2   **FUD** 090   J A2 80 50 ▢
AMA: 2002,Apr,13; 2002,May,7

28240 **Tenotomy, lengthening, or release, abductor hallucis muscle**
🔧 8.46   ✂ 12.9   **FUD** 090   J A2 50 ▢
AMA: 2002,Apr,13

28250 **Division of plantar fascia and muscle (eg, Steindler stripping) (separate procedure)**
🔧 11.6   ✂ 16.7   **FUD** 090   J A2 80 50 ▢
AMA: 2002,Apr,13; 1998,Nov,1

28260 **Capsulotomy, midfoot; medial release only (separate procedure)**
🔧 14.9   ✂ 20.2   **FUD** 090   J A2 80 50 ▢
AMA: 2002,Apr,13

28261 **with tendon lengthening**
🔧 27.0   ✂ 34.6   **FUD** 090   J A2 80 50 ▢
AMA: 2002,Apr,13

28262 **extensive, including posterior talotibial capsulotomy and tendon(s) lengthening (eg, resistant clubfoot deformity)**
🔧 32.5   ✂ 40.4   **FUD** 090   J A2 80 50 ▢
AMA: 2002,Apr,13; 1998,Nov,1

28264 **Capsulotomy, midtarsal (eg, Heyman type procedure)**
🔧 22.2   ✂ 29.1   **FUD** 090   J A2 80 50 ▢
AMA: 2002,Apr,13; 1998,Nov,1

28270   **Capsulotomy; metatarsophalangeal joint, with or without tenorrhaphy, each joint (separate procedure)**
📷 9.64   ⚕ 14.2   **FUD** 090   `J` `A2` `50` ▢
AMA: 2018,Jan,8; 2017,Jan,8; 2016,Jan,13

Tarsals
Cuneiform bones
Metatarsophalangeal joint
Medial   Lateral
Navicular   Intermediate
Phalanges
Proximal   Distal
Astragalus (talus)
Calcaneus
Cuboid
Metatarsals
Medial
Tarsometatarsal joint
Interphalangeal joints

Tenorrhaphy

28272   **interphalangeal joint, each joint (separate procedure)**
📷 7.25   ⚕ 11.2   **FUD** 090   `J` `P3` `50` ▢
AMA: 2018,Jan,8; 2017,Jan,8; 2016,Jan,13

28280   **Syndactylization, toes (eg, webbing or Kelikian type procedure)**
📷 10.0   ⚕ 14.8   **FUD** 090   `J` `A2` `80` `50` ▢
AMA: 2002,Apr,13; 1998,Nov,1

28285   **Correction, hammertoe (eg, interphalangeal fusion, partial or total phalangectomy)**
📷 10.9   ⚕ 15.5   **FUD** 090   `J` `A2` `50` ▢
AMA: 2018,Jan,8; 2017,Jan,8; 2016,Jun,8; 2016,Jan,13

28286   **Correction, cock-up fifth toe, with plastic skin closure (eg, Ruiz-Mora type procedure)**
📷 8.56   ⚕ 12.8   **FUD** 090   `J` `A2` `50` ▢
AMA: 2002,Apr,13; 1998,Nov,1

28288   **Ostectomy, partial, exostectomy or condylectomy, metatarsal head, each metatarsal head**
📷 12.4   ⚕ 17.5   **FUD** 090   `J` `A2` ▢
AMA: 2002,Apr,13; 1998,Nov,1

28289   **Hallux rigidus correction with cheilectomy, debridement and capsular release of the first metatarsophalangeal joint; without implant**
📷 13.2   ⚕ 20.5   **FUD** 090   `J` `A2` `80` `50` ▢
AMA: 2020,Aug,14; 2020,Jul,13; 2018,Jan,8; 2017,Jan,8; 2016,Dec,3; 2016,Jan,13

28291   **with implant**
📷 14.1   ⚕ 21.0   **FUD** 090   `J` `J8` `80` `50` ▢
AMA: 2020,Aug,14; 2018,Jan,8; 2017,Nov,10; 2017,Jan,8; 2016,Dec,3

28292   **Correction, hallux valgus (bunionectomy), with sesamoidectomy, when performed; with resection of proximal phalanx base, when performed, any method**
📷 13.9   ⚕ 21.3   **FUD** 090   `J` `A2` `80` `50` ▢
AMA: 2018,Jan,8; 2017,Jan,8; 2016,Dec,3; 2016,Jan,13

28295   *Resequenced code. See code following 28296.*

28296   **with distal metatarsal osteotomy, any method**
📷 14.8   ⚕ 26.1   **FUD** 090   `J` `A2` `80` `50` ▢
AMA: 2020,Jul,13; 2018,Sep,14; 2018,Jan,8; 2017,Jan,8; 2016,Dec,3; 2016,Jan,13

\#   **28295**   **with proximal metatarsal osteotomy, any method**
📷 16.1   ⚕ 28.5   **FUD** 090   `J` `62` `80` `50` ▢
AMA: 2018,Jan,8; 2017,Jan,8; 2016,Dec,3

28297   **with first metatarsal and medial cuneiform joint arthrodesis, any method**
📷 17.4   ⚕ 30.2   **FUD** 090   `J` `J8` `80` `50` ▢
AMA: 2018,Jan,8; 2017,Jan,8; 2016,Dec,3; 2016,Jan,13

28298   **with proximal phalanx osteotomy, any method**
INCLUDES   Akin procedure
📷 14.3   ⚕ 24.3   **FUD** 090   `J` `J8` `80` `50` ▢
AMA: 2018,Jan,8; 2017,Jan,8; 2016,Dec,3; 2016,Jan,13

28299   **with double osteotomy, any method**
📷 16.8   ⚕ 29.1   **FUD** 090   `J` `A2` `80` `50` ▢
AMA: 2018,Jan,8; 2017,Jan,8; 2016,Dec,3; 2016,Apr,8; 2016,Jan,13

Hallux valgus bunion
Medial eminence of metatarsal bone
Kirschner wires stabilize the osteotomies
A portion of the metatarsal head is resected
A wedge of the proximal phalanx is resected

28300   **Osteotomy; calcaneus (eg, Dwyer or Chambers type procedure), with or without internal fixation**
📷 18.7   ⚕ 18.7   **FUD** 090   `J` `J8` `80` `50` ▢
AMA: 2002,Apr,13; 1998,Nov,1

28302   **talus**
📷 20.6   ⚕ 20.6   **FUD** 090   `J` `A2` `80` `50` ▢
AMA: 2002,Apr,13

28304   **Osteotomy, tarsal bones, other than calcaneus or talus;**
📷 17.3   ⚕ 23.6   **FUD** 090   `J` `A2` `80` `50` ▢
AMA: 2002,Apr,13; 1998,Nov,1

28305   **with autograft (includes obtaining graft) (eg, Fowler type)**
📷 19.3   ⚕ 19.3   **FUD** 090   `J` `J8` `80` `50` ▢
AMA: 2002,Apr,13; 1998,Nov,1

28306   **Osteotomy, with or without lengthening, shortening or angular correction, metatarsal; first metatarsal**
📷 11.6   ⚕ 17.6   **FUD** 090   `J` `A2` `80` `50` ▢
AMA: 2018,Jan,8; 2017,Jan,8; 2016,Jan,13

28307   **first metatarsal with autograft (other than first toe)**
📷 11.9   ⚕ 17.9   **FUD** 090   `J` `A2` `80` `50` ▢
AMA: 2002,Apr,13; 1998,Nov,1

28308   **other than first metatarsal, each**
📷 10.9   ⚕ 16.4   **FUD** 090   `J` `A2` `80` `50` ▢
AMA: 2002,Apr,13; 1998,Nov,1

28309   **multiple (eg, Swanson type cavus foot procedure)**
📷 25.5   ⚕ 25.5   **FUD** 090   `J` `J8` `80` `50` ▢
AMA: 2018,Jan,8; 2017,Jan,8; 2016,Jan,13

28310   **Osteotomy, shortening, angular or rotational correction; proximal phalanx, first toe (separate procedure)**
📷 10.3   ⚕ 15.7   **FUD** 090   `J` `A2` `50` ▢
AMA: 2018,Jan,8; 2017,Jan,8; 2016,Jan,13

28312   **other phalanges, any toe**
📷 9.12   ⚕ 14.4   **FUD** 090   `J` `A2` ▢
AMA: 2002,Apr,13

28313 Reconstruction, angular deformity of toe, soft tissue procedures only (eg, overlapping second toe, fifth toe, curly toes)
🔧 10.2   ✂ 15.1   **FUD** 090   J A2 ▭
AMA: 2002,Apr,13; 1998,Nov,1

28315 Sesamoidectomy, first toe (separate procedure)
🔧 9.37   ✂ 13.9   **FUD** 090   J A2 50 ▭
AMA: 2002,Apr,13

28320 Repair, nonunion or malunion; tarsal bones
🔧 17.5   ✂ 17.5   **FUD** 090   J J8 80 50 ▭
AMA: 2002,Apr,13; 1998,Nov,1

28322 metatarsal, with or without bone graft (includes obtaining graft)
🔧 16.5   ✂ 22.5   **FUD** 090   J J8 80 ▭
AMA: 2002,Apr,13

28340 Reconstruction, toe, macrodactyly; soft tissue resection
🔧 11.8   ✂ 16.5   **FUD** 090   J A2 ▭
AMA: 2002,Apr,13

28341 requiring bone resection
🔧 14.1   ✂ 19.3   **FUD** 090   J A2 ▭
AMA: 2002,Apr,13

28344 Reconstruction, toe(s); polydactyly
🔧 8.04   ✂ 12.2   **FUD** 090   J A2 50 ▭
AMA: 2002,Apr,13

28345 syndactyly, with or without skin graft(s), each web
🔧 10.5   ✂ 14.9   **FUD** 090   J A2 80 ▭
AMA: 2002,Apr,13

28360 Reconstruction, cleft foot
🔧 31.4   ✂ 31.4   **FUD** 090   J G2 80 50 ▭
AMA: 2002,Apr,13

28400-28675 Treatment of Fracture/Dislocation of Foot/Toe

28400 Closed treatment of calcaneal fracture; without manipulation
🔧 6.55   ✂ 7.09   **FUD** 090   T A2 50 ▭
AMA: 2002,Apr,13

28405 with manipulation
INCLUDES   Bohler reduction
🔧 10.0   ✂ 11.1   **FUD** 090   T A2 80 50 ▭
AMA: 2002,Apr,13

28406 Percutaneous skeletal fixation of calcaneal fracture, with manipulation
🔧 15.1   ✂ 15.1   **FUD** 090   J A2 80 50 ▭
AMA: 2002,Apr,13

28415 Open treatment of calcaneal fracture, includes internal fixation, when performed;
🔧 32.2   ✂ 32.2   **FUD** 090   J J8 80 50 ▭
AMA: 2002,Apr,13

28420 with primary iliac or other autogenous bone graft (includes obtaining graft)
🔧 37.1   ✂ 37.1   **FUD** 090   J J8 80 50 ▭
AMA: 2002,Apr,13

28430 Closed treatment of talus fracture; without manipulation
🔧 6.03   ✂ 6.85   **FUD** 090   T P2 50 ▭
AMA: 2002,Apr,13

28435 with manipulation
🔧 9.31   ✂ 10.4   **FUD** 090   J A2 80 50 ▭
AMA: 2002,Apr,13

28436 Percutaneous skeletal fixation of talus fracture, with manipulation
🔧 12.9   ✂ 12.9   **FUD** 090   J G2 50 ▭
AMA: 2002,Apr,13

28445 Open treatment of talus fracture, includes internal fixation, when performed
🔧 30.2   ✂ 30.2   **FUD** 090   J J8 80 50 ▭
AMA: 2002,Apr,13

28446 Open osteochondral autograft, talus (includes obtaining graft[s])
INCLUDES   Osteotomy; fibula (27707)
  Osteotomy; tibia (27705)
EXCLUDES   *Arthroscopically aided osteochondral talus graft (29892)*
  Open osteochondral allograft or repairs with industrial grafts (28899)
🔧 35.1   ✂ 35.1   **FUD** 090   J G2 80 50 ▭
AMA: 2018,Jan,8; 2017,Jan,8; 2016,Jan,13

28450 Treatment of tarsal bone fracture (except talus and calcaneus); without manipulation, each
🔧 5.47   ✂ 6.07   **FUD** 090   T P2 ▭
AMA: 2018,Jan,8; 2017,Jan,8; 2016,Jan,13

28455 with manipulation, each
🔧 7.40   ✂ 8.27   **FUD** 090   J P3 80 ▭
AMA: 2002,Apr,13

28456 Percutaneous skeletal fixation of tarsal bone fracture (except talus and calcaneus), with manipulation, each
🔧 9.74   ✂ 9.74   **FUD** 090   J A2 ▭
AMA: 2002,Apr,13

28465 Open treatment of tarsal bone fracture (except talus and calcaneus), includes internal fixation, when performed, each
🔧 18.1   ✂ 18.1   **FUD** 090   J J8 ▭
AMA: 2019,Aug,10

28470 Closed treatment of metatarsal fracture; without manipulation, each
🔧 5.85   ✂ 6.26   **FUD** 090   T P2 ▭
AMA: 2002,Apr,13

28475 with manipulation, each
🔧 6.52   ✂ 7.37   **FUD** 090   T P2 ▭
AMA: 2002,Apr,13

28476 Percutaneous skeletal fixation of metatarsal fracture, with manipulation, each
🔧 10.5   ✂ 10.5   **FUD** 090   J A2 80 ▭
AMA: 2002,Apr,13

28485 Open treatment of metatarsal fracture, includes internal fixation, when performed, each
🔧 15.8   ✂ 15.8   **FUD** 090   J J8 ▭
AMA: 2019,Aug,10

28490 Closed treatment of fracture great toe, phalanx or phalanges; without manipulation
🔧 3.57   ✂ 4.12   **FUD** 090   T P3 50 ▭
AMA: 2002,Apr,13

28495 with manipulation
🔧 4.25   ✂ 5.10   **FUD** 090   T P2 50 ▭
AMA: 2002,Apr,13

28496 Percutaneous skeletal fixation of fracture great toe, phalanx or phalanges, with manipulation
🔧 6.93   ✂ 12.9   **FUD** 090   J A2 50 ▭
AMA: 2002,Apr,13

28505 Open treatment of fracture, great toe, phalanx or phalanges, includes internal fixation, when performed
🔧 14.3   ✂ 19.1   **FUD** 090   J A2 50 ▭
AMA: 2002,Apr,13

28510 Closed treatment of fracture, phalanx or phalanges, other than great toe; without manipulation, each
🔧 3.41   ✂ 3.47   **FUD** 090   T P3 ▭
AMA: 2002,Apr,13

28515 with manipulation, each
🔧 4.08   ✂ 4.67   **FUD** 090   T P2 ▭
AMA: 2002,Apr,13

28525 Open treatment of fracture, phalanx or phalanges, other than great toe, includes internal fixation, when performed, each
11.6   16.5   **FUD** 090   J A2 80
AMA: 2002,Apr,13

28530 Closed treatment of sesamoid fracture
2.88   3.30   **FUD** 090   T P3 80 50
AMA: 2002,Apr,13

28531 Open treatment of sesamoid fracture, with or without internal fixation
5.22   9.73   **FUD** 090   J A2 50
AMA: 2002,Apr,13

28540 Closed treatment of tarsal bone dislocation, other than talotarsal; without anesthesia
5.01   5.57   **FUD** 090   T P2 80 50
AMA: 2002,Apr,13

28545 requiring anesthesia
7.62   8.67   **FUD** 090   J G2 80 50
AMA: 2002,Apr,13

28546 Percutaneous skeletal fixation of tarsal bone dislocation, other than talotarsal, with manipulation
9.85   16.7   **FUD** 090   J A2 80 50
AMA: 2002,Apr,13

28555 Open treatment of tarsal bone dislocation, includes internal fixation, when performed
18.7   24.6   **FUD** 090   J J8 80 50
AMA: 2002,Apr,13

28570 Closed treatment of talotarsal joint dislocation; without anesthesia
5.52   6.57   **FUD** 090   T P2 80 50
AMA: 2002,Apr,13

28575 requiring anesthesia
9.57   10.6   **FUD** 090   J A2 80 50
AMA: 2002,Apr,13

28576 Percutaneous skeletal fixation of talotarsal joint dislocation, with manipulation
11.1   11.1   **FUD** 090   J A2 80 50
AMA: 2002,Apr,13

28585 Open treatment of talotarsal joint dislocation, includes internal fixation, when performed
19.6   25.0   **FUD** 090   J J8 80 50
AMA: 2018,Jan,8; 2017,Jan,8; 2016,Jan,13

28600 Closed treatment of tarsometatarsal joint dislocation; without anesthesia
5.35   6.26   **FUD** 090   T P2 80
AMA: 2002,Apr,13

28605 requiring anesthesia
8.57   9.58   **FUD** 090   T A2 80
AMA: 2002,Apr,13

28606 Percutaneous skeletal fixation of tarsometatarsal joint dislocation, with manipulation
11.1   11.1   **FUD** 090   J A2
AMA: 2002,Apr,13

28615 Open treatment of tarsometatarsal joint dislocation, includes internal fixation, when performed
23.4   23.4   **FUD** 090   J J8 80
AMA: 2002,Apr,13

28630 Closed treatment of metatarsophalangeal joint dislocation; without anesthesia
3.15   4.49   **FUD** 010   T P3 80
AMA: 2002,Apr,13

28635 requiring anesthesia
3.81   5.04   **FUD** 010   J A2 80
AMA: 2002,Apr,13

28636 Percutaneous skeletal fixation of metatarsophalangeal joint dislocation, with manipulation
5.74   8.98   **FUD** 010   J A2
AMA: 2002,Apr,13

28645 Open treatment of metatarsophalangeal joint dislocation, includes internal fixation, when performed
14.0   18.9   **FUD** 090   J A2
AMA: 2018,Jan,8; 2017,Jan,8; 2016,Jan,13

28660 Closed treatment of interphalangeal joint dislocation; without anesthesia
2.56   3.38   **FUD** 010   T P3
AMA: 2002,Apr,13

28665 requiring anesthesia
3.72   4.41   **FUD** 010   T A2 80
AMA: 2002,Apr,13

28666 Percutaneous skeletal fixation of interphalangeal joint dislocation, with manipulation
4.79   4.79   **FUD** 010   J A2
AMA: 2002,Apr,13

28675 Open treatment of interphalangeal joint dislocation, includes internal fixation, when performed
11.6   16.4   **FUD** 090   J A2
AMA: 2002,Apr,13

28705-28760 Arthrodesis of Foot/Toe

28705 Arthrodesis; pantalar
35.4   35.4   **FUD** 090   J J8 80 50
AMA: 2020,May,13

28715 triple
27.1   27.1   **FUD** 090   J J8 80 50
AMA: 2020,May,13

28725 subtalar
INCLUDES   Dunn arthrodesis
Grice arthrodesis
22.4   22.4   **FUD** 090   J J8 80 50
AMA: 2020,May,13; 2018,Jan,8; 2017,Jan,8; 2016,Jan,13

28730 Arthrodesis, midtarsal or tarsometatarsal, multiple or transverse;
INCLUDES   Lambrinudi arthrodesis
21.2   21.2   **FUD** 090   J J8 80 50
AMA: 2020,May,13

28735 with osteotomy (eg, flatfoot correction)
22.4   22.4   **FUD** 090   J J8 80 50
AMA: 2020,May,13; 2019,May,10

28737 Arthrodesis, with tendon lengthening and advancement, midtarsal, tarsal navicular-cuneiform (eg, Miller type procedure)
19.8   19.8   **FUD** 090   J J8 80 50
AMA: 2020,May,13

28740 Arthrodesis, midtarsal or tarsometatarsal, single joint
17.9   24.3   **FUD** 090   J J8 80 50
AMA: 2020,May,13; 2018,Jan,8; 2017,Jan,8; 2016,Jan,13

28750 Arthrodesis, great toe; metatarsophalangeal joint
16.8   22.9   **FUD** 090   J J8 80 50
AMA: 2020,May,13; 2018,Jan,8; 2017,Jan,8; 2016,Dec,3; 2016,Jan,13

28755 interphalangeal joint
9.56   14.7   **FUD** 090   J A2 50
AMA: 2020,May,13

28760 Arthrodesis, with extensor hallucis longus transfer to first metatarsal neck, great toe, interphalangeal joint (eg, Jones type procedure)
INCLUDES   Jones procedure
EXCLUDES   *Hammer toe repair or interphalangeal fusion (28285)*
16.6   22.5   **FUD** 090   J A2 80 50
AMA: 2020,May,13

28800-28825 Amputation Foot/Toe

28800 Amputation, foot; midtarsal (eg, Chopart type procedure)
🦴 15.4 ⚖ 15.4 **FUD** 090 C 80 50 ▭
AMA: 2002,Apr,13; 1998,Nov,1

28805 transmetatarsal
🦴 20.9 ⚖ 20.9 **FUD** 090 J 62 80 50 ▭
AMA: 2002,Apr,13; 1997,May,4

28810 Amputation, metatarsal, with toe, single
🦴 12.3 ⚖ 12.3 **FUD** 090 J A2 80 ▭
AMA: 2002,Apr,13

28820 Amputation, toe; metatarsophalangeal joint
🦴 11.3 ⚖ 16.1 **FUD** 090 J A2 ▭
AMA: 2002,Apr,13; 1997,May,4

28825 interphalangeal joint
🦴 10.6 ⚖ 15.4 **FUD** 090 J A2 ▭
AMA: 2002,Apr,13

28890-28899 Other/Unlisted Procedures Foot/Toe

28890 Extracorporeal shock wave, high energy, performed by a physician or other qualified health care professional, requiring anesthesia other than local, including ultrasound guidance, involving the plantar fascia
EXCLUDES Extracorporeal shock wave therapy integumentary system not otherwise specified, when performed on same treatment area ([0512T, 0513T])
Extracorporeal shock wave therapy musculoskeletal system not otherwise specified (0101T-0102T)
🦴 6.38 ⚖ 9.18 **FUD** 090 J P3 50 ▭
AMA: 2018,Dec,5; 2018,Dec,5; 2018,Jan,8; 2017,Jan,8; 2016,Jan,13

28899 Unlisted procedure, foot or toes
🦴 0.00 ⚖ 0.00 **FUD** YYY T 80 ▭
AMA: 2018,Oct,11; 2018,Jan,8; 2017,Nov,10; 2017,Sep,14; 2017,Jan,8; 2016,Dec,3; 2016,Jun,8; 2016,Jan,13

29000-29086 Casting: Arm/Shoulder/Torso

INCLUDES Cast removal without replacement by same provider
Cast replacement during or after global period
EXCLUDES Initial cast application performed with restorative treatment, report appropriate musculoskeletal system code
Orthotic supervision and training (97760-97763)
Removal cast by different provider (29700, 29705, 29710)
Code also cast material

29000 Application of halo type body cast (see 20661-20663 for insertion)
🦴 5.57 ⚖ 9.69 **FUD** 000 T G2 80 ▭
AMA: 2018,Jan,8; 2018,Jan,3; 2017,Jan,8; 2016,Jan,13

29010 Application of Risser jacket, localizer, body; only
🦴 4.58 ⚖ 7.63 **FUD** 000 T P2 80 ▭
AMA: 2018,Jan,8; 2018,Jan,3; 2017,Jan,8; 2016,Jan,13

29015 including head
🦴 5.18 ⚖ 8.22 **FUD** 000 T P2 80 ▭
AMA: 2018,Jan,8; 2018,Jan,3; 2017,Jan,8; 2016,Jan,13

29035 Application of body cast, shoulder to hips;
🦴 4.08 ⚖ 7.13 **FUD** 000 T P2 80 ▭
AMA: 2018,Jan,8; 2018,Jan,3; 2017,Jan,8; 2016,Jan,13

29040 including head, Minerva type
🦴 4.95 ⚖ 8.17 **FUD** 000 T G2 80 ▭
AMA: 2018,Jan,8; 2018,Jan,3; 2017,Jan,8; 2016,Jan,13

29044 including 1 thigh
🦴 4.78 ⚖ 8.01 **FUD** 000 T P2 80 ▭
AMA: 2018,Jan,8; 2018,Jan,3; 2017,Jan,8; 2016,Jan,13

29046 including both thighs
🦴 5.37 ⚖ 8.78 **FUD** 000 T G2 80 ▭
AMA: 2018,Jan,8; 2018,Jan,3; 2017,Jan,8; 2016,Jan,13

29049 Application, cast; figure-of-eight
🦴 2.00 ⚖ 2.79 **FUD** 000 T P3 80 ▭
AMA: 2018,Jan,3; 2018,Jan,8; 2017,Jan,8; 2016,Jan,13

29055 shoulder spica
🦴 3.93 ⚖ 6.22 **FUD** 000 T P2 80 ▭
AMA: 2018,Jan,8; 2018,Jan,3; 2017,Jan,8; 2016,Jan,13

29058 plaster Velpeau
🦴 2.71 ⚖ 3.51 **FUD** 000 T P3 80 ▭
AMA: 2018,Jan,8; 2018,Jan,3; 2017,Jan,8; 2016,Jan,13

29065 shoulder to hand (long arm)
🦴 1.95 ⚖ 2.70 **FUD** 000 T P3 50 ▭
AMA: 2018,Jan,8; 2018,Jan,3; 2017,Jan,8; 2016,Jan,13

29075 elbow to finger (short arm)
🦴 1.76 ⚖ 2.43 **FUD** 000 T P3 50 ▭
AMA: 2018,Jan,8; 2018,Jan,3; 2017,Jan,8; 2016,Jan,13

29085 hand and lower forearm (gauntlet)
🦴 1.92 ⚖ 2.68 **FUD** 000 T P3 50 ▭
AMA: 2018,Jan,3; 2018,Jan,8; 2017,Jan,8; 2016,Jan,13

29086 finger (eg, contracture)
🦴 1.47 ⚖ 2.22 **FUD** 000 T P3 50 ▭
AMA: 2018,Jan,8; 2018,Jan,3; 2017,Jan,8; 2016,Jan,13

29105-29280 Splinting and Strapping: Torso/Upper Extremities

INCLUDES Replacement splint or strapping during or after global period
EXCLUDES Initial splinting/strapping application performed with restorative treatment, report appropriate musculoskeletal system code
Orthotic supervision and training (97760-97763)
Code also splint/strapping material

29105 Application of long arm splint (shoulder to hand)
🦴 1.38 ⚖ 2.33 **FUD** 000 T P3 50 ▭
AMA: 2018,Jan,3; 2018,Jan,8; 2017,Jan,8; 2016,Jan,13

29125 Application of short arm splint (forearm to hand); static
🦴 1.13 ⚖ 1.82 **FUD** 000 01 N1 50 ▭
AMA: 2018,Jan,8; 2018,Jan,3; 2017,Jan,8; 2016,Jan,13

29126 dynamic
🦴 1.40 ⚖ 2.18 **FUD** 000 01 N1 50 ▭
AMA: 2018,Jan,8; 2018,Jan,3; 2017,Jan,8; 2016,Jan,13

29130 Application of finger splint; static
🦴 0.85 ⚖ 1.18 **FUD** 000 01 N1 50 ▭
AMA: 2018,Jan,8; 2018,Jan,3; 2017,Jan,8; 2016,Jan,13

29131 dynamic
🦴 0.98 ⚖ 1.48 **FUD** 000 01 N1 50 ▭
AMA: 2018,Jan,8; 2018,Jan,3; 2017,Jan,8; 2016,Jan,13

29200 Strapping; thorax
EXCLUDES Strapping of low back (29799)
🦴 0.54 ⚖ 0.93 **FUD** 000 T P3 ▭
AMA: 2018,Jan,8; 2018,Jan,3; 2017,Jan,8; 2016,Jan,13

29240 shoulder (eg, Velpeau)
🦴 0.54 ⚖ 0.87 **FUD** 000 01 N1 50 ▭
AMA: 2018,Jan,3; 2018,Jan,8; 2017,Jan,8; 2016,Jan,13

29260 elbow or wrist
🦴 0.56 ⚖ 0.86 **FUD** 000 01 N1 50 ▭
AMA: 2018,Jan,8; 2018,Jan,3; 2017,Jan,8; 2016,Jan,13

29280 hand or finger
🦴 0.60 ⚖ 0.88 **FUD** 000 01 N1 50 ▭
AMA: 2018,Jan,8; 2018,Jan,3; 2017,Jan,8; 2016,Jan,13

29305-29450 Casting: Legs

INCLUDES Cast removal without replacement by same provider
Cast replacement during or after global period
EXCLUDES Initial cast application performed with restorative treatment, report appropriate musculoskeletal system code
Orthotic supervision and training (97760-97763)
Removal cast by different provider (29700, 29705, 29710)
Code also cast material

29305 Application of hip spica cast; 1 leg
EXCLUDES Hip spica cast thighs only (29046)
🦴 4.53 ⚖ 6.93 **FUD** 000 T P2 80 ▭
AMA: 2018,Jan,8; 2018,Jan,3; 2017,Jan,8; 2016,Jan,13

29325 **1 and one-half spica or both legs**
EXCLUDES   *Hip spica cast thighs only (29046)*
🚗 5.11   ⚕ 7.75   **FUD** 000   [T] [P2] [80] [▢]
AMA: 2018,Jan,8; 2018,Jan,3; 2017,Jan,8; 2016,Jan,13

29345 **Application of long leg cast (thigh to toes);**
🚗 2.87   ⚕ 3.85   **FUD** 000   [T] [P3] [50] [▢]
AMA: 2018,Jan,3; 2018,Jan,8; 2017,Jan,8; 2016,Jan,13

29355 **walker or ambulatory type**
🚗 3.07   ⚕ 4.03   **FUD** 000   [T] [P3] [50] [▢]
AMA: 2018,Jan,3; 2018,Jan,8; 2017,Jan,8; 2016,Jan,13

29358 **Application of long leg cast brace**
🚗 2.96   ⚕ 4.51   **FUD** 000   [T] [P3] [50] [▢]
AMA: 2018,Jan,3; 2018,Jan,8; 2017,Jan,8; 2016,Jan,13

29365 **Application of cylinder cast (thigh to ankle)**
🚗 2.50   ⚕ 3.47   **FUD** 000   [T] [P3] [50] [▢]
AMA: 2018,Jan,3; 2018,Jan,8; 2017,Jan,8; 2016,Jan,13

29405 **Application of short leg cast (below knee to toes);**
🚗 1.69   ⚕ 2.26   **FUD** 000   [T] [P3] [50] [▢]
AMA: 2018,Jan,3; 2018,Jan,8; 2017,Jan,8; 2016,Jan,13

29425 **walking or ambulatory type**
🚗 1.59   ⚕ 2.17   **FUD** 000   [T] [P3] [50] [▢]
AMA: 2018,Jan,3; 2018,Jan,8; 2017,Jan,8; 2016,Jan,13

29435 **Application of patellar tendon bearing (PTB) cast**
🚗 2.35   ⚕ 3.25   **FUD** 000   [T] [P3] [50] [▢]
AMA: 2018,Jan,3; 2018,Jan,8; 2017,Jan,8; 2016,Jan,13

29440 **Adding walker to previously applied cast**
🚗 0.83   ⚕ 1.23   **FUD** 000   [T] [P3] [50] [▢]
AMA: 2018,Jan,8; 2018,Jan,3; 2017,Jan,8; 2016,Jan,13

29445 **Application of rigid total contact leg cast**
🚗 2.94   ⚕ 3.72   **FUD** 000   [T] [P3] [50] [▢]
AMA: 2018,Jan,3; 2018,Jan,8; 2017,Jan,8; 2016,Jan,13

29450 **Application of clubfoot cast with molding or manipulation, long or short leg**
🚗 3.26   ⚕ 4.11   **FUD** 000   [T] [P3] [50] [▢]
AMA: 2018,Jan,8; 2018,Jan,3; 2017,Jan,8; 2016,Jan,13

29505-29584 Splinting and Strapping Ankle/Foot/Leg/Toes

INCLUDES   Replacement splint or strapping during or after global period
EXCLUDES   *Initial splinting/strapping application performed with restorative treatment, report appropriate musculoskeletal system code*
Orthotic supervision and training (97760-97763)
Code also splint/strapping material

29505 **Application of long leg splint (thigh to ankle or toes)**
🚗 1.45   ⚕ 2.41   **FUD** 000   [T] [P3] [50] [▢]
AMA: 2018,Jan,3; 2018,Jan,8; 2017,Jan,8; 2016,Jan,13

29515 **Application of short leg splint (calf to foot)**
🚗 1.42   ⚕ 2.01   **FUD** 000   [T] [P3] [50] [▢]
AMA: 2019,Oct,10; 2018,Jan,8; 2018,Jan,3; 2017,Jan,8; 2016,Jan,13

29520 **Strapping; hip**
EXCLUDES   *For treatment in same extremity:*
Endovenous ablation therapy incompetent vein (36473-36479, [36482], [36483])
Sclerosal injection for incompetent vein(s) ([36465], [36466], 36468-36471)
🚗 0.55   ⚕ 1.00   **FUD** 000   [01] [N1] [80] [50] [▢]
AMA: 2018,Jan,8; 2018,Jan,3; 2017,Jan,8; 2016,Jan,13

29530 **knee**
EXCLUDES   *For treatment in same extremity:*
Endovenous ablation therapy incompetent vein (36473-36479, [36482], [36483])
Sclerosal injection for incompetent vein(s) ([36465], [36466], 36468-36471)
🚗 0.54   ⚕ 0.86   **FUD** 000   [01] [N1] [50] [▢]
AMA: 2018,Jan,3; 2018,Jan,8; 2017,Jan,8; 2016,Jan,13

29540 **ankle and/or foot**
EXCLUDES   *For treatment in same extremity:*
Endovenous ablation therapy incompetent vein (36473-36479, [36482, 36483])
Multi-layer compression system (29581)
Sclerosal injection for incompetent vein(s) ([36465], [36466], 36468-36471)
Unna boot (29580)
🚗 0.51   ⚕ 0.81   **FUD** 000   [T] [P3] [50] [▢]
AMA: 2018,Jan,3; 2018,Jan,8; 2017,Jan,8; 2016,Aug,3; 2016,Jan,13

29550 **toes**
EXCLUDES   *For treatment in same extremity:*
Endovenous ablation therapy incompetent vein (36473-36479, [36482, 36483])
Sclerosal injection for incompetent vein(s) ([36465], [36466], 36468-36471)
🚗 0.33   ⚕ 0.54   **FUD** 000   [01] [N1] [50] [▢]
AMA: 2018,Jan,8; 2018,Jan,3; 2017,Jan,8; 2016,Jan,13

29580 **Unna boot**
EXCLUDES   *Application multilayer compression system (29581)*
For treatment in same extremity:
Endovenous ablation therapy incompetent vein (36473-36479, [36482, 36483])
Sclerosal injection for incompetent vein(s) ([36465], [36466], 36468-36471)
Strapping ankle or foot (29540)
🚗 0.79   ⚕ 1.80   **FUD** 000   [T] [P3] [50] [▢]
AMA: 2018,Jan,3; 2018,Jan,8; 2017,Jan,8; 2016,Aug,3; 2016,Jan,13

29581 **Application of multi-layer compression system; leg (below knee), including ankle and foot**
EXCLUDES   *For treatment in same extremity:*
Endovenous ablation therapy incompetent vein (36473-36479, [36482, 36483])
Sclerosal injection for incompetent vein(s) ([36465], [36466], 36468-36471)
Strapping (29540, 29580)
🚗 0.80   ⚕ 2.54   **FUD** 000   [T] [P3] [80] [50] [▢]
AMA: 2018,Mar,3; 2018,Jan,8; 2018,Jan,3; 2017,Jan,8; 2016,Nov,3; 2016,Aug,3; 2016,Jan,13

29584 **upper arm, forearm, hand, and fingers**
EXCLUDES   *For treatment in same extremity:*
Endovenous ablation therapy incompetent vein (36473-36479, [36482], [36483])
Sclerosal injection for incompetent vein(s) ([36465], [36466], 36468-36471)
🚗 0.47   ⚕ 2.37   **FUD** 000   [T] [P2] [80] [50] [▢]
AMA: 2018,Jan,3; 2018,Jan,8; 2017,Jan,8; 2016,Aug,3; 2016,Jan,13

29700-29799 Casting Services Other Than Application

INCLUDES   Casts applied by treating individual
Removal casts applied by treating individual

29700 **Removal or bivalving; gauntlet, boot or body cast**
🚗 0.96   ⚕ 1.78   **FUD** 000   [T] [P3]
AMA: 2018,Jan,3; 2018,Jan,8; 2017,Jan,8; 2016,Jan,13

29705 **full arm or full leg cast**
🚗 1.31   ⚕ 1.82   **FUD** 000   [T] [P3] [50] [▢]
AMA: 2018,Jan,3; 2018,Jan,8; 2017,Jan,8; 2016,Jan,13

29710 **shoulder or hip spica, Minerva, or Risser jacket, etc.**
🚗 2.41   ⚕ 3.48   **FUD** 000   [T] [P3] [80] [50] [▢]
AMA: 2018,Jan,3; 2018,Jan,8; 2017,Jan,8; 2016,Jan,13

29720 **Repair of spica, body cast or jacket**
🚗 1.26   ⚕ 2.38   **FUD** 000   [T] [P3] [▢]
AMA: 2018,Jan,3; 2018,Jan,8; 2017,Jan,8; 2016,Jan,13

29730 **Windowing of cast**
🚗 1.25   ⚕ 1.76   **FUD** 000   [T] [P3] [▢]
AMA: 2018,Jan,3; 2018,Jan,8; 2017,Jan,8; 2016,Jan,13

29740   **Wedging of cast (except clubfoot casts)**
🦶 2.02   ⚕ 2.82   **FUD** 000   T P3 ▭
AMA: 2018,Jan,3; 2018,Jan,8; 2017,Jan,8; 2016,Jan,13

29750   **Wedging of clubfoot cast**
🦶 2.26   ⚕ 3.07   **FUD** 000   T P3 80 50 ▭
AMA: 2018,Jan,3; 2018,Jan,8; 2017,Jan,8; 2016,Jan,13

29799   **Unlisted procedure, casting or strapping**
🦶 0.00   ⚕ 0.00   **FUD** YYY   T 80 ▭
AMA: 2018,Jan,3; 2018,Jan,8; 2017,Jan,8; 2016,Aug,3;
2016,Jan,13

29800-29999 [29914, 29915, 29916] Arthroscopic Procedures

INCLUDES   Diagnostic arthroscopy with surgical arthroscopy
EXCLUDES   Reporting removal foreign or loose body(ies) smaller than arthroscopic
cannula diameter utilized for procedure
Code also modifier 51 when arthroscopy performed with arthrotomy

29800   **Arthroscopy, temporomandibular joint, diagnostic, with or
without synovial biopsy (separate procedure)**
🦶 15.2   ⚕ 15.2   **FUD** 090   J A2 80 50 ▭
AMA: 2018,Jan,8; 2017,Jan,8; 2016,Jan,13

29804   **Arthroscopy, temporomandibular joint, surgical**
EXCLUDES   Open surgery (21010)
🦶 17.7   ⚕ 17.7   **FUD** 090   J A2 80 50 ▭
AMA: 2018,Jan,8; 2017,Jan,8; 2016,Jan,13

29805   **Arthroscopy, shoulder, diagnostic, with or without synovial
biopsy (separate procedure)**
EXCLUDES   Open surgery (23065-23066, 23100-23101)
🦶 13.5   ⚕ 13.5   **FUD** 090   J A2 50 ▭
AMA: 2018,Jan,8; 2017,Jan,8; 2016,Jan,13

29806   **Arthroscopy, shoulder, surgical; capsulorrhaphy**
EXCLUDES   Open surgery (23450-23466)
Thermal capsulorrhaphy (29999)
🦶 30.5   ⚕ 30.5   **FUD** 090   J A2 50 ▭
AMA: 2020,Dec,8; 2018,Jun,11; 2018,Jan,8; 2017,Jan,8;
2016,Jan,13

29807   **repair of SLAP lesion**
🦶 29.8   ⚕ 29.8   **FUD** 090   J A2 50 ▭
AMA: 2018,Jan,8; 2017,Jan,8; 2016,Jan,13

29819   **with removal of loose body or foreign body**
EXCLUDES   Open surgery (23040-23044, 23107)
🦶 16.9   ⚕ 16.9   **FUD** 090   J A2 50 ▭
AMA: 2020,Dec,8; 2020,Dec,13; 2018,Jun,11; 2018,Jan,8;
2017,Jan,8; 2016,Jan,13

29820   **synovectomy, partial**
EXCLUDES   Open surgery (23105)
🦶 15.3   ⚕ 15.3   **FUD** 090   J A2 80 50 ▭
AMA: 2018,Jan,8; 2017,Jan,8; 2016,Jan,13

29821   **synovectomy, complete**
EXCLUDES   Open surgery (23105)
🦶 17.1   ⚕ 17.1   **FUD** 090   J A2 80 50 ▭
AMA: 2018,Jan,8; 2017,Jan,8; 2016,Jan,13

29822   **debridement, limited, 1 or 2 discrete structures (eg,
humeral bone, humeral articular cartilage, glenoid bone,
glenoid articular cartilage, biceps tendon, biceps anchor
complex, labrum, articular capsule, articular side of the
rotator cuff, bursal side of the rotator cuff, subacromial
bursa, foreign body[ies])**
EXCLUDES   Open surgery (see specific shoulder section)
🦶 16.6   ⚕ 16.6   **FUD** 090   J A2 80 50 ▭
AMA: 2020,Dec,8; 2018,Jan,8; 2018,Jan,7; 2017,Jan,8;
2016,Jan,13

29823   **debridement, extensive, 3 or more discrete structures (eg,
humeral bone, humeral articular cartilage, glenoid bone,
glenoid articular cartilage, biceps tendon, biceps anchor
complex, labrum, articular capsule, articular side of the
rotator cuff, bursal side of the rotator cuff, subacromial
bursa, foreign body[ies])**
EXCLUDES   Open surgery (see specific shoulder section)
🦶 18.1   ⚕ 18.1   **FUD** 090   J A2 80 50 ▭
AMA: 2020,Dec,8; 2018,Jan,8; 2018,Jan,7; 2017,Jan,8;
2016,Dec,16; 2016,Jan,13

29824   **distal claviculectomy including distal articular surface
(Mumford procedure)**
EXCLUDES   Open surgery (23120)
🦶 19.4   ⚕ 19.4   **FUD** 090   J A2 80 50 ▭
AMA: 2018,Jan,8; 2017,Jan,8; 2016,Jan,13

29825   **with lysis and resection of adhesions, with or without
manipulation**
EXCLUDES   Open surgery (see specific shoulder section)
🦶 16.9   ⚕ 16.9   **FUD** 090   J A2 80 50 ▭
AMA: 2018,Jan,8; 2017,Jan,8; 2016,Jan,13

+ **29826**   **decompression of subacromial space with partial
acromioplasty, with coracoacromial ligament (ie, arch)
release, when performed (List separately in addition to
code for primary procedure)**
EXCLUDES   Open surgery (23130, 23415)
Code first (29806-29825, 29827-29828)
🦶 5.07   ⚕ 5.07   **FUD** ZZZ   N N1 80 50 ▭
AMA: 2018,Jan,8; 2017,Jan,8; 2016,Jan,13

29827   **with rotator cuff repair**
EXCLUDES   Distal clavicle excision (29824)
Open surgery or mini open repair (23412)
Subacromial decompression (29826)
🦶 30.9   ⚕ 30.9   **FUD** 090   J A2 80 50 ▭
AMA: 2018,Jan,8; 2017,Jan,8; 2016,Jul,8; 2016,Jan,13

29828   **biceps tenodesis**
EXCLUDES   Arthroscopy, shoulder, diagnostic, with or without
synovial biopsy (29805)
Arthroscopy, shoulder, surgical; debridement, limited
(29822)
Arthroscopy, shoulder, surgical; synovectomy, partial
(29820)
Tenodesis long tendon biceps (23430)
🦶 26.5   ⚕ 26.5   **FUD** 090   J 62 80 50 ▭
AMA: 2018,Jan,8; 2017,Jan,8; 2016,Jul,8; 2016,Jan,13

29830   **Arthroscopy, elbow, diagnostic, with or without synovial
biopsy (separate procedure)**
🦶 13.1   ⚕ 13.1   **FUD** 090   J A2 50 ▭
AMA: 2018,Jan,8; 2017,Jan,8; 2016,Jan,13

29834   **Arthroscopy, elbow, surgical; with removal of loose body or
foreign body**
🦶 14.1   ⚕ 14.1   **FUD** 090   J A2 80 50 ▭
AMA: 2020,Dec,8; 2018,Jan,8; 2017,Jan,8; 2016,Jan,13

29835   **synovectomy, partial**
🦶 14.6   ⚕ 14.6   **FUD** 090   J A2 80 50 ▭
AMA: 2018,Jan,8; 2017,Jan,8; 2016,Jan,13

29836   **synovectomy, complete**
🦶 16.8   ⚕ 16.8   **FUD** 090   J A2 80 50 ▭
AMA: 2018,Jan,8; 2017,Jan,8; 2016,Jan,13

29837   **debridement, limited**
🦶 15.2   ⚕ 15.2   **FUD** 090   J A2 80 50 ▭
AMA: 2018,Jan,8; 2017,Jan,8; 2016,Jan,13

29838   **debridement, extensive**
🦶 17.0   ⚕ 17.0   **FUD** 090   J A2 80 50 ▭
AMA: 2018,Jan,8; 2017,Jan,8; 2016,Jan,13

29840   **Arthroscopy, wrist, diagnostic, with or without synovial
biopsy (separate procedure)**
🦶 12.9   ⚕ 12.9   **FUD** 090   J A2 80 50 ▭
AMA: 2018,Jan,8; 2017,Jan,8; 2016,Jan,13

| 26/TC PC/TC Only | A2-Z3 ASC Payment | 50 Bilateral | ♂ Male Only | ♀ Female Only | 🦶 Facility RVU | ⚕ Non-Facility RVU | ▭ CCI | ✖ CLIA |
| FUD Follow-up Days | CMS: IOM | AMA: CPT Asst | A-Y OPPSI | 80/80 Surg Assist Allowed / w/Doc | ▭ Lab Crosswalk | ▭ Radiology Crosswalk |

102   CPT © 2021 American Medical Association. All Rights Reserved.   © 2021 Optum360, LLC

29843 Arthroscopy, wrist, surgical; for infection, lavage and drainage
🚑 14.0   ⚖ 14.0   **FUD** 090   [J] [A2] [80] [50] [▯]
AMA: 2018,Jan,8; 2017,Jan,8; 2016,Jan,13

29844 synovectomy, partial
🚑 14.2   ⚖ 14.2   **FUD** 090   [J] [A2] [80] [50] [▯]
AMA: 2018,Jan,8; 2017,Jan,8; 2016,Jan,13

29845 synovectomy, complete
🚑 16.8   ⚖ 16.8   **FUD** 090   [J] [A2] [80] [50] [▯]
AMA: 2018,Jan,8; 2017,Jan,8; 2016,Jan,13

29846 excision and/or repair of triangular fibrocartilage and/or joint debridement
🚑 15.0   ⚖ 15.0   **FUD** 090   [J] [A2] [80] [50] [▯]
AMA: 2018,Jan,8; 2017,Jan,8; 2016,Jan,13

29847 internal fixation for fracture or instability
🚑 15.6   ⚖ 15.6   **FUD** 090   [J] [A2] [80] [50] [▯]
AMA: 2018,Jan,8; 2017,Jan,8; 2016,Jan,13

29848 Endoscopy, wrist, surgical, with release of transverse carpal ligament
EXCLUDES   Open surgery (64721)
Tissue expander, other than breast (11960)
🚑 14.7   ⚖ 14.7   **FUD** 090   [J] [A2] [50] [▯]
AMA: 2018,Apr,10; 2018,Jan,8; 2017,Jan,8; 2017,Jan,6; 2016,Jan,13

29850 Arthroscopically aided treatment of intercondylar spine(s) and/or tuberosity fracture(s) of the knee, with or without manipulation; without internal or external fixation (includes arthroscopy)
🚑 17.9   ⚖ 17.9   **FUD** 090   [J] [A2] [80] [50] [▯]
AMA: 2018,Jan,8; 2017,Jan,8; 2016,Jan,13

29851 with internal or external fixation (includes arthroscopy)
EXCLUDES   Bone graft (20900, 20902)
🚑 26.8   ⚖ 26.8   **FUD** 090   [J] [A2] [80] [50] [▯]
AMA: 2018,Jan,8; 2017,Jan,8; 2016,Jan,13

29855 Arthroscopically aided treatment of tibial fracture, proximal (plateau); unicondylar, includes internal fixation, when performed (includes arthroscopy)
EXCLUDES   Bone graft (20900, 20902)
🚑 22.5   ⚖ 22.5   **FUD** 090   [J] [J8] [80] [50] [▯]
AMA: 2019,Nov,13; 2018,Sep,14; 2018,Jan,8; 2017,Jan,8; 2016,Jan,13

29856 bicondylar, includes internal fixation, when performed (includes arthroscopy)
EXCLUDES   Bone graft (20900, 20902)
🚑 28.6   ⚖ 28.6   **FUD** 090   [J] [J8] [80] [50] [▯]
AMA: 2018,Jan,8; 2017,Jan,8; 2016,Jan,13

29860 Arthroscopy, hip, diagnostic with or without synovial biopsy (separate procedure)
🚑 19.2   ⚖ 19.2   **FUD** 090   [J] [A2] [80] [50] [▯]
AMA: 2018,Jan,8; 2017,Jan,8; 2016,Jan,13

29861 Arthroscopy, hip, surgical; with removal of loose body or foreign body
🚑 20.8   ⚖ 20.8   **FUD** 090   [J] [A2] [80] [50] [▯]
AMA: 2020,Dec,8; 2018,Jan,8; 2017,Jan,8; 2016,Jan,13

29862 with debridement/shaving of articular cartilage (chondroplasty), abrasion arthroplasty, and/or resection of labrum
🚑 23.4   ⚖ 23.4   **FUD** 090   [J] [A2] [80] [50] [▯]
AMA: 2018,Jan,8; 2017,Jan,8; 2016,Jan,13

29863 with synovectomy
🚑 23.2   ⚖ 23.2   **FUD** 090   [J] [A2] [80] [50] [▯]
AMA: 2018,Jan,8; 2017,Jan,8; 2016,Jan,13

\# **29914** with femoroplasty (ie, treatment of cam lesion)
INCLUDES   Chondroplasty (29862)
Synovectomy (29863)
🚑 28.7   ⚖ 28.7   **FUD** 090   [J] [G2] [80] [50] [▯]
AMA: 2018,Jan,8; 2017,Jan,8; 2016,Jan,13

\# **29915** with acetabuloplasty (ie, treatment of pincer lesion)
INCLUDES   Chondroplasty (29862)
Synovectomy (29863)
🚑 29.5   ⚖ 29.5   **FUD** 090   [J] [G2] [80] [50] [▯]
AMA: 2018,Jan,8; 2017,Jan,8; 2016,Jan,13

\# **29916** with labral repair
INCLUDES   Acetabuloplasty ([29915])
Chondroplasty (29862)
Synovectomy (29863)
🚑 29.5   ⚖ 29.5   **FUD** 090   [J] [G2] [80] [50] [▯]
AMA: 2018,Jan,8; 2017,Jan,8; 2016,Jan,13

29866 Arthroscopy, knee, surgical; osteochondral autograft(s) (eg, mosaicplasty) (includes harvesting of the autograft[s])
EXCLUDES   Open osteochondral autograft knee (27416)
Procedures performed at same surgical session (29870-29871, 29875, 29884)
Procedures performed in same compartment (29874, 29877, 29879, 29885-29887)
🚑 30.3   ⚖ 30.3   **FUD** 090   [J] [G2] [80] [50] [▯]
AMA: 2018,Jan,8; 2017,Jan,8; 2016,Jan,13

Cylindrical plugs of healthy bone are harvested, usually from a non-weight bearing area of the femur

The technique employs arthroscopy

Recipient holes are drilled and the grafts tamped into position

29867 osteochondral allograft (eg, mosaicplasty)
EXCLUDES   Procedures performed at same surgical session (27415, 27570, 29870-29871, 29875, 29884)
Procedures performed in same compartment (29874, 29877, 29879, 29885-29887)
🚑 36.9   ⚖ 36.9   **FUD** 090   [J] [J8] [80] [50] [▯]
AMA: 2018,Jan,8; 2017,Jan,8; 2016,Jan,13

29868 meniscal transplantation (includes arthrotomy for meniscal insertion), medial or lateral
EXCLUDES   Procedures performed at same surgical session (29870-29871, 29875, 29880, 29883-29884)
Procedures performed in same compartment (29874, 29877, 29881-29882)
🚑 48.4   ⚖ 48.4   **FUD** 090   [J] [G2] [80] [50] [▯]
AMA: 2018,Jan,8; 2017,Jan,8; 2016,Jan,13

29870 **Arthroscopy, knee, diagnostic, with or without synovial biopsy (separate procedure)**
> EXCLUDES Open procedure (27412)
> 🖐 11.7 ☌ 16.4 **FUD** 090 Ⓙ A2 50 ▭
> AMA: 2019,Nov,14; 2018,Jan,8; 2017,Jan,8; 2016,Jan,13

29871 **Arthroscopy, knee, surgical; for infection, lavage and drainage**
> EXCLUDES Injection contrast for knee arthrography (27369)
> Osteochondral graft (27412, 27415, 29866-29867)
> 🖐 14.8 ☌ 14.8 **FUD** 090 Ⓙ A2 50 ▭
> AMA: 2019,Aug,7; 2018,Jan,8; 2017,Jan,8; 2016,Jan,13

29873 **with lateral release**
> EXCLUDES Open procedure (27425)
> 🖐 15.2 ☌ 15.2 **FUD** 090 Ⓙ A2 50 ▭
> AMA: 2018,Jan,8; 2017,Jan,8; 2016,Jan,13

29874 **for removal of loose body or foreign body (eg, osteochondritis dissecans fragmentation, chondral fragmentation)**
> 🖐 15.5 ☌ 15.5 **FUD** 090 Ⓙ A2 80 50 ▭
> AMA: 2020,Dec,8; 2018,Jan,8; 2017,Jan,8; 2016,Jan,13

29875 **synovectomy, limited (eg, plica or shelf resection) (separate procedure)**
> 🖐 14.3 ☌ 14.3 **FUD** 090 Ⓙ A2 80 50 ▭
> AMA: 2018,Jan,8; 2017,Jan,8; 2016,Jan,13; 2016,Jan,11

29876 **synovectomy, major, 2 or more compartments (eg, medial or lateral)**
> 🖐 18.8 ☌ 18.8 **FUD** 090 Ⓙ A2 50 ▭
> AMA: 2018,Jan,8; 2017,Jan,8; 2016,Jan,13

29877 **debridement/shaving of articular cartilage (chondroplasty)**
> EXCLUDES Arthroscopy, knee, surgical; with meniscectomy (29880-29881)
> 🖐 17.9 ☌ 17.9 **FUD** 090 Ⓙ A2 80 50 ▭
> AMA: 2020,May,13; 2018,Jan,8; 2017,Jan,8; 2016,Jan,13

29879 **abrasion arthroplasty (includes chondroplasty where necessary) or multiple drilling or microfracture**
> 🖐 19.0 ☌ 19.0 **FUD** 090 Ⓙ A2 80 50 ▭
> AMA: 2018,Jan,8; 2017,Jan,8; 2016,Jan,13

29880 **with meniscectomy (medial AND lateral, including any meniscal shaving) including debridement/shaving of articular cartilage (chondroplasty), same or separate compartment(s), when performed**
> 🖐 16.1 ☌ 16.1 **FUD** 090 Ⓙ A2 80 50 ▭
> AMA: 2018,Jan,8; 2017,Jan,8; 2016,Jan,13

29881 **with meniscectomy (medial OR lateral, including any meniscal shaving) including debridement/shaving of articular cartilage (chondroplasty), same or separate compartment(s), when performed**
> 🖐 15.5 ☌ 15.5 **FUD** 090 Ⓙ A2 80 50 ▭
> AMA: 2020,Sep,14; 2020,May,13; 2019,Nov,14; 2018,Jan,8; 2017,Jan,8; 2016,Jan,13; 2016,Jan,11

29882 **with meniscus repair (medial OR lateral)**
> EXCLUDES Meniscus transplant (29868)
> 🖐 19.9 ☌ 19.9 **FUD** 090 Ⓙ A2 50 ▭
> AMA: 2019,May,10; 2018,Jan,8; 2017,Jan,8; 2016,Jan,13

29883 **with meniscus repair (medial AND lateral)**
> EXCLUDES Meniscus transplant (29868)
> 🖐 24.2 ☌ 24.2 **FUD** 090 Ⓙ A2 80 50 ▭
> AMA: 2018,Jan,8; 2017,Jan,8; 2016,Jan,13

29884 **with lysis of adhesions, with or without manipulation (separate procedure)**
> 🖐 17.8 ☌ 17.8 **FUD** 090 Ⓙ A2 80 50 ▭
> AMA: 2018,Jan,8; 2017,Jan,8; 2016,Jan,13

29885 **drilling for osteochondritis dissecans with bone grafting, with or without internal fixation (including debridement of base of lesion)**
> 🖐 21.7 ☌ 21.7 **FUD** 090 Ⓙ J8 80 50 ▭
> AMA: 2018,Jan,8; 2017,Jan,8; 2016,Jan,13

29886 **drilling for intact osteochondritis dissecans lesion**
> 🖐 18.3 ☌ 18.3 **FUD** 090 Ⓙ A2 50 ▭
> AMA: 2018,Jan,8; 2017,Jan,8; 2016,Jan,13

29887 **drilling for intact osteochondritis dissecans lesion with internal fixation**
> 🖐 21.6 ☌ 21.6 **FUD** 090 Ⓙ A2 80 50 ▭
> AMA: 2018,Jan,8; 2017,Jan,8; 2016,Jan,13

29888 **Arthroscopically aided anterior cruciate ligament repair/augmentation or reconstruction**
> 🖐 28.3 ☌ 28.3 **FUD** 090 Ⓙ J8 80 50 ▭
> AMA: 2018,Jan,8; 2017,Jan,8; 2016,Nov,9; 2016,Jan,13

29889 **Arthroscopically aided posterior cruciate ligament repair/augmentation or reconstruction**
> 🖐 35.3 ☌ 35.3 **FUD** 090 Ⓙ J8 80 50 ▭
> AMA: 2018,Jan,8; 2017,Jan,8; 2016,Jan,13

29891 **Arthroscopy, ankle, surgical, excision of osteochondral defect of talus and/or tibia, including drilling of the defect**
> 🖐 19.3 ☌ 19.3 **FUD** 090 Ⓙ A2 80 50 ▭
> AMA: 2018,Jan,8; 2017,Jan,8; 2016,Jan,13

29892 **Arthroscopically aided repair of large osteochondritis dissecans lesion, talar dome fracture, or tibial plafond fracture, with or without internal fixation (includes arthroscopy)**
> 🖐 18.7 ☌ 18.7 **FUD** 090 Ⓙ A2 80 50 ▭
> AMA: 2018,Jan,8; 2017,Jan,8; 2016,Jan,13

29893 **Endoscopic plantar fasciotomy**
> 🖐 12.3 ☌ 17.8 **FUD** 090 Ⓙ A2 50 ▭
> AMA: 2018,Jan,8; 2017,Jan,8; 2016,Jan,13

29894 **Arthroscopy, ankle (tibiotalar and fibulotalar joints), surgical; with removal of loose body or foreign body**
> 🖐 14.2 ☌ 14.2 **FUD** 090 Ⓙ A2 80 50 ▭
> AMA: 2020,Dec,8; 2018,Jan,8; 2017,Jan,8; 2016,Jan,13

29895 **synovectomy, partial**
> 🖐 13.4 ☌ 13.4 **FUD** 090 Ⓙ A2 80 50 ▭
> AMA: 2018,Jan,8; 2017,Jan,8; 2016,Jan,13

29897 **debridement, limited**
> 🖐 14.4 ☌ 14.4 **FUD** 090 Ⓙ A2 80 50 ▭
> AMA: 2018,Jan,8; 2017,Jan,8; 2016,Jan,13

29898 **debridement, extensive**
> 🖐 16.1 ☌ 16.1 **FUD** 090 Ⓙ A2 80 50 ▭
> AMA: 2018,Jan,8; 2017,Jan,8; 2016,Jan,13

29899 **with ankle arthrodesis**
> EXCLUDES Open procedure (27870)
> 🖐 29.7 ☌ 29.7 **FUD** 090 Ⓙ J8 80 50 ▭
> AMA: 2018,Jan,8; 2017,Jan,8; 2016,Jan,13

29900 **Arthroscopy, metacarpophalangeal joint, diagnostic, includes synovial biopsy**
> EXCLUDES Arthroscopy, metacarpophalangeal joint, surgical (29901-29902)
> 🖐 14.3 ☌ 14.3 **FUD** 090 Ⓙ A2 80 50 ▭
> AMA: 2018,Jan,8; 2017,Jan,8; 2016,Jan,13

29901 **Arthroscopy, metacarpophalangeal joint, surgical; with debridement**
> 🖐 15.4 ☌ 15.4 **FUD** 090 Ⓙ A2 80 50 ▭
> AMA: 2018,Jan,8; 2017,Jan,8; 2016,Jan,13

29902 **with reduction of displaced ulnar collateral ligament (eg, Stenar lesion)**
> 🖐 16.4 ☌ 16.4 **FUD** 090 Ⓙ A2 80 50 ▭
> AMA: 2018,Jan,8; 2017,Jan,8; 2016,Jan,13

26/TC PC/TC Only	A2-Z3 ASC Payment	50 Bilateral	♂ Male Only	♀ Female Only	🖐 Facility RVU	☌ Non-Facility RVU	▭ CCI	✖ CLIA
FUD Follow-up Days	CMS: IOM	AMA: CPT Asst	A-Y OPPSI	80/80 Surg Assist Allowed / w/Doc	▦ Lab Crosswalk	▦ Radiology Crosswalk

29904 **Arthroscopy, subtalar joint, surgical; with removal of loose body or foreign body**
    🛠 18.3   ⚒ 18.3   **FUD** 090   J 62 80 50 ▢
    AMA: 2020,Dec,8; 2018,Jan,8; 2017,Jan,8; 2016,Jan,13

29905 **with synovectomy**
    🛠 14.9   ⚒ 14.9   **FUD** 090   J 62 80 50 ▢
    AMA: 2018,Jan,8; 2017,Jan,8; 2016,Jan,13

29906 **with debridement**
    🛠 19.5   ⚒ 19.5   **FUD** 090   J 62 80 50 ▢
    AMA: 2018,Jan,8; 2017,Jan,8; 2016,Jan,13

29907 **with subtalar arthrodesis**
    🛠 25.3   ⚒ 25.3   **FUD** 090   J 62 80 50 ▢
    AMA: 2018,Jan,8; 2017,Jan,8; 2016,Jan,13

29914 **Resequenced code. See code following 29863.**

29915 **Resequenced code. See code following 29863.**

29916 **Resequenced code. See code before 29866.**

29999 **Unlisted procedure, arthroscopy**
    🛠 0.00   ⚒ 0.00   **FUD** YYY   T 80 50 ▢
    AMA: 2019,Dec,12; 2019,Nov,13; 2018,Jan,8; 2017,Apr,9; 2017,Jan,8; 2016,Dec,16; 2016,Jan,13

30000-30115 I&D, Biopsy, Excision Procedures of the Nose

30000 **Drainage abscess or hematoma, nasal, internal approach**

> *EXCLUDES* *Incision and drainage (10060, 10140)*

📖 3.38   🔧 7.18   **FUD** 010   [T] [P2] [80] 🖥

AMA: 2005,May,13-14; 1994,Spr,24

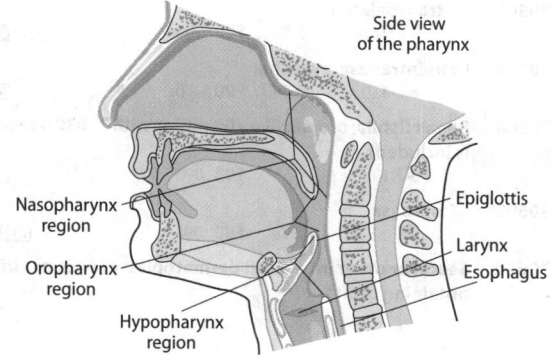

Side view of the pharynx

Nasopharynx region
Oropharynx region
Hypopharynx region
Epiglottis
Larynx
Esophagus

The nasopharynx is the membranous passage above the level of the soft palate; the oropharynx is the region between the soft palate and the upper edge of the epiglottis; the hypopharynx is the region of the epiglottis to the juncture of the larynx and esophagus; the three regions are collectively known as the pharynx

30020 **Drainage abscess or hematoma, nasal septum**

> *EXCLUDES* *Lateral rhinotomy incision (30118, 30320)*

📖 3.37   🔧 6.90   **FUD** 010   [T] [P3] 🖥

30100 **Biopsy, intranasal**

> *EXCLUDES* *Superficial biopsy nose (11102-11107)*

📖 1.91   🔧 4.03   **FUD** 000   [T] [P3] 🖥

AMA: 2019,Jan,9

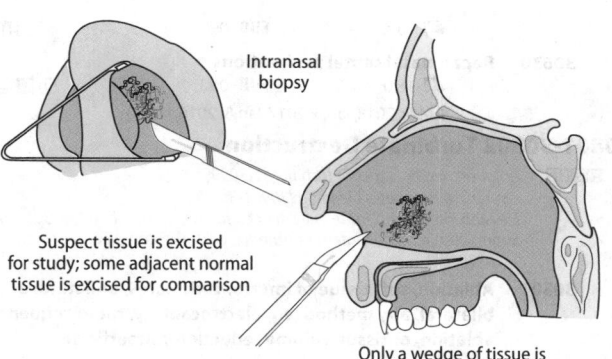

Intranasal biopsy

Suspect tissue is excised for study; some adjacent normal tissue is excised for comparison

Only a wedge of tissue is removed for larger lesions

30110 **Excision, nasal polyp(s), simple**

📖 3.70   🔧 6.82   **FUD** 010   [T] [P3] [50] 🖥

30115 **Excision, nasal polyp(s), extensive**

📖 12.7   🔧 12.7   **FUD** 090   [J] [A2] [50] 🖥

30117-30118 Destruction Procedures Nose

CMS: 100-03,140.5 Laser Procedures

30117 **Excision or destruction (eg, laser), intranasal lesion; internal approach**

📖 9.47   🔧 26.4   **FUD** 090   [J] [A2] 🖥

AMA: 2020,Sep,14; 2019,Nov,14; 2019,Jul,10

30118 **external approach (lateral rhinotomy)**

📖 22.0   🔧 22.0   **FUD** 090   [J] [A2] 🖥

30120-30140 Excision Procedures Nose, Turbinate

30120 **Excision or surgical planing of skin of nose for rhinophyma**

📖 12.3   🔧 14.6   **FUD** 090   [J] [A2] 🖥

AMA: 2018,Jan,8; 2017,Jan,8; 2016,Jan,13

30124 **Excision dermoid cyst, nose; simple, skin, subcutaneous**

📖 8.19   🔧 8.19   **FUD** 090   [T] [R2] 🖥

30125 **complex, under bone or cartilage**

📖 17.5   🔧 17.5   **FUD** 090   [J] [A2] [80] 🖥

30130 **Excision inferior turbinate, partial or complete, any method**

> *EXCLUDES* *Ablation, soft tissue inferior turbinates, unilateral or bilateral, any method (30801-30802)*
> *Excision middle/superior turbinate(s) (30999)*
> *Fracture nasal inferior turbinate(s), therapeutic (30930)*

📖 11.2   🔧 11.2   **FUD** 090   [J] [A2] [50] 🖥

AMA: 2018,Jan,8; 2017,Jan,8; 2016,Jan,13

30140 **Submucous resection inferior turbinate, partial or complete, any method**

> *EXCLUDES* *Ablation, soft tissue inferior turbinates, unilateral or bilateral, any method (30801-30802)*
> *Endoscopic resection concha bullosa middle turbinate (31240)*
> *Fracture nasal inferior turbinate(s), therapeutic (30930)*
> *Submucous resection:*
>   *Nasal septum (30520)*
>   *Superior or middle turbinate (30999)*

📖 5.12   🔧 7.92   **FUD** 000   [J] [A2] [50] 🖥

AMA: 2020,Jan,12; 2018,Jan,8; 2017,Jan,8; 2016,Jan,13

30150-30160 Surgical Removal: Nose

> *EXCLUDES* *Reconstruction and/or closure (primary or delayed primary intention) (13151-13160, 14060-14302, 15120-15121, 15260-15261, 15760, 20900-20912)*

30150 **Rhinectomy; partial**

📖 22.4   🔧 22.4   **FUD** 090   [J] [A2] 🖥

30160 **total**

📖 22.6   🔧 22.6   **FUD** 090   [J] [A2] [80] 🖥

30200-30320 Turbinate Injection, Removal Foreign Substance in the Nose

30200 **Injection into turbinate(s), therapeutic**

📖 1.66   🔧 3.18   **FUD** 000   [T] [P3] 🖥

AMA: 2018,Jan,8; 2017,Jan,8; 2016,Jan,13

30210 **Displacement therapy (Proetz type)**

📖 2.82   🔧 4.24   **FUD** 010   [T] [P3] 🖥

AMA: 2018,Jan,8; 2017,Jan,8; 2016,Jan,13

30220 **Insertion, nasal septal prosthesis (button)**

📖 3.55   🔧 8.60   **FUD** 010   [T] [A2] 🖥

30300 **Removal foreign body, intranasal; office type procedure**

📖 3.23   🔧 5.40   **FUD** 010   [01] [N1] 🖥

AMA: 2018,Jan,8; 2017,Jan,8; 2016,Jan,13

30310 **requiring general anesthesia**

📖 5.80   🔧 5.80   **FUD** 010   [J] [A2] [80] 🖥

30320 **by lateral rhinotomy**

📖 13.2   🔧 13.2   **FUD** 090   [T] [A2] [80] 🖥

30400-30630 Reconstruction or Repair of Nose

> *EXCLUDES* *Harvesting bone/tissue/fat grafts ([15769], 15773-15774, 20900-20924, 21210)*
> *Liposuction for autologous fat grafting (15773-15774)*

30400 **Rhinoplasty, primary; lateral and alar cartilages and/or elevation of nasal tip**

> *INCLUDES* *Carpue's operation*
> *EXCLUDES* *Reconstruction columella (13151-13153)*

📖 34.3   🔧 34.3   **FUD** 090   [J] [A2] [80] 🖥

30410 **complete, external parts including bony pyramid, lateral and alar cartilages, and/or elevation of nasal tip**

📖 39.8   🔧 39.8   **FUD** 090   [J] [A2] [80] 🖥

30420 including major septal repair

🔹 40.3 ⚕ 40.3 **FUD** 090 〔J〕〔A2〕🖳

AMA: 2018,Jan,8; 2017,Nov,11; 2017,Jan,8; 2016,Jul,8

30430 Rhinoplasty, secondary; minor revision (small amount of nasal tip work)

🔹 29.7 ⚕ 29.7 **FUD** 090 〔J〕〔A2〕〔80〕🖳

30435 intermediate revision (bony work with osteotomies)

🔹 37.6 ⚕ 37.6 **FUD** 090 〔J〕〔A2〕〔80〕🖳

30450 major revision (nasal tip work and osteotomies)

🔹 49.8 ⚕ 49.8 **FUD** 090 〔J〕〔A2〕〔80〕🖳

30460 Rhinoplasty for nasal deformity secondary to congenital cleft lip and/or palate, including columellar lengthening; tip only

🔹 23.5 ⚕ 23.5 **FUD** 090 〔J〕〔A2〕〔80〕🖳

AMA: 2018,Jan,8; 2017,Jan,8; 2016,Jan,13

Cleft lip and cleft palate are described according to length of cleft and whether bilateral or unilateral

Complete unilateral cleft lip

Hard palate

Nasal cavity

Nasal septum

Soft palate

Isolated unilateral complete cleft of palate

Bilateral complete cleft of lip and palate

30462 tip, septum, osteotomies

🔹 45.1 ⚕ 45.1 **FUD** 090 〔J〕〔A2〕〔80〕🖳

AMA: 2018,Jan,8; 2017,Jan,8; 2016,Jan,13

30465 Repair of nasal vestibular stenosis (eg, spreader grafting, lateral nasal wall reconstruction)

INCLUDES Bilateral procedure

EXCLUDES Harvesting ear cartilage graft, autogenous (21235)

Repair nasal valve or vestibular lateral wall collapse with implants same side during same operative session (30468)

Repair nasal vestibular stenosis without graft, implant, or reconstruction lateral wall (30999)

Code also modifier 52 for unilateral procedure

🔹 28.5 ⚕ 28.5 **FUD** 090 〔J〕〔A2〕〔80〕🖳

AMA: 2020,Sep,14

30468 Repair of nasal valve collapse with subcutaneous/submucosal lateral wall implant(s)

INCLUDES Bilateral procedure

EXCLUDES Repair nasal vestibular stenosis same side during same operative session (30465)

Repair nasal vestibular stenosis without graft, implant, or reconstruction lateral wall (30999)

Code also modifier 52 for unilateral procedure

🔹 4.87 ⚕ 83.9 **FUD** 000 〔J8〕〔50〕🖳

30520 Septoplasty or submucous resection, with or without cartilage scoring, contouring or replacement with graft

EXCLUDES Turbinate resection (30140)

🔹 18.4 ⚕ 18.4 **FUD** 090 〔J〕〔A2〕🖳

AMA: 2019,Jul,10; 2018,Jan,8; 2017,Jan,8; 2016,Jan,13

30540 Repair choanal atresia; intranasal

🔹 20.2 ⚕ 20.2 **FUD** 090 〔63〕〔J〕〔A2〕〔80〕🖳

30545 transpalatine

🔹 27.6 ⚕ 27.6 **FUD** 090 〔63〕〔J〕〔A2〕〔80〕🖳

30560 Lysis intranasal synechia

🔹 4.02 ⚕ 8.34 **FUD** 010 〔T〕〔A2〕🖳

30580 Repair fistula; oromaxillary (combine with 31030 if antrotomy is included)

🔹 13.6 ⚕ 17.8 **FUD** 090 〔J〕〔A2〕🖳

30600 oronasal

🔹 12.3 ⚕ 16.8 **FUD** 090 〔J〕〔A2〕〔80〕🖳

30620 Septal or other intranasal dermatoplasty (does not include obtaining graft)

Retraction suture

Access incision for lateral rhinotomy

Diseased septal mucosa is excised and graft is placed

🔹 18.2 ⚕ 18.2 **FUD** 090 〔J〕〔A2〕🖳

30630 Repair nasal septal perforations

🔹 18.0 ⚕ 18.0 **FUD** 090 〔J〕〔A2〕〔80〕🖳

AMA: 2018,Jan,8; 2017,Jan,8; 2016,Jan,13

30801-30802 Turbinate Destruction

EXCLUDES Ablation middle/superior turbinates (30999)

Cautery to stop nasal bleeding (30901-30906)

Excision inferior turbinate, partial or complete, any method (30130)

Submucous resection inferior turbinate, partial or complete, any method (30140)

30801 Ablation, soft tissue of inferior turbinates, unilateral or bilateral, any method (eg, electrocautery, radiofrequency ablation, or tissue volume reduction); superficial

EXCLUDES Submucosal ablation inferior turbinates (30802)

🔹 4.10 ⚕ 6.18 **FUD** 010 〔T〕〔A2〕🖳

AMA: 2019,Jul,10

30802 intramural (ie, submucosal)

EXCLUDES Superficial ablation inferior turbinates (30801)

🔹 5.58 ⚕ 7.86 **FUD** 010 〔T〕〔A2〕🖳

AMA: 2019,Jul,10; 2018,Jan,8; 2017,Jan,8; 2016,Jan,13

30901-30920 Control Nose Bleed

30901 Control nasal hemorrhage, anterior, simple (limited cautery and/or packing) any method

🔹 1.64 ⚕ 4.09 **FUD** 000 〔01〕〔N1〕〔50〕🖳

AMA: 2020,Oct,13; 2020,Jul,13

30903 Control nasal hemorrhage, anterior, complex (extensive cautery and/or packing) any method

🔹 2.28 ⚕ 6.49 **FUD** 000 〔T〕〔A2〕〔50〕🖳

AMA: 1990,Win,4

30905 Control nasal hemorrhage, posterior, with posterior nasal packs and/or cautery, any method; initial
🔧 3.07 ⚕ 9.64 **FUD** 000 T A2 🖾
AMA: 2018,Jan,8; 2017,Jan,8; 2016,Jan,13

30906 subsequent
🔧 3.92 ⚕ 10.0 **FUD** 000 T A2 🖾
AMA: 2002,May,7

30915 Ligation arteries; ethmoidal
EXCLUDES External carotid artery (37600)
🔧 16.7 ⚕ 16.7 **FUD** 090 T A2 🖾

30920 internal maxillary artery, transantral
EXCLUDES External carotid artery (37600)
🔧 24.3 ⚕ 24.3 **FUD** 090 T A2 🖾

30930-30999 Other and Unlisted Procedures of Nose

30930 Fracture nasal inferior turbinate(s), therapeutic
EXCLUDES Excision inferior turbinate, partial or complete, any method (30130)
Fracture superior or middle turbinate(s) (30999)
Submucous resection inferior turbinate, partial or complete, any method (30140)
🔧 3.43 ⚕ 3.43 **FUD** 010 J A2 🖾
AMA: 2018,Jan,8; 2017,Nov,11; 2017,Jan,8; 2016,Jul,8; 2016,Jan,13

30999 Unlisted procedure, nose
🔧 0.00 ⚕ 0.00 **FUD** YYY T 80 🖾
AMA: 2020,Sep,14; 2019,Nov,14; 2018,Jan,8; 2017,Jan,8; 2016,Jan,13

31000-31230 Opening Sinuses

31000 Lavage by cannulation; maxillary sinus (antrum puncture or natural ostium)
🔧 3.02 ⚕ 5.17 **FUD** 010 T P2 50 🖾
AMA: 2018,Jan,8; 2017,Jan,8; 2016,Jan,13

Schematic showing lateral wall of the nasal cavity (above) and coronal section showing nasal and paranasal sinuses (left)

Frontal sinus
Crista galli
Ethmoidal cells
Orbital cavity
Posterior ethmoidal cells
Sphenoid sinus
Nostril
Conchae (nasal cavity)
Hard palate
Maxillary sinus
Superior, middle, and inferior conchae
Caldwell-Luc approach

31002 sphenoid sinus
🔧 5.39 ⚕ 5.39 **FUD** 010 T J8 80 50 🖾

31020 Sinusotomy, maxillary (antrotomy); intranasal
🔧 10.4 ⚕ 13.6 **FUD** 090 J A2 50 🖾

31030 radical (Caldwell-Luc) without removal of antrochoanal polyps
🔧 14.7 ⚕ 18.4 **FUD** 090 J A2 50 🖾

31032 radical (Caldwell-Luc) with removal of antrochoanal polyps
🔧 16.5 ⚕ 16.5 **FUD** 090 J A2 50 🖾

31040 Pterygomaxillary fossa surgery, any approach
EXCLUDES Transantral ligation internal maxillary artery (30920)
🔧 22.0 ⚕ 22.0 **FUD** 090 J R2 50 🖾

31050 Sinusotomy, sphenoid, with or without biopsy;
🔧 14.1 ⚕ 14.1 **FUD** 090 J A2 50 🖾

31051 with mucosal stripping or removal of polyp(s)
🔧 19.0 ⚕ 19.0 **FUD** 090 J A2 50 🖾

31070 Sinusotomy frontal; external, simple (trephine operation)
INCLUDES Killian operation
EXCLUDES Intranasal frontal sinusotomy (31276)
🔧 12.9 ⚕ 12.9 **FUD** 090 J A2 50 🖾

31075 transorbital, unilateral (for mucocele or osteoma, Lynch type)
🔧 22.8 ⚕ 22.8 **FUD** 090 J A2 80 50 🖾

31080 obliterative without osteoplastic flap, brow incision (includes ablation)
INCLUDES Ridell sinusotomy
🔧 30.0 ⚕ 30.0 **FUD** 090 J A2 80 50 🖾

31081 obliterative, without osteoplastic flap, coronal incision (includes ablation)
🔧 32.3 ⚕ 32.3 **FUD** 090 J A2 80 50 🖾

31084 obliterative, with osteoplastic flap, brow incision
🔧 33.5 ⚕ 33.5 **FUD** 090 J A2 80 50 🖾

31085 obliterative, with osteoplastic flap, coronal incision
🔧 34.6 ⚕ 34.6 **FUD** 090 J J8 80 50 🖾

31086 nonobliterative, with osteoplastic flap, brow incision
🔧 32.6 ⚕ 32.6 **FUD** 090 J A2 80 50 🖾

31087 nonobliterative, with osteoplastic flap, coronal incision
🔧 31.2 ⚕ 31.2 **FUD** 090 J A2 80 50 🖾

31090 Sinusotomy, unilateral, 3 or more paranasal sinuses (frontal, maxillary, ethmoid, sphenoid)
🔧 30.3 ⚕ 30.3 **FUD** 090 J A2 50 🖾
AMA: 1998,Nov,1; 1997,Nov,1

31200 Ethmoidectomy; intranasal, anterior
🔧 16.7 ⚕ 16.7 **FUD** 090 J A2 50 🖾
AMA: 2018,Jan,8; 2017,Jan,8; 2016,Feb,10

31201 intranasal, total
🔧 21.9 ⚕ 21.9 **FUD** 090 J A2 50 🖾
AMA: 2018,Jan,8; 2017,Jan,8; 2016,Feb,10

31205 extranasal, total
🔧 26.3 ⚕ 26.3 **FUD** 090 J A2 80 50 🖾
AMA: 2018,Jan,8; 2017,Jan,8; 2016,Feb,10

31225 Maxillectomy; without orbital exenteration
🔧 52.1 ⚕ 52.1 **FUD** 090 C 80 50 🖾

31230 with orbital exenteration (en bloc)
EXCLUDES Orbital exenteration without maxillectomy (65110-65114)
Skin grafts (15120-15121)
🔧 58.3 ⚕ 58.3 **FUD** 090 C 80 50 🖾

31231-31235 Nasal Endoscopy, Diagnostic

INCLUDES Complete sinus exam (e.g., nasal cavity, turbinates, sphenoethmoidal recess)
Code also stereotactic navigation, when performed (61782)

31231 Nasal endoscopy, diagnostic, unilateral or bilateral (separate procedure)
🔧 1.82 ⚕ 5.48 **FUD** 000 T P2 🖾
AMA: 2018,Apr,3; 2018,Jan,8; 2017,Jul,7; 2017,Jan,8; 2017,Jan,6; 2016,Dec,13; 2016,Feb,10; 2016,Jan,13

31233 Nasal/sinus endoscopy, diagnostic; with maxillary sinusoscopy (via inferior meatus or canine fossa puncture)
EXCLUDES When performed on same side:
Dilation of maxillary sinus ostium (31295)
Maxillary antrostomy (31256, 31267)
🔧 3.87 ⚕ 7.41 **FUD** 000 T A2 80 50 🖾
AMA: 2018,Apr,3; 2018,Jan,8; 2017,Jan,8; 2016,Jan,13

31235 **with sphenoid sinusoscopy (via puncture of sphenoidal face or cannulation of ostium)**

> *EXCLUDES* *Insertion drug-eluting implant performed with biopsy, debridement, or polypectomy (31237)*
> *Insertion drug-eluting implant without other nasal/sinus endoscopic procedure (31299)*
> *When performed on same side:*
> *Sinus dilation (31297-31298)*
> *Sphenoidotomy (31287-31288)*
> *Total ethmoidectomy with sphenoidotomy ([31257, 31259])*

　　🔵 4.54　　🔧 8.49　　**FUD** 000　　　J A2 80 50 ▣

AMA: 2018,Apr,3; 2018,Jan,8; 2017,Jan,8; 2016,Jan,13

31237-31253 [31253] Nasal Endoscopy, Surgical

> *INCLUDES* Diagnostic nasal/sinus endoscopy
> Code also stereotactic navigation, when performed (61782)

31237 **Nasal/sinus endoscopy, surgical; with biopsy, polypectomy or debridement (separate procedure)**

> *EXCLUDES* *When performed on same side:*
> *Frontal sinus exploration (31276)*
> *Maxillary antrostomy (31256, 31267)*
> *Nasal hemorrhage control (31238)*
> *Optic nerve decompression (31294)*
> *Orbital wall decompression, medial and/or inferior (31292-31293)*
> *Other total ethmoidectomy procedures ([31253], 31255, [31257], [31259])*
> *Partial ethmoidectomy (31254)*
> *Repair CSF leak (31290-31291)*
> *Sphenoidotomy (31287-31288)*

　　🔵 4.54　　🔧 7.21　　**FUD** 000　　　J A2 50 ▣

AMA: 2020,Jan,12; 2019,Jul,7; 2019,Apr,10; 2018,Apr,3; 2018,Jan,8; 2017,Jan,8; 2016,Feb,10; 2016,Jan,13

31238 **with control of nasal hemorrhage**

> *EXCLUDES* *When performed on same side:*
> *Biopsy, polypectomy, or debridement (31237)*
> *Sphenopalatine artery ligation (31241)*

　　🔵 4.80　　🔧 7.17　　**FUD** 000　　　J A2 80 50 ▣

AMA: 2018,Apr,3; 2018,Jan,8; 2017,Jan,8; 2016,Jan,13

31239 **with dacryocystorhinostomy**

　　🔵 17.4　　🔧 17.4　　**FUD** 010　　　J A2 80 50 ▣

AMA: 2018,Apr,3; 2018,Jan,8; 2017,Jan,8; 2016,Jan,13

31240 **with concha bullosa resection**

　　🔵 4.52　　🔧 4.52　　**FUD** 000　　　J A2 80 50 ▣

AMA: 2018,Apr,3; 2018,Jan,8; 2017,Jan,8; 2016,Feb,10; 2016,Jan,13

31241 **with ligation of sphenopalatine artery**

> *EXCLUDES* *When performed on same side:*
> *Nasal hemorrhage control (31238)*

　　🔵 12.7　　🔧 12.7　　**FUD** 000　　　C G2 80 50 ▣

AMA: 2018,Apr,3

31253 Resequenced code. See code following 31255.

31254-31259 [31253, 31257, 31259] Nasal Endoscopy with Ethmoid Removal

> *INCLUDES* Diagnostic nasal/sinus endoscopy
> Sinusotomy, when applicable
> *EXCLUDES* *When performed on same side:*
> *Biopsy, polypectomy, or debridement (31237)*
> *Optic nerve decompression (31294)*
> *Orbital wall decompression, medial, and/or inferior (31292-31293)*
> *Repair CSF leak (31290-31291)*
> Code also stereotactic navigation, when performed (61782)

31254 **Nasal/sinus endoscopy, surgical with ethmoidectomy; partial (anterior)**

> *EXCLUDES* *When performed on same side:*
> *Other total ethmoidectomy procedures (31253, 31255, [31257], [31259])*

　　🔵 7.01　　🔧 11.7　　**FUD** 000　　　J A2 50 ▣

AMA: 2019,Apr,10; 2018,Apr,3; 2018,Jan,8; 2017,Jan,8; 2016,Feb,10; 2016,Jan,13

31255 **total (anterior and posterior)**

> *EXCLUDES* *When performed on same side:*
> *Frontal sinus exploration (31276)*
> *Other total ethmoidectomy procedures (31253, [31257], [31259])*
> *Partial ethmoidectomy (31254)*
> *Sphenoidotomy (31287-31288)*

　　🔵 9.31　　🔧 9.31　　**FUD** 000　　　J A2 50 ▣

AMA: 2019,Apr,10; 2018,Apr,3; 2018,Apr,10; 2018,Jan,8; 2017,Jan,8; 2016,Feb,10; 2016,Jan,13

 # 31253 **total (anterior and posterior), including frontal sinus exploration, with removal of tissue from frontal sinus, when performed**

> *EXCLUDES* *When performed on same side:*
> *Dilation sinus (31296, 31298)*
> *Frontal sinus exploration (31276)*
> *Partial ethmoidectomy (31254)*
> *Total ethmoidectomy (31255)*

　　🔵 14.4　　🔧 14.4　　**FUD** 000　　　J G2 50 ▣

AMA: 2019,Apr,10; 2018,Apr,10; 2018,Apr,3

 # 31257 **total (anterior and posterior), including sphenoidotomy**

> *EXCLUDES* *When performed on same side:*
> *Diagnostic sphenoid sinusoscopy (31235)*
> *Dilation sinus (31297-31298)*
> *Other total ethmoidectomy procedures (31255, [31259])*
> *Partial ethmoidectomy (31254)*
> *Sphenoidotomy (31287-31288)*

　　🔵 12.8　　🔧 12.8　　**FUD** 000　　　J G2 50 ▣

AMA: 2019,Apr,10; 2018,Apr,10; 2018,Apr,3

 # 31259 **total (anterior and posterior), including sphenoidotomy, with removal of tissue from the sphenoid sinus**

> *EXCLUDES* *When performed on same side:*
> *Diagnostic sphenoid sinusoscopy (31235)*
> *Dilation sinus (31297-31298)*
> *Other total ethmoidectomy procedures (31255, [31257])*
> *Partial ethmoidectomy (31254)*
> *Sphenoidotomy (31287-31288)*

　　🔵 13.6　　🔧 13.6　　**FUD** 000　　　J G2 50 ▣

AMA: 2019,Apr,10; 2018,Apr,3

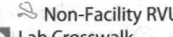

31256-31267 [31257, 31259] Nasal Endoscopy with Maxillary Procedures

INCLUDES Diagnostic nasal/sinus endoscopy
Sinusotomy, when applicable
EXCLUDES *When performed on same side:*
Biopsy, polypectomy, or debridement (31237)
Dilation maxillary sinus ostium (31295)
Maxillary sinusoscopy (31233)
Code also stereotactic navigation, when performed (61782)

31256 Nasal/sinus endoscopy, surgical, with maxillary antrostomy;

> **EXCLUDES** *When performed on the same side:*
> *Maxillary antrostomy with removal of tissue from maxillary sinus (31267)*
>
> 5.19 5.19 **FUD** 000   J A2 50
>
> **AMA:** 2019,Apr,10; 2018,Apr,3; 2018,Apr,10; 2018,Jan,8; 2017,Jan,8; 2016,Jan,13

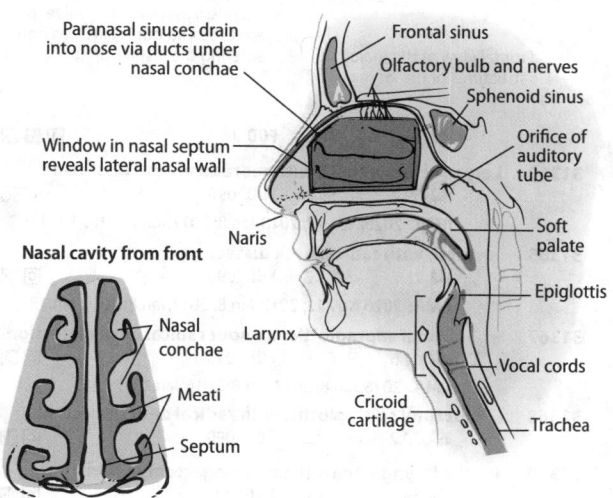

Paranasal sinuses drain into nose via ducts under nasal conchae
Frontal sinus
Olfactory bulb and nerves
Sphenoid sinus
Window in nasal septum reveals lateral nasal wall
Orifice of auditory tube
Naris
Soft palate
Epiglottis
Nasal conchae
Larynx
Vocal cords
Meati
Cricoid cartilage
Trachea
Septum
Nasal cavity from front

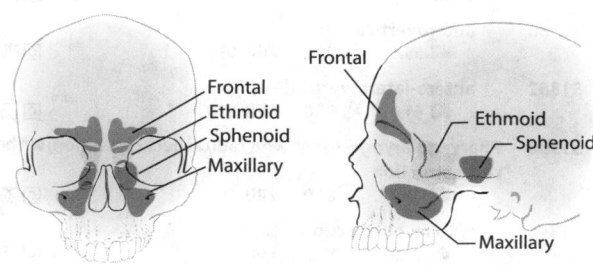

Frontal
Ethmoid
Sphenoid
Maxillary
Frontal
Ethmoid
Sphenoid
Maxillary

31257 Resequenced code. See code following 31255.

31259 Resequenced code. See code following 31255.

31267 with removal of tissue from maxillary sinus

> **EXCLUDES** *When performed on same side:*
> *Maxillary antrostomy without removal tissue (31256)*
>
> 7.61 7.61 **FUD** 000   J A2 50
>
> **AMA:** 2019,Apr,10; 2018,Apr,3; 2018,Jan,8; 2017,Jan,8; 2016,Jan,13

31276 Nasal Endoscopy with Frontal Sinus Examination

INCLUDES Diagnostic nasal/sinus endoscopy
Sinusotomy, when applicable
EXCLUDES *When performed on same side:*
Biopsy, polypectomy, or debridement (31237)
Dilation frontal or frontal and sphenoid sinus (31296, 31298)
Other total ethmoidectomy procedures (31253, 31255)
Code also stereotactic navigation, when performed (61782)

31276 Nasal/sinus endoscopy, surgical, with frontal sinus exploration, including removal of tissue from frontal sinus, when performed

> 10.9 10.9 **FUD** 000   J A2 50
>
> **AMA:** 2019,Apr,10; 2018,Apr,3; 2018,Apr,10; 2018,Jan,8; 2017,Jan,8; 2016,Jan,13

31287-31288 Nasal Endoscopy with Sphenoid Procedures

EXCLUDES *Sinus dilation (31297-31298)*
When performed on same side:
Biopsy, polypectomy, or debridement (31237)
Diagnostic sphenoid sinusoscopy (31235)
Optic nerve decompression (31294)
Other total ethmoidectomy procedures (31255, [31257], [31259])
Repair CSF leak (31291)
Code also stereotactic navigation, when performed (61782)

31287 Nasal/sinus endoscopy, surgical, with sphenoidotomy;

> **EXCLUDES** *When performed on same side:*
> *Sphenoidotomy with removal tissue (31288)*
>
> 5.78 5.78 **FUD** 000   J A2 80 50
>
> **AMA:** 2019,Apr,10; 2018,Apr,3; 2018,Jan,8; 2017,Jan,8; 2016,Jan,13

31288 with removal of tissue from the sphenoid sinus

> **EXCLUDES** *When performed on same side:*
> *Sphenoidotomy without removal tissue (31287)*
>
> 6.71 6.71 **FUD** 000   J A2 80 50
>
> **AMA:** 2019,Apr,10; 2018,Apr,3; 2018,Jan,8; 2017,Jan,8; 2016,Feb,10; 2016,Jan,13

31290-31294 Nasal Endoscopy with Repair and Decompression

INCLUDES Diagnostic nasal/sinus endoscopy
Sinusotomy, when applicable
EXCLUDES *When performed on same side:*
Biopsy, polypectomy, or debridement (31237)
Other total ethmoidectomy procedures ([31253], 31255, [31257], [31259])
Partial ethmoidectomy (31254)
Code also stereotactic navigation, when performed (61782)

31290 Nasal/sinus endoscopy, surgical, with repair of cerebrospinal fluid leak; ethmoid region

> 32.7 32.7 **FUD** 010   C 80 50
>
> **AMA:** 2018,Apr,3; 2018,Jan,8; 2017,Jan,8; 2016,Feb,10; 2016,Jan,13

31291 sphenoid region

> **EXCLUDES** *When performed on same side:*
> *Sphenoidotomy (31287-31288)*
>
> 34.9 34.9 **FUD** 010   C 80 50
>
> **AMA:** 2018,Apr,3; 2018,Jan,8; 2017,Jan,8; 2016,Jan,13

31292 Nasal/sinus endoscopy, surgical, with orbital decompression; medial or inferior wall

> **EXCLUDES** *When performed on same side:*
> *Dilation frontal sinus only (31296)*
> *Orbital wall decompression, medial and inferior (31293)*
>
> 28.4 28.4 **FUD** 010   J 62 80 50
>
> **AMA:** 2018,Apr,3; 2018,Jan,8; 2017,Jan,8; 2016,Jan,13

31293 medial and inferior wall

> **EXCLUDES** *When performed on same side:*
> *Orbital wall decompression, medial or inferior (31292)*
>
> 30.8 30.8 **FUD** 010   J 62 80 50
>
> **AMA:** 2018,Apr,3; 2018,Jan,8; 2017,Jan,8; 2016,Jan,13

Respiratory System

31294 — 31400

31294   **Nasal/sinus endoscopy, surgical, with optic nerve decompression**

> EXCLUDES   *When performed on same side:*
> *Sphenoidotomy (31287-31288)*

🔧 35.2   ✂ 35.2   **FUD** 010   J 62 80 50 ▭

AMA: 2018,Apr,3; 2018,Jan,8; 2017,Jan,8; 2016,Jan,13

31295-31298 Nasal Endoscopy with Sinus Ostia Dilation

> INCLUDES   Any method tissue displacement
> Fluoroscopy, when performed
> Code also stereotactic navigation, when performed (61782)

31295   **Nasal/sinus endoscopy, surgical, with dilation (eg, balloon dilation); maxillary sinus ostium, transnasal or via canine fossa**

> EXCLUDES   *When performed on same side:*
> *Maxillary antrostomy (31256-31267)*
> *Maxillary sinusoscopy (31233)*

🔧 4.55   ✂ 55.6   **FUD** 000   J P3 80 50 ▭

AMA: 2020,Jun,14; 2018,Apr,3; 2018,Jan,8; 2017,Jan,8; 2016,Jan,13

31296   **frontal sinus ostium**

> EXCLUDES   *When performed on same side:*
> *Frontal sinus exploration (31276)*
> *Dilation frontal and sphenoid sinus (31298)*
> *Dilation sphenoid sinus only (31297)*
> *Total ethmoidectomy (31253)*

🔧 5.15   ✂ 54.2   **FUD** 000   J P3 80 50 ▭

AMA: 2020,Jun,14; 2018,Apr,3; 2018,Jan,8; 2017,Jan,8; 2016,Jan,13

31297   **sphenoid sinus ostium**

> EXCLUDES   *When performed on same side:*
> *Diagnostic sphenoid sinusoscopy (31235)*
> *Dilation frontal and sphenoid sinus (31298)*
> *Dilation frontal sinus only (31296)*
> *Sphenoidotomy (31287-31288)*
> *Total ethmoidectomy procedures ([31257], [31259])*

🔧 4.12   ✂ 53.1   **FUD** 000   J P3 80 50 ▭

AMA: 2020,Jun,14; 2018,Apr,3; 2018,Jan,8; 2017,Jan,8; 2016,Jan,13

31298   **frontal and sphenoid sinus ostia**

> EXCLUDES   *When performed on same side:*
> *Diagnostic sphenoid sinusoscopy (31235)*
> *Dilation frontal sinus only (31296)*
> *Dilation sphenoid sinus only (31297)*
> *Frontal sinus exploration (31276)*
> *Other total ethmoidectomy procedures (31253, [31257], [31259])*
> *Sphenoidotomy (31287-31288)*

🔧 7.34   ✂ 102.   **FUD** 000   J P2 80 50 ▭

AMA: 2020,Jun,14; 2018,Apr,3

31299 Unlisted Procedures of Accessory Sinuses

CMS: 100-04,4,180.3 Unlisted Service or Procedure

> EXCLUDES   *Hypophysectomy (61546, 61548)*

31299   **Unlisted procedure, accessory sinuses**

🔧 0.00   ✂ 0.00   **FUD** YYY   T 80 ▭

AMA: 2019,Jul,7; 2019,Apr,10; 2018,Jan,8; 2017,Nov,11; 2017,Jan,8; 2016,Feb,10; 2016,Jan,13

31300-31502 Procedures of the Larynx

31300   **Laryngotomy (thyrotomy, laryngofissure), with removal of tumor or laryngocele, cordectomy**

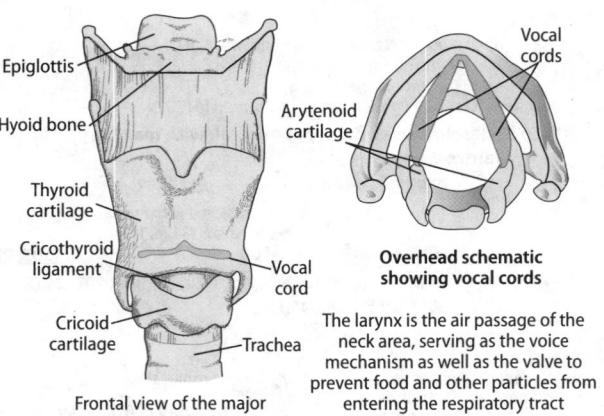

Epiglottis
Hyoid bone
Thyroid cartilage
Cricothyroid ligament
Cricoid cartilage
Vocal cord
Trachea

Frontal view of the major structures of the larynx

Vocal cords
Arytenoid cartilage

Overhead schematic showing vocal cords

The larynx is the air passage of the neck area, serving as the voice mechanism as well as the valve to prevent food and other particles from entering the respiratory tract

🔧 36.6   ✂ 36.6   **FUD** 090   J A2 80 ▭

31360   **Laryngectomy; total, without radical neck dissection**

🔧 59.2   ✂ 59.2   **FUD** 090   C 80 ▭

AMA: 2020,Nov,12; 2018,Jan,8; 2017,Jan,8; 2016,Jan,13

31365   **total, with radical neck dissection**

🔧 73.2   ✂ 73.2   **FUD** 090   C 80 ▭

AMA: 2020,Nov,12; 2018,Jan,8; 2017,Jan,8; 2016,Jan,13

31367   **subtotal supraglottic, without radical neck dissection**

🔧 62.6   ✂ 62.6   **FUD** 090   C 80 ▭

AMA: 2018,Jan,8; 2017,Jan,8; 2016,Jan,13

31368   **subtotal supraglottic, with radical neck dissection**

🔧 70.2   ✂ 70.2   **FUD** 090   C 80 ▭

31370   **Partial laryngectomy (hemilaryngectomy); horizontal**

🔧 59.4   ✂ 59.4   **FUD** 090   C 80 ▭

31375   **laterovertical**

🔧 55.8   ✂ 55.8   **FUD** 090   C 80 ▭

31380   **anterovertical**

🔧 55.6   ✂ 55.6   **FUD** 090   C 80 ▭

31382   **antero-latero-vertical**

🔧 61.0   ✂ 61.0   **FUD** 090   C 80 ▭

31390   **Pharyngolaryngectomy, with radical neck dissection; without reconstruction**

🔧 81.0   ✂ 81.0   **FUD** 090   C 80 ▭

31395   **with reconstruction**

🔧 86.5   ✂ 86.5   **FUD** 090   C 80 ▭

31400   **Arytenoidectomy or arytenoidopexy, external approach**

> EXCLUDES   *Endoscopic arytenoidectomy (31560)*

🔧 28.0   ✂ 28.0   **FUD** 090   J A2 80 ▭

31420 Epiglottidectomy

Epiglottis
Hyoid bone

Choanae

Parotid gland

Nasal septum

Root of tongue

Posterior cutaway view

Epiglottis

Aditus of larynx

Plane of view

🔧 23.4   🔨 23.4   **FUD** 090   J A2 80 ▱

31500 Intubation, endotracheal, emergency procedure

EXCLUDES *Chest x-ray performed to confirm endotracheal tube position*

🔧 4.14   🔨 4.14   **FUD** 000   T G2 ▱

AMA: 2018,Jan,8; 2017,Jan,8; 2016,Oct,8; 2016,May,3; 2016,Jan,13

31502 Tracheotomy tube change prior to establishment of fistula tract

🔧 1.01   🔨 1.01   **FUD** 000   T G2 ▱

AMA: 2020,Dec,11

31505-31541 Endoscopy of the Larynx

31505 Laryngoscopy, indirect; diagnostic (separate procedure)

🔧 1.39   🔨 2.48   **FUD** 000   T P3 ▱

AMA: 2018,Jan,8; 2017,Jan,8; 2016,Jan,13

31510 with biopsy

🔧 3.46   🔨 6.01   **FUD** 000   J A2 80 ▱

AMA: 2018,Jan,8; 2017,Jan,8; 2016,Jan,13

31511 with removal of foreign body

🔧 3.79   🔨 6.04   **FUD** 000   T A2 ▱

AMA: 2018,Jan,8; 2017,Jan,8; 2016,Jan,13

31512 with removal of lesion

🔧 3.70   🔨 5.92   **FUD** 000   J A2 80 ▱

AMA: 2018,Jan,8; 2017,Jan,8; 2016,Jan,13

31513 with vocal cord injection

🔧 3.76   🔨 3.76   **FUD** 000   T A2 80 ▱

AMA: 2018,Jan,8; 2017,Jan,8; 2016,Jan,13

31515 Laryngoscopy direct, with or without tracheoscopy; for aspiration

🔧 3.12   🔨 5.79   **FUD** 000   T A2 ▱

AMA: 2020,Dec,11

31520 diagnostic, newborn

🔧 4.44   🔨 4.44   **FUD** 000   A   63 T G2 80 ▱

AMA: 2020,Dec,11

31525 diagnostic, except newborn

🔧 4.56   🔨 7.15   **FUD** 000   J A2 ▱

AMA: 2020,Dec,11; 2018,Jan,8; 2017,Jan,8; 2016,Jan,13

31526 diagnostic, with operating microscope or telescope

INCLUDES Operating microscope (69990)

🔧 4.49   🔨 4.49   **FUD** 000   J A2 ▱

AMA: 2020,Dec,11; 2018,Jan,8; 2017,Jun,10; 2016,Feb,12

31527 with insertion of obturator

🔧 5.55   🔨 5.55   **FUD** 000   J A2 80 ▱

AMA: 2020,Dec,11

31528 with dilation, initial

🔧 4.09   🔨 4.09   **FUD** 000   J A2 80 ▱

AMA: 2020,Dec,11

31529 with dilation, subsequent

🔧 4.59   🔨 4.59   **FUD** 000   J A2 80 ▱

AMA: 2020,Dec,11

31530 Laryngoscopy, direct, operative, with foreign body removal;

🔧 5.70   🔨 5.70   **FUD** 000   J A2 ▱

AMA: 2020,Dec,11

31531 with operating microscope or telescope

INCLUDES Operating microscope (69990)

🔧 6.08   🔨 6.08   **FUD** 000   J A2 80 ▱

AMA: 2020,Dec,11; 2018,Jan,8; 2017,Jun,10; 2016,Feb,12

31535 Laryngoscopy, direct, operative, with biopsy;

🔧 5.39   🔨 5.39   **FUD** 000   J A2 ▱

AMA: 2020,Dec,11

31536 with operating microscope or telescope

INCLUDES Operating microscope (69990)

🔧 6.00   🔨 6.00   **FUD** 000   J A2 ▱

AMA: 2020,Dec,11; 2018,Jan,8; 2017,Jun,10; 2016,Feb,12

31540 Laryngoscopy, direct, operative, with excision of tumor and/or stripping of vocal cords or epiglottis;

🔧 6.89   🔨 6.89   **FUD** 000   J A2 ▱

AMA: 2020,Dec,11

31541 with operating microscope or telescope

INCLUDES Operating microscope (69990)

🔧 7.52   🔨 7.52   **FUD** 000   J A2 ▱

AMA: 2020,Dec,11; 2019,Sep,10; 2019,Jul,10; 2018,Jan,8; 2017,Jun,10; 2016,Feb,12

31545-31554 [31551, 31552, 31553, 31554] Endoscopy of Larynx with Reconstruction

INCLUDES Operating microscope (69990)

EXCLUDES *Laryngoscopy, direct, operative, with excision tumor and/or vocal cord or epiglottis stripping (31540-31541)*
Vocal cord reconstruction with allograft (31599)

31545 Laryngoscopy, direct, operative, with operating microscope or telescope, with submucosal removal of non-neoplastic lesion(s) of vocal cord; reconstruction with local tissue flap(s)

🔧 10.3   🔨 10.3   **FUD** 000   J A2 50 ▱

AMA: 2020,Dec,11; 2016,Feb,12

31546 reconstruction with graft(s) (includes obtaining autograft)

EXCLUDES *Autologous fat graft obtained by liposuction (15771-15774)*
Autologous soft tissue grafts obtained by direct excision ([15769])

🔧 15.7   🔨 15.7   **FUD** 000   J A2 50 ▱

AMA: 2020,Dec,11; 2018,Jan,8; 2017,Jan,8; 2016,Feb,12; 2016,Jan,13

31551	Resequenced code. See code following 31580.
31552	Resequenced code. See code following 31580.
31553	Resequenced code. See code following 31580.
31554	Resequenced code. See code following 31580.

31560-31571 Endoscopy of Larynx with Arytenoid Removal, Vocal Cord Injection

31560 Laryngoscopy, direct, operative, with arytenoidectomy;

🔧 8.97   🔨 8.97   **FUD** 000   J A2 80 ▱

AMA: 2020,Dec,11

31561 with operating microscope or telescope

INCLUDES Operating microscope (69990)

🔧 9.82   🔨 9.82   **FUD** 000   J A2 80 ▱

AMA: 2020,Dec,11; 2018,Jan,8; 2017,Jun,10; 2016,Feb,12

● New Code   ▲ Revised Code   ○ Reinstated   ● New Web Release   ▲ Revised Web Release   + Add-on   Unlisted   Not Covered   # Resequenced
50 Optum Mod 50 Exempt   Ⓝ AMA Mod 51 Exempt   51 Optum Mod 51 Exempt   63 Mod 63 Exempt   ⚲ Non-FDA Drug   ★ Telemedicine   M Maternity   A Age Edit

31570 Laryngoscopy, direct, with injection into vocal cord(s), therapeutic;

🔪 6.53   ⚕ 9.68   **FUD** 000   J A2 🖵

AMA: 2020,Dec,11; 2018,Jan,8; 2017,Jan,8; 2017,Jan,6; 2016,Jan,13

31571 with operating microscope or telescope

INCLUDES   Operating microscope (69990)

🔪 7.14   ⚕ 7.14   **FUD** 000   J A2 🖵

AMA: 2020,Dec,11; 2018,Jan,8; 2017,Jun,10; 2017,Jan,8; 2017,Jan,6; 2016,Feb,12; 2016,Jan,13

31572-31579 [31572, 31573, 31574] Endoscopy of Larynx, Flexible Fiberoptic

EXCLUDES   Evaluation by flexible fiberoptic endoscope:
     Sensory assessment (92614-92615)
     Swallowing (92612-92613)
     Swallowing and sensory assessment (92616-92617)
   Flexible fiberoptic endoscopic examination/testing by cine or video recording (92612-92617)

31572 Resequenced code. See code following 31578.

31573 Resequenced code. See code following 31578.

31574 Resequenced code. See code following 31578.

31575 Laryngoscopy, flexible; diagnostic

EXCLUDES   Diagnostic nasal endoscopy not through additional endoscope (31231)
   Procedure during same session ([31572, 31573, 31574], 31576-31578, 42975, 43197-43198, 92511, 92612, 92614, 92616)

🔪 1.90   ⚕ 3.49   **FUD** 000   T P2 🖵

AMA: 2020,Dec,11; 2018,Jan,8; 2017,Jul,7; 2017,Apr,8; 2017,Jan,8; 2016,Dec,13

31576 with biopsy(ies)

EXCLUDES   Destruction or excision lesion (31572, 31578)

🔪 3.38   ⚕ 7.63   **FUD** 000   J A2 🖵

AMA: 2018,Jan,8; 2017,Jul,7; 2017,Apr,8; 2017,Jan,8; 2016,Dec,13

31577 with removal of foreign body(s)

🔪 3.82   ⚕ 7.93   **FUD** 000   T A2 80 🖵

AMA: 2018,Jan,8; 2017,Jul,7; 2017,Apr,8; 2017,Jan,8; 2016,Dec,13

31578 with removal of lesion(s), non-laser

🔪 4.27   ⚕ 8.59   **FUD** 000   J A2 80 🖵

AMA: 2018,Jan,8; 2017,Jul,7; 2017,Apr,8; 2017,Jan,8; 2016,Dec,13

\# **31572** with ablation or destruction of lesion(s) with laser, unilateral

EXCLUDES   Biopsy or excision lesion (31576, 31578)

🔪 5.15   ⚕ 14.7   **FUD** 000   J 62 80 50 🖵

AMA: 2020,Dec,11; 2019,Sep,10; 2018,Jan,8; 2017,Jul,7; 2017,Apr,8; 2017,Jan,8; 2016,Dec,13

\# **31573** with therapeutic injection(s) (eg, chemodenervation agent or corticosteroid, injected percutaneous, transoral, or via endoscope channel), unilateral

🔪 4.27   ⚕ 7.61   **FUD** 000   J P3 80 50 🖵

AMA: 2020,Dec,11; 2018,May,7; 2018,Jan,8; 2017,Jul,7; 2017,Apr,8; 2017,Jan,8; 2016,Dec,13

\# **31574** with injection(s) for augmentation (eg, percutaneous, transoral), unilateral

🔪 4.27   ⚕ 28.7   **FUD** 000   J 62 80 50 🖵

AMA: 2020,Dec,11; 2018,May,7; 2018,Jan,8; 2017,Jul,7; 2017,Apr,8; 2017,Jan,8; 2016,Dec,13

31579 Laryngoscopy, flexible or rigid telescopic, with stroboscopy

🔪 3.41   ⚕ 5.46   **FUD** 000   T P3 🖵

AMA: 2018,Jan,8; 2017,Jul,7; 2017,Apr,8; 2017,Jan,8; 2016,Dec,13

31580-31599 [31551, 31552, 31553, 31554] Larynx Reconstruction

31580 Laryngoplasty; for laryngeal web, with indwelling keel or stent insertion

EXCLUDES   Keel or stent removal (31599)
   Tracheostomy (31600-31601, 31603, 31605, 31610)
   Treatment laryngeal stenosis (31551-31554)

🔪 35.7   ⚕ 35.7   **FUD** 090   J A2 80 🖵

AMA: 2018,Jan,8; 2017,Apr,5; 2017,Mar,10

\# **31551** for laryngeal stenosis, with graft, without indwelling stent placement, younger than 12 years of age   A

EXCLUDES   Cartilage graft obtained through same incision
   Procedure during same session (31552-31554, 31580)
   Tracheostomy (31600-31601, 31603, 31605, 31610)

🔪 41.2   ⚕ 41.2   **FUD** 090   J 62 80 🖵

AMA: 2020,Dec,11; 2018,Jan,8; 2017,Jul,7; 2017,Apr,5; 2017,Mar,10

\# **31552** for laryngeal stenosis, with graft, without indwelling stent placement, age 12 years or older   A

EXCLUDES   Cartilage graft obtained through same incision
   Procedure during same session (31551, 31553-31554, 31580)
   Tracheostomy (31600-31601, 31603, 31605, 31610)

🔪 42.0   ⚕ 42.0   **FUD** 090   J 62 80 🖵

AMA: 2020,Dec,11; 2018,Jan,8; 2017,Jul,7; 2017,Apr,5; 2017,Mar,10

\# **31553** for laryngeal stenosis, with graft, with indwelling stent placement, younger than 12 years of age   A

EXCLUDES   Cartilage graft obtained through same incision
   Procedure during same session (31551-31552, 31554, 31580)
   Stent removal (31599)
   Tracheostomy (31600-31601, 31603, 31605, 31610)

🔪 47.8   ⚕ 47.8   **FUD** 090   J 62 80 🖵

AMA: 2020,Dec,11; 2018,Jan,8; 2017,Jul,7; 2017,Apr,5; 2017,Mar,10

\# **31554** for laryngeal stenosis, with graft, with indwelling stent placement, age 12 years or older   A

EXCLUDES   Cartilage graft obtained through same incision
   Procedure during same session (31551-31553, 31580)
   Stent removal (31599)
   Tracheostomy (31600-31601, 31603, 31605, 31610)

🔪 47.8   ⚕ 47.8   **FUD** 090   J 62 80 🖵

AMA: 2020,Dec,11; 2018,Jan,8; 2017,Jul,7; 2017,Apr,5; 2017,Mar,10

31584 with open reduction and fixation of (eg, plating) fracture, includes tracheostomy, if performed

EXCLUDES   Cartilage graft obtained through same incision

🔪 39.6   ⚕ 39.6   **FUD** 090   J 62 80 🖵

AMA: 2018,Jan,8; 2017,Apr,5; 2017,Mar,10

31587 Laryngoplasty, cricoid split, without graft placement

EXCLUDES   Tracheostomy (31600-31601, 31603, 31605, 31610)

🔪 33.2   ⚕ 33.2   **FUD** 090   J 62 80 🖵

AMA: 2018,Jan,8; 2017,Apr,5; 2017,Mar,10

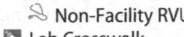

31590 Laryngeal reinnervation by neuromuscular pedicle
🔾 24.9 ⚖ 24.9 **FUD** 090 [J][A2][80]
AMA: 2018,Jan,8; 2017,Mar,10

Posterior lateral view

31591 Laryngoplasty, medialization, unilateral
🔾 30.7 ⚖ 30.7 **FUD** 090 [J][G2][80][50]
AMA: 2018,Jan,8; 2017,Jul,7; 2017,Apr,5; 2017,Mar,10

31592 Cricotracheal resection
EXCLUDES *Advancement or rotational flaps performed not*
requiring additional incision
Cartilage graft obtained through same incision
Tracheal stenosis excision/anastomosis (31780-31781)
Tracheostomy (31600-31601, 31603, 31605, 31610)
🔾 49.2 ⚖ 49.2 **FUD** 090 [J][G2][80]
AMA: 2018,Jan,8; 2017,Jul,7; 2017,Apr,5; 2017,Mar,10;
2017,Feb,14

31599 Unlisted procedure, larynx
🔾 0.00 ⚖ 0.00 **FUD** YYY [T][80]
AMA: 2018,Jan,8; 2017,Apr,5; 2017,Mar,10; 2017,Jan,8;
2017,Jan,6; 2016,Dec,13; 2016,Jan,13

31600-31610 Stoma Creation: Trachea
EXCLUDES *Aspiration trachea, direct vision (31515)*
Endotracheal intubation (31500)

31600 Tracheostomy, planned (separate procedure);
🔾 8.91 ⚖ 8.91 **FUD** 000 [J][G2]
AMA: 2020,Dec,11; 2019,Sep,10; 2017,Apr,5

31601 younger than 2 years [A]
🔾 12.9 ⚖ 12.9 **FUD** 000 [J][G2][80]
AMA: 2020,Dec,11; 2017,Apr,5

31603 Tracheostomy, emergency procedure; transtracheal
🔾 9.30 ⚖ 9.30 **FUD** 000 [T][A2]
AMA: 2020,Dec,11; 2017,Apr,5

31605 cricothyroid membrane
🔾 9.61 ⚖ 9.61 **FUD** 000 [T][G2]
AMA: 2017,Apr,5

31610 Tracheostomy, fenestration procedure with skin flaps
🔾 27.2 ⚖ 27.2 **FUD** 090 [J][G2]
AMA: 2020,Dec,11; 2017,Apr,5

31611-31614 Procedures of the Trachea

31611 Construction of tracheoesophageal fistula and subsequent insertion of an alaryngeal speech prosthesis (eg, voice button, Blom-Singer prosthesis)
🔾 15.1 ⚖ 15.1 **FUD** 090 [J][A2][80]

31612 Tracheal puncture, percutaneous with transtracheal aspiration and/or injection
EXCLUDES *Tracheal aspiration under direct vision (31515)*
🔾 1.37 ⚖ 2.46 **FUD** 000 [J][A2][80]
AMA: 1994,Win,1

31613 Tracheostoma revision; simple, without flap rotation
🔾 12.6 ⚖ 12.6 **FUD** 090 [J][A2]

31614 complex, with flap rotation
🔾 20.7 ⚖ 20.7 **FUD** 090 [J][A2]

31615 Endoscopy Through Tracheostomy
INCLUDES Diagnostic bronchoscopy
EXCLUDES *Endobronchial ultrasound [EBUS] guided biopsies mediastinal or hilar lymph*
nodes (31652-31653)
Tracheoscopy (31515-31578)
Code also endobronchial ultrasound [EBUS] during diagnostic/therapeutic peripheral
lesion intervention (31654)

31615 Tracheobronchoscopy through established tracheostomy incision
🔾 3.29 ⚖ 4.83 **FUD** 000 [T][A2]
AMA: 2020,Dec,11; 2018,Jan,8; 2017,Jan,8; 2016,Jan,13

31622-31654 [31651] Endoscopy of Lung
INCLUDES Diagnostic bronchoscopy with surgical bronchoscopy procedures
Fluoroscopic imaging guidance, when performed

31622 Bronchoscopy, rigid or flexible, including fluoroscopic guidance, when performed; diagnostic, with cell washing, when performed (separate procedure)
🔾 3.78 ⚖ 6.84 **FUD** 000 [J][A2]
AMA: 2018,Jan,8; 2017,Jan,8; 2016,Apr,5; 2016,Jan,13

31623 with brushing or protected brushings
🔾 3.82 ⚖ 7.66 **FUD** 000 [J][A2]
AMA: 2018,Jan,8; 2017,Jan,8; 2016,Apr,5; 2016,Jan,13

31624 with bronchial alveolar lavage
🔾 3.87 ⚖ 7.16 **FUD** 000 [J][A2]
AMA: 2018,Jan,8; 2017,Jun,10; 2017,Jan,8; 2016,Apr,5;
2016,Jan,13

31625 with bronchial or endobronchial biopsy(s), single or multiple sites
🔾 4.50 ⚖ 9.80 **FUD** 000 [J][A2]
AMA: 2018,Jan,8; 2017,Jan,8; 2016,Apr,5; 2016,Jan,13

31626 with placement of fiducial markers, single or multiple
Code also device
🔾 5.72 ⚖ 23.9 **FUD** 000 [J][G2][80]
AMA: 2018,Jan,8; 2017,Jun,10; 2017,Jan,8; 2016,Apr,5;
2016,Jan,13

+ 31627 with computer-assisted, image-guided navigation (List separately in addition to code for primary procedure[s])
INCLUDES 3D reconstruction (76376-76377)
Code first (31615, 31622-31626, 31628-31631, 31635-31636,
31638-31643)
🔾 2.78 ⚖ 36.3 **FUD** ZZZ [N][N1][80]
AMA: 2018,Jan,8; 2017,Jan,8; 2016,Jan,13

31628 with transbronchial lung biopsy(s), single lobe
INCLUDES All biopsies taken from lobe
EXCLUDES *Transbronchial biopsies by needle aspiration (31629,*
31633)
Code also transbronchial biopsies additional lobe(s) (31632)
🔾 5.06 ⚖ 10.4 **FUD** 000 [J][A2]
AMA: 2018,Jan,8; 2017,Jun,10; 2017,Jan,8; 2016,Apr,5;
2016,Jan,13

31629 with transbronchial needle aspiration biopsy(s), trachea, main stem and/or lobar bronchus(i)
INCLUDES All biopsies from same lobe or upper airway
EXCLUDES *Transbronchial biopsies lung (31628, 31632)*
Code also transbronchial needle biopsies additional lobe(s)
(31633)
🔾 5.37 ⚖ 12.8 **FUD** 000 [J][A2]
AMA: 2018,Jan,8; 2017,Jan,8; 2016,Apr,5; 2016,Jan,13

31630 with tracheal/bronchial dilation or closed reduction of fracture
🚑 5.72 ⚕ 5.72 **FUD** 000 J A2 ▣
AMA: 2018,Jan,8; 2017,Jan,8; 2016,Jan,13

31631 with placement of tracheal stent(s) (includes tracheal/bronchial dilation as required)
EXCLUDES Bronchial stent placement (31636-31637)
Revision bronchial or tracheal stent (31638)
🚑 6.58 ⚕ 6.58 **FUD** 000 J A2 ▣
AMA: 2018,Jan,8; 2017,Jan,8; 2016,Jan,13

+ **31632** with transbronchial lung biopsy(s), each additional lobe (List separately in addition to code for primary procedure)
INCLUDES All biopsies taken from additional lobe lung
Code first (31628)
🚑 1.43 ⚕ 1.82 **FUD** ZZZ N N1 ▣
AMA: 2018,Jan,8; 2017,Jan,8; 2016,Jan,13

+ **31633** with transbronchial needle aspiration biopsy(s), each additional lobe (List separately in addition to code for primary procedure)
INCLUDES All needle biopsies from another lobe or from trachea
Code first (31629)
🚑 1.82 ⚕ 2.26 **FUD** ZZZ N N1 ▣
AMA: 2018,Jan,8; 2017,Jan,8; 2016,Jan,13

31634 with balloon occlusion, with assessment of air leak, with administration of occlusive substance (eg, fibrin glue), if performed
EXCLUDES When performed during same operative session: Bronchoscopy, rigid or flexible, including fluoroscopic guidance; with balloon occlusio, assessment air leak, airway sizing, and insertion bronchial valve(s), initial lobe (31647, [31651])
🚑 5.53 ⚕ 49.4 **FUD** 000 J 62 80 ▣
AMA: 2018,Jan,8; 2017,Jan,8; 2016,Jan,13

31635 with removal of foreign body
EXCLUDES Removal implanted bronchial valves (31648-31649)
🚑 5.06 ⚕ 8.03 **FUD** 000 J A2 ▣
AMA: 2018,Jan,8; 2017,Jan,8; 2016,Jan,13

31636 with placement of bronchial stent(s) (includes tracheal/bronchial dilation as required), initial bronchus
🚑 6.33 ⚕ 6.33 **FUD** 000 J J8 ▣
AMA: 2018,Jan,8; 2017,Jan,8; 2016,Jan,13

+ **31637** each additional major bronchus stented (List separately in addition to code for primary procedure)
Code first (31636)
🚑 2.22 ⚕ 2.22 **FUD** ZZZ N N1 ▣
AMA: 2018,Jan,8; 2017,Jan,8; 2016,Jan,13

31638 with revision of tracheal or bronchial stent inserted at previous session (includes tracheal/bronchial dilation as required)
🚑 7.21 ⚕ 7.21 **FUD** 000 J A2 ▣
AMA: 2018,Jan,8; 2017,Jan,8; 2016,Jan,13

31640 with excision of tumor
🚑 7.21 ⚕ 7.21 **FUD** 000 J A2 ▣
AMA: 2018,Jan,8; 2017,Jan,8; 2016,Apr,5; 2016,Jan,13

31641 with destruction of tumor or relief of stenosis by any method other than excision (eg, laser therapy, cryotherapy)
Code also any photodynamic therapy via bronchoscopy (96570-96571)
🚑 7.39 ⚕ 7.39 **FUD** 000 J A2 ▣
AMA: 2018,Jan,8; 2017,Jan,8; 2016,Jan,13

31643 with placement of catheter(s) for intracavitary radioelement application
Code also when appropriate (77761-77763, 77770-77772)
🚑 5.04 ⚕ 5.04 **FUD** 000 J A2 ▣
AMA: 2018,Jan,8; 2017,Jan,8; 2016,Apr,5; 2016,Jan,13

31645 with therapeutic aspiration of tracheobronchial tree, initial (eg, drainage of lung abscess)
EXCLUDES Bedside aspiration trachea, bronchi (31725)
🚑 4.21 ⚕ 7.42 **FUD** 000 J A2 ▣
AMA: 2018,Jan,8; 2017,Jan,8; 2016,Apr,5; 2016,Jan,13

31646 with therapeutic aspiration of tracheobronchial tree, subsequent
EXCLUDES Bedside aspiration trachea, bronchi (31725)
🚑 4.08 ⚕ 4.08 **FUD** 000 T A2 ▣
AMA: 2018,Sep,3; 2018,Jan,8; 2017,Jan,8; 2016,Apr,5; 2016,Jan,13

31647 with balloon occlusion, when performed, assessment of air leak, airway sizing, and insertion of bronchial valve(s), initial lobe
🚑 6.10 ⚕ 6.10 **FUD** 000 J J8 ▣
AMA: 2018,Sep,3; 2018,Jan,8; 2017,Jan,8; 2016,Jan,13

+ # **31651** with balloon occlusion, when performed, assessment of air leak, airway sizing, and insertion of bronchial valve(s), each additional lobe (List separately in addition to code for primary procedure[s])
Code first (31647)
🚑 2.13 ⚕ 2.13 **FUD** ZZZ N N1 ▣
AMA: 2018,Sep,3; 2018,Jan,8; 2017,Jan,8; 2016,Jan,13

31648 with removal of bronchial valve(s), initial lobe
EXCLUDES Removal with reinsertion bronchial valve during same session (31647 and 31648) and ([31651])
🚑 5.80 ⚕ 5.80 **FUD** 000 J 62 ▣
AMA: 2018,Sep,3; 2018,Jan,8; 2017,Jan,8; 2016,Jan,13

+ **31649** with removal of bronchial valve(s), each additional lobe (List separately in addition to code for primary procedure)
Code first (31648)
🚑 1.94 ⚕ 1.94 **FUD** ZZZ 02 62 ▣
AMA: 2018,Sep,3; 2018,Jan,8; 2017,Jan,8; 2016,Jan,13

31651 **Resequenced code. See code following 31647.**

31652 with endobronchial ultrasound (EBUS) guided transtracheal and/or transbronchial sampling (eg, aspiration[s]/biopsy[ies]), one or two mediastinal and/or hilar lymph node stations or structures
EXCLUDES Procedures performed more than one time per session
🚑 6.38 ⚕ 31.2 **FUD** 000 J 62 ▣
AMA: 2018,Jan,8; 2017,Jan,8; 2016,Apr,5

31653 with endobronchial ultrasound (EBUS) guided transtracheal and/or transbronchial sampling (eg, aspiration[s]/biopsy[ies]), 3 or more mediastinal and/or hilar lymph node stations or structures
EXCLUDES Procedures performed more than one time per session
🚑 7.08 ⚕ 28.7 **FUD** 000 J 62 ▣
AMA: 2018,Jan,8; 2017,Jan,8; 2016,Apr,5

+ **31654** with transendoscopic endobronchial ultrasound (EBUS) during bronchoscopic diagnostic or therapeutic intervention(s) for peripheral lesion(s) (List separately in addition to code for primary procedure[s])
EXCLUDES Endobronchial ultrasound [EBUS] for mediastinal/hilar lymph node station/adjacent structure access (31652-31653)
Procedures performed more than one time per session
Code first (31622-31626, 31628-31629, 31640, 31643-31646)
🚑 1.94 ⚕ 3.48 **FUD** ZZZ N N1 ▣
AMA: 2018,Jan,8; 2017,Jan,8; 2016,Apr,5

31660-31661 Bronchial Thermoplasty
INCLUDES Fluoroscopic imaging guidance, when performed

31660 Bronchoscopy, rigid or flexible, including fluoroscopic guidance, when performed; with bronchial thermoplasty, 1 lobe
🚑 5.62 ⚕ 5.62 **FUD** 000 J J8 ▣
AMA: 2018,Jan,8; 2017,Jan,8; 2016,Jan,13

31661 with bronchial thermoplasty, 2 or more lobes
🚑 5.93 ⚕ 5.93 **FUD** 000 [J] [J8] [▣]
AMA: 2018,Jan,8; 2017,Jan,8; 2016,Jan,13

31717-31899 Respiratory Procedures

EXCLUDES Endotracheal intubation (31500)
Tracheal aspiration under direct vision (31515)

31717 Catheterization with bronchial brush biopsy
🚑 3.18 ⚕ 7.98 **FUD** 000 [T] [A2] [▣]
AMA: 2018,Jan,8; 2017,Jan,8; 2016,Jan,13

31720 Catheter aspiration (separate procedure); nasotracheal
🚑 1.59 ⚕ 1.59 **FUD** 000 [01] [N1] [▣]
AMA: 1994,Win,1

31725 tracheobronchial with fiberscope, bedside
🚑 2.27 ⚕ 2.27 **FUD** 000 [C] [▣]

31730 Transtracheal (percutaneous) introduction of needle wire dilator/stent or indwelling tube for oxygen therapy
🚑 4.33 ⚕ 33.8 **FUD** 000 [J] [A2] [▣]
AMA: 1992,Win,1

31750 Tracheoplasty; cervical
🚑 39.1 ⚕ 39.1 **FUD** 090 [J] [A2] [80] [▣]

31755 tracheopharyngeal fistulization, each stage
🚑 49.1 ⚕ 49.1 **FUD** 090 [J] [A2] [80] [▣]

31760 intrathoracic
🚑 39.6 ⚕ 39.6 **FUD** 090 [C] [80] [▣]

31766 Carinal reconstruction
🚑 51.3 ⚕ 51.3 **FUD** 090 [C] [80] [▣]

31770 Bronchoplasty; graft repair
EXCLUDES Bronchoplasty done with lobectomy (32501)
🚑 38.4 ⚕ 38.4 **FUD** 090 [C] [80] [▣]

31775 excision stenosis and anastomosis
EXCLUDES Bronchoplasty done with lobectomy (32501)
🚑 40.4 ⚕ 40.4 **FUD** 090 [C] [80] [▣]

31780 Excision tracheal stenosis and anastomosis; cervical
🚑 34.2 ⚕ 34.2 **FUD** 090 [C] [80] [▣]
AMA: 2018,Jan,8; 2017,Apr,5; 2017,Feb,14

31781 cervicothoracic
🚑 39.8 ⚕ 39.8 **FUD** 090 [C] [80] [▣]
AMA: 2018,Jan,8; 2017,Apr,5; 2017,Feb,14

31785 Excision of tracheal tumor or carcinoma; cervical
🚑 30.8 ⚕ 30.8 **FUD** 090 [J] [62] [80] [▣]
AMA: 2003,Jan,1

31786 thoracic
🚑 41.6 ⚕ 41.6 **FUD** 090 [C] [80] [▣]

31800 Suture of tracheal wound or injury; cervical
🚑 20.3 ⚕ 20.3 **FUD** 090 [C] [80] [▣]
AMA: 1994,Win,1

31805 intrathoracic
🚑 23.5 ⚕ 23.5 **FUD** 090 [C] [80] [▣]

31820 Surgical closure tracheostomy or fistula; without plastic repair
EXCLUDES Tracheoesophageal fistula repair (43305, 43312)
🚑 9.35 ⚕ 12.3 **FUD** 090 [J] [A2] [80] [▣]

31825 with plastic repair
EXCLUDES Tracheoesophageal fistula repair (43305, 43312)
🚑 13.6 ⚕ 17.1 **FUD** 090 [J] [A2] [80] [▣]

31830 Revision of tracheostomy scar

Any of a wide variety of scar revision techniques may be employed. A Z-plasty may be used to lengthen or realign the scar line. Revision also serves to neutralize contractures that occur along the scar line

Thyroid cartilage

Tracheostomies typically enter at the second, third, or fourth ring

Cricoid cartilage

1st ring

Example of a common Z-plasty where flaps are rotated to break scar line

2nd ring

A tracheostomy closure scar is revised, usually to make the scar less noticeable

3rd ring

🚑 10.0 ⚕ 13.2 **FUD** 090 [J] [A2] [80] [▣]

31899 Unlisted procedure, trachea, bronchi
🚑 0.00 ⚕ 0.00 **FUD** YYY [T] [80] [▣]
AMA: 2020,Dec,11; 2018,Jan,8; 2017,Jan,8; 2016,Jan,13

32035-32036 Procedures for Empyema

EXCLUDES Wound exploration without thoracotomy for penetrating chest wound (20101)

32035 Thoracostomy; with rib resection for empyema
🚑 21.0 ⚕ 21.0 **FUD** 090 [C] [80] [50] [▣]

32036 with open flap drainage for empyema
🚑 22.3 ⚕ 22.3 **FUD** 090 [C] [80] [50] [▣]

32096-32098 Open Biopsy of Chest and Pleura

INCLUDES Varying amounts lung tissue excised for analysis
Wedge technique with tissue obtained without precise margin consideration

EXCLUDES Core needle biopsy, lung or mediastinum (32408)
Percutaneous needle biopsy pleura (32400)
Thoracoscopy with:
Biopsy (32607-32609)
Diagnostic wedge resection resulting in anatomic lung resection (32507, 32668)

32096 Thoracotomy, with diagnostic biopsy(ies) of lung infiltrate(s) (eg, wedge, incisional), unilateral
EXCLUDES Procedure performed more than one time per lung
Removal lung (32440-32445, 32488)
Code also appropriate add-on code for more extensive procedure at same location when diagnostic wedge resection results in need for further surgery (32507, 32668)
🚑 23.1 ⚕ 23.1 **FUD** 090 [C] [80] [▣]
AMA: 2018,Jan,8; 2017,Jan,8; 2016,Jan,13

32097 **Thoracotomy, with diagnostic biopsy(ies) of lung nodule(s) or mass(es) (eg, wedge, incisional), unilateral**

> EXCLUDES　*Procedure performed more than one time per lung*
> *Removal lung (32440-32445, 32488)*
> Code also appropriate add-on code for more extensive procedure in same location when diagnostic wedge resection results in need for further surgery (32507, 32668)

🚑 23.1　🔧 23.1　**FUD** 090　　　C 80 🖵

AMA: 2018,Jan,8; 2017,Jan,8; 2016,Jan,13

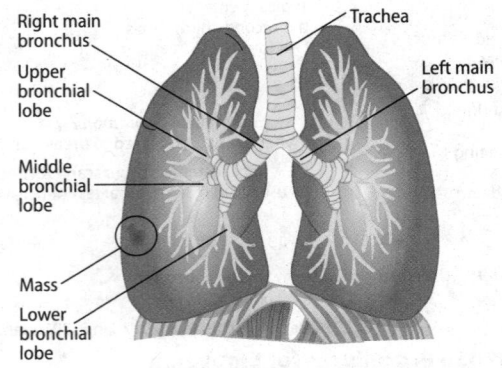

Right main bronchus　　　　　　　Trachea
Upper bronchial lobe　　　　　　　Left main bronchus
Middle bronchial lobe
Mass
Lower bronchial lobe

32098 **Thoracotomy, with biopsy(ies) of pleura**

🚑 21.9　🔧 21.9　**FUD** 090　　　C 80 🖵

AMA: 2018,Jan,8; 2017,Jan,8; 2016,Jan,13

32100-32160 Open Procedures: Chest

INCLUDES　Exploration penetrating chest wound
EXCLUDES　*Lung resection (32480-32504)*
　　　　　Wound exploration without thoracotomy for penetrating chest wound (20101)

32100 **Thoracotomy; with exploration**

> EXCLUDES　*Excision chest wall tumor, when performed (21601-21603)*
> *Extracorporeal membrane oxygenation (ECMO)/extracorporeal life support (ECLS) (33955-33957, [33963, 33964])*
> *Resection apical lung tumor (32503-32504)*

🚑 23.3　🔧 23.3　**FUD** 090　　　C 80 🖵

AMA: 2019,Dec,5; 2019,Dec,4; 2018,Jan,8; 2017,Jan,8; 2016,Jan,13

32110 **with control of traumatic hemorrhage and/or repair of lung tear**

🚑 42.4　🔧 42.4　**FUD** 090　　　C 80 🖵

AMA: 2018,Jan,8; 2017,Jan,8; 2016,Jan,13

32120 **for postoperative complications**

🚑 25.2　🔧 25.2　**FUD** 090　　　C 80 🖵

32124 **with open intrapleural pneumonolysis**

🚑 26.7　🔧 26.7　**FUD** 090　　　C 80 🖵

AMA: 2018,Jan,8; 2017,Jan,8; 2016,Jan,13

32140 **with cyst(s) removal, includes pleural procedure when performed**

🚑 28.5　🔧 28.5　**FUD** 090　　　C 80 🖵

AMA: 2018,Jan,8; 2017,Jan,8; 2016,Jan,13

32141 **with resection-plication of bullae, includes any pleural procedure when performed**

> EXCLUDES　*Lung volume reduction (32491)*

🚑 44.0　🔧 44.0　**FUD** 090　　　C 80 🖵

AMA: 2018,Jan,8; 2017,Jan,8; 2016,Jan,13

32150 **with removal of intrapleural foreign body or fibrin deposit**

🚑 28.9　🔧 28.9　**FUD** 090　　　C 80 🖵

AMA: 2018,Jan,8; 2017,Jan,8; 2016,Jan,13

32151 **with removal of intrapulmonary foreign body**

🚑 29.0　🔧 29.0　**FUD** 090　　　C 80 🖵

32160 **with cardiac massage**

🚑 22.9　🔧 22.9　**FUD** 090　　　C 80 🖵

32200-32320 Open Procedures: Lung

32200 **Pneumonostomy, with open drainage of abscess or cyst**

> EXCLUDES　*Image-guided, percutaneous drainage (eg, abscess, cyst) of lungs/mediastinum via catheter (49405)*

🔲 (75989)
🚑 32.7　🔧 32.7　**FUD** 090　　　C 80 🖵

AMA: 2013,Nov,9; 1997,Nov,1

32215 **Pleural scarification for repeat pneumothorax**

🚑 23.0　🔧 23.0　**FUD** 090　　　C 80 50 🖵

32220 **Decortication, pulmonary (separate procedure); total**

🚑 45.9　🔧 45.9　**FUD** 090　　　C 80 50 🖵

32225 **partial**

🚑 28.7　🔧 28.7　**FUD** 090　　　C 80 50 🖵

32310 **Pleurectomy, parietal (separate procedure)**

🚑 26.3　🔧 26.3　**FUD** 090　　　C 80 🖵

AMA: 1994,Win,1

32320 **Decortication and parietal pleurectomy**

🚑 46.1　🔧 46.1　**FUD** 090　　　C 80 🖵

AMA: 1994,Fall,1

32400-32408 Lung Biopsy

EXCLUDES　*Fine needle aspiration ([10004, 10005, 10006, 10007, 10008, 10009, 10010, 10011, 10012], 10021)*
　　　　　Open lung biopsy (32096-32097)
　　　　　Open mediastinal biopsy (39000-39010)
　　　　　Thoracoscopic (VATS) biopsy lung, pericardium, pleural, or mediastinal space (32604-32609)

32400 **Biopsy, pleura, percutaneous needle**

🔲 (76942, 77002, 77012, 77021)
🚑 2.48　🔧 4.56　**FUD** 090　　　J A2

AMA: 2019,Apr,4; 2018,Jan,8; 2017,Jan,8; 2016,Jan,13

32408 **Core needle biopsy, lung or mediastinum, percutaneous, including imaging guidance, when performed**

> INCLUDES　Imaging guidance performed during tsame session on same lesion (76942, 77002, 77012, 77021)
> Code also core needle biopsy performed during same operative session:
> 　Other anatomical site; report both codes and append modifier 59 on second code
> 　Same anatomical site, different lesion; report 32408 for each lesion biopsied and append modifier 59 on second code
> Code also FNA biopsy and core needle biopsy performed during same operative session:
> 　Different lesion, utilizing same or different imaging guidance; report both codes and append modifier 59 on either code
> 　Same lesion, utilizing different imaging guidance; report both image-guided biopsy codes and append modifier 59 on either code
> 　Same lesion, utilizing same imaging guidance; report both codes and append modifier 52 on either code

🚑 4.44　🔧 27.7　**FUD** 000　　　62 🖵

| 26/TC PC/TC Only | A2-Z3 ASC Payment | 50 Bilateral | ♂ Male Only | ♀ Female Only | 🚑 Facility RVU | 🔧 Non-Facility RVU | 🖵 CCI | ☒ CLIA |
| FUD Follow-up Days | CMS: IOM | AMA: CPT Asst | A-Y OPPSI | 80/80 Surg Assist Allowed / w/Doc | 🔬 Lab Crosswalk | 📻 Radiology Crosswalk | | |

118　　　　　　CPT © 2021 American Medical Association. All Rights Reserved.　　　　　　© 2021 Optum360, LLC

32440-32501 Lung Resection

32440   **Removal of lung, pneumonectomy;**
Code also excision chest wall tumor, when performed (21601-21603)
🚑 45.1   ✂ 45.1   **FUD** 090   [C] [80] ▣
AMA: 2018,Jan,8; 2017,Jan,8; 2016,Jan,13

Removal of entire lung

32442   **with resection of segment of trachea followed by broncho-tracheal anastomosis (sleeve pneumonectomy)**
Code also excision chest wall tumor, when performed (21601-21603)
🚑 88.9   ✂ 88.9   **FUD** 090   [C] [80] ▣
AMA: 2018,Jan,8; 2017,Jun,10; 2017,Jan,8; 2016,Jan,13

32445   **extrapleural**
Code also:
    Empyemectomy with extrapleural pneumonectomy (32540)
    Excision chest wall tumor, when performed (21601-21603)
🚑 102.   ✂ 102.   **FUD** 090   [C] [80] ▣
AMA: 2018,Jan,8; 2017,Jan,8; 2016,Jan,13

32480   **Removal of lung, other than pneumonectomy; single lobe (lobectomy)**
EXCLUDES   Lung removal with bronchoplasty (32501)
Code also:
    Decortication (32320)
    Excision chest wall tumor, when performed (21601-21603)
🚑 42.6   ✂ 42.6   **FUD** 090   [C] [80] ▣
AMA: 2018,Jan,8; 2017,Jan,8; 2016,Jan,13

32482   **2 lobes (bilobectomy)**
EXCLUDES   Lung removal with bronchoplasty (32501)
Code also:
    Decortication (32320)
    Excision chest wall tumor, when performed (21601-21603)
🚑 45.8   ✂ 45.8   **FUD** 090   [C] [80] ▣
AMA: 2018,Jan,8; 2017,Jan,8; 2016,Jan,13

32484   **single segment (segmentectomy)**
EXCLUDES   Lung removal with bronchoplasty (32501)
Code also:
    Decortication (32320)
    Excision chest wall tumor, when performed (21601-21603)
🚑 41.3   ✂ 41.3   **FUD** 090   [C] [80] ▣
AMA: 2018,Jan,8; 2017,Jan,8; 2016,Jan,13

32486   **with circumferential resection of segment of bronchus followed by broncho-bronchial anastomosis (sleeve lobectomy)**
Code also:
    Decortication (32320)
    Excision chest wall tumor, when performed (21601-21603)
🚑 68.1   ✂ 68.1   **FUD** 090   [C] [80] ▣
AMA: 2018,Jan,8; 2017,Jun,10; 2017,Jan,8; 2016,Jan,13

32488   **with all remaining lung following previous removal of a portion of lung (completion pneumonectomy)**
Code also:
    Decortication (32320)
    Excision chest wall tumor, when performed (21601-21603)
🚑 69.1   ✂ 69.1   **FUD** 090   [C] [80] ▣
AMA: 2018,Jan,8; 2017,Jan,8; 2016,Jan,13

32491   **with resection-plication of emphysematous lung(s) (bullous or non-bullous) for lung volume reduction, sternal split or transthoracic approach, includes any pleural procedure, when performed**
Code also:
    Decortication (32320)
    Excision chest wall tumor, when performed (21601-21603)
🚑 42.4   ✂ 42.4   **FUD** 090   [C] [80] [50] ▣
AMA: 2018,Jan,8; 2017,Jan,8; 2016,Jan,13

+ **32501**   **Resection and repair of portion of bronchus (bronchoplasty) when performed at time of lobectomy or segmentectomy (List separately in addition to code for primary procedure)**
INCLUDES   Plastic closure bronchus, not closure resected bronchus
Code first (32480-32484)
🚑 7.04   ✂ 7.04   **FUD** ZZZ   [C] [80] ▣
AMA: 1995,Win,1

32503-32504 Excision of Lung Neoplasm

EXCLUDES   Excision chest wall tumor (21601-21603)
    Thoracentesis, needle or catheter, aspiration pleural space (32554-32555)
    Thoracotomy; with exploration (32100)
    Tube thoracostomy (32551)

32503   **Resection of apical lung tumor (eg, Pancoast tumor), including chest wall resection, rib(s) resection(s), neurovascular dissection, when performed; without chest wall reconstruction(s)**
🚑 51.9   ✂ 51.9   **FUD** 090   [C] [80] ▣
AMA: 2019,Dec,4

32504   **with chest wall reconstruction**
🚑 59.1   ✂ 59.1   **FUD** 090   [C] [80] ▣
AMA: 2019,Dec,4

32505-32507 Thoracotomy with Wedge Resection

INCLUDES   Wedge technique with tissue obtained with precise consideration margins and complete resection
Code also resection chest wall tumor with lung resection, when performed (21601-21603)

32505   **Thoracotomy; with therapeutic wedge resection (eg, mass, nodule), initial**
EXCLUDES   Removal lung (32440, 32442, 32445, 32488)
Code also more extensive procedure lung when performed on contralateral lung or different lobe with modifier 59 despite intraoperative pathology consultation
🚑 26.9   ✂ 26.9   **FUD** 090   [C] [80] ▣
AMA: 2018,Jan,8; 2017,Jan,8; 2016,Jan,13

+ **32506**   **with therapeutic wedge resection (eg, mass or nodule), each additional resection, ipsilateral (List separately in addition to code for primary procedure)**
Code also more extensive procedure lung when performed on contralateral lung or different lobe with modifier 59 despite intraoperative pathology consultation
Code first (32505)
🚑 4.52   ✂ 4.52   **FUD** ZZZ   [C] [80] ▣
AMA: 2018,Jan,8; 2017,Jan,8; 2016,Jan,13

Respiratory System

32507 — 32652

+ **32507** **with diagnostic wedge resection followed by anatomic lung resection (List separately in addition to code for primary procedure)**
    - INCLUDES Classification as diagnostic wedge resection when intraoperative pathology consultation dictates more extensive resection in same anatomical area
    - EXCLUDES *Diagnostic wedge resection by thoracoscopy (32668)*
      Therapeutic wedge resection (32505-32506, 32666-32667)
      Code first (32440, 32442, 32445, 32480-32488, 32503-32504)
    - 🖪 4.52   ⚕ 4.52   **FUD** ZZZ   C 80 📷
    - **AMA:** 2018,Jan,8; 2017,Jan,8; 2016,Jan,13

32540 Removal of Empyema

32540 **Extrapleural enucleation of empyema (empyemectomy)**
- Code also appropriate removal lung code when done with lobectomy (32480-32488)
- 🖪 50.1   ⚕ 50.1   **FUD** 090   C 80 📷
- **AMA:** 1994,Fall,1

32550-32552 Chest Tube/Catheter

32550 **Insertion of indwelling tunneled pleural catheter with cuff**
- EXCLUDES *Procedures performed on same side chest with (32554-32557)*
- 🔁 (75989)
- 🖪 5.98   ⚕ 21.2   **FUD** 000   J 62 📷
- **AMA:** 2018,Jan,8; 2017,Jan,8; 2016,Jan,13

32551 **Tube thoracostomy, includes connection to drainage system (eg, water seal), when performed, open (separate procedure)**
- EXCLUDES *Procedures performed on same side chest with (33020, 33025)*
- 🖪 4.56   ⚕ 4.56   **FUD** 000   T 62 50 📷
- **AMA:** 2019,Dec,4; 2018,Jul,7; 2018,Jan,8; 2017,Jun,10; 2017,Jan,8; 2016,Jan,13

32552 **Removal of indwelling tunneled pleural catheter with cuff**
- 🖪 4.55   ⚕ 5.28   **FUD** 010   02 62 80 📷
- **AMA:** 2018,Jan,8; 2017,Jan,8; 2016,Jan,13

32553 Intrathoracic Placement Radiation Therapy Devices

EXCLUDES *Percutaneous placement interstitial device(s) for radiation therapy guidance: intra-abdominal, intrapelvic, and/or retroperitoneal (49411)*
Code also device

32553 **Placement of interstitial device(s) for radiation therapy guidance (eg, fiducial markers, dosimeter), percutaneous, intra-thoracic, single or multiple**
- 🔁 (76942, 77002, 77012, 77021)
- 🖪 5.17   ⚕ 15.1   **FUD** 000   S 62 80 📷
- **AMA:** 2018,Jan,8; 2017,Jan,8; 2016,Jun,3; 2016,Jan,13

32554-32557 Pleural Aspiration and Drainage

EXCLUDES *Chest x-ray performed to confirm chest tube position, complications, procedure adequacy*
Open tube thoracostomy (32551)
Placement indwelling tunneled pleural drainage catheter (cuffed) (32550)

32554 **Thoracentesis, needle or catheter, aspiration of the pleural space; without imaging guidance**
- EXCLUDES *Radiologic guidance (75989, 76942, 77002, 77012, 77021)*
- 🖪 2.58   ⚕ 6.01   **FUD** 000   T 62 50 📷
- **AMA:** 2019,Dec,4; 2018,Jan,8; 2017,Jan,8; 2016,Jan,13

32555 **with imaging guidance**
- INCLUDES Radiologic guidance (75989, 76942, 77002, 77012, 77021)
- 🖪 3.22   ⚕ 8.51   **FUD** 000   T 62 50 📷
- **AMA:** 2019,Dec,4; 2018,Jan,8; 2017,Jan,8; 2016,Jan,13

32556 **Pleural drainage, percutaneous, with insertion of indwelling catheter; without imaging guidance**
- EXCLUDES *Radiologic guidance (75989, 76942, 77002, 77012, 77021)*
- 🖪 3.55   ⚕ 17.4   **FUD** 000   J 62 50 📷
- **AMA:** 2018,Jan,8; 2017,Jan,8; 2016,Jan,13

32557 **with imaging guidance**
- INCLUDES Radiologic guidance (75989, 76942, 77002, 77012, 77021)
- 🖪 4.39   ⚕ 16.0   **FUD** 000   T 62 50 📷
- **AMA:** 2018,Jan,8; 2017,Jan,8; 2016,Jan,13

32560-32562 Instillation Drug/Chemical by Chest Tube

EXCLUDES *Insertion chest tube (32551)*

32560 **Instillation, via chest tube/catheter, agent for pleurodesis (eg, talc for recurrent or persistent pneumothorax)**
- 🖪 2.25   ⚕ 7.38   **FUD** 000   T 62 📷
- **AMA:** 2018,Jan,8; 2017,Jan,8; 2016,Jan,13

32561 **Instillation(s), via chest tube/catheter, agent for fibrinolysis (eg, fibrinolytic agent for break up of multiloculated effusion); initial day**
- EXCLUDES *Reporting code more than one time on initial treatment date*
- 🖪 1.95   ⚕ 2.66   **FUD** 000   T 62 80 📷
- **AMA:** 2018,Jan,8; 2017,Jan,8; 2016,Jan,13

32562 **subsequent day**
- EXCLUDES *Reporting code more than one time on each day subsequent treatment*
- 🖪 1.75   ⚕ 2.40   **FUD** 000   T 62 80 📷
- **AMA:** 2018,Jan,8; 2017,Jan,8; 2016,Jan,13

32601-32674 Thoracic Surgery: Video-Assisted (VATS)

INCLUDES Diagnostic thoracoscopy in surgical thoracoscopy

32601 **Thoracoscopy, diagnostic (separate procedure); lungs, pericardial sac, mediastinal or pleural space, without biopsy**
- 🖪 8.90   ⚕ 8.90   **FUD** 000   J 62 80 📷
- **AMA:** 2018,Jan,8; 2017,Jan,8; 2016,Jan,13

32604 **pericardial sac, with biopsy**
- EXCLUDES *Open biopsy pericardium (39010)*
- 🖪 13.8   ⚕ 13.8   **FUD** 000   J 62 80 📷
- **AMA:** 2018,Jan,8; 2017,Jan,8; 2016,Jan,13

32606 **mediastinal space, with biopsy**
- 🖪 13.3   ⚕ 13.3   **FUD** 000   J 62 80 📷
- **AMA:** 2018,Jan,8; 2017,Jan,8; 2016,Jan,13

32607 **Thoracoscopy; with diagnostic biopsy(ies) of lung infiltrate(s) (eg, wedge, incisional), unilateral**
- EXCLUDES *Removal lung (32440-32445, 32488)*
  Thoracoscopy, surgical; with removal lung (32671)
  Reporting code more than one time per lung
- 🖪 8.92   ⚕ 8.92   **FUD** 000   J 62 80 📷
- **AMA:** 2018,Jan,8; 2017,Jan,8; 2016,Jan,13

32608 **with diagnostic biopsy(ies) of lung nodule(s) or mass(es) (eg, wedge, incisional), unilateral**
- EXCLUDES *Removal lung (32440-32445, 32488)*
  Thoracoscopy, surgical; with removal lung (32671)
  Reporting code more than one time per lung
- 🖪 10.9   ⚕ 10.9   **FUD** 000   J 62 80 📷
- **AMA:** 2018,Jan,8; 2017,Jan,8; 2016,Jan,13

32609 **with biopsy(ies) of pleura**
- 🖪 7.43   ⚕ 7.43   **FUD** 000   J 62 80 📷
- **AMA:** 2018,Jan,8; 2017,Jan,8; 2016,Jan,13

32650 **Thoracoscopy, surgical; with pleurodesis (eg, mechanical or chemical)**
- 🖪 19.1   ⚕ 19.1   **FUD** 090   C 80 50 📷
- **AMA:** 2018,Jan,8; 2017,Jan,8; 2016,Jan,13

32651 **with partial pulmonary decortication**
- 🖪 31.6   ⚕ 31.6   **FUD** 090   C 80 50 📷
- **AMA:** 2018,Jan,8; 2017,Jan,8; 2016,Jan,13

32652 **with total pulmonary decortication, including intrapleural pneumonolysis**
- 🖪 47.9   ⚕ 47.9   **FUD** 090   C 80 50 📷
- **AMA:** 2018,Jan,8; 2017,Jan,8; 2016,Jan,13

2G/TC PC/TC Only   A2-Z3 ASC Payment   50 Bilateral   ♂ Male Only   ♀ Female Only   🖪 Facility RVU   ⚕ Non-Facility RVU   📋 CCI   ✖ CLIA
FUD Follow-up Days   CMS: IOM   AMA: CPT Asst   A-Y OPPSI   80/80 Surg Assist Allowed / w/Doc   📖 Lab Crosswalk   📷 Radiology Crosswalk

120   CPT © 2021 American Medical Association. All Rights Reserved.   © 2021 Optum360, LLC

32653 **with removal of intrapleural foreign body or fibrin deposit**
🚑 30.6 ⚕ 30.6 **FUD** 090   C 80 ▢
AMA: 2018,Jan,8; 2017,Jan,8; 2016,Jan,13

32654 **with control of traumatic hemorrhage**
🚑 33.5 ⚕ 33.5 **FUD** 090   C 80 50 ▢
AMA: 2018,Jan,8; 2017,Jan,8; 2016,Jan,13

32655 **with resection-plication of bullae, includes any pleural procedure when performed**
EXCLUDES *Thoracoscopic lung volume reduction surgery (32672)*
🚑 27.5 ⚕ 27.5 **FUD** 090   C 80 50 ▢
AMA: 2018,Jan,8; 2017,Jan,8; 2016,Jan,13

32656 **with parietal pleurectomy**
🚑 23.1 ⚕ 23.1 **FUD** 090   C 80 50 ▢
AMA: 2018,Jan,8; 2017,Jan,8; 2016,Jan,13

32658 **with removal of clot or foreign body from pericardial sac**
🚑 20.6 ⚕ 20.6 **FUD** 090   C 80 ▢
AMA: 2018,Jan,8; 2017,Jan,8; 2016,Jan,13

32659 **with creation of pericardial window or partial resection of pericardial sac for drainage**
🚑 21.1 ⚕ 21.1 **FUD** 090   C 80 ▢
AMA: 2018,Jan,8; 2017,Jan,8; 2016,Jan,13

32661 **with excision of pericardial cyst, tumor, or mass**
🚑 23.0 ⚕ 23.0 **FUD** 090   C 80 ▢
AMA: 2018,Jan,8; 2017,Jan,8; 2016,Jan,13

32662 **with excision of mediastinal cyst, tumor, or mass**
🚑 25.7 ⚕ 25.7 **FUD** 090   C 80 ▢
AMA: 2018,Jan,8; 2017,Jan,8; 2016,Jan,13

32663 **with lobectomy (single lobe)**
EXCLUDES *Thoracoscopic segmentectomy (32669)*
🚑 40.4 ⚕ 40.4 **FUD** 090   C 80 ▢
AMA: 2018,Jan,8; 2017,Jan,8; 2016,Jan,13

32664 **with thoracic sympathectomy**
🚑 24.4 ⚕ 24.4 **FUD** 090   C 80 50 ▢
AMA: 2018,Jan,8; 2017,Jan,8; 2016,Jan,13

32665 **with esophagomyotomy (Heller type)**
EXCLUDES *Exploratory thoracoscopy with and without biopsy (32601-32609)*
Peroral endoscopic myotomy (POEM) (43497)
🚑 35.2 ⚕ 35.2 **FUD** 090   C 80 ▢
AMA: 2018,Jan,8; 2017,Jan,8; 2016,Jan,13

32666 **with therapeutic wedge resection (eg, mass, nodule), initial unilateral**
EXCLUDES *Removal lung (32440-32445, 32488)*
Thoracoscopy, surgical; with removal lung (32671)
Code also more extensive procedure lung when performed on contralateral lung or different lobe with modifier 59 despite pathology consultation
🚑 25.0 ⚕ 25.0 **FUD** 090   C 80 50 ▢
AMA: 2018,Jan,8; 2017,Jan,8; 2016,Jan,13

+ **32667** **with therapeutic wedge resection (eg, mass or nodule), each additional resection, ipsilateral (List separately in addition to code for primary procedure)**
EXCLUDES *Removal lung (32440-32445, 32488)*
Thoracoscopy, surgical; with removal lung (32671)
Code also more extensive procedure lung when performed on contralateral lung or different lobe with modifier 59 despite intraoperative pathology consultation
Code first (32666)
🚑 4.53 ⚕ 4.53 **FUD** ZZZ   C 80 ▢
AMA: 2018,Jan,8; 2017,Jan,8; 2016,Jan,13

+ **32668** **with diagnostic wedge resection followed by anatomic lung resection (List separately in addition to code for primary procedure)**
INCLUDES Classification as diagnostic wedge resection when intraoperative pathology consultation dictates more extensive resection in same anatomical area
Code first (32440-32488, 32503-32504, 32663, 32669-32671)
🚑 4.54 ⚕ 4.54 **FUD** ZZZ   C 80 ▢
AMA: 2018,Jan,8; 2017,Jan,8; 2016,Jan,13

32669 **with removal of a single lung segment (segmentectomy)**
🚑 38.8 ⚕ 38.8 **FUD** 090   C 80 ▢
AMA: 2018,Jan,8; 2017,Jan,8; 2016,Jan,13

32670 **with removal of two lobes (bilobectomy)**
🚑 46.2 ⚕ 46.2 **FUD** 090   C 80 ▢
AMA: 2018,Jan,8; 2017,Jan,8; 2016,Jan,13

32671 **with removal of lung (pneumonectomy)**
🚑 51.1 ⚕ 51.1 **FUD** 090   C 80 ▢
AMA: 2018,Jan,8; 2017,Jan,8; 2016,Jan,13

32672 **with resection-plication for emphysematous lung (bullous or non-bullous) for lung volume reduction (LVRS), unilateral includes any pleural procedure, when performed**
🚑 44.0 ⚕ 44.0 **FUD** 090   C 80 ▢
AMA: 2018,Jan,8; 2017,Jan,8; 2016,Jan,13

32673 **with resection of thymus, unilateral or bilateral**
EXCLUDES *Exploratory thoracoscopy with and without biopsy (32601-32609)*
Open excision mediastinal cyst (39200)
Open excision mediastinal tumor (39220)
Open thymectomy (60520-60522)
🚑 35.1 ⚕ 35.1 **FUD** 090   C 80 ▢
AMA: 2018,Jan,8; 2017,Jan,8; 2016,Jan,13

Respiratory System

32674 — 32999

+   **32674**   **with mediastinal and regional lymphadenectomy (List separately in addition to code for primary procedure)**

INCLUDES   Mediastinal lymph nodes:
Left side:
Aortopulmonary window
Inferior pulmonary ligament
Paraesophageal
Subcarinal
Right side:
Inferior pulmonary ligament
Paraesophageal
Paratracheal
Subcarinal

EXCLUDES   *Mediastinal and regional lymphadenectomy by thoracotomy (38746)*

Code first (21601, 31760, 31766, 31786, 32096-32200, 32220-32320, 32440-32491, 32503-32505, 32601-32663, 32666, 32669-32673, 32815, 33025, 33030, 33050-33130, 39200-39220, 39560-39561, 43101, 43112, 43117-43118, 43122-43123, 43287-43288, 43351, 60270, 60505)

🔧 6.23   ✂ 6.23   **FUD** ZZZ   C 80 ▭

AMA: 2018,Jan,8; 2017,Jan,8; 2016,Jan,13

Mediastinum
Superior vena cava
Arch of aorta
Right lung
Left lung
Ribs (cut)
Heart
Diaphragm

32701 Target Delineation for Stereotactic Radiation Therapy

INCLUDES   Collaboration between radiation oncologist and surgeon
Correlation tumor and contiguous body structures
Determination borders and volume of tumor
Identification fiducial markers
Verification target when fiducial markers not used
EXCLUDES   *Fiducial marker insertion (31626, 32553)*
Procedure performed by same physician as radiation treatment management (77427-77499)
Radiation oncology services (77295, 77331, 77370, 77373, 77435)
Therapeutic radiology (77261-77799 [77295, 77385, 77386, 77387, 77424, 77425])

32701   **Thoracic target(s) delineation for stereotactic body radiation therapy (SRS/SBRT), (photon or particle beam), entire course of treatment**

🔧 6.21   ✂ 6.21   **FUD** XXX   B 80 26 ▭

AMA: 2018,Jan,8; 2017,Jan,8; 2016,Jan,13

32800-32820 Chest Repair and Reconstruction Procedures

32800   **Repair lung hernia through chest wall**
🔧 27.0   ✂ 27.0   **FUD** 090   C 80 ▭

32810   **Closure of chest wall following open flap drainage for empyema (Clagett type procedure)**
🔧 26.0   ✂ 26.0   **FUD** 090   C 80 ▭

32815   **Open closure of major bronchial fistula**
🔧 81.0   ✂ 81.0   **FUD** 090   C 80 ▭

32820   **Major reconstruction, chest wall (posttraumatic)**
🔧 38.3   ✂ 38.3   **FUD** 090   C 80 ▭

32850-32856 Lung Transplant Procedures

INCLUDES   Harvesting donor lung(s), cold preservation, preparation donor lung(s), transplantation into recipient
EXCLUDES   *Assessment marginal cadaver donor lungs (0494T-0496T)*
Repairs or resection donor lung(s) (32491, 32505-32507, 35216, 35276)

32850   **Donor pneumonectomy(s) (including cold preservation), from cadaver donor**
🔧 0.00   ✂ 0.00   **FUD** XXX   C ▭
AMA: 1993,Win,1

32851   **Lung transplant, single; without cardiopulmonary bypass**
🔧 94.8   ✂ 94.8   **FUD** 090   C 80 ▭
AMA: 1993,Win,1

32852   **with cardiopulmonary bypass**
🔧 103.   ✂ 103.   **FUD** 090   C 80 ▭
AMA: 2017,Dec,3

32853   **Lung transplant, double (bilateral sequential or en bloc); without cardiopulmonary bypass**
🔧 133.   ✂ 133.   **FUD** 090   C 80 ▭
AMA: 1993,Win,1

32854   **with cardiopulmonary bypass**
🔧 141.   ✂ 141.   **FUD** 090   C 80 ▭
AMA: 2017,Dec,3

32855   **Backbench standard preparation of cadaver donor lung allograft prior to transplantation, including dissection of allograft from surrounding soft tissues to prepare pulmonary venous/atrial cuff, pulmonary artery, and bronchus; unilateral**
🔧 0.00   ✂ 0.00   **FUD** XXX   C 80 ▭

32856   **bilateral**
🔧 0.00   ✂ 0.00   **FUD** XXX   C 80 ▭

32900-32997 [32994] Chest and Respiratory Procedures

32900   **Resection of ribs, extrapleural, all stages**
🔧 41.0   ✂ 41.0   **FUD** 090   C 80 ▭

32905   **Thoracoplasty, Schede type or extrapleural (all stages);**
🔧 38.5   ✂ 38.5   **FUD** 090   C 80 ▭

32906   **with closure of bronchopleural fistula**
EXCLUDES   *Open closure bronchial fistula (32815)*
Resection first rib for thoracic compression (21615-21616)
🔧 47.6   ✂ 47.6   **FUD** 090   C 80 ▭

32940   **Pneumonolysis, extraperiosteal, including filling or packing procedures**
🔧 35.4   ✂ 35.4   **FUD** 090   C 80 ▭

32960   **Pneumothorax, therapeutic, intrapleural injection of air**
🔧 2.62   ✂ 3.61   **FUD** 000   T 62 ▭

32994   **Resequenced code. See code following 32998.**

32997   **Total lung lavage (unilateral)**
EXCLUDES   *Broncho-alveolar lavage by bronchoscopy (31624)*
🔧 9.84   ✂ 9.84   **FUD** 000   C 50 ▭
AMA: 2018,Jan,8; 2017,Jan,8; 2016,Jan,13

32998-32999 [32994] Destruction of Lung Neoplasm

32998   **Ablation therapy for reduction or eradication of 1 or more pulmonary tumor(s) including pleura or chest wall when involved by tumor extension, percutaneous, including imaging guidance when performed, unilateral; radiofrequency**
🔧 12.7   ✂ 99.5   **FUD** 000   J 62 80 50 ▭
AMA: 2018,Jan,8; 2017,Nov,8

\#   **32994**   **cryoablation**
🔧 12.8   ✂ 155.   **FUD** 000   J J8 80 50 ▭
AMA: 2018,Jan,8; 2017,Nov,8

32999   **Unlisted procedure, lungs and pleura**
🔧 0.00   ✂ 0.00   **FUD** YYY   T ▭
AMA: 2018,Jan,8; 2017,Jan,8; 2016,Jan,13

33016-33050 Procedures of the Pericardial Sac

EXCLUDES Surgical thoracoscopy (video-assisted thoracic surgery [VATS]) procedures pericardium (32601, 32604, 32658-32659, 32661)

33016 **Pericardiocentesis, including imaging guidance, when performed**

INCLUDES Imaging guidance for needle placement:
Computed tomography (77012)
Fluoroscopy (77002)
Magnetic resonance (77021)
Ultrasound (76942)

EXCLUDES Echocardiography for pericardiocentesis guidance (93303-93325)

🚑 6.85   ⚕ 6.85   FUD 000   G2 ▣

AMA: 2020,Jan,7

33017 **Pericardial drainage with insertion of indwelling catheter, percutaneous, including fluoroscopy and/or ultrasound guidance, when performed; 6 years and older without congenital cardiac anomaly**

INCLUDES Catheters that remain in patient at procedure conclusion
Imaging guidance for needle placement:
Fluoroscopy (77002)
Magnetic resonance (77021)
Ultrasound (76942)

EXCLUDES CT guided pericardial drainage (33019)
Echocardiography for pericardiocentesis guidance (93303-93325)
Pericardial drainage for patients:
Any age with congenital cardiac anomaly (33018)
Younger than 6 years of age (33018)
Radiologically guided catheter placement for percutaneous drainage (75989)

🚑 7.10   ⚕ 7.10   FUD 000   ▣

AMA: 2020,Jan,7

33018 **birth through 5 years of age or any age with congenital cardiac anomaly**

INCLUDES Catheters that remain in patient at procedure conclusion
Imaging guidance for needle placement:
Fluoroscopy (77002)
Magnetic resonance (77021)
Ultrasound (76942)
Patient age birth to 5 years without congenital cardiac anomaly
Patient any age with congenital cardiac anomaly, such as heterotaxy, dextrocardia, mesocardia, or single ventricle anomaly, or 90 days following repair congenital cardiac anomaly

EXCLUDES CT guided pericardial drainage (33019)
Echocardiography for pericardiocentesis guidance (93303-93325)
Radiologically guided catheter placement for percutaneous drainage (75989)

🚑 8.09   ⚕ 8.09   FUD 000   ▣

AMA: 2020,Jan,7

33019 **Pericardial drainage with insertion of indwelling catheter, percutaneous, including CT guidance**

INCLUDES Catheters that remain in patient at procedure conclusion
Imaging guidance for needle placement:
Computed tomography (77012)
Fluoroscopy (77002)
Magnetic resonance (77021)
Ultrasound (76942)

EXCLUDES Radiologically guided catheter placement for percutaneous drainage (75989)

🚑 6.57   ⚕ 6.57   FUD 000   ▣

AMA: 2020,Jan,7

33020 **Pericardiotomy for removal of clot or foreign body (primary procedure)**

INCLUDES Tube thoracostomy when chest tube or pleural drain placed on same side (32551)

🚑 23.8   ⚕ 23.8   FUD 090   C 80 ▣

AMA: 1997,Nov,1

33025 **Creation of pericardial window or partial resection for drainage**

INCLUDES Tube thoracostomy when chest tube or pleural drain placed on same side (32551)

EXCLUDES Surgical thoracoscopy (video-assisted thoracic surgery [VATS]) creation of pericardial window (32659)

🚑 22.2   ⚕ 22.2   FUD 090   C 80 ▣

AMA: 1997,Nov,1

33030 **Pericardiectomy, subtotal or complete; without cardiopulmonary bypass**

INCLUDES Delorme pericardiectomy

🚑 57.8   ⚕ 57.8   FUD 090   C 80 ▣

AMA: 1997,Nov,1; 1994,Win,1

33031 **with cardiopulmonary bypass**

🚑 71.7   ⚕ 71.7   FUD 090   C 80 ▣

AMA: 2017,Dec,3

33050 **Resection of pericardial cyst or tumor**

EXCLUDES Open biopsy pericardium (39010)
Surgical thoracoscopy (video-assisted thoracic surgery [VATS]) resection of cyst, mass, or tumor pericardium (32661)

🚑 29.1   ⚕ 29.1   FUD 090   C 80 ▣

AMA: 1997,Nov,1

33120-33130 Neoplasms of Heart

Code also removal thrombus through separate heart incision, when performed (33310-33315); append modifier 59 to (33315)

33120 **Excision of intracardiac tumor, resection with cardiopulmonary bypass**

🚑 60.6   ⚕ 60.6   FUD 090   C 80 ▣

AMA: 2018,Jan,8; 2017,Dec,3; 2017,Jan,8; 2016,Jan,13

33130 **Resection of external cardiac tumor**

🚑 39.5   ⚕ 39.5   FUD 090   C 80 ▣

AMA: 2018,Jan,8; 2017,Jan,8; 2016,Jan,13

33140-33141 Transmyocardial Revascularization

33140 **Transmyocardial laser revascularization, by thoracotomy; (separate procedure)**

🚑 45.1   ⚕ 45.1   FUD 090   C 80 ▣

AMA: 2018,Jan,8; 2017,Jan,8; 2016,Jan,13

+ **33141** **performed at the time of other open cardiac procedure(s) (List separately in addition to code for primary procedure)**

Code first (33390-33391, 33404-33496, 33510-33536, 33542)

🚑 3.80   ⚕ 3.80   FUD ZZZ   C 80 ▣

AMA: 2018,Jan,8; 2017,Jan,8; 2016,Jan,13

33202-33203 Placement Epicardial Leads

CMS: 100-04,32,270 Implantable Cardiac Defibrillators (ICDs); 100-04,32,270.1 Coding Requirements for ICDs; 100-04,32,270.2 Special Editing for Inpatient Claims; 100-04,32,270.3 Denial Messaging

INCLUDES
   Imaging guidance:
      Fluoroscopy (76000)
      Ultrasound (76942, 76998, 93318)
      Temporary pacemaker (33210-33211)
   Code also insertion pulse generator when performed by same physician/same surgical session (33212-33213, [33221], 33230-33231, 33240)

33202   **Insertion of epicardial electrode(s); open incision (eg, thoracotomy, median sternotomy, subxiphoid approach)**

      22.3   22.3   **FUD** 090   C

      AMA: 2019,Mar,6; 2018,Jan,8; 2017,Jan,8; 2016,Aug,5; 2016,May,5; 2016,Jan,13

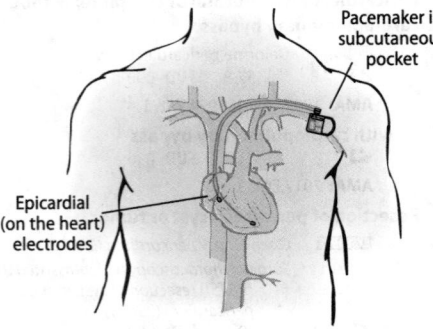

Pacemaker in subcutaneous pocket

Epicardial (on the heart) electrodes

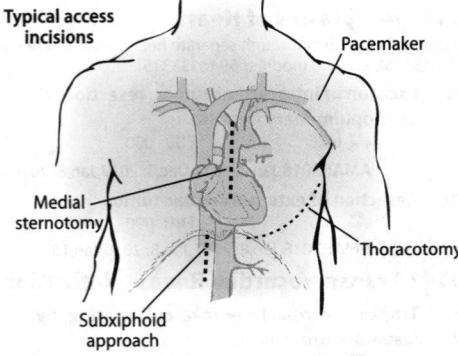

Typical access incisions

Pacemaker

Medial sternotomy

Thoracotomy

Subxiphoid approach

33203   **endoscopic approach (eg, thoracoscopy, pericardioscopy)**

      23.3   23.3   **FUD** 090   C

      AMA: 2019,Mar,6; 2018,Jan,8; 2017,Jan,8; 2016,Aug,5; 2016,May,5; 2016,Jan,13

33206-33214 [33221] Pacemakers

INCLUDES
   Device evaluation (93279-93298 [93260, 93261])
   Dual lead: device that paces and senses in two heart chambers
   Imaging guidance:
      Fluoroscopy (76000)
      Ultrasound (76942, 76998, 93318)
   Multiple lead: device that paces and senses in three or more heart chambers
   Radiological supervision and interpretation for pacemaker procedure
   Single lead: device that paces and senses in one heart chamber
   Skin pocket revision, when performed
   Temporary pacemaker (33210-33211)

EXCLUDES
   Electrode repositioning:
      Left ventricle (33226)
      Pacemaker (33215)
   Insertion lead for left ventricular (biventricular) pacing (33224-33225)
   Leadless pacemaker systems ([33274, 33275])
   Code also wound infection or hematoma incision/drainage, when performed (10140, 10180, 11042-11047 [11045, 11046])

33206   **Insertion of new or replacement of permanent pacemaker with transvenous electrode(s); atrial**

      INCLUDES   Pulse generator insertion/single transvenous electrode placement

      EXCLUDES   *Insertion transvenous electrode only (33216-33217)*
          Removal with immediate replacement pacemaker pulse generator only, single lead system ([33227])

      Code also removal old pacemaker pulse generator and electrode, when replacement entire system performed:
         Electrode (33234)
         Pulse generator (33233)

      13.1   13.1   **FUD** 090   J J8

      AMA: 2019,Oct,3; 2019,Mar,6; 2018,Jan,8; 2017,Jan,8; 2016,Aug,5; 2016,May,5; 2016,Jan,13

33207   **ventricular**

      INCLUDES   Pulse generator insertion/single transvenous electrode placement

      EXCLUDES   *Insertion transvenous electrode only (33216-33217)*
          Removal with immediate replacement pacemaker pulse generator only, single lead system ([33227])

      Code also removal old pacemaker pulse generator and electrode, when replacement entire system performed:
         Electrode (33234)
         Pulse generator (33233)

      13.9   13.9   **FUD** 090   J J8

      AMA: 2019,Oct,3; 2019,Mar,6; 2018,Jan,8; 2017,Jan,8; 2016,Aug,5; 2016,May,5; 2016,Jan,13

33208   **atrial and ventricular**

      INCLUDES   Pulse generator insertion/dual transvenous electrode placement

      EXCLUDES   *Insertion transvenous electrode(s) only (33216-33217)*
          Removal with immediate replacement pacemaker pulse generator only, dual or multiple lead system ([33228, 33229])

      Code also removal old pacemaker pulse generator and electrode, when replacement entire system performed:
         Electrodes (33235)
         Pulse generator (33233)

      15.1   15.1   **FUD** 090   J J8

      AMA: 2019,Oct,3; 2019,Mar,6; 2018,Jan,8; 2017,Jan,8; 2016,Aug,5; 2016,May,5; 2016,Jan,13

33210   **Insertion or replacement of temporary transvenous single chamber cardiac electrode or pacemaker catheter (separate procedure)**

      4.74   4.74   **FUD** 000   J G2

      AMA: 2019,Oct,3; 2019,Mar,6; 2018,Jan,8; 2017,Jan,8; 2016,Aug,5; 2016,May,5; 2016,Jan,13

33211   **Insertion or replacement of temporary transvenous dual chamber pacing electrodes (separate procedure)**

      4.90   4.90   **FUD** 000   J J8

      AMA: 2019,Oct,3; 2019,Mar,6; 2018,Jan,8; 2017,Jan,8; 2016,Aug,5; 2016,May,5; 2016,Jan,13

2G/TC PC/TC Only   A2-Z3 ASC Payment   50 Bilateral   ♂ Male Only   ♀ Female Only   Facility RVU   Non-Facility RVU   CCI   CLIA
FUD Follow-up Days   **CMS:** IOM   **AMA:** CPT Asst   A-Y OPPSI   80/80 Surg Assist Allowed / w/Doc   Lab Crosswalk   Radiology Crosswalk

124   CPT © 2021 American Medical Association. All Rights Reserved.   © 2021 Optum360, LLC

33212 **Insertion of pacemaker pulse generator only; with existing single lead**

> *EXCLUDES* *Insertion for replacement single lead pacemaker pulse generator ([33227])*
>
> *Insertion transvenous electrode(s) (33216-33217)*
>
> *Removal permanent pacemaker pulse generator only (33233)*
>
> Code also placement epicardial leads by same physician/same surgical session (33202-33203)

⚙ 9.31 ⚕ 9.31 **FUD** 090 [J] [J8] ▢

AMA: 2019,Oct,3; 2019,Mar,6; 2018,Jan,8; 2017,Jan,8; 2016,Aug,5; 2016,May,5; 2016,Jan,13

33213 **with existing dual leads**

> *EXCLUDES* *Insertion for replacement dual lead pacemaker pulse generator ([33228])*
>
> *Insertion transvenous electrode(s) (33216-33217)*
>
> *Removal permanent pacemaker pulse generator only (33233)*
>
> Code also placement epicardial leads by same physician/same surgical session (33202-33203)

⚙ 9.73 ⚕ 9.73 **FUD** 090 [J] [J8] ▢

AMA: 2019,Oct,3; 2019,Mar,6; 2018,Jan,8; 2017,Jan,8; 2016,Aug,5; 2016,May,5; 2016,Jan,13

**33221** **with existing multiple leads**

> *EXCLUDES* *Insertion for replacement multiple lead pacemaker pulse generator ([33229])*
>
> *Insertion transvenous electrode(s) (33216-33217)*
>
> *Removal permanent pacemaker pulse generator only (33233)*
>
> Code also placement epicardial leads by same physician/same surgical session (33202-33203)

⚙ 10.4 ⚕ 10.4 **FUD** 090 [J] [J8] ▢

AMA: 2019,Oct,3; 2019,Mar,6; 2018,Jan,8; 2017,Jan,8; 2016,Aug,5; 2016,May,5; 2016,Jan,13

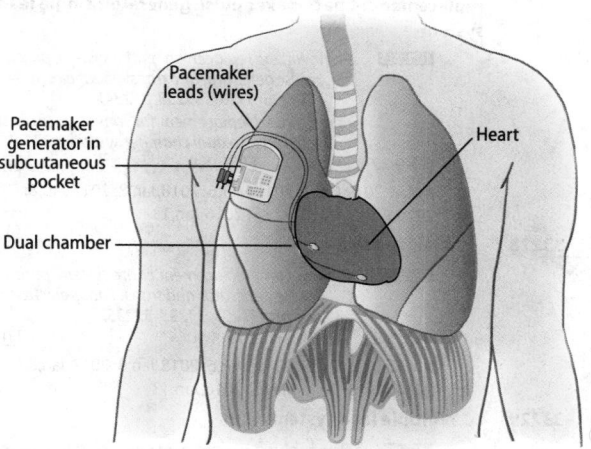

Pacemaker leads (wires)

Pacemaker generator in subcutaneous pocket

Heart

Dual chamber

33214 **Upgrade of implanted pacemaker system, conversion of single chamber system to dual chamber system (includes removal of previously placed pulse generator, testing of existing lead, insertion of new lead, insertion of new pulse generator)**

> *EXCLUDES* *Insertion transvenous electrode(s) (33216-33217)*
>
> *Removal and replacement pacemaker pulse generator (33227-33229)*

⚙ 13.8 ⚕ 13.8 **FUD** 090 [J] [J8] [80] ▢

AMA: 2019,Oct,3; 2019,Mar,6; 2018,Jan,8; 2017,Jan,8; 2016,Aug,5; 2016,May,5; 2016,Jan,13

33215-33249 [33221, 33227, 33228, 33229, 33230, 33231, 33262, 33263, 33264] Pacemakers/Implantable Defibrillator/Electrode Insertion/Replacement/Revision/Repair

> *INCLUDES* Device evaluation (93279-93298 [93260, 93261])
> Dual lead: device that paces and senses in two heart chambers
> Imaging guidance:
>   Fluoroscopy (76000)
>   Ultrasound (76942, 76998, 93318)
> Multiple lead: device that paces and senses in three or more heart chambers
> Radiological supervision and interpretation for pacemaker or pacing cardioverter-defibrillator procedure
> Single lead: device that paces and senses in one heart chamber
> Skin pocket revision, when performed
> Temporary pacemaker (33210-33211)
>
> *EXCLUDES* *Electrode repositioning:*
>   *Left ventricle (33226)*
>   *Pacemaker or implantable defibrillator (33215)*
> *Insertion lead for left ventricular (biventricular) pacing (33224-33225)*
> *Removal leadless pacemaker system ([33275])*
> *Removal subcutaneous implantable defibrillator electrode ([33272])*
> *Testing defibrillator threshold (DFT) during follow-up evaluation (93642-93644)*
> *Testing defibrillator threshold (DFT) during insertion/replacement (93640-93641)*
> Code also wound infection or hematoma incision/drainage, when performed (10140, 10180, 11042-11047 [11045, 11046])

33215 **Repositioning of previously implanted transvenous pacemaker or implantable defibrillator (right atrial or right ventricular) electrode**

⚙ 9.01 ⚕ 9.01 **FUD** 090 [T] [G2] ▢

AMA: 2019,Oct,3; 2019,Mar,6; 2018,Jan,8; 2017,Jan,8; 2016,Aug,5; 2016,May,5; 2016,Jan,13

33216 **Insertion of a single transvenous electrode, permanent pacemaker or implantable defibrillator**

> *EXCLUDES* *Insertion or replacement lead for cardiac venous system (33224-33225)*
>
> *Insertion or replacement permanent implantable defibrillator generator or system (33249)*
>
> *Removal and replacement permanent pacemaker or implantable defibrillator (33206-33208, 33212-33213, [33221], 33227-33229, 33230-33231, 33240, [33262, 33263, 33264])*

⚙ 10.7 ⚕ 10.7 **FUD** 090 [J] [J8] ▢

AMA: 2019,Oct,3; 2019,Mar,6; 2018,Jan,8; 2017,Jan,8; 2016,Aug,5; 2016,May,5; 2016,Jan,13

33217 **Insertion of 2 transvenous electrodes, permanent pacemaker or implantable defibrillator**

> *EXCLUDES* *Insertion or replacement lead for cardiac venous system (33224-33225)*
>
> *Insertion or replacement permanent implantable defibrillator generator or system (33249)*
>
> *Removal and replacement permanent pacemaker or implantable defibrillator (33206-33208, 33212-33213, [33221], 33227-33229, 33230-33231, 33240, [33262, 33263, 33264])*

⚙ 10.6 ⚕ 10.6 **FUD** 090 [J] [J8] ▢

AMA: 2019,Oct,3; 2019,Mar,6; 2018,Jan,8; 2017,Jan,8; 2016,Aug,5; 2016,May,5; 2016,Jan,13

33218 **Repair of single transvenous electrode, permanent pacemaker or implantable defibrillator**

> Code also removal old generator with insertion new generator replacement, when performed:
>   Implantable defibrillator ([33262, 33263, 33264])
>   Pacemaker ([33227, 33228, 33229])

⚙ 11.2 ⚕ 11.2 **FUD** 090 [T] [G2] ▢

AMA: 2019,Oct,3; 2019,Mar,6; 2018,Jan,8; 2017,Jan,8; 2016,Aug,5; 2016,May,5; 2016,Jan,13

33220 **Repair of 2 transvenous electrodes for permanent pacemaker or implantable defibrillator**

Code also modifier 52 Reduced services, when one electrode in two-chamber system repaired

Code also removal old generator with insertion new generator replacement, when performed:

Implantable defibrillator ([33263, 33264])

Pacemaker ([33228, 33229])

🚑 10.9   ⚖ 10.9   **FUD** 090   T J8 ▭

AMA: 2019,Oct,3; 2019,Mar,6; 2018,Jan,8; 2017,Jan,8; 2016,Aug,5; 2016,May,5; 2016,Jan,13

33221 **Resequenced code. See code following 33213.**

33222 **Relocation of skin pocket for pacemaker**

INCLUDES   Formation new pocket

Procedures related to existing pocket:

Accessing pocket

Incision/drainage abscess or hematoma (10140, 10180)

Pocket closure (13100-13102)

EXCLUDES   Debridement, subcutaneous tissue (11042-11047 [11045, 11046])

Code also removal and replacement existing generator

🚑 9.84   ⚖ 9.84   **FUD** 090   T A2 ▭

AMA: 2019,Oct,3; 2019,Mar,6; 2018,Jan,8; 2017,Jan,8; 2016,Aug,5; 2016,May,5; 2016,Jan,13

33223 **Relocation of skin pocket for implantable defibrillator**

INCLUDES   Formation new pocket

Procedures related to existing pocket:

Accessing pocket

Incision/drainage abscess or hematoma (10140, 10180)

Pocket closure (13100-13102)

EXCLUDES   Debridement, subcutaneous tissue (11042-11047 [11045, 11046])

Code also removal and replacement existing generator

🚑 11.8   ⚖ 11.8   **FUD** 090   T A2 80 ▭

AMA: 2019,Oct,3; 2019,Mar,6; 2018,Jan,8; 2017,Jan,8; 2016,Aug,5; 2016,Jan,13

33224 **Insertion of pacing electrode, cardiac venous system, for left ventricular pacing, with attachment to previously placed pacemaker or implantable defibrillator pulse generator (including revision of pocket, removal, insertion, and/or replacement of existing generator)**

Code also:

Body surface-activation mapping for optimization electrical synchrony when performed (0695T)

Placement epicardial electrode when appropriate (33202-33203)

🚑 14.9   ⚖ 14.9   **FUD** 000   J J8 ▭

AMA: 2019,Oct,3; 2019,Mar,6; 2018,Jan,8; 2017,Jan,8; 2016,Aug,5; 2016,May,5; 2016,Jan,13

+ **33225** **Insertion of pacing electrode, cardiac venous system, for left ventricular pacing, at time of insertion of implantable defibrillator or pacemaker pulse generator (eg, for upgrade to dual chamber system) (List separately in addition to code for primary procedure)**

Code also:

Body surface-activation mapping for optimization electrical synchrony when performed (0695T)

Placement epicardial electrode when appropriate (33202-33203)

Code first (33206-33208, 33212-33213, [33221], 33214, 33216-33217, 33223, 33228-33229, 33230-33231, 33233, 33234-33235, 33240, [33263, 33264], 33249)

Code first (33223) for relocation pocket for implantable defibrillator

Code first (33222) for relocation pocket for pacemaker pulse generator

🚑 13.6   ⚖ 13.6   **FUD** ZZZ   N N1 ▭

AMA: 2019,Oct,3; 2019,Mar,6; 2018,Jan,8; 2017,Jan,8; 2016,Aug,5; 2016,May,5; 2016,Jan,13

33226 **Repositioning of previously implanted cardiac venous system (left ventricular) electrode (including removal, insertion and/or replacement of existing generator)**

Code also body surface-activation mapping for optimization electrical synchrony when performed (0695T)

🚑 14.4   ⚖ 14.4   **FUD** 000   T 62 ▭

AMA: 2019,Oct,3; 2019,Mar,6; 2018,Jan,8; 2017,Jan,8; 2016,Aug,5; 2016,May,5; 2016,Jan,13

33227 **Resequenced code. See code following 33233.**

33228 **Resequenced code. See code following 33233.**

33229 **Resequenced code. See code before 33234.**

33230 **Resequenced code. See code following 33240.**

33231 **Resequenced code. See code before 33241.**

33233 **Removal of permanent pacemaker pulse generator only**

EXCLUDES   Removal with immediate replacement pacemaker pulse generator, without replacement electrode(s):

Dual lead system ([33228])

Multiple lead system ([33229])

Single lead system ([33227])

Code also insertion replacement pacemaker pulse generator with transvenous electrode(s) (total system), when performed:

Pacemaker and dual leads (33208)

Pacemaker and single atrial lead (33206)

Pacemaker and single ventricular lead (33207)

Code also removal electrode(s), when removal total system without replacement performed:

Dual leads (atrial and ventricular) (33235)

Single lead (atrial or ventricular) (33234)

🚑 6.68   ⚖ 6.68   **FUD** 090   Q2 J8 ▭

AMA: 2019,Oct,3; 2019,Mar,6; 2018,Jan,8; 2017,Jan,8; 2016,Aug,5; 2016,May,5; 2016,Jan,13

\# **33227** **Removal of permanent pacemaker pulse generator with replacement of pacemaker pulse generator; single lead system**

EXCLUDES   Removal and replacement entire system, pacemaker pulse generator and transvenous electrode, report (33206-33207, 33233, 33234)

Removal and replacement for conversion from single chamber to dual chamber system (33214)

🚑 9.82   ⚖ 9.82   **FUD** 090   J J8 ▭

AMA: 2019,Oct,3; 2019,Mar,6; 2018,Jan,8; 2017,Jan,8; 2016,Aug,5; 2016,May,5; 2016,Jan,13

\# **33228** **dual lead system**

EXCLUDES   Removal and replacement entire system, pacemaker pulse generator and transvenous electrode(s), report (33208, 33233, 33235)

🚑 10.2   ⚖ 10.2   **FUD** 090   J J8 ▭

AMA: 2019,Oct,3; 2019,Mar,6; 2018,Jan,8; 2017,Jan,8; 2016,Aug,5; 2016,May,5; 2016,Jan,13

\# **33229** **multiple lead system**

EXCLUDES   Removal and replacement entire system, pacemaker pulse generator and transvenous electrode(s), report (33208, 33233, 33235)

🚑 10.8   ⚖ 10.8   **FUD** 090   J J8 ▭

AMA: 2019,Oct,3; 2019,Mar,6; 2018,Jan,8; 2017,Jan,8; 2016,Aug,5; 2016,May,5; 2016,Jan,13

26/TC PC/TC Only   A2-Z3 ASC Payment   50 Bilateral   ♂ Male Only   ♀ Female Only   🚑 Facility RVU   ⚖ Non-Facility RVU   ▭ CCI   ✖ CLIA
FUD Follow-up Days   CMS: IOM   AMA: CPT Asst   A-Y OPPSI   80/80 Surg Assist Allowed / w/Doc   Lab Crosswalk   Radiology Crosswalk

126   CPT © 2021 American Medical Association. All Rights Reserved.   © 2021 Optum360, LLC

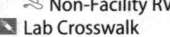

33234 **Removal of transvenous pacemaker electrode(s); single lead system, atrial or ventricular**

Code also pacing electrode insertion in cardiac venous system for pacing left ventricle during insertion pulse generator (pacemaker or implantable defibrillator) when performed (33225)

Code also removal old pacemaker pulse generator and insertion replacement pacemaker pulse generator with transvenous electrode (total system), when performed:
Insertion pacemaker and atrial lead (33206) OR
Insertion pacemaker and ventricular lead (33207) AND
Removal generator (33233)

Code also thoracotomy to remove electrode, when performed, for unsuccessful transvenous removal (33238)

🚑 14.0   🔪 14.0   **FUD** 090   02 J8 ▣

AMA: 2019,Oct,3; 2019,Mar,6; 2018,Jan,8; 2017,Jan,8; 2016,Aug,5; 2016,May,5; 2016,Jan,13

33235 **dual lead system**

Code also pacing electrode insertion in cardiac venous system for pacing left ventricle during insertion pulse generator (pacemaker or implantable defibrillator) when performed (33225)

Code also removal old pacemaker pulse generator and insertion replacement pacemaker pulse generator with transvenous electrodes (total system), when performed:
Insertion generator and dual leads (33208) AND
Insertion pacemaker and atrial lead (33206) OR
Insertion pacemaker and ventricular lead (33207) AND
Removal generator (33233)

Code also thoracotomy to remove electrode, when performed, for unsuccessful transvenous removal (33238)

🚑 18.5   🔪 18.5   **FUD** 090   02 J8 ▣

AMA: 2019,Oct,3; 2019,Mar,6; 2018,Jan,8; 2017,Jan,8; 2016,Aug,5; 2016,May,5; 2016,Jan,13

33236 **Removal of permanent epicardial pacemaker and electrodes by thoracotomy; single lead system, atrial or ventricular**

EXCLUDES *Removal implantable defibrillator electrode(s) by thoracotomy (33243)*
Removal transvenous electrodes by thoracotomy (33238)
Removal transvenous pacemaker electrodes, single or dual lead system; without thoracotomy (33234, 33235)

🚑 22.5   🔪 22.5   **FUD** 090   C 80 ▣

AMA: 2019,Oct,3; 2019,Mar,6; 2018,Jan,8; 2017,Jan,8; 2016,Aug,5; 2016,May,5; 2016,Jan,13

33237 **dual lead system**

EXCLUDES *Removal implantable defibrillator electrode(s) by thoracotomy (33243)*
Removal transvenous electrodes by thoracotomy (33238)
Removal transvenous pacemaker electrodes, single or dual lead system; without thoracotomy (33234, 33235)

🚑 24.1   🔪 24.1   **FUD** 090   C 80 ▣

AMA: 2019,Oct,3; 2019,Mar,6; 2018,Jan,8; 2017,Jan,8; 2016,Aug,5; 2016,May,5; 2016,Jan,13

33238 **Removal of permanent transvenous electrode(s) by thoracotomy**

EXCLUDES *Removal implantable defibrillator electrode(s) by thoracotomy (33243)*
Removal transvenous pacemaker electrodes, single or dual lead system; without thoracotomy (33234, 33235)

🚑 27.0   🔪 27.0   **FUD** 090   C 80 ▣

AMA: 2019,Oct,3; 2018,Jan,8; 2017,Jan,8; 2016,Aug,5; 2016,May,5; 2016,Jan,13

33240 **Insertion of implantable defibrillator pulse generator only; with existing single lead**

EXCLUDES *Insertion electrode(s) (33216-33217, [33271])*
Removal and replacement implantable defibrillator pulse generator only ([33262, 33263, 33264])

Code also placement epicardial leads by same physician/same surgical session as generator insertion (33202-33203)

🚑 10.5   🔪 10.5   **FUD** 090   J J8 ▣

AMA: 2019,Oct,3; 2018,Jan,8; 2017,Jan,8; 2016,Aug,5; 2016,Jan,13

33230 **with existing dual leads**

EXCLUDES *Insertion single transvenous electrode, permanent pacemaker or implantable defibrillator (33216-33217)*
Removal and replacement implantable defibrillator pulse generator only ([33262, 33263, 33264])

Code also placement epicardial leads by same physician/same surgical session as generator insertion (33202-33203)

🚑 11.0   🔪 11.0   **FUD** 090   J J8 ▣

AMA: 2019,Oct,3; 2019,Mar,6; 2018,Jan,8; 2017,Jan,8; 2016,Aug,5; 2016,Jan,13

33231 **with existing multiple leads**

EXCLUDES *Insertion single transvenous electrode, permanent pacemaker or implantable defibrillator (33216-33217)*
Removal and replacement implantable defibrillator pulse generator only ([33262, 33263, 33264])

Code also placement epicardial leads by same physician/same surgical session as generator placement (33202-33203)

🚑 11.6   🔪 11.6   **FUD** 090   J J8 ▣

AMA: 2019,Oct,3; 2019,Mar,6; 2018,Jan,8; 2017,Jan,8; 2016,Aug,5; 2016,Jan,13

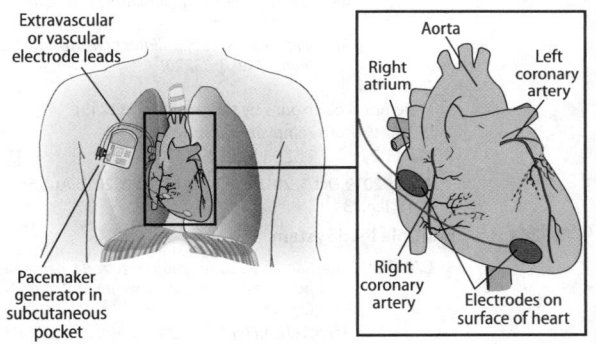

Extravascular or vascular electrode leads

Pacemaker generator in subcutaneous pocket

Aorta
Right atrium
Left coronary artery
Right coronary artery
Electrodes on surface of heart

33241 **Removal of implantable defibrillator pulse generator only**

EXCLUDES *Removal substernal implantable defibrillator pulse generator only (0580T)*
Removal with immediate replacement implantable defibrillator pulse generator only ([33262, 33263, 33264])

Code also removal electrode(s) and insertion replacement defibrillator with electrode(s) (total system), when performed:
Removal electrode(s) (33243-33244) AND
Insertion defibrillator system, single or dual (33249) OR
Removal subcutaneous electrode ([33272]) AND
Insertion subcutaneous defibrillator system ([33270])

Code also removal electrode(s), when total system removed without replacement:
Subcutaneous electrode ([33272])
Transvenous electrode(s) (33243)

🚑 6.20   🔪 6.20   **FUD** 090   02 62 ▣

AMA: 2019,Oct,3; 2018,Jan,8; 2017,Jan,8; 2016,Aug,5; 2016,Jan,13

**33262** **Removal of implantable defibrillator pulse generator with replacement of implantable defibrillator pulse generator; single lead system**

> *EXCLUDES* *Insertion electrode(s) (33216-33217, [33271])*
> *Removal and replacement implantable defibrillator pulse generator and electrode(s) (total system) (33241, 33243-33244, 33249)*
> *Removal and replacement subcutaneous defibrillator pulse generator and electrode(s) (total system) (33241, [33270], [33272])*
> *Removal and replacement substernal implantable defibrillator pulse generator ([0614T])*
> *Removal implantable defibrillator pulse generator only (33241)*
> *Repair implantable defibrillator pulse generator and/or leads (33218, 33220)*

Code also:
Electrode(s) removal by thoracotomy (33243)
Subcutaneous electrode removal ([33272])
Transvenous removal of electrode(s) (33244)

🚑 10.8   ≥ 10.8   **FUD** 090   J J8 ▭

AMA: 2019,Oct,3; 2018,Jan,8; 2017,Jan,8; 2016,Aug,5; 2016,Jan,13

**33263** **dual lead system**

> *EXCLUDES* *Insertion single transvenous electrode, permanent pacemaker or implantable defibrillator (33216-33217)*
> *Removal and replacement implantable defibrillator pulse generator and electrode(s) (total system) (33241, 33243-33244, 33249)*
> *Removal and replacement subcutaneous defibrillator pulse generator and electrode (total system) (33241, [33270], [33272])*
> *Removal implantable defibrillator pulse generator only (33241)*
> *Repair implantable defibrillator pulse generator and/or leads (33218, 33220)*

Code also:
Removal electrodes by thoracotomy (33243)
Transvenous removal electrodes (33244)

🚑 11.2   ≥ 11.2   **FUD** 090   J J8 ▭

AMA: 2019,Oct,3; 2018,Jan,8; 2017,Jan,8; 2016,Aug,5; 2016,Jan,13

**33264** **multiple lead system**

> *EXCLUDES* *Insertion single transvenous electrode, permanent pacemaker or implantable defibrillator (33216-33217)*
> *Removal and replacement implantable defibrillator pulse generator and electrode(s) (total system) (33241, 33243-33244, 33249)*
> *Removal and replacement subcutaneous defibrillator pulse generator and electrode(s) (total system) (33241, [33270], [33272])*
> *Removal implantable defibrillator pulse generator only (33241)*
> *Repair implantable defibrillator pulse generator and/or leads (33218, 33220)*

Code also:
Removal electrodes by thoracotomy (33243)
Transvenous removal electrodes (33244)

🚑 11.7   ≥ 11.7   **FUD** 090   J J8 ▭

AMA: 2019,Oct,3; 2018,Jan,8; 2017,Jan,8; 2016,Aug,5; 2016,Jan,13

33243 **Removal of single or dual chamber implantable defibrillator electrode(s); by thoracotomy**

> *EXCLUDES* *Transvenous removal defibrillator electrode(s) (33244)*

Code also removal implantable defibrillator pulse generator and insertion replacement defibrillator with electrodes (total system), when entire system replaced:
Insertion defibrillator system, single or dual (33249)
Removal generator (33241)
Code also removal implantable defibrillator pulse generator, when entire system removed without replacement (33241)
Code also replacement implantable defibrillator pulse generator, when performed:
Dual lead system ([33263])
Multiple lead system ([33264])
Single lead system ([33262])

🚑 39.6   ≥ 39.6   **FUD** 090   C 80 ▭

AMA: 2019,Oct,3; 2018,Jan,8; 2017,Jan,8; 2016,Aug,5; 2016,Jan,13

33244 **by transvenous extraction**

Code also removal implantable defibrillator pulse generator and insertion replacement defibrillator with electrodes (total system), when entire system replaced:
Insertion defibrillator system, single or dual (33249)
Removal generator (33241)
Code also removal implantable defibrillator pulse generator, when entire system removed without replacement (33241)
Code also replacement implantable defibrillator pulse generator, when performed:
Dual lead system ([33263])
Multiple lead system ([33264])
Single lead system ([33262])
Code also thoracotomy to remove electrode, when performed, if transvenous removal unsuccessful (33238, 33243)

🚑 25.1   ≥ 25.1   **FUD** 090   02 62 ▭

AMA: 2019,Oct,3; 2018,Jan,8; 2017,Jan,8; 2016,Aug,5; 2016,Jan,13

33249 **Insertion or replacement of permanent implantable defibrillator system, with transvenous lead(s), single or dual chamber**

> *EXCLUDES* *Insertion single transvenous electrode, permanent pacemaker or implantable defibrillator (33216-33217)*

Code also removal defibrillator generator when upgrading from single to dual-chamber system (33241)
Code also removal implantable defibrillator pulse generator and removal electrode(s), when entire system replaced:
Removal electrode(s) (33243-33244)
Removal generator (33241)

🚑 26.6   ≥ 26.6   **FUD** 090   J J8 ▭

AMA: 2019,Oct,3; 2018,Jan,8; 2017,Jan,8; 2016,Aug,5; 2016,Jan,13

26/TC PC/TC Only   A2-73 ASC Payment   50 Bilateral   ♂ Male Only   ♀ Female Only   🚑 Facility RVU   ≥ Non-Facility RVU   ▭ CCI   ✖ CLIA
FUD Follow-up Days   CMS: IOM   AMA: CPT Asst   A-Y OPPSI   80/80 Surg Assist Allowed / w/Doc   ▭ Lab Crosswalk   ▤ Radiology Crosswalk

128   CPT © 2021 American Medical Association. All Rights Reserved.   © 2021 Optum360, LLC

33270-33275 [33270, 33271, 33272, 33273, 33274, 33275] Subcutaneous Implantable Defibrillator

INCLUDES Programming and interrogation of:
Leadless pacemaker (93279, 93286, 93288, 93294, 93296)
Subcutaneous implantable defibrillator ([93260, 93261])

\# **33270** **Insertion or replacement of permanent subcutaneous implantable defibrillator system, with subcutaneous electrode, including defibrillation threshold evaluation, induction of arrhythmia, evaluation of sensing for arrhythmia termination, and programming or reprogramming of sensing or therapeutic parameters, when performed**

INCLUDES Electrophysiologic evaluation at initial insertion (93644)

EXCLUDES *Insertion subcutaneous implantable defibrillator electrode only ([33271])*

Insertion/replacement permanent implantable defibrillator system with substernal electrode (0571T)

Code also electrophysiologic evaluation following replacement subcutaneous implantable defibrillator, when performed (93644)

Code also removal subcutaneous implantable defibrillator and removal subcutaneous electrode, when entire system is being replaced:
Defibrillator (33241)
Electrode ([33272])

🔧 16.4   ⚗ 16.4   **FUD** 090   J J8 ▱

AMA: 2019,Oct,3; 2018,Jan,8; 2017,Jan,8; 2016,Aug,5; 2016,Jan,13

\# **33271** **Insertion of subcutaneous implantable defibrillator electrode**

EXCLUDES *Insertion implantable defibrillator pulse generator only, other than subcutaneous:*
Initial insertion (33240)
Removal/replacement ([33262])
Insertion subcutaneous implantable defibrillator and electrode (total system) ([33270])
Insertion substernal defibrillator electrode (0572T)

🔧 13.1   ⚗ 13.1   **FUD** 090   J J8 ▱

AMA: 2019,Oct,3; 2018,Jan,8; 2017,Jan,8; 2016,Aug,5; 2016,Jan,13

\# **33272** **Removal of subcutaneous implantable defibrillator electrode**

EXCLUDES *Removal substernal defibrillator electrode (0573T)*

Code also removal implantable defibrillator, when performed:
Removal with replacement ([33262])
Removal without replacement (33241)

Code also removal subcutaneous implantable defibrillator and insertion replacement implantable subcutaneous defibrillator with electrode (total system), when entire system is being replaced:
Insertion total system ([33270])
Removal defibrillator (33241)

🔧 10.0   ⚗ 10.0   **FUD** 090   02 62 ▱

AMA: 2019,Oct,3; 2018,Jan,8; 2017,Jan,8; 2016,Aug,5; 2016,Jan,13

\# **33273** **Repositioning of previously implanted subcutaneous implantable defibrillator electrode**

EXCLUDES *Repositioning substernal defibrillator electrode (0574T)*

🔧 11.5   ⚗ 11.5   **FUD** 090   T 62 ▱

AMA: 2019,Oct,3; 2018,Jan,8; 2017,Jan,8; 2016,Aug,5; 2016,Jan,13

\# **33274** **Transcatheter insertion or replacement of permanent leadless pacemaker, right ventricular, including imaging guidance (eg, fluoroscopy, venous ultrasound, ventriculography, femoral venography) and device evaluation (eg, interrogation or programming), when performed**

INCLUDES Cardiac catheterization for insertion leadless pacemaker (93451, 93453, 93456-93457, 93460-93461, 93593-93594, 93596-93598)
Femoral venography (75820)
Imaging guidance (76000, 76937, 77002)
Right ventriculography (93566)

EXCLUDES *Removal permanent leadless pacemaker ([33275])*
Services for pacemakers with leads (33202-33203, 33206-33208, 33212-33214[33221], 33215-33218, 33220, 33233-33237 [33227, 33228, 33229])

Code also intracardiac echocardiography, if performed (93662)

🔧 14.2   ⚗ 14.2   **FUD** 090   J8 ▱

AMA: 2019,Mar,6

\# **33275** **Transcatheter removal of permanent leadless pacemaker, right ventricular, including imaging guidance (eg, fluoroscopy, venous ultrasound, ventriculography, femoral venography), when performed**

INCLUDES Cardiac catheterization for insertion leadless pacemaker (93451, 93453, 93456-93457, 93460-93461, 93593-93594, 93596-93598)
Femoral venography (75820)
Imaging guidance (76000, 76937, 77002)
Right ventriculography (93566)

EXCLUDES *Insertion/replacement leadless pacemaker ([33274])*
Services for pacemakers with leads (33202-33203, 33206-33208, 33212-33214[33221], 33215-33218, 33220, 33233-33237 [33227, 33228, 33229])

Code also intracardiac echocardiography, if performed (93662)

🔧 15.4   ⚗ 15.4   **FUD** 090   J8 ▱

AMA: 2019,Mar,6

33250-33251 Surgical Ablation Arrhythmogenic Foci, Supraventricular

INCLUDES Procedures using cryotherapy, laser, microwave, radiofrequency, and ultrasound

33250 **Operative ablation of supraventricular arrhythmogenic focus or pathway (eg, Wolff-Parkinson-White, atrioventricular node re-entry), tract(s) and/or focus (foci); without cardiopulmonary bypass**

EXCLUDES *Pacing and mapping during surgery by other provider (93631)*

🔧 42.4   ⚗ 42.4   **FUD** 090   C 80 ▱

AMA: 2018,Jan,8; 2017,Jan,8; 2016,Jan,13

33251 **with cardiopulmonary bypass**

🔧 47.0   ⚗ 47.0   **FUD** 090   C 80 ▱

AMA: 2018,Jan,8; 2017,Dec,3; 2017,Jan,8; 2016,Jan,13

33254-33256 Surgical Ablation Arrhythmogenic Foci, Atrial (e.g., Maze)

INCLUDES Excision or isolation left atrial appendage
Procedures using cryotherapy, laser, microwave, radiofrequency, and ultrasound

EXCLUDES *Any procedure involving median sternotomy or cardiopulmonary bypass*
Aortic valve procedures (33390-33391, 33404-33415)
Aortoplasty (33417)
Ascending aorta graft (33858-33859, 33863-33864)
Coronary artery bypass (33510-33516, 33517-33523, 33533-33536)
Excision intracardiac tumor, resection (33120)
Mitral valve procedures (33418-33430)
Outflow tract augmentation (33478)
Prosthetic valve repair (33496)
Pulmonary artery embolectomy (33910-33920)
Pulmonary valve procedures (33471-33477)
Repair aberrant coronary artery anatomy (33500-33507)
Repair aberrant heart anatomy (33600-33853)
Resection external cardiac tumor (33130)
Temporary pacemaker (33210-33211)
Thoracotomy; with exploration (32100)
Tricuspid valve procedures (33460-33468)
Tube thoracostomy, includes connection to drainage system (32551)
Ventricular reconstruction (33542-33548)
Ventriculomyotomy (33416)

33254 Operative tissue ablation and reconstruction of atria, limited (eg, modified maze procedure)
39.0 ⚖ 39.0 **FUD** 090 C 80
AMA: 2018,Jan,8; 2017,Jan,8; 2016,Jan,13

33255 Operative tissue ablation and reconstruction of atria, extensive (eg, maze procedure); without cardiopulmonary bypass
47.3 ⚖ 47.3 **FUD** 090 C 80
AMA: 2018,Jan,8; 2017,Jan,8; 2016,Jan,13

33256 with cardiopulmonary bypass
56.1 ⚖ 56.1 **FUD** 090 C 80
AMA: 2018,Jan,8; 2017,Dec,3; 2017,Jan,8; 2016,Jan,13

33257-33259 Surgical Ablation Arrhythmogenic Foci, Atrial, with Other Heart Procedure(s)

EXCLUDES *Operative tissue ablation and reconstruction atria (without other cardiac procedure), limited or extensive:*
Endoscopic (33265-33266)
Open (33254-33256)
Temporary pacemaker (33210-33211)
Tube thoracostomy, includes connection to drainage system (32551)

+ **33257** Operative tissue ablation and reconstruction of atria, performed at the time of other cardiac procedure(s), limited (eg, modified maze procedure) (List separately in addition to code for primary procedure)
Code first (33120-33130, 33250-33251, 33261, 33300-33335, 33365, 33390-33391, 33404-33417 [33440], 33420-33430, 33460-33476, 33478, 33496, 33500-33507, 33510-33516, 33533-33548, 33600-33619, 33641-33697, 33702-33732, 33735-33767, 33770-33877, 33910-33922, 33925-33926, 33975-33983)
16.8 ⚖ 16.8 **FUD** ZZZ C 80

+ **33258** Operative tissue ablation and reconstruction of atria, performed at the time of other cardiac procedure(s), extensive (eg, maze procedure), without cardiopulmonary bypass (List separately in addition to code for primary procedure)
Code first, when performed without cardiopulmonary bypass (33130, 33250, 33300, 33310, 33320-33321, 33330, 33365, 33420, 33471, 33501-33503, 33510-33516, 33533-33536, 33690, 33735, 33737, 33750-33766, 33800-33813, 33820-33824, 33840-33852, 33875, 33877, 33915, 33925, 33981, 33982)
18.7 ⚖ 18.7 **FUD** ZZZ C 80

+ **33259** Operative tissue ablation and reconstruction of atria, performed at the time of other cardiac procedure(s), extensive (eg, maze procedure), with cardiopulmonary bypass (List separately in addition to code for primary procedure)
Code first, when performed with cardiopulmonary bypass (33120, 33251, 33261, 33305, 33315, 33322, 33335, 33390-33391, 33404-33410, 33411-33417, 33422-33430, 33460-33468, 33474-33478, 33496, 33500, 33504-33507, 33510-33516, 33533-33548, 33600-33688, 33692-33726, 33730, 33732, 33736, 33767, 33770, 33783, 33786-33788, 33814, 33853, 33858-33877, 33910, 33916-33922, 33926, 33975-33980, 33983)
24.3 ⚖ 24.3 **FUD** ZZZ C 80
AMA: 2017,Dec,3

33261-33264 [33262, 33263, 33264, 33267, 33268, 33269] Surgical Ablation Arrhythmogenic Foci, Ventricular

33261 Operative ablation of ventricular arrhythmogenic focus with cardiopulmonary bypass
46.7 ⚖ 46.7 **FUD** 090 C 80
AMA: 2018,Jan,8; 2017,Dec,3; 2017,Jan,8; 2016,Jan,13

Impulse centers that are causing arrhythmia are treated with ablation

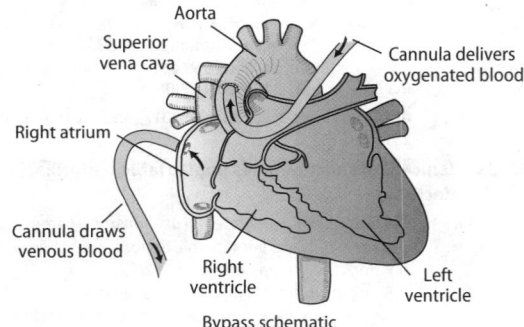

Bypass schematic

● # **33267** Exclusion of left atrial appendage, open, any method (eg, excision, isolation via stapling, oversewing, ligation, plication, clip)
EXCLUDES *Replacement, mitral valve (33430)*
Sternotomy/thoracotomy procedures performed during same operative session
Tissue ablation/reconstruction atria (33254-33259, 33265-33266)
Valvotomy, mitral valve (33420, 33422)
Valvuloplasty, mitral valve (33425-33427)
0.00 ⚖ 0.00 **FUD** 000

● + # **33268** Exclusion of left atrial appendage, open, performed at the time of other sternotomy or thoracotomy procedure(s), any method (eg, excision, isolation via stapling, oversewing, ligation, plication, clip) (List separately in addition to code for primary procedure)
EXCLUDES *Replacement, mitral valve (33430)*
Tissue ablation/reconstruction atria (33254-33259, 33265-33266)
Valvotomy, mitral valve (33420, 33422)
Valvuloplasty, mitral valve (33425-33427)
Code first primary procedure requiring sternotomy/thoracotomy
0.00 ⚖ 0.00 **FUD** 000

26/TC PC/TC Only   A2-Z3 ASC Payment   50 Bilateral   ♂ Male Only   ♀ Female Only   Facility RVU   ⚖ Non-Facility RVU   CCI   CLIA
FUD Follow-up Days   CMS: IOM   AMA: CPT Asst   A-Y OPPSI   80/80 Surg Assist Allowed / w/Doc   Lab Crosswalk   Radiology Crosswalk

130   CPT © 2021 American Medical Association. All Rights Reserved.   © 2021 Optum360, LLC

● # **33269** **Exclusion of left atrial appendage, thoracoscopic, any method (eg, excision, isolation via stapling, oversewing, ligation, plication, clip)**

> EXCLUDES *Replacement, mitral valve (33430)*
> *Tissue ablation/reconstruction atria (33254-33259, 33265-33266)*
> *Valvotomy, mitral valve (33420, 33422)*
> *Valvuloplasty, mitral valve (33425-33427)*
>
> 🔲 0.00 ⚖ 0.00 **FUD** 000

33262 Resequenced code. See code following 33241.

33263 Resequenced code. See code following 33241.

33264 Resequenced code. See code before 33243.

33265-33275 [33267, 33268, 33269, 33270, 33271, 33272, 33273, 33274, 33275] Surgical Ablation Arrhythmogenic Foci, Endoscopic

> EXCLUDES *Insertion or replacement temporary transvenous single chamber cardiac electrode or pacemaker catheter (separate procedure) (33210-33211)*
> *Tube thoracostomy, includes connection to drainage system (32551)*

33265 **Endoscopy, surgical; operative tissue ablation and reconstruction of atria, limited (eg, modified maze procedure), without cardiopulmonary bypass**

> 🔲 39.3 ⚖ 39.3 **FUD** 090 C 80 ▭
>
> **AMA:** 2018,Jan,8; 2017,Jan,8; 2016,Jan,13

33266 **operative tissue ablation and reconstruction of atria, extensive (eg, maze procedure), without cardiopulmonary bypass**

> 🔲 53.4 ⚖ 53.4 **FUD** 090 C 80 ▭
>
> **AMA:** 2018,Jan,8; 2017,Jan,8; 2016,Jan,13

33267 Resequenced code. See code following 33261.

33268 Resequenced code. See code following 33261.

33269 Resequenced code. See code following 33261.

33270 Resequenced code. See code following 33249.

33271 Resequenced code. See code following 33249.

33272 Resequenced code. See code following 33249.

33273 Resequenced code. See code following 33249.

33274 Resequenced code. See code following 33249.

33275 Resequenced code. See code following 33249.

33285-33289 Cardiac Rhythm Monitor System

33285 **Insertion, subcutaneous cardiac rhythm monitor, including programming**

> INCLUDES Implantation device into subcutaneous prepectoral pocket
> Initial programming
> EXCLUDES *Successive analysis and/or reprogramming (93285, 93291, 93298)*
>
> 🔲 2.57 ⚖ 142. **FUD** 000 J8 ▭
>
> **AMA:** 2019,Oct,3; 2019,Apr,3

33286 **Removal, subcutaneous cardiac rhythm monitor**

> 🔲 2.54 ⚖ 3.80 **FUD** 000 G2 ▭
>
> **AMA:** 2019,Apr,3

33289 **Transcatheter implantation of wireless pulmonary artery pressure sensor for long-term hemodynamic monitoring, including deployment and calibration of the sensor, right heart catheterization, selective pulmonary catheterization, radiological supervision and interpretation, and pulmonary artery angiography, when performed**

> INCLUDES Device implantation into subcutaneous pocket
> Fluoroscopy (76000)
> Pulmonary artery angiography/injection (75741, 75743, 75746, 93568)
> Pulmonary artery catheterization (36013-36015)
> Radiologic supervision and interpretation
> Remote monitoring (93264)
> Right heart catheterization (93451, 93453, 93456-93457, 93460-93461, 93593-93594, 93596-93598)
> Sensor deployment and calibration
>
> 🔲 9.55 ⚖ 9.55 **FUD** 000 80 ▭
>
> **AMA:** 2019,Jun,3

33300-33315 Procedures for Injury of the Heart

> INCLUDES Procedures with and without cardiopulmonary bypass
> Code also transvascular ventricular support, when performed:
> Balloon pump (33967, 33968, 33970-33974)
> Extracorporeal membrane oxygenation (ECMO)/extracorporeal life support (ECLS) (33946-33949)
> Ventricular assist device (33975-33983, [33995], 33990-33993 [33997])

33300 **Repair of cardiac wound; without bypass**

> 🔲 71.0 ⚖ 71.0 **FUD** 090 C 80 ▭
>
> **AMA:** 1997,Nov,1

33305 **with cardiopulmonary bypass**

> 🔲 118. ⚖ 118. **FUD** 090 C 80 ▭
>
> **AMA:** 2017,Dec,3

33310 **Cardiotomy, exploratory (includes removal of foreign body, atrial or ventricular thrombus); without bypass**

> EXCLUDES *Other cardiac procedures unless separate incision into heart necessary to remove thrombus*
>
> 🔲 33.7 ⚖ 33.7 **FUD** 090 C 80 ▭
>
> **AMA:** 1997,Nov,1

33315 **with cardiopulmonary bypass**

> EXCLUDES *Other cardiac procedures unless separate incision into heart necessary to remove thrombus*
> Code also excision thrombus with cardiopulmonary bypass and append modifier 59 when separate incision required with (33120, 33130, 33420-33430, 33460-33468, 33496, 33542, 33545, 33641-33647, 33670, 33681, 33975-33980)
>
> 🔲 55.3 ⚖ 55.3 **FUD** 090 C 80 ▭
>
> **AMA:** 2018,Jan,8; 2017,Dec,3; 2017,Jan,8; 2016,Jan,13

33320-33335 Procedures for Injury of the Aorta/Great Vessels

> Code also transvascular ventricular support, when performed:
> Balloon pump (33967, 33968, 33970-33974)
> Extracorporeal membrane oxygenation (ECMO)/extracorporeal life support (ECLS) (33946-33949)
> Ventricular assist device (33975-33983, [33995], 33990-33993 [33997])

33320 **Suture repair of aorta or great vessels; without shunt or cardiopulmonary bypass**

> 🔲 30.5 ⚖ 30.5 **FUD** 090 C 80 ▭
>
> **AMA:** 2018,Jun,11; 2018,Jan,8; 2017,Jan,8; 2016,Jan,13

33321 **with shunt bypass**

> 🔲 34.3 ⚖ 34.3 **FUD** 090 C 80 ▭
>
> **AMA:** 2018,Jun,11

33322 **with cardiopulmonary bypass**

> 🔲 40.2 ⚖ 40.2 **FUD** 090 C 80 ▭
>
> **AMA:** 2018,Jun,11; 2018,Jan,8; 2017,Dec,3; 2017,Jan,8; 2016,Jan,13

33330 **Insertion of graft, aorta or great vessels; without shunt, or cardiopulmonary bypass**

> 🔲 41.2 ⚖ 41.2 **FUD** 090 C 80 ▭
>
> **AMA:** 2018,Jun,11

● New Code ▲ Revised Code ○ Reinstated ● New Web Release ▲ Revised Web Release + Add-on Unlisted Not Covered # Resequenced
⑤⓪ Optum Mod 50 Exempt ⚖ AMA Mod 51 Exempt ⑤① Optum Mod 51 Exempt ⑥③ Mod 63 Exempt ⚕ Non-FDA Drug ★ Telemedicine Ⓜ Maternity Ⓐ Age Edit

© 2021 Optum360, LLC CPT © 2021 American Medical Association. All Rights Reserved. 131

33335   **with cardiopulmonary bypass**
🔷 54.6 ⚕ 54.6 **FUD** 090   C 80 ▢
AMA: 2018,Jun,11; 2017,Dec,3

33340 Closure Left Atrial Appendage

EXCLUDES *Cardiac catheterization except for reasons other than closure left atrial appendage (93451-93453, 93456, 93458-93461, 93462, 93593-93598)*
Code also intracardiac echocardiography, if performed (93662)
Code also transvascular ventricular support, when performed:
  Balloon pump (33967, 33968, 33970-33974)
  Extracorporeal membrane oxygenation (ECMO)/extracorporeal life support (ECLS) (33946-33949)
  Ventricular assist device (33975-33983, [33995], 33990-33993 [33997])

33340   **Percutaneous transcatheter closure of the left atrial appendage with endocardial implant, including fluoroscopy, transseptal puncture, catheter placement(s), left atrial angiography, left atrial appendage angiography, when performed, and radiological supervision and interpretation**
🔷 22.9 ⚕ 22.9 **FUD** 000   C 80 ▢
AMA: 2018,Jan,8; 2017,Jul,3

33361-33369 Transcatheter Aortic Valve Replacement

CMS: 100-03,20.32 Transcatheter Aortic Valve Replacement (TAVR); 100-04,32,290.3 Claims Processing TAVR Inpatient; 100-04,32,290.4 Payment of TAVR for MA Plan Participants

INCLUDES Access and implantation aortic valve (33361-33366)
    Access sheath placement
    Advancement valve delivery system
    Arteriotomy closure
    Balloon aortic valvuloplasty
    Cardiac or open arterial approach
    Deployment of valve
    Percutaneous access
    Radiology procedures:
      Angiography during and after procedure
      Assessment access site for closure
      Documentation intervention completion
      Guidance for valve placement
      Supervision and interpretation
    Temporary pacemaker
    Valve repositioning when necessary
EXCLUDES *Cardiac catheterization procedures included in TAVR/TAVI service (93452-93453, 93458-93461, 93567)*
    Percutaneous coronary interventional procedures
Code also cardiac catheterization services for purposes other than TAVR/TAVI
Code also diagnostic coronary angiography at different session from interventional procedure
Code also diagnostic coronary angiography same time as TAVR/TAVI when:
  Previous study available, but documentation states patient's condition has changed since previous study, visualization anatomy/pathology inadequate, or change occurs during procedure warranting additional evaluation outside current target area
  No previous catheter-based coronary angiography study available, and full diagnostic study performed, with decision to perform intervention based on that study
Code also modifier 59 when diagnostic coronary angiography procedures performed as separate and distinct procedural services on same day or session as TAVR/TAVI
Code also modifier 62 as all TAVI/TAVR procedures require work two physicians
Code also transvascular ventricular support, when performed:
  Balloon pump (33967, 33970, 33973)
  Ventricular assist device (33975-33976, [33995], 33990-33993 [33997])

33361   **Transcatheter aortic valve replacement (TAVR/TAVI) with prosthetic valve; percutaneous femoral artery approach**
Code also cardiopulmonary bypass when performed (33367-33369)
🔷 39.4 ⚕ 39.4 **FUD** 000   C 80 ▢
AMA: 2018,Jan,8; 2017,Jan,8; 2016,Jan,13

33362   **open femoral artery approach**
Code also cardiopulmonary bypass when performed (33367-33369)
🔷 43.1 ⚕ 43.1 **FUD** 000   C 80 ▢
AMA: 2018,Jan,8; 2017,Dec,3; 2017,Jan,8; 2016,Jan,13

33363   **open axillary artery approach**
Code also cardiopulmonary bypass when performed (33367-33369)
🔷 44.6 ⚕ 44.6 **FUD** 000   C 80 ▢
AMA: 2018,Jan,8; 2017,Dec,3; 2017,Jan,8; 2016,Jan,13

33364   **open iliac artery approach**
Code also cardiopulmonary bypass when performed (33367-33369)
🔷 46.1 ⚕ 46.1 **FUD** 000   C 80 ▢
AMA: 2018,Jan,8; 2017,Dec,3; 2017,Jan,8; 2016,Jan,13

33365   **transaortic approach (eg, median sternotomy, mediastinotomy)**
Code also cardiopulmonary bypass when performed (33367-33369)
🔷 51.8 ⚕ 51.8 **FUD** 000   C 80 ▢
AMA: 2018,Jan,8; 2017,Jan,8; 2016,Jan,13

33366   **transapical exposure (eg, left thoracotomy)**
Code also cardiopulmonary bypass when performed (33367-33369)
🔷 45.7 ⚕ 45.7 **FUD** 000   C 80 ▢
AMA: 2018,Jan,8; 2017,Jan,8; 2016,Jan,13

+ **33367**   **cardiopulmonary bypass support with percutaneous peripheral arterial and venous cannulation (eg, femoral vessels) (List separately in addition to code for primary procedure)**
EXCLUDES *Cardiopulmonary bypass support with open or central arterial and venous cannulation (33368-33369)*
    Cerebral embolic protection device (33370)
Code first (33361-33366, 33418, 33477, 0483T-0484T, 0544T, 0545T, [0643T], 0569T, 0570T, 0644T)
🔷 18.2 ⚕ 18.2 **FUD** ZZZ   C 80 ▢
AMA: 2018,Jan,8; 2017,Jan,8; 2016,Mar,5; 2016,Jan,13

+ **33368**   **cardiopulmonary bypass support with open peripheral arterial and venous cannulation (eg, femoral, iliac, axillary vessels) (List separately in addition to code for primary procedure)**
EXCLUDES *Cardiopulmonary bypass support with percutaneous or central arterial and venous cannulation (33367, 33369)*
Code first (33361-33366, 33418, 33477, 0483T-0484T, 0544T, 0545T, [0643T], 0569T, 0570T, 0644T)
🔷 21.7 ⚕ 21.7 **FUD** ZZZ   C 80 ▢
AMA: 2018,Jan,8; 2017,Jan,8; 2016,Mar,5; 2016,Jan,13

+ **33369**   **cardiopulmonary bypass support with central arterial and venous cannulation (eg, aorta, right atrium, pulmonary artery) (List separately in addition to code for primary procedure)**
EXCLUDES *Cardiopulmonary bypass support with percutaneous or open arterial and venous cannulation (33367-33368)*
Code first (33361-33366, 33418, 33477, 0483T-0484T, 0544T, 0545T, [0643T], 0569T-0570T, 0644T)
🔷 28.6 ⚕ 28.6 **FUD** ZZZ   C 80 ▢
AMA: 2018,Jan,8; 2017,Jan,8; 2016,Mar,5; 2016,Jan,13

33370 Cerebral Embolic Protection Device

● + **33370**   **Transcatheter placement and subsequent removal of cerebral embolic protection device(s), including arterial access, catheterization, imaging, and radiological supervision and interpretation, percutaneous (List separately in addition to code for primary procedure)**
INCLUDES Angiography (75710)
    Aortography (75600)
    Ultrasound guidance (76937)
EXCLUDES *Additional or multiple filter placement*
Code first transcatheter aortic valve replacement (TAVR/TAVI) (33361-33366)
🔷 0.00 ⚕ 0.00 **FUD** 000

26/TC PC/TC Only   A2-Z3 ASC Payment   50 Bilateral   ♂ Male Only   ♀ Female Only   🔷 Facility RVU   ⚕ Non-Facility RVU   ▢ CCI   ✖ CLIA
FUD Follow-up Days   CMS: IOM   AMA: CPT Asst   A-Y OPPSI   80/80 Surg Assist Allowed / w/Doc   ▢ Lab Crosswalk   ▣ Radiology Crosswalk

132   CPT © 2021 American Medical Association. All Rights Reserved.   © 2021 Optum360, LLC

33390-33415 [33440] Aortic Valve Procedures

Code also transvascular ventricular support, when performed:
Balloon pump (33967, 33968, 33970-33974)
Extracorporeal membrane oxygenation (ECMO)/extracorporeal life support (ECLS) (33946-33949)
Ventricular assist device (33975-33983, [33995], 33990-33993 [33997])

33390 Valvuloplasty, aortic valve, open, with cardiopulmonary bypass; simple (ie, valvotomy, debridement, debulking, and/or simple commissural resuspension)
🚗 55.8 ⚕ 55.8 **FUD** 090 [C] 80 ▢
AMA: 2018,Jan,8; 2017,Dec,3

33391 complex (eg, leaflet extension, leaflet resection, leaflet reconstruction, or annuloplasty)
INCLUDES Simple aortic valvuloplasty (33390)
🚗 66.4 ⚕ 66.4 **FUD** 090 [C] 80 ▢
AMA: 2018,Jan,8; 2017,Dec,3

33404 Construction of apical-aortic conduit
🚗 50.6 ⚕ 50.6 **FUD** 090 [C] 80 ▢
AMA: 2018,Jan,8; 2017,Dec,3; 2017,Jan,8; 2016,Jan,13

33405 Replacement, aortic valve, open, with cardiopulmonary bypass; with prosthetic valve other than homograft or stentless valve
🚗 65.7 ⚕ 65.7 **FUD** 090 [C] 80 ▢
AMA: 2019,Nov,9; 2019,Apr,6; 2018,Jan,8; 2017,Dec,3; 2017,Jan,8; 2016,Jan,13

33406 with allograft valve (freehand)
🚗 83.4 ⚕ 83.4 **FUD** 090 [C] 80 ▢
AMA: 2019,Nov,9; 2019,Apr,6; 2018,Jan,8; 2017,Dec,3; 2017,Jan,8; 2016,Jan,13

33410 with stentless tissue valve
🚗 73.6 ⚕ 73.6 **FUD** 090 [C] 80 ▢
AMA: 2019,Nov,9; 2019,Apr,6; 2018,Jan,8; 2017,Dec,3; 2017,Jan,8; 2016,Jan,13

 # 33440 Replacement, aortic valve; by translocation of autologous pulmonary valve and transventricular aortic annulus enlargement of the left ventricular outflow tract with valved conduit replacement of pulmonary valve (Ross-Konno procedure)
INCLUDES Open replacement aortic valve with aortic annulus enlargement (33411-33412)
Open replacement aortic valve with translocation pulmonary valve (33413)
EXCLUDES Aortoplasty for supravalvular stenosis (33417)
Open replacement aortic valve (33405-33406, 33410)
Repair complex cardiac anomaly (except pulmonary atresia) (33608)
Repair left ventricular outlet obstruction (33414)
Repair pulmonary atresia (33920)
Replacement pulmonary valve (33475)
Resection/incision subvalvular tissue for aortic stenosis (33416)
🚗 98.1 ⚕ 98.1 **FUD** 090 80 ▢
AMA: 2019,Apr,6

33411 with aortic annulus enlargement, noncoronary sinus
🚗 97.4 ⚕ 97.4 **FUD** 090 [C] 80 ▢
AMA: 2019,Nov,9; 2019,Apr,6; 2018,Jan,8; 2017,Dec,3; 2017,Jan,8; 2016,Jan,13

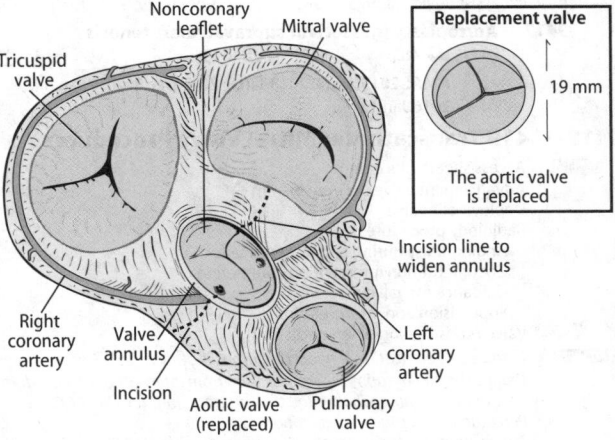

Overhead schematic of major heart valves

33412 with transventricular aortic annulus enlargement (Konno procedure)
EXCLUDES Replacement aortic valve by translocation pulmonary valve, aortic annulus enlargement, valved conduit pulmonary valve replacement ([33440])
Replacement aortic valve with translocation pulmonary valve (33413)
🚗 91.4 ⚕ 91.4 **FUD** 090 [C] 80 ▢
AMA: 2019,Nov,9; 2019,Apr,6; 2018,Jan,8; 2017,Dec,3; 2017,Jan,8; 2016,Jan,13

33413 by translocation of autologous pulmonary valve with allograft replacement of pulmonary valve (Ross procedure)
EXCLUDES Replacement aortic valve by translocation pulmonary valve, aortic annulus enlargement, valved conduit pulmonary valve replacement ([33440])
Replacement aortic valve with transventricular aortic annulus enlargement (33412)
🚗 92.7 ⚕ 92.7 **FUD** 090 [C] 80 ▢
AMA: 2019,Nov,9; 2019,Apr,6; 2018,Jan,8; 2017,Dec,3; 2017,Jan,8; 2016,Jan,13

33414 Repair of left ventricular outflow tract obstruction by patch enlargement of the outflow tract
🚗 62.2 ⚕ 62.2 **FUD** 090 [C] 80 ▢
AMA: 2019,Apr,6; 2018,Jan,8; 2017,Dec,3; 2017,Jan,8; 2016,Jan,13

33415 Resection or incision of subvalvular tissue for discrete subvalvular aortic stenosis
🚗 58.7 ⚕ 58.7 **FUD** 090 [C] 80 ▢
AMA: 2018,Jan,8; 2017,Dec,3; 2017,Jan,8; 2016,Jan,13

33416 Ventriculectomy

CMS: 100-03,20.26 Partial Ventriculectomy
EXCLUDES Percutaneous transcatheter septal reduction therapy (93583)
Code also transvascular ventricular support, when performed:
Balloon pump (33967, 33968, 33970-33974)
Extracorporeal membrane oxygenation (ECMO)/extracorporeal life support (ECLS) (33946-33949)
Ventricular assist device (33975-33983, [33995], 33990-33993 [33997])

33416 Ventriculomyotomy (-myectomy) for idiopathic hypertrophic subaortic stenosis (eg, asymmetric septal hypertrophy)
🚗 58.5 ⚕ 58.5 **FUD** 090 [C] 80 ▢
AMA: 2019,Apr,6; 2018,Jan,8; 2017,Dec,3; 2017,Jan,8; 2016,Jan,13

33417 Repair of Supravalvular Stenosis by Aortoplasty

Code also transvascular ventricular support, when performed:
Balloon pump (33967, 33968, 33970-33974)
Extracorporeal membrane oxygenation (ECMO)/extracorporeal life support (ECLS) (33946-33949)
Ventricular assist device (33975-33983, [33995], 33990-33993 [33997])

	33417	Aortoplasty (gusset) for supravalvular stenosis

🔧 48.2   ⚖ 48.2   **FUD** 090   C 80 ▭

AMA: 2019,Apr,6; 2018,Jan,8; 2017,Dec,3; 2017,Jan,8; 2016,Jan,13

33418-33419 Transcatheter Mitral Valve Procedures

INCLUDES   Access sheath placement
Advancement valve delivery system
Deployment valve
Radiology procedures:
   Angiography during and after procedure
   Documentation intervention completion
   Guidance for valve placement
   Supervision and interpretation
Valve repositioning when necessary

EXCLUDES   *Cardiac catheterization services for purposes other than TMVR*
Diagnostic angiography different session from interventional procedure
Percutaneous approach through the coronary sinus for TMVR (0345T)
Percutaneous coronary interventional procedures
Transcatheter mitral valve annulus reconstruction (0544T)
Transcatheter TMVI by percutaneous or transthoracic approach (0483T-0484T)

Code also cardiopulmonary bypass:
Central (33369)
Open peripheral (33368)
Percutaneous peripheral (33367)
Code also diagnostic coronary angiography and cardiac catheterization procedures when:
No previous study available and full diagnostic study performed
Previous study inadequate or patient's clinical indication for study changed prior to or during procedure
Report modifier 59 with cardiac catheterization procedures when on same day or same session as TMVR
Code also transvascular ventricular support, when performed:
Balloon pump (33967, 33970, 33973)
Ventricular assist device ([33995], 33990-33993 [33997])

	33418	Transcatheter mitral valve repair, percutaneous approach, including transseptal puncture when performed; initial prosthesis

Code also left heart catheterization when performed by transapical puncture (93462)
🔧 52.1   ⚖ 52.1   **FUD** 090   C 80 ▭

AMA: 2018,Jan,8; 2017,Jan,8; 2016,Jan,13

+	33419	additional prosthesis(es) during same session (List separately in addition to code for primary procedure)

EXCLUDES   *Procedures performed more than one time per session*
Code first (33418)
🔧 12.3   ⚖ 12.3   **FUD** ZZZ   N N1 80 ▭

AMA: 2018,Jan,8; 2017,Jan,8; 2016,Jan,13

33420-33440 [33440] Mitral Valve Procedures

Code also thrombus removal through separate heart incision, when performed (33310-33315); append modifier 59 to (33315)
Code also transvascular ventricular support, when performed:
Balloon pump (33967, 33968, 33970-33974)
Extracorporeal membrane oxygenation (ECMO)/extracorporeal life support (ECLS) (33946-33949)
Ventricular assist device (33975-33983, [33995], 33990-33993 [33997])

	33420	Valvotomy, mitral valve; closed heart

🔧 42.3   ⚖ 42.3   **FUD** 090   C ▭

AMA: 2018,Jan,8; 2017,Jan,8; 2016,Jan,13

	33422	open heart, with cardiopulmonary bypass

🔧 48.1   ⚖ 48.1   **FUD** 090   C 80 ▭

AMA: 2018,Jan,8; 2017,Dec,3; 2017,Jan,8; 2016,Jan,13

	33425	Valvuloplasty, mitral valve, with cardiopulmonary bypass;

🔧 79.1   ⚖ 79.1   **FUD** 090   C 80 ▭

AMA: 2018,Jan,8; 2017,Dec,3; 2017,Jan,8; 2016,Jan,13

	33426	with prosthetic ring

🔧 69.0   ⚖ 69.0   **FUD** 090   C 80 ▭

AMA: 2018,Jan,8; 2017,Dec,3; 2017,Jan,8; 2016,Jan,13

	33427	radical reconstruction, with or without ring

🔧 70.7   ⚖ 70.7   **FUD** 090   C 80 ▭

AMA: 2018,Jan,8; 2017,Dec,3; 2017,Jan,8; 2016,Jan,13

	33430	Replacement, mitral valve, with cardiopulmonary bypass

🔧 81.1   ⚖ 81.1   **FUD** 090   C 80 ▭

AMA: 2018,Jan,8; 2017,Dec,3; 2017,Jan,8; 2016,Jan,13

	33440	**Resequenced code. See code following 33410.**

33460-33468 Tricuspid Valve Procedures

EXCLUDES   *Transcatheter tricuspid valve annulus reconstruction (0545T)*
Transcatheter tricuspid valve implantation (TTVI)/replacement ([0646T])
Transcatheter tricuspid valve repair (0569T-0570T)

Code also thrombus removal through separate heart incision, when performed (33310-33315); append modifier 59 to (33315)
Code also transvascular ventricular support, when performed:
Balloon pump (33967, 33968, 33970-33974)
Extracorporeal membrane oxygenation (ECMO)/extracorporeal life support (ECLS) (33946-33949)
Ventricular assist device (33975-33983, [33995], 33990-33993 [33997])

	33460	Valvectomy, tricuspid valve, with cardiopulmonary bypass

🔧 69.6   ⚖ 69.6   **FUD** 090   C 80 ▭

AMA: 2018,Jan,8; 2017,Dec,3; 2017,Jan,8; 2016,Jan,13

	33463	Valvuloplasty, tricuspid valve; without ring insertion

🔧 89.4   ⚖ 89.4   **FUD** 090   C 80 ▭

AMA: 2018,Jan,8; 2017,Dec,3; 2017,Jan,8; 2016,Jan,13

	33464	with ring insertion

🔧 70.7   ⚖ 70.7   **FUD** 090   C 80 ▭

AMA: 2018,Jan,8; 2017,Dec,3; 2017,Jan,8; 2016,Jan,13

	33465	Replacement, tricuspid valve, with cardiopulmonary bypass

🔧 79.9   ⚖ 79.9   **FUD** 090   C 80 ▭

AMA: 2018,Jan,8; 2017,Dec,3; 2017,Jan,8; 2016,Jan,13

	33468	Tricuspid valve repositioning and plication for Ebstein anomaly

🔧 71.0   ⚖ 71.0   **FUD** 090   C 80 ▭

AMA: 2018,Jan,8; 2017,Dec,3; 2017,Jan,8; 2016,Jan,13

33470-33474 Pulmonary Valvotomy

INCLUDES   Brock's operation
Code also concurrent systemic-to-pulmonary artery shunt ligation/takedown (33924)
Code also transvascular ventricular support, when performed:
Balloon pump (33967, 33968, 33970-33974)
Extracorporeal membrane oxygenation (ECMO)/extracorporeal life support (ECLS) (33946-33949)
Ventricular assist device (33975-33983, [33995], 33990-33993 [33997])

	33470	~~Valvotomy, pulmonary valve, closed heart; transventricular~~

▲	33471	Valvotomy, pulmonary valve, closed heart, via pulmonary artery

EXCLUDES   *Percutaneous valvuloplasty pulmonary valve (92990)*
🔧 38.3   ⚖ 38.3   **FUD** 090   C 80 ▭

AMA: 2018,Jan,8; 2017,Jan,8; 2016,Jan,13

	33474	Valvotomy, pulmonary valve, open heart, with cardiopulmonary bypass

🔧 63.0   ⚖ 63.0   **FUD** 090   C 80 ▭

AMA: 2017,Dec,3

33475-33476 Other Procedures Pulmonary Valve

Code also concurrent systemic-to-pulmonary artery shunt ligation/takedown (33924)
Code also transvascular ventricular support, when performed:
Balloon pump (33967, 33968, 33970-33974)
Extracorporeal membrane oxygenation (ECMO)/extracorporeal life support (ECLS) (33946-33949)
Ventricular assist device (33975-33983, [33995], 33990-33993 [33997])

	33475	Replacement, pulmonary valve

🔧 67.5   ⚖ 67.5   **FUD** 090   C 80 ▭

AMA: 2019,Apr,6; 2018,Jan,8; 2017,Dec,3; 2017,Jan,8; 2016,Jan,13

26/TC PC/TC Only   A2-Z3 ASC Payment   50 Bilateral   ♂ Male Only   ♀ Female Only   🔧 Facility RVU   ⚖ Non-Facility RVU   ▭ CCI   ✖ CLIA
FUD Follow-up Days   **CMS:** IOM   **AMA:** CPT Asst   A-Y OPPSI   80/80 Surg Assist Allowed / w/Doc   Lab Crosswalk   Radiology Crosswalk

134   CPT © 2021 American Medical Association. All Rights Reserved.   © 2021 Optum360, LLC

33476 Right ventricular resection for infundibular stenosis, with or without commissurotomy

INCLUDES Brock's operation

🔧 44.0 ⚒ 44.0 **FUD** 090 C 80 ▣

AMA: 2018,Jan,8; 2017,Dec,3; 2017,Jan,8; 2016,Jan,13

33477 Transcatheter Pulmonary Valve Implantation

INCLUDES Procedures integral to TPVI:
Cardiac catheterization/angiography procedures (93451, 93453-93461, 93593-93594, 93596-93568)
Fluoroscopy (76000)
Injection procedures during cardiac catheterization (93563, 93566-93568)
Pulmonary artery angioplasty/valvuloplasty within treatment area (92997-92998)
Pulmonary artery stenting within treatment area (37236-37237)

EXCLUDES *Procedures performed at a separate session from TPVI:*
Diagnostic coronary angiography, when performed
Percutaneous coronary interventional procedures, when performed
Percutaneous interventions pulmonary artery branch, when performed
Procedures performed more than one time per session

Code also, when performed:
Balloon pump (33967, 33970, 33973)
Concurrent systemic-to-pulmonary artery shunt ligation/takedown (33924)
Diagnostic cardiac catheterization/angiography procedures, when performed distinctly separate from TPVI, if patient's condition (clinical indication) changed since intervention or prior study, no available prior catheter-based diagnostic study in treatment zone, or prior study not adequate (93451-93461, 93563-93564, 93568, 93593-93598)
Diagnostic cardiac catheterization procedures when performed distinctly separate from TPVI during same day/session, and append modifier 59 (93451-93461, 93593-93598)
Extracorporeal membrane oxygenation (ECMO)/extracorporeal life support (ECLS) (33946-33959, [33962], [33963], [33964], [33965], [33966], [33969], [33984], [33985], [33986], [33987], [33988], [33989])
Ventricular assist device ([33995], 33990-33993 [33997])

33477 Transcatheter pulmonary valve implantation, percutaneous approach, including pre-stenting of the valve delivery site, when performed

🔧 39.4 ⚒ 39.4 **FUD** 000 C 80 ▣

AMA: 2018,Jan,8; 2017,Jan,8; 2016,Aug,9; 2016,Mar,5

33478 Outflow Tract Augmentation

Code also for cavopulmonary anastomosis to second superior vena cava (33768)
Code also concurrent ligation/takedown systemic-to-pulmonary artery shunt (33924)
Code also transvascular ventricular support, when performed:
Balloon pump (33967, 33968, 33970-33974)
Extracorporeal membrane oxygenation (ECMO)/extracorporeal life support (ECLS) (33946-33949)
Ventricular assist device (33975-33983, [33995], 33990-33993 [33997])

33478 Outflow tract augmentation (gusset), with or without commissurotomy or infundibular resection

🔧 45.4 ⚒ 45.4 **FUD** 090 C 80 ▣

AMA: 2018,Jan,8; 2017,Dec,3; 2017,Jan,8; 2016,Jan,13

33496 Prosthetic Valve Repair

Code also thrombus removal through separate heart incision, when performed (33310-33315); append modifier 59 to (33315)
Code also reoperation if performed (33530)

33496 Repair of non-structural prosthetic valve dysfunction with cardiopulmonary bypass (separate procedure)

🔧 48.5 ⚒ 48.5 **FUD** 090 C 80 ▣

AMA: 2018,Jan,8; 2017,Dec,3; 2017,Jan,8; 2016,Jan,13

33500-33507 Repair Aberrant Coronary Artery Anatomy

INCLUDES Angioplasty and/or endarterectomy

33500 Repair of coronary arteriovenous or arteriocardiac chamber fistula; with cardiopulmonary bypass

🔧 45.0 ⚒ 45.0 **FUD** 090 C 80 ▣

AMA: 2017,Dec,3

33501 without cardiopulmonary bypass

🔧 32.2 ⚒ 32.2 **FUD** 090 C 80 ▣

AMA: 2007,Mar,1-3; 1997,Nov,1

33502 Repair of anomalous coronary artery from pulmonary artery origin; by ligation

🔧 36.9 ⚒ 36.9 **FUD** 090 63 C 80 ▣

AMA: 2017,Dec,3

33503 by graft, without cardiopulmonary bypass

🔧 38.3 ⚒ 38.3 **FUD** 090 63 C 80 ▣

AMA: 2007,Mar,1-3; 1997,Nov,1

33504 by graft, with cardiopulmonary bypass

🔧 42.3 ⚒ 42.3 **FUD** 090 C 80 ▣

AMA: 2017,Dec,3

33505 with construction of intrapulmonary artery tunnel (Takeuchi procedure)

🔧 59.8 ⚒ 59.8 **FUD** 090 63 C 80 ▣

AMA: 2017,Dec,3

33506 by translocation from pulmonary artery to aorta

🔧 57.8 ⚒ 57.8 **FUD** 090 63 C 80 ▣

AMA: 2017,Dec,3

33507 Repair of anomalous (eg, intramural) aortic origin of coronary artery by unroofing or translocation

🔧 49.8 ⚒ 49.8 **FUD** 090 C 80 ▣

AMA: 2018,Jan,8; 2017,Dec,3; 2017,Jan,8; 2016,Jan,13

33508-33509 Endoscopic Harvesting Bypass Grafts

INCLUDES Diagnostic endoscopy

+ **33508** Endoscopy, surgical, including video-assisted harvest of vein(s) for coronary artery bypass procedure (List separately in addition to code for primary procedure)

EXCLUDES *Harvesting upper extremity vein, open (35500)*
Harvesting femoropopliteal vein (35572)

Code first (33510-33523)

🔧 0.48 ⚒ 0.48 **FUD** ZZZ N N1 80 ▣

AMA: 1997,Nov,1

● **33509** Harvest of upper extremity artery, 1 segment, for coronary artery bypass procedure, endoscopic

EXCLUDES *Harvesting upper extremity artery, open (35600)*

🔧 0.00 ⚒ 0.00 **FUD** 000 ⊘ 50

33510-33523 Coronary Artery Bypass: Venous Grafts

INCLUDES Obtaining saphenous vein grafts

EXCLUDES *Percutaneous ventricular assist devices ([33995], 33990-33993 [33997])*

Code also:
Modifier 80 when assistant at surgery obtains grafts
Vein graft harvest (33508, 35500, 35572)

33510 Coronary artery bypass, vein only; single coronary venous graft

🔧 55.9 ⚒ 55.9 **FUD** 090 C 80 ▣

AMA: 2018,Jan,8; 2017,Dec,3; 2017,Jan,8; 2016,Jan,13

33511 2 coronary venous grafts

🔧 61.4 ⚒ 61.4 **FUD** 090 C 80 ▣

AMA: 2018,Jan,8; 2017,Dec,3; 2017,Jan,8; 2016,Jan,13

33512 3 coronary venous grafts

🔧 70.0 ⚒ 70.0 **FUD** 090 C 80 ▣

AMA: 2018,Jan,8; 2017,Dec,3; 2017,Jan,8; 2016,Jan,13

33513 4 coronary venous grafts

🔧 71.9 ⚒ 71.9 **FUD** 090 C 80 ▣

AMA: 2018,Jan,8; 2017,Dec,3; 2017,Jan,8; 2016,Jan,13

33514 5 coronary venous grafts

🔧 75.6 ⚒ 75.6 **FUD** 090 C 80 ▣

AMA: 2018,Jan,8; 2017,Dec,3; 2017,Jan,8; 2016,Jan,13

33516 6 or more coronary venous grafts

🔧 78.4 ⚒ 78.4 **FUD** 090 C 80 ▣

AMA: 2018,Jan,8; 2017,Dec,3; 2017,Jan,8; 2016,Jan,13

+ **33517** Coronary artery bypass, using venous graft(s) and arterial graft(s); single vein graft (List separately in addition to code for primary procedure)

Code first (33533-33536)

🔧 5.44 ⚒ 5.44 **FUD** ZZZ C 80 ▣

AMA: 2018,Jan,8; 2017,Jan,8; 2016,Jan,13

Cardiovascular, Hemic, and Lymphatic

33518 — 33606

+ 33518   **2 venous grafts (List separately in addition to code for primary procedure)**
Code first (33533-33536)
🔹 11.9   🔹 11.9   **FUD** ZZZ   C 80 ▯
AMA: 2018,Jan,8; 2017,Jan,8; 2016,Jan,13

+ 33519   **3 venous grafts (List separately in addition to code for primary procedure)**
Code first (33533-33536)
🔹 15.8   🔹 15.8   **FUD** ZZZ   C 80 ▯
AMA: 2018,Jan,8; 2017,Jan,8; 2016,Jan,13

+ 33521   **4 venous grafts (List separately in addition to code for primary procedure)**
Code first (33533-33536)
🔹 18.9   🔹 18.9   **FUD** ZZZ   C 80 ▯
AMA: 2018,Jan,8; 2017,Jan,8; 2016,Jan,13

Vein grafts

Aortic arch

Left coronary artery

Right coronary artery

Circumflex branch

Descending branch

+ 33522   **5 venous grafts (List separately in addition to code for primary procedure)**
Code first (33533-33536)
🔹 21.2   🔹 21.2   **FUD** ZZZ   C 80 ▯
AMA: 2018,Jan,8; 2017,Jan,8; 2016,Jan,13

+ 33523   **6 or more venous grafts (List separately in addition to code for primary procedure)**
Code first (33533-33536)
🔹 24.0   🔹 24.0   **FUD** ZZZ   C 80 ▯
AMA: 2018,Jan,8; 2017,Jan,8; 2016,Jan,13

33530 Reoperative Coronary Artery Bypass Graft or Valve Procedure

EXCLUDES   Percutaneous ventricular assist devices (33990-33993)
Code first (33390-33391, 33404-33496, 33510-33536, 33863)

+ 33530   **Reoperation, coronary artery bypass procedure or valve procedure, more than 1 month after original operation (List separately in addition to code for primary procedure)**
🔹 15.2   🔹 15.2   **FUD** ZZZ   C 80 ▯
AMA: 2018,Jan,8; 2017,Jan,8; 2016,Jan,13

33533-33536 Coronary Artery Bypass: Arterial Grafts

INCLUDES   Arterial grafts obtained from all sites except upper extremity (eg, epigastric, internal mammary, gastroepiploic and others)
EXCLUDES   Percutaneous ventricular assist devices ([33995], 33990-33993 [33997])
Venous bypass (33510-33516)
Code also:
   Arterial graft harvest, upper extremity (eg, radial artery): (33509, 35600)
   Combined arterial-venous grafts (33517-33523)
   Modifier 80 when assistant at surgery obtains grafts

33533   **Coronary artery bypass, using arterial graft(s); single arterial graft**
🔹 54.1   🔹 54.1   **FUD** 090   C 80 ▯
AMA: 2018,Jan,8; 2017,Dec,3; 2017,Jan,8; 2016,Jan,13

33534   **2 coronary arterial grafts**
🔹 63.6   🔹 63.6   **FUD** 090   C 80 ▯
AMA: 2018,Jan,8; 2017,Dec,3; 2017,Jan,8; 2016,Jan,13

33535   **3 coronary arterial grafts**
🔹 70.9   🔹 70.9   **FUD** 090   C 80 ▯
AMA: 2018,Jan,8; 2017,Dec,3; 2017,Jan,8; 2016,Jan,13

33536   **4 or more coronary arterial grafts**
🔹 76.1   🔹 76.1   **FUD** 090   C 80 ▯
AMA: 2018,Jan,8; 2017,Dec,3; 2017,Jan,8; 2016,Jan,13

33542-33548 Ventricular Reconstruction

EXCLUDES   Percutaneous ventricular assist devices ([33995], 33990-33993 [33997])

33542   **Myocardial resection (eg, ventricular aneurysmectomy)**
Code also thrombus removal through separate heart incision, when performed (33310-33315); append modifier 59 to (33315)
🔹 76.1   🔹 76.1   **FUD** 090   C 80 ▯
AMA: 2018,Jan,8; 2017,Dec,3; 2017,Jan,8; 2016,Jan,13

33545   **Repair of postinfarction ventricular septal defect, with or without myocardial resection**
Code also thrombus removal through separate heart incision, when performed (33310-33315); append modifier 59 to (33315)
🔹 89.0   🔹 89.0   **FUD** 090   C 80 ▯
AMA: 2018,Jan,8; 2017,Dec,3; 2017,Jan,8; 2016,Jan,13

33548   **Surgical ventricular restoration procedure, includes prosthetic patch, when performed (eg, ventricular remodeling, SVR, SAVER, Dor procedures)**
EXCLUDES   Batista procedure or pachopexy (33999)
Cardiotomy, exploratory (33310, 33315)
Implantation transcatheter left ventricular restoration device ([0643T])
Temporary pacemaker (33210-33211)
Tube thoracostomy (32551)
🔹 85.8   🔹 85.8   **FUD** 090   C 80 ▯
AMA: 2018,Jan,8; 2017,Dec,3; 2017,Jan,8; 2016,Jan,13

33572 Endarterectomy with CABG (LAD, RCA, Cx)

Code first (33510-33516, 33533-33536)

+ 33572   **Coronary endarterectomy, open, any method, of left anterior descending, circumflex, or right coronary artery performed in conjunction with coronary artery bypass graft procedure, each vessel (List separately in addition to primary procedure)**
🔹 6.67   🔹 6.67   **FUD** ZZZ   C 80 ▯
AMA: 1997,Nov,1; 1994,Win,1

33600-33622 Repair Aberrant Heart Anatomy

33600   **Closure of atrioventricular valve (mitral or tricuspid) by suture or patch**
🔹 49.8   🔹 49.8   **FUD** 090   C 80 ▯
AMA: 2018,Jan,8; 2017,Dec,3; 2017,Jan,8; 2016,Jan,13

33602   **Closure of semilunar valve (aortic or pulmonary) by suture or patch**
Code also concurrent systemic-to-pulmonary artery shunt ligation/takedown (33924)
🔹 48.2   🔹 48.2   **FUD** 090   C 80 ▯
AMA: 2017,Dec,3

33606   **Anastomosis of pulmonary artery to aorta (Damus-Kaye-Stansel procedure)**
Code also concurrent systemic-to-pulmonary artery shunt ligation/takedown (33924)
🔹 51.4   🔹 51.4   **FUD** 090   C 80
AMA: 2017,Dec,3

26/TC PC/TC Only   A2-Z3 ASC Payment   50 Bilateral   ♂ Male Only   ♀ Female Only   🔹 Facility RVU   🔹 Non-Facility RVU   ▯ CCI   ✖ CLIA
FUD Follow-up Days   **CMS:** IOM   **AMA:** CPT Asst   A-Y OPPSI   80/80 Surg Assist Allowed / w/Doc   🔹 Lab Crosswalk   🔹 Radiology Crosswalk

136   CPT © 2021 American Medical Association. All Rights Reserved.   © 2021 Optum360, LLC

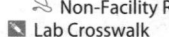

33608 Repair of complex cardiac anomaly other than pulmonary atresia with ventricular septal defect by construction or replacement of conduit from right or left ventricle to pulmonary artery

EXCLUDES *Unifocalization arborization anomalies pulmonary artery (33925, 33926)*

Code also concurrent systemic-to-pulmonary artery shunt ligation/takedown (33924)

🚑 52.2 ⚕ 52.2 **FUD** 090

🆑 C 80 ▭

AMA: 2019,Apr,6; 2017,Dec,3

33610 Repair of complex cardiac anomalies (eg, single ventricle with subaortic obstruction) by surgical enlargement of ventricular septal defect

Code also concurrent systemic-to-pulmonary artery shunt ligation/takedown (33924)

🚑 51.5 ⚕ 51.5 **FUD** 090

⑥³ C 80 ▭

AMA: 2017,Dec,3

33611 Repair of double outlet right ventricle with intraventricular tunnel repair;

Code also concurrent systemic-to-pulmonary artery shunt ligation/takedown (33924)

🚑 56.5 ⚕ 56.5 **FUD** 090

⑥³ C 80 ▭

AMA: 2017,Dec,3

33612 with repair of right ventricular outflow tract obstruction

Code also concurrent systemic-to-pulmonary artery shunt ligation/takedown (33924)

🚑 58.2 ⚕ 58.2 **FUD** 090

C 80 ▭

AMA: 2017,Dec,3

33615 Repair of complex cardiac anomalies (eg, tricuspid atresia) by closure of atrial septal defect and anastomosis of atria or vena cava to pulmonary artery (simple Fontan procedure)

Code also concurrent systemic-to-pulmonary artery shunt ligation/takedown (33924)

🚑 58.0 ⚕ 58.0 **FUD** 090

C 80 ▭

AMA: 2017,Dec,3

33617 Repair of complex cardiac anomalies (eg, single ventricle) by modified Fontan procedure

Code also:

Cavopulmonary anastomosis to second superior vena cava (33768)

Concurrent systemic-to-pulmonary artery shunt ligation/takedown (33924)

🚑 62.6 ⚕ 62.6 **FUD** 090

C 80 ▭

AMA: 2017,Dec,3

33619 Repair of single ventricle with aortic outflow obstruction and aortic arch hypoplasia (hypoplastic left heart syndrome) (eg, Norwood procedure)

🚑 79.3 ⚕ 79.3 **FUD** 090

⑥³ C 80 ▭

AMA: 2018,Jan,8; 2017,Dec,3; 2017,Jan,8; 2016,Jul,3; 2016,Jan,13

33620 Application of right and left pulmonary artery bands (eg, hybrid approach stage 1)

EXCLUDES *Banding main pulmonary artery related to septal defect (33690)*

Code also transthoracic insertion catheter for stent placement with catheter removal and closure when performed during same session (33621)

🚑 47.7 ⚕ 47.7 **FUD** 090

C 80 ▭

AMA: 2018,Jan,8; 2017,Dec,3; 2017,Jan,8; 2016,Jul,3; 2016,Jan,13

33621 Transthoracic insertion of catheter for stent placement with catheter removal and closure (eg, hybrid approach stage 1)

Code also:

Application right and left pulmonary artery bands when performed during same session (33620)

Stent placement (37236)

🚑 26.9 ⚕ 26.9 **FUD** 090

C 80 ▭

AMA: 2018,Jan,8; 2017,Dec,3; 2017,Jan,8; 2016,Jul,3; 2016,Jan,13

33622 Reconstruction of complex cardiac anomaly (eg, single ventricle or hypoplastic left heart) with palliation of single ventricle with aortic outflow obstruction and aortic arch hypoplasia, creation of cavopulmonary anastomosis, and removal of right and left pulmonary bands (eg, hybrid approach stage 2, Norwood, bidirectional Glenn, pulmonary artery debanding)

EXCLUDES *Excision coarctation aorta (33840, 33845, 33851)*

Repair hypoplastic or interrupted aortic arch (33853)

Repair patent ductus arteriosus (33822)

Repair pulmonary artery stenosis by reconstruction with patch or graft (33917)

Repair single ventricle with aortic outflow obstruction and aortic arch hypoplasia (33619)

Shunt; superior vena cava to pulmonary artery for flow to both lungs (33767)

Code also:

Anastomosis, cavopulmonary, second superior vena cava for bilateral bidirectional Glenn procedure (33768)

Concurrent systemic-to-pulmonary artery shunt ligation/takedown (33924)

🚑 100. ⚕ 100. **FUD** 090

C 80 ▭

AMA: 2018,Jan,8; 2017,Dec,3; 2017,Jan,8; 2016,Jul,3; 2016,Jan,13

33641-33645 Closure of Defect: Atrium

Code also thrombus removal through separate heart incision, when performed (33310-33315); append modifier 59 to (33315)

33641 Repair atrial septal defect, secundum, with cardiopulmonary bypass, with or without patch

🚑 47.3 ⚕ 47.3 **FUD** 090

C 80 ▭

AMA: 2018,Jan,8; 2017,Dec,3; 2017,Jan,8; 2016,Jan,13

33645 Direct or patch closure, sinus venosus, with or without anomalous pulmonary venous drainage

EXCLUDES *Repair isolated partial anomalous pulmonary venous return (33724)*

Repair pulmonary venous stenosis (33726)

🚑 49.8 ⚕ 49.8 **FUD** 090

C 80 ▭

AMA: 2017,Dec,3

33647 Closure of Septal Defect: Atrium AND Ventricle

EXCLUDES *Tricuspid atresia repair procedures (33615)*

Code also thrombus removal through separate heart incision, when performed (33310-33315); append modifier 59 to (33315)

33647 Repair of atrial septal defect and ventricular septal defect, with direct or patch closure

🚑 52.6 ⚕ 52.6 **FUD** 090

⑥³ C 80 ▭

AMA: 2017,Dec,3

33660-33670 Closure of Defect: Atrioventricular Canal

33660 Repair of incomplete or partial atrioventricular canal (ostium primum atrial septal defect), with or without atrioventricular valve repair

🚑 50.8 ⚕ 50.8 **FUD** 090

C 80 ▭

AMA: 2017,Dec,3

33665 Repair of intermediate or transitional atrioventricular canal, with or without atrioventricular valve repair

🚑 55.6 ⚕ 55.6 **FUD** 090

C 80 ▭

AMA: 2017,Dec,3

33670 Repair of complete atrioventricular canal, with or without prosthetic valve

Code also thrombus removal through separate heart incision, when performed (33310-33315); append modifier 59 to (33315)

🚑 57.4 ⚕ 57.4 **FUD** 090

⑥³ C 80 ▭

AMA: 2017,Dec,3

33675-33677 Closure of Multiple Septal Defects: Ventricle

EXCLUDES Closure single ventricular septal defect (33681, 33684, 33688)
Insertion or replacement temporary transvenous single chamber cardiac electrode or pacemaker catheter (33210)
Percutaneous closure (93581)
Thoracentesis (32554-32555)
Thoracotomy (32100)
Tube thoracostomy (32551)

33675 **Closure of multiple ventricular septal defects;**
🚑 57.1   ⚕ 57.1   **FUD** 090   C 80 ▭
AMA: 2018,Jan,8; 2017,Dec,3; 2017,Jan,8; 2016,Jan,13

33676 **with pulmonary valvotomy or infundibular resection (acyanotic)**
🚑 58.6   ⚕ 58.6   **FUD** 090   C 80 ▭
AMA: 2018,Jan,8; 2017,Dec,3; 2017,Jan,8; 2016,Jan,13

33677 **with removal of pulmonary artery band, with or without gusset**
🚑 60.9   ⚕ 60.9   **FUD** 090   C 80 ▭
AMA: 2018,Jan,8; 2017,Dec,3; 2017,Jan,8; 2016,Jan,13

33681-33688 Closure of Septal Defect: Ventricle

EXCLUDES Repair pulmonary vein that requires creating an atrial septal defect (33724)

33681 **Closure of single ventricular septal defect, with or without patch;**
Code also thrombus removal through separate heart incision, when performed (33310-33315); append modifier 59 to (33315)
🚑 53.0   ⚕ 53.0   **FUD** 090   C 80 ▭
AMA: 2018,Jan,8; 2017,Dec,3; 2017,Jan,8; 2016,Jan,13

33684 **with pulmonary valvotomy or infundibular resection (acyanotic)**
Code also concurrent systemic-to-pulmonary artery shunt ligation/takedown, if performed (33924)
🚑 54.8   ⚕ 54.8   **FUD** 090   C 80 ▭
AMA: 2017,Dec,3

33688 **with removal of pulmonary artery band, with or without gusset**
Code also concurrent systemic-to-pulmonary artery shunt ligation/takedown, if performed (33924)
🚑 54.8   ⚕ 54.8   **FUD** 090   C 80 ▭
AMA: 2017,Dec,3

33690 Reduce Pulmonary Overcirculation in Septal Defects

EXCLUDES Left and right pulmonary artery banding in single ventricle (33620)

33690 **Banding of pulmonary artery**
🚑 34.7   ⚕ 34.7   **FUD** 090   63 C 80 ▭
AMA: 2018,Jan,8; 2017,Jan,8; 2016,Jan,13

33692-33697 Repair of Defects of Tetralogy of Fallot

Code also concurrent systemic-to-pulmonary artery shunt ligation/takedown, when performed (33924)

33692 **Complete repair tetralogy of Fallot without pulmonary atresia;**
🚑 56.6   ⚕ 56.6   **FUD** 090   C 80 ▭
AMA: 2017,Dec,3

33694 **with transannular patch**
🚑 56.5   ⚕ 56.5   **FUD** 090   63 C 80 ▭
AMA: 2017,Dec,3

33697 **Complete repair tetralogy of Fallot with pulmonary atresia including construction of conduit from right ventricle to pulmonary artery and closure of ventricular septal defect**
🚑 59.7   ⚕ 59.7   **FUD** 090   C 80 ▭
AMA: 2018,Jan,8; 2017,Dec,3; 2017,Jan,8; 2016,Jan,13

33702-33722 Repair Anomalies Sinus of Valsalva

33702 **Repair sinus of Valsalva fistula, with cardiopulmonary bypass;**
🚑 44.8   ⚕ 44.8   **FUD** 090   C 80 ▭
AMA: 2018,Jan,8; 2017,Dec,3; 2017,Jan,8; 2016,Jan,13

33710 **with repair of ventricular septal defect**
🚑 59.6   ⚕ 59.6   **FUD** 090   C 80 ▭
AMA: 2017,Dec,3

33720 **Repair sinus of Valsalva aneurysm, with cardiopulmonary bypass**
🚑 44.7   ⚕ 44.7   **FUD** 090   C 80 ▭
AMA: 2017,Dec,3

~~33722~~ ~~Closure of aortico-left ventricular tunnel~~

33724-33732 Repair Aberrant Pulmonary Venous Connection

33724 **Repair of isolated partial anomalous pulmonary venous return (eg, Scimitar Syndrome)**
EXCLUDES Temporary pacemaker (33210-33211)
Tube thoracostomy (32551)
🚑 44.6   ⚕ 44.6   **FUD** 090   C 80 ▭ *
AMA: 2018,Jan,8; 2017,Dec,3; 2017,Jan,8; 2016,Jan,13

33726 **Repair of pulmonary venous stenosis**
EXCLUDES Temporary pacemaker (33210-33211)
Tube thoracostomy (32551)
🚑 58.8   ⚕ 58.8   **FUD** 090   C 80 ▭
AMA: 2018,Jan,8; 2017,Dec,3; 2017,Jan,8; 2016,Jan,13

33730 **Complete repair of anomalous pulmonary venous return (supracardiac, intracardiac, or infracardiac types)**
EXCLUDES Partial anomalous pulmonary venous return (33724)
Repair pulmonary venous stenosis (33726)
🚑 58.0   ⚕ 58.0   **FUD** 090   63 C 80 ▭
AMA: 2018,Jan,8; 2017,Dec,3; 2017,Jan,8; 2016,Jan,13

33732 **Repair of cor triatriatum or supravalvular mitral ring by resection of left atrial membrane**
🚑 47.6   ⚕ 47.6   **FUD** 090   63 C 80 ▭
AMA: 2018,Jan,8; 2017,Dec,3; 2017,Jan,8; 2016,Jan,13

33735-33737 Creation of Atrial Septal Defect

Code also concurrent systemic-to-pulmonary artery shunt ligation/takedown, when performed (33924)

33735 **Atrial septectomy or septostomy; closed heart (Blalock-Hanlon type operation)**
🚑 37.4   ⚕ 37.4   **FUD** 090   63 C 80 ▭
AMA: 2018,Jan,8; 2017,Jan,8; 2016,Jan,13

33736 **open heart with cardiopulmonary bypass**
🚑 40.7   ⚕ 40.7   **FUD** 090   63 C 80 ▭
AMA: 2017,Dec,3

33737 **open heart, with inflow occlusion**
🚑 37.6   ⚕ 37.6   **FUD** 090   C 80 ▭
AMA: 2020,Nov,7

33741-33746 Transcatheter Procedures

33741 **Transcatheter atrial septostomy (TAS) for congenital cardiac anomalies to create effective atrial flow, including all imaging guidance by the proceduralist, when performed, any method (eg, Rashkind, Sang-Park, balloon, cutting balloon, blade)**

INCLUDES Angiography to carry out procedure

Fluoroscopic and ultrasound guidance for access and intervention

Percutaneous access, access sheath placement, advancement transcatheter delivery system, creation effective intracardiac blood flow

EXCLUDES *Left heart catheterization via transseptal puncture (93462)*

Septostomy performed for noncongenital indications (93799)

Code also:

Diagnostic congenital cardiac catheterization procedures when patient's condition (clinical indication) changed since intervention or prior study, no available prior catheter-based diagnostic study in treatment zone, or prior study not adequate, and append modifier 59 (93593-93597)

Injection, diagnostic angiography, when performed separate from shunt creation and append modifier 59 (93563, 93565-93568)

🔧 22.1   ✂ 22.1   **FUD** 000   ⑥③ 80 ▣

33745 **Transcatheter intracardiac shunt (TIS) creation by stent placement for congenital cardiac anomalies to establish effective intracardiac flow, including all imaging guidance by the proceduralist, when performed, left and right heart diagnostic cardiac catheterization for congenital cardiac anomalies, and target zone angioplasty, when performed (eg, atrial septum, Fontan fenestration, right ventricular outflow tract, Mustard/Senning/Warden baffles); initial intracardiac shunt**

INCLUDES Angiography to carry out procedure

Balloon angioplasty(ies) and dilation(s) performed in target lesion

Diagnostic cardiac catheterization (93451-93453, 93456, 93458, 93460)

Fluoroscopic and ultrasound guidance for access and intervention

Intracardiac stent(s), including angioplasty before and after placement

Percutaneous access, access sheath placement, advancement transcatheter delivery system, creation effective intracardiac blood flow

EXCLUDES *Heart catheterization for congenital cardiac anomalies (93593-93597)*

Code also injection, diagnostic angiography when performed distinctly separate from shunt creation and append modifier 59 (93563, 93565-93568)

🔧 31.2   ✂ 31.2   **FUD** 000   80 ▣

+ 33746 **each additional intracardiac shunt location (List separately in addition to code for primary procedure)**

INCLUDES Balloon angioplasty(ies) and dilation(s) performed in target lesion

Intracardiac stent(s), including angioplasty before and after placement

EXCLUDES *Heart catheterization for congenital cardiac anomalies (93593-93597)*

Code also angioplasty performed in distinctly separate cardiac lesion

Code first (33745)

🔧 12.3   ✂ 12.3   **FUD** ZZZ   80 ▣

33750-33767 Systemic Vessel to Pulmonary Artery Shunts

Code also concurrent systemic-to-pulmonary artery shunt ligation/takedown, when performed (33924)

33750 **Shunt; subclavian to pulmonary artery (Blalock-Taussig type operation)**

🔧 36.5   ✂ 36.5   **FUD** 090   ⑥③ ⓒ 80 ▣

AMA: 2017,Dec,3

33755 **ascending aorta to pulmonary artery (Waterston type operation)**

🔧 38.0   ✂ 38.0   **FUD** 090   ⑥③ ⓒ 80 ▣

AMA: 2017,Dec,3

33762 **descending aorta to pulmonary artery (Potts-Smith type operation)**

🔧 37.1   ✂ 37.1   **FUD** 090   ⑥③ ⓒ 80 ▣

AMA: 2017,Dec,3

33764 **central, with prosthetic graft**

🔧 38.0   ✂ 38.0   **FUD** 090   ⓒ 80 ▣

AMA: 2017,Dec,3

33766 **superior vena cava to pulmonary artery for flow to 1 lung (classical Glenn procedure)**

🔧 38.6   ✂ 38.6   **FUD** 090   ⓒ 80 ▣

AMA: 2017,Dec,3

33767 **superior vena cava to pulmonary artery for flow to both lungs (bidirectional Glenn procedure)**

🔧 41.1   ✂ 41.1   **FUD** 090   ⓒ 80 ▣

AMA: 2018,Jan,8; 2017,Dec,3; 2017,Jan,8; 2016,Jul,3

33768 Cavopulmonary Anastomosis to Decrease Volume Load

EXCLUDES *Temporary pacemaker (33210-33211)*

Tube thoracostomy (32551)

Code first (33478, 33617, 33622, 33767)

+ 33768 **Anastomosis, cavopulmonary, second superior vena cava (List separately in addition to primary procedure)**

🔧 12.0   ✂ 12.0   **FUD** ZZZ   ⓒ 80 ▣

AMA: 2018,Jan,8; 2017,Jan,8; 2016,Jul,3; 2016,Jan,13

33770-33783 Repair Aberrant Anatomy: Transposition Great Vessels

Code also concurrent systemic-to-pulmonary artery shunt ligation/takedown, when performed (33924)

33770 **Repair of transposition of the great arteries with ventricular septal defect and subpulmonary stenosis; without surgical enlargement of ventricular septal defect**

🔧 61.3   ✂ 61.3   **FUD** 090   ⓒ 80 ▣

AMA: 2018,Jan,8; 2017,Dec,3; 2017,Jan,8; 2016,Jan,13

33771 **with surgical enlargement of ventricular septal defect**

🔧 63.1   ✂ 63.1   **FUD** 090   ⓒ 80 ▣

AMA: 2017,Dec,3

33774 **Repair of transposition of the great arteries, atrial baffle procedure (eg, Mustard or Senning type) with cardiopulmonary bypass;**

🔧 52.0   ✂ 52.0   **FUD** 090   ⓒ 80 ▣

AMA: 2017,Dec,3

33775 **with removal of pulmonary band**

🔧 53.6   ✂ 53.6   **FUD** 090   ⓒ 80 ▣

AMA: 2017,Dec,3

33776 **with closure of ventricular septal defect**

🔧 56.7   ✂ 56.7   **FUD** 090   ⓒ 80 ▣

AMA: 2017,Dec,3

33777 **with repair of subpulmonic obstruction**

🔧 54.9   ✂ 54.9   **FUD** 090   ⓒ 80 ▣

AMA: 2017,Dec,3

33778 **Repair of transposition of the great arteries, aortic pulmonary artery reconstruction (eg, Jatene type);**

🔧 68.0   ✂ 68.0   **FUD** 090   ⑥③ ⓒ 80 ▣

AMA: 2017,Dec,3

33779 **with removal of pulmonary band**

🔧 67.4   ✂ 67.4   **FUD** 090   ⓒ 80 ▣

AMA: 2017,Dec,3

33780 **with closure of ventricular septal defect**

🔧 68.6   ✂ 68.6   **FUD** 090   ⓒ 80 ▣

AMA: 2017,Dec,3

33781   **with repair of subpulmonic obstruction**
📁 67.0 ⚕ 67.0   **FUD** 090   C 80 ▭
AMA: 2018,Jan,8; 2017,Dec,3; 2017,Jan,8; 2016,Jan,13

33782   **Aortic root translocation with ventricular septal defect and pulmonary stenosis repair (ie, Nikaidoh procedure); without coronary ostium reimplantation**
EXCLUDES *Closure single ventricular septal defect (33681)*
Repair complex cardiac anomaly other than pulmonary atresia (33608)
Repair pulmonary atresia with ventricular septal defect (33920)
Repair transposition great arteries (33770-33771, 33778, 33780)
Replacement, aortic valve (33412-33413)
📁 94.0 ⚕ 94.0   **FUD** 090   C 80 ▭
AMA: 2017,Dec,3

33783   **with reimplantation of 1 or both coronary ostia**
📁 101. ⚕ 101.   **FUD** 090   C 80 ▭
AMA: 2017,Dec,3

33786-33788 Repair Aberrant Anatomy: Truncus Arteriosus

33786   **Total repair, truncus arteriosus (Rastelli type operation)**
Code also concurrent systemic-to-pulmonary artery shunt ligation/takedown, when performed (33924)
📁 66.0 ⚕ 66.0   **FUD** 090   ⑬ C 80 ▭
AMA: 2018,Jan,8; 2017,Dec,3; 2017,Jan,8; 2016,Jan,13

33788   **Reimplantation of an anomalous pulmonary artery**
EXCLUDES *Pulmonary artery banding (33690)*
📁 44.3 ⚕ 44.3   **FUD** 090   C 80 ▭
AMA: 2018,Jan,8; 2017,Dec,3; 2017,Jan,8; 2016,Jan,13

33800-33853 Repair Aberrant Anatomy: Aorta

33800   **Aortic suspension (aortopexy) for tracheal decompression (eg, for tracheomalacia) (separate procedure)**
📁 28.6 ⚕ 28.6   **FUD** 090   C 80 ▭
AMA: 2018,Jan,8; 2017,Jan,8; 2016,Jan,13

33802   **Division of aberrant vessel (vascular ring);**
📁 31.4 ⚕ 31.4   **FUD** 090   C 80 ▭
AMA: 2017,Dec,3

33803   **with reanastomosis**
📁 33.4 ⚕ 33.4   **FUD** 090   C 80 ▭
AMA: 2017,Dec,3

33813   **Obliteration of aortopulmonary septal defect; without cardiopulmonary bypass**
📁 35.8 ⚕ 35.8   **FUD** 090   C 80 ▭
AMA: 2007,Mar,1-3; 1997,Nov,1

33814   **with cardiopulmonary bypass**
📁 44.1 ⚕ 44.1   **FUD** 090   C 80 ▭
AMA: 2017,Dec,3

33820   **Repair of patent ductus arteriosus; by ligation**
EXCLUDES *Percutaneous transcatheter closure patent ductus arteriosus (93582)*
📁 27.9 ⚕ 27.9   **FUD** 090   C 80 ▭
AMA: 2018,Jan,8; 2017,Dec,3; 2017,Jan,8; 2016,Jan,13

33822   **by division, younger than 18 years**   A
EXCLUDES *Percutaneous transcatheter closure patent ductus arteriosus (93582)*
📁 29.6 ⚕ 29.6   **FUD** 090   C 80 ▭
AMA: 2018,Jan,8; 2017,Dec,3; 2017,Jan,8; 2016,Jul,3; 2016,Jan,13

33824   **by division, 18 years and older**
EXCLUDES *Percutaneous closure patent ductus arteriosus (93582)*
📁 34.2 ⚕ 34.2   **FUD** 090   C 80 ▭
AMA: 2017,Dec,3

33840   **Excision of coarctation of aorta, with or without associated patent ductus arteriosus; with direct anastomosis**
📁 35.8 ⚕ 35.8   **FUD** 090   C 80 ▭
AMA: 2018,Jan,8; 2017,Jan,8; 2016,Jul,3

33845   **with graft**
📁 38.5 ⚕ 38.5   **FUD** 090   C 80 ▭
AMA: 2018,Jan,8; 2017,Dec,3; 2017,Jan,8; 2016,Jul,3

33851   **repair using either left subclavian artery or prosthetic material as gusset for enlargement**
📁 36.8 ⚕ 36.8   **FUD** 090   C 80 ▭
AMA: 2018,Jan,8; 2017,Dec,3; 2017,Jan,8; 2016,Jul,3

33852   **Repair of hypoplastic or interrupted aortic arch using autogenous or prosthetic material; without cardiopulmonary bypass**
EXCLUDES *Hypoplastic left heart syndrome repair by excision coarctation of aorta (33619)*
📁 38.5 ⚕ 38.5   **FUD** 090   C 80 ▭
AMA: 2007,Mar,1-3; 1997,Nov,1

33853   **with cardiopulmonary bypass**
EXCLUDES *Hypoplastic left heart syndrome repair by excision coarctation of aorta (33619)*
📁 53.0 ⚕ 53.0   **FUD** 090   C 80 ▭
AMA: 2018,Jan,8; 2017,Dec,3; 2017,Jan,8; 2016,Jul,3; 2016,Jan,13

33858-33877 Aortic Graft Procedures

33858   **Ascending aorta graft, with cardiopulmonary bypass, includes valve suspension, when performed; for aortic dissection**
INCLUDES Treatment for aortic dissection
EXCLUDES *Ascending aorta graft:*
Treatment other aortic disease(s), such as aneurysm (33859)
With remodeling aortic root (33864)
With replacement aortic root (33863)
📁 98.5 ⚕ 98.5   **FUD** 090   80 ▭

33859   **for aortic disease other than dissection (eg, aneurysm)**
INCLUDES Treatment of aortic disease(s) other than dissection, such as aneurysm
EXCLUDES *Ascending aorta graft:*
Treatment other aortic dissection (33858)
With remodeling aortic root (33864)
With replacement aortic root (33863)
📁 70.7 ⚕ 70.7   **FUD** 090   80 ▭

33863   **Ascending aorta graft, with cardiopulmonary bypass, with aortic root replacement using valved conduit and coronary reconstruction (eg, Bentall)**
EXCLUDES *Ascending aorta graft:*
With remodeling aortic root (33864)
Without aortic root replacement or remodeling (33858-33859)
Replacement, aortic valve, with cardiopulmonary bypass (33405-33406, 33410-33413)
📁 91.4 ⚕ 91.4   **FUD** 090   C 80 ▭
AMA: 2019,Nov,9; 2018,Jan,8; 2017,Dec,3; 2017,Jan,8; 2016,Jan,13

26/TC PC/TC Only	A2-Z3 ASC Payment	50 Bilateral	♂ Male Only	♀ Female Only	📁 Facility RVU	⚕ Non-Facility RVU	▭ CCI	☒ CLIA
FUD Follow-up Days	**CMS:** IOM	**AMA:** CPT Asst	A-Y OPPSI	80/80 Surg Assist Allowed / w/Doc		◼ Lab Crosswalk		◼ Radiology Crosswalk

140   CPT © 2021 American Medical Association. All Rights Reserved.   © 2021 Optum360, LLC

33864 Ascending aorta graft, with cardiopulmonary bypass with valve suspension, with coronary reconstruction and valve-sparing aortic root remodeling (eg, David Procedure, Yacoub Procedure)

> EXCLUDES Ascending aorta graft:
> With replacement aortic root (33863)
> Without aortic root replacement or remodeling (33858-33859)
>
> 93.3   93.3   **FUD** 090
>
> C 80
>
> **AMA:** 2019,Nov,9; 2018,Jan,8; 2017,Dec,3; 2017,Jan,8; 2016,Jan,13

+ 33866 Aortic hemiarch graft including isolation and control of the arch vessels, beveled open distal aortic anastomosis extending under one or more of the arch vessels, and total circulatory arrest or isolated cerebral perfusion (List separately in addition to code for primary procedure)

> INCLUDES Procedure includes:
> Extension ascending aortic graft by beveled anastomosis creation to distal ascending aorta and aortic arch without crossclamp (open anastomosis)
> Incision into transverse arch that extends under one or more arch vessels (e.g., left common carotid, left subclavian, innominate artery)
> Total circulatory arrest or isolated cerebral perfusion (antegrade or retrograde)
>
> EXCLUDES Complete transverse arch graft (33871)
>
> Code first (33858-33859, 33863-33864)
>
> 26.7   26.7   **FUD** ZZZ
>
> N1 80
>
> **AMA:** 2019,Nov,9

33871 Transverse aortic arch graft, with cardiopulmonary bypass, with profound hypothermia, total circulatory arrest and isolated cerebral perfusion with reimplantation of arch vessel(s) (eg, island pedicle or individual arch vessel reimplantation)

> EXCLUDES Ascending aortic graft (33858-33859, 33863-33864)
> Hemiarch aortic graft performed in addition to ascending aorta graft (33866)
>
> 94.7   94.7   **FUD** 090
>
> 80

33875 Descending thoracic aorta graft, with or without bypass

> 79.5   79.5   **FUD** 090
>
> C 80
>
> **AMA:** 2017,Dec,3

33877 Repair of thoracoabdominal aortic aneurysm with graft, with or without cardiopulmonary bypass

> 105.   105.   **FUD** 090
>
> C 80
>
> **AMA:** 2017,Dec,3

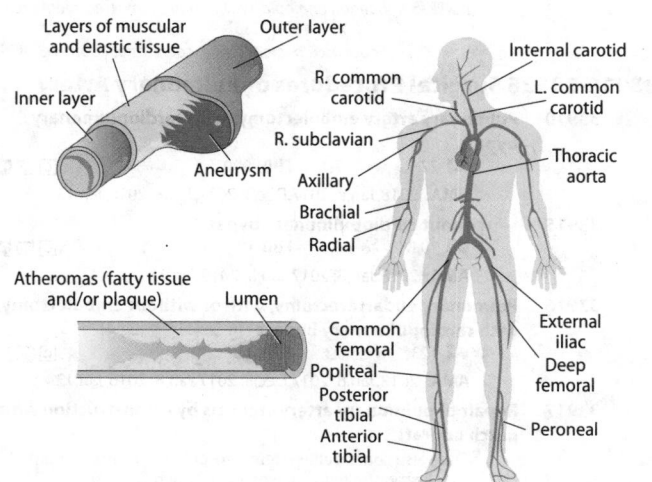

Layers of muscular and elastic tissue
Outer layer
Inner layer
Aneurysm

Internal carotid
R. common carotid
L. common carotid
R. subclavian
Axillary
Brachial
Radial
Thoracic aorta

Atheromas (fatty tissue and/or plaque)
Lumen

Common femoral
External iliac
Popliteal
Deep femoral
Posterior tibial
Anterior tibial
Peroneal

33880-33891 Endovascular Repair Aortic Aneurysm: Thoracic

> INCLUDES Balloon angioplasty
> Introduction, manipulation, placement, and device deployment
> Stent deployment
>
> EXCLUDES Additional interventional procedures provided during endovascular repair
> Carotid-carotid bypass (33891)
> Guidewire and catheter insertion (36140, 36200-36218)
> Open exposure artery/subsequent closure ([34812], 34714-34716 [34820, 34833, 34834])
> Stent deployment or balloon angioplasty, congenital coarctation or postsurgical recoarctation aorta (33894-33895, 33897)
> Subclavian to carotid artery transposition (33889)
> Substantial artery repair/replacement (35226, 35286)

33880 Endovascular repair of descending thoracic aorta (eg, aneurysm, pseudoaneurysm, dissection, penetrating ulcer, intramural hematoma, or traumatic disruption); involving coverage of left subclavian artery origin, initial endoprosthesis plus descending thoracic aortic extension(s), if required, to level of celiac artery origin

> INCLUDES Placement distal extensions in distal thoracic aorta
>
> EXCLUDES Proximal extensions
>
> (75956)
>
> 52.0   52.0   **FUD** 090
>
> C 80
>
> **AMA:** 2018,Jan,8; 2017,Dec,3; 2017,Jan;8; 2016,Jan,13

33881 not involving coverage of left subclavian artery origin, initial endoprosthesis plus descending thoracic aortic extension(s), if required, to level of celiac artery origin

> INCLUDES Placement distal extensions in distal thoracic aorta
>
> EXCLUDES Procedure where extension placement includes coverage left subclavian artery origin (33880)
> Proximal extensions
>
> (75957)
>
> 44.6   44.6   **FUD** 090
>
> C 80
>
> **AMA:** 2018,Jan,8; 2017,Dec,3; 2017,Jan,8; 2016,Jan,13

33883 Placement of proximal extension prosthesis for endovascular repair of descending thoracic aorta (eg, aneurysm, pseudoaneurysm, dissection, penetrating ulcer, intramural hematoma, or traumatic disruption); initial extension

> EXCLUDES Procedure where extension placement includes coverage left subclavian artery origin (33880)
>
> (75958)
>
> 32.3   32.3   **FUD** 090
>
> C 80
>
> **AMA:** 2018,Jan,8; 2017,Dec,3; 2017,Jan,8; 2016,Jan,13

+ 33884 each additional proximal extension (List separately in addition to code for primary procedure)

> Code first (33883)
>
> (75958)
>
> 11.5   11.5   **FUD** ZZZ
>
> C 80
>
> **AMA:** 2018,Jan,8; 2017,Dec,3; 2017,Jan,8; 2016,Jan,13

33886 **Placement of distal extension prosthesis(s) delayed after endovascular repair of descending thoracic aorta**

INCLUDES All modules deployed

EXCLUDES *Endovascular repair descending thoracic aorta (33880, 33881)*

⚙ (75959)

🚑 27.7   ⚷ 27.7   **FUD** 090   C 80 ▱

AMA: 2018,Jan,8; 2017,Dec,3; 2017,Jan,8; 2016,Jan,13

Celiac trunk
Original graft
Descending aorta
Aneurysm
Site of endoleak
Insert extension prosthesis within original graft
Extension prosthesis
Diaphragm

Repair of endoleak in descending thoracic aorta

33889 **Open subclavian to carotid artery transposition performed in conjunction with endovascular repair of descending thoracic aorta, by neck incision, unilateral**

EXCLUDES *Transposition and/or reimplantation; subclavian to carotid artery (35694)*

🚑 22.9   ⚷ 22.9   **FUD** 000   C 80 50 ▱

AMA: 2018,Jan,8; 2017,Jan,8; 2016,Jan,13

33891 **Bypass graft, with other than vein, transcervical retropharyngeal carotid-carotid, performed in conjunction with endovascular repair of descending thoracic aorta, by neck incision**

EXCLUDES *Bypass graft (35509, 35601)*

🚑 28.0   ⚷ 28.0   **FUD** 000   C 80 50 ▱

AMA: 2018,Jan,8; 2017,Jan,8; 2016,Jan,13

33894-33897 Repair Coarctation Aorta

INCLUDES Balloon angioplasty within targeted treatment area
Fluoroscopic guidance for all diagnostic and interventional procedures across the targeted treatment area
Temporay pacemaker insertion (33210)

EXCLUDES *Angiography other vascular structures*
Aortography (75600, 75605, 75625)
Endovascular repair infrarenal aorta and/or iliac artery(ies) by deployment of:
  Aorto-aortic tube endograft (34701-34702)
  Aorto-uni-iliac or aorto-bi-iliac endograft (34703-34706)
Heart catheterization for congenital heart defect(s) (93595-93597)
Injection during cardiac catheterization (93567)
Introduction catheter, aorta (36200)
Right heart catheterization for congenital heart defect(s), during same operative session (93593-93594)
Code also balloon angioplasty aorta, other than coarctation during same operative session, when performed (37246)

● **33894** **Endovascular stent repair of coarctation of the ascending, transverse, or descending thoracic or abdominal aorta, involving stent placement; across major side branches**

INCLUDES Stent(s) deployed over target and as extension from target area
Treatment across one or more major side branches of aorta: brachiocephalic, carotid, celiac, inferior/superior mesenteric, subclavian, and renal arteries

EXCLUDES *Balloon angioplasty within the same treatment area (33897, [37246], 37236)*
Injection during cardiac catheterization (93563-93566, 93568)
Code also interventions performed on other vessels (i.e., carotid, iliac, innomiante, pulmonary, subclavian, visceral), including balloon angioplasty, embolization, and stenting, during same operative session, when performed

● **33895**   **not crossing major side branches**

INCLUDES Stent(s) deployed over target and as extension from target area

EXCLUDES *Balloon angioplasty within the same treatment area (33897, [37246], 37236)*
Injection during cardiac catheterization (93563-93566, 93568)
Code also interventions performed on other vessels (i.e., carotid, iliac, innominate, pulmonary, subclavian, visceral), including balloon angioplasty, embolization, and stenting, during same operative session, when performed

● **33897** **Percutaneous transluminal angioplasty of native or recurrent coarctation of the aorta**

INCLUDES Dilation coarctation utilizing balloon angioplasty without stent deployment

EXCLUDES *Balloon angioplasty within the same treatment area ([37246], 37236)*
Endovascular stent repair, coarctation (33894-33895)

33910-33926 Surgical Procedures of Pulmonary Artery

33910 **Pulmonary artery embolectomy; with cardiopulmonary bypass**

🚑 77.1   ⚷ 77.1   **FUD** 090   C 80 ▱

AMA: 2018,Jan,8; 2017,Dec,3; 2017,Jan,8; 2016,Jan,13

33915   **without cardiopulmonary bypass**

🚑 39.8   ⚷ 39.8   **FUD** 090   C 80 ▱

AMA: 2018,Jan,8; 2017,Jan,8; 2016,Jan,13

33916 **Pulmonary endarterectomy, with or without embolectomy, with cardiopulmonary bypass**

🚑 123.   ⚷ 123.   **FUD** 090   C 80 ▱

AMA: 2018,Jan,8; 2017,Dec,3; 2017,Jan,8; 2016,Jan,13

33917 **Repair of pulmonary artery stenosis by reconstruction with patch or graft**

Code also concurrent systemic-to-pulmonary artery shunt ligation/takedown, when performed (33924)

🚑 42.1   ⚷ 42.1   **FUD** 090   C 80 ▱

AMA: 2018,Jan,8; 2017,Dec,3; 2017,Jan,8; 2016,Jul,3; 2016,Jan,13

33920 **Repair of pulmonary atresia with ventricular septal defect, by construction or replacement of conduit from right or left ventricle to pulmonary artery**

> EXCLUDES *Repair complicated cardiac anomalies by creating/replacing conduit from ventricle to pulmonary artery (33608)*
>
> Code also concurrent systemic-to-pulmonary artery shunt ligation/takedown, when performed (33924)
>
> 💰 52.4   ⚕ 52.4   **FUD** 090   C 80 🖵
>
> **AMA:** 2019,Apr,6; 2018,Jan,8; 2017,Dec,3; 2017,Jan,8; 2016,Jan,13

33922 **Transection of pulmonary artery with cardiopulmonary bypass**

> Code also concurrent systemic-to-pulmonary artery shunt ligation/takedown, when performed (33924)
>
> 💰 40.1   ⚕ 40.1   **FUD** 090   63 C 80 🖵
>
> **AMA:** 2017,Dec,3

+ 33924 **Ligation and takedown of a systemic-to-pulmonary artery shunt, performed in conjunction with a congenital heart procedure (List separately in addition to code for primary procedure)**

> Code first (33471-33478, 33600-33617, 33622, 33684-33688, 33692-33697, 33735-33767, 33770-33783, 33786, 33917, 33920-33922, 33925-33926, 33935, 33945)
>
> 💰 8.29   ⚕ 8.29   **FUD** ZZZ   C 80 🖵
>
> **AMA:** 1997,Nov,1; 1995,Win,1

33925 **Repair of pulmonary artery arborization anomalies by unifocalization; without cardiopulmonary bypass**

> Code also concurrent systemic-to-pulmonary artery shunt ligation/takedown, when performed (33924)
>
> 💰 49.7   ⚕ 49.7   **FUD** 090   C 80 🖵

33926 **with cardiopulmonary bypass**

> Code also concurrent systemic-to-pulmonary artery shunt ligation/takedown, when performed (33924)
>
> 💰 70.0   ⚕ 70.0   **FUD** 090   C 80 🖵
>
> **AMA:** 2017,Dec,3

33927-33945 Heart and Heart-Lung Transplants

> INCLUDES Backbench work to prepare donor heart and/or lungs for transplantation (33933, 33944)
> Harvesting donor organs with cold preservation (33930, 33940)
> Transplantation heart and/or lungs into recipient (33935, 33945)

33927 **Implantation of a total replacement heart system (artificial heart) with recipient cardiectomy**

> EXCLUDES *Implantation ventricular assist device:*
> *Extracorporeal (33975-33976)*
> *Intracorporeal (33979)*
> *Percutaneous ([33995], 33990-33991)*
>
> 💰 74.2   ⚕ 74.2   **FUD** XXX   C 80 🖵
>
> **AMA:** 2018,Jun,3

33928 **Removal and replacement of total replacement heart system (artificial heart)**

> EXCLUDES *Replacement or revision elements artificial heart (33999)*
>
> 💰 0.00   ⚕ 0.00   **FUD** XXX   C 80 🖵
>
> **AMA:** 2018,Jun,3

+ 33929 **Removal of a total replacement heart system (artificial heart) for heart transplantation (List separately in addition to code for primary procedure)**

> Code first (33945)
>
> 💰 0.00   ⚕ 0.00   **FUD** ZZZ   C 80 🖵
>
> **AMA:** 2018,Jun,3

33930 **Donor cardiectomy-pneumonectomy (including cold preservation)**

> 💰 0.00   ⚕ 0.00   **FUD** XXX   C 🖵
>
> **AMA:** 1997,Nov,1

33933 **Backbench standard preparation of cadaver donor heart/lung allograft prior to transplantation, including dissection of allograft from surrounding soft tissues to prepare aorta, superior vena cava, inferior vena cava, and trachea for implantation**

> 💰 0.00   ⚕ 0.00   **FUD** XXX   C 80 🖵
>
> **AMA:** 1997,Nov,1

33935 **Heart-lung transplant with recipient cardiectomy-pneumonectomy**

> Code also concurrent systemic-to-pulmonary artery shunt ligation/takedown, when performed (33924)
>
> 💰 143.   ⚕ 143.   **FUD** 090   C 80 🖵
>
> **AMA:** 2017,Dec,3

33940 **Donor cardiectomy (including cold preservation)**

> 💰 0.00   ⚕ 0.00   **FUD** XXX   C 🖵
>
> **AMA:** 2018,Jan,8; 2017,Jan,8; 2016,Jan,13

33944 **Backbench standard preparation of cadaver donor heart allograft prior to transplantation, including dissection of allograft from surrounding soft tissues to prepare aorta, superior vena cava, inferior vena cava, pulmonary artery, and left atrium for implantation**

> EXCLUDES *Procedures performed on donor heart (33300, 33310, 33320, 33390, 33463-33464, 33510, 33641, 35216, 35276, 35685)*
>
> 💰 0.00   ⚕ 0.00   **FUD** XXX   C 80 🖵
>
> **AMA:** 1997,Nov,1

33945 **Heart transplant, with or without recipient cardiectomy**

> Code also concurrent systemic-to-pulmonary artery shunt ligation/takedown, when performed (33924)
>
> 💰 141.   ⚕ 141.   **FUD** 090   C 80 🖵
>
> **AMA:** 2018,Jun,3; 2017,Dec,3

33946-33989 [33962, 33963, 33964, 33965, 33966, 33969, 33984, 33985, 33986, 33987, 33988, 33989] Extracorporeal Circulatory and Respiratory Support

> INCLUDES Cannula repositioning and cannula insertion performed during same procedure
> Multiple physician and nonphysician team collaboration
> Veno-arterial ECMO/ECLS for heart and lung support
> Veno-venous ECMO/ECLS for lung support

Code also:
> Extensive arterial repair/replacement (35266, 35286, 35371, 35665)
> Overall daily management services needed to manage patient; report appropriate observation, hospital inpatient, or critical care E/M codes

33946 **Extracorporeal membrane oxygenation (ECMO)/extracorporeal life support (ECLS) provided by physician; initiation, veno-venous**

> EXCLUDES *Daily ECMO/ECLS veno-venous management initial service date (33948)*
> *Repositioning ECMO/ECLS cannula initial service date (33957-33959 [33962, 33963, 33964])*
>
> Code also cannula insertion (33951-33956)
>
> 💰 8.95   ⚕ 8.95   **FUD** XXX   63 C 🖵
>
> **AMA:** 2018,Jan,8; 2017,Jan,8; 2016,Mar,5; 2016,Jan,13

33947 **initiation, veno-arterial**

> EXCLUDES *Daily ECMO/ECLS veno-venous management initial service date (33948)*
> *Repositioning ECMO/ECLS cannula initial service date (33957-33959 [33962, 33963, 33964])*
>
> Code also cannula insertion (33951-33956)
>
> 💰 9.99   ⚕ 9.99   **FUD** XXX   63 C 🖵
>
> **AMA:** 2018,Jan,8; 2017,Jan,8; 2016,Mar,5; 2016,Jan,13

33948 **daily management, each day, veno-venous**

> EXCLUDES *ECMO/ECLS initiation, veno-venous (33946)*
>
> 💰 6.94   ⚕ 6.94   **FUD** XXX   63 C 🖵
>
> **AMA:** 2018,Jan,8; 2017,Jan,8; 2016,Mar,5; 2016,Jan,13

33949 **daily management, each day, veno-arterial**

> EXCLUDES *ECMO/ECLS initiation, veno-arterial (33947)*
>
> 💰 6.73   ⚕ 6.73   **FUD** XXX   63 C 🖵
>
> **AMA:** 2018,Jan,8; 2017,Jan,8; 2016,Mar,5; 2016,Jan,13

33951 insertion of peripheral (arterial and/or venous) cannula(e), percutaneous, birth through 5 years of age (includes fluoroscopic guidance, when performed) Ⓐ

INCLUDES Cannula replacement same vessel
Cannula repositioning during same episode care

Code also:
Cannula removal when new cannula inserted in different vessel with ([33965, 33966, 33969, 33984, 33985, 33986])
ECMO/ECLS initiation or daily management (33946-33947, 33948-33949)

🚑 12.3   ⚕ 12.3   **FUD** 000   C 80 ▭

AMA: 2018,Jan,8; 2017,Jan,8; 2016,Mar,5; 2016,Jan,13

33952 insertion of peripheral (arterial and/or venous) cannula(e), percutaneous, 6 years and older (includes fluoroscopic guidance, when performed) Ⓐ

INCLUDES Cannula replacement same vessel
Cannula repositioning during same episode care

Code also:
Cannula removal when new cannula inserted in different vessel with ([33965, 33966, 33969, 33984, 33985, 33986])
ECMO/ECLS initiation or daily management (33946-33947, 33948-33949)

🚑 12.4   ⚕ 12.4   **FUD** 000   C 80 ▭

AMA: 2018,Jan,8; 2017,Jan,8; 2016,Mar,5; 2016,Jan,13

33953 insertion of peripheral (arterial and/or venous) cannula(e), open, birth through 5 years of age Ⓐ

INCLUDES Cannula replacement same vessel
Cannula repositioning during same episode care

EXCLUDES Open artery exposure for delivery/deployment endovascular prosthesis ([34812], 34714-34716 [34820, 34833, 34834], [34820])

Code also:
Cannula removal when new cannula inserted in different vessel with ([33965, 33966, 33969, 33984, 33985, 33986])
ECMO/ECLS initiation or daily management (33946-33947, 33948-33949)

🚑 13.8   ⚕ 13.8   **FUD** 000   C 80 ▭

AMA: 2018,Jan,8; 2017,Dec,3; 2017,Jan,8; 2016,Mar,5; 2016,Jan,13

33954 insertion of peripheral (arterial and/or venous) cannula(e), open, 6 years and older Ⓐ

INCLUDES Cannula replacement same vessel
Cannula repositioning during same episode care

EXCLUDES Open artery exposure for delivery/deployment endovascular prosthesis ([34812], 34714-34716 [34820, 34833, 34834])

Code also:
Cannula removal when new cannula inserted in different vessel with ([33965, 33966, 33969, 33984, 33985, 33986])
ECMO/ECLS initiation or daily management (33946-33947, 33948-33949)

🚑 13.8   ⚕ 13.8   **FUD** 000   C 80 ▭

AMA: 2018,Jan,8; 2017,Dec,3; 2017,Jan,8; 2016,Mar,5; 2016,Jan,13

33955 insertion of central cannula(e) by sternotomy or thoracotomy, birth through 5 years of age Ⓐ

INCLUDES Cannula replacement same vessel
Cannula repositioning during same episode care

EXCLUDES Mediastinotomy (39010)
Thoracotomy (32100)

Code also:
Cannula removal when new cannula inserted in different vessel with ([33965, 33966, 33969, 33984, 33985, 33986])
ECMO/ECLS initiation or daily management (33946-33947, 33948-33949)

🚑 24.0   ⚕ 24.0   **FUD** 000   C 80 ▭

AMA: 2018,Jan,8; 2017,Jan,8; 2016,Mar,5; 2016,Jan,13

33956 insertion of central cannula(e) by sternotomy or thoracotomy, 6 years and older Ⓐ

INCLUDES Cannula replacement same vessel
Cannula repositioning during same episode care

EXCLUDES Mediastinotomy (39010)
Thoracotomy (32100)

Code also:
Cannula removal when new cannula inserted in different vessel with ([33965, 33966, 33969, 33984, 33985, 33986])
ECMO/ECLS initiation or daily management (33946-33947, 33948-33949)

🚑 24.2   ⚕ 24.2   **FUD** 000   C 80 ▭

AMA: 2018,Jan,8; 2017,Jan,8; 2016,Mar,5; 2016,Jan,13

33957 reposition peripheral (arterial and/or venous) cannula(e), percutaneous, birth through 5 years of age (includes fluoroscopic guidance, when performed) Ⓐ

INCLUDES Fluoroscopic guidance

EXCLUDES ECMO/ECLS initiation, veno-arterial (33947)
ECMO/ECLS initiation, veno-venous (33946)
ECMO/ECLS insertion cannula (33951-33956)
Percutaneous access and closure femoral artery for endograft delivery (34713)

🚑 5.36   ⚕ 5.36   **FUD** 000   C 80 ▭

AMA: 2018,Jan,8; 2017,Jan,8; 2016,Mar,5; 2016,Jan,13

33958 reposition peripheral (arterial and/or venous) cannula(e), percutaneous, 6 years and older (includes fluoroscopic guidance, when performed) Ⓐ

INCLUDES Fluoroscopic guidance

EXCLUDES ECMO/ECLS initiation, veno-arterial (33947)
ECMO/ECLS initiation, veno-venous (33946)
ECMO/ECLS insertion of cannula (33951-33956)
Percutaneous access and closure femoral artery for endograft delivery (34713)

🚑 5.36   ⚕ 5.36   **FUD** 000   C 80 ▭

AMA: 2018,Jan,8; 2017,Jan,8; 2016,Mar,5; 2016,Jan,13

33959 reposition peripheral (arterial and/or venous) cannula(e), open, birth through 5 years of age (includes fluoroscopic guidance, when performed) Ⓐ

INCLUDES Fluoroscopic guidance

EXCLUDES ECMO/ECLS initiation, veno-arterial (33947)
ECMO/ECLS initiation, veno-venous (33946)
ECMO/ECLS insertion of cannula (33951-33956)
Open artery exposure for delivery/deployment endovascular prosthesis ([34812], 34714-34716 [34820, 34833, 34834])

🚑 6.84   ⚕ 6.84   **FUD** 000   C 80 ▭

AMA: 2018,Jan,8; 2017,Dec,3; 2017,Jan,8; 2016,Mar,5; 2016,Jan,13

33962 reposition peripheral (arterial and/or venous) cannula(e), open, 6 years and older (includes fluoroscopic guidance, when performed) Ⓐ

INCLUDES Fluoroscopic guidance

EXCLUDES ECMO/ECLS initiation, veno-arterial (33947)
ECMO/ECLS initiation, veno-venous (33946)
ECMO/ECLS insertion of cannula (33951-33956)
Open artery exposure for delivery/deployment endovascular prosthesis ([34812], 34714-34716 [34820, 34833, 34834])

🚑 6.79   ⚕ 6.79   **FUD** 000   C 80 ▭

AMA: 2018,Jan,8; 2017,Dec,3; 2017,Jan,8; 2016,Mar,5; 2016,Jan,13

2B/1B PC/TC Only   A2-Z3 ASC Payment   50 Bilateral   ♂ Male Only   ♀ Female Only   🚑 Facility RVU   ⚕ Non-Facility RVU   ▭ CCI   ✖ CLIA
FUD Follow-up Days   CMS: IOM   AMA: CPT Asst   A-Y OPPSI   80/80 Surg Assist Allowed / w/Doc   ▬ Lab Crosswalk   ✚ Radiology Crosswalk

144   CPT © 2021 American Medical Association. All Rights Reserved.   © 2021 Optum360, LLC

33963
reposition of central cannula(e) by sternotomy or thoracotomy, birth through 5 years of age (includes fluoroscopic guidance, when performed) Ⓐ

INCLUDES Fluoroscopic guidance

EXCLUDES ECMO/ECLS initiation, veno-arterial (33947)
ECMO/ECLS initiation, veno-venous (33946)
ECMO/ECLS insertion of cannula (33951-33956)
Open artery exposure for delivery/deployment endovascular prosthesis ([34812], 34714-34716 [34820, 34833, 34834])

🚑 13.5   ⚕ 13.5   **FUD** 000   Ⓒ 80 ▣

AMA: 2018,Jan,8; 2017,Jan,8; 2016,Mar,5; 2016,Jan,13

33964
reposition central cannula(e) by sternotomy or thoracotomy, 6 years and older (includes fluoroscopic guidance, when performed) Ⓐ

INCLUDES Fluoroscopic guidance

EXCLUDES ECMO/ECLS initiation, veno-arterial (33947)
ECMO/ECLS initiation, veno-venous (33946)
ECMO/ECLS insertion cannula (33951-33956)
Mediastinotomy (39010)
Thoracotomy (32100)

🚑 14.3   ⚕ 14.3   **FUD** 000   Ⓒ 80 ▣

AMA: 2018,Jan,8; 2017,Jan,8; 2016,Mar,5; 2016,Jan,13

33965
removal of peripheral (arterial and/or venous) cannula(e), percutaneous, birth through 5 years of age Ⓐ

Code also:
Extensive arterial repair/replacement, when performed (35266, 35286, 35371, 35665)
New cannula insertion into different vessel (33951-33956)

🚑 5.36   ⚕ 5.36   **FUD** 000   Ⓒ 80 ▣

AMA: 2018,Jan,8; 2017,Jan,8; 2016,Mar,5; 2016,Jan,13

33966
removal of peripheral (arterial and/or venous) cannula(e), percutaneous, 6 years and older Ⓐ

Code also:
Extensive arterial repair/replacement, when performed (35266, 35286, 35371, 35665)
New cannula insertion into different vessel (33951-33956)

🚑 6.87   ⚕ 6.87   **FUD** 000   Ⓒ 80 ▣

AMA: 2018,Jan,8; 2017,Jan,8; 2016,Mar,5; 2016,Jan,13

33969
removal of peripheral (arterial and/or venous) cannula(e), open, birth through 5 years of age Ⓐ

EXCLUDES Open artery exposure for delivery/deployment endovascular prosthesis ([34812], 34714-34716 [34820, 34833, 34834])
Repair blood vessel (35201, 35206, 35211, 35216, 35226)

Code also:
Extensive arterial repair/replacement, when performed (35266, 35286, 35371, 35665)
New cannula insertion into different vessel (33951-33956)

🚑 7.98   ⚕ 7.98   **FUD** 000   Ⓒ 80 ▣

AMA: 2018,Jan,8; 2017,Dec,3; 2017,Jan,8; 2016,Mar,5; 2016,Jan,13

33984
removal of peripheral (arterial and/or venous) cannula(e), open, 6 years and older Ⓐ

EXCLUDES Open artery exposure for delivery/deployment endovascular prosthesis ([34812], 34714-34716 [34820, 34833, 34834])
Repair blood vessel (35201, 35206, 35211, 35216, 35226)

🚑 8.25   ⚕ 8.25   **FUD** 000   Ⓒ 80 ▣

AMA: 2018,Jan,8; 2017,Dec,3; 2017,Jan,8; 2016,Mar,5; 2016,Jan,13

33985
removal of central cannula(e) by sternotomy or thoracotomy, birth through 5 years of age Ⓐ

EXCLUDES Repair blood vessel (35201, 35206, 35211, 35216, 35226)

Code also:
Extensive arterial repair/replacement, when performed (35266, 35286, 35371, 35665)
New cannula insertion into different vessel (33951-33956)

🚑 14.9   ⚕ 14.9   **FUD** 000   Ⓒ 80 ▣

AMA: 2018,Jan,8; 2017,Jan,8; 2016,Mar,5; 2016,Jan,13

33986
removal of central cannula(e) by sternotomy or thoracotomy, 6 years and older Ⓐ

EXCLUDES Repair blood vessel (35201, 35206, 35211, 35216, 35226)

Code also:
Extensive arterial repair/replacement, when performed (35266, 35286, 35371, 35665)
New cannula insertion into different vessel (33951-33956)

🚑 15.1   ⚕ 15.1   **FUD** 000   Ⓒ 80 ▣

AMA: 2018,Jan,8; 2017,Jan,8; 2016,Mar,5; 2016,Jan,13

+ # 33987
Arterial exposure with creation of graft conduit (eg, chimney graft) to facilitate arterial perfusion for ECMO/ECLS (List separately in addition to code for primary procedure)

EXCLUDES Open artery exposure for delivery/deployment endovascular prosthesis ([34812], 34714-34716 [34820, 34833, 34834])

Code first (33953-33956)

🚑 6.09   ⚕ 6.09   **FUD** ZZZ   Ⓒ 80 ▣

AMA: 2018,Jan,8; 2017,Dec,3; 2017,Jan,8; 2016,Mar,5; 2016,Jan,13

33988
Insertion of left heart vent by thoracic incision (eg, sternotomy, thoracotomy) for ECMO/ECLS

🚑 22.5   ⚕ 22.5   **FUD** 000   Ⓒ 80 ▣

AMA: 2018,Jan,8; 2017,Jan,8; 2016,Mar,5; 2016,Jan,13

33989
Removal of left heart vent by thoracic incision (eg, sternotomy, thoracotomy) for ECMO/ECLS

🚑 14.3   ⚕ 14.3   **FUD** 000   Ⓒ 80 ▣

AMA: 2018,Jan,8; 2017,Jan,8; 2016,Mar,5; 2016,Jan,13

33962-33999 [33962, 33963, 33964, 33965, 33966, 33969, 33984, 33985, 33986, 33987, 33988, 33989, 33995, 33997]
Mechanical Circulatory Support

EXCLUDES Insertion, removal, replacement, or repositioning permanently implantable aortic counterpulsation ventricular assist system (33999)

33962 **Resequenced code. See code following 33959.**

33963 **Resequenced code. See code following 33959.**

33964 **Resequenced code. See code following 33959.**

33965 **Resequenced code. See code following 33959.**

33966 **Resequenced code. See code following 33959.**

33967 **Insertion of intra-aortic balloon assist device, percutaneous**

🚑 7.51   ⚕ 7.51   **FUD** 000   Ⓒ 80 ▣

AMA: 2018,Jan,8; 2017,Jan,8; 2016,Mar,5; 2016,Jan,13

33968 **Removal of intra-aortic balloon assist device, percutaneous**

🚑 0.98   ⚕ 0.98   **FUD** 000   Ⓒ ▣

AMA: 2018,Jan,8; 2017,Jan,8; 2016,Mar,5; 2016,Jan,13

33969 **Resequenced code. See code following 33959.**

33970 **Insertion of intra-aortic balloon assist device through the femoral artery, open approach**

EXCLUDES Percutaneous insertion intra-aortic balloon assist device (33967)

🚑 10.2   ⚕ 10.2   **FUD** 000   Ⓒ 80 ▣

AMA: 2018,Jan,8; 2017,Jan,8; 2016,Mar,5; 2016,Jan,13

33971 **Removal of intra-aortic balloon assist device including repair of femoral artery, with or without graft**

🚑 20.3   ⚕ 20.3   **FUD** 090   Ⓒ ▣

AMA: 2018,Jan,8; 2017,Jan,8; 2016,Mar,5; 2016,Jan,13

33973 **Insertion of intra-aortic balloon assist device through the ascending aorta**

🚑 14.8   ⚕ 14.8   **FUD** 000   Ⓒ 80 ▣

AMA: 2018,Jan,8; 2017,Jan,8; 2016,Mar,5; 2016,Jan,13

33974 **Removal of intra-aortic balloon assist device from the ascending aorta, including repair of the ascending aorta, with or without graft**

🚑 25.7   ⚕ 25.7   **FUD** 090   Ⓒ ▣

AMA: 2018,Jan,8; 2017,Jan,8; 2016,Mar,5; 2016,Jan,13

33975   **Insertion of ventricular assist device; extracorporeal, single ventricle**

INCLUDES   Insertion new pump with de-airing, connection, and initiation

Removal old pump with replacement entire ventricular assist device system, including pump(s) and cannulas

Transthoracic approach

EXCLUDES   *Percutaneous approach ([33995], 33990-33991)*

Code also removal thrombus through separate heart incision, when performed (33310-33315); append modifier 59 to (33315)

🚑 37.8   ⚕ 37.8   **FUD** XXX   C 80 ▭

AMA: 2018,Jun,3; 2018,Jan,8; 2017,Dec,3; 2017,Jan,8; 2016,Mar,5; 2016,Jan,13

33976   **extracorporeal, biventricular**

INCLUDES   Insertion new pump with de-airing, connection, and initiation

Removal with replacement entire ventricular assist device system, including pump(s) and cannulas

Transthoracic approach

EXCLUDES   *Percutaneous approach ([33995], 33990-33991)*

Code also removal thrombus through separate heart incision, when performed (33310-33315); append modifier 59 to (33315)

🚑 46.0   ⚕ 46.0   **FUD** XXX   C 80 ▭

AMA: 2018,Jun,3; 2018,Jan,8; 2017,Dec,3; 2017,Jan,8; 2016,Mar,5; 2016,Jan,13

33977   **Removal of ventricular assist device; extracorporeal, single ventricle**

INCLUDES   Removal entire device and cannulas

EXCLUDES   *Removal ventricular assist device when performed same time as new device insertion*

Code also thrombus removal through separate heart incision, when performed (33310-33315); append modifier 59 to (33315)

🚑 32.6   ⚕ 32.6   **FUD** XXX   C 80 ▭

AMA: 2018,Jan,8; 2017,Dec,3; 2017,Jan,8; 2016,Mar,5; 2016,Jan,13

33978   **extracorporeal, biventricular**

INCLUDES   Removal entire device and cannulas

EXCLUDES   *Removal ventricular assist device when performed same time as new device insertion*

Code also thrombus removal through separate heart incision, when performed (33310-33315); append modifier 59 to (33315)

🚑 38.5   ⚕ 38.5   **FUD** XXX   C 80 ▭

AMA: 2018,Jan,8; 2017,Dec,3; 2017,Jan,8; 2016,Mar,5; 2016,Jan,13

33979   **Insertion of ventricular assist device, implantable intracorporeal, single ventricle**

INCLUDES   New pump insertion with connection, de-airing, and initiation

Removal with replacement entire ventricular assist device system, including pump(s) and cannulas

Transthoracic approach

EXCLUDES   *Percutaneous approach ([33995], 33990-33991)*

Code also thrombus removal through separate heart incision, when performed (33310-33315); append modifier 59 to (33315)

🚑 56.5   ⚕ 56.5   **FUD** XXX   C 80 ▭

AMA: 2018,Jun,3; 2018,Jan,8; 2017,Dec,3; 2017,Jan,8; 2016,Mar,5; 2016,Jan,13

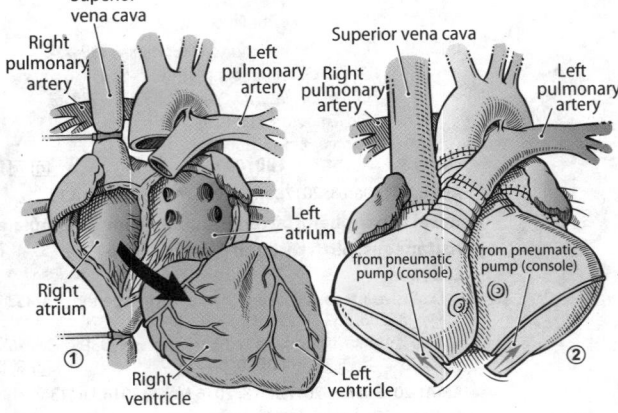

33980   **Removal of ventricular assist device, implantable intracorporeal, single ventricle**

INCLUDES   Removal entire device and cannulas

EXCLUDES   *Removal ventricular assist device when performed same time as new device insertion*

Code also thrombus removal through separate heart incision, when performed (33310-33315); append modifier 59 to (33315)

🚑 51.5   ⚕ 51.5   **FUD** XXX   C 80 ▭

AMA: 2018,Jan,8; 2017,Dec,3; 2017,Jan,8; 2016,Mar,5; 2016,Jan,13

33981   **Replacement of extracorporeal ventricular assist device, single or biventricular, pump(s), single or each pump**

INCLUDES   New pump insertion with de-airing, connection, and initiation

Removal old pump

🚑 24.3   ⚕ 24.3   **FUD** XXX   C 80 ▭

AMA: 2018,Jan,8; 2017,Jan,8; 2016,Mar,5; 2016,Jan,13

33982   **Replacement of ventricular assist device pump(s); implantable intracorporeal, single ventricle, without cardiopulmonary bypass**

INCLUDES   New pump insertion with connection, de-airing, and initiation

Removal old pump

🚑 57.1   ⚕ 57.1   **FUD** XXX   C 80 ▭

AMA: 2018,Jan,8; 2017,Jan,8; 2016,Mar,5; 2016,Jan,13

33983   **implantable intracorporeal, single ventricle, with cardiopulmonary bypass**

INCLUDES   Removal old pump

EXCLUDES   *Percutaneous transseptal approach (33999)*

🚑 67.0   ⚕ 67.0   **FUD** XXX   C 80 ▭

AMA: 2018,Jan,8; 2017,Dec,3; 2017,Jan,8; 2016,Mar,5; 2016,Jan,13

33984   **Resequenced code. See code following 33959.**

33985   **Resequenced code. See code following 33959.**

33986   **Resequenced code. See code following 33959.**

Cardiovascular, Hemic, and Lymphatic

33975 — 33986

33987 Resequenced code. See code following 33959.

33988 Resequenced code. See code following 33959.

33989 Resequenced code. See code following 33959.

33995 Insertion of ventricular assist device, percutaneous, including radiological supervision and interpretation; right heart, venous access only

> INCLUDES Initial insertion and replacement percutaneous ventricular assist device
>
> EXCLUDES Extensive artery repair/replacement (35226, 35286)
> Open arterial approach to aid insertion percutaneous ventricular assist device, when used ([34812], 34714-34716 [34820, 34833, 34834])
> Removal percutaneous ventricular assist device with entire system replacement (33992)
> Transthoracic approach (33975-33976, 33979)

> 🔁 10.6 　 ⚕ 10.6 　 **FUD** 000 　　　　　 80 ▣

> **AMA:** 2020,Dec,4

33990 left heart, arterial access only

> INCLUDES Initial insertion and replacement percutaneous ventricular assist device
>
> EXCLUDES Extensive artery repair/replacement (35226, 35286)
> Open arterial approach to aid insertion percutaneous ventricular assist device, when used ([34812], 34714-34716 [34820, 34833, 34834])
> Removal percutaneous ventricular assist device with entire system replacement (33992)
> Transthoracic approach (33975-33976, 33979)

> 🔁 12.4 　 ⚕ 12.4 　 **FUD** XXX 　　　　 C 80 ▣

> **AMA:** 2020,Dec,4; 2018,Jun,3; 2018,Jan,8; 2017,Dec,3; 2017,Jan,8; 2016,Mar,5; 2016,Jan,13

33991 left heart, both arterial and venous access, with transseptal puncture

> INCLUDES Initial insertion and replacement percutaneous ventricular assist device
>
> EXCLUDES Extensive artery repair/replacement (35226, 35286)
> Open arterial approach to aid with insertion percutaneous ventricular assist device, when performed (34812 [34812], 34714-34716 [34820, 34833, 34834])
> Removal percutaneous ventricular assist device with entire system replacement (33992)
> Transthoracic approach (33975-33976, 33979)

> 🔁 18.1 　 ⚕ 18.1 　 **FUD** XXX 　　　　 C 80 ▣

> **AMA:** 2020,Dec,4; 2018,Jun,3; 2018,Jan,8; 2017,Dec,3; 2017,Jan,8; 2016,Mar,5; 2016,Jan,13

33992 Removal of percutaneous left heart ventricular assist device, arterial or arterial and venous cannula(s), at separate and distinct session from insertion

> INCLUDES Removal device and cannulas
> Code also modifier 59 when percutaneous ventricular assist device removed on same day as insertion, but different session

> 🔁 5.80 　 ⚕ 5.80 　 **FUD** XXX 　　　　 C 80 ▣

> **AMA:** 2020,Dec,4; 2018,Jan,8; 2017,Jan,8; 2016,Mar,5; 2016,Jan,13

33997 Removal of percutaneous right heart ventricular assist device, venous cannula, at separate and distinct session from insertion

> 🔁 4.72 　 ⚕ 4.72 　 **FUD** 000 　　　　 80 ▣

> **AMA:** 2020,Dec,4

33993 Repositioning of percutaneous right or left heart ventricular assist device with imaging guidance at separate and distinct session from insertion

> EXCLUDES Repositioning percutaneous ventricular assist device without image guidance
> Repositioning percutaneous ventricular assist device same session as insertion (33990-33991)
> Code also modifier 59 when percutaneous ventricular assist device repositioned using imaging guidance on same day as insertion, but different session

> 🔁 5.09 　 ⚕ 5.09 　 **FUD** XXX 　　　　 C 80 ▣

> **AMA:** 2020,Dec,4; 2018,Jan,8; 2017,Jan,8; 2016,Mar,5; 2016,Jan,13

33995 Resequenced code. See code following 33983.

33997 Resequenced code. See code following 33992.

33999 Unlisted procedure, cardiac surgery

> 🔁 0.00 　 ⚕ 0.00 　 **FUD** YYY 　　　　 T 80 ▣

> **AMA:** 2019,Apr,10; 2019,Jan,14; 2018,Jun,3; 2018,Jan,8; 2017,Jan,8; 2016,May,5; 2016,Jan,13

34001-34530 Surgical Revascularization: Veins and Arteries

> INCLUDES Repair blood vessel
> Surgeon's component operative arteriogram

34001 Embolectomy or thrombectomy, with or without catheter; carotid, subclavian or innominate artery, by neck incision

> 🔁 27.8 　 ⚕ 27.8 　 **FUD** 090 　　 C 80 50 ▣

> **AMA:** 1997,Nov,1

Major arteries of the arm: Subclavian artery, Axillary artery, Brachial, Superior ulnar collateral, Radial artery, Posterior ulnar recurrent, Ulnar artery, Common interosseous. Major arteries of the leg: Aorto-femoral artery, Femoral and deep femoral branches, Popliteal artery, Peroneal artery, Anterior tibial artery, Posterior tibial artery. Arteries (red) are usually accompanied by at least one vein (blue)

34051 innominate, subclavian artery, by thoracic incision

> 🔁 28.6 　 ⚕ 28.6 　 **FUD** 090 　　 C 80 50 ▣

> **AMA:** 1997,Nov,1

34101 axillary, brachial, innominate, subclavian artery, by arm incision

> 🔁 17.3 　 ⚕ 17.3 　 **FUD** 090 　 T 62 80 50 ▣

> **AMA:** 1997,Nov,1

34111 radial or ulnar artery, by arm incision

> 🔁 17.3 　 ⚕ 17.3 　 **FUD** 090 　 T 62 80 50 ▣

> **AMA:** 1997,Nov,1

34151 renal, celiac, mesentery, aortoiliac artery, by abdominal incision

> 🔁 40.4 　 ⚕ 40.4 　 **FUD** 090 　　 C 80 50 ▣

> **AMA:** 1997,Nov,1

34201 femoropopliteal, aortoiliac artery, by leg incision

> 🔁 29.8 　 ⚕ 29.8 　 **FUD** 090 　 T 62 80 50 ▣

> **AMA:** 2018,Jan,8; 2017,Jan,8; 2016,Jan,13

34203 popliteal-tibio-peroneal artery, by leg incision

> 🔁 27.6 　 ⚕ 27.6 　 **FUD** 090 　 T 62 80 50 ▣

> **AMA:** 1997,Nov,1

34401 Thrombectomy, direct or with catheter; vena cava, iliac vein, by abdominal incision
🔧 42.4 ⚕ 42.4 **FUD** 090 C 80 50 ▢
AMA: 1997,Nov,1

34421 vena cava, iliac, femoropopliteal vein, by leg incision
🔧 21.5 ⚕ 21.5 **FUD** 090 T 62 80 50 ▢
AMA: 2018,Jan,8; 2017,Jan,8; 2016,Jan,13

34451 vena cava, iliac, femoropopliteal vein, by abdominal and leg incision
🔧 41.7 ⚕ 41.7 **FUD** 090 C 80 50 ▢
AMA: 1997,Nov,1

34471 subclavian vein, by neck incision
🔧 31.1 ⚕ 31.1 **FUD** 090 T 62 50 ▢
AMA: 1997,Nov,1

34490 axillary and subclavian vein, by arm incision
🔧 18.5 ⚕ 18.5 **FUD** 090 T 62 50 ▢
AMA: 1997,Nov,1

34501 Valvuloplasty, femoral vein
🔧 25.8 ⚕ 25.8 **FUD** 090 T 62 80 50 ▢
AMA: 1997,Nov,1

34502 Reconstruction of vena cava, any method
🔧 44.7 ⚕ 44.7 **FUD** 090 C 80 ▢
AMA: 1997,Nov,1

34510 Venous valve transposition, any vein donor
🔧 29.6 ⚕ 29.6 **FUD** 090 T 62 80 50 ▢
AMA: 1997,Nov,1

34520 Cross-over vein graft to venous system
🔧 28.7 ⚕ 28.7 **FUD** 090 T 62 80 50 ▢
AMA: 1997,Nov,1

34530 Saphenopopliteal vein anastomosis
🔧 27.2 ⚕ 27.2 **FUD** 090 T 62 80 50 ▢
AMA: 1997,Nov,1

34701-34713 [34717, 34718] Abdominal Aorta and Iliac Artery Repairs

INCLUDES Closure artery after endograft delivery using sheath size less than 12 French
Treatment with covered stent for:
  Aneurysm
  Aortic dissection
  Arteriovenous malformation
  Pseudoaneurysm
  Trauma
Treatment zones (vessel(s) in which endograft deployed):
  Iliac artery(ies) (34707-34708, [34717], [34718])
  Infrarenal aorta (34701-34702)
  Infrarenal aorta and both common iliac arteries (34705-34706)
  Infrarenal aorta and ipsilateral common iliac artery (34703-34704)

EXCLUDES *Treatment atherosclerotic occlusive disease with covered stent:*
  Aorta (37236-37237)
  Iliac artery(ies) (37221, 37223)

Code also:
  Open arterial exposure, when appropriate ([34812], 34714 [34820, 34833, 34834], 34715-34716)
  Percutaneous closure artery when endograft delivered through sheath 12 French or larger (34713)
  Selective catheterization arteries outside target treatment zone

34701 Endovascular repair of infrarenal aorta by deployment of an aorto-aortic tube endograft including pre-procedure sizing and device selection, all nonselective catheterization(s), all associated radiological supervision and interpretation, all endograft extension(s) placed in the aorta from the level of the renal arteries to the aortic bifurcation, and all angioplasty/stenting performed from the level of the renal arteries to the aortic bifurcation; for other than rupture (eg, for aneurysm, pseudoaneurysm, dissection, penetrating ulcer)
INCLUDES Nonselective catheterization
Code also intravascular ultrasound when performed (37252-37253)
🔧 36.1 ⚕ 36.1 **FUD** 090 C 80 ▢
AMA: 2019,Nov,6; 2018,Jan,8; 2017,Dec,3

34702 for rupture including temporary aortic and/or iliac balloon occlusion, when performed (eg, for aneurysm, pseudoaneurysm, dissection, penetrating ulcer, traumatic disruption)
INCLUDES Nonselective catheterization
Code also:
  Decompressive laparotomy for treatment abdominal compartment syndrome (49000)
  Intravascular ultrasound when performed (37252-37253)
🔧 53.9 ⚕ 53.9 **FUD** 090 C 80 ▢
AMA: 2019,Nov,6; 2018,Jan,8; 2017,Dec,3

34703 Endovascular repair of infrarenal aorta and/or iliac artery(ies) by deployment of an aorto-uni-iliac endograft including pre-procedure sizing and device selection, all nonselective catheterization(s), all associated radiological supervision and interpretation, all endograft extension(s) placed in the aorta from the level of the renal arteries to the iliac bifurcation, and all angioplasty/stenting performed from the level of the renal arteries to the iliac bifurcation; for other than rupture (eg, for aneurysm, pseudoaneurysm, dissection, penetrating ulcer)
INCLUDES Endograft extensions ending in common iliac arteries
  Nonselective catheterization
Code also intravascular ultrasound when performed (37252-37253)
🔧 39.8 ⚕ 39.8 **FUD** 090 C 80 ▢
AMA: 2019,Nov,6; 2018,Jan,8; 2017,Dec,3

34704 for rupture including temporary aortic and/or iliac balloon occlusion, when performed (eg, for aneurysm, pseudoaneurysm, dissection, penetrating ulcer, traumatic disruption)
INCLUDES Endograft extensions ending in common iliac arteries
  Nonselective catheterization
Code also:
  Decompressive laparotomy for treatment abdominal compartment syndrome (49000)
  Intravascular ultrasound when performed (37252-37253)
🔧 66.4 ⚕ 66.4 **FUD** 090 C 80 ▢
AMA: 2019,Nov,6; 2018,Jan,8; 2017,Dec,3

34705 Endovascular repair of infrarenal aorta and/or iliac artery(ies) by deployment of an aorto-bi-iliac endograft including pre-procedure sizing and device selection, all nonselective catheterization(s), all associated radiological supervision and interpretation, all endograft extension(s) placed in the aorta from the level of the renal arteries to the iliac bifurcation, and all angioplasty/stenting performed from the level of the renal arteries to the iliac bifurcation; for other than rupture (eg, for aneurysm, pseudoaneurysm, dissection, penetrating ulcer)
INCLUDES Endograft extensions ending in common iliac arteries
  Nonselective catheterization
Code also intravascular ultrasound when performed (37252-37253)
🔧 44.5 ⚕ 44.5 **FUD** 090 C 80 ▢
AMA: 2019,Nov,6; 2018,Jan,8; 2017,Dec,3

34706 for rupture including temporary aortic and/or iliac balloon occlusion, when performed (eg, for aneurysm, pseudoaneurysm, dissection, penetrating ulcer, traumatic disruption)
INCLUDES Endograft extensions ending in common iliac arteries
  Nonselective catheterization
Code also:
  Decompressive laparotomy for treatment abdominal compartment syndrome (49000)
  Intravascular ultrasound when performed (37252-37253)
🔧 67.1 ⚕ 67.1 **FUD** 090 C 80 ▢
AMA: 2019,Nov,6; 2018,Jan,8; 2017,Dec,3

34707 Endovascular repair of iliac artery by deployment of an ilio-iliac tube endograft including pre-procedure sizing and device selection, all nonselective catheterization(s), all associated radiological supervision and interpretation, and all endograft extension(s) proximally to the aortic bifurcation and distally to the iliac bifurcation, and treatment zone angioplasty/stenting, when performed, unilateral; for other than rupture (eg, for aneurysm, pseudoaneurysm, dissection, arteriovenous malformation)

> **INCLUDES** Endograft extensions ending in common iliac arteries
> Nonselective catheterization
> **EXCLUDES** *Deployment iliac branched endograft:*
> *At same time as aorto-iliac graft placement ([34717])*
> *Delayed/separate from aorto-iliac endograft deployment ([34718])*
> Code also intravascular ultrasound when performed (37252-37253)

🚑 33.7 ⚕ 33.7 **FUD** 090 Ⓒ 80 50 ▭

AMA: 2019,Nov,6; 2018,Jan,8; 2017,Dec,3

34708 for rupture including temporary aortic and/or iliac balloon occlusion, when performed (eg, for aneurysm, pseudoaneurysm, dissection, arteriovenous malformation, traumatic disruption)

> **INCLUDES** Endograft extensions ending in common iliac arteries
> Nonselective catheterization
> **EXCLUDES** *Deployment iliac branched endograft:*
> *At same time as aorto-iliac graft placement ([34717])*
> *Delayed/separate from aorto-iliac endograft deployment ([34718])*
> Code also:
> · Decompressive laparotomy for treatment abdominal compartment syndrome (49000)
> Intravascular ultrasound when performed (37252-37253)

🚑 53.8 ⚕ 53.8 **FUD** 090 Ⓒ 80 50 ▭

AMA: 2019,Nov,6; 2018,Jan,8; 2017,Dec,3

+ # 34717 Endovascular repair of iliac artery at the time of aorto-iliac artery endograft placement by deployment of an iliac branched endograft including pre-procedure sizing and device selection, all ipsilateral selective iliac artery catheterization(s), all associated radiological supervision and interpretation, and all endograft extension(s) proximally to the aortic bifurcation and distally in the internal iliac, external iliac, and common femoral artery(ies), and treatment zone angioplasty/stenting, when performed, for rupture or other than rupture (eg, for aneurysm, pseudoaneurysm, dissection, arteriovenous malformation, penetrating ulcer, traumatic disruption), unilateral (List separately in addition to code for primary procedure)

> **INCLUDES** Endograft extensions into internal and external iliac, and/or common femoral arteries
> **EXCLUDES** *Delayed deployment branched iliac endograft, separate from aorto-iliac endograft placement ([34718])*
> *Placement prosthesis extensions on same side (34709, 34710-34711)*
> *Reporting with modifier 50. Report once for each side when performed bilaterally*
> Code first (34703-34706)

🚑 12.9 ⚕ 12.9 **FUD** ZZZ 80 ▭

+ 34709 Placement of extension prosthesis(es) distal to the common iliac artery(ies) or proximal to the renal artery(ies) for endovascular repair of infrarenal abdominal aortic or iliac aneurysm, false aneurysm, dissection, penetrating ulcer, including pre-procedure sizing and device selection, all nonselective catheterization(s), all associated radiological supervision and interpretation, and treatment zone angioplasty/stenting, when performed, per vessel treated (List separately in addition to code for primary procedure)

> **EXCLUDES** *Placement covered stent (37236-37237)*
> *Placement iliac branched endograft ([34717], [34718])*
> *Reporting code more than one time for each vessel treated*
> Code first (34701-34708, 34845-34848)

🚑 9.42 ⚕ 9.42 **FUD** ZZZ Ⓒ 80 ▭

AMA: 2019,Nov,6; 2018,Jan,8; 2017,Dec,3

 # 34718 Endovascular repair of iliac artery, not associated with placement of an aorto-iliac artery endograft at the same session, by deployment of an iliac branched endograft, including pre-procedure sizing and device selection, all ipsilateral selective iliac artery catheterization(s), all associated radiological supervision and interpretation, and all endograft extension(s) proximally to the aortic bifurcation and distally in the internal iliac, external iliac, and common femoral artery(ies), and treatment zone angioplasty/stenting, when performed, for other than rupture (eg, for aneurysm, pseudoaneurysm, dissection, arteriovenous malformation, penetrating ulcer), unilateral

> **INCLUDES** Endograft extensions into internal and external iliac, and/or common femoral arteries
> **EXCLUDES** *Branched iliac endograft deployed same session as aorto-iliac endograft placement (34703-34706, [34717])*
> *Placement isolated iliac branched endograft, for rupture (37799)*
> *Placement prosthesis extensions on same side (34709, 34710-34711)*

🚑 36.0 ⚕ 36.0 **FUD** 090 80 ▭

34710 Delayed placement of distal or proximal extension prosthesis for endovascular repair of infrarenal abdominal aortic or iliac aneurysm, false aneurysm, dissection, endoleak, or endograft migration, including pre-procedure sizing and device selection, all nonselective catheterization(s), all associated radiological supervision and interpretation, and treatment zone angioplasty/stenting, when performed; initial vessel treated

> **EXCLUDES** *Fenestrated endograft repair (34841-34848)*
> *Initial endovascular repair by endograft (34701-34709)*
> *Reporting code more than one time per procedure*
> Code also decompressive laparotomy for treatment abdominal compartment syndrome (49000)

🚑 23.3 ⚕ 23.3 **FUD** 090 Ⓒ 80 ▭

AMA: 2019,Nov,6; 2018,Jan,8; 2017,Dec,3

+ 34711 each additional vessel treated (List separately in addition to code for primary procedure)

> **EXCLUDES** *Fenestrated endograft repair (34841-34848)*
> *Initial endovascular repair by endograft (34701-34709)*
> *Reporting code more than one time per procedure*
> Code first (34710)

🚑 8.68 ⚕ 8.68 **FUD** ZZZ Ⓒ 80 ▭

AMA: 2019,Nov,6; 2018,Jan,8; 2017,Dec,3

34712 Transcatheter delivery of enhanced fixation device(s) to the endograft (eg, anchor, screw, tack) and all associated radiological supervision and interpretation

> **EXCLUDES** *Reporting code more than one time per procedure*

🚑 19.2 ⚕ 19.2 **FUD** 090 Ⓒ 80 ▭

AMA: 2018,Jan,8; 2017,Dec,3

+ 34713 Percutaneous access and closure of femoral artery for delivery of endograft through a large sheath (12 French or larger), including ultrasound guidance, when performed, unilateral (List separately in addition to code for primary procedure)

> INCLUDES Ultrasound imaging guidance
> Unilateral procedure through large sheath 12 French or larger
>
> EXCLUDES *Reporting with modifier 50. Report once for each side when performed bilaterally*
>
> Code first (33880-33881, 33883-33884, 33886, 34701-34708, [34718], 34710, 34712, 34841-34848)
>
> 🚑 3.63   ⚕ 3.63   **FUD** ZZZ   N NI 80 ▣
>
> **AMA:** 2018,Jan,8; 2017,Dec,3

34812-34834 [34717, 34718, 34812, 34820, 34833, 34834]
Open Exposure for Endovascular Prosthesis Delivery

> INCLUDES Balloon angioplasty/stent deployment within target treatment zone
> Introduction, manipulation, placement, and device deployment
> Open exposure femoral or iliac artery/subsequent closure
> Thromboendarterectomy at site of aneurysm
>
> EXCLUDES *Additional interventional procedures outside target treatment zone*
> *Guidewire and catheter insertion (36140, 36200, 36245-36248)*
> *Substantial artery repair/replacement (35226, 35286)*

+ # 34812 Open femoral artery exposure for delivery of endovascular prosthesis, by groin incision, unilateral (List separately in addition to code for primary procedure)

> EXCLUDES *ECMO/ECLS insertion, removal or repositioning (33953-33954, 33959, [33962], [33969], [33984], [33987])*
> *Extensive repair femoral artery (35226, 35286, 35371)*
> *Reporting with modifier 50. Report once for each side when performed bilaterally*
>
> Code first (33880-33881, 33883-33884, 33886, 33990-33991, 34701-34708, [34718], 34710, 34712, 34841-34848)
>
> 🚑 6.01   ⚕ 6.01   **FUD** ZZZ   C 80 ▣
>
> **AMA:** 2018,Jan,8; 2017,Dec,3; 2017,Jan,8; 2016,Jan,13

+ 34714 Open femoral artery exposure with creation of conduit for delivery of endovascular prosthesis or for establishment of cardiopulmonary bypass, by groin incision, unilateral (List separately in addition to code for primary procedure)

> EXCLUDES *Delivery endovascular prosthesis via open femoral artery ([34812])*
> *ECMO/ECLS insertion, removal or repositioning on same side (33953-33954, 33959, [33962], [33969], [33984])*
> *Reporting with modifier 50. Report once for each side when performed bilaterally*
> *Transcatheter aortic valve replacement via open axillary artery (33362)*
>
> Code first (32852, 32854, 33031, 33120, 33251, 33256, 33259, 33261, 33305, 33315, 33322, 33335, 33390-33391, 33404-33406, 33410, 33440 [33440], 33411-33417, 33422, 33425-33427, 33430, 33460, 33463-33465, 33468, 33474-33476, 33478, 33496, 33500, 33502, 33504-33507, 33510-33516, 33533-33536, 33542, 33545, 33548, 33600-33688, 33692, 33694, 33697, 33702, 33710, 33720, 33724, 33726, 33730, 33732, 33736, 33750, 33755, 33762, 33764, 33766-33767, 33770-33783, 33786, 33788, 33802-33803, 33814, 33820, 33822, 33824, 33840, 33845, 33851, 33853, 33858-33859, 33863-33864, 33871, 33875, 33877, 33880-33881, 33883-33884, 33886, 33910, 33916-33917, 33920, 33922, 33926, 33935, 33945, 33975-33980, 33983, 33990-33991, 34701-34708, 34718 [34718], 34710, 34712, 34841-34848)
>
> 🚑 7.87   ⚕ 7.87   **FUD** ZZZ   N NI 80 ▣
>
> **AMA:** 2018,Jan,8; 2017,Dec,3

+ # 34820 Open iliac artery exposure for delivery of endovascular prosthesis or iliac occlusion during endovascular therapy, by abdominal or retroperitoneal incision, unilateral (List separately in addition to code for primary procedure)

> EXCLUDES *ECMO/ECLS insertion, removal or repositioning (33953-33954, 33959, [33962], [33969], [33984])*
> *Reporting with modifier 50. Report once for each side when performed bilaterally*
>
> Code first (33880-33881, 33883-33884, 33886, 33990-33991, 34701-34708, [34718], 34710, 34712, 34841-34848)
>
> 🚑 10.1   ⚕ 10.1   **FUD** ZZZ   C 80 ▣
>
> **AMA:** 2018,Jan,8; 2017,Dec,3; 2017,Jan,8; 2016,Jan,13

+ # 34833 Open iliac artery exposure with creation of conduit for delivery of endovascular prosthesis or for establishment of cardiopulmonary bypass, by abdominal or retroperitoneal incision, unilateral (List separately in addition to code for primary procedure)

> EXCLUDES *Delivery endovascular prosthesis via open iliac artery ([34820])*
> *ECMO/ECLS insertion, removal or repositioning on same side (33953-33954, 33959, [33962], [33969], [33984])*
> *Reporting with modifier 50. Report once for each side when performed bilaterally*
> *Transcatheter aortic valve replacement via open iliac artery (33364)*
>
> Code first (32852, 32854, 33031, 33256, 33259, 33261, 33305, 33315, 33322, 33335, 33390-33391, 33404-33406, 33410, [33440], 33411-33417, 33422, 33425-33427, 33430, 33460, 33463-33465, 33468, 33474-33476, 33478, 33496, 33500, 33502, 33504-33514, 33516, 33533-33536, 33542, 33545, 33548, 33600-33688, 33692, 33694, 33697, 33702, 33710, 33720, 33724, 33726, 33730, 33732, 33736, 33750, 33755, 33762, 33764, 33766-33767, 33770-33783, 33786, 33788, 33802-33803, 33814, 33820, 33822, 33824, 33840, 33845, 33851, 33853, 33858-33859, 33863-33864, 33871, 33875, 33877, 33880-33881, 33883-33884, 33886, 33910, 33916-33917, 33920, 33922, 33926, 33935, 33945, 33975-33980, 33983, 33990-33991, 34701-34708, [34718], 34710, 34712, 34841-34848)
>
> 🚑 11.7   ⚕ 11.7   **FUD** ZZZ   C 80 ▣
>
> **AMA:** 2018,Jan,8; 2017,Dec,3; 2017,Jan,8; 2016,Jan,13

+ # 34834 Open brachial artery exposure for delivery of endovascular prosthesis, unilateral (List separately in addition to code for primary procedure)

> EXCLUDES *ECMO/ECLS insertion, removal or repositioning (33953-33954, 33959, [33962], [33969], [33984])*
> *Reporting with modifier 50. Report once for each side when performed bilaterally*
>
> Code first (33880-33881, 33883-33884, 33886, 33990-33991, 34701-34708, [34718], 34710, 34712, 34841-34848)
>
> 🚑 3.75   ⚕ 3.75   **FUD** ZZZ   C 80 ▣
>
> **AMA:** 2018,Jan,8; 2017,Dec,3; 2017,Jan,8; 2016,Jan,13

+ 34715 Open axillary/subclavian artery exposure for delivery of endovascular prosthesis by infraclavicular or supraclavicular incision, unilateral (List separately in addition to code for primary procedure)

> EXCLUDES *ECMO/ECLS insertion, removal or repositioning on same side (33953-33954, 33959, [33962], [33969], [33984])*
> *Reporting with modifier 50. Report once for each side when performed bilaterally*
> *Transcatheter aortic valve replacement via open axillary artery (33363)*
>
> Code first (33880-33881, 33883-33884, 33886, 33990-33991, 34701-34708, [34718], 34710, 34712, 34841-34848)
>
> 🚑 8.72   ⚕ 8.72   **FUD** ZZZ   N NI 80 ▣
>
> **AMA:** 2018,Jan,8; 2017,Dec,3

26/TC PC/TC Only   A2-Z3 ASC Payment   50 Bilateral   ♂ Male Only   ♀ Female Only   🚑 Facility RVU   ⚕ Non-Facility RVU   ▣ CCI   ✖ CLIA
FUD Follow-up Days   CMS: IOM   AMA: CPT Asst   A-Y OPPSI   80/80 Surg Assist Allowed / w/Doc   ▣ Lab Crosswalk   ▣ Radiology Crosswalk

150   CPT © 2021 American Medical Association. All Rights Reserved.   © 2021 Optum360, LLC

+ **34716** Open axillary/subclavian artery exposure with creation of conduit for delivery of endovascular prosthesis or for establishment of cardiopulmonary bypass, by infraclavicular or supraclavicular incision, unilateral (List separately in addition to code for primary procedure)

> EXCLUDES *Reporting with modifier 50. Report once for each side when performed bilaterally*

Code first (32852, 32854, 33031, 33120, 33251, 33256, 33259, 33261, 33305, 33315, 33322, 33335, 33390-33391, 33404-33406, 33410, [33440], 33411-33417, 33422, 33425-33427, 33430, 33460, 33463-33465, 33468, 33474-33476, 33478, 33496, 33500, 33502, 33504-33514, 33516, 33533-33536, 33542, 33545, 33548, 33600-33688, 33692, 33694, 33697, 33702, 33710, 33720, 33724, 33726, 33730, 33732, 33736, 33750, 33755, 33762, 33764, 33766-33767, 33770-33783, 33786, 33788, 33802-33803, 33814, 33820, 33822, 33824, 33840, 33845, 33851, 33853, 33858-33859, 33863-33864, 33871, 33875, 33877, 33880-33881, 33883-33884, 33886, 33910, 33916-33917, 33920, 33922, 33926, 33935, 33945, 33975-33980, 33983, 33990-33991, 34701-34708, [34718], 34710, 34712, 34841-34848)

🔪 10.8   ⚖ 10.8   **FUD** ZZZ   N N1 80 ▭

AMA: 2018,Jan,8; 2017,Dec,3

34717	Resequenced code. See code following 34708.
34718	Resequenced code. See code following 34709.

+ **34808** Endovascular placement of iliac artery occlusion device (List separately in addition to code for primary procedure)

Code first (34701-34704, 34707-34708, 34709, 34710, 34813, 34841-34844)

🔪 5.81   ⚖ 5.81   **FUD** ZZZ   C 80 ▭

AMA: 2018,Jan,8; 2017,Jan,8; 2016,Jan,13

34812	Resequenced code. See code following 34713.

+ **34813** Placement of femoral-femoral prosthetic graft during endovascular aortic aneurysm repair (List separately in addition to code for primary procedure)

> EXCLUDES *Grafting femoral artery (35521, 35533, 35539, 35540, 35556, 35558, 35566, 35621, 35646, 35654-35661, 35666, 35700)*

Code first ([34812])

🔪 6.85   ⚖ 6.85   **FUD** ZZZ   C 80 ▭

AMA: 2018,Jan,8; 2017,Jan,8; 2016,Jan,13

34820	Resequenced code. See code following 34714.

34830 Open repair of infrarenal aortic aneurysm or dissection, plus repair of associated arterial trauma, following unsuccessful endovascular repair; tube prosthesis

🔪 51.2   ⚖ 51.2   **FUD** 090   C 80 ▭

AMA: 2018,Jan,8; 2017,Jan,8; 2016,Jan,13

A tube prosthesis is placed and any associated arterial trauma is repaired

34831 aorto-bi-iliac prosthesis

🔪 56.0   ⚖ 56.0   **FUD** 090   C 80 ▭

AMA: 2018,Jan,8; 2017,Jan,8; 2016,Jan,13

34832 aorto-bifemoral prosthesis

🔪 54.7   ⚖ 54.7   **FUD** 090   C 80 ▭

AMA: 2018,Jan,8; 2017,Jan,8; 2016,Jan,13

34833	Resequenced code. See code following 34714.
34834	Resequenced code. See code following 34714.

34839-34848 Repair Visceral Aorta with Fenestrated Endovascular Grafts

> INCLUDES Angiography
> Balloon angioplasty before and after graft deployment
> Fluoroscopic guidance
> Guidewire and catheter insertion vessels in target treatment zone
> Radiologic supervision and interpretation
> Visceral aorta (34841-34844)
> Visceral aorta and associated infrarenal abdominal aorta (34845-34848)

> EXCLUDES *Catheterization:*
> *Arterial families outside treatment zone*
> *Hypogastric arteries*
> *Distal extension prosthesis terminating in common femoral, external iliac, or internal iliac artery (34709-34711 [34718])*
> *Insertion bare metal or covered intravascular stents in visceral branches in target treatment zone (37236-37237)*
> *Interventional procedures outside treatment zone*
> *Open exposure access vessels (34713-34716 [34812, 34820, 34833, 34834])*
> *Placement distal extension prosthesis into internal/external iliac or common femoral artery (34709, [34718], 34710-34711)*
> *Repair abdominal aortic aneurysm without fenestrated graft (34701-34708)*
> *Substantial artery repair (35226, 35286)*

Code also associated endovascular repair descending thoracic aorta (33880-33886, 75956-75959)

34839 Physician planning of a patient-specific fenestrated visceral aortic endograft requiring a minimum of 90 minutes of physician time

> EXCLUDES *3D rendering with interpretation and image reporting (76376-76377)*
> *Endovascular repair procedure on day of or day after planning (34701-34706, 34841-34848)*
> *Planning on day of or day before endovascular repair procedure*
> *Total planning time less than 90 minutes*

🔪 0.00   ⚖   **FUD** YYY   B 80 ▭

34841 Endovascular repair of visceral aorta (eg, aneurysm, pseudoaneurysm, dissection, penetrating ulcer, intramural hematoma, or traumatic disruption) by deployment of a fenestrated visceral aortic endograft and all associated radiological supervision and interpretation, including target zone angioplasty, when performed; including one visceral artery endoprosthesis (superior mesenteric, celiac or renal artery)

> EXCLUDES *Endovascular repair aorta (34701-34706, 34845-34848)*
> *Physician planning patient-specific fenestrated visceral aortic endograft (34839)*

🔪 0.00   ⚖ 0.00   **FUD** YYY   C 80 ▭

AMA: 2018,Jan,8; 2017,Dec,3; 2017,Jul,3; 2017,Jan,8; 2016,Jan,13

34842 including two visceral artery endoprostheses (superior mesenteric, celiac and/or renal artery[s])

> INCLUDES Repairs extending from visceral aorta to one or more four visceral artery origins to infrarenal aorta level

> EXCLUDES *Endovascular repair aorta (34701-34706, 34845-34848)*
> *Physician planning patient-specific fenestrated visceral aortic endograft (34839)*

🔪 0.00   ⚖ 0.00   **FUD** YYY   C 80 ▭

AMA: 2018,Jan,8; 2017,Dec,3; 2017,Jul,3; 2017,Jan,8; 2016,Jan,13

34843 including three visceral artery endoprostheses (superior mesenteric, celiac and/or renal artery[s])

> INCLUDES Repairs extending from visceral aorta to one or more four visceral artery origins to infrarenal aorta level

> EXCLUDES *Endovascular repair aorta (34701-34706, 34845-34848)*
> *Physician planning patient-specific fenestrated visceral aortic endograft (34839)*

🔪 0.00   ⚖ 0.00   **FUD** YYY   C 80 ▭

AMA: 2018,Jan,8; 2017,Dec,3; 2017,Jul,3; 2017,Jan,8; 2016,Jan,13

34844 including four or more visceral artery endoprostheses (superior mesenteric, celiac and/or renal artery[s])

INCLUDES Repairs extending from visceral aorta to one or more four visceral artery origins to infrarenal aorta level

EXCLUDES Endovascular repair aorta (34701-34706, 34845-34848)

Physician planning patient-specific fenestrated visceral aortic endograft (34839)

🖰 0.00   ⚭ 0.00   **FUD** YYY   C 80 🖵

AMA: 2018,Jan,8; 2017,Dec,3; 2017,Jul,3; 2017,Jan,8; 2016,Jan,13

34845 **Endovascular repair of visceral aorta and infrarenal abdominal aorta (eg, aneurysm, pseudoaneurysm, dissection, penetrating ulcer, intramural hematoma, or traumatic disruption) with a fenestrated visceral aortic endograft and concomitant unibody or modular infrarenal aortic endograft and all associated radiological supervision and interpretation, including target zone angioplasty, when performed; including one visceral artery endoprosthesis (superior mesenteric, celiac or renal artery)**

INCLUDES Placement device and extensions into common iliac arteries

Repairs extending from visceral aorta to one or more four visceral artery origins to infrarenal aorta level

EXCLUDES Direct repair aneurysm (35081, 35102)

Endovascular repair aorta (34701-34706, 34845-34848)

Physician planning patient-specific fenestrated visceral aortic endograft (34839)

Code also iliac artery revascularization when performed outside target treatment zone (37220-37223)

🖰 0.00   ⚭ 0.00   **FUD** YYY   C 80 🖵

AMA: 2018,Jan,8; 2017,Dec,3; 2017,Jul,3; 2017,Jan,8; 2016,Jan,13

34846 including two visceral artery endoprostheses (superior mesenteric, celiac and/or renal artery[s])

INCLUDES Placement device and extensions into common iliac arteries

Repairs extending from visceral aorta to one or more four visceral artery origins to infrarenal aorta level

EXCLUDES Direct repair aneurysm (35081, 35102)

Endovascular repair aorta (34701-34706, 34841-34844)

Physician planning patient-specific fenestrated visceral aortic endograft (34839)

Code also iliac artery revascularization when performed outside target treatment zone (37220-37223)

🖰 0.00   ⚭ 0.00   **FUD** YYY   C 80 🖵

AMA: 2018,Jan,8; 2017,Dec,3; 2017,Jul,3; 2017,Jan,8; 2016,Jan,13

34847 including three visceral artery endoprostheses (superior mesenteric, celiac and/or renal artery[s])

INCLUDES Placement device and extensions into common iliac arteries

Repairs extending from visceral aorta to one or more four visceral artery origins to infrarenal aorta level

EXCLUDES Direct repair aneurysm (35081, 35102)

Endovascular repair aorta (34701-34706, 34841-34844)

Physician planning patient-specific fenestrated visceral aortic endograft (34839)

Code also iliac artery revascularization when performed outside target treatment zone (37220-37223)

🖰 0.00   ⚭ 0.00   **FUD** YYY   C 80 🖵

AMA: 2018,Jan,8; 2017,Dec,3; 2017,Jul,3; 2017,Jan,8; 2016,Jan,13

34848 including four or more visceral artery endoprostheses (superior mesenteric, celiac and/or renal artery[s])

INCLUDES Placement device and extensions into common iliac arteries

Repairs extending from visceral aorta to one or more four visceral artery origins to infrarenal aorta level

EXCLUDES Direct repair aneurysm (35081, 35102)

Endovascular repair aorta (34701-34706, 34841-34844)

Physician planning patient-specific fenestrated visceral aortic endograft (34839)

Code also iliac artery revascularization when performed outside target treatment zone (37220-37223)

🖰 0.00   ⚭ 0.00   **FUD** YYY   C 80 🖵

AMA: 2018,Jan,8; 2017,Dec,3; 2017,Aug,9; 2017,Jul,3; 2017,Jan,8; 2016,Jul,6; 2016,Jan,13

35001-35152 Repair Aneurysm, False Aneurysm, Related Arterial Disease

INCLUDES Endarterectomy procedures

EXCLUDES Endovascular repairs:

Abdominal aortic aneurysm (34701-34716 [34717, 34718, 34812, 34820, 34833, 34834])

Thoracic aortic aneurysm (33858-33859, 33863-33875)

Intracranial aneurysms (61697-61710)

Repairs related to occlusive disease only (35201-35286)

35001 **Direct repair of aneurysm, pseudoaneurysm, or excision (partial or total) and graft insertion, with or without patch graft; for aneurysm and associated occlusive disease, carotid, subclavian artery, by neck incision**

🖰 32.6   ⚭ 32.6   **FUD** 090   C 80 50 🖵

AMA: 2002,May,7; 2000,Dec,1

35002 for ruptured aneurysm, carotid, subclavian artery, by neck incision

🖰 33.0   ⚭ 33.0   **FUD** 090   C 80 50 🖵

AMA: 2002,May,7; 1997,Nov,1

35005 for aneurysm, pseudoaneurysm, and associated occlusive disease, vertebral artery

🖰 28.6   ⚭ 28.6   **FUD** 090   C 80 50 🖵

AMA: 2002,May,7; 1997,Nov,1

An incision is made in the back of the neck to directly approach an aneurysm or false aneurysm of the vertebral artery. The artery is either repaired directly or excised with a graft

Graft repair

Vertebral artery

Subclavian artery

35011 for aneurysm and associated occlusive disease, axillary-brachial artery, by arm incision

🖰 29.0   ⚭ 29.0   **FUD** 090   T 62 80 50 🖵

AMA: 2002,May,7; 1997,Nov,1

35013 for ruptured aneurysm, axillary-brachial artery, by arm incision

🖰 36.6   ⚭ 36.6   **FUD** 090   C 80 50 🖵

AMA: 2002,May,7; 1997,Nov,1

35021 for aneurysm, pseudoaneurysm, and associated occlusive disease, innominate, subclavian artery, by thoracic incision
🚑 36.4 ⚬ 36.4 **FUD** 090 C 80 50 ▢
AMA: 2002,May,7; 1997,Nov,1

35022 for ruptured aneurysm, innominate, subclavian artery, by thoracic incision
🚑 41.9 ⚬ 41.9 **FUD** 090 C 80 50 ▢
AMA: 2002,May,7; 1997,Nov,1

35045 for aneurysm, pseudoaneurysm, and associated occlusive disease, radial or ulnar artery
🚑 28.4 ⚬ 28.4 **FUD** 090 T 62 80 50 ▢
AMA: 2002,May,7; 1997,Nov,1

35081 for aneurysm, pseudoaneurysm, and associated occlusive disease, abdominal aorta
🚑 50.3 ⚬ 50.3 **FUD** 090 C 80 ▢
AMA: 2018,Jan,8; 2017,Jan,8; 2016,Jan,13

35082 for ruptured aneurysm, abdominal aorta
🚑 63.4 ⚬ 63.4 **FUD** 090 C 80 ▢
AMA: 2002,May,7; 1997,Nov,1

35091 for aneurysm, pseudoaneurysm, and associated occlusive disease, abdominal aorta involving visceral vessels (mesenteric, celiac, renal)
🚑 52.0 ⚬ 52.0 **FUD** 090 C 80 50 ▢
AMA: 2018,Jan,8; 2017,Jan,8; 2016,Jan,13

35092 for ruptured aneurysm, abdominal aorta involving visceral vessels (mesenteric, celiac, renal)
🚑 75.7 ⚬ 75.7 **FUD** 090 C 80 50 ▢
AMA: 2002,May,7; 1997,Nov,1

35102 for aneurysm, pseudoaneurysm, and associated occlusive disease, abdominal aorta involving iliac vessels (common, hypogastric, external)
🚑 54.6 ⚬ 54.6 **FUD** 090 C 80 50 ▢
AMA: 2018,Jan,8; 2017,Jan,8; 2016,Jan,13

35103 for ruptured aneurysm, abdominal aorta involving iliac vessels (common, hypogastric, external)
🚑 65.0 ⚬ 65.0 **FUD** 090 C 80 50 ▢
AMA: 2002,May,7; 1997,Nov,1

35111 for aneurysm, pseudoaneurysm, and associated occlusive disease, splenic artery
🚑 38.5 ⚬ 38.5 **FUD** 090 C 80 50 ▢
AMA: 2002,May,7; 1997,Nov,1

35112 for ruptured aneurysm, splenic artery
🚑 47.4 ⚬ 47.4 **FUD** 090 C 80 50 ▢
AMA: 2002,May,7; 1997,Nov,1

35121 for aneurysm, pseudoaneurysm, and associated occlusive disease, hepatic, celiac, renal, or mesenteric artery
🚑 45.9 ⚬ 45.9 **FUD** 090 C 80 50 ▢
AMA: 2002,May,7; 1997,Nov,1

35122 for ruptured aneurysm, hepatic, celiac, renal, or mesenteric artery
🚑 54.9 ⚬ 54.9 **FUD** 090 C 80 50 ▢
AMA: 2002,May,7; 1997,Nov,1

35131 for aneurysm, pseudoaneurysm, and associated occlusive disease, iliac artery (common, hypogastric, external)
🚑 40.2 ⚬ 40.2 **FUD** 090 C 80 50 ▢
AMA: 2018,Jan,8; 2017,Jan,8; 2016,Jan,13

35132 for ruptured aneurysm, iliac artery (common, hypogastric, external)
🚑 47.4 ⚬ 47.4 **FUD** 090 C 80 50 ▢
AMA: 2002,May,7; 1997,Nov,1

35141 for aneurysm, pseudoaneurysm, and associated occlusive disease, common femoral artery (profunda femoris, superficial femoral)
🚑 31.9 ⚬ 31.9 **FUD** 090 C 80 50 ▢
AMA: 2002,May,7; 1997,Nov,1

35142 for ruptured aneurysm, common femoral artery (profunda femoris, superficial femoral)
🚑 38.6 ⚬ 38.6 **FUD** 090 C 80 50 ▢
AMA: 2002,May,7; 1997,Nov,1

35151 for aneurysm, pseudoaneurysm, and associated occlusive disease, popliteal artery
🚑 35.9 ⚬ 35.9 **FUD** 090 C 80 50 ▢
AMA: 2002,May,7; 1997,Nov,1

35152 for ruptured aneurysm, popliteal artery
🚑 40.5 ⚬ 40.5 **FUD** 090 C 80 50 ▢
AMA: 2002,May,7; 1997,Nov,1

35180-35190 Surgical Repair Arteriovenous Fistula

35180 Repair, congenital arteriovenous fistula; head and neck
🚑 25.4 ⚬ 25.4 **FUD** 090 T 62 80 ▢
AMA: 2018,Jan,8; 2017,Jan,8; 2016,Jan,13

35182 thorax and abdomen
🚑 51.9 ⚬ 51.9 **FUD** 090 C 80 ▢
AMA: 2018,Jan,8; 2017,Jan,8; 2016,Jan,13

35184 extremities
🚑 27.9 ⚬ 27.9 **FUD** 090 T 62 80 ▢
AMA: 2018,Jan,8; 2017,Jan,8; 2016,Jan,13

35188 Repair, acquired or traumatic arteriovenous fistula; head and neck
🚑 36.9 ⚬ 36.9 **FUD** 090 T A2 80 ▢
AMA: 2018,Jan,8; 2017,Jan,8; 2016,Jan,13

35189 thorax and abdomen
🚑 43.8 ⚬ 43.8 **FUD** 090 C 80 ▢
AMA: 2018,Jan,8; 2017,Jan,8; 2016,Jan,13

35190 extremities
🚑 22.0 ⚬ 22.0 **FUD** 090 T 62 80 ▢
AMA: 2018,Jan,8; 2017,Jan,8; 2016,Jan,13

35201-35286 Surgical Repair Artery or Vein

EXCLUDES *Arteriovenous fistula repair (35180-35190)*
Primary open vascular procedures

35201 Repair blood vessel, direct; neck
EXCLUDES *Removal ECMO/ECLS cannula ([33969, 33984, 33985, 33986])*
🚑 27.3 ⚬ 27.3 **FUD** 090 T 62 80 50 ▢
AMA: 2019,Dec,5; 2018,Jan,8; 2017,Jan,8; 2016,Jan,13

35206 upper extremity
EXCLUDES *Removal ECMO/ECLS cannula ([33969, 33984, 33985, 33986])*
🚑 22.6 ⚬ 22.6 **FUD** 090 T 62 80 50 ▢
AMA: 2020,Dec,4; 2019,Dec,5; 2018,Jan,8; 2017,Jan,8; 2016,Jan,13

35207 hand, finger
🚑 21.7 ⚬ 21.7 **FUD** 090 T A2 50 ▢
AMA: 2019,Dec,5

35211 intrathoracic, with bypass
EXCLUDES *Removal ECMO/ECLS cannula ([33969, 33984, 33985, 33986])*
🚑 40.0 ⚬ 40.0 **FUD** 090 C 80 50 ▢
AMA: 2015,Jul,3; 2012,Apr,3-9

35216 intrathoracic, without bypass
EXCLUDES *Removal ECMO/ECLS cannula ([33969, 33984, 33985, 33986])*
🚑 60.0 ⚬ 60.0 **FUD** 090 C 80 50 ▢
AMA: 2018,Jan,8; 2017,Jan,8; 2016,Jan,13

35221 intra-abdominal
🚑 42.6 ⚬ 42.6 **FUD** 090 C 80 50 ▢
AMA: 2012,Apr,3-9; 2003,Feb,1

	lower extremity
35226	

EXCLUDES Removal ECMO/ECLS cannula ([33969, 33984, 33985, 33986])

🔷 24.1   ⚓ 24.1   **FUD** 090   T 62 80 50 ▣

AMA: 2020,Dec,4; 2019,Jul,10; 2018,Jan,8; 2017,Aug,10; 2017,Jul,3; 2017,Jan,8; 2016,Jul,6; 2016,Jan,13

35231   Repair blood vessel with vein graft; neck

🔷 36.3   ⚓ 36.3   **FUD** 090   T 62 80 50 ▣

AMA: 2019,Dec,5

35236   upper extremity

🔷 29.1   ⚓ 29.1   **FUD** 090   T 62 80 50 ▣

AMA: 2019,Dec,5; 2018,Jan,8; 2017,Jan,8; 2016,Jan,13

35241   intrathoracic, with bypass

🔷 41.5   ⚓ 41.5   **FUD** 090   C 80 50 ▣

AMA: 2012,Apr,3-9; 2003,Feb,1

35246   intrathoracic, without bypass

🔷 45.2   ⚓ 45.2   **FUD** 090   C 80 50 ▣

AMA: 2012,Apr,3-9; 2003,Feb,1

35251   intra-abdominal

🔷 50.7   ⚓ 50.7   **FUD** 090   C 80 50 ▣

AMA: 2012,Apr,3-9; 2003,Feb,1

35256   lower extremity

🔷 29.7   ⚓ 29.7   **FUD** 090   T 62 80 50 ▣

AMA: 2019,Dec,5

35261   Repair blood vessel with graft other than vein; neck

🔷 28.4   ⚓ 28.4   **FUD** 090   T 62 80 50 ▣

AMA: 2019,Dec,5

35266   upper extremity

🔷 25.1   ⚓ 25.1   **FUD** 090   T 62 80 50 ▣

AMA: 2019,Dec,5; 2018,Jan,8; 2017,Jan,8; 2016,Jan,13

35271   intrathoracic, with bypass

🔷 39.9   ⚓ 39.9   **FUD** 090   C 80 50 ▣

AMA: 2012,Apr,3-9; 2003,Feb,1

35276   intrathoracic, without bypass

🔷 42.1   ⚓ 42.1   **FUD** 090   C 80 50 ▣

AMA: 2012,Apr,3-9; 2003,Feb,1

35281   intra-abdominal

🔷 47.3   ⚓ 47.3   **FUD** 090   C 80 50 ▣

AMA: 2012,Apr,3-9; 2003,Feb,1

35286   lower extremity

🔷 26.9   ⚓ 26.9   **FUD** 090   T 62 80 50 ▣

AMA: 2020,Dec,4; 2019,Dec,5; 2019,Jul,10; 2018,Jan,8; 2017,Aug,10; 2017,Jul,3; 2017,Jan,8; 2016,Jul,6; 2016,Jan,13

35301-35372 Surgical Thromboendarterectomy Peripheral and Visceral Arteries

INCLUDES Obtaining saphenous or arm vein for graft
Thrombectomy/embolectomy

EXCLUDES Coronary artery bypass procedures (33510-33536, 33572)
Thromboendarterectomy for vascular occlusion on different vessel during same session

35301   Thromboendarterectomy, including patch graft, if performed; carotid, vertebral, subclavian, by neck incision

🔷 32.7   ⚓ 32.7   **FUD** 090   C 80 50 ▣

AMA: 2018,Jan,8; 2017,Jan,8; 2016,Jan,13

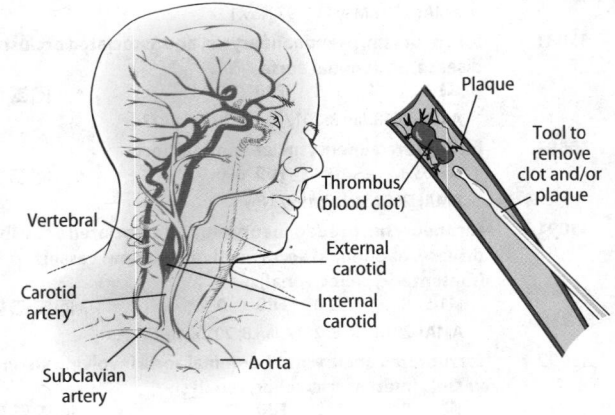

Plaque

Tool to remove clot and/or plaque

Thrombus (blood clot)

Vertebral

External carotid

Internal carotid

Carotid artery

Aorta

Subclavian artery

35302   superficial femoral artery

EXCLUDES Revascularization, endovascular, open or percutaneous, femoral, popliteal artery(s) (37225, 37227)

🔷 32.6   ⚓ 32.6   **FUD** 090   C 80 50 ▣

AMA: 2018,Jan,8; 2017,Jan,8; 2016,Jan,13

35303   popliteal artery

EXCLUDES Revascularization, endovascular, open or percutaneous, femoral, popliteal artery(s) (37225, 37227)

🔷 36.0   ⚓ 36.0   **FUD** 090   C 80 50 ▣

AMA: 2018,Jan,8; 2017,Jan,8; 2016,Jan,13

35304   tibioperoneal trunk artery

EXCLUDES Revascularization, endovascular, open or percutaneous, tibial/peroneal artery (37229, 37231, 37233, 37235)

🔷 37.0   ⚓ 37.0   **FUD** 090   C 80 50 ▣

AMA: 2018,Jan,8; 2017,Jan,8; 2016,Jan,13

35305   tibial or peroneal artery, initial vessel

EXCLUDES Revascularization, endovascular, open or percutaneous, tibial/peroneal artery (37229, 37231, 37233, 37235)

🔷 35.6   ⚓ 35.6   **FUD** 090   C 80 50 ▣

AMA: 2018,Jan,8; 2017,Jan,8; 2016,Jan,13

+ 35306   each additional tibial or peroneal artery (List separately in addition to code for primary procedure)

EXCLUDES Revascularization, endovascular, open or percutaneous, tibial/peroneal artery (37229, 37231, 37233, 37235)

Code first (35305)

🔷 12.9   ⚓ 12.9   **FUD** ZZZ   C 80 ▣

AMA: 2018,Jan,8; 2017,Jan,8; 2016,Jan,13

35311   subclavian, innominate, by thoracic incision

🔷 45.1   ⚓ 45.1   **FUD** 090   C 80 50 ▣

AMA: 1997,Nov,1

35321   axillary-brachial

🔷 25.9   ⚓ 25.9   **FUD** 090   T 62 80 50 ▣

AMA: 1997,Nov,1

35331   abdominal aorta

🔷 42.2   ⚓ 42.2   **FUD** 090   C 80 50 ▣

AMA: 1997,Nov,1

28/ TC PC/TC Only   **A2-Z3** ASC Payment   **50** Bilateral   ♂ Male Only   ♀ Female Only   🔷 Facility RVU   ⚓ Non-Facility RVU   ▣ CCI   ❌ CLIA
FUD Follow-up Days   **CMS:** IOM   **AMA:** CPT Asst   **A-Y** OPPSI   **80/80** Surg Assist Allowed / w/Doc   📘 Lab Crosswalk   📕 Radiology Crosswalk

154   CPT © 2021 American Medical Association. All Rights Reserved.   © 2021 Optum360, LLC

35341   **mesenteric, celiac, or renal**
    🚑 39.9   ⚕ 39.9   **FUD** 090   C 80 50 ▣
    AMA: 1997,Nov,1

35351   **iliac**
    🚑 37.3   ⚕ 37.3   **FUD** 090   C 80 50 ▣
    AMA: 1997,Nov,1

35355   **iliofemoral**
    🚑 29.9   ⚕ 29.9   **FUD** 090   C 80 50 ▣
    AMA: 1997,Nov,1

35361   **combined aortoiliac**
    🚑 44.2   ⚕ 44.2   **FUD** 090   C 80 50 ▣
    AMA: 1997,Nov,1

35363   **combined aortoiliofemoral**
    🚑 47.1   ⚕ 47.1   **FUD** 090   C 80 50 ▣
    AMA: 1997,Nov,1

35371   **common femoral**
    🚑 23.7   ⚕ 23.7   **FUD** 090   C 80 50 ▣
    AMA: 2020,Dec,4; 2018,Jan,8; 2017,Aug,10; 2017,Jul,3; 2017,Jan,8; 2016,Jan,13

35372   **deep (profunda) femoral**
    🚑 28.4   ⚕ 28.4   **FUD** 090   C 80 50 ▣
    AMA: 2018,Jan,8; 2017,Jan,8; 2016,Jan,13

35390 Surgical Thromboendarterectomy: Carotid Reoperation
Code first (35301)

+   **35390**   **Reoperation, carotid, thromboendarterectomy, more than 1 month after original operation (List separately in addition to code for primary procedure)**
    🚑 4.65   ⚕ 4.65   **FUD** ZZZ   C 80 ▣
    AMA: 1997,Nov,1; 1993,Win,1

35400 Endoscopic Visualization of Vessels
Code first therapeutic intervention

+   **35400**   **Angioscopy (noncoronary vessels or grafts) during therapeutic intervention (List separately in addition to code for primary procedure)**
    🚑 4.32   ⚕ 4.32   **FUD** ZZZ   C 80 ▣
    AMA: 1997,Dec,1; 1997,Nov,1

35500 Obtain Arm Vein for Graft
EXCLUDES   *Endoscopic harvest (33508)*
    Harvesting multiple vein segments (35682, 35683)
Code first (33510-33536, 35556, 35566, 35570-35571, 35583-35587)

+   **35500**   **Harvest of upper extremity vein, 1 segment, for lower extremity or coronary artery bypass procedure (List separately in addition to code for primary procedure)**
    🚑 9.29   ⚕ 9.29   **FUD** ZZZ   N 80 ▣
    AMA: 2018,Jan,8; 2017,Jan,8; 2016,Jan,13

35501-35571 Arterial Bypass Using Vein Grafts
INCLUDES   *Obtaining saphenous vein grafts*
EXCLUDES   *Obtaining multiple vein segments (35682, 35683)*
    Obtaining vein grafts, upper extremity or femoropopliteal (35500, 35572)
    Treatment different sites with different bypass procedures during same operative session

35501   **Bypass graft, with vein; common carotid-ipsilateral internal carotid**
    🚑 42.4   ⚕ 42.4   **FUD** 090   C 80 50 ▣
    AMA: 2018,Jan,8; 2017,Jan,8; 2016,Jan,13

35506   **carotid-subclavian or subclavian-carotid**
    🚑 37.0   ⚕ 37.0   **FUD** 090   C 80 50 ▣
    AMA: 2018,Jan,8; 2017,Jan,8; 2016,Jan,13

35508   **carotid-vertebral**
    INCLUDES   Endoscopic procedure
    🚑 38.5   ⚕ 38.5   **FUD** 090   C 80 50 ▣
    AMA: 1999,Mar,6; 1999,Apr,11

35509   **carotid-contralateral carotid**
    🚑 40.6   ⚕ 40.6   **FUD** 090   C 80 50 ▣
    AMA: 2018,Jan,8; 2017,Jan,8; 2016,Jan,13

35510   **carotid-brachial**
    🚑 35.7   ⚕ 35.7   **FUD** 090   C 80 50 ▣
    AMA: 2018,Jan,8; 2017,Jan,8; 2016,Jan,13

35511   **subclavian-subclavian**
    🚑 32.5   ⚕ 32.5   **FUD** 090   C 80 50 ▣
    AMA: 2018,Jan,8; 2017,Jan,8; 2016,Jan,13

35512   **subclavian-brachial**
    🚑 35.0   ⚕ 35.0   **FUD** 090   C 80 50 ▣
    AMA: 2018,Jan,8; 2017,Jan,8; 2016,Jan,13

35515   **subclavian-vertebral**
    🚑 38.5   ⚕ 38.5   **FUD** 090   C 80 50 ▣
    AMA: 1999,Mar,6; 1999,Apr,11

35516   **subclavian-axillary**
    🚑 35.4   ⚕ 35.4   **FUD** 090   C 80 50 ▣
    AMA: 1999,Mar,6; 1999,Apr,11

35518   **axillary-axillary**
    🚑 33.1   ⚕ 33.1   **FUD** 090   C 80 50 ▣
    AMA: 2018,Jan,8; 2017,Jan,8; 2016,Jan,13

35521   **axillary-femoral**
    EXCLUDES   *Synthetic graft (35621)*
    🚑 35.6   ⚕ 35.6   **FUD** 090   C 80 50 ▣
    AMA: 2018,Jan,8; 2017,Jan,8; 2016,Jan,13

35522   **axillary-brachial**
    🚑 35.3   ⚕ 35.3   **FUD** 090   C 80 50 ▣
    AMA: 2018,Jan,8; 2017,Jan,8; 2016,Jan,13

35523   **brachial-ulnar or -radial**
    EXCLUDES   *Bypass graft using synthetic conduit (37799)*
    Bypass graft, with vein; brachial-brachial (35525)
    Distal revascularization and interval ligation (DRIL), upper extremity hemodialysis access (steal syndrome) (36838)
    Harvest upper extremity vein, 1 segment, for lower extremity or coronary artery bypass procedure (35500)
    Repair blood vessel, direct; upper extremity (35206)
    🚑 37.1   ⚕ 37.1   **FUD** 090   C 80 50 ▣

35525   **brachial-brachial**
    🚑 33.0   ⚕ 33.0   **FUD** 090   C 80 50 ▣
    AMA: 2018,Jan,8; 2017,Jan,8; 2016,Jan,13

35526   **aortosubclavian, aortoinnominate, or aortocarotid**
    EXCLUDES   *Synthetic graft (35626)*
    🚑 50.1   ⚕ 50.1   **FUD** 090   C 80 50 ▣
    AMA: 1999,Mar,6; 1999,Apr,11

35531   **aortoceliac or aortomesenteric**
    🚑 56.6   ⚕ 56.6   **FUD** 090   C 80 50 ▣
    AMA: 1999,Mar,6; 1999,Apr,11

35533   **axillary-femoral-femoral**
    EXCLUDES   *Synthetic graft (35654)*
    🚑 43.7   ⚕ 43.7   **FUD** 090   C 80 50 ▣
    AMA: 2012,Apr,3-9; 1999,Mar,6

35535   **hepatorenal**
    EXCLUDES   *Bypass graft (35536, 35560, 35631, 35636)*
    Harvest upper extremity vein, 1 segment, for lower extremity or coronary artery bypass procedure (35500)
    Repair blood vessel (35221, 35251, 35281)
    🚑 55.3   ⚕ 55.3   **FUD** 090   C 80 50 ▣

35536   **splenorenal**
    🚑 49.1   ⚕ 49.1   **FUD** 090   C 80 50 ▣
    AMA: 2018,Jan,8; 2017,Jan,8; 2016,Jan,13

35537   **aortoiliac**
    EXCLUDES   *Bypass graft, with vein; aortobi-iliac (35538)*
    Synthetic graft (35637)
    🚑 60.6   ⚕ 60.6   **FUD** 090   C 80 ▣
    AMA: 2018,Jan,8; 2017,Jan,8; 2016,Jan,13

● New Code   ▲ Revised Code   ○ Reinstated   ● New Web Release   ▲ Revised Web Release   + Add-on   Unlisted   Not Covered   # Resequenced
50 Optum Mod 50 Exempt   ⊘ AMA Mod 51 Exempt   51 Optum Mod 51 Exempt   63 Mod 63 Exempt   ✗ Non-FDA Drug   ★ Telemedicine   M Maternity   A Age Edit

35538

35538 aortobi-iliac
EXCLUDES Bypass graft, with vein; aortoiliac (35537)
Synthetic graft (35638)
⚕ 67.9   ⚖ 67.9   **FUD** 090   C 80
AMA: 2018,Jan,8; 2017,Jan,8; 2016,Jan,13

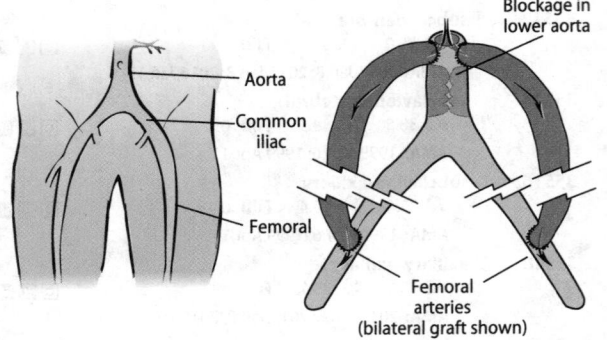

Blockage in lower aorta
Aorta
Common iliac
Femoral
Femoral arteries (bilateral graft shown)

35539 aortofemoral
EXCLUDES Bypass graft, with vein; aortobifemoral (35540)
Synthetic graft (35647)
⚕ 63.7   ⚖ 63.7   **FUD** 090   C 80 50
AMA: 2018,Jan,8; 2017,Jan,8; 2016,Jan,13

35540 aortobifemoral
EXCLUDES Bypass graft, with vein; aortofemoral (35539)
Synthetic graft (35646)
⚕ 70.6   ⚖ 70.6   **FUD** 090   C 50
AMA: 2018,Jan,8; 2017,Jan,8; 2016,Jan,13

35556 femoral-popliteal
⚕ 40.7   ⚖ 40.7   **FUD** 090   C 80 50
AMA: 2018,Jan,8; 2017,Jan,8; 2016,Jan,13

35558 femoral-femoral
⚕ 35.7   ⚖ 35.7   **FUD** 090   C 80 50
AMA: 2012,Apr,3-9; 1999,Mar,6

35560 aortorenal
⚕ 49.2   ⚖ 49.2   **FUD** 090   C 80 50
AMA: 2018,Jan,8; 2017,Jan,8; 2016,Jan,13

35563 ilioiliac
⚕ 38.4   ⚖ 38.4   **FUD** 090   C 80 50
AMA: 1999,Mar,6; 1999,Apr,11

35565 iliofemoral
⚕ 38.1   ⚖ 38.1   **FUD** 090   C 80 50
AMA: 2012,Apr,3-9; 2004,Oct,6

35566 femoral-anterior tibial, posterior tibial, peroneal artery or other distal vessels
⚕ 48.6   ⚖ 48.6   **FUD** 090   C 80 50
AMA: 2018,Jan,8; 2017,Jan,8; 2016,Jan,13

35570 tibial-tibial, peroneal-tibial, or tibial/peroneal trunk-tibial
EXCLUDES Repair blood vessel with graft (35256, 35286)
⚕ 42.8   ⚖ 42.8   **FUD** 090   C 80 50
AMA: 2018,Jan,8; 2017,Jan,8; 2016,Jan,13

35571 popliteal-tibial, -peroneal artery or other distal vessels
⚕ 38.5   ⚖ 38.5   **FUD** 090   C 80 50
AMA: 2018,Jan,8; 2017,Jan,8; 2016,Jan,13

35572 Obtain Femoropopliteal Vein for Graft
EXCLUDES Reporting with modifier 50. Report once for each side when performed bilaterally
Code first (33510-33523, 33533-33536, 34502, 34520, 35001-35002, 35011-35022, 35102-35103, 35121-35152, 35231-35256, 35501-35587, 35879-35907)

+ 35572 Harvest of femoropopliteal vein, 1 segment, for vascular reconstruction procedure (eg, aortic, vena caval, coronary, peripheral artery) (List separately in addition to code for primary procedure)
⚕ 10.0   ⚖ 10.0   **FUD** ZZZ   N M 80
AMA: 2018,Jan,8; 2017,Jan,8; 2016,Jan,13

35583-35587 Lower Extremity Revascularization: In-situ Vein Bypass
INCLUDES Obtaining saphenous vein grafts
EXCLUDES Obtaining multiple vein segments (35682, 35683)
Obtaining vein graft, upper extremity or femoropopliteal (35500, 35572)

35583 In-situ vein bypass; femoral-popliteal
Code also:
Aortobifemoral bypass graft other than vein for aortobifemoral bypass using synthetic conduit and femoral-popliteal bypass with vein conduit in situ (35646)
Concurrent aortofemoral bypass for aortofemoral bypass graft with synthetic conduit and femoral-popliteal bypass with vein conduit in-situ (35647)
Concurrent aortofemoral bypass (vein) for aortofemoral bypass using vein conduit or femoral-popliteal bypass with vein conduit in-situ (35539)
⚕ 41.8   ⚖ 41.8   **FUD** 090   C 80 50
AMA: 2018,Jan,8; 2017,Jan,8; 2016,Jan,13

35585 femoral-anterior tibial, posterior tibial, or peroneal artery
⚕ 48.6   ⚖ 48.6   **FUD** 090   C 80 50
AMA: 2018,Jan,8; 2017,Jan,8; 2016,Jan,13

35587 popliteal-tibial, peroneal
⚕ 39.6   ⚖ 39.6   **FUD** 090   C 80 50
AMA: 2018,Jan,8; 2017,Jan,8; 2016,Jan,13

35600 Obtain Arm Artery for Coronary Bypass
EXCLUDES Transposition and/or reimplantation arteries (35691-35695)

▲ 35600 Harvest of upper extremity artery, 1 segment, for coronary artery bypass procedure, open
EXCLUDES Endoscopic approach (33508-33509, 37500)
⚕ 7.43   ⚖ 7.43   **FUD** ZZZ   ⊘ C 80 50
AMA: 2018,Jan,8; 2017,Jan,8; 2016,Jan,13

Median
Ulnar
Radial
An upper extremity artery or segment is harvested for a coronary artery bypass procedure

35601-35671 Arterial Bypass: Grafts Other Than Veins

EXCLUDES *Transposition and/or reimplantation arteries (35691-35695)*

35601 **Bypass graft, with other than vein; common carotid-ipsilateral internal carotid**

EXCLUDES *Open transcervical common carotid-common carotid bypass with endovascular repair descending thoracic aorta (33891)*

🚗 40.4   ⚕ 40.4   **FUD** 090   C 80 50 ▢

AMA: 2018,Jan,8; 2017,Jan,8; 2016,Jan,13

35606 **carotid-subclavian**

EXCLUDES *Open subclavian to carotid artery transposition performed with endovascular thoracic aneurysm repair via neck incision (33889)*

🚗 34.0   ⚕ 34.0   **FUD** 090   C 80 50 ▢

AMA: 1997,Nov,1

35612 **subclavian-subclavian**

🚗 30.3   ⚕ 30.3   **FUD** 090   C 80 50 ▢

AMA: 1997,Nov,1

35616 **subclavian-axillary**

🚗 32.0   ⚕ 32.0   **FUD** 090   C 80 50 ▢

AMA: 1997,Nov,1

35621 **axillary-femoral**

🚗 31.8   ⚕ 31.8   **FUD** 090   C 80 50 ▢

AMA: 2018,Jan,8; 2017,Jan,8; 2016,Jan,13

35623 **axillary-popliteal or -tibial**

🚗 38.1   ⚕ 38.1   **FUD** 090   C 80 50 ▢

AMA: 2012,Apr,3-9; 1997,Nov,1

35626 **aortosubclavian, aortoinnominate, or aortocarotid**

🚗 46.1   ⚕ 46.1   **FUD** 090   C 80 50 ▢

AMA: 1997,Nov,1

35631 **aortoceliac, aortomesenteric, aortorenal**

🚗 53.8   ⚕ 53.8   **FUD** 090   C 80 50 ▢

AMA: 1997,Nov,1

Vena cava and renal veins · Celiac trunk · Abdominal aorta · Superior mesenteric · Renal · Abdominal aorta as it exits diaphragm · Synthetic graft · Blockage

35632 **ilio-celiac**

EXCLUDES *Bypass graft (35531, 35631)*
Repair blood vessel (35221, 35251, 35281)

🚗 52.5   ⚕ 52.5   **FUD** 090   C 80 50 ▢

35633 **ilio-mesenteric**

EXCLUDES *Bypass graft (35531, 35631)*
Repair blood vessel (35221, 35251, 35281)

🚗 57.6   ⚕ 57.6   **FUD** 090   C 80 50 ▢

35634 **iliorenal**

EXCLUDES *Bypass graft (35536, 35560, 35631)*
Repair blood vessel (35221, 35251, 35281)

🚗 51.4   ⚕ 51.4   **FUD** 090   C 80 50 ▢

35636 **splenorenal (splenic to renal arterial anastomosis)**

🚗 46.3   ⚕ 46.3   **FUD** 090   C 80 50 ▢

AMA: 1997,Nov,1; 1994,Win,1

35637 **aortoiliac**

EXCLUDES *Bypass graft (35638, 35646)*

🚗 47.9   ⚕ 47.9   **FUD** 090   C 80 ▢

AMA: 2018,Jan,8; 2017,Jan,8; 2016,Jan,13

35638 **aortobi-iliac**

EXCLUDES *Bypass graft (35637, 35646)*
Open placement aorto-bi-iliac prosthesis after failed endovascular repair (34831)

🚗 50.7   ⚕ 50.7   **FUD** 090   C 80 ▢

AMA: 2018,Jan,8; 2017,Jan,8; 2016,Jan,13

35642 **carotid-vertebral**

🚗 28.6   ⚕ 28.6   **FUD** 090   C 80 50 ▢

AMA: 1997,Nov,1

35645 **subclavian-vertebral**

🚗 27.4   ⚕ 27.4   **FUD** 090   C 80 50 ▢

AMA: 1997,Nov,1

35646 **aortobifemoral**

EXCLUDES *Bypass graft using vein graft (35540)*
Open placement aorto-bi-iliac prosthesis after failed endovascular repair (34831)

🚗 49.9   ⚕ 49.9   **FUD** 090   C 80 ▢

AMA: 2018,Jan,8; 2017,Jan,8; 2016,Jan,13

35647 **aortofemoral**

EXCLUDES *Bypass graft using vein graft (35539)*

🚗 44.9   ⚕ 44.9   **FUD** 090   C 80 50 ▢

AMA: 2018,Jan,8; 2017,Jan,8; 2016,Jan,13

35650 **axillary-axillary**

🚗 29.6   ⚕ 29.6   **FUD** 090   C 80 50 ▢

AMA: 1997,Nov,1

35654 **axillary-femoral-femoral**

🚗 39.8   ⚕ 39.8   **FUD** 090   C 80 ▢

AMA: 2018,Jan,8; 2017,Jan,8; 2016,Jan,13

35656 **femoral-popliteal**

🚗 31.4   ⚕ 31.4   **FUD** 090   C 80 50 ▢

AMA: 2018,Jan,8; 2017,Jan,8; 2016,Jan,13

35661 **femoral-femoral**

🚗 31.5   ⚕ 31.5   **FUD** 090   C 80 50 ▢

AMA: 2018,Jan,8; 2017,Jan,8; 2016,Jan,13

35663 **ilioiliac**

🚗 35.3   ⚕ 35.3   **FUD** 090   C 80 50 ▢

AMA: 1997,Nov,1

35665 **iliofemoral**

🚗 34.1   ⚕ 34.1   **FUD** 090   C 80 50 ▢

AMA: 2018,Jan,8; 2017,Jan,8; 2016,Jan,13

35666 **femoral-anterior tibial, posterior tibial, or peroneal artery**

🚗 37.0   ⚕ 37.0   **FUD** 090   C 80 50 ▢

AMA: 2018,Jan,8; 2017,Jan,8; 2016,Jan,13

35671 **popliteal-tibial or -peroneal artery**

🚗 32.2   ⚕ 32.2   **FUD** 090   C 80 50 ▢

AMA: 2012,Apr,3-9; 1997,Nov,1

35681-35683 Arterial Bypass Using Combination Synthetic and Donor Graft

INCLUDES Acquiring multiple vein segments from sites other than extremity for which arterial bypass performed
Anastomosis vein segments to create bypass graft conduits

+ **35681** **Bypass graft; composite, prosthetic and vein (List separately in addition to code for primary procedure)**

EXCLUDES *Bypass graft (35682, 35683)*
Code first primary procedure

🚗 2.36   ⚕ 2.36   **FUD** ZZZ   C 80 ▢

AMA: 2018,Jan,8; 2017,Jan,8; 2016,Jan,13

● New Code   ▲ Revised Code   ○ Reinstated   ● New Web Release   ▲ Revised Web Release   + Add-on   Unlisted   Not Covered   # Resequenced

🔄 Optum Mod 50 Exempt   ⊘ AMA Mod 51 Exempt   🔄 Optum Mod 51 Exempt   ⑥³ Mod 63 Exempt   ✗ Non-FDA Drug   ★ Telemedicine   Ⓜ Maternity   Ⓐ Age Edit

© 2021 Optum360, LLC   CPT © 2021 American Medical Association. All Rights Reserved.   157

+ 35682 autogenous composite, 2 segments of veins from 2 locations (List separately in addition to code for primary procedure)

> EXCLUDES *Bypass graft (35681, 35683)*
> Code first (35556, 35566, 35570-35571, 35583-35587)
> 🗐 10.2 ⚕ 10.2 **FUD** ZZZ   C 80 ▭
> **AMA:** 2018,Jan,8; 2017,Jan,8; 2016,Jan,13

+ 35683 autogenous composite, 3 or more segments of vein from 2 or more locations (List separately in addition to code for primary procedure)

> EXCLUDES *Bypass graft (35681-35682)*
> Code first (35556, 35566, 35570-35571, 35583-35587)
> 🗐 11.8 ⚕ 11.8 **FUD** ZZZ   C 80 ▭
> **AMA:** 2018,Jan,8; 2017,Jan,8; 2016,Jan,13

35685-35686 Supplemental Procedures

> INCLUDES Additional procedures needed with bypass graft to increase graft patency
> EXCLUDES *Composite grafts (35681-35683)*

+ 35685 Placement of vein patch or cuff at distal anastomosis of bypass graft, synthetic conduit (List separately in addition to code for primary procedure)

> INCLUDES Connection vein segment (cuff or patch) between distal portion synthetic graft and native artery
> Code first (35656, 35666, 35671)
> 🗐 5.78 ⚕ 5.78 **FUD** ZZZ   N 80 ▭
> **AMA:** 2018,Jan,8; 2017,Jan,8; 2016,Jan,13

+ 35686 Creation of distal arteriovenous fistula during lower extremity bypass surgery (non-hemodialysis) (List separately in addition to code for primary procedure)

> INCLUDES Creation fistula between peroneal or tibial artery and vein at or past distal anastomosis site
> Code first (35556, 35566, 35570-35571, 35583-35587, 35623, 35656, 35666, 35671)
> 🗐 4.68 ⚕ 4.68 **FUD** ZZZ   N 80 ▭
> **AMA:** 2018,Jan,8; 2017,Jan,8; 2016,Jan,13

35691-35697 Arterial Translocation

> CMS: 100-03,160.8 Electroencephalographic Monitoring During Cerebral Vasculature Surgery

35691 Transposition and/or reimplantation; vertebral to carotid artery

> 🗐 27.2 ⚕ 27.2 **FUD** 090   C 80 50 ▭
> **AMA:** 1997,Nov,1; 1993,Win,1

35693 vertebral to subclavian artery

> 🗐 23.6 ⚕ 23.6 **FUD** 090   C 80 50 ▭
> **AMA:** 1997,Nov,1; 1994,Sum,29

35694 subclavian to carotid artery

> EXCLUDES *Subclavian to carotid artery transposition procedure (open) with concurrent repair descending thoracic aorta (endovascular) (33889)*
> 🗐 28.4 ⚕ 28.4 **FUD** 090   C 80 50 ▭
> **AMA:** 1997,Nov,1; 1993,Win,1

35695 carotid to subclavian artery

> 🗐 29.7 ⚕ 29.7 **FUD** 090   C 80 50 ▭
> **AMA:** 1997,Nov,1; 1993,Win,1

+ 35697 Reimplantation, visceral artery to infrarenal aortic prosthesis, each artery (List separately in addition to code for primary procedure)

> EXCLUDES *Repair thoracoabdominal aortic aneurysm with graft (33877)*
> Code first primary procedure
> 🗐 4.29 ⚕ 4.29 **FUD** ZZZ   C 80 ▭
> **AMA:** 1997,Nov,1

35700 Reoperative Bypass Lower Extremities

> Code first (35556, 35566, 35570-35571, 35583, 35585, 35587, 35656, 35666, 35671)

+ 35700 Reoperation, femoral-popliteal or femoral (popliteal)-anterior tibial, posterior tibial, peroneal artery, or other distal vessels, more than 1 month after original operation (List separately in addition to code for primary procedure)

> 🗐 4.44 ⚕ 4.44 **FUD** ZZZ   C 80 ▭
> **AMA:** 2018,Jan,8; 2017,Jan,8; 2016,Jan,13

35701-35703 Arterial Exploration without Repair

> EXCLUDES *Exploration to identify recipient artery for microvascular free graft/flap anastomosis:*
> *Bone (20955-20962)*
> *Jejunum (43496)*
> *Muscle, skin or fascia (15756-15758)*
> *Omentum (49906)*
> *Osteocutaneous (20969-20973)*
> *Exploration without surgical repair:*
> *Abdominal artery (49000)*
> *Chest artery (32100)*
> *Other arteries not in neck, upper or lower extremities, chest, abdomen, or retroperitoneum (37799)*
> *Retroperitoneal artery (49010)*
> Code also nonvascular surgical procedures performed in addition to exploration when exploration through separate incision

35701 Exploration not followed by surgical repair, artery; neck (eg, carotid, subclavian)

> EXCLUDES *Exploration for postoperative hemorrhage, thrombosis or infection (35800)*
> *Repair blood vessel on same side neck (35201, 35231, 35261)*
> 🗐 12.6 ⚕ 12.6 **FUD** 090   C 80 50 ▭
> **AMA:** 2019,Dec,5

35702 upper extremity (eg, axillary, brachial, radial, ulnar)

> EXCLUDES *Exploration for postoperative hemorrhage, thrombosis or infection in same extremity (35860)*
> *Repair blood vessel in same extremity (35206-35207, 35236, 35266)*
> 🗐 11.9 ⚕ 11.9 **FUD** 090   80 50 ▭
> **AMA:** 2019,Dec,5

35703 lower extremity (eg, common femoral, deep femoral, superficial femoral, popliteal, tibial, peroneal)

> EXCLUDES *Exploration for postoperative hemorrhage, thrombosis or infection in same extremity (35860)*
> *Repair blood vessel in same extremity (35256, 35286)*
> 🗐 12.0 ⚕ 12.0 **FUD** 090   80 50 ▭
> **AMA:** 2019,Dec,5

35800-35860 Arterial Exploration for Postoperative Complication

> INCLUDES Return to operating room for postoperative hemorrhage

35800 Exploration for postoperative hemorrhage, thrombosis or infection; neck

> 🗐 20.8 ⚕ 20.8 **FUD** 090   C 80 ▭
> **AMA:** 2019,Dec,5

35820 chest

> 🗐 58.2 ⚕ 58.2 **FUD** 090   C 80 ▭
> **AMA:** 1997,Nov,1

35840 abdomen

> 🗐 34.8 ⚕ 34.8 **FUD** 090   C 80 ▭
> **AMA:** 1997,May,4; 1997,Nov,1

35860 extremity

> 🗐 24.2 ⚕ 24.2 **FUD** 090   T 62 80 ▭
> **AMA:** 2019,Dec,5; 2018,Jan,8; 2017,Jan,8; 2016,Jan,13

35870 Repair Secondary Aortoenteric Fistula

35870 Repair of graft-enteric fistula

> 🗐 36.1 ⚕ 36.1 **FUD** 090   C 80 ▭
> **AMA:** 1997,Nov,1

35875-35876 Removal of Thrombus from Graft

> EXCLUDES *Thrombectomy dialysis fistula or graft (36831, 36833)*
> *Thrombectomy with blood vessel repair, lower extremity, vein graft (35256)*
> *Thrombectomy with blood vessel repair, lower extremity, with/without patch angioplasty (35226)*

35875 Thrombectomy of arterial or venous graft (other than hemodialysis graft or fistula);

> 🗐 17.3 ⚕ 17.3 **FUD** 090   T A2
> **AMA:** 2018,Jan,8; 2017,Jan,8; 2016,Jan,13

35876 with revision of arterial or venous graft

> 🗐 27.5 ⚕ 27.5 **FUD** 090   T A2 80 ▭
> **AMA:** 1999,Mar,6; 1999,Nov,1

| 26/TC PC/TC Only | A2-Z3 ASC Payment | 50 Bilateral | ♂ Male Only | ♀ Female Only | 🗐 Facility RVU | ⚕ Non-Facility RVU | ▭ CCI | ☒ CLIA |
| FUD Follow-up Days | CMS: IOM | AMA: CPT Asst | A-Y OPPSI | 80/80 Surg Assist Allowed / w/Doc | | 🔲 Lab Crosswalk | | 🔳 Radiology Crosswalk |

  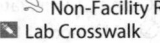

158   CPT © 2021 American Medical Association. All Rights Reserved.   © 2021 Optum360, LLC

35879-35884 Revision Lower Extremity Bypass Graft

EXCLUDES *Removal infected graft (35901-35907)*
Revascularization following removal infected graft(s)
Thrombectomy dialysis fistula or graft (36831, 36833)
Thrombectomy with blood vessel repair, lower extremity, vein graft (35256)
Thrombectomy with blood vessel repair, lower extremity, with/without patch angioplasty (35226)
Thrombectomy with graft revision (35876)

35879 **Revision, lower extremity arterial bypass, without thrombectomy, open; with vein patch angioplasty**
🔧 26.8 ⚕ 26.8 **FUD** 090 [T] [G2] [80] [50] ▣
AMA: 2018,Jan,8; 2017,Jan,8; 2016,Jan,13

35881 **with segmental vein interposition**
EXCLUDES *Revision femoral anastomosis synthetic arterial bypass graft (35883-35884)*
🔧 29.6 ⚕ 29.6 **FUD** 090 [T] [G2] [80] [50] ▣
AMA: 2018,Jan,8; 2017,Jan,8; 2016,Jan,13

35883 **Revision, femoral anastomosis of synthetic arterial bypass graft in groin, open; with nonautogenous patch graft (eg, Dacron, ePTFE, bovine pericardium)**
EXCLUDES *Reoperation, femoral-popliteal or femoral (popliteal)-anterior tibial, posterior tibial, peroneal artery, or other distal vessels (35700)*
Revision, femoral anastomosis synthetic arterial bypass graft in groin, open; with autogenous vein patch graft (35884)
Thrombectomy arterial or venous graft (35875)
🔧 34.8 ⚕ 34.8 **FUD** 090 [T] [G2] [80] [50] ▣
AMA: 2018,Jan,8; 2017,Jan,8; 2016,Jan,13

35884 **with autogenous vein patch graft**
EXCLUDES *Reoperation, femoral-popliteal or femoral (popliteal)-anterior tibial, posterior tibial, peroneal artery, or other distal vessels (35700)*
Revision, femoral anastomosis synthetic arterial bypass graft in groin, open; with autogenous vein patch graft (35883)
Thrombectomy arterial or venous graft (35875-35876)
🔧 36.0 ⚕ 36.0 **FUD** 090 [T] [G2] [80] [50] ▣
AMA: 2018,Jan,8; 2017,Jan,8; 2016,Jan,13

35901-35907 Removal of Infected Graft

35901 **Excision of infected graft; neck**
🔧 13.6 ⚕ 13.6 **FUD** 090 [C] [80] ▣
AMA: 1997,Nov,1; 1993,Win,1

The physician removes an infected graft from the neck and repairs the blood vessel. If a new graft is placed, report the appropriate revascularization code

35903 **extremity**
🔧 16.4 ⚕ 16.4 **FUD** 090 [T] [G2] [80] ▣
AMA: 2018,Aug,10

35905 **thorax**
🔧 48.5 ⚕ 48.5 **FUD** 090 [C] [80] ▣
AMA: 1997,Nov,1; 1993,Win,1

35907 **abdomen**
🔧 55.3 ⚕ 55.3 **FUD** 090 [C] [80] ▣
AMA: 1997,Nov,1; 1993,Win,1

36000 Intravenous Access Established

INCLUDES Venous access for phlebotomy, prophylactic intravenous access, infusion therapy, chemotherapy, hydration, transfusion, drug administration, etc., included in primary procedure work value

36000 **Introduction of needle or intracatheter, vein**
🔧 0.26 ⚕ 0.79 **FUD** XXX [N] [N1] ▣
AMA: 2019,Aug,8; 2018,Mar,3; 2018,Jan,8; 2017,Jan,8; 2016,Nov,3; 2016,Jan,13

36002 Injection Treatment of Pseudoaneurysm

INCLUDES Insertion needle or catheter, local anesthesia, contrast injection, power injections, and all pre- and postinjection care provided

EXCLUDES *Arteriotomy site sealant*
Compression repair pseudoaneurysm, ultrasound guided (76936)
Medications, contrast material, catheters

36002 **Injection procedures (eg, thrombin) for percutaneous treatment of extremity pseudoaneurysm**
🔗 (76942, 77002, 77012, 77021)
🔧 3.04 ⚕ 4.43 **FUD** 000 [T] [G2] [50] ▣
AMA: 2018,Mar,3; 2018,Jan,8; 2017,Jan,8; 2016,Nov,3; 2016,Jan,13

36005-36015 Insertion Needle or Intracatheter: Venous

INCLUDES Insertion needle or catheter, local anesthesia, contrast injection, power injections, and all pre- and postinjection care provided

EXCLUDES *Medications, contrast materials, catheters*
Code also:
Catheterization second order vessels (or higher) supplied by same first order branch, same vascular family (36012)
Each vascular family (e.g., bilateral procedures are separate vascular families)

36005 **Injection procedure for extremity venography (including introduction of needle or intracatheter)**
🔗 (75820, 75822)
🔧 1.38 ⚕ 8.44 **FUD** 000 [N] [N1] [80] [50] ▣
AMA: 2018,Mar,3; 2018,Jan,8; 2017,Jan,8; 2016,Nov,3; 2016,Jul,6; 2016,Jan,13

36010 **Introduction of catheter, superior or inferior vena cava**
🔧 3.19 ⚕ 15.0 **FUD** XXX [N] [N1] [50] ▣
AMA: 2018,Jan,8; 2017,Feb,14; 2017,Jan,8; 2016,Jul,6; 2016,Jan,13

36011 **Selective catheter placement, venous system; first order branch (eg, renal vein, jugular vein)**
🔧 4.54 ⚕ 24.0 **FUD** XXX [N] [N1] [50] ▣
AMA: 2018,Jan,8; 2017,Jan,8; 2016,Jul,6; 2016,Jan,13

36012 **second order, or more selective, branch (eg, left adrenal vein, petrosal sinus)**
🔧 5.04 ⚕ 25.0 **FUD** XXX [N] [N1] [50] ▣
AMA: 2018,Oct,3; 2018,Jan,8; 2017,Jan,8; 2016,Jul,6; 2016,Jan,13

36013 **Introduction of catheter, right heart or main pulmonary artery**
🔧 3.53 ⚕ 22.7 **FUD** XXX [N] [N1] ▣
AMA: 2019,Jun,3; 2018,Jan,8; 2017,Jan,8; 2016,Jul,6; 2016,Jan,13

36014 **Selective catheter placement, left or right pulmonary artery**
🔧 4.41 ⚕ 23.7 **FUD** XXX [N] [N1] [50] ▣
AMA: 2019,Jun,3; 2018,Jan,8; 2017,Jan,8; 2016,Jul,6; 2016,Jan,13

36015 **Selective catheter placement, segmental or subsegmental pulmonary artery**
EXCLUDES *Placement Swan Ganz/other flow directed catheter for monitoring (93503)*
Selective blood sampling, specific organs (36500)
🔧 5.00 ⚕ 25.7 **FUD** XXX [N] [N1] [50] ▣
AMA: 2019,Jun,3; 2018,Jan,8; 2017,Jan,8; 2016,Jul,6; 2016,Jan,13

36100-36218 Insertion Needle or Intracatheter: Arterial

INCLUDES Introduction catheter and catheterization all lesser order vessels used for approach

Local anesthesia, placement catheter/needle, contrast injection, power injections, all pre- and postinjection care

EXCLUDES Angiography (36222-36228, 75600-75774)
Angioplasty ([37246, 37247])
Chemotherapy injections (96401-96549)
Injection procedures for cardiac catheterizations (93454-93461, 93564, 93593-93597)
Internal mammary artery angiography without left heart catheterization (36216, 36217)
Medications, contrast, catheters
Transcatheter interventions (37200, 37211, 37213-37214, 37241-37244, 61624, 61626)

Code also:
Additional first order or higher catheterization for vascular families when vascular family supplied by first order vessel different from one already coded
Catheterization second and third order vessels supplied by same first order branch, same vascular family (36218, 36248)

36100 Introduction of needle or intracatheter, carotid or vertebral artery
⚕ 4.54 ⚖ 14.8 **FUD** XXX N N1 50
AMA: 2000,Oct,4; 1998,Apr,1

36140 Introduction of needle or intracatheter, upper or lower extremity artery
EXCLUDES Arteriovenous cannula insertion (36810-36821)
⚕ 2.60 ⚖ 13.6 **FUD** XXX N N1
AMA: 2018,Jan,8; 2017,Jan,8; 2016,Jan,13

36160 Introduction of needle or intracatheter, aortic, translumbar
⚕ 3.59 ⚖ 14.6 **FUD** XXX N N1
AMA: 2018,Jan,8; 2017,Jan,8; 2016,Jan,13

36200 Introduction of catheter, aorta
EXCLUDES Nonselective angiography extracranial carotid and/or cerebral vessels and cervicocerebral arch (36221)
⚕ 4.06 ⚖ 16.8 **FUD** 000 N N1 50
AMA: 2018,Jan,8; 2017,Mar,3; 2017,Jan,8; 2016,Jul,6; 2016,Jan,13

36215 Selective catheter placement, arterial system; each first order thoracic or brachiocephalic branch, within a vascular family
INCLUDES Introduction catheter into aorta (36200)
EXCLUDES Placement catheter for coronary angiography (93454-93461)
⚕ 6.13 ⚖ 30.7 **FUD** 000 N N1
AMA: 2018,Jan,8; 2017,Mar,3; 2017,Jan,8; 2016,Jul,6; 2016,Jan,13

36216 initial second order thoracic or brachiocephalic branch, within a vascular family
⚕ 7.90 ⚖ 32.5 **FUD** 000 N N1
AMA: 2018,Jan,8; 2017,Jan,8; 2016,Jul,6; 2016,Jan,13

36217 initial third order or more selective thoracic or brachiocephalic branch, within a vascular family
⚕ 9.52 ⚖ 53.9 **FUD** 000 N N1
AMA: 2018,Jan,8; 2017,Jan,8; 2016,Jul,6; 2016,Jan,13

+ 36218 additional second order, third order, and beyond, thoracic or brachiocephalic branch, within a vascular family (List in addition to code for initial second or third order vessel as appropriate)
Code also transcatheter therapy procedures (37200, 37211, 37213-37214, 37236-37239, 37241-37244, 61624, 61626)
Code first (36216-36217, 36225-36226)
⚕ 1.51 ⚖ 6.89 **FUD** ZZZ N N1
AMA: 2018,Oct,3; 2018,Jan,8; 2017,Jan,8; 2016,Jul,6; 2016,Jan,13

36221-36228 Diagnostic Studies: Aortic Arch/Carotid/Vertebral Arteries

INCLUDES Accessing vessel
Arterial contrast injection including arterial, capillary, and venous phase imaging, when performed
Arteriotomy closure (pressure or closure device)
Catheter placement
Radiologic supervision and interpretation
Reporting selective catheter placement based on service intensity in following hierarchy:
36226>36225
36224>36223>36222

EXCLUDES 3D rendering when performed (76376-76377)
Interventional procedures
Ultrasound guidance (76937)
Code also diagnostic angiography upper extremities/other vascular beds during same session, when performed (75774)

36221 Non-selective catheter placement, thoracic aorta, with angiography of the extracranial carotid, vertebral, and/or intracranial vessels, unilateral or bilateral, and all associated radiological supervision and interpretation, includes angiography of the cervicocerebral arch, when performed
EXCLUDES Selective catheter placement, common carotid or innominate artery (36222-36226)
Transcatheter intravascular stent placement common carotid or innominate artery on same side (37217)
⚕ 5.80 ⚖ 29.3 **FUD** 000 02 N1
AMA: 2018,Jan,8; 2017,Jan,8; 2016,Mar,3; 2016,Jan,13

36222 Selective catheter placement, common carotid or innominate artery, unilateral, any approach, with angiography of the ipsilateral extracranial carotid circulation and all associated radiological supervision and interpretation, includes angiography of the cervicocerebral arch, when performed
EXCLUDES Transcatheter placement intravascular stent(s) (37215-37218)
Code also modifier 59 when different territories on both sides body studied
⚕ 8.22 ⚖ 34.7 **FUD** 000 02 N1 50
AMA: 2018,Jan,8; 2017,Jan,8; 2016,Mar,3; 2016,Jan,13

36223 Selective catheter placement, common carotid or innominate artery, unilateral, any approach, with angiography of the ipsilateral intracranial carotid circulation and all associated radiological supervision and interpretation, includes angiography of the extracranial carotid and cervicocerebral arch, when performed
EXCLUDES Transcatheter placement intravascular stent(s) (37215-37218)
Code also modifier 59 when different territories on both sides body studied
⚕ 9.18 ⚖ 43.9 **FUD** 000 02 N1 50
AMA: 2018,Jan,8; 2017,Jan,8; 2016,Mar,3; 2016,Jan,13

36224 Selective catheter placement, internal carotid artery, unilateral, with angiography of the ipsilateral intracranial carotid circulation and all associated radiological supervision and interpretation, includes angiography of the extracranial carotid and cervicocerebral arch, when performed
EXCLUDES Transcatheter placement intravascular stent(s) (37215-37218)
Code also modifier 59 when different territories on both sides body studied
⚕ 10.4 ⚖ 56.8 **FUD** 000 02 N1 50
AMA: 2018,Jan,8; 2017,Jan,8; 2016,Mar,3; 2016,Jan,13

36225 Selective catheter placement, subclavian or innominate artery, unilateral, with angiography of the ipsilateral vertebral circulation and all associated radiological supervision and interpretation, includes angiography of the cervicocerebral arch, when performed
EXCLUDES Transcatheter placement intravascular stent(s) (37217)
⚕ 9.16 ⚖ 42.3 **FUD** 000 02 N1 50
AMA: 2018,Jan,8; 2017,Jan,8; 2016,Mar,3; 2016,Jan,13

36226 Selective catheter placement, vertebral artery, unilateral, with angiography of the ipsilateral vertebral circulation and all associated radiological supervision and interpretation, includes angiography of the cervicocerebral arch, when performed

EXCLUDES *Transcatheter placement intravascular stent(s) (37217)*

10.3   53.7   **FUD** 000   02 N1 ▣ 50 ▣

AMA: 2018,Jan,8; 2017,Jan,8; 2016,Mar,3; 2016,Jan,13

+ 36227 Selective catheter placement, external carotid artery, unilateral, with angiography of the ipsilateral external carotid circulation and all associated radiological supervision and interpretation (List separately in addition to code for primary procedure)

EXCLUDES *Reporting with modifier 50. Report once for each side when performed bilaterally*
Transcatheter placement intravascular stent(s) (37217)

Code first (36222-36224)

3.41   7.23   **FUD** ZZZ   N N1 50 ▣

AMA: 2018,Jan,8; 2017,Jan,8; 2016,Jan,13

+ 36228 Selective catheter placement, each intracranial branch of the internal carotid or vertebral arteries, unilateral, with angiography of the selected vessel circulation and all associated radiological supervision and interpretation (eg, middle cerebral artery, posterior inferior cerebellar artery) (List separately in addition to code for primary procedure)

EXCLUDES *Procedure performed more than two times per side*
Reporting with modifier 50. Report once for each side when performed bilaterally

Code first (36223-36226)

7.03   37.6   **FUD** ZZZ   N N1 50 ▣

AMA: 2018,Jan,8; 2017,Jan,8; 2016,Jan,13

36245-36254 Catheter Placement: Arteries of the Lower Body

INCLUDES Introduction catheter and catheterization all lesser order vessels used for approach
Local anesthesia, placement catheter/needle, contrast injection, power injections

EXCLUDES *Angiography (36222-36228, 75600-75774)*
Chemotherapy injections (96401-96549)
Injection procedures for cardiac catheterizations (93454-93461, 93564, 93593-93597)
Internal mammary artery angiography without left heart catheterization (36216-36217)
Medications, contrast, catheters
Transcatheter procedures (37200, 37211, 37213-37214, 37236-37239, 37241-37244, 61624, 61626)

Code also:
Additional first order or higher catheterization for vascular families when vascular family supplied by first order vessel different from one already coded
Catheterization second and third order vessels supplied by same first order branch, same vascular family (36218, 36248)

(75600-75774)

36245 Selective catheter placement, arterial system; each first order abdominal, pelvic, or lower extremity artery branch, within a vascular family

6.89   38.1   **FUD** XXX   N N1 50 ▣

AMA: 2018,Jan,8; 2017,Jan,8; 2016,Jul,6; 2016,Jan,13

36246 initial second order abdominal, pelvic, or lower extremity artery branch, within a vascular family

7.35   24.5   **FUD** 000   N N1 50 ▣

AMA: 2018,Jan,8; 2017,Jan,8; 2016,Jul,6; 2016,Jan,13

36247 initial third order or more selective abdominal, pelvic, or lower extremity artery branch, within a vascular family

8.75   43.2   **FUD** 000   N N1 50 ▣

AMA: 2020,Sep,14; 2018,Jan,8; 2017,Jan,8; 2016,Jul,6; 2016,Jan,13

+ 36248 additional second order, third order, and beyond, abdominal, pelvic, or lower extremity artery branch, within a vascular family (List in addition to code for initial second or third order vessel as appropriate)

Code first (36246, 36247)

1.41   3.92   **FUD** ZZZ   N N1 ▣

AMA: 2018,Oct,3; 2018,Jan,8; 2017,Jan,8; 2016,Jul,6; 2016,Jan,13

36251 Selective catheter placement (first-order), main renal artery and any accessory renal artery(s) for renal angiography, including arterial puncture and catheter placement(s), fluoroscopy, contrast injection(s), image postprocessing, permanent recording of images, and radiological supervision and interpretation, including pressure gradient measurements when performed, and flush aortogram when performed; unilateral

INCLUDES Closure device placement at vascular access site

EXCLUDES *Transcatheter renal sympathetic denervation, percutaneous approach (0338T-0339T)*

7.51   39.7   **FUD** 000   02 N1 ▣

AMA: 2018,Jan,8; 2017,Jan,8; 2016,Jan,13

36252 bilateral

INCLUDES Closure device placement at vascular access site

EXCLUDES *Transcatheter renal sympathetic denervation, percutaneous approach (0338T-0339T)*

10.4   42.8   **FUD** 000   02 N1 ▣

AMA: 2018,Jan,8; 2017,Jan,8; 2016,Jan,13

36253 Superselective catheter placement (one or more second order or higher renal artery branches) renal artery and any accessory renal artery(s) for renal angiography, including arterial puncture, catheterization, fluoroscopy, contrast injection(s), image postprocessing, permanent recording of images, and radiological supervision and interpretation, including pressure gradient measurements when performed, and flush aortogram when performed; unilateral

INCLUDES Closure device placement at vascular access site

EXCLUDES *Procedure performed on same kidney with (36251)*
Transcatheter renal sympathetic denervation, percutaneous approach (0338T-0339T)

10.3   62.9   **FUD** 000   02 N1 ▣

AMA: 2018,Jan,8; 2017,Jan,8; 2016,Jan,13

36254 bilateral

INCLUDES Closure device placement at vascular access site

EXCLUDES *Selective catheter placement (first-order), main renal artery and any accessory renal artery(s) for renal angiography (36252)*
Transcatheter renal sympathetic denervation, percutaneous approach (0338T-0339T)

12.0   61.6   **FUD** 000   02 N1 ▣

AMA: 2018,Jan,8; 2017,Jan,8; 2016,Jan,13

36260-36299 Implanted Infusion Pumps: Intra-arterial

36260 Insertion of implantable intra-arterial infusion pump (eg, for chemotherapy of liver)

18.8   18.8   **FUD** 090   T A2 ▣

AMA: 2018,Jan,8; 2017,Jan,8; 2016,Jan,13

36261 Revision of implanted intra-arterial infusion pump

11.7   11.7   **FUD** 090   T J8 80 ▣

AMA: 2000,Oct,4; 1997,Nov,1

36262 Removal of implanted intra-arterial infusion pump

8.96   8.96   **FUD** 090   02 G2 ▣

AMA: 2000,Oct,4; 1997,Nov,1

36299 Unlisted procedure, vascular injection

0.00   0.00   **FUD** YYY   N 80 ▣

AMA: 2000,Oct,4; 1997,Nov,1

36400-36425 Specimen Collection: Phlebotomy

EXCLUDES *Specimen collection from:*
Completely implantable device (36591)
Established catheter (36592)

36400 Venipuncture, younger than age 3 years, necessitating the skill of a physician or other qualified health care professional, not to be used for routine venipuncture; femoral or jugular vein A

🏥 0.53 ⚕ 0.75 **FUD** XXX N N1 ▣
AMA: 2018,Jan,8; 2017,Jan,8; 2016,Jan,13

36405 scalp vein A

🏥 0.44 ⚕ 0.66 **FUD** XXX N N1 ▣
AMA: 2018,Jan,8; 2017,Jan,8; 2016,Jan,13

36406 other vein A

🏥 0.25 ⚕ 0.47 **FUD** XXX N N1 ▣
AMA: 2018,Jan,8; 2017,Jan,8; 2016,Jan,13

36410 Venipuncture, age 3 years or older, necessitating the skill of a physician or other qualified health care professional (separate procedure), for diagnostic or therapeutic purposes (not to be used for routine venipuncture) A

🏥 0.27 ⚕ 0.49 **FUD** XXX N N1 ▣
AMA: 2019,Aug,8; 2018,Mar,3; 2018,Jan,8; 2017,Jan,8; 2016,Nov,3; 2016,Jan,13

36415 Collection of venous blood by venipuncture

🏥 0.00 ⚕ 0.00 **FUD** XXX 63 Q ▣
AMA: 2019,Aug,8; 2018,Jan,8; 2017,Jan,8; 2016,Jan,13

36416 Collection of capillary blood specimen (eg, finger, heel, ear stick)

🏥 0.00 ⚕ 0.00 **FUD** XXX N N1 ▣
AMA: 2008,Apr,-9; 2003,Feb,7

36420 Venipuncture, cutdown; younger than age 1 year A

🏥 1.35 ⚕ 1.35 **FUD** XXX 63 01 N1 80 ▣
AMA: 2018,Jan,8; 2017,Jan,8; 2016,Jan,13

36425 age 1 or over A

EXCLUDES *Endovenous ablation therapy incompetent vein, extremity (36475-36476, 36478-36479)*

🏥 1.15 ⚕ 1.15 **FUD** XXX 01 N1 ▣
AMA: 2018,Mar,3; 2018,Jan,8; 2017,Jan,8; 2016,Nov,3; 2016,Jan,13

36430-36460 Transfusions

CMS: 100-01,3,20.5 Blood Deductibles; 100-03,110.16 Transfusion in Kidney Transplants; 100-03,110.7 Blood Transfusions; 100-03,110.8 Blood Platelet Transfusions

36430 Transfusion, blood or blood components

EXCLUDES *Infant partial exchange transfusion (36456)*

🏥 0.99 ⚕ 0.99 **FUD** XXX S P3 ▣
AMA: 2020,Jun,14; 2019,Jun,5; 2018,Jan,8; 2017,Jul,3; 2017,Jan,8; 2016,Jan,13

36440 Push transfusion, blood, 2 years or younger A

EXCLUDES *Infant partial exchange transfusion (36456)*

🏥 1.46 ⚕ 1.46 **FUD** XXX S R2 80 ▣
AMA: 2018,Jan,8; 2017,Jul,3; 2017,Jan,8; 2016,Jan,13

36450 Exchange transfusion, blood; newborn A

EXCLUDES *Automated red cell exchange (36512)*
Infant partial exchange transfusion (36456)

🏥 4.93 ⚕ 4.93 **FUD** XXX 63 S R2 80 ▣
AMA: 2018,Jan,8; 2017,Jul,3

36455 other than newborn A

EXCLUDES *Automated red cell exchange (36512)*

🏥 3.68 ⚕ 3.68 **FUD** XXX S 62 ▣
AMA: 2003,Apr,7; 1997,Nov,1

36456 Partial exchange transfusion, blood, plasma or crystalloid necessitating the skill of a physician or other qualified health care professional, newborn A

EXCLUDES *Automated red cell exchange (36512)*
Transfusions other types (36430-36450)

🏥 2.93 ⚕ 2.93 **FUD** XXX 63 S 80 ▣
AMA: 2018,Jan,8; 2017,Jul,3

36460 Transfusion, intrauterine, fetal A ♀

🔗 (76941)
🏥 10.1 ⚕ 10.1 **FUD** XXX 63 S 62 80 ▣
AMA: 2003,Apr,7; 1997,Nov,1

36465-36466 [36465, 36466] Destruction Spider Veins

INCLUDES All supplies, equipment, compression stockings or bandages when performed in physician office

EXCLUDES *Multi-layer compression system applied to leg (29581, 29584)*
Strapping leg: ankle, foot, hip, knee, toes same extremity (29520, 29530, 29540, 29550)
Unna boot (29580)
Reporting code more than one time for each extremity treated
Vascular embolization and occlusion (37241-37244)
Vascular embolization vein in same operative field (37241)

36465 Resequenced code. See code following 36471.

36466 Resequenced code. See code following 36471.

36468 Injection(s) of sclerosant for spider veins (telangiectasia), limb or trunk

🔗 (76942)
🏥 0.00 ⚕ 0.00 **FUD** 000 01 N1 80 ▣
AMA: 2018,Mar,3; 2018,Jan,8; 2017,Jan,8; 2016,Nov,3; 2016,Jan,13

36470 Injection of sclerosant; single incompetent vein (other than telangiectasia)

EXCLUDES *Injection foam sclerosant with ultrasound guidance for compression maneuvers (36465-36466)*

🔗 (76942)
🏥 1.10 ⚕ 3.10 **FUD** 000 T P3 50 ▣
AMA: 2018,Dec,10; 2018,Dec,10; 2018,Mar,3; 2018,Jan,8; 2017,Jan,8; 2016,Nov,3; 2016,Jan,13

36471 multiple incompetent veins (other than telangiectasia), same leg

EXCLUDES *Injection foam sclerosant with ultrasound guidance for compression maneuvers (36465-36466)*

🔗 (76942)
🏥 2.22 ⚕ 5.59 **FUD** 000 T P3 50 ▣
AMA: 2018,Dec,10; 2018,Dec,10; 2018,Mar,3; 2018,Jan,8; 2017,Jan,8; 2016,Nov,3; 2016,Jan,13

\# **36465** Injection of non-compounded foam sclerosant with ultrasound compression maneuvers to guide dispersion of the injectate, inclusive of all imaging guidance and monitoring; single incompetent extremity truncal vein (eg, great saphenous vein, accessory saphenous vein)

EXCLUDES *Ablation vein using chemical adhesive ([36482, 36483])*
Injection foam sclerosant with ultrasound guidance for compression maneuvers (36465-36466)

🏥 3.48 ⚕ 42.9 **FUD** 000 T P2 50 ▣
AMA: 2019,Feb,9; 2018,Dec,10; 2018,Dec,10; 2018,Mar,3

\# **36466** multiple incompetent truncal veins (eg, great saphenous vein, accessory saphenous vein), same leg

EXCLUDES *Ablation vein using chemical adhesive ([36482, 36483])*
Injection foam sclerosant with ultrasound guidance for compression maneuvers (36465-36466)

🏥 4.46 ⚕ 47.6 **FUD** 000 T P2 50 ▣
AMA: 2019,Feb,9; 2018,Dec,10; 2018,Dec,10; 2018,Mar,3

26/TC PC/TC Only   A2-Z3 ASC Payment   50 Bilateral   ♂ Male Only   ♀ Female Only   🏥 Facility RVU   ⚕ Non-Facility RVU   ▣ CCI   ☒ CLIA
FUD Follow-up Days   **CMS:** IOM   **AMA:** CPT Asst   A-Y OPPSI   80/80 Surg Assist Allowed / w/Doc   ▣ Lab Crosswalk   ▣ Radiology Crosswalk

36473-36483 [36482, 36483] Vein Ablation

INCLUDES
Multi-layer compression system applied to leg (29581, 29584)
Patient monitoring
Radiological guidance (76000, 76937, 76942, 76998, 77002)
Venous access/injections (36000-36005, 36410, 36425)

EXCLUDES
Duplex scans (93970-93971)
Strapping leg: ankle, foot, hip, knee, toes same extremity (29520, 29530, 29540, 29550)
Transcatheter embolization (75894)
Unna boot (29580)
Vascular embolization vein in same operative field (37241)

36473 Endovenous ablation therapy of incompetent vein, extremity, inclusive of all imaging guidance and monitoring, percutaneous, mechanochemical; first vein treated

INCLUDES Local anesthesia

EXCLUDES Laser ablation incompetent vein (36478-36479)
Radiofrequency ablation incompetent vein (36475-36476)

5.18   40.4   **FUD** 000   T P3 50

AMA: 2019,Feb,9; 2018,Mar,3; 2018,Jan,8; 2017,Jan,8; 2016,Nov,3

+ 36474 subsequent vein(s) treated in a single extremity, each through separate access sites (List separately in addition to code for primary procedure)

INCLUDES Local anesthesia

EXCLUDES Laser ablation incompetent vein (36478-36479)
Radiofrequency ablation incompetent vein (36475-36476)
Reporting code more than one time per extremity

Code first (36473)

2.60   8.23   **FUD** ZZZ   N N1 50

AMA: 2019,Feb,9; 2018,Mar,3; 2018,Jan,8; 2017,Jan,8; 2016,Nov,3

36475 Endovenous ablation therapy of incompetent vein, extremity, inclusive of all imaging guidance and monitoring, percutaneous, radiofrequency; first vein treated

INCLUDES Tumescent anesthesia

EXCLUDES Ablation vein using chemical adhesive ([36482, 36483])
Endovenous ablation therapy incompetent vein (36478-36479)

8.09   38.9   **FUD** 000   T A2 50

AMA: 2018,Mar,3; 2018,Jan,8; 2017,Jan,8; 2016,Nov,3; 2016,Aug,3; 2016,Jan,13

+ 36476 subsequent vein(s) treated in a single extremity, each through separate access sites (List separately in addition to code for primary procedure)

INCLUDES Tumescent anesthesia

EXCLUDES Ablation vein using chemical adhesive ([36482, 36483])
Endovenous ablation therapy incompetent vein (36478-36479)
Reporting code more than one time per extremity
Vascular embolization or occlusion (37242-37244)

Code first (36475)

3.92   8.81   **FUD** ZZZ   N N1 50

AMA: 2018,Mar,3; 2018,Jan,8; 2017,Jan,8; 2016,Nov,3; 2016,Aug,3; 2016,Jan,13

36478 Endovenous ablation therapy of incompetent vein, extremity, inclusive of all imaging guidance and monitoring, percutaneous, laser; first vein treated

INCLUDES Tumescent anesthesia

EXCLUDES Ablation vein using chemical adhesive ([36482, 36483])
Endovenous ablation therapy incompetent vein (36478-36479)

8.06   30.2   **FUD** 000   T A2 50

AMA: 2020,May,13; 2018,Mar,3; 2018,Jan,8; 2017,Jan,8; 2016,Nov,3; 2016,Aug,3; 2016,Jan,13

+ 36479 subsequent vein(s) treated in a single extremity, each through separate access sites (List separately in addition to code for primary procedure)

INCLUDES Tumescent anesthesia

EXCLUDES Ablation vein using chemical adhesive ([36482, 36483])
Endovenous ablation therapy incompetent vein (36478-36479)
Vascular embolization or occlusion (37241)

Code first (36478)

3.96   9.28   **FUD** ZZZ   N N1 50

AMA: 2020,May,13; 2018,Mar,3; 2018,Jan,8; 2017,Jan,8; 2016,Nov,3; 2016,Aug,3; 2016,Jan,13

 # 36482 Endovenous ablation therapy of incompetent vein, extremity, by transcatheter delivery of a chemical adhesive (eg, cyanoacrylate) remote from the access site, inclusive of all imaging guidance and monitoring, percutaneous; first vein treated

INCLUDES Local anesthesia

EXCLUDES Laser ablation incompetent vein (36478-36479)
Radiofrequency ablation incompetent vein (36475-36476)

5.20   54.0   **FUD** 000   T P3 50

AMA: 2019,Feb,9; 2018,Mar,3

+ # 36483 subsequent vein(s) treated in a single extremity, each through separate access sites (List separately in addition to code for primary procedure)

INCLUDES Local anesthesia

EXCLUDES Laser ablation incompetent vein (36478-36479)
Radiofrequency ablation incompetent vein (36475-36476)
Reporting code more than one time per extremity

Code first ([36482])

2.61   4.45   **FUD** ZZZ   N N1 50

AMA: 2019,Feb,9; 2018,Mar,3

36481-36510 [36482, 36483] Other Venous Catheterization Procedures

EXCLUDES
Specimen collection from:
Completely implantable device (36591)
Established catheter (36592)

36481 Percutaneous portal vein catheterization by any method

(75885, 75887)

9.56   54.6   **FUD** 000   N N1

AMA: 2018,Jan,8; 2017,Jan,8; 2016,Jan,13

36482 Resequenced code. See code following 36479.

36483 Resequenced code. See code following 36479.

36500 Venous catheterization for selective organ blood sampling

EXCLUDES Inferior or superior vena cava catheterization (36010)

(75893)

5.30   5.30   **FUD** 000   N N1

AMA: 2014,Jan,11; 1997,Nov,1

36510 Catheterization of umbilical vein for diagnosis or therapy, newborn   A

EXCLUDES Specimen collection from:
Capillary blood (36416)
Venipuncture (36415)

1.55   2.36   **FUD** 000   63 N N1 80

AMA: 2018,Jan,8; 2017,Jan,8; 2016,May,3; 2016,Jan,13

36511-36516 Apheresis

CMS: 100-03,110.14 Apheresis (Therapeutic Pheresis); 100-04,4,231.9 Billing for Pheresis and Apheresis Services

EXCLUDES Specimen collection for therapeutic treatment from:
Completely implantable device (36591)
Established catheter (36592)

36511 Therapeutic apheresis; for white blood cells

3.15   3.15   **FUD** 000   S 62

AMA: 2018,Jan,8; 2017,Jan,8; 2016,Jan,13

36512   **for red blood cells**

> _EXCLUDES_   _Manual red cell exchange (36450, 36455, 36456)_
> 📠 3.12   ⚕ 3.12   **FUD** 000   [S] [G2] [▭]
> **AMA:** 2018,Jan,8; 2017,Jan,8; 2016,Jan,13

36513   **for platelets**

> _EXCLUDES_   _Collection platelets from donors_
> 📠 3.15   ⚕ 3.15   **FUD** 000   [S] [R2] [▭]
> **AMA:** 2018,Jan,8; 2017,Jan,8; 2016,Jan,13

36514   **for plasma pheresis**

> 📠 2.75   ⚕ 19.1   **FUD** 000   [S] [G2] [▭]
> **AMA:** 2018,May,10; 2018,Jan,8; 2017,Jan,8; 2016,Jan,13

36516   **with extracorporeal immunoadsorption, selective adsorption or selective filtration and plasma reinfusion**

> Code also modifier 26 for professional evaluation
> 📠 2.44   ⚕ 55.4   **FUD** 000   [S] [P3] [▭]
> **AMA:** 2018,Jan,8; 2017,Jan,8; 2016,Jan,13

36522 Extracorporeal Photopheresis

CMS: 100-03,110.4 Extracorporeal Photopheresis; 100-04,32,190 Billing for Extracorporeal Photopheresis; 100-04,32,190.2 Healthcare Common Procedural Coding System (HCPCS), Applicable Diagnosis Codes and Procedure Code; 100-04,32,190.3 Medicare Summary Notices (MSNs), Remittance Advice Remark Codes (RAs) and Claim Adjustment Reason Code; 100-04,4,231.9 Billing for Pheresis and Apheresis Services

> _EXCLUDES_   _Dialysis (90935-90999)_
> _Therapeutic apheresis (36511-36514, 36516)_
> _Therapeutic ultrafiltration (0692T)_

36522   **Photopheresis, extracorporeal**

> 📠 2.79   ⚕ 61.2   **FUD** 000   [S] [G2] [▭]
> **AMA:** 2018,May,10; 2018,Jan,8; 2017,Jan,8; 2016,Jan,13

36555-36573 [36572, 36573] Placement of Implantable Venous Access Device

> _INCLUDES_   Devices accessed by exposed catheter, or subcutaneous port or pump
> Devices inserted via cutdown or percutaneous access:
>   Centrally (eg, femoral, jugular, subclavian veins, or inferior vena cava)
>   Peripherally (e.g., basilic, cephalic, saphenous vein)
> Devices terminating in brachiocephalic (innominate), iliac, subclavian veins, vena cava, or right atrium
> _EXCLUDES_   _Insertion midline catheter (36400, 36406, 36410)_
> _Maintenance/refilling implantable pump/reservoir (96522)_
> Code also removal central venous access device (if code available) when new device placed through separate venous access

36555   **Insertion of non-tunneled centrally inserted central venous catheter; younger than 5 years of age**   [A]

> _EXCLUDES_   _Peripheral insertion (36568)_
> 🩻 (76937, 77001)
> 📠 2.44   ⚕ 5.35   **FUD** 000   [T] [A2] [▭]
> **AMA:** 2019,May,3; 2018,Jan,8; 2017,Jan,8; 2016,Jan,13

Direct CVC

A non-tunneled centrally inserted CVC is inserted

36556   **age 5 years or older**   [A]

> _EXCLUDES_   _Peripheral insertion (36569)_
> 🩻 (76937, 77001)
> 📠 2.46   ⚕ 6.08   **FUD** 000   [T] [A2] [▭]
> **AMA:** 2019,May,3; 2018,Nov,11; 2018,Jan,8; 2017,Jan,8; 2016,Jan,13

36557   **Insertion of tunneled centrally inserted central venous catheter, without subcutaneous port or pump; younger than 5 years of age**   [A]

> 🩻 (76937, 77001)
> 📠 9.25   ⚕ 31.3   **FUD** 010   [T] [A2] [80] [50] [▭]
> **AMA:** 2018,Jan,8; 2017,Jan,8; 2016,Jan,13

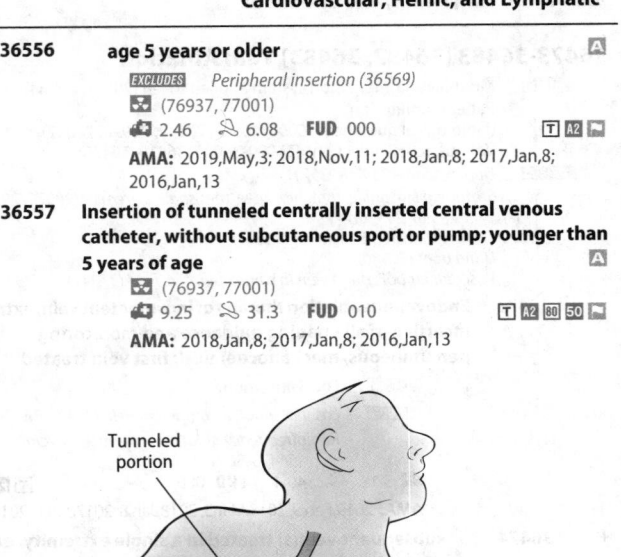

Tunneled portion

A tunneled centrally inserted CVC is inserted

36558   **age 5 years or older**   [A]

> _EXCLUDES_   _Peripheral insertion (36571)_
> 🩻 (76937, 77001)
> 📠 7.55   ⚕ 23.1   **FUD** 010   [T] [A2] [80] [50] [▭]
> **AMA:** 2018,Jan,8; 2017,Jan,8; 2016,Jan,13

36560   **Insertion of tunneled centrally inserted central venous access device, with subcutaneous port; younger than 5 years of age**   [A]

> _EXCLUDES_   _Peripheral insertion (36570)_
> 🩻 (76937, 77001)
> 📠 11.0   ⚕ 37.4   **FUD** 010   [T] [G2] [80] [50] [▭]
> **AMA:** 2018,Jan,8; 2017,Jan,8; 2016,Jan,13

36561   **age 5 years or older**   [A]

> _EXCLUDES_   _Peripheral insertion (36571)_
> 🩻 (76937, 77001)
> 📠 9.74   ⚕ 30.6   **FUD** 010   [T] [A2] [80] [50] [▭]
> **AMA:** 2018,Jan,8; 2017,Jan,8; 2016,Jan,13

36563   **Insertion of tunneled centrally inserted central venous access device with subcutaneous pump**

> 🩻 (76937, 77001)
> 📠 10.6   ⚕ 33.9   **FUD** 010   [T] [A2] [80] [▭]
> **AMA:** 2018,Jan,8; 2017,Jan,8; 2016,Jan,13

36565   **Insertion of tunneled centrally inserted central venous access device, requiring 2 catheters via 2 separate venous access sites; without subcutaneous port or pump (eg, Tesio type catheter)**

> 🩻 (76937, 77001)
> 📠 9.71   ⚕ 25.0   **FUD** 010   [T] [A2] [80] [50] [▭]
> **AMA:** 2018,Jan,8; 2017,Jan,8; 2016,Jan,13

36566   **with subcutaneous port(s)**

> 🩻 (76937, 77001)
> 📠 10.4   ⚕ 132.   **FUD** 010   [T] [A2] [80] [50] [▭]
> **AMA:** 2018,Jan,8; 2017,Jan,8; 2016,Jan,13

36568 Insertion of peripherally inserted central venous catheter (PICC), without subcutaneous port or pump, without imaging guidance; younger than 5 years of age `A`

    EXCLUDES   *Centrally inserted placement (36555)*
            Imaging guidance (76937, 77001)
            Peripherally inserted ([36572])
            PICC line removal with codes for removal tunneled central venous catheters; report appropriate E/M code
    2.65   2.65   **FUD** 000   `T` `A2`
    AMA: 2019,May,3; 2018,Jan,8; 2017,Jan,8; 2016,Jan,13

36569 age 5 years or older `A`

    EXCLUDES   *Centrally inserted placement (36556)*
            Imaging guidance (76937, 77001)
            Peripherally inserted ([36573])
            PICC line removal with codes for removal tunneled central venous catheters; report appropriate E/M code
    2.73   2.73   **FUD** 000   `T` `A2`
    AMA: 2019,May,3; 2018,Jan,8; 2017,Jan,8; 2016,Jan,13

**36572** Insertion of peripherally inserted central venous catheter (PICC), without subcutaneous port or pump, including all imaging guidance, image documentation, and all associated radiological supervision and interpretation required to perform the insertion; younger than 5 years of age `A`

    INCLUDES   Verification site catheter tip (71045-71048)
    EXCLUDES   *Centrally inserted placement (36555)*
            Imaging guidance (76937, 77001)
            Peripherally inserted without imaging guidance (36568)
    2.62   12.3   **FUD** 000   `G2`
    AMA: 2019,May,3; 2019,Mar,10

**36573** age 5 years or older `A`

    INCLUDES   Verification site catheter tip (71045-71048)
    EXCLUDES   *Centrally inserted placement (36556)*
            Imaging guidance (76937, 77001)
            Peripherally inserted without imaging guidance (36569)
    2.45   11.3   **FUD** 000   `G2`
    AMA: 2019,May,3; 2019,Mar,10

36570 Insertion of peripherally inserted central venous access device, with subcutaneous port; younger than 5 years of age `A`

    EXCLUDES   *Centrally inserted placement (36560)*
    9.61   42.3   **FUD** 010   `T` `A2` `80` `50`
    AMA: 2018,Jan,8; 2017,Jan,8; 2016,Jan,13

36571 age 5 years or older `A`

    EXCLUDES   *Centrally inserted placement (36561)*
    9.03   37.0   **FUD** 010   `T` `A2` `80` `50`
    AMA: 2018,Jan,8; 2017,Jan,8; 2016,Jan,13

36572   **Resequenced code. See code following 36569.**

36573   **Resequenced code. See code following 36569.**

36575-36590 Repair, Removal, and Replacement Implantable Venous Access Device

    EXCLUDES   *Mechanical removal obstructive material, pericatheter/intraluminal (36595, 36596)*
    Code also frequency of two for procedures involving both catheters from multicatheter device

36575 Repair of tunneled or non-tunneled central venous access catheter, without subcutaneous port or pump, central or peripheral insertion site

    INCLUDES   Repair device without replacing any parts
    1.01   4.57   **FUD** 000   `T` `A2` `80`
    AMA: 2018,Jan,8; 2017,Jan,8; 2016,Jan,13

36576 Repair of central venous access device, with subcutaneous port or pump, central or peripheral insertion site

    INCLUDES   Repair device without replacing any parts
    5.33   9.31   **FUD** 010   `T` `A2` `80`
    AMA: 2018,Jan,8; 2017,Jan,8; 2016,Jan,13

36578 Replacement, catheter only, of central venous access device, with subcutaneous port or pump, central or peripheral insertion site

    INCLUDES   Partial replacement (catheter only)
    EXCLUDES   *Total replacement entire device using same venous access sites (36582-36583)*
    5.89   13.4   **FUD** 010   `T` `A2` `80`
    AMA: 2018,Jan,8; 2017,Jan,8; 2016,Jan,13

36580 Replacement, complete, of a non-tunneled centrally inserted central venous catheter, without subcutaneous port or pump, through same venous access

    INCLUDES   Complete replacement (replace all components/same access site)
    1.91   6.22   **FUD** 000   `T` `J8`
    AMA: 2018,Jan,8; 2017,Jan,8; 2016,Jan,13

36581 Replacement, complete, of a tunneled centrally inserted central venous catheter, without subcutaneous port or pump, through same venous access

    INCLUDES   Complete replacement (replace all components/same access site)
    EXCLUDES   *Removal old device and insertion new device using separate venous access site*
    5.30   22.9   **FUD** 010   `T` `A2` `80`
    AMA: 2018,Jan,8; 2017,Jan,8; 2016,Jan,13

36582 Replacement, complete, of a tunneled centrally inserted central venous access device, with subcutaneous port, through same venous access

    INCLUDES   Complete replacement (replace all components/same access site)
    EXCLUDES   *Removal old device and insertion new device using separate venous access site*
    8.40   28.2   **FUD** 010   `T` `A2` `80`
    AMA: 2018,Jan,8; 2017,Jan,8; 2016,Jan,13

36583 Replacement, complete, of a tunneled centrally inserted central venous access device, with subcutaneous pump, through same venous access

    INCLUDES   Complete replacement (replace all components/same access site)
    EXCLUDES   *Removal old device and insertion new device using separate venous access site*
    9.45   35.9   **FUD** 010   `T` `G2` `80`
    AMA: 2018,Jan,8; 2017,Jan,8; 2016,Jan,13

36584 Replacement, complete, of a peripherally inserted central venous catheter (PICC), without subcutaneous port or pump, through same venous access, including all imaging guidance, image documentation, and all associated radiological supervision and interpretation required to perform the replacement

    INCLUDES   Complete replacement (replace all components/same access site)
            Imaging guidance (76937, 77001)
            Verification site catheter tip (71045-71048)
    EXCLUDES   *Replacement PICC line without imaging guidance (37799)*
    1.73   9.92   **FUD** 000   `T` `A2`
    AMA: 2019,May,3; 2019,Mar,10; 2018,Jan,8; 2017,Jan,8; 2016,Jan,13

36585 Replacement, complete, of a peripherally inserted central venous access device, with subcutaneous port, through same venous access

    INCLUDES   Complete replacement (replace all components/same access site)
    7.86   31.4   **FUD** 010   `T` `A2` `80`
    AMA: 2018,Jan,8; 2017,Jan,8; 2016,Jan,13

36589 Removal of tunneled central venous catheter, without subcutaneous port or pump
> INCLUDES Complete removal/all components
> EXCLUDES Non-tunneled central venous catheter removal; report appropriate E/M code
> 🔲 3.97 ⚕ 4.76 **FUD** 010   Q2 A2 80 🔲
> **AMA:** 2018;Jan,8; 2017,Jan,8; 2016,Jan,13

36590 Removal of tunneled central venous access device, with subcutaneous port or pump, central or peripheral insertion
> INCLUDES Complete removal/all components
> EXCLUDES Non-tunneled central venous catheter removal; report appropriate E/M code
> 🔲 5.51 ⚕ 6.40 **FUD** 010   Q2 A2 80 🔲
> **AMA:** 2018,Jan,8; 2017,Jan,8; 2016,Jan,13

36591-36592 Obtain Blood Specimen from Implanted Device or Catheter
> EXCLUDES Reporting code with any other service except laboratory services

36591 Collection of blood specimen from a completely implantable venous access device
> EXCLUDES Collection:
> Capillary blood specimen (36416)
> Venous blood specimen by venipuncture (36415)
> 🔲 0.70 ⚕ 0.70 **FUD** XXX   Q1 N1 80 TC 🔲
> **AMA:** 2019,Aug,8; 2018,Jan,8; 2017,Jan,8; 2016,Jan,13

36592 Collection of blood specimen using established central or peripheral catheter, venous, not otherwise specified
> EXCLUDES Collection blood from established arterial catheter (37799)
> 🔲 0.77 ⚕ 0.77 **FUD** XXX   Q1 N1 80 TC 🔲
> **AMA:** 2018,Jan,8; 2017,Jan,8; 2016,Jan,13

36593-36596 Restore Patency of Occluded Catheter or Device
> EXCLUDES Venous catheterization (36010-36012)

36593 Declotting by thrombolytic agent of implanted vascular access device or catheter
> 🔲 0.89 ⚕ 0.89 **FUD** XXX   T P3 80 TC 🔲
> **AMA:** 2018,Jan,8; 2017,Jan,8; 2016,Jan,13

36595 Mechanical removal of pericatheter obstructive material (eg, fibrin sheath) from central venous device via separate venous access
> EXCLUDES Declotting by thrombolytic agent (36593)
> 🔀 (75901)
> 🔲 5.30 ⚕ 17.3 **FUD** 000   T J8 🔲
> **AMA:** 2018,Jan,8; 2017,Jan,8; 2016,Jan,13

36596 Mechanical removal of intraluminal (intracatheter) obstructive material from central venous device through device lumen
> EXCLUDES Declotting by thrombolytic agent (36593)
> 🔀 (75902)
> 🔲 1.26 ⚕ 3.47 **FUD** 000   T G2 🔲
> **AMA:** 2018,Jan,8; 2017,Jan,8; 2016,Jan,13

36597-36598 Repositioning or Assessment of In Situ Venous Access Device

36597 Repositioning of previously placed central venous catheter under fluoroscopic guidance
> 🔀 (76000)
> 🔲 1.75 ⚕ 3.79 **FUD** 000   T G2 🔲
> **AMA:** 2018,Jan,8; 2017,Jan,8; 2016,Jan,13

36598 Contrast injection(s) for radiologic evaluation of existing central venous access device, including fluoroscopy, image documentation and report
> EXCLUDES Complete venography studies (75820, 75825, 75827)
> Fluoroscopy (76000)
> Mechanical removal pericatheter obstructive material (36595-36596)
> 🔲 1.07 ⚕ 3.44 **FUD** 000   T P3 80 50 🔲
> **AMA:** 2014,Jan,11

36600-36660 Insertion Needle or Catheter: Artery

36600 Arterial puncture, withdrawal of blood for diagnosis
> EXCLUDES Critical care services
> 🔲 0:45 ⚕ 0.86 **FUD** XXX   Q1 N1 🔲
> **AMA:** 2019,Aug,8; 2018,Jan,8; 2017,Jan,8; 2016,Jan,13

36620 Arterial catheterization or cannulation for sampling, monitoring or transfusion (separate procedure); percutaneous
> 🔲 1.28 ⚕ 1.28 **FUD** 000   N N1 🔲
> **AMA:** 2018,Jan,8; 2017,Jan,8; 2016,Jan,13

36625 cutdown
> 🔲 3.06 ⚕ 3.06 **FUD** 000   N N1 🔲
> **AMA:** 2018,Jan,8; 2017,Jan,8; 2016,Jan,13

36640 Arterial catheterization for prolonged infusion therapy (chemotherapy), cutdown
> EXCLUDES Intra-arterial chemotherapy (96420-96425)
> Transcatheter embolization (75894)
> 🔲 3.31 ⚕ 3.31 **FUD** 000   T A2 🔲
> **AMA:** 2018,Jan,8; 2017,Jan,8; 2016,Jan,13

36660 Catheterization, umbilical artery, newborn, for diagnosis or therapy   A
> 🔲 1.97 ⚕ 1.97 **FUD** 000   63 C 80 🔲
> **AMA:** 2018,Jan,8; 2017,Jan,8; 2016,Jan,13

36680 Percutaneous Placement of Catheter/Needle into Bone Marrow Cavity

36680 Placement of needle for intraosseous infusion
> 🔲 1.74 ⚕ 1.74 **FUD** 000   Q1 N1 80 🔲
> **AMA:** 2018,Jan,8; 2017,Jan,8; 2016,Jan,13

36800-36821 Vascular Access for Hemodialysis

36800 Insertion of cannula for hemodialysis, other purpose (separate procedure); vein to vein
> 🔲 3.55 ⚕ 3.55 **FUD** 000   T G2 🔲
> **AMA:** 2018,Jan,8; 2017,Jan,8; 2016,Jan,13

36810 arteriovenous, external (Scribner type)
> 🔲 6.11 ⚕ 6.11 **FUD** 000   T A2 🔲
> **AMA:** 2018,Jan,8; 2017,Jan,8; 2016,Jan,13

36815 arteriovenous, external revision, or closure
> 🔲 3.91 ⚕ 3.91 **FUD** 000   T A2 🔲
> **AMA:** 2018,Jan,8; 2017,Jan,8; 2016,Jan,13

36818 Arteriovenous anastomosis, open; by upper arm cephalic vein transposition
> INCLUDES Two incisions in upper arm: medial incision over brachial artery and lateral incision for exposure to portion of cephalic vein
> EXCLUDES When performed unilaterally with:
> Arteriovenous anastomosis, open (36819-36820)
> Creation arteriovenous fistula by other than direct arteriovenous anastomosis (36830)
> Code also modifier 50 or 59, as appropriate, for bilateral procedure
> 🔲 20.1 ⚕ 20.1 **FUD** 090   T A2 80 🔲
> **AMA:** 2018,Jan,8; 2017,Mar,3; 2017,Jan,8; 2016,Mar,10; 2016,Jan,13

36819   by upper arm basilic vein transposition
EXCLUDES When performed unilaterally with:
Arteriovenous anastomosis, open (36818, 36820-36821)
Creation arteriovenous fistula by other than direct arteriovenous anastomosis (36830)
Code also modifier 50 or 59, as appropriate, for bilateral procedure
21.2   21.2   **FUD** 090   T A2 80
AMA: 2018,Jan,8; 2017,Mar,3; 2017,Jan,8; 2016,Jan,13

36820   by forearm vein transposition
21.2   21.2   **FUD** 090   T A2 80 50
AMA: 2018,Jan,8; 2017,Mar,3; 2017,Jan,8; 2016,Jan,13

36821   direct, any site (eg, Cimino type) (separate procedure)
19.3   19.3   **FUD** 090   T A2 80
AMA: 2018,Jan,8; 2017,Mar,3; 2017,Jan,8; 2016,Jan,13

36823 Vascular Access for Extracorporeal Circulation
INCLUDES Chemotherapy perfusion
EXCLUDES Chemotherapy administration (96409-96425)
Maintenance for extracorporeal circulation (33946-33949)

36823   Insertion of arterial and venous cannula(s) for isolated extracorporeal circulation including regional chemotherapy perfusion to an extremity, with or without hyperthermia, with removal of cannula(s) and repair of arteriotomy and venotomy sites
40.5   40.5   **FUD** 090   C
AMA: 2018,Jan,8; 2017,Mar,3

36825-36835 Permanent Vascular Access Procedures

36825   Creation of arteriovenous fistula by other than direct arteriovenous anastomosis (separate procedure); autogenous graft
EXCLUDES Direct arteriovenous (AV) anastomosis (36821)
23.0   23.0   **FUD** 090   T A2 80
AMA: 2018,Jan,8; 2017,Mar,3; 2017,Jan,8; 2016,Jan,13

Artery and vein connected by a vein graft in an end-to-side manner, creating an arteriovenous fistula
Radial artery
Radial artery
Graft
Basilic vein
Basilic vein
Artery and vein connected by a synthetic graft

36830   nonautogenous graft (eg, biological collagen, thermoplastic graft)
EXCLUDES Direct arteriovenous (AV) anastomosis (36821)
19.4   19.4   **FUD** 090   T A2 80
AMA: 2018,Jan,8; 2017,Mar,3; 2017,Jan,8; 2016,Jan,13

36831   Thrombectomy, open, arteriovenous fistula without revision, autogenous or nonautogenous dialysis graft (separate procedure)
17.9   17.9   **FUD** 090   T A2 80
AMA: 2018,Jan,8; 2017,Mar,3; 2017,Jan,8; 2016,Jan,13

36832   Revision, open, arteriovenous fistula; without thrombectomy, autogenous or nonautogenous dialysis graft (separate procedure)
INCLUDES Revision arteriovenous access fistula or graft
21.9   21.9   **FUD** 090   T A2 80
AMA: 2018,Jan,8; 2017,Mar,3; 2017,Jan,8; 2016,Jan,13

36833   with thrombectomy, autogenous or nonautogenous dialysis graft (separate procedure)
EXCLUDES Hemodialysis circuit procedures (36901-36906)
23.5   23.5   **FUD** 090   T A2 80
AMA: 2018,Jan,8; 2017,Mar,3; 2017,Jan,8; 2016,Jan,13

36835   Insertion of Thomas shunt (separate procedure)
13.8   13.8   **FUD** 090   T J8
AMA: 2014,Jan,11; 1997,Nov,1

36838 DRIL Procedure for Ischemic Steal Syndrome
EXCLUDES Bypass graft, with vein (35512, 35522-35523)
Ligation (37607, 37618)
Revision, open, arteriovenous fistula (36832)

36838   Distal revascularization and interval ligation (DRIL), upper extremity hemodialysis access (steal syndrome)
33.3   33.3   **FUD** 090   T 62 80 50
AMA: 2014,Jan,11; 1997,Nov,1

36860-36861 Restore Patency of Occluded Cannula or Arteriovenous Fistula

36860   External cannula declotting (separate procedure); without balloon catheter
(76000)
3.23   7.05   **FUD** 000   T A2
AMA: 2018,Jan,8; 2017,Jan,8; 2016,Jan,13

36861   with balloon catheter
(76000)
4.05   4.05   **FUD** 000   T A2
AMA: 2018,Jan,8; 2017,Jan,8; 2016,Jan,13

36901-36909 Hemodialysis Circuit Procedures
EXCLUDES Arteriography to assess inflow to hemodialysis circuit when performed (76937)

36901   Introduction of needle(s) and/or catheter(s), dialysis circuit, with diagnostic angiography of the dialysis circuit, including all direct puncture(s) and catheter placement(s), injection(s) of contrast, all necessary imaging from the arterial anastomosis and adjacent artery through entire venous outflow including the inferior or superior vena cava, fluoroscopic guidance, radiological supervision and interpretation and image documentation and report;
INCLUDES Access
Catheter advancement (e.g., imaging of accessory veins, assess all circuit sections)
Contrast injection
EXCLUDES Balloon angioplasty peripheral segment (36902)
Open revision with thrombectomy arteriovenous fistula (36833)
Percutaneous transluminal procedures peripheral segment (36904-36906)
Stent placement in peripheral segment (36903)
Reporting code more than one time per procedure
4.88   18.3   **FUD** 000   T P2
AMA: 2018,Jan,8; 2017,Mar,3

36902   with transluminal balloon angioplasty, peripheral dialysis segment, including all imaging and radiological supervision and interpretation necessary to perform the angioplasty
EXCLUDES Open revision with thrombectomy arteriovenous fistula (36833)
Percutaneous transluminal procedures peripheral segment (36904-36906)
Stent placement in peripheral segment (36903)
Reporting code more than one time per procedure
6.94   36.9   **FUD** 000   J 62
AMA: 2018,Jan,8; 2017,Jul,3; 2017,Mar,3

36903 with transcatheter placement of intravascular stent(s), peripheral dialysis segment, including all imaging and radiological supervision and interpretation necessary to perform the stenting, and all angioplasty within the peripheral dialysis segment

INCLUDES Balloon angioplasty peripheral segment (36902)

EXCLUDES Central hemodialysis circuit procedures (36907-36908)
Open revision with thrombectomy arteriovenous fistula (36833)
Percutaneous transluminal procedures peripheral segment (36904-36906)
Reporting code more than one time per procedure

🖪 9.20   ⅀ 146.   **FUD** 000   J J8 🖵

AMA: 2018,Jan,8; 2017,Jul,3; 2017,Mar,3

36904 Percutaneous transluminal mechanical thrombectomy and/or infusion for thrombolysis, dialysis circuit, any method, including all imaging and radiological supervision and interpretation, diagnostic angiography, fluoroscopic guidance, catheter placement(s), and intraprocedural pharmacological thrombolytic injection(s);

EXCLUDES Open thrombectomy arteriovenous fistula with/without revision (36831, 36833)
Reporting code more than one time per procedure

🖪 10.7   ⅀ 54.7   **FUD** 000   J 62 🖵

AMA: 2018,Jan,8; 2017,Jul,3; 2017,Mar,3

36905 with transluminal balloon angioplasty, peripheral dialysis segment, including all imaging and radiological supervision and interpretation necessary to perform the angioplasty

INCLUDES Percutaneous mechanical thrombectomy (36904)

EXCLUDES Reporting code more than one time per procedure

🖪 12.8   ⅀ 68.7   **FUD** 000   J 62 🖵

AMA: 2018,Jan,8; 2017,Jul,3; 2017,Mar,3

36906 with transcatheter placement of intravascular stent(s), peripheral dialysis segment, including all imaging and radiological supervision and interpretation necessary to perform the stenting, and all angioplasty within the peripheral dialysis circuit

INCLUDES Percutaneous transluminal balloon angioplasty (36905)
Percutaneous transluminal thrombectomy (36904)

EXCLUDES Hemodialysis circuit procedures provided by catheter or needle access (36901-36903)
Reporting code more than one time per procedure

Code also:
Balloon angioplasty central veins, when performed (36907)
Stent placement in central veins, when performed (36908)

🖪 14.9   ⅀ 186.   **FUD** 000   J J8 🖵

AMA: 2018,Jan,8; 2017,Jul,3; 2017,Mar,3

+ 36907 Transluminal balloon angioplasty, central dialysis segment, performed through dialysis circuit, including all imaging and radiological supervision and interpretation required to perform the angioplasty (List separately in addition to code for primary procedure)

INCLUDES All central hemodialysis segment angiography

EXCLUDES Angiography with stent placement (36908)

Code first (36818-36833, 36901-36906)

🖪 4.25   ⅀ 19.6   **FUD** ZZZ   N N1 🖵

AMA: 2018,Jan,8; 2017,Jul,3; 2017,Mar,3

+ 36908 Transcatheter placement of intravascular stent(s), central dialysis segment, performed through dialysis circuit, including all imaging and radiological supervision and interpretation required to perform the stenting, and all angioplasty in the central dialysis segment (List separately in addition to code for primary procedure)

INCLUDES All central hemodialysis segment stent(s) placed
Balloon angioplasty central dialysis segment (36907)

Code first when performed (36818-36833, 36901-36906)

🖪 6.02   ⅀ 59.6   **FUD** ZZZ   N N1 🖵

AMA: 2018,Jan,8; 2017,Jul,3; 2017,Mar,3

+ 36909 Dialysis circuit permanent vascular embolization or occlusion (including main circuit or any accessory veins), endovascular, including all imaging and radiological supervision and interpretation necessary to complete the intervention (List separately in addition to code for primary procedure)

INCLUDES All embolization/occlusion procedures performed in hemodialysis circuit

EXCLUDES Banding/ligation arteriovenous fistula (37607)
Reporting code more than one time per day

Code first (36901-36906)

🖪 5.83   ⅀ 56.8   **FUD** ZZZ   N N1 🖵

AMA: 2018,Jan,8; 2017,Mar,3

37140-37181 Open Decompression of Portal Circulation

EXCLUDES Peritoneal-venous shunt (49425)

37140 Venous anastomosis, open; portocaval

🖪 67.7   ⅀ 67.7   **FUD** 090   C 🖵

AMA: 2014,Jan,11; 1997,Nov,1

37145 renoportal

🖪 62.7   ⅀ 62.7   **FUD** 090   C 80 🖵

AMA: 2014,Jan,11; 1997,Nov,1

37160 caval-mesenteric

🖪 64.4   ⅀ 64.4   **FUD** 090   C 80 🖵

AMA: 2014,Jan,11; 1997,Nov,1

37180 splenorenal, proximal

🖪 61.9   ⅀ 61.9   **FUD** 090   C 80 🖵

AMA: 2014,Jan,11; 1997,Nov,1

37181 splenorenal, distal (selective decompression of esophagogastric varices, any technique)

EXCLUDES Percutaneous procedure (37182)

🖪 67.7   ⅀ 67.7   **FUD** 090   C 80 🖵

AMA: 2014,Jan,11; 1997,Nov,1

37182-37183 Transvenous Decompression of Portal Circulation

INCLUDES Percutaneous transhepatic portography (75885, 75887)

37182 Insertion of transvenous intrahepatic portosystemic shunt(s) (TIPS) (includes venous access, hepatic and portal vein catheterization, portography with hemodynamic evaluation, intrahepatic tract formation/dilatation, stent placement and all associated imaging guidance and documentation)

EXCLUDES Open procedure (37140)

🖪 23.7   ⅀ 23.7   **FUD** 000   C 80 🖵

AMA: 2018,Jan,8; 2017,Jan,8; 2016,Jan,13

37183 Revision of transvenous intrahepatic portosystemic shunt(s) (TIPS) (includes venous access, hepatic and portal vein catheterization, portography with hemodynamic evaluation, intrahepatic tract recanulization/dilatation, stent placement and all associated imaging guidance and documentation)

EXCLUDES Arteriovenous (AV) aneurysm repair (36832)

🖪 10.8   ⅀ 176.   **FUD** 000   J J8 80 🖵

AMA: 2018,Jan,8; 2017,Jan,8; 2016,Jan,13

26/TC PC/TC Only   A2-Z3 ASC Payment   50 Bilateral   ♂ Male Only   ♀ Female Only   🖪 Facility RVU   ⅀ Non-Facility RVU   🖵 CCI   ❌ CLIA
FUD Follow-up Days   **CMS:** IOM   **AMA:** CPT Asst   A-Y OPPSI   80/80 Surg Assist Allowed / w/Doc   🄽 Lab Crosswalk   🅡 Radiology Crosswalk

168   CPT © 2021 American Medical Association. All Rights Reserved.   © 2021 Optum360, LLC

37184-37188 Removal of Thrombus from Vessel: Percutaneous

INCLUDES Fluoroscopic guidance (76000)
Injection(s) thrombolytics during procedure
Postprocedure evaluation
Pretreatment planning

EXCLUDES *Catheter placement*
Continuous infusion thrombolytics prior to and after procedure (37211-37214)
Diagnostic studies
Intracranial arterial mechanical thrombectomy or infusion (61645)
Mechanical thrombectomy, coronary (92973)
Other interventions performed percutaneously (e.g., balloon angioplasty)
Radiological supervision/interpretation

37184 **Primary percutaneous transluminal mechanical thrombectomy, noncoronary, non-intracranial, arterial or arterial bypass graft, including fluoroscopic guidance and intraprocedural pharmacological thrombolytic injection(s); initial vessel**

EXCLUDES *Intracranial arterial mechanical thrombectomy (61645)*
Mechanical thrombectomy another vascular family/separate access site, append modifier 59 to primary service
Mechanical thrombectomy for embolus/thrombus complicating another percutaneous interventional procedure (37186)
Therapeutic, prophylactic, or diagnostic injection (96374)

  12.9 60.2 **FUD** 000   J J8 50

AMA: 2019,Sep,5; 2018,Jan,8; 2017,Jan,8; 2016,Jul,6; 2016,Mar,3; 2016,Jan,13

+ **37185** **second and all subsequent vessel(s) within the same vascular family (List separately in addition to code for primary mechanical thrombectomy procedure)**

INCLUDES Treatment second and all succeeding vessel(s) in same vascular family

EXCLUDES *Intravenous drug injections administered subsequent to initial service*
Mechanical thrombectomy another vascular family/separate access site, append modifier 59 to primary service
Therapeutic, prophylactic, or diagnostic injection (96375)

Code first (37184)

  4.77 16.9 **FUD** ZZZ   N N1

AMA: 2019,Sep,5; 2018,Jan,8; 2017,Jan,8; 2016,Jul,6; 2016,Jan,13

+ **37186** **Secondary percutaneous transluminal thrombectomy (eg, nonprimary mechanical, snare basket, suction technique), noncoronary, non-intracranial, arterial or arterial bypass graft, including fluoroscopic guidance and intraprocedural pharmacological thrombolytic injections, provided in conjunction with another percutaneous intervention other than primary mechanical thrombectomy (List separately in addition to code for primary procedure)**

INCLUDES Removal small emboli/thrombi prior to or after another percutaneous procedure

EXCLUDES *Primary percutaneous transluminal mechanical thrombectomy, noncoronary, non-intracranial (37184-37185)*
Therapeutic, prophylactic, or diagnostic injection (96375)

Code first primary procedure

  7.10 37.4 **FUD** ZZZ   N N1

AMA: 2019,Sep,5; 2018,Jan,8; 2017,Jan,8; 2016,Jul,6; 2016,Jan,13

37187 **Percutaneous transluminal mechanical thrombectomy, vein(s), including intraprocedural pharmacological thrombolytic injections and fluoroscopic guidance**

INCLUDES Secondary or subsequent intravenous injection after another initial service

EXCLUDES *Therapeutic, prophylactic, or diagnostic injection (96375)*

  11.4 55.0 **FUD** 000   J J8 50

AMA: 2018,Jan,8; 2017,Jan,8; 2016,Jul,6; 2016,Mar,3; 2016,Jan,13

37188 **Percutaneous transluminal mechanical thrombectomy, vein(s), including intraprocedural pharmacological thrombolytic injections and fluoroscopic guidance, repeat treatment on subsequent day during course of thrombolytic therapy**

EXCLUDES *Therapeutic, prophylactic, or diagnostic injection (96375)*

  8.10 46.3 **FUD** 000   T G2 50

AMA: 2018,Jan,8; 2017,Jan,8; 2016,Jul,6; 2016,Mar,3; 2016,Jan,13

37191-37193 Vena Cava Filters

37191 **Insertion of intravascular vena cava filter, endovascular approach including vascular access, vessel selection, and radiological supervision and interpretation, intraprocedural roadmapping, and imaging guidance (ultrasound and fluoroscopy), when performed**

EXCLUDES *Open ligation inferior vena cava via laparotomy or retroperitoneal approach (37619)*

  6.48 68.0 **FUD** 000   T J8

AMA: 2018,Jan,8; 2017,Feb,14; 2017,Jan,8; 2016,May,11; 2016,Jan,13

Renal vein

Filter

Inferior vena cava

Clot

37192 **Repositioning of intravascular vena cava filter, endovascular approach including vascular access, vessel selection, and radiological supervision and interpretation, intraprocedural roadmapping, and imaging guidance (ultrasound and fluoroscopy), when performed**

EXCLUDES *Insertion intravascular vena cava filter (37191)*

  10.0 38.2 **FUD** 000   T J8

AMA: 2018,Jan,8; 2017,Jan,8; 2016,May,11; 2016,Jan,13

37193 **Retrieval (removal) of intravascular vena cava filter, endovascular approach including vascular access, vessel selection, and radiological supervision and interpretation, intraprocedural roadmapping, and imaging guidance (ultrasound and fluoroscopy), when performed**

EXCLUDES *Transcatheter retrieval intravascular foreign body, percutaneous (37197)*

  10.1 44.0 **FUD** 000   T G2

AMA: 2018,Jan,8; 2017,Jan,8; 2016,May,11; 2016,Jan,13

37195 Intravenous Cerebral Thrombolysis

37195 **Thrombolysis, cerebral, by intravenous infusion**

  0.00 0.00 **FUD** XXX   T G2 80

AMA: 2020,Jan,12

37197-37214 Transcatheter Procedures: Infusions, Biopsy, Foreign Body Removal

37197 Transcatheter retrieval, percutaneous, of intravascular foreign body (eg, fractured venous or arterial catheter), includes radiological supervision and interpretation, and imaging guidance (ultrasound or fluoroscopy), when performed

EXCLUDES *Percutaneous vena cava filter retrieval (37193)*
Removal leadless pacemaker system ([33275])

⚕ 8.78   ⚗ 43.4   **FUD** 000   T G2 ▢

AMA: 2018,Jan,8; 2017,Feb,14; 2017,Jan,8; 2016,May,11; 2016,Jan,13

37200 Transcatheter biopsy

⊞ (75970)

⚕ 6.30   ⚗ 6.30   **FUD** 000   T G2 ▢

AMA: 2014,Jan,11; 1998,Nov,1

37211 Transcatheter therapy, arterial infusion for thrombolysis other than coronary or intracranial, any method, including radiological supervision and interpretation, initial treatment day

INCLUDES Catheter change or position change
E/M services on day of and related to thrombolysis
First day transcatheter thrombolytic infusion
Fluoroscopic guidance
Follow-up arteriography or venography
Radiologic supervision and interpretation

EXCLUDES *Angiography through existing catheter for follow-up study for transcatheter therapy, embolization, or infusion, other than for thrombolysis (75898)*
Catheter placement
Declotting implanted catheter or vascular access device by thrombolytic agent (36593)
Diagnostic studies
Intracranial arterial mechanical thrombectomy or infusion (61645)
Percutaneous interventions
Procedure performed more than one time per date of service
Ultrasound guidance (76937)
Code also significant, separately identifiable E/M service on day of thrombolysis using modifier 25

⚕ 11.2   ⚗ 11.2   **FUD** 000   T G2 50 ▢

AMA: 2019,Sep,6; 2018,Jan,8; 2017,Jan,8; 2016,Jul,6; 2016,Mar,3; 2016,Jan,13

37212 Transcatheter therapy, venous infusion for thrombolysis, any method, including radiological supervision and interpretation, initial treatment day

INCLUDES Catheter change or position change
E/M services on day of and related to thrombolysis
First day transcatheter thrombolytic infusion
Fluoroscopic guidance
Follow-up arteriography or venography
Initiation and completion thrombolysis on same date of service
Radiologic supervision and interpretation

EXCLUDES *Angiography through existing catheter for follow-up study for transcatheter therapy, embolization, or infusion, other than for thrombolysis (75898)*
Catheter placement
Declotting implanted catheter or vascular access device by thrombolytic agent (36593)
Diagnostic studies
Percutaneous interventions
Procedure performed more than one time per date of service
Ultrasound guidance (76937)
Code also significant, separately identifiable E/M service on day of thrombolysis using modifier 25

⚕ 9.81   ⚗ 9.81   **FUD** 000   T G2 50 ▢

AMA: 2019,Sep,6; 2018,Jan,8; 2017,Jan,8; 2016,Jul,6; 2016,Mar,3; 2016,Jan,13

37213 Transcatheter therapy, arterial or venous infusion for thrombolysis other than coronary, any method, including radiological supervision and interpretation, continued treatment on subsequent day during course of thrombolytic therapy, including follow-up catheter contrast injection, position change, or exchange, when performed;

INCLUDES Continued thrombolytic infusions on subsequent days besides initial and last days of treatment
E/M services on day of and related to thrombolysis
Fluoroscopic guidance
Radiologic supervision and interpretation

EXCLUDES *Angiography through existing catheter for follow-up study for transcatheter therapy, embolization, or infusion, other than for thrombolysis (75898)*
Catheter placement
Declotting implanted catheter or vascular access device by thrombolytic agent (36593)
Diagnostic studies
Percutaneous interventions
Procedure performed more than one time per date of service
Ultrasound guidance (76937)
Code also significant, separately identifiable E/M service on day of thrombolysis using modifier 25

⚕ 6.76   ⚗ 6.76   **FUD** 000   T G2 ▢

AMA: 2019,Sep,6; 2018,Jan,8; 2017,Jan,8; 2016,Jul,6; 2016,Mar,3; 2016,Jan,13

37214 cessation of thrombolysis including removal of catheter and vessel closure by any method

INCLUDES E/M services on day of and related to thrombolysis
Fluoroscopic guidance
Last day transcatheter thrombolytic infusions
Radiologic supervision and interpretation

EXCLUDES *Angiography through existing catheter for follow-up study for transcatheter therapy, embolization, or infusion, other than for thrombolysis (75898)*
Catheter placement
Declotting implanted catheter or vascular access device by thrombolytic agent (36593)
Diagnostic studies
Percutaneous interventions
Procedure performed more than one time per date of service
Ultrasound guidance (76937)
Code also significant, separately identifiable E/M service on day of thrombolysis using modifier 25

⚕ 3.57   ⚗ 3.57   **FUD** 000   T G2 ▢

AMA: 2019,Sep,6; 2018,Jan,8; 2017,Jan,8; 2016,Jul,6; 2016,Mar,3; 2016,Jan,13

26/TC PC/TC Only   A2-Z3 ASC Payment   50 Bilateral   ♂ Male Only   ♀ Female Only   ⚕ Facility RVU   ⚗ Non-Facility RVU   ▢ CCI   ☒ CLIA
FUD Follow-up Days   CMS: IOM   AMA: CPT Asst   A-Y OPPSI   80/80 Surg Assist Allowed / w/Doc   ▦ Lab Crosswalk   ⊞ Radiology Crosswalk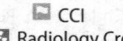

170   CPT © 2021 American Medical Association. All Rights Reserved.   © 2021 Optum360, LLC

37215-37216 Stenting of Cervical Carotid Artery with/without Insertion Distal Embolic Protection Device

INCLUDES
Carotid stenting, if required
Ipsilateral cerebral and cervical carotid diagnostic imaging/supervision and interpretation
Ipsilateral selective carotid catheterization

EXCLUDES
Carotid catheterization and imaging, if carotid stenting not required
Selective catheter placement, common carotid or innominate artery (36222-36224)
Transcatheter placement extracranial vertebral artery stents, open or percutaneous (0075T, 0076T)

37215 **Transcatheter placement of intravascular stent(s), cervical carotid artery, open or percutaneous, including angioplasty, when performed, and radiological supervision and interpretation; with distal embolic protection**

⏰ 29.0   ✂ 29.0   **FUD** 090   C 80 50 ▣

AMA: 2018,Jan,8; 2017,Jul,3; 2017,Jan,8; 2016,Jan,13

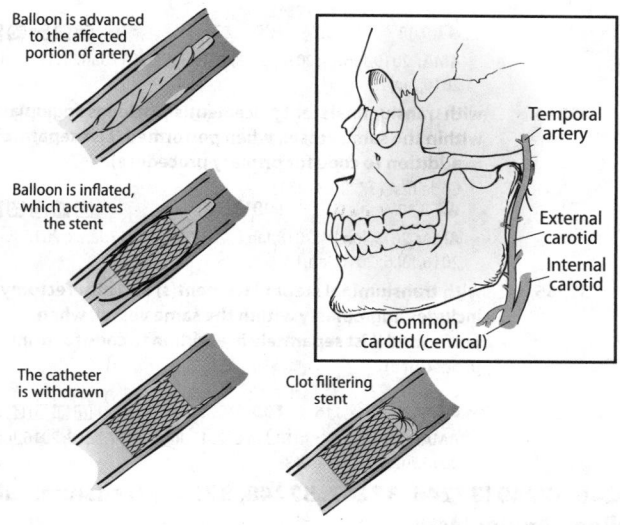

Balloon is advanced to the affected portion of artery

Balloon is inflated, which activates the stent

The catheter is withdrawn

Temporal artery

External carotid

Internal carotid

Common carotid (cervical)

Clot filitering stent

37216 **without distal embolic protection**

⏰ 28.2   ✂ 28.2   **FUD** 090   E ▣

AMA: 2018,Jan,8; 2017,Jul,3; 2017,Jan,8; 2016,Jan,13

37217-37218 Stenting of Intrathoracic Carotid Artery/Innominate Artery

INCLUDES
Access to vessel (open)
Arteriotomy closure by suture
Catheterization vessel (selective) (36222-36227)
Imaging during and after procedure
Radiological supervision and interpretation

EXCLUDES
Carotid artery revascularization procedures when performed during same session
Transcatheter insertion extracranial vertebral artery stents, open or percutaneous (0075T-0076T)
Transcatheter insertion intracranial stents (61635)
Transcatheter insertion intravascular cervical carotid artery stents, open or percutaneous (37215-37216)

37217 **Transcatheter placement of intravascular stent(s), intrathoracic common carotid artery or innominate artery by retrograde treatment, open ipsilateral cervical carotid artery exposure, including angioplasty, when performed, and radiological supervision and interpretation**

INCLUDES
When performed on same side:
Direct repair blood vessel, neck (35201)
Nonselective catheterization, thoracic aorta (36221)
Transluminal balloon angioplasty (37246-37247 [37246, 37247])

⏰ 31.3   ✂ 31.3   **FUD** 090   C 80 50 ▣

AMA: 2018,Jan,8; 2017,Jul,3; 2017,Jan,8; 2016,Jan,13

37218 **Transcatheter placement of intravascular stent(s), intrathoracic common carotid artery or innominate artery, open or percutaneous antegrade approach, including angioplasty, when performed, and radiological supervision and interpretation**

EXCLUDES
Selective catheter placement, common carotid or innominate artery (36222-36224)

⏰ 23.7   ✂ 23.7   **FUD** 090   C 80 50 ▣

AMA: 2018,Jan,8; 2017,Jul,3; 2017,Jan,8; 2016,Jan,13

37220-37235 Endovascular Revascularization Lower Extremities

INCLUDES
Percutaneous and open interventional and associated procedures for lower extremity occlusive disease; unilateral
Accessing vessel
Arteriotomy closure by suturing puncture or pressure with arterial closure device application
Atherectomy (e.g., directional, laser, rotational)
Balloon angioplasty (e.g., cryoplasty, cutting balloon, low-profile)
Catheterization vessel (selective)
Embolic protection
Imaging once procedure complete
Radiological supervision and interpretation
Stenting (e.g., bare metal, balloon-expandable, covered, drug-eluting, self-expanding)
Traversing lesion
Reporting most comprehensive treatment in given vessel according to following hierarchy:
1. Stent and atherectomy
2. Atherectomy
3. Stent
4. PTA
Revascularization procedures for three arterial vascular territories:
Femoral/popliteal vascular territory including common, deep, and superficial femoral arteries, and popliteal artery (one extremity = a single vessel) (37224-37227)
Iliac vascular territory: common iliac, external iliac, internal iliac (37220-37223)
Tibial/peroneal territory: includes anterior tibial, peroneal artery, posterior tibial (37228-37235)

EXCLUDES
Assignment more than one code from this family for each lower extremity vessel treated
Assignment more than one code when multiple vessels are treated in femoral/popliteal territory (report most complex service for more than one lesion in territory); when contiguous lesion that spans from one territory to another can be opened with single procedure; or when more than one stent deployed in same vessel
Extensive repair or replacement artery (35226, 35286)
Mechanical thrombectomy and/or thrombolysis

Code also:
Add-on codes for different vessels, but not different lesions in same vessel; and for multiple territories in same leg
Modifier 59 if same territory(ies) both legs are treated during same surgical session
Code first one primary code for initial service in each leg

37220 **Revascularization, endovascular, open or percutaneous, iliac artery, unilateral, initial vessel; with transluminal angioplasty**

Code also only when transluminal angioplasty performed outside treatment target zone of (34701-34708, 34709, [34718], 34710-34711, 34845-34848)

⏰ 11.6   ✂ 82.1   **FUD** 000   J 62 50 ▣

AMA: 2019,Jun,14; 2018,Jan,8; 2017,Jul,3; 2017,Jan,8; 2016,Jul,8; 2016,Jan,13

37221 **with transluminal stent placement(s), includes angioplasty within the same vessel, when performed**

Code also only when transluminal angioplasty performed outside treatment target zone of (34701-34708, 34709, [34718], 34710-34711, 34845-34848)

⏰ 14.4   ✂ 118.   **FUD** 000   J J8 80 50 ▣

AMA: 2019,Jun,14; 2018,Jan,8; 2017,Dec,3; 2017,Jul,3; 2017,Jan,8; 2016,Jul,6; 2016,Jul,8; 2016,Jan,13

Cardiovascular, Hemic, and Lymphatic

37222 — 37246

+ **37222** **Revascularization, endovascular, open or percutaneous, iliac artery, each additional ipsilateral iliac vessel; with transluminal angioplasty (List separately in addition to code for primary procedure)**

　　Code also only when transluminal angioplasty performed outside treatment target zone of (34701-34708, 34709, [34718], 34710-34711, 34845-34848)
　　Code first (37220-37221)
　　📷 5.42　　♒ 21.2　　**FUD** ZZZ　　　　Ⓝ Ⓝ1 80 50 ▱
　　AMA: 2019,Jun,14; 2018,Jan,8; 2017,Jul,3; 2017,Jan,8; 2016,Jul,8; 2016,Jan,13

+ **37223** **with transluminal stent placement(s), includes angioplasty within the same vessel, when performed (List separately in addition to code for primary procedure)**

　　Code also only when transluminal angioplasty performed outside treatment target zone of (34701-34708, 34709, [34718], 34710-34711, 34845-34848)
　　Code first (37221)
　　📷 6.20　　♒ 62.6　　**FUD** ZZZ　　　　Ⓝ Ⓝ1 80 50 ▱
　　AMA: 2019,Jun,14; 2018,Jan,8; 2017,Dec,3; 2017,Jul,3; 2017,Jan,8; 2016,Jul,8; 2016,Jul,6; 2016,Jan,13

37224 **Revascularization, endovascular, open or percutaneous, femoral, popliteal artery(s), unilateral; with transluminal angioplasty**

　　EXCLUDES *Revascularization with intravascular stent grafts in femoral-popliteal segment (0505T)*
　　📷 12.9　　♒ 97.6　　**FUD** 000　　　　Ⓙ J8 80 50 ▱
　　AMA: 2019,Jun,14; 2018,Jan,8; 2017,Jul,3; 2017,Jan,8; 2016,Jul,8; 2016,Jan,13

37225 **with atherectomy, includes angioplasty within the same vessel, when performed**

　　EXCLUDES *Revascularization with intravascular stent grafts in femoral-popliteal segment (0505T)*
　　📷 17.5　　♒ 320.　　**FUD** 000　　　　Ⓙ J8 80 50 ▱
　　AMA: 2019,Jun,14; 2018,Jan,8; 2017,Jul,3; 2017,Jan,8; 2016,Jul,8; 2016,Jan,13

37226 **with transluminal stent placement(s), includes angioplasty within the same vessel, when performed**

　　EXCLUDES *Revascularization with intravascular stent grafts in femoral-popliteal segment (0505T)*
　　📷 15.1　　♒ 285.　　**FUD** 000　　　　Ⓙ J8 80 50 ▱
　　AMA: 2019,Jun,14; 2018,Jan,8; 2017,Jul,3; 2017,Jan,8; 2016,Jul,6; 2016,Jul,8; 2016,Jan,13

37227 **with transluminal stent placement(s) and atherectomy, includes angioplasty within the same vessel, when performed**

　　EXCLUDES *Revascularization with intravascular stent grafts in femoral-popliteal segment (0505T)*
　　📷 21.1　　♒ 444.　　**FUD** 000　　　　Ⓙ J8 80 50 ▱
　　AMA: 2019,Jun,14; 2018,Jan,8; 2017,Jul,3; 2017,Jan,8; 2016,Jul,6; 2016,Jul,8; 2016,Jan,13

37228 **Revascularization, endovascular, open or percutaneous, tibial, peroneal artery, unilateral, initial vessel; with transluminal angioplasty**

　　📷 15.7　　♒ 140.　　**FUD** 000　　　　Ⓙ J8 80 50 ▱
　　AMA: 2019,Jun,14; 2018,Jan,8; 2017,Jul,3; 2017,Jan,8; 2016,Jul,8; 2016,Jan,13

37229 **with atherectomy, includes angioplasty within the same vessel, when performed**

　　📷 20.4　　♒ 322.　　**FUD** 000　　　　Ⓙ J8 80 50 ▱
　　AMA: 2019,Jun,14; 2018,Jan,8; 2017,Jul,3; 2017,Jan,8; 2016,Jul,8; 2016,Jan,13

37230 **with transluminal stent placement(s), includes angioplasty within the same vessel, when performed**

　　📷 20.3　　♒ 289.　　**FUD** 000　　　　Ⓙ J8 80 50 ▱
　　AMA: 2020,Jul,13; 2019,Jun,14; 2018,Jan,8; 2017,Jul,3; 2017,Jan,8; 2016,Jul,6; 2016,Jul,8; 2016,Jan,13

37231 **with transluminal stent placement(s) and atherectomy, includes angioplasty within the same vessel, when performed**

　　📷 22.0　　♒ 401.　　**FUD** 000　　　　Ⓙ J8 80 50 ▱
　　AMA: 2019,Jun,14; 2018,Jan,8; 2017,Jul,3; 2017,Jan,8; 2016,Jul,8; 2016,Jul,6; 2016,Jan,13

+ **37232** **Revascularization, endovascular, open or percutaneous, tibial/peroneal artery, unilateral, each additional vessel; with transluminal angioplasty (List separately in addition to code for primary procedure)**

　　Code first (37228-37231)
　　📷 5.83　　♒ 29.0　　**FUD** ZZZ　　　　Ⓝ Ⓝ1 80 50 ▱
　　AMA: 2019,Jun,14; 2018,Jan,8; 2017,Jul,3; 2017,Jan,8; 2016,Jul,8; 2016,Jan,13

+ **37233** **with atherectomy, includes angioplasty within the same vessel, when performed (List separately in addition to code for primary procedure)**

　　Code first (37229, 37231)
　　📷 9.48　　♒ 35.7　　**FUD** ZZZ　　　　Ⓝ Ⓝ1 80 50 ▱
　　AMA: 2019,Jun,14; 2018,Jan,8; 2017,Jul,3; 2017,Jan,8; 2016,Jul,8; 2016,Jan,13

+ **37234** **with transluminal stent placement(s), includes angioplasty within the same vessel, when performed (List separately in addition to code for primary procedure)**

　　Code first (37229-37231)
　　📷 8.30　　♒ 110.　　**FUD** ZZZ　　　　Ⓝ Ⓝ1 80 50 ▱
　　AMA: 2019,Jun,14; 2018,Jan,8; 2017,Jul,3; 2017,Jan,8; 2016,Jul,8; 2016,Jul,6; 2016,Jan,13

+ **37235** **with transluminal stent placement(s) and atherectomy, includes angioplasty within the same vessel, when performed (List separately in addition to code for primary procedure)**

　　Code first (37231)
　　📷 11.7　　♒ 116.　　**FUD** ZZZ　　　　Ⓝ Ⓝ1 80 50 ▱
　　AMA: 2019,Jun,14; 2018,Jan,8; 2017,Jul,3; 2017,Jan,8; 2016,Jul,6; 2016,Jul,8; 2016,Jan,13

37246-37249 [37246, 37247, 37248, 37249] Transluminal Balloon Angioplasty

　　INCLUDES Open and percutaneous balloon angioplasty
　　　　　　Radiological supervision and interpretation (37220-37235)
　　EXCLUDES *Angioplasty other vessels:*
　　　　　　Aortic/visceral arteries (with endovascular repair) (34841-34848)
　　　　　　Coronary artery (92920-92944)
　　　　　　Intracranial artery (61630, 61635)
　　　　　　Performed in hemodialysis circuit (36901-36909)
　　　　　　Infusion thrombolytics (37211-37214)
　　　　　　Mechanical thrombectomy (37184-37188)
　　　　　　Pulmonary artery (92997-92998)
　　　　　　Reporting codes more than one time for all services performed in single vessel or treatable with one angioplasty procedure
　　Code also:
　　　　Angioplasty different vessel, when performed ([37247], [37249])
　　　　Extensive artery repair or replacement, when performed (35226, 35286)
　　　　Intravascular ultrasound, when performed (37252-37253)

\# **37246** **Transluminal balloon angioplasty (except lower extremity artery(ies) for occlusive disease, intracranial, coronary, pulmonary, or dialysis circuit), open or percutaneous, including all imaging and radiological supervision and interpretation necessary to perform the angioplasty within the same artery; initial artery**

　　EXCLUDES *Intravascular stent placement except lower extremities (37236-37237)*
　　　　　　Revascularization lower extremities (37220-37235)
　　　　　　Stent placement:
　　　　　　Cervical carotid artery (37215-37216)
　　　　　　Intrathoracic carotid or innominate artery (37217-37218)
　　📷 10.1　　♒ 58.3　　**FUD** 000　　　　Ⓙ 62 50 ▱
　　AMA: 2018,Jan,8; 2017,Aug,10; 2017,Jul,3

| 26/TC | PC/TC Only | A2-Z3 | ASC Payment | 50 | Bilateral | ♂ Male Only | ♀ Female Only | 📷 Facility RVU | ♒ Non-Facility RVU | ▱ CCI | ☒ CLIA |
| **FUD** Follow-up Days | | **CMS:** IOM | | **AMA:** CPT Asst | | A-Y OPPSI | | 80/80 Surg Assist Allowed / w/Doc | | ▧ Lab Crosswalk | ▦ Radiology Crosswalk |

172　　　　　　　　　　CPT © 2021 American Medical Association. All Rights Reserved.　　　　　　　　© 2021 Optum360, LLC

+ # 37247 each additional artery (List separately in addition to code for primary procedure)

> *EXCLUDES*
> *Intravascular stent placement except lower extremities (37236-37237)*
> *Revascularization lower extremities (37220-37235)*
> *Stent placement:*
> *Cervical carotid artery (37215-37216)*
> *Intrathoracic carotid or innominate artery (37217-37218)*

Code first ([37246])

🔧 4.97 ⚕ 20.5 **FUD** ZZZ   N N1 50 ▣

AMA: 2018,Jan,8; 2017,Aug,10; 2017,Jul,3

 # 37248 Transluminal balloon angioplasty (except dialysis circuit), open or percutaneous, including all imaging and radiological supervision and interpretation necessary to perform the angioplasty within the same vein; initial vein

> *EXCLUDES*
> *Endovascular venous arterialization with intravascular stent graft(s) in tibial-peroneal segment (0620T)*
> *Placement intravascular (venous) stent in same vein, same session as (37238-37239)*
> *Revascularization with intravascular stent grafts in femoral-popliteal segment (0505T)*

🔧 8.64 ⚕ 42.9 **FUD** 000   J 62 50 ▣

AMA: 2018,Jan,8; 2017,Aug,10; 2017,Jul,3; 2017,Mar,3

+ # 37249 each additional vein (List separately in addition to code for primary procedure)

> *EXCLUDES*
> *Endovascular venous arterialization with intravascular stent graft(s) in tibial-peroneal segment (0620T)*
> *Placement intravascular (venous) stent in same vein, same session as (37238-37239)*
> *Revascularization with intravascular stent grafts in femoral-popliteal segment (0505T)*

Code first ([37248])

🔧 4.24 ⚕ 15.6 **FUD** ZZZ   N N1 50 ▣

AMA: 2018,Jan,8; 2017,Aug,10; 2017,Jul,3; 2017,Mar,3

37236-37239 Endovascular Revascularization Excluding Lower Extremities

> *INCLUDES*
> Arteriotomy closure by suturing puncture, pressure, or arterial closure device application
> Balloon angioplasty
> Post-dilation after stent deployment
> Predilation performed as primary or secondary angioplasty
> Treatment lesion inside same vessel but outside stented portion
> Treatment using different-sized balloons to accomplish procedure
> Endovascular revascularization arteries and veins other than carotid, coronary, extracranial, intracranial, lower extremities
> Imaging once procedure complete
> Radiological supervision and interpretation
> Stent placement provided as only treatment

> *EXCLUDES*
> *Angioplasty in unrelated vessel*
> *Extensive repair or replacement artery (35226, 35286)*
> *Insertion multiple stents in single vessel using more than one code*
> *Intravascular ultrasound (37252-37253)*
> *Mechanical thrombectomy (37184-37188)*
> *Selective and nonselective catheterization (36005, 36010-36015, 36200, 36215-36218, 36245-36248)*
> *Stent placement in:*
> *Cervical carotid artery (37215-37216)*
> *Extracranial vertebral (0075T-0076T)*
> *Hemodialysis circuit (36903, 36905, 36908)*
> *Intracoronary (92928-92929, 92933-92934, 92937-92938, 92941, 92943-92944)*
> *Intracranial (61635)*
> *Intrathoracic common carotid or innominate artery, retrograde or antegrade approach (37218)*
> *Lower extremity arteries for occlusive disease (37221, 37223, 37226-37227, 37230-37231, 37234-37235)*
> *Visceral arteries with fenestrated aortic repair (34841-34848)*
> *Thrombolytic therapy (37211-37214)*
> *Ultrasound guidance (76937)*

Code also add-on codes for different vessels treated during same operative session

37236 Transcatheter placement of an intravascular stent(s) (except lower extremity artery(s) for occlusive disease, cervical carotid, extracranial vertebral or intrathoracic carotid, intracranial, or coronary), open or percutaneous, including radiological supervision and interpretation and including all angioplasty within the same vessel, when performed; initial artery

> *EXCLUDES*
> *Procedures in same target treatment zone with (34841-34848)*

🔧 12.9 ⚕ 101. **FUD** 000   J J8 80 50 ▣

AMA: 2018,Jan,8; 2017,Dec,3; 2017,Jul,3; 2017,Jan,8; 2016,Jul,3; 2016,Jul,6; 2016,Mar,5; 2016,Jan,13

+ 37237 each additional artery (List separately in addition to code for primary procedure)

> *EXCLUDES*
> *Procedures in same target treatment zone with (34841-34848)*

Code first (37236)

🔧 6.18 ⚕ 53.2 **FUD** ZZZ   N N1 80 50 ▣

AMA: 2018,Jan,8; 2017,Dec,3; 2017,Jul,3; 2017,Jan,8; 2016,Jul,6; 2016,Mar,5; 2016,Jan,13

37238 Transcatheter placement of an intravascular stent(s), open or percutaneous, including radiological supervision and interpretation and including angioplasty within the same vessel, when performed; initial vein

> *EXCLUDES*
> *Endovascular venous arterialization with intravascular stent graft(s) in tibial-peroneal segment (0620T)*
> *Revascularization with intravascular stent grafts in femoral-popliteal segment (0505T)*

🔧 8.88 ⚕ 90.3 **FUD** 000   J J8 80 50 ▣

AMA: 2018,Jan,8; 2017,Jul,3; 2017,Mar,3; 2017,Jan,8; 2016,Jul,6; 2016,Jun,8

+ **37239** **each additional vein (List separately in addition to code for primary procedure)**

> *EXCLUDES* *Endovascular venous arterialization with intravascular stent graft(s) in tibial-peroneal segment (0620T)*
> *Revascularization with intravascular stent grafts in femoral-popliteal segment (0505T)*

Code first (37238)

🏥 4.43   ≥ 41.8   **FUD** ZZZ   N N1 80 50

AMA: 2018,Jan,8; 2017,Jul,3; 2017,Mar,3; 2017,Jan,8; 2016,Jul,6

37241-37249 [37246, 37247, 37248, 37249] Therapeutic Vascular Embolization/Occlusion

> *INCLUDES* Embolization or occlusion arteries, lymphatics, and veins except for head/neck and central nervous system
> Imaging once procedure complete
> Intraprocedural guidance
> Radiological supervision and interpretation
> Roadmapping
> Stent placement provided as support for embolization

> *EXCLUDES* *Embolization code assigned more than once per operative field*
> *Head, neck, or central nervous system embolization (61624, 61626, 61710)*
> *Multiple codes for indications that overlap, code only indication needing most immediate attention*
> *Stent deployment as primary aneurysm management, pseudoaneurysm, or vascular extravasation*
> *Vein destruction with sclerosing solution (36468-36471)*

Code also:

> Additional embolization procedure(s) and appropriate modifiers (e.g., modifier 59) when embolization procedures performed in multiple operative fields
> Diagnostic angiography and catheter placement; append modifier 59 when appropriate

37241 **Vascular embolization or occlusion, inclusive of all radiological supervision and interpretation, intraprocedural roadmapping, and imaging guidance necessary to complete the intervention; venous, other than hemorrhage (eg, congenital or acquired venous malformations, venous and capillary hemangiomas, varices, varicoceles)**

> *EXCLUDES* *Embolization side branch(es) outflow vein from hemodialysis access (36909)*
> *Procedure in same operative field with:*
> *Endovenous ablation therapy incompetent vein (36475-36479)*
> *Injection sclerosing solution; single vein (36470-36471)*
> *Transcatheter embolization procedures (75894, 75898)*
> *Vein destruction (36468-36479 [36465, 36466])*

🏥 12.7   ≥ 140.   **FUD** 000   J P2

AMA: 2019,Sep,6; 2018,Mar,3; 2018,Jan,8; 2017,Mar,3; 2017,Jan,8; 2016,Nov,3; 2016,Jan,13

37242 **arterial, other than hemorrhage or tumor (eg, congenital or acquired arterial malformations, arteriovenous malformations, arteriovenous fistulas, aneurysms, pseudoaneurysms)**

> *EXCLUDES* *Percutaneous treatment pseudoaneurysm extremity (36002)*

🏥 13.8   ≥ 211.   **FUD** 000   J J8

AMA: 2019,Sep,6; 2018,Jul,14; 2018,Mar,3; 2018,Jan,8; 2017,Jan,8; 2016,Jan,13

37243 **for tumors, organ ischemia, or infarction**

> *INCLUDES* Embolization uterine fibroids (37244)

> *EXCLUDES* *Procedure in same operative field:*
> *Angiography (75898)*
> *Transcatheter embolization in same operative field (75894)*

Code also:

> Chemotherapy when provided with embolization procedure (96420-96425)
> Injection radioisotopes when provided with embolization procedure (79445)

🏥 16.3   ≥ 273.   **FUD** 000   J 62

AMA: 2019,Sep,6; 2018,Mar,3; 2018,Jan,8; 2017,Jan,8; 2016,Jan,13

37244 **for arterial or venous hemorrhage or lymphatic extravasation**

> *INCLUDES* Embolization uterine arteries for hemorrhage

🏥 19.3   ≥ 200.   **FUD** 000   J J8

AMA: 2019,Sep,6; 2018,Jul,14; 2018,Mar,3; 2018,Jan,8; 2017,Oct,9; 2017,Jan,8; 2016,Jan,13

37246	Resequenced code. See code following 37235.
37247	Resequenced code. See code following 37235.
37248	Resequenced code. See code following 37235.
37249	Resequenced code. See code following 37235.

37252-37253 Intravascular Ultrasound: Noncoronary

> *INCLUDES* Manipulation and repositioning transducer prior to and after therapeutic interventional procedures

> *EXCLUDES* *Selective or non-selective catheter placement for access (36005-36248)*
> *Transcatheter procedures (37200, 37236-37239, 37241-37244, 61624, 61626)*
> *Vena cava filter procedures (37191-37193, 37197)*

Code first (33361-33369, 33477, 33880-33886, 34701-34708, 34709, [34718], 34710-34711, 34712, 34841-34848, 36010-36015, 36100-36218, 36221-36228, 36245-36248, 36251-36254, 36481, 36555-36571 [36572, 36573], 36578, 36580-36585, 36595, 36901-36909, 37184-37188, 37200, 37211-37218, 37220-37239 [37246, 37247, 37248, 37249], 37241-37244, 61623, 75600-75635, 75705-75774, 75805, 75807, 75810, 75820-75833, 75860-75872, 75885-75898, 75901-75902, 75956-75959, 75970, 76000, 77001, 0075T-0076T, 0234T-0238T, 0338T)

+ **37252** **Intravascular ultrasound (noncoronary vessel) during diagnostic evaluation and/or therapeutic intervention, including radiological supervision and interpretation; initial noncoronary vessel (List separately in addition to code for primary procedure)**

Code first primary procedure

🏥 2.63   ≥ 33.2   **FUD** ZZZ   N N1 80

AMA: 2019,Nov,6; 2018,Jan,8; 2017,Dec,3; 2017,Aug,10; 2017,Mar,3; 2017,Jan,8; 2016,Jul,6; 2016,May,11

+ **37253** **each additional noncoronary vessel (List separately in addition to code for primary procedure)**

Code first (37252)

🏥 2.11   ≥ 5.38   **FUD** ZZZ   N N1 80

AMA: 2019,Nov,6; 2018,Jan,8; 2017,Dec,3; 2017,Aug,10; 2017,Mar,3; 2017,Jan,8; 2016,Jul,6; 2016,May,11

37500-37501 Vascular Endoscopic Procedures

> *INCLUDES* Diagnostic endoscopy
> *EXCLUDES* *Open procedure (37760)*

37500 **Vascular endoscopy, surgical, with ligation of perforator veins, subfascial (SEPS)**

🏥 18.3   ≥ 18.3   **FUD** 090   T A2 50

AMA: 2018,Jan,8; 2017,Jan,8; 2016,Jan,13

37501 **Unlisted vascular endoscopy procedure**

🏥 0.00   ≥ 0.00   **FUD** YYY   T 50

AMA: 2014,Jan,11; 1997,Nov,1

37565-37606 Ligation Procedures: Jugular Vein, Carotid Arteries

CMS: 100-03,160.8 Electroencephalographic Monitoring During Cerebral Vasculature Surgery

> *EXCLUDES* *Arterial balloon occlusion, endovascular, temporary (61623)*
> *Suture arteries and veins (35201-35286)*
> *Transcatheter arterial embolization/occlusion, permanent (61624-61626)*
> *Treatment intracranial aneurysm (61703)*

37565 **Ligation, internal jugular vein**

🏥 20.7   ≥ 20.7   **FUD** 090   T 62 80 50

AMA: 2014,Jan,11; 1997,Nov,1

37600 Ligation; external carotid artery
🔧 21.2 ✂ 21.2 **FUD** 090   T G2 80 ▣
AMA: 2014,Jan,11; 1997,Nov,1

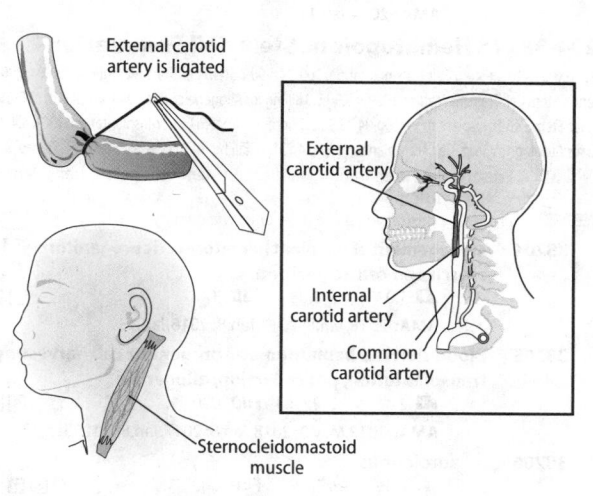

External carotid artery is ligated

External carotid artery

Internal carotid artery

Common carotid artery

Sternocleidomastoid muscle

37605 internal or common carotid artery
🔧 21.4 ✂ 21.4 **FUD** 090   T G2 80 ▣
AMA: 2014,Jan,11; 1997,Nov,1

37606 internal or common carotid artery, with gradual occlusion, as with Selverstone or Crutchfield clamp
🔧 20.7 ✂ 20.7 **FUD** 090   T G2 80 ▣
AMA: 2014,Jan,11; 1997,Nov,1

37607-37609 Ligation Hemodialysis Angioaccess or Temporal Artery
EXCLUDES Suture arteries and veins (35201-35286)

37607 Ligation or banding of angioaccess arteriovenous fistula
🔧 10.8 ✂ 10.8 **FUD** 090   T A2 ▣
AMA: 2014,Jan,11; 1997,Nov,1

37609 Ligation or biopsy, temporal artery
🔧 5.94 ✂ 8.94 **FUD** 010   J A2 50 ▣
AMA: 2014,Jan,11; 1997,Nov,1

37615-37618 Arterial Ligation, Major Vessel, for Injury/Rupture
EXCLUDES Suture arteries and veins (35201-35286)

37615 Ligation, major artery (eg, post-traumatic, rupture); neck
INCLUDES Touroff ligation
🔧 15.3 ✂ 15.3 **FUD** 090   T G2 80 ▣
AMA: 2014,Jan,11; 1997,Nov,1

37616 chest
INCLUDES Bardenheuer operation
🔧 32.0 ✂ 32.0 **FUD** 090   C 80 ▣
AMA: 2014,Jan,11; 1997,Nov,1

37617 abdomen
🔧 38.6 ✂ 38.6 **FUD** 090   C 80 ▣
AMA: 2018,Jan,8; 2017,Jan,8; 2016,Jan,13

37618 extremity
🔧 11.2 ✂ 11.2 **FUD** 090   C 80 ▣
AMA: 2014,Jan,11; 1997,Nov,1

37619 Ligation Inferior Vena Cava
EXCLUDES Suture arteries and veins (35201-35286)
Endovascular delivery inferior vena cava filter (37191)

37619 Ligation of inferior vena cava
🔧 50.0 ✂ 50.0 **FUD** 090   T G2 80 ▣
AMA: 2018,Jan,8; 2017,Jan,8; 2016,Jan,13

37650-37660 Venous Ligation, Femoral and Common Iliac
EXCLUDES Suture arteries and veins (35201-35286)

37650 Ligation of femoral vein
🔧 13.2 ✂ 13.2 **FUD** 090   T A2 50 ▣
AMA: 2014,Jan,11; 1997,Nov,1

37660 Ligation of common iliac vein
🔧 38.3 ✂ 38.3 **FUD** 090   C 80 50 ▣
AMA: 2014,Jan,11; 1997,Nov,1

37700-37785 Treatment of Varicose Veins of Legs
EXCLUDES Suture arteries and veins (35201-35286)

37700 Ligation and division of long saphenous vein at saphenofemoral junction, or distal interruptions
INCLUDES Babcock operation
EXCLUDES Ligation, division, and stripping vein (37718, 37722)
🔧 7.08 ✂ 7.08 **FUD** 090   T A2 50 ▣
AMA: 2018,Mar,3; 2018,Jan,8; 2017,Jan,8; 2016,Jan,13

37718 Ligation, division, and stripping, short saphenous vein
EXCLUDES Ligation, division, and stripping vein (37700, 37735, 37780)
🔧 12.2 ✂ 12.2 **FUD** 090   T A2 50 ▣
AMA: 2018,Mar,3; 2018,Jan,8; 2017,Jan,8

37722 Ligation, division, and stripping, long (greater) saphenous veins from saphenofemoral junction to knee or below
EXCLUDES Ligation, division, and stripping vein (37700, 37718, 37735)
🔧 13.6 ✂ 13.6 **FUD** 090   T A2 50 ▣
AMA: 2018,Mar,3; 2018,Jan,8; 2017,Jan,8

37735 Ligation and division and complete stripping of long or short saphenous veins with radical excision of ulcer and skin graft and/or interruption of communicating veins of lower leg, with excision of deep fascia
EXCLUDES Ligation, division, and stripping vein (37700, 37718, 37722, 37780)
🔧 16.8 ✂ 16.8 **FUD** 090   T A2 50 ▣
AMA: 2018,Mar,3; 2018,Jan,8; 2017,Jan,8; 2016,Jan,13

37760 Ligation of perforator veins, subfascial, radical (Linton type), including skin graft, when performed, open,1 leg
EXCLUDES Duplex scan extremity veins (93971)
Ligation subfascial perforator veins, endoscopic (37500)
Ultrasonic guidance (76937, 76942, 76998)
🔧 18.1 ✂ 18.1 **FUD** 090   T A2 50 ▣
AMA: 2018,Mar,3; 2018,Jan,8; 2017,Jan,8; 2016,Jan,13

37761 Ligation of perforator vein(s), subfascial, open, including ultrasound guidance, when performed, 1 leg
INCLUDES Ultrasonic guidance (76937, 76942, 76998)
EXCLUDES Duplex scan extremity veins (93971)
Ligation subfascial perforator veins, endoscopic (37500)
🔧 15.7 ✂ 15.7 **FUD** 090   T R2 80 50 ▣
AMA: 2018,Mar,3; 2018,Jan,8; 2017,Jan,8; 2016,Jan,13

37765 Stab phlebectomy of varicose veins, 1 extremity; 10-20 stab incisions
EXCLUDES Fewer than 10 incisions (37799)
More than 20 incisions (37766)
🔧 7.88 ✂ 12.6 **FUD** 010   T P3 50 ▣
AMA: 2018,Mar,3; 2018,Jan,8; 2017,Jan,8; 2016,Nov,3; 2016,Jan,13

37766 more than 20 incisions
EXCLUDES Fewer than 10 incisions (37799)
10-20 incisions (37765)
🔧 9.65 ✂ 14.8 **FUD** 010   T P3 50 ▣
AMA: 2018,Mar,3; 2018,Jan,8; 2017,Jan,8; 2016,Nov,3; 2016,Jan,13

37780 Ligation and division of short saphenous vein at saphenopopliteal junction (separate procedure)
🔧 6.75 ✂ 6.75 **FUD** 090   T A2 50 ▣
AMA: 2018,Jan,8; 2017,Jan,8; 2016,Jan,13

37785 Ligation, division, and/or excision of varicose vein cluster(s), 1 leg

⚕ 7.45　✂ 10.0　**FUD** 090　　　T A2 50 ▭

AMA: 2018,Jan,8; 2017,Jan,8; 2016,Jan,13

37788-37790 Treatment of Vascular Disease of the Penis

37788 Penile revascularization, artery, with or without vein graft　♂

⚕ 36.5　✂ 36.5　**FUD** 090　　　C 80 ▭

AMA: 2014,Jan,11; 1997,Nov,1

37790 Penile venous occlusive procedure

⚕ 14.0　✂ 14.0　**FUD** 090　　　J A2 80 ▭

AMA: 2014,Jan,11; 1997,Nov,1

37799 Unlisted Vascular Surgery Procedures

CMS: 100-04,32,161 Intracranial Percutaneous Transluminal Angioplasty (PTA) With Stenting; 100-04,4,180.3 Unlisted Service or Procedure

37799 Unlisted procedure, vascular surgery

⚕ 0.00　✂ 0.00　**FUD** YYY　　　T 80 ▭

AMA: 2019,Dec,5; 2019,Nov,6; 2018,Nov,11; 2018,Jan,8; 2017,Jan,8; 2016,Nov,3; 2016,Jan,13

38100-38200 Splenic Procedures

38100 Splenectomy; total (separate procedure)

⚕ 33.5　✂ 33.5　**FUD** 090　　　C 80 ▭

AMA: 2018,Jan,8; 2017,Jan,8; 2016,Jan,13

Short gastric vessels ligated

Ligated splenic artery

Splenic vein

Pancreas

Gastro-splenic ligament

Ruptured spleen

38101 partial (separate procedure)

⚕ 33.5　✂ 33.5　**FUD** 090　　　C 80 ▭

AMA: 2018,Jan,8; 2017,Jan,8; 2016,Jan,13

+ **38102** total, en bloc for extensive disease, in conjunction with other procedure (List in addition to code for primary procedure)

Code first primary procedure

⚕ 7.63　✂ 7.63　**FUD** ZZZ　　　C 80 ▭

AMA: 2018,Jan,8; 2017,Jan,8; 2016,Jan,13

38115 Repair of ruptured spleen (splenorrhaphy) with or without partial splenectomy

⚕ 37.1　✂ 37.1　**FUD** 090　　　C 80 ▭

AMA: 2018,Jan,8; 2017,Jan,8; 2016,Jan,13

38120 Laparoscopy, surgical, splenectomy

INCLUDES Diagnostic laparoscopy (49320)

⚕ 30.6　✂ 30.6　**FUD** 090　　　J 62 80 ▭

AMA: 2018,Jan,8; 2017,Jan,8; 2016,Jan,13

38129 Unlisted laparoscopy procedure, spleen

⚕ 0.00　✂ 0.00　**FUD** YYY　　　J 80 ▭

AMA: 2018,Jan,8; 2017,Jan,8; 2016,Jan,13

38200 Injection procedure for splenoportography

⚕⚕ (75810)

⚕ 3.85　✂ 3.85　**FUD** 000　　　N N1 80 ▭

AMA: 2014,Jan,11

38204-38215 Hematopoietic Stem Cell Preparation

CMS: 100-03,110.23 Stem Cell Transplantation; 100-04,3,90.3 Stem Cell Transplantation; 100-04,3,90.3.1 Allogeneic Stem Cell Transplantation; 100-04,3,90.3.3 Billing for Allogeneic Stem Cell Transplants; 100-04,32,90 Billing for Stem Cell Transplantation; 100-04,32,90.2.1 Coding for Stem Cell Transplantation; 100-04,4,231.10 Billing for Autologous Stem Cell Transplants; 100-04,4,231.11 Billing for Allogeneic Stem Cell Transplants

INCLUDES Preservation, preparation, purification stem cells before transplant or reinfusion

EXCLUDES *Procedure performed more than one time per day*

38204 Management of recipient hematopoietic progenitor cell donor search and cell acquisition

⚕ 3.03　✂ 3.03　**FUD** XXX　　　N N1 ▭

AMA: 2018,Jan,8; 2017,Jan,8; 2016,Jan,13

38205 Blood-derived hematopoietic progenitor cell harvesting for transplantation, per collection; allogeneic

⚕ 2.44　✂ 2.44　**FUD** 000　　　B 80 ▭

AMA: 2018,May,3; 2018,Jan,8; 2017,Jan,8; 2016,Jan,13

38206 autologous

⚕ 2.39　✂ 2.39　**FUD** 000　　　S G2 80 ▭

AMA: 2018,May,3; 2018,Jan,8; 2017,Jan,8; 2016,Jan,13

38207 Transplant preparation of hematopoietic progenitor cells; cryopreservation and storage

EXCLUDES *Flow cytometry (88182, 88184-88189)*

📷 (88240)

⚕ 1.31　✂ 1.31　**FUD** XXX　　　S G2 ▭

AMA: 2018,Jan,8; 2017,Jan,8; 2016,Jan,13

38208 thawing of previously frozen harvest, without washing, per donor

EXCLUDES *Flow cytometry (88182, 88184-88189)*

📷 (88241)

⚕ 0.83　✂ 0.83　**FUD** XXX　　　S G2 ▭

AMA: 2018,Jan,8; 2017,Jan,8; 2016,Jan,13

38209 thawing of previously frozen harvest, with washing, per donor

EXCLUDES *Flow cytometry (88182, 88184-88189)*

⚕ 0.35　✂ 0.35　**FUD** XXX　　　S G2 ▭

AMA: 2018,Jan,8; 2017,Jan,8; 2016,Jan,13

38210 specific cell depletion within harvest, T-cell depletion

EXCLUDES *Flow cytometry (88182, 88184-88189)*

⚕ 2.29　✂ 2.29　**FUD** XXX　　　S G2 ▭

AMA: 2018,Jan,8; 2017,Jan,8; 2016,Jan,13

38211 tumor cell depletion

EXCLUDES *Flow cytometry (88182, 88184-88189)*

⚕ 2.08　✂ 2.08　**FUD** XXX　　　S G2 ▭

AMA: 2018,Jan,8; 2017,Jan,8; 2016,Jan,13

38212 red blood cell removal

EXCLUDES *Flow cytometry (88182, 88184-88189)*

⚕ 1.39　✂ 1.39　**FUD** XXX　　　S G2 ▭

AMA: 2018,Jan,8; 2017,Jan,8; 2016,Jan,13

38213 platelet depletion

EXCLUDES *Flow cytometry (88182, 88184-88189)*

⚕ 0.35　✂ 0.35　**FUD** XXX　　　S G2 ▭

AMA: 2018,Jan,8; 2017,Jan,8; 2016,Jan,13

38214 plasma (volume) depletion

EXCLUDES *Flow cytometry (88182, 88184-88189)*

⚕ 1.23　✂ 1.23　**FUD** XXX　　　S G2 ▭

AMA: 2018,Jan,8; 2017,Jan,8; 2016,Jan,13

38215 cell concentration in plasma, mononuclear, or buffy coat layer

EXCLUDES *Flow cytometry (88182, 88184-88189)*

⚕ 1.39　✂ 1.39　**FUD** XXX　　　S G2 ▭

AMA: 2018,Jan,8; 2017,Jan,8; 2016,Jan,13

| 26/TC PC/TC Only | A2-Z3 ASC Payment | 50 Bilateral | ♂ Male Only | ♀ Female Only | ⚕ Facility RVU | ✂ Non-Facility RVU | ▭ CCI | ✖ CLIA |
| FUD Follow-up Days | CMS: IOM | AMA: CPT Asst | A-Y OPPSI | | 80/80 Surg Assist Allowed / w/Doc | 📷 Lab Crosswalk | | 📷 Radiology Crosswalk |

176　　　CPT © 2021 American Medical Association. All Rights Reserved.　　　© 2021 Optum360, LLC

38220-38232 Bone Marrow Procedures

CMS: 100-03,110.23 Stem Cell Transplantation; 100-04,3,90.3 Stem Cell Transplantation; 100-04,32,90 Billing for Stem Cell Transplantation; 100-04,4,231.11 Billing for Allogeneic Stem Cell Transplants

38220 **Diagnostic bone marrow; aspiration(s)**

EXCLUDES *Aspiration bone marrow for spinal graft (20939)*
Bone marrow biopsy (38221)
Bone marrow for platelet rich stem cell injection (0232T)
Code also biopsy bone marrow during same session (38222)

🚑 1.99 ⚕ 4.71 **FUD** XXX [J] [P3] [80] [50] [≡]

AMA: 2018,May,3; 2018,Jan,8; 2017,Jan,8; 2016,Jan,13

38221 **biopsy(ies)**

EXCLUDES *Aspiration and biopsy during same session (38222)*
Aspiration bone marrow (38220)

◣ (88305)

🚑 2.00 ⚕ 4.47 **FUD** XXX [J] [P3] [80] [50] [≡]

AMA: 2018,May,3; 2018,Jan,8; 2017,Jan,8; 2016,Jan,13

38222 **biopsy(ies) and aspiration(s)**

EXCLUDES *Aspiration bone marrow only (38221)*
Biopsy bone marrow only (38220)

◣ (88305)

🚑 2.24 ⚕ 4.94 **FUD** XXX [J] [G2] [80] [50] [≡]

AMA: 2018,May,3

38230 **Bone marrow harvesting for transplantation; allogeneic**

EXCLUDES *Aspiration bone marrow for platelet rich stem cell injection (0232T)*
Harvesting blood-derived hematopoietic progenitor cells for transplant (allogeneic) (38205)

🚑 5.92 ⚕ 5.92 **FUD** 000 [S] [G2] [80] [≡]

AMA: 2018,Jan,8; 2017,Jan,8; 2016,Jan,13

38232 **autologous**

EXCLUDES *Aspiration bone marrow (38220, 38222)*
Aspiration bone marrow for platelet rich stem cell injection (0232T)
Aspiration bone marrow for spinal graft (20939)
Harvesting blood-derived peripheral stem cells for transplant (allogenic/autologous) (38205-38206)

🚑 5.76 ⚕ 5.76 **FUD** 000 [S] [G2] [80] [≡]

AMA: 2018,Jan,8; 2017,Jan,8; 2016,Jan,13

38240-38243 [38243] Hematopoietic Progenitor Cell Transplantation

CMS: 100-03,110.23 Stem Cell Transplantation; 100-04,3,90.3 Stem Cell Transplantation; 100-04,3,90.3.1 Allogeneic Stem Cell Transplantation; 100-04,3,90.3.2 Autologous Stem Cell Transplantation (AuSCT); 100-04,3,90.3.3 Billing for Allogeneic Stem Cell Transplants; 100-04,32,90 Billing for Stem Cell Transplantation; 100-04,32,90.2 Allogeneic Stem Cell Transplantation; 100-04,32,90.2.1 Coding for Stem Cell Transplantation; 100-04,32,90.3 Autologous Stem Cell Transplantation; 100-04,32,90.4 Edits Stem Cell Transplant; 100-04,32,90.6 Clinical Trials for Stem Cell Transplant for Myelodysplastic Syndrome (; 100-04,4,231.10 Billing for Autologous Stem Cell Transplants; 100-04,4,231.11 Billing for Allogeneic Stem Cell Transplants

INCLUDES Evaluation patient prior to, during, and after infusion
Management uncomplicated adverse reactions such as hives or nausea
Monitoring physiological parameters
Physician presence during infusion
Supervision clinical staff

EXCLUDES *Administration fluids for transplant or incidental hydration separately*
Concurrent administration medications with infusion for transplant
Cryopreservation, freezing, and storage hematopoietic progenitor cells for transplant (38207)
Human leukocyte antigen (HLA) testing (81379-81383, 86812-86821)
Modification, treatment, processing hematopoietic progenitor cell specimens for transplant (38210-38215)
Thawing and expansion hematopoietic progenitor cells for transplant (38208-38209)

Code also:

Administration medications and/or fluids not related to transplant, append modifier 59

E/M service for treatment more complicated adverse reactions after infusion, as appropriate

Separately identifiable E/M service on same date, appending modifier 25 as appropriate (99211-99215, 99217-99220, [99224, 99225, 99226], 99221-99223, 99231-99239, 99471-99472, 99475-99476)

38240 **Hematopoietic progenitor cell (HPC); allogeneic transplantation per donor**

EXCLUDES *Allogeneic lymphocyte infusions on same date of service with (38242)*
Hematopoietic progenitor cell (HPC); HPC boost on same date of service with ([38243])

🚑 6.78 ⚕ 6.78 **FUD** XXX [J] [G2] [80] [≡]

AMA: 2018,Jan,8; 2017,Jan,8; 2016,Jan,13

38241 **autologous transplantation**

🚑 5.02 ⚕ 5.02 **FUD** XXX [S] [G2] [80] [≡]

AMA: 2018,Jan,8; 2017,Jan,8; 2016,Jan,13

\# **38243** **HPC boost**

EXCLUDES *Allogeneic lymphocyte infusions on same date of service with (38242)*
Hematopoietic progenitor cell (HPC); allogeneic transplantation per donor on same date of service with (38240)

🚑 3.47 ⚕ 3.47 **FUD** 000 [S] [R2] [80] [≡]

AMA: 2018,Jan,8; 2017,Jan,8; 2016,Jan,13

38242 **Allogeneic lymphocyte infusions**

EXCLUDES *Aspiration bone marrow (38220, 38222)*
Aspiration bone marrow for platelet rich stem cell injection (0232T)
Aspiration bone marrow for spinal graft (20939)
Hematopoietic progenitor cell (HPC); allogeneic transplantation per donor on same date of service with (38240)
Hematopoietic progenitor cell (HPC); HPC boost on same service date with ([38243])

◣ (81379-81383, 86812-86813, 86816-86817, 86821)

🚑 3.63 ⚕ 3.63 **FUD** 000 [S] [R2] [80] [≡]

AMA: 2018,Jan,8; 2017,Jan,8; 2016,Jan,13

38243 **Resequenced code. See code following 38241.**

38300-38382 Incision Lymphatic Vessels

38300 **Drainage of lymph node abscess or lymphadenitis; simple**

🚑 5.91 ⚕ 9.40 **FUD** 010 [J] [A2] [≡]

AMA: 2014,Jan,11

38305 **extensive**

🚑 14.1 ⚕ 14.1 **FUD** 090 [J] [A2] [≡]

AMA: 2014,Jan,11

 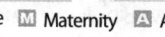

38308 Lymphangiotomy or other operations on lymphatic channels
🚑 13.0 ⚕ 13.0 **FUD** 090   J A2 80 ▣
AMA: 2014,Jan,11

38380 Suture and/or ligation of thoracic duct; cervical approach
🚑 16.3 ⚕ 16.3 **FUD** 090   C 80 ▣
AMA: 2014,Jan,11

38381 thoracic approach
🚑 23.2 ⚕ 23.2 **FUD** 090   C 80 ▣
AMA: 2014,Jan,11

38382 abdominal approach
🚑 19.4 ⚕ 19.4 **FUD** 090   C 80 ▣
AMA: 2014,Jan,11

38500-38555 Biopsy/Excision Lymphatic Vessels

EXCLUDES Injection for sentinel node identification (38792)
Percutaneous needle biopsy retroperitoneal mass (49180)

38500 Biopsy or excision of lymph node(s); open, superficial
EXCLUDES Lymphadenectomy (38700-38780)
🚑 7.38 ⚕ 9.68 **FUD** 010   J A2 50 ▣
AMA: 2019,Feb,8; 2018,Jan,8; 2017,Jan,8; 2016,Jan,13

38505 by needle, superficial (eg, cervical, inguinal, axillary)
EXCLUDES Fine needle aspiration (10004-10012, 10021)
📥 (88172-88173)
📤 (76942, 77002, 77012, 77021)
🚑 2.02 ⚕ 3.55 **FUD** 000   J A2 50 ▣
AMA: 2019,Feb,8; 2018,Jan,8; 2017,Jan,8; 2016,Jan,13

38510 open, deep cervical node(s)
🚑 12.0 ⚕ 14.9 **FUD** 010   J A2 50 ▣
AMA: 2020,Dec,11; 2019,Feb,8; 2018,Jan,8; 2017,Jan,8; 2016,Jan,13

38520 open, deep cervical node(s) with excision scalene fat pad
🚑 13.4 ⚕ 13.4 **FUD** 090   J A2 50 ▣
AMA: 2019,Feb,8; 2018,Jan,8; 2017,Jan,8; 2016,Jan,13

38525 open, deep axillary node(s)
🚑 12.6 ⚕ 12.6 **FUD** 090   J A2 50 ▣
AMA: 2019,Feb,8; 2018,Jan,8; 2017,Jan,8; 2016,Jan,13

38530 open, internal mammary node(s)
EXCLUDES Fine needle aspiration (10005-10012)
Lymphadenectomy (38720-38746)
🚑 16.3 ⚕ 16.3 **FUD** 090   J A2 80 50 ▣
AMA: 2019,Feb,8; 2018,Jan,8; 2017,Jan,8; 2016,Jan,13

38531 open, inguinofemoral node(s)
🚑 12.5 ⚕ 12.5 **FUD** 090   62 80 50 ▣
AMA: 2019,Feb,8

38542 Dissection, deep jugular node(s)
EXCLUDES Complete cervical lymphadenectomy (38720)
🚑 14.8 ⚕ 14.8 **FUD** 090   J A2 80 50 ▣
AMA: 2019,Feb,8; 2018,Jan,8; 2017,Jan,8; 2016,Jan,13

38550 Excision of cystic hygroma, axillary or cervical; without deep neurovascular dissection
🚑 14.7 ⚕ 14.7 **FUD** 090   J A2 80 ▣
AMA: 2014,Jan,11; 1994,Win,1

38555 with deep neurovascular dissection
🚑 29.5 ⚕ 29.5 **FUD** 090   J A2 80 ▣
AMA: 2014,Jan,11; 1994,Win,1

38562-38564 Limited Lymphadenectomy: Staging

38562 Limited lymphadenectomy for staging (separate procedure); pelvic and para-aortic
EXCLUDES Prostatectomy (55812, 55842)
Radioactive substance inserted into prostate (55862)
🚑 20.4 ⚕ 20.4 **FUD** 090   C 80 ▣
AMA: 2019,Feb,8; 2018,Jan,8; 2017,Jan,8; 2016,Jan,13

38564 retroperitoneal (aortic and/or splenic)
🚑 20.4 ⚕ 20.4 **FUD** 090   C 80 ▣
AMA: 2019,Feb,8

38570-38589 Laparoscopic Lymph Node Procedures

INCLUDES Diagnostic laparoscopy (49320)
EXCLUDES Laparoscopy with draining lymphocele to peritoneal cavity (49323)
Limited lymphadenectomy:
Pelvic (38562)
Retroperitoneal (38564)

38570 Laparoscopy, surgical; with retroperitoneal lymph node sampling (biopsy), single or multiple
🚑 14.7 ⚕ 14.7 **FUD** 010   J A2 80 ▣
AMA: 2019,Feb,8; 2018,Jan,8; 2017,Jan,8; 2016,Jan,13

38571 with bilateral total pelvic lymphadenectomy
🚑 19.1 ⚕ 19.1 **FUD** 010   J A2 80 ▣
AMA: 2019,Feb,8; 2018,Jan,8; 2017,Jan,8; 2016,Jan,13

38572 with bilateral total pelvic lymphadenectomy and peri-aortic lymph node sampling (biopsy), single or multiple
EXCLUDES Lymphocele drainage into peritoneal cavity (49323)
🚑 26.3 ⚕ 26.3 **FUD** 010   J A2 80 ▣
AMA: 2019,Feb,8; 2018,Jan,8; 2017,Jan,8; 2016,Jan,13

38573 with bilateral total pelvic lymphadenectomy and peri-aortic lymph node sampling, peritoneal washings, peritoneal biopsy(ies), omentectomy, and diaphragmatic washings, including diaphragmatic and other serosal biopsy(ies), when performed
EXCLUDES Laparoscopic hysterectomy procedures (58541-58554)
Laparoscopic omentopexy (separate procedure) (49326)
Laparoscopy abdomen, diagnostic (separate procedure)(49320)
Laparoscopy unlisted (38589)
Laparoscopy without omentectomy (38570-38572)
Lymphadenectomy for staging (38562-38564)
Omentectomy (separate procedure) (49255)
Pelvic lymphadenectomy external iliac, hypogastric, and obturator nodes (38770)
Retroperitoneal lymphadenectomy aortic, pelvic, and renal nodes (separate procedure) (38780)
🚑 33.5 ⚕ 33.5 **FUD** 010   J 62 80 ▣
AMA: 2019,Mar,5; 2018,Apr,10

38589 Unlisted laparoscopy procedure, lymphatic system
🚑 0.00 ⚕ 0.00 **FUD** YYY   J 80 50 ▣
AMA: 2018,Apr,10; 2018,Jan,8; 2017,Jan,8; 2016,Jan,13

38700-38780 Lymphadenectomy Procedures

INCLUDES Lymph node biopsy/excision (38500)
EXCLUDES Excision lymphedematous skin and subcutaneous tissue (15004-15005)
Limited lymphadenectomy
Pelvic (38562)
Retroperitoneal (38564)
Repair lymphedematous skin and tissue (15570-15650)

38700 Suprahyoid lymphadenectomy
🚑 23.1 ⚕ 23.1 **FUD** 090   J 62 80 50 ▣
AMA: 2020,Dec,11; 2019,Feb,8; 2018,Jan,8; 2017,Jan,8; 2016,Jan,13

38720 Cervical lymphadenectomy (complete)
🚑 38.5 ⚕ 38.5 **FUD** 090   J 62 80 50 ▣
AMA: 2020,Apr,10; 2019,Feb,8; 2018,Jan,8; 2017,Jan,8; 2016,Jan,13

38724 Cervical lymphadenectomy (modified radical neck dissection)
🚑 41.5 ⚕ 41.5 **FUD** 090   C 80 50 ▣
AMA: 2020,Dec,11; 2019,Mar,10; 2019,Feb,8; 2018,Jan,8; 2017,Jan,8; 2016,Jan,13

38740 Axillary lymphadenectomy; superficial
🚑 20.2 ⚕ 20.2 **FUD** 090   J A2 80 50 ▣
AMA: 2019,Feb,8; 2018,Jan,8; 2017,Jan,8; 2016,Jan,13

38745 **complete**
🔧 25.4   ✂ 25.4   **FUD** 090   J A2 80 50 ▣
AMA: 2019,Feb,8

+ **38746** **Thoracic lymphadenectomy by thoracotomy, mediastinal and regional lymphadenectomy (List separately in addition to code for primary procedure)**
INCLUDES   Left side
   Aortopulmonary window
   Inferior pulmonary ligament
   Paraesophageal
   Subcarinal
   Right side
   Inferior pulmonary ligament
   Paraesophageal
   Paratracheal
   Subcarinal
EXCLUDES   *Thoracoscopic mediastinal and regional lymphadenectomy (32674)*
Code first (21601, 31760, 31766, 31786, 32096-32200, 32220-32320, 32440-32491, 32503-32505, 33025, 33030, 33050-33130, 39200-39220, 39560-39561, 43101, 43112, 43117-43118, 43122-43123, 43351, 60270, 60505)
🔧 6.22   ✂ 6.22   **FUD** ZZZ   C 80 ▣
AMA: 2019,Feb,8; 2018,Jan,8; 2017,Jan,8; 2016,Jan,13

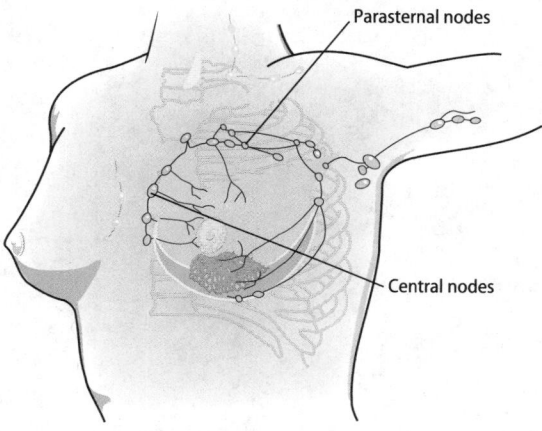

Parasternal nodes

Central nodes

+ **38747** **Abdominal lymphadenectomy, regional, including celiac, gastric, portal, peripancreatic, with or without para-aortic and vena caval nodes (List separately in addition to code for primary procedure)**
Code first primary procedure
🔧 7.77   ✂ 7.77   **FUD** ZZZ   C 80 ▣
AMA: 2020,Apr,10; 2019,Feb,8

38760 **Inguinofemoral lymphadenectomy, superficial, including Cloquet's node (separate procedure)**
🔧 24.2   ✂ 24.2   **FUD** 090   J A2 80 50 ▣
AMA: 2019,Feb,8; 2018,Jan,8; 2017,Jan,8; 2016,Jan,13

38765 **Inguinofemoral lymphadenectomy, superficial, in continuity with pelvic lymphadenectomy, including external iliac, hypogastric, and obturator nodes (separate procedure)**
🔧 37.7   ✂ 37.7   **FUD** 090   C 80 50 ▣
AMA: 2019,Feb,8; 2018,Jan,8; 2017,Jan,8; 2016,Jan,13

38770 **Pelvic lymphadenectomy, including external iliac, hypogastric, and obturator nodes (separate procedure)**
🔧 23.2   ✂ 23.2   **FUD** 090   C 80 50 ▣
AMA: 2019,Feb,8

38780 **Retroperitoneal transabdominal lymphadenectomy, extensive, including pelvic, aortic, and renal nodes (separate procedure)**
🔧 29.9   ✂ 29.9   **FUD** 090   C 80 ▣
AMA: 2019,Feb,8

38790-38999 Cannulation/Injection/Other Procedures

38790 **Injection procedure; lymphangiography**
🔲 (75801-75807)
🔧 2.36   ✂ 2.36   **FUD** 000   N N1 50 ▣
AMA: 2014,Jan,11; 1999,Jul,6

38792 **radioactive tracer for identification of sentinel node**
EXCLUDES   *Sentinel node excision (38500-38542)*
   Sentinel node(s) identification (mapping) intraoperative with nonradioactive dye injection (38900)
🔲 (78195)
🔧 0.97   ✂ 2.37   **FUD** 000   01 N1 50 ▣
AMA: 2019,Feb,8; 2018,Jan,8; 2017,Jan,8; 2016,Jan,13

38794 **Cannulation, thoracic duct**
🔧 8.52   ✂ 8.52   **FUD** 090   N N1 80 ▣
AMA: 2014,Jan,11

+ **38900** **Intraoperative identification (eg, mapping) of sentinel lymph node(s) includes injection of non-radioactive dye, when performed (List separately in addition to code for primary procedure)**
EXCLUDES   *Injection tracer for sentinel node identification (38792)*
Code first (19302, 19307, 38500, 38510, 38520, 38525, 38530-38531, 38542, 38562-38564, 38570-38572, 38740, 38745, 38760, 38765, 38770, 38780, 56630-56634, 56637, 56640)
🔧 4.03   ✂ 4.03   **FUD** ZZZ   N N1 80 50 ▣
AMA: 2019,Feb,8; 2018,Jan,8; 2017,Jan,8; 2016,Jan,13

38999 **Unlisted procedure, hemic or lymphatic system**
🔧 0.00   ✂ 0.00   **FUD** YYY   S 80 ▣
AMA: 2020,Dec,11; 2018,Jan,8; 2017,Jan,8; 2016,Jan,13

39000-39499 Surgical Procedures: Mediastinum

39000 **Mediastinotomy with exploration, drainage, removal of foreign body, or biopsy; cervical approach**
🔧 14.3   ✂ 14.3   **FUD** 090   C 80 ▣
AMA: 2014,Jan,11; 1994,Win,1

39010 **transthoracic approach, including either transthoracic or median sternotomy**
EXCLUDES   *ECMO/ECLS insertion or reposition cannula (33955-33956, [33963, 33964])*
   Video-assisted thoracic surgery (VATS) pericardial biopsy (32604)
🔧 22.7   ✂ 22.7   **FUD** 090   C 80 ▣
AMA: 2018,Jan,8; 2017,Jan,8; 2016,Jan,13

39200 **Resection of mediastinal cyst**
🔧 25.2   ✂ 25.2   **FUD** 090   C 80 ▣
AMA: 2014,Jan,11; 2012,Oct,9-11

39220 **Resection of mediastinal tumor**
EXCLUDES   *Thymectomy (60520)*
   Thyroidectomy, substernal (60270)
   Video-assisted thoracic surgery (VATS) resection cyst, mass, or tumor of mediastinum (32662)
🔧 32.7   ✂ 32.7   **FUD** 090   C 80 ▣
AMA: 2014,Jan,11; 2012,Oct,9-11

39401 **Mediastinoscopy; includes biopsy(ies) of mediastinal mass (eg, lymphoma), when performed**
🔧 8.93   ✂ 8.93   **FUD** 000   J 62 ▣
AMA: 2018,Jan,8; 2017,Jan,8; 2016,Jun,4

39402 **with lymph node biopsy(ies) (eg, lung cancer staging)**
🔧 11.7   ✂ 11.7   **FUD** 000   J 62 ▣
AMA: 2018,Jan,8; 2017,Jan,8; 2016,Jun,4

39499 **Unlisted procedure, mediastinum**
🔧 0.00   ✂ 0.00   **FUD** YYY   C 80 ▣
AMA: 2014,Jan,11

39501-39599 Surgical Procedures: Diaphragm

EXCLUDES Esophagogastric fundoplasty, with fundic patch (43325)
Repair diaphragmatic (esophageal) hernias:
Laparoscopic with fundoplication (43280-43282)
Laparotomy (43332-43333)
Thoracoabdominal (43336-43337)
Thoracotomy (43334-43335)

39501 **Repair, laceration of diaphragm, any approach**
📇 24.6   ⚕ 24.6   **FUD** 090   C 80 ▭
AMA: 2018,Jan,8; 2017,Jan,8; 2016,Jan,13

39503 **Repair, neonatal diaphragmatic hernia, with or without chest tube insertion and with or without creation of ventral hernia** A
📇 173.   ⚕ 173.   **FUD** 090   63 C 80 ▭
AMA: 2018,Jan,8; 2017,Jan,8; 2016,Jan,13

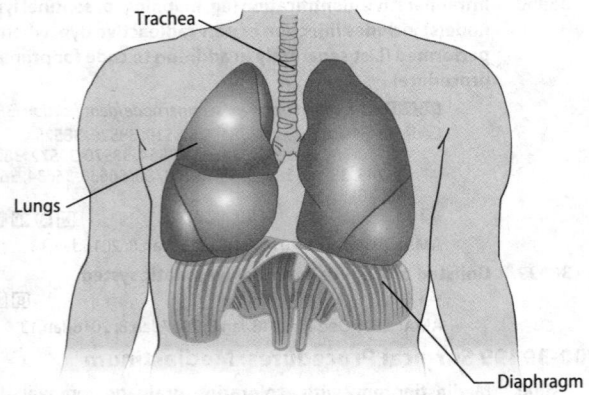

Trachea

Lungs

Diaphragm

A defect of the diaphragm can allow abdominal
contents to herniate into the thoracic cavity

39540 **Repair, diaphragmatic hernia (other than neonatal), traumatic; acute**
📇 25.3   ⚕ 25.3   **FUD** 090   C 80 ▭
AMA: 2018,Jan,8; 2017,Jan,8; 2016,Jan,13

39541 **chronic**
📇 27.3   ⚕ 27.3   **FUD** 090   C 80 ▭
AMA: 2018,Jan,8; 2017,Jan,8; 2016,Jan,13

39545 **Imbrication of diaphragm for eventration, transthoracic or transabdominal, paralytic or nonparalytic**
📇 25.8   ⚕ 25.8   **FUD** 090   C 80 ▭
AMA: 2018,Jan,8; 2017,Jan,8; 2016,Jan,13

39560 **Resection, diaphragm; with simple repair (eg, primary suture)**
📇 23.1   ⚕ 23.1   **FUD** 090   C 80 ▭
AMA: 2018,Jan,8; 2017,Jan,8; 2016,Jan,13

39561 **with complex repair (eg, prosthetic material, local muscle flap)**
📇 35.9   ⚕ 35.9   **FUD** 090   C 80 ▭
AMA: 2018,Jan,8; 2017,Jan,8; 2016,Jan,13

39599 **Unlisted procedure, diaphragm**
EXCLUDES Insertion/replacement diaphragmatic stimulation
system (0674T-0675T, 0680T)
📇 0.00   ⚕ 0.00   **FUD** YYY   C 80 ▭
AMA: 2014,Jan,11

40490-40799 Resection and Repair Procedures of the Lips

EXCLUDES *Procedures on skin of lips — see integumentary section codes*

40490 **Biopsy of lip**
🔧 2.03 ⚕ 3.55 **FUD** 000 [T] [P3] [▢]
AMA: 2019,Jan,9

40500 **Vermilionectomy (lip shave), with mucosal advancement**
🔧 10.4 ⚕ 14.7 **FUD** 090 [J] [A2] [▢]
AMA: 2014,Jan,11; 2000,Sep,11

40510 **Excision of lip; transverse wedge excision with primary closure**
EXCLUDES *Excision mucous lesions (40810-40816)*
🔧 10.0 ⚕ 13.9 **FUD** 090 [J] [A2] [▢]
AMA: 2014,Jan,11

40520 **V-excision with primary direct linear closure**
EXCLUDES *Excision mucous lesions (40810-40816)*
🔧 10.2 ⚕ 14.2 **FUD** 090 [J] [A2] [▢]
AMA: 2014,Jan,11; 2000,Sep,11

40525 **full thickness, reconstruction with local flap (eg, Estlander or fan)**
🔧 15.8 ⚕ 15.8 **FUD** 090 [J] [A2] [▢]
AMA: 2014,Jan,11

40527 **full thickness, reconstruction with cross lip flap (Abbe-Estlander)**
INCLUDES *Cleft lip repair with cross lip pedicle flap (Abbe-Estlander type), without pedicle sectioning and insertion*
EXCLUDES *Cleft lip repair with cross lip pedicle flap (Abbe-Estlander type), with pedicle sectioning and insertion (40761)*
🔧 17.7 ⚕ 17.7 **FUD** 090 [J] [A2] [80] [▢]
AMA: 2014,Jan,11

40530 **Resection of lip, more than one-fourth, without reconstruction**
EXCLUDES *Reconstruction (13131-13153)*
🔧 11.4 ⚕ 15.6 **FUD** 090 [J] [A2] [▢]
AMA: 2014,Jan,11

40650 **Repair lip, full thickness; vermilion only**
🔧 8.79 ⚕ 13.2 **FUD** 090 [T] [A2] [80] [▢]
AMA: 2018,Jan,8; 2017,Jan,8; 2016,Nov,7; 2016,Jan,13

40652 **up to half vertical height**
🔧 10.2 ⚕ 14.5 **FUD** 090 [T] [A2] [80] [▢]
AMA: 2018,Jan,8; 2017,Jan,8; 2016,Nov,7; 2016,Jan,13

40654 **over one-half vertical height, or complex**
🔧 12.1 ⚕ 16.5 **FUD** 090 [T] [A2] [▢]
AMA: 2018,Jan,8; 2017,Jan,8; 2016,Nov,7

40700 **Plastic repair of cleft lip/nasal deformity; primary, partial or complete, unilateral**
EXCLUDES *Cleft lip repair with cross lip pedicle flap (Abbe-Estlander type):*
With pedicle sectioning and insertion (40761)
Without pedicle sectioning and insertion (40527)
Rhinoplasty for nasal deformity secondary to congenital cleft lip (30460, 30462)
🔧 29.2 ⚕ 29.2 **FUD** 090 [J] [A2] [80] [▢]
AMA: 2018,Jan,8; 2017,Jan,8; 2016,Jan,13

40701 **primary bilateral, 1-stage procedure**
EXCLUDES *Cleft lip repair with cross lip pedicle flap (Abbe-Estlander type):*
With pedicle sectioning and insertion (40761)
Without pedicle sectioning and insertion (40527)
Rhinoplasty for nasal deformity secondary to congenital cleft lip (30460, 30462)
🔧 34.6 ⚕ 34.6 **FUD** 090 [J] [A2] [80] [▢]
AMA: 2018,Jan,8; 2017,Jan,8; 2016,Jan,13

Bilateral cleft lip

Cleft margins on both sides are incised

Margins are closed, correcting cleft

40702 **primary bilateral, 1 of 2 stages**
EXCLUDES *Cleft lip repair with cross lip pedicle flap (Abbe-Estlander type):*
With pedicle sectioning and insertion (40761)
Without pedicle sectioning and insertion (40527)
Rhinoplasty for nasal deformity secondary to congenital cleft lip (30460, 30462)
🔧 29.0 ⚕ 29.0 **FUD** 090 [J] [R2] [80] [▢]
AMA: 2018,Jan,8; 2017,Jan,8; 2016,Jan,13

40720 **secondary, by recreation of defect and reclosure**
EXCLUDES *Cleft lip repair with cross lip pedicle flap (Abbe-Estlander type):*
With pedicle sectioning and insertion (40761)
Without pedicle sectioning and insertion (40527)
Rhinoplasty for nasal deformity secondary to congenital cleft lip (30460, 30462)
🔧 29.8 ⚕ 29.8 **FUD** 090 [J] [A2] [80] [50] [▢]
AMA: 2018,Jan,8; 2017,Jan,8; 2016,Jan,13

40761 **with cross lip pedicle flap (Abbe-Estlander type), including sectioning and inserting of pedicle**
EXCLUDES *Cleft lip repair with cross lip pedicle flap (Abbe-Estlander type) without sectioning and insertion pedicle (40527)*
Cleft palate repair (42200-42225)
Other reconstructive procedures (14060-14061, 15120-15261, 15574, 15576, 15630)
🔧 31.3 ⚕ 31.3 **FUD** 090 [J] [A2]
AMA: 2014,Jan,11

40799 **Unlisted procedure, lips**
🔧 0.00 ⚕ 0.00 **FUD** YYY [T] [80] [▢]
AMA: 2014,Jan,11

40800-40819 Incision and Resection of Buccal Cavity

INCLUDES *Mucosal/submucosal tissue of lips/cheeks*
Oral cavity outside dentoalveolar structures

40800 **Drainage of abscess, cyst, hematoma, vestibule of mouth; simple**
🔧 3.56 ⚕ 5.96 **FUD** 010 [T] [P3] [▢]
AMA: 2014,Jan,11

40801 **complicated**
🔧 5.96 ⚕ 8.59 **FUD** 010 [T] [A2] [▢]
AMA: 2014,Jan,11

40804 **Removal of embedded foreign body, vestibule of mouth; simple**
🔧 3.37 ⚕ 5.48 **FUD** 010 [Q1] [N1] [80] [▢]
AMA: 2014,Jan,11

40490 — 40804

Digestive System

40805 — 41018

40805   **complicated**
6.43   8.91   **FUD** 010   T P3
AMA: 2014,Jan,11

40806   **Incision of labial frenum (frenotomy)**
0.87   2.84   **FUD** 000   T P3 80
AMA: 2014,Jan,11

40808   **Biopsy, vestibule of mouth**
2.47   4.54   **FUD** 010   T P3
AMA: 2019,Jan,9

40810   **Excision of lesion of mucosa and submucosa, vestibule of mouth; without repair**
3.64   5.99   **FUD** 010   J P3
AMA: 2014,Jan,11

40812   **with simple repair**
5.63   8.30   **FUD** 010   J P3
AMA: 2014,Jan,11

40814   **with complex repair**
8.41   10.8   **FUD** 090   J A2
AMA: 2014,Jan,11

40816   **complex, with excision of underlying muscle**
8.81   11.4   **FUD** 090   J A2
AMA: 2014,Jan,11

40818   **Excision of mucosa of vestibule of mouth as donor graft**
7.78   10.4   **FUD** 090   T A2 80
AMA: 2014,Jan,11

40819   **Excision of frenum, labial or buccal (frenumectomy, frenulectomy, frenectomy)**
6.79   9.05   **FUD** 090   T A2 80
AMA: 2020,Aug,14

40820 Destruction of Lesion of Buccal Cavity

CMS: 100-03,140.5 Laser Procedures
INCLUDES   Mucosal/submucosal tissue lips/cheeks
Oral cavity outside dentoalveolar structures

40820   **Destruction of lesion or scar of vestibule of mouth by physical methods (eg, laser, thermal, cryo, chemical)**
4.78   7.42   **FUD** 010   J P3
AMA: 2014,Jan,11; 1997,Nov,1

40830-40899 Repair Procedures of the Buccal Cavity

INCLUDES   Mucosal/submucosal tissue lips/cheeks
Oral cavity outside dentoalveolar structures
EXCLUDES   Skin grafts (15002-15630)

40830   **Closure of laceration, vestibule of mouth; 2.5 cm or less**
4.84   7.98   **FUD** 010   T G2 80
AMA: 2014,Jan,11

40831   **over 2.5 cm or complex**
6.64   10.1   **FUD** 010   T A2 80
AMA: 2014,Jan,11

40840   **Vestibuloplasty; anterior**
18.0   23.5   **FUD** 090   J A2 80
AMA: 2014,Jan,11

40842   **posterior, unilateral**
19.5   26.2   **FUD** 090   J A2 80
AMA: 2014,Jan,11

40843   **posterior, bilateral**
23.6   30.1   **FUD** 090   J A2 80
AMA: 2014,Jan,11

40844   **entire arch**
34.2   42.9   **FUD** 090   J A2 80
AMA: 2014,Jan,11

40845   **complex (including ridge extension, muscle repositioning)**
35.2   42.2   **FUD** 090   J A2 80
AMA: 2014,Jan,11

40899   **Unlisted procedure, vestibule of mouth**
0.00   0.00   **FUD** YYY   T 80
AMA: 2014,Jan,11

41000-41018 Surgical Incision of Floor of Mouth or Tongue

EXCLUDES   Frenoplasty (41520)

41000   **Intraoral incision and drainage of abscess, cyst, or hematoma of tongue or floor of mouth; lingual**
3.13   4.54   **FUD** 010   T P3
AMA: 2014,Jan,11

A small incision is made in the floor of the mouth; the cyst is opened and the fluid is drained

Cyst and line of incision

41005   **sublingual, superficial**
3.30   6.20   **FUD** 010   T A2 80
AMA: 2014,Jan,11

41006   **sublingual, deep, supramylohyoid**
6.85   9.81   **FUD** 090   T A2 80
AMA: 2014,Jan,11

41007   **submental space**
6.64   9.63   **FUD** 090   T A2 80
AMA: 2014,Jan,11

41008   **submandibular space**
7.45   10.9   **FUD** 090   J A2 80
AMA: 2014,Jan,11

41009   **masticator space**
8.19   11.8   **FUD** 090   T A2 80
AMA: 2014,Jan,11

41010   **Incision of lingual frenum (frenotomy)**
3.09   5.97   **FUD** 010   T A2 80
AMA: 2020,Aug,14; 2018,Jan,8; 2017,Nov,10; 2017,Sep,14

41015   **Extraoral incision and drainage of abscess, cyst, or hematoma of floor of mouth; sublingual**
8.92   11.6   **FUD** 090   T A2 80
AMA: 2014,Jan,11

41016   **submental**
9.92   13.0   **FUD** 090   J A2 80
AMA: 2014,Jan,11

41017   **submandibular**
9.86   12.9   **FUD** 090   J A2 80
AMA: 2014,Jan,11

41018   **masticator space**
11.4   14.5   **FUD** 090   T A2 80
AMA: 2014,Jan,11

26/TC PC/TC Only   A2-Z3 ASC Payment   50 Bilateral   ♂ Male Only   ♀ Female Only   Facility RVU   Non-Facility RVU   CCI   CLIA
FUD Follow-up Days   **CMS:** IOM   **AMA:** CPT Asst   A-Y OPPSI   80/80 Surg Assist Allowed / w/Doc   Lab Crosswalk   Radiology Crosswalk

182   CPT © 2021 American Medical Association. All Rights Reserved.   © 2021 Optum360, LLC

41019 Placement of Devices for Brachytherapy

EXCLUDES *Application interstitial radioelements (77770-77772, 77778)*
Intracranial brachytherapy radiation sources with stereotactic insertion (61770)

41019 Placement of needles, catheters, or other device(s) into the head and/or neck region (percutaneous, transoral, or transnasal) for subsequent interstitial radioelement application
(76942, 77002, 77012, 77021)
13.9 13.9 **FUD** 000
J G2 80
AMA: 2018,Jan,8; 2017,Jan,8; 2016,Jan,13

41100-41599 Resection and Repair of the Tongue

41100 Biopsy of tongue; anterior two-thirds
3.07 4.94 **FUD** 010
T P3
AMA: 2019,Jan,9

Anterior (front) two-thirds of tongue makes up most of the easily visible portions

Anterior two-thirds

Lesion and elliptical incision

41105 posterior one-third
3.11 5.05 **FUD** 010
J P3
AMA: 2014,Jan,11

41108 Biopsy of floor of mouth
2.52 4.43 **FUD** 010
J P3
AMA: 2019,Jan,9

41110 Excision of lesion of tongue without closure
3.73 6.29 **FUD** 010
J P3
AMA: 2014,Jan,11

41112 Excision of lesion of tongue with closure; anterior two-thirds
7.03 9.57 **FUD** 090
J A2
AMA: 2014,Jan,11

41113 posterior one-third
7.98 10.5 **FUD** 090
J A2
AMA: 2014,Jan,11

41114 with local tongue flap
INCLUDES *Excision lesion tongue with closure anterior/posterior two-thirds (41112-41113)*
17.7 17.7 **FUD** 090
J A2 80
AMA: 2014,Jan,11

41115 Excision of lingual frenum (frenectomy)
4.16 7.25 **FUD** 010
T P3 80
AMA: 2018,Jan,8; 2017,Nov,10; 2017,Sep,14

41116 Excision, lesion of floor of mouth
6.18 9.50 **FUD** 090
J A2
AMA: 2014,Jan,11

41120 Glossectomy; less than one-half tongue
30.3 30.3 **FUD** 090
J A2 80
AMA: 2018,Jan,8; 2017,Jan,8; 2016,Jan,13

41130 hemiglossectomy
38.0 38.0 **FUD** 090
C 80
AMA: 2018,Jan,8; 2017,Jan,8; 2016,Jan,13

41135 partial, with unilateral radical neck dissection
62.0 62.0 **FUD** 090
C 80
AMA: 2018,Jan,8; 2017,Jan,8; 2016,Jan,13

41140 complete or total, with or without tracheostomy, without radical neck dissection
INCLUDES *Regnoli's excision*
62.3 62.3 **FUD** 090
C 80
AMA: 2018,Jan,8; 2017,Jan,8; 2016,Jan,13

41145 complete or total, with or without tracheostomy, with unilateral radical neck dissection
78.9 78.9 **FUD** 090
C 80
AMA: 2018,Jan,8; 2017,Jan,8; 2016,Jan,13

41150 composite procedure with resection floor of mouth and mandibular resection, without radical neck dissection
62.8 62.8 **FUD** 090
C 80
AMA: 2018,Jan,8; 2017,Jan,8; 2016,Jan,13

41153 composite procedure with resection floor of mouth, with suprahyoid neck dissection
68.8 68.8 **FUD** 090
C 80
AMA: 2018,Jan,8; 2017,Jan,8; 2016,Jan,13

41155 composite procedure with resection floor of mouth, mandibular resection, and radical neck dissection (Commando type)
86.1 86.1 **FUD** 090
C 80
AMA: 2018,Jan,8; 2017,Jan,8; 2016,Jan,13

41250 Repair of laceration 2.5 cm or less; floor of mouth and/or anterior two-thirds of tongue
4.43 7.98 **FUD** 010
Q1 N1 80
AMA: 2014,Jan,11

41251 posterior one-third of tongue
5.27 8.83 **FUD** 010
T A2 80
AMA: 2014,Jan,11

41252 Repair of laceration of tongue, floor of mouth, over 2.6 cm or complex
6.01 9.18 **FUD** 010
T A2 80
AMA: 2014,Jan,11

41510 Suture of tongue to lip for micrognathia (Douglas type procedure)
13.0 13.0 **FUD** 090
J A2 80
AMA: 2018,Jan,8; 2017,Jan,8; 2016,Jan,13

41512 Tongue base suspension, permanent suture technique
EXCLUDES *Suture tongue to lip for micrognathia (41510)*
18.8 18.8 **FUD** 090
J G2 80
AMA: 2018,Jan,8; 2017,Jan,8; 2016,Jan,13

41520 Frenoplasty (surgical revision of frenum, eg, with Z-plasty)
EXCLUDES *Frenotomy (40806, 41010)*
7.11 10.1 **FUD** 090
J A2 80
AMA: 2020,Aug,14; 2018,Jan,8; 2017,Nov,10; 2017,Sep,14

41530 Submucosal ablation of the tongue base, radiofrequency, 1 or more sites, per session
10.7 27.4 **FUD** 000
J P3 80
AMA: 2018,Jan,8; 2017,Jan,8; 2016,Jan,13

41599 Unlisted procedure, tongue, floor of mouth
0.00 0.00 **FUD** YYY
T 80
AMA: 2018,Jan,8; 2017,Jan,8; 2016,Jan,13

41800-41899 Procedures of the Teeth and Supporting Structures

41800 Drainage of abscess, cyst, hematoma from dentoalveolar structures
4.35 8.29 **FUD** 010
Q1 N1
AMA: 2014,Jan,11

41805 Removal of embedded foreign body from dentoalveolar structures; soft tissues
5.42 8.45 **FUD** 010
T P3 80
AMA: 2014,Jan,11

41806 bone
7.86 11.4 **FUD** 010
T P3 80
AMA: 2014,Jan,11

Digestive System

41820 — 42225

41820 Gingivectomy, excision gingiva, each quadrant
🔶 0.00 🔧 0.00 **FUD** 000 [J] [R2] [80] 🔲
AMA: 2014,Jan,11

Gingival recession

Excessive mucosal growth

Gingivitis is an inflammatory response to bacteria on the teeth; it is characterized by tender, red, swollen gums and can lead to gingival recession

41821 Operculectomy, excision pericoronal tissues
🔶 0.00 🔧 0.00 **FUD** 000 [T] [G2] [80] 🔲
AMA: 2014,Jan,11

41822 Excision of fibrous tuberosities, dentoalveolar structures
🔶 5.71 🔧 9.88 **FUD** 010 [T] [P3] [80] 🔲
AMA: 2014,Jan,11

41823 Excision of osseous tuberosities, dentoalveolar structures
🔶 10.2 🔧 14.5 **FUD** 090 [J] [P3] [80] 🔲
AMA: 2014,Jan,11

41825 Excision of lesion or tumor (except listed above), dentoalveolar structures; without repair
EXCLUDES Lesion destruction nonexcisional (41850)
🔶 3.43 🔧 6.19 **FUD** 010 [J] [P3] 🔲
AMA: 2014,Jan,11

41826 with simple repair
EXCLUDES Lesion destruction nonexcisional (41850)
🔶 5.88 🔧 8.96 **FUD** 010 [J] [P3] 🔲
AMA: 2014,Jan,11

41827 with complex repair
EXCLUDES Lesion destruction nonexcisional (41850)
🔶 8.59 🔧 12.7 **FUD** 090 [J] [A2] 🔲
AMA: 2014,Jan,11

41828 Excision of hyperplastic alveolar mucosa, each quadrant (specify)
🔶 6.43 🔧 9.95 **FUD** 010 [J] [P3] [80] 🔲
AMA: 2014,Jan,11; 1994,Win,1

41830 Alveolectomy, including curettage of osteitis or sequestrectomy
🔶 8.91 🔧 13.0 **FUD** 010 [J] [P3] [80] 🔲
AMA: 2014,Jan,11

41850 Destruction of lesion (except excision), dentoalveolar structures
🔶 0.00 🔧 0.00 **FUD** 000 [T] [R2] [80] 🔲
AMA: 2014,Jan,11

41870 Periodontal mucosal grafting
🔶 0.00 🔧 0.00 **FUD** 000 [J] [G2] [80] 🔲
AMA: 2014,Jan,11

41872 Gingivoplasty, each quadrant (specify)
🔶 8.54 🔧 12.8 **FUD** 090 [J] [P3] [80] 🔲
AMA: 2014,Jan,11; 1994,Win,1

41874 Alveoloplasty, each quadrant (specify)
EXCLUDES Fracture reduction (21421-21490)
Laceration closure (40830-40831)
Maxilla osteotomy, segmental (21206)
🔶 7.21 🔧 11.2 **FUD** 090 [J] [P3] [80] 🔲
AMA: 2014,Jan,11; 1994,Win,1

41899 Unlisted procedure, dentoalveolar structures
🔶 0.00 🔧 0.00 **FUD** YYY [T] [80] 🔲
AMA: 2014,Jan,11

42000-42299 Procedures of the Palate and Uvula

42000 Drainage of abscess of palate, uvula
🔶 2.98 🔧 4.49 **FUD** 010 [T] [A2] [80] 🔲
AMA: 2014,Jan,11

42100 Biopsy of palate, uvula
🔶 3.08 🔧 4.22 **FUD** 010 [T] [P3] 🔲
AMA: 2014,Jan,11

42104 Excision, lesion of palate, uvula; without closure
🔶 3.90 🔧 6.20 **FUD** 010 [J] [P3] 🔲
AMA: 2014,Jan,11

42106 with simple primary closure
🔶 4.86 🔧 7.62 **FUD** 010 [J] [P3] 🔲
AMA: 2014,Jan,11

42107 with local flap closure
EXCLUDES Mucosal graft (40818)
Skin graft (14040-14302)
🔶 9.73 🔧 13.2 **FUD** 090 [J] [A2] 🔲
AMA: 2014,Jan,11

42120 Resection of palate or extensive resection of lesion
EXCLUDES Palate reconstruction using extraoral tissue (14040-14302, 15050, 15120, 15240, 15576)
🔶 28.7 🔧 28.7 **FUD** 090 [J] [A2] [80] 🔲
AMA: 2014,Jan,11; 1991,Fall,1

42140 Uvulectomy, excision of uvula
🔶 4.46 🔧 8.04 **FUD** 090 [J] [A2] 🔲
AMA: 2014,Jan,11

42145 Palatopharyngoplasty (eg, uvulopalatopharyngoplasty, uvulopharyngoplasty)
EXCLUDES Excision maxillary torus palatinus (21032)
Excision torus mandibularis (21031)
🔶 19.8 🔧 19.8 **FUD** 090 [J] [A2] 🔲
AMA: 2018,Jan,8; 2017,Jan,8; 2016,Jan,13

42160 Destruction of lesion, palate or uvula (thermal, cryo or chemical)
🔶 4.15 🔧 6.71 **FUD** 010 [J] [P3] [80] 🔲
AMA: 2018,Jan,8; 2017,Jan,8; 2016,Jan,13

42180 Repair, laceration of palate; up to 2 cm
🔶 5.28 🔧 7.17 **FUD** 010 [T] [A2] [80] 🔲
AMA: 2014,Jan,11

42182 over 2 cm or complex
🔶 7.34 🔧 9.34 **FUD** 010 [J] [A2] [80] 🔲
AMA: 2014,Jan,11

42200 Palatoplasty for cleft palate, soft and/or hard palate only
🔶 27.2 🔧 27.2 **FUD** 090 [J] [A2] [80] 🔲
AMA: 2018,Jan,8; 2017,Jan,8; 2016,Jan,13

42205 Palatoplasty for cleft palate, with closure of alveolar ridge; soft tissue only
🔶 28.4 🔧 28.4 **FUD** 090 [J] [A2] [80] 🔲
AMA: 2014,Jan,11

42210 with bone graft to alveolar ridge (includes obtaining graft)
🔶 31.7 🔧 31.7 **FUD** 090 [J] [J8] [80] 🔲
AMA: 2014,Jan,11

42215 Palatoplasty for cleft palate; major revision
🔶 20.7 🔧 20.7 **FUD** 090 [J] [A2] [80] 🔲
AMA: 2014,Jan,11

42220 secondary lengthening procedure
🔶 17.0 🔧 17.0 **FUD** 090 [J] [A2] [80] 🔲
AMA: 2014,Jan,11

42225 attachment pharyngeal flap
🔶 28.2 🔧 28.2 **FUD** 090 [J] [G2] [80] 🔲
AMA: 2018,Jan,8; 2017,Jan,8; 2016,Jan,13

42226 **Lengthening of palate, and pharyngeal flap**
  25.3   25.3   **FUD** 090   J A2 80 ▭
  AMA: 2014,Jan,11

42227 **Lengthening of palate, with island flap**
  23.6   23.6   **FUD** 090   J G2 80 ▭
  AMA: 2014,Jan,11

42235 **Repair of anterior palate, including vomer flap**
  EXCLUDES Oronasal fistula repair (30600)
  20.7   20.7   **FUD** 090   J A2 80 ▭
  AMA: 2018,Jan,8; 2017,Jan,8; 2016,Jan,13

42260 **Repair of nasolabial fistula**
  EXCLUDES Cleft lip repair (40700-40761)
  18.9   23.8   **FUD** 090   J A2 80 ▭
  AMA: 2014,Jan,11

42280 **Maxillary impression for palatal prosthesis**
  3.12   5.08   **FUD** 010   T P3 80 ▭
  AMA: 2014,Jan,11

42281 **Insertion of pin-retained palatal prosthesis**
  4.64   6.51   **FUD** 010   J G2 80 ▭
  AMA: 2014,Jan,11

42299 **Unlisted procedure, palate, uvula**
  0.00   0.00   **FUD** YYY   T 80 ▭
  AMA: 2018,Jan,8; 2017,Jan,8; 2016,Jan,13

42300-42699 Procedures of the Salivary Ducts and Glands

42300 **Drainage of abscess; parotid, simple**
  4.39   6.10   **FUD** 010   T A2 ▭
  AMA: 2014,Jan,11

42305 **parotid, complicated**
  12.2   12.2   **FUD** 090   J A2 80 ▭
  AMA: 2014,Jan,11

42310 **Drainage of abscess; submaxillary or sublingual, intraoral**
  3.81   4.99   **FUD** 010   T A2 80 ▭
  AMA: 2014,Jan,11

42320 **submaxillary, external**
  5.03   7.31   **FUD** 010   T A2 80 ▭
  AMA: 2014,Jan,11

42330 **Sialolithotomy; submandibular (submaxillary), sublingual or parotid, uncomplicated, intraoral**
  4.69   6.63   **FUD** 010   J P3 ▭
  AMA: 2014,Jan,11

42335 **submandibular (submaxillary), complicated, intraoral**
  7.37   11.5   **FUD** 090   J P3 ▭
  AMA: 2014,Jan,11

42340 **parotid, extraoral or complicated intraoral**
  9.65   14.1   **FUD** 090   J A2 80 50 ▭
  AMA: 2014,Jan,11

42400 **Biopsy of salivary gland; needle**
  EXCLUDES Fine needle aspiration (10021, [10004, 10005, 10006, 10007, 10008, 10009, 10010, 10011, 10012])
   (76942, 77002, 77012, 77021)
   (88172-88173)
  1.54   2.95   **FUD** 000   T P3 ▭
  AMA: 2019,Apr,4

42405 **incisional**
   (76942, 77002, 77012, 77021)
  6.48   8.61   **FUD** 010   J A2 ▭
  AMA: 2014,Jan,11

42408 **Excision of sublingual salivary cyst (ranula)**
  10.0   15.0   **FUD** 090   J A2 80 ▭
  AMA: 2014,Jan,11

42409 **Marsupialization of sublingual salivary cyst (ranula)**
  6.42   10.4   **FUD** 090   J A2 80 ▭
  AMA: 2014,Jan,11

42410 **Excision of parotid tumor or parotid gland; lateral lobe, without nerve dissection**
  EXCLUDES Facial nerve suture or graft (64864, 64865, 69740, 69745)
  17.9   17.9   **FUD** 090   J A2 80 50 ▭
  AMA: 2014,Jan,11

42415 **lateral lobe, with dissection and preservation of facial nerve**
  EXCLUDES Facial nerve suture or graft (64864, 64865, 69740, 69745)
  30.2   30.2   **FUD** 090   J A2 80 50 ▭
  AMA: 2014,Jan,11

42420 **total, with dissection and preservation of facial nerve**
  EXCLUDES Facial nerve suture or graft (64864, 64865, 69740, 69745)
  33.9   33.9   **FUD** 090   J A2 80 50 ▭
  AMA: 2014,Jan,11; 2010,Aug,3-7

42425 **total, en bloc removal with sacrifice of facial nerve**
  EXCLUDES Facial nerve suture or graft (64864, 64865, 69740, 69745)
  23.9   23.9   **FUD** 090   J A2 80 50 ▭
  AMA: 2014,Jan,11

42426 **total, with unilateral radical neck dissection**
  EXCLUDES Facial nerve suture or graft (64864, 64865, 69740, 69745)
  38.8   38.8   **FUD** 090   C 80 50 ▭
  AMA: 2018,Jan,8; 2017,Jan,8; 2016,Jan,13

42440 **Excision of submandibular (submaxillary) gland**
  11.8   11.8   **FUD** 090   J A2 80 50 ▭
  AMA: 2014,Jan,11

42450 **Excision of sublingual gland**
  10.3   13.1   **FUD** 090   J A2 ▭
  AMA: 2014,Jan,11

42500 **Plastic repair of salivary duct, sialodochoplasty; primary or simple**
  9.71   12.4   **FUD** 090   J A2 80 ▭
  AMA: 2014,Jan,11

42505 **secondary or complicated**
  12.9   15.9   **FUD** 090   J A2
  AMA: 2014,Jan,11

42507 **Parotid duct diversion, bilateral (Wilke type procedure);**
  14.4   14.4   **FUD** 090   J A2 80 ▭
  AMA: 2014,Jan,11

42509 **with excision of both submandibular glands**
  23.6   23.6   **FUD** 090   J A2 80 ▭
  AMA: 2014,Jan,11

42510 **with ligation of both submandibular (Wharton's) ducts**
  17.5   17.5   **FUD** 090   J A2 80 ▭
  AMA: 2014,Jan,11

42550 **Injection procedure for sialography**
   (70390)
  1.83   4.39   **FUD** 000   N N1 ▭
  AMA: 2014,Jan,11

42600 **Closure salivary fistula**
  9.99   14.5   **FUD** 090   J A2 80 ▭
  AMA: 2014,Jan,11

42650 **Dilation salivary duct**
  1.65   2.25   **FUD** 000   T P3 ▭
  AMA: 2014,Jan,11

42660 **Dilation and catheterization of salivary duct, with or without injection**
  2.52   3.52   **FUD** 000   T P3 80 ▭
  AMA: 2014,Jan,11

42665 **Ligation salivary duct, intraoral**
  5.97   9.82   **FUD** 090   J A2 80 ▭
  AMA: 2014,Jan,11

Digestive System

42699   **Unlisted procedure, salivary glands or ducts**
🚑 0.00   ⚕ 0.00   **FUD** YYY   [T] [80] [CCI]
AMA: 2014,Jan,11

42700-42999 Procedures of the Adenoids/Throat/Tonsils

42700   **Incision and drainage abscess; peritonsillar**
🚑 3.88   ⚕ 5.43   **FUD** 010   [T] [A2] [CCI]
AMA: 2014,Jan,11

42720   **retropharyngeal or parapharyngeal, intraoral approach**
🚑 11.1   ⚕ 12.9   **FUD** 010   [J] [A2] [80] [CCI]
AMA: 2014,Jan,11

42725   **retropharyngeal or parapharyngeal, external approach**
🚑 23.0   ⚕ 23.0   **FUD** 090   [J] [A2] [80] [CCI]
AMA: 2014,Jan,11

42800   **Biopsy; oropharynx**
EXCLUDES   *Laryngoscopy with biopsy (31510, 31535-31536)*
🚑 3.22   ⚕ 4.49   **FUD** 010   [J] [P3] [CCI]
AMA: 2014,Jan,11

42804   **nasopharynx, visible lesion, simple**
EXCLUDES   *Laryngoscopy with biopsy (31510, 31535-31536)*
🚑 3.27   ⚕ 5.65   **FUD** 010   [J] [A2] [CCI]
AMA: 2014,Jan,11

42806   **nasopharynx, survey for unknown primary lesion**
EXCLUDES   *Laryngoscopy with biopsy (31510, 31535-31536)*
🚑 3.81   ⚕ 6.33   **FUD** 010   [J] [A2] [CCI]
AMA: 2014,Jan,11

42808   **Excision or destruction of lesion of pharynx, any method**
🚑 4.66   ⚕ 6.53   **FUD** 010   [J] [A2] [CCI]
AMA: 2014,Jan,11

42809   **Removal of foreign body from pharynx**
🚑 3.56   ⚕ 5.76   **FUD** 010   [Q1] [N1] [CCI]
AMA: 2014,Jan,11

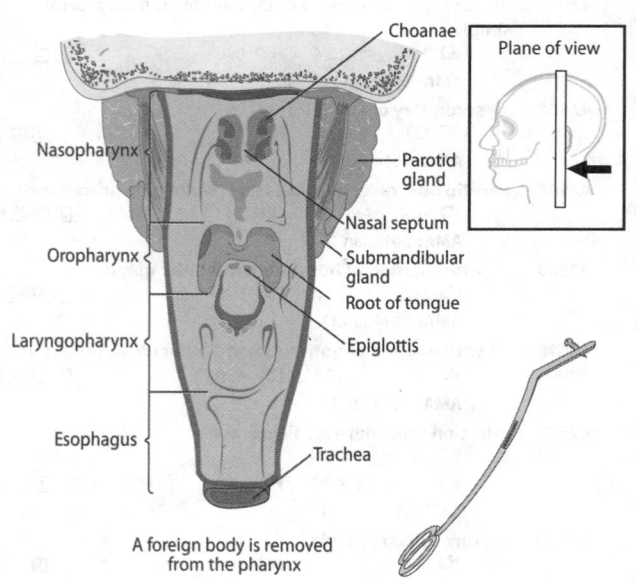

Choanae
Nasopharynx
Parotid gland
Nasal septum
Oropharynx
Submandibular gland
Root of tongue
Laryngopharynx
Epiglottis
Esophagus
Trachea

Plane of view

A foreign body is removed from the pharynx

42810   **Excision branchial cleft cyst or vestige, confined to skin and subcutaneous tissues**
🚑 8.10   ⚕ 11.0   **FUD** 090   [J] [A2] [80] [50] [CCI]
AMA: 2014,Jan,11

42815   **Excision branchial cleft cyst, vestige, or fistula, extending beneath subcutaneous tissues and/or into pharynx**
🚑 15.6   ⚕ 15.6   **FUD** 090   [J] [A2] [80] [50] [CCI]
AMA: 2014,Jan,11

42820   **Tonsillectomy and adenoidectomy; younger than age 12**   [A]
🚑 8.26   ⚕ 8.26   **FUD** 090   [J] [A2] [80] [CCI]
AMA: 2018,Jan,8; 2017,Jan,8; 2016,Jan,13

42821   **age 12 or over**   [A]
🚑 8.62   ⚕ 8.62   **FUD** 090   [J] [A2] [80] [CCI]
AMA: 2018,Jan,8; 2017,Jan,8; 2016,Jan,13

42825   **Tonsillectomy, primary or secondary; younger than age 12**   [A]
🚑 7.52   ⚕ 7.52   **FUD** 090   [J] [A2] [80] [CCI]
AMA: 2018,Jan,8; 2017,Jan,8; 2016,Jan,13

42826   **age 12 or over**   [A]
🚑 7.20   ⚕ 7.20   **FUD** 090   [J] [A2] [CCI]
AMA: 2018,Jan,8; 2017,Jan,8; 2016,Jan,13

42830   **Adenoidectomy, primary; younger than age 12**   [A]
🚑 5.95   ⚕ 5.95   **FUD** 090   [J] [A2] [80] [CCI]
AMA: 2018,Jan,8; 2017,Jan,8; 2016,Jan,13

42831   **age 12 or over**   [A]
🚑 6.44   ⚕ 6.44   **FUD** 090   [J] [A2] [80] [CCI]
AMA: 2018,Jan,8; 2017,Jan,8; 2016,Jan,13

42835   **Adenoidectomy, secondary; younger than age 12**   [A]
🚑 5.51   ⚕ 5.51   **FUD** 090   [J] [A2] [80] [CCI]
AMA: 2018,Jan,8; 2017,Jan,8; 2016,Jan,13

42836   **age 12 or over**   [A]
🚑 6.89   ⚕ 6.89   **FUD** 090   [J] [A2] [80] [CCI]
AMA: 2018,Jan,8; 2017,Jan,8; 2016,Jan,13

42842   **Radical resection of tonsil, tonsillar pillars, and/or retromolar trigone; without closure**
🚑 28.7   ⚕ 28.7   **FUD** 090   [J] [G2] [80] [CCI]
AMA: 2018,Jan,8; 2017,Jan,8; 2016,Jan,13

42844   **closure with local flap (eg, tongue, buccal)**
🚑 39.9   ⚕ 39.9   **FUD** 090   [J] [G2] [80] [CCI]
AMA: 2018,Jan,8; 2017,Jan,8; 2016,Jan,13

42845   **closure with other flap**
Code also:
Closure with other flap(s)
Radical neck dissection when combined (38720)
🚑 63.9   ⚕ 63.9   **FUD** 090   [C] [80]
AMA: 2018,Jan,8; 2017,Jan,8; 2016,Jan,13

42860   **Excision of tonsil tags**
🚑 5.40   ⚕ 5.40   **FUD** 090   [J] [A2] [80] [CCI]
AMA: 2014,Jan,11

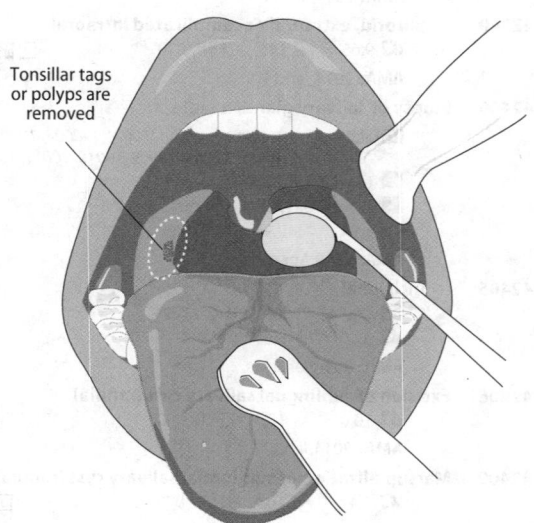

Tonsillar tags or polyps are removed

26/[TC] PC/TC Only   [A2]-[Z3] ASC Payment   [50] Bilateral   ♂ Male Only   ♀ Female Only   🚑 Facility RVU   ⚕ Non-Facility RVU   [CCI] CCI   [X] CLIA
FUD Follow-up Days   **CMS:** IOM   **AMA:** CPT Asst   [A]-[Y] OPPSI   80/[80] Surg Assist Allowed / w/Doc   Lab Crosswalk   Radiology Crosswalk

186   CPT © 2021 American Medical Association. All Rights Reserved.   © 2021 Optum360, LLC

42870 Excision or destruction lingual tonsil, any method (separate procedure)

> EXCLUDES *Nasopharynx resection (juvenile angiofibroma) by transzygomatic/bicoronal approach (61586, 61600)*
>
> 🔾 17.0 🔾 17.0 **FUD** 090 J A2 80 □
>
> AMA: 2014,Jan,11

42890 Limited pharyngectomy

> Code also radical neck dissection when combined (38720)
>
> 🔾 40.7 🔾 40.7 **FUD** 090 J A2 80 □
>
> AMA: 2014,Jan,11; 2010,Aug,3-7

42892 Resection of lateral pharyngeal wall or pyriform sinus, direct closure by advancement of lateral and posterior pharyngeal walls

> Code also radical neck dissection when combined (38720)
>
> 🔾 53.6 🔾 53.6 **FUD** 090 J A2 80 □
>
> AMA: 2018,Jan,8; 2017,Jan,8; 2016,Jan,13

42894 Resection of pharyngeal wall requiring closure with myocutaneous or fasciocutaneous flap or free muscle, skin, or fascial flap with microvascular anastomosis

> EXCLUDES *Flap used for reconstruction (15730, 15733-15734, 15756-15758)*
>
> Code also radical neck dissection when combined (38720)
>
> 🔾 67.7 🔾 67.7 **FUD** 090 C 80 □
>
> AMA: 2018,Jan,8; 2017,Jan,8; 2016,Jan,13

42900 Suture pharynx for wound or injury

> 🔾 9.56 🔾 9.56 **FUD** 010 T J8 80 □
>
> AMA: 2014,Jan,11

42950 Pharyngoplasty (plastic or reconstructive operation on pharynx)

> EXCLUDES *Pharyngeal flap (42225)*
>
> 🔾 22.8 🔾 22.8 **FUD** 090 J A2 80 □
>
> AMA: 2019,Oct,10; 2018,Jan,8; 2017,Jan,8; 2016,Apr,8

42953 Pharyngoesophageal repair

> Code also closure using myocutaneous or other flap
>
> 🔾 27.3 🔾 27.3 **FUD** 090 C 80 □
>
> AMA: 2014,Jan,11

42955 Pharyngostomy (fistulization of pharynx, external for feeding)

> 🔾 21.7 🔾 21.7 **FUD** 090 T A2 80 □
>
> AMA: 2014,Jan,11

42960 Control oropharyngeal hemorrhage, primary or secondary (eg, post-tonsillectomy); simple

> 🔾 4.83 🔾 4.83 **FUD** 010 T A2 80 □
>
> AMA: 2014,Jan,11

42961 complicated, requiring hospitalization

> 🔾 11.9 🔾 11.9 **FUD** 090 C 80 □
>
> AMA: 2014,Jan,11

42962 with secondary surgical intervention

> 🔾 14.7 🔾 14.7 **FUD** 090 J A2 □
>
> AMA: 2014,Jan,11

42970 Control of nasopharyngeal hemorrhage, primary or secondary (eg, postadenoidectomy); simple, with posterior nasal packs, with or without anterior packs and/or cautery

> 🔾 11.7 🔾 11.7 **FUD** 090 T R2 □
>
> AMA: 2014,Jan,11; 2002,May,7

42971 complicated, requiring hospitalization

> 🔾 12.9 🔾 12.9 **FUD** 090 C 80 □
>
> AMA: 2014,Jan,11

42972 with secondary surgical intervention

> 🔾 14.5 🔾 14.5 **FUD** 090 J A2 80 □
>
> AMA: 2014,Jan,11

● **42975** Drug-induced sleep endoscopy, with dynamic evaluation of velum, pharynx, tongue base, and larynx for evaluation of sleep-disordered breathing, flexible, diagnostic

> EXCLUDES *Diagnostic flexible laryngoscopy (31575)*
>
> *Nasal endoscopy, diagnostic, unless different type endoscope used and for different condition (31231)*
>
> *Nasopharyngoscopy with endoscope (92511)*

42999 Unlisted procedure, pharynx, adenoids, or tonsils

> 🔾 0.00 🔾 0.00 **FUD** YYY T 80 □
>
> AMA: 2018,Jan,8; 2017,Jan,8; 2016,Jan,13

43020-43135 Incision/Resection of Esophagus

43020 Esophagotomy, cervical approach, with removal of foreign body

> EXCLUDES *Laparotomy with esophageal intubation (43510)*
>
> 🔾 16.2 🔾 16.2 **FUD** 090 T 62 80 □
>
> AMA: 2014,Jan,11

43030 Cricopharyngeal myotomy

> EXCLUDES *Laparotomy with esophageal intubation (43510)*
>
> 🔾 14.8 🔾 14.8 **FUD** 090 J 62 80 □
>
> AMA: 2020,Nov,12; 2020,Jul,13

43045 Esophagotomy, thoracic approach, with removal of foreign body

> EXCLUDES *Laparotomy with esophageal intubation (43510)*
>
> 🔾 37.6 🔾 37.6 **FUD** 090 C 80 □
>
> AMA: 2014,Jan,11; 1994,Win,1

43100 Excision of lesion, esophagus, with primary repair; cervical approach

> EXCLUDES *Gastrointestinal reconstruction for previous esophagectomy (43360-43361)*
>
> *Wide excision malignant lesion cervical esophagus, with total laryngectomy:*
>
> *With radical neck dissection (31365, 43107, 43116, 43124)*
>
> *Without radical neck dissection (31360, 43107, 43116, 43124)*
>
> 🔾 18.0 🔾 18.0 **FUD** 090 C 80 □
>
> AMA: 2014,Jan,11; 1994,Win,1

43101 thoracic or abdominal approach

> EXCLUDES *Gastrointestinal reconstruction for previous esophagectomy (43360-43361)*
>
> *Wide excision malignant lesion cervical esophagus, with total laryngectomy:*
>
> *With radical neck dissection (31365, 43107, 43116, 43124)*
>
> *Without radical neck dissection (31360, 43107, 43116, 43124)*
>
> 🔾 29.1 🔾 29.1 **FUD** 090 C 80 □
>
> AMA: 2018,Jan,8; 2017,Jan,8; 2016,Jan,13

43107 Total or near total esophagectomy, without thoracotomy; with pharyngogastrostomy or cervical esophagogastrostomy, with or without pyloroplasty (transhiatal)

> EXCLUDES *Gastrointestinal reconstruction for previous esophagectomy (43360-43361)*
>
> 🔾 86.5 🔾 86.5 **FUD** 090 C 80 □
>
> AMA: 2014,Jan,11; 2010,Aug,3-7

43108 with colon interposition or small intestine reconstruction, including intestine mobilization, preparation and anastomosis(es)

> EXCLUDES *Gastrointestinal reconstruction for previous esophagectomy (43360-43361)*
>
> 🔾 129. 🔾 129. **FUD** 090 C 80 □
>
> AMA: 2014,Jan,11; 2002,May,7

Digestive System

43112 — 43193

43112 **Total or near total esophagectomy, with thoracotomy; with pharyngogastrostomy or cervical esophagogastrostomy, with or without pyloroplasty (ie, McKeown esophagectomy or tri-incisional esophagectomy)**

> EXCLUDES Gastrointestinal reconstruction for previous esophagectomy (43360-43361)
> 🚑 101. ⚕ 101. **FUD** 090 C 80 ▭
> **AMA:** 2018,Jul,7; 2018,Jan,8; 2017,Jan,8; 2016,Jan,13

43113 **with colon interposition or small intestine reconstruction, including intestine mobilization, preparation, and anastomosis(es)**

> EXCLUDES Gastrointestinal reconstruction for previous esophagectomy (43360-43361)
> 🚑 126. ⚕ 126. **FUD** 090 C 80 ▭
> **AMA:** 2014,Jan,11; 2002,May,7

43116 **Partial esophagectomy, cervical, with free intestinal graft, including microvascular anastomosis, obtaining the graft and intestinal reconstruction**

> INCLUDES Operating microscope (69990)
> EXCLUDES Free jejunal graft with microvascular anastomosis performed by different physician (43496)
> Gastrointestinal reconstruction for previous esophagectomy (43360-43361)
> Code also modifier 52 when intestinal or free jejunal graft with microvascular anastomosis performed by another physician
> 🚑 145. ⚕ 145. **FUD** 090 C 80 ▭
> **AMA:** 2016,Feb,12

43117 **Partial esophagectomy, distal two-thirds, with thoracotomy and separate abdominal incision, with or without proximal gastrectomy; with thoracic esophagogastrostomy, with or without pyloroplasty (Ivor Lewis)**

> EXCLUDES Esophagogastrectomy (lower third) and vagotomy (43122)
> Gastrointestinal reconstruction for previous esophagectomy (43360-43361)
> Total esophagectomy with gastropharyngostomy (43107, 43124)
> 🚑 94.3 ⚕ 94.3 **FUD** 090 C 80 ▭
> **AMA:** 2014,Jan,11; 1994,Win,1

43118 **with colon interposition or small intestine reconstruction, including intestine mobilization, preparation, and anastomosis(es)**

> EXCLUDES Esophagogastrectomy (lower third) and vagotomy (43122)
> Gastrointestinal reconstruction for previous esophagectomy (43360-43361)
> Total esophagectomy with gastropharyngostomy (43107, 43124)
> 🚑 105. ⚕ 105. **FUD** 090 C 80 ▭
> **AMA:** 2014,Jan,11; 2002,May,7

43121 **Partial esophagectomy, distal two-thirds, with thoracotomy only, with or without proximal gastrectomy, with thoracic esophagogastrostomy, with or without pyloroplasty**

> EXCLUDES Gastrointestinal reconstruction for previous esophagectomy (43360-43361)
> 🚑 82.8 ⚕ 82.8 **FUD** 090 C 80 ▭
> **AMA:** 2014,Jan,11; 1994,Win,1

43122 **Partial esophagectomy, thoracoabdominal or abdominal approach, with or without proximal gastrectomy; with esophagogastrostomy, with or without pyloroplasty**

> EXCLUDES Gastrointestinal reconstruction for previous esophagectomy (43360-43361)
> 🚑 74.3 ⚕ 74.3 **FUD** 090 C 80 ▭
> **AMA:** 2014,Jan,11; 1994,Win,1

43123 **with colon interposition or small intestine reconstruction, including intestine mobilization, preparation, and anastomosis(es)**

> EXCLUDES Gastrointestinal reconstruction for previous esophagectomy (43360-43361)
> 🚑 131. ⚕ 131. **FUD** 090 C 80 ▭
> **AMA:** 2014,Jan,11; 2002,May,7

43124 **Total or partial esophagectomy, without reconstruction (any approach), with cervical esophagostomy**

> EXCLUDES Gastrointestinal reconstruction for previous esophagectomy (43360-43361)
> 🚑 110. ⚕ 110. **FUD** 090 C 80 ▭
> **AMA:** 2018,Jan,8; 2017,Jan,8; 2016,Jan,13

43130 **Diverticulectomy of hypopharynx or esophagus, with or without myotomy; cervical approach**

> EXCLUDES Diverticulectomy hypopharynx or cervical esophagus, endoscopic (43180)
> Gastrointestinal reconstruction for previous esophagectomy (43360-43361)
> 🚑 22.6 ⚕ 22.6 **FUD** 090 J 62 80 ▭
> **AMA:** 2018,Jan,8; 2017,Jan,8; 2016,Jan,13

43135 **thoracic approach**

> EXCLUDES Diverticulectomy hypopharynx or cervical esophagus, endoscopic (43180)
> Gastrointestinal reconstruction for previous esophagectomy (43360-43361)
> 🚑 42.6 ⚕ 42.6 **FUD** 090 C 80 ▭
> **AMA:** 2018,Jan,8; 2017,Jan,8; 2016,Jan,13

43180-43233 [43210, 43211, 43212, 43213, 43214, 43233] Endoscopic Procedures: Esophagus

> INCLUDES Control bleeding due to endoscopic procedure during same operative session
> Diagnostic endoscopy with surgical endoscopy
> Examination upper esophageal sphincter (cricopharyngeus muscle) to/including gastroesophageal junction
> Retroflexion examination proximal region stomach

43180 **Esophagoscopy, rigid, transoral with diverticulectomy of hypopharynx or cervical esophagus (eg, Zenker's diverticulum), with cricopharyngeal myotomy, includes use of telescope or operating microscope and repair, when performed**

> INCLUDES Operating microscope (69990)
> EXCLUDES Esophagogastroduodenoscopy, flexible, transoral; with esophagogastric fundoplasty (43210)
> Open diverticulectomy hypopharynx or esophagus (43130-43135)
> 🚑 15.6 ⚕ 15.6 **FUD** 090 J 62 ▭
> **AMA:** 2018,Jan,8; 2017,Jan,8; 2016,Feb,12; 2016,Jan,13

43191 **Esophagoscopy, rigid, transoral; diagnostic, including collection of specimen(s) by brushing or washing when performed (separate procedure)**

> EXCLUDES Esophagogastroduodenoscopy, flexible, transoral; with esophagogastric fundoplasty (43210)
> Esophagoscopy:
> Flexible, transnasal (43197-43198)
> Flexible, transoral (43200)
> Rigid, transoral (43192-43196)
> Myotomy, transoral lower esophageal (43497)
> 🚑 4.45 ⚕ 4.45 **FUD** 000 J 62 ▭
> **AMA:** 2018,Jan,8; 2017,Jan,8; 2016,Jan,13

43192 **with directed submucosal injection(s), any substance**

> EXCLUDES Esophagoscopy:
> Flexible, transnasal (43197-43198)
> Flexible, transoral (43201)
> Rigid, transoral (43191)
> Injection sclerosis of esophageal varices:
> Flexible, transoral (43204)
> Rigid, transoral (43499)
> 🚑 4.88 ⚕ 4.88 **FUD** 000 J 62 ▭
> **AMA:** 2018,Jan,8; 2017,Jan,8; 2016,Jan,13

43193 **with biopsy, single or multiple**

> EXCLUDES Esophagoscopy:
> Flexible, transnasal (43197-43198)
> Flexible, transoral (43202)
> Rigid, transoral (43191)
> 🚑 4.85 ⚕ 4.85 **FUD** 000 J 62 ▭
> **AMA:** 2018,Jan,8; 2017,Jan,8; 2016,Jan,13

43194 **with removal of foreign body(s)**

EXCLUDES Esophagoscopy:
Flexible, transnasal (43197-43198)
Flexible, transoral (43215)
Rigid, transoral (43191)

⊞ (76000)

🚑 5.55 ⚕ 5.55 **FUD** 000   J G2 🖵

AMA: 2018,Jan,8; 2017,Jan,8; 2016,Jan,13

43195 **with balloon dilation (less than 30 mm diameter)**

EXCLUDES Dilation of esophagus:
Flexible, with balloon diameter 30 mm or larger
(43214, 43233)
Flexible, with balloon diameter less than 30 mm
(43220)
Without endoscopic visualization (43450-43453)
Esophagoscopy:
Flexible, transnasal (43197-43198)
Rigid, transoral (43191)

⊞ (74360)

🚑 5.28 ⚕ 5.28 **FUD** 000   J G2 🖵

AMA: 2018,Jan,8; 2017,Jan,8; 2016,Jan,13

43196 **with insertion of guide wire followed by dilation over guide wire**

EXCLUDES Esophagoscopy:
Flexible, transnasal (43197-43198)
Flexible, transoral (43226)
Rigid, transoral (43191)

⊞ (74360)

🚑 5.63 ⚕ 5.63 **FUD** 000   J G2 🖵

AMA: 2018,Jan,8; 2017,Jan,8; 2016,Jan,13

43197 **Esophagoscopy, flexible, transnasal; diagnostic, including collection of specimen(s) by brushing or washing, when performed (separate procedure)**

EXCLUDES Esophagogastroduodenoscopy, flexible, transnasal
(0652T-0654T)
Esophagogastroduodenoscopy, flexible, transoral
(43235-43259 [43233, 43266, 43270])
Esophagoscopy:
Flexible, transnasal; with biopsy, single or multiple
(43198)
Flexible, transoral (43200-43232 [43211, 43212,
43213, 43214])
Rigid, transoral (43191-43196)
Laryngoscopy, flexible fiberoptic; diagnostic (31575)
Myotomy, transoral lower esophageal (43497)
Nasal endoscopy, diagnostic, unless different type
endoscope used (31231)
Nasopharyngoscopy with endoscope (92511)

🚑 2.40 ⚕ 5.34 **FUD** 000   T P3 🖵

AMA: 2018,Jan,8; 2017,Jul,7; 2017,Jan,8; 2016,Dec,13;
2016,Sep,6; 2016,Jan,13

43198 **with biopsy, single or multiple**

EXCLUDES Esophagogastroduodenoscopy, flexible, transnasal
(0652T-0654T)
Esophagogastroduodenoscopy, flexible, transoral
(43235-43259 [43233, 43266, 43270])
Esophagoscopy:
Flexible, transnasal (43197)
Flexible, transoral (43200-43232 [43211, 43212,
43213, 43214])
Rigid, transoral (43191-43196)
Laryngoscopy, flexible fiberoptic; diagnostic (31575)
Nasal endoscopy, diagnostic, unless different type
endoscope used (31231)
Nasopharyngoscopy with endoscope (92511)

🚑 2.86 ⚕ 6.08 **FUD** 000   T P3 🖵

AMA: 2018,Jan,8; 2017,Jul,7; 2017,Jan,8; 2016,Dec,13;
2016,Sep,6; 2016,Jan,13

43200 **Esophagoscopy, flexible, transoral; diagnostic, including collection of specimen(s) by brushing or washing, when performed (separate procedure)**

EXCLUDES Esophagogastroduodenoscopy, flexible, transoral
(43235)
Esophagoscopy:
Flexible, transnasal (43197-43198)
Flexible, transoral (43201-43232 [43211, 43212,
43213, 43214])
Rigid, transoral (43191)
Myotomy, transoral lower esophageal (43497)

🚑 2.53 ⚕ 6.50 **FUD** 000   T A2 🖵

AMA: 2018,Jan,8; 2017,Jan,8; 2016,Jan,13

43201 **with directed submucosal injection(s), any substance**

EXCLUDES Esophagoscopy:
Flexible, transnasal (43197-43198)
Flexible, transoral, on same lesion (43200, 43204,
43211, 43227)
Injection sclerosis esophageal varices:
Flexible, transoral (43204)
Rigid, transoral (43192, 43499)

🚑 2.98 ⚕ 6.89 **FUD** 000   J A2 🖵

AMA: 2018,Jan,8; 2017,Jan,8; 2016,Jan,13

43202 **with biopsy, single or multiple**

EXCLUDES Esophagoscopy:
Flexible, transnasal (43197-43198)
Flexible, transoral; diagnostic (43200)
Flexible, transoral, on same lesion (43211)
Rigid, transoral (43193)

🚑 2.97 ⚕ 9.64 **FUD** 000   J A2 🖵

AMA: 2018,Jan,8; 2017,Jan,8; 2016,Jan,13

43204 **with injection sclerosis of esophageal varices**

EXCLUDES Band ligation non-variceal bleeding (43227)
Esophagoscopy:
Flexible, transnasal or transoral; diagnostic
(43197-43198, 43200)
Flexible, transoral; with control bleeding, any method,
on same lesion (43227)
Flexible, transoral; with directed submucosal
injection(s), any substance, on same lesion
(43201)
Rigid, transoral, with injection esophageal varices
(43499)

🚑 3.90 ⚕ 3.90 **FUD** 000   J A2 🖵

AMA: 2018,Jan,8; 2017,Jan,8; 2016,Jan,13

43205 **with band ligation of esophageal varices**

EXCLUDES Band ligation non-variceal bleeding on same lesion
(43227)
Esophagoscopy, flexible, transnasal or transoral;
diagnostic (43197-43198, 43200)

🚑 4.07 ⚕ 4.07 **FUD** 000   J A2 🖵

AMA: 2018,Jan,8; 2017,Jan,8; 2016,Jan,13

43206 **with optical endomicroscopy**

EXCLUDES Esophagoscopy, flexible, transnasal or transoral;
diagnostic (43197-43198, 43200)
Optical endomicroscopic image(s), interpretation and
report (88375)
Code also contrast agent

🚑 3.90 ⚕ 7.85 **FUD** 000   J G2 🖵

AMA: 2018,Jan,8; 2017,Nov,10; 2017,Jan,8; 2016,Jan,13

43210	**Resequenced code. See code following 43259.**
43211	**Resequenced code. See code following 43217.**
43212	**Resequenced code. See code following 43217.**
43213	**Resequenced code. See code following 43220.**
43214	**Resequenced code. See code following 43220.**

Digestive System

43215 — 43229

43215 with removal of foreign body(s)

Esophagoscopy:
Flexible, transnasal or transoral; diagnostic (43197-43198, 43200)
Rigid, transoral (43194)

(76000)

4.14   10.5   **FUD** 000   J A2

AMA: 2018,Jan,8; 2017,Jan,8; 2016,Jan,13

43216 with removal of tumor(s), polyp(s), or other lesion(s) by hot biopsy forceps

EXCLUDES *Esophagoscopy, flexible, transnasal or transoral; diagnostic (43197-43198, 43200)*

3.86   11.1   **FUD** 000   J A2

AMA: 2018,Jan,8; 2017,Jan,8; 2016,Jan,13

43217 with removal of tumor(s), polyp(s), or other lesion(s) by snare technique

EXCLUDES *Esophagogastroduodenoscopy, flexible, transoral (43251)*
Esophagoscopy:
Flexible, transnasal or transoral; diagnostic (43197-43198, 43200)
Flexible, transoral; with endoscopic mucosal resection, on same lesion (43211)

4.62   11.4   **FUD** 000   J A2

AMA: 2020,May,13; 2018,Jan,8; 2017,Jan,8; 2016,Jan,13

 # 43211 with endoscopic mucosal resection

EXCLUDES *Esophagoscopy:*
Flexible, transnasal or transoral; diagnostic (43197-43198, 43200)
Flexible, transoral; with directed submucosal injection(s), on same lesion (43201-43202)
Flexible, transoral; with removal tumor(s), polyp(s), or other lesion(s) by snare technique, on same lesion (43217)

6.77   6.77   **FUD** 000   J G2

AMA: 2019,Dec,14; 2018,Jan,8; 2017,Nov,10; 2017,Jan,8; 2016,Jan,13

 # 43212 with placement of endoscopic stent (includes pre- and post-dilation and guide wire passage, when performed)

EXCLUDES *Esophagogastroduodenoscopy, flexible, transoral; with insertion of intraluminal tube or catheter (43241)*
Esophagoscopy:
Flexible, transnasal or transoral; diagnostic (43197-43198, 43200)
Flexible, transoral; with insertion guide wire followed by passage dilator(s) over guide wire (43226)
Flexible, transoral; with transendoscopic balloon dilation (43220)

(74360)

5.48   5.48   **FUD** 000   J J8

AMA: 2018,Jan,8; 2017,Jan,8; 2016,Jan,13

43220 with transendoscopic balloon dilation (less than 30 mm diameter)

EXCLUDES *Dilation esophagus:*
Rigid, with balloon diameter 30 mm or larger (43214)
Rigid, with balloon diameter less than 30mm (43195)
Without endoscopic visualization (43450, 43453)
Esophagoscopy:
Flexible, transnasal; diagnostic (43197-43198)
Flexible, transoral (43200, 43212, 43226, 43229)

(74360)

3.43   29.5   **FUD** 000   J A2

AMA: 2018,Jan,8; 2017,Jan,8; 2016,Jan,13

 # 43213 with dilation of esophagus, by balloon or dilator, retrograde (includes fluoroscopic guidance, when performed)

INCLUDES Fluoroscopy (76000)

EXCLUDES *Esophagoscopy, flexible, transnasal or transoral; diagnostic (43197-43198, 43200)*
Intraluminal dilation of strictures and/or obstructions (eg, esophagus), radiological supervision and interpretation (74360)

Code also each additional stricture treated in same operative session with modifier 59 and (43213)

7.48   34.9   **FUD** 000   J G2

AMA: 2018,Jan,8; 2017,Jan,8; 2016,Jan,13

 # 43214 with dilation of esophagus with balloon (30 mm diameter or larger) (includes fluoroscopic guidance, when performed)

INCLUDES Fluoroscopy (76000)

EXCLUDES *Esophagoscopy, flexible, transnasal or transoral; diagnostic (43197-43198, 43200)*
Intraluminal dilation strictures and/or obstructions (eg, esophagus), radiological supervision and interpretation (74360)

5.61   5.61   **FUD** 000   J G2

AMA: 2018,Jan,8; 2017,Jan,8; 2016,Jan,13

43226 with insertion of guide wire followed by passage of dilator(s) over guide wire

EXCLUDES *Esophagoscopy:*
Flexible, transnasal or transoral; diagnostic (43197-43198, 43200)
Flexible, transoral; with ablation tumor(s), polyp(s), or other lesion(s), on same lesion (43229)
Flexible, transoral; with placement endoscopic stent (43212)
Flexible, transoral; with transendoscopic balloon dilation (43220)
Rigid, transoral (43196)

(74360)

3.75   10.1   **FUD** 000   J A2

AMA: 2018,Jan,8; 2017,Jan,8; 2016,Jan,13

43227 with control of bleeding, any method

EXCLUDES *Esophagoscopy:*
Flexible, transnasal or transoral; diagnostic (43197-43198, 43200)
Flexible, transoral; with directed submucosal injection(s), on same lesion (43201)
Flexible, transoral; with injection sclerosis esophageal varices, on same lesion (43204-43205)

4.75   17.6   **FUD** 000   J A2

AMA: 2018,Jan,8; 2017,Jan,8; 2016,Jan,13

43229 with ablation of tumor(s), polyp(s), or other lesion(s) (includes pre- and post-dilation and guide wire passage, when performed)

EXCLUDES *Esophagoscopy:*
Flexible, transnasal or transoral; diagnostic (43197-43198, 43200)
Flexible, transoral; with insertion guide wire followed by passage dilator(s) over guide wire, on same lesion (43226)
Flexible, transoral; with transendoscopic balloon dilation, on same lesion (43220)

Code also esophagoscopic photodynamic therapy, when performed (96570-96571)

5.70   19.8   **FUD** 000   J J8

AMA: 2018,Jan,8; 2017,Jan,8; 2016,Jan,13

26/TC PC/TC Only   A2-Z3 ASC Payment   50 Bilateral   ♂ Male Only   ♀ Female Only   Facility RVU   Non-Facility RVU   CCI   CLIA
FUD Follow-up Days   CMS: IOM   AMA: CPT Asst   A-Y OPPSI   80/80 Surg Assist Allowed / w/Doc   Lab Crosswalk   Radiology Crosswalk

190   CPT © 2021 American Medical Association. All Rights Reserved.   © 2021 Optum360, LLC

43231   **with endoscopic ultrasound examination**

INCLUDES Gastrointestinal endoscopic ultrasound, supervision, and interpretation (76975)

EXCLUDES *Esophagoscopy:*

Flexible, transnasal or transoral; diagnostic (43197-43198, 43200)

Flexible, transoral; with transendoscopic ultrasound-guided intramural or transmural fine needle aspiration/biopsy(s) (43232)

Procedure performed more than one time per operative session

🚑 4.59   ⚕ 4.59   **FUD** 000   J A2 ▢

AMA: 2018,Jan,8; 2017,Jan,8; 2016,Jan,13

43232   **with transendoscopic ultrasound-guided intramural or transmural fine needle aspiration/biopsy(s)**

INCLUDES Gastrointestinal endoscopic ultrasound, supervision and interpretation (76975)

Ultrasonic guidance (76942)

EXCLUDES *Esophagoscopy:*

Flexible, transnasal or transoral; diagnostic (43197-43198, 43200)

Flexible, transoral; with endoscopic ultrasound examination (43231)

Procedure performed more than one time per operative session

🚑 5.75   ⚕ 5.75   **FUD** 000   J A2 ▢

AMA: 2018,Jan,8; 2017,Jan,8; 2016,Jan,13

43233   Resequenced code. See code following 43249.

43235-43210 [43210, 43233, 43266, 43270] Endoscopic Procedures: Esophagogastroduodenoscopy (EGD)

INCLUDES Control bleeding due to endoscopic procedure during same operative session

Diagnostic endoscopy with surgical endoscopy

Exam jejunum distal to anastomosis in surgically altered stomach, including post-gastroenterostomy (Billroth II) and gastric bypass (43235-43259 [43233, 43266, 43270])

EXCLUDES *Exam upper esophageal sphincter (cricopharyngeus muscle) to/including gastroesophageal junction and/or retroflexion exam proximal region stomach (43197-43232 [43211; 43212, 43213, 43214])*

Code also:

Modifier 52 when duodenum not examined either deliberately or due to significant issues and repeat procedure will not be performed

Modifier 53 when duodenum not examined either deliberately or due to significant issues and repeat procedure is planned

43235   **Esophagogastroduodenoscopy, flexible, transoral; diagnostic, including collection of specimen(s) by brushing or washing, when performed (separate procedure)**

EXCLUDES *Endoscopy small intestine (44360-44379)*

Esophagogastroduodenoscopy, flexible, transoral; with esophagogastric fundoplasty (43210)

Esophagoscopy, flexible, transnasal; diagnostic (43197-43198)

Myotomy, transoral lower esophageal (43497)

Procedure performed with surgical endoscopy (43236-43259 [43233, 43266, 43270])

🚑 3.54   ⚕ 7.98   **FUD** 000   T A2 ▢

AMA: 2019,Oct,10; 2018,Jul,14; 2018,Jan,8; 2017,Jul,10; 2017,Jan,8; 2016,Jan,13

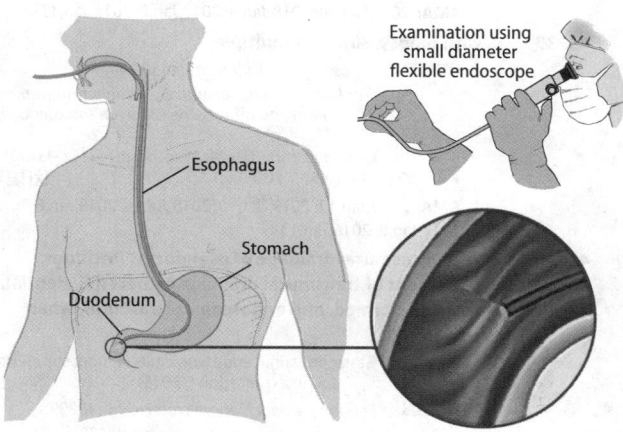

Examination using small diameter flexible endoscope

Esophagus

Stomach

Duodenum

43236   **with directed submucosal injection(s), any substance**

EXCLUDES *Endoscopy small intestine (44360-44379)*

Esophagogastroduodenoscopy, on same lesion:

Flexible, transoral; with control bleeding, any method (43255)

Flexible, transoral; with endoscopic mucosal resection (43254)

Flexible, transoral; with injection sclerosis esophageal/gastric varices (43243)

Esophagoscopy, flexible, transnasal or transoral; diagnostic (43197-43198, 43235)

Injection sclerosis varices, esophageal/gastric (43243)

🚑 4.05   ⚕ 10.0   **FUD** 000   T A2 ▢

AMA: 2019,Oct,10; 2018,Jan,8; 2017,Jan,8; 2016,Jan,13

● New Code   ▲ Revised Code   ○ Reinstated   ● New Web Release   ▲ Revised Web Release   + Add-on   Unlisted   Not Covered   # Resequenced

50 Optum Mod 50 Exempt   ⊘ AMA Mod 51 Exempt   51 Optum Mod 51 Exempt   63 Mod 63 Exempt   ✗ Non-FDA Drug   ★ Telemedicine   M Maternity   A Age Edit

© 2021 Optum360, LLC   CPT © 2021 American Medical Association. All Rights Reserved.   191

43237 with endoscopic ultrasound examination limited to the esophagus, stomach or duodenum, and adjacent structures

INCLUDES   Ultrasonic guidance (76942, 76975)

EXCLUDES   *Endoscopy of small intestine (44360-44379)*
Esophagogastroduodenoscopy, flexible, transoral (43238, 43242, 43253, 43259)
Esophagoscopy, flexible, transnasal; diagnostic (43197-43198)
Procedure performed more than one time per operative session

🖩 5.73   ⚕ 5.73   **FUD** 000   J A2 ▭

AMA: 2019,Oct,10; 2018,Jan,8; 2017,Jan,8; 2016,Jan,13; 2016,Jan,11

43238 with transendoscopic ultrasound-guided intramural or transmural fine needle aspiration/biopsy(s), (includes endoscopic ultrasound examination limited to the esophagus, stomach or duodenum, and adjacent structures)

INCLUDES   Gastrointestinal endoscopic ultrasound, supervision and interpretation (76975)
Ultrasonic guidance (76942)

EXCLUDES   *Endoscopy small intestine (44360-44379)*
Esophagogastroduodenoscopy, flexible, transoral (43237, 43242)
Esophagoscopy, flexible, transnasal (43197-43198)
Procedure performed more than one time per operative session

🖩 6.70   ⚕ 6.70   **FUD** 000   J A2 ▭

AMA: 2019,Oct,10; 2018,Jan,8; 2017,Jan,8; 2016,Jan,13

43239 with biopsy, single or multiple

EXCLUDES   *Endoscopy small intestine (44360-44379)*
Esophagogastroduodenoscopy, flexible, transoral; with endoscopic mucosal resection on same lesion (43254)
Esophagoscopy, flexible, transnasal (43197-43198)

🖩 3.99   ⚕ 10.6   **FUD** 000   T A2 ▭

AMA: 2020,Jan,12; 2019,Oct,10; 2018,Jul,14; 2018,Jan,8; 2017,Jan,8; 2016,Jan,13

43240 with transmural drainage of pseudocyst (includes placement of transmural drainage catheter[s]/stent[s], when performed, and endoscopic ultrasound, when performed)

INCLUDES   Gastrointestinal endoscopic ultrasound, supervision and interpretation (76975)

EXCLUDES   *Endoscopic pancreatic necrosectomy (48999)*
Endoscopy small intestine (44360-44379)
Esophagogastroduodenoscopy:
Flexible, transoral (43242, [43266], 43259)
Flexible, transoral; with transendoscopic ultrasound-guided transmural injection diagnostic or therapeutic substance(s), on same lesion (43253)
Esophagoscopy, flexible, transnasal (43197-43198)
Procedure performed more than one time per operative session

🖩 11.5   ⚕ 11.5   **FUD** 000   J J8 ▭

AMA: 2019,Oct,10; 2018,Jan,8; 2017,Jan,8; 2016,Jan,13

43241 with insertion of intraluminal tube or catheter

EXCLUDES   *Endoscopy small intestine (44360-44379)*
Esophagogastroduodenoscopy, flexible, transoral ([43266])
Esophagoscopy, flexible, transnasal or transoral (43197-43198, 43212)
Insertion long gastrointestinal tube (44500, 74340)
Naso or oro-gastric requiring professional skill and fluoroscopic guidance (43752)

🖩 4.17   ⚕ 4.17   **FUD** 000   J A2 ▭

AMA: 2019,Oct,10; 2018,Jan,8; 2017,Jan,8; 2016,Jan,13

43242 with transendoscopic ultrasound-guided intramural or transmural fine needle aspiration/biopsy(s) (includes endoscopic ultrasound examination of the esophagus, stomach, and either the duodenum or a surgically altered stomach where the jejunum is examined distal to the anastomosis)

INCLUDES   Gastrointestinal endoscopic ultrasound, supervision and interpretation (76975)
Ultrasonic guidance (76942)

EXCLUDES   *Endoscopy small intestine (44360-44379)*
Esophagogastroduodenoscopy, flexible, transoral (43237-43238, 43240, 43259)
Esophagoscopy, flexible, transnasal (43197-43198)
Procedure performed more than one time per operative session
Transmural fine needle biopsy/aspiration with ultrasound guidance, transendoscopic, esophagus/stomach/duodenum/neighboring structure (43238)

▣ 88172-88173

🖩 7.58   ⚕ 7.58   **FUD** 000   J A2 ▭

AMA: 2019,Oct,10; 2018,Jan,8; 2017,Jan,8; 2016,Jan,13

43243 with injection sclerosis of esophageal/gastric varices

EXCLUDES   *Endoscopy small intestine (44360-44379)*
Esophagogastroduodenoscopy, flexible, transoral on same lesion (43236, 43255)
Esophagoscopy, flexible, transnasal (43197-43198)

🖩 6.85   ⚕ 6.85   **FUD** 000   J A2 ▭

AMA: 2019,Oct,10; 2018,Jan,8; 2017,Jan,8; 2016,Jan,13

43244 with band ligation of esophageal/gastric varices

EXCLUDES   *Band ligation, non-variceal bleeding (43255)*
Endoscopy small intestine (44360-44379)
Esophagoscopy, flexible, transnasal (43197-43198)

🖩 7.08   ⚕ 7.08   **FUD** 000   J A2 ▭

AMA: 2019,Oct,10; 2018,Jan,8; 2017,Jan,8; 2016,Jan,13

43245 with dilation of gastric/duodenal stricture(s) (eg, balloon, bougie)

EXCLUDES   *Endoscopy small intestine (44360-44379)*
Esophagogastroduodenoscopy, flexible, transoral ([43266])
Esophagoscopy, flexible, transnasal (43197-43198)

▣ (74360)

🖩 5.08   ⚕ 16.7   **FUD** 000   J A2 ▭

AMA: 2019,Oct,10; 2018,Jan,8; 2017,Jan,8; 2016,Jan,13

43246 with directed placement of percutaneous gastrostomy tube

> EXCLUDES Endoscopy small intestine (44360-44372, 44376-44379)
> Esophagoscopy, flexible, transnasal (43197-43198)
> Gastrostomy tube replacement without endoscopy or imaging (43762-43763)
> Percutaneous insertion gastrostomy tube (49440)

🚗 5.86 ⚕ 5.86 **FUD** 000 　 J A2 80 ▢

AMA: 2019,Oct,10; 2019,Feb,5; 2018,Jan,8; 2017,Jan,8; 2016,Jan,13

Endoscope
Esophagus
Gastrostomy tube (PEG)
Stomach
Duodenum

43247 with removal of foreign body(s)

> EXCLUDES Endoscopy small intestine (44360-44379)
> Esophagoscopy, flexible, transnasal (43197-43198)

📷 (76000)

🚗 5.11 ⚕ 10.5 **FUD** 000 　 T A2 ▢

AMA: 2019,Oct,10; 2018,Jan,8; 2017,Jan,8; 2016,Jan,13

43248 with insertion of guide wire followed by passage of dilator(s) through esophagus over guide wire

> EXCLUDES Endoscopy small intestine (44360-44379)
> Esophagogastroduodenoscopy, flexible, transoral ([43266], [43270])
> Esophagoscopy, flexible, transnasal (43197-43198)

📷 (74360)

🚗 4.78 ⚕ 11.0 **FUD** 000 　 T A2 ▢

AMA: 2019,Oct,10; 2018,Jan,8; 2017,Jul,10; 2017,Jan,8; 2016,Jan,13

43249 with transendoscopic balloon dilation of esophagus (less than 30 mm diameter)

> EXCLUDES Endoscopy small intestine (44360-44379)
> Esophagogastroduodenoscopy:
>   Ablation lesion/tumor/polyp, when performed on same lesion ([43270])
>   With placement endoscopic stent ([43266])
> Esophagoscopy, flexible, transnasal (43197-43198)

📷 (74360)

🚗 4.42 ⚕ 31.0 **FUD** 000 　 J A2 ▢

AMA: 2019,Oct,10; 2018,Jul,14; 2018,Jan,8; 2017,Jan,8; 2016,Jan,13

#　43233 with dilation of esophagus with balloon (30 mm diameter or larger) (includes fluoroscopic guidance, when performed)

> INCLUDES Fluoroscopy (76000)
> EXCLUDES Endoscopy small intestine (44360-44379)
> Esophagoscopy, flexible, transnasal (43197-43198)
> Intraluminal dilation strictures and/or obstructions (e.g., esophagus), radiological supervision and interpretation (74360)

🚗 6.62 ⚕ 6.62 **FUD** 000 　 J G2 ▢

AMA: 2019,Oct,10; 2018,Jan,8; 2017,Jan,8; 2016,Jan,13

43250 with removal of tumor(s), polyp(s), or other lesion(s) by hot biopsy forceps

> EXCLUDES Endoscopy small intestine (44360-44379)
> Esophagoscopy, flexible, transnasal (43197-43198)

🚗 4.97 ⚕ 11.8 **FUD** 000 　 J A2 ▢

AMA: 2019,Oct,10; 2018,Jan,8; 2017,Jan,8; 2016,Jan,13

43251 with removal of tumor(s), polyp(s), or other lesion(s) by snare technique

> EXCLUDES Endoscopic mucosal resection when performed on same lesion (43254)
> Endoscopy small intestine (44360-44379)
> Esophagoscopy, flexible, transnasal (43197-43198)

🚗 5.66 ⚕ 13.5 **FUD** 000 　 J A2 ▢

AMA: 2019,Oct,10; 2018,Jan,8; 2017,Jan,8; 2016,Jan,13

43252 with optical endomicroscopy

> EXCLUDES Endoscopy small intestine (44360-44379)
> Esophagoscopy, flexible, transnasal (43197-43198)
> Optical endomicroscopic image(s), interpretation and report (88375)

Code also contrast agent

🚗 4.95 ⚕ 8.96 **FUD** 000 　 J G2 ▢

AMA: 2019,Oct,10; 2018,Jan,8; 2017,Jan,8; 2016,Jan,13

43253 with transendoscopic ultrasound-guided transmural injection of diagnostic or therapeutic substance(s) (eg, anesthetic, neurolytic agent) or fiducial marker(s) (includes endoscopic ultrasound examination of the esophagus, stomach, and either the duodenum or a surgically altered stomach where the jejunum is examined distal to the anastomosis)

> INCLUDES Gastrointestinal endoscopic ultrasound, supervision and interpretation (76975)
> Ultrasonic guidance (76942)
> EXCLUDES Endoscopy small intestine (44360-44379)
> Esophagogastroduodenoscopy:
>   Flexible, transoral (43237, 43259)
>   Flexible, transoral; with transmural drainage pseudocyst on same lesion with (43240)
> Esophagoscopy, flexible, transnasal (43197-43198)
> Procedure performed more than one time per operative session
> Transmural fine needle biopsy/aspiration with ultrasound guidance, transendoscopic, esophagus/stomach/duodenum/neighboring structures (43238, 43242)

🚗 7.70 ⚕ 7.70 **FUD** 000 　 J G2 ▢

AMA: 2019,Oct,10; 2018,Apr,10; 2018,Jan,8; 2017,Jan,8; 2016,Jan,13

43254 with endoscopic mucosal resection

> EXCLUDES Endoscopy small intestine (44360-44379)
> Esophagogastroduodenoscopy, flexible, transoral, on same lesion (43236, 43239, 43251)
> Esophagoscopy, flexible, transnasal (43197-43198)

🚗 7.80 ⚕ 7.80 **FUD** 000 　 J G2 ▢

AMA: 2019,Dec,14; 2019,Oct,10; 2018,Jan,8; 2017,Jan,8; 2016,Jan,13

43255 with control of bleeding, any method

> EXCLUDES Endoscopy small intestine (44360-44379)
> Esophagogastroduodenoscopy, flexible, transoral, on same lesion (43236, 43243-43244)
> Esophagoscopy, flexible, transnasal (43197-43198)

🚗 5.79 ⚕ 18.6 **FUD** 000 　 J A2 ▢

AMA: 2019,Oct,10; 2018,Jan,8; 2017,Jan,8; 2016,Jan,13

Digestive System

43266 — 43262

with placement of endoscopic stent (includes pre- and post-dilation and guide wire passage, when performed)

43266

INCLUDES When performed:
  Balloon dilation esophagus (43249)
  Dilation gastric/duodenal stricture (43245)
  Insertion guidewire/dilator (43248)

EXCLUDES *Endoscopy small intestine (44360-44379)*
  Esophagogastroduodenoscopy:
  Insertion intraluminal tube or catheter (43241)
  Transmural drainage pseudocyst (43240)
  Esophagoscopy, flexible, transnasal (43197-43198)

  (74360)

  6.39   6.39   **FUD** 000   J J8

  AMA: 2019,Oct,10; 2018,Jan,8; 2017,Jan,8; 2016,Jan,13

43257 with delivery of thermal energy to the muscle of lower esophageal sphincter and/or gastric cardia, for treatment of gastroesophageal reflux disease

EXCLUDES *Endoscopy small intestine (44360-44379)*
  Esophageal lesion ablation (43229, [43270])
  Esophagoscopy, flexible, transnasal (43197-43198)

  6.74   6.74   **FUD** 000   J A2

  AMA: 2019,Oct,10; 2018,Jan,8; 2017,Jan,8; 2016,Jan,13

43270 with ablation of tumor(s), polyp(s), or other lesion(s) (includes pre- and post-dilation and guide wire passage, when performed)

INCLUDES Endoscopic dilation performed on same lesion (43248-43249)

EXCLUDES *Endoscopy small intestine (44360-44379)*
  Esophagoscopy, flexible, transnasal (43197-43198)

  Code also photodynamic therapy, when performed (96570-96571)

  6.48   20.3   **FUD** 000   J G2

  AMA: 2019,Oct,10; 2018,Jan,8; 2017,Jan,8; 2016,Jan,13

43259 with endoscopic ultrasound examination, including the esophagus, stomach, and either the duodenum or a surgically altered stomach where the jejunum is examined distal to the anastomosis

INCLUDES Gastrointestinal endoscopic ultrasound, supervision and interpretation (76975)

EXCLUDES *Endoscopy small intestine (44360-44379)*
  Esophagogastroduodenoscopy, flexible, transoral (43237, 43240, 43242, 43253)
  Esophagoscopy, flexible, transnasal (43197-43198)
  Procedure performed more than one time per operative session

  6.53   6.53   **FUD** 000   J A2

  AMA: 2019,Oct,10; 2018,Jan,8; 2017,Jan,8; 2016,Jan,13; 2016,Jan,11

43210 with esophagogastric fundoplasty, partial or complete, includes duodenoscopy when performed

EXCLUDES *Esophagogastroduodenoscopy:*
  Flexible, transnasal (43197)
  Rigid, transoral (43180, 43191)
  Esophagoscopy, flexible, transoral (43200)

  12.5   12.5   **FUD** 000   J G2

  AMA: 2018,Jan,8; 2017,Jan,8; 2016,Jan,13

43260-43278 [43266, 43270, 43274, 43275, 43276, 43277, 43278] Endoscopic Procedures: ERCP

INCLUDES Diagnostic endoscopy with surgical endoscopy
  Pancreaticobiliary system:
  Biliary tree (right and left hepatic ducts, cystic duct/gallbladder, and common bile ducts)
  Pancreas (major and minor ducts)

EXCLUDES *ERCP via Roux-en-Y anatomy (for instance post-gastric or bariatric bypass or post total gastrectomy) or via gastrostomy (open or laparoscopic) (47999, 48999)*
  Optical endomicroscopy biliary tract and pancreas, report one time per session (0397T)
  Percutaneous biliary catheter procedures (47490-47544)

Code also:
  Appropriate endoscopy each anatomic site examined
  ERCP procedure when performed on altered postoperative anatomy (i.e., Billroth II gastroenterostomy) (43260, 43262-43265, [43274], [43275], [43276], [43277], [43278], 43273)
  Sphincteroplasty or ductal stricture dilation, when necessary to access debris/stones ([43277])

  (74328-74330)

43260 Endoscopic retrograde cholangiopancreatography (ERCP); diagnostic, including collection of specimen(s) by brushing or washing, when performed (separate procedure)

EXCLUDES *Endoscopic retrograde cholangiopancreatography (ERCP), therapeutic (43261-43265, 43274-43278 [43274, 43275, 43276, 43277, 43278])*

  9.31   9.31   **FUD** 000   J A2

  AMA: 2018,Jan,8; 2017,Jan,8; 2016,Jan,13

43261 with biopsy, single or multiple

INCLUDES Endoscopic retrograde cholangiopancreatography (ERCP); diagnostic (43260)

EXCLUDES *Percutaneous endoluminal biopsy biliary tree (47543)*

  9.92   9.92   **FUD** 000   J A2

  AMA: 2018,Jan,8; 2017,Jan,8; 2016,Jan,13

43262 with sphincterotomy/papillotomy

INCLUDES Endoscopic retrograde cholangiopancreatography (ERCP), diagnostic (43260)

EXCLUDES *Endoscopic retrograde cholangiopancreatography (ERCP):*
  With exchange/insertion/removal stent in same location ([43274], [43276])
  With trans-endoscopic balloon dilation ampulla/biliary or pancreatic ducts ([43277])
  Percutaneous balloon dilation biliary duct or ampulla (47542)

  Code also procedure performed with sphincterotomy (43261, 43263-43265, [43275], [43278])

  10.3   10.3   **FUD** 000   J A2

  AMA: 2018,Jan,8; 2017,Jan,8; 2016,Jan,13

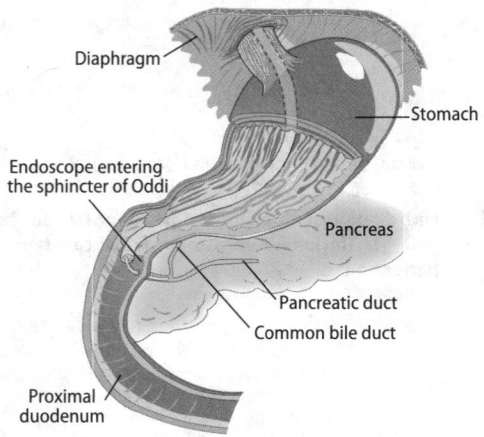

An endoscope is fed through the stomach and into the duodenum Usually a smaller sub-scope is fed up the sphincter of Oddi and into the ducts that drain the pancreas and the gallbladder (common bile)

43263 **with pressure measurement of sphincter of Oddi**

INCLUDES Endoscopic retrograde cholangiopancreatography (ERCP); diagnostic (43260)

EXCLUDES *Procedure performed more than one time per session*

🖐 10.4   ✂ 10.4   **FUD** 000   J A2 ▭

AMA: 2018,Jan,8; 2017,Jan,8; 2016,Jan,13

43264 **with removal of calculi/debris from biliary/pancreatic duct(s)**

INCLUDES Endoscopic retrograde cholangiopancreatography (ERCP); diagnostic (43260)

Incidental dilation due to instrument passage

EXCLUDES *Endoscopic retrograde cholangiopancreatography (ERCP) with calculi destruction (43265)*

Findings without debris or calculi, even when balloon used

Percutaneous calculus/debris removal (47544)

Code also sphincteroplasty when dilation necessary to access debris/stones ([43277])

🖐 10.4   ✂ 10.4   **FUD** 000   J A2 ▭

AMA: 2018,Jan,8; 2017,Jan,8; 2016,Jan,13

43265 **with destruction of calculi, any method (eg, mechanical, electrohydraulic, lithotripsy)**

INCLUDES Endoscopic retrograde cholangiopancreatography (ERCP); diagnostic (43260)

Incidental dilation due to instrument passage

Stone removal in same ductal system

EXCLUDES *Endoscopic retrograde cholangiopancreatography (ERCP) with removal of calculi/debris from biliary/pancreatic duct(s) (43264)*

Findings without debris or calculi, even when balloon used

Percutaneous calculus/debris removal (47544)

Code also sphincteroplasty when dilation necessary to access debris/stones ([43277])

🖐 12.5   ✂ 12.5   **FUD** 000   J A2 ▭

AMA: 2018,Jan,8; 2017,Jan,8; 2016,Jan,13

43266 **Resequenced code. See code following 43255.**

43270 **Resequenced code. See code following 43257.**

\# **43274** **with placement of endoscopic stent into biliary or pancreatic duct, including pre- and post-dilation and guide wire passage, when performed, including sphincterotomy, when performed, each stent**

INCLUDES Balloon dilation in same duct

Endoscopic retrograde cholangiopancreatography (ERCP); diagnostic (43260)

Tube placement for naso-pancreatic or naso-biliary drainage

EXCLUDES *Percutaneous placement biliary stent (47538-47540)*

Procedures for stent placement or exchange in same duct (43262, [43275], [43276], [43277])

Code also for each additional stent placement in different ducts or side by side in same duct same session/day, using modifier 59 with ([43274])

🖐 13.3   ✂ 13.3   **FUD** 000   J G2 ▭

AMA: 2018,Jan,8; 2017,Jan,8; 2016,Jan,13

\# **43275** **with removal of foreign body(s) or stent(s) from biliary/pancreatic duct(s)**

INCLUDES Endoscopic retrograde cholangiopancreatography (ERCP); diagnostic (43260)

EXCLUDES *Endoscopic retrograde cholangiopancreatography (ERCP) with exchange, placement, or removal of stent ([43274], [43276])*

Pancreatic or biliary duct stent removal without ERCP (43247)

Percutaneous calculus/debris removal (47544)

Procedure performed more than one time per session

🖐 11.0   ✂ 11.0   **FUD** 000   J G2 ▭

AMA: 2018,Jan,8; 2017,Jan,8; 2016,Jan,13

\# **43276** **with removal and exchange of stent(s), biliary or pancreatic duct, including pre- and post-dilation and guide wire passage, when performed, including sphincterotomy, when performed, each stent exchanged**

INCLUDES Balloon dilation in same duct

Endoscopic retrograde cholangiopancreatography (ERCP); diagnostic (43260)

Stent placement or exchange one stent

EXCLUDES *Endoscopic retrograde cholangiopancreatography (ERCP) with removal foreign body(s) or stent(s) ([43275])*

Procedures for stent insertion or exchange stent in same duct (43262, [43274])

Code also each additional stent exchanged same session/day, using modifier 59 with ([43276])

🖐 13.9   ✂ 13.9   **FUD** 000   J G2 ▭

AMA: 2018,Jan,8; 2017,Jan,8; 2016,Jan,13

\# **43277** **with trans-endoscopic balloon dilation of biliary/pancreatic duct(s) or of ampulla (sphincteroplasty), including sphincterotomy, when performed, each duct**

INCLUDES Endoscopic retrograde cholangiopancreatography (ERCP); diagnostic (43260)

EXCLUDES *Endoscopic retrograde cholangiopancreatography (ERCP):*

With ablation tumor(s), polyp(s), or other lesion(s) for same lesion ([43278])

With sphincterotomy/papillotomy (43262)

With stent exchange/removal same biliary/pancreatic duct ([43276])

With stent placement into same biliary/pancreatic duct ([43274])

Percutaneous dilation biliary duct/ampulla (47542)

Removal stone/debris, dilation incidental to instrument passage (43264-43265)

Code also:

Both right and left hepatic duct (bilateral) balloon dilation, using ([43277]); append modifier 59 to second procedure

Each additional balloon dilation in different ducts or side by side in same duct same session/day, appending modifier 59 to ([43277])

Sphincterotomy without sphincteroplasty during same operative session in different duct, appending modifier 59 to (43262)

🖐 10.9   ✂ 10.9   **FUD** 000   J G2 ▭

AMA: 2018,Jan,8; 2017,Jan,8; 2016,Jan,13

\# **43278** **with ablation of tumor(s), polyp(s), or other lesion(s), including pre- and post-dilation and guide wire passage, when performed**

INCLUDES Endoscopic retrograde cholangiopancreatography (ERCP); diagnostic (43260)

EXCLUDES *Ampullectomy (43254)*

Endoscopic retrograde cholangiopancreatography (ERCP); with trans-endoscopic balloon dilation biliary/pancreatic duct(s) or ampulla (sphincteroplasty) in same lesion with ([43277])

🖐 12.5   ✂ 12.5   **FUD** 000   J G2 ▭

AMA: 2018,Jan,8; 2017,Jan,8; 2016,Jan,13

\+ **43273** **Endoscopic cannulation of papilla with direct visualization of pancreatic/common bile duct(s) (List separately in addition to code(s) for primary procedure)**

EXCLUDES *Procedure performed more than one time per session*

Code first (43260-43265, [43274], [43275], [43276], [43277], [43278])

🖐 3.47   ✂ 3.47   **FUD** ZZZ   N N1 80 ▭

AMA: 2018,Jan,8; 2017,Jan,8; 2016,Jan,13

43274 **Resequenced code. See code following code 43270.**

43275 **Resequenced code. See code following code 43270.**

43276 **Resequenced code. See code following code 43270.**

43277 **Resequenced code. See code following code 43270.**

43278 **Resequenced code. See code following code 43270.**

● New Code ▲ Revised Code ○ Reinstated ● New Web Release ▲ Revised Web Release + Add-on Unlisted Not Covered \# Resequenced

50 Optum Mod 50 Exempt ⊘ AMA Mod 51 Exempt 51 Optum Mod 51 Exempt 63 Mod 63 Exempt ✗ Non-FDA Drug ★ Telemedicine M Maternity A Age Edit

© 2021 Optum360, LLC   CPT © 2021 American Medical Association. All Rights Reserved.   **195**

43279-43289 Laparoscopic Procedures of Esophagus

INCLUDES Diagnostic laparoscopy with surgical laparoscopy (49320)

43279 **Laparoscopy, surgical, esophagomyotomy (Heller type), with fundoplasty, when performed**

EXCLUDES *Esophagomyotomy, open method (43330–43331)*

Laparoscopy, surgical, esophagogastric fundoplasty (43280)

🛏 37.5 ⚕ 37.5 **FUD** 090 C 80 ▣

AMA: 2018,Jan,8; 2017,Aug,6; 2017,Jan,8; 2016,Jan,13

43280 **Laparoscopy, surgical, esophagogastric fundoplasty (eg, Nissen, Toupet procedures)**

EXCLUDES *Esophagogastric fundoplasty, open method (43327–43328)*

Esophagogastroduodenoscopy fundoplasty, transoral (43210)

Laparoscopy, surgical, esophageal sphincter augmentation (43284–43285)

Laparoscopy, surgical, esophagomyotomy (43279)

Laparoscopy, surgical, fundoplasty (43281–43282)

🛏 31.4 ⚕ 31.4 **FUD** 090 J 62 80 ▣

AMA: 2018,Jan,8; 2017,Aug,6; 2017,Jan,8; 2016,Jan,13

Esophagus

Diaphragm

Fundus of stomach

Normal stomach   After surgery

43281 **Laparoscopy, surgical, repair of paraesophageal hernia, includes fundoplasty, when performed; without implantation of mesh**

EXCLUDES *Dilation esophagus (43450, 43453)*

Implantation mesh or other prosthesis (49568)

Laparoscopy, surgical, esophagogastric fundoplasty (43280)

Transabdominal repair paraesophageal hiatal hernia (43332–43333)

Transthoracic repair diaphragmatic hernia (43334–43335)

🛏 44.7 ⚕ 44.7 **FUD** 090 J 62 80 ▣

AMA: 2018,Nov,11; 2018,Sep,14; 2018,Jan,8; 2017,Aug,6; 2017,Jan,8; 2016,Jan,13

43282 **with implantation of mesh**

EXCLUDES *Dilation esophagus (43450, 43453)*

Laparoscopy, surgical, esophagogastric fundoplasty (43280)

Transabdominal paraesophageal hernia repair (43332–43333)

Transthoracic paraesophageal hernia repair (43334–43335)

🛏 50.6 ⚕ 50.6 **FUD** 090 J 62 80 ▣

AMA: 2018,Jan,8; 2017,Aug,6; 2017,Jan,8; 2016,Aug,9; 2016,Jan,13

+ 43283 **Laparoscopy, surgical, esophageal lengthening procedure (eg, Collis gastroplasty or wedge gastroplasty) (List separately in addition to code for primary procedure)**

Code first (43280–43282)

🛏 4.60 ⚕ 4.60 **FUD** ZZZ C 80 ▣

AMA: 2018,Jan,8; 2017,Jan,8; 2016,Jan,13

43284 **Laparoscopy, surgical, esophageal sphincter augmentation procedure, placement of sphincter augmentation device (ie, magnetic band), including cruroplasty when performed**

EXCLUDES *Performed during same session (43279–43282)*

🛏 18.9 ⚕ 18.9 **FUD** 090 J J8 80 ▣

AMA: 2019,Apr,10; 2018,Sep,14; 2018,Jan,8; 2017,Aug,6

43285 **Removal of esophageal sphincter augmentation device**

🛏 19.5 ⚕ 19.5 **FUD** 090 02 62 80 ▣

AMA: 2018,Jan,8; 2017,Aug,6

43286 **Esophagectomy, total or near total, with laparoscopic mobilization of the abdominal and mediastinal esophagus and proximal gastrectomy, with laparoscopic pyloric drainage procedure if performed, with open cervical pharyngogastrostomy or esophagogastrostomy (ie, laparoscopic transhiatal esophagectomy)**

🛏 90.9 ⚕ 90.9 **FUD** 090 C 80 ▣

AMA: 2018,Jul,7

43287 **Esophagectomy, distal two-thirds, with laparoscopic mobilization of the abdominal and lower mediastinal esophagus and proximal gastrectomy, with laparoscopic pyloric drainage procedure if performed, with separate thoracoscopic mobilization of the middle and upper mediastinal esophagus and thoracic esophagogastrostomy (ie, laparoscopic thoracoscopic esophagectomy, Ivor Lewis esophagectomy)**

EXCLUDES *Right tube thoracostomy (32551)*

🛏 104. ⚕ 104. **FUD** 090 C 80 ▣

AMA: 2018,Jul,7

43288 **Esophagectomy, total or near total, with thoracoscopic mobilization of the upper, middle, and lower mediastinal esophagus, with separate laparoscopic proximal gastrectomy, with laparoscopic pyloric drainage procedure if performed, with open cervical pharyngogastrostomy or esophagogastrostomy (ie, thoracoscopic, laparoscopic and cervical incision esophagectomy, McKeown esophagectomy, tri-incisional esophagectomy)**

EXCLUDES *Right tube thoracostomy (32551)*

🛏 109. ⚕ 109. **FUD** 090 C 80 ▣

AMA: 2018,Jul,7

43289 **Unlisted laparoscopy procedure, esophagus**

🛏 0.00 ⚕ 0.00 **FUD** YYY J 80 50 ▣

AMA: 2018,Jul,7; 2018,Jan,8; 2017,Jan,8; 2016,Jan,13

26/TC PC/TC Only   A2-Z3 ASC Payment   50 Bilateral   ♂ Male Only   ♀ Female Only   🛏 Facility RVU   ⚕ Non-Facility RVU   ▣ CCI   ☒ CLIA

FUD Follow-up Days   **CMS:** IOM   **AMA:** CPT Asst   A-Y OPPSI   80/80 Surg Assist Allowed / w/Doc   ▣ Lab Crosswalk   ▣ Radiology Crosswalk

196   CPT © 2021 American Medical Association. All Rights Reserved.   © 2021 Optum360, LLC

43300-43425 Open Esophageal Repair Procedures

43300 Esophagoplasty (plastic repair or reconstruction), cervical approach; without repair of tracheoesophageal fistula
🚗 17.6 🔪 17.6 **FUD** 090 C 80 ▢
AMA: 2014,Jan,11; 2013,Jan,11-12

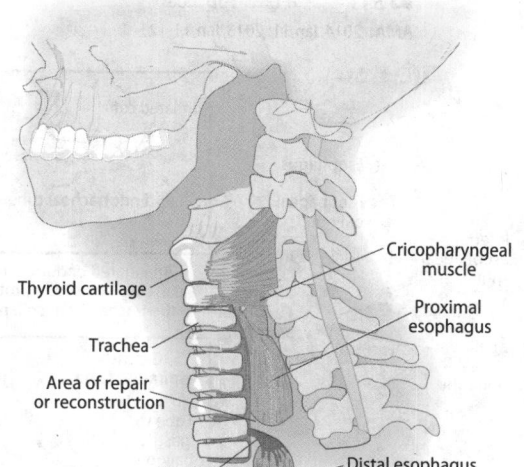

Cricopharyngeal muscle
Thyroid cartilage
Proximal esophagus
Trachea
Area of repair or reconstruction
Fistula
Distal esophagus

Example of esophageal atresia where the proximal esophagus fails to communicate with the lower portion; note that a fistula has developed from the trachea

43305 with repair of tracheoesophageal fistula
🚗 31.3 🔪 31.3 **FUD** 090 C 80 ▢
AMA: 2014,Jan,11; 2013,Jan,11-12

43310 Esophagoplasty (plastic repair or reconstruction), thoracic approach; without repair of tracheoesophageal fistula
🚗 42.9 🔪 42.9 **FUD** 090 C 80 ▢
AMA: 2014,Jan,11; 2013,Jan,11-12

43312 with repair of tracheoesophageal fistula
🚗 46.1 🔪 46.1 **FUD** 090 C 80 ▢
AMA: 2014,Jan,11; 2013,Jan,11-12

43313 Esophagoplasty for congenital defect (plastic repair or reconstruction), thoracic approach; without repair of congenital tracheoesophageal fistula
🚗 79.3 🔪 79.3 **FUD** 090 63 C 80 ▢
AMA: 2014,Jan,11; 2013,Jan,11-12

43314 with repair of congenital tracheoesophageal fistula
🚗 85.2 🔪 85.2 **FUD** 090 63 C 80 ▢
AMA: 2014,Jan,11; 2013,Jan,11-12

43320 Esophagogastrostomy (cardioplasty), with or without vagotomy and pyloroplasty, transabdominal or transthoracic approach
EXCLUDES *Laparoscopic approach (43280)*
🚗 40.7 🔪 40.7 **FUD** 090 C 80 ▢
AMA: 2014,Jan,11; 2013,Jan,11-12

43325 Esophagogastric fundoplasty, with fundic patch (Thal-Nissen procedure)
EXCLUDES *Myotomy, cricopharyngeal (43030)*
🚗 39.6 🔪 39.6 **FUD** 090 C 80 ▢
AMA: 2014,Jan,11; 2013,Jan,11-12

43327 Esophagogastric fundoplasty partial or complete; laparotomy
🚗 23.9 🔪 23.9 **FUD** 090 C 80 ▢
AMA: 2018,Jan,8; 2017,Jan,8; 2016,Jan,13

43328 thoracotomy
EXCLUDES *Esophagogastroduodenoscopy fundoplasty, transoral (43210)*
🚗 32.6 🔪 32.6 **FUD** 090 C 80 ▢
AMA: 2018,Jan,8; 2017,Jan,8; 2016,Jan,13

43330 Esophagomyotomy (Heller type); abdominal approach
EXCLUDES *Esophagomyotomy, laparoscopic method (43279)*
🚗 38.9 🔪 38.9 **FUD** 090 C 80 ▢
AMA: 2018,Jan,8; 2017,Jan,8; 2016,Jan,13

43331 thoracic approach
EXCLUDES *Thoracoscopy with esophagomyotomy (32665)*
🚗 38.7 🔪 38.7 **FUD** 090 C 80 ▢
AMA: 2018,Jan,8; 2017,Jan,8; 2016,Jan,13

43332 Repair, paraesophageal hiatal hernia (including fundoplication), via laparotomy, except neonatal; without implantation of mesh or other prosthesis
EXCLUDES *Neonatal diaphragmatic hernia repair (39503)*
🚗 33.7 🔪 33.7 **FUD** 090 C 80 ▢
AMA: 2018,Jan,8; 2017,Jan,8; 2016,Jan,13

43333 with implantation of mesh or other prosthesis
EXCLUDES *Neonatal diaphragmatic hernia repair (39503)*
🚗 36.8 🔪 36.8 **FUD** 090 C 80 ▢
AMA: 2018,Jan,8; 2017,Jan,8; 2016,Jan,13

43334 Repair, paraesophageal hiatal hernia (including fundoplication), via thoracotomy, except neonatal; without implantation of mesh or other prosthesis
EXCLUDES *Neonatal diaphragmatic hernia repair (39503)*
🚗 36.2 🔪 36.2 **FUD** 090 C 80 ▢
AMA: 2018,Jan,8; 2017,Jan,8; 2016,Jan,13

43335 with implantation of mesh or other prosthesis
EXCLUDES *Neonatal diaphragmatic hernia repair (39503)*
🚗 38.7 🔪 38.7 **FUD** 090 C 80 ▢
AMA: 2018,Jan,8; 2017,Jan,8; 2016,Jan,13

43336 Repair, paraesophageal hiatal hernia, (including fundoplication), via thoracoabdominal incision, except neonatal; without implantation of mesh or other prosthesis
EXCLUDES *Neonatal diaphragmatic hernia repair (39503)*
🚗 42.0 🔪 42.0 **FUD** 090 C 80 ▢
AMA: 2018,Jan,8; 2017,Jan,8; 2016,Jan,13

43337 with implantation of mesh or other prosthesis
EXCLUDES *Neonatal diaphragmatic hernia repair (39503)*
🚗 44.8 🔪 44.8 **FUD** 090 C 80 ▢
AMA: 2018,Jan,8; 2017,Jan,8; 2016,Jan,13

+ **43338** Esophageal lengthening procedure (eg, Collis gastroplasty or wedge gastroplasty) (List separately in addition to code for primary procedure)
Code first (43280, 43327-43337)
🚗 3.37 🔪 3.37 **FUD** ZZZ C 80 ▢
AMA: 2018,Jan,8; 2017,Jan,8; 2016,Jan,13

43340 Esophagojejunostomy (without total gastrectomy); abdominal approach
🚗 40.0 🔪 40.0 **FUD** 090 C 80 ▢
AMA: 2014,Jan,11; 2013,Jan,11-12

43341 thoracic approach
🚗 40.5 🔪 40.5 **FUD** 090 C 80 ▢
AMA: 2014,Jan,11; 2013,Jan,11-12

43351 Esophagostomy, fistulization of esophagus, external; thoracic approach
🚗 38.0 🔪 38.0 **FUD** 090 C 80 ▢
AMA: 2014,Jan,11; 2013,Jan,11-12

43352 cervical approach
🚗 30.8 🔪 30.8 **FUD** 090 C 80 ▢
AMA: 2014,Jan,11; 2013,Jan,11-12

43360 Gastrointestinal reconstruction for previous esophagectomy, for obstructing esophageal lesion or fistula, or for previous esophageal exclusion; with stomach, with or without pyloroplasty
🚗 65.3 🔪 65.3 **FUD** 090 C 80 ▢
AMA: 2014,Jan,11; 2013,Jan,11-12

Digestive System

43361 — 43520

43361   **with colon interposition or small intestine reconstruction, including intestine mobilization, preparation, and anastomosis(es)**
📋 78.6   ⚕ 78.6   **FUD** 090   C 80 ▭
AMA: 2014,Jan,11; 2013,Jan,11-12

43400   **Ligation, direct, esophageal varices**
📋 44.4   ⚕ 44.4   **FUD** 090   C 80 ▭
AMA: 2014,Jan,11; 2013,Jan,11-12

43405   **Ligation or stapling at gastroesophageal junction for pre-existing esophageal perforation**
📋 42.1   ⚕ 42.1   **FUD** 090   C 80 ▭
AMA: 2014,Jan,11; 2013,Jan,11-12

43410   **Suture of esophageal wound or injury; cervical approach**
📋 29.3   ⚕ 29.3   **FUD** 090   C 80 ▭
AMA: 2018,Jan,8; 2017,Jan,8; 2016,Jan,13

43415   **transthoracic or transabdominal approach**
📋 74.5   ⚕ 74.5   **FUD** 090   C 80 ▭
AMA: 2014,Jan,11; 2013,Jan,11-12

43420   **Closure of esophagostomy or fistula; cervical approach**
EXCLUDES   *Paraesophageal hiatal hernia repair:*
        Transabdominal (43332-43333)
        Transthoracic (43334-43335)
📋 29.1   ⚕ 29.1   **FUD** 090   J 62 80 ▭
AMA: 2014,Jan,11; 2013,Jan,11-12

43425   **transthoracic or transabdominal approach**
EXCLUDES   *Paraesophageal hiatal hernia repair:*
        Transabdominal (43332-43333)
        Transthoracic (43334-43335)
📋 41.8   ⚕ 41.8   **FUD** 090   C 80 ▭
AMA: 2014,Jan,11; 2013,Jan,11-12

43450-43453 Esophageal Dilation

43450   **Dilation of esophagus, by unguided sound or bougie, single or multiple passes**
📷 (74220, 74360)
📋 2.27   ⚕ 4.87   **FUD** 000   T A2 ▭
AMA: 2018,Jan,8; 2017,Jul,10; 2017,Jan,8; 2016,Jan,13

43453   **Dilation of esophagus, over guide wire**
EXCLUDES   *Dilation performed with endoscopic visualization (43195, 43226)*
        Endoscopic dilation by dilator or balloon:
        Balloon diameter 30 mm or larger (43214, 43233)
        Balloon diameter less than 30 mm (43195, 43220, 43249)
📷 (74220, 74360)
📋 2.50   ⚕ 25.4   **FUD** 000   J A2 ▭
AMA: 2018,Jan,8; 2017,Jan,8; 2016,Jan,13

43460-43499 Other/Unlisted Esophageal Procedures

43460   **Esophagogastric tamponade, with balloon (Sengstaken type)**
EXCLUDES   *Removal foreign body esophagus with balloon catheter (43499, 74235)*
📷 (74220)
📋 6.13   ⚕ 6.13   **FUD** 000   C ▭
AMA: 2014,Jan,11; Jan,11-12

[Anatomical illustration with labels: Esophagus, Esophageal balloon, Inferior esophageal sphincter, Diaphragm, Gastric balloon and aspiration tube, Fundus of stomach, Inflated cuff, Endotracheal tube, "An inflated endotracheal cuff may be used to protect the trachea from collapse", Gastric aspiration tube, Tube to gastric balloon, Tube to esophageal balloon]

Cutaway view of Sengstaken-type esophagogastric tamponade with balloons inflated

43496   **Free jejunum transfer with microvascular anastomosis**
INCLUDES   Operating microscope (69990)
📋 0.00   ⚕ 0.00   **FUD** 090   C 80 ▭
AMA: 2019,Dec,5; 2018,Jan,8; 2017,Jan,8; 2016,Feb,12; 2016,Jan,13

● **43497**   **Lower esophageal myotomy, transoral (ie, peroral endoscopic myotomy [POEM])**
EXCLUDES   *Esophagogastroduodenoscopy, flexible, transoral (43235)*
        Esophagoscopy:
        Flexible, transnasal (43197)
        Flexible, transoral (43200)
        Rigid, transoral (43191)
        Thoracoscopy with esophagomyotomy (32665)

43499   **Unlisted procedure, esophagus**
📋 0.00   ⚕ 0.00   **FUD** YYY   T ▭
AMA: 2018,Jul,7; 2018,Jan,8; 2017,Jan,8; 2016,Jan,13

43500-43641 Open Gastric Incisional and Resection Procedures

43500   **Gastrotomy; with exploration or foreign body removal**
📋 22.7   ⚕ 22.7   **FUD** 090   C 80 ▭
AMA: 2014,Jan,11; 2013,Jan,11-12

43501   **with suture repair of bleeding ulcer**
📋 39.2   ⚕ 39.2   **FUD** 090   C 80 ▭
AMA: 2014,Jan,11; 2013,Jan,11-12

43502   **with suture repair of pre-existing esophagogastric laceration (eg, Mallory-Weiss)**
📋 44.5   ⚕ 44.5   **FUD** 090   C 80 ▭
AMA: 2014,Jan,11; 2013,Jan,11-12

43510   **with esophageal dilation and insertion of permanent intraluminal tube (eg, Celestin or Mousseaux-Barbin)**
📋 27.6   ⚕ 27.6   **FUD** 090   T 62 80 ▭
AMA: 2014,Jan,11; 2013,Jan,11-12

43520   **Pyloromyotomy, cutting of pyloric muscle (Fredet-Ramstedt type operation)**
📋 19.9   ⚕ 19.9   **FUD** 090   63 C 80 ▭
AMA: 2014,Jan,11; 2013,Jan,11-12

26/TC PC/TC Only	A2-Z3 ASC Payment	50 Bilateral	♂ Male Only	♀ Female Only	📋 Facility RVU	⚕ Non-Facility RVU	▭ CCI	✖ CLIA
FUD Follow-up Days	CMS: IOM	AMA: CPT Asst	A-Y OPPSI		80/80 Surg Assist Allowed / w/Doc	📷 Lab Crosswalk		📷 Radiology Crosswalk

198   CPT © 2021 American Medical Association. All Rights Reserved.   © 2021 Optum360, LLC

43605 **Biopsy of stomach, by laparotomy**
🚑 24.4   ⚕ 24.4   **FUD** 090   C 80 ▣
AMA: 2014,Jan,11; 2013,Jan,11-12

43610 **Excision, local; ulcer or benign tumor of stomach**
🚑 28.5   ⚕ 28.5   **FUD** 090   C 80 ▣
AMA: 2014,Jan,11; 2013,Jan,11-12

43611 **malignant tumor of stomach**
🚑 35.6   ⚕ 35.6   **FUD** 090   C 80 ▣
AMA: 2014,Jan,11; 2013,Jan,11-12

43620 **Gastrectomy, total; with esophagoenterostomy**
🚑 57.8   ⚕ 57.8   **FUD** 090   C 80 ▣
AMA: 2014,Jan,11; 2013,Jan,11-12

43621 **with Roux-en-Y reconstruction**
🚑 66.2   ⚕ 66.2   **FUD** 090   C 80 ▣
AMA: 2014,Jan,11; 2013,Jan,11-12

43622 **with formation of intestinal pouch, any type**
🚑 67.5   ⚕ 67.5   **FUD** 090   C 80 ▣
AMA: 2014,Jan,11; 2013,Jan,11-12

43631 **Gastrectomy, partial, distal; with gastroduodenostomy**
INCLUDES Billroth operation
🚑 42.0   ⚕ 42.0   **FUD** 090   C 80 ▣
AMA: 2014,Jan,11; 2013,Jan,11-12

43632 **with gastrojejunostomy**
INCLUDES Polya anastomosis
🚑 59.3   ⚕ 59.3   **FUD** 090   C 80 ▣
AMA: 2014,Jan,11; 2013,Jan,11-12

43633 **with Roux-en-Y reconstruction**
🚑 56.1   ⚕ 56.1   **FUD** 090   C 80 ▣
AMA: 2014,Jan,11; 2013,Jan,11-12

43634 **with formation of intestinal pouch**
🚑 62.0   ⚕ 62.0   **FUD** 090   C 80 ▣
AMA: 2014,Jan,11; 2013,Jan,11-12

+ **43635** **Vagotomy when performed with partial distal gastrectomy (List separately in addition to code[s] for primary procedure)**
Code first as appropriate (43631-43634)
🚑 3.29   ⚕ 3.29   **FUD** ZZZ   C 80 ▣
AMA: 2014,Jan,11; 2013,Jan,11-12

43640 **Vagotomy including pyloroplasty, with or without gastrostomy; truncal or selective**
EXCLUDES Pyloroplasty (43800)
          Vagotomy (64755, 64760)
🚑 34.1   ⚕ 34.1   **FUD** 090   C 80 ▣
AMA: 2014,Jan,11; 2013,Jan,11-12

43641 **parietal cell (highly selective)**
EXCLUDES Upper gastrointestinal endoscopy (43235-43259 [43233, 43266, 43270])
🚑 34.9   ⚕ 34.9   **FUD** 090   C 80 ▣
AMA: 2014,Jan,11; 2013,Jan,11-12

43644-43645 Laparoscopic Gastric Bypass with Small Bowel Resection

CMS: 100-03,100.1 Bariatric Surgery for Treatment Co-morbid Conditions Due to Morbid Obesity; 100-04,32,150.1 Bariatric Surgery: Treatment of Co-Morbid Conditions Due to Morbid Obesity; 100-04,32,150.2 HCPCS Procedure Codes for Bariatric Surgery; 100-04,32,150.5 ICD Diagnosis Codes for BMI ≥35; 100-04,32,150.6 Bariatric Surgery Claims Guidance

INCLUDES Diagnostic laparoscopy (49320)
EXCLUDES Endoscopy, upper gastrointestinal, (esophagus/stomach/duodenum/jejunum) (43235-43259 [43233, 43266, 43270])

43644 **Laparoscopy, surgical, gastric restrictive procedure; with gastric bypass and Roux-en-Y gastroenterostomy (roux limb 150 cm or less)**
EXCLUDES Roux limb less than 150 cm (43846)
          Roux limb greater than 150 cm (43645)
🚑 50.6   ⚕ 50.6   **FUD** 090   C 80 ▣
AMA: 2014,Jan,11; 2013,Jan,11-12

43645 **with gastric bypass and small intestine reconstruction to limit absorption**
EXCLUDES Roux limb less than 150 cm (43847)
🚑 53.9   ⚕ 53.9   **FUD** 090   C 80 ▣
AMA: 2018,Jan,8; 2017,Jan,8; 2016,Jan,13

43647-43659 Other and Unlisted Laparoscopic Gastric Procedures

INCLUDES Diagnostic laparoscopy (49320)
EXCLUDES Endoscopy, upper gastrointestinal, (esophagus/stomach/duodenum/jejunum) (43235-43259 [43233, 43266, 43270])

43647 **Laparoscopy, surgical; implantation or replacement of gastric neurostimulator electrodes, antrum**
EXCLUDES Electronic analysis/programming gastric neurostimulator (95980-95982)
          Insertion gastric neurostimulator pulse generator, incisional (64590)
          Laparoscopy with implantation, removal, or revision gastric neurostimulator electrodes on lesser curvature stomach (43659)
          Open method (43881)
          Vagus nerve blocking pulse generator and/or neurostimulator electrode array implantation, reprogramming, replacement, revision, or removal at esophagogastric junction performed laparoscopically (0312T-0317T)
🚑 0.00   ⚕ 0.00   **FUD** YYY   J J8 80 ▣
AMA: 2019,Feb,6; 2018,Jan,8; 2017,Jan,8; 2016,Jan,13

43648 **revision or removal of gastric neurostimulator electrodes, antrum**
EXCLUDES Electronic analysis/programming gastric neurostimulator (95980-95982)
          Laparoscopy with implantation, removal, or revision gastric neurostimulator electrodes on lesser curvature stomach (43659)
          Open method (43882)
          Removal or revision gastric neurostimulator pulse generator (64595)
          Vagus nerve blocking pulse generator and/or neurostimulator electrode array implantation, reprogramming, replacement, revision, or removal at esophagogastric junction performed laparoscopically (0312T-0317T)
🚑 0.00   ⚕ 0.00   **FUD** YYY   J G2 80 ▣
AMA: 2019,Feb,6; 2018,Jan,8; 2017,Jan,8; 2016,Jan,13

43651 **Laparoscopy, surgical; transection of vagus nerves, truncal**
🚑 19.0   ⚕ 19.0   **FUD** 090   J G2 80 ▣
AMA: 2018,Jan,8; 2017,Jan,8; 2016,Jan,13

43652 **transection of vagus nerves, selective or highly selective**
🚑 22.2   ⚕ 22.2   **FUD** 090   J G2 80 ▣
AMA: 2018,Jan,8; 2017,Jan,8; 2016,Jan,13

43653 **gastrostomy, without construction of gastric tube (eg, Stamm procedure) (separate procedure)**
🚑 16.6   ⚕ 16.6   **FUD** 090   J A2 80 ▣
AMA: 2018,Jan,8; 2017,Jan,8; 2016,Jan,13

43659 **Unlisted laparoscopy procedure, stomach**
🚑 0.00   ⚕ 0.00   **FUD** YYY   J 80 50 ▣
AMA: 2018,Jul,7; 2018,Jan,8; 2017,Jan,8; 2016,Jan,13

43752-43763 Nonsurgical Gastric Tube Procedures

43752 **Naso- or oro-gastric tube placement, requiring physician's skill and fluoroscopic guidance (includes fluoroscopy, image documentation and report)**

> *EXCLUDES* *Critical care services (99291-99292)*
> *Initial inpatient neonatal/pediatric critical care, per day (99468-99469, 99471-99472)*
> *Insertion long gastrointestinal tube (44500, 74340)*
> *Percutaneous insertion gastrostomy tube (43246, 49440)*
> *Subsequent intensive care, per day, for low birth weight infant (99478-99479)*

> 🔧 1.18   ⚕ 1.18   **FUD** 000   Q1 G2 🖵

> **AMA:** 2019,Aug,8; 2018,Mar,11; 2018,Jan,8; 2017,Jan,8; 2016,Jan,13

43753 **Gastric intubation and aspiration(s) therapeutic, necessitating physician's skill (eg, for gastrointestinal hemorrhage), including lavage if performed**

> 🔧 0.63   ⚕ 0.63   **FUD** 000   Q1 N1 80 🖵

> **AMA:** 2019,Aug,8; 2018,Jan,8; 2017,Jan,8; 2016,Jan,13

43754 **Gastric intubation and aspiration, diagnostic; single specimen (eg, acid analysis)**

> *EXCLUDES* *Analysis gastric acid (82930)*
> *Naso- or oro-gastric tube placement using fluoroscopic guidance (43752)*

> 🔧 1.03   ⚕ 5.18   **FUD** 000   Q1 N1 80 🖵

> **AMA:** 2018,Jan,8; 2017,Jan,8; 2016,Jan,13

43755 **collection of multiple fractional specimens with gastric stimulation, single or double lumen tube (gastric secretory study) (eg, histamine, insulin, pentagastrin, calcium, secretin), includes drug administration**

> *EXCLUDES* *Analysis gastric acid (82930)*
> *Naso- or oro-gastric tube placement using fluoroscopic guidance (43752)*
> Code also drugs or substances administered

> 🔧 1.74   ⚕ 4.43   **FUD** 000   S G2 80 🖵

> **AMA:** 2018,Jan,8; 2017,Jan,8; 2016,Jan,13

43756 **Duodenal intubation and aspiration, diagnostic, includes image guidance; single specimen (eg, bile study for crystals or afferent loop culture)**

> Code also drugs or substances administered
> 📡 (89049-89240)

> 🔧 1.46   ⚕ 7.11   **FUD** 000   Q1 G2 80 🖵

> **AMA:** 2018,Jan,8; 2017,Jan,8; 2016,Jan,13

43757 **collection of multiple fractional specimens with pancreatic or gallbladder stimulation, single or double lumen tube, includes drug administration**

> Code also drugs or substances administered
> 📡 (89049-89240)

> 🔧 2.20   ⚕ 9.76   **FUD** 000   T G2 80 🖵

> **AMA:** 2018,Jan,8; 2017,Jan,8; 2016,Jan,13

43761 **Repositioning of a naso- or oro-gastric feeding tube, through the duodenum for enteric nutrition**

> *EXCLUDES* *Conversion gastrostomy tube to gastro-jejunostomy tube, percutaneous (49446)*
> *Gastrostomy tube converted endoscopically to jejunostomy tube (44373)*
> *Insertion long gastrointestinal tube (44500, 74340)*
> 🔧 (76000)

> 🔧 3.01   ⚕ 3.50   **FUD** 000   T A2 🖵

> **AMA:** 2018,Jan,8; 2017,Jan,8; 2016,Jan,13

43762 **Replacement of gastrostomy tube, percutaneous, includes removal, when performed, without imaging or endoscopic guidance; not requiring revision of gastrostomy tract**

> 🔧 1.10   ⚕ 6.45   **FUD** 000   G2 🖵

> **AMA:** 2019,Feb,5

43763 **requiring revision of gastrostomy tract**

> *EXCLUDES* *Gastrostomy tube replacement using fluoroscopy (49450)*
> *Percutaneous insertion gastrostomy tube (43246)*

> 🔧 2.44   ⚕ 9.64   **FUD** 000   G2 🖵

> **AMA:** 2019,Oct,10; 2019,Feb,5

43770-43775 Laparoscopic Bariatric Procedures

CMS: 100-03,100.1 Bariatric Surgery for Treatment Co-morbid Conditions Due to Morbid Obesity; 100-04,32,150.1 Bariatric Surgery: Treatment of Co-Morbid Conditions Due to Morbid Obesity; 100-04,32,150.2 HCPCS Procedure Codes for Bariatric Surgery; 100-04,32,150.5 ICD Diagnosis Codes for BMI ≥35; 100-04,32,150.6 Bariatric Surgery Claims Guidance

> *INCLUDES* Diagnostic laparoscopy (49320)
> Stomach/duodenum/jejunum/ileum
> Subsequent band adjustments (change gastric band component diameter by injection/aspiration fluid through subcutaneous port component) during postoperative period

43770 **Laparoscopy, surgical, gastric restrictive procedure; placement of adjustable gastric restrictive device (eg, gastric band and subcutaneous port components)**

> Code also modifier 52 for placement individual component
> 🔧 32.8   ⚕ 32.8   **FUD** 090   J J8 80 🖵

> **AMA:** 2018,Jan,8; 2017,Jan,8; 2016,Jan,13

43771 **revision of adjustable gastric restrictive device component only**

> 🔧 37.2   ⚕ 37.2   **FUD** 090   C 80 🖵

> **AMA:** 2018,Jan,8; 2017,Jan,8; 2016,Jan,13

43772 **removal of adjustable gastric restrictive device component only**

> 🔧 27.4   ⚕ 27.4   **FUD** 090   J G2 80 🖵

> **AMA:** 2018,Jan,8; 2017,Jan,8; 2016,Jan,13

43773 **removal and replacement of adjustable gastric restrictive device component only**

> *EXCLUDES* *Laparoscopy, surgical, gastric restrictive procedure; removal adjustable gastric restrictive device component only (43772)*

> 🔧 37.2   ⚕ 37.2   **FUD** 090   J G2 80 🖵

> **AMA:** 2018,Jan,8; 2017,Jan,8; 2016,Jan,13

43774 **removal of adjustable gastric restrictive device and subcutaneous port components**

> *EXCLUDES* *Removal/replacement subcutaneous port components and gastric band (43659)*

> 🔧 28.0   ⚕ 28.0   **FUD** 090   J G2 80 🖵

> **AMA:** 2018,Jan,8; 2017,Jan,8; 2016,Jan,13

43775 **longitudinal gastrectomy (ie, sleeve gastrectomy)**

> *EXCLUDES* *Open gastric restrictive procedure for morbid obesity, without gastric bypass, other than vertical-banded gastroplasty (43843)*
> *Vagus nerve blocking pulse generator and/or neurostimulator electrode array implantation, reprogramming, replacement, revision, or removal at esophagogastric junction performed laparoscopically (0312T-0317T)*

> 🔧 32.5   ⚕ 32.5   **FUD** 090   C 80 🖵

> **AMA:** 2019,Oct,10

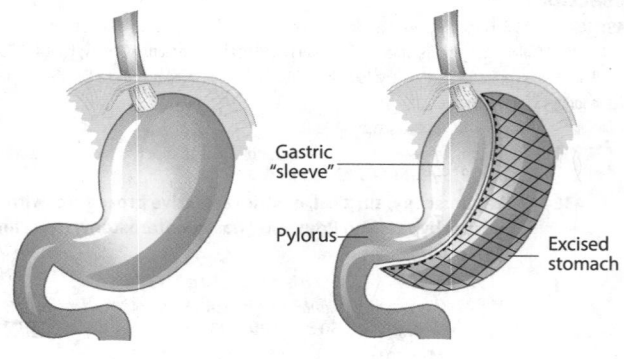

Gastric "sleeve"

Pylorus

Excised stomach

| 26/TC PC/TC Only | A2-Z3 ASC Payment | 50 Bilateral | ♂ Male Only | ♀ Female Only | 🔧 Facility RVU | ⚕ Non-Facility RVU | 🖵 CCI | ✖ CLIA |
| FUD Follow-up Days | CMS: IOM | AMA: CPT Asst | A-Y OPPSI | 80/80 Surg Assist Allowed / w/Doc | | 📡 Lab Crosswalk | 🔧 Radiology Crosswalk | |

200   CPT © 2021 American Medical Association. All Rights Reserved.   © 2021 Optum360, LLC

43800-43840 Open Gastric Incisional/Repair/Resection Procedures

43800 **Pyloroplasty**

EXCLUDES *Vagotomy with pyloroplasty (43640)*
🔪 27.2 ✂ 27.2 **FUD** 090   C 80 ▢
AMA: 2014,Jan,11; 2013,Jan,11-12

43810 **Gastroduodenostomy**
🔪 29.7 ✂ 29.7 **FUD** 090   C 80 ▢
AMA: 2014,Jan,11; 2013,Jan,11-12

43820 **Gastrojejunostomy; without vagotomy**
🔪 39.1 ✂ 39.1 **FUD** 090   C 80 ▢
AMA: 2014,Jan,11; 2013,Jan,11-12

43825 **with vagotomy, any type**
🔪 38.0 ✂ 38.0 **FUD** 090   C 80 ▢
AMA: 2014,Jan,11; 2013,Jan,11-12

43830 **Gastrostomy, open; without construction of gastric tube (eg, Stamm procedure) (separate procedure)**
🔪 20.4 ✂ 20.4 **FUD** 090   J 62 80 ▢
AMA: 2019,Feb,5; 2018,Jan,8; 2017,Jan,8; 2016,Jan,13

43831 **neonatal, for feeding**   A
EXCLUDES *Change gastrostomy tube (43762-43763)*
Gastrostomy tube replacement using fluoroscopy (49450)
🔪 17.5 ✂ 17.5 **FUD** 090   63 T 62 80 ▢
AMA: 2019,Feb,5; 2018,Jan,8; 2017,Jan,8; 2016,Jan,13

43832 **with construction of gastric tube (eg, Janeway procedure)**
EXCLUDES *Endoscopic placement percutaneous gastrostomy tube (43246)*
🔪 30.3 ✂ 30.3 **FUD** 090   C 80 ▢
AMA: 2018,Jan,8; 2017,Jan,8; 2016,Jan,13

43840 **Gastrorrhaphy, suture of perforated duodenal or gastric ulcer, wound, or injury**
🔪 39.4 ✂ 39.4 **FUD** 090   C 80 ▢
AMA: 2014,Jan,11; 2013,Jan,11-12

43842-43848 Open Bariatric Procedures for Morbid Obesity

CMS: 100-03,100.1 Bariatric Surgery for Treatment Co-morbid Conditions Due to Morbid Obesity; 100-04,32,150.1 Bariatric Surgery: Treatment of Co-Morbid Conditions Due to Morbid Obesity; 100-04,32,150.2 HCPCS Procedure Codes for Bariatric Surgery; 100-04,32,150.5 ICD Diagnosis Codes for BMI ≥35; 100-04,32,150.6 Bariatric Surgery Claims Guidance

43842 **Gastric restrictive procedure, without gastric bypass, for morbid obesity; vertical-banded gastroplasty**
🔪 33.4 ✂ 33.4 **FUD** 090   E ▢
AMA: 2018,Jan,8; 2017,Jan,8; 2016,Jan,13

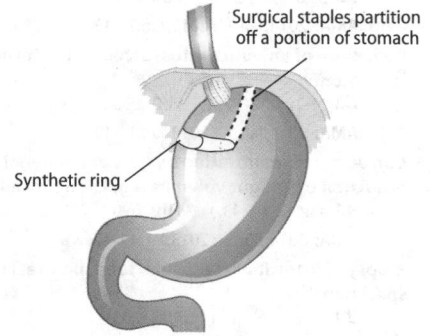

Surgical staples partition off a portion of stomach

Synthetic ring

The stomach is surgically restricted to treat morbid obesity; a vertical-banded partitioning technique gives the patient a sensation of fullness, thus decreasing daily caloric intake

43843 **other than vertical-banded gastroplasty**
EXCLUDES *Laparoscopic longitudinal gastrectomy (e.g., sleeve gastrectomy) (43775)*
🔪 37.4 ✂ 37.4 **FUD** 090   C 80 ▢
AMA: 2018,Jan,8; 2017,Jan,8; 2016,Jan,13

43845 **Gastric restrictive procedure with partial gastrectomy, pylorus-preserving duodenoileostomy and ileoileostomy (50 to 100 cm common channel) to limit absorption (biliopancreatic diversion with duodenal switch)**
EXCLUDES *Enteroenterostomy, anastomosis intestine (44130)*
Exploratory laparotomy, exploratory celiotomy (49000)
Gastrectomy, partial, distal; with Roux-en-Y reconstruction (43633)
Gastric restrictive procedure, with gastric bypass for morbid obesity; with small intestine reconstruction (43847)
🔪 56.8 ✂ 56.8 **FUD** 090   C 80 ▢
AMA: 2018,Jan,8; 2017,Jan,8; 2016,Jan,13

43846 **Gastric restrictive procedure, with gastric bypass for morbid obesity; with short limb (150 cm or less) Roux-en-Y gastroenterostomy**
EXCLUDES *Performed laparoscopically (43644)*
Roux limb more than 150 cm (43847)
🔪 47.3 ✂ 47.3 **FUD** 090   C 80 ▢
AMA: 2018,Jan,8; 2017,Jan,8; 2016,Jan,13

43847 **with small intestine reconstruction to limit absorption**
EXCLUDES *Performed laparoscopically (43645)*
🔪 52.1 ✂ 52.1 **FUD** 090   C 80 ▢
AMA: 2018,Jan,8; 2017,Jan,8; 2016,Jan,13

43848 **Revision, open, of gastric restrictive procedure for morbid obesity, other than adjustable gastric restrictive device (separate procedure)**
EXCLUDES *Gastric restrictive port procedures (43886-43888)*
Procedures for adjustable gastric restrictive devices (43770-43774)
🔪 55.9 ✂ 55.9 **FUD** 090   C 80 ▢
AMA: 2018,Jan,8; 2017,Jan,8; 2016,Jan,13

43850-43882 Open Gastric Procedures: Closure/Implantation/Replacement/Revision

43850 ~~Revision of gastroduodenal anastomosis (gastroduodenostomy) with reconstruction; without vagotomy~~

43855 ~~with vagotomy~~

43860 **Revision of gastrojejunal anastomosis (gastrojejunostomy) with reconstruction, with or without partial gastrectomy or intestine resection; without vagotomy**
🔪 47.7 ✂ 47.7 **FUD** 090   C 80 ▢
AMA: 2014,Jan,11; 2013,Jan,11-12

43865 **with vagotomy**
🔪 49.9 ✂ 49.9 **FUD** 090   C 80 ▢
AMA: 2014,Jan,11; 2013,Jan,11-12

43870 **Closure of gastrostomy, surgical**
🔪 20.6 ✂ 20.6 **FUD** 090   J A2 80 ▢
AMA: 2018,Jul,14

43880 **Closure of gastrocolic fistula**
🔪 46.1 ✂ 46.1 **FUD** 090   C 80 ▢
AMA: 2014,Jan,11; 2013,Jan,11-12

Digestive System

43881 — 44110

43881 Implantation or replacement of gastric neurostimulator electrodes, antrum, open

> EXCLUDES Electronic analysis and programming (95980-95982)
> Implantation/removal/revision gastric neurostimulator electrodes, lesser curvature or vagal trunk (EGJ):
> Laparoscopically (43659)
> Open, lesser curvature (43999)
> Implantation/replacement performed laparoscopically (43647)
> Insertion gastric neurostimulator pulse generator (64590)
> Vagus nerve blocking pulse generator and/or neurostimulator electrode array implantation, reprogramming, replacement, revision, or removal at esophagogastric junction performed laparoscopically (0312T-0317T)
>
> 🚑 0.00   ⚕ 0.00   **FUD** YYY   C 80 ▱
>
> **AMA:** 2019,Feb,6; 2018,Jan,8; 2017,Jan,8; 2016,Jan,13

43882 Revision or removal of gastric neurostimulator electrodes, antrum, open

> EXCLUDES Electronic analysis and programming (95980-95982)
> Implantation/removal/revision gastric neurostimulator electrodes, lesser curvature or vagal trunk (EGJ):
> Laparoscopic (43659)
> Open, lesser curvature (43999)
> Revision/removal gastric neurostimulator electrodes, antrum, performed laparoscopically (43648)
> Revision/removal gastric neurostimulator pulse generator (64595)
> Vagus nerve blocking pulse generator and/or neurostimulator electrode array implantation, reprogramming, replacement, revision, or removal at esophagogastric junction performed laparoscopically (0312T-0317T)
>
> 🚑 0.00   ⚕ 0.00   **FUD** YYY   C 80 ▱
>
> **AMA:** 2019,Feb,6; 2018,Jan,8; 2017,Jan,8; 2016,Jan,13

43886-43999 Bariatric Procedures: Removal/Replacement/Revision Port Components

CMS: 100-04,32,150.1 Bariatric Surgery: Treatment of Co-Morbid Conditions Due to Morbid Obesity; 100-04,32,150.2 HCPCS Procedure Codes for Bariatric Surgery; 100-04,32,150.5 ICD Diagnosis Codes for BMI ≥35; 100-04,32,150.6 Bariatric Surgery Claims Guidance

43886 Gastric restrictive procedure, open; revision of subcutaneous port component only

> 🚑 10.5   ⚕ 10.5   **FUD** 090   T 62 80 ▱
>
> **AMA:** 2018,Jan,8; 2017,Jan,8; 2016,Jan,13

43887 removal of subcutaneous port component only

> EXCLUDES Gastric band and subcutaneous port components:
> Removal and replacement performed laparoscopically (43659)
> Removal performed laparoscopically (43774)
>
> 🚑 9.52   ⚕ 9.52   **FUD** 090   02 62 80 ▱
>
> **AMA:** 2018,Jan,8; 2017,Jan,8; 2016,Jan,13

43888 removal and replacement of subcutaneous port component only

> EXCLUDES Gastric band and subcutaneous port components:
> Removal and replacement performed laparoscopically (43659)
> Removal performed laparoscopically (43774)
> Gastric restrictive procedure, open; removal subcutaneous port component only (43887)
>
> 🚑 13.4   ⚕ 13.4   **FUD** 090   T 62 80 ▱
>
> **AMA:** 2018,Jan,8; 2017,Jan,8; 2016,Jan,13

43999 Unlisted procedure, stomach

> 🚑 0.00   ⚕ 0.00   **FUD** YYY   T 80 ▱
>
> **AMA:** 2018,Dec,10; 2018,Dec,10; 2018,Jul,14; 2018,Jan,8; 2017,Jan,8; 2016,Jan,13

44005-44130 Incisional and Resection Procedures of Bowel

44005 Enterolysis (freeing of intestinal adhesion) (separate procedure)

> EXCLUDES Enterolysis performed laparoscopically (44180)
> Excision ileoanal reservoir with ileostomy (45136)
>
> 🚑 31.7   ⚕ 31.7   **FUD** 090   C 80 ▱
>
> **AMA:** 2018,Feb,11; 2018,Jan,8; 2017,Jan,8; 2016,Jan,13

44010 Duodenotomy, for exploration, biopsy(s), or foreign body removal

> 🚑 24.8   ⚕ 24.8   **FUD** 090   C 80 ▱
>
> **AMA:** 2014,Jan,11; 2013,Jan,11-12

The duodenum is surgically accessed and explored
A foreign body may be removed and/or a biopsy specimen taken

+ 44015 Tube or needle catheter jejunostomy for enteral alimentation, intraoperative, any method (List separately in addition to primary procedure)

> Code first primary procedure
>
> 🚑 4.15   ⚕ 4.15   **FUD** ZZZ   C 80 ▱
>
> **AMA:** 2018,Jan,8; 2017,Jan,8; 2016,Jan,13

44020 Enterotomy, small intestine, other than duodenum; for exploration, biopsy(s), or foreign body removal

> 🚑 28.2   ⚕ 28.2   **FUD** 090   C 80 ▱
>
> **AMA:** 2014,Jan,11; 2013,Jan,11-12

44021 for decompression (eg, Baker tube)

> 🚑 28.3   ⚕ 28.3   **FUD** 090   C 80 ▱
>
> **AMA:** 2014,Jan,11; 2013,Jan,11-12

44025 Colotomy, for exploration, biopsy(s), or foreign body removal

> INCLUDES Amussat's operation
> EXCLUDES Intestine exteriorization (Mikulicz resection with crushing of spur) (44602-44605)
>
> 🚑 28.6   ⚕ 28.6   **FUD** 090   C 80 ▱
>
> **AMA:** 2014,Jan,11; 2013,Jan,11-12

44050 Reduction of volvulus, intussusception, internal hernia, by laparotomy

> 🚑 27.2   ⚕ 27.2   **FUD** 090   C 80 ▱
>
> **AMA:** 2014,Jan,11; 2013,Jan,11-12

44055 Correction of malrotation by lysis of duodenal bands and/or reduction of midgut volvulus (eg, Ladd procedure)

> 🚑 43.4   ⚕ 43.4   **FUD** 090   63 C 80 ▱
>
> **AMA:** 2014,Jan,11; 2013,Jan,11-12

44100 Biopsy of intestine by capsule, tube, peroral (1 or more specimens)

> 🚑 3.11   ⚕ 3.11   **FUD** 000   T A2 ▱
>
> **AMA:** 2014,Jan,11; 2013,Jan,11-12

44110 Excision of 1 or more lesions of small or large intestine not requiring anastomosis, exteriorization, or fistulization; single enterotomy

> 🚑 24.6   ⚕ 24.6   **FUD** 090   C 80 ▱
>
> **AMA:** 2014,Jan,11; 2013,Jan,11-12

44111   multiple enterotomies
    28.5   28.5   **FUD** 090   C 80
    AMA: 2014,Jan,11; 2013,Jan,11-12

44120   Enterectomy, resection of small intestine; single resection and anastomosis
    35.6   35.6   **FUD** 090   C 80
    AMA: 2018,Nov,11; 2018,Jan,8; 2017,Jan,8; 2016,Jan,13

+ **44121**   each additional resection and anastomosis (List separately in addition to code for primary procedure)
    Code first (44120)
    7.04   7.04   **FUD** ZZZ   C 80
    AMA: 2014,Jan,11; 2013,Jan,11-12

44125   with enterostomy
    34.3   34.3   **FUD** 090   C 80
    AMA: 2014,Jan,11; 2013,Jan,11-12

44126   Enterectomy, resection of small intestine for congenital atresia, single resection and anastomosis of proximal segment of intestine; without tapering
    71.7   71.7   **FUD** 090   63 C 80
    AMA: 2014,Jan,11; 2013,Jan,11-12

44127   with tapering
    83.3   83.3   **FUD** 090   63 C 80
    AMA: 2014,Jan,11; 2013,Jan,11-12

+ **44128**   each additional resection and anastomosis (List separately in addition to code for primary procedure)
    Code first single resection small intestine (44126, 44127)
    7.10   7.10   **FUD** ZZZ   63 C 80
    AMA: 2014,Jan,11; 2013,Jan,11-12

44130   Enteroenterostomy, anastomosis of intestine, with or without cutaneous enterostomy (separate procedure)
    38.2   38.2   **FUD** 090   C 80
    AMA: 2014,Jan,11; 2013,Jan,11-12

44132-44137 Intestine Transplant Procedures

CMS: 100-03,260.5 Intestinal and Multi-Visceral Transplantation; 100-04,3,90.6 Intestinal and Multi-Visceral Transplants

44132   Donor enterectomy (including cold preservation), open; from cadaver donor
    INCLUDES   Graft:
      Cold preservation
      Harvest
    EXCLUDES   Preparation/reconstruction backbench intestinal graft (44715, 44720-44721)
    0.00   0.00   **FUD** XXX   C 80
    AMA: 2014,Jan,11; 2013,Jan,11-12

44133   partial, from living donor
    INCLUDES   Donor care
      Graft:
      Cold preservation
      Harvest
    EXCLUDES   Preparation/reconstruction backbench intestinal graft (44715, 44720-44721)
    0.00   0.00   **FUD** XXX   C 80
    AMA: 2014,Jan,11; 2013,Jan,11-12

44135   Intestinal allotransplantation; from cadaver donor
    INCLUDES   Allograft transplantation
      Recipient care
    0.00   0.00   **FUD** XXX   C 80
    AMA: 2014,Jan,11; 2013,Jan,11-12

44136   from living donor
    INCLUDES   Allograft transplantation
      Recipient care
    0.00   0.00   **FUD** XXX   C 80
    AMA: 2014,Jan,11; 2013,Jan,11-12

44137   Removal of transplanted intestinal allograft, complete
    EXCLUDES   Partial removal transplant allograft (44120-44121, 44140)
    0.00   0.00   **FUD** XXX   C 80
    AMA: 2014,Jan,11; 2013,Jan,11-12

44139-44160 Colon Resection Procedures

+ **44139**   Mobilization (take-down) of splenic flexure performed in conjunction with partial colectomy (List separately in addition to primary procedure)
    Code first partial colectomy (44140-44147)
    3.52   3.52   **FUD** ZZZ   C 80
    AMA: 2014,Jan,11; 2013,Jan,11-12

44140   Colectomy, partial; with anastomosis
    EXCLUDES   Laparoscopic method (44204)
    39.0   39.0   **FUD** 090   C 80
    AMA: 2020,Apr,10; 2018,Jan,8; 2017,Jan,8; 2016,Jan,13

44141   with skin level cecostomy or colostomy
    52.9   52.9   **FUD** 090   C 80
    AMA: 2018,Jan,8; 2017,Jan,8; 2016,Jan,13

44143   with end colostomy and closure of distal segment (Hartmann type procedure)
    EXCLUDES   Laparoscopic method (44206)
    48.4   48.4   **FUD** 090   C 80
    AMA: 2018,Jan,8; 2017,Jan,8; 2016,Jan,13

44144   with resection, with colostomy or ileostomy and creation of mucofistula
    51.4   51.4   **FUD** 090   C 80
    AMA: 2018,Jan,8; 2017,Jan,8; 2016,Jan,13

44145   with coloproctostomy (low pelvic anastomosis)
    EXCLUDES   Laparoscopic method (44207)
    48.0   48.0   **FUD** 090   C 80
    AMA: 2014,Jan,11; 2013,Jan,11-12

44146   with coloproctostomy (low pelvic anastomosis), with colostomy
    EXCLUDES   Laparoscopic method (44208)
    61.2   61.2   **FUD** 090   C 80
    AMA: 2018,Jun,11; 2018,Jan,8; 2017,Jan,8; 2016,Jan,13

44147   abdominal and transanal approach
    56.3   56.3   **FUD** 090   C 80
    AMA: 2018,Jan,8; 2017,Jan,8; 2016,Jan,13

44150   Colectomy, total, abdominal, without proctectomy; with ileostomy or ileoproctostomy
    INCLUDES   Lane's operation
    EXCLUDES   Laparoscopic method (44210)
    54.0   54.0   **FUD** 090   C 80
    AMA: 2014,Jan,11; 2013,Jan,11-12

44151   with continent ileostomy
    62.9   62.9   **FUD** 090   C 80
    AMA: 2014,Jan,11; 2013,Jan,11-12

44155   Colectomy, total, abdominal, with proctectomy; with ileostomy
    INCLUDES   Miles' colectomy
    EXCLUDES   Laparoscopic method (44212)
    60.0   60.0   **FUD** 090   C 80
    AMA: 2014,Jan,11; 2013,Jan,11-12

44156   with continent ileostomy
    67.4   67.4   **FUD** 090   C 80
    AMA: 2014,Jan,11; 2013,Jan,11-12

44157   with ileoanal anastomosis, includes loop ileostomy, and rectal mucosectomy, when performed
    63.9   63.9   **FUD** 090   C 80
    AMA: 2014,Jan,11; 2013,Jan,11-12

44158   with ileoanal anastomosis, creation of ileal reservoir (S or J), includes loop ileostomy, and rectal mucosectomy, when performed

> EXCLUDES   *Laparoscopic method (44211)*
> 🖐 65.5   ✂ 65.5   **FUD** 090   C 80 ▭
> **AMA:** 2014,Jan,11; 2013,Jan,11-12

44160   Colectomy, partial, with removal of terminal ileum with ileocolostomy

> EXCLUDES   *Laparoscopic method (44205)*
> 🖐 36.0   ✂ 36.0   **FUD** 090   C 80 ▭
> **AMA:** 2018,Jan,8; 2017,Jan,8; 2016,Jan,13

44180 Laparoscopic Enterolysis

> INCLUDES   Diagnostic laparoscopy (49320)
> EXCLUDES   *Laparoscopic salpingolysis/ovariolysis (58660)*

44180   Laparoscopy, surgical, enterolysis (freeing of intestinal adhesion) (separate procedure)

> 🖐 26.6   ✂ 26.6   **FUD** 090   J 62 80 ▭
> **AMA:** 2018,Feb,11; 2018,Jan,8; 2017,Jan,8; 2016,Jan,13

44186-44238 Laparoscopic Enterostomy Procedures

> INCLUDES   Diagnostic laparoscopy (49320)

44186   Laparoscopy, surgical; jejunostomy (eg, for decompression or feeding)

> 🖐 18.9   ✂ 18.9   **FUD** 090   J 62 80 ▭
> **AMA:** 2018,Jan,8; 2017,Jan,8; 2016,Jan,13

44187   ileostomy or jejunostomy, non-tube

> EXCLUDES   *Open method (44310)*
> 🖐 31.8   ✂ 31.8   **FUD** 090   C 80 ▭
> **AMA:** 2019,Sep,10; 2018,Jan,8; 2017,Jan,8; 2016,Jan,13

44188   Laparoscopy, surgical, colostomy or skin level cecostomy

> EXCLUDES   *Laparoscopy, surgical, appendectomy (44970)*
>   *Open method (44320)*
> 🖐 35.4   ✂ 35.4   **FUD** 090   C 80 ▭
> **AMA:** 2018,Jan,8; 2017,Jan,8; 2016,Jan,13

44202   Laparoscopy, surgical; enterectomy, resection of small intestine, single resection and anastomosis

> EXCLUDES   *Open method (44120)*
> 🖐 40.1   ✂ 40.1   **FUD** 090   C 80 ▭
> **AMA:** 2020,Jul,13; 2018,Jan,8; 2017,Jan,8; 2016,Jan,13

+   44203   each additional small intestine resection and anastomosis (List separately in addition to code for primary procedure)

> EXCLUDES   *Open method (44121)*
> Code first single resection small intestine (44202)
> 🖐 7.00   ✂ 7.00   **FUD** ZZZ   C 80 ▭
> **AMA:** 2018,Jan,8; 2017,Jan,8; 2016,Jan,13

44204   colectomy, partial, with anastomosis

> EXCLUDES   *Open method (44140)*
> 🖐 44.7   ✂ 44.7   **FUD** 090   C 80 ▭
> **AMA:** 2018,Jan,8; 2017,Dec,14; 2017,Jan,8; 2016,Jan,13

44205   colectomy, partial, with removal of terminal ileum with ileocolostomy

> EXCLUDES   *Open method (44160)*
> 🖐 38.8   ✂ 38.8   **FUD** 090   C 80 ▭
> **AMA:** 2018,Jan,8; 2017,Jan,8; 2016,Jan,13

44206   colectomy, partial, with end colostomy and closure of distal segment (Hartmann type procedure)

> EXCLUDES   *Open method (44143)*
> 🖐 50.7   ✂ 50.7   **FUD** 090   C 80 ▭
> **AMA:** 2018,Jan,8; 2017,Jan,8; 2016,Jan,13

44207   colectomy, partial, with anastomosis, with coloproctostomy (low pelvic anastomosis)

> EXCLUDES   *Open method (44145)*
> 🖐 52.6   ✂ 52.6   **FUD** 090   C 80 ▭
> **AMA:** 2018,Jan,8; 2017,Jan,8; 2016,Jan,13

44208   colectomy, partial, with anastomosis, with coloproctostomy (low pelvic anastomosis) with colostomy

> EXCLUDES   *Open method (44146)*
> 🖐 57.4   ✂ 57.4   **FUD** 090   C 80 ▭
> **AMA:** 2018,Jan,8; 2017,Jan,8; 2016,Jan,13

44210   colectomy, total, abdominal, without proctectomy, with ileostomy or ileoproctostomy

> EXCLUDES   *Open method (44150)*
> 🖐 51.3   ✂ 51.3   **FUD** 090   C 80 ▭
> **AMA:** 2018,Jan,8; 2017,Jan,8; 2016,Jan,13

44211   colectomy, total, abdominal, with proctectomy, with ileoanal anastomosis, creation of ileal reservoir (S or J), with loop ileostomy, includes rectal mucosectomy, when performed

> EXCLUDES   *Open method (44157-44158)*
> 🖐 61.2   ✂ 61.2   **FUD** 090   C 80 ▭
> **AMA:** 2018,Jan,8; 2017,Jan,8; 2016,Jan,13

44212   colectomy, total, abdominal, with proctectomy, with ileostomy

> EXCLUDES   *Open method (44155)*
> 🖐 59.0   ✂ 59.0   **FUD** 090   C 80 ▭
> **AMA:** 2018,Jan,8; 2017,Jan,8; 2016,Jan,13

+   44213   Laparoscopy, surgical, mobilization (take-down) of splenic flexure performed in conjunction with partial colectomy (List separately in addition to primary procedure)

> EXCLUDES   *Open method (44139)*
> Code first partial colectomy (44204-44208)
> 🖐 5.43   ✂ 5.43   **FUD** ZZZ   C 80 ▭
> **AMA:** 2018,Jan,8; 2017,Jan,8; 2016,Jan,13

44227   Laparoscopy, surgical, closure of enterostomy, large or small intestine, with resection and anastomosis

> EXCLUDES   *Open method (44625-44626)*
> 🖐 48.4   ✂ 48.4   **FUD** 090   C 80 ▭
> **AMA:** 2018,Jan,8; 2017,Jan,8; 2016,Jan,13

44238   Unlisted laparoscopy procedure, intestine (except rectum)

> 🖐 0.00   ✂ 0.00   **FUD** YYY   J 80 50 ▭
> **AMA:** 2020,Jul,13; 2019,Oct,10; 2018,Jan,8; 2017,Jul,10; 2017,Jan,8; 2016,Jan,13

44300-44346 Open Enterostomy Procedures

44300   Placement, enterostomy or cecostomy, tube open (eg, for feeding or decompression) (separate procedure)

> EXCLUDES   *Intraoperative lavage, colon (44701)*
>   *Other gastrointestinal tube(s) placed percutaneously with fluoroscopic imaging guidance (49441-49442)*
> 🖐 24.5   ✂ 24.5   **FUD** 090   C 80 ▭
> **AMA:** 2018,Jan,8; 2017,Jan,8; 2016,Jan,13

44310   Ileostomy or jejunostomy, non-tube

> EXCLUDES   *Colectomy, partial; with resection, with colostomy or ileostomy and creation mucofistula (44144)*
>   *Colectomy, total, abdominal (44150-44151, 44155-44156)*
>   *Excision ileoanal reservoir with ileostomy (45136)*
>   *Laparoscopic method (44187)*
>   *Proctectomy (45113, 45119)*
> 🖐 30.2   ✂ 30.2   **FUD** 090   C 80 ▭
> **AMA:** 2018,Jan,8; 2017,Jan,8; 2016,Jan,13

44312   Revision of ileostomy; simple (release of superficial scar) (separate procedure)

> 🖐 17.1   ✂ 17.1   **FUD** 090   T A2 80 ▭
> **AMA:** 2014,Jan,11; 2013,Jan,11-12

44314   complicated (reconstruction in-depth) (separate procedure)

> 🖐 29.1   ✂ 29.1   **FUD** 090   C 80 ▭
> **AMA:** 2014,Jan,11; 2013,Jan,11-12

26/TC PC/TC Only   A2-Z4 ASC Payment   50 Bilateral   ♂ Male Only   ♀ Female Only   🖐 Facility RVU   ✂ Non-Facility RVU   ▭ CCI   ✖ CLIA
FUD Follow-up Days   **CMS:** IOM   **AMA:** CPT Asst   A-Y OPPSI   80/80 Surg Assist Allowed / w/Doc   ▨ Lab Crosswalk   ▨ Radiology Crosswalk

204   CPT © 2021 American Medical Association. All Rights Reserved.   © 2021 Optum360, LLC

44316 Continent ileostomy (Kock procedure) (separate procedure)
> EXCLUDES *Fiberoptic evaluation (44385)*
> 🚗 41.2   🔪 41.2   **FUD** 090   C 80 ▢
> AMA: 2014,Jan,11; 2013,Jan,11-12

44320 Colostomy or skin level cecostomy;
> EXCLUDES *Closure fistula (45805, 45825, 57307)*
> *Colectomy, partial (44141, 44144, 44146)*
> *Exploration, repair, and presacral drainage (45563)*
> *Laparoscopic method (44188)*
> *Pelvic exenteration (45126, 51597, 58240)*
> *Proctectomy (45110, 45119)*
> *Suture large intestine (44605)*
> *Ureterosigmoidostomy (50810)*
> 🚗 34.9   🔪 34.9   **FUD** 090   C 80 ▢
> AMA: 2018,Jan,8; 2017,Jan,8; 2016,Jan,13

44322 with multiple biopsies (eg, for congenital megacolon) (separate procedure)
> 🚗 29.2   🔪 29.2   **FUD** 090   C 80 ▢
> AMA: 2014,Jan,11; 2013,Jan,11-12

44340 Revision of colostomy; simple (release of superficial scar) (separate procedure)
> 🚗 18.0   🔪 18.0   **FUD** 090   T A2 ▢
> AMA: 2014,Jan,11; 2013,Jan,11-12

44345 complicated (reconstruction in-depth) (separate procedure)
> 🚗 30.4   🔪 30.4   **FUD** 090   C 80 ▢
> AMA: 2014,Jan,11; 2013,Jan,11-12

44346 with repair of paracolostomy hernia (separate procedure)
> 🚗 34.2   🔪 34.2   **FUD** 090   C 80 ▢
> AMA: 2018,Jan,8; 2017,Jan,8; 2016,Jan,13

Skin

Herniations that have formed around the site of a colostomy are repaired

The colon is mobilized, trimmed if necessary, and a new stoma is often created

44360-44379 Endoscopy of Small Intestine
> INCLUDES Control bleeding due to endoscopic procedure during same operative session

44360 Small intestinal endoscopy, enteroscopy beyond second portion of duodenum, not including ileum; diagnostic, including collection of specimen(s) by brushing or washing, when performed (separate procedure)
> EXCLUDES *Esophagogastroduodenoscopy, flexible, transoral (43235-43259 [43233, 43266, 43270])*
> 🚗 4.14   🔪 4.14   **FUD** 000   J A2 ▢
> AMA: 2019,Oct,10; 2018,Jan,8; 2017,Jan,8; 2016,Jan,13

44361 with biopsy, single or multiple
> EXCLUDES *Esophagogastroduodenoscopy, flexible, transoral (43235-43259 [43233, 43266, 43270])*
> 🚗 4.65   🔪 4.65   **FUD** 000   J A2 ▢
> AMA: 2019,Oct,10

44363 with removal of foreign body(s)
> EXCLUDES *Esophagogastroduodenoscopy, flexible, transoral (43235-43259 [43233, 43266, 43270])*
> 🚗 5.54   🔪 5.54   **FUD** 000   J A2 80 ▢
> AMA: 2019,Oct,10

44364 with removal of tumor(s), polyp(s), or other lesion(s) by snare technique
> EXCLUDES *Esophagogastroduodenoscopy, flexible, transoral (43235-43259 [43233, 43266, 43270])*
> 🚗 5.90   🔪 5.90   **FUD** 000   J A2 80 ▢
> AMA: 2019,Oct,10

44365 with removal of tumor(s), polyp(s), or other lesion(s) by hot biopsy forceps or bipolar cautery
> EXCLUDES *Esophagogastroduodenoscopy, flexible, transoral (43235-43259 [43233, 43266, 43270])*
> 🚗 5.24   🔪 5.24   **FUD** 000   J A2 80 ▢
> AMA: 2019,Oct,10

44366 with control of bleeding (eg, injection, bipolar cautery, unipolar cautery, laser, heater probe, stapler, plasma coagulator)
> EXCLUDES *Esophagogastroduodenoscopy, flexible, transoral (43235-43259 [43233, 43266, 43270])*
> 🚗 6.93   🔪 6.93   **FUD** 000   J A2
> AMA: 2019,Oct,10; 2018,Jan,8; 2017,Jan,8; 2016,Jan,13

44369 with ablation of tumor(s), polyp(s), or other lesion(s) not amenable to removal by hot biopsy forceps, bipolar cautery or snare technique
> EXCLUDES *Esophagogastroduodenoscopy, flexible, transoral (43235-43259 [43233, 43266, 43270])*
> 🚗 7.10   🔪 7.10   **FUD** 000   J A2 80 ▢
> AMA: 2019,Oct,10

44370 with transendoscopic stent placement (includes predilation)
> EXCLUDES *Esophagogastroduodenoscopy, flexible, transoral (43235-43259 [43233, 43266, 43270])*
> 🚗 7.80   🔪 7.80   **FUD** 000   J J8 80 ▢
> AMA: 2019,Oct,10; 2018,Jan,8; 2017,Jan,8; 2016,Jan,13

44372 with placement of percutaneous jejunostomy tube
> EXCLUDES *Esophagogastroduodenoscopy, flexible, transoral (43235-43259 [43233, 43266, 43270])*
> 🚗 7.02   🔪 7.02   **FUD** 000   J A2 ▢
> AMA: 2019,Oct,10; 2018,Jan,8; 2017,Jan,8; 2016,Jan,13

44373 with conversion of percutaneous gastrostomy tube to percutaneous jejunostomy tube
> EXCLUDES *Esophagogastroduodenoscopy, flexible, transoral (43235-43259 [43233, 43266, 43270])*
> 🚗 5.62   🔪 5.62   **FUD** 000   J A2 ▢
> AMA: 2019,Oct,10; 2018,Jan,8; 2017,Jan,8; 2016,Jan,13

44376 Small intestinal endoscopy, enteroscopy beyond second portion of duodenum, including ileum; diagnostic, with or without collection of specimen(s) by brushing or washing (separate procedure)
> EXCLUDES *Small intestinal endoscopy, enteroscopy (44360-44373)*
> 🚗 8.33   🔪 8.33   **FUD** 000   J A2 80 ▢
> AMA: 2018,Jan,8; 2017,Jan,8; 2016,Jan,13

44377 with biopsy, single or multiple
> EXCLUDES *Small intestinal endoscopy, enteroscopy (44360-44373)*
> 🚗 8.63   🔪 8.63   **FUD** 000   J A2 80 ▢
> AMA: 2018,Jan,8; 2017,Jan,8; 2016,Jan,13

44378 with control of bleeding (eg, injection, bipolar cautery, unipolar cautery, laser, heater probe, stapler, plasma coagulator)
> EXCLUDES *Small intestinal endoscopy, enteroscopy (44360-44373)*
> 🚗 11.2   🔪 11.2   **FUD** 000   J A2 80 ▢
> AMA: 2018,Jan,8; 2017,Jan,8; 2016,Jan,13

44379 — 44401

44379   with transendoscopic stent placement (includes predilation)

> EXCLUDES   *Small intestinal endoscopy, enteroscopy (44360-44373)*

🔧 11.8   ✂ 11.8   **FUD** 000   J A2 80 ▭

AMA: 2018,Jan,8; 2017,Jan,8; 2016,Jan,13

44380-44384 [44381] Ileoscopy Via Stoma

> INCLUDES   Control bleeding due to endoscopic procedure during same operative session

> EXCLUDES   *Computed tomographic colonography (74261-74263)*

Code also exam nonfunctional distal colon/rectum, when performed, with:
Anoscopy (46600, 46604-46606, 46608-46615)
Proctosigmoidoscopy (45300-45327)
Sigmoidoscopy (45330-45347 [45346])

44380   Ileoscopy, through stoma; diagnostic, including collection of specimen(s) by brushing or washing, when performed (separate procedure)

> EXCLUDES   *Ileoscopy, through stoma (44382-44384 [44381])*

🔧 1.61   ✂ 5.20   **FUD** 000   T A2 ▭

AMA: 2018,Jan,8; 2017,Jan,8; 2016,Jan,13

44381   Resequenced code. See code following 44382.

44382   with biopsy, single or multiple

> EXCLUDES   *Ileoscopy, through stoma; diagnostic (44380)*

🔧 2.10   ✂ 8.14   **FUD** 000   T A2 ▭

AMA: 2018,Jan,8; 2017,Jan,8; 2016,Jan,13

\#   **44381**   **with transendoscopic balloon dilation**

> EXCLUDES   *Ileoscopy, through stoma (44380, 44384)*

Code also each additional stricture dilated in same session, using modifier 59 with (44381)

🔧 (74360)

🔧 2.46   ✂ 26.3   **FUD** 000   J G2 ▭

AMA: 2018,Jan,8; 2017,Jan,8; 2016,Jan,13

44384   with placement of endoscopic stent (includes pre- and post-dilation and guide wire passage, when performed)

> EXCLUDES   *Ileoscopy, through stoma (44380-44381)*

🔧 (74360)

🔧 4.44   ✂ 4.44   **FUD** 000   J G2 ▭

AMA: 2018,Jan,8; 2017,Jan,8; 2016,Jan,13

44385-44386 Endoscopy of Small Intestinal Pouch

> INCLUDES   Control bleeding due to endoscopic procedure during same operative session

> EXCLUDES   *Computed tomographic colonography (74261-74263)*

44385   Endoscopic evaluation of small intestinal pouch (eg, Kock pouch, ileal reservoir [S or J]); diagnostic, including collection of specimen(s) by brushing or washing, when performed (separate procedure)

> EXCLUDES   *Endoscopic evaluation small intestinal pouch (44386)*

🔧 2.09   ✂ 5.60   **FUD** 000   T A2 ▭

AMA: 2018,Jan,8; 2017,Jan,8; 2016,Jan,13

44386   with biopsy, single or multiple

> EXCLUDES   *Endoscopic evaluation small intestinal pouch (44385)*

🔧 2.57   ✂ 8.54   **FUD** 000   T A2 ▭

AMA: 2018,Jan,8; 2017,Jan,8; 2016,Jan,13

44388-44408 [44401] Colonoscopy Via Stoma

> INCLUDES   Control bleeding due to endoscopic procedure during same operative session

> EXCLUDES   *Colonoscopy via rectum (45378, 45392-45393 [45390, 45398])*
> *Computed tomographic colonography (74261-74263)*

Code also exam nonfunctional distal colon/rectum, when performed, with:
Anoscopy (46600, 46604-46606, 46608-46615)
Proctosigmoidoscopy (45300-45327)
Sigmoidoscopy (45330-45347 [45346])

44388   Colonoscopy through stoma; diagnostic, including collection of specimen(s) by brushing or washing, when performed (separate procedure)

> EXCLUDES   *Colonoscopy through stoma (44389-44408 [44401])*

Code also modifier 53 when planned total colonoscopy cannot be completed

🔧 4.56   ✂ 8.42   **FUD** 000   T A2 ▭

AMA: 2018,Jan,8; 2017,Jan,8; 2016,Jan,13

44389   with biopsy, single or multiple

> EXCLUDES   *Colonoscopy through stoma; diagnostic (44388)*
> *Colonoscopy through stoma; with endoscopic mucosal resection on same lesion (44403)*

Code also modifier 52 when colonoscope fails to reach junction small intestine

🔧 4.97   ✂ 11.4   **FUD** 000   T A2 ▭

AMA: 2018,Jan,8; 2017,Jan,8; 2016,Jan,13

44390   with removal of foreign body(s)

> EXCLUDES   *Colonoscopy through stoma; diagnostic (44388)*

Code also modifier 52 when colonoscope fails to reach junction small intestine

🔧 (76000)

🔧 6.07   ✂ 11.2   **FUD** 000   T A2 ▭

AMA: 2018,Jan,8; 2017,Jan,8; 2016,Jan,13

44391   with control of bleeding, any method

> EXCLUDES   *Colonoscopy through stoma; diagnostic (44388)*
> *Colonoscopy through stoma; with directed submucosal injection(s) in same lesion (44404)*

Code also modifier 52 when colonoscope fails to reach junction small intestine

🔧 6.65   ✂ 19.2   **FUD** 000   T A2 ▭

AMA: 2018,Jan,8; 2017,Jan,8; 2016,Jan,13

44392   with removal of tumor(s), polyp(s), or other lesion(s) by hot biopsy forceps

> EXCLUDES   *Colonoscopy through stoma; diagnostic (44388)*

Code also modifier 52 when colonoscope fails to reach junction small intestine

🔧 5.82   ✂ 10.2   **FUD** 000   T A2 ▭

AMA: 2018,Jan,8; 2017,Jan,8; 2016,Jan,13

\#   **44401**   **with ablation of tumor(s), polyp(s), or other lesion(s) (includes pre-and post-dilation and guide wire passage, when performed)**

> EXCLUDES   *Colonoscopy through stoma; diagnostic (44388)*
> *Colonoscopy through stoma; with transendoscopic balloon dilation for same lesion (44405)*

Code also modifier 52 when colonoscope fails to reach junction small intestine

🔧 7.00   ✂ 80.2   **FUD** 000   T G2 ▭

AMA: 2018,Jan,8; 2017,Jan,8; 2016,Jan,13

44394   with removal of tumor(s), polyp(s), or other lesion(s) by snare technique

> EXCLUDES   *Colonoscopy through stoma; diagnostic (44388)*
> *Colonoscopy through stoma; with directed submucosal injection(s) same lesion (44403)*

Code also modifier 52 when colonoscope fails to reach junction small intestine

🔧 6.60   ✂ 11.7   **FUD** 000   T A2 ▭

AMA: 2018,Jan,8; 2017,Jan,8; 2016,Jan,13

44401   Resequenced code. See code following 44392.

26/TC PC/TC Only   A2-Z3 ASC Payment   50 Bilateral   ♂ Male Only   ♀ Female Only   🔧 Facility RVU   ✂ Non-Facility RVU   ▭ CCI   ✖ CLIA
FUD Follow-up Days   CMS: IOM   AMA: CPT Asst   A-Y OPPSI   80/80 Surg Assist Allowed / w/Doc   ▪ Lab Crosswalk   🔧 Radiology Crosswalk

206   CPT © 2021 American Medical Association. All Rights Reserved.   © 2021 Optum360, LLC

44402 **with endoscopic stent placement (including pre- and post-dilation and guide wire passage, when performed)**

EXCLUDES *Colonoscopy through stoma (44388, 44405)*

Code also modifier 52 when colonoscope fails to reach junction small intestine

(74360)

🚑 7.56 ⚖ 7.56 **FUD** 000 [J] [J8] [▣]

AMA: 2018,Jan,8; 2017,Jan,8; 2016,Jan,13

44403 **with endoscopic mucosal resection**

EXCLUDES *Colonoscopy through stoma; diagnostic (44388)*
Colonoscopy through stoma for same lesion (44389, 44394, 44404)

Code also modifier 52 when colonoscope fails to reach junction small intestine

🚑 8.77 ⚖ 8.77 **FUD** 000 [T] [G2] [▣]

AMA: 2019,Dec,14; 2018,Jan,8; 2017,Jan,8; 2016,Jan,13

44404 **with directed submucosal injection(s), any substance**

EXCLUDES *Colonoscopy through stoma; diagnostic (44388)*
Colonoscopy through stoma for same lesion (44391, 44403)

Code also modifier 52 when colonoscope fails to reach small intestine junction

🚑 4.97 ⚖ 11.3 **FUD** 000 [T] [G2] [▣]

AMA: 2018,Jan,8; 2017,Jan,8; 2016,Jan,13

44405 **with transendoscopic balloon dilation**

EXCLUDES *Colonoscopy through stoma (44388, [44401], 44402)*

Code also:

Each additional stricture dilated same session, appending modifier 59 to (44405)

Modifier 52 when colonoscope fails to reach small intestine junction

(74360)

🚑 5.28 ⚖ 15.9 **FUD** 000 [T] [G2] [▣]

AMA: 2018,Jan,8; 2017,Jan,8; 2016,Jan,13

44406 **with endoscopic ultrasound examination, limited to the sigmoid, descending, transverse, or ascending colon and cecum and adjacent structures**

INCLUDES *Gastrointestinal endoscopic ultrasound, supervision and interpretation (76975)*

EXCLUDES *Colonoscopy through stoma (44388, 44407)*
Procedure performed more than one time per operative session

Code also modifier 52 when colonoscope fails to reach small intestine junction

🚑 6.62 ⚖ 6.62 **FUD** 000 [T] [G2] [▣]

AMA: 2018,Jan,8; 2017,Jan,8; 2016,Jan,13

44407 **with transendoscopic ultrasound guided intramural or transmural fine needle aspiration/biopsy(s), includes endoscopic ultrasound examination limited to the sigmoid, descending, transverse, or ascending colon and cecum and adjacent structures**

INCLUDES *Gastrointestinal endoscopic ultrasound, supervision and interpretation (76975)*
Ultrasonic guidance (76942)

EXCLUDES *Colonoscopy through stoma (44388, 44406)*
Procedure performed more than one time per operative session

Code also modifier 52 when colonoscope fails to reach small intestine junction

🚑 8.11 ⚖ 8.11 **FUD** 000 [T] [G2] [▣]

AMA: 2018,Jan,8; 2017,Jan,8; 2016,Jan,13

44408 **with decompression (for pathologic distention) (eg, volvulus, megacolon), including placement of decompression tube, when performed**

EXCLUDES *Colonoscopy through stoma; diagnostic (44388)*
Procedure performed more than one time per operative session

🚑 6.68 ⚖ 6.68 **FUD** 000 [T] [R2] [▣]

AMA: 2018,Jan,8; 2017,Jan,8; 2016,Jan,13

44500 Gastrointestinal Intubation

44500 **Introduction of long gastrointestinal tube (eg, Miller-Abbott) (separate procedure)**

EXCLUDES *Placement oro- or naso-gastric tube (43752)*

(74340)

🚑 0.56 ⚖ 0.56 **FUD** 000 [⊘] [T] [G2] [80] [▣]

AMA: 2020,Aug,9; 2018,Jan,8; 2017,Jan,8; 2016,Sep,9; 2016,Jan,13

44602-44680 Open Repair Procedures of Intestines

44602 **Suture of small intestine (enterorrhaphy) for perforated ulcer, diverticulum, wound, injury or rupture; single perforation**

🚑 41.0 ⚖ 41.0 **FUD** 090 [C] [80] [▣]

AMA: 2020,Feb,13

44603 **multiple perforations**

🚑 47.1 ⚖ 47.1 **FUD** 090 [C] [80] [▣]

AMA: 2014,Jan,11; 2013,Dec,3

44604 **Suture of large intestine (colorrhaphy) for perforated ulcer, diverticulum, wound, injury or rupture (single or multiple perforations); without colostomy**

🚑 30.7 ⚖ 30.7 **FUD** 090 [C] [80] [▣]

AMA: 2014,Jan,11; 2013,Dec,3

44605 **with colostomy**

🚑 37.7 ⚖ 37.7 **FUD** 090 [C] [80] [▣]

AMA: 2014,Jan,11; 2013,Dec,3

44615 **Intestinal stricturoplasty (enterotomy and enterorrhaphy) with or without dilation, for intestinal obstruction**

🚑 31.1 ⚖ 31.1 **FUD** 090 [C] [80] [▣]

AMA: 2014,Jan,11; 2013,Dec,3

44620 **Closure of enterostomy, large or small intestine;**

EXCLUDES *Laparoscopic method (44227)*

🚑 25.1 ⚖ 25.1 **FUD** 090 [C] [80] [▣]

AMA: 2014,Jan,11; 2013,Dec,3

44625 **with resection and anastomosis other than colorectal**

EXCLUDES *Laparoscopic method (44227)*

🚑 29.3 ⚖ 29.3 **FUD** 090 [C] [80] [▣]

AMA: 2014,Jan,11; 2013,Dec,3

44626 **with resection and colorectal anastomosis (eg, closure of Hartmann type procedure)**

EXCLUDES *Laparoscopic method (44227)*

🚑 46.5 ⚖ 46.5 **FUD** 090 [C] [80] [▣]

AMA: 2014,Jan,11; 2013,Dec,3

44640 **Closure of intestinal cutaneous fistula**

🚑 40.6 ⚖ 40.6 **FUD** 090 [C] [80] [▣]

AMA: 2014,Jan,11; 2013,Dec,3

44650 **Closure of enteroenteric or enterocolic fistula**

🚑 42.0 ⚖ 42.0 **FUD** 090 [C] [80] [▣]

AMA: 2014,Jan,11; 2013,Dec,3

44660 **Closure of enterovesical fistula; without intestinal or bladder resection**

EXCLUDES *Closure fistula:*
Gastrocolic (43880)
Rectovesical (45800, 45805)
Renocolic (50525-50526)

🚑 38.7 ⚖ 38.7 **FUD** 090 [C] [80] [▣]

AMA: 2014,Jan,11; 2013,Dec,3

44661 **with intestine and/or bladder resection**

EXCLUDES *Closure fistula:*
Gastrocolic (43880)
Rectovesical (45800, 45805)
Renocolic (50525-50526)

🚑 45.0 ⚖ 45.0 **FUD** 090 [C] [80] [▣]

AMA: 2014,Jan,11; 2013,Dec,3

Digestive System

44680 — 45100

44680   Intestinal plication (separate procedure)
         INCLUDES   Noble intestinal plication
         ⊕ 30.8   ⅜ 30.8   **FUD** 090   C 80 ▭
         AMA: 2014,Jan,11; 2013,Dec,3

44700-44705 Other Intestinal Procedures

44700   Exclusion of small intestine from pelvis by mesh or other
         prosthesis, or native tissue (eg, bladder or omentum)
         EXCLUDES   Therapeutic radiation clinical treatment (77261-77799
                     [77295, 77385, 77386, 77387, 77424, 77425])
         ⊕ 29.1   ⅜ 29.1   **FUD** 090   C 80 ▭
         AMA: 2014,Jan,11; 2013,Dec,3

+ 44701   Intraoperative colonic lavage (List separately in addition to
            code for primary procedure)
            EXCLUDES   Appendectomy (44950-44960)
            Code first as appropriate (44140, 44145, 44150, 44604)
            ⊕ 4.94   ⅜ 4.94   **FUD** ZZZ   N M1 80 ▭
            AMA: 2014,Jan,11; 2013,Dec,3

44705   Preparation of fecal microbiota for instillation, including
         assessment of donor specimen
         EXCLUDES   Fecal instillation by enema or oro-nasogastric tube
                     (44799)
                     Therapeutic enema (74283)
         ⊕ 2.16   ⅜ 3.25   **FUD** XXX   B ▭
         AMA: 2018,Jan,8; 2017,Jan,8; 2016,Jan,13

44715-44799 Backbench Transplant Procedures
CMS: 100-04,3,90.6 Intestinal and Multi-Visceral Transplants

44715   Backbench standard preparation of cadaver or living donor
         intestine allograft prior to transplantation, including
         mobilization and fashioning of the superior mesenteric artery
         and vein
         INCLUDES   Mobilization/fashioning of superior mesenteric
                     vein/artery
         ⊕ 0.00   ⅜ 0.00   **FUD** XXX   C 80 ▭
         AMA: 2014,Jan,11; 2013,Dec,3

44720   Backbench reconstruction of cadaver or living donor intestine
         allograft prior to transplantation; venous anastomosis,
         each
         ⊕ 8.02   ⅜ 8.02   **FUD** XXX   C 80 ▭
         AMA: 2014,Jan,11; 2013,Dec,3

44721   arterial anastomosis, each
         ⊕ 11.2   ⅜ 11.2   **FUD** XXX   C 80 ▭
         AMA: 2018,Jan,8; 2017,Jan,8; 2016,Jan,13

44799   Unlisted procedure, small intestine
         EXCLUDES   Unlisted colon procedure (45399)
                     Unlisted intestinal procedure performed
                     laparoscopically (44238)
                     Unlisted rectal procedure (45499, 45999)
         ⊕ 0.00   ⅜ 0.00   **FUD** YYY   T ▭
         AMA: 2018,Jan,8; 2017,Jan,8; 2016,Jan,13

44800-44899 Meckel's Diverticulum and Mesentery Procedures

44800   Excision of Meckel's diverticulum (diverticulectomy) or
         omphalomesenteric duct
         ⊕ 22.3   ⅜ 22.3   **FUD** 090   C 80 ▭
         AMA: 2014,Jan,11; 2013,Dec,3

44820   Excision of lesion of mesentery (separate procedure)
         EXCLUDES   Resection intestine (44120-44128, 44140-44160)
         ⊕ 24.3   ⅜ 24.3   **FUD** 090   C 80 ▭
         AMA: 2014,Jan,11; 2013,Dec,3

44850   Suture of mesentery (separate procedure)
         EXCLUDES   Internal hernia repair/reduction (44050)
         ⊕ 21.7   ⅜ 21.7   **FUD** 090   C 80 ▭
         AMA: 2014,Jan,11; 2013,Dec,3

44899   Unlisted procedure, Meckel's diverticulum and the
         mesentery
         ⊕ 0.00   ⅜ 0.00   **FUD** YYY   C 80 ▭
         AMA: 2020,Jul,13

44900-44979 Open and Endoscopic Appendix Procedures

44900   Incision and drainage of appendiceal abscess, open
         EXCLUDES   Image guided percutaneous catheter drainage (49406)
         ⊕ 22.4   ⅜ 22.4   **FUD** 090   C 80 ▭
         AMA: 2014,Jan,11; 2013,Nov,9

44950   Appendectomy;
         INCLUDES   Battle's operation
         EXCLUDES   Procedure performed with other intra-abdominal
                     procedure(s) when appendectomy incidental
         ⊕ 18.7   ⅜ 18.7   **FUD** 090   J 62 80 ▭
         AMA: 2018,Jan,8; 2017,Jan,8; 2016,Jan,13

Cecum

Swollen and
inflamed appendix

+ 44955   when done for indicated purpose at time of other major
            procedure (not as separate procedure) (List separately in
            addition to code for primary procedure)
            Code first primary procedure
            ⊕ 2.45   ⅜ 2.45   **FUD** ZZZ   N M1 80 ▭
            AMA: 2018,Jan,8; 2017,Jan,8; 2016,Jan,13

44960   for ruptured appendix with abscess or generalized
         peritonitis
         INCLUDES   Battle's operation
         ⊕ 25.5   ⅜ 25.5   **FUD** 090   C 80 ▭
         AMA: 2019,Dec,12; 2018,Jan,8; 2017,Jan,8; 2016,Jan,13

44970   Laparoscopy, surgical, appendectomy
         INCLUDES   Diagnostic laparoscopy
         ⊕ 17.4   ⅜ 17.4   **FUD** 090   J 62 80 ▭
         AMA: 2019,Dec,12; 2018,Jan,8; 2017,Jan,8; 2016,Jan,13

44979   Unlisted laparoscopy procedure, appendix
         ⊕ 0.00   ⅜ 0.00   **FUD** YYY   J 80 50 ▭
         AMA: 2018,Jan,8; 2017,Jan,8; 2016,Jan,13

45000-45190 Open and Transrectal Procedures of Rectum

45000   Transrectal drainage of pelvic abscess
         EXCLUDES   Image guided transrectal catheter drainage (49407)
         ⊕ 12.2   ⅜ 12.2   **FUD** 090   T A2 ▭
         AMA: 2014,Jan,11; 2013,Nov,9

45005   Incision and drainage of submucosal abscess, rectum
         ⊕ 4.69   ⅜ 8.38   **FUD** 010   T A2 ▭
         AMA: 2014,Jan,11; 2013,Dec,3

45020   Incision and drainage of deep supralevator, pelvirectal, or
         retrorectal abscess
         EXCLUDES   Incision and drainage perianal, ischiorectal, intramural
                     abscess (46050, 46060)
         ⊕ 16.5   ⅜ 16.5   **FUD** 090   J A2 ▭
         AMA: 2014,Jan,11; 2013,Dec,3

45100   Biopsy of anorectal wall, anal approach (eg, congenital
         megacolon)
         EXCLUDES   Biopsy performed endoscopically (45305)
         ⊕ 8.65   ⅜ 8.65   **FUD** 090   J A2 ▭
         AMA: 2014,Jan,11; 2013,Dec,3

45108 **Anorectal myomectomy**
🔧 10.7 ⚕ 10.7 **FUD** 090   J A2 ▣
AMA: 2014,Jan,11; 2013,Dec,3

45110 **Proctectomy; complete, combined abdominoperineal, with colostomy**
EXCLUDES   *Laparoscopic method (45395)*
🔧 53.1 ⚕ 53.1 **FUD** 090   C 80 ▣
AMA: 2014,Jan,11; 2013,Dec,3

45111 **partial resection of rectum, transabdominal approach**
🔧 31.4 ⚕ 31.4 **FUD** 090   C 80 ▣
AMA: 2014,Jan,11; 2013,Dec,3

45112 **Proctectomy, combined abdominoperineal, pull-through procedure (eg, colo-anal anastomosis)**
EXCLUDES   *Proctectomy for colo-anal anastomosis with colonic pouch or reservoir creation (45119)*
🔧 53.9 ⚕ 53.9 **FUD** 090   C 80 ▣
AMA: 2014,Jan,11; 2013,Dec,3

45113 **Proctectomy, partial, with rectal mucosectomy, ileoanal anastomosis, creation of ileal reservoir (S or J), with or without loop ileostomy**
🔧 54.7 ⚕ 54.7 **FUD** 090   C 80 ▣
AMA: 2014,Jan,11; 2013,Dec,3

45114 **Proctectomy, partial, with anastomosis; abdominal and transsacral approach**
🔧 53.0 ⚕ 53.0 **FUD** 090   C 80 ▣
AMA: 2014,Jan,11; 2013,Dec,3

45116 **transsacral approach only (Kraske type)**
🔧 45.1 ⚕ 45.1 **FUD** 090   C 80 ▣
AMA: 2014,Jan,11; 2013,Dec,3

45119 **Proctectomy, combined abdominoperineal pull-through procedure (eg, colo-anal anastomosis), with creation of colonic reservoir (eg, J-pouch), with diverting enterostomy when performed**
EXCLUDES   *Laparoscopic method (45397)*
🔧 55.9 ⚕ 55.9 **FUD** 090   C 80 ▣
AMA: 2018,Jan,8; 2017,Jan,8; 2016,Jan,13

45120 **Proctectomy, complete (for congenital megacolon), abdominal and perineal approach; with pull-through procedure and anastomosis (eg, Swenson, Duhamel, or Soave type operation)**
🔧 46.5 ⚕ 46.5 **FUD** 090   C 80 ▣
AMA: 2014,Jan,11; 2013,Dec,3

45121 **with subtotal or total colectomy, with multiple biopsies**
🔧 50.5 ⚕ 50.5 **FUD** 090   C 80 ▣
AMA: 2014,Jan,11; 2013,Dec,3

45123 **Proctectomy, partial, without anastomosis, perineal approach**
🔧 32.4 ⚕ 32.4 **FUD** 090   C 80 ▣
AMA: 2014,Jan,11; 2013,Dec,3

45126 **Pelvic exenteration for colorectal malignancy, with proctectomy (with or without colostomy), with removal of bladder and ureteral transplantations, and/or hysterectomy, or cervicectomy, with or without removal of tube(s), with or without removal of ovary(s), or any combination thereof**
🔧 80.1 ⚕ 80.1 **FUD** 090   C 80 ▣
AMA: 2014,Jan,11; 2013,Dec,3

45130 **Excision of rectal procidentia, with anastomosis; perineal approach**
INCLUDES   Altemeier procedure
🔧 31.3 ⚕ 31.3 **FUD** 090   C 80 ▣
AMA: 2014,Jan,11; 2013,Dec,3

45135 **abdominal and perineal approach**
INCLUDES   Altemeier procedure
🔧 37.6 ⚕ 37.6 **FUD** 090   C 80 ▣
AMA: 2014,Jan,11; 2013,Dec,3

45136 **Excision of ileoanal reservoir with ileostomy**
EXCLUDES   *Enterolysis (44005)*
       Ileostomy or jejunostomy, non-tube (44310)
🔧 51.8 ⚕ 51.8 **FUD** 090   C 80 ▣
AMA: 2014,Jan,11; 2013,Dec,3

45150 **Division of stricture of rectum**
🔧 12.1 ⚕ 12.1 **FUD** 090   T A2 80 ▣
AMA: 2014,Jan,11; 2013,Dec,3

45160 **Excision of rectal tumor by proctotomy, transsacral or transcoccygeal approach**
🔧 29.7 ⚕ 29.7 **FUD** 090   J A2 80 ▣
AMA: 2014,Jan,11; 2013,Dec,3

45171 **Excision of rectal tumor, transanal approach; not including muscularis propria (ie, partial thickness)**
EXCLUDES   *Transanal destruction rectal tumor (45190)*
       Transanal endoscopic microsurgical tumor excision (TEMS) (0184T)
🔧 17.5 ⚕ 17.5 **FUD** 090   J G2 80 ▣
AMA: 2018,Jan,8; 2017,Jan,8; 2016,Jan,13

45172 **including muscularis propria (ie, full thickness)**
EXCLUDES   *Transanal destruction rectal tumor (45190)*
       Transanal endoscopic microsurgical tumor excision (TEMS) (0184T)
🔧 23.5 ⚕ 23.5 **FUD** 090   J G2 80 ▣
AMA: 2018,Feb,11; 2018,Jan,8; 2017,Jan,8; 2016,Jan,13

45190 **Destruction of rectal tumor (eg, electrodesiccation, electrosurgery, laser ablation, laser resection, cryosurgery) transanal approach**
EXCLUDES   *Transanal endoscopic microsurgical tumor excision (TEMS) (0184T)*
       Transanal excision rectal tumor (45171-45172)
🔧 20.2 ⚕ 20.2 **FUD** 090   J A2 ▣
AMA: 2018,Jan,8; 2017,Jan,8; 2016,Jan,13

45300-45327 Rigid Proctosigmoidoscopy Procedures

INCLUDES   Control bleeding due to endoscopic procedure during same operative session
     Exam:
       Entire rectum
       Portion sigmoid colon
EXCLUDES   *Computed tomographic colonography (74261-74263)*
Code also examination colon through stoma:
   Colonoscopy via stoma (44388-44408 [44401])
   Ileoscopy via stoma (44380-44384 [44381])

45300 **Proctosigmoidoscopy, rigid; diagnostic, with or without collection of specimen(s) by brushing or washing (separate procedure)**
📷 (74360)
🔧 1.38 ⚕ 3.52 **FUD** 000   T P3 ▣
AMA: 2018,Jan,8; 2017,Jan,8; 2016,Jan,13

45303 **with dilation (eg, balloon, guide wire, bougie)**
📷 (74360)
🔧 2.45 ⚕ 27.2 **FUD** 000   T P2 ▣
AMA: 2018,Jan,8; 2017,Jan,8; 2016,Jan,13

45305 **with biopsy, single or multiple**
🔧 2.10 ⚕ 4.63 **FUD** 000   T A2 ▣
AMA: 2018,Jan,8; 2017,Jan,8; 2016,Jan,13

45307 **with removal of foreign body**
🔧 2.81 ⚕ 5.33 **FUD** 000   J A2 80 ▣
AMA: 2018,Jan,8; 2017,Jan,8; 2016,Jan,13

45308 with removal of single tumor, polyp, or other lesion by hot biopsy forceps or bipolar cautery

🚗 2.44 ⚕ 5.25 **FUD** 000 J A2 ▭

AMA: 2018,Jan,8; 2017,Jan,8; 2016,Jan,13

Hot biopsy forceps or cautery

Rectal tumor

Rectal polyp

Sigmoid flexure

Rigid scope

Sigmoid

A rigid proctosigmoid procedure of the rectum and sigmoid is performed

45309 with removal of single tumor, polyp, or other lesion by snare technique

🚗 2.60 ⚕ 5.43 **FUD** 000 T A2 ▭

AMA: 2018,Jan,8; 2017,Jan,8; 2016,Jan,13

45315 with removal of multiple tumors, polyps, or other lesions by hot biopsy forceps, bipolar cautery or snare technique

🚗 3.08 ⚕ 5.93 **FUD** 000 T A2 ▭

AMA: 2018,Jan,8; 2017,Jan,8; 2016,Jan,13

45317 with control of bleeding (eg, injection, bipolar cautery, unipolar cautery, laser, heater probe, stapler, plasma coagulator)

🚗 3.24 ⚕ 5.52 **FUD** 000 T A2 ▭

AMA: 2018,Jan,8; 2017,Jan,8; 2016,Jan,13

45320 with ablation of tumor(s), polyp(s), or other lesion(s) not amenable to removal by hot biopsy forceps, bipolar cautery or snare technique (eg, laser)

🚗 3.05 ⚕ 5.78 **FUD** 000 J A2 ▭

AMA: 2018,Jan,8; 2017,Jan,8; 2016,Jan,13

45321 with decompression of volvulus

🚗 3.01 ⚕ 3.01 **FUD** 000 J A2 ▭

AMA: 2018,Jan,8; 2017,Jan,8; 2016,Jan,13

45327 with transendoscopic stent placement (includes predilation)

🚗 3.41 ⚕ 3.41 **FUD** 000 J J8 ▭

AMA: 2018,Jan,8; 2017,Jan,8; 2016,Jan,13

45330-45350 [45346] Flexible Sigmoidoscopy Procedures

INCLUDES Control bleeding due to endoscopic procedure during same operative session
Exam:
Entire rectum
Entire sigmoid colon
Portion descending colon (when performed)
EXCLUDES Computed tomographic colonography (74261-74263)
Code also examination colon through stoma when appropriate:
Colonoscopy (44388-44408 [44401])
Ileoscopy (44380-44384 [44381])

45330 Sigmoidoscopy, flexible; diagnostic, including collection of specimen(s) by brushing or washing, when performed (separate procedure)

EXCLUDES Sigmoidoscopy, flexible (45331-45350 [45346])

🚗 1.61 ⚕ 4.98 **FUD** 000 T P3 ▭

AMA: 2018,Jan,8; 2017,Jan,8; 2016,Feb,13; 2016,Jan,13

45331 with biopsy, single or multiple

EXCLUDES Sigmoidoscopy, flexible; with endoscopic mucosal resection same lesion (45349)

🚗 2.08 ⚕ 7.60 **FUD** 000 T A2 ▭

AMA: 2018,Jan,8; 2017,Jan,8; 2016,Feb,13; 2016,Jan,13

45332 with removal of foreign body(s)

EXCLUDES Sigmoidoscopy, flexible; diagnostic (45330)

🔬 (76000)

🚗 3.06 ⚕ 7.36 **FUD** 000 T A2 ▭

AMA: 2018,Jan,8; 2017,Jan,8; 2016,Feb,13; 2016,Jan,13

45333 with removal of tumor(s), polyp(s), or other lesion(s) by hot biopsy forceps

EXCLUDES Sigmoidoscopy, flexible; diagnostic (45330)

🚗 2.71 ⚕ 8.92 **FUD** 000 T A2 ▭

AMA: 2018,Jan,8; 2017,Jan,8; 2016,Feb,13; 2016,Jan,13

45334 with control of bleeding, any method

EXCLUDES Sigmoidoscopy, flexible; diagnostic (45330)
Sigmoidoscopy, flexible; with band ligation same lesion (45350)
Sigmoidoscopy, flexible; with directed submucosal injection same lesion (45335)

🚗 3.44 ⚕ 15.3 **FUD** 000 T A2 ▭

AMA: 2018,Jan,8; 2017,Jan,8; 2016,Feb,13; 2016,Jan,13

45335 with directed submucosal injection(s), any substance

EXCLUDES Sigmoidoscopy, flexible; diagnostic (45330)
Sigmoidoscopy, flexible; with control bleeding same lesion (45334)
Sigmoidoscopy, flexible; with endoscopic mucosal resection same lesion (45349)

🚗 1.91 ⚕ 7.58 **FUD** 000 T A2 ▭

AMA: 2018,Jan,8; 2017,Jan,8; 2016,Feb,13; 2016,Jan,13

45337 with decompression (for pathologic distention) (eg, volvulus, megacolon), including placement of decompression tube, when performed

EXCLUDES Procedure performed more than one time per operative session
Sigmoidoscopy, flexible; diagnostic (45330)

🚗 3.37 ⚕ 3.37 **FUD** 000 T A2 ▭

AMA: 2018,Jan,8; 2017,Jan,8; 2016,Feb,13; 2016,Jan,13

45338 with removal of tumor(s), polyp(s), or other lesion(s) by snare technique

EXCLUDES Sigmoidoscopy, flexible; diagnostic (45330)
Sigmoidoscopy, flexible; with endoscopic mucosal resection same lesion (45349)

🚗 3.47 ⚕ 8.07 **FUD** 000 T A2 ▭

AMA: 2018,Jan,8; 2017,Jan,8; 2016,Feb,13; 2016,Jan,13

45346 with ablation of tumor(s), polyp(s), or other lesion(s) (includes pre- and post-dilation and guide wire passage, when performed)

EXCLUDES Sigmoidoscopy, flexible; diagnostic (45330)
Sigmoidoscopy, flexible; with transendoscopic balloon dilation same lesion (45340)

🚗 4.72 ⚕ 87.4 **FUD** 000 T G2 ▭

AMA: 2018,Jan,8; 2017,Jan,8; 2016,Feb,13; 2016,Jan,13

45340 with transendoscopic balloon dilation

EXCLUDES Sigmoidoscopy, flexible (45330, [45346], 45347)
Code also each additional stricture dilated same session, using modifier 59 with (45340)

🔬 (74360)

🚗 2.24 ⚕ 12.9 **FUD** 000 T A2 ▭

AMA: 2018,Jan,8; 2017,Jan,8; 2016,Feb,13; 2016,Jan,13

26/TC PC/TC Only   A2-Z3 ASC Payment   50 Bilateral   ♂ Male Only   ♀ Female Only   🚗 Facility RVU   ⚕ Non-Facility RVU   ▭ CCI   ❌ CLIA
FUD Follow-up Days   CMS: IOM   AMA: CPT Asst   A-Y OPPSI   80/80 Surg Assist Allowed / w/Doc   🔬 Lab Crosswalk   🔬 Radiology Crosswalk

210   CPT © 2021 American Medical Association. All Rights Reserved.   © 2021 Optum360, LLC

45341   **with endoscopic ultrasound examination**

INCLUDES Gastrointestinal endoscopic ultrasound, supervision, and interpretation (76975)
Ultrasound, transrectal (76872)

EXCLUDES *Procedure performed more than one time per operative session*
Sigmoidoscopy, flexible (45330, 45342)

3.57   3.57 **FUD** 000   T A2 ▣

AMA: 2018,Jan,8; 2017,Jan,8; 2016,Feb,13; 2016,Jan,13

45342   **with transendoscopic ultrasound guided intramural or transmural fine needle aspiration/biopsy(s)**

INCLUDES Gastrointestinal endoscopic ultrasound, supervision and interpretation (76975)
Ultrasonic guidance (76942)
Ultrasound, transrectal (76872)

EXCLUDES *Procedure performed more than one time per operative session*
Sigmoidoscopy, flexible (45330, 45341)

4.89   4.89 **FUD** 000   T A2 ▣

AMA: 2018,Jan,8; 2017,Jan,8; 2016,Feb,13; 2016,Jan,13

45346   **Resequenced code. See code following 45338.**

45347   **with placement of endoscopic stent (includes pre- and post-dilation and guide wire passage, when performed)**

EXCLUDES *Sigmoidoscopy, flexible (45330, 45340)*

☒ (74360)

4.44   4.44 **FUD** 000   J J8 ▣

AMA: 2018,Jan,8; 2017,Jan,8; 2016,Feb,13; 2016,Jan,13

45349   **with endoscopic mucosal resection**

EXCLUDES *Procedure performed same lesion with (45331, 45335, 45338, 45350)*
Sigmoidoscopy, flexible; diagnostic (45330)

5.73   5.73 **FUD** 000   T G2 ▣

AMA: 2020,May,13; 2019,Dec,14; 2018,Jan,8; 2017,Jan,8; 2016,Jan,13

45350   **with band ligation(s) (eg, hemorrhoids)**

EXCLUDES *Hemorrhoidectomy, internal, by rubber band ligation (46221)*
Procedure performed more than one time per operative session
Sigmoidoscopy, flexible; diagnostic (45330)
Sigmoidoscopy, flexible; with control bleeding same lesion (45334)
Sigmoidoscopy, flexible; with endoscopic mucosal resection (45349)

2.92   17.8 **FUD** 000   T G2 ▣

AMA: 2020,Feb,11; 2018,Jan,8; 2017,Jan,8; 2016,Jan,13

45378-45398 [45388, 45390, 45398] Flexible and Rigid Colonoscopy Procedures

INCLUDES Control bleeding due to endoscopic procedure during same operative session
Exam:
  Entire colon (rectum to cecum)
  Terminal ileum (when performed)

EXCLUDES *Computed tomographic colonography (74261-74263)*
Code also modifier 53 (physician), or 73, 74 (facility) for incomplete colonoscopy

45378   **Colonoscopy, flexible; diagnostic, including collection of specimen(s) by brushing or washing, when performed (separate procedure)**

EXCLUDES *Colonoscopy, flexible (45379-45393 [45388, 45390, 45398])*
Decompression for pathological distention (45393)

5.35   9.42 **FUD** 000   T A2 ▣

AMA: 2018,Jan,7; 2018,Jan,8; 2017,Sep,14; 2017,Jan,8; 2016,Jan,13

45379   **with removal of foreign body(s)**

EXCLUDES *Colonoscopy, flexible; diagnostic (45378)*
Code also modifier 52 when colonoscope fails to reach small intestine junction

☒ (76000)

6.91   12.1 **FUD** 000   T A2 ▣

AMA: 2018,Jan,8; 2017,Jan,8; 2016,Jan,13

45380   **with biopsy, single or multiple**

EXCLUDES *Colonoscopy, flexible; diagnostic (45378)*
Colonoscopy, flexible; with endoscopic mucosal resection same lesion (45390)
Code also modifier 52 when colonoscope fails to reach small intestine junction

5.87   11.7 **FUD** 000   T A2 ▣

AMA: 2018,Jan,8; 2017,Jan,8; 2016,Jan,13

45381   **with directed submucosal injection(s), any substance**

EXCLUDES *Colonoscopy, flexible; diagnostic (45378)*
Colonoscopy, flexible; with control bleeding same lesion (45382)
Colonoscopy, flexible; with endoscopic mucosal resection same lesion (45390)
Code also modifier 52 when colonoscope fails to reach small intestine junction

5.87   11.5 **FUD** 000   T A2 ▣

AMA: 2018,Jan,8; 2017,Jan,8; 2017,Jan,6; 2016,Jan,13

45382   **with control of bleeding, any method**

EXCLUDES *Colonoscopy, flexible; diagnostic (45378)*
Colonoscopy, flexible; with band ligation same lesion ([45398])
Colonoscopy, flexible; with directed submucosal injection same lesion (45381)
Code also modifier 52 when colonoscope fails to reach small intestine junction

7.48   20.0 **FUD** 000   T A2 ▣

AMA: 2018,Jan,8; 2017,Jan,8; 2016,Jan,13

\# **45388**   **with ablation of tumor(s), polyp(s), or other lesion(s) (includes pre- and post-dilation and guide wire passage, when performed)**

EXCLUDES *Colonoscopy, flexible (45378, 45386)*

7.83   82.9 **FUD** 000   T G2 ▣

AMA: 2018,Jan,8; 2017,Jan,8; 2016,Jan,13

45384   **with removal of tumor(s), polyp(s), or other lesion(s) by hot biopsy forceps**

EXCLUDES *Colonoscopy, flexible; diagnostic (45378)*
Code also modifier 52 when colonoscope fails to reach small intestine junction

6.68   13.1 **FUD** 000   T A2 ▣

AMA: 2018,Jan,8; 2017,Jan,8; 2016,Jan,13

45385   **with removal of tumor(s), polyp(s), or other lesion(s) by snare technique**

EXCLUDES *Colonoscopy, flexible; diagnostic (45378)*
Colonoscopy, flexible; with endoscopic mucosal resection same lesion (45390)
7.35   12.6 **FUD** 000   T A2 ▣

AMA: 2018,Jan,8; 2017,Jan,8; 2017,Jan,6; 2016,Jan,13

45386   **with transendoscopic balloon dilation**

EXCLUDES *Colonoscopy, flexible (45378, [45388], 45389)*
Code also each additional stricture dilated same operative session, using modifier 59 with (45386)

☒ (74360)

6.20   17.0 **FUD** 000   T A2 ▣

AMA: 2018,Jan,8; 2017,Jan,8; 2016,Jan,13

45388   **Resequenced code. See code following 45382.**

45389   **with endoscopic stent placement (includes pre- and post-dilation and guide wire passage, when performed)**

EXCLUDES *Colonoscopy, flexible (45378, 45386)*

☒ (74360)

8.37   8.37 **FUD** 000   J J8 ▣

AMA: 2018,Jan,8; 2017,Jan,8; 2016,Jan,13

45390   **Resequenced code. See code following 45392.**

● New Code ▲ Revised Code ○ Reinstated ● New Web Release ▲ Revised Web Release + Add-on Unlisted Not Covered # Resequenced
50 Optum Mod 50 Exempt 51 AMA Mod 51 Exempt 51 Optum Mod 51 Exempt 63 Mod 63 Exempt ✗ Non-FDA Drug ★ Telemedicine M Maternity A Age Edit

© 2021 Optum360, LLC   CPT © 2021 American Medical Association. All Rights Reserved.   **211**

45391 **with endoscopic ultrasound examination limited to the rectum, sigmoid, descending, transverse, or ascending colon and cecum, and adjacent structures**

INCLUDES *Gastrointestinal endoscopic ultrasound, supervision and interpretation (76975)*
Ultrasound, transrectal (76872)

EXCLUDES *Colonoscopy, flexible (45378, 45392)*
Procedure performed more than one time per operative session

🚑 7.43   🔾 7.43   **FUD** 000   T A2 ▭

AMA: 2018,Jan,8; 2017,Jan,8; 2016,Jan,13

45392 **with transendoscopic ultrasound guided intramural or transmural fine needle aspiration/biopsy(s), includes endoscopic ultrasound examination limited to the rectum, sigmoid, descending, transverse, or ascending colon and cecum, and adjacent structures**

INCLUDES *Gastrointestinal endoscopic ultrasound, supervision and interpretation (76975)*
Ultrasonic guidance (76942)
Ultrasound, transrectal (76872)

EXCLUDES *Colonoscopy, flexible (45378, 45391)*
Procedure performed more than one time per operative session

🚑 8.78   🔾 8.78   **FUD** 000   T A2 ▭

AMA: 2018,Jan,8; 2017,Jan,8; 2016,Jan,13

\# **45390** **with endoscopic mucosal resection**

EXCLUDES *Colonoscopy, flexible; diagnostic (45378)*
Colonoscopy, flexible; with band ligation same lesion ([45398])
Colonoscopy, flexible; with biopsy same lesion (45380-45381)
Colonoscopy, flexible; with removal tumor(s), polyp(s), or other lesion(s) by snare technique same lesion (45385)

🚑 9.79   🔾 9.79   **FUD** 000   T 62 ▭

AMA: 2020,May,13; 2019,Dec,14; 2018,Jan,8; 2017,Jan,6; 2017,Jan,8; 2016,Jan,13

45393 **with decompression (for pathologic distention) (eg, volvulus, megacolon), including placement of decompression tube, when performed**

EXCLUDES *Colonoscopy, flexible; diagnostic (45378)*
Procedure performed more than one time per operative session

🚑 7.31   🔾 7.31   **FUD** 000   T 62 ▭

AMA: 2018,Jan,8; 2017,Jan,8; 2016,Jan,13

\# **45398** **with band ligation(s) (eg, hemorrhoids)**

EXCLUDES *Bleeding control by band ligation (45382)*
Colonoscopy, flexible (45378, 45390)
Hemorrhoidectomy, internal, by rubber band ligation (46221)
Procedure performed more than one time per operative session

Code also modifier 52 when colonoscope fails to reach small intestine junction

🚑 6.83   🔾 22.3   **FUD** 000   T 62 ▭

AMA: 2020,Feb,11; 2018,Jan,8; 2018,Jan,7; 2017,Sep,14; 2017,Jan,8; 2016,Jan,13

45395-45499 [45398, 45399] Laparoscopic Procedures of Rectum

INCLUDES Diagnostic laparoscopy

45395 **Laparoscopy, surgical; proctectomy, complete, combined abdominoperineal, with colostomy**

EXCLUDES *Open method (45110)*

🚑 56.8   🔾 56.8   **FUD** 090   C 80 ▭

AMA: 2018,Jan,8; 2017,Jan,8; 2016,Jan,13

45397 **proctectomy, combined abdominoperineal pull-through procedure (eg, colo-anal anastomosis), with creation of colonic reservoir (eg, J-pouch), with diverting enterostomy, when performed**

EXCLUDES *Open method (45119)*

🚑 61.8   🔾 61.8   **FUD** 090   C 80 ▭

AMA: 2018,Jan,8; 2017,Jan,8; 2016,Jan,13

45398 Resequenced code. See code following 45393.

45399 Resequenced code. See code before 45990.

45400 **Laparoscopy, surgical; proctopexy (for prolapse)**

EXCLUDES *Open method (45540-45541)*

🚑 32.8   🔾 32.8   **FUD** 090   C 80 ▭

AMA: 2018,Jan,8; 2017,Jan,8; 2016,Jan,13

45402 **proctopexy (for prolapse), with sigmoid resection**

EXCLUDES *Open method (45550)*

🚑 43.8   🔾 43.8   **FUD** 090   C 80 ▭

AMA: 2018,Jan,8; 2017,Jan,8; 2016,Jan,13

45499 **Unlisted laparoscopy procedure, rectum**

EXCLUDES *Unlisted rectal procedure performed via open technique (45999)*

🚑 0.00   🔾 0.00   **FUD** YYY   J 80 ▭

AMA: 2014,Jan,11; 2013,Jan,11-12

45500-45825 Open Repairs of Rectum

45500 **Proctoplasty; for stenosis**

🚑 16.3   🔾 16.3   **FUD** 090   J A2 80 ▭

AMA: 2014,Jan,11; 2013,Jan,11-12

45505 **for prolapse of mucous membrane**

🚑 17.2   🔾 17.2   **FUD** 090   J A2 ▭

AMA: 2018,Jan,8; 2017,Jan,8; 2016,Jan,13

45520 **Perirectal injection of sclerosing solution for prolapse**

🚑 1.16   🔾 4.41   **FUD** 000   01 N1 ▭

AMA: 2018,Jan,8; 2017,Jan,8; 2016,Jan,13

45540 **Proctopexy (eg, for prolapse); abdominal approach**

EXCLUDES *Laparoscopic method (45400)*

🚑 30.6   🔾 30.6   **FUD** 090   C 80 ▭

AMA: 2014,Jan,11; 2013,Jan,11-12

45541 **perineal approach**

🚑 27.3   🔾 27.3   **FUD** 090   J 62 80 ▭

AMA: 2014,Jan,11; 2013,Jan,11-12

45550 **with sigmoid resection, abdominal approach**

INCLUDES Frickman proctopexy
EXCLUDES *Laparoscopic method (45402)*

🚑 42.3   🔾 42.3   **FUD** 090   C 80 ▭

AMA: 2014,Jan,11; 2013,Jan,11-12

45560 **Repair of rectocele (separate procedure)**

EXCLUDES *Posterior colporrhaphy with rectocele repair (57250)*

🚑 19.7   🔾 19.7   **FUD** 090   J A2 80 ▭

AMA: 2014,Jan,11; 2013,Jan,11-12

Urethra   Posterior vaginal wall

The posterior wall of the vagina is opened directly over the rectocele; the walls of both structures are repaired; a rectocele is a herniated protrusion of part of the rectum into the vagina

45562	Exploration, repair, and presacral drainage for rectal injury;

    🔧 32.7   ✂ 32.7   **FUD** 090   C 80 ▭

    AMA: 2014,Jan,11; 2013,Jan,11-12

45563   **with colostomy**

    INCLUDES   Maydl colostomy

    🔧 48.3   ✂ 48.3   **FUD** 090   C 80 ▭

    AMA: 2014,Jan,11; 2013,Jan,11-12

45800   **Closure of rectovesical fistula;**

    🔧 36.7   ✂ 36.7   **FUD** 090   C 80 ▭

    AMA: 2014,Jan,11; 2013,Jan,11-12

45805   **with colostomy**

    🔧 42.8   ✂ 42.8   **FUD** 090   C 80 ▭

    AMA: 2014,Jan,11; 2013,Jan,11-12

45820   **Closure of rectourethral fistula;**

    EXCLUDES   *Closure fistula, rectovaginal (57300-57308)*

    🔧 37.0   ✂ 37.0   **FUD** 090   C 80 ▭

    AMA: 2014,Jan,11; 2013,Jan,11-12

45825   **with colostomy**

    EXCLUDES   *Closure fistula, rectovaginal (57300-57308)*

    🔧 44.4   ✂ 44.4   **FUD** 090   C 80 ▭

    AMA: 2014,Jan,11; 2013,Jan,11-12

45900-45999 [45399] Closed Procedures of Rectum With Anesthesia

45900   **Reduction of procidentia (separate procedure) under anesthesia**

    🔧 6.14   ✂ 6.14   **FUD** 010   T A2 80 ▭

    AMA: 2014,Jan,11; 2013,Jan,11-12

45905   **Dilation of anal sphincter (separate procedure) under anesthesia other than local**

    🔧 4.86   ✂ 4.86   **FUD** 010   T A2 ▭

    AMA: 2014,Jan,11; 2013,Jan,11-12

45910   **Dilation of rectal stricture (separate procedure) under anesthesia other than local**

    🔧 5.54   ✂ 5.54   **FUD** 010   T A2 ▭

    AMA: 2014,Jan,11; 2013,Jan,11-12

45915   **Removal of fecal impaction or foreign body (separate procedure) under anesthesia**

    🔧 6.65   ✂ 9.90   **FUD** 010   T A2 ▭

    AMA: 2018,Jan,8; 2017,Jan,8; 2016,Jan,13

\#   **45399**   **Unlisted procedure, colon**

    🔧 0.00   ✂ 0.00   **FUD** YYY   T ▭

    AMA: 2018,Jan,8; 2017,Jan,8; 2016,Jan,13

45990   **Anorectal exam, surgical, requiring anesthesia (general, spinal, or epidural), diagnostic**

    INCLUDES   Diagnostic:
           Anoscopy
           Proctoscopy, rigid
        Exam:
           Pelvic (when performed)
           Perineal, external
           Rectal, digital

    EXCLUDES   *Anogenital examination (99170)*
         Anoscopy; diagnostic (46600)
         Pelvic examination under anesthesia (57410)
         Proctosigmoidoscopy, rigid (45300-45327)

    🔧 3.09   ✂ 3.09   **FUD** 000   J A2 80 ▭

    AMA: 2018,Jan,8; 2017,Jan,8; 2016,Jan,13

45999   **Unlisted procedure, rectum**

    EXCLUDES   *Unlisted rectal procedure performed laparoscopically (45499)*

    🔧 0.00   ✂ 0.00   **FUD** YYY   T 80 ▭

    AMA: 2018,Jan,8; 2017,Jan,8; 2016,Jan,13

46020-46083 Surgical Incision of Anus

EXCLUDES   *Cryosurgical destruction hemorrhoid(s) (46999)*
    Fistulotomy, subcutaneous (46270)
    Hemorrhoidopexy ([46947])
    Injection hemorrhoid(s) (46500)
    Thermal energy destruction internal hemorrhoid(s) (46930)

46020   **Placement of seton**

    EXCLUDES   *Anoscopy; diagnostic (46600)*
         Incision and drainage ischiorectal or intramural abscess (46060)
         Surgical anal fistula treatment (46280)

    🔧 6.82   ✂ 8.10   **FUD** 010   J A2 ▭

    AMA: 2014,Jan,11; 2013,Jan,11-12

46030   **Removal of anal seton, other marker**

    🔧 2.59   ✂ 4.13   **FUD** 010   T A2 80 ▭

    AMA: 2014,Jan,11; 2013,Jan,11-12

46040   **Incision and drainage of ischiorectal and/or perirectal abscess (separate procedure)**

    🔧 12.1   ✂ 15.7   **FUD** 090   T A2 ▭

    AMA: 2014,Jan,11; 2013,Jan,11-12

46045   **Incision and drainage of intramural, intramuscular, or submucosal abscess, transanal, under anesthesia**

    🔧 12.6   ✂ 12.6   **FUD** 090   J A2 ▭

    AMA: 2014,Jan,11; 2013,Jan,11-12

46050   **Incision and drainage, perianal abscess, superficial**

    EXCLUDES   *Incision and drainage abscess:*
         Ischiorectal/intramural (46060)
         Supralevator/pelvirectal/retrorectal (45020)

    🔧 2.85   ✂ 6.27   **FUD** 010   T A2 ▭

    AMA: 2014,Jan,11; 2013,Jan,11-12

46060   **Incision and drainage of ischiorectal or intramural abscess, with fistulectomy or fistulotomy, submuscular, with or without placement of seton**

    EXCLUDES   *Incision and drainage abscess:*
         Supralevator/pelvirectal/retrorectal (45020)
         Placement seton (46020)

    🔧 13.8   ✂ 13.8   **FUD** 090   J A2 ▭

    AMA: 2014,Jan,11; 2013,Jan,11-12

46070   **Incision, anal septum (infant)**   A

    EXCLUDES   *Anoplasty (46700-46705)*

    🔧 7.52   ✂ 7.52   **FUD** 090   63 J G2 80 ▭

    AMA: 2014,Jan,11; 2013,Jan,11-12

46080   **Sphincterotomy, anal, division of sphincter (separate procedure)**

    🔧 4.59   ✂ 7.41   **FUD** 010   J A2 ▭

    AMA: 2014,Jan,11; 2013,Jan,11-12

46083   **Incision of thrombosed hemorrhoid, external**

    🔧 3.08   ✂ 5.24   **FUD** 010   T P2 ▭

    AMA: 2018,Jan,8; 2017,Jan,8; 2016,Jan,13

46200-46262 [46220, 46320, 46945, 46946, 46948] Anal Resection and Hemorrhoidectomies

EXCLUDES   *Cryosurgical destruction hemorrhoid(s) (46999)*
    Hemorrhoidopexy ([46947])
    Injection hemorrhoid(s) (46500)
    Thermal energy destruction internal hemorrhoid(s) (46930)

46200   **Fissurectomy, including sphincterotomy, when performed**

    🔧 9.45   ✂ 13.0   **FUD** 090   J A2 ▭

    AMA: 2014,Jan,11; 2013,Jan,11-12

46220   **Resequenced code. See code before 46230.**

46221   **Hemorrhoidectomy, internal, by rubber band ligation(s)**

    EXCLUDES   *Colonoscopy or sigmoidoscopy, flexible; with band ligation (45350, [45398])*
         Transanal hemorrhoidal dearterialization, two or more columns/groups ([46948])

    🔧 5.51   ✂ 7.77   **FUD** 010   T P3 ▭

    AMA: 2020,Feb,11; 2018,Jan,8; 2018,Jan,7; 2017,Sep,14; 2017,Jan,8; 2016,Jan,13

● New Code   ▲ Revised Code   ○ Reinstated   ● New Web Release   ▲ Revised Web Release   + Add-on   Unlisted   Not Covered   # Resequenced
50 Optum Mod 50 Exempt   Ⓝ AMA Mod 51 Exempt   51 Optum Mod 51 Exempt   63 Mod 63 Exempt   ∕ Non-FDA Drug   ★ Telemedicine   M Maternity   A Age Edit

Digestive System

46945 — 46505

 # 46945 Hemorrhoidectomy, internal, by ligation other than rubber band; single hemorrhoid column/group, without imaging guidance

> EXCLUDES *Transanal hemorrhoidal dearterialization, two or more columns/groups ([46948])*
> *Ultrasonic guidance (76942)*
> *Ultrasonic guidance, intraoperative (76998)*
> *Ultrasound, transrectal (76872)*

🔪 6.54   ✂ 9.08   **FUD** 090   J R2 ▭

AMA: 2020,Feb,11; 2018,Jan,8; 2017,Jan,8; 2016,Jan,13

 # 46946 2 or more hemorrhoid columns/groups, without imaging guidance

> EXCLUDES *Transanal hemorrhoidal dearterialization, two or more columns/groups ([46948])*
> *Ultrasonic guidance (76942)*
> *Ultrasonic guidance, intraoperative (76998)*
> *Ultrasound, transrectal (76872)*

🔪 6.50   ✂ 9.17   **FUD** 090   J A2 ▭

AMA: 2020,Feb,11; 2018,Jan,8; 2017,Jan,8; 2016,Jan,13

 # 46948 Hemorrhoidectomy, internal, by transanal hemorrhoidal dearterialization, 2 or more hemorrhoid columns/groups, including ultrasound guidance, with mucopexy, when performed

> INCLUDES Ultrasonic guidance (76872, 76942, 76998)
> EXCLUDES *Transanal hemorrhoidal dearterialization, single column/group (46999)*

🔪 12.7   ✂ 12.7   **FUD** 090   G2 ▭

AMA: 2020,Feb,11

 # 46220 Excision of single external papilla or tag, anus

🔪 3.43   ✂ 6.54   **FUD** 010   T A2 ▭

AMA: 2014,Jan,11; 2013,Jan,11-12

46230 Excision of multiple external papillae or tags, anus

🔪 5.00   ✂ 8.43   **FUD** 010   J A2 ▭

AMA: 2014,Jan,11; 2013,Jan,11-12

 # 46320 Excision of thrombosed hemorrhoid, external

🔪 3.22   ✂ 5.65   **FUD** 010   T P3 ▭

AMA: 2014,Jan,11; 2013,Jan,11-12

46250 Hemorrhoidectomy, external, 2 or more columns/groups

> EXCLUDES *Hemorrhoidectomy, external, single column/group (46999)*
> *Transanal hemorrhoidal dearterialization, two or more columns/groups ([46948])*

🔪 9.19   ✂ 13.6   **FUD** 090   J A2 ▭

AMA: 2014,Jan,11; 2013,Jan,11-12

46255 Hemorrhoidectomy, internal and external, single column/group;

> EXCLUDES *Transanal hemorrhoidal dearterialization, two or more columns/groups ([46948])*

🔪 10.3   ✂ 14.8   **FUD** 090   J A2 ▭

AMA: 2018,Jan,8; 2017,Jan,8; 2016,Jan,13

46257 with fissurectomy

> EXCLUDES *Transanal hemorrhoidal dearterialization, two or more columns/groups ([46948])*

🔪 12.3   ✂ 12.3   **FUD** 090   J A2 ▭

AMA: 2014,Jan,11; 2013,Jan,11-12

46258 with fistulectomy, including fissurectomy, when performed

> EXCLUDES *Transanal hemorrhoidal dearterialization, two or more columns/groups ([46948])*

🔪 13.7   ✂ 13.7   **FUD** 090   J A2 80 ▭

AMA: 2014,Jan,11; 2013,Jan,11-12

46260 Hemorrhoidectomy, internal and external, 2 or more columns/groups;

> INCLUDES Whitehead hemorrhoidectomy
> EXCLUDES *Transanal hemorrhoidal dearterialization, two or more columns/groups ([46948])*

🔪 13.8   ✂ 13.8   **FUD** 090   J A2 ▭

AMA: 2014,Jan,11; 2013,Jan,11-12

46261 with fissurectomy

> EXCLUDES *Transanal hemorrhoidal dearterialization, two or more columns/groups ([46948])*

🔪 15.1   ✂ 15.1   **FUD** 090   J A2 ▭

AMA: 2014,Jan,11; 2013,Jan,11-12

46262 with fistulectomy, including fissurectomy, when performed

> EXCLUDES *Transanal hemorrhoidal dearterialization, two or more columns/groups ([46948])*

🔪 16.0   ✂ 16.0   **FUD** 090   J A2 ▭

AMA: 2018,Jan,8; 2017,Jan,8; 2016,Jan,13

46270-46320 [46320] Resection of Anal Fistula

46270 Surgical treatment of anal fistula (fistulectomy/fistulotomy); subcutaneous

🔪 11.3   ✂ 14.8   **FUD** 090   J A2 ▭

AMA: 2014,Jan,11; 2013,Jan,11-12

46275 intersphincteric

🔪 11.9   ✂ 15.6   **FUD** 090   J A2 ▭

AMA: 2014,Jan,11; 2013,Jan,11-12

46280 transsphincteric, suprasphincteric, extrasphincteric or multiple, including placement of seton, when performed

> EXCLUDES *Placement seton (46020)*

🔪 13.7   ✂ 13.7   **FUD** 090   J A2 ▭

AMA: 2014,Jan,11; 2013,Jan,11-12

46285 second stage

🔪 12.0   ✂ 15.7   **FUD** 090   J A2 ▭

AMA: 2014,Jan,11; 2013,Jan,11-12

46288 Closure of anal fistula with rectal advancement flap

🔪 15.8   ✂ 15.8   **FUD** 090   J A2 ▭

AMA: 2014,Jan,11; 2013,Jan,11-12

46320 Resequenced code. See code following 46230.

46500 Other Hemorrhoid Procedures

> EXCLUDES *Anoscopic injection bulking agent, submucosal, for fecal incontinence (46999)*

46500 Injection of sclerosing solution, hemorrhoids

🔪 5.20   ✂ 8.54   **FUD** 010   T P3 ▭

AMA: 2018,Jan,8; 2017,Jan,8; 2016,Jan,13

Internal hemorrhoids
Internal anal sphincter
External hemorrhoids
External anal sphincter
Dentate line

A sclerosing agent is injected into the tissues underlying hemorrhoids

46505 Chemodenervation Anal Sphincter

> EXCLUDES *Chemodenervation:*
> *Extremity muscles (64642-64645)*
> *Muscles/facial nerve (64612)*
> *Neck muscles (64616)*
> *Other peripheral nerve/branch (64640)*
> *Pudendal nerve (64630)*
> *Trunk muscles (64646-64647)*

Code also drug(s)/substance(s) given

46505 Chemodenervation of internal anal sphincter

🔪 7.00   ✂ 8.55   **FUD** 010   T G2 50 ▭

AMA: 2019,Apr,9; 2018,Jan,8; 2017,Jan,8; 2016,Jan,13

26/TC PC/TC Only   A2-Z3 ASC Payment   50 Bilateral   ♂ Male Only   ♀ Female Only   🔪 Facility RVU   ✂ Non-Facility RVU   ▭ CCI   ✖ CLIA
FUD Follow-up Days   CMS: IOM   AMA: CPT Asst   A-Y OPPSI   80/80 Surg Assist Allowed / w/Doc   Lab Crosswalk   Radiology Crosswalk

214   CPT © 2021 American Medical Association. All Rights Reserved.   © 2021 Optum360, LLC

46600-46615 Anoscopic Procedures

EXCLUDES Delivery thermal energy via anoscope to anal canal muscle (46999)
Injection bulking agent, submucosal, for fecal incontinence (46999)

46600 **Anoscopy; diagnostic, including collection of specimen(s) by brushing or washing, when performed (separate procedure)**

EXCLUDES Excision rectal tumor, transanal endoscopic microsurgical approach (i.e., TEMS) (0184T)
High-resolution anoscopy (HRA), diagnostic (46601)
Surgical incision anus (46020-46761 [46220, 46320, 46320, 46945, 46946, 46947, 46948])

🔧 1.17 ⚕ 2.94 **FUD** 000 〔Q1〕〔N1〕🖮

AMA: 2018,Jan,7; 2018,Jan,8; 2017,Jan,8; 2016,Jan,13

46601 **diagnostic, with high-resolution magnification (HRA) (eg, colposcope, operating microscope) and chemical agent enhancement, including collection of specimen(s) by brushing or washing, when performed**

INCLUDES Operating microscope (69990)

🔧 2.72 ⚕ 3.88 **FUD** 000 〔Q1〕〔N1〕🖮

AMA: 2018,Oct,11; 2016,Feb,12

46604 **with dilation (eg, balloon, guide wire, bougie)**

🔧 1.90 ⚕ 18.3 **FUD** 000 〔T〕〔P2〕🖮

AMA: 2018,Jan,8; 2017,Jan,8; 2016,Jan,13

46606 **with biopsy, single or multiple**

EXCLUDES High resolution anoscopy (HRA) with biopsy (46607)

🔧 2.17 ⚕ 7.31 **FUD** 000 〔T〕〔P3〕🖮

AMA: 2019,Sep,10; 2018,Jan,8; 2017,Jan,8; 2016,Jan,13

46607 **with high-resolution magnification (HRA) (eg, colposcope, operating microscope) and chemical agent enhancement, with biopsy, single or multiple**

INCLUDES Operating microscope (69990)

🔧 3.65 ⚕ 5.75 **FUD** 000 〔T〕〔G2〕🖮

AMA: 2019,Dec,12; 2018,Oct,11; 2016,Feb,12

46608 **with removal of foreign body**

🔧 2.44 ⚕ 7.68 **FUD** 000 〔T〕〔A2〕🖮

AMA: 2018,Jan,8; 2017,Jan,8; 2016,Jan,13

46610 **with removal of single tumor, polyp, or other lesion by hot biopsy forceps or bipolar cautery**

🔧 2.34 ⚕ 7.30 **FUD** 000 〔J〕〔A2〕🖮

AMA: 2018,Jan,8; 2017,Jan,8; 2016,Jan,13

46611 **with removal of single tumor, polyp, or other lesion by snare technique**

🔧 2.31 ⚕ 5.78 **FUD** 000 〔T〕〔A2〕🖮

AMA: 2018,Jan,8; 2017,Jan,8; 2016,Jan,13

46612 **with removal of multiple tumors, polyps, or other lesions by hot biopsy forceps, bipolar cautery or snare technique**

🔧 2.76 ⚕ 8.90 **FUD** 000 〔J〕〔A2〕🖮

AMA: 2018,Jan,8; 2017,Jan,8; 2016,Jan,13

46614 **with control of bleeding (eg, injection, bipolar cautery, unipolar cautery, laser, heater probe, stapler, plasma coagulator)**

🔧 1.85 ⚕ 4.21 **FUD** 000 〔T〕〔P3〕🖮

AMA: 2018,Jan,8; 2017,Jan,8; 2016,Jan,13

46615 **with ablation of tumor(s), polyp(s), or other lesion(s) not amenable to removal by hot biopsy forceps, bipolar cautery or snare technique**

🔧 2.64 ⚕ 4.34 **FUD** 000 〔J〕〔A2〕🖮

AMA: 2018,Jan,8; 2017,Jan,8; 2016,Jan,13

46700-46947 [46947] Anal Repairs and Stapled Hemorrhoidopexy

46700 **Anoplasty, plastic operation for stricture; adult**

🔧 18.9 ⚕ 18.9 **FUD** 090 〔J〕〔A2〕🖮

AMA: 2014,Jan,11; 2013,Jan,11-12

46705 **infant** 〔A〕

EXCLUDES Anal septum incision (46070)

🔧 16.1 ⚕ 16.1 **FUD** 090 〔63〕〔C〕〔80〕🖮

AMA: 2014,Jan,11; 2013,Jan,11-12

46706 **Repair of anal fistula with fibrin glue**

🔧 5.14 ⚕ 5.14 **FUD** 010 〔J〕〔A2〕🖮

AMA: 2014,Jan,11; 2013,Jan,11-12

46707 **Repair of anorectal fistula with plug (eg, porcine small intestine submucosa [SIS])**

🔧 14.4 ⚕ 14.4 **FUD** 090 〔J〕〔J8〕〔80〕🖮

AMA: 2018,Jan,8; 2017,Jan,8; 2016,Jan,13

46710 **Repair of ileoanal pouch fistula/sinus (eg, perineal or vaginal), pouch advancement; transperineal approach**

🔧 32.3 ⚕ 32.3 **FUD** 090 〔C〕〔80〕🖮

AMA: 2018,Jan,8; 2017,Jan,8; 2016,Jan,13

46712 **combined transperineal and transabdominal approach**

🔧 65.0 ⚕ 65.0 **FUD** 090 〔C〕〔80〕🖮

AMA: 2018,Jan,8; 2017,Jan,8; 2016,Jan,13

46715 **Repair of low imperforate anus; with anoperineal fistula (cut-back procedure)**

🔧 15.9 ⚕ 15.9 **FUD** 090 〔63〕〔C〕〔80〕🖮

AMA: 2014,Jan,11; 2013,Jan,11-12

46716 **with transposition of anoperineal or anovestibular fistula**

🔧 35.4 ⚕ 35.4 **FUD** 090 〔63〕〔C〕〔80〕🖮

AMA: 2014,Jan,11; 2013,Jan,11-12

46730 **Repair of high imperforate anus without fistula; perineal or sacroperineal approach**

🔧 57.4 ⚕ 57.4 **FUD** 090 〔63〕〔C〕〔80〕🖮

AMA: 2014,Jan,11; 2013,Jan,11-12

46735 **combined transabdominal and sacroperineal approaches**

🔧 66.2 ⚕ 66.2 **FUD** 090 〔63〕〔C〕〔80〕🖮

AMA: 2014,Jan,11; 2013,Jan,11-12

46740 **Repair of high imperforate anus with rectourethral or rectovaginal fistula; perineal or sacroperineal approach**

🔧 62.7 ⚕ 62.7 **FUD** 090 〔63〕〔C〕〔80〕🖮

AMA: 2014,Jan,11; 2013,Jan,11-12

46742 **combined transabdominal and sacroperineal approaches**

🔧 72.7 ⚕ 72.7 **FUD** 090 〔63〕〔C〕〔80〕🖮

AMA: 2014,Jan,11; 2013,Jan,11-12

46744 **Repair of cloacal anomaly by anorectovaginoplasty and urethroplasty, sacroperineal approach** ♀

🔧 103. ⚕ 103. **FUD** 090 〔63〕〔C〕〔80〕🖮

AMA: 2014,Jan,11; 2013,Jan,11-12

46746 **Repair of cloacal anomaly by anorectovaginoplasty and urethroplasty, combined abdominal and sacroperineal approach;** ♀

🔧 113. ⚕ 113. **FUD** 090 〔C〕〔80〕🖮

AMA: 2014,Jan,11; 2013,Jan,11-12

46748 **with vaginal lengthening by intestinal graft or pedicle flaps** ♀

🔧 122. ⚕ 122. **FUD** 090 〔C〕〔80〕🖮

AMA: 2014,Jan,11; 2013,Jan,11-12

46750 **Sphincteroplasty, anal, for incontinence or prolapse; adult**

🔧 21.7 ⚕ 21.7 **FUD** 090 〔J〕〔A2〕〔80〕🖮

AMA: 2014,Jan,11; 2013,Jan,11-12

46751 **child** 〔A〕

🔧 19.2 ⚕ 19.2 **FUD** 090 〔C〕〔80〕🖮

AMA: 2014,Jan,11; 2013,Jan,11-12

46753 **Graft (Thiersch operation) for rectal incontinence and/or prolapse**

🔧 17.7 ⚕ 17.7 **FUD** 090 〔J〕〔A2〕🖮

AMA: 2014,Jan,11; 2013,Jan,11-12

● New Code   ▲ Revised Code   ○ Reinstated   ● New Web Release   ▲ Revised Web Release   + Add-on   Unlisted   Not Covered   # Resequenced
㊿ Optum Mod 50 Exempt   ⚕ AMA Mod 51 Exempt   �91 Optum Mod 51 Exempt   �63 Mod 63 Exempt   ✗ Non-FDA Drug   ★ Telemedicine   Ⓜ Maternity   Ⓐ Age Edit

Digestive System

46754 — 47135

46754 Removal of Thiersch wire or suture, anal canal
🔧 6.76　🔨 9.30　**FUD** 010　　　　　J A2 80 ▢
AMA: 2014,Jan,11; 2013,Jan,11-12

46760 Sphincteroplasty, anal, for incontinence, adult; muscle transplant
🔧 31.6　🔨 31.6　**FUD** 090　　　　　J A2 80 ▢
AMA: 2014,Jan,11; 2013,Jan,11-12

46761 levator muscle imbrication (Park posterior anal repair)
🔧 26.6　🔨 26.6　**FUD** 090　　　　　J A2 80 ▢
AMA: 2014,Jan,11; 2013,Jan,11-12

\# **46947** Hemorrhoidopexy (eg, for prolapsing internal hemorrhoids) by stapling
🔧 11.1　🔨 11.1　**FUD** 090　　　　　J A2 ▢
AMA: 2018,Jan,8; 2017,Jan,8; 2016,Jan,13

46900-46999 [46945, 46946, 46947, 46948] Destruction Procedures: Anus

46900 Destruction of lesion(s), anus (eg, condyloma, papilloma, molluscum contagiosum, herpetic vesicle), simple; chemical
🔧 3.92　🔨 6.76　**FUD** 010　　　　　T P3 ▢
AMA: 2014,Jan,11; 2013,Jan,11-12

46910 electrodesiccation
🔧 3.84　🔨 7.39　**FUD** 010　　　　　T P3 ▢
AMA: 2019,Dec,12

46916 cryosurgery
🔧 4.06　🔨 7.00　**FUD** 010　　　　　T P2 ▢
AMA: 2014,Jan,11; 2013,Jan,11-12

46917 laser surgery
🔧 3.68　🔨 11.9　**FUD** 010　　　　　J A2 ▢
AMA: 2014,Jan,11; 2013,Jan,11-12

46922 surgical excision
🔧 3.92　🔨 8.00　**FUD** 010　　　　　J A2 ▢
AMA: 2014,Jan,11; 2013,Jan,11-12

46924 Destruction of lesion(s), anus (eg, condyloma, papilloma, molluscum contagiosum, herpetic vesicle), extensive (eg, laser surgery, electrosurgery, cryosurgery, chemosurgery)
🔧 5.21　🔨 15.1　**FUD** 010　　　　　J A2 ▢
AMA: 2014,Jan,11; 2013,Jan,11-12

46930 Destruction of internal hemorrhoid(s) by thermal energy (eg, infrared coagulation, cautery, radiofrequency)
　　EXCLUDES Other hemorrhoid procedures:
　　　　Cryosurgery destruction (46999)
　　　　Excision ([46320], 46250-46262)
　　　　Hemorrhoidopexy ([46947])
　　　　Incision (46083)
　　　　Injection sclerosing solution (46500)
　　　　Ligation (46221, [46945, 46946])
🔧 4.33　🔨 6.12　**FUD** 090　　　　　T P3 80 ▢
AMA: 2018,Jan,8; 2017,Jan,8; 2016,Jul,8; 2016,Jan,13

46940 Curettage or cautery of anal fissure, including dilation of anal sphincter (separate procedure); initial
🔧 4.20　🔨 6.79　**FUD** 010　　　　　J P3 ▢
AMA: 2014,Jan,11; 2013,Jan,11-12

46942 subsequent
🔧 3.74　🔨 6.72　**FUD** 010　　　　　T P3 80 ▢
AMA: 2014,Jan,11; 2013,Jan,11-12

46945 Resequenced code. See code following 46221.

46946 Resequenced code. See code following resequenced code 46945.

46947 Resequenced code. See code following 46761.

46948 Resequenced code. See code before resequenced code 46220.

46999 Unlisted procedure, anus
🔧 0.00　🔨 0.00　**FUD** YYY　　　　　T 80 ▢
AMA: 2020,Feb,11; 2018,Oct,11; 2018,Jan,8; 2017,Jan,8; 2016,Jan,13

47000-47001 Needle Biopsy of Liver

　EXCLUDES Fine needle aspiration (10021, [10004, 10005, 10006, 10007, 10008, 10009, 10010, 10011, 10012])

47000 Biopsy of liver, needle; percutaneous
　🔀 (76942, 77002, 77012, 77021)
　🔀 (88172-88173)
🔧 2.56　🔨 8.85　**FUD** 000　　　　　J A2 ▢
AMA: 2019,Apr,4; 2018,Jan,8; 2017,Jan,8; 2016,Jan,13

\+ **47001** when done for indicated purpose at time of other major procedure (List separately in addition to code for primary procedure)
Code first primary procedure
　🔀 (76942, 77002)
　🔀 (88172-88173)
🔧 3.04　🔨 3.04　**FUD** ZZZ　　　　　N N1 ▢
AMA: 2018,Jan,8; 2017,Jan,8; 2016,Jan,13

47010-47130 Open Incisional and Resection Procedures of Liver

47010 Hepatotomy, for open drainage of abscess or cyst, 1 or 2 stages
　EXCLUDES Image guided percutaneous catheter drainage (49505)
🔧 35.2　🔨 35.2　**FUD** 090　　　　　C 80 ▢
AMA: 2014,Jan,11; 2013,Nov,9

47015 Laparotomy, with aspiration and/or injection of hepatic parasitic (eg, amoebic or echinococcal) cyst(s) or abscess(es)
🔧 33.9　🔨 33.9　**FUD** 090　　　　　C 80 ▢
AMA: 2014,Jan,11; 2013,Jan,11-12

47100 Biopsy of liver, wedge
🔧 24.6　🔨 24.6　**FUD** 090　　　　　C 80 ▢
AMA: 2014,Jan,11; 2013,Jan,11-12

47120 Hepatectomy, resection of liver; partial lobectomy
🔧 68.0　🔨 68.0　**FUD** 090　　　　　C 80 ▢
AMA: 2018,Jan,8; 2017,Jan,8; 2016,Oct,11; 2016,Jan,13

47122 trisegmentectomy
🔧 100.　🔨 100.　**FUD** 090　　　　　C 80 ▢
AMA: 2014,Jan,11; 2013,Jan,11-12

47125 total left lobectomy
🔧 89.8　🔨 89.8　**FUD** 090　　　　　C 80 ▢
AMA: 2014,Jan,11; 2013,Jan,11-12

47130 total right lobectomy
🔧 96.4　🔨 96.4　**FUD** 090　　　　　C 80 ▢
AMA: 2014,Jan,11; 2013,Jan,11-12

47133-47147 Liver Transplant Procedures

CMS: 100-03,260.1 Adult Liver Transplantation; 100-03,260.2 Pediatric Liver Transplantation; 100-04,3,90.4 Liver Transplants; 100-04,3,90.4.1 Standard Liver Acquisition Charge; 100-04,3,90.4.2 Billing for Liver Transplant and Acquisition Services; 100-04,3,90.6 Intestinal and Multi-Visceral Transplants

47133 Donor hepatectomy (including cold preservation), from cadaver donor
　INCLUDES Graft:
　　　Cold preservation
　　　Harvest
🔧 0.00　🔨 0.00　**FUD** XXX　　　　　C ▢
AMA: 2014,Jan,11; 2013,Jan,11-12

47135 Liver allotransplantation, orthotopic, partial or whole, from cadaver or living donor, any age
　INCLUDES Partial/whole recipient hepatectomy
　　　Partial/whole transplant allograft
　　　Recipient care
🔧 157.　🔨 157.　**FUD** 090　　　　　C 80 ▢
AMA: 2018,Jan,8; 2017,Jan,8; 2016,Jan,13

26/TC PC/TC Only　　A2-Z3 ASC Payment　　50 Bilateral　　♂ Male Only　　♀ Female Only　　🔧 Facility RVU　　🔨 Non-Facility RVU　　▢ CCI　　☒ CLIA
FUD Follow-up Days　　CMS: IOM　　AMA: CPT Asst　　A-Y OPPSI　　80/80 Surg Assist Allowed / w/Doc　　🔀 Lab Crosswalk　　🔀 Radiology Crosswalk

216　　　　　　　　　　　CPT © 2021 American Medical Association. All Rights Reserved.　　　　　　　　　　© 2021 Optum360, LLC

47140 Donor hepatectomy (including cold preservation), from living donor; left lateral segment only (segments II and III)

INCLUDES Donor care
Graft:
Cold preservation
Harvest

103. 103. **FUD** 090 C 80

AMA: 2018,Jan,8; 2017,Jan,8; 2016,Jan,13

47141 total left lobectomy (segments II, III and IV)

INCLUDES Donor care
Graft:
Cold preservation
Harvest

124. 124. **FUD** 090 C 80

AMA: 2014,Jan,11; 2013,Jan,11-12

47142 total right lobectomy (segments V, VI, VII and VIII)

INCLUDES Donor care
Graft:
Cold preservation
Harvest

136. 136. **FUD** 090 C 80

AMA: 2014,Jan,11; 2013,Jan,11-12

47143 Backbench standard preparation of cadaver donor whole liver graft prior to allotransplantation, including cholecystectomy, if necessary, and dissection and removal of surrounding soft tissues to prepare the vena cava, portal vein, hepatic artery, and common bile duct for implantation; without trisegment or lobe split

EXCLUDES *Cholecystectomy (47600, 47610)*
Hepatectomy (47120-47125)

0.00 0.00 **FUD** XXX C 80

AMA: 2018,Jan,8; 2017,Jan,8; 2016,Jan,13

47144 with trisegment split of whole liver graft into 2 partial liver grafts (ie, left lateral segment [segments II and III] and right trisegment [segments I and IV through VIII])

EXCLUDES *Cholecystectomy (47600, 47610)*
Hepatectomy (47120-47125)

0.00 0.00 **FUD** 090 C 80

AMA: 2014,Jan,11; 2013,Jan,11-12

47145 with lobe split of whole liver graft into 2 partial liver grafts (ie, left lobe [segments II, III, and IV] and right lobe [segments I and V through VIII])

EXCLUDES *Cholecystectomy (47600, 47610)*
Hepatectomy (47120-47125)

0.00 0.00 **FUD** XXX C 80

AMA: 2014,Jan,11; 2013,Jan,11-12

47146 Backbench reconstruction of cadaver or living donor liver graft prior to allotransplantation; venous anastomosis, each

EXCLUDES *Cholecystectomy (47600, 47610)*
Hepatectomy (47120-47125)

9.57 9.57 **FUD** XXX C 80

AMA: 2014,Jan,11; 2013,Jan,11-12

47147 arterial anastomosis, each

EXCLUDES *Cholecystectomy (47600, 47610)*
Hepatectomy (47120-47125)

11.1 11.1 **FUD** XXX C 80

AMA: 2014,Jan,11; 2013,Jan,11-12

47300-47362 Open Repair of Liver

47300 Marsupialization of cyst or abscess of liver

32.9 32.9 **FUD** 090 C 80

AMA: 2014,Jan,11; 2013,Jan,11-12

Anterior abdominal skin — Hepatic cyst

Cutaway view of liver

Marsupialization of cyst

A liver cyst or abscess is marsupialized; this method involves surgical access to the cyst and making an incision into it; the edges of the cyst are sutured to the abdominal wall and drainage, open or closed, is placed into the cyst

47350 Management of liver hemorrhage; simple suture of liver wound or injury

39.7 39.7 **FUD** 090 C 80

AMA: 2020,Oct,14

47360 complex suture of liver wound or injury, with or without hepatic artery ligation

54.8 54.8 **FUD** 090 C 80

AMA: 2020,Oct,14

47361 exploration of hepatic wound, extensive debridement, coagulation and/or suture, with or without packing of liver

88.0 88.0 **FUD** 090 C 80

AMA: 2020,Oct,14

47362 re-exploration of hepatic wound for removal of packing

42.1 42.1 **FUD** 090 C 80

AMA: 2020,Jan,6

47370-47379 Laparoscopic Ablation Liver Tumors

INCLUDES Diagnostic laparoscopy (49320)

47370 Laparoscopy, surgical, ablation of 1 or more liver tumor(s); radiofrequency

(76940)

36.4 36.4 **FUD** 090 J 62 80

AMA: 2018,Jan,8; 2017,Jan,8; 2016,Jan,13

47371 cryosurgical

(76940)

36.5 36.5 **FUD** 090 J 62 80

AMA: 2014,Jan,11; 2013,Jan,11-12

47379 Unlisted laparoscopic procedure, liver

0.00 0.00 **FUD** YYY J 80

AMA: 2018,Aug,10; 2018,Jan,8; 2017,Jan,8; 2016,Jan,13

47380-47399 Open/Percutaneous Ablation Liver Tumors

47380 Ablation, open, of 1 or more liver tumor(s); radiofrequency

(76940)

42.1 42.1 **FUD** 090 C 80

AMA: 2018,Jan,8; 2017,Jan,8; 2016,Jan,13

47381   cryosurgical
          ⚕ (76940)
          🏥 43.2   ⚗ 43.2   **FUD** 090   C 80 ▢
          AMA: 2014,Jan,11; 2013,Jan,11-12

47382   Ablation, 1 or more liver tumor(s), percutaneous, radiofrequency
          ⚕ (76940, 77013, 77022)
          🏥 21.4   ⚗ 125.   **FUD** 010   J G2 ▢
          AMA: 2018,Jan,8; 2017,Jan,8; 2016,Jan,13

47383   Ablation, 1 or more liver tumor(s), percutaneous, cryoablation
          ⚕ (76940, 77013, 77022)
          🏥 13.1   ⚗ 195.   **FUD** 010   J J8 ▢
          AMA: 2018,Jan,8; 2017,Jan,8; 2016,Jan,13

47399   Unlisted procedure, liver
          🏥 0.00   ⚗ 0.00   **FUD** YYY   T ▢
          AMA: 2018,Jan,8; 2017,Mar,10; 2017,Jan,8; 2016,Jan,13

47400-47490 Biliary Tract Procedures

47400   Hepaticotomy or hepaticostomy with exploration, drainage, or removal of calculus
          🏥 62.9   ⚗ 62.9   **FUD** 090   C 80 ▢
          AMA: 2014,Jan,11; 2013,Jan,11-12

47420   Choledochotomy or choledochostomy with exploration, drainage, or removal of calculus, with or without cholecystotomy; without transduodenal sphincterotomy or sphincteroplasty
          🏥 39.1   ⚗ 39.1   **FUD** 090   C 80 ▢
          AMA: 2014,Jan,11; 2013,Jan,11-12

47425   with transduodenal sphincterotomy or sphincteroplasty
          🏥 39.9   ⚗ 39.9   **FUD** 090   C 80 ▢
          AMA: 2014,Jan,11; 2013,Jan,11-12

47460   Transduodenal sphincterotomy or sphincteroplasty, with or without transduodenal extraction of calculus (separate procedure)
          🏥 37.0   ⚗ 37.0   **FUD** 090   C 80 ▢
          AMA: 2014,Jan,11; 2013,Jan,11-12

47480   Cholecystotomy or cholecystostomy, open, with exploration, drainage, or removal of calculus (separate procedure)
          EXCLUDES   *Percutaneous cholecystostomy (47490)*
          🏥 25.4   ⚗ 25.4   **FUD** 090   C 80 ▢
          AMA: 2018,Jan,8; 2017,Jan,8; 2016,Jan,13

47490   Cholecystostomy, percutaneous, complete procedure, including imaging guidance, catheter placement, cholecystogram when performed, and radiological supervision and interpretation
          INCLUDES   Radiological guidance (75989, 76942, 77002, 77012, 77021)
          EXCLUDES   *Injection procedure for cholangiography (47531-47532)*
                   Open cholecystostomy (47480)
          🏥 9.56   ⚗ 9.56   **FUD** 010   J G2 ▢
          AMA: 2018,Jan,8; 2017,Jan,8; 2016,Jan,13

Percutaneous catheter passed through liver to gallbladder

Common hepatic duct
Gallstone impacted in cystic duct
Inflamed thick walled gallbladder

47531-47532 Injection/Insertion Procedures of Biliary Tract

INCLUDES   Contrast material injection
         Radiologic supervision and interpretation
EXCLUDES   *Intraoperative cholangiography (74300-74301)*
         Procedures performed via same access (47490, 47533-47541)

47531   Injection procedure for cholangiography, percutaneous, complete diagnostic procedure including imaging guidance (eg, ultrasound and/or fluoroscopy) and all associated radiological supervision and interpretation; existing access
          🏥 2.06   ⚗ 9.89   **FUD** 000   02 N1 ▢
          AMA: 2018,Jan,8; 2017,Jan,8

47532   new access (eg, percutaneous transhepatic cholangiogram)
          🏥 6.18   ⚗ 23.2   **FUD** 000   02 N1 ▢
          AMA: 2018,Jan,8; 2017,Jan,8

47533-47544 Percutaneous Procedures of the Biliary Tract

47533   Placement of biliary drainage catheter, percutaneous, including diagnostic cholangiography when performed, imaging guidance (eg, ultrasound and/or fluoroscopy), and all associated radiological supervision and interpretation; external
          EXCLUDES   *Conversion to internal-external drainage catheter (47535)*
                   Percutaneous placement stent bile duct (47538)
                   Placement stent bile duct, new access (47540)
                   Replacement existing internal drainage catheter (47536)
          🏥 7.74   ⚗ 35.2   **FUD** 000   J G2 ▢
          AMA: 2018,Jan,8; 2017,Jan,8

47534   internal-external
          EXCLUDES   *Conversion to external only drainage catheter (47536)*
                   Percutaneous placement stent bile duct (47538)
                   Placement stent bile duct, new access (47540)
          🏥 10.8   ⚗ 41.8   **FUD** 000   J G2 ▢
          AMA: 2018,Jan,8; 2017,Jan,8

47535 Conversion of external biliary drainage catheter to internal-external biliary drainage catheter, percutaneous, including diagnostic cholangiography when performed, imaging guidance (eg, fluoroscopy), and all associated radiological supervision and interpretation

🔲 5.75   ⚖ 28.4   **FUD** 000   [J] [62] [▭]

AMA: 2018,Jan,8; 2017,Jan,8

47536 Exchange of biliary drainage catheter (eg, external, internal-external, or conversion of internal-external to external only), percutaneous, including diagnostic cholangiography when performed, imaging guidance (eg, fluoroscopy), and all associated radiological supervision and interpretation

INCLUDES   Exchange one drainage catheter

EXCLUDES   *Placement stent(s) into bile duct, percutaneous (47538)*

Code also exchange additional catheters same session with modifier 59 (47536)

🔲 3.84   ⚖ 19.5   **FUD** 000   [J] [62] [▭]

AMA: 2018,Jan,8; 2017,Jan,8

47537 Removal of biliary drainage catheter, percutaneous, requiring fluoroscopic guidance (eg, with concurrent indwelling biliary stents), including diagnostic cholangiography when performed, imaging guidance (eg, fluoroscopy), and all associated radiological supervision and interpretation

EXCLUDES   *Placement stent(s) into bile duct via same access (47538)*
            Removal without fluoroscopic guidance; report with appropriate E/M service code

🔲 2.79   ⚖ 11.5   **FUD** 000   [02] [62] [▭]

AMA: 2018,Jan,8; 2017,Jan,8

47538 Placement of stent(s) into a bile duct, percutaneous, including diagnostic cholangiography, imaging guidance (eg, fluoroscopy and/or ultrasound), balloon dilation, catheter exchange(s) and catheter removal(s) when performed, and all associated radiological supervision and interpretation; existing access

EXCLUDES   *Drainage catheter inserted following stent placement (47536)*
            Procedures performed via same access (47536-47537)
            Treatment same lesion same operative session ([43277], 47542, 47555-47556)

Code also multiple stents placed during same session when: (47538-47540)
    Serial stents placed within same bile duct
    Stent placement via two or more percutaneous access sites or space between two other stents
    Two or more stents inserted through same percutaneous access

🔲 6.88   ⚖ 122.   **FUD** 000   [J] [J8] [▭]

AMA: 2018,Jan,8; 2017,Jan,8; 2016,Mar,10

Expandable metal stent: bile drains through stent
Liver
Common bile duct
Gallbladder
Bile drains to duodenum

47539 new access, without placement of separate biliary drainage catheter

EXCLUDES   *Treatment same lesion same operative session ([43277], 47542, 47555-47556)*

Code also multiple stents placed during same session when: (47538-47540)
    Serial stents placed within same bile duct
    Stent placement via two or more percutaneous access sites or space between two other stents
    Two or more stents inserted through same percutaneous access

🔲 12.4   ⚖ 136.   **FUD** 000   [J] [62] [▭]

AMA: 2018,Jan,8; 2017,Jan,8; 2016,Mar,10

47540 new access, with placement of separate biliary drainage catheter (eg, external or internal-external)

EXCLUDES   *Procedures performed via same access (47533-47534)*
            Treatment same lesion same operative session ([43277], 47542, 47555-47556)

Code also multiple stents placed during same session when: (47538-47540)
    Serial stents placed within same bile duct
    Stent placement via two or more percutaneous access sites or space between two other stents
    Two or more stents inserted through same percutaneous access

🔲 12.8   ⚖ 137.   **FUD** 000   [J] [J8] [▭]

AMA: 2018,Jan,8; 2017,Jan,8; 2016,Mar,10

47541 Placement of access through the biliary tree and into small bowel to assist with an endoscopic biliary procedure (eg, rendezvous procedure), percutaneous, including diagnostic cholangiography when performed, imaging guidance (eg, ultrasound and/or fluoroscopy), and all associated radiological supervision and interpretation, new access

EXCLUDES   *Access through biliary tree into small bowel for endoscopic biliary procedure (47535-47537)*
            Conversion, exchange, or removal external biliary drainage catheter (47535-47537)
            Injection procedure for cholangiography (47531-47532)
            Placement biliary drainage catheter (47533-47534)
            Placement stent(s) into bile duct (47538-47540)
            Procedure performed when previous catheter access exists

🔲 9.64   ⚖ 33.8   **FUD** 000   [J] [62] [▭]

AMA: 2018,Jan,8; 2017,Jan,8

+ 47542 Balloon dilation of biliary duct(s) or of ampulla (sphincteroplasty), percutaneous, including imaging guidance (eg, fluoroscopy), and all associated radiological supervision and interpretation, each duct (List separately in addition to code for primary procedure)

EXCLUDES   *Biliary endoscopy, with dilation of biliary duct stricture (47555-47556)*
            Endoscopic balloon dilation ([43277], 47555-47556)
            Endoscopic retrograde cholangiopancreatography (ERCP) (43262, [43277])
            Placement stent(s) into a bile duct (47538-47540)
            Procedure performed with balloon to remove calculi, debris, sludge without dilation (47544)

Code also one additional dilation code when more than one dilation performed same session, using modifier 59 with (47542)

Code first (47531-47537, 47541)

🔲 3.94   ⚖ 13.9   **FUD** ZZZ   [N] [N1] [▭]

AMA: 2018,Jan,8; 2017,Jan,8

Digestive System

47543 — 47740

+ **47543** Endoluminal biopsy(ies) of biliary tree, percutaneous, any method(s) (eg, brush, forceps, and/or needle), including imaging guidance (eg, fluoroscopy), and all associated radiological supervision and interpretation, single or multiple (List separately in addition to code for primary procedure)

> EXCLUDES Endoscopic biopsy (46261, 47553)
> Endoscopic brushings (43260, 47552)
> Procedure performed more than one time per session
> Code first (47531-47540)

    🔧 4.20   ⚕ 13.3   **FUD** ZZZ   N N1 ▭

AMA: 2018,Jan,8; 2017,Jan,8

+ **47544** Removal of calculi/debris from biliary duct(s) and/or gallbladder, percutaneous, including destruction of calculi by any method (eg, mechanical, electrohydraulic, lithotripsy) when performed, imaging guidance (eg, fluoroscopy), and all associated radiological supervision and interpretation (List separately in addition to code for primary procedure)

> EXCLUDES Device deployment without finding calculi/debris
> Endoscopic calculi removal/destruction (43264-43265, 47554)
> Endoscopic retrograde cholangiopancreatography (ERCP); with removal calculi/debris from biliary/pancreatic duct(s) (43264)
> Procedures with removal incidental debris (47531-47543)
> Code first when debris removal not incidental, as appropriate (47531-47540)

    🔧 4.65   ⚕ 30.5   **FUD** ZZZ   N N1 ▭

AMA: 2018,Jan,8; 2017,Jan,8

47550-47556 Endoscopic Procedures of the Biliary Tract

INCLUDES Diagnostic endoscopy (49320)
EXCLUDES Endoscopic retrograde cholangiopancreatography (ERCP) (43260-43265, [43274], [43275], [43276], [43277], [43278], 74328-74330, 74363)

+ **47550** Biliary endoscopy, intraoperative (choledochoscopy) (List separately in addition to code for primary procedure)

> Code first primary procedure

    🔧 4.80   ⚕ 4.80   **FUD** ZZZ   C 80 ▭

AMA: 2014,Jan,11; 2013,Jan,11-12

47552 Biliary endoscopy, percutaneous via T-tube or other tract; diagnostic, with collection of specimen(s) by brushing and/or washing, when performed (separate procedure)

    🔧 9.01   ⚕ 9.01   **FUD** 000   J A2 ▭

AMA: 2018,Jan,8; 2017,Jan,8; 2016,Jan,13

47553 with biopsy, single or multiple

    🔧 8.91   ⚕ 8.91   **FUD** 000   J A2 ▭

AMA: 2018,Jan,8; 2017,Jan,8; 2016,Jan,13

47554 with removal of calculus/calculi

    🔧 14.9   ⚕ 14.9   **FUD** 000   J A2 ▭

AMA: 2018,Jan,8; 2017,Jan,8; 2016,Jan,13

47555 with dilation of biliary duct stricture(s) without stent

> 🔲 (74363)

    🔧 9.46   ⚕ 9.46   **FUD** 000   J A2 ▭

AMA: 2018,Jan,8; 2017,Jan,8; 2016,Jan,13

47556 with dilation of biliary duct stricture(s) with stent

> 🔲 (74363)

    🔧 10.7   ⚕ 10.7   **FUD** 000   J J8 ▭

AMA: 2018,Jan,8; 2017,Jan,8; 2016,Jan,13

47562-47579 Laparoscopic Gallbladder Procedures

INCLUDES Diagnostic laparoscopy (49320)

47562 Laparoscopy, surgical; cholecystectomy

    🔧 19.0   ⚕ 19.0   **FUD** 090   J 62 80 ▭

AMA: 2020,Aug,14; 2018,Jan,8; 2017,Jan,8; 2016,Jan,13

47563 cholecystectomy with cholangiography

> EXCLUDES Percutaneous cholangiography (47531-47532)
> Code also intraoperative radiology supervision and interpretation (74300-74301)

    🔧 20.7   ⚕ 20.7   **FUD** 090   J 62 80 ▭

AMA: 2019,Mar,10; 2018,Jan,8; 2017,Jan,8; 2016,Jan,13

47564 cholecystectomy with exploration of common duct

    🔧 32.2   ⚕ 32.2   **FUD** 090   J 62 80 ▭

AMA: 2018,Jan,8; 2017,Jan,8; 2016,Jan,13

47570 cholecystoenterostomy

    🔧 22.5   ⚕ 22.5   **FUD** 090   C 80 ▭

AMA: 2018,Jan,8; 2017,Jan,8; 2016,Jan,13

47579 Unlisted laparoscopy procedure, biliary tract

    🔧 0.00   ⚕ 0.00   **FUD** YYY   J 80 50 ▭

AMA: 2018,Jan,8; 2017,Jan,8; 2016,Jan,13

47600-47620 Open Gallbladder Procedures

47600 Cholecystectomy;

> EXCLUDES Laparoscopic method (47562-47564)

    🔧 30.9   ⚕ 30.9   **FUD** 090   C 80 ▭

AMA: 2018,Jan,8; 2017,Jan,8; 2016,Jan,13

47605 with cholangiography

> EXCLUDES Laparoscopic method (47563-47564)

    🔧 32.6   ⚕ 32.6   **FUD** 090   C 80 ▭

AMA: 2018,Jan,8; 2017,Jan,8; 2016,Jan,13

47610 Cholecystectomy with exploration of common duct;

> EXCLUDES Laparoscopic method (47564)
> Code also biliary endoscopy when performed in conjunction with cholecystectomy with exploration common duct (47550)

    🔧 36.3   ⚕ 36.3   **FUD** 090   C 80 ▭

AMA: 2018,Jan,8; 2017,Jan,8; 2016,Jan,13

47612 with choledochoenterostomy

    🔧 36.6   ⚕ 36.6   **FUD** 090   C 80 ▭

AMA: 2014,Jan,11; 2013,Jan,11-12

47620 with transduodenal sphincterotomy or sphincteroplasty, with or without cholangiography

    🔧 40.0   ⚕ 40.0   **FUD** 090   C 80 ▭

AMA: 2014,Jan,11; 2013,Jan,11-12

47700-47999 Open Resection and Repair of Biliary Tract

47700 Exploration for congenital atresia of bile ducts, without repair, with or without liver biopsy, with or without cholangiography

    🔧 30.6   ⚕ 30.6   **FUD** 090   63 C 80 ▭

AMA: 2014,Jan,11; 2013,Jan,11-12

47701 Portoenterostomy (eg, Kasai procedure)

    🔧 50.4   ⚕ 50.4   **FUD** 090   63 C 80 ▭

AMA: 2014,Jan,11; 2013,Jan,11-12

47711 Excision of bile duct tumor, with or without primary repair of bile duct; extrahepatic

> EXCLUDES Anastomosis (47760-47800)

    🔧 45.1   ⚕ 45.1   **FUD** 090   C 80 ▭

AMA: 2014,Jan,11; 2013,Jan,11-12

47712 intrahepatic

> EXCLUDES Anastomosis (47760-47800)

    🔧 58.1   ⚕ 58.1   **FUD** 090   C 80 ▭

AMA: 2014,Jan,11; 2013,Jan,11-12

47715 Excision of choledochal cyst

    🔧 38.6   ⚕ 38.6   **FUD** 090   C 80 ▭

AMA: 2018,Jan,8; 2017,Jan,8; 2016,Jan,13

47720 Cholecystoenterostomy; direct

> EXCLUDES Laparoscopic method (47570)

    🔧 33.4   ⚕ 33.4   **FUD** 090   C 80 ▭

AMA: 2018,Jan,8; 2017,Jan,8; 2016,Jan,13

47721 with gastroenterostomy

    🔧 39.3   ⚕ 39.3   **FUD** 090   C 80 ▭

AMA: 2014,Jan,11; 2013,Jan,11-12

47740 Roux-en-Y

    🔧 37.7   ⚕ 37.7   **FUD** 090   C 80 ▭

AMA: 2014,Jan,11; 2013,Jan,11-12

26/TC PC/TC Only   A2-Z3 ASC Payment   50 Bilateral   ♂ Male Only   ♀ Female Only   🔧 Facility RVU   ⚕ Non-Facility RVU   ▭ CCI   ✖ CLIA
FUD Follow-up Days   CMS: IOM   AMA: CPT Asst   A-Y OPPSI   80/80 Surg Assist Allowed / w/Doc   🔲 Lab Crosswalk   🔲 Radiology Crosswalk

220   CPT © 2021 American Medical Association. All Rights Reserved.   © 2021 Optum360, LLC

47741   **Roux-en-Y with gastroenterostomy**
     42.8   42.8   **FUD** 090   C 80 ▣
    AMA: 2014,Jan,11; 2013,Jan,11-12

47760   **Anastomosis, of extrahepatic biliary ducts and gastrointestinal tract**
     65.4   65.4   **FUD** 090   C 80 ▣
    AMA: 2014,Jan,11; 2013,Jan,11-12

47765   **Anastomosis, of intrahepatic ducts and gastrointestinal tract**
    INCLUDES   Longmire anastomosis
     87.9   87.9   **FUD** 090   C 80 ▣
    AMA: 2014,Jan,11; 2013,Jan,11-12

47780   **Anastomosis, Roux-en-Y, of extrahepatic biliary ducts and gastrointestinal tract**
     71.8   71.8   **FUD** 090   C 80 ▣
    AMA: 2014,Jan,11; 2013,Jan,11-12

47785   **Anastomosis, Roux-en-Y, of intrahepatic biliary ducts and gastrointestinal tract**
     94.4   94.4   **FUD** 090   C 80 ▣
    AMA: 2014,Jan,11; 2013,Jan,11-12

47800   **Reconstruction, plastic, of extrahepatic biliary ducts with end-to-end anastomosis**
     45.5   45.5   **FUD** 090   C 80 ▣
    AMA: 2014,Jan,11; 2013,Jan,11-12

47801   **Placement of choledochal stent**
     32.3   32.3   **FUD** 090   C 80 ▣
    AMA: 2018,Jan,8; 2017,Jan,8; 2016,Jan,13

47802   **U-tube hepaticoenterostomy**
     44.3   44.3   **FUD** 090   C 80 ▣
    AMA: 2014,Jan,11; 2013,Jan,11-12

47900   **Suture of extrahepatic biliary duct for pre-existing injury (separate procedure)**
     39.7   39.7   **FUD** 090   C 80 ▣
    AMA: 2014,Jan,11; 2013,Jan,11-12

47999   **Unlisted procedure, biliary tract**
     0.00   0.00   **FUD** YYY   T ▣
    AMA: 2018,Jan,8; 2017,Jan,8; 2016,Jan,13

48000-48548 Open Procedures of the Pancreas

EXCLUDES   *Peroral pancreatic procedures performed endoscopically (43260-43265, [43274], [43275], [43276], [43277], [43278])*

48000   **Placement of drains, peripancreatic, for acute pancreatitis;**
     54.7   54.7   **FUD** 090   C 80 ▣
    AMA: 2014,Jan,11; 2013,Jan,11-12

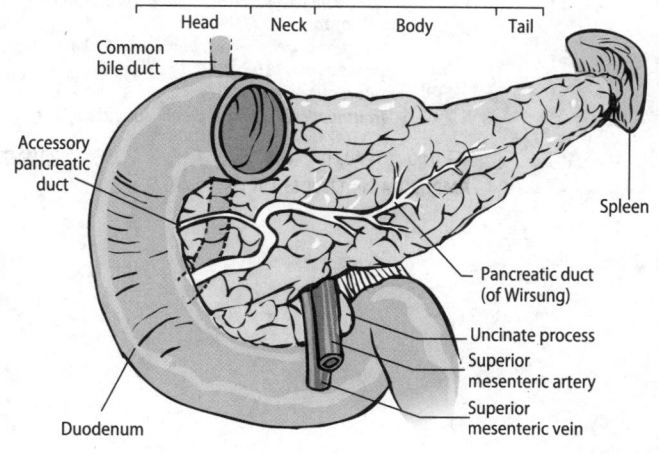

48001   **with cholecystostomy, gastrostomy, and jejunostomy**
     67.1   67.1   **FUD** 090   C 80 ▣
    AMA: 2014,Jan,11; 2013,Jan,11-12

48020   **Removal of pancreatic calculus**
     34.1   34.1   **FUD** 090   C 80 ▣
    AMA: 2014,Jan,11; 2013,Jan,11-12

48100   **Biopsy of pancreas, open (eg, fine needle aspiration, needle core biopsy, wedge biopsy)**
     25.8   25.8   **FUD** 090   C 80 ▣
    AMA: 2014,Jan,11; 2013,Jan,11-12

Pancreas tissue may be defined by placing surgical staples

Example of wedge biopsy

Pancreas tissue is collected in an open surgical session for biopsy purposes

Biopsy needle for fine needle aspiration or percutaneous removal

48102   **Biopsy of pancreas, percutaneous needle**
    EXCLUDES   *Fine needle aspiration ([10005, 10006, 10007, 10008, 10009, 10010, 10011, 10012])*
     (76942, 77002, 77012, 77021)
     (88172-88173)
     6.97   15.1   **FUD** 010   J A2 ▣
    AMA: 2019,Apr,4

48105   **Resection or debridement of pancreas and peripancreatic tissue for acute necrotizing pancreatitis**
     82.4   82.4   **FUD** 090   C 80 ▣
    AMA: 2014,Jan,11; 2013,Jan,11-12

48120   **Excision of lesion of pancreas (eg, cyst, adenoma)**
     32.0   32.0   **FUD** 090   C 80 ▣
    AMA: 2014,Jan,11; 2013,Jan,11-12

48140   **Pancreatectomy, distal subtotal, with or without splenectomy; without pancreaticojejunostomy**
     45.4   45.4   **FUD** 090   C 80 ▣
    AMA: 2018,Jan,8; 2017,Jul,10

48145   **with pancreaticojejunostomy**
     47.4   47.4   **FUD** 090   C 80 ▣
    AMA: 2014,Jan,11; 2013,Jan,11-12

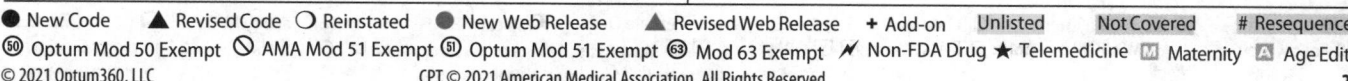

48146 — 48551

Digestive System

48146 **Pancreatectomy, distal, near-total with preservation of duodenum (Child-type procedure)**
🔲 54.5   ⚕ 54.5   **FUD** 090   C 80 🔲
AMA: 2014,Jan,11; 2013,Jan,11-12

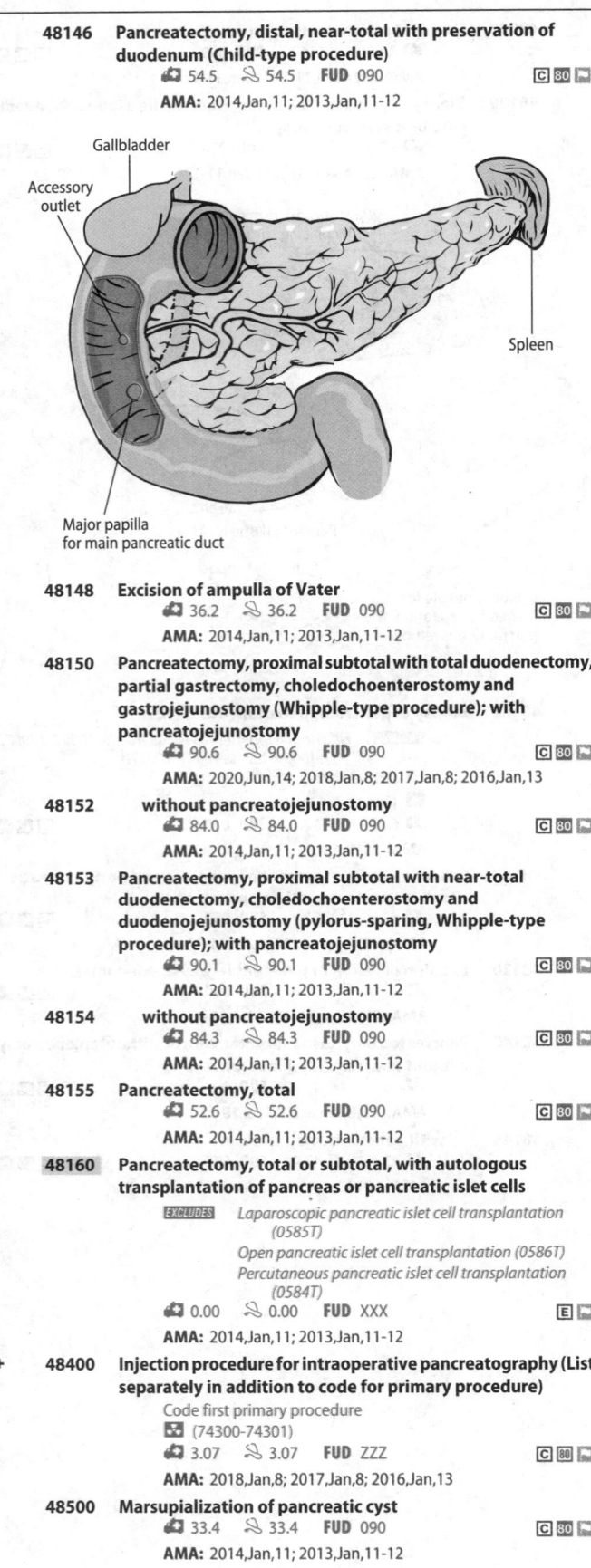

Gallbladder

Accessory outlet

Spleen

Major papilla for main pancreatic duct

48148 **Excision of ampulla of Vater**
🔲 36.2   ⚕ 36.2   **FUD** 090   C 80 🔲
AMA: 2014,Jan,11; 2013,Jan,11-12

48150 **Pancreatectomy, proximal subtotal with total duodenectomy, partial gastrectomy, choledochoenterostomy and gastrojejunostomy (Whipple-type procedure); with pancreatojejunostomy**
🔲 90.6   ⚕ 90.6   **FUD** 090   C 80 🔲
AMA: 2020,Jun,14; 2018,Jan,8; 2017,Jan,8; 2016,Jan,13

48152 **without pancreatojejunostomy**
🔲 84.0   ⚕ 84.0   **FUD** 090   C 80 🔲
AMA: 2014,Jan,11; 2013,Jan,11-12

48153 **Pancreatectomy, proximal subtotal with near-total duodenectomy, choledochoenterostomy and duodenojejunostomy (pylorus-sparing, Whipple-type procedure); with pancreatojejunostomy**
🔲 90.1   ⚕ 90.1   **FUD** 090   C 80 🔲
AMA: 2014,Jan,11; 2013,Jan,11-12

48154 **without pancreatojejunostomy**
🔲 84.3   ⚕ 84.3   **FUD** 090   C 80 🔲
AMA: 2014,Jan,11; 2013,Jan,11-12

48155 **Pancreatectomy, total**
🔲 52.6   ⚕ 52.6   **FUD** 090   C 80 🔲
AMA: 2014,Jan,11; 2013,Jan,11-12

48160 **Pancreatectomy, total or subtotal, with autologous transplantation of pancreas or pancreatic islet cells**
    EXCLUDES   *Laparoscopic pancreatic islet cell transplantation (0585T)*
           Open pancreatic islet cell transplantation (0586T)
           Percutaneous pancreatic islet cell transplantation (0584T)
🔲 0.00   ⚕ 0.00   **FUD** XXX   E 🔲
AMA: 2014,Jan,11; 2013,Jan,11-12

+ 48400 **Injection procedure for intraoperative pancreatography (List separately in addition to code for primary procedure)**
    Code first primary procedure
    🔲 (74300-74301)
🔲 3.07   ⚕ 3.07   **FUD** ZZZ   C 80 🔲
AMA: 2018,Jan,8; 2017,Jan,8; 2016,Jan,13

48500 **Marsupialization of pancreatic cyst**
🔲 33.4   ⚕ 33.4   **FUD** 090   C 80 🔲
AMA: 2014,Jan,11; 2013,Jan,11-12

48510 **External drainage, pseudocyst of pancreas, open**
    EXCLUDES   *Image guided percutaneous catheter drainage (49405)*
🔲 31.7   ⚕ 31.7   **FUD** 090   C 80 🔲
AMA: 2014,Jan,11; 2013,Nov,9

48520 **Internal anastomosis of pancreatic cyst to gastrointestinal tract; direct**
🔲 31.5   ⚕ 31.5   **FUD** 090   C 80 🔲
AMA: 2014,Jan,11; 2013,Jan,11-12

48540 **Roux-en-Y**
🔲 37.8   ⚕ 37.8   **FUD** 090   C 80 🔲
AMA: 2014,Jan,11; 2013,Jan,11-12

48545 **Pancreatorrhaphy for injury**
🔲 38.9   ⚕ 38.9   **FUD** 090   C 80 🔲
AMA: 2014,Jan,11; 2013,Jan,11-12

48547 **Duodenal exclusion with gastrojejunostomy for pancreatic injury**
🔲 52.1   ⚕ 52.1   **FUD** 090   C 80 🔲
AMA: 2014,Jan,11; 2013,Jan,11-12

48548 **Pancreaticojejunostomy, side-to-side anastomosis (Puestow-type operation)**
🔲 48.2   ⚕ 48.2   **FUD** 090   C 80 🔲
AMA: 2014,Jan,11; 2013,Jan,11-12

48550-48999 Pancreas Transplant Procedures

CMS: 100-03,260.3 Pancreas Transplants; 100-04,3,90.5 Pancreas Transplants with Kidney Transplants; 100-04,3,90.5.1 Pancreas Transplants Alone

48550 **Donor pancreatectomy (including cold preservation), with or without duodenal segment for transplantation**
    INCLUDES   Graft:
           Cold preservation
           Harvest (with or without duodenal segment)
🔲 0.00   ⚕ 0.00   **FUD** XXX   E 🔲
AMA: 2018,Jan,8; 2017,Jan,8; 2016,Jan,13

48551 **Backbench standard preparation of cadaver donor pancreas allograft prior to transplantation, including dissection of allograft from surrounding soft tissues, splenectomy, duodenotomy, ligation of bile duct, ligation of mesenteric vessels, and Y-graft arterial anastomoses from iliac artery to superior mesenteric artery and to splenic artery**
    EXCLUDES   *Biopsy pancreas (48100-48102)*
           Bypass graft, with vein (35531, 35563)
           Duodenotomy (44010)
           Endoscopic procedures biliary tract (47550-47556)
           Excision lesion mesentery (44820)
           Excision lesion pancreas (48120)
           Pancreatorrhaphy for injury (48545)
           Placement vein patch or cuff at distal anastomosis bypass graft (35685)
           Resection or debridement pancreas (48105)
           Splenectomy (38100-38102)
           Suture mesentery (44850)
           Transduodenal sphincterotomy, sphincteroplasty (47460)
🔲 0.00   ⚕ 0.00   **FUD** XXX   C 80 🔲
AMA: 2014,Jan,11; 2013,Jan,11-12

26/TC PC/TC Only   A2-Z3 ASC Payment   50 Bilateral   ♂ Male Only   ♀ Female Only   🔲 Facility RVU   ⚕ Non-Facility RVU   🔲 CCI   ❌ CLIA
FUD Follow-up Days   **CMS:** IOM   **AMA:** CPT Asst   A-Y OPPSI   80/80 Surg Assist Allowed / w/Doc   🔲 Lab Crosswalk   🔲 Radiology Crosswalk

222   CPT © 2021 American Medical Association. All Rights Reserved.   © 2021 Optum360, LLC

48552 Backbench reconstruction of cadaver donor pancreas allograft prior to transplantation, venous anastomosis, each

EXCLUDES
Biopsy pancreas (48100-48102)
Bypass graft, with vein (35531, 35563)
Duodenotomy (44010)
Endoscopic procedures biliary tract (47550-47556)
Excision lesion mesentery (44820)
Excision lesion pancreas (48120)
Pancreatorrhaphy for injury (48545)
Placement vein patch or cuff at distal anastomosis bypass graft (35685)
Resection or debridement pancreas (48105)
Splenectomy (38100-38102)
Suture mesentery (44850)
Transduodenal sphincterotomy, sphincteroplasty (47460)

6.87   6.87   **FUD** XXX   C 80

AMA: 2014,Jan,11; 2013,Jan,11-12

48554 Transplantation of pancreatic allograft

INCLUDES
Allograft transplant
Recipient care

74.4   74.4   **FUD** 090   C 80

AMA: 2014,Jan,11; 2013,Jan,11-12

48556 Removal of transplanted pancreatic allograft

37.1   37.1   **FUD** 090   C 80

AMA: 2014,Jan,11; 2013,Jan,11-12

48999 Unlisted procedure, pancreas

0.00   0.00   **FUD** YYY   T 80

AMA: 2018,Jan,8; 2017,Jan,8; 2016,Jan,13

49000-49084 Exploratory and Drainage Procedures: Abdomen/Peritoneum

49000 Exploratory laparotomy, exploratory celiotomy with or without biopsy(s) (separate procedure)

EXCLUDES
Exploration penetrating wound without laparotomy (20102)

22.3   22.3   **FUD** 090   C 80

AMA: 2020,Jan,6; 2019,Dec,5; 2018,Jan,8; 2017,Dec,3; 2017,Jan,8; 2016,Jan,13

49002 Reopening of recent laparotomy

EXCLUDES
Hepatic wound re-exploration for packing removal (47362)
Pelvic wound re-exploration for packing removal/repacking (49014)

30.4   30.4   **FUD** 090   C 80

AMA: 2020,Jan,6; 2018,Jan,8; 2017,Jan,8; 2016,Jan,13

49010 Exploration, retroperitoneal area with or without biopsy(s) (separate procedure)

EXCLUDES
Exploration penetrating wound without laparotomy (20102)

26.8   26.8   **FUD** 090   C 80

AMA: 2020,Jan,6; 2019,Dec,5

49013 Preperitoneal pelvic packing for hemorrhage associated with pelvic trauma, including local exploration

12.7   12.7   **FUD** 000

AMA: 2020,Jan,6

49014 Re-exploration of pelvic wound with removal of preperitoneal pelvic packing, including repacking, when performed

10.5   10.5   **FUD** 000

AMA: 2020,Jan,6

49020 Drainage of peritoneal abscess or localized peritonitis, exclusive of appendiceal abscess, open

EXCLUDES
Appendiceal abscess (44900)
Image-guided percutaneous catheter drainage abscess/peritonitis via catheter (49406)
Image-guided transrectal/transvaginal drainage peritoneal abscess via catheter (49407)

46.3   46.3   **FUD** 090   C 80

AMA: 2014,Jan,11; 2013,Nov,9

49040 Drainage of subdiaphragmatic or subphrenic abscess, open

EXCLUDES
Image-guided percutaneous drainage subdiaphragmatic/subphrenic abscess via catheter (49406)

29.1   29.1   **FUD** 090   C 80

AMA: 2014,Jan,11; 2013,Nov,9

49060 Drainage of retroperitoneal abscess, open

EXCLUDES
Image-guided percutaneous drainage retroperitoneal abscess via catheter (49406)
Transrectal/transvaginal image-guided drainage retroperitoneal abscess via catheter (49407)

32.0   32.0   **FUD** 090   C

AMA: 2018,Jan,8; 2017,Jan,8; 2016,Jan,13

49062 Drainage of extraperitoneal lymphocele to peritoneal cavity, open

EXCLUDES
Drainage lymphocele to peritoneal cavity, laparoscopic (49323)
Image-guided percutaneous drainage retroperitoneal lymphocele via catheter (49406)

21.3   21.3   **FUD** 090   C 80

AMA: 2018,Jan,8; 2017,Jan,8; 2016,Jan,13

49082 Abdominal paracentesis (diagnostic or therapeutic); without imaging guidance

2.12   5.67   **FUD** 000   T 62

AMA: 2018,Jan,8; 2017,Jan,8; 2016,Jan,13

49083 with imaging guidance

INCLUDES
Radiological guidance (76942, 77002, 77012, 77021)

EXCLUDES
Image-guided percutaneous drainage retroperitoneal abscess via catheter (49406)

3.11   8.44   **FUD** 000   T 62

AMA: 2018,Jan,8; 2017,Jan,8; 2016,Jan,13

49084 Peritoneal lavage, including imaging guidance, when performed

INCLUDES
Radiological guidance (76942, 77002, 77012, 77021)

EXCLUDES
Image-guided percutaneous drainage retroperitoneal abscess via catheter (49406)

3.16   3.16   **FUD** 000   T 62

AMA: 2018,Jan,8; 2017,Jan,8; 2016,Jan,13

49180 Biopsy of Mass: Abdomen/Retroperitoneum

EXCLUDES
Fine needle aspiration (10021, [10004, 10005, 10006, 10007, 10008, 10009, 10010, 10011, 10012])
Lysis intestinal adhesions (44005)

49180 Biopsy, abdominal or retroperitoneal mass, percutaneous needle

(76942, 77002, 77012, 77021)
(88172-88173)

2.43   4.86   **FUD** 000   J A2

AMA: 2019,Feb,8; 2019,Apr,4; 2018,Jan,8; 2017,Jan,8; 2016,Jan,13

Digestive System

49185 — 49329

49185 Sclerotherapy of a Fluid Collection

49185 Sclerotherapy of a fluid collection (eg, lymphocele, cyst, or seroma), percutaneous, including contrast injection(s), sclerosant injection(s), diagnostic study, imaging guidance (eg, ultrasound, fluoroscopy) and radiological supervision and interpretation when performed

INCLUDES   Multiple lesions treated via same access

EXCLUDES   *Contrast injection for assessment abscess or cyst (49424)*
Pleurodesis (32560)
Radiologic examination, abscess, fistula or sinus tract stud (76080)
Sclerosis veins/endovenous ablation incompetent veins extremity (36468, 36470-36471, 36475-36476, 36478-36479)
Sclerotherapy lymphatic/vascular malformation (37241)

Code also:
Access or drainage via needle or catheter (10030, 10160, 49405-49407, 50390)
Existing catheter exchange pre- or post-sclerosant injection (49423, 75984)
Modifier 59 for treatment multiple lesions same session via separate access

🖥 3.47   ⚕ 33.4   **FUD** 000   T 62 ▭

AMA: 2018,Jan,8; 2017,Jan,8; 2016,Mar,10

49203-49205 Open Destruction or Excision: Abdominal Tumors

EXCLUDES   *Ablation, open, one or more renal mass lesion(s), cryosurgical*
Biopsy kidney or ovary (50205, 58900)
Cryoablation renal tumor (50250, 50593)
Excision perinephric cyst (50290)
Excision presacral or sacrococcygeal tumor (49215)
Exploration, renal or retroperitoneal area (49010, 50010)
Exploratory laparotomy (49000)
Laparotomy, for staging or restaging ovarian, tubal, or primary peritoneal malignancy (58960)
Nephrectomy (50225, 50236)
Oophorectomy (58940-58958)
Ovarian cystectomy (58925)
Pelvic or retroperitoneal lymphadenectomy (38770, 38780)
Primary, recurrent ovarian, uterine, or tubal resection (58957-58958)
Wedge resection or bisection ovary (58920)

Code also:
Colectomy (44140)
Nephrectomy (50220, 50240)
Small bowel resection (44120)
Vena caval resection with reconstruction (37799)

49203 Excision or destruction, open, intra-abdominal tumors, cysts or endometriomas, 1 or more peritoneal, mesenteric, or retroperitoneal primary or secondary tumors; largest tumor 5 cm diameter or less

🖥 34.7   ⚕ 34.7   **FUD** 090   C 80 ▭

AMA: 2018,Jan,8; 2017,Jan,8; 2016,Jan,13

49204 largest tumor 5.1-10.0 cm diameter

🖥 44.2   ⚕ 44.2   **FUD** 090   C 80 ▭

AMA: 2018,Jan,8; 2017,Jan,8; 2016,Jan,13

49205 largest tumor greater than 10.0 cm diameter

🖥 50.6   ⚕ 50.6   **FUD** 090   C 80 ▭

AMA: 2018,Jan,8; 2017,Jan,8; 2016,Jan,13

49215 Resection Presacral/Sacrococcygeal Tumor

49215 Excision of presacral or sacrococcygeal tumor

🖥 64.2   ⚕ 64.2   **FUD** 090   63 C 80 ▭

AMA: 2014,Jan,11; 2013,Jan,11-12

49250-49255 Other Open Abdominal Procedures

EXCLUDES   *Lysis intestinal adhesions (44005)*

49250 Umbilectomy, omphalectomy, excision of umbilicus (separate procedure)

🖥 17.0   ⚕ 17.0   **FUD** 090   J A2 ▭

AMA: 2014,Jan,11; 2013,Jan,11-12

49255 Omentectomy, epiploectomy, resection of omentum (separate procedure)

🖥 22.8   ⚕ 22.8   **FUD** 090   C 80 ▭

AMA: 2018,Mar,11; 2018,Jan,8; 2017,Jan,8; 2016,Jan,13

49320-49329 Laparoscopic Procedures of the Abdomen/Peritoneum/Omentum

INCLUDES   Diagnostic laparoscopy (49320)

EXCLUDES   *Fulguration/excision lesions ovary/pelvic viscera/peritoneal surface, performed laparoscopically (58662)*

49320 Laparoscopy, abdomen, peritoneum, and omentum, diagnostic, with or without collection of specimen(s) by brushing or washing (separate procedure)

🖥 9.54   ⚕ 9.54   **FUD** 010   J A2 80 ▭

AMA: 2018,Jan,8; 2017,Apr,7; 2017,Jan,8; 2016,Jan,13

49321 Laparoscopy, surgical; with biopsy (single or multiple)

🖥 10.0   ⚕ 10.0   **FUD** 010   J A2 80 ▭

AMA: 2018,Aug,10; 2018,Jan,8; 2017,Jan,8; 2016,Jan,13

49322 with aspiration of cavity or cyst (eg, ovarian cyst) (single or multiple)

🖥 10.8   ⚕ 10.8   **FUD** 010   J A2 80 ▭

AMA: 2018,Jan,8; 2017,Jan,8; 2016,Jan,13

49323 with drainage of lymphocele to peritoneal cavity

EXCLUDES   *Open drainage lymphocele to peritoneal cavity (49062)*

🖥 18.3   ⚕ 18.3   **FUD** 090   J 62 80 ▭

AMA: 2018,Jan,8; 2017,Jan,8; 2016,Jan,13

49324 with insertion of tunneled intraperitoneal catheter

EXCLUDES   *Open approach (49421)*

Code also insertion subcutaneous extension to intraperitoneal cannula with remote chest exit site, when appropriate (49435)

🖥 11.3   ⚕ 11.3   **FUD** 010   J 62 80 ▭

AMA: 2014,Jan,11; 2013,Jan,11-12

49325 with revision of previously placed intraperitoneal cannula or catheter, with removal of intraluminal obstructive material if performed

🖥 12.1   ⚕ 12.1   **FUD** 010   J 62 80 ▭

AMA: 2014,Jan,11; 2013,Jan,11-12

+ **49326** with omentopexy (omental tacking procedure) (List separately in addition to code for primary procedure)

Code first laparoscopy with permanent intraperitoneal cannula or catheter insertion or revision previously placed catheter/cannula (49324, 49325)

🖥 5.52   ⚕ 5.52   **FUD** ZZZ   N N1 80 ▭

AMA: 2014,Jan,11; 2013,Jan,11-12

+ **49327** with placement of interstitial device(s) for radiation therapy guidance (eg, fiducial markers, dosimeter), intra-abdominal, intrapelvic, and/or retroperitoneum, including imaging guidance, if performed, single or multiple (List separately in addition to code for primary procedure)

EXCLUDES   *Open approach (49412)*
Percutaneous approach (49411)

Code first laparoscopic abdominal, pelvic or retroperitoneal procedures

🖥 3.81   ⚕ 3.81   **FUD** ZZZ   N N1 80 ▭

AMA: 2014,Jan,11; 2013,Jan,11-12

49329 Unlisted laparoscopy procedure, abdomen, peritoneum and omentum

🖥 0.00   ⚕ 0.00   **FUD** YYY   J 80 50 ▭

AMA: 2020,Feb,13; 2019,Mar,10; 2018,Jan,8; 2017,Jan,8; 2016,Jan,13

26/TC PC/TC Only   A2-Z3 ASC Payment   50 Bilateral   ♂ Male Only   ♀ Female Only   🖥 Facility RVU   ⚕ Non-Facility RVU   ▭ CCI   ☒ CLIA
FUD Follow-up Days   CMS: IOM   AMA: CPT Asst   A-Y OPPSI   80/80 Surg Assist Allowed / w/Doc   ◼ Lab Crosswalk   ☒ Radiology Crosswalk

224   CPT © 2021 American Medical Association. All Rights Reserved.   © 2021 Optum360, LLC

49400-49436 Peritoneal and Visceral Procedures: Drainage/Insertion/Modifications/Removal

49400 Injection of air or contrast into peritoneal cavity (separate procedure)
(74190)
2.68 3.93 **FUD** 000 N N1
AMA: 2018,Jan,8; 2017,Jan,8; 2016,Jan,13

49402 Removal of peritoneal foreign body from peritoneal cavity
EXCLUDES Enterolysis (44005)
Percutaneous or open drainage or lavage (49020, 49040, 49082-49084, 49406)
Percutaneous tunneled intraperitoneal catheter insertion without subcutaneous port (49418)
24.9 24.9 **FUD** 090 J A2
AMA: 2014,Jan,11; 2013,Jan,11-12

49405 Image-guided fluid collection drainage by catheter (eg, abscess, hematoma, seroma, lymphocele, cyst); visceral (eg, kidney, liver, spleen, lung/mediastinum), percutaneous
INCLUDES Radiological guidance (75989, 76942, 77002-77003, 77012, 77021)
EXCLUDES Open drainage (47010, 48510, 50020)
Percutaneous cholecystostomy (47490)
Percutaneous pleural drainage (32556-32557)
Pneumonostomy (32200)
Thoracentesis (32554-32555)
Code also each individual collection drained per separate catheter
5.71 25.1 **FUD** 000 J G2
AMA: 2020,Feb,13; 2018,Jan,8; 2017,Jan,8; 2016,Jan,13

49406 peritoneal or retroperitoneal, percutaneous
INCLUDES Radiological guidance (75989, 76942, 77002-77003, 77012, 77021)
EXCLUDES Diagnostic or therapeutic percutaneous abdominal paracentesis (49082-49083)
Open peritoneal/retroperitoneal drainage (44900, 49020-49062, 49084, 50020, 58805, 58822)
Open transrectal drainage pelvic abscess (45000)
Percutaneous tunneled intraperitoneal catheter insertion without subcutaneous port (49418)
Transrectal/transvaginal image-guided peritoneal/retroperitoneal drainage via catheter (49407)
Code also each individual collection drained per separate catheter
5.70 25.1 **FUD** 000 J G2
AMA: 2020,Feb,13; 2018,Jan,8; 2017,Jan,8; 2016,Jan,13

49407 peritoneal or retroperitoneal, transvaginal or transrectal
INCLUDES Radiological guidance (75989, 76942, 77002-77003, 77012, 77021)
EXCLUDES Image-guided percutaneous catheter drainage soft tissue (eg, abdominal wall, neck, extremity) (10030)
Open transrectal/transvaginal drainage (45000, 58800, 58820)
Percutaneous pleural drainage (32556-32557)
Peritoneal drainage or lavage, open or percutaneous (49020, 49040, 49060)
Thoracentesis (32554-32555)
Code also each individual collection drained per separate catheter
6.05 20.6 **FUD** 000 J G2
AMA: 2018,Jan,8; 2017,Jan,8; 2016,Jan,13

49411 Placement of interstitial device(s) for radiation therapy guidance (eg, fiducial markers, dosimeter), percutaneous, intra-abdominal, intra-pelvic (except prostate), and/or retroperitoneum, single or multiple
EXCLUDES Placement (percutaneous) interstitial device(s) for intrathoracic radiation therapy guidance (32553)
Code also supply device
(76942, 77002, 77012, 77021)
5.33 13.9 **FUD** 000 S P3 80
AMA: 2018,Jan,8; 2017,Jan,8; 2016,Jun,3; 2016,Jan,13

+ 49412 Placement of interstitial device(s) for radiation therapy guidance (eg, fiducial markers, dosimeter), open, intra-abdominal, intrapelvic, and/or retroperitoneum, including image guidance, if performed, single or multiple (List separately in addition to code for primary procedure)
EXCLUDES Laparoscopic approach (49327)
Percutaneous approach (49411)
Code first open abdominal, pelvic or retroperitoneal procedure(s)
2.41 2.41 **FUD** ZZZ C 80
AMA: 2014,Jan,11; 2013,Jan,11-12

49418 Insertion of tunneled intraperitoneal catheter (eg, dialysis, intraperitoneal chemotherapy instillation, management of ascites), complete procedure, including imaging guidance, catheter placement, contrast injection when performed, and radiological supervision and interpretation, percutaneous
5.88 34.1 **FUD** 000 J G2 80
AMA: 2014,Jan,11; 2013,Nov,9

49419 Insertion of tunneled intraperitoneal catheter, with subcutaneous port (ie, totally implantable)
EXCLUDES Removal catheter/cannula (49422)
12.5 12.5 **FUD** 090 T A2
AMA: 2014,Jan,11; 2013,Jan,11-12

49421 Insertion of tunneled intraperitoneal catheter for dialysis, open
EXCLUDES Laparoscopic approach (49324)
Code also insertion subcutaneous extension to intraperitoneal cannula with remote chest exit site, when appropriate (49435)
6.65 6.65 **FUD** 000 J G2
AMA: 2018,Jan,8; 2017,Jan,8; 2016,Jan,13

49422 Removal of tunneled intraperitoneal catheter
EXCLUDES Removal temporary catheter or cannula (Report appropriate E/M code)
6.46 6.46 **FUD** 000 02 A2
AMA: 2014,Jan,11; 2013,Jan,11-12

49423 Exchange of previously placed abscess or cyst drainage catheter under radiological guidance (separate procedure)
(75984)
2.05 16.9 **FUD** 000 J G2 80
AMA: 2018,Jan,8; 2017,Jan,8; 2016,Jan,13

49424 Contrast injection for assessment of abscess or cyst via previously placed drainage catheter or tube (separate procedure)
(76080)
1.10 4.35 **FUD** 000 N N1 80
AMA: 2018,Jan,8; 2017,Jan,8; 2016,Jan,13

49425 Insertion of peritoneal-venous shunt
20.7 20.7 **FUD** 090 C 80
AMA: 2014,Jan,11; 2013,Jan,11-12

49426 Revision of peritoneal-venous shunt
EXCLUDES Shunt patency test (78291)
19.4 19.4 **FUD** 090 J A2
AMA: 2014,Jan,11; 2013,Jan,11-12

49427 Injection procedure (eg, contrast media) for evaluation of previously placed peritoneal-venous shunt
(75809, 78291)
1.13 1.13 **FUD** 000 N N1 80
AMA: 2014,Jan,11; 2013,Jan,11-12

49428   **Ligation of peritoneal-venous shunt**
📋 12.5   ⚖ 12.5   **FUD** 010   C 🔲
AMA: 2014,Jan,11; 2013,Jan,11-12

49429   **Removal of peritoneal-venous shunt**
📋 13.3   ⚖ 13.3   **FUD** 010   02 G2 🔲
AMA: 2014,Jan,11; 2013,Jan,11-12

+   **49435**   **Insertion of subcutaneous extension to intraperitoneal cannula or catheter with remote chest exit site (List separately in addition to code for primary procedure)**
Code first permanent insertion intraperitoneal catheter/cannula (49324, 49421)
📋 3.50   ⚖ 3.50   **FUD** ZZZ   N N1 80 🔲
AMA: 2014,Jan,11; 2013,Jan,11-12

49436   **Delayed creation of exit site from embedded subcutaneous segment of intraperitoneal cannula or catheter**
📋 5.42   ⚖ 5.42   **FUD** 010   J G2 80 🔲
AMA: 2014,Jan,11; 2013,Jan,11-12

49440-49442 Insertion of Percutaneous Gastrointestinal Tube

EXCLUDES   *Naso- or oro-gastric tube placement (43752)*

49440   **Insertion of gastrostomy tube, percutaneous, under fluoroscopic guidance including contrast injection(s), image documentation and report**
INCLUDES   Needle placement with fluoroscopic guidance (77002)
Code also gastrostomy to gastro-jejunostomy tube conversion with initial gastrostomy tube insertion, when performed (49446)
📋 5.93   ⚖ 26.6   **FUD** 010   J G2 80 🔲
AMA: 2018,Jan,8; 2017,Jan,8; 2016,Jan,13

49441   **Insertion of duodenostomy or jejunostomy tube, percutaneous, under fluoroscopic guidance including contrast injection(s), image documentation and report**
EXCLUDES   *Gastrostomy tube to gastrojejunostomy tube conversion (49446)*
📋 7.00   ⚖ 30.6   **FUD** 010   J G2 80 🔲
AMA: 2018,Jan,8; 2017,Jan,8; 2016,Jan,13

49442   **Insertion of cecostomy or other colonic tube, percutaneous, under fluoroscopic guidance including contrast injection(s), image documentation and report**
📋 6.00   ⚖ 25.2   **FUD** 010   T G2 80 🔲
AMA: 2018,Jan,8; 2017,Jan,8; 2016,Jan,13

49446 Percutaneous Conversion: Gastrostomy to Gastro-jejunostomy Tube

EXCLUDES   *Code also initial gastrostomy tube insertion (49440) when conversion performed same time*

49446   **Conversion of gastrostomy tube to gastro-jejunostomy tube, percutaneous, under fluoroscopic guidance including contrast injection(s), image documentation and report**
📋 4.30   ⚖ 25.6   **FUD** 000   J G2 80 🔲
AMA: 2018,Jan,8; 2017,Jan,8; 2016,Jan,13

49450-49452 Replacement Gastrointestinal Tube

EXCLUDES   *Placement new tube whether gastrostomy, jejunostomy, duodenostomy, gastro-jejunostomy, or cecostomy different percutaneous site (49440-49442)*

49450   **Replacement of gastrostomy or cecostomy (or other colonic) tube, percutaneous, under fluoroscopic guidance including contrast injection(s), image documentation and report**
EXCLUDES   *Change gastrostomy tube, percutaneous, without imaging or endoscopic guidance (43762-43763)*
📋 1.91   ⚖ 18.7   **FUD** 000   T G2 80 🔲
AMA: 2019,Feb,5; 2018,Jan,8; 2017,Jan,8; 2016,Jan,13

49451   **Replacement of duodenostomy or jejunostomy tube, percutaneous, under fluoroscopic guidance including contrast injection(s), image documentation and report**
📋 2.61   ⚖ 20.3   **FUD** 000   T G2 80 🔲
AMA: 2018,Jan,8; 2017,Jan,8; 2016,Jan,13

49452   **Replacement of gastro-jejunostomy tube, percutaneous, under fluoroscopic guidance including contrast injection(s), image documentation and report**
📋 4.01   ⚖ 25.1   **FUD** 000   T G2 80 🔲
AMA: 2018,Jan,8; 2017,Jan,8; 2016,Jan,13

49460-49465 Removal of Obstruction/Injection for Contrast Through Gastrointestinal Tube

49460   **Mechanical removal of obstructive material from gastrostomy, duodenostomy, jejunostomy, gastro-jejunostomy, or cecostomy (or other colonic) tube, any method, under fluoroscopic guidance including contrast injection(s), if performed, image documentation and report**
INCLUDES   Contrast injection (49465)
EXCLUDES   *Replacement gastrointestinal tube (49450-49452)*
📋 1.39   ⚖ 20.4   **FUD** 000   T G2 80 🔲
AMA: 2018,Jan,8; 2017,Jan,8; 2016,Jan,13

49465   **Contrast injection(s) for radiological evaluation of existing gastrostomy, duodenostomy, jejunostomy, gastro-jejunostomy, or cecostomy (or other colonic) tube, from a percutaneous approach including image documentation and report**
EXCLUDES   *Mechanical removal obstructive material from gastrointestinal tube (49460)*
Replacement gastrointestinal tube (49450-49452)
📋 0.89   ⚖ 4.48   **FUD** 000   01 G2 80 🔲
AMA: 2018,Jan,8; 2017,Jan,8; 2016,Jan,13

49491-49492 Inguinal Hernia Repair on Premature Infant

INCLUDES   Hernia repairs done on preterm infants younger than or equal to 50 weeks postconception age and younger than 6 months
Initial repair: no previous repair required
Mesh or other prosthesis
EXCLUDES   *Abdominal wall debridement (11042, 11043)*
Intra-abdominal hernia repair/reduction (44050)
Code also repair or excision testicle(s), intestine, ovaries, when performed (44120, 54520, 58940)

49491   **Repair, initial inguinal hernia, preterm infant (younger than 37 weeks gestation at birth), performed from birth up to 50 weeks postconception age, with or without hydrocelectomy; reducible**   A
📋 23.2   ⚖ 23.2   **FUD** 090   63 J G2 80 50 🔲
AMA: 2018,Jan,8; 2017,Jan,8; 2016,Jan,13

49492   **incarcerated or strangulated**   A
📋 27.9   ⚖ 27.9   **FUD** 090   63 J G2 80 50 🔲
AMA: 2018,Jan,8; 2017,Jan,8; 2016,Jan,13

49495-49557 Hernia Repair: Femoral/Inguinal /Lumbar

INCLUDES   Initial repair: no previous repair required
Mesh or other prosthesis
Recurrent repair: required previous repair(s)
EXCLUDES   *Abdominal wall debridement (11042, 11043)*
Intra-abdominal hernia repair/reduction (44050)
Code also repair or excision testicle(s), intestine, ovaries, when performed (44120, 54520, 58940)

49495   **Repair, initial inguinal hernia, full term infant younger than age 6 months, or preterm infant older than 50 weeks postconception age and younger than age 6 months at the time of surgery, with or without hydrocelectomy; reducible**   A
INCLUDES   Hernia repairs done on preterm infants older than 50 weeks postconception age and younger than 6 months
📋 11.8   ⚖ 11.8   **FUD** 090   63 J A2 80 50 🔲
AMA: 2018,Jan,8; 2017,Jan,8; 2016,Jan,13

49496   **incarcerated or strangulated**   A
INCLUDES   Hernia repairs done on preterm infants older than 50 weeks postconception age and younger than 6 months
📋 17.7   ⚖ 17.7   **FUD** 090   63 J A2 80 50 🔲
AMA: 2018,Jan,8; 2017,Jan,8; 2016,Jan,13

49500 Repair initial inguinal hernia, age 6 months to younger than 5 years, with or without hydrocelectomy; reducible [A]

INCLUDES   Repairs performed on patients 6 months to younger than 5 years old

⚙ 11.9   ⚖ 11.9   **FUD** 090   [J] [A2] [80] [50] [▢]

AMA: 2018,Jan,8; 2017,Jan,8; 2016,Jan,13

49501 incarcerated or strangulated [A]

INCLUDES   Repairs performed on patients 6 months to younger than 5 years old

⚙ 17.6   ⚖ 17.6   **FUD** 090   [J] [A2] [80] [50] [▢]

AMA: 2018,Jan,8; 2017,Jan,8; 2016,Jan,13

49505 Repair initial inguinal hernia, age 5 years or older; reducible [A]

INCLUDES   MacEwen hernia repair

Code also when performed:
   Excision hydrocele (55040)
   Excision spermatocele (54840)
   Simple orchiectomy (54520)

⚙ 15.0   ⚖ 15.0   **FUD** 090   [J] [A2] [80] [50] [▢]

AMA: 2018,Jan,8; 2017,Jan,8; 2016,Jan,13

49507 incarcerated or strangulated [A]

Code also when performed:
   Excision hydrocele (55040)
   Excision spermatocele (54840)
   Simple orchiectomy (54520)

⚙ 17.0   ⚖ 17.0   **FUD** 090   [J] [A2] [80] [50] [▢]

AMA: 2018,Jan,8; 2017,Jan,8; 2016,Jan,13

49520 Repair recurrent inguinal hernia, any age; reducible

⚙ 18.3   ⚖ 18.3   **FUD** 090   [J] [A2] [80] [50] [▢]

AMA: 2018,Jan,8; 2017,Jan,8; 2016,Jan,13

49521 incarcerated or strangulated

⚙ 20.8   ⚖ 20.8   **FUD** 090   [J] [A2] [80] [50] [▢]

AMA: 2018,Jan,8; 2017,Jan,8; 2016,Jan,13

49525 Repair inguinal hernia, sliding, any age

EXCLUDES   Inguinal hernia repair, incarcerated/strangulated (49496, 49501, 49507, 49521)

⚙ 16.7   ⚖ 16.7   **FUD** 090   [J] [A2] [80] [50] [▢]

AMA: 2018,Jan,8; 2017,Jan,8; 2016,Jan,13

Peritoneal lining is forced through a defect in the inguinal wall

A peritoneal sac is created

Because the bowel is attached to the peritoneum, it is pulled through the abdominal defect as well

Sliding inguinal hernia

Anterior inguinal wall

Spermatic cord

Inguinal ligament

Femoral sheath

49540 Repair lumbar hernia

⚙ 19.5   ⚖ 19.5   **FUD** 090   [J] [A2] [80] [50] [▢]

AMA: 2018,Jan,8; 2017,Jan,8; 2016,Jan,13

49550 Repair initial femoral hernia, any age; reducible

⚙ 16.7   ⚖ 16.7   **FUD** 090   [J] [A2] [80] [50] [▢]

AMA: 2018,Jan,8; 2017,Jan,8; 2016,Jan,13

49553 incarcerated or strangulated

⚙ 18.3   ⚖ 18.3   **FUD** 090   [J] [A2] [80] [50] [▢]

AMA: 2018,Jan,8; 2017,Jan,8; 2016,Jan,13

49555 Repair recurrent femoral hernia; reducible

⚙ 17.5   ⚖ 17.5   **FUD** 090   [J] [A2] [80] [50] [▢]

AMA: 2018,Jan,8; 2017,Jan,8; 2016,Jan,13

49557 incarcerated or strangulated

⚙ 21.0   ⚖ 21.0   **FUD** 090   [J] [A2] [80] [50] [▢]

AMA: 2018,Jan,8; 2017,Jan,8; 2016,Jan,13

49560-49568 Hernia Repair: Incisional/Ventral

INCLUDES   Initial repair: no previous repair required
           Recurrent repair: required previous repair(s)
EXCLUDES   Abdominal wall debridement (11042, 11043)
           Intra-abdominal hernia repair/reduction (44050)
Code also repair or excision testicle(s), intestine, ovaries, when performed (44120, 54520, 58940)

49560 Repair initial incisional or ventral hernia; reducible

Code also implantation mesh or other prosthesis, when performed (49568)

⚙ 21.5   ⚖ 21.5   **FUD** 090   [J] [A2] [80] [50] [▢]

AMA: 2019,Nov,14; 2018,Jan,8; 2017,Jan,8; 2016,Jan,13

49561 incarcerated or strangulated

Code also implantation mesh or other prosthesis, when performed (49568)

⚙ 27.0   ⚖ 27.0   **FUD** 090   [J] [A2] [80] [50] [▢]

AMA: 2019,Nov,14; 2018,Jul,14; 2018,Mar,11; 2018,Jan,8; 2017,Jan,8; 2016,Jan,13

49565 Repair recurrent incisional or ventral hernia; reducible

Code also implantation mesh or other prosthesis, when performed (49568)

⚙ 22.3   ⚖ 22.3   **FUD** 090   [J] [A2] [80] [50] [▢]

AMA: 2019,Nov,14; 2018,Jan,8; 2017,Jan,8; 2016,Jan,13

49566 incarcerated or strangulated

Code also implantation mesh or other prosthesis, when performed (49568)

⚙ 27.3   ⚖ 27.3   **FUD** 090   [J] [A2] [80] [50] [▢]

AMA: 2019,Nov,14; 2018,Jan,8; 2017,Jan,8; 2016,Jan,13

+ **49568** Implantation of mesh or other prosthesis for open incisional or ventral hernia repair or mesh for closure of debridement for necrotizing soft tissue infection (List separately in addition to code for the incisional or ventral hernia repair)

EXCLUDES   Reporting with modifier 50. Report once for each side when performed bilaterally

Code first (11004-11006, 49560-49566)

⚙ 7.77   ⚖ 7.77   **FUD** ZZZ   [N] [N1] [80] [▢]

AMA: 2019,Nov,14; 2018,Jan,8; 2017,Jan,8; 2016,Jan,13

49570-49590 Hernia Repair: Epigastric/Lateral Ventral/Umbilical

INCLUDES   Mesh or other prosthesis
EXCLUDES   Abdominal wall debridement (11042, 11043)
           Intra-abdominal hernia repair/reduction (44050)
Code also repair or excision testicle(s), intestine, ovaries, when performed (44120, 54520, 58940)

49570 Repair epigastric hernia (eg, preperitoneal fat); reducible (separate procedure)

⚙ 12.1   ⚖ 12.1   **FUD** 090   [J] [A2] [80] [50] [▢]

AMA: 2018,Jan,8; 2017,Jan,8; 2016,Jan,13

49572 incarcerated or strangulated

⚙ 14.9   ⚖ 14.9   **FUD** 090   [J] [A2] [80] [50] [▢]

AMA: 2018,Jan,8; 2017,Jan,8; 2016,Jan,13

49580 Repair umbilical hernia, younger than age 5 years; reducible [A]

⚙ 9.69   ⚖ 9.69   **FUD** 090   [J] [A2] [80] [▢]

AMA: 2018,Jan,8; 2017,Jan,8; 2016,Jan,13

49582 incarcerated or strangulated [A]

⚙ 14.0   ⚖ 14.0   **FUD** 090   [J] [A2] [80] [▢]

AMA: 2018,Jan,8; 2017,Jan,8; 2016,Jan,13

49585 Repair umbilical hernia, age 5 years or older; reducible [A]

INCLUDES   Mayo hernia repair

⚙ 12.9   ⚖ 12.9   **FUD** 090   [J] [A2] [80] [▢]

AMA: 2018,Jan,8; 2017,Jan,8; 2016,Jan,13

49587 incarcerated or strangulated [A]

⚙ 13.7   ⚖ 13.7   **FUD** 090   [J] [A2] [80] [▢]

AMA: 2018,Jan,8; 2017,Jan,8; 2016,Jan,13

Digestive System

49590 Repair spigelian hernia
🚑 16.5　✂ 16.5　**FUD** 090　　　　J A2 80 50 ▭
AMA: 2018,Jan,8; 2017,Jan,8; 2016,Jan,13

49600-49611 Repair Birth Defect Abdominal Wall: Omphalocele/Gastroschisis

INCLUDES Mesh or other prosthesis
EXCLUDES Abdominal wall debridement (11042, 11043)
Intra-abdominal hernia repair/reduction (44050)
Repair:
Diaphragmatic or hiatal hernia (39503, 43332-43337)
Omentum (49999)

49600 Repair of small omphalocele, with primary closure
🚑 21.0　✂ 21.0　**FUD** 090　　　63 J A2 80 ▭
AMA: 2018,Jan,8; 2017,Jan,8; 2016,Jan,13

49605 Repair of large omphalocele or gastroschisis; with or without prosthesis
🚑 144.　✂ 144.　**FUD** 090　　　63 C 80 ▭
AMA: 2018,Jan,8; 2017,Jan,8; 2016,Jan,13

49606 with removal of prosthesis, final reduction and closure, in operating room
🚑 32.9　✂ 32.9　**FUD** 090　　　63 C 80 ▭
AMA: 2018,Jan,8; 2017,Jan,8; 2016,Jan,13

49610 Repair of omphalocele (Gross type operation); first stage
🚑 20.1　✂ 20.1　**FUD** 090　　　63 C 80 ▭
AMA: 2018,Jan,8; 2017,Jan,8; 2016,Jan,13

49611 second stage
🚑 17.7　✂ 17.7　**FUD** 090　　　63 C 80 ▭
AMA: 2018,Jan,8; 2017,Jan,8; 2016,Jan,13

49650-49659 Laparoscopic Hernia Repair

INCLUDES Diagnostic laparoscopy (49320)
Mesh or other prosthesis (49568)

49650 Laparoscopy, surgical; repair initial inguinal hernia
🚑 12.5　✂ 12.5　**FUD** 090　　　J A2 80 50 ▭
AMA: 2018,Jan,8; 2017,Jan,8; 2016,Jan,13

49651 repair recurrent inguinal hernia
🚑 16.2　✂ 16.2　**FUD** 090　　　J A2 80 50 ▭
AMA: 2018,Jan,8; 2017,Jan,8; 2016,Jan,13

49652 Laparoscopy, surgical, repair, ventral, umbilical, spigelian or epigastric hernia (includes mesh insertion, when performed); reducible
INCLUDES Laparoscopy, surgical, enterolysis (44180)
🚑 21.5　✂ 21.5　**FUD** 090　　　J 62 80 50 ▭
AMA: 2014,Jan,11; 2013,Jan,11-12

49653 incarcerated or strangulated
INCLUDES Laparoscopy, surgical, enterolysis (44180)
🚑 27.0　✂ 27.0　**FUD** 090　　　J 62 80 50 ▭
AMA: 2014,Jan,11; 2013,Jan,11-12

49654 Laparoscopy, surgical, repair, incisional hernia (includes mesh insertion, when performed); reducible
INCLUDES Laparoscopy, surgical, enterolysis (44180)
🚑 24.6　✂ 24.6　**FUD** 090　　　J 62 80 50 ▭
AMA: 2018,Jan,7

49655 incarcerated or strangulated
INCLUDES Laparoscopy, surgical, enterolysis (44180)
🚑 29.9　✂ 29.9　**FUD** 090　　　J 62 80 50 ▭
AMA: 2018,Jan,7

49656 Laparoscopy, surgical, repair, recurrent incisional hernia (includes mesh insertion, when performed); reducible
INCLUDES Laparoscopy, surgical, enterolysis (44180)
🚑 26.7　✂ 26.7　**FUD** 090　　　J 62 80 50 ▭
AMA: 2014,Jan,11; 2013,Jan,11-12

49657 incarcerated or strangulated
INCLUDES Laparoscopy, surgical, enterolysis (44180)
🚑 38.2　✂ 38.2　**FUD** 090　　　J 62 80 50 ▭
AMA: 2014,Jan,11; 2013,Jan,11-12

49659 Unlisted laparoscopy procedure, hernioplasty, herniorrhaphy, herniotomy
🚑 0.00　✂ 0.00　**FUD** YYY　　　J 80 50 ▭
AMA: 2018,Jan,8; 2017,Jul,10; 2017,Jan,8; 2016,Jan,13

49900 Surgical Repair Abdominal Wall

EXCLUDES Abdominal wall debridement (11042, 11043)
Suture ruptured diaphragm (39540-39541)

49900 Suture, secondary, of abdominal wall for evisceration or dehiscence
🚑 23.7　✂ 23.7　**FUD** 090　　　C 80 ▭
AMA: 2018,Jan,8; 2017,Jan,8; 2016,Jan,13

49904-49999 Harvesting of Omental Flap

49904 Omental flap, extra-abdominal (eg, for reconstruction of sternal and chest wall defects)
INCLUDES Harvest and transfer
EXCLUDES Omental flap harvest by second surgeon: both surgeons report code with modifier 62
🚑 40.5　✂ 40.5　**FUD** 090　　　C ▭
AMA: 2014,Jan,11; 2013,Jan,11-12

+ **49905** Omental flap, intra-abdominal (List separately in addition to code for primary procedure)
EXCLUDES Exclusion small intestine from pelvis by mesh, other prosthesis, or native tissue (44700)
Code first primary procedure
🚑 10.3　✂ 10.3　**FUD** ZZZ　　　C 80 ▭
AMA: 2020,Feb,13; 2018,Jan,8; 2017,Jan,8; 2016,Jan,13

49906 Free omental flap with microvascular anastomosis
INCLUDES Operating microscope (69990)
🚑 0.00　✂ 0.00　**FUD** 090　　　C ▭
AMA: 2019,Dec,5; 2018,Jan,8; 2017,Jan,8; 2016,Feb,12; 2016,Jan,13

49999 Unlisted procedure, abdomen, peritoneum and omentum
🚑 0.00　✂ 0.00　**FUD** YYY　　　T ▭
AMA: 2020,Jun,14; 2019,Nov,14; 2018,Jan,8; 2017,Jan,8; 2016,Jan,13

50010-50045 Kidney Procedures for Exploration or Drainage

EXCLUDES *Donor nephrectomy performed laparoscopically (50547)*
Retroperitoneal
 Abscess drainage (49060)
 Exploration (49010)
 Tumor/cyst excision (49203-49205)

50010 **Renal exploration, not necessitating other specific procedures**

EXCLUDES *Laparoscopic ablation mass lesions of kidney (50542)*

🔧 21.2 ✂ 21.2 **FUD** 090 [C] [80] [50] 📄

AMA: 2014,Jan,11; 2008,Aug,7-9

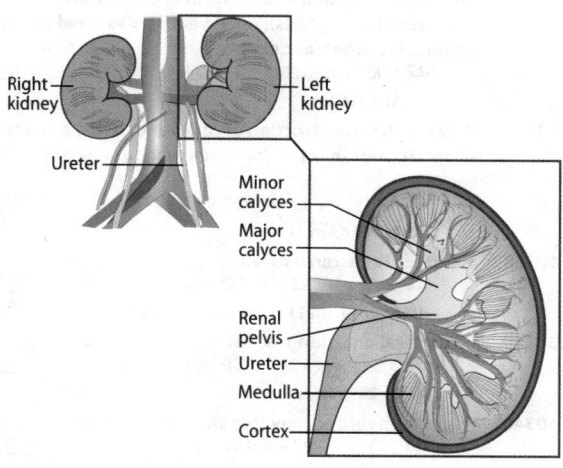

Right kidney — Left kidney
Ureter
Minor calyces
Major calyces
Renal pelvis
Ureter
Medulla
Cortex

50020 **Drainage of perirenal or renal abscess, open**

EXCLUDES *Image-guided percutaneous drainage perirenal or renal abscess (49405)*

🔧 29.2 ✂ 29.2 **FUD** 090 [J] [62] 📄

AMA: 2018,Jan,8; 2017,Jan,8; 2016,Jan,13

50040 **Nephrostomy, nephrotomy with drainage**

🔧 26.6 ✂ 26.6 **FUD** 090 [C] [50] 📄

AMA: 2018,Jan,8; 2017,Jan,8; 2016,Jan,13

50045 **Nephrotomy, with exploration**

EXCLUDES *Renal endoscopy through nephrotomy (50570-50580)*

🔧 26.9 ✂ 26.9 **FUD** 090 [C] [80] [50] 📄

AMA: 2018,Jan,8; 2017,Jan,8; 2016,Jan,13

50060-50081 Treatment of Kidney Stones

CMS: 100-03,230.1 NCD for Treatment of Kidney Stones

EXCLUDES *Retroperitoneal:*
 Abscess drainage (49060)
 Exploration (49010)
 Tumor/cyst excision (49203-49205)

50060 **Nephrolithotomy; removal of calculus**

🔧 32.9 ✂ 32.9 **FUD** 090 [C] [80] [50] 📄

AMA: 2018,Jan,8; 2017,Jan,8; 2016,Jan,13

50065 **secondary surgical operation for calculus**

🔧 34.9 ✂ 34.9 **FUD** 090 [C] [80] [50] 📄

AMA: 2018,Jan,8; 2017,Jan,8; 2016,Jan,13

50070 **complicated by congenital kidney abnormality**

🔧 34.2 ✂ 34.2 **FUD** 090 [C] [80] [50] 📄

AMA: 2018,Jan,8; 2017,Jan,8; 2016,Jan,13

50075 **removal of large staghorn calculus filling renal pelvis and calyces (including anatrophic pyelolithotomy)**

🔧 42.1 ✂ 42.1 **FUD** 090 [C] [80] [50] 📄

AMA: 2018,Jan,8; 2017,Jan,8; 2016,Jan,13

50080 **Percutaneous nephrostolithotomy or pyelostolithotomy, with or without dilation, endoscopy, lithotripsy, stenting, or basket extraction; up to 2 cm**

EXCLUDES *Dilation existing tract by same provider ([50436, 50437])*
Nephrostomy without nephrostolithotomy (50040, [50432, 50433], 52334)

📷 (76000)

🔧 25.0 ✂ 25.0 **FUD** 090 [J] [62] [50] 📄

AMA: 2018,Jan,8; 2017,Jan,8; 2016,Jan,13

50081 **over 2 cm**

EXCLUDES *Dilation existing tract by same provider ([50436, 50437])*
Nephrostomy without nephrostolithotomy (50040, [50432, 50433], 52334)

📷 (76000)

🔧 36.9 ✂ 36.9 **FUD** 090 [J] [62] [80] [50] 📄

AMA: 2018,Jan,8; 2017,Jan,8; 2016,Jan,13

50100 Repair of Anomalous Vessels of the Kidney

EXCLUDES *Retroperitoneal:*
 Abscess drainage (49060)
 Exploration (49010)
 Tumor/cyst excision (49203-49205)

50100 **Transection or repositioning of aberrant renal vessels (separate procedure)**

🔧 31.4 ✂ 31.4 **FUD** 090 [C] [80] [50] 📄

AMA: 2018,Jan,8; 2017,Jan,8; 2016,Jan,13

50120-50135 Procedures of Renal Pelvis

EXCLUDES *Retroperitoneal:*
 Abscess drainage (49060)
 Exploration (49010)
 Tumor/cyst excision (49203-49205)

50120 **Pyelotomy; with exploration**

INCLUDES *Gol-Vernet pyelotomy*

EXCLUDES *Renal endoscopy through pyelotomy (50570-50580)*

🔧 27.4 ✂ 27.4 **FUD** 090 [C] [80] [50] 📄

AMA: 2018,Jan,8; 2017,Jan,8; 2016,Jan,13

50125 **with drainage, pyelostomy**

🔧 28.3 ✂ 28.3 **FUD** 090 [C] [80] [50] 📄

AMA: 2018,Jan,8; 2017,Jan,8; 2016,Jan,13

50130 **with removal of calculus (pyelolithotomy, pelviolithotomy, including coagulum pyelolithotomy)**

🔧 29.8 ✂ 29.8 **FUD** 090 [C] [80] [50] 📄

AMA: 2018,Jan,8; 2017,Jan,8; 2016,Jan,13

50135 **complicated (eg, secondary operation, congenital kidney abnormality)**

🔧 32.4 ✂ 32.4 **FUD** 090 [C] [80] [50] 📄

AMA: 2018,Jan,8; 2017,Jan,8; 2016,Jan,13

50200-50205 Biopsy of Kidney

EXCLUDES *Laparoscopic renal mass lesion ablation (50542)*
Retroperitoneal tumor/cyst excision (49203-49205)

50200 **Renal biopsy; percutaneous, by trocar or needle**

EXCLUDES *Fine needle aspiration ([10005, 10006,*10007, 10008, 10009, 10010, 10011, 10012])*

📷 (76942, 77002, 77012, 77021)

🔬 (88172-88173)

🔧 3.70 ✂ 15.4 **FUD** 000 [J] [A2] [50] 📄

AMA: 2019,Apr,4; 2018,Jan,8; 2017,Jan,8; 2016,Jan,13

50205 **by surgical exposure of kidney**

🔧 21.9 ✂ 21.9 **FUD** 090 [C] [80] [50] 📄

AMA: 2018,Jan,8; 2017,Jan,8; 2016,Jan,13

50220-50240 Nephrectomy Procedures

EXCLUDES *Laparoscopic renal mass lesion ablation (50542)*
Retroperitoneal tumor/cyst excision (49203-49205)

50220 **Nephrectomy, including partial ureterectomy, any open approach including rib resection;**

🔧 30.3 ✂ 30.3 **FUD** 090 [C] [80] [50] 📄

AMA: 2018,Jan,8; 2017,Jan,8; 2016,Jan,13

Urinary System

50225 — 50382

50225   complicated because of previous surgery on same kidney

🗀 34.7   ⚕ 34.7   **FUD** 090   C 80 50 ▭

AMA: 2018,Jan,8; 2017,Jan,8; 2016,Jan,13

50230   radical, with regional lymphadenectomy and/or vena caval thrombectomy

EXCLUDES   *Vena caval resection with reconstruction (37799)*

🗀 37.0   ⚕ 37.0   **FUD** 090   C 80 50 ▭

AMA: 2018,Jan,8; 2017,Jan,8; 2016,Jan,13

50234   Nephrectomy with total ureterectomy and bladder cuff; through same incision

🗀 37.6   ⚕ 37.6   **FUD** 090   C 80 50 ▭

AMA: 2018,Jan,8; 2017,Jan,8; 2016,Jan,13

50236   through separate incision

🗀 42.3   ⚕ 42.3   **FUD** 090   C 80 50 ▭

AMA: 2018,Jan,8; 2017,Jan,8; 2016,Jan,13

50240   Nephrectomy, partial

EXCLUDES   *Laparoscopic partial nephrectomy (50543)*

🗀 38.2   ⚕ 38.2   **FUD** 090   C 80 50 ▭

AMA: 2018,Jan,8; 2017,Jan,8; 2016,Jan,13

50250-50290 Open Removal Kidney Lesions

EXCLUDES   *Open destruction or excision intra-abdominal tumors (49203-49205)*

50250   Ablation, open, 1 or more renal mass lesion(s), cryosurgical, including intraoperative ultrasound guidance and monitoring, if performed

EXCLUDES   *Laparoscopic renal mass lesion ablation (50542)*
             Percutaneous renal tumor ablation (50592-50593)

🗀 35.1   ⚕ 35.1   **FUD** 090   C 80 ▭

AMA: 2018,Jan,8; 2017,Jan,8; 2016,Jan,13

50280   Excision or unroofing of cyst(s) of kidney

EXCLUDES   *Renal cyst laparoscopic ablation (50541)*

🗀 27.6   ⚕ 27.6   **FUD** 090   C 80 50 ▭

AMA: 2018,Jan,8; 2017,Jan,8; 2016,Jan,13

50290   Excision of perinephric cyst

🗀 25.9   ⚕ 25.9   **FUD** 090   C 80 ▭

AMA: 2018,Jan,8; 2017,Jan,8; 2016,Jan,13

50300-50380 Kidney Transplant Procedures

CMS: 100-04,3,90.1 Kidney Transplant - General; 100-04,3,90.1.1 Standard Kidney Acquisition Charge; 100-04,3,90.1.2 Billing for Kidney Transplant and Acquisition Services; 100-04,3,90.5 Pancreas Transplants with Kidney Transplants

EXCLUDES   *Dialysis procedures (90935-90999)*
             Lymphocele drainage to peritoneal cavity performed laparoscopically (49323)

50300   Donor nephrectomy (including cold preservation); from cadaver donor, unilateral or bilateral

INCLUDES   Graft:
             Cold preservation
             Harvesting

EXCLUDES   *Donor nephrectomy performed laparoscopically (50547)*

🗀 0.00   ⚕ 0.00   **FUD** XXX   C ▭

AMA: 2018,Jan,8; 2017,Jan,8; 2016,Jan,13

50320   open, from living donor

INCLUDES   Donor care
             Graft:
             Cold preservation
             Harvesting

EXCLUDES   *Donor nephrectomy performed laparoscopically (50547)*

🗀 43.7   ⚕ 43.7   **FUD** 090   C 80 50 ▭

AMA: 2018,Jan,8; 2017,Jan,8; 2016,Jan,13

50323   Backbench standard preparation of cadaver donor renal allograft prior to transplantation, including dissection and removal of perinephric fat, diaphragmatic and retroperitoneal attachments, excision of adrenal gland, and preparation of ureter(s), renal vein(s), and renal artery(s), ligating branches, as necessary

EXCLUDES   *Adrenalectomy (60540, 60545)*

🗀 0.00   ⚕ 0.00   **FUD** XXX   C 80 ▭

AMA: 2018,Jan,8; 2017,Jan,8; 2016,Jan,13

50325   Backbench standard preparation of living donor renal allograft (open or laparoscopic) prior to transplantation, including dissection and removal of perinephric fat and preparation of ureter(s), renal vein(s), and renal artery(s), ligating branches, as necessary

🗀 0.00   ⚕ 0.00   **FUD** XXX   C 80 ▭

AMA: 2014,Jan,11

50327   Backbench reconstruction of cadaver or living donor renal allograft prior to transplantation; venous anastomosis, each

🗀 6.29   ⚕ 6.29   **FUD** XXX   C 80 ▭

AMA: 2014,Jan,11

50328   arterial anastomosis, each

🗀 5.53   ⚕ 5.53   **FUD** XXX   C 80 ▭

AMA: 2014,Jan,11

50329   ureteral anastomosis, each

🗀 5.24   ⚕ 5.24   **FUD** XXX   C 80 ▭

AMA: 2014,Jan,11

50340   Recipient nephrectomy (separate procedure)

🗀 27.4   ⚕ 27.4   **FUD** 090   C 80 50 ▭

AMA: 2014,Jan,11

50360   Renal allotransplantation, implantation of graft; without recipient nephrectomy

INCLUDES   Allograft transplantation
             Recipient care
         Code also:
             Backbench work (50323, 50325, 50327-50329)
             Donor nephrectomy (cadaver or living donor) (50300, 50320, 50547)

🗀 70.0   ⚕ 70.0   **FUD** 090   C 80 ▭

AMA: 2014,Jan,11; 1994,Win,1

50365   with recipient nephrectomy

INCLUDES   Allograft transplantation
             Recipient care

🗀 83.5   ⚕ 83.5   **FUD** 090   C 80 50 ▭

AMA: 2018,Jan,8; 2017,Jan,8; 2016,Jan,13

50370   Removal of transplanted renal allograft

🗀 35.0   ⚕ 35.0   **FUD** 090   C 80 ▭

AMA: 2014,Jan,11; 2002,Oct,5

50380   Renal autotransplantation, reimplantation of kidney

INCLUDES   Reimplantation autograft

EXCLUDES   *Secondary procedures:*
             Nephrolithotomy (50060-50075)
             Partial nephrectomy (50240, 50543)

🗀 58.4   ⚕ 58.4   **FUD** 090   C 80 ▭

AMA: 2019,Sep,10; 2018,Jan,8; 2017,Jan,8; 2016,Jan,13

50382-50386 Removal With/Without Replacement Internal Ureteral Stent

INCLUDES   Radiological supervision and interpretation

50382   Removal (via snare/capture) and replacement of internally dwelling ureteral stent via percutaneous approach, including radiological supervision and interpretation

EXCLUDES   *Dilation existing tract, percutaneous for endourologic procedure ([50436, 50437])*
             Removal and replacement internally dwelling ureteral stent using transurethral approach (50385)

🗀 7.46   ⚕ 31.3   **FUD** 000   J 62 50 ▭

AMA: 2018,Jan,8; 2017,Jan,8; 2016,Jan,13; 2016,Jan,3

26/TC PC/TC Only   A2-Z3 ASC Payment   50 Bilateral   ♂ Male Only   ♀ Female Only   🗀 Facility RVU   ⚕ Non-Facility RVU   ▭ CCI   ✖ CLIA

FUD Follow-up Days   **CMS:** IOM   **AMA:** CPT Asst   A-Y OPPSI   80/80 Surg Assist Allowed / w/Doc   ▭ Lab Crosswalk   ▪ Radiology Crosswalk

230   CPT © 2021 American Medical Association. All Rights Reserved.   © 2021 Optum360, LLC

50384 Removal (via snare/capture) of internally dwelling ureteral stent via percutaneous approach, including radiological supervision and interpretation

> EXCLUDES Dilation existing tract, percutaneous for endourologic procedure ([50436, 50437])
> Removal internally dwelling ureteral stent using transurethral approach (50386)

🔧 6.68 ⚕ 25.0 **FUD** 000 [02] [62] [50] 🔲

AMA: 2018,Jan,8; 2017,Jan,8; 2016,Jan,13; 2016,Jan,3

50385 Removal (via snare/capture) and replacement of internally dwelling ureteral stent via transurethral approach, without use of cystoscopy, including radiological supervision and interpretation

🔧 6.34 ⚕ 30.7 **FUD** 000 [J] [62] [80] [50] 🔲

AMA: 2018,Jan,8; 2017,Jan,8; 2016,Jan,13; 2016,Jan,3

50386 Removal (via snare/capture) of internally dwelling ureteral stent via transurethral approach, without use of cystoscopy, including radiological supervision and interpretation

🔧 4.70 ⚕ 20.3 **FUD** 000 [02] [P3] [80] [50] 🔲

AMA: 2018,Jan,8; 2017,Jan,8; 2016,Jan,3; 2016,Jan,13

50387 Remove/Replace Accessible Ureteral Stent

> EXCLUDES Removal and replacement ureteral stent through ureterostomy tube or ileal conduit (50688)
> Removal without replacement externally accessible ureteral stent without fluoroscopic guidance, report with appropriate E/M code

50387 Removal and replacement of externally accessible nephroureteral catheter (eg, external/internal stent) requiring fluoroscopic guidance, including radiological supervision and interpretation

🔧 2.43 ⚕ 14.6 **FUD** 000 [J] [62] [80] [50] 🔲

AMA: 2018,Jan,8; 2017,Jan,8; 2016,Mar,10; 2016,Jan,13; 2016,Jan,3

50389-50435 [50430, 50431, 50432, 50433, 50434, 50435, 50436, 50437] Percutaneous and Injection Procedures With/Without Indwelling Tube/Catheter Access

50389 Removal of nephrostomy tube, requiring fluoroscopic guidance (eg, with concurrent indwelling ureteral stent)

> EXCLUDES Nephrostomy tube removal without fluoroscopic guidance, report with appropriate E/M code

🔧 1.56 ⚕ 9.49 **FUD** 000 [02] [62] [50] 🔲

AMA: 2018,Jan,8; 2017,Jan,8; 2016,Jan,13; 2016,Jan,3

50390 Aspiration and/or injection of renal cyst or pelvis by needle, percutaneous

> EXCLUDES Antegrade nephrostogram/pyelogram ([50430, 50431])
> 🔲 (74425, 74470, 76942, 77002, 77012, 77021)

🔧 2.78 ⚕ 2.78 **FUD** 000 [T] [A2] [50] 🔲

AMA: 2018,Jan,8; 2017,Jan,8; 2016,Jan,13

50391 Instillation(s) of therapeutic agent into renal pelvis and/or ureter through established nephrostomy, pyelostomy or ureterostomy tube (eg, anticarcinogenic or antifungal agent)

Code also therapeutic agent

🔧 2.84 ⚕ 3.52 **FUD** 000 [T] [P3] [50] 🔲

AMA: 2018,Jan,8; 2017,Jan,8; 2016,Jan,13

 # 50436 Dilation of existing tract, percutaneous, for an endourologic procedure including imaging guidance (eg, ultrasound and/or fluoroscopy) and all associated radiological supervision and interpretation, with postprocedure tube placement, when performed

> EXCLUDES Percutaneous nephrostolithotomy (50080-50081)
> Procedure performed for same renal collecting system/ureter ([50430, 50431, 50432, 50433], 52334, 74485)
> Removal, replacement internally dwelling ureteral stent (50382, 50384)

🔧 4.35 ⚕ 4.35 **FUD** 000 [62] [50] 🔲

 # 50437 including new access into the renal collecting system

> EXCLUDES Percutaneous nephrostolithotomy (50080-50081)
> Procedure performed for same renal collecting system/ureter ([50430, 50431, 50432, 50433], 52334, 74485)
> Removal, replacement internally dwelling ureteral stent (50382, 50384)

🔧 7.29 ⚕ 7.29 **FUD** 000 [62] [50] 🔲

50396 Manometric studies through nephrostomy or pyelostomy tube, or indwelling ureteral catheter

🔲 (74425)

🔧 3.38 ⚕ 3.38 **FUD** 000 [J] [A2] [80] [50] 🔲

AMA: 2018,Jan,8; 2017,Jan,8; 2016,Jan,13

 # 50430 Injection procedure for antegrade nephrostogram and/or ureterogram, complete diagnostic procedure including imaging guidance (eg, ultrasound and fluoroscopy) and all associated radiological supervision and interpretation; new access

> INCLUDES Renal pelvis and associated ureter as single element
> EXCLUDES Procedure performed for same renal collecting system/ureter ([50432, 50433, 50434, 50435], 50693-50695, 74425)

🔧 4.46 ⚕ 14.5 **FUD** 000 [02] [N1] [80] [50] 🔲

AMA: 2018,Jan,8; 2017,Jan,8; 2016,Jan,3; 2016,Jan,13

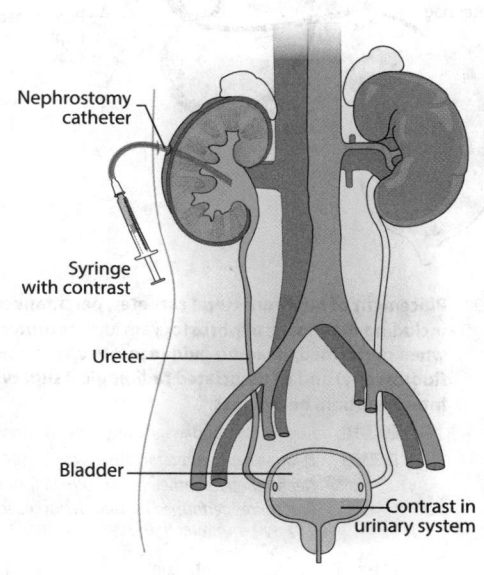

Nephrostomy catheter

Syringe with contrast

Ureter

Bladder

Contrast in urinary system

 # 50431 existing access

> INCLUDES Renal pelvis and associated ureter as single element
> EXCLUDES Procedure performed for same renal collecting system/ureter ([50432, 50433, 50434, 50435], 50693-50695, 74425)

🔧 1.91 ⚕ 4.64 **FUD** 000 [02] [N1] [50] 🔲

AMA: 2018,Jan,8; 2017,Jan,8; 2016,Jan,3; 2016,Jan,13

Urinary System

50432 — 50520

\# **50432** **Placement of nephrostomy catheter, percutaneous, including diagnostic nephrostogram and/or ureterogram when performed, imaging guidance (eg, ultrasound and/or fluoroscopy) and all associated radiological supervision and interpretation**

> INCLUDES   Renal pelvis and associated ureter as single element
>
> EXCLUDES   *Dilation nephroureteral catheter tract ([50436, 50437])*
> *Procedure performed for same renal collecting system/ureter ([50430, 50431], [50433], 50694-50695, 74425)*
>
> 🔲 5.98   ⚕ 23.5   **FUD** 000   J 62 50 ▭
>
> **AMA:** 2018,Mar,11; 2018,Jan,8; 2017,Jan,8; 2016,Jan,3; 2016,Jan,13

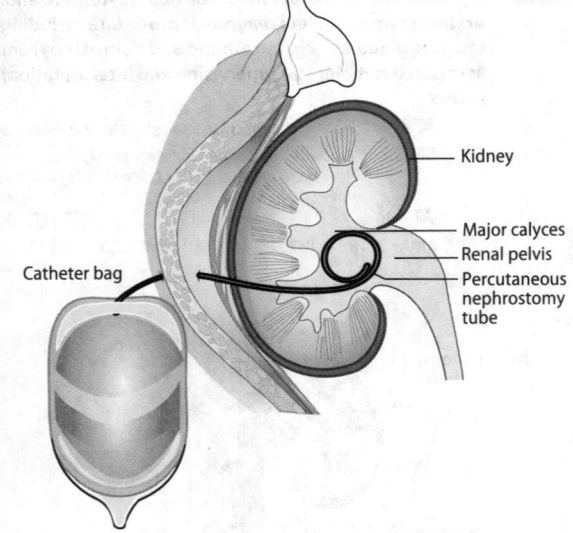

Kidney
Major calyces
Renal pelvis
Percutaneous nephrostomy tube
Catheter bag

\# **50433** **Placement of nephroureteral catheter, percutaneous, including diagnostic nephrostogram and/or ureterogram when performed, imaging guidance (eg, ultrasound and/or fluoroscopy) and all associated radiological supervision and interpretation, new access**

> INCLUDES   Renal pelvis and associated ureter as single element
>
> EXCLUDES   *Dilation nephroureteral catheter tract ([50436, 50437])*
> *Nephroureteral catheter removal/replacement (50387)*
> *Procedures performed for same renal collecting system/ureter ([50430, 50431, 50432], 50693-50695, 74425)*
>
> 🔲 7.44   ⚕ 31.2   **FUD** 000   J 62 50 ▭
>
> **AMA:** 2018,Mar,11; 2018,Jan,8; 2017,Jan,8; 2016,Jan,3; 2016,Jan,13

\# **50434** **Convert nephrostomy catheter to nephroureteral catheter, percutaneous, including diagnostic nephrostogram and/or ureterogram when performed, imaging guidance (eg, ultrasound and/or fluoroscopy) and all associated radiological supervision and interpretation, via pre-existing nephrostomy tract**

> INCLUDES   Renal pelvis and associated ureter as single element
>
> EXCLUDES   *Procedure performed for same renal collecting system/ureter ([50430, 50431], [50435], 50684, 50693, 74425)*
>
> 🔲 5.60   ⚕ 24.6   **FUD** 000   J 62 50 ▭
>
> **AMA:** 2018,Jan,8; 2017,Jan,8; 2016,Jan,3; 2016,Jan,13

\# **50435** **Exchange nephrostomy catheter, percutaneous, including diagnostic nephrostogram and/or ureterogram when performed, imaging guidance (eg, ultrasound and/or fluoroscopy) and all associated radiological supervision and interpretation**

> INCLUDES   Renal pelvis and associated ureter as single element
>
> EXCLUDES   *Procedure performed for same renal collecting system/ureter ([50430, 50431], [50434], 50693, 74425)*
> *Removal nephrostomy catheter requiring fluoroscopic guidance (50389)*
>
> 🔲 2.90   ⚕ 14.6   **FUD** 000   J 62 50 ▭
>
> **AMA:** 2018,Mar,11; 2018,Jan,8; 2017,Jan,8; 2016,Jan,3; 2016,Jan,13

50400-50540 [50430, 50431, 50432, 50433, 50434, 50435, 50436, 50437] Open Surgical Procedures of Kidney

50400 **Pyeloplasty (Foley Y-pyeloplasty), plastic operation on renal pelvis, with or without plastic operation on ureter, nephropexy, nephrostomy, pyelostomy, or ureteral splinting; simple**

> EXCLUDES   *Laparoscopic pyeloplasty (50544)*
>
> 🔲 33.5   ⚕ 33.5   **FUD** 090   C 80 50 ▭
>
> **AMA:** 2018,Jan,8; 2017,Jan,8; 2016,Jan,13

50405 **complicated (congenital kidney abnormality, secondary pyeloplasty, solitary kidney, calycoplasty)**

> EXCLUDES   *Laparoscopic pyeloplasty (50544)*
>
> 🔲 40.3   ⚕ 40.3   **FUD** 090   C 80 50 ▭
>
> **AMA:** 2018,Jan,8; 2017,Jan,8; 2016,Jan,13

50430 Resequenced code. See code following 50396.

50431 Resequenced code. See code following 50396.

50432 Resequenced code. See code following 50396.

50433 Resequenced code. See code following 50396.

50434 Resequenced code. See code following 50396.

50435 Resequenced code. See code following 50396.

50436 Resequenced code. See code following 50391.

50437 Resequenced code. See code following 50391.

50500 **Nephrorrhaphy, suture of kidney wound or injury**

> 🔲 37.3   ⚕ 37.3   **FUD** 090   C 80 ▭
>
> **AMA:** 2014,Jan,11

Periaortic lymph nodes
Adrenal gland
Kidney
Aorta
Upper ureter
Bladder
Major renal vessels
Renal pelvis
Glomerulus
Capillaries
Vein
Artery
Bowman's capsule
Collecting tubule
Schematic of nephron

50520 **Closure of nephrocutaneous or pyelocutaneous fistula**

> 🔲 33.6   ⚕ 33.6   **FUD** 090   C 80 ▭
>
> **AMA:** 2014,Jan,11; 2000,Oct,8

26/TC PC/TC Only   A2-Z3 ASC Payment   50 Bilateral   ♂ Male Only   ♀ Female Only   🔲 Facility RVU   ⚕ Non-Facility RVU   ▭ CCI   ✖ CLIA
FUD Follow-up Days   **CMS:** IOM   **AMA:** CPT Asst   A-Y OPPSI   80/80 Surg Assist Allowed / w/Doc   Lab Crosswalk   Radiology Crosswalk

232   CPT © 2021 American Medical Association. All Rights Reserved.   © 2021 Optum360, LLC

50525 Closure of nephrovisceral fistula (eg, renocolic), including visceral repair; abdominal approach
  42.6 ⚗ 42.6 **FUD** 090   C 80 ▣
  AMA: 2014,Jan,11

50526 thoracic approach
  45.9 ⚗ 45.9 **FUD** 090   C 80 ▣
  AMA: 2014,Jan,11

50540 Symphysiotomy for horseshoe kidney with or without pyeloplasty and/or other plastic procedure, unilateral or bilateral (1 operation)
  33.1 ⚗ 33.1 **FUD** 090   C 80 ▣
  AMA: 2014,Jan,11; 2000,Oct,8

50541-50549 Laparoscopic Surgical Procedures of the Kidney

INCLUDES Diagnostic laparoscopy (49320)
EXCLUDES *Laparoscopic drainage lymphocele to peritoneal cavity (49323)*

50541 Laparoscopy, surgical; ablation of renal cysts
  26.5 ⚗ 26.5 **FUD** 090   J G2 80 50 ▣
  AMA: 2018,Jan,8; 2017,Jan,8; 2016,Jan,13

50542 ablation of renal mass lesion(s), including intraoperative ultrasound guidance and monitoring, when performed
  EXCLUDES *Open ablation renal mass lesions (50250)*
           Percutaneous ablation renal tumors (50592-50593)
  33.7 ⚗ 33.7 **FUD** 090   J G2 80 50 ▣
  AMA: 2018,Jan,8; 2017,Jan,8; 2016,Jan,13

50543 partial nephrectomy
  EXCLUDES *Partial nephrectomy, open approach (50240)*
  43.0 ⚗ 43.0 **FUD** 090   J G2 80 50 ▣
  AMA: 2018,Jan,8; 2017,Jan,8; 2016,Jan,13

50544 pyeloplasty
  36.0 ⚗ 36.0 **FUD** 090   J G2 80 50 ▣
  AMA: 2018,Jan,8; 2017,Jan,8; 2016,Jan,13

50545 radical nephrectomy (includes removal of Gerota's fascia and surrounding fatty tissue, removal of regional lymph nodes, and adrenalectomy)
  EXCLUDES *Radical nephrectomy, open approach (50230)*
  38.7 ⚗ 38.7 **FUD** 090   C 80 50 ▣
  AMA: 2018,Jan,8; 2017,Jan,8; 2016,Jan,13

50546 nephrectomy, including partial ureterectomy
  34.7 ⚗ 34.7 **FUD** 090   C 80 50 ▣
  AMA: 2018,Jan,8; 2017,Jan,8; 2016,Jan,13

50547 donor nephrectomy (including cold preservation), from living donor
  INCLUDES Donor care
           Graft:
             Cold preservation
             Harvesting
  EXCLUDES *Backbench reconstruction renal allograft prior to transplantation (50327-50329)*
           Backbench standard preparation living donor renal allograft prior to transplantation (50325)
           Donor nephrectomy, open approach (50320)
  46.4 ⚗ 46.4 **FUD** 090   C 80 50 ▣
  AMA: 2018,Jan,8; 2017,Jan,8; 2016,Jan,13

50548 nephrectomy with total ureterectomy
  EXCLUDES *Nephrectomy, open approach (50234, 50236)*
  38.9 ⚗ 38.9 **FUD** 090   C 80 50 ▣
  AMA: 2018,Jan,8; 2017,Jan,8; 2016,Jan,13

50549 Unlisted laparoscopy procedure, renal
  0.00 ⚗ 0.00 **FUD** YYY   J 80 50 ▣
  AMA: 2018,Jan,8; 2017,Jan,8; 2016,Jan,13

50551-50562 Endoscopic Procedures of Kidney via Established Nephrostomy/Pyelostomy Access

50551 Renal endoscopy through established nephrostomy or pyelostomy, with or without irrigation, instillation, or ureteropyelography, exclusive of radiologic service;
  8.54 ⚗ 10.4 **FUD** 000   J A2 80 50 ▣
  AMA: 2018,Jan,8; 2017,Jan,8; 2016,Jan,13

50553 with ureteral catheterization, with or without dilation of ureter
  EXCLUDES *Image-guided ureter dilation without endoscopic guidance (50706)*
  9.09 ⚗ 11.1 **FUD** 000   J A2 50 ▣
  AMA: 2018,Jan,8; 2017,Jan,8; 2016,Jan,3; 2016,Jan,13

50555 with biopsy
  EXCLUDES *Image-guided biopsy ureter/renal pelvis without endoscopic guidance (50606)*
  9.88 ⚗ 11.9 **FUD** 000   J A2 80 50 ▣
  AMA: 2018,Jan,8; 2017,Jan,8; 2016,Jan,3; 2016,Jan,13

50557 with fulguration and/or incision, with or without biopsy
  10.0 ⚗ 12.1 **FUD** 000   J A2 80 50 ▣
  AMA: 2018,Jan,8; 2017,Jan,8; 2016,Jan,13

50561 with removal of foreign body or calculus
  11.3 ⚗ 13.6 **FUD** 000   J A2 80 50 ▣
  AMA: 2018,Jan,8; 2017,Jan,8; 2016,Jan,13

50562 with resection of tumor
  16.8 ⚗ 16.8 **FUD** 090   J G2 80 ▣
  AMA: 2018,Jan,8; 2017,Jan,8; 2016,Jan,13

50570-50580 Endoscopic Procedures of Kidney via Nephrotomy/Pyelotomy Access

Code also when provided service significant and identifiable (50045, 50120)

50570 Renal endoscopy through nephrotomy or pyelotomy, with or without irrigation, instillation, or ureteropyelography, exclusive of radiologic service;
  14.2 ⚗ 14.2 **FUD** 000   J G2 80 50 ▣
  AMA: 2018,Jan,8; 2017,Jan,8; 2016,Jan,13

50572 with ureteral catheterization, with or without dilation of ureter
  EXCLUDES *Image-guided ureter dilation without endoscopic guidance (50706)*
  15.4 ⚗ 15.4 **FUD** 000   T G2 80 50 ▣
  AMA: 2018,Jan,8; 2017,Jan,8; 2016,Jan,3; 2016,Jan,13

50574 with biopsy
  EXCLUDES *Image-guide ureter/renal pelvis biopsy without endoscopic guidance (50606)*
  16.3 ⚗ 16.3 **FUD** 000   J G2 80 50 ▣
  AMA: 2018,Jan,8; 2017,Jan,8; 2016,Jan,3; 2016,Jan,13

50575 with endopyelotomy (includes cystoscopy, ureteroscopy, dilation of ureter and ureteral pelvic junction, incision of ureteral pelvic junction and insertion of endopyelotomy stent)
  20.6 ⚗ 20.6 **FUD** 000   J G2 50 ▣
  AMA: 2018,Jan,8; 2017,Jan,8; 2016,Jan,13

50576 with fulguration and/or incision, with or without biopsy
  16.3 ⚗ 16.3 **FUD** 000   J G2 80 50 ▣
  AMA: 2018,Jan,8; 2017,Jan,8; 2016,Jan,13

50580 with removal of foreign body or calculus
  17.5 ⚗ 17.5 **FUD** 000   J G2 80 50 ▣
  AMA: 2018,Jan,8; 2017,Jan,8; 2016,Jan,13

● New Code ▲ Revised Code ○ Reinstated ● New Web Release ▲ Revised Web Release + Add-on Unlisted Not Covered # Resequenced
50 Optum Mod 50 Exempt ⊘ AMA Mod 51 Exempt 51 Optum Mod 51 Exempt 63 Mod 63 Exempt ✗ Non-FDA Drug ★ Telemedicine M Maternity A Age Edit

50590-50593 Noninvasive and Minimally Invasive Procedures of the Kidney

50590 **Lithotripsy, extracorporeal shock wave**
🔧 16.4 ⚕ 20.8 **FUD** 090   J 62 50 ▢
AMA: 2018,Jan,8; 2017,Jan,8; 2016,Jan,13

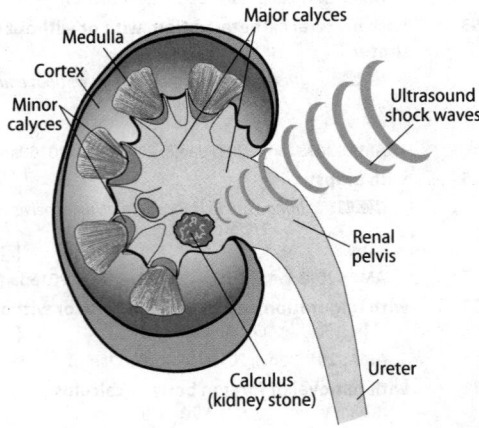

Major calyces
Medulla
Cortex
Minor calyces
Ultrasound shock waves
Renal pelvis
Ureter
Calculus (kidney stone)

50592 **Ablation, 1 or more renal tumor(s), percutaneous, unilateral, radiofrequency**
☒ (76940, 77013, 77022)
🔧 9.93 ⚕ 92.3 **FUD** 010   J 62 50 ▢
AMA: 2014,Jan,11

50593 **Ablation, renal tumor(s), unilateral, percutaneous, cryotherapy**
☒ (76940, 77013, 77022)
🔧 13.3 ⚕ 125. **FUD** 010   J J8 80 50 ▢
AMA: 2018,Jan,8

50600-50940 Open and Injection Procedures of Ureter

50600 **Ureterotomy with exploration or drainage (separate procedure)**
Code also ureteral endoscopy through ureterotomy when procedures constitute significant identifiable service (50970-50980)
🔧 27.1 ⚕ 27.1 **FUD** 090   C 80 50 ▢
AMA: 2014,Jan,11; 2000,Oct,8

50605 **Ureterotomy for insertion of indwelling stent, all types**
🔧 28.6 ⚕ 28.6 **FUD** 090   C 80 50 ▢
AMA: 2018,Jan,8; 2017,Jan,8; 2016,Jan,13

+ **50606** **Endoluminal biopsy of ureter and/or renal pelvis, non-endoscopic, including imaging guidance (eg, ultrasound and/or fluoroscopy) and all associated radiological supervision and interpretation (List separately in addition to code for primary procedure)**
INCLUDES   Renal pelvis and associated ureter as single element
EXCLUDES   *Procedure performed for same renal collecting system/associated ureter with (50555, 50574, 50955, 50974, 52007, 74425)*
Code first (50382-50389, [50430, 50431, 50432, 50433, 50434, 50435], 50684, 50688, 50690, 50693-50695, 51610)
🔧 4.43 ⚕ 18.8 **FUD** ZZZ   N N1 50 ▢
AMA: 2018,Jan,8; 2017,Jan,8; 2016,Jan,3

50610 **Ureterolithotomy; upper one-third of ureter**
EXCLUDES   *Cystotomy with calculus basket extraction ureteral calculus (51065)*
Transvesical ureterolithotomy (51060)
Ureteral calculus manipulation/extraction performed endoscopically (50080-50081, 50561, 50961, 50980, 52320-52330, 52352-52353, [52356])
Ureterolithotomy performed laparoscopically (50945)
🔧 27.3 ⚕ 27.3 **FUD** 090   C 80 50 ▢
AMA: 2018,Jan,8; 2017,Jan,8; 2016,Jan,13

50620 **middle one-third of ureter**
EXCLUDES   *Cystotomy with calculus basket extraction ureteral calculus (51065)*
Transvesical ureterolithotomy (51060)
Ureteral calculus manipulation/extraction performed endoscopically (50080-50081, 50561, 50961, 50980, 52320-52330, 52352-52353, [52356])
Ureterolithotomy performed laparoscopically (50945)
🔧 26.1 ⚕ 26.1 **FUD** 090   C 80 50 ▢
AMA: 2018,Jan,8; 2017,Jan,8; 2016,Jan,13

50630 **lower one-third of ureter**
EXCLUDES   *Cystotomy with calculus basket extraction ureteral calculus (51065)*
Transvesical ureterolithotomy (51060)
Ureteral calculus manipulation/extraction performed endoscopically (50080-50081, 50561, 50961, 50980, 52320-52330, 52352-52353, [52356])
Ureterolithotomy performed laparoscopically (50945)
🔧 25.8 ⚕ 25.8 **FUD** 090   C 80 50 ▢
AMA: 2018,Jan,8; 2017,Jan,8; 2016,Jan,13

50650 **Ureterectomy, with bladder cuff (separate procedure)**
EXCLUDES   *Ureterocele (51535, 52300)*
🔧 30.0 ⚕ 30.0 **FUD** 090   C 80 50 ▢
AMA: 2014,Jan,11

50660 **Ureterectomy, total, ectopic ureter, combination abdominal, vaginal and/or perineal approach**
EXCLUDES   *Ureterocele (51535, 52300)*
🔧 33.0 ⚕ 33.0 **FUD** 090   C 80 ▢
AMA: 2014,Jan,11

50684 **Injection procedure for ureterography or ureteropyelography through ureterostomy or indwelling ureteral catheter**
EXCLUDES   *Placement nephroureteral catheter ([50433, 50434])*
Placement ureteral stent (50693-50695)
☒ (74425)
🔧 1.45 ⚕ 3.10 **FUD** 000   N N1 50 ▢
AMA: 2018,Jan,8; 2017,Jan,8; 2016,Jan,3

50686 **Manometric studies through ureterostomy or indwelling ureteral catheter**
🔧 2.54 ⚕ 4.03 **FUD** 000   S P2 80 ▢
AMA: 2014,Jan,11

50688 **Change of ureterostomy tube or externally accessible ureteral stent via ileal conduit**
☒ (75984)
🔧 2.25 ⚕ 2.25 **FUD** 010   J A2
AMA: 2018,Jan,8; 2017,Jan,8; 2016,Jan,3

50690 **Injection procedure for visualization of ileal conduit and/or ureteropyelography, exclusive of radiologic service**
☒ (74420, 74425)
🔧 2.02 ⚕ 2.87 **FUD** 000   N N1 ▢
AMA: 2018,Jan,8; 2017,Jan,8; 2016,Jan,3

26/TC PC/TC Only   A2-Z3 ASC Payment   50 Bilateral   ♂ Male Only   ♀ Female Only   🔧 Facility RVU   ⚕ Non-Facility RVU   ▢ CCI   ☒ CLIA
FUD Follow-up Days   **CMS:** IOM   **AMA:** CPT Asst   A-Y OPPSI   80/80 Surg Assist Allowed / w/Doc   Lab Crosswalk   Radiology Crosswalk

234

50693 Placement of ureteral stent, percutaneous, including diagnostic nephrostogram and/or ureterogram when performed, imaging guidance (eg, ultrasound and/or fluoroscopy), and all associated radiological supervision and interpretation; pre-existing nephrostomy tract

INCLUDES Renal pelvis and associated ureter as single element

EXCLUDES *Procedure performed for same renal collecting system/ureter ([50430, 50431, 50432, 50433, 50434, 50435], 50684, 74425)*

🔧 5.94 ✂ 28.7 **FUD** 000 [J] [G2] [50] ▣

AMA: 2018,Jan,8; 2017,Jan,8; 2016,Jan,3; 2016,Jan,13

Proximal curl of stent in kidney

Indwelling stent

Catheter

Ureter

Distal curl of stent in bladder

Bladder

50694 new access, without separate nephrostomy catheter

INCLUDES Renal pelvis and associated ureter as single element

EXCLUDES *Procedure performed for same renal collecting system/ureter ([50430, 50431, 50432, 50433, 50434, 50435], 50684, 74425)*

🔧 7.77 ✂ 31.7 **FUD** 000 [J] [G2] [50] ▣

AMA: 2018,Jan,8; 2017,Jan,8; 2016,Jan,3; 2016,Jan,13

50695 new access, with separate nephrostomy catheter

INCLUDES Placement separate ureteral stent and nephrostomy catheter into ureter/associated renal pelvis through new access

Renal pelvis and associated ureter as single element

EXCLUDES *Procedure performed for same renal collecting system/ureter ([50430, 50431, 50432, 50433, 50434, 50435], 50684, 74425)*

🔧 9.96 ✂ 37.8 **FUD** 000 [J] [G2] [50] ▣

AMA: 2018,Jan,8; 2017,Jan,8; 2016,Jan,3; 2016,Jan,13

50700 Ureteroplasty, plastic operation on ureter (eg, stricture)

🔧 26.7 ✂ 26.7 **FUD** 090 [C] [80] [50] ▣

AMA: 2014,Jan,11

+ 50705 Ureteral embolization or occlusion, including imaging guidance (eg, ultrasound and/or fluoroscopy) and all associated radiological supervision and interpretation (List separately in addition to code for primary procedure)

INCLUDES Renal pelvis and associated ureter as single element

Code also when performed:
Additional catheter insertions
Diagnostic pyelography/ureterography
Other interventions

Code first (50382-50389, [50430, 50431, 50432, 50433, 50434, 50435], 50684, 50688, 50690, 50693-50695, 51610)

🔧 5.69 ✂ 56.8 **FUD** ZZZ [N] [N1] [50] ▣

AMA: 2018,Jan,8; 2017,Jan,8; 2016,Jan,3

+ 50706 Balloon dilation, ureteral stricture, including imaging guidance (eg, ultrasound and/or fluoroscopy) and all associated radiological supervision and interpretation (List separately in addition to code for primary procedure)

INCLUDES Dilation nephrostomy, ureters, or urethra (74485)
Renal pelvis and associated ureter as single element

EXCLUDES *Cystourethroscopy (52341, 52344-52345)*
Renal endoscopy (50553, 50572)
Ureteral endoscopy (50953, 50972)

Code also when performed:
Additional catheter insertions
Diagnostic pyelography/ureterography
Other interventions

Code first (50382-50389, [50430, 50431, 50432, 50433, 50434, 50435], 50684, 50688, 50690, 50693-50695, 51610)

🔧 5.31 ✂ 27.4 **FUD** ZZZ [N] [N1] [50] ▣

AMA: 2018,Jan,8; 2017,Jan,8; 2016,Jan,3

50715 Ureterolysis, with or without repositioning of ureter for retroperitoneal fibrosis

🔧 35.2 ✂ 35.2 **FUD** 090 [C] [80] [50] ▣

AMA: 2014,Jan,11

50722 Ureterolysis for ovarian vein syndrome ♀

🔧 29.8 ✂ 29.8 **FUD** 090 [C] [80] ▣

AMA: 2014,Jan,11

50725 Ureterolysis for retrocaval ureter, with reanastomosis of upper urinary tract or vena cava

🔧 31.9 ✂ 31.9 **FUD** 090 [C] [80] ▣

AMA: 2014,Jan,11

50727 Revision of urinary-cutaneous anastomosis (any type urostomy);

🔧 14.7 ✂ 14.7 **FUD** 090 [J] [G2] [80] ▣

AMA: 2014,Jan,11; 1992,Win,1

50728 with repair of fascial defect and hernia

🔧 21.2 ✂ 21.2 **FUD** 090 [C] [80] ▣

AMA: 2014,Jan,11; 1992,Win,1

50740 Ureteropyelostomy, anastomosis of ureter and renal pelvis

🔧 35.4 ✂ 35.4 **FUD** 090 [C] [80] [50] ▣

AMA: 2018,Jan,8; 2017,Jan,8; 2016,Jan,13

50750 Ureterocalycostomy, anastomosis of ureter to renal calyx

🔧 33.3 ✂ 33.3 **FUD** 090 [C] [80] [50] ▣

AMA: 2018,Jan,8; 2017,Jan,8; 2016,Jan,13

50760 Ureteroureterostomy

🔧 32.6 ✂ 32.6 **FUD** 090 [C] [80] [50] ▣

AMA: 2018,Jan,8; 2017,Jan,8; 2016,Jan,13

50770 Transureteroureterostomy, anastomosis of ureter to contralateral ureter

🔧 33.3 ✂ 33.3 **FUD** 090 [C] [80] ▣

AMA: 2014,Jan,11

50780 Ureteroneocystostomy; anastomosis of single ureter to bladder

INCLUDES Minor procedures to prevent vesicoureteral reflux

EXCLUDES *Cystourethroplasty with ureteroneocystostomy (51820)*

🔧 31.9 ✂ 31.9 **FUD** 090 [C] [80] [50] ▣

AMA: 2018,Feb,11; 2018,Jan,8; 2017,Jan,8; 2016,Jan,13

50782 anastomosis of duplicated ureter to bladder

INCLUDES Minor procedures to prevent vesicoureteral reflux

🔧 31.1 ✂ 31.1 **FUD** 090 [C] [80] [50] ▣

AMA: 2018,Jan,8; 2017,Jan,8; 2016,Jan,13

50783 with extensive ureteral tailoring

INCLUDES Minor procedures to prevent vesicoureteral reflux

🔧 32.6 ✂ 32.6 **FUD** 090 [C] [80] [50] ▣

AMA: 2018,Jan,8; 2017,Jan,8; 2016,Jan,13

50785 with vesico-psoas hitch or bladder flap

INCLUDES Minor procedures to prevent vesicoureteral reflux

🔧 35.1 ✂ 35.1 **FUD** 090 [C] [80] [50] ▣

AMA: 2018,Jan,8; 2017,Jan,8; 2016,Jan,13

50800   Ureteroenterostomy, direct anastomosis of ureter to intestine

> EXCLUDES   *Cystectomy with ureterosigmoidostomy/ureteroileal conduit (51580-51595)*

> 🔧 26.8   ⚕ 26.8   **FUD** 090   C 80 50 ▭

> **AMA:** 2018,Jan,8; 2017,Jan,8; 2016,Jan,13

50810   Ureterosigmoidostomy, with creation of sigmoid bladder and establishment of abdominal or perineal colostomy, including intestine anastomosis

> EXCLUDES   *Cystectomy with ureterosigmoidostomy/ureteroileal conduit (51580-51595)*

> 🔧 40.8   ⚕ 40.8   **FUD** 090   C 80 ▭

> **AMA:** 2018,Jan,8; 2017,Jan,8; 2016,Jan,13

50815   Ureterocolon conduit, including intestine anastomosis

> EXCLUDES   *Cystectomy with ureterosigmoidostomy/ureteroileal conduit (51580-51595)*

> 🔧 35.3   ⚕ 35.3   **FUD** 090   C 80 50 ▭

> **AMA:** 2018,Jan,8; 2017,Jan,8; 2016,Jan,13

50820   Ureteroileal conduit (ileal bladder), including intestine anastomosis (Bricker operation)

> EXCLUDES   *Cystectomy with ureterosigmoidostomy/ureteroileal conduit (51580-51595)*

> 🔧 38.0   ⚕ 38.0   **FUD** 090   C 80 50 ▭

> **AMA:** 2018,Jan,8; 2017,Jan,8; 2016,Jan,13

50825   Continent diversion, including intestine anastomosis using any segment of small and/or large intestine (Kock pouch or Camey enterocystoplasty)

> 🔧 47.8   ⚕ 47.8   **FUD** 090   C 80 ▭

> **AMA:** 2018,Jan,8; 2017,Jan,8; 2016,Jan,13

50830   Urinary undiversion (eg, taking down of ureteroileal conduit, ureterosigmoidostomy or ureteroenterostomy with ureteroureterostomy or ureteroneocystostomy)

> 🔧 52.1   ⚕ 52.1   **FUD** 090   C 80 ▭

> **AMA:** 2018,Jan,8; 2017,Jan,8; 2016,Jan,13

50840   Replacement of all or part of ureter by intestine segment, including intestine anastomosis

> 🔧 35.5   ⚕ 35.5   **FUD** 090   C 80 50 ▭

> **AMA:** 2018,Jan,8; 2017,Jan,8; 2016,Jan,13

50845   Cutaneous appendico-vesicostomy

> INCLUDES   Mitrofanoff operation

> 🔧 36.1   ⚕ 36.1   **FUD** 090   C 80 ▭

> **AMA:** 2014,Jan,11; 1993,Win,1

50860   Ureterostomy, transplantation of ureter to skin

> 🔧 27.3   ⚕ 27.3   **FUD** 090   C 80 50 ▭

> **AMA:** 2014,Jan,11; 2001,Oct,8

50900   Ureterorrhaphy, suture of ureter (separate procedure)

> 🔧 24.3   ⚕ 24.3   **FUD** 090   C 80 50 ▭

> **AMA:** 2014,Jan,11; 2001,Oct,8

50920   Closure of ureterocutaneous fistula

> 🔧 25.5   ⚕ 25.5   **FUD** 090   C 80 ▭

> **AMA:** 2014,Jan,11; 2001,Oct,8

50930   Closure of ureterovisceral fistula (including visceral repair)

> 🔧 31.8   ⚕ 31.8   **FUD** 090   C 80 ▭

> **AMA:** 2014,Jan,11; 2001,Oct,8

50940   Deligation of ureter

> EXCLUDES   *Ureteroplasty/ureterolysis (50700-50860)*

> 🔧 25.6   ⚕ 25.6   **FUD** 090   C 80 50 ▭

> **AMA:** 2014,Jan,11; 2001,Oct,8

50945-50949 Laparoscopic Procedures of Ureter

> INCLUDES   Diagnostic laparoscopy (49320)

> EXCLUDES   *Ureteroneocystostomy, open approach (50780-50785)*

50945   Laparoscopy, surgical; ureterolithotomy

> 🔧 28.1   ⚕ 28.1   **FUD** 090   J 02 80 50 ▭

> **AMA:** 2018,Jan,8; 2017,Jan,8; 2016,Jan,13

50947   ureteroneocystostomy with cystoscopy and ureteral stent placement

> 🔧 40.1   ⚕ 40.1   **FUD** 090   J A2 80 50 ▭

> **AMA:** 2018,Jan,8; 2017,Jan,8; 2016,Jan,13

50948   ureteroneocystostomy without cystoscopy and ureteral stent placement

> 🔧 36.7   ⚕ 36.7   **FUD** 090   J A2 80 50 ▭

> **AMA:** 2018,Jan,8; 2017,Jan,8; 2016,Jan,13

50949   Unlisted laparoscopy procedure, ureter

> 🔧 0.00   ⚕ 0.00   **FUD** YYY   J 80 50 ▭

> **AMA:** 2018,Jan,8; 2017,Jan,8; 2016,Jan,13

50951-50961 Endoscopic Procedures of Ureter via Established Ureterostomy Access

50951   Ureteral endoscopy through established ureterostomy, with or without irrigation, instillation, or ureteropyelography, exclusive of radiologic service;

> 🔧 8.89   ⚕ 10.9   **FUD** 000   J A2 80 50 ▭

> **AMA:** 2018,Jan,8; 2017,Jan,8; 2016,Jan,13

50953   with ureteral catheterization, with or without dilation of ureter

> EXCLUDES   *Image-guided ureter dilation without endoscopic guidance (50706)*

> 🔧 9.46   ⚕ 11.5   **FUD** 000   J A2 80 50 ▭

> **AMA:** 2018,Jan,8; 2017,Jan,8; 2016,Jan,13; 2016,Jan,3

50955   with biopsy

> EXCLUDES   *Image-guided biopsy of ureter and/or renal pelvis without endoscopic guidance (50606)*

> 🔧 10.2   ⚕ 12.3   **FUD** 000   J A2 80 50 ▭

> **AMA:** 2018,Jan,8; 2017,Jan,8; 2016,Jan,13; 2016,Jan,3

50957   with fulguration and/or incision, with or without biopsy

> 🔧 10.2   ⚕ 12.4   **FUD** 000   J A2 80 50 ▭

> **AMA:** 2018,Jan,8; 2017,Jan,8; 2016,Jan,13

50961   with removal of foreign body or calculus

> 🔧 9.17   ⚕ 11.1   **FUD** 000   J A2 80 50 ▭

> **AMA:** 2018,Jan,8; 2017,Jan,8; 2016,Jan,13

50970-50980 Endoscopic Procedures of Ureter via Ureterotomy

> EXCLUDES   *Ureterotomy (50600)*

50970   Ureteral endoscopy through ureterotomy, with or without irrigation, instillation, or ureteropyelography, exclusive of radiologic service;

> 🔧 10.7   ⚕ 10.7   **FUD** 000   J A2 80 50 ▭

> **AMA:** 2018,Jan,8; 2017,Jan,8; 2016,Jan,13

50972   with ureteral catheterization, with or without dilation of ureter

> EXCLUDES   *Image-guided ureter dilation without endoscopic guidance (50706)*

> 🔧 10.3   ⚕ 10.3   **FUD** 000   J A2 80 50 ▭

> **AMA:** 2018,Jan,8; 2017,Jan,8; 2016,Jan,3; 2016,Jan,13

50974   with biopsy

> EXCLUDES   *Image-guided biopsy of ureter and/or renal pelvis without endoscopic guidance (50606)*

> 🔧 13.6   ⚕ 13.6   **FUD** 000   J A2 80 50 ▭

> **AMA:** 2018,Jan,8; 2017,Jan,8; 2016,Jan,3; 2016,Jan,13

50976   with fulguration and/or incision, with or without biopsy

> 🔧 13.5   ⚕ 13.5   **FUD** 000   J A2 80 50 ▭

> **AMA:** 2018,Jan,8; 2017,Jan,8; 2016,Jan,13

50980   with removal of foreign body or calculus

> 🔧 10.3   ⚕ 10.3   **FUD** 000   J A2 80 50 ▭

> **AMA:** 2018,Jan,8; 2017,Jan,8; 2016,Jan,13

51020-51080 Open Incisional Procedures of Bladder

51020   Cystotomy or cystostomy; with fulguration and/or insertion of radioactive material

> 🔧 13.5   ⚕ 13.5   **FUD** 090   J A2 80 ▭

> **AMA:** 2014,Jan,11

51030 with cryosurgical destruction of intravesical lesion
🔧 13.6 ⚖ 13.6 **FUD** 090 J A2 80 ▢
AMA: 2014,Jan,11

51040 Cystostomy, cystotomy with drainage
🔧 8.36 ⚖ 8.36 **FUD** 090 J A2 80 ▢
AMA: 2014,Jan,11

51045 Cystotomy, with insertion of ureteral catheter or stent (separate procedure)
🔧 14.4 ⚖ 14.4 **FUD** 090 J A2 80 ▢
AMA: 2014,Jan,11

51050 Cystolithotomy, cystotomy with removal of calculus, without vesical neck resection
🔧 13.6 ⚖ 13.6 **FUD** 090 J A2 80 ▢
AMA: 2014,Jan,11

51060 Transvesical ureterolithotomy
🔧 16.8 ⚖ 16.8 **FUD** 090 J G2 80 ▢
AMA: 2014,Jan,11

51065 Cystotomy, with calculus basket extraction and/or ultrasonic or electrohydraulic fragmentation of ureteral calculus
🔧 16.7 ⚖ 16.7 **FUD** 090 J A2 80 ▢
AMA: 2014,Jan,11; 2002,May,7

51080 Drainage of perivesical or prevesical space abscess
EXCLUDES *Image-guided percutaneous catheter drainage (49406)*
🔧 11.8 ⚖ 11.8 **FUD** 090 J A2 80 ▢
AMA: 2014,Jan,11

51100-51102 Bladder Aspiration Procedures

51100 Aspiration of bladder; by needle
▦ (76942, 77002, 77012)
🔧 1.13 ⚖ 1.84 **FUD** 000 T P3 ▢
AMA: 2018,Jan,8; 2017,Jan,8; 2016,Jan,13

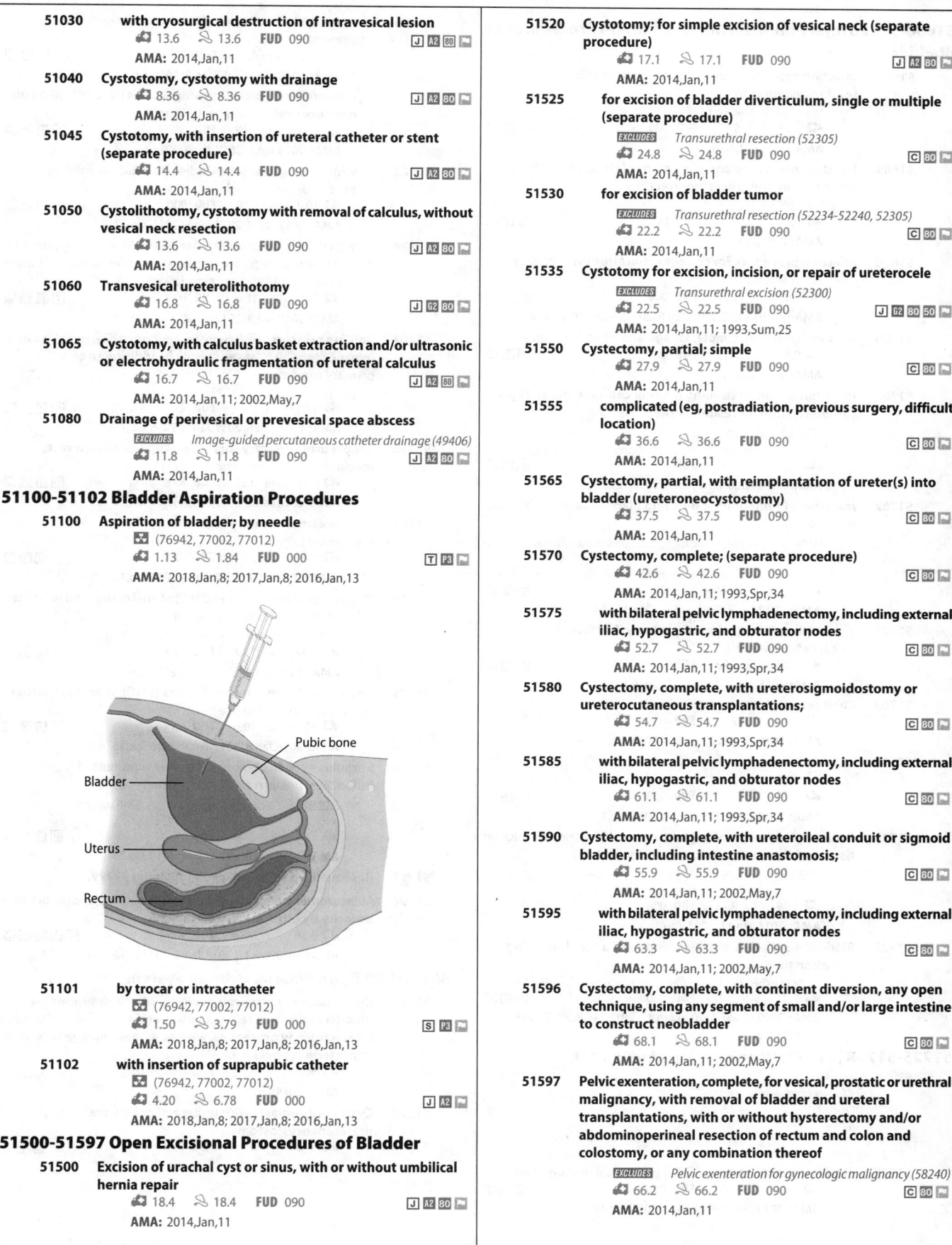

Pubic bone
Bladder
Uterus
Rectum

51101 by trocar or intracatheter
▦ (76942, 77002, 77012)
🔧 1.50 ⚖ 3.79 **FUD** 000 S P3 ▢
AMA: 2018,Jan,8; 2017,Jan,8; 2016,Jan,13

51102 with insertion of suprapubic catheter
▦ (76942, 77002, 77012)
🔧 4.20 ⚖ 6.78 **FUD** 000 J A2 ▢
AMA: 2018,Jan,8; 2017,Jan,8; 2016,Jan,13

51500-51597 Open Excisional Procedures of Bladder

51500 Excision of urachal cyst or sinus, with or without umbilical hernia repair
🔧 18.4 ⚖ 18.4 **FUD** 090 J A2 80 ▢
AMA: 2014,Jan,11

51520 Cystotomy; for simple excision of vesical neck (separate procedure)
🔧 17.1 ⚖ 17.1 **FUD** 090 J A2 80 ▢
AMA: 2014,Jan,11

51525 for excision of bladder diverticulum, single or multiple (separate procedure)
EXCLUDES *Transurethral resection (52305)*
🔧 24.8 ⚖ 24.8 **FUD** 090 C 80 ▢
AMA: 2014,Jan,11

51530 for excision of bladder tumor
EXCLUDES *Transurethral resection (52234-52240, 52305)*
🔧 22.2 ⚖ 22.2 **FUD** 090 C 80 ▢
AMA: 2014,Jan,11

51535 Cystotomy for excision, incision, or repair of ureterocele
EXCLUDES *Transurethral excision (52300)*
🔧 22.5 ⚖ 22.5 **FUD** 090 J G2 80 50 ▢
AMA: 2014,Jan,11; 1993,Sum,25

51550 Cystectomy, partial; simple
🔧 27.9 ⚖ 27.9 **FUD** 090 C 80 ▢
AMA: 2014,Jan,11

51555 complicated (eg, postradiation, previous surgery, difficult location)
🔧 36.6 ⚖ 36.6 **FUD** 090 C 80 ▢
AMA: 2014,Jan,11

51565 Cystectomy, partial, with reimplantation of ureter(s) into bladder (ureteroneocystostomy)
🔧 37.5 ⚖ 37.5 **FUD** 090 C 80 ▢
AMA: 2014,Jan,11

51570 Cystectomy, complete; (separate procedure)
🔧 42.6 ⚖ 42.6 **FUD** 090 C 80 ▢
AMA: 2014,Jan,11; 1993,Spr,34

51575 with bilateral pelvic lymphadenectomy, including external iliac, hypogastric, and obturator nodes
🔧 52.7 ⚖ 52.7 **FUD** 090 C 80 ▢
AMA: 2014,Jan,11; 1993,Spr,34

51580 Cystectomy, complete, with ureterosigmoidostomy or ureterocutaneous transplantations;
🔧 54.7 ⚖ 54.7 **FUD** 090 C 80 ▢
AMA: 2014,Jan,11; 1993,Spr,34

51585 with bilateral pelvic lymphadenectomy, including external iliac, hypogastric, and obturator nodes
🔧 61.1 ⚖ 61.1 **FUD** 090 C 80 ▢
AMA: 2014,Jan,11; 1993,Spr,34

51590 Cystectomy, complete, with ureteroileal conduit or sigmoid bladder, including intestine anastomosis;
🔧 55.9 ⚖ 55.9 **FUD** 090 C 80 ▢
AMA: 2014,Jan,11; 2002,May,7

51595 with bilateral pelvic lymphadenectomy, including external iliac, hypogastric, and obturator nodes
🔧 63.3 ⚖ 63.3 **FUD** 090 C 80 ▢
AMA: 2014,Jan,11; 2002,May,7

51596 Cystectomy, complete, with continent diversion, any open technique, using any segment of small and/or large intestine to construct neobladder
🔧 68.1 ⚖ 68.1 **FUD** 090 C 80 ▢
AMA: 2014,Jan,11; 2002,May,7

51597 Pelvic exenteration, complete, for vesical, prostatic or urethral malignancy, with removal of bladder and ureteral transplantations, with or without hysterectomy and/or abdominoperineal resection of rectum and colon and colostomy, or any combination thereof
EXCLUDES *Pelvic exenteration for gynecologic malignancy (58240)*
🔧 66.2 ⚖ 66.2 **FUD** 090 C 80 ▢
AMA: 2014,Jan,11

51600-51720 Injection/Insertion/Instillation Procedures of Bladder

51600 Injection procedure for cystography or voiding urethrocystography
🔀 (74430, 74455)
🏥 1.29 ⚖ 5.57 **FUD** 000 N N1 🖵
AMA: 2019,Oct,10

51605 Injection procedure and placement of chain for contrast and/or chain urethrocystography
🔀 (74430)
🏥 1.11 ⚖ 1.11 **FUD** 000 N N1 🖵
AMA: 2014,Jan,11

51610 Injection procedure for retrograde urethrocystography
🔀 (74450)
🏥 1.85 ⚖ 3.21 **FUD** 000 N N1 🖵
AMA: 2019,Oct,10; 2018,Jan,8; 2017,Jan,8; 2016,Jan,3

51700 Bladder irrigation, simple, lavage and/or instillation
🏥 0.87 ⚖ 2.12 **FUD** 000 T P3 🖵
AMA: 2014,Jan,11

51701 Insertion of non-indwelling bladder catheter (eg, straight catheterization for residual urine)
EXCLUDES Catheterization for specimen collection (P9612)
Insertion catheter as another procedure component
🏥 0.73 ⚖ 1.27 **FUD** 000 Q1 N1 🖵
AMA: 2018,Jan,8; 2017,Jan,8; 2016,Jan,13

51702 Insertion of temporary indwelling bladder catheter; simple (eg, Foley)
EXCLUDES Focused ultrasound ablation uterine leiomyomata (0071T-0072T)
Insertion catheter as another procedure component
🏥 0.74 ⚖ 1.74 **FUD** 000 Q1 N1 🖵
AMA: 2018,Jan,8; 2017,Jan,8; 2016,Jan,13

51703 complicated (eg, altered anatomy, fractured catheter/balloon)
🏥 2.23 ⚖ 3.98 **FUD** 000 S P2 🖵
AMA: 2018,Jan,8; 2017,Jan,8; 2016,Jan,13

51705 Change of cystostomy tube; simple
🏥 1.50 ⚖ 2.67 **FUD** 000 T P3 🖵
AMA: 2018,Jan,8; 2017,Jan,8; 2016,Jan,13

51710 complicated
🔀 (75984)
🏥 2.28 ⚖ 3.77 **FUD** 000 T A2 🖵
AMA: 2018,Jan,8; 2017,Jan,8; 2016,Jan,13

51715 Endoscopic injection of implant material into the submucosal tissues of the urethra and/or bladder neck
EXCLUDES Injection bulking agent (submucosal) for fecal incontinence, via anoscope (46999)
🏥 5.79 ⚖ 9.78 **FUD** 000 J J8 🖵
AMA: 2014,Jan,11; 1993,Win,1

51720 Bladder instillation of anticarcinogenic agent (including retention time)
Code also bacillus Calmette-Guerin vaccine (BCG) (90586)
🏥 1.27 ⚖ 2.40 **FUD** 000 T P3 🖵
AMA: 2020,NovSE,1; 2020,Jan,11; 2018,Jan,8; 2017,Jan,8; 2016,Jan,13

51725-51798 [51797] Uroflowmetric Evaluations

INCLUDES Equipment
Fees for technician services
Medications
Supplies
Code also modifier 26 when physician/other qualified health care professional provides only interpretation results and/or operates equipment

51725 Simple cystometrogram (CMG) (eg, spinal manometer)
🏥 6.04 ⚖ 6.04 **FUD** 000 T P2 🖵
AMA: 2018,Jan,8; 2017,Jan,8; 2016,Jan,13

51726 Complex cystometrogram (ie, calibrated electronic equipment);
🏥 8.23 ⚖ 8.23 **FUD** 000 T A2 🖵
AMA: 2018,Jan,8; 2017,Jan,8; 2016,Jan,13

51727 with urethral pressure profile studies (ie, urethral closure pressure profile), any technique
🏥 9.39 ⚖ 9.39 **FUD** 000 T P3 80 🖵
AMA: 2018,Jan,8; 2017,Jan,8; 2016,Jan,13

51728 with voiding pressure studies (ie, bladder voiding pressure), any technique
🏥 10.0 ⚖ 10.0 **FUD** 000 T P3 80 🖵
AMA: 2018,Jan,8; 2017,Jan,8; 2016,Jan,13

51729 with voiding pressure studies (ie, bladder voiding pressure) and urethral pressure profile studies (ie, urethral closure pressure profile), any technique
🏥 10.6 ⚖ 10.6 **FUD** 000 T P3 80 🖵
AMA: 2018,Jan,8; 2017,Jan,8; 2016,Jan,13

+ # 51797 Voiding pressure studies, intra-abdominal (ie, rectal, gastric, intraperitoneal) (List separately in addition to code for primary procedure)
Code first (51728-51729)
🏥 4.61 ⚖ 4.61 **FUD** ZZZ N N1 80 🖵
AMA: 2018,Jan,8; 2017,Jan,8; 2016,Jan,13

51736 Simple uroflowmetry (UFR) (eg, stop-watch flow rate, mechanical uroflowmeter)
🏥 0.39 ⚖ 0.39 **FUD** XXX Q1 N1 80 🖵
AMA: 2018,Jan,8; 2017,Jan,8; 2016,Jan,13

51741 Complex uroflowmetry (eg, calibrated electronic equipment)
🏥 0.41 ⚖ 0.41 **FUD** XXX Q1 N1 🖵
AMA: 2018,Jan,8; 2017,Jan,8; 2016,Jan,13

51784 Electromyography studies (EMG) of anal or urethral sphincter, other than needle, any technique
EXCLUDES Stimulus evoked response (51792)
🏥 1.92 ⚖ 1.92 **FUD** XXX S P3 🖵
AMA: 2018,Jan,8; 2017,Jan,8; 2016,Jan,13

51785 Needle electromyography studies (EMG) of anal or urethral sphincter, any technique
🏥 10.6 ⚖ 10.6 **FUD** XXX T A2 80 🖵
AMA: 2018,Jan,8; 2017,Jan,8; 2016,Jan,13

51792 Stimulus evoked response (eg, measurement of bulbocavernosus reflex latency time)
EXCLUDES Electromyography studies (EMG) anal or urethral sphincter (51784)
🏥 7.04 ⚖ 7.04 **FUD** 000 Q1 N1 80 🖵
AMA: 2018,Jan,8; 2017,Jan,8; 2016,Jan,13

51797 Resequenced code. See code following 51729.

51798 Measurement of post-voiding residual urine and/or bladder capacity by ultrasound, non-imaging
🏥 0.36 ⚖ 0.36 **FUD** XXX Q1 N1 80 TC 🖵
AMA: 2018,Jun,11; 2018,Jan,8; 2017,Jan,8; 2016,Jan,13

51800-51980 Open Repairs Urinary System

51800 Cystoplasty or cystourethroplasty, plastic operation on bladder and/or vesical neck (anterior Y-plasty, vesical fundus resection), any procedure, with or without wedge resection of posterior vesical neck
🏥 30.3 ⚖ 30.3 **FUD** 090 C 80 🖵
AMA: 2014,Jan,11

51820 Cystourethroplasty with unilateral or bilateral ureteroneocystostomy
🏥 31.3 ⚖ 31.3 **FUD** 090 C 80 🖵
AMA: 2014,Jan,11

51840   Anterior vesicourethropexy, or urethropexy (eg, Marshall-Marchetti-Krantz, Burch); simple
EXCLUDES   *Pereyra type urethropexy (57289)*
🚗 19.3   ⚕ 19.3   **FUD** 090   ⃞C ⃞80 ⃞
AMA: 2018,Jan,8; 2017,Jan,8; 2016,Jan,13

51841   complicated (eg, secondary repair)
EXCLUDES   *Pereyra type urethropexy (57289)*
🚗 22.4   ⚕ 22.4   **FUD** 090   ⃞C ⃞80 ⃞
AMA: 2018,Jan,8; 2017,Jan,8; 2016,Jan,13

51845   Abdomino-vaginal vesical neck suspension, with or without endoscopic control (eg, Stamey, Raz, modified Pereyra) ♀
🚗 16.8   ⚕ 16.8   **FUD** 090   ⃞J ⃞G2 ⃞80 ⃞
AMA: 2018,Jan,8; 2017,Jan,8; 2016,Jan,13

51860   Cystorrhaphy, suture of bladder wound, injury or rupture; simple
🚗 21.5   ⚕ 21.5   **FUD** 090   ⃞J ⃞G2 ⃞80 ⃞
AMA: 2014,Jan,11

51865   complicated
🚗 25.9   ⚕ 25.9   **FUD** 090   ⃞C ⃞80 ⃞
AMA: 2014,Jan,11

51880   Closure of cystostomy (separate procedure)
🚗 13.5   ⚕ 13.5   **FUD** 090   ⃞J ⃞A2 ⃞80 ⃞
AMA: 2014,Jan,11

Physician removes a cystostomy tube

51900   Closure of vesicovaginal fistula, abdominal approach ♀
EXCLUDES   *Vesicovaginal fistula closure, vaginal approach (57320-57330)*
🚗 23.8   ⚕ 23.8   **FUD** 090   ⃞C ⃞80 ⃞
AMA: 2014,Jan,11

51920   Closure of vesicouterine fistula; ♀
EXCLUDES   *Enterovesical fistula closure (44660-44661)*
Rectovesical fistula closure (45800-45805)
🚗 22.0   ⚕ 22.0   **FUD** 090   ⃞C ⃞80 ⃞
AMA: 2014,Jan,11

51925   with hysterectomy ♀
EXCLUDES   *Enterovesical fistula closure (44660-44661)*
Rectovesical fistula closure (45800-45805)
🚗 29.5   ⚕ 29.5   **FUD** 090   ⃞C ⃞80 ⃞
AMA: 2014,Jan,11

51940   Closure, exstrophy of bladder
EXCLUDES   *Epispadias reconstruction with exstrophy bladder (54390)*
🚗 47.5   ⚕ 47.5   **FUD** 090   ⃞C ⃞80 ⃞
AMA: 2014,Jan,11; 2002,May,7

51960   Enterocystoplasty, including intestinal anastomosis
🚗 40.0   ⚕ 40.0   **FUD** 090   ⃞C ⃞80 ⃞
AMA: 2014,Jan,11; 2002,May,7

51980   Cutaneous vesicostomy
🚗 20.6   ⚕ 20.6   **FUD** 090   ⃞C ⃞80 ⃞
AMA: 2014,Jan,11

51990-51999 Laparoscopic Procedures of Urinary System

CMS: 100-03,230.10 Incontinence Control Devices
INCLUDES   Diagnostic laparoscopy (49320)

51990   Laparoscopy, surgical; urethral suspension for stress incontinence
🚗 21.6   ⚕ 21.6   **FUD** 090   ⃞J ⃞G2 ⃞80 ⃞
AMA: 2019,Feb,10; 2018,Jan,8; 2017,Jan,8; 2016,Jan,13

51992   sling operation for stress incontinence (eg, fascia or synthetic)
EXCLUDES   *Removal/revision sling for stress incontinence (57287)*
Sling operation for stress incontinence, open approach (57288)
🚗 24.0   ⚕ 24.0   **FUD** 090   ⃞J ⃞J8 ⃞80 ⃞
AMA: 2019,Feb,10; 2018,Jan,8; 2017,Jan,8; 2016,Jan,13

51999   Unlisted laparoscopy procedure, bladder
🚗 0.00   ⚕ 0.00   **FUD** YYY   ⃞J ⃞80 ⃞
AMA: 2018,Jan,8; 2017,Dec,14

52000-52318 Endoscopic Procedures via Urethra: Bladder and Urethra

INCLUDES   Diagnostic and therapeutic endoscopy bowel segments utilized as replacements for native bladder

52000   Cystourethroscopy (separate procedure)
EXCLUDES   *Cystourethroscopy (52001, 52320, 52325, 52327, 52330, 52332, 52334, 52341-52343, [52356], 57240, 57260, 57265)*
🚗 2.34   ⚕ 5.39   **FUD** 000   ⃞T ⃞A2 ⃞
AMA: 2019,Feb,10; 2018,Nov,10; 2018,Jan,8; 2017,Oct,9; 2017,Jan,8; 2016,Jan,13

52001   Cystourethroscopy with irrigation and evacuation of multiple obstructing clots
INCLUDES   Cystourethroscopy (separate procedure) (52000)
🚗 8.31   ⚕ 11.3   **FUD** 000   ⃞J ⃞A2 ⃞
AMA: 2014,Jan,11; 2001,May,5

52005   Cystourethroscopy, with ureteral catheterization, with or without irrigation, instillation, or ureteropyelography, exclusive of radiologic service;
INCLUDES   Howard test
🚗 3.84   ⚕ 8.05   **FUD** 000   ⃞J ⃞A2 ⃞
AMA: 2019,Mar,10; 2018,Jan,8; 2017,Jan,8; 2016,Jan,13

52007   with brush biopsy of ureter and/or renal pelvis
EXCLUDES   *Image-guided ureter/renal pelvis biopsy without endoscopic guidance (50606)*
🚗 4.80   ⚕ 13.1   **FUD** 000   ⃞J ⃞A2 ⃞50 ⃞
AMA: 2018,Jan,8; 2017,Jan,8; 2016,Jan,13; 2016,Jan,3

52010   Cystourethroscopy, with ejaculatory duct catheterization, with or without irrigation, instillation, or duct radiography, exclusive of radiologic service ♂
📷 (74440)
🚗 4.79   ⚕ 10.9   **FUD** 000   ⃞T ⃞A2 ⃞
AMA: 2018,Jan,8; 2017,Jan,8; 2016,Jan,13

52204   Cystourethroscopy, with biopsy(s)
🚗 4.08   ⚕ 10.8   **FUD** 000   ⃞J ⃞A2 ⃞
AMA: 2018,Jan,8; 2017,Jan,8; 2016,May,12; 2016,Jan,13

52214 Cystourethroscopy, with fulguration (including cryosurgery or laser surgery) of trigone, bladder neck, prostatic fossa, urethra, or periurethral glands

Code also modifier 78 when performed by same physician:
During postoperative period (52601, 52630)
During postoperative period related surgical procedure
For postoperative bleeding

⏣ 5.10 ⚕ 20.0 **FUD** 000 [J] [A2] ▭

AMA: 2018,Jan,8; 2017,Jan,8; 2016,May,12; 2016,Jan,13

52224 Cystourethroscopy, with fulguration (including cryosurgery or laser surgery) or treatment of MINOR (less than 0.5 cm) lesion(s) with or without biopsy

⏣ 5.89 ⚕ 20.9 **FUD** 000 [J] [A2] ▭

AMA: 2018,Jan,8; 2017,Jan,8; 2016,May,12; 2016,Jan,13

52234 Cystourethroscopy, with fulguration (including cryosurgery or laser surgery) and/or resection of; SMALL bladder tumor(s) (0.5 up to 2.0 cm)

EXCLUDES *Bladder tumor excision through cystotomy (51530)*

⏣ 7.12 ⚕ 7.12 **FUD** 000 [J] [A2] ▭

AMA: 2018,Jan,8; 2017,Jan,8; 2016,May,12; 2016,Jan,13

52235 MEDIUM bladder tumor(s) (2.0 to 5.0 cm)

EXCLUDES *Bladder tumor excision through cystotomy (51530)*

⏣ 8.34 ⚕ 8.34 **FUD** 000 [J] [A2] ▭

AMA: 2018,Jan,8; 2017,Jan,8; 2016,May,12; 2016,Jan,13

52240 LARGE bladder tumor(s)

EXCLUDES *Bladder tumor excision through cystotomy (51530)*

⏣ 11.3 ⚕ 11.3 **FUD** 000 [J] [A2] ▭

AMA: 2018,Jan,8; 2017,Jan,8; 2016,May,12; 2016,Jan,13

52250 Cystourethroscopy with insertion of radioactive substance, with or without biopsy or fulguration

⏣ 6.92 ⚕ 6.92 **FUD** 000 [J] [A2] ▭

AMA: 2018,Jan,8; 2017,Jan,8; 2016,Jan,13

52260 Cystourethroscopy, with dilation of bladder for interstitial cystitis; general or conduction (spinal) anesthesia

⏣ 6.07 ⚕ 6.07 **FUD** 000 [J] [A2] ▭

AMA: 2018,Jan,8; 2017,Jan,8; 2016,Jan,13

52265 local anesthesia

⏣ 4.67 ⚕ 10.6 **FUD** 000 [J] [P3] ▭

AMA: 2018,Jan,8; 2017,Jan,8; 2016,Jan,13

52270 Cystourethroscopy, with internal urethrotomy; female ♀

⏣ 5.27 ⚕ 10.9 **FUD** 000 [J] [A2] ▭

AMA: 2018,Jan,8; 2017,Jan,8; 2016,Jan,13

52275 male ♂

⏣ 7.19 ⚕ 14.4 **FUD** 000 [J] [A2] ▭

AMA: 2018,Jan,8; 2017,Jan,8; 2016,Jan,13

52276 Cystourethroscopy with direct vision internal urethrotomy

⏣ 7.65 ⚕ 7.65 **FUD** 000 [J] [A2] ▭

AMA: 2019,Feb,10; 2018,Jan,8; 2017,Jan,8; 2016,Jan,13

52277 Cystourethroscopy, with resection of external sphincter (sphincterotomy)

⏣ 9.35 ⚕ 9.35 **FUD** 000 [J] [A2] [80] ▭

AMA: 2018,Jan,8; 2017,Jan,8; 2016,Jan,13

52281 Cystourethroscopy, with calibration and/or dilation of urethral stricture or stenosis, with or without meatotomy, with or without injection procedure for cystography, male or female

EXCLUDES *Urethral delivery therapeutic drug (0499T)*

⏣ 4.40 ⚕ 8.53 **FUD** 000 [J] [A2] ▭

AMA: 2018,Jan,8; 2017,Oct,9; 2017,Jan,8; 2016,Jan,13

52282 Cystourethroscopy, with insertion of permanent urethral stent

EXCLUDES *Placement temporary prostatic urethral stent (53855)*

⏣ 9.76 ⚕ 9.76 **FUD** 000 [J] [A2] ▭

AMA: 2018,Jan,8; 2017,Jan,8; 2016,Jan,13

52283 Cystourethroscopy, with steroid injection into stricture

⏣ 5.83 ⚕ 8.68 **FUD** 000 [J] [A2] ▭

AMA: 2019,Feb,10; 2018,Jan,8; 2017,Jan,8; 2016,Jan,13

52285 Cystourethroscopy for treatment of the female urethral syndrome with any or all of the following: urethral meatotomy, urethral dilation, internal urethrotomy, lysis of urethrovaginal septal fibrosis, lateral incisions of the bladder neck, and fulguration of polyp(s) of urethra, bladder neck, and/or trigone ♀

⏣ 5.66 ⚕ 8.66 **FUD** 000 [J] [A2] ▭

AMA: 2018,Jan,8; 2017,Jan,8; 2016,Jan,13

52287 Cystourethroscopy, with injection(s) for chemodenervation of the bladder

Code also supply chemodenervation agent

⏣ 4.89 ⚕ 9.65 **FUD** 000 [J] [G2] ▭

AMA: 2019,Apr,9

52290 Cystourethroscopy; with ureteral meatotomy, unilateral or bilateral

⏣ 7.07 ⚕ 7.07 **FUD** 000 [J] [A2] ▭

AMA: 2018,Jan,8; 2017,Jan,8; 2016,Jan,13

52300 with resection or fulguration of orthotopic ureterocele(s), unilateral or bilateral

⏣ 8.09 ⚕ 8.09 **FUD** 000 [J] [A2] [80] ▭

AMA: 2018,Jan,8; 2017,Jan,8; 2016,Jan,13

52301 with resection or fulguration of ectopic ureterocele(s), unilateral or bilateral

⏣ 8.38 ⚕ 8.38 **FUD** 000 [J] [A2] [80] ▭

AMA: 2018,Jan,8; 2017,Jan,8; 2016,Jan,13

52305 with incision or resection of orifice of bladder diverticulum, single or multiple

⏣ 8.06 ⚕ 8.06 **FUD** 000 [J] [A2] ▭

AMA: 2018,Jan,8; 2017,Jan,8; 2016,Jan,13

52310 Cystourethroscopy, with removal of foreign body, calculus, or ureteral stent from urethra or bladder (separate procedure); simple

Code also modifier 58 for removal self-retaining, indwelling ureteral stent

⏣ 4.38 ⚕ 7.68 **FUD** 000 [J] [A2] ▭

AMA: 2018,Jan,8; 2017,Jan,8; 2016,Jan,13

52315 complicated

Code also modifier 58 for removal self-retaining, indwelling ureteral stent

⏣ 7.94 ⚕ 12.6 **FUD** 000 [J] [A2] ▭

AMA: 2018,Jan,8; 2017,Jan,8; 2016,Jan,13

52317 Litholapaxy: crushing or fragmentation of calculus by any means in bladder and removal of fragments; simple or small (less than 2.5 cm)

⏣ 10.0 ⚕ 24.1 **FUD** 000 [J] [A2] ▭

AMA: 2018,Jan,8; 2017,Jan,8; 2016,Jan,13

52318 complicated or large (over 2.5 cm)

⏣ 13.7 ⚕ 13.7 **FUD** 000 [J] [A2] ▭

AMA: 2018,Jan,8; 2017,Jan,8; 2016,Jan,13

52320-52356 [52356] Endoscopic Procedures via Urethra: Renal Pelvis and Ureter

INCLUDES Diagnostic cystourethroscopy when performed with therapeutic cystourethroscopy
Insertion/removal temporary ureteral catheter (52005)

EXCLUDES *Self-retaining/indwelling ureteral stent removal by cystourethroscope, with modifier 58 when appropriate (52310, 52315)*

Code also insertion indwelling stent performed in addition to other procedures within this section (52332)

52320 Cystourethroscopy (including ureteral catheterization); with removal of ureteral calculus

INCLUDES Cystourethroscopy (separate procedure) (52000)

⏣ 7.13 ⚕ 7.13 **FUD** 000 [J] [A2] [50] ▭

AMA: 2018,Jan,8; 2017,Jan,8; 2016,Jan,13

CPT © 2021 American Medical Association. All Rights Reserved.

52325 **with fragmentation of ureteral calculus (eg, ultrasonic or electro-hydraulic technique)**
> INCLUDES Cystourethroscopy (separate procedure) (52000)
> 🚑 9.27 ⚕ 9.27 **FUD** 000 [J] [A2] [50] 🖿
> **AMA:** 2018,Jan,8; 2017,Jan,8; 2016,Jan,13

52327 **with subureteric injection of implant material**
> INCLUDES Cystourethroscopy (separate procedure) (52000)
> 🚑 7.59 ⚕ 7.59 **FUD** 000 [J] [J8] [50] 🖿
> **AMA:** 2018,Jan,8; 2017,Jan,8; 2016,Jan,13

52330 **with manipulation, without removal of ureteral calculus**
> INCLUDES Cystourethroscopy (separate procedure) (52000)
> 🚑 7.63 ⚕ 15.4 **FUD** 000 [J] [A2] [50] 🖿
> **AMA:** 2018,Jan,8; 2017,Jan,8; 2016,Jan,13

52332 **Cystourethroscopy, with insertion of indwelling ureteral stent (eg, Gibbons or double-J type)**
> INCLUDES Cystourethroscopy (separate procedure) (52000)
> EXCLUDES *Cystourethroscopy, with ureteroscopy and/or pyeloscopy; with lithotripsy when performed on same side with (52353, [52356])*
> 🚑 4.50 ⚕ 13.5 **FUD** 000 [J] [A2] [50] 🖿
> **AMA:** 2019,Dec,12; 2018,Jan,8; 2017,Jan,8; 2016,Jan,13

52334 **Cystourethroscopy with insertion of ureteral guide wire through kidney to establish a percutaneous nephrostomy, retrograde**
> INCLUDES Cystourethroscopy (separate procedure) (52000)
> EXCLUDES *Cystourethroscopy with incision/fulguration/resection congenital posterior urethral valves/obstructive hypertrophic mucosal folds (52400)*
> *Cystourethroscopy with pyeloscopy and/or ureteroscopy (52351-52353 [52356])*
> *Dilation nephroureteral catheter tract ([50436], [50437])*
> *Nephrostomy tract establishment only ([50432, 50433])*
> *Percutaneous nephrostolithotomy (50080, 50081)*
> 🚑 5.30 ⚕ 5.30 **FUD** 000 [J] [A2] 🖿
> **AMA:** 2018,Jan,8; 2017,Jan,8; 2016,Jan,13

52341 **Cystourethroscopy; with treatment of ureteral stricture (eg, balloon dilation, laser, electrocautery, and incision)**
> INCLUDES Diagnostic cystourethroscopy (52351)
> EXCLUDES *Balloon dilation with imaging guidance (50706)*
> *Cystourethroscopy, separate procedure (52000)*
> 🔧 (74485)
> 🚑 8.21 ⚕ 8.21 **FUD** 000 [J] [A2] [50] 🖿
> **AMA:** 2018,Jan,8; 2017,Jan,8; 2016,Jan,13; 2016,Jan,3

52342 **with treatment of ureteropelvic junction stricture (eg, balloon dilation, laser, electrocautery, and incision)**
> INCLUDES Diagnostic cystourethroscopy (52351)
> EXCLUDES *Balloon dilation with imaging guidance (50706)*
> *Cystourethroscopy (separate procedure) (52000)*
> 🔧 (74485)
> 🚑 8.93 ⚕ 8.93 **FUD** 000 [J] [A2] [50] 🖿
> **AMA:** 2018,Jan,8; 2017,Jan,8; 2016,Jan,13

52343 **with treatment of intra-renal stricture (eg, balloon dilation, laser, electrocautery, and incision)**
> INCLUDES Diagnostic cystourethroscopy (52351)
> EXCLUDES *Balloon dilation with imaging guidance (50706)*
> *Cystourethroscopy (separate procedure) (52000)*
> 🔧 (74485)
> 🚑 9.96 ⚕ 9.96 **FUD** 000 [J] [A2] [50] 🖿
> **AMA:** 2018,Jan,8; 2017,Jan,8; 2016,Jan,13

52344 **Cystourethroscopy with ureteroscopy; with treatment of ureteral stricture (eg, balloon dilation, laser, electrocautery, and incision)**
> INCLUDES Diagnostic cystourethroscopy (52351)
> EXCLUDES *Balloon dilation, ureteral stricture (50706)*
> *Cystourethroscopy with transurethral resection or incision ejaculatory ducts (52402)*
> 🔧 (74485)
> 🚑 10.6 ⚕ 10.6 **FUD** 000 [J] [A2] [50] 🖿
> **AMA:** 2018,Jan,8; 2017,Jan,8; 2016,Jan,13; 2016,Jan,3

52345 **with treatment of ureteropelvic junction stricture (eg, balloon dilation, laser, electrocautery, and incision)**
> INCLUDES Diagnostic cystourethroscopy (52351)
> EXCLUDES *Balloon dilation, ureteral stricture (50706)*
> *Cystourethroscopy with transurethral resection or incision ejaculatory ducts (52402)*
> 🔧 (74485)
> 🚑 11.4 ⚕ 11.4 **FUD** 000 [J] [A2] [80] [50] 🖿
> **AMA:** 2018,Jan,8; 2017,Jan,8; 2016,Jan,13; 2016,Jan,3

52346 **with treatment of intra-renal stricture (eg, balloon dilation, laser, electrocautery, and incision)**
> INCLUDES Diagnostic cystourethroscopy (52351)
> EXCLUDES *Balloon dilation with imaging guidance (50706)*
> *Cystourethroscopy with transurethral resection or incision ejaculatory ducts (52402)*
> 🔧 (74485)
> 🚑 12.9 ⚕ 12.9 **FUD** 000 [J] [A2] [80] [50] 🖿
> **AMA:** 2018,Jan,8; 2017,Jan,8; 2016,Jan,13

52351 **Cystourethroscopy, with ureteroscopy and/or pyeloscopy; diagnostic**
> EXCLUDES *Cystourethroscopy (52341-52346, 52352-52353 [52356])*
> 🚑 8.75 ⚕ 8.75 **FUD** 000 [J] [A2]
> **AMA:** 2018,Jan,8; 2017,Jan,8; 2016,Jan,13

52352 **with removal or manipulation of calculus (ureteral catheterization is included)**
> INCLUDES Diagnostic cystourethroscopy (52351)
> 🚑 10.2 ⚕ 10.2 **FUD** 000 [J] [A2] [50] 🖿
> **AMA:** 2018,Jan,8; 2017,Jan,8; 2016,Jan,13

Right kidney — Left kidney — Stone basket — Calculus — Ureters — Bladder — Cystourethroscope

52353 **with lithotripsy (ureteral catheterization is included)**
> INCLUDES Diagnostic cystourethroscopy (52351)
> EXCLUDES *Cystourethroscopy when performed on same side (52332, [52356])*
> 🚑 11.3 ⚕ 11.3 **FUD** 000 [J] [A2] [50] 🖿
> **AMA:** 2019,Dec,12; 2018,Jan,8; 2017,Jan,8; 2016,Jan,13

| 52356 with lithotripsy including insertion of indwelling ureteral stent (eg, Gibbons or double-J type)

> INCLUDES Diagnostic cystourethroscopy (52351)
>
> EXCLUDES Cystourethroscopy (separate procedure) (52000)
> When performed on same side:
> Cystourethroscopy, with insertion indwelling ureteral stent (e.g., Gibbons or double-J type) (52332)
> Cystourethroscopy, with ureteroscopy and/or pyeloscopy; with lithotripsy (ureteral catheterization is included) (52353)

🔹 12.0   ⚕ 12.0   **FUD** 000   J 62 50 ▭

AMA: 2019,Dec,12; 2018,Jan,8; 2017,Jan,8; 2016,Jan,13

52354 with biopsy and/or fulguration of ureteral or renal pelvic lesion

> INCLUDES Diagnostic cystourethroscopy (52351)
>
> EXCLUDES Image guided biopsy without endoscopic guidance (50606)

🔹 12.0   ⚕ 12.0   **FUD** 000   J A2 50 ▭

AMA: 2018,Jan,8; 2017,Jan,8; 2016,Jan,13

52355 with resection of ureteral or renal pelvic tumor

> INCLUDES Diagnostic cystourethroscopy (52351)

🔹 13.5   ⚕ 13.5   **FUD** 000   J A2 50 ▭

AMA: 2018,Jan,8; 2017,Jan,8; 2016,Jan,13

52356   Resequenced code. See code following 52353.

52400-52700 Endoscopic Procedures via Urethra: Prostate and Vesical Neck

52400 Cystourethroscopy with incision, fulguration, or resection of congenital posterior urethral valves, or congenital obstructive hypertrophic mucosal folds

🔹 13.8   ⚕ 13.8   **FUD** 090   J A2 ▭

AMA: 2018,Jan,8; 2017,Jan,8; 2016,Jan,13

52402 Cystourethroscopy with transurethral resection or incision of ejaculatory ducts ♂

🔹 7.73   ⚕ 7.73   **FUD** 000   J A2 ▭

AMA: 2014,Jan,11; 2001,Apr,4

52441 Cystourethroscopy, with insertion of permanent adjustable transprostatic implant; single implant

🔹 6.58   ⚕ 35.7   **FUD** 000   B ▭

AMA: 2018,Jan,8; 2017,Jan,8; 2016,Jan,13

+ ### 52442 each additional permanent adjustable transprostatic implant (List separately in addition to code for primary procedure)

> EXCLUDES Permanent urethral stent insertion (52282)
> Removal stent, calculus, or foreign body (implant) (52310)
> Temporary prostatic urethral stent insertion (53855)
> Code first (52441)

🔹 1.75   ⚕ 27.4   **FUD** ZZZ   B ▭

AMA: 2018,Jan,8; 2017,Jan,8; 2016,Jan,13

52450 Transurethral incision of prostate ♂

🔹 13.5   ⚕ 13.5   **FUD** 090   J A2 ▭

AMA: 2018,Jan,8; 2017,Jan,8; 2016,Jan,13

52500 Transurethral resection of bladder neck (separate procedure)

🔹 14.1   ⚕ 14.1   **FUD** 090   J A2 ▭

AMA: 2018,Jan,8; 2017,Jan,8; 2016,Jan,13

52601 Transurethral electrosurgical resection of prostate, including control of postoperative bleeding, complete (vasectomy, meatotomy, cystourethroscopy, urethral calibration and/or dilation, and internal urethrotomy are included) ♂

> INCLUDES Stage 1 partial transurethral resection prostate
>
> EXCLUDES Ablation by waterjet (0421T)
> Excision prostate (55801-55845)
> Transurethral fulguration prostate (52214)
> Code also modifier 58 for stage 2 partial transurethral resection prostate

🔹 21.0   ⚕ 21.0   **FUD** 090   J A2 ▭

AMA: 2018,Jan,8; 2017,Jan,8; 2016,Jan,13

52630 Transurethral resection; residual or regrowth of obstructive prostate tissue including control of postoperative bleeding, complete (vasectomy, meatotomy, cystourethroscopy, urethral calibration and/or dilation, and internal urethrotomy are included) ♂

> EXCLUDES Ablation by waterjet (0421T)
> Excision prostate (55801-55845)
> Code also modifier 78 when performed by same physician within postoperative period related procedure

🔹 11.5   ⚕ 11.5   **FUD** 090   J A2 ▭

AMA: 2018,Jan,8; 2017,Jan,8; 2016,Jan,13

52640 of postoperative bladder neck contracture

> EXCLUDES Excision prostate (55801-55845)

🔹 9.12   ⚕ 9.12   **FUD** 090   J A2 ▭

AMA: 2018,Jan,8; 2017,Jan,8; 2016,Jan,13

52647 Laser coagulation of prostate, including control of postoperative bleeding, complete (vasectomy, meatotomy, cystourethroscopy, urethral calibration and/or dilation, and internal urethrotomy are included if performed) ♂

🔹 18.7   ⚕ 46.2   **FUD** 090   J A2 ▭

AMA: 2018,Jan,8; 2017,Jan,8; 2016,Jan,13

52648 Laser vaporization of prostate, including control of postoperative bleeding, complete (vasectomy, meatotomy, cystourethroscopy, urethral calibration and/or dilation, internal urethrotomy and transurethral resection of prostate are included if performed) ♂

🔹 19.9   ⚕ 47.7   **FUD** 090   J A2 ▭

AMA: 2018,Jan,8; 2017,Jan,8; 2016,Jan,13

52649 Laser enucleation of the prostate with morcellation, including control of postoperative bleeding, complete (vasectomy, meatotomy, cystourethroscopy, urethral calibration and/or dilation, internal urethrotomy and transurethral resection of prostate are included if performed) ♂

> INCLUDES Cystourethroscopy (52000, 52276, 52281)
> Laser coagulation prostate (52647-52648)
> Meatotomy (53020)
> Transurethral resection of prostate (52601)
> Vasectomy (55250)

🔹 23.8   ⚕ 23.8   **FUD** 090   J 62 80 ▭

AMA: 2018,Jan,8; 2017,Jan,8; 2016,Jan,13

26/TC PC/TC Only   A2-Z3 ASC Payment   50 Bilateral   ♂ Male Only   ♀ Female Only   🔹 Facility RVU   ⚕ Non-Facility RVU   ▭ CCI   ☒ CLIA
FUD Follow-up Days   CMS: IOM   AMA: CPT Asst   A-Y OPPSI   80/80 Surg Assist Allowed / w/Doc   Lab Crosswalk   Radiology Crosswalk

© 2021 Optum360, LLC

52700 Transurethral drainage of prostatic abscess ♂
EXCLUDES Litholapaxy (52317, 52318)
🚑 12.7 ✂ 12.7 **FUD** 090 J A2 80 ▢
AMA: 2018,Jan,8; 2017,Jan,8; 2016,Jan,13

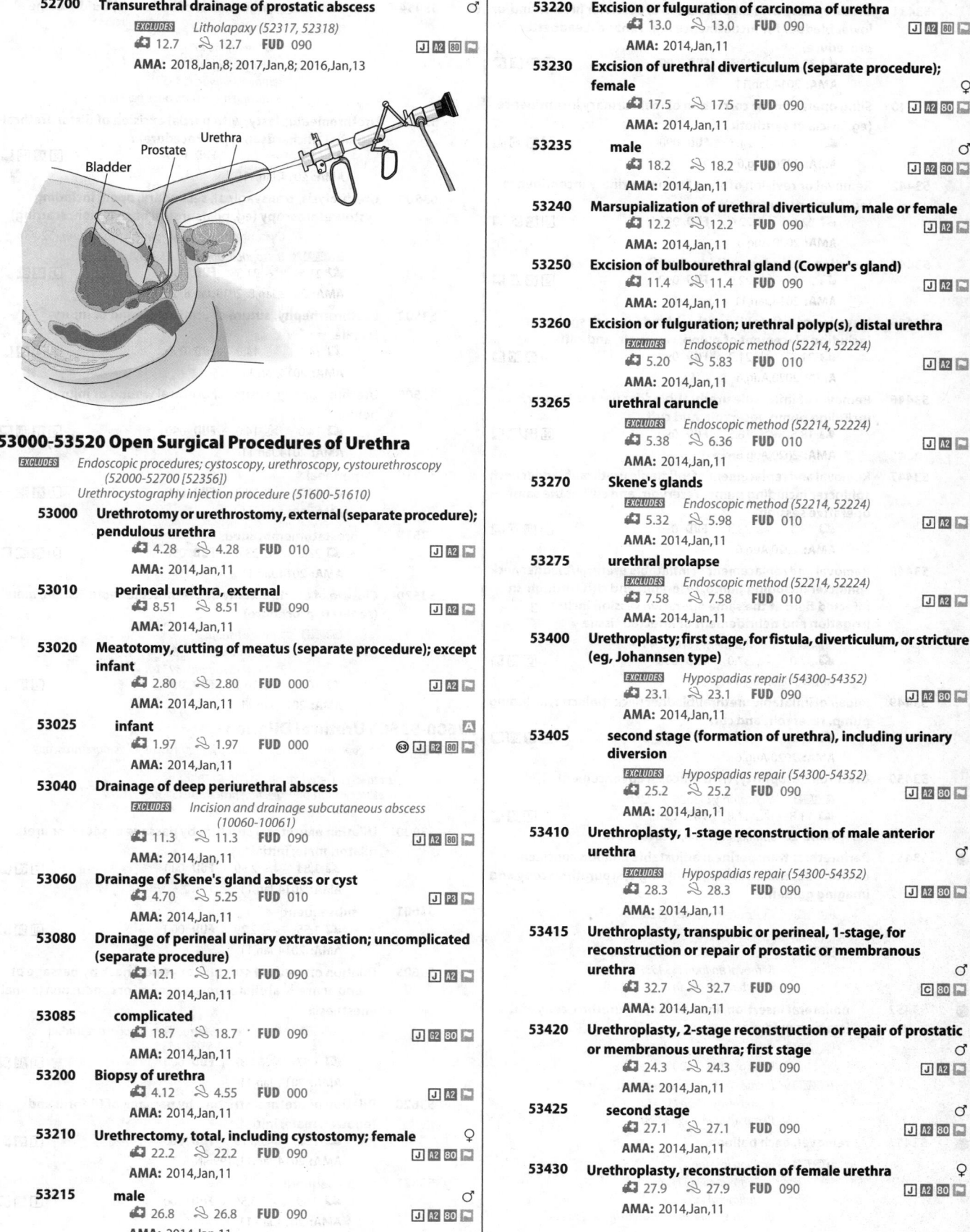

Bladder • Prostate • Urethra

53000-53520 Open Surgical Procedures of Urethra

EXCLUDES Endoscopic procedures; cystoscopy, urethroscopy, cystourethroscopy
(52000-52700 [52356])
Urethrocystography injection procedure (51600-51610)

53000 Urethrotomy or urethrostomy, external (separate procedure); pendulous urethra
🚑 4.28 ✂ 4.28 **FUD** 010 J A2 ▢
AMA: 2014,Jan,11

53010 perineal urethra, external
🚑 8.51 ✂ 8.51 **FUD** 090 J A2 ▢
AMA: 2014,Jan,11

53020 Meatotomy, cutting of meatus (separate procedure); except infant
🚑 2.80 ✂ 2.80 **FUD** 000 J A2 ▢
AMA: 2014,Jan,11

53025 infant A
🚑 1.97 ✂ 1.97 **FUD** 000 63 J R2 80 ▢
AMA: 2014,Jan,11

53040 Drainage of deep periurethral abscess
EXCLUDES Incision and drainage subcutaneous abscess (10060-10061)
🚑 11.3 ✂ 11.3 **FUD** 090 A2 80 ▢
AMA: 2014,Jan,11

53060 Drainage of Skene's gland abscess or cyst
🚑 4.70 ✂ 5.25 **FUD** 010 J P3 ▢
AMA: 2014,Jan,11

53080 Drainage of perineal urinary extravasation; uncomplicated (separate procedure)
🚑 12.1 ✂ 12.1 **FUD** 090 J A2 ▢
AMA: 2014,Jan,11

53085 complicated
🚑 18.7 ✂ 18.7 **FUD** 090 J G2 80 ▢
AMA: 2014,Jan,11

53200 Biopsy of urethra
🚑 4.12 ✂ 4.55 **FUD** 000 J A2 ▢
AMA: 2014,Jan,11

53210 Urethrectomy, total, including cystostomy; female ♀
🚑 22.2 ✂ 22.2 **FUD** 090 J A2 80 ▢
AMA: 2014,Jan,11

53215 male ♂
🚑 26.8 ✂ 26.8 **FUD** 090 J A2 80 ▢
AMA: 2014,Jan,11

53220 Excision or fulguration of carcinoma of urethra
🚑 13.0 ✂ 13.0 **FUD** 090 J A2 80 ▢
AMA: 2014,Jan,11

53230 Excision of urethral diverticulum (separate procedure); female ♀
🚑 17.5 ✂ 17.5 **FUD** 090 J A2 80 ▢
AMA: 2014,Jan,11

53235 male ♂
🚑 18.2 ✂ 18.2 **FUD** 090 J A2 80 ▢
AMA: 2014,Jan,11

53240 Marsupialization of urethral diverticulum, male or female
🚑 12.2 ✂ 12.2 **FUD** 090 J A2 ▢
AMA: 2014,Jan,11

53250 Excision of bulbourethral gland (Cowper's gland)
🚑 11.4 ✂ 11.4 **FUD** 090 J A2 ▢
AMA: 2014,Jan,11

53260 Excision or fulguration; urethral polyp(s), distal urethra
EXCLUDES Endoscopic method (52214, 52224)
🚑 5.20 ✂ 5.83 **FUD** 010 J A2 ▢
AMA: 2014,Jan,11

53265 urethral caruncle
EXCLUDES Endoscopic method (52214, 52224)
🚑 5.38 ✂ 6.36 **FUD** 010 J A2 ▢
AMA: 2014,Jan,11

53270 Skene's glands
EXCLUDES Endoscopic method (52214, 52224)
🚑 5.32 ✂ 5.98 **FUD** 010 J A2 ▢
AMA: 2014,Jan,11

53275 urethral prolapse
EXCLUDES Endoscopic method (52214, 52224)
🚑 7.58 ✂ 7.58 **FUD** 010 J A2 ▢
AMA: 2014,Jan,11

53400 Urethroplasty; first stage, for fistula, diverticulum, or stricture (eg, Johannsen type)
EXCLUDES Hypospadias repair (54300-54352)
🚑 23.1 ✂ 23.1 **FUD** 090 J A2 80 ▢
AMA: 2014,Jan,11

53405 second stage (formation of urethra), including urinary diversion
EXCLUDES Hypospadias repair (54300-54352)
🚑 25.2 ✂ 25.2 **FUD** 090 J A2 80 ▢
AMA: 2014,Jan,11

53410 Urethroplasty, 1-stage reconstruction of male anterior urethra ♂
EXCLUDES Hypospadias repair (54300-54352)
🚑 28.3 ✂ 28.3 **FUD** 090 J A2 80 ▢
AMA: 2014,Jan,11

53415 Urethroplasty, transpubic or perineal, 1-stage, for reconstruction or repair of prostatic or membranous urethra ♂
🚑 32.7 ✂ 32.7 **FUD** 090 C 80 ▢
AMA: 2014,Jan,11

53420 Urethroplasty, 2-stage reconstruction or repair of prostatic or membranous urethra; first stage ♂
🚑 24.3 ✂ 24.3 **FUD** 090 J A2 ▢
AMA: 2014,Jan,11

53425 second stage ♂
🚑 27.1 ✂ 27.1 **FUD** 090 J A2 80 ▢
AMA: 2014,Jan,11

53430 Urethroplasty, reconstruction of female urethra ♀
🚑 27.9 ✂ 27.9 **FUD** 090 J A2 80 ▢
AMA: 2014,Jan,11

● New Code ▲ Revised Code ○ Reinstated ● New Web Release ▲ Revised Web Release + Add-on Unlisted Not Covered # Resequenced
⑨⓪ Optum Mod 50 Exempt Ⓝ AMA Mod 51 Exempt ⑤① Optum Mod 51 Exempt ⑥③ Mod 63 Exempt ∕ Non-FDA Drug ★ Telemedicine Ⓜ Maternity Ⓐ Age Edit

Urinary System

53431   **Urethroplasty with tubularization of posterior urethra and/or lower bladder for incontinence (eg, Tenago, Leadbetter procedure)**
  🖥 33.4   ✂ 33.4   **FUD** 090   J A2 80 ▣
AMA: 2014,Jan,11

53440   **Sling operation for correction of male urinary incontinence (eg, fascia or synthetic)** ♂
  🖥 21.7   ✂ 21.7   **FUD** 090   J J8 80 ▣
AMA: 2020,Aug,6

53442   **Removal or revision of sling for male urinary incontinence (eg, fascia or synthetic)** ♂
  🖥 22.6   ✂ 22.6   **FUD** 090   J A2 80 ▣
AMA: 2020,Aug,6

53444   **Insertion of tandem cuff (dual cuff)**
  🖥 22.9   ✂ 22.9   **FUD** 090   J J8 80 ▣
AMA: 2014,Jan,11

53445   **Insertion of inflatable urethral/bladder neck sphincter, including placement of pump, reservoir, and cuff**
  🖥 21.7   ✂ 21.7   **FUD** 090   J J8 80 ▣
AMA: 2020,Aug,6

53446   **Removal of inflatable urethral/bladder neck sphincter, including pump, reservoir, and cuff**
  🖥 18.5   ✂ 18.5   **FUD** 090   Q2 A2 80 ▣
AMA: 2020,Aug,6

53447   **Removal and replacement of inflatable urethral/bladder neck sphincter including pump, reservoir, and cuff at the same operative session**
  🖥 23.3   ✂ 23.3   **FUD** 090   J J8 80 ▣
AMA: 2020,Aug,6

53448   **Removal and replacement of inflatable urethral/bladder neck sphincter including pump, reservoir, and cuff through an infected field at the same operative session including irrigation and debridement of infected tissue**
  INCLUDES   Debridement (11042, 11043)
  🖥 37.0   ✂ 37.0   **FUD** 090   C 80 ▣
AMA: 2020,Aug,6

53449   **Repair of inflatable urethral/bladder neck sphincter, including pump, reservoir, and cuff**
  🖥 17.6   ✂ 17.6   **FUD** 090   J A2 80 ▣
AMA: 2020,Aug,6

53450   **Urethromeatoplasty, with mucosal advancement**
  EXCLUDES   Meatotomy (53020, 53025)
  🖥 11.8   ✂ 11.8   **FUD** 090   J A2 ▣
AMA: 2018,Jan,8; 2017,Jan,8; 2016,Jan,13

● **53451**   **Periurethral transperineal adjustable balloon continence device; bilateral insertion, including cystourethroscopy and imaging guidance**
  INCLUDES   Cystourethroscopy (52000)
                Fluoroscopy (76000)
  EXCLUDES   Balloon(s) fluid volume adjustment (53454)
                Removal balloon (53453)
                Unilateral insertion only (53452)

● **53452**   **unilateral insertion, including cystourethroscopy and imaging guidance**
  INCLUDES   Cystourethroscopy (52000)
                Fluoroscopy (76000)
  EXCLUDES   Balloon(s) fluid volume adjustment (53454)
                Bilateral insertion (53452)
                Removal balloon (53453)

● **53453**   **removal, each balloon**
  EXCLUDES   Balloon insertion:
                Bilateral (53451)
                Unilateral (53452)
                Balloon(s) fluid volume adjustment (53454)

● **53454**   **percutaneous adjustment of balloon(s) fluid volume**
  EXCLUDES   Balloon insertion:
                Bilateral (53451)
                Unilateral (53452)
              Removal balloon (53453)
              Reporting more than once per encounter

53460   **Urethromeatoplasty, with partial excision of distal urethral segment (Richardson type procedure)**
  🖥 13.2   ✂ 13.2   **FUD** 090   J A2 80 ▣
AMA: 2014,Jan,11

53500   **Urethrolysis, transvaginal, secondary, open, including cystourethroscopy (eg, postsurgical obstruction, scarring)**
  INCLUDES   Cystourethroscopy (separate procedure) (52000)
  EXCLUDES   Retropubic approach (53899)
  🖥 21.5   ✂ 21.5   **FUD** 090   J 62 80 ▣
AMA: 2018,Jan,8; 2017,Jan,8; 2016,Jan,13

53502   **Urethrorrhaphy, suture of urethral wound or injury, female** ♀
  🖥 14.0   ✂ 14.0   **FUD** 090   J A2 ▣
AMA: 2014,Jan,11

53505   **Urethrorrhaphy, suture of urethral wound or injury; penile** ♂
  🖥 14.0   ✂ 14.0   **FUD** 090   J A2 80 ▣
AMA: 2014,Jan,11

53510   **perineal** ♂
  🖥 18.2   ✂ 18.2   **FUD** 090   J A2 80 ▣
AMA: 2014,Jan,11

53515   **prostatomembranous** ♂
  🖥 23.0   ✂ 23.0   **FUD** 090   J A2 80 ▣
AMA: 2014,Jan,11

53520   **Closure of urethrostomy or urethrocutaneous fistula, male (separate procedure)** ♂
  EXCLUDES   Closure fistula:
                Urethrorectal (45820, 45825)
                Urethrovaginal (57310)
  🖥 16.1   ✂ 16.1   **FUD** 090   J A2 ▣
AMA: 2014,Jan,11

53600-53665 Urethral Dilation

EXCLUDES   Endoscopic procedures; cystoscopy, urethroscopy, cystourethroscopy (52000-52700 [52356])
         Urethral catheterization (51701-51703)
         Urethrocystography injection procedure (51600-51610)
         (74485)

53600   **Dilation of urethral stricture by passage of sound or urethral dilator, male; initial** ♂
  🖥 1.84   ✂ 2.39   **FUD** 000   T P3 ▣
AMA: 2014,Jan,11

53601   **subsequent** ♂
  🖥 1.55   ✂ 2.29   **FUD** 000   Q1 N1 ▣
AMA: 2014,Jan,11

53605   **Dilation of urethral stricture or vesical neck by passage of sound or urethral dilator, male, general or conduction (spinal) anesthesia** ♂
  EXCLUDES   Procedure performed under local anesthesia (53600-53601, 53620-53621)
  🖥 1.87   ✂ 1.87   **FUD** 000   J A2 ▣
AMA: 2014,Jan,11

53620   **Dilation of urethral stricture by passage of filiform and follower, male; initial** ♂
  🖥 2.52   ✂ 3.79   **FUD** 000   T P3 ▣
AMA: 2014,Jan,11; 1996,Nov,1

53621   **subsequent** ♂
  🖥 2.09   ✂ 3.56   **FUD** 000   T P3 ▣
AMA: 2014,Jan,11

2G/TC PC/TC Only   A2-Z3 ASC Payment   50 Bilateral   ♂ Male Only   ♀ Female Only   🖥 Facility RVU   ✂ Non-Facility RVU   ▣ CCI   ✖ CLIA
FUD Follow-up Days   CMS: IOM   **AMA:** CPT Asst   A-Y OPPSI   80/80 Surg Assist Allowed / w/Doc   Lab Crosswalk   Radiology Crosswalk

244   CPT © 2021 American Medical Association. All Rights Reserved.   © 2021 Optum360, LLC

53660 **Dilation of female urethra including suppository and/or instillation; initial** ♀

🚑 1.20 👤 1.99 **FUD** 000 S P3 ▢

AMA: 2014,Jan,11

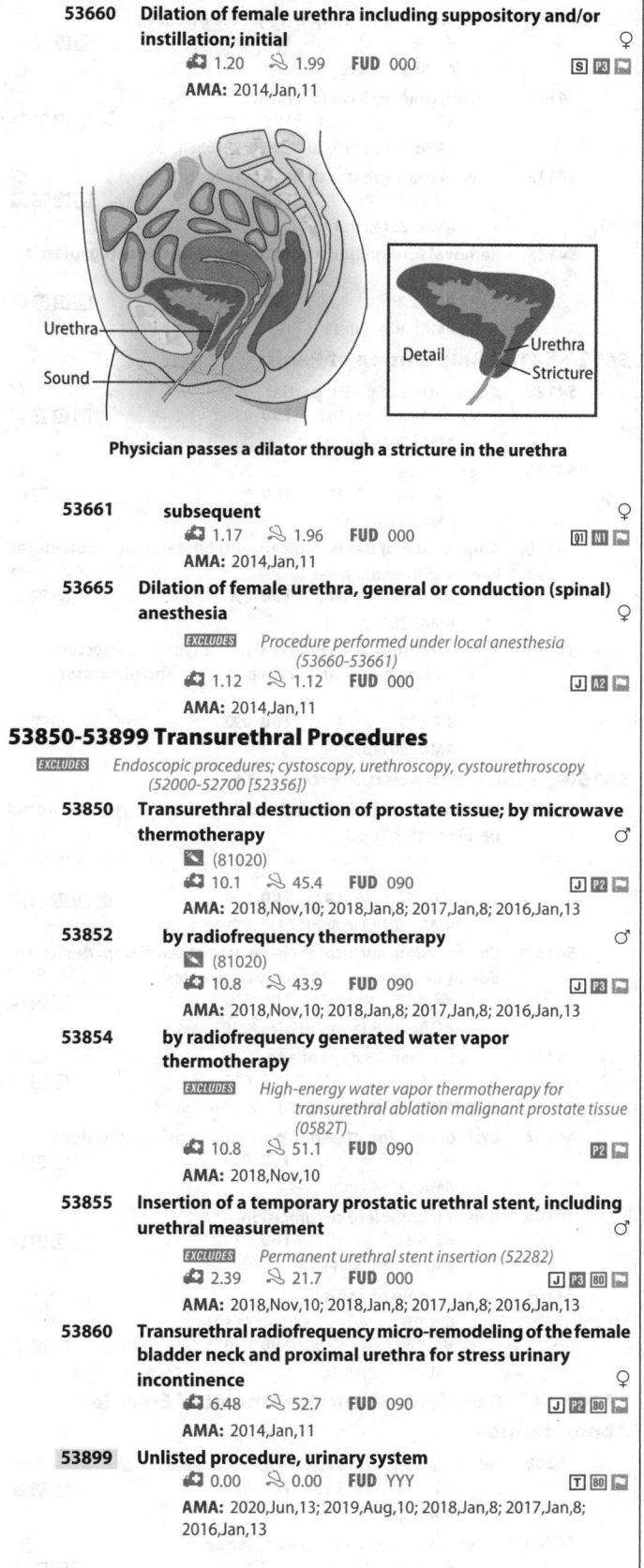

Urethra

Sound

Detail

Urethra

Stricture

Physician passes a dilator through a stricture in the urethra

53661 **subsequent** ♀

🚑 1.17 👤 1.96 **FUD** 000 01 N1 ▢

AMA: 2014,Jan,11

53665 **Dilation of female urethra, general or conduction (spinal) anesthesia** ♀

EXCLUDES *Procedure performed under local anesthesia (53660-53661)*

🚑 1.12 👤 1.12 **FUD** 000 J A2 ▢

AMA: 2014,Jan,11

53850-53899 Transurethral Procedures

EXCLUDES *Endoscopic procedures; cystoscopy, urethroscopy, cystourethroscopy (52000-52700 [52356])*

53850 **Transurethral destruction of prostate tissue; by microwave thermotherapy** ♂

🔬 (81020)

🚑 10.1 👤 45.4 **FUD** 090 J P2 ▢

AMA: 2018,Nov,10; 2018,Jan,8; 2017,Jan,8; 2016,Jan,13

53852 **by radiofrequency thermotherapy** ♂

🔬 (81020)

🚑 10.8 👤 43.9 **FUD** 090 J P3 ▢

AMA: 2018,Nov,10; 2018,Jan,8; 2017,Jan,8; 2016,Jan,13

53854 **by radiofrequency generated water vapor thermotherapy**

EXCLUDES *High-energy water vapor thermotherapy for transurethral ablation malignant prostate tissue (0582T)*

🚑 10.8 👤 51.1 **FUD** 090 P2 ▢

AMA: 2018,Nov,10

53855 **Insertion of a temporary prostatic urethral stent, including urethral measurement** ♂

EXCLUDES *Permanent urethral stent insertion (52282)*

🚑 2.39 👤 21.7 **FUD** 000 J P3 80 ▢

AMA: 2018,Nov,10; 2018,Jan,8; 2017,Jan,8; 2016,Jan,13

53860 **Transurethral radiofrequency micro-remodeling of the female bladder neck and proximal urethra for stress urinary incontinence** ♀

🚑 6.48 👤 52.7 **FUD** 090 J P2 80 ▢

AMA: 2014,Jan,11

53899 **Unlisted procedure, urinary system**

🚑 0.00 👤 0.00 **FUD** YYY T 80 ▢

AMA: 2020,Jun,13; 2019,Aug,10; 2018,Jan,8; 2017,Jan,8; 2016,Jan,13

● New Code ▲ Revised Code ○ Reinstated ● New Web Release ▲ Revised Web Release + Add-on Unlisted Not Covered # Resequenced
50 Optum Mod 50 Exempt Ⓢ AMA Mod 51 Exempt 51 Optum Mod 51 Exempt 63 Mod 63 Exempt ✗ Non-FDA Drug ★ Telemedicine M Maternity A Age Edit

54000-54015 Procedures of Penis: Incisional

EXCLUDES   *Debridement abdominal perineal gangrene (11004-11006)*

54000   **Slitting of prepuce, dorsal or lateral (separate procedure); newborn**   A ♂
   📋 3.14   ✂ 4.40   **FUD** 010   63 J A2 80 ▢
   AMA: 2014,Jan,11

54001   **except newborn**   ♂
   📋 4.02   ✂ 5.44   **FUD** 010   J A2 ▢
   AMA: 2014,Jan,11

54015   **Incision and drainage of penis, deep**   ♂
   EXCLUDES   *Abscess, skin/subcutaneous (10060-10160)*
   📋 8.92   ✂ 8.92   **FUD** 010   J A2 80 ▢
   AMA: 2014,Jan,11

Urethra
Hematoma or abscess
Hematoma or abscess

A postoperative drain may be placed. Sutures are required to repair the operative site

The physician incises the penis to drain an abscess or hematoma

54050-54065 Destruction of Penis Lesions: Multiple Methods

EXCLUDES   *Excision/destruction other lesions (11420-11426, 11620-11626, 17000-17250, 17270-17276)*

54050   **Destruction of lesion(s), penis (eg, condyloma, papilloma, molluscum contagiosum, herpetic vesicle), simple; chemical**   ♂
   📋 3.05   ✂ 3.80   **FUD** 010   Q1 N1 ▢
   AMA: 2014,Jan,11; 1997,Nov,1

54055   **electrodesiccation**   ♂
   📋 2.69   ✂ 3.49   **FUD** 010   T P3 ▢
   AMA: 2014,Jan,11; 1997,Nov,1

54056   **cryosurgery**   ♂
   📋 3.18   ✂ 4.03   **FUD** 010   Q1 N1 ▢
   AMA: 2014,Jan,11; 1997,Nov,1

54057   **laser surgery**   ♂
   📋 2.72   ✂ 3.94   **FUD** 010   T A2 ▢
   AMA: 2014,Jan,11; 1997,Nov,1

54060   **surgical excision**   ♂
   📋 3.76   ✂ 5.29   **FUD** 010   T A2 ▢
   AMA: 2014,Jan,11

54065   **Destruction of lesion(s), penis (eg, condyloma, papilloma, molluscum contagiosum, herpetic vesicle), extensive (eg, laser surgery, electrosurgery, cryosurgery, chemosurgery)**   ♂
   📋 4.97   ✂ 6.31   **FUD** 010   T A2 ▢
   AMA: 2014,Jan,11; 1997,Nov,1

54100-54115 Procedures of Penis: Excisional

54100   **Biopsy of penis; (separate procedure)**   ♂
   📋 3.64   ✂ 5.71   **FUD** 000   J A2 ▢
   AMA: 2019,Jan,9; 2018,Jan,8; 2017,Jan,8; 2016,Jan,13

54105   **deep structures**   ♂
   📋 6.16   ✂ 7.68   **FUD** 010   J A2 ▢
   AMA: 2014,Jan,11

54110   **Excision of penile plaque (Peyronie disease);**   ♂
   📋 18.0   ✂ 18.0   **FUD** 090   J A2 80 ▢
   AMA: 2014,Jan,11

54111   **with graft to 5 cm in length**   ♂
   📋 23.1   ✂ 23.1   **FUD** 090   J A2 80 ▢
   AMA: 2018,Jan,8; 2017,Jan,8; 2016,Jan,13

54112   **with graft greater than 5 cm in length**   ♂
   📋 27.1   ✂ 27.1   **FUD** 090   J A2 80 ▢
   AMA: 2014,Jan,11

54115   **Removal foreign body from deep penile tissue (eg, plastic implant)**   ♂
   📋 12.2   ✂ 13.0   **FUD** 090   J A2 80 ▢
   AMA: 2014,Jan,11

54120-54135 Amputation of Penis

54120   **Amputation of penis; partial**   ♂
   📋 18.2   ✂ 18.2   **FUD** 090   J A2 80 ▢
   AMA: 2014,Jan,11

54125   **complete**   ♂
   📋 23.5   ✂ 23.5   **FUD** 090   C 80 ▢
   AMA: 2014,Jan,11

54130   **Amputation of penis, radical; with bilateral inguinofemoral lymphadenectomy**   ♂
   📋 34.5   ✂ 34.5   **FUD** 090   C 80 ▢
   AMA: 2014,Jan,11

54135   **in continuity with bilateral pelvic lymphadenectomy, including external iliac, hypogastric and obturator nodes**   ♂
   📋 43.7   ✂ 43.7   **FUD** 090   C 80 ▢
   AMA: 2014,Jan,11

54150-54164 Circumcision Procedures

54150   **Circumcision, using clamp or other device with regional dorsal penile or ring block**   ♂
   Code also modifier 52 when performed without dorsal penile or ring block
   📋 2.83   ✂ 4.42   **FUD** 000   63 J A2 80 ▢
   AMA: 2018,Jan,8; 2017,Jan,8; 2016,Jan,13

54160   **Circumcision, surgical excision other than clamp, device, or dorsal slit; neonate (28 days of age or less)**   A ♂
   📋 4.17   ✂ 6.32   **FUD** 010   63 J A2 ▢
   AMA: 2018,Jan,8; 2017,Jan,8; 2016,Jan,13

54161   **older than 28 days of age**   A ♂
   📋 5.70   ✂ 5.70   **FUD** 010   J A2 ▢
   AMA: 2018,Jan,8; 2017,Jan,8; 2016,Jan,13

54162   **Lysis or excision of penile post-circumcision adhesions**   ♂
   📋 5.77   ✂ 7.42   **FUD** 010   J A2 ▢
   AMA: 2014,Jan,11

54163   **Repair incomplete circumcision**   ♂
   📋 6.31   ✂ 6.31   **FUD** 010   J A2 ▢
   AMA: 2014,Jan,11

54164   **Frenulotomy of penis**   ♂
   EXCLUDES   *Circumcision (54150-54163)*
   📋 5.60   ✂ 5.60   **FUD** 010   J A2 ▢
   AMA: 2014,Jan,11

54200-54250 Evaluation and Treatment of Erectile Abnormalities

54200   **Injection procedure for Peyronie disease;**   ♂
   📋 2.42   ✂ 3.13   **FUD** 010   T P3 ▢
   AMA: 2014,Jan,11

54205   **with surgical exposure of plaque**   ♂
   📋 15.4   ✂ 15.4   **FUD** 090   J A2 80 ▢
   AMA: 2014,Jan,11

| 26/TC PC/TC Only | A2-Z3 ASC Payment | 50 Bilateral | ♂ Male Only | ♀ Female Only | 📋 Facility RVU | ✂ Non-Facility RVU | ▢ CCI | ✕ CLIA |
| FUD Follow-up Days | CMS: IOM | AMA: CPT Asst | A-Y OPPSI | 80/80 Surg Assist Allowed / w/Doc | | Lab Crosswalk | Radiology Crosswalk |

54220 Irrigation of corpora cavernosa for priapism ♂
🚗 3.87 ⚕ 5.97 **FUD** 000 T A2 📷
AMA: 2014,Jan,11

54230 Injection procedure for corpora cavernosography ♂
📷 (74445)
🚗 2.30 ⚕ 2.82 **FUD** 000 N N1 📷
AMA: 2014,Jan,11

54231 Dynamic cavernosometry, including intracavernosal injection of vasoactive drugs (eg, papaverine, phentolamine) ♂
🚗 3.36 ⚕ 4.08 **FUD** 000 J P3 📷
AMA: 2014,Jan,11; 1994,Sum,29

54235 Injection of corpora cavernosa with pharmacologic agent(s) (eg, papaverine, phentolamine) ♂
🚗 2.11 ⚕ 2.56 **FUD** 000 T P3 📷
AMA: 2018,Jan,8; 2017,Jan,8; 2016,Jan,13

54240 Penile plethysmography ♂
🚗 2.94 ⚕ 2.94 **FUD** 000 S P3 80 📷
AMA: 2014,Jan,11

54250 Nocturnal penile tumescence and/or rigidity test ♂
🚗 3.50 ⚕ 3.50 **FUD** 000 T P3 80 📷
AMA: 2014,Jan,11

54300-54390 Hypospadias Repair and Related Procedures

EXCLUDES Other urethroplasties (53400-53430)
Revascularization penis (37788)

54300 Plastic operation of penis for straightening of chordee (eg, hypospadias), with or without mobilization of urethra ♂
🚗 18.6 ⚕ 18.6 **FUD** 090 J A2 80 📷
AMA: 2018,Jan,8; 2017,Jan,8; 2016,Jan,13

54304 Plastic operation on penis for correction of chordee or for first stage hypospadias repair with or without transplantation of prepuce and/or skin flaps ♂
🚗 21.6 ⚕ 21.6 **FUD** 090 J A2 80 📷
AMA: 2014,Jan,11

Chordee

Urethra Penis

Urethral opening

The foreskin is used in either a free graft or a flap graft to cover the ventral skin defects created to correct the chordee

54308 Urethroplasty for second stage hypospadias repair (including urinary diversion); less than 3 cm ♂
🚗 20.6 ⚕ 20.6 **FUD** 090 J A2 80 📷
AMA: 2014,Jan,11

54312 greater than 3 cm ♂
🚗 23.6 ⚕ 23.6 **FUD** 090 J A2 80 📷
AMA: 2014,Jan,11

54316 Urethroplasty for second stage hypospadias repair (including urinary diversion) with free skin graft obtained from site other than genitalia ♂
🚗 28.8 ⚕ 28.8 **FUD** 090 J A2 80 📷
AMA: 2014,Jan,11

54318 Urethroplasty for third stage hypospadias repair to release penis from scrotum (eg, third stage Cecil repair) ♂
🚗 20.5 ⚕ 20.5 **FUD** 090 J A2 80 📷
AMA: 2014,Jan,11

54322 1-stage distal hypospadias repair (with or without chordee or circumcision); with simple meatal advancement (eg, Magpi, V-flap) ♂
🚗 22.6 ⚕ 22.6 **FUD** 090 J A2 80 📷
AMA: 2014,Jan,11

54324 with urethroplasty by local skin flaps (eg, flip-flap, prepucial flap) ♂
INCLUDES Browne's operation
🚗 28.0 ⚕ 28.0 **FUD** 090 J A2 80 📷
AMA: 2014,Jan,11

54326 with urethroplasty by local skin flaps and mobilization of urethra ♂
🚗 27.3 ⚕ 27.3 **FUD** 090 J A2 80 📷
AMA: 2014,Jan,11

54328 with extensive dissection to correct chordee and urethroplasty with local skin flaps, skin graft patch, and/or island flap ♂
EXCLUDES Urethroplasty/straightening chordee (54308)
🚗 27.1 ⚕ 27.1 **FUD** 090 J A2 80 📷
AMA: 2018,Jan,8; 2017,Jan,8; 2016,Jan,13

54332 1-stage proximal penile or penoscrotal hypospadias repair requiring extensive dissection to correct chordee and urethroplasty by use of skin graft tube and/or island flap ♂
🚗 29.3 ⚕ 29.3 **FUD** 090 J 62 80 📷
AMA: 2018,Jan,8; 2017,Jan,8; 2016,Jan,13

54336 1-stage perineal hypospadias repair requiring extensive dissection to correct chordee and urethroplasty by use of skin graft tube and/or island flap ♂
🚗 34.4 ⚕ 34.4 **FUD** 090 J 62 80 📷
AMA: 2018,Jan,8; 2017,Jan,8; 2016,Jan,13

▲ **54340** Repair of hypospadias complication(s) (ie, fistula, stricture, diverticula); by closure, incision, or excision, simple ♂
🚗 16.4 ⚕ 16.4 **FUD** 090 J A2 80 📷
AMA: 2014,Jan,11

▲ **54344** requiring mobilization of skin flaps and urethroplasty with flap or patch graft ♂
🚗 27.4 ⚕ 27.4 **FUD** 090 J A2 80 📷
AMA: 2014,Jan,11

▲ **54348** requiring extensive dissection, and urethroplasty with flap, patch or tubed graft (including urinary diversion, when performed) ♂
🚗 29.3 ⚕ 29.3 **FUD** 090 J A2 80 📷
AMA: 2014,Jan,11

▲ 54352 **Revision of prior hypospadias repair requiring extensive dissection and excision of previously constructed structures including re-release of chordee and reconstruction of urethra and penis by use of local skin as grafts and island flaps and skin brought in as flaps or grafts** ♂

EXCLUDES Application skin substitute graft (15275)
Excision urethral diverticulum (53235)
Hypospadias repair:
Complications (54340, 54344, 54348)
Extensive dissection to correct chordee and urethroplasty, 1-stage perineal (54336)
Island pedicle flap (15740)
Plastic repair:
Angulation (54360)
Chordee (54300)
Tubed pedicle formation (15574)
Urethroplasty, 1-stage reconstruction male anterior urethra (53410)

🗲 41.0   ⚕ 41.0   **FUD** 090   J A2 80 ▭

AMA: 2014,Jan,11

54360 **Plastic operation on penis to correct angulation** ♂

🗲 20.8   ⚕ 20.8   **FUD** 090   J A2 80 ▭

AMA: 2014,Jan,11

54380 **Plastic operation on penis for epispadias distal to external sphincter;** ♂

INCLUDES Lowsley's operation

🗲 23.1   ⚕ 23.1   **FUD** 090   J A2 80 ▭

AMA: 2014,Jan,11

54385 **with incontinence** ♂

🗲 26.8   ⚕ 26.8   **FUD** 090   J A2 80 ▭

AMA: 2014,Jan,11

54390 **with exstrophy of bladder** ♂

🗲 35.9   ⚕ 35.9   **FUD** 090   C 80 ▭

AMA: 2014,Jan,11

54400-54417 Procedures to Treat Impotence

CMS: 100-03,230.4 Diagnosis and Treatment of Impotence

EXCLUDES Other urethroplasties (53400-53430)
Revascularization penis (37788)

54400 **Insertion of penile prosthesis; non-inflatable (semi-rigid)** ♂

EXCLUDES Replacement/removal penile prosthesis (54415, 54416)

🗲 15.3   ⚕ 15.3   **FUD** 090   J J8 ▭

AMA: 2014,Jan,11

54401 **inflatable (self-contained)** ♂

EXCLUDES Replacement/removal penile prosthesis (54415, 54416)

🗲 18.9   ⚕ 18.9   **FUD** 090   J J8 ▭

AMA: 2014,Jan,11

54405 **Insertion of multi-component, inflatable penile prosthesis, including placement of pump, cylinders, and reservoir** ♂

Code also modifier 52 for reduced services

🗲 23.4   ⚕ 23.4   **FUD** 090   J J8 80 ▭

AMA: 2014,Jan,11

54406 **Removal of all components of a multi-component, inflatable penile prosthesis without replacement of prosthesis** ♂

Code also modifier 52 for reduced services

🗲 21.1   ⚕ 21.1   **FUD** 090   02 A2 80 ▭

AMA: 2014,Jan,11

54408 **Repair of component(s) of a multi-component, inflatable penile prosthesis** ♂

🗲 22.8   ⚕ 22.8   **FUD** 090   J A2 80 ▭

AMA: 2014,Jan,11

54410 **Removal and replacement of all component(s) of a multi-component, inflatable penile prosthesis at the same operative session** ♂

🗲 24.8   ⚕ 24.8   **FUD** 090   J J8 80 ▭

AMA: 2014,Jan,11

54411 **Removal and replacement of all components of a multi-component inflatable penile prosthesis through an infected field at the same operative session, including irrigation and debridement of infected tissue** ♂

INCLUDES Debridement (11042, 11043)

Code also modifier 52 for reduced services

🗲 29.7   ⚕ 29.7   **FUD** 090   J J8 80 ▭

AMA: 2014,Jan,11

54415 **Removal of non-inflatable (semi-rigid) or inflatable (self-contained) penile prosthesis, without replacement of prosthesis** ♂

🗲 15.3   ⚕ 15.3   **FUD** 090   02 A2 80 ▭

AMA: 2014,Jan,11

54416 **Removal and replacement of non-inflatable (semi-rigid) or inflatable (self-contained) penile prosthesis at the same operative session** ♂

🗲 20.5   ⚕ 20.5   **FUD** 090   J J8 80 ▭

AMA: 2014,Jan,11

54417 **Removal and replacement of non-inflatable (semi-rigid) or inflatable (self-contained) penile prosthesis through an infected field at the same operative session, including irrigation and debridement of infected tissue** ♂

INCLUDES Debridement (11042, 11043)

🗲 26.0   ⚕ 26.0   **FUD** 090   J J8 80 ▭

AMA: 2014,Jan,11

54420-54450 Other Procedures of the Penis

EXCLUDES Other urethroplasties (53400-53430)
Revascularization penis (37788)

54420 **Corpora cavernosa-saphenous vein shunt (priapism operation), unilateral or bilateral** ♂

🗲 20.3   ⚕ 20.3   **FUD** 090   J A2 80 ▭

AMA: 2014,Jan,11

54430 **Corpora cavernosa-corpus spongiosum shunt (priapism operation), unilateral or bilateral** ♂

🗲 18.5   ⚕ 18.5   **FUD** 090   C 80 ▭

AMA: 2014,Jan,11

Cross section of penis

Corpus cavernosum

Corpus cavernosum

Corpus cavernosum

Corpus spongiosum

Communication

The physician creates a communication between the corpus cavernosum and the corpus spongiosum

54435 **Corpora cavernosa-glans penis fistulization (eg, biopsy needle, Winter procedure, rongeur, or punch) for priapism** ♂

🗲 12.0   ⚕ 12.0   **FUD** 090   J A2 ▭

AMA: 2014,Jan,11

54437 **Repair of traumatic corporeal tear(s)** ♂

EXCLUDES Urethral repair (53410, 53415)

🗲 19.4   ⚕ 19.4   **FUD** 090   J G2 80 ▭

26/TC PC/TC Only   A2-Z3 ASC Payment   50 Bilateral   ♂ Male Only   ♀ Female Only   🗲 Facility RVU   ⚕ Non-Facility RVU   ▭ CCI   ✖ CLIA
FUD Follow-up Days   CMS: IOM   AMA: CPT Asst   A-Y OPPSI   80/80 Surg Assist Allowed / w/Doc   Lab Crosswalk   Radiology Crosswalk

248   CPT © 2021 American Medical Association. All Rights Reserved.   © 2021 Optum360, LLC

54438 Replantation, penis, complete amputation including urethral repair ♂

> EXCLUDES Replantation/repair corporeal tear in incomplete amputation penis (54437)
> Replantation/urethral repair in incomplete amputation penis (53410-53415)

🔧 38.7 ⚕ 38.7 **FUD** 090 [C] [80] 🖵

54440 Plastic operation of penis for injury ♂

🔧 0.00 ⚕ 0.00 **FUD** 090 [J] [A2] [80] 🖵

AMA: 2014,Jan,11

54450 Foreskin manipulation including lysis of preputial adhesions and stretching ♂

🔧 1.67 ⚕ 1.99 **FUD** 000 [T] [A2] 🖵

AMA: 2014,Jan,11

54500-54560 Testicular Procedures: Incisional

> EXCLUDES Debridement abdominal perineal gangrene (11004-11006)

54500 Biopsy of testis, needle (separate procedure) ♂

> EXCLUDES Fine needle aspiration (10021, [10004, 10005, 10006, 10007, 10008, 10009, 10010, 10011, 10012])
> 🔬 (88172-88173)

🔧 2.16 ⚕ 2.16 **FUD** 000 [J] [A2] [80] [50] 🖵

AMA: 2019,Apr,4

54505 Biopsy of testis, incisional (separate procedure) ♂

Code also when combined with epididymogram, seminal vesiculogram or vasogram (55300)

🔧 6.07 ⚕ 6.07 **FUD** 010 [J] [A2] [80] [50] 🖵

AMA: 2018,Jan,8; 2017,Jan,8; 2016,Jan,13

54512 Excision of extraparenchymal lesion of testis ♂

🔧 15.6 ⚕ 15.6 **FUD** 090 [J] [A2] [50] 🖵

AMA: 2018,Jan,8; 2017,Jan,8; 2016,Jan,13

54520 Orchiectomy, simple (including subcapsular), with or without testicular prosthesis, scrotal or inguinal approach ♂

> INCLUDES Huggins' orchiectomy
> EXCLUDES Lymphadenectomy, radical retroperitoneal (38780)
> Code also hernia repair, when performed (49505, 49507)

🔧 9.45 ⚕ 9.45 **FUD** 090 [J] [A2] [50] 🖵

AMA: 2018,Jan,8; 2017,Jan,8; 2016,Jan,13

54522 Orchiectomy, partial ♂

> EXCLUDES Lymphadenectomy, radical retroperitoneal (38780)

🔧 17.0 ⚕ 17.0 **FUD** 090 [J] [A2] [80] [50] 🖵

AMA: 2018,Jan,8; 2017,Jan,8; 2016,Jan,13

54530 Orchiectomy, radical, for tumor; inguinal approach ♂

> EXCLUDES Lymphadenectomy, radical retroperitoneal (38780)

🔧 14.6 ⚕ 14.6 **FUD** 090 [J] [A2] [80] [50] 🖵

AMA: 2018,Jan,8; 2017,Jan,8; 2016,Jan,13

54535 with abdominal exploration ♂

> EXCLUDES Lymphadenectomy, radical retroperitoneal (38780)

🔧 21.5 ⚕ 21.5 **FUD** 090 [G2] [80] [50] 🖵

AMA: 2018,Jan,8; 2017,Jan,8; 2016,Jan,13

54550 Exploration for undescended testis (inguinal or scrotal area) ♂

🔧 14.2 ⚕ 14.2 **FUD** 090 [J] [A2] [80] [50] 🖵

AMA: 2018,Jan,8; 2017,Mar,10; 2017,Jan,8; 2016,Jan,13

54560 Exploration for undescended testis with abdominal exploration ♂

🔧 19.8 ⚕ 19.8 **FUD** 090 [J] [G2] [80] [50] 🖵

AMA: 2018,Jan,8; 2017,Jan,8; 2016,Jan,13

54600-54699 Open and Laparoscopic Testicular Procedures

54600 Reduction of torsion of testis, surgical, with or without fixation of contralateral testis ♂

🔧 13.1 ⚕ 13.1 **FUD** 090 [J] [A2] [50] 🖵

AMA: 2018,Jan,8; 2017,Jan,8; 2016,Jan,13

Normal testes   Torsion of testis

54620 Fixation of contralateral testis (separate procedure) ♂

🔧 8.66 ⚕ 8.66 **FUD** 010 [J] [A2] [50] 🖵

AMA: 2014,Jan,11

54640 Orchiopexy, inguinal or scrotal approach ♂

> INCLUDES Bevan's operation
> Koop inguinal orchiopexy
> Prentice orchiopexy
> EXCLUDES Repair inguinal hernia with inguinal orchiopexy (49495-49525)

🔧 13.8 ⚕ 13.8 **FUD** 090 [J] [A2] [80] [50] 🖵

AMA: 2018,Jan,8; 2017,Mar,10; 2017,Jan,8; 2016,Jan,13

54650 Orchiopexy, abdominal approach, for intra-abdominal testis (eg, Fowler-Stephens) ♂

> EXCLUDES Laparoscopic orchiopexy (54692)

🔧 20.5 ⚕ 20.5 **FUD** 090 [J] [G2] [80] [50] 🖵

AMA: 2018,Jan,8; 2017,Jan,8; 2016,Jan,13

54660 Insertion of testicular prosthesis (separate procedure) ♂

🔧 10.3 ⚕ 10.3 **FUD** 090 [J] [J8] [80] [50] 🖵

AMA: 2018,Jan,8; 2017,Jan,8; 2016,Jan,13

54670 Suture or repair of testicular injury ♂

🔧 11.7 ⚕ 11.7 **FUD** 090 [J] [A2] [80] [50] 🖵

AMA: 2018,Jan,8; 2017,Jan,8; 2016,Jan,13

54680 Transplantation of testis(es) to thigh (because of scrotal destruction) ♂

🔧 22.7 ⚕ 22.7 **FUD** 090 [J] [A2] [80] [50] 🖵

AMA: 2018,Jan,8; 2017,Jan,8; 2016,Jan,13

54690 Laparoscopy, surgical; orchiectomy ♂

> INCLUDES Diagnostic laparoscopy (49320)

🔧 19.0 ⚕ 19.0 **FUD** 090 [J] [A2] [80] [50] 🖵

AMA: 2019,Feb,10; 2018,Jan,8; 2017,Jan,8; 2016,Jan,13

54692 orchiopexy for intra-abdominal testis ♂

> INCLUDES Diagnostic laparoscopy (49320)

🔧 21.9 ⚕ 21.9 **FUD** 090 [J] [G2] [50] 🖵

AMA: 2018,Jan,8; 2017,Jan,8; 2016,Jan,13

54699 Unlisted laparoscopy procedure, testis ♂

🔧 0.00 ⚕ 0.00 **FUD** YYY [J] [80] [50] 🖵

AMA: 2018,Jan,8; 2017,Jan,8; 2016,Jan,13

54700-54901 Open Procedures of the Epididymis

54700 Incision and drainage of epididymis, testis and/or scrotal space (eg, abscess or hematoma) ♂

> EXCLUDES Debridement genitalia for necrotizing soft tissue infection (11004-11006)

🔧 6.16 ⚕ 6.16 **FUD** 010 [J] [A2] [50] 🖵

AMA: 2018,Jan,8; 2017,Jan,8; 2016,Jan,13

54800 Biopsy of epididymis, needle ♂

> **EXCLUDES** *Fine needle aspiration (10021, [10004, 10005, 10006, 10007, 10008, 10009, 10010, 10011, 10012])*

📧 88172-88173

📥 3.64   ⚕ 3.64   **FUD** 000   J A2 80 50 ▭

AMA: 2019,Apr,4; 2018,Jan,8; 2017,Jan,8; 2016,Jan,13

54830 Excision of local lesion of epididymis ♂

📥 10.7   ⚕ 10.7   **FUD** 090   J A2 80 50 ▭

AMA: 2018,Jan,8; 2017,Jan,8; 2016,Jan,13

54840 Excision of spermatocele, with or without epididymectomy ♂

📥 9.29   ⚕ 9.29   **FUD** 090   J A2 50 ▭

AMA: 2018,Jan,8; 2017,Jan,8; 2016,Jan,13

54860 Epididymectomy; unilateral ♂

📥 12.1   ⚕ 12.1   **FUD** 090   J A2 ▭

AMA: 2014,Jan,11

54861 bilateral ♂

📥 16.3   ⚕ 16.3   **FUD** 090   J A2 80 ▭

AMA: 2014,Jan,11

54865 Exploration of epididymis, with or without biopsy ♂

📥 10.3   ⚕ 10.3   **FUD** 090   J A2 80 ▭

AMA: 2014,Jan,11; 2007,Jul,5

54900 Epididymovasostomy, anastomosis of epididymis to vas deferens; unilateral ♂

> **EXCLUDES** *Operating microscope (69990)*

📥 23.1   ⚕ 23.1   **FUD** 090   J A2 80 ▭

AMA: 2018,Jan,8; 2017,Jan,8; 2016,Jan,13

54901 bilateral ♂

> **EXCLUDES** *Operating microscope (69990)*

📥 30.5   ⚕ 30.5   **FUD** 090   J A2 80 ▭

AMA: 2018,Jan,8; 2017,Jan,8; 2016,Jan,13

55000-55180 Procedures of the Tunica Vaginalis and Scrotum

55000 Puncture aspiration of hydrocele, tunica vaginalis, with or without injection of medication ♂

📥 2.44   ⚕ 3.39   **FUD** 000   T P3 50 ▭

AMA: 2014,Jan,11

Normal   Noncommunicating hydrocele   Communicating hydrocele   Hydrocele of the cord

Testicle
Scrotum

55040 Excision of hydrocele; unilateral ♂

> **EXCLUDES** *Repair hernia with hydrocelectomy (49495-49501)*

📥 9.77   ⚕ 9.77   **FUD** 090   J A2 ▭

AMA: 2018,Jan,8; 2017,Nov,10; 2017,Jan,8; 2016,Jan,13

55041 bilateral ♂

> **EXCLUDES** *Repair hernia with hydrocelectomy (49495-49501)*

📥 14.7   ⚕ 14.7   **FUD** 090   J A2 ▭

AMA: 2014,Jan,11

55060 Repair of tunica vaginalis hydrocele (Bottle type) ♂

📥 11.0   ⚕ 11.0   **FUD** 090   J A2 80 50 ▭

AMA: 2018,Jan,8; 2017,Jan,8; 2016,Jan,13

55100 Drainage of scrotal wall abscess ♂

> **EXCLUDES** *Debridement genitalia for necrotizing soft tissue infection (11004-11006)*
> *Incision and drainage scrotal space (54700)*

📥 4.80   ⚕ 6.43   **FUD** 010   J A2 ▭

AMA: 2014,Jan,11

55110 Scrotal exploration ♂

📥 11.1   ⚕ 11.1   **FUD** 090   J A2 ▭

AMA: 2014,Jan,11

55120 Removal of foreign body in scrotum ♂

📥 10.1   ⚕ 10.1   **FUD** 090   J A2 80 ▭

AMA: 2014,Jan,11

55150 Resection of scrotum ♂

> **EXCLUDES** *Lesion excision skin, scrotum (11420-11426, 11620-11626)*

📥 14.2   ⚕ 14.2   **FUD** 090   J A2 80 ▭

AMA: 2014,Jan,11

55175 Scrotoplasty; simple ♂

📥 10.5   ⚕ 10.5   **FUD** 090   J A2 80 ▭

AMA: 2018,Jan,8; 2017,Jan,8; 2016,Jan,13

55180 complicated ♂

📥 20.0   ⚕ 20.0   **FUD** 090   J A2 80 ▭

AMA: 2014,Jan,11

55200-55680 Procedures of Other Male Genital Ducts and Glands

55200 Vasotomy, cannulization with or without incision of vas, unilateral or bilateral (separate procedure) ♂

📥 8.00   ⚕ 11.7   **FUD** 090   J A2 80 ▭

AMA: 2014,Jan,11

55250 Vasectomy, unilateral or bilateral (separate procedure), including postoperative semen examination(s) ♂

📥 6.58   ⚕ 10.6   **FUD** 090   J A2

AMA: 2018,Jan,8; 2017,Jan,8; 2016,Jan,13

55300 Vasotomy for vasograms, seminal vesiculograms, or epididymograms, unilateral or bilateral ♂

Code also biopsy testis and modifier 51 when combined (54505)

📷 (74440)

📥 5.39   ⚕ 5.39   **FUD** 000   N N1 80 ▭

AMA: 2014,Jan,11

55400 Vasovasostomy, vasovasorrhaphy ♂

> **EXCLUDES** *Operating microscope (69990)*

📥 14.4   ⚕ 14.4   **FUD** 090   J A2 80 50 ▭

AMA: 2018,Jan,8; 2017,Jan,8; 2016,Jan,13

55500 Excision of hydrocele of spermatic cord, unilateral (separate procedure) ♂

📥 11.3   ⚕ 11.3   **FUD** 090   J A2 80 50 ▭

AMA: 2018,Jan,8; 2017,Jan,8; 2016,Jan,13

55520 Excision of lesion of spermatic cord (separate procedure) ♂

📥 13.2   ⚕ 13.2   **FUD** 090   J A2 80 50 ▭

AMA: 2018,Jan,8; 2017,Jan,8; 2016,Jan,13

55530 Excision of varicocele or ligation of spermatic veins for varicocele; (separate procedure) ♂

📥 10.1   ⚕ 10.1   **FUD** 090   J A2 50 ▭

AMA: 2018,Jan,8; 2017,Jan,8; 2016,Jan,13

55535 abdominal approach ♂

📥 12.4   ⚕ 12.4   **FUD** 090   J A2 80 50 ▭

AMA: 2018,Jan,8; 2017,Jan,8; 2016,Jan,13

55540 with hernia repair ♂

📥 16.0   ⚕ 16.0   **FUD** 090   J A2 50 ▭

AMA: 2018,Jan,8; 2017,Jan,8; 2016,Jan,13

26/TC PC/TC Only   A2-Z3 ASC Payment   50 Bilateral   ♂ Male Only   ♀ Female Only   📥 Facility RVU   ⚕ Non-Facility RVU   ▭ CCI   ✖ CLIA
FUD Follow-up Days   CMS: IOM   AMA: CPT Asst   A-Y OPPSI   80/80 Surg Assist Allowed / w/Doc   📧 Lab Crosswalk   📷 Radiology Crosswalk

250   CPT © 2021 American Medical Association. All Rights Reserved.   © 2021 Optum360, LLC

55550 **Laparoscopy, surgical, with ligation of spermatic veins for varicocele** ♂

INCLUDES Diagnostic laparoscopy (49320)

🔧 12.3 ⚕ 12.3 **FUD** 090 J A2 80 50 ▣

AMA: 2018,Jan,8; 2017,Jan,8; 2016,Jan,13

55559 **Unlisted laparoscopy procedure, spermatic cord** ♂

🔧 0.00 ⚕ 0.00 **FUD** YYY J 80 50 ▣

AMA: 2018,Jan,8; 2017,Jan,8; 2016,Jan,13

55600 **Vesiculotomy;** ♂

🔧 12.1 ⚕ 12.1 **FUD** 090 J R2 80 50 ▣

AMA: 2014,Jan,11

55605 **complicated** ♂

🔧 15.0 ⚕ 15.0 **FUD** 090 C 80 50 ▣

AMA: 2014,Jan,11

55650 **Vesiculectomy, any approach** ♂

🔧 20.7 ⚕ 20.7 **FUD** 090 C 80 50 ▣

AMA: 2014,Jan,11

55680 **Excision of Mullerian duct cyst** ♂

EXCLUDES Injection procedure (52010, 55300)

🔧 9.99 ⚕ 9.99 **FUD** 090 J A2 80 50 ▣

AMA: 2014,Jan,11

55700-55725 Procedures of Prostate: Incisional

55700 **Biopsy, prostate; needle or punch, single or multiple, any approach** ♂

EXCLUDES Fine needle aspiration (10021, [10004, 10005, 10006, 10007, 10008, 10009, 10010, 10011, 10012])
Needle biopsy prostate, saturation sampling for prostate mapping (55706)

📷 (76942, 77002, 77012, 77021)
🔬 (88172-88173)

🔧 3.77 ⚕ 7.12 **FUD** 000 J A2

AMA: 2018,Jul,11; 2018,Jan,8; 2017,Jan,8; 2016,Jan,13

55705 **incisional, any approach** ♂

🔧 7.67 ⚕ 7.67 **FUD** 010 J A2 ▣

AMA: 2014,Jan,11

55706 **Biopsies, prostate, needle, transperineal, stereotactic template guided saturation sampling, including imaging guidance** ♂

EXCLUDES Biopsy, prostate; needle or punch (55700)

🔧 10.7 ⚕ 10.7 **FUD** 010 J 62 80 ▣

AMA: 2018,Jan,8; 2017,Jan,8; 2016,Jan,13

55720 **Prostatotomy, external drainage of prostatic abscess, any approach; simple** ♂

EXCLUDES Drainage prostatic abscess, transurethral (52700)

🔧 13.0 ⚕ 13.0 **FUD** 090 J A2 80 ▣

AMA: 2014,Jan,11

55725 **complicated** ♂

EXCLUDES Drainage prostatic abscess, transurethral (52700)

🔧 17.1 ⚕ 17.1 **FUD** 090 J A2 80 ▣

AMA: 2014,Jan,11

55801-55845 Open Prostatectomy

EXCLUDES Limited pelvic lymphadenectomy for staging (separate procedure) (38562)
Node dissection, independent (38770-38780)
Transurethral prostate:
Destruction (53850-53852)
Resection (52601-52640)

55801 **Prostatectomy, perineal, subtotal (including control of postoperative bleeding, vasectomy, meatotomy, urethral calibration and/or dilation, and internal urethrotomy)** ♂

🔧 31.6 ⚕ 31.6 **FUD** 090 C 80 ▣

AMA: 2014,Jan,11; 2003,Jun,6

55810 **Prostatectomy, perineal radical;** ♂

INCLUDES Walsh modified radical prostatectomy

🔧 37.8 ⚕ 37.8 **FUD** 090 C 80 ▣

AMA: 2014,Jan,11; 2003,Jun,6

55812 **with lymph node biopsy(s) (limited pelvic lymphadenectomy)** ♂

🔧 46.4 ⚕ 46.4 **FUD** 090 C 80 ▣

AMA: 2014,Jan,11

55815 **with bilateral pelvic lymphadenectomy, including external iliac, hypogastric and obturator nodes** ♂

EXCLUDES When performed on separate days, report:
Pelvic lymphadenectomy, bilateral, and append modifier 50 (38770)
Perineal radical prostatectomy (55810)

🔧 50.9 ⚕ 50.9 **FUD** 090 C 80 ▣

AMA: 2014,Jan,11

55821 **Prostatectomy (including control of postoperative bleeding, vasectomy, meatotomy, urethral calibration and/or dilation, and internal urethrotomy); suprapubic, subtotal, 1 or 2 stages** ♂

🔧 25.2 ⚕ 25.2 **FUD** 090 C 80 ▣

AMA: 2014,Jan,11; 2003,Jun,6

55831 **retropubic, subtotal** ♂

🔧 27.3 ⚕ 27.3 **FUD** 090 C 80 ▣

AMA: 2014,Jan,11; 2003,Jun,6

55840 **Prostatectomy, retropubic radical, with or without nerve sparing;** ♂

EXCLUDES Prostatectomy, radical retropubic, performed laparoscopically (55866)

🔧 33.8 ⚕ 33.8 **FUD** 090 C 80 ▣

AMA: 2014,Jan,11; 2003,Jun,6

55842 **with lymph node biopsy(s) (limited pelvic lymphadenectomy)** ♂

EXCLUDES Prostatectomy, retropubic radical, performed laparoscopically (55866)

🔧 33.8 ⚕ 33.8 **FUD** 090 C 80 ▣

AMA: 2014,Jan,11; 2003,Jun,6

55845 **with bilateral pelvic lymphadenectomy, including external iliac, hypogastric, and obturator nodes** ♂

EXCLUDES Prostatectomy, retropubic radical, performed laparoscopically (55866)
When performed on separate days, report:
Pelvic lymphadenectomy, bilateral, and append modifier 50 (38770)
Radical prostatectomy, retropubic, with or without nerve sparing (55840)

🔧 39.3 ⚕ 39.3 **FUD** 090 C 80 ▣

AMA: 2014,Jan,11; 2003,Jun,6

55860-55865 Prostate Exposure for Radiation Source Application

55860 Exposure of prostate, any approach, for insertion of radioactive substance; ♂

EXCLUDES *Interstitial radioelement application (77770-77772, 77778)*

🔲 25.2 🔲 25.2 **FUD** 090 [J] [G2] [▢]
AMA: 2014,Jan,11

55862 with lymph node biopsy(s) (limited pelvic lymphadenectomy) ♂

🔲 31.6 🔲 31.6 **FUD** 090 [C] [80] [▢]
AMA: 2014,Jan,11

55865 with bilateral pelvic lymphadenectomy, including external iliac, hypogastric and obturator nodes ♂

🔲 38.5 🔲 38.5 **FUD** 090 [C] [80] [▢]
AMA: 2014,Jan,11

55866 Laparoscopic Prostatectomy

55866 Laparoscopy, surgical prostatectomy, retropubic radical, including nerve sparing, includes robotic assistance, when performed ♂

INCLUDES *Diagnostic laparoscopy (49320)*
EXCLUDES *Open method (55840)*

🔲 41.6 🔲 41.6 **FUD** 090 [J] [G2] [80] [▢]
AMA: 2018,Jan,8; 2017,Jan,8; 2016,Jan,13

55870-55899 Miscellaneous Prostate Procedures

55870 Electroejaculation ♂

EXCLUDES *Artificial insemination (58321-58322)*

🔲 4.10 🔲 5.04 **FUD** 000 [T] [P3] [▢]
AMA: 2014,Jan,11; 1991,Win,1

55873 Cryosurgical ablation of the prostate (includes ultrasonic guidance and monitoring) ♂

🔲 22.0 🔲 175. **FUD** 090 [J] [J8] [▢]
AMA: 2019,Sep,10; 2018,Jan,8; 2017,Jan,8; 2016,Jan,13

55874 Transperineal placement of biodegradable material, peri-prostatic, single or multiple injection(s), including image guidance, when performed ♂

INCLUDES *Ultrasound guidance (76942)*

🔲 4.77 🔲 87.0 **FUD** 000 [T] [J8] [▢]

55875 Transperineal placement of needles or catheters into prostate for interstitial radioelement application, with or without cystoscopy ♂

EXCLUDES *Placement needles/catheters for interstitial radioelement application, pelvic organs/genitalia, except prostate (55920)*
Code also interstitial radioelement application (77770-77772, 77778)
⭐ (76965)

🔲 22.2 🔲 22.2 **FUD** 090 [J] [A2] [80] [▢]
AMA: 2018,Jan,8; 2017,Jan,8; 2016,Jan,13

55876 Placement of interstitial device(s) for radiation therapy guidance (eg, fiducial markers, dosimeter), prostate (via needle, any approach), single or multiple ♂

Code also supply device
⭐ (76942, 77002, 77012, 77021)

🔲 2.91 🔲 4.16 **FUD** 000 [S] [P3] [▢]
AMA: 2018,Jan,8; 2017,Jan,8; 2016,Jun,3; 2016,Jan,13

55880 Ablation of malignant prostate tissue, transrectal, with high intensity-focused ultrasound (HIFU), including ultrasound guidance ♂

🔲 28.5 🔲 28.5 **FUD** 090 [G2] [▢]

55899 Unlisted procedure, male genital system ♂

🔲 0.00 🔲 0.00 **FUD** YYY [T] [80] [▢]
AMA: 2020,Aug,6; 2019,Dec,12; 2019,Jun,14; 2018,Jan,8; 2017,Jan,8; 2017,Jan,6; 2016,Jan,13

55920 Insertion Brachytherapy Catheters/Needles Pelvis/Genitalia, Male/Female

55920 Placement of needles or catheters into pelvic organs and/or genitalia (except prostate) for subsequent interstitial radioelement application

EXCLUDES *Insertion Heyman capsules for brachytherapy (58346)*
Insertion vaginal ovoids and/or uterine tandems for brachytherapy (57155)
Placement catheters or needles, prostate (55875)

🔲 13.0 🔲 13.0 **FUD** 000 [J] [G2] [80] [▢]
AMA: 2018,Jan,8; 2017,Jan,8; 2016,Jan,13

55970-55980 Transsexual Surgery

CMS: 100-02,16,10 Exclusions from Coverage; 100-02,16,180 Services Related to Noncovered Procedures

55970 Intersex surgery; male to female ♂

🔲 0.00 🔲 0.00 **FUD** YYY [J] [G2] [▢]
AMA: 2014,Jan,11

55980 female to male ♀

🔲 0.00 🔲 0.00 **FUD** YYY [J] [G2] [▢]
AMA: 2014,Jan,11

56405-56420 Incision and Drainage of Abscess

EXCLUDES *Incision and drainage Skene's gland cyst/abscess (53060)*
Incision and drainage subcutaneous abscess/cyst/furuncle (10040, 10060, 10061)

56405 Incision and drainage of vulva or perineal abscess ♀

🔲 3.43 🔲 3.69 **FUD** 010 [T] [P3] [▢]
AMA: 2019,Jul,6

56420 Incision and drainage of Bartholin's gland abscess ♀

🔲 2.97 🔲 4.47 **FUD** 010 [T] [P2] [▢]
AMA: 2019,Jul,6

56440-56442 Other Female Genital Incisional Procedures

EXCLUDES *Incision and drainage subcutaneous abscess/cyst/furuncle (10040, 10060, 10061)*

56440 Marsupialization of Bartholin's gland cyst ♀

🔲 5.25 🔲 5.25 **FUD** 010 [J] [A2] [▢]
AMA: 2019,Jul,6

56441 Lysis of labial adhesions ♀

🔲 4.09 🔲 4.33 **FUD** 010 [J] [A2] [80] [▢]
AMA: 2019,Jul,6

56442 Hymenotomy, simple incision ♀

🔲 1.36 🔲 1.36 **FUD** 000 [J] [A2] [80] [▢]
AMA: 2019,Jul,6

56501-56515 Destruction of Vulvar Lesions, Any Method

EXCLUDES Excision/fulguration/destruction:
Skene's glands (53270)
Urethral caruncle (53265)

56501 **Destruction of lesion(s), vulva; simple (eg, laser surgery, electrosurgery, cryosurgery, chemosurgery)** ♀
3.60   4.69   **FUD** 010   T P3 ▣
AMA: 2019,Aug,10; 2019,Jul,6

56515 **extensive (eg, laser surgery, electrosurgery, cryosurgery, chemosurgery)** ♀
5.97   7.25   **FUD** 010   T A2 ▣
AMA: 2019,Aug,10; 2019,Jul,6

56605-56606 Vulvar and Perineal Biopsies

EXCLUDES Excision local lesion (11420-11426, 11620-11626)

56605 **Biopsy of vulva or perineum (separate procedure); 1 lesion** ♀
1.71   2.43   **FUD** 000   T P3 ▣
AMA: 2019,Jul,6; 2019,Jan,9; 2018,Jan,8; 2017,Jan,8; 2016,Jan,13

+ **56606** **each separate additional lesion (List separately in addition to code for primary procedure)** ♀
Code first (56605)
0.86   1.11   **FUD** ZZZ   N N1 ▣
AMA: 2019,Jul,6; 2019,Jan,9

56620-56640 Vulvectomy Procedures

INCLUDES Removal:
Greater than 80% vulvar area - complete procedure
Less than 80% vulvar area - partial procedure
Skin and deep subcutaneous tissue - radical procedure
Skin and superficial subcutaneous tissues - simple procedure
EXCLUDES Skin graft (15004-15005, 15120-15121, 15240-15241)

56620 **Vulvectomy simple; partial** ♀
15.9   15.9   **FUD** 090   J A2 80 ▣
AMA: 2019,Jul,6; 2019,Jan,14; 2018,Jan,8; 2017,Jan,8; 2016,Jan,13

56625 **complete** ♀
18.6   18.6   **FUD** 090   J A2 80 ▣
AMA: 2019,Jul,6

56630 **Vulvectomy, radical, partial;** ♀
Code also lymph node biopsy/excision when partial radical vulvectomy with inguinofemoral lymph node biopsy without inguinofemoral lymphadenectomy performed (38531)
27.0   27.0   **FUD** 090   C 80 ▣
AMA: 2019,Jul,6; 2019,Feb,8

56631 **with unilateral inguinofemoral lymphadenectomy** ♀
INCLUDES Bassett's operation
34.4   34.4   **FUD** 090   C 80 ▣
AMA: 2019,Jul,6; 2019,Feb,8

56632 **with bilateral inguinofemoral lymphadenectomy** ♀
INCLUDES Bassett's operation
40.2   40.2   **FUD** 090   C 80 ▣
AMA: 2019,Jul,6; 2019,Feb,8

56633 **Vulvectomy, radical, complete;** ♀
INCLUDES Bassett's operation
34.9   34.9   **FUD** 090   C 80 ▣
AMA: 2019,Jul,6; 2019,Feb,8

56634 **with unilateral inguinofemoral lymphadenectomy** ♀
INCLUDES Bassett's operation
36.8   36.8   **FUD** 090   C 80 ▣
AMA: 2019,Jul,6; 2019,Feb,8

56637 **with bilateral inguinofemoral lymphadenectomy** ♀
INCLUDES Bassett's operation
Code also lymph node biopsy/excision when complete radical vulvectomy with inguinofemoral lymph node biopsy without inguinofemoral lymphadenectomy performed (38531)
43.9   43.9   **FUD** 090   C 80 ▣
AMA: 2019,Jul,6; 2019,Feb,8

56640 **Vulvectomy, radical, complete, with inguinofemoral, iliac, and pelvic lymphadenectomy** ♀
INCLUDES Bassett's operation
EXCLUDES Lymphadenectomy (38760-38780)
43.3   43.3   **FUD** 090   C 80 50 ▣
AMA: 2019,Jul,6; 2019,Feb,8

56700-56740 Other Excisional Procedures: External Female Genitalia

56700 **Partial hymenectomy or revision of hymenal ring** ♀
5.38   5.38   **FUD** 010   J A2 80 ▣
AMA: 2019,Jul,6

56740 **Excision of Bartholin's gland or cyst** ♀
EXCLUDES Excision/fulguration/marsupialization:
Skene's glands (53270)
Urethral carcinoma (53220)
Urethral caruncle (53265)
Urethral diverticulum (53230, 53240)
8.92   8.92   **FUD** 010   J A2 50 ▣
AMA: 2019,Jul,6

56800-56810 Repair/Reconstruction External Female Genitalia

EXCLUDES Repair urethra for mucosal prolapse (53275)

56800 **Plastic repair of introitus** ♀
INCLUDES Emmet's operation
7.17   7.17   **FUD** 010   J A2 80 ▣
AMA: 2019,Jul,6

56805 **Clitoroplasty for intersex state** ♀
33.6   33.6   **FUD** 090   J 62 80 ▣
AMA: 2019,Jul,6

56810 **Perineoplasty, repair of perineum, nonobstetrical (separate procedure)** ♀
INCLUDES Emmet's operation
EXCLUDES Genitalia wound repair (12001-12007, 12041-12047, 13131-13133)
Introitus plastic repair (56800)
Sphincteroplasty, anal (46750-46751)
Vaginal/perineum recent injury repair, nonobstetrical (57210)
7.72   7.72   **FUD** 010   J A2 80 ▣
AMA: 2019,Jul,6

56820-56821 Vulvar Colposcopy with/without Biopsy

EXCLUDES Colposcopic procedures and/or examinations:
Cervix (57452-57461)
Vagina (57420-57421)

56820 **Colposcopy of the vulva;** ♀
2.46   3.28   **FUD** 000   T P3 ▣
AMA: 2019,Jul,6; 2018,Jan,8; 2017,Jan,8; 2016,Jan,13

56821 **with biopsy(s)** ♀
3.28   4.36   **FUD** 000   T P3 ▣
AMA: 2019,Jul,6; 2018,Jan,8; 2017,Jan,8; 2016,Jan,13

57000-57023 Incisional Procedures: Vagina

57000 **Colpotomy; with exploration** ♀
5.44   5.44   **FUD** 010   J A2 80 ▣
AMA: 2019,Jul,6; 2018,Jan,8; 2017,Jan,8; 2016,Jan,13

Genital System

57010 — 57230

57010   **with drainage of pelvic abscess** ♀
INCLUDES   Laroyenne operation
⚕ 12.4   ⚕ 12.4   **FUD** 090   J A2 80 ▢
AMA: 2019,Jul,6

57020   **Colpocentesis (separate procedure)** ♀
⚕ 2.29   ⚕ 2.77   **FUD** 000   J A2 80 ▢
AMA: 2019,Jul,6

Speculum   Bladder

Fluid in pelvis

Vagina   Rectum

The physician aspirates matter from the pelvis through a needle inserted through the vaginal wall

57022   **Incision and drainage of vaginal hematoma; obstetrical/postpartum** ♀
⚕ 4.86   ⚕ 4.86   **FUD** 010   J R2 80 ▢
AMA: 2019,Jul,6

57023   **non-obstetrical (eg, post-trauma, spontaneous bleeding)** ♀
⚕ 8.83   ⚕ 8.83   **FUD** 010   J A2 80 ▢
AMA: 2019,Jul,6

57061-57065 Destruction of Vaginal Lesions, Any Method

CMS: 100-03,140.5 Laser Procedures

57061   **Destruction of vaginal lesion(s); simple (eg, laser surgery, electrosurgery, cryosurgery, chemosurgery)** ♀
⚕ 2.92   ⚕ 3.52   **FUD** 000   J P3 ▢
AMA: 2019,Jul,6; 2018,Jan,8; 2017,Jan,8; 2016,Jan,13

57065   **extensive (eg, laser surgery, electrosurgery, cryosurgery, chemosurgery)** ♀
⚕ 5.08   ⚕ 5.88   **FUD** 010   J A2 ▢
AMA: 2019,Jul,6; 2018,Jan,8; 2017,Jan,8; 2016,Jan,13

57100-57135 Excisional Procedures: Vagina

57100   **Biopsy of vaginal mucosa; simple (separate procedure)** ♀
⚕ 1.91   ⚕ 2.64   **FUD** 000   T P3 ▢
AMA: 2019,Jul,6

57105   **extensive, requiring suture (including cysts)** ♀
⚕ 3.75   ⚕ 4.19   **FUD** 010   J A2 ▢
AMA: 2019,Jul,6

57106   **Vaginectomy, partial removal of vaginal wall;** ♀
⚕ 14.5   ⚕ 14.5   **FUD** 090   J G2 80 ▢
AMA: 2019,Jul,6; 2018,Jan,8; 2017,Jan,8; 2016,Jan,13

57107   **with removal of paravaginal tissue (radical vaginectomy)** ♀
⚕ 41.9   ⚕ 41.9   **FUD** 090   J G2 80 ▢
AMA: 2019,Jul,6; 2018,Jan,8; 2017,Jan,8; 2016,Jan,13

57109   **with removal of paravaginal tissue (radical vaginectomy) with bilateral total pelvic lymphadenectomy and para-aortic lymph node sampling (biopsy)** ♀
⚕ 51.1   ⚕ 51.1   **FUD** 090   J G2 80 ▢
AMA: 2019,Jul,6; 2018,Jan,8; 2017,Jan,8; 2016,Jan,13

57110   **Vaginectomy, complete removal of vaginal wall;** ♀
⚕ 25.3   ⚕ 25.3   **FUD** 090   C 80 ▢
AMA: 2019,Jul,6; 2018,Jan,8; 2017,Jan,8; 2016,Jan,13

57111   **with removal of paravaginal tissue (radical vaginectomy)** ♀
⚕ 51.1   ⚕ 51.1   **FUD** 090   C 80 ▢
AMA: 2019,Jul,6; 2018,Jan,8; 2017,Jan,8; 2016,Jan,13

57120   **Colpocleisis (Le Fort type)** ♀
⚕ 14.6   ⚕ 14.6   **FUD** 090   J G2 80 ▢
AMA: 2019,Jul,6

57130   **Excision of vaginal septum** ♀
⚕ 4.60   ⚕ 5.32   **FUD** 010   J A2 80 ▢
AMA: 2019,Jul,6

57135   **Excision of vaginal cyst or tumor** ♀
⚕ 5.05   ⚕ 5.80   **FUD** 010   J A2 ▢
AMA: 2019,Jul,6

57150-57180 Irrigation/Insertion/Introduction Vaginal Medication or Supply

57150   **Irrigation of vagina and/or application of medicament for treatment of bacterial, parasitic, or fungoid disease** ♀
⚕ 0.75   ⚕ 1.38   **FUD** 000   Q1 N1 ▢
AMA: 2019,Jul,6

57155   **Insertion of uterine tandem and/or vaginal ovoids for clinical brachytherapy** ♀
EXCLUDES   Insertion radioelement sources or ribbons (77761-77763, 77770-77772)
Placement needles or catheters into pelvic organs and/or genitalia (except prostate) for interstitial radioelement application (55920)
⚕ 8.09   ⚕ 10.6   **FUD** 000   J A2 ▢
AMA: 2019,Jul,6; 2018,Jan,8; 2017,Jan,8; 2016,Jan,13

57156   **Insertion of a vaginal radiation afterloading apparatus for clinical brachytherapy** ♀
⚕ 4.27   ⚕ 5.92   **FUD** 000   T G2 80 ▢
AMA: 2019,Jul,6

57160   **Fitting and insertion of pessary or other intravaginal support device** ♀
⚕ 1.33   ⚕ 1.79   **FUD** 000   T P3 ▢
AMA: 2019,Jul,6; 2018,Jan,8; 2017,Jan,8; 2016,Jan,13

57170   **Diaphragm or cervical cap fitting with instructions** ♀
⚕ 1.37   ⚕ 1.85   **FUD** 000   T P3 80 ▢
AMA: 2019,Jul,6

57180   **Introduction of any hemostatic agent or pack for spontaneous or traumatic nonobstetrical vaginal hemorrhage (separate procedure)** ♀
⚕ 3.11   ⚕ 4.37   **FUD** 010   T A2 ▢
AMA: 2019,Jul,6; 2018,Jan,8; 2017,Jan,8; 2016,Jan,13

57200-57335 Vaginal Repair and Reconstruction

EXCLUDES   Marshall-Marchetti-Kranz type urethral suspension, abdominal approach (51840-51841)
Urethral suspension performed laparoscopically (51990)

57200   **Colporrhaphy, suture of injury of vagina (nonobstetrical)** ♀
⚕ 8.87   ⚕ 8.87   **FUD** 090   J A2 80 ▢
AMA: 2019,Jul,6

57210   **Colpoperineorrhaphy, suture of injury of vagina and/or perineum (nonobstetrical)** ♀
⚕ 10.6   ⚕ 10.6   **FUD** 090   J A2 80 ▢
AMA: 2019,Jul,6

57220   **Plastic operation on urethral sphincter, vaginal approach (eg, Kelly urethral plication)** ♀
⚕ 9.24   ⚕ 9.24   **FUD** 090   J A2 80 ▢
AMA: 2019,Jul,6

57230   **Plastic repair of urethrocele** ♀
⚕ 11.3   ⚕ 11.3   **FUD** 090   J A2 80 ▢
AMA: 2019,Jul,6

26/TC PC/TC Only   A2-Z3 ASC Payment   50 Bilateral   ♂ Male Only   ♀ Female Only   ⚕ Facility RVU   ⚕ Non-Facility RVU   ▢ CCI   ✖ CLIA
FUD Follow-up Days   **CMS:** IOM   **AMA:** CPT Asst   A-Y OPPSI   80/80 Surg Assist Allowed / w/Doc   Lab Crosswalk   Radiology Crosswalk

254   CPT © 2021 American Medical Association. All Rights Reserved.   © 2021 Optum360, LLC

57240 **Anterior colporrhaphy, repair of cystocele with or without repair of urethrocele, including cystourethroscopy, when performed** ♀

INCLUDES Cystourethroscopy (52000)

🔧 17.0 ⚕ 17.0 **FUD** 090 J A2 80 ▢

AMA: 2019,Jul,6; 2018,Jan,8; 2017,Jan,8; 2016,Jan,13

57250 **Posterior colporrhaphy, repair of rectocele with or without perineorrhaphy** ♀

INCLUDES Rectocele repair (separate procedure) without posterior colporrhaphy (45560)

🔧 17.0 ⚕ 17.0 **FUD** 090 J A2 80 ▢

AMA: 2019,Jul,6; 2018,Jan,8; 2017,Jan,8; 2016,Jan,13

57260 **Combined anteroposterior colporrhaphy, including cystourethroscopy, when performed;** ♀

INCLUDES Cystourethroscopy (52000)

🔧 21.7 ⚕ 21.7 **FUD** 090 J A2 80 ▢

AMA: 2019,Jul,6; 2018,Jan,8; 2017,Jan,8; 2016,Jan,13

57265 **with enterocele repair** ♀

INCLUDES Cystourethroscopy (52000)

🔧 24.4 ⚕ 24.4 **FUD** 090 J A2 80 ▢

AMA: 2019,Jul,6; 2018,Jan,8; 2017,Jan,8; 2016,Jan,13

+ 57267 **Insertion of mesh or other prosthesis for repair of pelvic floor defect, each site (anterior, posterior compartment), vaginal approach (List separately in addition to code for primary procedure)** ♀

Code first (45560, 57240-57265, 57285)

🔧 7.25 ⚕ 7.25 **FUD** ZZZ N N1 80 ▢

AMA: 2019,Jul,6; 2018,Jan,8; 2017,Jan,8; 2016,Jan,13

57268 **Repair of enterocele, vaginal approach (separate procedure)** ♀

🔧 13.9 ⚕ 13.9 **FUD** 090 J A2 80 ▢

AMA: 2019,Jul,6; 2018,Jan,8; 2017,Jan,8; 2016,Jan,13

57270 **Repair of enterocele, abdominal approach (separate procedure)** ♀

🔧 23.0 ⚕ 23.0 **FUD** 090 C 80 ▢

AMA: 2019,Jul,6; 2018,Jan,8; 2017,Jan,8; 2016,Jan,13

57280 **Colpopexy, abdominal approach** ♀

🔧 27.2 ⚕ 27.2 **FUD** 090 C 80 ▢

AMA: 2019,Jul,6; 2018,Jan,8; 2017,Jan,8; 2016,Jan,13

57282 **Colpopexy, vaginal; extra-peritoneal approach (sacrospinous, iliococcygeus)** ♀

🔧 15.1 ⚕ 15.1 **FUD** 090 J G2 80 ▢

AMA: 2019,Jul,6; 2018,Jan,8; 2017,Jan,8; 2016,Jan,13

57283 **intra-peritoneal approach (uterosacral, levator myorrhaphy)** ♀

EXCLUDES Excision cervical stump (57556)
Vaginal hysterectomy (58263, 58270, 58280, 58292, 58294)

🔧 19.6 ⚕ 19.6 **FUD** 090 J G2 80 ▢

AMA: 2019,Jul,6; 2018,Jan,8; 2017,Jan,8; 2016,Jan,13

57284 **Paravaginal defect repair (including repair of cystocele, if performed); open abdominal approach** ♀

EXCLUDES Anterior colporrhaphy (57240)
Anterior vesicourethropexy (51840-51841)
Combined anteroposterior colporrhaphy (57260-57265)
Hysterectomy (58152, 58267)
Laparoscopy, surgical; urethral suspension for stress incontinence (51990)

🔧 23.8 ⚕ 23.8 **FUD** 090 J G2 80 ▢

AMA: 2019,Jul,6; 2018,Jan,8; 2017,Jan,8; 2016,Jan,13

57285 **vaginal approach** ♀

EXCLUDES Anterior colporrhaphy (57240)
Combined anteroposterior colporrhaphy (57260-57265)
Laparoscopy, surgical; urethral suspension for stress incontinence (51990)
Vaginal hysterectomy (58267)

🔧 19.8 ⚕ 19.8 **FUD** 090 J G2 80 ▢

AMA: 2019,Jul,6; 2018,Jan,8; 2017,Jan,8; 2016,Jan,13

57287 **Removal or revision of sling for stress incontinence (eg, fascia or synthetic)** ♀

🔧 20.6 ⚕ 20.6 **FUD** 090 Q2 G2 80 ▢

AMA: 2019,Jul,6; 2018,Jan,8; 2017,Jan,8; 2016,Jan,13

57288 **Sling operation for stress incontinence (eg, fascia or synthetic)** ♀

INCLUDES Millin-Read operation

EXCLUDES Sling operation for stress incontinence performed laparoscopically (51992)

🔧 21.1 ⚕ 21.1 **FUD** 090 J J8 80 ▢

AMA: 2019,Jul,6; 2019,Feb,10; 2018,Jan,8; 2017,Jan,8; 2016,Jan,13

57289 **Pereyra procedure, including anterior colporrhaphy** ♀

🔧 22.6 ⚕ 22.6 **FUD** 090 J A2 80 ▢

AMA: 2019,Jul,6; 2018,Jan,8; 2017,Jan,8; 2016,Jan,13

57291 **Construction of artificial vagina; without graft** ♀

INCLUDES McIndoe vaginal construction

🔧 15.6 ⚕ 15.6 **FUD** 090 J A2 80 ▢

AMA: 2019,Jul,6

57292 **with graft** ♀

🔧 23.9 ⚕ 23.9 **FUD** 090 J G2 80 ▢

AMA: 2019,Jul,6

57295 **Revision (including removal) of prosthetic vaginal graft; vaginal approach** ♀

EXCLUDES Laparoscopic approach (57426)

🔧 14.2 ⚕ 14.2 **FUD** 090 J G2 80 ▢

AMA: 2019,Jul,6

57296 **open abdominal approach** ♀

EXCLUDES Laparoscopic approach (57426)

🔧 27.4 ⚕ 27.4 **FUD** 090 C 80 ▢

AMA: 2019,Jul,6

57300 **Closure of rectovaginal fistula; vaginal or transanal approach** ♀

🔧 17.0 ⚕ 17.0 **FUD** 090 J A2 ▢

AMA: 2019,Jul,6

57305 **abdominal approach** ♀

🔧 27.9 ⚕ 27.9 **FUD** 090 C 80 ▢

AMA: 2019,Jul,6

57307 **abdominal approach, with concomitant colostomy** ♀

🔧 30.3 ⚕ 30.3 **FUD** 090 C 80 ▢

AMA: 2019,Jul,6

57308 **transperineal approach, with perineal body reconstruction, with or without levator plication** ♀

🔧 19.0 ⚕ 19.0 **FUD** 090 C 80 ▢

AMA: 2019,Jul,6

57310 **Closure of urethrovaginal fistula;** ♀

🔧 13.8 ⚕ 13.8 **FUD** 090 J G2 80 ▢

AMA: 2019,Jul,6

57311 **with bulbocavernosus transplant** ♀

🔧 15.6 ⚕ 15.6 **FUD** 090 C 80 ▢

AMA: 2019,Jul,6

57320 **Closure of vesicovaginal fistula; vaginal approach** ♀

EXCLUDES Cystostomy, concomitant (51020-51040, 51101-51102)

🔧 15.8 ⚕ 15.8 **FUD** 090 J G2 80 ▢

AMA: 2019,Jul,6

Genital System

57330 — 57456

57330   **transvesical and vaginal approach**   ♀

> EXCLUDES *Vesicovaginal fistula closure, abdominal approach (51900)*

🔲 21.8   ⚗ 21.8   **FUD** 090   J 62 80 ▭

AMA: 2019,Jul,6

57335   **Vaginoplasty for intersex state**   ♀

🔲 33.9   ⚗ 33.9   **FUD** 090   J 62 80 ▭

AMA: 2019,Jul,6

57400-57415 Treatment of Vaginal Disorders Under Anesthesia

57400   **Dilation of vagina under anesthesia (other than local)**   ♀

🔲 3.78   ⚗ 3.78   **FUD** 000   J A2 80 ▭

AMA: 2019,Jul,6

57410   **Pelvic examination under anesthesia (other than local)**   ♀

🔲 3.05   ⚗ 3.05   **FUD** 000   J A2 ▭

AMA: 2019,Jul,6; 2018,Jan,8; 2017,Jan,8; 2016,Jan,13

57415   **Removal of impacted vaginal foreign body (separate procedure) under anesthesia (other than local)**   ♀

> EXCLUDES *Removal impacted vaginal foreign body without anesthesia, report with appropriate E/M code*

🔲 4.89   ⚗ 4.89   **FUD** 010   J A2 80 ▭

AMA: 2019,Jul,6

57420-57426 Endoscopic Vaginal Procedures

57420   **Colposcopy of the entire vagina, with cervix if present;**   ♀

> EXCLUDES *Colposcopic procedures and/or examinations:*
> *Cervix (57452-57461)*
> *Vulva (56820-56821)*

Code also:
> Computer-aided cervical mapping during colposcopy (57465)
> Endometrial sampling (biopsy) performed same time as colposcopy (58110)
> Modifier 51 for colposcopic procedures different sites, as appropriate

🔲 2.62   ⚗ 3.61   **FUD** 000   T P3 ▭

AMA: 2020,Dec,10; 2019,Jul,6; 2018,Jan,8; 2017,Jan,8; 2016,Jan,13

57421   **with biopsy(s) of vagina/cervix**   ♀

> EXCLUDES *Colposcopic procedures and/or examinations:*
> *Cervix (57452-57461)*
> *Vulva (56820-56821)*

Code also:
> Computer-aided cervical mapping during colposcopy (57465)
> Endometrial sampling (biopsy) performed same time as colposcopy (58110)
> Modifier 51 for colposcopic procedures different sites, as appropriate

🔲 3.55   ⚗ 4.86   **FUD** 000   T P3 ▭

AMA: 2020,Dec,10; 2019,Jul,6; 2018,Jan,8; 2017,Jan,8; 2016,Jan,13

57423   **Paravaginal defect repair (including repair of cystocele, if performed), laparoscopic approach**   ♀

> EXCLUDES *Anterior colporrhaphy (57240)*
> *Anterior vesicourethropexy (51840-51841)*
> *Combined anteroposterior colporrhaphy (57260)*
> *Diagnostic laparoscopy (49320)*
> *Hysterectomy (58152, 58267)*
> *Laparoscopy, surgical; urethral suspension for stress incontinence (51990)*

🔲 26.8   ⚗ 26.8   **FUD** 090   J 62 80 ▭

AMA: 2019,Jul,6; 2018,Jan,8; 2017,Jan,8; 2016,Jan,13

57425   **Laparoscopy, surgical, colpopexy (suspension of vaginal apex)**   ♀

🔲 27.6   ⚗ 27.6   **FUD** 090   J 62 80 ▭

AMA: 2019,Jul,6

57426   **Revision (including removal) of prosthetic vaginal graft, laparoscopic approach**   ♀

> EXCLUDES *Open abdominal approach (57296)*
> *Vaginal approach (57295)*

🔲 24.8   ⚗ 24.8   **FUD** 090   J 62 80 ▭

AMA: 2019,Jul,6

57452-57465 Endoscopic Cervical Procedures

> EXCLUDES *Colposcopic procedures and/or examinations:*
> *Vagina (57420-57421)*
> *Vulva (56820-56821)*

Code also endometrial sampling (biopsy) performed same time as colposcopy (58110)

57452   **Colposcopy of the cervix including upper/adjacent vagina;**   ♀

Code also computer-aided cervical mapping during colposcopy (57465)

🔲 2.64   ⚗ 3.45   **FUD** 000   T P3 ▭

AMA: 2020,Dec,10; 2019,Jul,6; 2018,Jan,8; 2017,Jan,8; 2016,Jan,13

Speculum
Light beam
Uterus
Cervix
Vagina
Colposcope

57454   **with biopsy(s) of the cervix and endocervical curettage**   ♀

> INCLUDES Colposcopy cervix (57452)

Code also computer-aided cervical mapping during colposcopy (57465)

🔲 3.89   ⚗ 4.71   **FUD** 000   T P3 ▭

AMA: 2020,Dec,10; 2019,Jul,6; 2018,Jan,8; 2017,Jan,8; 2016,Jan,13

57455   **with biopsy(s) of the cervix**   ♀

> INCLUDES Colposcopy cervix (57452)

Code also computer-aided cervical mapping during colposcopy (57465)

🔲 3.19   ⚗ 4.44   **FUD** 000   T P3 ▭

AMA: 2020,Dec,10; 2019,Jul,6; 2018,Jan,8; 2017,Jan,8; 2016,Jan,13

57456   **with endocervical curettage**   ♀

> INCLUDES Colposcopy cervix (57452)

> EXCLUDES *Colposcopy cervix including upper/adjacent vagina; with loop electrode conization cervix (57461)*

Code also computer-aided cervical mapping during colposcopy (57465)

🔲 2.90   ⚗ 3.95   **FUD** 000   T P3 ▭

AMA: 2020,Dec,10; 2019,Jul,6; 2018,Jan,8; 2017,Jan,8; 2016,Jan,13

57460   **with loop electrode biopsy(s) of the cervix** ♀

INCLUDES   Colposcopy cervix (57452)

Code also computer-aided cervical mapping during colposcopy (57465)

4.66   8.78   **FUD** 000   J P3

AMA: 2020,Dec,10; 2019,Jul,6; 2018,Jan,8; 2017,Jan,8; 2016,Jan,13

Loop electrocautery device guided by colposcope

Cervix

Vaginal lining

57461   **with loop electrode conization of the cervix** ♀

INCLUDES   Colposcopy cervix (57452)

EXCLUDES   Colposcopy cervix including upper/adjacent vagina; with endocervical curettage (57456)

Code also computer-aided cervical mapping during colposcopy (57465)

5.39   9.85   **FUD** 000   J P3

AMA: 2020,Dec,10; 2019,Jul,6; 2018,Jan,8; 2017,Jan,8; 2016,Jan,13

+ 57465   **Computer-aided mapping of cervix uteri during colposcopy, including optical dynamic spectral imaging and algorithmic quantification of the acetowhitening effect (List separately in addition to code for primary procedure)** ♀

Code first (57420-57421, 57452-57461)

1.27   1.66   **FUD** ZZZ   80

AMA: 2020,Dec,10

57500-57556 Cervical Procedures: Multiple Techniques

EXCLUDES   Radical surgical procedures (58200-58240)

57500   **Biopsy of cervix, single or multiple, or local excision of lesion, with or without fulguration (separate procedure)** ♀

2.17   4.11   **FUD** 000   T P3

AMA: 2019,Jul,6

57505   **Endocervical curettage (not done as part of a dilation and curettage)** ♀

2.90   3.69   **FUD** 010   T P3

AMA: 2019,Jul,6; 2018,Jan,8; 2017,Jan,8; 2016,Jan,13

57510   **Cautery of cervix; electro or thermal** ♀

3.29   4.33   **FUD** 010   J P3

AMA: 2019,Jul,6

57511   **cryocautery, initial or repeat** ♀

3.73   4.12   **FUD** 010   T P3

AMA: 2019,Jul,6

57513   **laser ablation** ♀

4.05   5.08   **FUD** 010   J A2

AMA: 2019,Jul,6

57520   **Conization of cervix, with or without fulguration, with or without dilation and curettage, with or without repair; cold knife or laser** ♀

EXCLUDES   Dilation and curettage, diagnostic/therapeutic, nonobstetrical (58120)

8.23   9.59   **FUD** 090   J A2

AMA: 2019,Jul,6; 2018,Jan,8; 2017,Jan,8; 2016,Jan,13

57522   **loop electrode excision** ♀

7.21   8.25   **FUD** 090   J A2

AMA: 2019,Jul,6; 2018,Jan,8; 2017,Jan,8; 2016,Jan,13

57530   **Trachelectomy (cervicectomy), amputation of cervix (separate procedure)** ♀

10.0   10.0   **FUD** 090   J A2 80

AMA: 2019,Jul,6

57531   **Radical trachelectomy, with bilateral total pelvic lymphadenectomy and para-aortic lymph node sampling biopsy, with or without removal of tube(s), with or without removal of ovary(s)** ♀

EXCLUDES   Radical hysterectomy (58210)

52.9   52.9   **FUD** 090   C 80

AMA: 2019,Jul,6

57540   **Excision of cervical stump, abdominal approach;** ♀

22.8   22.8   **FUD** 090   C 80

AMA: 2019,Jul,6

57545   **with pelvic floor repair** ♀

24.0   24.0   **FUD** 090   C 80

AMA: 2019,Jul,6

57550   **Excision of cervical stump, vaginal approach;** ♀

12.1   12.1   **FUD** 090   J A2 80

AMA: 2019,Jul,6

57555   **with anterior and/or posterior repair** ♀

17.7   17.7   **FUD** 090   J G2 80

AMA: 2019,Jul,6

57556   **with repair of enterocele** ♀

EXCLUDES   Insertion hemostatic agent/pack for spontaneous/traumatic nonobstetrical vaginal hemorrhage (57180)

Intrauterine device insertion (58300)

16.8   16.8   **FUD** 090   J A2 80

AMA: 2019,Jul,6

57558-57800 Cervical Procedures: Dilation, Suturing, or Instrumentation

57558   **Dilation and curettage of cervical stump** ♀

EXCLUDES   Radical surgical procedures (58200-58240)

3.33   3.80   **FUD** 010   J A2

AMA: 2019,Jul,6

57700   **Cerclage of uterine cervix, nonobstetrical** ♀

INCLUDES   McDonald cerclage

Shirodker operation

9.13   9.13   **FUD** 090   J A2 80

AMA: 2019,Jul,6

57720   **Trachelorrhaphy, plastic repair of uterine cervix, vaginal approach** ♀

INCLUDES   Emmet operation

9.33   9.33   **FUD** 090   J A2 80

AMA: 2019,Jul,6

57800   **Dilation of cervical canal, instrumental (separate procedure)** ♀

1.39   2.01   **FUD** 000   J P3

AMA: 2019,Jul,6

58100-58120 Procedures Involving the Endometrium

58100   **Endometrial sampling (biopsy) with or without endocervical sampling (biopsy), without cervical dilation, any method (separate procedure)** ♀

EXCLUDES   Endocervical curettage only (57505)

Endometrial sampling (biopsy) performed in conjunction with colposcopy (58110)

1.86   2.80   **FUD** 000   T P3

AMA: 2019,Jul,6

● New Code   ▲ Revised Code   ○ Reinstated   ● New Web Release   ▲ Revised Web Release   + Add-on   Unlisted   Not Covered   # Resequenced

50 Optum Mod 50 Exempt   ⊘ AMA Mod 51 Exempt   51 Optum Mod 51 Exempt   63 Mod 63 Exempt   ✗ Non-FDA Drug   ★ Telemedicine   M Maternity   A Age Edit

© 2021 Optum360, LLC   CPT © 2021 American Medical Association. All Rights Reserved.   257

Genital System

58110 — 58267

+ **58110** **Endometrial sampling (biopsy) performed in conjunction with colposcopy (List separately in addition to code for primary procedure)** ♀
  Code first colposcopy (57420-57421, 57452-57461)
  📷 1.19 ⚕ 1.46 **FUD** ZZZ   N N1 80 📄
  AMA: 2019,Jul,6; 2018,Jan,8; 2017,Jan,8; 2016,Jan,13

58120 **Dilation and curettage, diagnostic and/or therapeutic (nonobstetrical)** ♀
  EXCLUDES Postpartum hemorrhage (59160)
  📷 6.35 ⚕ 7.66 **FUD** 010   J A2 📄
  AMA: 2019,Jul,6; 2018,Jan,8; 2017,Jan,8; 2016,Jan,13

Uterus
Endometrial lining
Cervix and cervical canal
Curette
Vaginal canal
Dilator expands cervical opening

58140-58146 Myomectomy Procedures

58140 **Myomectomy, excision of fibroid tumor(s) of uterus, 1 to 4 intramural myoma(s) with total weight of 250 g or less and/or removal of surface myomas; abdominal approach** ♀
  📷 26.9 ⚕ 26.9 **FUD** 090   C 80 📄
  AMA: 2019,Jul,6; 2018,Jan,8; 2017,Jan,8; 2016,Jan,13

58145 **vaginal approach** ♀
  📷 16.2 ⚕ 16.2 **FUD** 090   J A2 80 📄
  AMA: 2019,Jul,6

58146 **Myomectomy, excision of fibroid tumor(s) of uterus, 5 or more intramural myomas and/or intramural myomas with total weight greater than 250 g, abdominal approach** ♀
  EXCLUDES Hysterectomy (58150-58240)
          Myomectomy procedures (58140-58145)
  📷 33.5 ⚕ 33.5 **FUD** 090   C 80 📄
  AMA: 2019,Jul,6; 2018,Jan,8; 2017,Jan,8; 2016,Jan,13

58150-58294 Abdominal and Vaginal Hysterectomies
CMS: 100-03,230.3 Sterilization
  EXCLUDES Destruction/excision endometriomas, open method (49203-49205, 58957-58958)
          Paracentesis (49082-49083)
          Pelvic laparotomy (49000)
          Secondary closure disruption evisceration abdominal wall (49900)

58150 **Total abdominal hysterectomy (corpus and cervix), with or without removal of tube(s), with or without removal of ovary(s);** ♀
  📷 29.2 ⚕ 29.2 **FUD** 090   C 80 📄
  AMA: 2019,Jul,6; 2018,Jan,8; 2017,Jan,8; 2016,Jan,13

58152 **with colpo-urethrocystopexy (eg, Marshall-Marchetti-Krantz, Burch)** ♀
  EXCLUDES Urethrocystopexy without hysterectomy (51840-51841)
  📷 36.3 ⚕ 36.3 **FUD** 090   C 80 📄
  AMA: 2019,Jul,6; 2018,Jan,8; 2017,Jan,8; 2016,Jan,13

58180 **Supracervical abdominal hysterectomy (subtotal hysterectomy), with or without removal of tube(s), with or without removal of ovary(s)** ♀
  📷 27.3 ⚕ 27.3 **FUD** 090   C 80 📄
  AMA: 2019,Jul,6

58200 **Total abdominal hysterectomy, including partial vaginectomy, with para-aortic and pelvic lymph node sampling, with or without removal of tube(s), with or without removal of ovary(s)** ♀
  📷 39.0 ⚕ 39.0 **FUD** 090   C 80 📄
  AMA: 2019,Jul,6

58210 **Radical abdominal hysterectomy, with bilateral total pelvic lymphadenectomy and para-aortic lymph node sampling (biopsy), with or without removal of tube(s), with or without removal of ovary(s)** ♀
  INCLUDES Wertheim hysterectomy
  EXCLUDES Chemotherapy (96401-96549)
          Hysterectomy, radical, with transposition ovary(s) (58825)
  📷 53.4 ⚕ 53.4 **FUD** 090   C 80 📄
  AMA: 2019,Jul,6; 2018,Jan,8; 2017,Jan,8; 2016,Jan,13

58240 **Pelvic exenteration for gynecologic malignancy, with total abdominal hysterectomy or cervicectomy, with or without removal of tube(s), with or without removal of ovary(s), with removal of bladder and ureteral transplantations, and/or abdominoperineal resection of rectum and colon and colostomy, or any combination thereof** ♀
  EXCLUDES Chemotherapy (96401-96549)
          Pelvic exenteration for male genital malignancy or lower urinary tract (51597)
  📷 83.8 ⚕ 83.8 **FUD** 090   C 80 📄
  AMA: 2019,Jul,6

58260 **Vaginal hysterectomy, for uterus 250 g or less;** ♀
  📷 24.2 ⚕ 24.2 **FUD** 090   J G2 80 📄
  AMA: 2019,Jul,6; 2018,Jan,8; 2017,Jan,8; 2016,Jan,13

58262 **with removal of tube(s), and/or ovary(s)** ♀
  📷 26.1 ⚕ 26.1 **FUD** 090   J G2 80 📄
  AMA: 2019,Jul,6

58263 **with removal of tube(s), and/or ovary(s), with repair of enterocele** ♀
  📷 28.8 ⚕ 28.8 **FUD** 090   J G2 80 📄
  AMA: 2019,Jul,6

58267 **with colpo-urethrocystopexy (Marshall-Marchetti-Krantz type, Pereyra type) with or without endoscopic control** ♀
  📷 30.9 ⚕ 30.9 **FUD** 090   C 80 📄
  AMA: 2019,Jul,6; 2018,Jan,8; 2017,Jan,8; 2016,Jan,13

58270 **with repair of enterocele** ♀

> EXCLUDES *Vaginal hysterectomy with repair enterocele and removal tubes and/or ovaries (58263)*
> 🔧 25.8 ✂ 25.8 **FUD** 090 [J] [G2] [80] 🔲
> **AMA:** 2019,Jul,6

Uterus is removed vaginally

Ovary · Round ligament · Excision around cervix · Broad ligament · Cervix · Protruding intestine (enterocele) · Posterior wall of vagina (site of protrusion)

Repair of enterocele — Posterior vaginal wall

58275 **Vaginal hysterectomy, with total or partial vaginectomy;** ♀
🔧 28.6 ✂ 28.6 **FUD** 090 [C] [80] 🔲
AMA: 2019,Jul,6

58280 **with repair of enterocele** ♀
🔧 29.7 ✂ 29.7 **FUD** 090 [C] [80] 🔲
AMA: 2019,Jul,6

58285 **Vaginal hysterectomy, radical (Schauta type operation)** ♀
🔧 41.8 ✂ 41.8 **FUD** 090 [C] [80] 🔲
AMA: 2019,Jul,6; 2018,Jan,8; 2017,Jan,8; 2016,Jan,13

58290 **Vaginal hysterectomy, for uterus greater than 250 g;** ♀
🔧 33.4 ✂ 33.4 **FUD** 090 [J] [G2] [80] 🔲
AMA: 2019,Jul,6

58291 **with removal of tube(s) and/or ovary(s)** ♀
🔧 36.2 ✂ 36.2 **FUD** 090 [J] [G2] [80] 🔲
AMA: 2019,Jul,6

58292 **with removal of tube(s) and/or ovary(s), with repair of enterocele** ♀
🔧 38.2 ✂ 38.2 **FUD** 090 [J] [G2] [80] 🔲
AMA: 2019,Jul,6

58294 **with repair of enterocele** ♀
🔧 34.3 ✂ 34.3 **FUD** 090 [J] [G2] [80] 🔲
AMA: 2019,Jul,6

58300-58323 Contraception and Reproduction Procedures

58300 **Insertion of intrauterine device (IUD)** ♀
> EXCLUDES *Insertion and/or removal implantable contraceptive capsules (11976, 11981-11983)*
> 🔧 1.49 ✂ 2.60 **FUD** XXX [E] 🔲
> **AMA:** 2019,Jul,6; 2018,Jan,8; 2017,Jan,8; 2016,Jan,13

58301 **Removal of intrauterine device (IUD)** ♀
> EXCLUDES *Insertion and/or removal implantable contraceptive capsules (11976, 11981-11983)*
> 🔧 1.95 ✂ 2.91 **FUD** 000 [02] [P3] [80] 🔲
> **AMA:** 2019,Jul,6; 2018,Jan,8; 2017,Jan,8; 2016,Jan,13

58321 **Artificial insemination; intra-cervical** ♀
🔧 1.40 ✂ 2.26 **FUD** 000 [T] [P3] [80] 🔲
AMA: 2019,Jul,6

58322 **intra-uterine** ♀
🔧 1.70 ✂ 2.56 **FUD** 000 [T] [P3] [80] 🔲
AMA: 2019,Jul,6

58323 **Sperm washing for artificial insemination** ♀
🔧 0.37 ✂ 0.45 **FUD** 000 [T] [P3] [80] 🔲
AMA: 2019,Jul,6

58340-58350 Fallopian Tube Patency and Brachytherapy Procedures

58340 **Catheterization and introduction of saline or contrast material for saline infusion sonohysterography (SIS) or hysterosalpingography** ♀
🔧 (74740, 76831)
🔧 1.65 ✂ 5.53 **FUD** 000 [N] [N1] 🔲
AMA: 2019,Jul,6; 2018,Jan,8; 2017,Jan,8; 2016,Jan,13

58345 **Transcervical introduction of fallopian tube catheter for diagnosis and/or re-establishing patency (any method), with or without hysterosalpingography** ♀
🔧 (74742)
🔧 8.27 ✂ 8.27 **FUD** 010 [J] [R2] [80] [50] 🔲
AMA: 2019,Jul,6; 2018,Jan,8; 2017,Jan,8; 2016,Jan,13

58346 **Insertion of Heyman capsules for clinical brachytherapy** ♀
> EXCLUDES *Insertion radioelement sources or ribbons (77761-77763, 77770-77772)*
> *Placement needles or catheters into pelvic organs and/or genitalia (except prostate) for interstitial radioelement application (55920)*
> 🔧 13.2 ✂ 13.2 **FUD** 090 [J] [A2] 🔲
> **AMA:** 2019,Jul,6; 2018,Jan,8; 2017,Jan,8; 2016,Jan,13

58350 **Chromotubation of oviduct, including materials** ♀
🔧 2.51 ✂ 3.62 **FUD** 010 [J] [A2] [50] 🔲
AMA: 2019,Jul,6; 2018,Jan,8; 2017,Jan,8; 2016,Jan,13

58353-58356 Ablation of Endometrium

> EXCLUDES *Destruction/excision endometriomas, open method (49203-49205)*

58353 **Endometrial ablation, thermal, without hysteroscopic guidance** ♀
> EXCLUDES *Endometrial ablation performed hysteroscopically (58563)*
> 🔧 6.54 ✂ 28.5 **FUD** 010 [J] [A2] 🔲
> **AMA:** 2019,Jul,6; 2018,Jan,8; 2017,Jan,8; 2016,Jan,13

58356 **Endometrial cryoablation with ultrasonic guidance, including endometrial curettage, when performed** ♀
> EXCLUDES *Dilation and curettage (58120)*
> *Endometrial biopsy (58100)*
> *Hysterosalpingography (58340)*
> *Ultrasound (76700, 76856)*
> 🔧 10.2 ✂ 52.0 **FUD** 010 [J] [P3] [80] 🔲
> **AMA:** 2019,Jul,6

58400-58540 Uterine Repairs: Vaginal and Abdominal

58400 **Uterine suspension, with or without shortening of round ligaments, with or without shortening of sacrouterine ligaments; (separate procedure)** ♀
> INCLUDES Alexander's operation
> Baldy-Webster operation
> Manchester colporrhaphy
> EXCLUDES *Anastomosis tubes to uterus (58752)*
> 🔧 13.1 ✂ 13.1 **FUD** 090 [C] [80] 🔲
> **AMA:** 2019,Jul,6

58410 **with presacral sympathectomy** ♀
> INCLUDES Alexander's operation
> EXCLUDES *Anastomosis tubes to uterus (58752)*
> 🔧 23.5 ✂ 23.5 **FUD** 090 [C] [80] 🔲
> **AMA:** 2019,Jul,6; 2018,Jan,8; 2017,Jan,8; 2016,Jan,13

58520   **Hysterorrhaphy, repair of ruptured uterus (nonobstetrical)** ♀
  📋 23.0   ⅀ 23.0   **FUD** 090   C 80 ▭
  AMA: 2019,Jul,6

58540   **Hysteroplasty, repair of uterine anomaly (Strassman type)** ♀
  INCLUDES   Strassman type
  EXCLUDES   Vesicouterine fistula closure (51920)
  📋 26.5   ⅀ 26.5   **FUD** 090   C 80 ▭
  AMA: 2019,Jul,6

58674-58554 [58674] Laparoscopic Procedures of the Uterus
  INCLUDES   Diagnostic laparoscopy
  EXCLUDES   Hysteroscopy (58555-58565)

58674   **Laparoscopy, surgical, ablation of uterine fibroid(s) including intraoperative ultrasound guidance and monitoring, radiofrequency** ♀
  INCLUDES   Intraoperative ultrasound (76998)
  EXCLUDES   Laparoscopy (49320, 58541-58554, 58570-58573)
  📋 23.6   ⅀ 23.6   **FUD** 090   J G2 80 ▭
  AMA: 2019,Jul,6; 2018,Jan,8; 2017,Apr,7; 2017,Feb,14

58541   **Laparoscopy, surgical, supracervical hysterectomy, for uterus 250 g or less;** ♀
  EXCLUDES   Colpotomy (57000)
           Hysteroscopy (58561)
           Laparoscopy (49320, 58545-58546, 58661, 58670-58671)
           Myomectomy procedures (58140-58146)
           Pelvic examination under anesthesia (57410)
           Treatment nonobstetrical vaginal hemorrhage (57180)
  📋 21.0   ⅀ 21.0   **FUD** 090   J G2 80 ▭
  AMA: 2019,Jul,6; 2018,Jan,8; 2017,Apr,7; 2017,Jan,8; 2016,Jan,13

58542   **with removal of tube(s) and/or ovary(s)** ♀
  EXCLUDES   Colpotomy (57000)
           Hysteroscopy (58561)
           Laparoscopy (49320, 58545-58546, 58661, 58670-58671)
           Myomectomy procedures (58140-58146)
           Pelvic examination under anesthesia (57410)
           Treatment nonobstetrical vaginal hemorrhage (57180)
  📋 23.9   ⅀ 23.9   **FUD** 090   J G2 80 ▭
  AMA: 2019,Jul,6; 2018,Jan,8; 2017,Apr,7; 2017,Jan,8; 2016,Jan,13

58543   **Laparoscopy, surgical, supracervical hysterectomy, for uterus greater than 250 g;** ♀
  EXCLUDES   Colpotomy (57000)
           Hysteroscopy (58561)
           Laparoscopy (49320, 58545-58546, 58661, 58670-58671)
           Myomectomy procedures (58140-58146)
           Pelvic examination under anesthesia (57410)
           Treatment nonobstetrical vaginal hemorrhage (57180)
  📋 24.3   ⅀ 24.3   **FUD** 090   J G2 80 ▭
  AMA: 2019,Jul,6; 2018,Jan,8; 2017,Apr,7; 2017,Jan,8; 2016,Jan,13

58544   **with removal of tube(s) and/or ovary(s)** ♀
  EXCLUDES   Colpotomy (57000)
           Hysteroscopy (58561)
           Laparoscopy (49320, 58545-58546, 58661, 58670-58671)
           Myomectomy procedures (58140-58146)
           Pelvic examination under anesthesia (57410)
           Treatment nonobstetrical vaginal hemorrhage (57180)
  📋 26.2   ⅀ 26.2   **FUD** 090   J G2 80 ▭
  AMA: 2019,Jul,6; 2018,Jan,8; 2017,Apr,7; 2017,Jan,8; 2016,Jan,13

58545   **Laparoscopy, surgical, myomectomy, excision; 1 to 4 intramural myomas with total weight of 250 g or less and/or removal of surface myomas** ♀
  📋 26.0   ⅀ 26.0   **FUD** 090   J A2 80 ▭
  AMA: 2019,Jul,6; 2017,Apr,7

58546   **5 or more intramural myomas and/or intramural myomas with total weight greater than 250 g** ♀
  📋 31.6   ⅀ 31.6   **FUD** 090   J A2 80 ▭
  AMA: 2019,Jul,6; 2018,Jan,8; 2017,Apr,7; 2017,Jan,8; 2016,Jan,13

58548   **Laparoscopy, surgical, with radical hysterectomy, with bilateral total pelvic lymphadenectomy and para-aortic lymph node sampling (biopsy), with removal of tube(s) and ovary(s), if performed** ♀
  EXCLUDES   Laparoscopy (38570-38572, 58550-58554)
           Radical hysterectomy (58210, 58285)
  📋 53.9   ⅀ 53.9   **FUD** 090   C 80 ▭
  AMA: 2019,Jul,6; 2019,Mar,5; 2018,Jan,8; 2017,Apr,7; 2017,Jan,8; 2016,Jan,13

58550   **Laparoscopy, surgical, with vaginal hysterectomy, for uterus 250 g or less;** ♀
  EXCLUDES   Colpotomy (57000)
           Hysteroscopy (58561)
           Laparoscopy (49320, 58545-58546, 58661, 58670-58671)
           Myomectomy procedures (58140-58146)
           Pelvic examination under anesthesia (57410)
           Treatment nonobstetrical vaginal hemorrhage (57180)
  📋 25.5   ⅀ 25.5   **FUD** 090   J A2 80 ▭
  AMA: 2019,Jul,6; 2018,Jan,8; 2017,Apr,7; 2017,Jan,8; 2016,Jan,13

58552   **with removal of tube(s) and/or ovary(s)** ♀
  EXCLUDES   Colpotomy (57000)
           Hysteroscopy (58561)
           Laparoscopy (49320, 58545-58546, 58661, 58670-58671)
           Myomectomy procedures (58140-58146)
           Pelvic examination under anesthesia (57410)
           Treatment nonobstetrical vaginal hemorrhage (57180)
  📋 28.0   ⅀ 28.0   **FUD** 090   J G2 80 ▭
  AMA: 2019,Jul,6; 2018,Jan,8; 2017,Apr,7; 2017,Jan,8; 2016,Jan,13

58553   **Laparoscopy, surgical, with vaginal hysterectomy, for uterus greater than 250 g;** ♀
  EXCLUDES   Colpotomy (57000)
           Hysteroscopy (58561)
           Laparoscopy (49320, 58545-58546, 58661, 58670-58671)
           Myomectomy procedures (58140-58146)
           Pelvic examination under anesthesia (57410)
           Treatment nonobstetrical vaginal hemorrhage (57180)
  📋 31.8   ⅀ 31.8   **FUD** 090   J G2 80 ▭
  AMA: 2019,Jul,6; 2018,Jan,8; 2017,Apr,7

58554   **with removal of tube(s) and/or ovary(s)** ♀
  EXCLUDES   Colpotomy (57000)
           Hysteroscopy (58561)
           Laparoscopy (49320, 58545-58546, 58661, 58670-58671)
           Myomectomy procedures (58140-58146)
           Pelvic examination under anesthesia (57410)
           Treatment nonobstetrical vaginal hemorrhage (57180)
  📋 38.1   ⅀ 38.1   **FUD** 090   J G2 80 ▭
  AMA: 2019,Jul,6; 2018,Jan,8; 2017,Apr,7

26/TC PC/TC Only   A2-Z3 ASC Payment   50 Bilateral   ♂ Male Only   ♀ Female Only   📋 Facility RVU   ⅀ Non-Facility RVU   ▭ CCI   ☒ CLIA
FUD Follow-up Days   **CMS:** IOM   **AMA:** CPT Asst   A-Y OPPSI   80/80 Surg Assist Allowed / w/Doc   ▪ Lab Crosswalk   ▪ Radiology Crosswalk

© 2021 Optum360, LLC

58555-58565 Hysteroscopy

INCLUDES Diagnostic hysteroscopy (58555)
EXCLUDES Laparoscopy (58541-58554, 58570-58578)

58555   Hysteroscopy, diagnostic (separate procedure) ♀
🚑 4.35   ⚕ 8.40   **FUD** 000   J A2 80 ▣
AMA: 2019,Jul,6; 2018,Jan,8; 2017,Jan,8; 2016,Jan,13

Hysteroscope
Bladder
Uterus
Ovary
Spine
Vagina
Cervix

58558   Hysteroscopy, surgical; with sampling (biopsy) of endometrium and/or polypectomy, with or without D & C ♀
🚑 6.74   ⚕ 39.6   **FUD** 000   J A2 ▣
AMA: 2019,Jul,6; 2018,Jan,8; 2017,Jan,8; 2016,Jan,13

58559   with lysis of intrauterine adhesions (any method) ♀
🚑 8.33   ⚕ 8.33   **FUD** 000   J A2 ▣
AMA: 2019,Jul,6; 2018,Jan,8; 2017,Jan,8; 2016,Jan,13

58560   with division or resection of intrauterine septum (any method) ♀
🚑 9.16   ⚕ 9.16   **FUD** 000   J A2 80 ▣
AMA: 2019,Jul,6; 2018,Jan,8; 2017,Jan,8; 2016,Jan,13

58561   with removal of leiomyomata ♀
🚑 10.4   ⚕ 10.4   **FUD** 000   J A2 80 ▣
AMA: 2019,Jul,6; 2018,Jan,8; 2017,Jan,8; 2016,Jan,13

58562   with removal of impacted foreign body ♀
🚑 6.34   ⚕ 10.3   **FUD** 000   J A2 ▣
AMA: 2019,Jul,6; 2018,Jan,8; 2017,Jan,8; 2016,Jan,13

58563   with endometrial ablation (eg, endometrial resection, electrosurgical ablation, thermoablation) ♀
🚑 7.18   ⚕ 55.6   **FUD** 000   J A2 80 ▣
AMA: 2019,Jul,6; 2018,Jan,8; 2017,Jan,8; 2016,Jan,13

58565   with bilateral fallopian tube cannulation to induce occlusion by placement of permanent implants ♀
EXCLUDES Diagnostic hysteroscopy (58555)
          Dilation cervical canal (57800)
Code also modifier 52 when unilateral procedure performed
🚑 12.9   ⚕ 51.6   **FUD** 090   J A2 ▣
AMA: 2019,Jul,6; 2018,Jan,8; 2017,Jan,8; 2016,Jan,13

58570-58579 Other Uterine Endoscopy

INCLUDES Diagnostic laparoscopy
EXCLUDES Hysteroscopy (58555-58565)

58570   Laparoscopy, surgical, with total hysterectomy, for uterus 250 g or less; ♀
EXCLUDES Colpotomy (57000)
          Hysteroscopy (58561)
          Laparoscopy (49320, 58545-58546, 58661, 58670-58671)
          Myomectomy procedures (58140-58146)
          Pelvic examination under anesthesia (57410)
          Total abdominal hysterectomy (58150)
          Treatment nonobstetrical vaginal hemorrhage (57180)
🚑 22.9   ⚕ 22.9   **FUD** 090   J 62 80 ▣
AMA: 2019,Jul,6; 2018,Jan,8; 2017,Apr,7

58571   with removal of tube(s) and/or ovary(s) ♀
EXCLUDES Colpotomy (57000)
          Hysteroscopy (58561)
          Laparoscopy (49320, 58545-58546, 58661, 58670-58671)
          Myomectomy procedures (58140-58146)
          Pelvic examination under anesthesia (57410)
          Total abdominal hysterectomy (58150)
          Treatment nonobstetrical vaginal hemorrhage (57180)
🚑 25.9   ⚕ 25.9   **FUD** 090   J 62 80 ▣
AMA: 2019,Jul,6; 2018,Feb,11; 2018,Jan,8; 2017,Apr,7; 2017,Jan,8; 2016,Jan,13

58572   Laparoscopy, surgical, with total hysterectomy, for uterus greater than 250 g; ♀
EXCLUDES Colpotomy (57000)
          Hysteroscopy (58561)
          Laparoscopy (49320, 58545-58546, 58661, 58670-58671)
          Myomectomy procedures (58140-58146)
          Pelvic examination under anesthesia (57410)
          Total abdominal hysterectomy (58150)
          Treatment nonobstetrical vaginal hemorrhage (57180)
🚑 29.3   ⚕ 29.3   **FUD** 090   J 62 80 ▣
AMA: 2019,Jul,6; 2018,Jan,8; 2017,Apr,7

58573   with removal of tube(s) and/or ovary(s) ♀
EXCLUDES Colpotomy (57000)
          Hysteroscopy (58561)
          Laparoscopy (49320, 58545-58546, 58661, 58670-58671)
          Myomectomy procedures (58140-58146)
          Pelvic examination under anesthesia (57410)
          Total abdominal hysterectomy (58150)
          Treatment nonobstetrical vaginal hemorrhage (57180)
🚑 35.0   ⚕ 35.0   **FUD** 090   J 62 80 ▣
AMA: 2019,Jul,6; 2019,Mar,5; 2018,Apr,10; 2018,Feb,11; 2018,Jan,8; 2017,Apr,7; 2017,Jan,8; 2016,Jan,13

58575   Laparoscopy, surgical, total hysterectomy for resection of malignancy (tumor debulking), with omentectomy including salpingo-oophorectomy, unilateral or bilateral, when performed ♀
EXCLUDES Laparoscopy (49320-49321, 58570-58573, 58661)
          Omentectomy (49255)
🚑 54.9   ⚕ 54.9   **FUD** 090   C 80 ▣
AMA: 2019,Jul,6; 2019,Mar,5

58578   Unlisted laparoscopy procedure, uterus ♀
🚑 0.00   ⚕ 0.00   **FUD** YYY   J 80 50 ▣
AMA: 2019,Jul,6; 2018,Jan,8; 2017,Jan,8; 2016,Jan,13

58579   Unlisted hysteroscopy procedure, uterus ♀
🚑 0.00   ⚕ 0.00   **FUD** YYY   T 80 50 ▣
AMA: 2019,Jul,6; 2018,Jan,8; 2017,Jan,8; 2016,Jan,13

58600-58615 Sterilization by Tubal Interruption

CMS: 100-03,230.3 Sterilization
EXCLUDES Destruction/excision endometriomas, open method (49203-49205)

58600   Ligation or transection of fallopian tube(s), abdominal or vaginal approach, unilateral or bilateral ♀
INCLUDES Madlener operation
🚑 10.6   ⚕ 10.6   **FUD** 090   J 62 80 ▣
AMA: 2019,Jul,6; 2018,Jan,8; 2017,Jan,8; 2016,Jan,13

58605   Ligation or transection of fallopian tube(s), abdominal or vaginal approach, postpartum, unilateral or bilateral, during same hospitalization (separate procedure) ♀
EXCLUDES Laparoscopic methods (58670-58671)
🚑 9.65   ⚕ 9.65   **FUD** 090   C 80 ▣
AMA: 2019,Jul,6; 2018,Jan,8; 2017,Jan,8; 2016,Jan,13

● New Code   ▲ Revised Code   ○ Reinstated   ● New Web Release   ▲ Revised Web Release   + Add-on   Unlisted   Not Covered   # Resequenced
50 Optum Mod 50 Exempt   ⚕ AMA Mod 51 Exempt   51 Optum Mod 51 Exempt   63 Mod 63 Exempt   ✗ Non-FDA Drug   ★ Telemedicine   M Maternity   A Age Edit

CPT © 2021 American Medical Association. All Rights Reserved.

Genital System

58611 — 58825

+ **58611** Ligation or transection of fallopian tube(s) when done at the time of cesarean delivery or intra-abdominal surgery (not a separate procedure) (List separately in addition to code for primary procedure) ♀
Code first primary procedure
2.24   2.24   **FUD** ZZZ   C 80
AMA: 2019,Jul,6

58615 Occlusion of fallopian tube(s) by device (eg, band, clip, Falope ring) vaginal or suprapubic approach ♀
EXCLUDES Laparoscopic method (58671)
Lysis adnexal adhesions (58740)
7.24   7.24   **FUD** 010   J 62 80
AMA: 2019,Jul,6; 2018,Jan,8; 2017,Jan,8; 2016,Jan,13

58660-58679 [58674] Endoscopic Procedures Fallopian Tubes and/or Ovaries
CMS: 100-03,230.3 Sterilization
INCLUDES Diagnostic laparoscopy (49320)
EXCLUDES Laparoscopy with biopsy fallopian tube or ovary (49321)
Laparoscopy with ovarian cyst aspiration (49322)

58660 Laparoscopy, surgical; with lysis of adhesions (salpingolysis, ovariolysis) (separate procedure) ♀
19.6   19.6   **FUD** 090   J A2 80
AMA: 2019,Jul,6; 2018,Jan,8; 2017,Jan,8; 2016,Jan,13

58661 with removal of adnexal structures (partial or total oophorectomy and/or salpingectomy) ♀
18.8   18.8   **FUD** 010   J A2 80 50
AMA: 2020,Jan,12; 2019,Jul,6; 2018,Jan,8; 2017,Jan,8; 2016,Jan,13

58662 with fulguration or excision of lesions of the ovary, pelvic viscera, or peritoneal surface by any method ♀
20.6   20.6   **FUD** 090   J A2 80
AMA: 2019,Jul,6; 2018,Jan,8; 2017,Dec,14; 2017,Jan,8; 2016,Jan,13

58670 with fulguration of oviducts (with or without transection) ♀
10.3   10.3   **FUD** 090   J A2
AMA: 2019,Jul,6; 2018,Jan,8; 2017,Jan,8; 2016,Jan,13

58671 with occlusion of oviducts by device (eg, band, clip, or Falope ring) ♀
10.6   10.6   **FUD** 090   J A2
AMA: 2019,Jul,6; 2018,Jan,8; 2017,Jan,8; 2016,Jan,13

58672 with fimbrioplasty ♀
21.3   21.3   **FUD** 090   J A2 80 50
AMA: 2019,Jul,6; 2018,Jan,8; 2017,Jan,8; 2016,Jan,13

58673 with salpingostomy (salpingoneostomy) ♀
23.1   23.1   **FUD** 090   J A2 80 50
AMA: 2019,Jul,6; 2018,Jan,8; 2017,Jan,8; 2016,Jan,13

58674 Resequenced code. See code before 58541.

58679 Unlisted laparoscopy procedure, oviduct, ovary ♀
0.00   0.00   **FUD** YYY   J 80 50
AMA: 2019,Jul,6; 2018,Jan,8; 2017,Jan,8; 2016,Jan,13

58700-58770 Open Procedures Fallopian Tubes, with/without Ovaries
EXCLUDES Destruction/excision endometriomas, open method (49203-49205)

58700 Salpingectomy, complete or partial, unilateral or bilateral (separate procedure) ♀
22.3   22.3   **FUD** 090   C 80
AMA: 2019,Jul,6; 2018,Sep,14

58720 Salpingo-oophorectomy, complete or partial, unilateral or bilateral (separate procedure) ♀
21.5   21.5   **FUD** 090   C 80
AMA: 2019,Jul,6; 2018,Jan,8; 2017,Jan,8; 2016,Jan,13

58740 Lysis of adhesions (salpingolysis, ovariolysis) ♀
EXCLUDES Excision/fulguration lesions performed laparoscopically (58662)
Laparoscopic method (58660)
25.9   25.9   **FUD** 090   C 80
AMA: 2019,Jul,6; 2018,Jan,8; 2017,Jan,8; 2016,Jan,13

58750 Tubotubal anastomosis ♀
26.3   26.3   **FUD** 090   C 80 50
AMA: 2019,Jul,6

Occluded section of tube is excised
Ovary
Tube ends are sutured

58752 Tubouterine implantation ♀
25.4   25.4   **FUD** 090   C 80 50
AMA: 2019,Jul,6

58760 Fimbrioplasty ♀
EXCLUDES Laparoscopic method (58672)
23.7   23.7   **FUD** 090   C 80 50
AMA: 2019,Jul,6; 2018,Jan,8; 2017,Jan,8; 2016,Jan,13

58770 Salpingostomy (salpingoneostomy) ♀
EXCLUDES Laparoscopic method (58673)
24.9   24.9   **FUD** 090   J 62 80 50
AMA: 2019,Jul,6; 2018,Jan,8; 2017,Jan,8; 2016,Jan,13

58800-58925 Open Procedures: Ovary
CMS: 100-03,230.3 Sterilization
EXCLUDES Destruction/excision endometriomas, open method (49203-49205)

58800 Drainage of ovarian cyst(s), unilateral or bilateral (separate procedure); vaginal approach ♀
8.92   9.96   **FUD** 090   J A2
AMA: 2019,Jul,6

58805 abdominal approach ♀
12.1   12.1   **FUD** 090   J 62 80
AMA: 2019,Jul,6

58820 Drainage of ovarian abscess; vaginal approach, open ♀
EXCLUDES Transrectal fluid drainage using catheter, image guided (49407)
9.02   9.02   **FUD** 090   J A2 80 50
AMA: 2019,Jul,6

58822 abdominal approach ♀
EXCLUDES Transrectal fluid drainage using catheter, image guided (49407)
19.8   19.8   **FUD** 090   C 80 50
AMA: 2019,Jul,6

58825 Transposition, ovary(s) ♀
20.4   20.4   **FUD** 090   C 80
AMA: 2019,Jul,6

26/TC PC/TC Only   A2-Z3 ASC Payment   50 Bilateral   ♂ Male Only   ♀ Female Only   Facility RVU   Non-Facility RVU   CCI   CLIA
FUD Follow-up Days   **CMS:** IOM   **AMA:** CPT Asst   A-Y OPPSI   80/80 Surg Assist Allowed / w/Doc   Lab Crosswalk   Radiology Crosswalk

58900 Biopsy of ovary, unilateral or bilateral (separate procedure) ♀
    EXCLUDES *Laparoscopy with biopsy fallopian tube or ovary (49321)*
    ⚕ 11.8   ⚕ 11.8   **FUD** 090   J A2 80 ▣
    AMA: 2019,Jul,6; 2018,Jan,8; 2017,Jan,8; 2016,Jan,13

58920 Wedge resection or bisection of ovary, unilateral or bilateral ♀
    ⚕ 19.8   ⚕ 19.8   **FUD** 090   J 62 80 ▣
    AMA: 2019,Jul,6

58925 Ovarian cystectomy, unilateral or bilateral ♀
    ⚕ 21.9   ⚕ 21.9   **FUD** 090   J 62 80 ▣
    AMA: 2019,Jul,6

58940-58960 Removal Ovary(s) with/without Multiple Procedures for Malignancy

CMS: 100-03,230.3 Sterilization

EXCLUDES *Chemotherapy (96401-96549)*
Destruction/excision tumors, cysts, or endometriomas, open method (49203-49205)

58940 Oophorectomy, partial or total, unilateral or bilateral; ♀
    EXCLUDES *Oophorectomy with tumor debulking for ovarian malignancy (58952)*
    ⚕ 15.3   ⚕ 15.3   **FUD** 090   C 80 ▣
    AMA: 2019,Jul,6; 2018,Jan,8; 2017,Jan,8; 2016,Jan,13

58943 for ovarian, tubal or primary peritoneal malignancy, with para-aortic and pelvic lymph node biopsies, peritoneal washings, peritoneal biopsies, diaphragmatic assessments, with or without salpingectomy(s), with or without omentectomy ♀
    ⚕ 33.6   ⚕ 33.6   **FUD** 090   C 80 ▣
    AMA: 2019,Jul,6

58950 Resection (initial) of ovarian, tubal or primary peritoneal malignancy with bilateral salpingo-oophorectomy and omentectomy; ♀
    EXCLUDES *Resection/tumor debulking recurrent ovarian/tubal/primary peritoneal/uterine malignancy (58957-58958)*
    ⚕ 32.6   ⚕ 32.6   **FUD** 090   C 80 ▣
    AMA: 2019,Jul,6

58951 with total abdominal hysterectomy, pelvic and limited para-aortic lymphadenectomy ♀
    EXCLUDES *Resection/tumor debulking recurrent ovarian/tubal/primary peritoneal/uterine malignancy (58957-58958)*
    ⚕ 42.1   ⚕ 42.1   **FUD** 090   C 80 ▣
    AMA: 2019,Jul,6; 2018,Jan,8; 2017,Jan,8; 2016,Jan,13

58952 with radical dissection for debulking (ie, radical excision or destruction, intra-abdominal or retroperitoneal tumors) ♀
    EXCLUDES *Resection/tumor debulking recurrent ovarian/tubal/primary peritoneal/uterine malignancy (58957-58958)*
    ⚕ 46.9   ⚕ 46.9   **FUD** 090   C 80 ▣
    AMA: 2019,Jul,6; 2018,Jan,8; 2017,Jan,8; 2016,Jan,13

58953 Bilateral salpingo-oophorectomy with omentectomy, total abdominal hysterectomy and radical dissection for debulking; ♀
    ⚕ 58.7   ⚕ 58.7   **FUD** 090   C 80 ▣
    AMA: 2019,Jul,6; 2018,Jan,8; 2017,Jan,8; 2016,Jan,13

58954 with pelvic lymphadenectomy and limited para-aortic lymphadenectomy ♀
    ⚕ 62.4   ⚕ 62.4   **FUD** 090   C 80 ▣
    AMA: 2019,Jul,6; 2018,Jan,8; 2017,Jan,8; 2016,Jan,13

58956 Bilateral salpingo-oophorectomy with total omentectomy, total abdominal hysterectomy for malignancy ♀
    EXCLUDES *Biopsy ovary (58900)*
Hysterectomy (58150, 58180, 58262-58263)
Laparoscopy (58550, 58661)
Omentectomy (49255)
Oophorectomy (58940)
Ovarian cystectomy (58925)
Resection malignancy (58957-58958)
Salpingectomy salpingo-oophorectomy, (58700, 58720)
    ⚕ 39.1   ⚕ 39.1   **FUD** 090   C 80 ▣
    AMA: 2019,Jul,6; 2018,Jan,8; 2017,Jan,8; 2016,Jan,13

58957 Resection (tumor debulking) of recurrent ovarian, tubal, primary peritoneal, uterine malignancy (intra-abdominal, retroperitoneal tumors), with omentectomy, if performed; ♀
    EXCLUDES *Biopsy ovary (58900)*
Destruction, excision cysts, endometriomas, or tumors (49203-49215)
Enterolysis (44005)
Exploratory laparotomy (49000)
Lymphadenectomy (38770, 38780)
Omentectomy (49255)
    ⚕ 46.2   ⚕ 46.2   **FUD** 090   C 80 ▣
    AMA: 2019,Jul,6

58958 with pelvic lymphadenectomy and limited para-aortic lymphadenectomy ♀
    EXCLUDES *Biopsy ovary (58900)*
Destruction, excision cysts, endometriomas, or tumors (49203-49215)
Enterolysis (44005)
Exploratory laparotomy (49000)
Lymphadenectomy (38770, 38780)
Omentectomy (49255)
    ⚕ 51.2   ⚕ 51.2   **FUD** 090   C 80 ▣
    AMA: 2019,Jul,6

58960 Laparotomy, for staging or restaging of ovarian, tubal, or primary peritoneal malignancy (second look), with or without omentectomy, peritoneal washing, biopsy of abdominal and pelvic peritoneum, diaphragmatic assessment with pelvic and limited para-aortic lymphadenectomy ♀
    EXCLUDES *Resection malignancy (58957-58958)*
    ⚕ 27.9   ⚕ 27.9   **FUD** 090   C 80 ▣
    AMA: 2019,Jul,6

58970-58999 Procedural Components: In Vitro Fertilization

58970 Follicle puncture for oocyte retrieval, any method M ♀
    ⊞ (76948)
    ⚕ 5.74   ⚕ 6.75   **FUD** 000   T A2 80 ▣
    AMA: 2019,Jul,6

58974 Embryo transfer, intrauterine M ♀
    ⚕ 0.00   ⚕ 0.00   **FUD** 000   T A2 80 ▣
    AMA: 2019,Jul,6

58976 Gamete, zygote, or embryo intrafallopian transfer, any method M ♀
    EXCLUDES *Adnexal procedures performed laparoscopically (58660-58673)*
    ⚕ 6.20   ⚕ 7.33   **FUD** 000   T A2 80 ▣
    AMA: 2019,Jul,6; 2018,Jan,8; 2017,Jan,8; 2016,Jan,13

58999 Unlisted procedure, female genital system (nonobstetrical) ♀
    ⚕ 0.00   ⚕ 0.00   **FUD** YYY   T ▣
    AMA: 2019,Jul,6; 2018,Jan,8; 2017,Jan,8; 2016,Jan,13

59000-59001 Aspiration of Amniotic Fluid

EXCLUDES   *Intrauterine fetal transfusion (36460)*
Unlisted fetal invasive procedure (59897)

59000   **Amniocentesis; diagnostic**   M ♀
    (76946)
    2.33   3.47   **FUD** 000   T P3
    AMA: 2019,Jul,6; 2018,Jan,8; 2017,Jan,8; 2016,Jan,13

59001   **therapeutic amniotic fluid reduction (includes ultrasound guidance)**   M ♀
    5.18   5.18   **FUD** 000   T R2
    AMA: 2019,Jul,6; 2018,Jan,8; 2017,Jan,8; 2016,Jan,13

59012-59076 Fetal Testing and Treatment

EXCLUDES   *Intrauterine fetal transfusion (36460)*
Unlisted fetal invasive procedures (59897)

59012   **Cordocentesis (intrauterine), any method**   M ♀
    (76941)
    5.87   5.87   **FUD** 000   T G2 80
    AMA: 2019,Jul,6

59015   **Chorionic villus sampling, any method**   M ♀
    (76945)
    3.82   4.51   **FUD** 000   T P3 80
    AMA: 2019,Jul,6; 2018,Jan,8; 2017,Jan,8; 2016,Jan,13

59020   **Fetal contraction stress test**   M ♀
    2.00   2.00   **FUD** 000   T P3 80
    AMA: 2019,Jul,6; 2018,Jan,8; 2017,Jan,8; 2016,Jan,13

59025   **Fetal non-stress test**   M ♀
    1.37   1.37   **FUD** 000   T P3 80
    AMA: 2019,Jul,6; 2018,Jan,8; 2017,Jan,8; 2016,Jan,13

59030   **Fetal scalp blood sampling**   M ♀
    Code also modifier 76 or 77, as appropriate, for repeat fetal scalp blood sampling
    3.28   3.28   **FUD** 000   T G2 80
    AMA: 2019,Jul,6

59050   **Fetal monitoring during labor by consulting physician (ie, non-attending physician) with written report; supervision and interpretation**   M ♀
    1.49   1.49   **FUD** XXX   M 80
    AMA: 2019,Jul,6

59051   **interpretation only**   M ♀
    1.23   1.23   **FUD** XXX   B 80
    AMA: 2019,Jul,6

59070   **Transabdominal amnioinfusion, including ultrasound guidance**   M ♀
    8.99   11.6   **FUD** 000   T G2 80
    AMA: 2019,Jul,6; 2018,Jan,8; 2017,Jan,8; 2016,Jan,13

59072   **Fetal umbilical cord occlusion, including ultrasound guidance**   M ♀
    15.2   15.2   **FUD** 000   T J8
    AMA: 2019,Jul,6; 2018,Jan,8; 2017,Jan,8; 2016,Jan,13

59074   **Fetal fluid drainage (eg, vesicocentesis, thoracocentesis, paracentesis), including ultrasound guidance**   M ♀
    8.92   11.1   **FUD** 000   T G2 80
    AMA: 2019,Jul,6; 2018,Jan,8; 2017,Jan,8; 2016,Jan,13

59076   **Fetal shunt placement, including ultrasound guidance**   M ♀
    15.2   15.2   **FUD** 000   T G2 80
    AMA: 2019,Jul,6; 2018,Jan,8; 2017,Jan,8; 2016,Jan,13

59100-59151 Tubal Pregnancy/Hysterotomy Procedures

CMS: 100-03,230.3 Sterilization

59100   **Hysterotomy, abdominal (eg, for hydatidiform mole, abortion)**   M ♀
    Code also ligation fallopian tubes when performed same time as hysterotomy (58611)
    24.1   24.1   **FUD** 090   J R2 80
    AMA: 2019,Jul,6

59120   **Surgical treatment of ectopic pregnancy; tubal or ovarian, requiring salpingectomy and/or oophorectomy, abdominal or vaginal approach**   M ♀
    23.4   23.4   **FUD** 090   C 80
    AMA: 2019,Jul,6

59121   **tubal or ovarian, without salpingectomy and/or oophorectomy**   M ♀
    23.0   23.0   **FUD** 090   C 80
    AMA: 2019,Jul,6

59130   **abdominal pregnancy**   M ♀
    26.8   26.8   **FUD** 090   C 80
    AMA: 2019,Jul,6

59135   ~~**interstitial, uterine pregnancy requiring total hysterectomy**~~

59136   **interstitial, uterine pregnancy with partial resection of uterus**   M ♀
    25.9   25.9   **FUD** 090   C 80
    AMA: 2019,Jul,6

59140   **cervical, with evacuation**   M ♀
    11.9   11.9   **FUD** 090   C 80
    AMA: 2019,Jul,6

59150   **Laparoscopic treatment of ectopic pregnancy; without salpingectomy and/or oophorectomy**   M ♀
    22.7   22.7   **FUD** 090   J G2 80
    AMA: 2019,Jul,6; 2018,Jan,8; 2017,Jan,8; 2016,Jan,13

59151   **with salpingectomy and/or oophorectomy**   M ♀
    21.7   21.7   **FUD** 090   J G2 80
    AMA: 2019,Jul,6

59160-59200 Procedures of Uterus Prior To/After Delivery

59160   **Curettage, postpartum**   M ♀
    5.11   6.21   **FUD** 010   J A2 80
    AMA: 2019,Jul,6; 2018,Jan,8; 2017,Jan,8; 2016,Jan,13

59200   **Insertion of cervical dilator (eg, laminaria, prostaglandin) (separate procedure)**   M ♀
    EXCLUDES   *Fetal transfusion, intrauterine (36460)*
        Hypertonic solution/prostaglandin introduction for labor initiation (59850-59857)
    1.30   2.56   **FUD** 000   T P3
    AMA: 2019,Jul,6; 2018,Jan,8; 2017,Dec,14; 2017,Jan,8; 2016,Jan,13

59300-59350 Postpartum Vaginal/Cervical/Uterine Repairs

EXCLUDES   *Nonpregnancy-related cerclage (57700)*

59300   **Episiotomy or vaginal repair, by other than attending**   M ♀
    4.26   6.15   **FUD** 000   J P3 80
    AMA: 2019,Jul,6

26/TC PC/TC Only   A2-Z3 ASC Payment   50 Bilateral   ♂ Male Only   ♀ Female Only   Facility RVU   Non-Facility RVU   CCI   CLIA
FUD Follow-up Days   **CMS:** IOM   **AMA:** CPT Asst   A-Y OPPSI   80/80 Surg Assist Allowed / w/Doc   Lab Crosswalk   Radiology Crosswalk

264   CPT © 2021 American Medical Association. All Rights Reserved.   © 2021 Optum360, LLC

59320   **Cerclage of cervix, during pregnancy; vaginal**   M ♀
   4.37   4.37   **FUD** 000   J A2 80
AMA: 2019,Jul,6; 2018,Jan,8; 2017,Jan,8; 2016,Jan,13

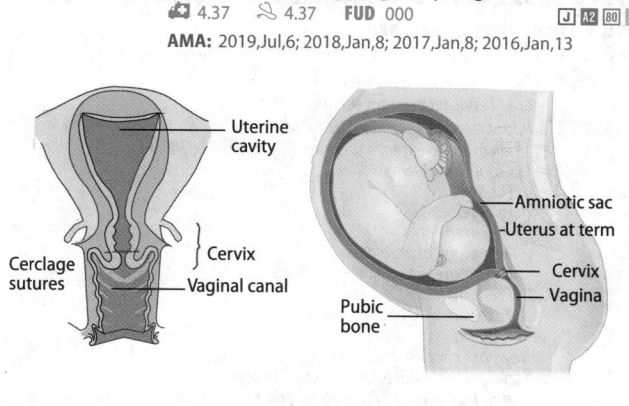

Uterine cavity
Cerclage sutures
Cervix
Vaginal canal
Amniotic sac
Uterus at term
Cervix
Vagina
Pubic bone

59325   **abdominal**   M ♀
   6.96   6.96   **FUD** 000   C 80
AMA: 2019,Jul,6; 2018,Jan,8; 2017,Jan,8; 2016,Jan,13

59350   **Hysterorrhaphy of ruptured uterus**   M ♀
   8.08   8.08   **FUD** 000   C 80
AMA: 2019,Jul,6

59400-59410 Vaginal Delivery: Comprehensive and Component Services

CMS: 100-02,15,180 Nurse-Midwife (CNM) Services; 100-02,15,20.1 Physician Expense for Surgery, Childbirth, and Treatment for Infertility

INCLUDES   Care provided for uncomplicated pregnancy including delivery, antepartum, and postpartum care:
     Admission history
     Admission to hospital
     Artificial rupture membranes
     Management uncomplicated labor
     Physical exam
     Vaginal delivery with or without episiotomy or forceps

EXCLUDES   *Medical complications pregnancy, labor, and delivery:*
     Cardiac problems
     Diabetes
     Hyperemesis
     Hypertension
     Neurological problems
     Premature rupture membranes
     Pre-term labor
     Toxemia
     Trauma
   Newborn circumcision (54150, 54160)
   Services incidental to or unrelated to pregnancy

59400   **Routine obstetric care including antepartum care, vaginal delivery (with or without episiotomy, and/or forceps) and postpartum care**   M ♀

INCLUDES   Fetal heart tones
     Hospital/office visits following cesarean section or vaginal delivery
     Initial/subsequent history
     Physical exams
     Recording weight/blood pressures
     Routine chemical urinalysis
     Routine prenatal visits:
       Each month up to 28 weeks gestation
       Every other week from 29 to 36 weeks gestation
       Weekly from 36 weeks until delivery
   60.4   60.4   **FUD** MMM   B
AMA: 2019,Jul,6; 2018,Jan,8; 2017,Jan,8; 2016,Jan,13

59409   **Vaginal delivery only (with or without episiotomy and/or forceps);**   M ♀
   Code also inpatient management after delivery/discharge services (99217-99239 [99224, 99225, 99226])
   23.3   23.3   **FUD** MMM   J G2 80
AMA: 2019,Jul,6; 2018,Jan,8; 2017,Jan,8; 2016,Jan,13

59410   **including postpartum care**   M ♀
INCLUDES   Hospital/office visits following cesarean section or vaginal delivery
   29.9   29.9   **FUD** MMM   B
AMA: 2019,Jul,6

59412-59414 Other Maternity Services

CMS: 100-02,15,180 Nurse-Midwife (CNM) Services; 100-02,15,20.1 Physician Expense for Surgery, Childbirth, and Treatment for Infertility

59412   **External cephalic version, with or without tocolysis**   M ♀
   Code also delivery code(s)
   2.95   2.95   **FUD** MMM   J G2 80
AMA: 2019,Jul,6

Complete breech presentation at term

The physician feels for the baby's head and bottom externally

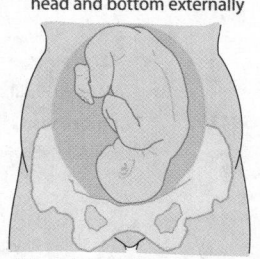

Turning the baby by applying external pressure

Baby is in cephalic presentation, engaged for normal delivery

59414   **Delivery of placenta (separate procedure)**   M ♀
   2.65   2.65   **FUD** MMM   J G2 80
AMA: 2019,Jul,6; 2018,Jan,8; 2017,Jan,8; 2016,Jan,13

Genital System

59425-59430 Prenatal and Postpartum Visits

CMS: 100-02,15,180 Nurse-Midwife (CNM) Services; 100-02,15,20.1 Physician Expense for Surgery, Childbirth, and Treatment for Infertility

INCLUDES Physician/other qualified health care professional providing all or portion antepartum/postpartum care, but no delivery due to:
Referral to another physician for delivery
Termination pregnancy by abortion

EXCLUDES Antepartum care, one to three visits, report with appropriate E/M service code
Medical complications pregnancy, labor, and delivery:
Cardiac problems
Diabetes
Hyperemesis
Hypertension
Neurological problems
Premature rupture membranes
Pre-term labor
Toxemia
Trauma
Newborn circumcision (54150, 54160)
Services incidental to or unrelated to pregnancy

59425   **Antepartum care only; 4-6 visits**   M ♀

INCLUDES Fetal heart tones
Initial/subsequent history
Physical exams
Recording weight/blood pressures
Routine chemical urinalysis
Routine prenatal visits:
Each month up to 28 weeks gestation
Every other week from 29 to 36 weeks gestation
Weekly from 36 weeks until delivery

10.2   13.1   **FUD** MMM   B 80

AMA: 2019,Jul,6; 2018,Jan,8; 2017,Jan,8; 2016,Jan,13

59426   **7 or more visits**   M ♀

INCLUDES Biweekly visits to 36 weeks gestation
Fetal heart tones
Initial/subsequent history
Monthly visits up to 28 weeks gestation
Physical exams
Recording weight/blood pressures
Routine chemical urinalysis
Weekly visits until delivery

17.9   23.5   **FUD** MMM   B 80

AMA: 2019,Jul,6; 2018,Jan,8; 2017,Jan,8; 2016,Jan,13

59430   **Postpartum care only (separate procedure)**   M ♀

INCLUDES Office/other outpatient visits following cesarean section or vaginal delivery

3.97   5.57   **FUD** MMM   B

AMA: 2019,Jul,6; 2018,Jan,8; 2017,Jan,8; 2016,Jan,13

59510-59525 Cesarean Section Delivery: Comprehensive and Components of Care

CMS: 100-02,15,20.1 Physician Expense for Surgery, Childbirth, and Treatment for Infertility

INCLUDES Classic cesarean section
Low cervical cesarean section

EXCLUDES Infant standby attendance (99360)
Medical complications pregnancy, labor, and delivery:
Cardiac problems
Diabetes
Hyperemesis
Hypertension
Neurological problems
Premature rupture membranes
Pre-term labor
Toxemia
Trauma
Newborn circumcision (54150, 54160)
Services incidental to or unrelated to pregnancy
Vaginal delivery after prior cesarean section (59610-59614)

59510   **Routine obstetric care including antepartum care, cesarean delivery, and postpartum care**   M ♀

INCLUDES Admission history
Admission to hospital
Cesarean delivery
Fetal heart tones
Hospital/office visits following cesarean section
Initial/subsequent history
Management uncomplicated labor
Physical exam
Recording weight/blood pressures
Routine chemical urinalysis
Routine prenatal visits:
Each month up to 28 weeks gestation
Every other week 29 to 36 weeks gestation
Weekly from 36 weeks until delivery

67.0   67.0   **FUD** MMM   B

AMA: 2019,Jul,6; 2018,Jan,8; 2017,Jan,8; 2016,Jan,13

Types of Cesarean section are classified by uterine incision

Body of uterus / Tube / Classical / Low vertical / Low transverse / Amniotic sac / Uterus at term / Cervix / Vagina / Pubic bone

59514   **Cesarean delivery only;**   M ♀

INCLUDES Admission history
Admission to hospital
Cesarean delivery
Management uncomplicated labor
Physical exam
Code also inpatient management after delivery/discharge services (99217-99239 [99224, 99225, 99226])

26.3   26.3   **FUD** MMM   C 80

AMA: 2019,Jul,6; 2018,Jan,8; 2017,Jan,8; 2016,Jan,13

59515   **including postpartum care**   M ♀

INCLUDES Admission history
Admission to hospital
Cesarean delivery
Hospital/office visits following cesarean section or vaginal delivery
Management uncomplicated labor
Physical exam

36.4   36.4   **FUD** MMM   B

AMA: 2019,Jul,6; 2018,Jan,8; 2017,Jan,8; 2016,Jan,13

+ **59525** **Subtotal or total hysterectomy after cesarean delivery (List separately in addition to code for primary procedure)** M ♀

Code first cesarean delivery (59510, 59514, 59515, 59618, 59620, 59622)

🚑 13.9 ⚕ 13.9 **FUD** ZZZ C 80 ▭

AMA: 2019,Jul,6

59610-59614 Vaginal Delivery After Prior Cesarean Section: Comprehensive and Components of Care

CMS: 100-02,15,180 Nurse-Midwife (CNM) Services; 100-02,15,20.1 Physician Expense for Surgery, Childbirth, and Treatment for Infertility

INCLUDES
Admission history
Admission to hospital
Management uncomplicated labor
Patients with previous cesarean delivery who present with vaginal delivery expectation
Physical exam
Successful vaginal delivery after previous cesarean delivery (VBAC)
Vaginal delivery with or without episiotomy or forceps

EXCLUDES
Elective cesarean delivery (59510, 59514, 59515)
Medical complications pregnancy, labor, and delivery:
Cardiac problems
Diabetes
Hyperemesis
Hypertension
Neurological problems
Premature rupture membranes
Pre-term labor
Toxemia
Trauma
Newborn circumcision (54150, 54160)
Services incidental to or unrelated to pregnancy

59610 **Routine obstetric care including antepartum care, vaginal delivery (with or without episiotomy, and/or forceps) and postpartum care, after previous cesarean delivery** M ♀

INCLUDES
Fetal heart tones
Hospital/office visits following cesarean section or vaginal delivery
Initial/subsequent history
Physical exams
Recording weight/blood pressures
Routine chemical urinalysis
Routine prenatal visits:
Each month up to 28 weeks gestation
Every other week 29 to 36 weeks gestation
Weekly from 36 weeks until delivery

🚑 63.4 ⚕ 63.4 **FUD** MMM B 80 ▭

AMA: 2019,Jul,6; 2018,Jan,8; 2017,Jan,8; 2016,Jan,13

59612 **Vaginal delivery only, after previous cesarean delivery (with or without episiotomy and/or forceps);** M ♀

Code also inpatient management after delivery/discharge services (99217-99239 [99224, 99225, 99226])

🚑 26.3 ⚕ 26.3 **FUD** MMM J 62 80 ▭

AMA: 2019,Jul,6; 2018,Jan,8; 2017,Jan,8; 2016,Jan,13

59614 **including postpartum care** M ♀

INCLUDES
Hospital/office visits following cesarean section or vaginal delivery

🚑 32.7 ⚕ 32.7 **FUD** MMM B 80 ▭

AMA: 2019,Jul,6; 2018,Jan,8; 2017,Jan,8; 2016,Jan,13

59618-59622 Cesarean Section After Attempted Vaginal Birth/Prior C-Section

CMS: 100-02,15,20.1 Physician Expense for Surgery, Childbirth, and Treatment for Infertility

INCLUDES
Admission history
Admission to hospital
Cesarean delivery
Cesarean delivery following unsuccessful vaginal delivery attempt after previous cesarean delivery
Management uncomplicated labor
Patients with previous cesarean delivery who present with vaginal delivery expectation
Physical exam

EXCLUDES
Elective cesarean delivery (59510, 59514, 59515)
Medical complications of pregnancy, labor, and delivery:
Cardiac problems
Diabetes
Hyperemesis
Hypertension
Neurological problems
Premature rupture of membranes
Pre-term labor
Toxemia
Trauma
Newborn circumcision (54150, 54160)
Services incidental to or unrelated to the pregnancy

59618 **Routine obstetric care including antepartum care, cesarean delivery, and postpartum care, following attempted vaginal delivery after previous cesarean delivery** M ♀

INCLUDES
Fetal heart tones
Hospital/office visits following cesarean section or vaginal delivery
Initial/subsequent history
Physical exams
Recording weight/blood pressures
Routine chemical urinalysis
Routine prenatal visits:
Each month up to 28 weeks gestation
Every two weeks 29 to 36 weeks gestation
Weekly from 36 weeks until delivery

🚑 67.8 ⚕ 67.8 **FUD** MMM B 80 ▭

AMA: 2019,Jul,6; 2018,Jan,8; 2017,Jan,8; 2016,Jan,13

59620 **Cesarean delivery only, following attempted vaginal delivery after previous cesarean delivery;** M ♀

Code also inpatient management after delivery/discharge services (99217-99239 [99224, 99225, 99226])

🚑 27.2 ⚕ 27.2 **FUD** MMM C 80 ▭

AMA: 2019,Jul,6; 2018,Jan,8; 2017,Jan,8; 2016,Jan,13

59622 **including postpartum care** M ♀

INCLUDES
Hospital/office visits following cesarean section or vaginal delivery

🚑 37.4 ⚕ 37.4 **FUD** MMM B 80 ▭

AMA: 2019,Jul,6; 2018,Jan,8; 2017,Jan,8; 2016,Jan,13

59812-59830 Treatment of Miscarriage

CMS: 100-02,15,20.1 Physician Expense for Surgery, Childbirth, and Treatment for Infertility

EXCLUDES
Medical treatment spontaneous complete abortion, any trimester (99202-99233 [99224, 99225, 99226])

59812 **Treatment of incomplete abortion, any trimester, completed surgically** M ♀

INCLUDES
Surgical treatment spontaneous abortion

🚑 8.59 ⚕ 9.37 **FUD** 090 J A2 ▭

AMA: 2019,Jul,6; 2018,Jan,8; 2017,Jan,8; 2016,Jan,13

59820 **Treatment of missed abortion, completed surgically; first trimester** M ♀

🚑 10.4 ⚕ 11.2 **FUD** 090 J A2 ▭

AMA: 2019,Jul,6; 2018,Jan,8; 2017,Jan,8; 2016,Jan,13

59821 **second trimester** M ♀

🚑 10.3 ⚕ 11.2 **FUD** 090 J A2 80 ▭

AMA: 2019,Jul,6; 2018,Jan,8; 2017,Jan,8; 2016,Jan,13

59830 **Treatment of septic abortion, completed surgically** M ♀

🚑 13.1 ⚕ 13.1 **FUD** 090 C 80 ▭

AMA: 2019,Jul,6; 2018,Jan,8; 2017,Jan,8; 2016,Jan,13

Genital System

59840 — 59899

59840-59866 Elective Abortions

CMS: 100-02,1,90 Termination of Pregnancy; 100-02,15,20.1 Physician Expense for Surgery, Childbirth, and Treatment for Infertility; 100-03,140.1 Abortion; 100-04,3,100.1 Billing for Abortion Services

59840 **Induced abortion, by dilation and curettage** Ⓜ ♀
🚗 6.08 ⚕ 6.50 **FUD** 010 Ⓙ A2 80 📶
AMA: 2019,Jul,6; 2018,Jan,8; 2017,Jan,8; 2016,Jan,13

59841 **Induced abortion, by dilation and evacuation** Ⓜ ♀
🚗 10.4 ⚕ 11.2 **FUD** 010 Ⓙ A2 80 📶
AMA: 2019,Jul,6; 2018,Jan,8; 2017,Jan,8; 2016,Jan,13

59850 **Induced abortion, by 1 or more intra-amniotic injections (amniocentesis-injections), including hospital admission and visits, delivery of fetus and secundines;** Ⓜ ♀
EXCLUDES *Cervical dilator insertion (59200)*
🚗 10.1 ⚕ 10.1 **FUD** 090 Ⓒ 80 📶
AMA: 2019,Jul,6; 2018,Jan,8; 2017,Jan,8; 2016,Jan,13

59851 **with dilation and curettage and/or evacuation** Ⓜ ♀
EXCLUDES *Cervical dilator insertion (59200)*
🚗 10.9 ⚕ 10.9 **FUD** 090 Ⓒ 80 📶
AMA: 2019,Jul,6; 2018,Jan,8; 2017,Jan,8; 2016,Jan,13

59852 **with hysterotomy (failed intra-amniotic injection)** Ⓜ ♀
EXCLUDES *Cervical dilator insertion (59200)*
🚗 16.5 ⚕ 16.5 **FUD** 090 Ⓒ 80 📶
AMA: 2019,Jul,6; 2018,Jan,8; 2017,Jan,8; 2016,Jan,13

59855 **Induced abortion, by 1 or more vaginal suppositories (eg, prostaglandin) with or without cervical dilation (eg, laminaria), including hospital admission and visits, delivery of fetus and secundines;** Ⓜ ♀
🚗 12.2 ⚕ 12.2 **FUD** 090 Ⓒ 80 📶
AMA: 2019,Jul,6

59856 **with dilation and curettage and/or evacuation** Ⓜ ♀
🚗 14.3 ⚕ 14.3 **FUD** 090 Ⓒ 80 📶
AMA: 2019,Jul,6

59857 **with hysterotomy (failed medical evacuation)** Ⓜ ♀
🚗 16.8 ⚕ 16.8 **FUD** 090 Ⓒ 80 📶
AMA: 2019,Jul,6

59866 **Multifetal pregnancy reduction(s) (MPR)** Ⓜ ♀
🚗 6.22 ⚕ 6.22 **FUD** 000 Ⓣ 62 80 📶
AMA: 2019,Jul,6

59870-59899 Miscellaneous Obstetrical Procedures

CMS: 100-02,15,20.1 Physician Expense for Surgery, Childbirth, and Treatment for Infertility

59870 **Uterine evacuation and curettage for hydatidiform mole** Ⓜ ♀
🚗 14.7 ⚕ 14.7 **FUD** 090 Ⓙ A2 80 📶
AMA: 2019,Jul,6; 2018,Jan,8; 2017,Jan,8; 2016,Jan,13

59871 **Removal of cerclage suture under anesthesia (other than local)** Ⓜ ♀
🚗 3.83 ⚕ 3.83 **FUD** 000 02 A2 80 📶
AMA: 2019,Jul,6; 2018,Jan,8; 2017,Jan,8; 2016,Jan,13

59897 **Unlisted fetal invasive procedure, including ultrasound guidance, when performed** Ⓜ ♀
🚗 0.00 ⚕ 0.00 **FUD** YYY Ⓣ 📶
AMA: 2019,Jul,6

59898 **Unlisted laparoscopy procedure, maternity care and delivery** Ⓜ ♀
🚗 0.00 ⚕ 0.00 **FUD** YYY Ⓙ 80 50 📶
AMA: 2019,Jul,6; 2018,Jan,8; 2017,Jan,8; 2016,Jan,13

59899 **Unlisted procedure, maternity care and delivery** Ⓜ ♀
🚗 0.00 ⚕ 0.00 **FUD** YYY Ⓣ 80 📶
AMA: 2019,Jul,6; 2018,Jan,8; 2017,Jan,8; 2016,Jan,13

60000 I&D of Infected Thyroglossal Cyst

60000 **Incision and drainage of thyroglossal duct cyst, infected**
🚑 4.37 ⚕ 4.99 **FUD** 010 [T] [A2] [80] ▣
AMA: 2014,Jan,11; 2002,May,7

60100 Core Needle Biopsy: Thyroid

EXCLUDES *Fine needle aspiration (10021, [10004, 10005, 10006, 10007, 10008, 10009, 10010, 10011, 10012])*

60100 **Biopsy thyroid, percutaneous core needle**
🔀 (76942, 77002, 77012, 77021)
🔀 (88172-88173)
🚑 2.25 ⚕ 3.18 **FUD** 000 [T] [P3] ▣
AMA: 2019,Apr,4; 2018,Jan,8; 2017,Jan,8; 2016,Jan,13

60200 Surgical Removal Thyroid Cyst or Mass; Division of Isthmus

60200 **Excision of cyst or adenoma of thyroid, or transection of isthmus**
🚑 19.0 ⚕ 19.0 **FUD** 090 [J] [A2] [80] ▣
AMA: 2018,Jan,8; 2017,Jan,8; 2016,Jan,13

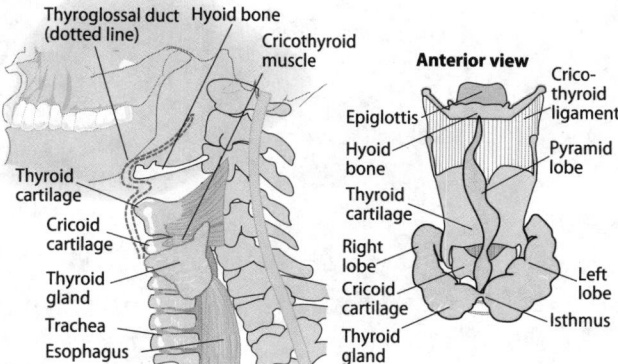

Lateral view
Thyroglossal duct (dotted line) Hyoid bone
Cricothyroid muscle
Thyroid cartilage
Cricoid cartilage
Thyroid gland
Trachea
Esophagus

Anterior view
Crico-thyroid ligament
Epiglottis
Hyoid bone
Pyramid lobe
Thyroid cartilage
Right lobe
Cricoid cartilage
Thyroid gland
Left lobe
Isthmus

60210-60225 Subtotal Thyroidectomy

60210 **Partial thyroid lobectomy, unilateral; with or without isthmusectomy**
🚑 20.3 ⚕ 20.3 **FUD** 090 [J] [62] [80] ▣
AMA: 2018,Jan,8; 2017,Jan,8; 2016,Jan,13

60212 **with contralateral subtotal lobectomy, including isthmusectomy**
🚑 29.0 ⚕ 29.0 **FUD** 090 [J] [62] [80] ▣
AMA: 2018,Jan,8; 2017,Jan,8; 2016,Jan,13

60220 **Total thyroid lobectomy, unilateral; with or without isthmusectomy**
🚑 20.3 ⚕ 20.3 **FUD** 090 [J] [62] [80] ▣
AMA: 2020,Aug,14; 2018,Jan,8; 2017,Jan,8; 2016,Jan,13

60225 **with contralateral subtotal lobectomy, including isthmusectomy**
🚑 26.8 ⚕ 26.8 **FUD** 090 [J] [62] [80] ▣
AMA: 2018,Jan,8; 2017,Jan,8; 2016,Jan,13

60240-60271 Complete Thyroidectomy Procedures

60240 **Thyroidectomy, total or complete**
EXCLUDES *Subtotal or partial thyroidectomy (60271)*
🚑 26.4 ⚕ 26.4 **FUD** 090 [J] [62] [80] ▣
AMA: 2018,Jan,8; 2017,Jan,8; 2016,Jan,13

60252 **Thyroidectomy, total or subtotal for malignancy; with limited neck dissection**
🚑 38.0 ⚕ 38.0 **FUD** 090 [J] [62] [80] ▣
AMA: 2018,Jan,8; 2017,Jan,8; 2016,Jan,13

60254 **with radical neck dissection**
🚑 48.2 ⚕ 48.2 **FUD** 090 [C] [80] ▣
AMA: 2018,Jan,8; 2017,Jan,8; 2016,Jan,13

60260 **Thyroidectomy, removal of all remaining thyroid tissue following previous removal of a portion of thyroid**
🚑 31.4 ⚕ 31.4 **FUD** 090 [J] [62] [80] [50] ▣
AMA: 2018,Jan,8; 2017,Jan,8; 2016,Jan,13

60270 **Thyroidectomy, including substernal thyroid; sternal split or transthoracic approach**
🚑 39.4 ⚕ 39.4 **FUD** 090 [C] [80] ▣
AMA: 2018,Jan,8; 2017,Jan,8; 2016,Jan,13

60271 **cervical approach**
🚑 30.4 ⚕ 30.4 **FUD** 090 [J] [62] [80] ▣
AMA: 2020,Aug,14; 2018,Jan,8; 2017,Jan,8; 2016,Jan,13

60280-60300 Treatment of Cyst/Sinus of Thyroid

60280 **Excision of thyroglossal duct cyst or sinus;**
EXCLUDES *Thyroid ultrasound (76536)*
🚑 12.6 ⚕ 12.6 **FUD** 090 [J] [A2] [80] ▣
AMA: 2014,Jan,11

60281 **recurrent**
EXCLUDES *Thyroid ultrasound (76536)*
🚑 16.8 ⚕ 16.8 **FUD** 090 [J] [A2] [80] ▣
AMA: 2014,Jan,11; 1994,Win,1

60300 **Aspiration and/or injection, thyroid cyst**
EXCLUDES *Fine needle aspiration (10021, [10004, 10005, 10006, 10007, 10008, 10009, 10010, 10011, 10012])*
🔀 (76942, 77012)
🚑 1.42 ⚕ 3.24 **FUD** 000 [T] [P3] ▣
AMA: 2014,Jan,11

60500-60512 Parathyroid Procedures

60500 **Parathyroidectomy or exploration of parathyroid(s);**
🚑 27.9 ⚕ 27.9 **FUD** 090 [J] [62] [80] ▣
AMA: 2018,Jan,8; 2017,Jan,8; 2016,Jan,13

Epiglottis
Pharynx
Thyroid gland
Parathyroid gland

Posterior view of pharynx, thyroid glands, and parathyroid glands

60502 **re-exploration**
🚑 37.5 ⚕ 37.5 **FUD** 090 [J] [62] [80] ▣
AMA: 2018,Jan,8; 2017,Jan,8; 2016,Jan,13

60505 **with mediastinal exploration, sternal split or transthoracic approach**
🚑 40.1 ⚕ 40.1 **FUD** 090 [C] [80] ▣
AMA: 2018,Jan,8; 2017,Jan,8; 2016,Jan,13

+ **60512** **Parathyroid autotransplantation (List separately in addition to code for primary procedure)**
Code first (60212, 60225, 60240, 60252, 60254, 60260, 60270-60271, 60500, 60502, 60505)
🚑 7.03 ⚕ 7.03 **FUD** ZZZ [N] [N1] [80] ▣
AMA: 2018,Jan,8; 2017,Jan,8; 2017,Jan,6; 2016,Jan,13

60520-60522 Thymus Procedures

EXCLUDES Surgical thoracoscopy (video-assisted thoracic surgery (VATS) thymectomy (32673))

60520 **Thymectomy, partial or total; transcervical approach (separate procedure)**
  🔪 30.4 ⚕ 30.4 **FUD** 090 J 62 80 ▣
  AMA: 2019,Mar,10

60521 **sternal split or transthoracic approach, without radical mediastinal dissection (separate procedure)**
  🔪 32.4 ⚕ 32.4 **FUD** 090 C 80 ▣
  AMA: 2018,Jan,8; 2017,Jan,8; 2016,Jan,13

60522 **sternal split or transthoracic approach, with radical mediastinal dissection (separate procedure)**
  🔪 39.5 ⚕ 39.5 **FUD** 090 C 80 ▣
  AMA: 2014,Jan,11; 2012,Oct,9-11

60540-60545 Adrenal Gland Procedures

EXCLUDES Laparoscopic approach (60650)
  Removal remote or disseminated pheochromocytoma (49203-49205)
  Standard backbench preparation cadaver donor (50323)

60540 **Adrenalectomy, partial or complete, or exploration of adrenal gland with or without biopsy, transabdominal, lumbar or dorsal (separate procedure);**
  🔪 31.0 ⚕ 31.0 **FUD** 090 C 80 50 ▣
  AMA: 2014,Jan,11; 1998,Nov,1

60545 **with excision of adjacent retroperitoneal tumor**
  🔪 35.7 ⚕ 35.7 **FUD** 090 C 80 50 ▣
  AMA: 2014,Jan,11; 1998,Nov,1

60600-60605 Carotid Body Procedures

60600 **Excision of carotid body tumor; without excision of carotid artery**
  🔪 39.7 ⚕ 39.7 **FUD** 090 C 80 ▣
  AMA: 2014,Jan,11

60605 **with excision of carotid artery**
  🔪 47.9 ⚕ 47.9 **FUD** 090 C 80 ▣
  AMA: 2018,Sep,9; 2017,Sep,13; 2016,Nov,8; 2016,Oct,10; 2016,Sep,8; 2016,Jul,10

60650-60699 Laparoscopic and Unlisted Procedures

INCLUDES Diagnostic laparoscopy (49320)

60650 **Laparoscopy, surgical, with adrenalectomy, partial or complete, or exploration of adrenal gland with or without biopsy, transabdominal, lumbar or dorsal**
  EXCLUDES Peritoneoscopy performed as separate procedure (49320)
  🔪 34.6 ⚕ 34.6 **FUD** 090 C 80 50 ▣
  AMA: 2018,Jan,8; 2017,Jan,8; 2016,Jan,13

60659 **Unlisted laparoscopy procedure, endocrine system**
  🔪 0.00 ⚕ 0.00 **FUD** YYY J 80 50 ▣
  AMA: 2018,Jan,8; 2017,Jan,8; 2016,Jan,13

60699 **Unlisted procedure, endocrine system**
  🔪 0.00 ⚕ 0.00 **FUD** YYY J 80 ▣
  AMA: 2018,Jan,8; 2017,Jan,8; 2016,Jan,13

61000-61253 Transcranial Access via Puncture, Burr Hole, Twist Hole, or Trephine

EXCLUDES *Injection for cerebral angiography (36100-36218)*

61000 **Subdural tap through fontanelle, or suture, infant, unilateral or bilateral; initial** A

EXCLUDES *Injection for:*
Pneumoencephalography (61055)
Ventriculography (61026, 61120)

🚑 3.25 ⚕ 3.25 **FUD** 000 T R2 ▭

AMA: 2014,Jan,11

Overhead view of newborn skull

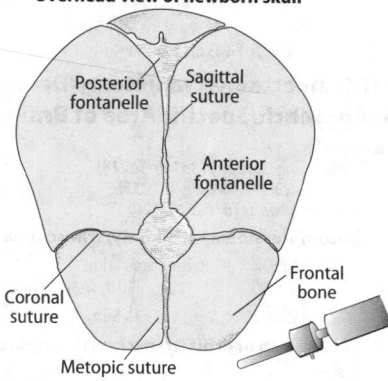

Posterior fontanelle
Sagittal suture
Anterior fontanelle
Coronal suture
Frontal bone
Metopic suture

An initial tap through to the subdural level is performed on an infant via a fontanelle or suture, either unilateral or bilateral

61001 **subsequent taps** A

🚑 3.09 ⚕ 3.09 **FUD** 000 T R2 ▭

AMA: 2014,Jan,11

61020 **Ventricular puncture through previous burr hole, fontanelle, suture, or implanted ventricular catheter/reservoir; without injection**

🚑 2.87 ⚕ 2.87 **FUD** 000 T A2 ▭

AMA: 2014,Jan,11

61026 **with injection of medication or other substance for diagnosis or treatment**

INCLUDES Injection for ventriculography

🚑 3.05 ⚕ 3.05 **FUD** 000 T A2 ▭

AMA: 2014,Jan,11; 2002,May,7

61050 **Cisternal or lateral cervical (C1-C2) puncture; without injection (separate procedure)**

🚑 2.44 ⚕ 2.44 **FUD** 000 T A2 80 ▭

AMA: 2014,Jan,11; 1991,Win,1

61055 **with injection of medication or other substance for diagnosis or treatment**

INCLUDES Injection for pneumoencephalography

EXCLUDES *Myelography via lumbar injection (62302-62305)*
Radiology procedures except when furnished by different provider

🚑 3.62 ⚕ 3.62 **FUD** 000 T A2 ▭

AMA: 2020,Oct,3

61070 **Puncture of shunt tubing or reservoir for aspiration or injection procedure**

🔀 (75809)

🚑 1.63 ⚕ 1.63 **FUD** 000 T A2 ▭

AMA: 2020,Oct,3; 2018,Jan,8; 2017,Jan,8; 2016,Jan,13

61105 **Twist drill hole for subdural or ventricular puncture**

🚑 13.5 ⚕ 13.5 **FUD** 090 C 80 ▭

AMA: 2014,Jan,11

61107 **Twist drill hole(s) for subdural, intracerebral, or ventricular puncture; for implanting ventricular catheter, pressure recording device, or other intracerebral monitoring device**

Code also intracranial neuroendoscopic ventricular catheter insertion or reinsertion, when performed (62160)

🚑 9.08 ⚕ 9.08 **FUD** 000 ⊘ C ▭

AMA: 2014,Jan,11; 2007,Jun,10-11

61108 **for evacuation and/or drainage of subdural hematoma**

🚑 25.8 ⚕ 25.8 **FUD** 090 C ▭

AMA: 2014,Jan,11

61120 **Burr hole(s) for ventricular puncture (including injection of gas, contrast media, dye, or radioactive material)**

INCLUDES Injection for ventriculography

🚑 21.8 ⚕ 21.8 **FUD** 090 C 80 ▭

AMA: 2014,Jan,11

61140 **Burr hole(s) or trephine; with biopsy of brain or intracranial lesion**

🚑 36.9 ⚕ 36.9 **FUD** 090 C 80 ▭

AMA: 2014,Jan,11

61150 **with drainage of brain abscess or cyst**

🚑 39.0 ⚕ 39.0 **FUD** 090 C ▭

AMA: 2014,Jan,11

61151 **with subsequent tapping (aspiration) of intracranial abscess or cyst**

🚑 29.1 ⚕ 29.1 **FUD** 090 C ▭

AMA: 2014,Jan,11

61154 **Burr hole(s) with evacuation and/or drainage of hematoma, extradural or subdural**

🚑 36.6 ⚕ 36.6 **FUD** 090 C 80 50 ▭

AMA: 2014,Jan,11

61156 **Burr hole(s); with aspiration of hematoma or cyst, intracerebral**

🚑 36.5 ⚕ 36.5 · **FUD** 090 C 80 ▭

AMA: 2014,Jan,11

61210 **for implanting ventricular catheter, reservoir, EEG electrode(s), pressure recording device, or other cerebral monitoring device (separate procedure)**

Code also intracranial neuroendoscopic ventricular catheter insertion or reinsertion, when performed (62160)

🚑 10.6 ⚕ 10.6 **FUD** 090 C ▭

AMA: 2018,Jan,8; 2017,Jan,8; 2016,Jan,13

61215 **Insertion of subcutaneous reservoir, pump or continuous infusion system for connection to ventricular catheter**

EXCLUDES *Chemotherapy (96450)*
Refilling and maintenance implantable infusion pump (95990)

🚑 14.8 ⚕ 14.8 **FUD** 090 J A2 ▭

AMA: 2018,Jan,8; 2017,Jan,8; 2016,Jan,13

61250 **Burr hole(s) or trephine, supratentorial, exploratory, not followed by other surgery**

EXCLUDES *Burr hole or trephine followed by craniotomy same operative session (61304-61321)*

🚑 25.4 ⚕ 25.4 **FUD** 090 C 80 50 ▭

AMA: 2014,Jan,11

61253 **Burr hole(s) or trephine, infratentorial, unilateral or bilateral**

EXCLUDES *Burr hole or trephine followed by craniotomy same operative session (61304-61321)*

🚑 29.1 ⚕ 29.1 **FUD** 090 C 80 ▭

AMA: 2018,Jan,8; 2017,Jan,8; 2016,Jan,13

61304-61323 Craniectomy/Craniotomy: By Indication/Specific Area of Brain

EXCLUDES Injection for:
Cerebral angiography (36100-36218)
Pneumoencephalography (61055)
Ventriculography (61026, 61120)

61304 Craniectomy or craniotomy, exploratory; supratentorial

EXCLUDES Other craniectomy/craniotomy procedures when performed same anatomical site and during same surgical encounter

⚕ 48.1   ☁ 48.1   **FUD** 090   C 80 ▱

AMA: 2014,Jan,11; 2002,Sep,10

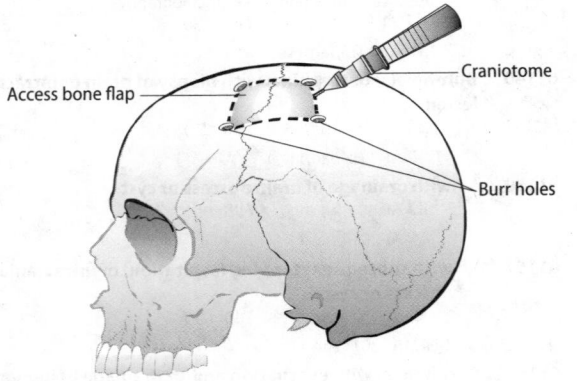

Access bone flap — Craniotome
— Burr holes

61305 infratentorial (posterior fossa)

EXCLUDES Other craniectomy/craniotomy procedures when performed same anatomical site and during same surgical encounter

⚕ 58.6   ☁ 58.6   **FUD** 090   C 80 ▱

AMA: 2014,Jan,11; 2002,Sep,10

61312 Craniectomy or craniotomy for evacuation of hematoma, supratentorial; extradural or subdural

⚕ 60.8   ☁ 60.8   **FUD** 090   C 80 ▱

AMA: 2018,Jan,8; 2017,Jan,8; 2016,Jan,13

61313 intracerebral

⚕ 57.2   ☁ 57.2   **FUD** 090   C 80 ▱

AMA: 2014,Jan,11; 2002,Sep,10

61314 Craniectomy or craniotomy for evacuation of hematoma, infratentorial; extradural or subdural

⚕ 53.2   ☁ 53.2   **FUD** 090   C 80 ▱

AMA: 2014,Jan,11; 2002,Sep,10

61315 intracerebellar

⚕ 60.4   ☁ 60.4   **FUD** 090   C 80 ▱

AMA: 2014,Jan,11; 2002,Sep,10

+ **61316** Incision and subcutaneous placement of cranial bone graft (List separately in addition to code for primary procedure)

Code first (61304, 61312-61313, 61322-61323, 61340, 61570-61571, 61680-61705)

⚕ 2.54   ☁ 2.54   **FUD** ZZZ   C

AMA: 2014,Jan,11; 2002,Sep,10

61320 Craniectomy or craniotomy, drainage of intracranial abscess; supratentorial

⚕ 54.8   ☁ 54.8   **FUD** 090   C 80 ▱

AMA: 2014,Jan,11; 2002,Sep,10

61321 infratentorial

⚕ 62.7   ☁ 62.7   **FUD** 090   C 80 ▱

AMA: 2014,Jan,11; 2002,Sep,10

61322 Craniectomy or craniotomy, decompressive, with or without duraplasty, for treatment of intracranial hypertension, without evacuation of associated intraparenchymal hematoma; without lobectomy

EXCLUDES Craniectomy or craniotomy for evacuation hematoma (61313)
Subtemporal decompression (61340)

⚕ 69.7   ☁ 69.7   **FUD** 090   C 80 ▱

AMA: 2020,May,13; 2018,Aug,10

61323 with lobectomy

EXCLUDES Craniectomy or craniotomy for evacuation hematoma (61313)
Subtemporal decompression (61340)

⚕ 69.8   ☁ 69.8   **FUD** 090   C 80 ▱

AMA: 2014,Jan,11; 1991,Sum,4

61330-61530 Craniectomy/Craniotomy/Decompression Brain By Surgical Approach/Specific Area of Brain

EXCLUDES Injection for:
Cerebral angiography (36100-36218)
Pneumoencephalography (61055)
Ventriculography (61026, 61120)

61330 Decompression of orbit only, transcranial approach

INCLUDES Naffziger operation

⚕ 52.2   ☁ 52.2   **FUD** 090   J 62 80 50 ▱

AMA: 2014,Jan,11; 1991,Sum,4

61333 Exploration of orbit (transcranial approach); with removal of lesion

⚕ 59.6   ☁ 59.6   **FUD** 090   C 80 50 ▱

AMA: 2014,Jan,11; 1991,Sum,4

61340 Subtemporal cranial decompression (pseudotumor cerebri, slit ventricle syndrome)

EXCLUDES Decompression craniotomy or craniectomy for intracranial hypertension, without hematoma removal (61322-61323)

⚕ 41.4   ☁ 41.4   **FUD** 090   C 80 50 ▱

AMA: 2020,May,13

61343 Craniectomy, suboccipital with cervical laminectomy for decompression of medulla and spinal cord, with or without dural graft (eg, Arnold-Chiari malformation)

⚕ 63.4   ☁ 63.4   **FUD** 090   C 80 ▱

AMA: 2014,Jan,11; 1991,Sum,4

61345 Other cranial decompression, posterior fossa

EXCLUDES Kroenlein procedure
Orbital decompression using lateral wall approach (67445)

⚕ 60.1   ☁ 60.1   **FUD** 090   C 80 ▱

AMA: 2014,Jan,11; 1991,Sum,4

61450 Craniectomy, subtemporal, for section, compression, or decompression of sensory root of gasserian ganglion

INCLUDES Frazier-Spiller procedure
Hartley-Krause
Krause decompression
Taarnhoj procedure

⚕ 56.6   ☁ 56.6   **FUD** 090   C 80 ▱

AMA: 2014,Jan,11; 1991,Sum,4

61458 Craniectomy, suboccipital; for exploration or decompression of cranial nerves

INCLUDES Jannetta decompression

⚕ 58.8   ☁ 58.8   **FUD** 090   C 80 ▱

AMA: 2014,Jan,11; 1991,Sum,4

61460 for section of 1 or more cranial nerves

🔧 61.7 ✂ 61.7 **FUD** 090   © 80 ▭

AMA: 2014,Jan,11; 1991,Sum,4

61520 cerebellopontine angle tumor

🔧 110. ✂ 110. **FUD** 090   © 80 ▭

AMA: 2014,Jan,11; 1991,Sum,4

Olfactory nerve (I)
Optic nerve (II)
Oculomotor nerve (III)
Trochlear nerve (IV)
Trigeminal nerve (V)
Abducens nerve (VI)
Facial nerve (VII)
Vestibulocochlear nerve (VIII)
Glossopharyngeal nerve (IX)
Vagus nerve (X)
Hypoglossal nerve (XII)
Accessory nerve (XI)
Pons

Central sulcus
Parietal lobe
Frontal lobe
Occipital lobe
Lateral sulcus
Temporal lobe
Cerebellum
Pons
Medulla oblongata

61500 Craniectomy; with excision of tumor or other bone lesion of skull

🔧 38.2 ✂ 38.2 **FUD** 090   © 80 ▭

AMA: 2018,Jan,8; 2017,Jan,8; 2016,Jan,13

61501 for osteomyelitis

🔧 33.1 ✂ 33.1 **FUD** 090   © 80 ▭

AMA: 2018,Jan,8; 2017,Jan,8; 2016,Jan,13

61510 Craniectomy, trephination, bone flap craniotomy; for excision of brain tumor, supratentorial, except meningioma

🔧 64.0 ✂ 64.0 **FUD** 090   © 80 ▭

AMA: 2014,Jan,11; 1991,Sum,4

61512 for excision of meningioma, supratentorial

🔧 74.8 ✂ 74.8 **FUD** 090   © 80 ▭

AMA: 2014,Jan,11; 1991,Sum,4

61514 for excision of brain abscess, supratentorial

🔧 55.9 ✂ 55.9 **FUD** 090   © 80 ▭

AMA: 2014,Jan,11; 1991,Sum,4

61516 for excision or fenestration of cyst, supratentorial

EXCLUDES   Craniopharyngioma (61545)
Pituitary tumor removal (61546, 61548)

🔧 54.4 ✂ 54.4 **FUD** 090   © 80 ▭

AMA: 2014,Jan,11; 1991,Sum,4

+ 61517 Implantation of brain intracavitary chemotherapy agent (List separately in addition to code for primary procedure)

EXCLUDES   Intracavity radioelement source or ribbon implantation (77770-77772)
Code first (61510, 61518)

🔧 2.59 ✂ 2.59 **FUD** ZZZ   © ▭

AMA: 2014,Jan,11; 1991,Sum,4

61518 Craniectomy for excision of brain tumor, infratentorial or posterior fossa; except meningioma, cerebellopontine angle tumor, or midline tumor at base of skull

🔧 81.0 ✂ 81.0 **FUD** 090   © 80 ▭

AMA: 2014,Jan,11; 1991,Sum,4

61519 meningioma

🔧 85.4 ✂ 85.4 **FUD** 090   © 80 ▭

AMA: 2014,Jan,11; 1991,Sum,4

61521 midline tumor at base of skull

🔧 94.2 ✂ 94.2 **FUD** 090   © 80 ▭

AMA: 2018,Jan,8; 2017,Jan,8; 2016,Jan,13

61522 Craniectomy, infratentorial or posterior fossa; for excision of brain abscess

🔧 62.9 ✂ 62.9 **FUD** 090   © 80 ▭

AMA: 2014,Jan,11; 1991,Sum,4

61524 for excision or fenestration of cyst

🔧 60.8 ✂ 60.8 **FUD** 090   © 80 ▭

AMA: 2014,Jan,11; 1991,Sum,4

61526 Craniectomy, bone flap craniotomy, transtemporal (mastoid) for excision of cerebellopontine angle tumor;

🔧 97.9 ✂ 97.9 **FUD** 090   © ▭

AMA: 2018,Mar,11; 2018,Jan,8; 2017,Jan,8; 2016,Jan,13

61530 combined with middle/posterior fossa craniotomy/craniectomy

🔧 91.0 ✂ 91.0 **FUD** 090   © ▭

AMA: 2014,Jan,11; 1991,Sum,4

61531-61545 Procedures for Seizures/Implanted Electrodes/Choroid Plexus/Craniopharyngioma

EXCLUDES   Craniotomy for:
Multiple subpial transections during procedure (61567)
Selective amygdalohippocampectomy (61566)
Injection for:
Cerebral angiography (36100-36218)
Pneumoencephalography (61055)
Ventriculography (61026, 61120)

61531 Subdural implantation of strip electrodes through 1 or more burr or trephine hole(s) for long-term seizure monitoring

EXCLUDES   Continuous EEG observation ([95700, 95705, 95706, 95707, 95708, 95709, 95710, 95711, 95712, 95713, 95714, 95715, 95716, 95717, 95718, 95719, 95720, 95721, 95722, 95723, 95724, 95725, 95726])
Craniotomy for intracranial arteriovenous malformation removal (61680-61692)
Stereotactic insertion electrodes (61760)

🔧 35.2 ✂ 35.2 **FUD** 090   © 80 ▭

AMA: 2019,Jul,10

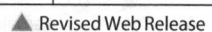

Nervous System

61533 — 61570

61533 Craniotomy with elevation of bone flap; for subdural implantation of an electrode array, for long-term seizure monitoring

> EXCLUDES Continuous EEG monitoring ([95700, 95705, 95706, 95707, 95708, 95709, 95710, 95711, 95712, 95713, 95714, 95715, 95716, 95717, 95718, 95719, 95720, 95721, 95722, 95723, 95724, 95725, 95726])

> 📁 44.4   ✂ 44.4   **FUD** 090   C 80 📠
> **AMA:** 2014,Jan,11; 1993,Sum,25

61534 for excision of epileptogenic focus without electrocorticography during surgery

> 📁 47.4   ✂ 47.4   **FUD** 090   C 80 📠
> **AMA:** 2014,Jan,11; 1991,Sum,4

61535 for removal of epidural or subdural electrode array, without excision of cerebral tissue (separate procedure)

> 📁 29.1   ✂ 29.1   **FUD** 090   C 80 📠
> **AMA:** 2019,Jul,10

61536 for excision of cerebral epileptogenic focus, with electrocorticography during surgery (includes removal of electrode array)

> 📁 76.1   ✂ 76.1   **FUD** 090   C 80 📠
> **AMA:** 2014,Jan,11; 1991,Sum,4

61537 for lobectomy, temporal lobe, without electrocorticography during surgery

> 📁 72.4   ✂ 72.4   **FUD** 090   C 80 📠
> **AMA:** 2014,Jan,11; 1991,Sum,4

61538 for lobectomy, temporal lobe, with electrocorticography during surgery

> 📁 78.2   ✂ 78.2   **FUD** 090   C 80 📠
> **AMA:** 2019,Mar,6

61539 for lobectomy, other than temporal lobe, partial or total, with electrocorticography during surgery

> 📁 69.6   ✂ 69.6   **FUD** 090   C 80 📠
> **AMA:** 2019,Mar,6

61540 for lobectomy, other than temporal lobe, partial or total, without electrocorticography during surgery

> 📁 64.2   ✂ 64.2   **FUD** 090   C 80 📠
> **AMA:** 2014,Jan,11; 1991,Sum,4

61541 for transection of corpus callosum

> 📁 63.3   ✂ 63.3   **FUD** 090   C 80 📠
> **AMA:** 2014,Jan,11; 1991,Sum,4

61543 for partial or subtotal (functional) hemispherectomy

> 📁 64.0   ✂ 64.0   **FUD** 090   C 80 📠
> **AMA:** 2014,Jan,11; 1991,Sum,4

61544 for excision or coagulation of choroid plexus

> 📁 54.8   ✂ 54.8   **FUD** 090   C 80 📠
> **AMA:** 2014,Jan,11; 1991,Sum,4

61545 for excision of craniopharyngioma

> 📁 92.3   ✂ 92.3   **FUD** 090   C 80 📠
> **AMA:** 2014,Jan,11; 1991,Sum,4

61546-61548 Removal Pituitary Gland/Tumor

> EXCLUDES Injection for:
> Cerebral angiography (36100-36218)
> Pneumoencephalography (61055)
> Ventriculography (61026, 61120)

61546 Craniotomy for hypophysectomy or excision of pituitary tumor, intracranial approach

> 📁 66.6   ✂ 66.6   **FUD** 090   C 80 📠
> **AMA:** 2014,Jan,11; 1991,Sum,4

61548 Hypophysectomy or excision of pituitary tumor, transnasal or transseptal approach, nonstereotactic

> INCLUDES Operating microscope (69990)
> 📁 45.8   ✂ 45.8   **FUD** 090   C 80 📠
> **AMA:** 2019,Dec,12; 2016,Feb,12

61550-61559 Craniosynostosis Procedures

> EXCLUDES Injection for:
> Cerebral angiography (36100-36218)
> Pneumoencephalography (61055)
> Ventriculography (61026, 61120)
> Orbital hypertelorism reconstruction (21260-21263)
> Reconstruction (21172-21180)

61550 Craniectomy for craniosynostosis; single cranial suture

> 📁 32.1   ✂ 32.1   **FUD** 090   C 80 📠
> **AMA:** 2018,Jan,8; 2017,Jan,8; 2016,Jan,13

61552 multiple cranial sutures

> 📁 43.5   ✂ 43.5   **FUD** 090   C 80 📠
> **AMA:** 2018,Jan,8; 2017,Jan,8; 2016,Jan,13

61556 Craniotomy for craniosynostosis; frontal or parietal bone flap

> 📁 49.2   ✂ 49.2   **FUD** 090   C 80 📠
> **AMA:** 2018,Jan,8; 2017,Jan,8; 2016,Jan,13

61557 bifrontal bone flap

> 📁 49.4   ✂ 49.4   **FUD** 090   C 80 📠
> **AMA:** 2018,Jan,8; 2017,Jan,8; 2016,Jan,13

61558 Extensive craniectomy for multiple cranial suture craniosynostosis (eg, cloverleaf skull); not requiring bone grafts

> 📁 54.2   ✂ 54.2   **FUD** 090   C 80 📠
> **AMA:** 2018,Jan,8; 2017,Jan,8; 2016,Jan,13

61559 recontouring with multiple osteotomies and bone autografts (eg, barrel-stave procedure) (includes obtaining grafts)

> 📁 69.1   ✂ 69.1   **FUD** 090   C 80 📠
> **AMA:** 2018,Jan,8; 2017,Jan,8; 2016,Jan,13

61563-61564 Removal Cranial Bone Tumor With/Without Optic Nerve Decompression

> EXCLUDES Injection for:
> Cerebral angiography (36100-36218)
> Pneumoencephalography (61055)
> Ventriculography (61026, 61120)
> Reconstruction (21181-21183)

61563 Excision, intra and extracranial, benign tumor of cranial bone (eg, fibrous dysplasia); without optic nerve decompression

> 📁 57.5   ✂ 57.5   **FUD** 090   C 80 📠
> **AMA:** 2014,Jan,11; 1991,Sum,4

61564 with optic nerve decompression

> 📁 69.5   ✂ 69.5   **FUD** 090   C 80 50 📠
> **AMA:** 2014,Jan,11; 1991,Sum,4

61566-61567 Craniotomy for Seizures

> EXCLUDES Injection for:
> Cerebral angiography (36100-36218)
> Pneumoencephalography (61055)
> Ventriculography (61026, 61120)

61566 Craniotomy with elevation of bone flap; for selective amygdalohippocampectomy

> 📁 66.1   ✂ 66.1   **FUD** 090   C 80 📠
> **AMA:** 2018,Nov,7

61567 for multiple subpial transections, with electrocorticography during surgery

> 📁 73.9   ✂ 73.9   **FUD** 090   C 80 📠
> **AMA:** 2014,Jan,11; 1991,Sum,4

61570-61571 Removal of Foreign Body from Brain

> EXCLUDES Injection for:
> Cerebral angiography (36100-36218)
> Pneumoencephalography (61055)
> Ventriculography (61026, 61120)
> Sequestrectomy for osteomyelitis (61501)

61570 Craniectomy or craniotomy; with excision of foreign body from brain

> 📁 53.9   ✂ 53.9   **FUD** 090   C 80 📠
> **AMA:** 2014,Jan,11; 1991,Sum,4

26/TC PC/TC Only   A2-Z3 ASC Payment   50 Bilateral   ♂ Male Only   ♀ Female Only   📁 Facility RVU   ✂ Non-Facility RVU   CCI   CLIA
FUD Follow-up Days   **CMS:** IOM   **AMA:** CPT Asst   A-Y OPPSI   80/80 Surg Assist Allowed / w/Doc   Lab Crosswalk   Radiology Crosswalk

61571 with treatment of penetrating wound of brain
📋 57.4 ⚕ 57.4 **FUD** 090 [C] [80] ▣
AMA: 2014,Jan,11; 1991,Sum,4

61575-61576 Transoral Approach Posterior Cranial Fossa/Upper Cervical Cord

EXCLUDES Arthrodesis (22548)
Injection for:
Cerebral angiography (36100-36218)
Pneumoencephalography (61055)
Ventriculography (61026, 61120)

61575 Transoral approach to skull base, brain stem or upper spinal cord for biopsy, decompression or excision of lesion;
📋 72.4 ⚕ 72.4 **FUD** 090 [C] [80] ▣
AMA: 2014,Jan,11; 1991,Sum,4

61576 requiring splitting of tongue and/or mandible (including tracheostomy)
📋 121. ⚕ 121. **FUD** 090 [C] [80] ▣
AMA: 2014,Jan,11; 1991,Sum,4

61580-61598 Surgical Approach: Cranial Fossae

EXCLUDES Definitive surgery (61600-61616)
Dural repair and/or reconstruction (61618-61619)
Injection for:
Cerebral angiography (36100-36218)
Pneumoencephalography (61055)
Ventriculography (61026, 61120)
Primary closure (15730, 15733, 15756-15758)

61580 Craniofacial approach to anterior cranial fossa; extradural, including lateral rhinotomy, ethmoidectomy, sphenoidectomy, without maxillectomy or orbital exenteration
📋 70.5 ⚕ 70.5 **FUD** 090 [C] [50] ▣
AMA: 2018,Jan,8; 2017,Jan,8; 2016,Jan,13

61581 extradural, including lateral rhinotomy, orbital exenteration, ethmoidectomy, sphenoidectomy and/or maxillectomy
📋 76.6 ⚕ 76.6 **FUD** 090 [C] [50] ▣
AMA: 2018,Jan,8; 2017,Jan,8; 2016,Jan,13

61582 extradural, including unilateral or bifrontal craniotomy, elevation of frontal lobe(s), osteotomy of base of anterior cranial fossa
📋 88.5 ⚕ 88.5 **FUD** 090 [C] [80] ▣
AMA: 2018,Jan,8; 2017,Jan,8; 2016,Jan,13

61583 intradural, including unilateral or bifrontal craniotomy, elevation or resection of frontal lobe, osteotomy of base of anterior cranial fossa
📋 84.2 ⚕ 84.2 **FUD** 090 [C] [80] ▣
AMA: 2018,Jan,8; 2017,Dec,13; 2017,Jan,8; 2016,Jan,13

61584 Orbitocranial approach to anterior cranial fossa, extradural, including supraorbital ridge osteotomy and elevation of frontal and/or temporal lobe(s); without orbital exenteration
📋 83.7 ⚕ 83.7 **FUD** 090 [C] [80] [50] ▣
AMA: 2018,Jan,8; 2017,Jan,8; 2016,Jan,13

61585 with orbital exenteration
📋 95.1 ⚕ 95.1 **FUD** 090 [C] [80] [50] ▣
AMA: 2018,Jan,8; 2017,Jan,8; 2016,Jan,13

61586 Bicoronal, transzygomatic and/or LeFort I osteotomy approach to anterior cranial fossa with or without internal fixation, without bone graft
📋 71.2 ⚕ 71.2 **FUD** 090 [C] [80] ▣
AMA: 2014,Jan,11; 1997,Nov,1

61590 Infratemporal pre-auricular approach to middle cranial fossa (parapharyngeal space, infratemporal and midline skull base, nasopharynx), with or without disarticulation of the mandible, including parotidectomy, craniotomy, decompression and/or mobilization of the facial nerve and/or petrous carotid artery
📋 87.6 ⚕ 87.6 **FUD** 090 [C] [80] [50] ▣
AMA: 2020,Apr,10; 2018,Jan,8; 2017,Jan,8; 2016,Jan,13

61591 Infratemporal post-auricular approach to middle cranial fossa (internal auditory meatus, petrous apex, tentorium, cavernous sinus, parasellar area, infratemporal fossa) including mastoidectomy, resection of sigmoid sinus, with or without decompression and/or mobilization of contents of auditory canal or petrous carotid artery
📋 89.1 ⚕ 89.1 **FUD** 090 [C] [80] [50] ▣
AMA: 2018,Jan,8; 2017,Jan,8; 2016,Jan,13

61592 Orbitocranial zygomatic approach to middle cranial fossa (cavernous sinus and carotid artery, clivus, basilar artery or petrous apex) including osteotomy of zygoma, craniotomy, extra- or intradural elevation of temporal lobe
📋 91.7 ⚕ 91.7 **FUD** 090 [C] [80] [50] ▣
AMA: 2018,Jan,8; 2017,Jan,8; 2016,Jan,13

61595 Transtemporal approach to posterior cranial fossa, jugular foramen or midline skull base, including mastoidectomy, decompression of sigmoid sinus and/or facial nerve, with or without mobilization
📋 68.1 ⚕ 68.1 **FUD** 090 [C] [50] ▣
AMA: 2018,Mar,11; 2018,Jan,8; 2017,Jan,8; 2016,Jan,13

61596 Transcochlear approach to posterior cranial fossa, jugular foramen or midline skull base, including labyrinthectomy, decompression, with or without mobilization of facial nerve and/or petrous carotid artery
📋 70.0 ⚕ 70.0 **FUD** 090 [C] [80] [50] ▣
AMA: 2018,Jan,8; 2017,Jan,8; 2016,Jan,13

61597 Transcondylar (far lateral) approach to posterior cranial fossa, jugular foramen or midline skull base, including occipital condylectomy, mastoidectomy, resection of C1-C3 vertebral body(s), decompression of vertebral artery, with or without mobilization
📋 84.9 ⚕ 84.9 **FUD** 090 [C] [80] [50] ▣
AMA: 2018,Jan,8; 2017,Jan,8; 2016,Jan,13

61598 Transpetrosal approach to posterior cranial fossa, clivus or foramen magnum, including ligation of superior petrosal sinus and/or sigmoid sinus
📋 82.4 ⚕ 82.4 **FUD** 090 [C] [80] ▣
AMA: 2018,Jan,8; 2017,Jan,8; 2016,Jan,13

61600-61616 Definitive Procedures: Cranial Fossae

EXCLUDES Dural repair and/or reconstruction (61618-61619)
Injection for:
Cerebral angiography (36100-36218)
Pneumoencephalography (61055)
Ventriculography (61026, 61120)
Primary closure (15730, 15733, 15756-15758)
Surgical approach (61580-61598)

61600 Resection or excision of neoplastic, vascular or infectious lesion of base of anterior cranial fossa; extradural
📋 61.5 ⚕ 61.5 **FUD** 090 [C] [80] ▣
AMA: 2018,Jan,8; 2017,Jan,8; 2016,Jan,13

61601 intradural, including dural repair, with or without graft
📋 69.6 ⚕ 69.6 **FUD** 090 [C] [80] ▣
AMA: 2018,Jan,8; 2017,Jan,8; 2016,Jan,13

61605 Resection or excision of neoplastic, vascular or infectious lesion of infratemporal fossa, parapharyngeal space, petrous apex; extradural
📋 62.2 ⚕ 62.2 **FUD** 090 [C] [80] ▣
AMA: 2020,Apr,10; 2018,Jan,8; 2017,Jan,8; 2016,Jan,13

Nervous System

61571 — 61605

Nervous System

61606 — 61630

61606   **intradural, including dural repair, with or without graft**
🔧 84.8   ✂ 84.8   **FUD** 090   C 80 ▣
AMA: 2018,Jan,8; 2017,Jan,8; 2016,Jan,13

61607   **Resection or excision of neoplastic, vascular or infectious lesion of parasellar area, cavernous sinus, clivus or midline skull base; extradural**
🔧 77.8   ✂ 77.8   **FUD** 090   C 80 ▣
AMA: 2018,Jan,8; 2017,Jan,8; 2016,Jan,13

61608   **intradural, including dural repair, with or without graft**
🔧 95.7   ✂ 95.7   **FUD** 090   C 80 ▣
AMA: 2018,Jan,8; 2017,Jan,8; 2016,Jan,13

+ 61611   **Transection or ligation, carotid artery in petrous canal; without repair (List separately in addition to code for primary procedure)**
Code first (61605-61608)
🔧 13.8   ✂ 13.8   **FUD** ZZZ   C 80 ▣
AMA: 2018,Jan,8; 2017,Jan,8; 2016,Jan,13

61613   **Obliteration of carotid aneurysm, arteriovenous malformation, or carotid-cavernous fistula by dissection within cavernous sinus**
🔧 96.9   ✂ 96.9   **FUD** 090   C 80 50 ▣
AMA: 2018,Jan,8; 2017,Jan,8; 2016,Jan,13

61615   **Resection or excision of neoplastic, vascular or infectious lesion of base of posterior cranial fossa, jugular foramen, foramen magnum, or C1-C3 vertebral bodies; extradural**
🔧 82.3   ✂ 82.3   **FUD** 090   C 80 ▣
AMA: 2018,Jan,8; 2017,Jan,8; 2016,Jan,13

61616   **intradural, including dural repair, with or without graft**
🔧 97.3   ✂ 97.3   **FUD** 090   C 80 ▣
AMA: 2018,Mar,11; 2018,Jan,8; 2017,Jan,8; 2016,Jan,13

61618-61619 Reconstruction Post-Surgical Cranial Fossae Defects

EXCLUDES   *Definitive surgery (61600-61616)*
Injection for:
   Cerebral angiography (36100-36218)
   Pneumoencephalography (61055)
   Ventriculography (61026, 61120)
   Primary closure (15730, 15733, 15756-15758)
   Surgical approach (61580-61598)

61618   **Secondary repair of dura for cerebrospinal fluid leak, anterior, middle or posterior cranial fossa following surgery of the skull base; by free tissue graft (eg, pericranium, fascia, tensor fascia lata, adipose tissue, homologous or synthetic grafts)**
🔧 37.5   ✂ 37.5   **FUD** 090   C 80 ▣
AMA: 2018,Jan,8; 2017,Jan,8; 2016,Jan,13

61619   **by local or regionalized vascularized pedicle flap or myocutaneous flap (including galea, temporalis, frontalis or occipitalis muscle)**
🔧 41.3   ✂ 41.3   **FUD** 090   C 80 ▣
AMA: 2018,Jan,8; 2017,Jan,8; 2016,Jan,13

61623-61651 Neurovascular Interventional Procedures

61623   **Endovascular temporary balloon arterial occlusion, head or neck (extracranial/intracranial) including selective catheterization of vessel to be occluded, positioning and inflation of occlusion balloon, concomitant neurological monitoring, and radiologic supervision and interpretation of all angiography required for balloon occlusion and to exclude vascular injury post occlusion**

EXCLUDES   *Diagnostic angiography target artery just before temporary occlusion; report only radiological supervision and interpretation*
Selective catheterization and angiography artery besides the target artery; report catheterization and radiological supervision and interpretation codes as appropriate
🔧 16.6   ✂ 16.6   **FUD** 000   J J8 ▣
AMA: 2018,Jan,8; 2017,Jan,8; 2016,Jan,13

Pericallosal artery

Posterior cerebral artery

Superior cerebellar artery

Right anterior cerebral artery

Basilar artery

Left vertebral artery

61624   **Transcatheter permanent occlusion or embolization (eg, for tumor destruction, to achieve hemostasis, to occlude a vascular malformation), percutaneous, any method; central nervous system (intracranial, spinal cord)**

EXCLUDES   *Non-central nervous system transcatheter occlusion or embolization other than head or neck (37241-37244)*
⊞ (75894)
🔧 33.7   ✂ 33.7   **FUD** 000   C ▣
AMA: 2019,Sep,6; 2018,Jan,8; 2017,Jan,8; 2016,Jan,13

61626   **non-central nervous system, head or neck (extracranial, brachiocephalic branch)**

EXCLUDES   *Non-central nervous system transcatheter occlusion or embolization other than head or neck (37241-37244)*
⊞ (75894)
🔧 25.5   ✂ 25.5   **FUD** 000   J J8 ▣
AMA: 2019,Sep,6; 2018,Jan,8; 2017,Jan,8; 2016,Jan,13

61630   **Balloon angioplasty, intracranial (eg, atherosclerotic stenosis), percutaneous**

INCLUDES   Diagnostic arteriogram when stent or angioplasty necessary
Radiology services for arteriography target vascular territory
Selective catheterization target vascular territory

EXCLUDES   *Diagnostic arteriogram when stent or angioplasty not necessary (report applicable code for selective catheterization and radiology services)*
Percutaneous arterial transluminal mechanical thrombectomy and/or infusion for thrombolysis performed same vascular territory (61645)
🔧 40.6   ✂ 40.6   **FUD** XXX   C 80 ▣
AMA: 2018,Jan,8; 2017,Jul,3; 2017,Apr,9; 2017,Jan,8; 2016,Mar,3; 2016,Jan,13

26/TC PC/TC Only   A2-Z3 ASC Payment   50 Bilateral   ♂ Male Only   ♀ Female Only   🔧 Facility RVU   ✂ Non-Facility RVU   ▣ CCI   ✖ CLIA
FUD Follow-up Days   **CMS:** IOM   **AMA:** CPT Asst   A-Y OPPSI   80/80 Surg Assist Allowed / w/Doc   ◼ Lab Crosswalk   ⊞ Radiology Crosswalk

276   CPT © 2021 American Medical Association. All Rights Reserved.   © 2021 Optum360, LLC

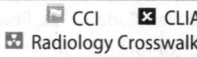

61635 Transcatheter placement of intravascular stent(s), intracranial (eg, atherosclerotic stenosis), including balloon angioplasty, if performed

INCLUDES
Diagnostic arteriogram when stent or angioplasty necessary
Radiology services for arteriography target vascular territory
Selective catheterization target vascular territory

EXCLUDES
Diagnostic arteriogram when stent or angioplasty not necessary (report applicable code for selective catheterization and radiology services)
Percutaneous arterial transluminal mechanical thrombectomy and/or infusion for thrombolysis performed same vascular territory (61645)

🚑 42.6   🔪 42.6   **FUD** XXX   [C] [80] 🖥

AMA: 2018,Jan,8; 2017,Jul,3; 2017,Jan,8; 2016,Mar,3; 2016,Jan,13

61640 Balloon dilatation of intracranial vasospasm, percutaneous; initial vessel

INCLUDES
Angiography after dilation vessel
Fluoroscopic guidance
Injection contrast material
Roadmapping
Selective catheterization target vessel
Vessel analysis

EXCLUDES
Endovascular intracranial prolonged administration pharmacologic agent performed same vascular territory (61650-61651)

🚑 14.0   🔪 14.0   **FUD** 000   [E] 🖥

AMA: 2018,Jan,8; 2017,Jan,8; 2016,Mar,3; 2016,Jan,13

+ 61641 each additional vessel in same vascular territory (List separately in addition to code for primary procedure)

INCLUDES
Angiography after dilation vessel
Fluoroscopic guidance
Injection contrast material
Roadmapping
Selective catheterization target vessel
Vessel analysis

EXCLUDES
Endovascular intracranial prolonged administration pharmacologic agent performed same vascular territory (61640)

Code first (61640)
🚑 4.92   🔪 4.92   **FUD** ZZZ   [E] 🖥

AMA: 2018,Jan,8; 2017,Jan,8; 2016,Mar,3; 2016,Jan,13

+ 61642 each additional vessel in different vascular territory (List separately in addition to code for primary procedure))

INCLUDES
Angiography after dilation vessel
Fluoroscopic guidance
Injection contrast material
Roadmapping
Selective catheterization target vessel
Vessel analysis

EXCLUDES
Endovascular intracranial prolonged administration pharmacologic agent performed same vascular territory (61650-61651)

Code first (61640)
🚑 9.84   🔪 9.84   **FUD** ZZZ   [E] 🖥

AMA: 2018,Jan,8; 2017,Jan,8; 2016,Mar,3; 2016,Jan,13

61645 Percutaneous arterial transluminal mechanical thrombectomy and/or infusion for thrombolysis, intracranial, any method, including diagnostic angiography, fluoroscopic guidance, catheter placement, and intraprocedural pharmacological thrombolytic injection(s)

INCLUDES
Interventions performed in intracranial artery including:
Angiography with radiologic supervision and interpretation (diagnostic and subsequent)
Closure arteriotomy by any method
Fluoroscopy
Patient monitoring
Procedures performed in vascular territories:
Left carotid
Right carotid
Vertebro-basilar

EXCLUDES
Procedure performed same vascular target area:
Balloon angioplasty, intracranial (61630)
Diagnostic studies: aortic arch, carotid, and vertebral arteries (36221-36226)
Endovascular intracranial prolonged administration pharmacologic agent (61650-61651)
Transcatheter placement intravascular stent (61635)
Transluminal thrombectomy (37184, 37186)
Reporting code more than one time for treatment each intracranial vascular territory
Venous thrombectomy or thrombolysis (37187-37188, 37212, 37214)

🚑 24.3   🔪 24.3   **FUD** 000   [C] [80] [50] 🖥

AMA: 2019,Sep,6; 2019,Sep,5; 2018,Jan,8; 2017,Jan,8; 2016,Mar,3; 2016,Jan,13

61650 Endovascular intracranial prolonged administration of pharmacologic agent(s) other than for thrombolysis, arterial, including catheter placement, diagnostic angiography, and imaging guidance; initial vascular territory

INCLUDES
Interventions performed in intracranial artery, including:
Angiography with radiologic supervision and interpretation (diagnostic and subsequent)
Closure arteriotomy by any method
Fluoroscopy
Patient monitoring
Procedures performed in vascular territories:
Left carotid
Right carotid
Vertebro-basilar
Prolonged (at least 10 minutes) arterial administration nonthrombolytic agents

EXCLUDES
Procedure performed same vascular target area:
Balloon dilatation intracranial vasospasm (61640-61642)
Chemotherapy administration (96420-96425)
Diagnostic studies: aortic arch, carotid, and vertebral arteries (36221-36228)
Transluminal thrombectomy (37184, 37186, 61645)
Reporting code more than one time for treatment each intracranial vascular territory
Treatment iatrogenic condition
Venous thrombectomy or thrombolysis

🚑 16.1   🔪 16.1   **FUD** 000   [C] 🖥

AMA: 2019,Sep,6; 2018,Jan,8; 2017,Jan,8; 2016,Mar,3; 2016,Jan,13

Nervous System

61651 — 61710

+ 61651 **each additional vascular territory (List separately in addition to code for primary procedure)**

INCLUDES Interventions performed in intracranial artery, including:
Angiography with radiologic supervision and interpretation (diagnostic and subsequent)
Closure arteriotomy by any method
Fluoroscopy
Patient monitoring
Procedures performed in vascular territories:
Left carotid
Right carotid
Vertebro-basilar
Prolonged (at least 10 minutes) arterial administration nonthrombolytic agents

EXCLUDES *Procedure performed same vascular target area:*
Balloon dilatation intracranial vasospasm (61640-61642)
Chemotherapy administration (96420-96425)
Diagnostic studies: aortic arch, carotid, and vertebral arteries (36221-36228)
Transluminal thrombectomy (37184, 37186, 61645)
Reporting code more than one time for treatment each intracranial vascular territory
Treatment iatrogenic condition
Venous thrombectomy or thrombolysis

Code first (61650)
🚑 7.01　　🔾 7.01　　**FUD** ZZZ　　　　　　C ▣
AMA: 2019,Sep,6; 2018,Jan,8; 2017,Jan,8; 2016,Mar,3; 2016,Jan,13

61680-61692 Surgical Treatment of Arteriovenous Malformation of the Brain

INCLUDES Craniotomy

61680 **Surgery of intracranial arteriovenous malformation; supratentorial, simple**
🚑 66.1　　🔾 66.1　　**FUD** 090　　　　　C 80 ▣
AMA: 2014,Jan,11

61682 **supratentorial, complex**
🚑 123.　　🔾 123.　　**FUD** 090　　　　　C 80 ▣
AMA: 2018,Jan,8; 2017,Jan,8; 2016,Jan,13

61684 **infratentorial, simple**
🚑 83.1　　🔾 83.1　　**FUD** 090　　　　　C 80 ▣
AMA: 2014,Jan,11

61686 **infratentorial, complex**
🚑 136.　　🔾 136.　　**FUD** 090　　　　　C 80 ▣
AMA: 2018,Jan,8; 2017,Jan,8; 2016,Jan,13

61690 **dural, simple**
🚑 63.6　　🔾 63.6　　**FUD** 090　　　　　C 80 ▣
AMA: 2014,Jan,11

61692 **dural, complex**
🚑 108.　　🔾 108.　　**FUD** 090　　　　　C 80 ▣
AMA: 2018,Jan,8; 2017,Jan,8; 2016,Jan,13

61697-61703 Surgical Treatment Brain Aneurysm

INCLUDES Craniotomy

61697 **Surgery of complex intracranial aneurysm, intracranial approach; carotid circulation**
INCLUDES Aneurysms bigger than 15 mm
Calcification aneurysm neck
Inclusion normal vessels in aneurysm neck
Surgery needing temporary vessel occlusion, trapping, or cardiopulmonary bypass to treat aneurysm
🚑 125.　　🔾 125.　　**FUD** 090　　　　　C 80 ▣
AMA: 2018,Jan,8; 2017,Dec,13

61698 **vertebrobasilar circulation**
INCLUDES Aneurysm bigger than 15 mm
Calcification aneurysm neck
Inclusion normal vessels in aneurysm neck
Surgery needing temporary vessel occlusion, trapping, or cardiopulmonary bypass to treat aneurysm
🚑 140.　　🔾 140.　　**FUD** 090　　　　　C 80 ▣
AMA: 2014,Jan,11

61700 **Surgery of simple intracranial aneurysm, intracranial approach; carotid circulation**
🚑 100.　　🔾 100.　　**FUD** 090　　　　　C 80 ▣
AMA: 2018,Jan,8; 2017,Dec,13; 2017,Jan,8; 2016,Jan,13

61702 **vertebrobasilar circulation**
🚑 118.　　🔾 118.　　**FUD** 090　　　　　C 80 ▣
AMA: 2014,Jan,11

Berry aneurysm

Berry aneurysms form at the site of a weakness in an arterial wall, often at a junction

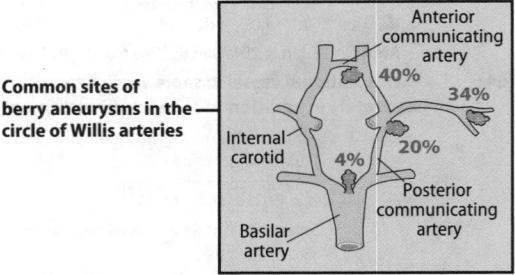

Common sites of berry aneurysms in the circle of Willis arteries

Anterior communicating artery 40%
34%
Internal carotid 4%　20%
Posterior communicating artery
Basilar artery

61703 **Surgery of intracranial aneurysm, cervical approach by application of occluding clamp to cervical carotid artery (Selverstone-Crutchfield type)**
EXCLUDES *Cervical approach for direct ligation carotid artery (37600-37606)*
🚑 39.9　　🔾 39.9　　**FUD** 090　　　　　C 80 ▣
AMA: 2014,Jan,11

61705-61710 Other Procedures for Aneurysm, Arteriovenous Malformation, and Carotid-Cavernous Fistula

INCLUDES Craniotomy

61705 **Surgery of aneurysm, vascular malformation or carotid-cavernous fistula; by intracranial and cervical occlusion of carotid artery**
🚑 73.6　　🔾 73.6　　**FUD** 090　　　　　C 80 ▣
AMA: 2014,Jan,11

61708 **by intracranial electrothrombosis**
EXCLUDES *Ligation or gradual occlusion internal or common carotid artery (37605-37606)*
🚑 75.1　　🔾 75.1　　**FUD** 090　　　　　C 80 ▣
AMA: 2014,Jan,11; 2000,Sep,11

61710 **by intra-arterial embolization, injection procedure, or balloon catheter**
🚑 62.0　　🔾 62.0　　**FUD** 090　　　　　C 80 ▣
AMA: 2018,Jan,8; 2017,Jan,8; 2016,Jan,13

61711 Extracranial-Intracranial Bypass

CMS: 100-02,16,10 Exclusions from Coverage; 100-03,20.2 Extracranial-intracranial (EC-IC) Arterial Bypass Surgery

INCLUDES Craniotomy

EXCLUDES Carotid or vertebral thromboendarterectomy (35301)

Code also operating microscope when appropriate (69990)

61711 **Anastomosis, arterial, extracranial-intracranial (eg, middle cerebral/cortical) arteries**
74.9 74.9 **FUD** 090   C 80
AMA: 2014,Jan,11

61720-61791 Stereotactic Procedures of the Brain

61720 **Creation of lesion by stereotactic method, including burr hole(s) and localizing and recording techniques, single or multiple stages; globus pallidus or thalamus**
37.3 37.3 **FUD** 090   J G2
AMA: 2018,Jan,8; 2017,Jan,8; 2016,Jan,13

61735 **subcortical structure(s) other than globus pallidus or thalamus**
46.8 46.8 **FUD** 090   C
AMA: 2014,Jul,8; 2014,Jan,11

● **61736** **Laser interstitial thermal therapy (LITT) of lesion, intracranial, including burr hole(s), with magnetic resonance imaging guidance, when performed; single trajectory for 1 simple lesion**
INCLUDES MRI (70551-70553, 70557-70559, 77021-77022)
EXCLUDES Application cranial tongs, caliper, or stereotactic frame (20660)
Laser interstitial thermal therapy (LITT), multiple trajectories (61737)
Stereotactic computer-assisted navigation, cranial/intradural (61781)

● **61737** **multiple trajectories for multiple or complex lesion(s)**
INCLUDES MRI (70551-70553, 70557-70559, 77021-77022)
EXCLUDES Application cranial tongs, caliper, stereotactic frame (20660)
Laser interstitial thermal therapy (LITT), single trajectory (61736)
Stereotactic computer-assisted navigation, cranial/intradural (61781)

61750 **Stereotactic biopsy, aspiration, or excision, including burr hole(s), for intracranial lesion;**
41.4 41.4 **FUD** 090   C
AMA: 2018,Jan,8; 2017,Jan,8; 2016,Jan,13

61751 **with computed tomography and/or magnetic resonance guidance**
(70450, 70460, 70470, 70551-70553)
39.7 39.7 **FUD** 090   C
AMA: 2018,Jan,8; 2017,Jan,8; 2016,Jan,13

61760 **Stereotactic implantation of depth electrodes into the cerebrum for long-term seizure monitoring**
46.0 46.0 **FUD** 090   C
AMA: 2014,Jul,8; 2014,Jan,11

61770 **Stereotactic localization, including burr hole(s), with insertion of catheter(s) or probe(s) for placement of radiation source**
47.7 47.7 **FUD** 090   J G2
AMA: 2018,Jan,8; 2017,Jan,8; 2016,Jan,13

+ **61781** **Stereotactic computer-assisted (navigational) procedure; cranial, intradural (List separately in addition to code for primary procedure)**
EXCLUDES Creation lesion by stereotactic method (61720-61791)
Extradural stereotactic computer-assisted procedure for same surgical session by same individual (61782)
Radiation treatment delivery, stereotactic radiosurgery (SRS) (77371-77373)
Stereotactic implantation neurostimulator electrode array (61863-61868)
Stereotactic radiation treatment management (77432)
Stereotactic radiosurgery (61796-61799)
Ventriculocisternostomy (62201)
Code first primary procedure
6.94 6.94 **FUD** ZZZ   N N1 80
AMA: 2018,Jan,8; 2017,Jan,8; 2016,Jan,13

Stereotactic guide in place

Computer assistance determines precise coordinates for a stereotactic intracranial procedure

CT or MRI scan

+ **61782** **cranial, extradural (List separately in addition to code for primary procedure)**
EXCLUDES Intradural stereotactic computer-assisted procedure for same surgical session by same individual (61781)
Stereotactic radiosurgery (61796-61799)
Code first primary procedure
5.02 5.02 **FUD** ZZZ   N N1 80
AMA: 2018,Apr,3; 2018,Jan,8; 2017,Jan,8; 2016,Jan,13

+ **61783** **spinal (List separately in addition to code for primary procedure)**
EXCLUDES Stereotactic radiosurgery (61796-61799, 63620-63621)
Code first primary procedure
6.80 6.80 **FUD** ZZZ   N N1 80
AMA: 2018,Jan,8; 2017,Jan,8; 2016,Jan,13

61790 **Creation of lesion by stereotactic method, percutaneous, by neurolytic agent (eg, alcohol, thermal, electrical, radiofrequency); gasserian ganglion**
25.7 25.7 **FUD** 090   J A2 50
AMA: 2014,Jul,8; 2014,Jan,11

61791 **trigeminal medullary tract**
33.0 33.0 **FUD** 090   J A2 80 50
AMA: 2018,Jan,8; 2017,Jan,8; 2016,Jan,13

Nervous System

61796 — 61880

61796-61800 Stereotactic Radiosurgery (SRS): Brain

INCLUDES   Planning, dosimetry, targeting, positioning, or blocking performed by neurosurgeon

EXCLUDES   *Application cranial tongs, caliper, or stereotactic frame (20660)*
Intensity modulated beam delivery plan and treatment (77301, 77385-77386)
Radiation treatment management and radiosurgery by same provider (77427-77435)
Stereotactic body radiation therapy (77373, 77435)
Stereotactic radiosurgery more than once per lesion per treatment course
Treatment planning, physics and dosimetry, and treatment delivery performed by radiation oncologist

61796   Stereotactic radiosurgery (particle beam, gamma ray, or linear accelerator); 1 simple cranial lesion

INCLUDES   Lesions < 3.5 cm

EXCLUDES   *Reporting code more than one time per treatment course*
Stereotactic computer-assisted procedures (61781-61783)
Stereotactic radiosurgery (61798)
Treatment complex lesions: (61798-61799)
     Arteriovenous malformations (AVM)
     Brainstem lesions
     Cavernous sinus/parasellar/petroclival tumors, glomus tumors, pituitary tumors, and tumors pineal region
     Lesions located <= 5 mm from optic nerve, chasm, or tract
     Schwannomas

Code also stereotactic headframe application, when performed (61800)

🔧 29.7   ⚕ 29.7   **FUD** 090   B 80 ▱

AMA: 2018,Jan,8; 2017,Jan,8; 2016,Jan,13

+ 61797   each additional cranial lesion, simple (List separately in addition to code for primary procedure)

INCLUDES   Lesions < 3.5 cm

EXCLUDES   *Reporting code for additional stereotactic radiosurgery more than four times in total per treatment course when used alone or in combination with (61799)*
Stereotactic computer-assisted procedures (61781-61783)
Treatment complex lesions: (61798-61799)
     Arteriovenous malformations (AVM)
     Brainstem lesion
     Cavernous sinus/parasellar/petroclival tumors, glomus tumors, pituitary tumors, and tumors pineal region
     Lesions located <= 5 mm from optic nerve, chasm, or tract
     Schwannomas

Code first (61796, 61798)

🔧 6.52   ⚕ 6.52   **FUD** ZZZ   B 80 ▱

AMA: 2018,Jan,8; 2017,Jan,8; 2016,Jan,13

61798   1 complex cranial lesion

INCLUDES   All therapeutic lesion creation procedures
Treatment complex lesions:
     Arteriovenous malformations (AVM)
     Brainstem lesions
     Cavernous sinus, parasellar, petroclival, glomus, pineal region, and pituitary tumors
     Lesions located <= 5 mm from optic nerve, chasm, or tract
     Lesions >= 3.5 cm
     Schwannomas
     Treatment multiple lesions when at least one considered complex

EXCLUDES   *Reporting code more than one time per treatment course*
Stereotactic computer-assisted procedures (61781-61783)
Stereotactic radiosurgery (61796)

Code also stereotactic headframe application, when performed (61800)

🔧 40.5   ⚕ 40.5   **FUD** 090   B 80 ▱

AMA: 2018,Jan,8; 2017,Jan,8; 2016,Jan,13

+ 61799   each additional cranial lesion, complex (List separately in addition to code for primary procedure)

INCLUDES   All therapeutic lesion creation procedures
Treatment complex lesions:
     Arteriovenous malformations (AVM)
     Brainstem lesions
     Cavernous sinus, parasellar, petroclival, glomus, pineal region, and pituitary tumors
     Lesions located <= 5 mm from optic nerve, chasm, or tract
     Lesions >= 3.5 cm
     Schwannomas

EXCLUDES   *Reporting code for additional stereotactic radiosurgery more than four times in total per treatment course when used alone or in combination with (61797)*
Stereotactic computer-assisted procedures (61781-61783)

Code first (61798)

🔧 8.98   ⚕ 8.98   **FUD** ZZZ   B 80 ▱

AMA: 2018,Jan,8; 2017,Jan,8; 2016,Jan,13

+ 61800   Application of stereotactic headframe for stereotactic radiosurgery (List separately in addition to code for primary procedure)

Code first (61796, 61798)

🔧 4.40   ⚕ 4.40   **FUD** ZZZ   B 80 ▱

AMA: 2018,Jan,8; 2017,Jan,8; 2016,Jan,13

61850-61888 Intracranial Neurostimulation

INCLUDES   Analysis system at implantation (95970)
Microelectrode recording by operating surgeon

EXCLUDES   *Electronic analysis and reprogramming neurostimulator pulse generator (95970, 95976-95977, [95983, 95984])*
Neurophysiological mapping by another physician/qualified health care professional (95961-95962)

61850   Twist drill or burr hole(s) for implantation of neurostimulator electrodes, cortical

🔧 28.8   ⚕ 28.8   **FUD** 090   C 80 ▱

AMA: 2019,Feb,6; 2018,Jan,8; 2017,Jan,8; 2016,Jan,13

61860   Craniectomy or craniotomy for implantation of neurostimulator electrodes, cerebral, cortical

🔧 45.7   ⚕ 45.7   **FUD** 090   C 80 ▱

AMA: 2019,Feb,6; 2018,Jan,8; 2017,Jan,8; 2016,Jan,13

61863   Twist drill, burr hole, craniotomy, or craniectomy with stereotactic implantation of neurostimulator electrode array in subcortical site (eg, thalamus, globus pallidus, subthalamic nucleus, periventricular, periaqueductal gray), without use of intraoperative microelectrode recording; first array

🔧 43.9   ⚕ 43.9   **FUD** 090   C 80 50 ▱

AMA: 2019,Feb,6; 2018,Jan,8; 2017,Jan,8; 2016,Jan,13

+ 61864   each additional array (List separately in addition to primary procedure)

Code first (61863)

🔧 8.36   ⚕ 8.36   **FUD** ZZZ   C 80 ▱

AMA: 2019,Feb,6

61867   Twist drill, burr hole, craniotomy, or craniectomy with stereotactic implantation of neurostimulator electrode array in subcortical site (eg, thalamus, globus pallidus, subthalamic nucleus, periventricular, periaqueductal gray), with use of intraoperative microelectrode recording; first array

🔧 66.8   ⚕ 66.8   **FUD** 090   C 80 50 ▱

AMA: 2019,Feb,6

+ 61868   each additional array (List separately in addition to primary procedure)

Code first (61867)

🔧 14.7   ⚕ 14.7   **FUD** ZZZ   C 80 ▱

AMA: 2019,Feb,6; 2018,Jan,8; 2017,Jan,8; 2016,Jan,13

61880   Revision or removal of intracranial neurostimulator electrodes

🔧 16.6   ⚕ 16.6   **FUD** 090   02 62 80 50 ▱

AMA: 2019,Feb,6

26/TC PC/TC Only   A2-Z3 ASC Payment   50 Bilateral   ♂ Male Only   ♀ Female Only   🔧 Facility RVU   ⚕ Non-Facility RVU   ▱ CCI   ✖ CLIA
FUD Follow-up Days   **CMS:** IOM   **AMA:** CPT Asst   A-Y OPPSI   80/80 Surg Assist Allowed / w/Doc   Lab Crosswalk   Radiology Crosswalk

280   CPT © 2021 American Medical Association. All Rights Reserved.   © 2021 Optum360, LLC

61885 Insertion or replacement of cranial neurostimulator pulse generator or receiver, direct or inductive coupling; with connection to a single electrode array

EXCLUDES Percutaneous procedure to place cranial nerve neurostimulator electrode(s) (64553)
Revision or replacement cranial nerve neurostimulator electrode array (64569)

🚗 14.9   ⚖ 14.9   **FUD** 090   J J8 80 50 📖

AMA: 2019,Feb,6; 2018,Jan,8; 2017,Jan,8; 2016,Jan,13

61886 with connection to 2 or more electrode arrays

EXCLUDES Percutaneous procedure to place cranial nerve neurostimulator electrode(s) (64553)
Revision or replacement cranial nerve neurostimulator electrode array (64569)

🚗 24.5   ⚖ 24.5   **FUD** 090   J J8 80 📖

AMA: 2019,Feb,6; 2018,Jan,8; 2017,Jan,8; 2016,Jan,13

61888 Revision or removal of cranial neurostimulator pulse generator or receiver

EXCLUDES Insertion or replacement cranial neurostimulator pulse generator or receiver (61885-61886)

🚗 11.3   ⚖ 11.3   **FUD** 010   J J8 50 📖

AMA: 2019,Feb,6; 2018,Jan,8; 2017,Jan,8; 2016,Jan,13

62000-62148 Repair of Skull and/or Cerebrospinal Fluid Leaks

62000 Elevation of depressed skull fracture; simple, extradural

🚗 30.2   ⚖ 30.2   **FUD** 090   J 62 📖

AMA: 2014,Jan,11

62005 compound or comminuted, extradural

🚗 37.2   ⚖ 37.2   **FUD** 090   C 80 📖

AMA: 2014,Jan,11

62010 with repair of dura and/or debridement of brain

🚗 44.7   ⚖ 44.7   **FUD** 090   C 80 📖

AMA: 2014,Jan,11

62100 Craniotomy for repair of dural/cerebrospinal fluid leak, including surgery for rhinorrhea/otorrhea

EXCLUDES Repair spinal fluid leak (63707, 63709)

🚗 45.6   ⚖ 45.6   **FUD** 090   C 80 📖

AMA: 2014,Jan,11; 2002,May,7

62115 Reduction of craniomegalic skull (eg, treated hydrocephalus); not requiring bone grafts or cranioplasty

🚗 49.2   ⚖ 49.2   **FUD** 090   C 80 📖

AMA: 2014,Jan,11

62117 requiring craniotomy and reconstruction with or without bone graft (includes obtaining grafts)

🚗 57.8   ⚖ 57.8   **FUD** 090   C 80 📖

AMA: 2014,Jan,11

62120 Repair of encephalocele, skull vault, including cranioplasty

🚗 61.9   ⚖ 61.9   **FUD** 090   C 80 📖

AMA: 2014,Jan,11

62121 Craniotomy for repair of encephalocele, skull base

🚗 45.7   ⚖ 45.7   **FUD** 090   C 80 📖

AMA: 2014,Jan,11

62140 Cranioplasty for skull defect; up to 5 cm diameter

🚗 29.9   ⚖ 29.9   **FUD** 090   C 80 📖

AMA: 2018,Jan,8; 2017,Jan,8; 2016,Jan,13

62141 larger than 5 cm diameter

🚗 33.1   ⚖ 33.1   **FUD** 090   C 80 📖

AMA: 2018,Jan,8; 2017,Jan,8; 2016,Jan,13

62142 Removal of bone flap or prosthetic plate of skull

🚗 25.8   ⚖ 25.8   **FUD** 090   C 80 📖

AMA: 2018,Jan,8; 2017,Jan,8; 2016,Jan,13

62143 Replacement of bone flap or prosthetic plate of skull

🚗 30.3   ⚖ 30.3   **FUD** 090   C 80 📖

AMA: 2018,Jan,8; 2017,Jan,8; 2016,Jan,13

62145 Cranioplasty for skull defect with reparative brain surgery

🚗 41.0   ⚖ 41.0   **FUD** 090   C 80 📖

AMA: 2018,Jan,8; 2017,Jan,8; 2016,Jan,13

62146 Cranioplasty with autograft (includes obtaining bone grafts); up to 5 cm diameter

🚗 34.2   ⚖ 34.2   **FUD** 090   C 80 📖

AMA: 2018,Jan,8; 2017,Jan,8; 2016,Jan,13

62147 larger than 5 cm diameter

🚗 41.0   ⚖ 41.0   **FUD** 090   C 80 📖

AMA: 2018,Jan,8; 2017,Jan,8; 2016,Jan,13

+ 62148 Incision and retrieval of subcutaneous cranial bone graft for cranioplasty (List separately in addition to code for primary procedure)

Code first (62140-62147)

🚗 3.73   ⚖ 3.73   **FUD** ZZZ   C 📖

AMA: 2014,Jan,11

62160-62165 Neuroendoscopic Brain Procedures

INCLUDES Diagnostic endoscopy

+ 62160 Neuroendoscopy, intracranial, for placement or replacement of ventricular catheter and attachment to shunt system or external drainage (List separately in addition to code for primary procedure)

Code first (61107, 61210, 62220-62230, 62258)

🚗 5.61   ⚖ 5.61   **FUD** ZZZ   N M 📖

AMA: 2018,Jan,8; 2017,Jan,8; 2016,Jan,13

62161 Neuroendoscopy, intracranial; with dissection of adhesions, fenestration of septum pellucidum or intraventricular cysts (including placement, replacement, or removal of ventricular catheter)

🚗 44.1   ⚖ 44.1   **FUD** 090   C 80 📖

AMA: 2014,Jan,11

62162 with fenestration or excision of colloid cyst, including placement of external ventricular catheter for drainage

🚗 55.3   ⚖ 55.3   **FUD** 090   C 80 📖

AMA: 2014,Jan,11

62164 with excision of brain tumor, including placement of external ventricular catheter for drainage

🚗 60.3   ⚖ 60.3   **FUD** 090   C 80 📖

AMA: 2014,Jan,11

62165 with excision of pituitary tumor, transnasal or trans-sphenoidal approach

🚗 44.6   ⚖ 44.6   **FUD** 090   C 80 📖

AMA: 2019,Dec,12; 2018,Jan,8; 2017,Dec,14

62180-62258 Cerebrospinal Fluid Diversion Procedures

62180 Ventriculocisternostomy (Torkildsen type operation)

🚗 47.0   ⚖ 47.0   **FUD** 090   C 80 📖

AMA: 2014,Jan,11

62190 **Creation of shunt; subarachnoid/subdural-atrial, -jugular, -auricular**
　　26.6　　26.6　　**FUD** 090　　　　　　　C ▢
　　AMA: 2014,Jan,11; 2000,Dec,12

Origin of shunt is
subarachnoid/subdural

Shunt to jugular,
atria, or auricle

Shunt to pleura,
peritoneum,
or other site

62192 **subarachnoid/subdural-peritoneal, -pleural, other terminus**
　　28.3　　28.3　　**FUD** 090　　　　　　C 80 ▢
　　AMA: 2014,Jan,11

62194 **Replacement or irrigation, subarachnoid/subdural catheter**
　　14.2　　14.2　　**FUD** 010　　　　J A2 80 ▢
　　AMA: 2018,Jan,8; 2017,Jan,8; 2016,Jan,13

62200 **Ventriculocisternostomy, third ventricle;**
　　INCLUDES　　Dandy ventriculocisternostomy
　　39.7　　39.7　　**FUD** 090　　　　　C 80 ▢
　　AMA: 2014,Jan,11

62201 **stereotactic, neuroendoscopic method**
　　EXCLUDES　　Intracranial neuroendoscopic surgery (62161-62165)
　　34.8　　34.8　　**FUD** 090　　　　　C ▢
　　AMA: 2018,Jan,8; 2017,Jan,8; 2016,Jan,13

62220 **Creation of shunt; ventriculo-atrial, -jugular, -auricular**
　　Code also intracranial neuroendoscopic ventricular catheter
　　　insertion, when performed (62160)
　　28.4　　28.4　　**FUD** 090　　　　　C 80 ▢
　　AMA: 2014,Jan,11; 2007,Jun,10-11

62223 **ventriculo-peritoneal, -pleural, other terminus**
　　Code also intracranial neuroendoscopic ventricular catheter
　　　insertion, when performed (62160)
　　30.0　　30.0　　**FUD** 090　　　　　C 80 ▢
　　AMA: 2014,Jan,11; 2007,Jun,10-11

62225 **Replacement or irrigation, ventricular catheter**
　　Code also intracranial neuroendoscopic ventricular catheter
　　　insertion, when performed (62160)
　　15.1　　15.1　　**FUD** 090　　　　　J A2 ▢
　　AMA: 2018,Jan,8; 2017,Jan,8; 2016,Jan,13

62230 **Replacement or revision of cerebrospinal fluid shunt, obstructed valve, or distal catheter in shunt system**
　　Code also:
　　　Intracranial neuroendoscopic ventricular catheter insertion,
　　　　when performed (62160)
　　　Proximal catheter and valve replacement, when performed
　　　　(62225)
　　24.2　　24.2　　**FUD** 090　　　　J A2 80 ▢
　　AMA: 2018,Jan,8; 2017,Jan,8; 2016,Jan,13

62252 **Reprogramming of programmable cerebrospinal shunt**
　　2.31　　2.31　　**FUD** XXX　　　　S P3 80 ▢
　　AMA: 2014,Jan,11; 2002,May,7

62256 **Removal of complete cerebrospinal fluid shunt system; without replacement**
　　EXCLUDES　　Reprogramming cerebrospinal fluid (CSF) shunt (62252)
　　17.5　　17.5　　**FUD** 090　　　　　C 80 ▢
　　AMA: 2014,Jan,11; 2002,May,7

62258 **with replacement by similar or other shunt at same operation**
　　EXCLUDES　　Aspiration or irrigation shunt reservoir (61070)
　　　　　　　　Reprogramming cerebrospinal fluid (CSF) shunt (62252)
　　Code also intracranial neuroendoscopic ventricular catheter
　　　insertion, when performed (62160)
　　32.0　　32.0　　**FUD** 090　　　　　C 80 ▢
　　AMA: 2018,Jan,8; 2017,Jan,8; 2016,Jan,13

62263-62264 Lysis of Epidural Lesions with Injection of Solution/Mechanical Methods

　　INCLUDES　　Fluoroscopic guidance (77003)
　　　　　　　　Percutaneous mechanical lysis

62263 **Percutaneous lysis of epidural adhesions using solution injection (eg, hypertonic saline, enzyme) or mechanical means (eg, catheter) including radiologic localization (includes contrast when administered), multiple adhesiolysis sessions; 2 or more days**
　　INCLUDES　　All adhesiolysis treatments, injections, and infusions
　　　　　　　　during treatment course
　　　　　　　　Percutaneous epidural catheter insertion and removal
　　　　　　　　for neurolytic agent injections during treatment
　　　　　　　　sessions series
　　EXCLUDES　　Procedure performed more than one time for complete
　　　　　　　　series spanning two or more treatment days
　　8.92　　17.1　　**FUD** 010　　　　　T A2 ▢
　　AMA: 2018,Jan,8; 2017,Jan,8; 2016,Jan,13

62264 **1 day**
　　INCLUDES　　Multiple treatment sessions performed same day
　　EXCLUDES　　Percutaneous lysis epidural adhesions using solution
　　　　　　　　injection, two or more treatment days (62263)
　　6.89　　12.2　　**FUD** 010　　　　　T A2 ▢
　　AMA: 2018,Jan,8; 2017,Jan,8; 2016,Jan,13

62267-62269 Percutaneous Procedures of Spinal Cord

62267 **Percutaneous aspiration within the nucleus pulposus, intervertebral disc, or paravertebral tissue for diagnostic purposes**
　　EXCLUDES　　Bone biopsy (20225)
　　　　　　　　Decompression intervertebral disc (62287)
　　　　　　　　Fine needle aspiration ([10005, 10006, 10007, 10008,
　　　　　　　　　10009, 10010, 10011, 10012]
　　　　　　　　Injection for discography (62290-62291)
　　Code also fluoroscopic guidance (77003)
　　4.55　　7.34　　**FUD** 000　　　　T 62 80 ▢
　　AMA: 2019,Apr,4; 2018,Jan,8; 2017,Feb,12; 2017,Jan,8;
　　2016,Jan,13

62268 **Percutaneous aspiration, spinal cord cyst or syrinx**
　　⊞ (76942, 77002, 77012)
　　7.44　　7.44　　**FUD** 000　　　　　T A2 ▢
　　AMA: 2018,Jan,8; 2017,Dec,13

62269 **Biopsy of spinal cord, percutaneous needle**
　　EXCLUDES　　Fine needle aspiration [(10005, 1006, 1007, 1008, 1009,
　　　　　　　　　10010, 10011, 10012)]
　　⊞ (76942, 77002, 77012)
　　◣ (88172-88173)
　　7.66　　7.66　　**FUD** 000　　　　J A2 80 ▢
　　AMA: 2019,Apr,4

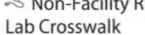

62270-62329 [62328, 62329] Spinal Puncture, Subarachnoid Space, Diagnostic/Therapeutic

62270   Spinal puncture, lumbar, diagnostic;

> **EXCLUDES** *Radiological guidance (77003, 77012)*
> Code also ultrasound or MRI guidance (76942, 77021)
> 🚑 1.79   ⚕ 3.97   **FUD** 000   T A2 📷
> **AMA:** 2020,Jun,10; 2018,Jan,8; 2017,Jan,8; 2016,Jan,13

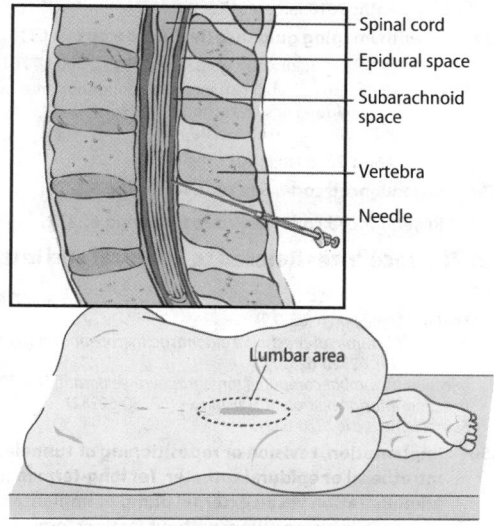

Spinal cord
Epidural space
Subarachnoid space
Vertebra
Needle

Lumbar area

Common position to access vertebral interspace

62328   with fluoroscopic or CT guidance

> **INCLUDES** Radiological guidance (77003, 77012)
> Code also ultrasound or MRI guidance (76942, 77021)
> 🚑 2.59   ⚕ 7.40   **FUD** 000   G2 📷
> **AMA:** 2020,Jun,10

62272   Spinal puncture, therapeutic, for drainage of cerebrospinal fluid (by needle or catheter);

> **EXCLUDES** *Radiological guidance (77003, 77012)*
> Code also ultrasound or MRI guidance (76942, 77021)
> 🚑 2.54   ⚕ 5.22   **FUD** 000   T A2 📷
> **AMA:** 2020,Jun,10; 2018,Jan,8; 2017,Jan,8; 2016,Jan,13

62329   with fluoroscopic or CT guidance

> **INCLUDES** Radiological guidance (77003, 77012)
> Code also ultrasound or MRI guidance (76942, 77021)
> 🚑 3.26   ⚕ 9.19   **FUD** 000   G2 📷
> **AMA:** 2020,Jul,15; 2020,Jun,10

62273 Epidural Blood Patch

CMS: 100-03,10.5 NCD for Autogenous Epidural Blood Graft (10.5)
> **EXCLUDES** *Injection diagnostic or therapeutic material (62320-62327)*
> Code also fluoroscopic guidance (77003)

62273   Injection, epidural, of blood or clot patch

> 🚑 3.26   ⚕ 4.93   **FUD** 000   T A2 📷
> **AMA:** 2018,Jan,8; 2017,Jan,8; 2016,Jan,13

62280-62282 Neurolysis

> **INCLUDES** Contrast injection during fluoroscopic guidance/localization
> **EXCLUDES** *Injection diagnostic or therapeutic material only (62320-62327)*
> Code also fluoroscopic guidance and localization unless formal contrast study performed (77003)

62280   Injection/infusion of neurolytic substance (eg, alcohol, phenol, iced saline solutions), with or without other therapeutic substance; subarachnoid

> 🚑 4.76   ⚕ 9.45   **FUD** 010   T A2 📷
> **AMA:** 2018,Jan,8; 2017,Jan,8; 2016,Jan,13

62281   epidural, cervical or thoracic

> 🚑 4.58   ⚕ 6.83   **FUD** 010   T A2 📷
> **AMA:** 2018,Jan,8; 2017,Jan,8; 2016,Jan,13

62282   epidural, lumbar, sacral (caudal)

> 🚑 4.13   ⚕ 8.76   **FUD** 010   T A2 📷
> **AMA:** 2018,Jan,8; 2017,Jan,8; 2016,Jan,13

62284-62294 Injection/Aspiration of Spine, Diagnostic/Therapeutic

62284   Injection procedure for myelography and/or computed tomography, lumbar

> **EXCLUDES** *Injection C1-C2 (61055)*
> *Myelography (62302-62305, 72240, 72255, 72265, 72270)*
> Code also fluoroscopic guidance (77003)
> 🚑 2.50   ⚕ 5.66   **FUD** 000   N N1 📷
> **AMA:** 2018,Jan,8; 2017,Jan,8; 2016,Jan,13

62287   Decompression procedure, percutaneous, of nucleus pulposus of intervertebral disc, any method utilizing needle based technique to remove disc material under fluoroscopic imaging or other form of indirect visualization, with discography and/or epidural injection(s) at the treated level(s), when performed, single or multiple levels, lumbar

> **INCLUDES** Endoscopic approach
> **EXCLUDES** *Injection for discography (62290)*
> *Injection diagnostic or therapeutic substance(s) (62322)*
> *Lumbar discography (72295)*
> *Percutaneous aspiration, diagnostic (62267)*
> *Percutaneous decompression nucleus pulposus intervertebral disc, non-needle based technique (0274T-0275T)*
> *Radiological guidance (77003, 77012)*
> 🚑 16.7   ⚕ 16.7   **FUD** 090   J A2 📷
> **AMA:** 2019,Dec,12; 2018,Jan,8; 2017,Feb,12; 2017,Jan,8; 2016,Jan,13

Posterior
Posterolateral
Lateral
Nucleus pulposus

62290   Injection procedure for discography, each level; lumbar

> 🔁 (72295)
> 🚑 4.81   ⚕ 9.62   **FUD** 000   N N1 📷
> **AMA:** 2018,Jan,8; 2017,Feb,12; 2017,Jan,8; 2016,Jan,13

62291   cervical or thoracic

> 🔁 (72285)
> 🚑 4.57   ⚕ 9.55   **FUD** 000   N N1 📷
> **AMA:** 2018,Jan,8; 2017,Jan,8; 2016,Jan,13

62292   Injection procedure for chemonucleolysis, including discography, intervertebral disc, single or multiple levels, lumbar

> 🚑 16.6   ⚕ 16.6   **FUD** 090   J R2 80 📷
> **AMA:** 2018,Jan,8; 2017,Jan,8; 2016,Jan,13

62294   Injection procedure, arterial, for occlusion of arteriovenous malformation, spinal

> 🚑 27.3   ⚕ 27.3   **FUD** 090   T A2 📷
> **AMA:** 2014,Jan,11; 2000,Jan,1

62302-62305 Myelography

EXCLUDES
Injection C1-C2 (61055)
Lumbar myelogram furnished by other providers (62284, 72240, 72255, 72265, 72270)

62302   Myelography via lumbar injection, including radiological supervision and interpretation; cervical

> EXCLUDES   *Myelography (62303-62305)*
> 🖫 3.53   ⚘ 6.91   **FUD** 000   02 N1 ▢

62303   thoracic

> EXCLUDES   *Myelography (62302, 62304-62305)*
> 🖫 3.53   ⚘ 7.07   **FUD** 000   02 N1 ▢

62304   lumbosacral

> EXCLUDES   *Myelography (62302-62303, 62305)*
> 🖫 3.46   ⚘ 6.82   **FUD** 000   02 N1 ▢

62305   2 or more regions (eg, lumbar/thoracic, cervical/thoracic, lumbar/cervical, lumbar/thoracic/cervical)

> EXCLUDES   *Myelography (62302-62305)*
> 🖫 3.60   ⚘ 7.65   **FUD** 000   02 N1 ▢

62320-62329 [62328, 62329] Injection/Infusion Diagnostic/Therapeutic Material

EXCLUDES
Reporting code more than one time even when catheter tip or injected drug travels into different spinal area
Transforaminal epidural injection (64479-64484)

62320   Injection(s), of diagnostic or therapeutic substance(s) (eg, anesthetic, antispasmodic, opioid, steroid, other solution), not including neurolytic substances, including needle or catheter placement, interlaminar epidural or subarachnoid, cervical or thoracic; without imaging guidance

> 🖫 2.85   ⚘ 4.68   **FUD** 000   T G2 ▢
> **AMA:** 2020,Oct,3; 2018,Jan,8; 2017,Sep,6

62321   with imaging guidance (ie, fluoroscopy or CT)

> INCLUDES   *Radiologic guidance (76942, 77003, 77012)*
> 🖫 3.07   ⚘ 7.19   **FUD** 000   T G2 ▢
> **AMA:** 2020,Oct,3; 2018,Jan,8; 2017,Sep,6

62322   Injection(s), of diagnostic or therapeutic substance(s) (eg, anesthetic, antispasmodic, opioid, steroid, other solution), not including neurolytic substances, including needle or catheter placement, interlaminar epidural or subarachnoid, lumbar or sacral (caudal); without imaging guidance

> 🖫 2.46   ⚘ 4.36   **FUD** 000   T G2 ▢
> **AMA:** 2020,Oct,3; 2018,Jan,8; 2017,Sep,6; 2017,Feb,12

62323   with imaging guidance (ie, fluoroscopy or CT)

> INCLUDES   *Radiologic guidance (76942, 77003, 77012)*
> 🖫 2.84   ⚘ 7.11   **FUD** 000   T G2 ▢
> **AMA:** 2020,Oct,3; 2018,Jan,8; 2017,Sep,6

62324   Injection(s), including indwelling catheter placement, continuous infusion or intermittent bolus, of diagnostic or therapeutic substance(s) (eg, anesthetic, antispasmodic, opioid, steroid, other solution), not including neurolytic substances, interlaminar epidural or subarachnoid, cervical or thoracic; without imaging guidance

> Code also hospital management continuous infusion drug, epidural or subarachnoid (01996)
> 🖫 2.60   ⚘ 4.12   **FUD** 000   T G2 ▢
> **AMA:** 2018,Jan,8; 2017,Sep,6

62325   with imaging guidance (ie, fluoroscopy or CT)

> INCLUDES   *Radiologic guidance (76942, 77003, 77012)*
> Code also hospital management continuous infusion drug, epidural or subarachnoid (01996)
> 🖫 3.08   ⚘ 6.67   **FUD** 000   T G2 ▢
> **AMA:** 2018,Jan,8; 2017,Sep,6

62326   Injection(s), including indwelling catheter placement, continuous infusion or intermittent bolus, of diagnostic or therapeutic substance(s) (eg, anesthetic, antispasmodic, opioid, steroid, other solution), not including neurolytic substances, interlaminar epidural or subarachnoid, lumbar or sacral (caudal); without imaging guidance

> Code also hospital management continuous infusion drug, epidural or subarachnoid (01996)
> 🖫 2.56   ⚘ 4.28   **FUD** 000   T 02 ▢
> **AMA:** 2018,Jan,8; 2017,Sep,6

62327   with imaging guidance (ie, fluoroscopy or CT)

> INCLUDES   *Radiologic guidance (76942, 77003, 77012)*
> Code also hospital management continuous infusion drug, epidural or subarachnoid (01996)
> 🖫 2.78   ⚘ 6.69   **FUD** 000   T 02 ▢
> **AMA:** 2018,Jan,8; 2017,Sep,6

62328   Resequenced code. See code following 62270.

62329   Resequenced code. See code following 62272.

62350-62370 Procedures Related to Epidural and Intrathecal Catheters

EXCLUDES
Epidural blood patch (62273)
Injection epidural/subarachnoid diagnostic/therapeutic drugs ([62328], [62329], 62320-62327)
Injection for lumbar computed tomography/myelography (62284)
Injection/infusion neurolytic substances (62280-62282)
Spinal puncture (62270-62272)

62350   Implantation, revision or repositioning of tunneled intrathecal or epidural catheter, for long-term medication administration via an external pump or implantable reservoir/infusion pump; without laminectomy

> EXCLUDES   *Maintenance and refilling infusion pumps for CNS drug therapy (95990-95991)*
> 🖫 11.5   ⚘ 11.5   **FUD** 010   J J8 ▢
> **AMA:** 2018,Jan,8; 2017,Jan,8; 2016,Jan,13

62351   with laminectomy

> EXCLUDES   *Maintenance and refilling infusion pumps for CNS drug therapy (95990-95991)*
> 🖫 25.1   ⚘ 25.1   **FUD** 090   J G2 80 ▢
> **AMA:** 2018,Jan,8; 2017,Jan,8; 2016,Jan,13

62355   Removal of previously implanted intrathecal or epidural catheter

> 🖫 7.79   ⚘ 7.79   **FUD** 010   02 A2 80 ▢
> **AMA:** 2014,Jan,11; 1995,Win,1

62360   Implantation or replacement of device for intrathecal or epidural drug infusion; subcutaneous reservoir

> 🖫 9.13   ⚘ 9.13   **FUD** 010   J J8 80 ▢
> **AMA:** 2014,Jan,11; 1995,Win,1

62361   nonprogrammable pump

> 🖫 12.5   ⚘ 12.5   **FUD** 010   J J8 80 ▢
> **AMA:** 2014,Jan,11; 1995,Win,1

62362   programmable pump, including preparation of pump, with or without programming

> 🖫 11.0   ⚘ 11.0   **FUD** 010   J J8 80 ▢
> **AMA:** 2018,Jan,8; 2017,Jan,8; 2016,Jan,13

62365   Removal of subcutaneous reservoir or pump, previously implanted for intrathecal or epidural infusion

> 🖫 8.48   ⚘ 8.48   **FUD** 010   02 A2 80 ▢
> **AMA:** 2014,Jan,11; 1995,Win,1

62367   Electronic analysis of programmable, implanted pump for intrathecal or epidural drug infusion (includes evaluation of reservoir status, alarm status, drug prescription status); without reprogramming or refill

> EXCLUDES   *Maintenance and refilling infusion pumps for CNS drug therapy (95990-95991)*
> 🖫 0.72   ⚘ 1.14   **FUD** XXX   S P3 ▢
> **AMA:** 2018,Jan,8; 2017,Jan,8; 2016,Jan,13

62368 **with reprogramming**

EXCLUDES *Maintenance and refilling infusion pumps for CNS drug therapy (95990-95991)*

📷 1.01 ⚕ 1.57 **FUD** XXX [S] [P3] ▭

AMA: 2018,Jan,8; 2017,Jan,8; 2016,Jan,13

62369 **with reprogramming and refill**

EXCLUDES *Maintenance and refilling infusion pumps for CNS drug therapy (95990-95991)*

📷 1.01 ⚕ 3.34 **FUD** XXX [S] [P3] ▭

AMA: 2018,Jan,8; 2017,Jan,8; 2016,Jan,13

62370 **with reprogramming and refill (requiring skill of a physician or other qualified health care professional)**

EXCLUDES *Maintenance and refilling infusion pumps for CNS drug therapy (95990-95991)*

📷 1.33 ⚕ 3.47 **FUD** XXX [S] [P3] ▭

AMA: 2018,Jan,8; 2017,Jan,8; 2016,Jan,13

62380 Endoscopic Decompression/Laminectomy/Laminotomy

EXCLUDES *Open decompression (63030, 63056)*
Percutaneous decompression (62267, 0274T-0275T)

62380 **Endoscopic decompression of spinal cord, nerve root(s), including laminotomy, partial facetectomy, foraminotomy, discectomy and/or excision of herniated intervertebral disc, 1 interspace, lumbar**

📷 0.00 ⚕ 0.00 **FUD** 090 [J] [62] [80] [50] ▭

AMA: 2018,Jan,8; 2017,Feb,12

63001-63053 [63052, 63053] Posterior Midline Approach: Laminectomy/Laminotomy/Decompression

INCLUDES Endoscopic assistance through open and direct visualization
EXCLUDES *Arthrodesis (22590-22614)*
Percutaneous decompression (62287, 0274T, 0275T)

63001 **Laminectomy with exploration and/or decompression of spinal cord and/or cauda equina, without facetectomy, foraminotomy or discectomy (eg, spinal stenosis), 1 or 2 vertebral segments; cervical**

📷 35.7 ⚕ 35.7 **FUD** 090 [J] [62] [80] ▭

AMA: 2018,Jan,8; 2017,Mar,7; 2017,Jan,8; 2016,Jan,13

63003 **thoracic**

📷 35.7 ⚕ 35.7 **FUD** 090 [J] [62] [80] ▭

AMA: 2018,Jan,8; 2017,Mar,7; 2017,Jan,8; 2016,Jan,13

63005 **lumbar, except for spondylolisthesis**

📷 34.4 ⚕ 34.4 **FUD** 090 [J] [62] [80] ▭

AMA: 2018,Jan,8; 2017,Mar,7; 2017,Feb,9; 2017,Jan,8; 2016,Jan,13

63011 **sacral**

📷 31.6 ⚕ 31.6 **FUD** 090 [J] [62] [80] ▭

AMA: 2018,Jan,8; 2017,Mar,7; 2017,Jan,8; 2016,Jan,13

63012 **Laminectomy with removal of abnormal facets and/or pars inter-articularis with decompression of cauda equina and nerve roots for spondylolisthesis, lumbar (Gill type procedure)**

📷 34.6 ⚕ 34.6 **FUD** 090 [J] [62] [80] ▭

AMA: 2019,Dec,12; 2018,Jan,8; 2017,Mar,7; 2017,Feb,9; 2017,Jan,8; 2016,Jan,13

63015 **Laminectomy with exploration and/or decompression of spinal cord and/or cauda equina, without facetectomy, foraminotomy or discectomy (eg, spinal stenosis), more than 2 vertebral segments; cervical**

📷 42.7 ⚕ 42.7 **FUD** 090 [J] [62] [80] ▭

AMA: 2018,Jan,8; 2017,Mar,7; 2017,Jan,8; 2016,Jan,13

63016 **thoracic**

📷 44.3 ⚕ 44.3 **FUD** 090 [J] [62] [80] ▭

AMA: 2018,Jan,8; 2017,Mar,7; 2017,Jan,8; 2016,Jan,13

63017 **lumbar**

📷 36.7 ⚕ 36.7 **FUD** 090 [J] [62] [80] ▭

AMA: 2018,Jan,8; 2017,Mar,7; 2017,Feb,9; 2017,Jan,8; 2016,Jan,13

Nerve root problems in C5 through C7 cause paralysis of the upper limb

C1 to C4
C5 to C7

Atlas (C1)
Axis (C2)

The specialized atlas allows for rotary motion, which turns the head

63020 **Laminotomy (hemilaminectomy), with decompression of nerve root(s), including partial facetectomy, foraminotomy and/or excision of herniated intervertebral disc; 1 interspace, cervical**

📷 33.4 ⚕ 33.4 **FUD** 090 [J] [62] [80] [50] ▭

AMA: 2018,Jan,8; 2017,Mar,7; 2017,Jan,8; 2016,Jan,13

63030 **1 interspace, lumbar**

EXCLUDES *Laminectomy at same session as posterior interbody fusion for:*
Decompression nerves or spinal components ([63052])
Preparation of interspace (22630, 22633)

📷 28.2 ⚕ 28.2 **FUD** 090 [J] [62] [80] [50] ▭

AMA: 2020,May,13; 2019,Nov,14; 2018,Jan,8; 2017,Mar,7; 2017,Feb,12; 2017,Feb,9; 2017,Jan,8; 2016,May,13; 2016,Jan,13

+ **63035** **each additional interspace, cervical or lumbar (List separately in addition to code for primary procedure)**

EXCLUDES *Laminectomy at same session as posterior interbody fusion for:*
Decompression nerves or spinal components ([63053])
Preparation of interspace (22632, 22634)
Reporting with modifier 50. Report once for each side when performed bilaterally

Code first (63020-63030)

📷 5.55 ⚕ 5.55 **FUD** ZZZ [N] [M1] [80] ▭

AMA: 2018,Jan,8; 2017,Feb,9; 2017,Jan,8; 2016,Jan,13

63040 **Laminotomy (hemilaminectomy), with decompression of nerve root(s), including partial facetectomy, foraminotomy and/or excision of herniated intervertebral disc, reexploration, single interspace; cervical**

📷 40.4 ⚕ 40.4 **FUD** 090 [J] [62] [80] [50] ▭

AMA: 2020,May,13; 2018,Jan,8; 2017,Mar,7; 2017,Jan,8; 2016,Jan,13

63042 **lumbar**

EXCLUDES *Laminectomy at same session as posterior interbody fusion for:*
Decompression nerves or spinal components ([63052])
Preparation of interspace (22630, 22633)

📷 37.5 ⚕ 37.5 **FUD** 090 [J] [62] [80] [50] ▭

AMA: 2020,May,13; 2018,Jan,8; 2017,Mar,7; 2017,Feb,9; 2017,Jan,8; 2016,Jan,13

+ **63043** each additional cervical interspace (List separately in addition to code for primary procedure)

> EXCLUDES Reporting with modifier 50. Report once for each side when performed bilaterally

Code first (63040)

🔪 0.00 ⚕ 0.00 **FUD** ZZZ N N1 80 ▭

AMA: 2020,May,13; 2018,Jan,8; 2017,Jan,8; 2016,Jan,13

+ **63044** each additional lumbar interspace (List separately in addition to code for primary procedure)

> EXCLUDES Laminectomy at same session as posterior interbody fusion for:
> Decompression nerves or spinal components ([63053])
> Preparation of interspace (22632, 22634)
> Reporting with modifier 50. Report once for each side when performed bilaterally

Code first (63042)

🔪 0.00 ⚕ 0.00 **FUD** ZZZ N N1 80 ▭

AMA: 2020,May,13; 2018,Jan,8; 2017,Feb,9; 2017,Jan,8; 2016,Jan,13

63045 Laminectomy, facetectomy and foraminotomy (unilateral or bilateral with decompression of spinal cord, cauda equina and/or nerve root[s], [eg, spinal or lateral recess stenosis]), single vertebral segment; cervical

🔪 37.1 ⚕ 37.1 **FUD** 090 J 62 80 ▭

AMA: 2018,Jan,8; 2017,Mar,7; 2017,Jan,8; 2016,Jan,13

63046 thoracic

🔪 35.4 ⚕ 35.4 **FUD** 090 J 62 80 ▭

AMA: 2018,Jan,8; 2017,Mar,7; 2017,Jan,8; 2016,Jan,13

63047 lumbar

> EXCLUDES Laminectomy, facetectomy or foraminotomy at same session as posterior interbody fusion for:
> Decompression nerves or spinal components ([63052])
> Preparation of interspace (22630, 22633)

🔪 31.9 ⚕ 31.9 **FUD** 090 J 62 80 ▭

AMA: 2020,May,13; 2019,Dec,12; 2018,May,10; 2018,May,9; 2018,Jan,8; 2017,Mar,7; 2017,Feb,9; 2017,Feb,12; 2017,Jan,8; 2016,Oct,11; 2016,Jan,13

▲ + **63048** each additional vertebral segment, cervical, thoracic, or lumbar (List separately in addition to code for primary procedure)

> EXCLUDES Laminectomy, facetectomy or foraminotomy at same session as posterior interbody fusion for:
> Decompression nerves or spinal components ([63053])
> Preparation of interspace (22632, 22634)

Code first (63045-63047)

🔪 6.13 ⚕ 6.13 **FUD** ZZZ N N1 80 ▭

AMA: 2018,Jan,8; 2017,Feb,9; 2017,Jan,8; 2016,Jan,13

● + # **63052** Laminectomy, facetectomy, or foraminotomy (unilateral or bilateral with decompression of spinal cord, cauda equina and/or nerve root[s] [eg, spinal or lateral recess stenosis]), during posterior interbody arthrodesis, lumbar; single vertebral segment (List separately in addition to code for primary procedure)

Code first (22630-22634)

🔪 0.00 ⚕ 0.00 **FUD** 000

● + # **63053** each additional segment (List separately in addition to code for primary procedure)

Code first (22630-22634, [63052])

🔪 0.00 ⚕ 0.00 **FUD** 000

63050-63051 Cervical Laminoplasty: Posterior Midline Approach

> EXCLUDES Procedure performed on same vertebral segment(s) (22600, 22614, 22840-22842, 63001, 63015, 63045, 63048, 63295)

63050 Laminoplasty, cervical, with decompression of the spinal cord, 2 or more vertebral segments;

🔪 43.5 ⚕ 43.5 **FUD** 090 C 80 ▭

AMA: 2018,Jan,8; 2017,Mar,7; 2017,Jan,8; 2016,Jan,13

63051 with reconstruction of the posterior bony elements (including the application of bridging bone graft and non-segmental fixation devices [eg, wire, suture, mini-plates], when performed)

🔪 49.3 ⚕ 49.3 **FUD** 090 C 80 ▭

AMA: 2018,Jan,8; 2017,Mar,7; 2017,Jan,8; 2016,Jan,13

63052-63066 [63052, 63053] Spinal Cord/Nerve Root Decompression: Costovertebral or Transpedicular Approach

63052 Resequenced code. See code following 63048.

63053 Resequenced code. See code following 63048.

63055 Transpedicular approach with decompression of spinal cord, equina and/or nerve root(s) (eg, herniated intervertebral disc), single segment; thoracic

🔪 47.0 ⚕ 47.0 **FUD** 090 J 62 80 ▭

AMA: 2018,Jan,8; 2017,Mar,7; 2017,Jan,8; 2016,Jan,13

63056 lumbar (including transfacet, or lateral extraforaminal approach) (eg, far lateral herniated intervertebral disc)

> EXCLUDES Discectomy at same session as posterior interbody fusion for:
> Decompression nerves or spinal components ([63052])
> Preparation of interspace (22630, 22633)

🔪 43.0 ⚕ 43.0 **FUD** 090 J 62 80 ▭

AMA: 2019,Nov,14; 2018,Jan,8; 2017,Mar,7; 2017,Feb,12; 2017,Jan,8; 2016,Jan,13

+ **63057** each additional segment, thoracic or lumbar (List separately in addition to code for primary procedure)

> EXCLUDES Discectomy at same session as posterior interbody fusion for:
> Decompression nerves or spinal components ([63053])
> Preparation of interspace (22632, 22634)

Code first (63055-63056)

🔪 9.28 ⚕ 9.28 **FUD** ZZZ N N1 80 ▭

AMA: 2018,Jan,8; 2017,Jan,8; 2016,Jan,13

63064 Costovertebral approach with decompression of spinal cord or nerve root(s) (eg, herniated intervertebral disc), thoracic; single segment

> EXCLUDES Laminectomy with intraspinal thoracic lesion removal (63266, 63271, 63276, 63281, 63286)

🔪 51.5 ⚕ 51.5 **FUD** 090 J 62 80 ▭

AMA: 2018,Jan,8; 2017,Mar,7; 2017,Jan,8; 2016,Jan,13

+ **63066** each additional segment (List separately in addition to code for primary procedure)

> EXCLUDES Laminectomy with intraspinal thoracic lesion removal (63266, 63271, 63276, 63281, 63286)

Code first (63064)

🔪 5.97 ⚕ 5.97 **FUD** ZZZ N N1 80 ▭

AMA: 2014,Jan,11; 1996,Feb,6

63075-63078 Discectomy: Anterior or Anterolateral Approach

> INCLUDES Operating microscope (69990)

63075 Discectomy, anterior, with decompression of spinal cord and/or nerve root(s), including osteophytectomy; cervical, single interspace

> EXCLUDES Anterior cervical discectomy and anterior interbody fusion at same level during same operative session (22551)
> Anterior interbody arthrodesis (even by another provider) (22554)

🔪 39.1 ⚕ 39.1 **FUD** 090 J 62 80 ▭

AMA: 2018,Jan,8; 2017,Mar,7; 2017,Jan,8; 2016,Feb,12; 2016,Jan,13

+ 63076 cervical, each additional interspace (List separately in addition to code for primary procedure)

EXCLUDES *Anterior cervical discectomy and anterior interbody fusion at same level during same operative session (22552)*

Anterior interbody arthrodesis (even by another provider) (22554)

Code first (63075)

⚙ 7.20 ⚖ 7.20 **FUD** ZZZ N N1 80 ▣

AMA: 2018,Jan,8; 2017,Jan,8; 2016,Feb,12; 2016,Jan,13

63077 thoracic, single interspace

⚙ 44.2 ⚖ 44.2 **FUD** 090 C 80 ▣

AMA: 2018,Jan,8; 2017,Mar,7; 2017,Jan,8; 2016,Feb,12; 2016,Jan,13

+ 63078 thoracic, each additional interspace (List separately in addition to code for primary procedure)

Code first (63077)

⚙ 6.01 ⚖ 6.01 **FUD** ZZZ C 80 ▣

AMA: 2018,Jan,8; 2017,Jan,8; 2016,Feb,12; 2016,Jan,13

63081-63091 Vertebral Corpectomy, All Levels, Anterior Approach

INCLUDES Disc removal level below and/or above vertebral segment
Partial removal:
Cervical: Removal ≥ 1/2 vertebral body
Lumbar: Removal ≥ 1/3 vertebral body
Thoracic: Removal ≥ 1/3 vertebral body

EXCLUDES *Arthrodesis (22548-22812)*

Code also reconstruction (20930-20938, 22548-22812, 22840-22855 [22859])

63081 Vertebral corpectomy (vertebral body resection), partial or complete, anterior approach with decompression of spinal cord and/or nerve root(s); cervical, single segment

EXCLUDES *Transoral approach (61575-61576)*

⚙ 50.9 ⚖ 50.9 **FUD** 090 C 80 ▣

AMA: 2018,Jan,8; 2017,Mar,7; 2017,Jan,8; 2016,Apr,8; 2016,Jan,13

+ 63082 cervical, each additional segment (List separately in addition to code for primary procedure)

EXCLUDES *Transoral approach (61575-61576)*

Code first (63081)

⚙ 7.72 ⚖ 7.72 **FUD** ZZZ C 80 ▣

AMA: 2018,Jan,8; 2017,Jan,8; 2016,Apr,8; 2016,Jan,13

63085 Vertebral corpectomy (vertebral body resection), partial or complete, transthoracic approach with decompression of spinal cord and/or nerve root(s); thoracic, single segment

⚙ 55.7 ⚖ 55.7 **FUD** 090 C 80 ▣

AMA: 2018,Jan,8; 2017,Mar,7; 2017,Jan,8; 2016,Apr,8; 2016,Jan,13

+ 63086 thoracic, each additional segment (List separately in addition to code for primary procedure)

Code first (63085)

⚙ 5.53 ⚖ 5.53 **FUD** ZZZ C 80 ▣

AMA: 2018,Jan,8; 2017,Jan,8; 2016,Apr,8; 2016,Jan,13

63087 Vertebral corpectomy (vertebral body resection), partial or complete, combined thoracolumbar approach with decompression of spinal cord, cauda equina or nerve root(s), lower thoracic or lumbar; single segment

⚙ 69.8 ⚖ 69.8 **FUD** 090 C 80 ▣

AMA: 2018,Jan,8; 2017,Mar,7; 2017,Jan,8; 2016,Apr,8; 2016,Jan,13

+ 63088 each additional segment (List separately in addition to code for primary procedure)

Code first (63087)

⚙ 7.43 ⚖ 7.43 **FUD** ZZZ C 80 ▣

AMA: 2018,Jan,8; 2017,Jan,8; 2016,Apr,8; 2016,Jan,13

63090 Vertebral corpectomy (vertebral body resection), partial or complete, transperitoneal or retroperitoneal approach with decompression of spinal cord, cauda equina or nerve root(s), lower thoracic, lumbar, or sacral; single segment

⚙ 56.8 ⚖ 56.8 **FUD** 090 C 80 ▣

AMA: 2018,Jan,8; 2017,Mar,7; 2017,Jan,8; 2016,Apr,8; 2016,Jan,13

+ 63091 each additional segment (List separately in addition to code for primary procedure)

Code first (63090)

⚙ 5.18 ⚖ 5.18 **FUD** ZZZ C 80 ▣

AMA: 2018,Jan,8; 2017,Jan,8; 2016,Apr,8; 2016,Jan,13

63101-63103 Corpectomy: Lateral Extracavitary Approach

INCLUDES Partial removal:
Cervical: Removal ≥ 1/2 vertebral body
Lumbar: Removal ≥ 1/3 vertebral body
Thoracic: Removal ≥ 1/3 vertebral body

63101 Vertebral corpectomy (vertebral body resection), partial or complete, lateral extracavitary approach with decompression of spinal cord and/or nerve root(s) (eg, for tumor or retropulsed bone fragments); thoracic, single segment

⚙ 67.2 ⚖ 67.2 **FUD** 090 C 80 ▣

AMA: 2018,Jan,8; 2017,Mar,7; 2017,Jan,8; 2016,Jan,13

63102 lumbar, single segment

⚙ 65.5 ⚖ 65.5 **FUD** 090 C 80 ▣

AMA: 2018,Jan,8; 2017,Mar,7; 2017,Jan,8; 2016,Jan,13

+ 63103 thoracic or lumbar, each additional segment (List separately in addition to code for primary procedure)

Code first (63101-63102)

⚙ 8.53 ⚖ 8.53 **FUD** ZZZ C 80 ▣

AMA: 2014,Jan,11

63170-63295 Laminectomies

63170 Laminectomy with myelotomy (eg, Bischof or DREZ type), cervical, thoracic, or thoracolumbar

⚙ 45.9 ⚖ 45.9 **FUD** 090 C 80 ▣

AMA: 2018,Jan,8; 2017,Mar,7; 2017,Jan,8; 2016,Jan,13

63172 Laminectomy with drainage of intramedullary cyst/syrinx; to subarachnoid space

⚙ 40.0 ⚖ 40.0 **FUD** 090 C 80 ▣

AMA: 2018,Jan,8; 2017,Mar,7; 2017,Jan,8; 2016,Jan,13

63173 to peritoneal or pleural space

⚙ 49.7 ⚖ 49.7 **FUD** 090 C 80 ▣

AMA: 2018,Jan,8; 2017,Mar,7; 2017,Jan,8; 2016,Jan,13

63185 Laminectomy with rhizotomy; 1 or 2 segments

INCLUDES Dana rhizotomy
Stoffel rhizotomy

⚙ 33.1 ⚖ 33.1 **FUD** 090 C 80 ▣

AMA: 2018,Jan,8; 2017,Mar,7; 2017,Jan,8; 2016,Jan,13

63190 more than 2 segments

⚙ 36.0 ⚖ 36.0 **FUD** 090 C 80 ▣

AMA: 2018,Jan,8; 2017,Mar,7; 2017,Jan,8; 2016,Jan,13

63191 Laminectomy with section of spinal accessory nerve

EXCLUDES *Division sternocleidomastoid muscle for torticollis (21720)*

⚙ 39.7 ⚖ 39.7 **FUD** 090 C 80 50 ▣

AMA: 2018,Jan,8; 2017,Mar,7; 2017,Jan,8; 2016,Jan,13

63194 ~~Laminectomy with cordotomy, with section of 1 spinothalamic tract, 1 stage; cervical~~

63195 ~~thoracic~~

63196 ~~Laminectomy with cordotomy, with section of both spinothalamic tracts, 1 stage; cervical~~

▲ 63197 Laminectomy with cordotomy, with section of both spinothalamic tracts, 1 stage, thoracic

⚙ 49.3 ⚖ 49.3 **FUD** 090 C 80 ▣

AMA: 2018,Jan,8; 2017,Mar,7; 2017,Jan,8; 2016,Jan,13

63198 Laminectomy with cordotomy with section of both spinothalamic tracts, 2 stages within 14 days; cervical

63199 thoracic

63200 Laminectomy, with release of tethered spinal cord, lumbar
📊 44.1 ⚗ 44.1 **FUD** 090 Ⓒ 80 ▭
AMA: 2018,Jan,8; 2017,Mar,7; 2017,Jan,8; 2016,Jan,13

63250 Laminectomy for excision or occlusion of arteriovenous malformation of spinal cord; cervical
📊 87.8 ⚗ 87.8 **FUD** 090 Ⓒ 80 ▭
AMA: 2018,Jan,8; 2017,Mar,7; 2017,Jan,8; 2016,Jan,13

Cervical C1 to C7

Thoracic T1 to T12

Lumbar L1 to L5

Sacrum

Dura mater
Nerve roots
Pia mater
Arachnoid
White matter
Gray matter

Schematic of spinal cord layers

63251 thoracic
📊 87.8 ⚗ 87.8 **FUD** 090 Ⓒ 80 ▭
AMA: 2018,Jan,8; 2017,Mar,7; 2017,Jan,8; 2016,Jan,13

63252 thoracolumbar
📊 87.8 ⚗ 87.8 **FUD** 090 Ⓒ 80 ▭
AMA: 2018,Jan,8; 2017,Mar,7; 2017,Jan,8; 2016,Jan,13

63265 Laminectomy for excision or evacuation of intraspinal lesion other than neoplasm, extradural; cervical
📊 48.2 ⚗ 48.2 **FUD** 090 Ⓒ 80 ▭
AMA: 2018,Jan,8; 2017,Mar,7; 2017,Jan,8; 2016,Jan,13

63266 thoracic
📊 49.7 ⚗ 49.7 **FUD** 090 Ⓒ 80 ▭
AMA: 2017,Mar,7

63267 lumbar
📊 39.6 ⚗ 39.6 **FUD** 090 Ⓒ 80 ▭
AMA: 2018,Jan,8; 2017,Mar,7; 2017,Jan,8; 2016,Jan,13

63268 sacral
📊 40.9 ⚗ 40.9 **FUD** 090 Ⓒ 80 ▭
AMA: 2018,Jan,8; 2017,Mar,7; 2017,Jan,8; 2016,Jan,13

63270 Laminectomy for excision of intraspinal lesion other than neoplasm, intradural; cervical
📊 60.4 ⚗ 60.4 **FUD** 090 Ⓒ 80 ▭
AMA: 2018,Jan,8; 2017,Mar,7; 2017,Jan,8; 2016,Jan,13

63271 thoracic
📊 59.8 ⚗ 59.8 **FUD** 090 Ⓒ 80 ▭
AMA: 2018,Jan,8; 2017,Mar,7; 2017,Jan,8; 2016,Jan,13

63272 lumbar
📊 54.5 ⚗ 54.5 **FUD** 090 Ⓒ 80 ▭
AMA: 2018,Jan,8; 2017,Mar,7; 2017,Jan,8; 2016,Jan,13

63273 sacral
📊 53.8 ⚗ 53.8 **FUD** 090 Ⓒ 80 ▭
AMA: 2018,Jan,8; 2017,Mar,7; 2017,Jan,8; 2016,Jan,13

63275 Laminectomy for biopsy/excision of intraspinal neoplasm; extradural, cervical
📊 52.1 ⚗ 52.1 **FUD** 090 Ⓒ 80 ▭
AMA: 2018,Jan,8; 2017,Mar,7; 2017,Jan,8; 2016,Jan,13

63276 extradural, thoracic
📊 51.7 ⚗ 51.7 **FUD** 090 Ⓒ 80 ▭
AMA: 2018,Jan,8; 2017,Mar,7; 2017,Jan,8; 2016,Jan,13

63277 extradural, lumbar
📊 45.0 ⚗ 45.0 **FUD** 090 Ⓒ 80 ▭
AMA: 2018,Jan,8; 2017,Mar,7; 2017,Jan,8; 2016,Jan,13

63278 extradural, sacral
📊 45.9 ⚗ 45.9 **FUD** 090 Ⓒ 80 ▭
AMA: 2018,Jan,8; 2017,Mar,7; 2017,Jan,8; 2016,Jan,13

63280 intradural, extramedullary, cervical
📊 61.2 ⚗ 61.2 **FUD** 090 Ⓒ 80 ▭
AMA: 2018,Jan,8; 2017,Mar,7; 2017,Jan,8; 2016,Jan,13

63281 intradural, extramedullary, thoracic
📊 60.5 ⚗ 60.5 **FUD** 090 Ⓒ 80 ▭
AMA: 2018,Jan,8; 2017,Mar,7; 2017,Jan,8; 2016,Jan,13

63282 intradural, extramedullary, lumbar
📊 57.7 ⚗ 57.7 **FUD** 090 Ⓒ 80 ▭
AMA: 2018,Jan,8; 2017,Mar,7; 2017,Jan,8; 2016,Jan,13

63283 intradural, sacral
📊 55.3 ⚗ 55.3 **FUD** 090 Ⓒ 80 ▭
AMA: 2018,Jan,8; 2017,Mar,7; 2017,Jan,8; 2016,Jan,13

63285 intradural, intramedullary, cervical
📊 77.2 ⚗ 77.2 **FUD** 090 Ⓒ 80 ▭
AMA: 2018,Jan,8; 2017,Mar,7; 2017,Jan,8; 2016,Jan,13

63286 intradural, intramedullary, thoracic
📊 74.7 ⚗ 74.7 **FUD** 090 Ⓒ 80 ▭
AMA: 2018,Jan,8; 2017,Mar,7; 2017,Jan,8; 2016,Jan,13

63287 intradural, intramedullary, thoracolumbar
📊 80.1 ⚗ 80.1 **FUD** 090 Ⓒ 80 ▭
AMA: 2018,Jan,8; 2017,Mar,7; 2017,Jan,8; 2016,Jan,13

63290 combined extradural-intradural lesion, any level
EXCLUDES *Drainage intramedullary cyst or syrinx (63172-63173)*
📊 80.7 ⚗ 80.7 **FUD** 090 Ⓒ 80 ▭
AMA: 2018,Jan,8; 2017,Mar,7; 2017,Jan,8; 2016,Jan,13

+ 63295 Osteoplastic reconstruction of dorsal spinal elements, following primary intraspinal procedure (List separately in addition to code for primary procedure)
EXCLUDES *Procedure performed same vertebral segment(s) (22590-22614, 22840-22844, 63050-63051)*
Code first (63172-63173, 63185, 63190, 63200-63290)
📊 9.76 ⚗ 9.76 **FUD** ZZZ Ⓒ 80 ▭
AMA: 2014,Jan,11

63300-63308 Vertebral Corpectomy for Intraspinal Lesion: Anterior/Anterolateral Approach

INCLUDES Partial removal:
Cervical: Removal ≥ 1/2 vertebral body
Lumbar: Removal ≥ 1/3 vertebral body
Thoracic: Removal ≥ 1/3 vertebral body
EXCLUDES *Arthrodesis (22548-22585)*
Spinal reconstruction (20930-20938)

63300 Vertebral corpectomy (vertebral body resection), partial or complete, for excision of intraspinal lesion, single segment; extradural, cervical
📊 53.1 ⚗ 53.1 **FUD** 090 Ⓒ 80 ▭
AMA: 2018,Jan,8; 2017,Mar,7; 2017,Jan,8; 2016,Jan,13

63301 extradural, thoracic by transthoracic approach
📊 63.7 ⚗ 63.7 **FUD** 090 Ⓒ 80 ▭
AMA: 2018,Jan,8; 2017,Mar,7; 2017,Jan,8; 2016,Jan,13

63302 extradural, thoracic by thoracolumbar approach
📊 62.9 ⚗ 62.9 **FUD** 090 Ⓒ 80 ▭
AMA: 2018,Jan,8; 2017,Mar,7; 2017,Jan,8; 2016,Jan,13

63303 **extradural, lumbar or sacral by transperitoneal or retroperitoneal approach**
🚗 63.1 ⚖ 63.1 **FUD** 090 C 80 ▨
AMA: 2018,Jan,8; 2017,Mar,7; 2017,Jan,8; 2016,Jan,13

63304 **intradural, cervical**
🚗 67.8 ⚖ 67.8 **FUD** 090 C 80 ▨
AMA: 2018,Jan,8; 2017,Mar,7; 2017,Jan,8; 2016,Jan,13

63305 **intradural, thoracic by transthoracic approach**
🚗 73.7 ⚖ 73.7 **FUD** 090 C 80 ▨
AMA: 2018,Jan,8; 2017,Mar,7; 2017,Jan,8; 2016,Jan,13

63306 **intradural, thoracic by thoracolumbar approach**
🚗 71.0 ⚖ 71.0 **FUD** 090 C 80 ▨
AMA: 2018,Jan,8; 2017,Mar,7; 2017,Jan,8; 2016,Jan,13

63307 **intradural, lumbar or sacral by transperitoneal or retroperitoneal approach**
🚗 69.5 ⚖ 69.5 **FUD** 090 C 80 ▨
AMA: 2018,Jan,8; 2017,Mar,7; 2017,Jan,8; 2016,Jan,13

+ 63308 **each additional segment (List separately in addition to codes for single segment)**
Code first (63300-63307)
🚗 9.37 ⚖ 9.37 **FUD** ZZZ C 80 ▨
AMA: 2014,Jan,11; 2002,Feb,4

63600-63610 Stereotactic Procedures of the Spinal Cord

63600 **Creation of lesion of spinal cord by stereotactic method, percutaneous, any modality (including stimulation and/or recording)**
🚗 32.0 ⚖ 32.0 **FUD** 090 J A2 80 ▨
AMA: 2014,Jan,11; 2000,Dec,12

63610 **Stereotactic stimulation of spinal cord, percutaneous, separate procedure not followed by other surgery**
🚗 17.1 ⚖ 17.1 **FUD** 000 J J8 80 ▨
AMA: 2014,Jan,11

63620-63621 Stereotactic Radiosurgery (SRS): Spine

INCLUDES Computer assisted planning
Planning dosimetry, targeting, positioning, or blocking by neurosurgeon
EXCLUDES *Arteriovenous malformations (see Radiation Oncology Section)*
Intensity modulated beam delivery plan and treatment (77301, 77385-77386)
Radiation treatment management by same provider (77427-77432)
Stereotactic body radiation therapy (77373, 77435)
Stereotactic computer-assisted procedures (61781-61783)
Treatment planning, physics, dosimetry, treatment delivery and management provided by radiation oncologist (77261-77790 [77295, 77385, 77386, 77387, 77424, 77425])

63620 **Stereotactic radiosurgery (particle beam, gamma ray, or linear accelerator); 1 spinal lesion**
EXCLUDES *Reporting code more than one time per entire treatment course*
🚗 32.2 ⚖ 32.2 **FUD** 090 B 80 ▨
AMA: 2018,Jan,8; 2017,Jan,8; 2016,Jan,13

+ 63621 **each additional spinal lesion (List separately in addition to code for primary procedure)**
EXCLUDES *Reporting code more than one time per lesion*
Reporting code more than two times per entire treatment course
Code first (63620)
🚗 7.30 ⚖ 7.30 **FUD** ZZZ B 80 ▨
AMA: 2018,Jan,8; 2017,Jan,8; 2016,Jan,13

63650-63688 Spinal Neurostimulation

INCLUDES Analysis system at implantation (95970)
Complex and simple neurostimulators
EXCLUDES *Analysis and programming neurostimulator pulse generator (95970-95972)*

63650 **Percutaneous implantation of neurostimulator electrode array, epidural**
INCLUDES Neurostimulator system components:
Multiple contacts which four or more provide electrical stimulation in epidural space
Contacts on catheter-type lead (array)
Extension
External controller
Implanted neurostimulator
🚗 11.9 ⚖ 54.1 **FUD** 010 J J8 ▨
AMA: 2019,Feb,6; 2018,Oct,11; 2018,Jan,8; 2017,Dec,13; 2017,Jan,8; 2016,Jan,13; 2016,Jan,11

63655 **Laminectomy for implantation of neurostimulator electrodes, plate/paddle, epidural**
INCLUDES Neurostimulator system components:
Multiple contacts which four or more provide electrical stimulation in epidural space
Contacts on catheter-type lead (array)
Extension
External controller
Implanted neurostimulator
🚗 24.0 ⚖ 24.0 **FUD** 090 J J8 80 ▨
AMA: 2020,Dec,13; 2019,Feb,6; 2018,Jan,8; 2017,Jan,8; 2016,Jan,13

63661 **Removal of spinal neurostimulator electrode percutaneous array(s), including fluoroscopy, when performed**
INCLUDES Neurostimulator system components:
Multiple contacts which four or more provide electrical stimulation in epidural space
Contacts on catheter-type lead (array)
Extension
External controller
Implanted neurostimulator
EXCLUDES *Reporting code when removing or replacing temporary array placed percutaneously for external generator*
🚗 9.33 ⚖ 18.3 **FUD** 010 Q2 62 80 ▨
AMA: 2019,Feb,6; 2018,Jan,8; 2017,Jan,8; 2016,Jan,13

63662 **Removal of spinal neurostimulator electrode plate/paddle(s) placed via laminotomy or laminectomy, including fluoroscopy, when performed**
INCLUDES Neurostimulator system components:
Multiple contacts which four or more provide electrical stimulation in epidural space
Contacts on catheter-type lead (array)
Extension
External controller
Implanted neurostimulator
🚗 24.3 ⚖ 24.3 **FUD** 090 Q2 62 80 ▨
AMA: 2020,Dec,13; 2019,Feb,6; 2018,Jan,8; 2017,Jan,8; 2016,Jan,13

63663 **Revision including replacement, when performed, of spinal neurostimulator electrode percutaneous array(s), including fluoroscopy, when performed**
INCLUDES Neurostimulator system components:
Multiple contacts which four or more provide electrical stimulation in epidural space
Contacts on catheter-type lead (array)
Extension
External controller
Implanted neurostimulator
EXCLUDES *Removal of spinal neurostimulator electrode percutaneous array(s), plate/paddle(s) at same level (63661-63662)*
Reporting code when removing or replacing temporary array placed percutaneously for external generator
🚗 12.9 ⚖ 23.4 **FUD** 010 J J8 80 ▨
AMA: 2019,Feb,6; 2018,Jan,8; 2017,Jan,8; 2016,Jan,13

63664 Revision including replacement, when performed, of spinal neurostimulator electrode plate/paddle(s) placed via laminotomy or laminectomy, including fluoroscopy, when performed

> INCLUDES Neurostimulator system components:
> Multiple contacts which four or more provide electrical stimulation in epidural space
> Contacts on catheter-type lead (array)
> Extension
> External controller
> Implanted neurostimulator
>
> EXCLUDES Removal spinal neurostimulator electrode percutaneous array(s), plate/paddle(s) at same level (63661-63662)

📓 25.2 ⅗ 25.2 **FUD** 090 ☐ J J8 80 ☐

AMA: 2019,Feb,6; 2018,Jan,8; 2017,Jan,8; 2016,Jan,13

63685 Insertion or replacement of spinal neurostimulator pulse generator or receiver, direct or inductive coupling

> EXCLUDES Reporting code for insertion/replacement with code for revision/removal (63688)

📓 10.3 ⅗ 10.3 **FUD** 010 ☐ J J8 80 ☐

AMA: 2019,Feb,6; 2018,Jan,8; 2017,Dec,13; 2017,Jan,8; 2016,Jan,13

63688 Revision or removal of implanted spinal neurostimulator pulse generator or receiver

> EXCLUDES Reporting code for revision/removal with code for insertion/replacement (63685)

📓 10.7 ⅗ 10.7 **FUD** 010 ☐ 02 A2 ☐

AMA: 2019,Feb,6; 2018,Jan,8; 2017,Jan,8; 2016,Jan,13

63700-63706 Repair Congenital Neural Tube Defects

> EXCLUDES Complex skin repair (see appropriate integumentary closure code)

63700 Repair of meningocele; less than 5 cm diameter

📓 37.6 ⅗ 37.6 **FUD** 090 63 C 80 ☐

AMA: 2014,Jan,11

Most children with severe spina bifida also have hydrocephalus, which is excessive fluid in the skull

Cervical
Thoracic
Lumbar

A fluid-filled herniation that protrudes is spina bifida cystica, or meningocele

If nerves protrude into the defect, it is called rachischisis, or meningomyelocele

Dura mater
Spinal cord
Vertebra

63702 larger than 5 cm diameter

📓 41.8 ⅗ 41.8 **FUD** 090 63 C 80 ☐

AMA: 2014,Jan,11

63704 Repair of myelomeningocele; less than 5 cm diameter

📓 47.7 ⅗ 47.7 **FUD** 090 63 C 80 ☐

AMA: 2014,Jan,11

63706 larger than 5 cm diameter

📓 53.1 ⅗ 53.1 **FUD** 090 63 C 80 ☐

AMA: 2014,Jan,11

63707-63710 Repair Dural Cerebrospinal Fluid Leak

63707 Repair of dural/cerebrospinal fluid leak, not requiring laminectomy

📓 26.8 ⅗ 26.8 **FUD** 090 C 80 ☐

AMA: 2014,Jan,11; 2002,May,7

63709 Repair of dural/cerebrospinal fluid leak or pseudomeningocele, with laminectomy

📓 32.0 ⅗ 32.0 **FUD** 090 C 80 ☐

AMA: 2014,Jan,11; 2002,May,7

63710 Dural graft, spinal

📓 31.6 ⅗ 31.6 **FUD** 090 C 80 ☐

AMA: 2014,Jan,11

63740-63746 Cerebrospinal Fluid (CSF) Shunt: Lumbar

> EXCLUDES Placement subarachnoid catheter with reservoir and/or pump:
> Not requiring laminectomy (62350, 62360-62362)
> With laminectomy (62351, 62360-62362)

63740 Creation of shunt, lumbar, subarachnoid-peritoneal, -pleural, or other; including laminectomy

📓 28.1 ⅗ 28.1 **FUD** 090 C 80 ☐

AMA: 2014,Jan,11; 2000,Dec,12

63741 percutaneous, not requiring laminectomy

📓 19.7 ⅗ 19.7 **FUD** 090 J J8 80 ☐

AMA: 2014,Jan,11; 1990,Win,4

63744 Replacement, irrigation or revision of lumbosubarachnoid shunt

📓 19.5 ⅗ 19.5 **FUD** 090 J J8 80 ☐

AMA: 2014,Jan,11

63746 Removal of entire lumbosubarachnoid shunt system without replacement

📓 17.3 ⅗ 17.3 **FUD** 090 02 A2 80 ☐

AMA: 2014,Jan,11

64400-64484 [64461, 64462, 64463] Nerve Blocks and Transforaminal Injections

> EXCLUDES Epidural or subarachnoid injection (62320-62327)
> Nerve destruction (62280-62282, 64600-64681 [64624, 64625, 64633, 64634, 64635, 64636])
> Reporting code more than one time per encounter when multiple injections required to block nerve and branches
> Code also imaging guidance and localization, when performed, except with (64451, 64454, 64479-64480, 64483-64484)

64400 Injection(s), anesthetic agent(s) and/or steroid; trigeminal nerve, each branch (ie, ophthalmic, maxillary, mandibular)

📓 1.44 ⅗ 3.05 **FUD** 000 T P3 50 ☐

AMA: 2018,Jan,8; 2017,Jan,8; 2016,Jan,13

64405 greater occipital nerve

📓 1.55 ⅗ 2.07 **FUD** 000 T P3 50 ☐

AMA: 2018,Jan,8; 2017,Jan,8; 2016,Oct,11; 2016,Jan,13

64408 vagus nerve

📓 2.44 ⅗ 3.35 **FUD** 000 T P3 80 50 ☐

AMA: 2018,Jan,8; 2017,Jan,8; 2016,Jan,13

64415 brachial plexus

📓 1.83 ⅗ 3.22 **FUD** 000 T A2 50 ☐

AMA: 2018,Jan,8; 2017,Jan,8; 2016,Jan,13

64416 brachial plexus, continuous infusion by catheter (including catheter placement)

> EXCLUDES Management epidural or subarachnoid continuous drug administration (01996)

📓 1.85 ⅗ 1.85 **FUD** 000 T 62 50 ☐

AMA: 2018,Jan,8; 2017,Jan,8; 2016,Jan,13

64417 axillary nerve

📓 2.02 ⅗ 3.76 **FUD** 000 T A2 50 ☐

AMA: 2018,Jan,8; 2017,Jan,8; 2016,Jan,13

64418 suprascapular nerve

📓 1.64 ⅗ 2.42 **FUD** 000 T P3 50 ☐

AMA: 2018,Jan,8; 2017,Jan,8; 2016,Jan,13

Nervous System

63664 — 64418

64420 **intercostal nerve, single level**
🔷 1.72 🔶 2.85 **FUD** 000 [T] [A2] [50] 🔲
AMA: 2018,Jan,8; 2017,Jan,8; 2016,Jan,9; 2016,Jan,13

+ 64421 **intercostal nerve, each additional level (List separately in addition to code for primary procedure)**
EXCLUDES *Reporting with modifier 50. Report once for each side when performed bilaterally*
Code first (64420)
🔷 0.73 🔶 0.97 **FUD** ZZZ [T] [A2] 🔲
AMA: 2018,Jan,8; 2017,Jan,8; 2016,Jan,9; 2016,Jan,13

64425 **ilioinguinal, iliohypogastric nerves**
🔷 1.60 🔶 3.19 **FUD** 000 [T] [P3] [50] 🔲
AMA: 2018,Jan,8; 2017,Jan,8; 2016,Jan,13

64430 **pudendal nerve**
🔷 2.30 🔶 4.14 **FUD** 000 [T] [A2] [50] 🔲
AMA: 2018,Jan,8; 2017,Jan,8; 2016,Jan,13

64435 **paracervical (uterine) nerve** ♀
🔷 1.26 🔶 2.09 **FUD** 000 [T] [P3] [50] 🔲
AMA: 2018,Jan,8; 2017,Jan,8; 2016,Jan,13

64445 **sciatic nerve**
🔷 2.09 🔶 3.89 **FUD** 000 [T] [P3] [50] 🔲
AMA: 2018,Jan,8; 2017,Jan,8; 2016,Jan,13

64446 **sciatic nerve, continuous infusion by catheter (including catheter placement)**
EXCLUDES *Management epidural or subarachnoid continuous drug administration (01996)*
🔷 2.28 🔶 2.28 **FUD** 000 [T] [G2] [50] 🔲
AMA: 2018,Jan,8; 2017,Jan,8; 2016,Jan,13

64447 **femoral nerve**
EXCLUDES *Injection genicular nerve branches (64454)*
Management epidural or subarachnoid continuous drug administration (01996)
🔷 1.91 🔶 3.46 **FUD** 000 [T] [P3] [50] 🔲
AMA: 2018,Jan,8; 2017,Jan,8; 2016,Jan,13

64448 **femoral nerve, continuous infusion by catheter (including catheter placement)**
EXCLUDES *Injection genicular nerve branches (64454)*
Management epidural or subarachnoid continuous drug administration (01996)
🔷 2.05 🔶 2.05 **FUD** 000 [T] [G2] [50] 🔲
AMA: 2018,Jan,8; 2017,Jan,8; 2016,Jan,13

64449 **lumbar plexus, posterior approach, continuous infusion by catheter (including catheter placement)**
EXCLUDES *Management epidural or subarachnoid continuous drug administration (01996)*
🔷 1.79 🔶 1.79 **FUD** 000 [T] [G2] [50] 🔲
AMA: 2018,Jan,8; 2017,Jan,8; 2016,Jan,13

64450 **other peripheral nerve or branch**
EXCLUDES *Injection genicular nerve branches (64454)*
Injection nerves innervating the sacroiliac joint (64451)
🔷 1.28 🔶 2.19 **FUD** 000 [T] [P3] [50] 🔲
AMA: 2019,Nov,14; 2018,Nov,10; 2018,Jan,8; 2017,Jan,8; 2016,Oct,11; 2016,Jan,13

64451 **nerves innervating the sacroiliac joint, with image guidance (ie, fluoroscopy or computed tomography)**
INCLUDES Imaging guidance and any contrast injection
EXCLUDES *Injection nerves innervating paravertebral facet joint (64493-64495)*
Injection with ultrasound (76999)
🔷 2.29 🔶 5.99 **FUD** 000 [G2] [50] 🔲
AMA: 2020,Jul,13

64454 **genicular nerve branches, including imaging guidance, when performed**
INCLUDES Articular branches of the following innervating the knee joint:
Common peroneal
Femoral
Obturator
Saphenous
Tibial
Imaging guidance and any contrast injection
Code also modifier 52 for injection fewer than following all genicular nerve branches: superolateral, superomedial, and inferomedial
🔷 2.36 🔶 6.05 **FUD** 000 [P3] [50] 🔲
AMA: 2020,Dec,13; 2019,Dec,8

64455 **plantar common digital nerve(s) (eg, Morton's neuroma)**
INCLUDES Single or multiple injections on the same site
EXCLUDES *Destruction by neurolytic agent; plantar common digital nerve (64632)*
Code also imaging guidance and localization, when performed
🔷 1.00 🔶 1.36 **FUD** 000 [T] [P3] [80] [50] 🔲
AMA: 2018,Jan,8; 2017,Jan,8; 2016,Jan,13

64461 **Resequenced code. See code following 64484.**

64462 **Resequenced code. See code following 64484.**

64463 **Resequenced code. See code following 64484.**

64479 **transforaminal epidural, with imaging guidance (fluoroscopy or CT), cervical or thoracic, single level**
INCLUDES Imaging guidance (fluoroscopy or CT) and contrast injection
Single or multiple injections same site
Transforaminal epidural injection T12-L1 level
🔷 3.76 🔶 6.95 **FUD** 000 [T] [A2] [50] 🔲
AMA: 2018,Jan,8; 2017,Jan,8; 2016,Jan,13; 2016,Jan,9

Thoracic vertebra (superior view)

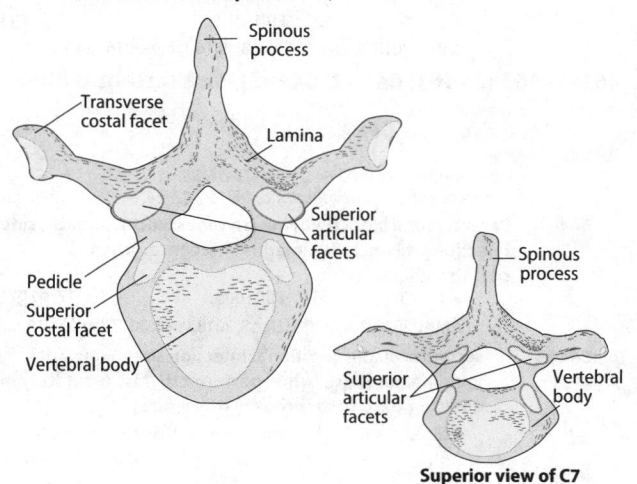

Superior view of C7

Nervous System

64480 — 64495

+ **64480** **transforaminal epidural, with imaging guidance (fluoroscopy or CT), cervical or thoracic, each additional level (List separately in addition to code for primary procedure)**

> INCLUDES Imaging guidance (fluoroscopy or CT) and contrast injection
> Single or multiple injections same site
> EXCLUDES *Destruction genicular nerve branches ([64624])*
> *Injection genicular nerve branches (64454)*
> *Reporting with modifier 50. Report once for each side when performed bilaterally*
> *Transforaminal epidural injection T12-L1 level*
> Code first (64479)
> 🔧 1.80 ⚕ 3.42 **FUD** ZZZ   N N1 ▢
> **AMA:** 2018,Jan,8; 2017,Jan,8; 2016,Jan,9; 2016,Jan,13

64483 **transforaminal epidural, with imaging guidance (fluoroscopy or CT), lumbar or sacral, single level**

> INCLUDES Imaging guidance (fluoroscopy or CT) and contrast injection
> Single or multiple injections same site
> EXCLUDES *Destruction genicular nerve branches ([64624])*
> *Injection genicular nerve branches (64454)*
> 🔧 3.19 ⚕ 6.44 **FUD** 000   T A2 50 ▢
> **AMA:** 2018,Jan,8; 2017,Jan,8; 2016,Oct,11; 2016,Jan,13; 2016,Jan,9

+ **64484** **transforaminal epidural, with imaging guidance (fluoroscopy or CT), lumbar or sacral, each additional level (List separately in addition to code for primary procedure)**

> INCLUDES Imaging guidance (fluoroscopy or CT) and contrast injection
> Single or multiple injections same site
> EXCLUDES *Destruction genicular nerve branches ([64624])*
> *Injection genicular nerve branches (64454)*
> *Reporting with modifier 50. Report once for each side when performed bilaterally*
> Code first (64483)
> 🔧 1.49 ⚕ 2.62 **FUD** ZZZ   N N1 ▢
> **AMA:** 2018,Jan,8; 2017,Jan,8; 2016,Jan,9; 2016,Jan,13

64461-64463 [64461, 64462, 64463] Paravertebral Blocks

> INCLUDES Contrast injection
> Imaging guidance (76942, 77002-77003)
> EXCLUDES *Injection:*
> *Anesthetic agent (64420-64421, 64479-64480)*
> *Diagnostic or therapeutic substance (62320, 62324, 64490-64492)*

64461 **Paravertebral block (PVB) (paraspinous block), thoracic; single injection site (includes imaging guidance, when performed)**

> 🔧 2.33 ⚕ 3.96 **FUD** 000   T 62 50 ▢
> **AMA:** 2018,Dec,8; 2018,Dec,8; 2018,Jan,8; 2017,Jan,8; 2016,Jan,9

+ # **64462** **second and any additional injection site(s) (includes imaging guidance, when performed) (List separately in addition to code for primary procedure)**

> EXCLUDES *Procedure performed more than one time per day*
> *Reporting with modifier 50. Report once for each side when performed bilaterally*
> Code first (64461)
> 🔧 1.47 ⚕ 2.20 **FUD** ZZZ   N N1 50 ▢
> **AMA:** 2018,Dec,8; 2018,Dec,8; 2018,Jan,8; 2017,Jan,8; 2016,Jan,9

64463 **continuous infusion by catheter (includes imaging guidance, when performed)**

> 🔧 2.42 ⚕ 5.13 **FUD** 000   T 62 50 ▢
> **AMA:** 2018,Dec,8; 2018,Dec,8; 2018,Jan,8; 2017,Jan,8; 2016,Jan,9

64486-64489 Transversus Abdominis Plane (TAP) Block

> INCLUDES Imaging guidance and any contrast injection

64486 **Transversus abdominis plane (TAP) block (abdominal plane block, rectus sheath block) unilateral; by injection(s) (includes imaging guidance, when performed)**

> 🔧 1.61 ⚕ 3.12 **FUD** 000   N N1 50 ▢
> **AMA:** 2018,Jan,8; 2017,Jan,8; 2016,Jan,13

64487 **by continuous infusion(s) (includes imaging guidance, when performed)**

> 🔧 1.91 ⚕ 3.80 **FUD** 000   N N1 50 ▢
> **AMA:** 2018,Jan,8; 2017,Jan,8; 2016,Jan,13

64488 **Transversus abdominis plane (TAP) block (abdominal plane block, rectus sheath block) bilateral; by injections (includes imaging guidance, when performed)**

> 🔧 2.05 ⚕ 3.83 **FUD** 000   N N1 ▢
> **AMA:** 2018,Jan,8; 2017,Jan,8; 2016,Jan,13

64489 **by continuous infusions (includes imaging guidance, when performed)**

> 🔧 2.28 ⚕ 5.19 **FUD** 000   N N1 ▢
> **AMA:** 2018,Jan,8; 2017,Jan,8; 2016,Jan,13

64490-64495 Paraspinal Nerve Injections

> INCLUDES Image guidance (CT or fluoroscopy) and any contrast injection
> EXCLUDES *Injection without imaging (20552-20553)*
> *Ultrasonic guidance (0213T-0218T)*

64490 **Injection(s), diagnostic or therapeutic agent, paravertebral facet (zygapophyseal) joint (or nerves innervating that joint) with image guidance (fluoroscopy or CT), cervical or thoracic; single level**

> INCLUDES Injection T12-L1 joint and nerves that innervate joint
> 🔧 3.04 ⚕ 5.38 **FUD** 000   T 62 80 50 ▢
> **AMA:** 2018,Jan,8; 2017,Jan,8; 2016,Jan,9; 2016,Jan,13

+ **64491** **second level (List separately in addition to code for primary procedure)**

> EXCLUDES *Reporting with modifier 50. Report once for each side when performed bilaterally*
> Code first (64490)
> 🔧 1.72 ⚕ 2.68 **FUD** ZZZ   N N1 80 ▢
> **AMA:** 2018,Jan,8; 2017,Jan,8; 2016,Jan,9; 2016,Jan,13

+ **64492** **third and any additional level(s) (List separately in addition to code for primary procedure)**

> EXCLUDES *Procedure performed more than one time per day*
> *Reporting with modifier 50. Report once for each side when performed bilaterally*
> Code also when appropriate (64491)
> Code first (64490)
> 🔧 1.74 ⚕ 2.70 **FUD** ZZZ   N N1 80 ▢
> **AMA:** 2018,Jan,8; 2017,Jan,8; 2016,Jan,9; 2016,Jan,13

64493 **Injection(s), diagnostic or therapeutic agent, paravertebral facet (zygapophyseal) joint (or nerves innervating that joint) with image guidance (fluoroscopy or CT), lumbar or sacral; single level**

> EXCLUDES *Injection nerves innervating sacroiliac joint (64451)*
> 🔧 2.58 ⚕ 4.91 **FUD** 000   T 62 80 50 ▢
> **AMA:** 2020,Jul,13; 2018,May,10; 2018,Jan,8; 2017,Jan,8; 2016,Jan,13

+ **64494** **second level (List separately in addition to code for primary procedure)**

> EXCLUDES *Reporting with modifier 50. Report once for each side when performed bilaterally*
> Code first (64493)
> 🔧 1.49 ⚕ 2.49 **FUD** ZZZ   N N1 80 ▢
> **AMA:** 2020,Jul,13; 2018,May,10; 2018,Jan,8; 2017,Jan,8; 2016,Jan,13

+ **64495** **third and any additional level(s) (List separately in addition to code for primary procedure)**

> EXCLUDES *Procedure performed more than one time per day*
> *Reporting with modifier 50. Report once for each side when performed bilaterally*
> Code also when appropriate (64494)
> Code first (64493)
> 🔧 1.51 ⚕ 2.49 **FUD** ZZZ   N N1 80 ▢
> **AMA:** 2018,May,10; 2018,Jan,8; 2017,Jan,8; 2016,Jan,13

64505-64530 Sympathetic Nerve Blocks

64505 **Injection, anesthetic agent; sphenopalatine ganglion**
🚗 2.69 ⚕ 3.36 **FUD** 000   T P3 50 ▱
AMA: 2018,Jan,8; 2017,Jan,8; 2016,Jan,13

64510 **stellate ganglion (cervical sympathetic)**
🚗 2.13 ⚕ 3.78 **FUD** 000   T A2 50 ▱
AMA: 2018,Jan,8; 2017,Jan,8; 2016,Jan,13

64517 **superior hypogastric plexus**
🚗 3.60 ⚕ 5.47 **FUD** 000   T A2 ▱
AMA: 2018,Jan,8; 2017,Jan,8; 2016,Jan,13

64520 **lumbar or thoracic (paravertebral sympathetic)**
🚗 2.34 ⚕ 5.75 **FUD** 000   T A2 50 ▱
AMA: 2018,Jan,8; 2017,Jan,8; 2016,Jan,13

64530 **celiac plexus, with or without radiologic monitoring**
EXCLUDES *Transmural anesthetic injection with transendoscopic ultrasound-guidance (43253)*
🚗 2.63 ⚕ 5.73 **FUD** 000   T A2 ▱
AMA: 2018,Jan,8; 2017,Jan,8; 2016,Jan,13

64553-64570 Electrical Nerve Stimulation: Insertion/Replacement/Removal/Revision

INCLUDES Analysis system at implantation (95970)
Simple and complex neurostimulators
EXCLUDES *Analysis and programming neurostimulator pulse generator (95970-95972, 0589T-0590T)*
TENS therapy (97014, 97032)

64553 **Percutaneous implantation of neurostimulator electrode array; cranial nerve**
INCLUDES Temporary and permanent percutaneous array placement
EXCLUDES *Open procedure (61885-61886)*
Percutaneous electrical stimulation peripheral nerve with needle or needle electrodes (64999)
🚗 10.1 ⚕ 48.8 **FUD** 010   J J8 80 ▱
AMA: 2019,Feb,6; 2018,Oct,8; 2018,Jan,8; 2017,Jan,8; 2016,Jan,13

64555 **peripheral nerve (excludes sacral nerve)**
INCLUDES Temporary and permanent percutaneous array placement
EXCLUDES *Percutaneous electrical stimulation cranial nerve with needle or needle electrodes (64999)*
Posterior tibial neurostimulation (64566, 0587T-0588T)
🚗 9.85 ⚕ 44.3 **FUD** 010   J J8 ▱
AMA: 2019,Feb,6; 2018,Oct,8; 2018,Aug,10; 2018,Jan,8; 2017,Dec,13; 2017,Jan,8; 2016,Feb,13; 2016,Jan,13

64561 **sacral nerve (transforaminal placement) including image guidance, if performed**
INCLUDES Temporary and permanent percutaneous array placement
EXCLUDES *Percutaneous electrical stimulation or neuromodulation with needle or needle electrodes (64999)*
🚗 8.75 ⚕ 20.9 **FUD** 010   J J8 50 ▱
AMA: 2019,Feb,6; 2018,Oct,8; 2018,Jan,8; 2017,Jan,8; 2016,Jan,13

64566 **Posterior tibial neurostimulation, percutaneous needle electrode, single treatment, includes programming**
EXCLUDES *Electronic analysis implanted neurostimulator pulse generator system (95970-95972)*
Percutaneous implantation neurostimulator electrode array; peripheral nerve (64555)
Posterior tibial neurostimulation (0587T-0588T)
🚗 0.87 ⚕ 3.62 **FUD** 000   T P3 80 ▱
AMA: 2019,Feb,6; 2018,Oct,8; 2018,Jan,8; 2017,Jan,8; 2016,Jan,13

▲ **64568** **Open implantation of cranial nerve (eg, vagus nerve) neurostimulator electrode array and pulse generator**
EXCLUDES *Insertion, replacement cranial neurostimulator pulse generator or receiver (61885-61886)*
Removal neurostimulator electrode array and pulse generator (64570)
🚗 18.4 ⚕ 18.4 **FUD** 090   J J8 80 50 ▱
AMA: 2019,Feb,6; 2018,Mar,9; 2018,Jan,8; 2017,Jan,8; 2016,Nov,6; 2016,Jan,13

64569 **Revision or replacement of cranial nerve (eg, vagus nerve) neurostimulator electrode array, including connection to existing pulse generator**
EXCLUDES *Removal neurostimulator electrode array and pulse generator (64570)*
Replacement pulse generator (61885)
Revision, removal pulse generator (61888)
🚗 22.1 ⚕ 22.1 **FUD** 090   J J8 80 50 ▱
AMA: 2019,Feb,6; 2018,Mar,9; 2018,Jan,8; 2017,Jan,8; 2016,Nov,6; 2016,Jan,13

64570 **Removal of cranial nerve (eg, vagus nerve) neurostimulator electrode array and pulse generator**
EXCLUDES *Laparoscopic revision, replacement, removal, or implantation vagus nerve blocking neurostimulator pulse generator and/or electrode array at esophagogastric junction (0312T-0317T)*
Revision, removal pulse generator (61888)
🚗 21.4 ⚕ 21.4 **FUD** 090   02 62 80 50 ▱
AMA: 2019,Feb,6; 2018,Mar,9; 2018,Jan,8; 2017,Jan,8; 2016,Nov,6; 2016,Jan,13

64575-64595 Implantation/Revision/Removal Neurostimulators: Incisional

INCLUDES Simple and complex neurostimulators
EXCLUDES *Analysis and programming neurostimulator pulse generator (95970-95972, 0589T-0590T)*

▲ **64575** **Open implantation of neurostimulator electrode array; peripheral nerve (excludes sacral nerve)**
EXCLUDES *Posterior tibial neurostimulation (0587T-0588T)*
🚗 9.80 ⚕ 9.80 **FUD** 090   J J8 ▱
AMA: 2019,Feb,6

▲ **64580** **neuromuscular**
🚗 8.97 ⚕ 8.97 **FUD** 090   J J8 80 ▱
AMA: 2019,Feb,6

▲ **64581** **sacral nerve (transforaminal placement)**
🚗 19.0 ⚕ 19.0 **FUD** 090   J J8 ▱
AMA: 2019,Feb,6; 2018,Jan,8; 2017,Jan,8; 2016,Jan,13

● **64582** **Open implantation of hypoglossal nerve neurostimulator array, pulse generator, and distal respiratory sensor electrode or electrode array**

● **64583** **Revision or replacement of hypoglossal nerve neurostimulator array and distal respiratory sensor electrode or electrode array, including connection to existing pulse generator**
EXCLUDES *Implantation neurostimulator array (64582)*
Removal neurostimulator array, pulse generator, and distal respiratory sensor (64584)
Replacement pulse generator (61886)
Code also modifier 52 for revision or replacement of neurostimulator array or distal respiratory sensor only

● **64584** **Removal of hypoglossal nerve neurostimulator array, pulse generator, and distal respiratory sensor electrode or electrode array**
Code also modifier 52 for removal of only one or two components

64585 **Revision or removal of peripheral neurostimulator electrode array**
🚗 4.14 ⚕ 7.03 **FUD** 010   02 A2 ▱
AMA: 2019,Feb,6

Nervous System

64590   —   64612

64590   **Insertion or replacement of peripheral or gastric neurostimulator pulse generator or receiver, direct or inductive coupling**

> **EXCLUDES** *Posterior tibial neurostimulation (0587T-0588T)*
> *Revision, removal neurostimulator pulse generator (64595)*

📋 4.64   ✂ 7.60   **FUD** 010   J J8 ▭

AMA: 2019,Feb,6; 2018,Aug,10; 2018,Jan,8; 2017,Dec,13; 2017,Jan,8; 2016,Jan,13

64595   **Revision or removal of peripheral or gastric neurostimulator pulse generator or receiver**

> **EXCLUDES** *Insertion, replacement neurostimulator pulse generator (64590)*

📋 3.63   ✂ 6.89   **FUD** 010   Q2 A2 ▭

AMA: 2019,Feb,6; 2018,Jan,8; 2017,Jan,8; 2016,Jan,13

64600-64610 Chemical Denervation Trigeminal Nerve

INCLUDES Injection therapeutic medication
EXCLUDES *Electromyography or muscle electric stimulation guidance (95873-95874)*
Nerve destruction:
   Anal sphincter (46505)
   Bladder (52287)
   Strabismus involving extraocular muscles (67345)
   Treatments that do not destroy target nerve (64999)
Code also chemodenervation agent

64600   **Destruction by neurolytic agent, trigeminal nerve; supraorbital, infraorbital, mental, or inferior alveolar branch**

📋 6.66   ✂ 12.3   **FUD** 010   T A2 ▭

AMA: 2020,Dec,13; 2019,Apr,9; 2018,Jan,8; 2017,Jan,8; 2016,Jan,13

64605   **second and third division branches at foramen ovale**

📋 10.0   ✂ 16.8   **FUD** 010   J A2 80 50 ▭

AMA: 2020,Dec,13; 2019,Apr,9; 2018,Jan,8; 2017,Jan,8; 2016,Jan,13

64610   **second and third division branches at foramen ovale under radiologic monitoring**

📋 14.2   ✂ 22.0   **FUD** 010   J A2 50 ▭

AMA: 2020,Dec,13; 2019,Apr,9; 2018,Jan,8; 2017,Apr,9; 2017,Jan,8; 2016,Jan,13

64624 [64624] Chemical Denervation Genicular Nerve Branches

**64624**   **Destruction by neurolytic agent, genicular nerve branches including imaging guidance, when performed**

> **EXCLUDES** *Injection genicular nerve branches (64454)*

Code also modifier 52 for destruction fewer than all genicular nerve branches: superolateral, superomedial, and inferomedial

📋 4.23   ✂ 11.5   **FUD** 010   G2 80 50 ▭

AMA: 2020,Dec,13; 2019,Dec,8

64625-64629 [64625, 64628, 64629] Radiofrequency Ablation Sacroiliac Joint Nerves

**64625**   **Radiofrequency ablation, nerves innervating the sacroiliac joint, with image guidance (ie, fluoroscopy or computed tomography)**

> **INCLUDES** CT needle guidance (77012)
> Electrical stimulation or needle electromyelograph for guidance (95873-95874)
> Fluoroscopic needle guidance or localization (77002-77003)
> **EXCLUDES** *Destruction by neurolytic agent, paravertebral facet joint nerve ([64635])*
> *Radiofrequency ablation with ultrasound (76999)*

📋 5.59   ✂ 14.1   **FUD** 010   G2 50 ▭

AMA: 2020,Dec,13; 2020,Jun,14; 2019,Dec,8

● **#** **64628**   **Thermal destruction of intraosseous basivertebral nerve, including all imaging guidance; first 2 vertebral bodies, lumbar or sacral**

> **INCLUDES** CT needle guidance (77012)
> Fluoroscopic needle guidance and localization (77003)

📋 0.00   ✂ 0.00   **FUD** 000

● + **#** **64629**   **each additional vertebral body, lumbar or sacral (List separately in addition to code for primary procedure)**

> **INCLUDES** CT needle guidance (77012)
> Fluoroscopic needle guidance and localization (77003)

Code first ([64628])

📋 0.00   ✂ 0.00   **FUD** 000

64611-64617 Chemical Denervation Procedures Head and Neck

INCLUDES Injection therapeutic medication
EXCLUDES *Electromyography or muscle electric stimulation guidance (95873-95874)*
Nerve destruction:
   Anal sphincter (46505)
   Bladder (52287)
   Extraocular muscles to treat strabismus (67345)
   Treatments that do not destroy target nerve (64999)

64611   **Chemodenervation of parotid and submandibular salivary glands, bilateral**

Code also modifier 52 for injection of fewer than four salivary glands

📋 3.03   ✂ 3.45   **FUD** 010   T P3 80 ▭

AMA: 2020,Dec,13; 2019,Apr,9; 2018,Jan,8; 2017,Jan,8; 2016,Jan,13

64612   **Chemodenervation of muscle(s); muscle(s) innervated by facial nerve, unilateral (eg, for blepharospasm, hemifacial spasm)**

📋 3.39   ✂ 3.83   **FUD** 010   T P3 50 ▭

AMA: 2020,Dec,13; 2019,Apr,9; 2018,Jan,8; 2017,Jan,8; 2016,Jan,13

64615   **muscle(s) innervated by facial, trigeminal, cervical spinal and accessory nerves, bilateral (eg, for chronic migraine)**

> *EXCLUDES*   *Chemodenervation (64612, 64616-64617, 64642-64647)*
> *Procedure performed more than one time per session*
> Code also any guidance by muscle electrical stimulation or needle electromyography but report only once (95873-95874)

📷 3.58   ⚖ 4.27   **FUD** 010   T P3 🔲

AMA: 2020,Dec,13; 2019,Apr,9; 2018,Jan,8; 2017,Jan,8; 2016,Jan,13

64616   **neck muscle(s), excluding muscles of the larynx, unilateral (eg, for cervical dystonia, spasmodic torticollis)**

> Code also guidance by muscle electrical stimulation or needle electromyography, but report only once (95873-95874)

📷 3.18   ⚖ 3.80   **FUD** 010   T P3 50 🔲

AMA: 2020,Dec,13; 2019,Apr,9; 2018,Jan,8; 2017,Jan,8; 2016,Jan,13

64617   **larynx, unilateral, percutaneous (eg, for spasmodic dysphonia), includes guidance by needle electromyography, when performed**

> *EXCLUDES*   *Chemodenervation larynx via direct laryngoscopy (31570-31571)*
> *Diagnostic needle electromyography larynx (95865)*
> *Electrical stimulation guidance for chemodenervation (95873-95874)*

📷 3.14   ⚖ 4.62   **FUD** 010   T P3 50 🔲

AMA: 2020,Dec,13; 2019,Apr,9; 2018,Jan,8; 2017,Jan,8; 2016,Jan,13

64620-64640 [64624, 64625, 64628, 64629, 64633, 64634, 64635, 64636] Chemical Denervation Intercostal, Facet Joint, Plantar, and Pudendal Nerve(s)

> *INCLUDES*   Injection therapeutic medication

64620   **Destruction by neurolytic agent, intercostal nerve**

📷 5.00   ⚖ 5.91   **FUD** 010   T A2 🔲

AMA: 2020,Dec,13; 2019,Nov,14; 2019,Apr,9; 2018,Jan,8; 2017,Jan,8; 2016,Jan,13

64624   **Resequenced code. See code following 64610.**

64625   **Resequenced code. See code before 64611.**

64628   **Resequenced code. See code before 64611.**

64629   **Resequenced code. See code before 64611.**

\#   **64633**   **Destruction by neurolytic agent, paravertebral facet joint nerve(s), with imaging guidance (fluoroscopy or CT); cervical or thoracic, single facet joint**

> *INCLUDES*   Paravertebral facet destruction T12-L1 joint or nerve(s) that innervate joint
> Radiological guidance (77003, 77012)
> *EXCLUDES*   *Denervation performed using chemical, low grade thermal, or pulsed radiofrequency methods (64999)*
> *Destruction paravertebral facet joint nerve(s) without imaging guidance (64999)*

📷 6.43   ⚖ 11.8   **FUD** 010   J 62 50 🔲

AMA: 2020,Dec,13; 2019,Apr,9; 2018,Jan,8; 2017,Jan,8; 2016,Jan,13

+ \#   **64634**   **cervical or thoracic, each additional facet joint (List separately in addition to code for primary procedure)**

> *INCLUDES*   Radiological guidance (77003, 77012)
> *EXCLUDES*   *Denervation performed using chemical, low grade thermal, or pulsed radiofrequency methods (64999)*
> *Destruction paravertebral facet joint nerve(s) without imaging guidance (64999)*
> *Reporting with modifier 50. Report once for each side when performed bilaterally*
> Code first ([64633])

📷 1.95   ⚖ 5.34   **FUD** ZZZ   N N1 🔲

AMA: 2020,Dec,13; 2019,Apr,9; 2018,Jan,8; 2017,Jan,8; 2016,Jan,13

\#   **64635**   **lumbar or sacral, single facet joint**

> *INCLUDES*   Radiological guidance (77003, 77012)
> *EXCLUDES*   *Denervation performed using chemical, low grade thermal, or pulsed radiofrequency methods (64999)*
> *Destruction individual nerves, sacroiliac joint, by neurolytic agent (64640)*
> *Destruction paravertebral facet joint nerve(s) without imaging guidance (64999)*

📷 6.34   ⚖ 11.7   **FUD** 010   J 62 50 🔲

AMA: 2020,Dec,13; 2020,May,13; 2019,Dec,8; 2019,Apr,9; 2018,Jan,8; 2017,Jan,8; 2016,Jan,13

+ \#   **64636**   **lumbar or sacral, each additional facet joint (List separately in addition to code for primary procedure)**

> *INCLUDES*   Radiological guidance (77003, 77012)
> *EXCLUDES*   *Denervation performed using chemical, low grade thermal, or pulsed radiofrequency methods (64999)*
> *Destruction individual nerves, sacroiliac joint, by neurolytic agent (64640)*
> *Destruction paravertebral facet joint nerve(s) without imaging guidance (64999)*
> *Radiofrequency ablation nerves innervating sacroiliac joint with imaging ([64625])*
> *Reporting with modifier 50. Report once for each side when performed bilaterally*
> Code first ([64635])

📷 1.71   ⚖ 4.85   **FUD** ZZZ   N N1 🔲

AMA: 2020,Dec,13; 2020,May,13; 2019,Apr,9; 2018,Jan,8; 2017,Jan,8; 2016,Jan,13

64630   **Destruction by neurolytic agent; pudendal nerve**

📷 5.47   ⚖ 6.77   **FUD** 010   T A2 80 🔲

AMA: 2020,Dec,13; 2019,Apr,9; 2018,Jan,8; 2017,Oct,9; 2017,Jan,8; 2016,Jan,13

64632   **plantar common digital nerve**

> *EXCLUDES*   *Injection(s), anesthetic agent and/or steroid (64455)*

📷 1.96   ⚖ 2.45   **FUD** 010   T P3 80 50 🔲

AMA: 2020,Dec,13; 2019,Apr,9; 2018,Jan,8; 2017,Oct,9; 2017,Jan,8; 2016,Jan,13

64633   **Resequenced code. See code following 64620.**

64634   **Resequenced code. See code following 64620.**

64635   **Resequenced code. See code following 64620.**

64636   **Resequenced code. See code before 64630.**

64640   **other peripheral nerve or branch**

> *INCLUDES*   Neurolytic destruction of nerves of sacroiliac joint

📷 2.69   ⚖ 3.86   **FUD** 010   T P3 50 🔲

AMA: 2020,Dec,13; 2019,Apr,9; 2018,Jan,8; 2018,Jan,7; 2017,Oct,9; 2017,Jan,8; 2016,Jan,13

64642-64645 Chemical Denervation Extremity Muscles

> *INCLUDES*   Somatic muscles except the erector spinae, paraspinal, rectus abdominus, or oblique trunk muscles
> *EXCLUDES*   *Chemodenervation with needle-guided electromyography or with guidance provided by muscle electrical stimulation (95873-95874)*
> *Procedure performed more than once per extremity*
> Code also other extremities when appropriate, up to total four units per patient (when all extremities injected) (64642-64645)

64642   **Chemodenervation of one extremity; 1-4 muscle(s)**

> *EXCLUDES*   *Reporting more than one base code per session (64642)*

📷 3.12   ⚖ 4.15   **FUD** 000   T P3 🔲

AMA: 2019,Aug,10; 2019,Apr,9; 2018,Jan,8; 2017,Jan,8; 2016,Jan,13

+   **64643**   **each additional extremity, 1-4 muscle(s) (List separately in addition to code for primary procedure)**

> Code first (64642, 64644)

📷 2.08   ⚖ 2.65   **FUD** ZZZ   N N1 🔲

AMA: 2019,Aug,10; 2019,Apr,9; 2018,Jan,8; 2017,Jan,8; 2016,Jan,13

Nervous System

64644 — 64760

64644   **Chemodenervation of one extremity; 5 or more muscles**

> EXCLUDES   *Reporting more than one base code per session (64644)*
>
> 3.42   4.82   **FUD** 000   T P3
>
> **AMA:** 2019,Aug,10; 2019,Apr,9; 2018,Jan,8; 2017,Jan,8; 2016,Jan,13

+ 64645   **each additional extremity, 5 or more muscles (List separately in addition to code for primary procedure)**

> Code first (64644)
>
> 2.40   3.33   **FUD** ZZZ   N N1
>
> **AMA:** 2019,Aug,10; 2019,Apr,9; 2018,Jan,8; 2017,Jan,8; 2016,Jan,13

64646-64647 Chemical Denervation Trunk Muscles

> INCLUDES   Trunk muscles include erector spinae, paraspinal, rectus abdominus and oblique muscles
>
> EXCLUDES   *Procedure performed more than once per session*

64646   **Chemodenervation of trunk muscle(s); 1-5 muscle(s)**

> 3.34   4.35   **FUD** 000   T P3
>
> **AMA:** 2019,Apr,9; 2018,Jan,8; 2017,Jan,8; 2016,Jan,13

64647   **6 or more muscles**

> 3.96   5.12   **FUD** 000   T P3
>
> **AMA:** 2019,Apr,9; 2018,Jan,8; 2017,Jan,8; 2016,Jan,13

64650-64653 Chemical Denervation Eccrine Glands

> INCLUDES   Injection therapeutic medication
>
> EXCLUDES   *Bladder chemodenervation (52287)*
>   *Chemodenervation extremities (64999)*
>
> Code also drugs or other substances used

64650   **Chemodenervation of eccrine glands; both axillae**

> 1.21   2.25   **FUD** 000   T P3 80
>
> **AMA:** 2019,Apr,9; 2018,Jan,8; 2017,Jan,8; 2016,Jan,13

64653   **other area(s) (eg, scalp, face, neck), per day**

> 1.55   2.76   **FUD** 000   T P3 80
>
> **AMA:** 2019,Apr,9; 2018,Jan,8; 2017,Jan,8; 2016,Jan,13

64680-64681 Neurolysis: Celiac Plexus, Superior Hypogastric Plexus

> INCLUDES   Injection therapeutic medication

64680   **Destruction by neurolytic agent, with or without radiologic monitoring; celiac plexus**

> EXCLUDES   *Transmural neurolytic agent injection with transendoscopic ultrasound guidance (43253)*
>
> 4.66   9.07   **FUD** 010   T A2
>
> **AMA:** 2019,Apr,9; 2018,Jan,8; 2017,Jan,8; 2016,Jan,13

64681   **superior hypogastric plexus**

> 7.87   16.4   **FUD** 010   T A2
>
> **AMA:** 2019,Apr,9; 2018,Jan,8; 2017,Jan,8; 2016,Jan,13

64702-64727 Decompression and/or Transposition of Nerve

> INCLUDES   External neurolysis and/or transposition to repair or restore nerve
>   Neuroplasty with nerve wrapping
>   Surgical decompression/freeing nerve from scar tissue
>
> EXCLUDES   *Facial nerve decompression (69720)*
>   *Percutaneous neurolysis (62263-62264, 62280-62282)*
>   *Reporting with tissue expander insertion (11960)*

64702   **Neuroplasty; digital, 1 or both, same digit**

> 14.3   14.3   **FUD** 090   J A2
>
> **AMA:** 2018,Jan,8; 2017,Jan,8; 2016,Jan,13

64704   **nerve of hand or foot**

> 9.23   9.23   **FUD** 090   J A2 80
>
> **AMA:** 2018,Jan,8; 2017,Jan,8; 2016,Jan,13

64708   **Neuroplasty, major peripheral nerve, arm or leg, open; other than specified**

> 14.4   14.4   **FUD** 090   J G2 80
>
> **AMA:** 2018,Jan,8; 2017,Nov,10; 2016,Jan,13

64712   **sciatic nerve**

> 16.7   16.7   **FUD** 090   J G2 80 50
>
> **AMA:** 2018,Jan,8; 2017,Jan,8; 2016,Jan,13

64713   **brachial plexus**

> 22.1   22.1   **FUD** 090   J G2 80 50
>
> **AMA:** 2018,Jan,8; 2017,Jan,8; 2016,Jan,13

64714   **lumbar plexus**

> 20.8   20.8   **FUD** 090   J G2 80 50
>
> **AMA:** 2018,Jan,8; 2017,Jan,8; 2016,Jan,13

64716   **Neuroplasty and/or transposition; cranial nerve (specify)**

> 15.0   15.0   **FUD** 090   J A2 80
>
> **AMA:** 2018,Jan,8; 2017,Jan,8; 2016,Jan,13

64718   **ulnar nerve at elbow**

> 17.0   17.0   **FUD** 090   J A2 80 50
>
> **AMA:** 2020,Jun,14; 2018,Jan,8; 2017,Jan,8; 2016,Jan,13

64719   **ulnar nerve at wrist**

> 11.5   11.5   **FUD** 090   J A2 50
>
> **AMA:** 2018,Jan,8; 2017,Jan,8; 2016,Jan,13

64721   **median nerve at carpal tunnel**

> EXCLUDES   *Endoscopic procedure (29848)*
>
> 12.3   12.4   **FUD** 090   J A2 50
>
> **AMA:** 2018,Jan,8; 2017,Jan,8; 2016,Jan,13

64722   **Decompression; unspecified nerve(s) (specify)**

> 10.3   10.3   **FUD** 090   J A2 80
>
> **AMA:** 2018,Jan,8; 2017,Jan,8; 2016,Jan,13

64726   **plantar digital nerve**

> 7.80   7.80   **FUD** 090   J A2
>
> **AMA:** 2018,Jan,8; 2017,Jan,8; 2016,Jan,13

+ 64727   **Internal neurolysis, requiring use of operating microscope (List separately in addition to code for neuroplasty) (Neuroplasty includes external neurolysis)**

> INCLUDES   Operating microscope (69990)
>
> Code first neuroplasty (64702-64721)
>
> 5.31   5.31   **FUD** ZZZ   N N1
>
> **AMA:** 2018,Jan,8; 2017,Jan,8; 2016,Feb,12; 2016,Jan,13

64732-64772 Surgical Avulsion/Transection of Nerve

> EXCLUDES   *Stereotactic lesion gasserian ganglion (61790)*

64732   **Transection or avulsion of; supraorbital nerve**

> 12.8   12.8   **FUD** 090   J A2 80 50
>
> **AMA:** 2018,Jan,8; 2017,Jan,8; 2016,Jan,13

64734   **infraorbital nerve**

> 14.5   14.5   **FUD** 090   J A2 80 50
>
> **AMA:** 2014,Jan,11

64736   **mental nerve**

> 10.0   10.0   **FUD** 090   J A2 80 50
>
> **AMA:** 2014,Jan,11

64738   **inferior alveolar nerve by osteotomy**

> 13.3   13.3   **FUD** 090   J A2 80 50
>
> **AMA:** 2014,Jan,11

64740   **lingual nerve**

> 14.0   14.0   **FUD** 090   J A2 80 50
>
> **AMA:** 2014,Jan,11

64742   **facial nerve, differential or complete**

> 14.1   14.1   **FUD** 090   J A2 80 50
>
> **AMA:** 2014,Jan,11

64744   **greater occipital nerve**

> 14.2   14.2   **FUD** 090   J A2 80 50
>
> **AMA:** 2014,Jan,11

64746   **phrenic nerve**

> 12.4   12.4   **FUD** 090   J A2 80 50
>
> **AMA:** 2014,Jan,11

64755   **vagus nerves limited to proximal stomach (selective proximal vagotomy, proximal gastric vagotomy, parietal cell vagotomy, supra- or highly selective vagotomy)**

> EXCLUDES   *Laparoscopic procedure (43652)*
>
> 26.3   26.3   **FUD** 090   C 80
>
> **AMA:** 2018,Jan,8; 2017,Jan,8; 2016,Jan,13

64760   **vagus nerve (vagotomy), abdominal**

> EXCLUDES   *Laparoscopic procedure (43651)*
>
> 14.9   14.9   **FUD** 090   C 80
>
> **AMA:** 2018,Jan,8; 2017,Jan,8; 2016,Jan,13

26/TC PC/TC Only   A2-Z3 ASC Payment   50 Bilateral   ♂ Male Only   ♀ Female Only   Facility RVU   Non-Facility RVU   CCI   CLIA

FUD Follow-up Days   **CMS:** IOM   **AMA:** CPT Asst   A-Y OPPSI   80/80 Surg Assist Allowed / w/Doc   Lab Crosswalk   Radiology Crosswalk

64763 Transection or avulsion of obturator nerve, extrapelvic, with or without adductor tenotomy
🔧 14.7 ⚕ 14.7 **FUD** 090   J G2 80 50 ▭
AMA: 2014,Jan,11

64766 Transection or avulsion of obturator nerve, intrapelvic, with or without adductor tenotomy
🔧 17.8 ⚕ 17.8 **FUD** 090   J G2 80 50 ▭
AMA: 2014,Jan,11

64771 Transection or avulsion of other cranial nerve, extradural
🔧 17.0 ⚕ 17.0 **FUD** 090   J A2 80 ▭
AMA: 2014,Jan,11

64772 Transection or avulsion of other spinal nerve, extradural
EXCLUDES   Removal tender scar and soft tissue including neuroma when necessary (11400-11446, 13100-13153)
🔧 16.2 ⚕ 16.2 **FUD** 090   J A2 80 ▭
AMA: 2018,Jan,8; 2017,Jan,8; 2016,Jan,13

64774-64823 Excisional Nerve Procedures
EXCLUDES   Morton neuroma excision (28080)

64774 Excision of neuroma; cutaneous nerve, surgically identifiable
🔧 11.7 ⚕ 11.7 **FUD** 090   J A2 ▭
AMA: 2014,Jan,11

64776 digital nerve, 1 or both, same digit
🔧 11.1 ⚕ 11.1 **FUD** 090   J A2 80 ▭
AMA: 2014,Jan,11

+ **64778** digital nerve, each additional digit (List separately in addition to code for primary procedure)
Code first (64776)
🔧 5.30 ⚕ 5.30 **FUD** ZZZ   N N1 ▭
AMA: 2014,Jan,11

64782 hand or foot, except digital nerve
🔧 13.2 ⚕ 13.2 **FUD** 090   J A2 ▭
AMA: 2014,Jan,11

+ **64783** hand or foot, each additional nerve, except same digit (List separately in addition to code for primary procedure)
Code first (64782)
🔧 6.33 ⚕ 6.33 **FUD** ZZZ   N N1 ▭
AMA: 2014,Jan,11

64784 major peripheral nerve, except sciatic
🔧 20.9 ⚕ 20.9 **FUD** 090   J A2 80 ▭
AMA: 2014,Jan,11

64786 sciatic nerve
🔧 28.9 ⚕ 28.9 **FUD** 090   J A2 80 50 ▭
AMA: 2014,Jan,11

+ **64787** Implantation of nerve end into bone or muscle (List separately in addition to neuroma excision)
Code also, when appropriate (64774-64786)
🔧 6.96 ⚕ 6.96 **FUD** ZZZ   N N1 80 ▭
AMA: 2014,Jan,11

64788 Excision of neurofibroma or neurolemmoma; cutaneous nerve
🔧 11.5 ⚕ 11.5 **FUD** 090   J A2 ▭
AMA: 2018,Jan,8; 2017,Jan,8; 2016,Apr,3

64790 major peripheral nerve
🔧 24.1 ⚕ 24.1 **FUD** 090   J A2 80 ▭
AMA: 2018,Jan,8; 2017,Jan,8; 2016,Apr,3

64792 extensive (including malignant type)
EXCLUDES   Destruction neurofibroma skin (0419T-0420T)
🔧 31.4 ⚕ 31.4 **FUD** 090   J A2 80 ▭
AMA: 2018,Jan,8; 2017,Jan,8; 2016,Apr,3

64795 Biopsy of nerve
🔧 5.64 ⚕ 5.64 **FUD** 000   J A2 ▭
AMA: 2014,Jan,11

64802 Sympathectomy, cervical
🔧 24.3 ⚕ 24.3 **FUD** 090   J A2 80 50 ▭
AMA: 2014,Jan,11

64804 Sympathectomy, cervicothoracic
🔧 34.1 ⚕ 34.1 **FUD** 090   J G2 80 50 ▭
AMA: 2014,Jan,11

64809 Sympathectomy, thoracolumbar
INCLUDES   Leriche sympathectomy
🔧 31.0 ⚕ 31.0 **FUD** 090   C 80 50 ▭
AMA: 2014,Jan,11

64818 Sympathectomy, lumbar
🔧 22.5 ⚕ 22.5 **FUD** 090   C 80 50 ▭
AMA: 2014,Jan,11

64820 Sympathectomy; digital arteries, each digit
INCLUDES   Operating microscope (69990)
🔧 20.5 ⚕ 20.5 **FUD** 090   J G2 ▭
AMA: 2018,Jan,8; 2017,Jan,8; 2016,Feb,12; 2016,Jan,13

64821 radial artery
INCLUDES   Operating microscope (69990)
🔧 20.0 ⚕ 20.0 **FUD** 090   J A2 50 ▭
AMA: 2016,Feb,12

64822 ulnar artery
INCLUDES   Operating microscope (69990)
🔧 20.0 ⚕ 20.0 **FUD** 090   J G2 50 ▭
AMA: 2016,Feb,12

64823 superficial palmar arch
INCLUDES   Operating microscope (69990)
🔧 22.7 ⚕ 22.7 **FUD** 090   J G2 50 ▭
AMA: 2016,Feb,12

64831-64907 Nerve Repair: Suture and Nerve Grafts

64831 Suture of digital nerve, hand or foot; 1 nerve
🔧 19.7 ⚕ 19.7 **FUD** 090   J A2 50 ▭
AMA: 2018,Jan,8; 2017,Jan,8; 2016,Jan,13

+ **64832** each additional digital nerve (List separately in addition to code for primary procedure)
Code first (64831)
🔧 9.73 ⚕ 9.73 **FUD** ZZZ   N N1 80 ▭
AMA: 2018,Jan,8; 2017,Jan,8; 2016,Jan,13

64834 Suture of 1 nerve; hand or foot, common sensory nerve
🔧 21.3 ⚕ 21.3 **FUD** 090   J A2 80 50 ▭
AMA: 2014,Jan,11

64835 median motor thenar
🔧 23.5 ⚕ 23.5 **FUD** 090   J A2 80 50 ▭
AMA: 2014,Jan,11

64836 ulnar motor
🔧 23.5 ⚕ 23.5 **FUD** 090   J A2 80 50 ▭
AMA: 2014,Jan,11

+ **64837** Suture of each additional nerve, hand or foot (List separately in addition to code for primary procedure)
Code first (64834-64836)
🔧 10.6 ⚕ 10.6 **FUD** ZZZ   N N1 80 ▭
AMA: 2014,Jan,11

64840 Suture of posterior tibial nerve
🔧 27.8 ⚕ 27.8 **FUD** 090   J A2 80 50 ▭
AMA: 2014,Jan,11

64856 Suture of major peripheral nerve, arm or leg, except sciatic; including transposition
🔧 29.2 ⚕ 29.2 **FUD** 090   J A2 ▭
AMA: 2014,Jan,11

64857 without transposition
🔧 30.4 ⚕ 30.4 **FUD** 090   J A2 80 ▭
AMA: 2014,Jan,11

64858 Suture of sciatic nerve
🔧 34.0 ⚕ 34.0 **FUD** 090   J J8 80 50 ▭
AMA: 2014,Jan,11

● New Code   ▲ Revised Code   ○ Reinstated   ● New Web Release   ▲ Revised Web Release   + Add-on   Unlisted   Not Covered   # Resequenced
50 Optum Mod 50 Exempt   ⊘ AMA Mod 51 Exempt   51 Optum Mod 51 Exempt   63 Mod 63 Exempt   ⫫ Non-FDA Drug   ★ Telemedicine   M Maternity   A Age Edit

Nervous System

64859 — 64911

+ **64859** Suture of each additional major peripheral nerve (List separately in addition to code for primary procedure)
Code first (64856-64857)
🔧 7.23 ⚕ 7.23 **FUD** ZZZ   N N1 80 ▣
AMA: 2014,Jan,11

64861 Suture of; brachial plexus
🔧 44.5 ⚕ 44.5 **FUD** 090   J A2 80 50 ▣
AMA: 2014,Jan,11

64862 lumbar plexus
🔧 39.8 ⚕ 39.8 **FUD** 090   J A2 80 50 ▣
AMA: 2014,Jan,11

64864 Suture of facial nerve; extracranial
🔧 24.8 ⚕ 24.8 **FUD** 090   J A2 80 ▣
AMA: 2014,Jan,11

64865 infratemporal, with or without grafting
🔧 31.4 ⚕ 31.4 **FUD** 090   J A2 80 ▣
AMA: 2014,Jan,11

64866 Anastomosis; facial-spinal accessory
🔧 36.7 ⚕ 36.7 **FUD** 090   C 80 ▣
AMA: 2014,Jan,11

64868 facial-hypoglossal
INCLUDES   Korte-Ballance anastomosis
🔧 28.8 ⚕ 28.8 **FUD** 090   C 80 ▣
AMA: 2014,Jan,11

+ **64872** Suture of nerve; requiring secondary or delayed suture (List separately in addition to code for primary neurorrhaphy)
Code first (64831-64865)
🔧 3.39 ⚕ 3.39 **FUD** ZZZ   N N1 80 ▣
AMA: 2014,Jan,11

+ **64874** requiring extensive mobilization, or transposition of nerve (List separately in addition to code for nerve suture)
Code first (64831-64865)
🔧 5.05 ⚕ 5.05 **FUD** ZZZ   N N1 80 ▣
AMA: 2014,Jan,11

+ **64876** requiring shortening of bone of extremity (List separately in addition to code for nerve suture)
Code first (64831-64865)
🔧 5.71 ⚕ 5.71 **FUD** ZZZ   N N1 80 ▣
AMA: 2014,Jan,11; 2003,Jan,1

64885 Nerve graft (includes obtaining graft), head or neck; up to 4 cm in length
🔧 32.1 ⚕ 32.1 **FUD** 090   J A2 80 ▣
AMA: 2018,Jan,8; 2017,Dec,12; 2017,Jan,8; 2016,Jan,13

64886 more than 4 cm length
🔧 37.2 ⚕ 37.2 **FUD** 090   J J8 80 ▣
AMA: 2018,Jan,8; 2017,Dec,12; 2017,Jan,8; 2016,Jan,13

64890 Nerve graft (includes obtaining graft), single strand, hand or foot; up to 4 cm length
🔧 31.2 ⚕ 31.2 **FUD** 090   J A2 80 ▣
AMA: 2018,Jan,8; 2017,Dec,12; 2017,Jan,8; 2016,Jan,13

64891 more than 4 cm length
🔧 33.2 ⚕ 33.2 **FUD** 090   J J8 80 ▣
AMA: 2018,Jan,8; 2017,Dec,12

64892 Nerve graft (includes obtaining graft), single strand, arm or leg; up to 4 cm length
🔧 30.4 ⚕ 30.4 **FUD** 090   J A2 80 ▣
AMA: 2018,Jan,8; 2017,Dec,12

64893 more than 4 cm length
🔧 32.4 ⚕ 32.4 **FUD** 090   J G2 80 ▣
AMA: 2018,Jan,8; 2017,Dec,12

64895 Nerve graft (includes obtaining graft), multiple strands (cable), hand or foot; up to 4 cm length
🔧 38.4 ⚕ 38.4 **FUD** 090   J A2 80 ▣
AMA: 2018,Jan,8; 2017,Dec,12; 2017,Jan,8; 2016,Jan,13

64896 more than 4 cm length
🔧 41.4 ⚕ 41.4 **FUD** 090   J A2 80 ▣
AMA: 2018,Jan,8; 2017,Dec,12; 2017,Jan,8; 2016,Jan,13

64897 Nerve graft (includes obtaining graft), multiple strands (cable), arm or leg; up to 4 cm length
🔧 36.7 ⚕ 36.7 **FUD** 090   J G2 80 ▣
AMA: 2018,Jan,8; 2017,Dec,12; 2017,Jan,8; 2016,Jan,13

64898 more than 4 cm length
🔧 39.7 ⚕ 39.7 **FUD** 090   J A2 80 ▣
AMA: 2018,Jan,8; 2017,Dec,12; 2017,Jan,8; 2016,Jan,13

+ **64901** Nerve graft, each additional nerve; single strand (List separately in addition to code for primary procedure)
Code first (64885-64893)
🔧 17.4 ⚕ 17.4 **FUD** ZZZ   N N1 80 ▣
AMA: 2018,Jan,8; 2017,Dec,12; 2017,Jan,8; 2016,Jan,13

+ **64902** multiple strands (cable) (List separately in addition to code for primary procedure)
Code first (64885-64886, 64895-64898)
🔧 20.1 ⚕ 20.1 **FUD** ZZZ   N N1 80 ▣
AMA: 2018,Jan,8; 2017,Dec,12; 2017,Jan,8; 2016,Jan,13

64905 Nerve pedicle transfer; first stage
🔧 29.4 ⚕ 29.4 **FUD** 090   J A2 80 ▣
AMA: 2018,Jan,8; 2017,Dec,12

64907 second stage
🔧 37.7 ⚕ 37.7 **FUD** 090   J A2 80 ▣
AMA: 2018,Jan,8; 2017,Dec,12

64910-64999 Nerve Repair: Synthetic and Vein Grafts

64910 Nerve repair; with synthetic conduit or vein allograft (eg, nerve tube), each nerve
INCLUDES   Operating microscope (69990)
🔧 22.7 ⚕ 22.7 **FUD** 090   J J8 80 ▣
AMA: 2018,Jan,8; 2017,Dec,12; 2017,Jan,8; 2016,Jan,13

Damaged nerve

Healthy nerve

Artificial nerve conduit

A synthetic "bridge" is affixed to each end of a severed nerve with sutures
The procedure is performed using an operating microscope

64911 with autogenous vein graft (includes harvest of vein graft), each nerve
INCLUDES   Operating microscope (69990)
🔧 29.5 ⚕ 29.5 **FUD** 090   J G2 80 ▣
AMA: 2018,Jan,8; 2017,Dec,12; 2017,Jan,8; 2016,Jan,13

64912   **with nerve allograft, each nerve, first strand (cable)**

       [INCLUDES]   Operating microscope (69990)

       🚑 26.3   ⚕ 26.3   **FUD** 090   [J] [J8] [80] [▭]

       AMA: 2018,Jan,8; 2017,Dec,12

+   **64913**   **with nerve allograft, each additional strand (List separately in addition to code for primary procedure)**

       [INCLUDES]   Operating microscope (69990)

       Code first (64912)

       🚑 5.16   ⚕ 5.16   **FUD** ZZZ   [N] [N1] [80] [▭]

       AMA: 2018,Jan,8; 2017,Dec,12

64999   **Unlisted procedure, nervous system**

       🚑 0.00   ⚕ 0.00   **FUD** YYY   [T] [80]

       AMA: 2020,Dec,13; 2020,Jun,14; 2020,Feb,13; 2019,Dec,12; 2019,Jul,10; 2019,May,10; 2019,Apr,9; 2018,Dec,8; 2018,Dec,8; 2018,Oct,8; 2018,Oct,11; 2018,Aug,10; 2018,Mar,9; 2018,Jan,8; 2018,Jan,7; 2017,Dec,14; 2017,Dec,12; 2017,Dec,13; 2017,Jan,8; 2016,Nov,6; 2016,Oct,11; 2016,Feb,13; 2016,Jan,13

65091-65093 Surgical Removal of Eyeball Contents

INCLUDES Operating microscope (69990)

65091 **Evisceration of ocular contents; without implant**
⚕ 18.4 ⚕ 18.4 **FUD** 090   J A2 80 50 ▣
AMA: 2016,Feb,12

Evisceration involves removal of the contents of the eyeball: the vitreous; retina; choroid; lens; iris; and ciliary muscle. Only the scleral shell remains. A temporary or permanent implant is usually inserted

Enucleation involves severing the extraorbital muscles and optic nerve with removal of the eyeball. An implant is usually inserted and, if permanent, may involve attachment to the severed extraorbital muscles

65093 **with implant**
⚕ 19.3 ⚕ 19.3 **FUD** 090   J A2 50 ▣
AMA: 2016,Feb,12

65101-65105 Surgical Removal of Eyeball

INCLUDES Operating microscope (69990)
EXCLUDES Conjunctivoplasty following enucleation (68320-68328)

65101 **Enucleation of eye; without implant**
⚕ 21.3 ⚕ 21.3 **FUD** 090   J A2 50 ▣
AMA: 2016,Feb,12

65103 **with implant, muscles not attached to implant**
⚕ 23.3 ⚕ 23.3 **FUD** 090   J A2 50 ▣
AMA: 2016,Feb,12

65105 **with implant, muscles attached to implant**
⚕ 24.4 ⚕ 24.4 **FUD** 090   J A2 80 50 ▣
AMA: 2016,Feb,12

65110-65114 Surgical Removal of Orbital Contents

INCLUDES Operating microscope (69990)
EXCLUDES Free full thickness graft (15260-15261)
Repair more extensive than skin (67930-67975)
Skin graft (15120-15121)

65110 **Exenteration of orbit (does not include skin graft), removal of orbital contents; only**
⚕ 36.0 ⚕ 36.0 **FUD** 090   J A2 80 50 ▣
AMA: 2016,Feb,12

65112 **with therapeutic removal of bone**
⚕ 41.5 ⚕ 41.5 **FUD** 090   J A2 80 50 ▣
AMA: 2016,Feb,12

65114 **with muscle or myocutaneous flap**
⚕ 43.4 ⚕ 43.4 **FUD** 090   J A2 80 50 ▣
AMA: 2016,Feb,12

65125-65175 Implant Procedures: Insertion, Removal, and Revision

INCLUDES Ocular implant procedures (inside muscle cone)
Operating microscope (69990)
EXCLUDES Orbital implant insertion (outside muscle cone) (67550)
Orbital implant removal or revision (outside muscle cone) (67560)

65125 **Modification of ocular implant with placement or replacement of pegs (eg, drilling receptacle for prosthesis appendage) (separate procedure)**
⚕ 8.26 ⚕ 12.9 **FUD** 090   J 62 50 ▣
AMA: 2016,Feb,12

65130 **Insertion of ocular implant secondary; after evisceration, in scleral shell**
⚕ 21.1 ⚕ 21.1 **FUD** 090   J A2 50 ▣
AMA: 2016,Feb,12

65135 **after enucleation, muscles not attached to implant**
⚕ 21.4 ⚕ 21.4 **FUD** 090   J A2 50 ▣
AMA: 2016,Feb,12

65140 **after enucleation, muscles attached to implant**
⚕ 23.3 ⚕ 23.3 **FUD** 090   J A2 50 ▣
AMA: 2016,Feb,12

65150 **Reinsertion of ocular implant; with or without conjunctival graft**
⚕ 18.0 ⚕ 18.0 **FUD** 090   J A2 80 50 ▣
AMA: 2016,Feb,12

65155 **with use of foreign material for reinforcement and/or attachment of muscles to implant**
⚕ 25.6 ⚕ 25.6 **FUD** 090   J A2 50 ▣
AMA: 2016,Feb,12

65175 **Removal of ocular implant**
⚕ 19.0 ⚕ 19.0 **FUD** 090   J A2 50 ▣
AMA: 2016,Feb,12

65205-65265 Foreign Body Removal By Area of Eye

INCLUDES Operating microscope (69990)
EXCLUDES Removal foreign body:
Eyelid (67938)
Lacrimal system (68530)
Orbit:
Frontal approach (67413)
Lateral approach (67430)
Removal implant:
Anterior segment (65920)
Ocular (65175)
Orbital (67560)
Posterior segment (67120)

65205 **Removal of foreign body, external eye; conjunctival superficial**
📷 (70030, 76529)
⚕ 1.02 ⚕ 1.31 **FUD** 000   01 N1 50 ▣
AMA: 2018,Jan,8; 2017,Jan,8; 2016,Feb,12; 2016,Jan,13

65210 **conjunctival embedded (includes concretions), subconjunctival, or scleral nonperforating**
📷 (70030, 76529)
⚕ 1.04 ⚕ 1.30 **FUD** 000   01 N1 50 ▣
AMA: 2016,Feb,12

65220 **corneal, without slit lamp**
EXCLUDES Repair corneal wound with foreign body (65275)
📷 (70030, 76529)
⚕ 1.19 ⚕ 1.70 **FUD** 000   01 N1 50 ▣
AMA: 2018,Jan,8; 2017,Jan,8; 2016,Feb,12; 2016,Jan,13

65222 **corneal, with slit lamp**
EXCLUDES Repair corneal wound with foreign body (65275)
📷 (70030, 76529)
⚕ 1.46 ⚕ 1.93 **FUD** 000   01 N1 50 ▣
AMA: 2018,Jan,8; 2017,Jan,8; 2016,Feb,12; 2016,Jan,13

65235 **Removal of foreign body, intraocular; from anterior chamber of eye or lens**
EXCLUDES Removal implanted material from anterior segment (65920)
📷 (70030, 76529)
⚕ 20.2 ⚕ 20.2 **FUD** 090   J A2 80 50 ▣
AMA: 2018,Jan,8; 2017,Jan,8; 2016,Feb,12; 2016,Jan,13

65260 **from posterior segment, magnetic extraction, anterior or posterior route**
EXCLUDES Removal implanted material from posterior segment (67120)
📷 (70030, 76529)
⚕ 27.5 ⚕ 27.5 **FUD** 090   J A2 80 50 ▣
AMA: 2016,Feb,12

65265 **from posterior segment, nonmagnetic extraction**

> EXCLUDES   Removal implanted material from posterior segment
> (67120)
>
> ⊡ (70030, 76529)
>
> 🖥 30.9   ⚖ 30.9   **FUD** 090   [J] [A2] [80] [50] [▣]
>
> **AMA:** 2016,Feb,12

65270-65290 Laceration Repair External Eye

> INCLUDES   Conjunctival flap
> Operating microscope (69990)
> Restoration anterior chamber with air or saline injection
>
> EXCLUDES   Repair:
> Ciliary body or iris (66680)
> Eyelid laceration (12011-12018, 12051-12057, 13151-13160, 67930, 67935)
> Lacrimal system injury (68700)
> Surgical wound (66250)
> Treatment orbit fracture (21385-21408)

65270 **Repair of laceration; conjunctiva, with or without nonperforating laceration sclera, direct closure**

> 🖥 3.99   ⚖ 7.94   **FUD** 010   [J] [A2] [80] [50] [▣]
>
> **AMA:** 2018,Jan,8; 2017,Jan,8; 2016,Feb,12; 2016,Jan,13

65272 **conjunctiva, by mobilization and rearrangement, without hospitalization**

> 🖥 10.0   ⚖ 14.5   **FUD** 090   [J] [A2] [50] [▣]
>
> **AMA:** 2016,Feb,12

65273 **conjunctiva, by mobilization and rearrangement, with hospitalization**

> 🖥 10.8   ⚖ 10.8   **FUD** 090   [C] [50] [▣]
>
> **AMA:** 2016,Feb,12

65275 **cornea, nonperforating, with or without removal foreign body**

> 🖥 13.1   ⚖ 16.5   **FUD** 090   [J] [A2] [80] [50] [▣]
>
> **AMA:** 2016,Feb,12

65280 **cornea and/or sclera, perforating, not involving uveal tissue**

> EXCLUDES   Procedure performed for surgical wound repair
>
> 🖥 19.1   ⚖ 19.1   **FUD** 090   [J] [A2] [80] [50] [▣]
>
> **AMA:** 2018,Jan,8; 2017,Jan,8; 2016,Feb,12; 2016,Jan,13

65285 **cornea and/or sclera, perforating, with reposition or resection of uveal tissue**

> EXCLUDES   Procedure performed for surgical wound repair
>
> 🖥 31.4   ⚖ 31.4   **FUD** 090   [J] [A2] [50] [▣]
>
> **AMA:** 2018,Jan,8; 2017,Jan,8; 2016,Feb,12; 2016,Jan,13

65286 **application of tissue glue, wounds of cornea and/or sclera**

> 🖥 14.1   ⚖ 20.0   **FUD** 090   [J] [P3] [50] [▣]
>
> **AMA:** 2018,Jan,8; 2017,Jan,8; 2016,Feb,12; 2016,Jan,13

65290 **Repair of wound, extraocular muscle, tendon and/or Tenon's capsule**

> 🖥 13.9   ⚖ 13.9   **FUD** 090   [J] [A2] [50] [▣]
>
> **AMA:** 2016,Feb,12

65400-65600 Removal Corneal Lesions

> INCLUDES   Operating microscope (69990)

65400 **Excision of lesion, cornea (keratectomy, lamellar, partial), except pterygium**

> 🖥 17.0   ⚖ 19.4   **FUD** 090   [T] [A2] [50] [▣]
>
> **AMA:** 2018,Jan,8; 2017,Jan,8; 2016,Feb,12; 2016,Jan,13

65410 **Biopsy of cornea**

> 🖥 2.96   ⚖ 4.11   **FUD** 000   [J] [A2] [80] [50] [▣]
>
> **AMA:** 2018,Jan,8; 2017,Jan,8; 2016,Feb,12; 2016,Jan,13

65420 **Excision or transposition of pterygium; without graft**

> 🖥 10.6   ⚖ 15.0   **FUD** 090   [J] [A2] [50] [▣]
>
> **AMA:** 2018,Jan,8; 2017,Jan,8; 2016,Feb,12; 2016,Jan,13

The conjunctiva is subject to numerous acute and chronic irritations and disorders

Labels: Conjunctiva, Cornea, Lens, Posterior chamber, Iris, Anterior chamber, Pterygium

65426 **with graft**

> 🖥 13.6   ⚖ 18.7   **FUD** 090   [J] [A2] [50] [▣]
>
> **AMA:** 2018,May,10; 2018,Jan,8; 2017,Jan,8; 2016,Feb,12; 2016,Jan,13

65430 **Scraping of cornea, diagnostic, for smear and/or culture**

> 🖥 2.90   ⚖ 3.28   **FUD** 000   [01] [N1] [50] [▣]
>
> **AMA:** 2016,Feb,12

65435 **Removal of corneal epithelium; with or without chemocauterization (abrasion, curettage)**

> EXCLUDES   Collagen cross-linking, cornea (0402T)
>
> 🖥 1.98   ⚖ 2.33   **FUD** 000   [T] [P3] [50] [▣]
>
> **AMA:** 2018,Jan,8; 2017,Jan,8; 2016,Feb,12; 2016,Jan,13

65436 **with application of chelating agent (eg, EDTA)**

> 🖥 10.5   ⚖ 11.0   **FUD** 090   [J] [P3] [50] [▣]
>
> **AMA:** 2016,Feb,12

65450 **Destruction of lesion of cornea by cryotherapy, photocoagulation or thermocauterization**

> 🖥 9.15   ⚖ 9.30   **FUD** 090   [T] [62] [50] [▣]
>
> **AMA:** 2016,Feb,12

65600 **Multiple punctures of anterior cornea (eg, for corneal erosion, tattoo)**

> 🖥 9.61   ⚖ 11.7   **FUD** 090   [J] [P3] [50] [▣]
>
> **AMA:** 2016,Feb,12

65710-65757 Corneal Transplants

> **CMS:** 100-03,80.7 Refractive Keratoplasty
>
> INCLUDES   Operating microscope (69990)
>
> EXCLUDES   Computerized corneal topography (92025)
> Processing, preserving, and transporting corneal tissue (V2785)

65710 **Keratoplasty (corneal transplant); anterior lamellar**

> INCLUDES   Use and preparation fresh or preserved graft
>
> EXCLUDES   Refractive keratoplasty surgery (65760-65767)
>
> 🖥 31.7   ⚖ 31.7   **FUD** 090   [J] [A2] [80] [50] [▣]
>
> **AMA:** 2018,Jan,8; 2017,Jan,8; 2016,Feb,12; 2016,Jan,13

65730 **penetrating (except in aphakia or pseudophakia)**

> INCLUDES   Use and preparation fresh or preserved graft
>
> EXCLUDES   Refractive keratoplasty surgery (65760-65767)
>
> 🖥 35.1   ⚖ 35.1   **FUD** 090   [J] [A2] [80] [50] [▣]
>
> **AMA:** 2018,Jan,8; 2017,Jan,8; 2016,Feb,12; 2016,Jan,13

65750 **penetrating (in aphakia)**

> INCLUDES   Use and preparation fresh or preserved graft
>
> EXCLUDES   Refractive keratoplasty surgery (65760-65767)
>
> 🖥 35.3   ⚖ 35.3   **FUD** 090   [J] [A2] [80] [50] [▣]
>
> **AMA:** 2018,Jan,8; 2017,Jan,8; 2016,Feb,12; 2016,Jan,13

65755 **penetrating (in pseudophakia)**

> INCLUDES   Use and preparation fresh or preserved graft
>
> EXCLUDES   Refractive keratoplasty surgery (65760-65767)
>
> 🖥 35.1   ⚖ 35.1   **FUD** 090   [J] [A2] [80] [50] [▣]
>
> **AMA:** 2018,Jan,8; 2017,Jan,8; 2016,Feb,12; 2016,Jan,13

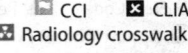

65756 endothelial

> *EXCLUDES* *Refractive keratoplasty surgery (65760-65767)*
>
> Code also:
>   Backbench preparation, when appropriate (65757)
>   Donor material
> 🚗 33.4 ⚕ 33.4 **FUD** 090 [J] [G2] [80] [50] [▣]
>
> **AMA:** 2018,Jan,8; 2017,Jan,8; 2016,Feb,12; 2016,Jan,8

+ 65757 Backbench preparation of corneal endothelial allograft prior to transplantation (List separately in addition to code for primary procedure)

> Code first (65756)
> 🚗 0.00 ⚕ 0.00 **FUD** ZZZ [N] [N1] [80] [▣]
>
> **AMA:** 2018,Jan,8; 2017,Jan,8; 2016,Feb,12; 2016,Jan,13

65760-65785 Corneal Refractive Procedures

CMS: 100-03,80.7 Refractive Keratoplasty

INCLUDES Operating microscope (69990)
EXCLUDES Unlisted corneal procedures (66999)

65760 Keratomileusis

> *EXCLUDES* *Computerized corneal topography (92025)*
> 🚗 0.00 ⚕ 0.00 **FUD** XXX [E] [▣]
>
> **AMA:** 2016,Feb,12

65765 Keratophakia

> *EXCLUDES* *Computerized corneal topography (92025)*
> 🚗 0.00 ⚕ 0.00 **FUD** XXX [E] [▣]
>
> **AMA:** 2016,Feb,12

65767 Epikeratoplasty

> *EXCLUDES* *Computerized corneal topography (92025)*
> 🚗 0.00 ⚕ 0.00 **FUD** XXX [E] [▣]
>
> **AMA:** 2016,Feb,12

65770 Keratoprosthesis

> *EXCLUDES* *Computerized corneal topography (92025)*
> 🚗 39.5 ⚕ 39.5 **FUD** 090 [J] [J8] [80] [50] [▣]
>
> **AMA:** 2016,Feb,12

65771 Radial keratotomy

> *EXCLUDES* *Computerized corneal topography (92025)*
> 🚗 0.00 ⚕ 0.00 **FUD** XXX [E] [▣]
>
> **AMA:** 2016,Feb,12

65772 Corneal relaxing incision for correction of surgically induced astigmatism

> 🚗 11.5 ⚕ 12.8 **FUD** 090 [T] [A2] [50] [▣]
>
> **AMA:** 2016,Feb,12

65775 Corneal wedge resection for correction of surgically induced astigmatism

> *EXCLUDES* *Fitting contact lens to treat disease (92071-92072)*
> 🚗 15.8 ⚕ 15.8 **FUD** 090 [J] [A2] [50] [▣]
>
> **AMA:** 2018,Jan,8; 2017,Jan,8; 2016,Feb,12; 2016,Jan,13

65778 Placement of amniotic membrane on the ocular surface; without sutures

> *EXCLUDES* *Ocular surface reconstruction (65780)*
> *Removal corneal epithelium (65435)*
> *Scraping cornea, diagnostic (65430)*
> *Using tissue glue to place amniotic membrane (66999)*
> 🚗 1.58 ⚕ 40.0 **FUD** 000 [02] [N1] [80] [50] [▣]
>
> **AMA:** 2018,Feb,11; 2018,Jan,8; 2017,Jan,8; 2016,Feb,12; 2016,Jan,13

65779 single layer, sutured

> *EXCLUDES* *Ocular surface reconstruction (65780)*
> *Removal corneal epithelium (65435)*
> *Scraping cornea, diagnostic (65430)*
> *Using tissue glue to place amniotic membrane (66999)*
> 🚗 4.32 ⚕ 34.5 **FUD** 000 [02] [N1] [80] [50] [▣]
>
> **AMA:** 2018,Feb,11; 2018,Jan,8; 2017,Jan,8; 2016,Feb,12; 2016,Jan,13

65780 Ocular surface reconstruction; amniotic membrane transplantation, multiple layers

> *EXCLUDES* *Placement amniotic membrane without reconstruction without sutures or single layer sutures (65778-65779)*
> 🚗 18.9 ⚕ 18.9 **FUD** 090 [J] [A2] [50] [▣]
>
> **AMA:** 2018,Feb,11; 2018,Jan,8; 2017,Jan,8; 2016,Feb,12; 2016,Jan,13

65781 limbal stem cell allograft (eg, cadaveric or living donor)

> 🚗 37.9 ⚕ 37.9 **FUD** 090 [J] [J8] [80] [50] [▣]
>
> **AMA:** 2018,Jan,8; 2017,Jan,8; 2016,Feb,12; 2016,Jan,13

65782 limbal conjunctival autograft (includes obtaining graft)

> *EXCLUDES* *Conjunctival allograft harvest from living donor (68371)*
> 🚗 32.6 ⚕ 32.6 **FUD** 090 [J] [A2] [50] [▣]
>
> **AMA:** 2018,Jan,8; 2017,Jan,8; 2016,Feb,12; 2016,Jan,13

65785 Implantation of intrastromal corneal ring segments

> 🚗 12.5 ⚕ 69.5 **FUD** 090 [J] [P2] [50] [▣]
>
> **AMA:** 2016,Feb,12

65800-66030 Anterior Segment Procedures

INCLUDES Operating microscope (69990)
EXCLUDES Unlisted procedures anterior segment (66999)

65800 Paracentesis of anterior chamber of eye (separate procedure); with removal of aqueous

> *EXCLUDES* *Insertion ocular telescope prosthesis (0308T)*
> 🚗 2.59 ⚕ 3.42 **FUD** 000 [J] [A2] [50] [▣]
>
> **AMA:** 2018,Jan,8; 2017,Jan,8; 2016,Feb,12; 2016,Jan,13

65810 with removal of vitreous and/or discission of anterior hyaloid membrane, with or without air injection

> *EXCLUDES* *Insertion ocular telescope prosthesis (0308T)*
> 🚗 13.2 ⚕ 13.2 **FUD** 090 [J] [A2] [50] [▣]
>
> **AMA:** 2018,Jan,8; 2017,Jan,8; 2016,Feb,12; 2016,Jan,13

65815 with removal of blood, with or without irrigation and/or air injection

> *EXCLUDES* *Injection only (66020-66030)*
> *Insertion ocular telescope prosthesis (0308T)*
> *Removal blood clot only (65930)*
> 🚗 13.5 ⚕ 18.2 **FUD** 090 [J] [A2] [50] [▣]
>
> **AMA:** 2018,Jan,8; 2017,Jan,8; 2016,Feb,12; 2016,Jan,13

65820 Goniotomy

> *INCLUDES* Barkan's operation
> Code also ophthalmic endoscope if used (66990)
> 🚗 21.5 ⚕ 21.5 **FUD** 090 [63] [J] [A2] [80] [50] [▣]
>
> **AMA:** 2019,Sep,10; 2018,Dec,8; 2018,Dec,8; 2018,Jul,3; 2018,Jan,8; 2017,Jan,8; 2016,Feb,12; 2016,Jan,13

65850 Trabeculotomy ab externo

> 🚗 23.8 ⚕ 23.8 **FUD** 090 [J] [A2] [50] [▣]
>
> **AMA:** 2016,Feb,12

65855 Trabeculoplasty by laser surgery

> *EXCLUDES* *Severing adhesions anterior segment (65860-65880)*
> *Trabeculectomy ab externo (66170)*
> 🚗 5.91 ⚕ 7.01 **FUD** 010 [T] [P3] [50] [▣]
>
> **AMA:** 2018,Jan,8; 2017,Jan,8; 2016,Feb,12; 2016,Jan,13

65860 Severing adhesions of anterior segment, laser technique (separate procedure)

> 🚗 7.18 ⚕ 8.81 **FUD** 090 [T] [P3] [80] [50] [▣]
>
> **AMA:** 2016,Feb,12

65865 Severing adhesions of anterior segment of eye, incisional technique (with or without injection of air or liquid) (separate procedure); goniosynechiae

> *EXCLUDES* *Laser trabeculectomy (65855)*
> 🚗 13.4 ⚕ 13.4 **FUD** 090 [J] [A2] [50] [▣]
>
> **AMA:** 2016,Feb,12

65870 anterior synechiae, except goniosynechiae

> 🚗 16.7 ⚕ 16.7 **FUD** 090 [J] [A2] [50] [▣]
>
> **AMA:** 2016,Feb,12

65875 **posterior synechiae**
Code also ophthalmic endoscope when used (66990)
🔲 17.9   ⚕ 17.9   **FUD** 090
AMA: 2018,Jan,8; 2017,Jan,8; 2016,Feb,12; 2016,Jan,13

65880 **corneovitreal adhesions**
EXCLUDES   Laser procedure (66821)
🔲 18.8   ⚕ 18.8   **FUD** 090   J A2 50
AMA: 2016,Feb,12

65900 **Removal of epithelial downgrowth, anterior chamber of eye**
🔲 27.6   ⚕ 27.6   **FUD** 090   J A2 80 50
AMA: 2016,Feb,12

65920 **Removal of implanted material, anterior segment of eye**
Code also ophthalmic endoscope when used (66990)
🔲 22.3   ⚕ 22.3   **FUD** 090   J A2 50
AMA: 2018,Jan,8; 2017,Jan,8; 2016,Feb,12; 2016,Jan,13

65930 **Removal of blood clot, anterior segment of eye**
🔲 18.0   ⚕ 18.0   **FUD** 090   J A2 50
AMA: 2016,Feb,12

66020 **Injection, anterior chamber of eye (separate procedure); air or liquid**
EXCLUDES   Insertion ocular telescope prosthesis (0308T)
🔲 3.74   ⚕ 5.43   **FUD** 010   J A2 50
AMA: 2018,Jan,8; 2017,Jan,8; 2016,Feb,12; 2016,Jan,13

66030 **medication**
EXCLUDES   Insertion ocular telescope prosthesis (0308T)
🔲 3.16   ⚕ 4.87   **FUD** 010   J A2 50
AMA: 2016,Feb,12

66130 Excision Scleral Lesion
INCLUDES   Operating microscope (69990)
EXCLUDES   Removal intraocular foreign body (65235)
Surgery on posterior sclera (67250, 67255)

66130 **Excision of lesion, sclera**
🔲 16.1   ⚕ 19.9   **FUD** 090   J A2 80 50
AMA: 2016,Feb,12

66150-66185 Procedures for Glaucoma
INCLUDES   Operating microscope (69990)
EXCLUDES   Removal intraocular foreign body (65235)
Surgery on posterior sclera (67250, 67255)

66150 **Fistulization of sclera for glaucoma; trephination with iridectomy**
🔲 24.9   ⚕ 24.9   **FUD** 090   J A2 50
AMA: 2018,Jul,3; 2016,Feb,12

66155 **thermocauterization with iridectomy**
🔲 24.9   ⚕ 24.9   **FUD** 090   J A2 50
AMA: 2018,Jul,3; 2016,Feb,12

66160 **sclerectomy with punch or scissors, with iridectomy**
INCLUDES   Knapp's operation
🔲 27.9   ⚕ 27.9   **FUD** 090   J A2 50
AMA: 2018,Jul,3; 2016,Feb,12

66170 **trabeculectomy ab externo in absence of previous surgery**
EXCLUDES   Repair surgical wound (66250)
Trabeculectomy ab externo (65850)
🔲 31.1   ⚕ 31.1   **FUD** 090   J A2 80 50
AMA: 2018,Dec,8; 2018,Dec,10; 2018,Dec,8; 2018,Dec,10; 2018,Jul,3; 2018,Jan,8; 2017,Jan,8; 2016,Feb,12; 2016,Jan,13

66172 **trabeculectomy ab externo with scarring from previous ocular surgery or trauma (includes injection of antifibrotic agents)**
🔲 33.9   ⚕ 33.9   **FUD** 090   J A2 80 50
AMA: 2019,Apr,7; 2018,Dec,10; 2018,Dec,10; 2018,Jul,3; 2018,Jan,8; 2017,Jan,8; 2016,Feb,12; 2016,Jan,13

66174 **Transluminal dilation of aqueous outflow canal; without retention of device or stent**
EXCLUDES   Goniotomy (65820)
🔲 26.9   ⚕ 26.9   **FUD** 090   J A2 80 50
AMA: 2019,Sep,10; 2018,Dec,8; 2018,Dec,8; 2016,Feb,12

66175 **with retention of device or stent**
🔲 28.2   ⚕ 28.2   **FUD** 090   J A2 80 50
AMA: 2016,Feb,12

66179 **Aqueous shunt to extraocular equatorial plate reservoir, external approach; without graft**
🔲 30.6   ⚕ 30.6   **FUD** 090   J G2 80 50
AMA: 2018,Jul,3; 2018,Jan,8; 2017,Jan,8; 2016,Feb,12; 2016,Jan,13

66180 **with graft**
EXCLUDES   Scleral reinforcement (67255)
🔲 32.3   ⚕ 32.3   **FUD** 090   J J8 80 50
AMA: 2018,Jul,3; 2018,Jan,8; 2017,Jan,8; 2016,Feb,12; 2016,Jan,13

66183 **Insertion of anterior segment aqueous drainage device, without extraocular reservoir, external approach**
🔲 29.2   ⚕ 29.2   **FUD** 090   J J8 80 50
AMA: 2020,Jun,14; 2018,Jul,3; 2018,Jan,8; 2017,Jan,8; 2016,Feb,12; 2016,Jan,13

66184 **Revision of aqueous shunt to extraocular equatorial plate reservoir; without graft**
🔲 22.3   ⚕ 22.3   **FUD** 090   J G2 80 50
AMA: 2018,Jan,8; 2017,Jan,8; 2016,Feb,12; 2016,Jan,13

66185 **with graft**
EXCLUDES   Removal implanted shunt (67120)
Scleral reinforcement (67255)
🔲 24.0   ⚕ 24.0   **FUD** 090   J A2 80 50
AMA: 2018,Jan,8; 2017,Jan,8; 2016,Feb,12; 2016,Jan,13

66225 Staphyloma Repair
INCLUDES   Operating microscope (69990)
EXCLUDES   Scleral procedures with retinal procedures (67101-67228)
Scleral reinforcement (67250, 67255)

66225 **Repair of scleral staphyloma; with graft**
🔲 26.4   ⚕ 26.4   **FUD** 090   J G2 50
AMA: 2016,Feb,12

66250 Anterior Segment Operative Wound Revision or Repair
INCLUDES   Operating microscope (69990)
EXCLUDES   Unlisted procedures anterior sclera (66999)

66250 **Revision or repair of operative wound of anterior segment, any type, early or late, major or minor procedure**
🔲 15.8   ⚕ 21.4   **FUD** 090   J A2 50
AMA: 2018,Dec,8; 2018,Dec,8; 2018,Jan,8; 2017,Jan,8; 2016,Feb,12; 2016,Jan,13

66500-66505 Iridotomy With/Without Transfixion
INCLUDES   Operating microscope (69990)
EXCLUDES   Photocoagulation iridotomy (66761)

66500 **Iridotomy by stab incision (separate procedure); except transfixion**
🔲 10.2   ⚕ 10.2   **FUD** 090   J A2 50
AMA: 2016,Feb,12

66505 **with transfixion as for iris bombe**
🔲 11.1   ⚕ 11.1   **FUD** 090   J A2 50
AMA: 2016,Feb,12

66600-66635 Iridectomy Procedures
INCLUDES   Operating microscope (69990)
EXCLUDES   Insertion ocular telescope prosthesis (0308T)
Photocoagulation coreoplasty (66762)

66600 **Iridectomy, with corneoscleral or corneal section; for removal of lesion**
🔲 23.9   ⚕ 23.9   **FUD** 090   J A2 50
AMA: 2016,Feb,12

66605   with cyclectomy
🚑 30.3   ✂ 30.3   **FUD** 090   J A2 50 ▭
AMA: 2016,Feb,12

66625   peripheral for glaucoma (separate procedure)
🚑 12.2   ✂ 12.2   **FUD** 090   J A2 50 ▭
AMA: 2016,Feb,12

66630   sector for glaucoma (separate procedure)
🚑 16.1   ✂ 16.1   **FUD** 090   J A2 50 ▭
AMA: 2016,Feb,12

66635   optical (separate procedure)
🚑 16.3   ✂ 16.3   **FUD** 090   J A2 50 ▭
AMA: 2016,Feb,12

66680-66770 Other Procedures of the Uveal Tract

INCLUDES   Operating microscope (69990)
EXCLUDES   *Unlisted procedures ciliary body or iris (66999)*

66680   **Repair of iris, ciliary body (as for iridodialysis)**
EXCLUDES   *Resection/repositioning uveal tissue for perforating
laceration, cornea and/or sclera (65285)*
🚑 14.7   ✂ 14.7   **FUD** 090   J A2 50 ▭
AMA: 2016,Feb,12

66682   **Suture of iris, ciliary body (separate procedure) with retrieval
of suture through small incision (eg, McCannel suture)**
🚑 18.3   ✂ 18.3   **FUD** 090   J A2 50 ▭
AMA: 2016,Feb,12

66700   **Ciliary body destruction; diathermy**
INCLUDES   Heine's operation
🚑 11.1   ✂ 12.8   **FUD** 090   J A2 80 50 ▭
AMA: 2016,Feb,12

66710   cyclophotocoagulation, transscleral
🚑 11.1   ✂ 12.6   **FUD** 090   J A2 50 ▭
AMA: 2018,Jan,8; 2017,Jan,8; 2016,Feb,12; 2016,Jan,13

66711   cyclophotocoagulation, endoscopic, without concomitant
removal of crystalline lens
EXCLUDES   *Endoscopic cyclophotocoagulation performed in
conjunction with extracapsular cataract removal
with insertion lens ([66987], [66988])*
🚑 18.2   ✂ 18.2   **FUD** 090   J A2 50 ▭
AMA: 2019,Dec,6; 2018,Jan,8; 2017,Jan,8; 2016,Feb,12;
2016,Jan,13

66720   cryotherapy
🚑 11.6   ✂ 13.1   **FUD** 090   J A2 50 ▭
AMA: 2016,Feb,12

66740   cyclodialysis
🚑 11.1   ✂ 12.5   **FUD** 090   J A2 50 ▭
AMA: 2016,Feb,12

66761   **Iridotomy/iridectomy by laser surgery (eg, for glaucoma) (per
session)**
EXCLUDES   *Insertion ocular telescope prosthesis (0308T)*
🚑 6.68   ✂ 8.49   **FUD** 010   T P3 50 ▭
AMA: 2018,Jan,8; 2017,Jan,8; 2016,Feb,12; 2016,Jan,13

66762   **Iridoplasty by photocoagulation (1 or more sessions) (eg, for
improvement of vision, for widening of anterior chamber
angle)**
🚑 12.0   ✂ 13.5   **FUD** 090   T P2 50 ▭
AMA: 2018,Jan,8; 2017,Jan,8; 2016,Feb,12; 2016,Jan,13

66770   **Destruction of cyst or lesion iris or ciliary body (nonexcisional
procedure)**
EXCLUDES   *Excision:
Epithelial downgrowth (65900)
Iris, ciliary body lesion (66600-66605)*
🚑 13.7   ✂ 15.0   **FUD** 090   T P2 50 ▭
AMA: 2016,Feb,12

66820-66825 Post-Cataract Surgery Procedures

INCLUDES   Operating microscope (69990)

66820   **Discission of secondary membranous cataract (opacified
posterior lens capsule and/or anterior hyaloid); stab incision
technique (Ziegler or Wheeler knife)**
🚑 11.4   ✂ 11.4   **FUD** 090   J G2 50 ▭
AMA: 2016,Feb,12

Cataract   Iris

Lens

Artificial lens   Cornea

Opaque lens   Iris
capsule

An after-cataract is a cataract that
develops in a lens tissue that remains
after most of the lens has already been removed

66821   laser surgery (eg, YAG laser) (1 or more stages)
🚑 8.85   ✂ 9.42   **FUD** 090   T A2 50 ▭
AMA: 2016,Feb,12

66825   **Repositioning of intraocular lens prosthesis, requiring an
incision (separate procedure)**
EXCLUDES   *Insertion ocular telescope prosthesis (0308T)*
🚑 21.8   ✂ 21.8   **FUD** 090   J A2 80 50 ▭
AMA: 2016,Feb,12

 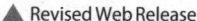

66830-66940 Cataract Extraction; Without Insertion Intraocular Lens

CMS: 100-03,80.10 Phacoemulsification Procedure--Cataract Extraction

INCLUDES Anterior and/or posterior capsulotomy
Enzymatic zonulysis
Iridectomy/iridotomy
Lateral canthotomy
Medications
Operating microscope (69990)
Subconjunctival injection
Subtenon injection
Using viscoelastic material

EXCLUDES *Removal intralenticular foreign body without lens excision (65235)*
Repair surgical laceration (66250)

66830 **Removal of secondary membranous cataract (opacified posterior lens capsule and/or anterior hyaloid) with corneo-scleral section, with or without iridectomy (iridocapsulotomy, iridocapsulectomy)**

INCLUDES Graefe's operation
🗂 20.1 ⚕ 20.1 **FUD** 090 ⬚ J A2 50 ⬚
AMA: 2016,Feb,12

Cataract
Iris
Lens
Coloboma

A congenital keyhole pupil is also called a coloboma of the iris

66840 **Removal of lens material; aspiration technique, 1 or more stages**

INCLUDES Fukala's operation
🗂 19.7 ⚕ 19.7 **FUD** 090 ⬚ J A2 50 ⬚
AMA: 2018,Jan,8; 2017,Jan,8; 2016,Sep,9; 2016,Jun,6; 2016,Apr,8; 2016,Feb,12; 2016,Jan,13

66850 **phacofragmentation technique (mechanical or ultrasonic) (eg, phacoemulsification), with aspiration**

🗂 22.5 ⚕ 22.5 **FUD** 090 ⬚ J A2 50 ⬚
AMA: 2018,Jan,8; 2017,Jan,8; 2016,Jun,6; 2016,Feb,12; 2016,Jan,13

66852 **pars plana approach, with or without vitrectomy**

🗂 23.9 ⚕ 23.9 **FUD** 090 ⬚ J A2 80 50 ⬚
AMA: 2018,Jan,8; 2017,Jan,8; 2016,Jun,6; 2016,Feb,12; 2016,Jan,13

66920 **intracapsular**

🗂 21.4 ⚕ 21.4 **FUD** 090 ⬚ J A2 80 50 ⬚
AMA: 2018,Jan,8; 2017,Jan,8; 2016,Feb,12; 2016,Jan,13

66930 **intracapsular, for dislocated lens**

🗂 24.3 ⚕ 24.3 **FUD** 090 ⬚ J A2 80 50 ⬚
AMA: 2018,Jan,8; 2017,Jan,8; 2016,Feb,12; 2016,Jan,13

66940 **extracapsular (other than 66840, 66850, 66852)**

🗂 22.2 ⚕ 22.2 **FUD** 090 ⬚ J A2 80 50 ⬚
AMA: 2018,Jan,8; 2017,Jan,8; 2016,Jun,6; 2016,Feb,12; 2016,Jan,13

66982-66988 [66987, 66988, 66989, 66991] Cataract Extraction: With Insertion Intraocular Lens

INCLUDES Anterior or posterior capsulotomy
Enzymatic zonulysis
Iridectomy/iridotomy
Lateral canthotomy
Medications
Operating microscope (69990)
Subconjunctival injection
Subtenon injection
Using viscoelastic material

EXCLUDES *Implanted material removal from anterior segment (65920)*
Insertion ocular telescope prosthesis (0308T)
Secondary fixation (66682)
Supply intraocular lens

66982 **Extracapsular cataract removal with insertion of intraocular lens prosthesis (1-stage procedure), manual or mechanical technique (eg, irrigation and aspiration or phacoemulsification), complex, requiring devices or techniques not generally used in routine cataract surgery (eg, iris expansion device, suture support for intraocular lens, or primary posterior capsulorrhexis) or performed on patients in the amblyogenic developmental stage; without endoscopic cyclophotocoagulation**

EXCLUDES *Complex extracapsular cataract removal in conjunction with aqueous drainage device insertion ([66989])*
Complex extracapsular cataract removal in conjunction with endoscopic cyclophotocoagulation ([66987])

🔲 (76519)
🗂 22.5 ⚕ 22.5 **FUD** 090 ⬚ J A2 50 ⬚
AMA: 2019,Dec,6; 2018,Dec,6; 2018,Dec,6; 2018,Jan,8; 2017,Dec,14; 2017,Jan,8; 2016,Mar,10; 2016,Feb,12; 2016,Jan,13

● # **66989** **with insertion of intraocular (eg, trabecular meshwork, supraciliary, suprachoroidal) anterior segment aqueous drainage device, without extraocular reservoir, internal approach, one or more**

EXCLUDES *Complex extracapsular cataract removal without aqueous drainage device insertion during same operative session (66982)*
Insertion anterior segment aqueous drainage device only ([0671T])

🗂 0.00 ⚕ 0.00 **FUD** 000

66987 **with endoscopic cyclophotocoagulation**

EXCLUDES *Complex extracapsular cataract removal without endoscopic cyclophotocoagulation (66982)*
🗂 0.00 ⚕ 0.00 **FUD** 090 ⬚ J8 80 50 ⬚
AMA: 2019,Dec,6

66983 **Intracapsular cataract extraction with insertion of intraocular lens prosthesis (1 stage procedure)**

🔲 (76519)
🗂 21.0 ⚕ 21.0 **FUD** 090 ⬚ J A2 50 ⬚
AMA: 2019,Dec,6; 2018,Jan,8; 2017,Jan,8; 2016,Feb,12; 2016,Jan,13

66984 **Extracapsular cataract removal with insertion of intraocular lens prosthesis (1 stage procedure), manual or mechanical technique (eg, irrigation and aspiration or phacoemulsification); without endoscopic cyclophotocoagulation**

EXCLUDES *Complex extracapsular cataract removal (66982)*
Complex extracapsular cataract removal in conjunction with aqueous drainage device insertion ([66989])
Extracapsular cataract removal in conjunction with endoscopic cyclophotocoagulation ([66988])
Insertion anterior segment aqueous drainage device only ([0671T])

🔲 (76519)
🗂 18.1 ⚕ 18.1 **FUD** 090 ⬚ J A2 50 ⬚
AMA: 2020,Dec,13; 2019,Dec,6; 2018,Dec,6; 2018,Dec,6; 2018,Jan,8; 2017,Jan,8; 2016,Feb,12; 2016,Jan,13

● # **66991** **with insertion of intraocular (eg, trabecular meshwork, supraciliary, suprachoroidal) anterior segment aqueous drainage device, without extraocular reservoir, internal approach, one or more**

EXCLUDES *Extracapsular cataract removal without aqueous drainage device insertion during same operative session (66984)*
Insertion anterior segment aqueous drainage device only ([0671T])
🚗 0.00 ⚕ 0.00 **FUD** 000

66988 **with endoscopic cyclophotocoagulation**

EXCLUDES *Complex extracapsular cataract removal in conjunction with endoscopic cyclophotocoagulation ([66987])*
Extracapsular cataract removal without endoscopic cyclophotocoagulation (66984)
🚗 0.00 ⚕ 0.00 **FUD** 090　J8 80 50 🔲
AMA: 2019,Dec,6

66985-66989 [66987, 66988, 66989] Secondary Insertion or Replacement of Intraocular Lens

INCLUDES Operating microscope (69990)
EXCLUDES *Implanted material removal from anterior segment (65920)*
Insertion ocular telescope prosthesis (0308T)
Secondary fixation (66682)
Supply intraocular lens
Code also ophthalmic endoscope if used (66990)

66985 **Insertion of intraocular lens prosthesis (secondary implant), not associated with concurrent cataract removal**

EXCLUDES *Implanted material removal from anterior segment (65920)*
Insertion lens at time of cataract procedure (66982-66984)
Insertion ocular telescope prosthesis (0308T)
Secondary fixation (66682)
Supply intraocular lens
🔲 (76519)
🚗 21.8 ⚕ 21.8 **FUD** 090　J A2 50 🔲
AMA: 2018,Jan,8; 2017,Jan,8; 2016,Feb,12; 2016,Jan,13

66986 **Exchange of intraocular lens**
🔲 (76519)
🚗 25.8 ⚕ 25.8 **FUD** 090　J A2 50 🔲
AMA: 2018,Jan,8; 2017,Jan,8; 2016,Feb,12; 2016,Jan,13

66987 **Resequenced code. See code following resequenced code 66989.**

66988 **Resequenced code. See code following resequenced code 66991.**

66989 **Resequenced code. See code following resequenced code 66982.**

66990-66999 [66991] Ophthalmic Endoscopy

INCLUDES Operating microscope (69990)

+ **66990** **Use of ophthalmic endoscope (List separately in addition to code for primary procedure)**
Code first (65820, 65875, 65920, 66985-66986, 67036, 67039-67043, 67113)
🚗 2.56 ⚕ 2.56 **FUD** ZZZ　N N1 🔲
AMA: 2018,Jul,3; 2018,Jan,8; 2017,Jan,8; 2016,Sep,5; 2016,Feb,12; 2016,Jan,13

66991 **Resequenced code. See code following 66984.**

66999 **Unlisted procedure, anterior segment of eye**
🚗 0.00 ⚕ 0.00 **FUD** YYY　J 80 50 🔲
AMA: 2018,Jan,8; 2017,Jan,8; 2016,Apr,8; 2016,Feb,12; 2016,Jan,13

67005-67015 Vitrectomy: Partial and Subtotal

INCLUDES Operating microscope (69990)

67005 **Removal of vitreous, anterior approach (open sky technique or limbal incision); partial removal**
EXCLUDES *Anterior chamber vitrectomy by paracentesis (65810)*
Severing corneovitreal adhesions (65880)
🚗 13.4 ⚕ 13.4 **FUD** 090　J A2 50 🔲
AMA: 2018,Jan,8; 2017,Jan,8; 2016,Feb,12; 2016,Jan,13

67010 **subtotal removal with mechanical vitrectomy**
EXCLUDES *Anterior chamber vitrectomy by paracentesis (65810)*
Severing corneovitreal adhesions (65880)
🚗 15.4 ⚕ 15.4 **FUD** 090　J A2 50 🔲
AMA: 2018,Jan,8; 2017,Jan,8; 2016,Feb,12; 2016,Jan,13

67015 **Aspiration or release of vitreous, subretinal or choroidal fluid, pars plana approach (posterior sclerotomy)**
🚗 16.5 ⚕ 16.5 **FUD** 090　J A2 50 🔲
AMA: 2018,Jan,8; 2017,Jan,8; 2016,Sep,5; 2016,Jun,6; 2016,Feb,12

67025-67028 Intravitreal Injection/Implantation

INCLUDES Operating microscope (69990)

67025 **Injection of vitreous substitute, pars plana or limbal approach (fluid-gas exchange), with or without aspiration (separate procedure)**
🚗 17.9 ⚕ 20.8 **FUD** 090　J A2 50 🔲
AMA: 2019,Aug,10; 2018,Feb,3; 2016,Feb,12

67027 **Implantation of intravitreal drug delivery system (eg, ganciclovir implant), includes concomitant removal of vitreous**
EXCLUDES *Removal drug delivery system (67121)*
🚗 24.2 ⚕ 24.2 **FUD** 090　J A2 80 50 🔲
AMA: 2018,Feb,3; 2018,Jan,8; 2017,Jan,8; 2016,Feb,12; 2016,Jan,13

67028 **Intravitreal injection of a pharmacologic agent (separate procedure)**
🚗 2.79 ⚕ 2.86 **FUD** 000　S P3 50 🔲
AMA: 2018,Feb,3; 2018,Jan,8; 2017,Jan,8; 2016,Feb,12; 2016,Jan,13

67030-67031 Incision of Vitreous Strands/Membranes

INCLUDES Operating microscope (69990)

67030 **Discission of vitreous strands (without removal), pars plana approach**
🚗 15.2 ⚕ 15.2 **FUD** 090　J A2 50 🔲
AMA: 2016,Feb,12

67031 **Severing of vitreous strands, vitreous face adhesions, sheets, membranes or opacities, laser surgery (1 or more stages)**
🚗 10.1 ⚕ 11.1 **FUD** 090　T A2 50 🔲
AMA: 2016,Feb,12

67036-67043 Pars Plana Mechanical Vitrectomy

INCLUDES Operating microscope (69990)
EXCLUDES *Lens removal (66850)*
Removal foreign body (65260, 65265)
Unlisted vitreal procedures (67299)
Vitrectomy in retinal detachment (67108, 67113)
Code also ophthalmic endoscope if used (66990)

67036 **Vitrectomy, mechanical, pars plana approach;**
🚗 25.6 ⚕ 25.6 **FUD** 090　J A2 80 50 🔲
AMA: 2018,Jan,8; 2017,Jan,8; 2016,Sep,5; 2016,Feb,12; 2016,Jan,13

67039 **with focal endolaser photocoagulation**
🚗 27.4 ⚕ 27.4 **FUD** 090　J A2 80 50 🔲
AMA: 2018,Jan,8; 2017,Jan,8; 2016,Sep,5; 2016,Feb,12; 2016,Jan,13

67040 **with endolaser panretinal photocoagulation**
🚗 29.6 ⚕ 29.6 **FUD** 090　J A2 80 50 🔲
AMA: 2018,Jan,8; 2017,Jan,8; 2016,Sep,5; 2016,Feb,12; 2016,Jan,13

67041 **with removal of preretinal cellular membrane (eg, macular pucker)**
🚗 32.7 ⚕ 32.7 **FUD** 090　J G2 80 50 🔲
AMA: 2018,Jan,8; 2017,Jan,8; 2016,Sep,5; 2016,Feb,12; 2016,Jan,13

67042   with removal of internal limiting membrane of retina (eg, for repair of macular hole, diabetic macular edema), includes, if performed, intraocular tamponade (ie, air, gas or silicone oil)

    📋 32.7   ✂ 32.7   **FUD** 090   J 62 80 50 ▣

    AMA: 2018,Jan,8; 2017,Jan,8; 2016,Sep,5; 2016,Feb,12; 2016,Jan,13

67043   with removal of subretinal membrane (eg, choroidal neovascularization), includes, if performed, intraocular tamponade (ie, air, gas or silicone oil) and laser photocoagulation

    📋 34.3   ✂ 34.3   **FUD** 090   J 62 80 50 ▣

    AMA: 2018,Jan,8; 2017,Jan,8; 2016,Sep,5; 2016,Feb,12; 2016,Jan,13

67101-67115 Detached Retina Repair

INCLUDES   Operating microscope (69990)
Primary technique when cryotherapy and/or diathermy and/or photocoagulation are used in combination

67101   Repair of retinal detachment, including drainage of subretinal fluid when performed; cryotherapy

    📋 8.10   ✂ 9.40   **FUD** 010   J P3 50 ▣

    AMA: 2018,Jan,8; 2017,Feb,14; 2017,Jan,8; 2016,Sep,5; 2016,Jun,6; 2016,Feb,12; 2016,Jan,13

Optic nerve

Vitreous

Optic disc

Choroid

Sclera

Retina

Posterior chamber   Pars plana

67105   photocoagulation

    📋 7.82   ✂ 8.45   **FUD** 010   T P3 50 ▣

    AMA: 2018,Jan,8; 2017,Feb,14; 2017,Jan,8; 2016,Sep,5; 2016,Jun,6; 2016,Feb,12; 2016,Jan,13

67107   Repair of retinal detachment; scleral buckling (such as lamellar scleral dissection, imbrication or encircling procedure), including, when performed, implant, cryotherapy, photocoagulation, and drainage of subretinal fluid

    INCLUDES   Gonin's operation

    📋 31.9   ✂ 31.9   **FUD** 090   J 62 80 50 ▣

    AMA: 2019,Aug,10; 2018,Jan,8; 2017,Jan,8; 2016,Sep,5; 2016,Jun,6; 2016,Feb,12

67108   with vitrectomy, any method, including, when performed, air or gas tamponade, focal endolaser photocoagulation, cryotherapy, drainage of subretinal fluid, scleral buckling, and/or removal of lens by same technique

    📋 34.1   ✂ 34.1   **FUD** 090   J 62 80 50 ▣

    AMA: 2018,Jan,8; 2017,Jan,8; 2016,Sep,5; 2016,Jun,6; 2016,Feb,12; 2016,Jan,13

67110   by injection of air or other gas (eg, pneumatic retinopexy)

    📋 23.1   ✂ 25.0   **FUD** 090   J P3 50 ▣

    AMA: 2018,Jan,8; 2017,Jan,8; 2016,Sep,5; 2016,Jun,6; 2016,Feb,12

67113   Repair of complex retinal detachment (eg, proliferative vitreoretinopathy, stage C-1 or greater, diabetic traction retinal detachment, retinopathy of prematurity, retinal tear of greater than 90 degrees), with vitrectomy and membrane peeling, including, when performed, air, gas, or silicone oil tamponade, cryotherapy, endolaser photocoagulation, drainage of subretinal fluid, scleral buckling, and/or removal of lens

    EXCLUDES   Vitrectomy for other than retinal detachment, pars plana approach (67036-67043)
    Code also ophthalmic endoscope if used (66990)

    📋 38.0   ✂ 38.0   **FUD** 090   J 62 80 50 ▣

    AMA: 2018,Jan,8; 2017,Jan,8; 2016,Sep,5; 2016,Jun,6; 2016,Feb,12; 2016,Jan,13

67115   Release of encircling material (posterior segment)

    📋 14.1   ✂ 14.1   **FUD** 090   J A2 50 ▣

    AMA: 2016,Feb,12

67120-67121 Removal of Previously Implanted Prosthetic Device

INCLUDES   Operating microscope (69990)
EXCLUDES   Foreign body removal (65260, 65265)
Removal implanted material anterior segment (65920)

67120   Removal of implanted material, posterior segment; extraocular

    📋 15.8   ✂ 18.8   **FUD** 090   J A2 50 ▣

    AMA: 2016,Feb,12

67121   intraocular

    📋 25.6   ✂ 25.6   **FUD** 090   J A2 80 50 ▣

    AMA: 2016,Feb,12

67141-67145 Retinal Detachment: Preventative Procedures

INCLUDES   Operating microscope (69990)
Treatment at one or more sessions that may occur at different encounters
EXCLUDES   Procedure performed more than one time during defined period of treatment

▲ **67141**   Prophylaxis of retinal detachment (eg, retinal break, lattice degeneration) without drainage; cryotherapy, diathermy

    📋 13.8   ✂ 14.9   **FUD** 090   T A2 50 ▣

    AMA: 2018,Jan,8; 2017,Jan,8; 2016,Sep,5; 2016,Feb,12; 2016,Jan,13

▲ **67145**   photocoagulation

    📋 14.1   ✂ 15.0   **FUD** 090   T P2 50 ▣

    AMA: 2018,Jan,8; 2017,Jan,8; 2016,Sep,5; 2016,Feb,12; 2016,Jan,13

67208-67218 Destruction of Retinal Lesions

INCLUDES   Operating microscope (69990)
Treatment at one or more sessions that may occur at different encounters
EXCLUDES   Procedure performed more than one time during defined period of treatment
Unlisted retinal procedures (67299)

67208   Destruction of localized lesion of retina (eg, macular edema, tumors), 1 or more sessions; cryotherapy, diathermy

    📋 16.4   ✂ 17.0   **FUD** 090   T P2 50 ▣

    AMA: 2018,Jan,8; 2017,Jan,8; 2016,Feb,12; 2016,Jan,13

67210   photocoagulation

    📋 14.1   ✂ 14.6   **FUD** 090   T P2 50 ▣

    AMA: 2018,Jan,8; 2017,Jan,8; 2016,Feb,12; 2016,Jan,13

67218   radiation by implantation of source (includes removal of source)

    📋 39.4   ✂ 39.4   **FUD** 090   J A2 50 ▣

    AMA: 2018,Jan,8; 2017,Jan,8; 2016,Feb,12; 2016,Jan,13

26/TC PC/TC Only   A2-Z3 ASC Payment   50 Bilateral   ♂ Male Only   ♀ Female Only   📋 Facility RVU   ✂ Non-Facility RVU   ▣ CCI   ✖ CLIA
FUD Follow-up Days   **CMS:** IOM   **AMA:** CPT Asst   A-Y OPPSI   80/80 Surg Assist Allowed / w/Doc   ◪ Lab crosswalk   ◪ Radiology crosswalk

308   CPT © 2021 American Medical Association. All Rights Reserved.   © 2021 Optum360, LLC

67220-67225 Destruction of Choroidal Lesions

INCLUDES Operating microscope (69990)

67220 Destruction of localized lesion of choroid (eg, choroidal neovascularization); photocoagulation (eg, laser), 1 or more sessions

INCLUDES Treatment at one or more sessions that may occur at different encounters
EXCLUDES Procedure performed more than one time during defined period of treatment

🔧 14.1 🔨 15.0 **FUD** 090 [T] [P2] [50] 🔲

AMA: 2018,Jan,8; 2017,Jan,8; 2016,Feb,12; 2016,Jan,13

67221 photodynamic therapy (includes intravenous infusion)

🔧 6.05 🔨 8.07 **FUD** 000 [T] [P3] 🔲

AMA: 2018,Feb,10; 2018,Jan,8; 2017,Jan,8; 2016,Feb,12; 2016,Jan,13

+ 67225 photodynamic therapy, second eye, at single session (List separately in addition to code for primary eye treatment)

Code first (67221)

🔧 0.81 🔨 0.85 **FUD** ZZZ [N] [N1] 🔲

AMA: 2018,Jan,8; 2017,Jan,8; 2016,Feb,12; 2016,Jan,13

67227-67229 Destruction Retinopathy

INCLUDES Operating microscope (69990)
EXCLUDES Unlisted retinal procedures (67299)

67227 Destruction of extensive or progressive retinopathy (eg, diabetic retinopathy), cryotherapy, diathermy

🔧 7.24 🔨 8.33 **FUD** 010 [J] [P3] [50] 🔲

AMA: 2018,Jan,8; 2017,Jan,8; 2016,Feb,12; 2016,Jan,13

67228 Treatment of extensive or progressive retinopathy (eg, diabetic retinopathy), photocoagulation

🔧 8.64 🔨 9.67 **FUD** 010 [T] [P3] [50] 🔲

AMA: 2018,Jan,8; 2017,Jan,8; 2016,Feb,12; 2016,Jan,13

67229 Treatment of extensive or progressive retinopathy, 1 or more sessions, preterm infant (less than 37 weeks gestation at birth), performed from birth up to 1 year of age (eg, retinopathy of prematurity), photocoagulation or cryotherapy

INCLUDES Treatment at one or more sessions that may occur at different encounters
EXCLUDES Procedure performed more than one time during defined period of treatment

🔧 33.1 🔨 33.1 **FUD** 090 [T] [R2] [50] 🔲

AMA: 2018,Jan,8; 2017,Jan,8; 2016,Feb,12; 2016,Jan,13

67250-67255 Reinforcement of Posterior Sclera

INCLUDES Operating microscope (69990)
EXCLUDES Removal scleral lesion (66130)
Repair scleral staphyloma (66225)

67250 Scleral reinforcement (separate procedure); without graft

🔧 22.6 🔨 22.6 **FUD** 090 [J] [A2] [50] 🔲

AMA: 2016,Feb,12

67255 with graft

EXCLUDES Aqueous shunt to extraocular equatorial plate reservoir (66180)
Revision aqueous shunt to extraocular equatorial plate reservoir; with graft (66185)

🔧 19.3 🔨 19.3 **FUD** 090 [J] [A2] [80] [50] 🔲

AMA: 2018,Jan,8; 2017,Jan,8; 2016,Feb,12; 2016,Jan,13

67299 Unlisted Posterior Segment Procedure

CMS: 100-04,4,180.3 Unlisted Service or Procedure
INCLUDES Operating microscope (69990)

67299 Unlisted procedure, posterior segment

🔧 0.00 🔨 0.00 **FUD** YYY [J] [80] [50] 🔲

AMA: 2018,Jan,8; 2017,Jan,8; 2016,Feb,12; 2016,Jan,13

67311-67334 Strabismus Procedures on Extraocular Muscles

INCLUDES Operating microscope (69990)
Code also adjustable sutures (67335)

67311 Strabismus surgery, recession or resection procedure; 1 horizontal muscle

🔧 16.8 🔨 16.8 **FUD** 090 [J] [A2] [50] 🔲

AMA: 2018,Jan,8; 2017,Jan,8; 2017,Jan,6; 2016,Feb,12; 2016,Jan,13

Muscles of the eyeball (right eye shown)

67312 2 horizontal muscles

🔧 20.3 🔨 20.3 **FUD** 090 [J] [A2] [50] 🔲

AMA: 2018,Jan,8; 2017,Jan,8; 2016,Feb,12; 2016,Jan,13

67314 1 vertical muscle (excluding superior oblique)

🔧 19.1 🔨 19.1 **FUD** 090 [J] [A2] [50] 🔲

AMA: 2018,Jan,8; 2017,Jan,8; 2016,Feb,12; 2016,Jan,13

67316 2 or more vertical muscles (excluding superior oblique)

🔧 22.7 🔨 22.7 **FUD** 090 [J] [A2] [80] [50] 🔲

AMA: 2018,Jan,8; 2017,Jan,8; 2016,Feb,12; 2016,Jan,13

67318 Strabismus surgery, any procedure, superior oblique muscle

🔧 20.0 🔨 20.0 **FUD** 090 [J] [A2] [50] 🔲

AMA: 2018,Jan,8; 2017,Jan,8; 2016,Feb,12; 2016,Jan,13

+ 67320 Transposition procedure (eg, for paretic extraocular muscle), any extraocular muscle (specify) (List separately in addition to code for primary procedure)

Code first (67311-67318)

🔧 9.17 🔨 9.17 **FUD** ZZZ [N] [N1] 🔲

AMA: 2018,Jan,8; 2017,Jan,8; 2016,Feb,12; 2016,Jan,13

+ 67331 Strabismus surgery on patient with previous eye surgery or injury that did not involve the extraocular muscles (List separately in addition to code for primary procedure)

Code first (67311-67318)

🔧 8.70 🔨 8.70 **FUD** ZZZ [N] [N1] [50] 🔲

AMA: 2018,Jan,8; 2017,Jan,8; 2016,Feb,12; 2016,Jan,13

+ 67332 Strabismus surgery on patient with scarring of extraocular muscles (eg, prior ocular injury, strabismus or retinal detachment surgery) or restrictive myopathy (eg, dysthyroid ophthalmopathy) (List separately in addition to code for primary procedure)

Code first (67311-67318)

🔧 9.37 🔨 9.37 **FUD** ZZZ [N] [N1] [50] 🔲

AMA: 2018,Jan,8; 2017,Jan,8; 2016,Feb,12; 2016,Jan,13

+ 67334 Strabismus surgery by posterior fixation suture technique, with or without muscle recession (List separately in addition to code for primary procedure)

Code first (67311-67318)

🔧 8.52 🔨 8.52 **FUD** ZZZ [N] [N1] [50] 🔲

AMA: 2018,Jan,8; 2017,Jan,8; 2016,Feb,12; 2016,Jan,13

● New Code ▲ Revised Code ○ Reinstated ● New Web Release ▲ Revised Web Release + Add-on Unlisted Not Covered # Resequenced
50 Optum Mod 50 Exempt ⊘ AMA Mod 51 Exempt 51 Optum Mod 51 Exempt 63 Mod 63 Exempt ✔ Non-FDA Drug ★ Telemedicine Ⓜ Maternity Ⓐ Age Edit

67335-67399 Other Procedures of Extraocular Muscles

INCLUDES   Operating microscope (69990)

+   67335   Placement of adjustable suture(s) during strabismus surgery, including postoperative adjustment(s) of suture(s) (List separately in addition to code for specific strabismus surgery)
Code first (67311-67334)
🔧 4.21   ⚕ 4.21   **FUD** ZZZ   N N1 50 ▣
AMA: 2018,Jan,8; 2017,Jan,8; 2016,Feb,12; 2016,Jan,13

+   67340   Strabismus surgery involving exploration and/or repair of detached extraocular muscle(s) (List separately in addition to code for primary procedure)
INCLUDES   Hummelsheim operation
Code first (67311-67334)
🔧 10.1   ⚕ 10.1   **FUD** ZZZ   N N1 80 ▣
AMA: 2018,Jan,8; 2017,Jan,8; 2016,Feb,12; 2016,Jan,13

67343   Release of extensive scar tissue without detaching extraocular muscle (separate procedure)
Code also when performed on other than affected muscle (67311-67340)
🔧 18.5   ⚕ 18.5   **FUD** 090   J A2 50 ▣
AMA: 2018,Jan,8; 2017,Jan,8; 2016,Feb,12; 2016,Jan,13

67345   Chemodenervation of extraocular muscle
EXCLUDES   Nerve destruction for blepharospasm and other neurological disorders (64612, 64616)
🔧 6.22   ⚕ 6.96   **FUD** 010   T P3 50 ▣
AMA: 2019,Apr,9; 2018,Jan,8; 2017,Jan,8; 2016,Feb,12; 2016,Jan,13

67346   Biopsy of extraocular muscle
EXCLUDES   Repair laceration extraocular muscle, tendon, or Tenon's capsule (65290)
🔧 5.50   ⚕ 5.50   **FUD** 000   J A2 80 50 ▣
AMA: 2016,Feb,12

67399   Unlisted procedure, extraocular muscle
🔧 0.00   ⚕ 0.00   **FUD** YYY   T 80 50 ▣
AMA: 2018,Jan,8; 2017,Jul,10; 2016,Feb,12

67400-67415 Frontal Orbitotomy

INCLUDES   Operating microscope (69990)

67400   Orbitotomy without bone flap (frontal or transconjunctival approach); for exploration, with or without biopsy
🔧 26.7   ⚕ 26.7   **FUD** 090   J A2 50 ▣
AMA: 2016,Feb,12

67405   with drainage only
🔧 22.8   ⚕ 22.8   **FUD** 090   J A2 50 ▣
AMA: 2018,Jan,8; 2017,Jan,8; 2016,Feb,12; 2016,Jan,13

67412   with removal of lesion
🔧 26.1   ⚕ 26.1   **FUD** 090   J A2 50 ▣
AMA: 2016,Feb,12

67413   with removal of foreign body
🔧 25.8   ⚕ 25.8   **FUD** 090   J A2 80 50 ▣
AMA: 2016,Feb,12

67414   with removal of bone for decompression
🔧 38.1   ⚕ 38.1   **FUD** 090   J G2 80 50 ▣
AMA: 2018,Jan,8; 2017,Jan,8; 2016,Feb,12; 2016,Jan,13

67415   Fine needle aspiration of orbital contents
EXCLUDES   Decompression optic nerve (67570)
          Exenteration, enucleation, and repair (65101-65175)
🔧 2.97   ⚕ 2.97   **FUD** 000   J A2 80 50 ▣
AMA: 2016,Feb,12

67420-67450 Lateral Orbitotomy

INCLUDES   Operating microscope (69990)
EXCLUDES   Orbital implant (67550, 67560)
          Surgical removal all or some orbital contents or repair after removal (65091-65175)
          Transcranial approach orbitotomy (61330, 61333)

67420   Orbitotomy with bone flap or window, lateral approach (eg, Kroenlein); with removal of lesion
🔧 47.5   ⚕ 47.5   **FUD** 090   J A2 80 50 ▣
AMA: 2016,Feb,12

67430   with removal of foreign body
🔧 37.3   ⚕ 37.3   **FUD** 090   J A2 80 50 ▣
AMA: 2016,Feb,12

67440   with drainage
🔧 36.1   ⚕ 36.1   **FUD** 090   J A2 80 50 ▣
AMA: 2016,Feb,12

67445   with removal of bone for decompression
EXCLUDES   Decompression optic nerve sheath (67570)
🔧 41.6   ⚕ 41.6   **FUD** 090   J A2 80 50 ▣
AMA: 2019,Dec,14; 2016,Feb,12

67450   for exploration, with or without biopsy
🔧 36.1   ⚕ 36.1   **FUD** 090   J A2 80 50 ▣
AMA: 2016,Feb,12

67500-67515 Eye Injections

INCLUDES   Operating microscope (69990)

67500   Retrobulbar injection; medication (separate procedure, does not include supply of medication)
🔧 1.74   ⚕ 2.07   **FUD** 000   T P3 50 ▣
AMA: 2018,Jan,8; 2017,Jan,8; 2016,Feb,12; 2016,Jan,13

67505   alcohol
🔧 2.03   ⚕ 2.38   **FUD** 000   T P3 50 ▣
AMA: 2016,Feb,12

67515   Injection of medication or other substance into Tenon's capsule
EXCLUDES   Subconjunctival injection (68200)
🔧 2.06   ⚕ 2.24   **FUD** 000   T P3 50 ▣
AMA: 2018,Jan,8; 2017,Jan,8; 2016,Feb,12; 2016,Jan,13

67550-67560 Orbital Implant

INCLUDES   Operating microscope (69990)
EXCLUDES   Fracture repair malar area, orbit (21355-21408)
          Ocular implant inside muscle cone (65093-65105, 65130-65175)

67550   Orbital implant (implant outside muscle cone); insertion
🔧 29.0   ⚕ 29.0   **FUD** 090   J A2 50 ▣
AMA: 2016,Feb,12

67560   removal or revision
🔧 28.5   ⚕ 28.5   **FUD** 090   J A2 80 50 ▣
AMA: 2016,Feb,12

67570-67599 Other and Unlisted Orbital Procedures

INCLUDES   Operating microscope (69990)

67570   Optic nerve decompression (eg, incision or fenestration of optic nerve sheath)
🔧 35.6   ⚕ 35.6   **FUD** 090   J A2 80 50 ▣
AMA: 2016,Feb,12

67599   Unlisted procedure, orbit
🔧 0.00   ⚕ 0.00   **FUD** YYY   T 80 50 ▣
AMA: 2016,Feb,12

67700-67810 [67810] Incisional Procedures of Eyelids

INCLUDES   Operating microscope (69990)

67700   Blepharotomy, drainage of abscess, eyelid
🔧 3.31   ⚕ 7.82   **FUD** 010   T P2 50 ▣
AMA: 2018,Jan,8; 2017,Jan,8; 2016,Feb,12; 2016,Jan,13

67710   Severing of tarsorrhaphy
🔧 2.75   ⚕ 6.68   **FUD** 010   T P3 50 ▣
AMA: 2018,Jan,8; 2017,Jan,8; 2016,Feb,12; 2016,Jan,13

26/TC PC/TC Only   A2-Z3 ASC Payment   50 Bilateral   ♂ Male Only   ♀ Female Only   🔧 Facility RVU   ⚕ Non-Facility RVU   ▣ CCI   ✖ CLIA
FUD Follow-up Days   **CMS:** IOM   **AMA:** CPT Asst   A-Y OPPSI   80/80 Surg Assist Allowed / w/Doc   Lab crosswalk   Radiology crosswalk

310   CPT © 2021 American Medical Association. All Rights Reserved.   © 2021 Optum360, LLC

67715 **Canthotomy (separate procedure)**

EXCLUDES *Canthoplasty (67950)*
Symblepharon division (68340)

🚑 3.08 ✂ 7.07 **FUD** 010 `J` `A2` `50` ▢

AMA: 2018,Jan,8; 2017,Jan,8; 2016,Feb,12; 2016,Jan,13

\# **67810** **Incisional biopsy of eyelid skin including lid margin**

EXCLUDES *Biopsy eyelid skin (11102-11107)*

🚑 2.03 ✂ 4.99 **FUD** 000 `T` `P2` `50` ▢

AMA: 2019,Jan,9; 2018,Jan,8; 2017,Jan,8; 2016,Feb,12; 2016,Jan,13

67800-67808 Excision of Chalazion (Meibomian Cyst)

INCLUDES Lesion removal requiring more than skin:
Lid margin
Palpebral conjunctiva
Tarsus
Operating microscope (69990)

EXCLUDES *Blepharoplasty, graft, or reconstructive procedures (67930-67975)*
Excision/destruction skin lesion eyelid (11310-11313, 11440-11446, 11640-11646, 17000-17004)

67800 **Excision of chalazion; single**

🚑 2.91 ✂ 3.64 **FUD** 010 `T` `P3` ▢

AMA: 2018,Jan,8; 2017,Jan,8; 2016,Feb,12; 2016,Jan,13

67801 **multiple, same lid**

🚑 3.74 ✂ 4.61 **FUD** 010 `T` `P3` ▢

AMA: 2016,Feb,12

67805 **multiple, different lids**

🚑 4.63 ✂ 5.72 **FUD** 010 `T` `P3` ▢

AMA: 2018,Jan,8; 2017,Jan,8; 2016,Feb,12; 2016,Jan,13

67808 **under general anesthesia and/or requiring hospitalization, single or multiple**

🚑 10.4 ✂ 10.4 **FUD** 090 `J` `A2`

AMA: 2016,Feb,12

67810-67850 [67810] Other Eyelid Procedures

INCLUDES Operating microscope (69990)

67810 **Resequenced code. See code following 67715.**

67820 **Correction of trichiasis; epilation, by forceps only**

🚑 0.99 ✂ 0.93 **FUD** 000 `01` `N1` `50` ▢

AMA: 2018,Jan,8; 2017,Jan,8; 2016,Feb,12; 2016,Jan,13

67825 **epilation by other than forceps (eg, by electrosurgery, cryotherapy, laser surgery)**

🚑 3.46 ✂ 3.71 **FUD** 010 `T` `P3` `50` ▢

AMA: 2018,Jan,8; 2017,Jan,8; 2016,Feb,12; 2016,Jan,13

67830 **incision of lid margin**

🚑 3.92 ✂ 7.64 **FUD** 010 `T` `A2` `50` ▢

AMA: 2016,Feb,12

67835 **incision of lid margin, with free mucous membrane graft**

🚑 12.4 ✂ 12.4 **FUD** 090 `J` `A2` `80` `50` ▢

AMA: 2016,Feb,12

67840 **Excision of lesion of eyelid (except chalazion) without closure or with simple direct closure**

EXCLUDES *Eyelid resection and reconstruction (67961, 67966)*

🚑 4.49 ✂ 7.91 **FUD** 010 `T` `P3` `50` ▢

AMA: 2019,Jan,14; 2016,Feb,12

67850 **Destruction of lesion of lid margin (up to 1 cm)**

EXCLUDES *Mohs micro procedures (17311-17315)*
Topical chemotherapy (99202-99215)

🚑 3.75 ✂ 6.12 **FUD** 010 `T` `P3` `50` ▢

AMA: 2016,Feb,12

67875-67882 Suturing of the Eyelids

INCLUDES Operating microscope (69990)

EXCLUDES *Canthoplasty (67950)*
Canthotomy (67715)
Severing of tarsorrhaphy (67710)

67875 **Temporary closure of eyelids by suture (eg, Frost suture)**

🚑 2.75 ✂ 4.96 **FUD** 000 `T` `G2` `50` ▢

AMA: 2016,Feb,12

67880 **Construction of intermarginal adhesions, median tarsorrhaphy, or canthorrhaphy;**

🚑 10.4 ✂ 13.1 **FUD** 090 `J` `A2` `50` ▢

AMA: 2016,Feb,12

67882 **with transposition of tarsal plate**

🚑 13.3 ✂ 16.1 **FUD** 090 `J` `A2` `50` ▢

AMA: 2016,Feb,12

67900-67912 Repair of Ptosis/Retraction Eyelids, Eyebrows

INCLUDES Operating microscope (69990)

67900 **Repair of brow ptosis (supraciliary, mid-forehead or coronal approach)**

EXCLUDES *Forehead rhytidectomy (15824)*

🚑 14.4 ✂ 18.2 **FUD** 090 `J` `A2` `50` ▢

AMA: 2018,Jan,8; 2017,Jan,8; 2016,Feb,12; 2016,Jan,13

67901 **Repair of blepharoptosis; frontalis muscle technique with suture or other material (eg, banked fascia)**

🚑 16.5 ✂ 21.9 **FUD** 090 `J` `A2` `50` ▢

AMA: 2018,Jan,8; 2017,Jul,10; 2017,Jan,8; 2016,Feb,12; 2016,Jan,13

67902 **frontalis muscle technique with autologous fascial sling (includes obtaining fascia)**

🚑 20.5 ✂ 20.5 **FUD** 090 `J` `A2` `50` ▢

AMA: 2018,Jan,8; 2017,Jan,8; 2016,Feb,12; 2016,Jan,13

67903 **(tarso) levator resection or advancement, internal approach**

🚑 13.7 ✂ 16.9 **FUD** 090 `J` `A2` `50` ▢

AMA: 2018,Jan,8; 2017,Jan,8; 2016,Feb,12; 2016,Jan,13

67904 **(tarso) levator resection or advancement, external approach**

INCLUDES Everbusch's operation

🚑 16.9 ✂ 20.9 **FUD** 090 `J` `A2` `50` ▢

AMA: 2018,Jan,8; 2017,Jan,8; 2016,Feb,12; 2016,Jan,13

67906 **superior rectus technique with fascial sling (includes obtaining fascia)**

🚑 14.4 ✂ 14.4 **FUD** 090 `J` `A2` `50` ▢

AMA: 2018,Jan,8; 2017,Jan,8; 2016,Feb,12; 2016,Jan,13

67908 **conjunctivo-tarso-Muller's muscle-levator resection (eg, Fasanella-Servat type)**

🚑 12.1 ✂ 14.1 **FUD** 090 `J` `A2` `50` ▢

AMA: 2018,Jan,8; 2017,Jan,8; 2016,Feb,12; 2016,Jan,13

67909 **Reduction of overcorrection of ptosis**

🚑 12.4 ✂ 15.3 **FUD** 090 `J` `A2` `50` ▢

AMA: 2018,Jan,8; 2017,Jan,8; 2016,Feb,12; 2016,Jan,13

Eye, Ocular Adnexa, and Ear

67911 Correction of lid retraction

EXCLUDES Autologous graft harvest ([15769], 20920, 20922)
Lid defect correction using fat obtained via liposuction (15773-15774)
Mucous membrane graft repair trichiasis (67835)

🔪 15.9   🔪 15.9   **FUD** 090   J A2 50 ▣

AMA: 2018,Jan,8; 2017,Jan,8; 2016,Feb,12; 2016,Jan,13

67912 Correction of lagophthalmos, with implantation of upper eyelid lid load (eg, gold weight)

🔪 13.8   🔪 25.4   **FUD** 090   J A2 50 ▣

AMA: 2018,Jan,8; 2017,Jan,8; 2016,Feb,12; 2016,Jan,13

67914-67924 Repair Ectropion/Entropion

INCLUDES Operating microscope (69990)
EXCLUDES Cicatricial ectropion or entropion with scar excision or graft (67961-67966)

67914 Repair of ectropion; suture

INCLUDES Canthoplasty (67950)

🔪 9.29   🔪 13.5   **FUD** 090   J A2 50 ▣

AMA: 2018,Jan,8; 2017,Jan,8; 2016,Feb,12; 2016,Jan,13

67915 thermocauterization

🔪 5.62   🔪 8.52   **FUD** 090   J P3 50 ▣

AMA: 2018,Jan,8; 2017,Jan,8; 2016,Feb,12; 2016,Jan,13

67916 excision tarsal wedge

🔪 12.2   🔪 17.0   **FUD** 090   J A2 50 ▣

AMA: 2018,Jan,8; 2017,Jan,8; 2016,Feb,12; 2016,Jan,13

67917 extensive (eg, tarsal strip operations)

EXCLUDES Repair everted punctum (68705)

🔪 13.0   🔪 17.3   **FUD** 090   J A2 50 ▣

AMA: 2020,Feb,13; 2018,Jan,8; 2017,Jan,8; 2016,Feb,12; 2016,Jan,13

67921 Repair of entropion; suture

🔪 8.82   🔪 13.2   **FUD** 090   J A2 50 ▣

AMA: 2018,Jan,8; 2017,Jan,8; 2016,Feb,12; 2016,Jan,13

67922 thermocauterization

🔪 5.52   🔪 8.42   **FUD** 090   J P3 50 ▣

AMA: 2018,Jan,8; 2017,Jan,8; 2016,Feb,12; 2016,Jan,13

67923 excision tarsal wedge

🔪 12.1   🔪 17.1   **FUD** 090   J A2 50 ▣

AMA: 2018,Jan,8; 2017,Jan,8; 2016,Feb,12; 2016,Jan,13

67924 extensive (eg, tarsal strip or capsulopalpebral fascia repairs operation)

INCLUDES Canthoplasty (67950)

🔪 12.9   🔪 18.2   **FUD** 090   J A2 50 ▣

AMA: 2018,Jan,8; 2017,Jan,8; 2016,Feb,12; 2016,Jan,13

67930-67935 Repair Eyelid Wound

INCLUDES Operating microscope (69990)
Repairs involving more than skin:
  Lid margin
  Palpebral conjunctiva
  Tarsus
EXCLUDES Blepharoplasty for entropion or ectropion (67916-67917, 67923-67924)
Correction lid retraction and blepharoptosis (67901-67911)
Free graft (15120-15121, 15260-15261)
Graft preparation (15004)
Plastic repair lacrimal canaliculi (68700)
Removal eyelid lesion (67800 [67810], 67840-67850)
Repair blepharochalasis (15820-15823)
Repair involving eyelid skin (12011-12018, 12051-12057, 13151-13153)
Skin adjacent tissue transfer (14060-14061)
Tarsorrhaphy, canthorrhaphy (67880, 67882)

67930 Suture of recent wound, eyelid, involving lid margin, tarsus, and/or palpebral conjunctiva direct closure; partial thickness

🔪 6.78   🔪 10.4   **FUD** 010   J P3 50 ▣

AMA: 2016,Feb,12

67935 full thickness

🔪 12.5   🔪 16.9   **FUD** 090   J A2 50 ▣

AMA: 2016,Feb,12

67938-67999 Eyelid Reconstruction/Repair/Removal Deep Foreign Body

INCLUDES Operating microscope (69990)
EXCLUDES Blepharoplasty for entropion or ectropion (67916-67917, 67923-67924)
Correction lid retraction and blepharoptosis (67901-67911)
Free graft (15120-15121, 15260-15261)
Graft preparation (15004)
Plastic repair lacrimal canaliculi (68700)
Removal eyelid lesion (67800-67808, 67840-67850)
Repair blepharochalasis (15820-15823)
Repair involving eyelid skin (12011-12018, 12051-12057, 13151-13153)
Skin adjacent tissue transfer (14060-14061)
Tarsorrhaphy, canthorrhaphy (67880, 67882)

67938 Removal of embedded foreign body, eyelid

🔪 3.28   🔪 7.36   **FUD** 010   T P2 50 ▣

AMA: 2018,Jan,8; 2017,Jan,8; 2016,Feb,12; 2016,Jan,13

67950 Canthoplasty (reconstruction of canthus)

🔪 13.1   🔪 16.4   **FUD** 090   J A2 50 ▣

AMA: 2016,Feb,12

67961 Excision and repair of eyelid, involving lid margin, tarsus, conjunctiva, canthus, or full thickness, may include preparation for skin graft or pedicle flap with adjacent tissue transfer or rearrangement; up to one-fourth of lid margin

INCLUDES Canthoplasty (67950)
EXCLUDES Delay flap (15630)
Flap attachment (15650)
Free skin grafts (15120-15121, 15260-15261)
Tubed pedicle flap preparation (15576)

🔪 12.9   🔪 16.4   **FUD** 090   J A2 80 50 ▣

AMA: 2018,Jan,8; 2017,Jan,8; 2016,Feb,12; 2016,Jan,13

67966 over one-fourth of lid margin

INCLUDES Canthoplasty (67950)
EXCLUDES Delay flap (15630)
Flap attachment (15650)
Free skin grafts (15120-15121, 15260-15261)
Tubed pedicle flap preparation (15576)

🔪 18.7   🔪 21.9   **FUD** 090   J A2 50 ▣

AMA: 2018,Jan,8; 2017,Jan,8; 2016,Feb,12; 2016,Jan,13

67971 Reconstruction of eyelid, full thickness by transfer of tarsoconjunctival flap from opposing eyelid; up to two-thirds of eyelid, 1 stage or first stage

INCLUDES Dupuy-Dutemp reconstruction
Landboldt's operation

🔪 20.4   🔪 20.4   **FUD** 090   J A2 50 ▣

AMA: 2016,Feb,12

67973 total eyelid, lower, 1 stage or first stage

INCLUDES Landboldt's operation

🔪 26.3   🔪 26.3   **FUD** 090   J A2 80 50 ▣

AMA: 2016,Feb,12

67974 total eyelid, upper, 1 stage or first stage

INCLUDES Landboldt's operation

🔪 26.2   🔪 26.2   **FUD** 090   J A2 80 50 ▣

AMA: 2016,Feb,12

67975 second stage

INCLUDES Landboldt's operation

🔪 19.4   🔪 19.4   **FUD** 090   J A2 50 ▣

AMA: 2016,Feb,12

67999 Unlisted procedure, eyelids

🔪 0.00   🔪 0.00   **FUD** YYY   T 80 50 ▣

AMA: 2018,Jan,8; 2017,Jul,10; 2017,Jan,8; 2016,Feb,12; 2016,Jan,13

26/TC PC/TC Only   A2-Z3 ASC Payment   50 Bilateral   ♂ Male Only   ♀ Female Only   🔪 Facility RVU   🔪 Non-Facility RVU   ▣ CCI   ✖ CLIA
FUD Follow-up Days   CMS: IOM   AMA: CPT Asst   A-Y OPPSI   80/80 Surg Assist Allowed / w/Doc   Lab crosswalk   Radiology crosswalk

68020-68200 Conjunctival Biopsy/Injection/Treatment of Lesions

INCLUDES   Operating microscope (69990)
EXCLUDES   Foreign body removal (65205-65265)

68020   **Incision of conjunctiva, drainage of cyst**
🔾 3.11   ⚕ 3.41   **FUD** 010   T P3 50 ▣
AMA: 2016,Feb,12

68040   **Expression of conjunctival follicles (eg, for trachoma)**
EXCLUDES   Automated evacuation meibomian glands with heat/pressure (0207T)
Manual evacuation meibomian glands ([0563T])
🔾 1.40   ⚕ 1.78   **FUD** 000   T P3 50 ▣
AMA: 2018,Jan,8; 2017,Jan,8; 2016,Feb,12; 2016,Jan,13

68100   **Biopsy of conjunctiva**
🔾 2.75   ⚕ 4.97   **FUD** 000   J P3 50 ▣
AMA: 2019,Jan,9; 2016,Feb,12

68110   **Excision of lesion, conjunctiva; up to 1 cm**
🔾 4.18   ⚕ 6.63   **FUD** 010   J P3 50 ▣
AMA: 2018,Feb,11; 2018,Jan,8; 2017,Jan,6; 2016,Feb,12

68115   **over 1 cm**
🔾 5.18   ⚕ 9.19   **FUD** 010   J A2 50 ▣
AMA: 2018,Feb,11; 2016,Feb,12

68130   **with adjacent sclera**
🔾 11.6   ⚕ 15.5   **FUD** 090   J A2 50 ▣
AMA: 2016,Feb,12

68135   **Destruction of lesion, conjunctiva**
🔾 4.24   ⚕ 4.46   **FUD** 010   J P3 50 ▣
AMA: 2016,Feb,12

68200   **Subconjunctival injection**
EXCLUDES   Retrobulbar or Tenon's capsule injection (67500-67515)
🔾 0.99   ⚕ 1.19   **FUD** 000   Q1 N1 50 ▣
AMA: 2018,Jan,8; 2017,Jan,8; 2016,Feb,12; 2016,Jan,13

68320-68340 Conjunctivoplasty Procedures

INCLUDES   Operating microscope (69990)
EXCLUDES   Conjunctival foreign body removal (65205, 65210)
Laceration repair (65270-65273)

68320   **Conjunctivoplasty; with conjunctival graft or extensive rearrangement**
🔾 15.3   ⚕ 20.8   **FUD** 090   J A2 50 ▣
AMA: 2018,Jan,8; 2017,Jan,8; 2016,Feb,12; 2016,Jan,13

68325   **with buccal mucous membrane graft (includes obtaining graft)**
🔾 18.5   ⚕ 18.5   **FUD** 090   J A2 50 ▣
AMA: 2016,Feb,12

68326   **Conjunctivoplasty, reconstruction cul-de-sac; with conjunctival graft or extensive rearrangement**
🔾 18.2   ⚕ 18.2   **FUD** 090   J A2 50 ▣
AMA: 2016,Feb,12

68328   **with buccal mucous membrane graft (includes obtaining graft)**
🔾 20.1   ⚕ 20.1   **FUD** 090   J A2 80 50 ▣
AMA: 2016,Feb,12

68330   **Repair of symblepharon; conjunctivoplasty, without graft**
🔾 13.0   ⚕ 17.4   **FUD** 090   J A2 80 50 ▣
AMA: 2016,Feb,12

68335   **with free graft conjunctiva or buccal mucous membrane (includes obtaining graft)**
🔾 18.2   ⚕ 18.2   **FUD** 090   J A2 50 ▣
AMA: 2016,Feb,12

68340   **division of symblepharon, with or without insertion of conformer or contact lens**
🔾 11.2   ⚕ 16.4   **FUD** 090   J A2 80 50 ▣
AMA: 2016,Feb,12

68360-68399 Conjunctival Flaps and Unlisted Procedures

INCLUDES   Operating microscope (69990)

68360   **Conjunctival flap; bridge or partial (separate procedure)**
EXCLUDES   Conjunctival flap for injury (65280, 65285)
Conjunctival foreign body removal (65205, 65210)
Surgical wound repair (66250)
🔾 11.7   ⚕ 15.3   **FUD** 090   J A2 50 ▣
AMA: 2016,Feb,12

68362   **total (such as Gunderson thin flap or purse string flap)**
EXCLUDES   Conjunctival flap for injury (65280, 65285)
Conjunctival foreign body removal (65205, 65210)
Surgical wound repair (66250)
🔾 18.5   ⚕ 18.5   **FUD** 090   J A2 50 ▣
AMA: 2018,Jan,8; 2017,Jan,8; 2016,Feb,12; 2016,Jan,13

68371   **Harvesting conjunctival allograft, living donor**
🔾 11.7   ⚕ 11.7   **FUD** 010   J A2 50 ▣
AMA: 2018,Jan,8; 2017,Jan,8; 2016,Feb,12; 2016,Jan,13

68399   **Unlisted procedure, conjunctiva**
🔾 0.00   ⚕ 0.00   **FUD** YYY   T 80 50 ▣
AMA: 2018,Jan,8; 2017,Jan,8; 2016,Feb,12; 2016,Jan,13

68400-68899 Nasolacrimal System Procedures

INCLUDES   Operating microscope (69990)

68400   **Incision, drainage of lacrimal gland**
🔾 3.71   ⚕ 8.30   **FUD** 010   T P3 50 ▣
AMA: 2016,Feb,12

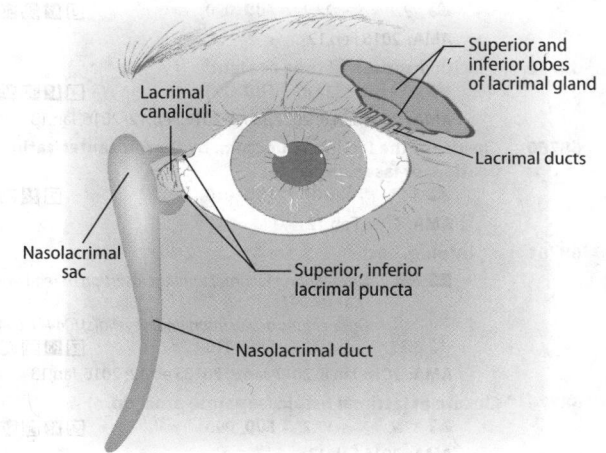

68420   **Incision, drainage of lacrimal sac (dacryocystotomy or dacryocystostomy)**
🔾 4.78   ⚕ 9.28   **FUD** 010   J P3 50 ▣
AMA: 2016,Feb,12

68440   **Snip incision of lacrimal punctum**
🔾 2.80   ⚕ 2.92   **FUD** 010   T P3 50 ▣
AMA: 2016,Feb,12

68500   **Excision of lacrimal gland (dacryoadenectomy), except for tumor; total**
🔾 28.6   ⚕ 28.6   **FUD** 090   J A2 50 ▣
AMA: 2016,Feb,12

68505   **partial**
🔾 28.5   ⚕ 28.5   **FUD** 090   J A2 50 ▣
AMA: 2016,Feb,12

68510   **Biopsy of lacrimal gland**
🔾 8.26   ⚕ 12.9   **FUD** 000   J A2 80 50 ▣
AMA: 2016,Feb,12

68520   **Excision of lacrimal sac (dacryocystectomy)**
🔾 20.0   ⚕ 20.0   **FUD** 090   J A2 80 50 ▣
AMA: 2016,Feb,12

68525 Biopsy of lacrimal sac
🖥 7.52 ⚕ 7.52 **FUD** 000 ☐ J A2 50 ☐
AMA: 2016,Feb,12

68530 Removal of foreign body or dacryolith, lacrimal passages
INCLUDES Meller's excision
🖥 7.23 ⚕ 12.2 **FUD** 010 ☐ T P2 50 ☐
AMA: 2016,Feb,12

68540 Excision of lacrimal gland tumor; frontal approach
🖥 27.0 ⚕ 27.0 **FUD** 090 ☐ J A2 50 ☐
AMA: 2016,Feb,12

68550 involving osteotomy
🖥 33.3 ⚕ 33.3 **FUD** 090 ☐ J A2 50 ☐
AMA: 2016,Feb,12

68700 Plastic repair of canaliculi
🖥 17.0 ⚕ 17.0 **FUD** 090 ☐ J A2 50 ☐
AMA: 2016,Feb,12

68705 Correction of everted punctum, cautery
🖥 4.68 ⚕ 7.19 **FUD** 010 ☐ T P2 50 ☐
AMA: 2020,Feb,13; 2018,Jan,8; 2017,Jan,8; 2016,Feb,12; 2016,Jan,13

68720 Dacryocystorhinostomy (fistulization of lacrimal sac to nasal cavity)
🖥 22.1 ⚕ 22.1 **FUD** 090 ☐ J A2 80 50 ☐
AMA: 2018,Jan,8; 2017,Jan,8; 2016,Feb,12; 2016,Jan,13

68745 Conjunctivorhinostomy (fistulization of conjunctiva to nasal cavity); without tube
🖥 22.2 ⚕ 22.2 **FUD** 090 ☐ J A2 80 50 ☐
AMA: 2016,Feb,12

68750 with insertion of tube or stent
🖥 22.4 ⚕ 22.4 **FUD** 090 ☐ J A2 80 50 ☐
AMA: 2018,Jan,8; 2017,Jan,8; 2016,Feb,12; 2016,Jan,13

68760 Closure of the lacrimal punctum; by thermocauterization, ligation, or laser surgery
🖥 4.11 ⚕ 6.07 **FUD** 010 ☐ T P2 50 ☐
AMA: 2016,Feb,12

68761 by plug, each
EXCLUDES Drug-eluting lacrimal implant insertion or removal (68841)
Drug-eluting ocular insert under eyelid(s) (0444T-0445T)
🖥 3.32 ⚕ 4.20 **FUD** 010 ☐ T P3 80 50 ☐
AMA: 2018,Jan,8; 2017,Jan,8; 2016,Feb,12; 2016,Jan,13

68770 Closure of lacrimal fistula (separate procedure)
🖥 17.7 ⚕ 17.7 **FUD** 090 ☐ J A2 80 50 ☐
AMA: 2016,Feb,12

68801 Dilation of lacrimal punctum, with or without irrigation
🖥 2.18 ⚕ 2.60 **FUD** 010 ☐ 01 N1 50 ☐
AMA: 2016,Feb,12

68810 Probing of nasolacrimal duct, with or without irrigation;
EXCLUDES Ophthalmological exam under anesthesia (92018)
🖥 3.64 ⚕ 4.47 **FUD** 010 ☐ T A2 50 ☐
AMA: 2018,Jan,8; 2017,Jan,8; 2016,Feb,12; 2016,Jan,13

68811 requiring general anesthesia
EXCLUDES Ophthalmological exam under anesthesia (92018)
🖥 3.82 ⚕ 3.82 **FUD** 010 ☐ J A2 50 ☐
AMA: 2018,Jan,8; 2017,Jan,8; 2016,Feb,12; 2016,Jan,13

68815 with insertion of tube or stent
EXCLUDES Drug-eluting lacrimal implant insertion or removal (68841)
Drug-eluting ocular insert under eyelid(s) (0444T-0445T)
Ophthalmological exam under anesthesia (92018)
🖥 6.27 ⚕ 11.0 **FUD** 010 ☐ J A2 50 ☐
AMA: 2018,Jan,8; 2017,Jan,8; 2016,Feb,12; 2016,Jan,13

68816 with transluminal balloon catheter dilation
EXCLUDES Probing nasolacrimal duct (68810-68811, 68815)
🖥 4.45 ⚕ 22.2 **FUD** 010 ☐ J C2 50 ☐
AMA: 2018,Jan,8; 2017,Jan,8; 2016,Feb,12; 2016,Jan,13

68840 Probing of lacrimal canaliculi, with or without irrigation
🖥 3.27 ⚕ 3.70 **FUD** 010 ☐ T P3 50 ☐
AMA: 2016,Feb,12

● **68841 Insertion of drug-eluting implant, including punctal dilation when performed, into lacrimal canaliculus, each**
EXCLUDES Drug-eluting ocular insert under eyelid(s) (0444T-0445T)
Code also drug-eluting implant with 99070 or other appropriate supply code

68850 Injection of contrast medium for dacryocystography
📷 (70170, 78660)
🖥 1.59 ⚕ 1.80 **FUD** 000 ☐ N N1 50 ☐
AMA: 2018,Jan,8; 2017,Jan,8; 2016,Feb,12; 2016,Jan,13

68899 Unlisted procedure, lacrimal system
🖥 0.00 ⚕ 0.00 **FUD** YYY ☐ T 80 50 ☐
AMA: 2014,Jan,11; 1991,Sum,17

69000-69020 Treatment External Abscess/Hematoma

69000 Drainage external ear, abscess or hematoma; simple
🖥 3.47 ⚕ 5.34 **FUD** 010 ☐ T P3 50 ☐
AMA: 2018,Jan,8; 2017,Jan,8; 2016,Jan,13

An incision is made to drain the contents of an abscess or hematoma

69005 complicated
🖥 4.50 ⚕ 6.13 **FUD** 010 ☐ J P3 50 ☐
AMA: 2014,Jan,11; 1999,Oct,10

69020 Drainage external auditory canal, abscess
🖥 4.03 ⚕ 6.57 **FUD** 010 ☐ T P3 50 ☐
AMA: 2018,Jan,8; 2017,Jan,8; 2016,Jan,13

69090 Cosmetic Ear Piercing

CMS: 100-02,16,10 Exclusions from Coverage; 100-02,16,120 Cosmetic Procedures

69090 Ear piercing
🖥 0.00 ⚕ 0.00 **FUD** XXX ☐ E ☐
AMA: 2014,Jan,11; 1999,Oct,10

69100-69222 External Ear/Auditory Canal Procedures

EXCLUDES Reconstruction ear (see integumentary section codes)

69100 Biopsy external ear
🖥 1.37 ⚕ 2.79 **FUD** 000 ☐ T P3 ☐
AMA: 2019,Jan,9

69105 Biopsy external auditory canal
🖥 1.78 ⚕ 4.00 **FUD** 000 ☐ T P3 50 ☐
AMA: 2014,Jan,11; 1999,Oct,10

69110 Excision external ear; partial, simple repair
🖥 9.28 ⚕ 13.1 **FUD** 090 ☐ J A2 50 ☐
AMA: 2014,Jan,11; 1999,Oct,10

69120 complete amputation
🖥 11.1 ⚕ 11.1 **FUD** 090 ☐ J A2 ☐
AMA: 2014,Jan,11; 1999,Oct,10

69140 Excision exostosis(es), external auditory canal
🚗 24.8 ⚖ 24.8 **FUD** 090 [J] [A2] [80] [50] [▭]
AMA: 2014,Jan,11; 1999,Oct,10

69145 Excision soft tissue lesion, external auditory canal
🚗 7.04 ⚖ 11.1 **FUD** 090 [J] [A2] [50] [▭]
AMA: 2019,Dec,14

69150 Radical excision external auditory canal lesion; without neck dissection
EXCLUDES Skin graft (15004-15261)
Temporal bone resection (69535)
🚗 29.5 ⚖ 29.5 **FUD** 090 [J] [A2] [▭]
AMA: 2014,Jan,11; 2003,Jan,1

69155 with neck dissection
EXCLUDES Skin graft (15004-15261)
Temporal bone resection (69535)
🚗 47.0 ⚖ 47.0 **FUD** 090 [C] [80] [▭]
AMA: 2014,Jan,11; 1999,Oct,10

69200 Removal foreign body from external auditory canal; without general anesthesia
🚗 1.35 ⚖ 2.31 **FUD** 000 [01] [N1] [50] [▭]
AMA: 2014,Jan,11; 1999,Oct,10

69205 with general anesthesia
🚗 2.77 ⚖ 2.77 **FUD** 010 [J] [A2] [50] [▭]
AMA: 2018,Jan,8; 2017,Jan,8; 2016,Jan,13

69209 Removal impacted cerumen using irrigation/lavage, unilateral
EXCLUDES Removal impacted cerumen using instrumentation (69210)
Removal nonimpacted cerumen (see appropriate E/M code(s)) (99202-99233 [99224, 99225, 99226], 99241-99255, 99281-99285, 99304-99318, 99324-99337, 99341-99350)
🚗 0.40 ⚖ 0.40 **FUD** 000 [01] [N1] [50] [▭]
AMA: 2018,Jan,8; 2017,Jan,8; 2016,Mar,10; 2016,Feb,13; 2016,Jan,7

69210 Removal impacted cerumen requiring instrumentation, unilateral
EXCLUDES Removal impacted cerumen using irrigation or lavage (69209)
Removal nonimpacted cerumen (see appropriate E/M code(s)) (99202-99233 [99224, 99225, 99226], 99241-99255, 99281-99285, 99304-99318, 99324-99337, 99341-99350)
🚗 0.96 ⚖ 1.36 **FUD** 000 [01] [N1] [▭]
AMA: 2018,Jan,8; 2017,Jan,8; 2016,Mar,10; 2016,Feb,13; 2016,Jan,13; 2016,Jan,7

69220 Debridement, mastoidectomy cavity, simple (eg, routine cleaning)
🚗 1.46 ⚖ 2.25 **FUD** 000 [01] [N1] [50] [▭]
AMA: 2014,Jan,11; 1999,Oct,10

69222 Debridement, mastoidectomy cavity, complex (eg, with anesthesia or more than routine cleaning)
🚗 3.81 ⚖ 6.02 **FUD** 010 [T] [P3] [50] [▭]
AMA: 2014,Jan,11; 1999,Oct,10

69300 Plastic Surgery for Prominent Ears

CMS: 100-02,16,120 Cosmetic Procedures; 100-02,16,180 Services Related to Noncovered Procedures
EXCLUDES Suture laceration external ear (12011-14302)

69300 Otoplasty, protruding ear, with or without size reduction
🚗 13.1 ⚖ 17.6 **FUD** YYY [J] [A2] [80] [50] [▭]
AMA: 2014,Jan,11; 1999,Oct,10

69310-69399 Reconstruction Auditory Canal: Postaural Approach

EXCLUDES Suture laceration external ear (12011-14302)

69310 Reconstruction of external auditory canal (meatoplasty) (eg, for stenosis due to injury, infection) (separate procedure)
🚗 30.9 ⚖ 30.9 **FUD** 090 [J] [A2] [50] [▭]
AMA: 2018,Jan,8; 2017,Jan,8; 2016,Jan,13

69320 Reconstruction external auditory canal for congenital atresia, single stage
EXCLUDES Other reconstruction surgery with graft (13151-15760, 21230-21235)
Tympanoplasty (69631, 69641)
🚗 43.4 ⚖ 43.4 **FUD** 090 [J] [A2] [80] [50] [▭]
AMA: 2014,Jan,11; 1999,Oct,10

69399 Unlisted procedure, external ear
EXCLUDES Otoscopy under general anesthesia (92502)
🚗 0.00 ⚖ 0.00 **FUD** YYY [T] [80] [▭]
AMA: 2014,Jan,11; 1999,Oct,10

69420-69450 Ear Drum Procedures

69420 Myringotomy including aspiration and/or eustachian tube inflation
🚗 3.39 ⚖ 5.31 **FUD** 010 [T] [P2] [50] [▭]
AMA: 2018,Jan,8; 2017,Jan,8; 2016,Jan,13

69421 Myringotomy including aspiration and/or eustachian tube inflation requiring general anesthesia
🚗 4.21 ⚖ 4.21 **FUD** 010 [J] [A2] [50] [▭]
AMA: 2018,Jan,8; 2017,Jan,8; 2016,Jan,13

69424 Ventilating tube removal requiring general anesthesia
EXCLUDES Cochlear device implantation (69930)
Eardrum repair (69610-69646)
Foreign body removal (69205)
Implantation, replacement electromagnetic bone conduction hearing device in temporal bone (69710-69745)
Labyrinth procedures (69801-69915)
Mastoid obliteration (69670)
Myringotomy (69420-69421)
Polyp, glomus tumor removal (69535-69554)
Removal impacted cerumen requiring instrumentation (69210)
Repair window (69666-69667)
Revised mastoidectomy (69601-69604)
Stapes procedures (69650-69662)
Transmastoid excision (69501-69530)
Tympanic neurectomy (69676)
Tympanostomy, tympanolysis (69433-69450)
🚗 1.73 ⚖ 3.62 **FUD** 000 [02] [P3] [50] [▭]
AMA: 2018,Jan,8; 2017,Jan,8; 2016,Jan,13

Eye, Ocular Adnexa, and Ear

69433 — 69633

69433 **Tympanostomy (requiring insertion of ventilating tube), local or topical anesthesia**

> *EXCLUDES* *Tympanostomy with tube insertion using iontophoresis and automated tube delivery system (0583T)*
>
> 🔹 3.72 ⚕ 5.62 **FUD** 010   T P3 50 ▭
>
> **AMA:** 2018,Feb,11; 2018,Jan,8; 2017,Jan,8; 2016,Jan,13

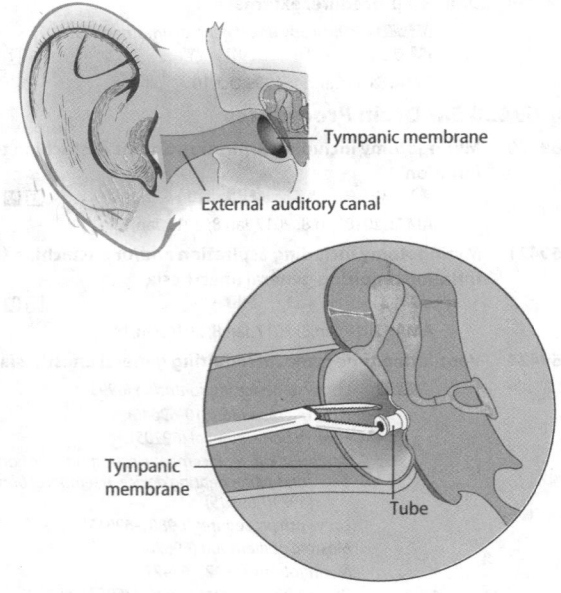

Tympanic membrane

External auditory canal

Tympanic membrane

Tube

69436 **Tympanostomy (requiring insertion of ventilating tube), general anesthesia**

> 🔹 4.51 ⚕ 4.51 **FUD** 010   T A2 50 ▭
>
> **AMA:** 2018,Feb,11; 2018,Jan,8; 2017,Jan,8; 2016,Jan,13

69440 **Middle ear exploration through postauricular or ear canal incision**

> *EXCLUDES* *Atticotomy (69601-69604)*
>
> 🔹 19.5 ⚕ 19.5 **FUD** 090   J A2 50 ▭
>
> **AMA:** 2014,Jan,11; 2008,Sep,10 -11

69450 **Tympanolysis, transcanal**

> 🔹 15.4 ⚕ 15.4 **FUD** 090   J A2 80 50 ▭
>
> **AMA:** 2014,Jan,11; 2008,Sep,10 -11

69501-69530 Transmastoid Excision

> *EXCLUDES* *Mastoidectomy cavity debridement (69220, 69222)*
> *Skin graft (15004-15770)*

69501 **Transmastoid antrotomy (simple mastoidectomy)**

> 🔹 20.3 ⚕ 20.3 **FUD** 090   J A2 50 ▭
>
> **AMA:** 2018,Jan,8; 2017,Jan,8; 2016,Jan,13

69502 **Mastoidectomy; complete**

> 🔹 27.3 ⚕ 27.3 **FUD** 090   J A2 80 50 ▭
>
> **AMA:** 2018,Jan,8; 2017,Jan,8; 2016,Jan,13

69505 **modified radical**

> 🔹 34.2 ⚕ 34.2 **FUD** 090   J A2 80 50 ▭
>
> **AMA:** 2018,Jan,8; 2017,Jan,8; 2016,Jan,13

69511 **radical**

> 🔹 35.0 ⚕ 35.0 **FUD** 090   J A2 80 50 ▭
>
> **AMA:** 2018,Jan,8; 2017,Jan,8; 2016,Jan,13

69530 **Petrous apicectomy including radical mastoidectomy**

> 🔹 47.1 ⚕ 47.1 **FUD** 090   J A2 80 50 ▭
>
> **AMA:** 2014,Jan,11; 1999,Oct,10

69535-69554 Polyp and Glomus Tumor Removal

69535 **Resection temporal bone, external approach**

> *EXCLUDES* *Middle fossa approach (69950-69970)*
>
> 🔹 75.4 ⚕ 75.4 **FUD** 090   C 50 ▭
>
> **AMA:** 2014,Jan,11; 1999,Oct,10

69540 **Excision aural polyp**

> 🔹 3.58 ⚕ 5.83 **FUD** 010   T P3 50 ▭
>
> **AMA:** 2014,Jan,11; 1999,Oct,10

69550 **Excision aural glomus tumor; transcanal**

> 🔹 29.5 ⚕ 29.5 **FUD** 090   J A2 80 50 ▭
>
> **AMA:** 2014,Jan,11; 1999,Oct,10

69552 **transmastoid**

> 🔹 44.6 ⚕ 44.6 **FUD** 090   J A2 80 50 ▭
>
> **AMA:** 2014,Jan,11; 1999,Oct,10

69554 **extended (extratemporal)**

> 🔹 71.5 ⚕ 71.5 **FUD** 090   C 80 50 ▭
>
> **AMA:** 2014,Jan,11; 1999,Oct,10

69601-69604 Revised Mastoidectomy

> *EXCLUDES* *Skin graft (15120-15121, 15260-15261)*

69601 **Revision mastoidectomy; resulting in complete mastoidectomy**

> 🔹 29.5 ⚕ 29.5 **FUD** 090   J A2 80 50 ▭
>
> **AMA:** 2018,Jan,8; 2017,Jan,8; 2016,Jan,13

69602 **resulting in modified radical mastoidectomy**

> 🔹 30.8 ⚕ 30.8 **FUD** 090   J A2 80 50 ▭
>
> **AMA:** 2018,Jan,8; 2017,Jan,8; 2016,Jan,13

69603 **resulting in radical mastoidectomy**

> 🔹 35.9 ⚕ 35.9 **FUD** 090   J A2 80 50 ▭
>
> **AMA:** 2018,Jan,8; 2017,Jan,8; 2016,Jan,13

69604 **resulting in tympanoplasty**

> *EXCLUDES* *Secondary tympanoplasty following mastoidectomy (69631-69632)*
>
> 🔹 31.5 ⚕ 31.5 **FUD** 090   J A2 50 ▭
>
> **AMA:** 2018,Jan,8; 2017,Jan,8; 2016,Jan,13

69610-69646 Eardrum Repair with/without Other Procedures

69610 **Tympanic membrane repair, with or without site preparation of perforation for closure, with or without patch**

> 🔹 8.27 ⚕ 10.8 **FUD** 010   J P3 50 ▭
>
> **AMA:** 2018,Jan,8; 2017,Jan,8; 2016,Jan,13

69620 **Myringoplasty (surgery confined to drumhead and donor area)**

> 🔹 13.9 ⚕ 20.0 **FUD** 090   J A2 50 ▭
>
> **AMA:** 2018,Jan,8; 2017,Jan,8; 2016,Jan,13

69631 **Tympanoplasty without mastoidectomy (including canalplasty, atticotomy and/or middle ear surgery), initial or revision; without ossicular chain reconstruction**

> 🔹 25.0 ⚕ 25.0 **FUD** 090   J A2 50 ▭
>
> **AMA:** 2018,Jan,8; 2017,Jan,8; 2016,Jan,13

69632 **with ossicular chain reconstruction (eg, postfenestration)**

> 🔹 30.5 ⚕ 30.5 **FUD** 090   J A2 50 ▭
>
> **AMA:** 2018,Jan,8; 2017,Jan,8; 2016,Jan,13

69633 **with ossicular chain reconstruction and synthetic prosthesis (eg, partial ossicular replacement prosthesis [PORP], total ossicular replacement prosthesis [TORP])**

> 🔹 29.6 ⚕ 29.6 **FUD** 090   J A2 50 ▭
>
> **AMA:** 2018,Jan,8; 2017,Jan,8; 2016,Jan,13

69635 Tympanoplasty with antrotomy or mastoidotomy (including canalplasty, atticotomy, middle ear surgery, and/or tympanic membrane repair); without ossicular chain reconstruction
35.3 ⚕ 35.3 **FUD** 090 J A2 50 ▭
AMA: 2018,Jan,8; 2017,Jan,8; 2016,Jan,13

Helix
Scaphoid fossa
Ossicular chain
Semicircular canals
Cochlear nerve
External acoustic canal
Concha
Tympanic membrane (eardrum)
Cochlea
Lobule
Malleus
Incus
Stapes
Detail of ossicular chain

69636 with ossicular chain reconstruction
39.2 ⚕ 39.2 **FUD** 090 J A2 80 50 ▭
AMA: 2018,Jan,8; 2017,Jan,8; 2016,Jan,13

69637 with ossicular chain reconstruction and synthetic prosthesis (eg, partial ossicular replacement prosthesis [PORP], total ossicular replacement prosthesis [TORP])
39.9 ⚕ 39.9 **FUD** 090 J A2 80 50 ▭
AMA: 2018,Jan,8; 2017,Jan,8; 2016,Jan,13

69641 Tympanoplasty with mastoidectomy (including canalplasty, middle ear surgery, tympanic membrane repair); without ossicular chain reconstruction
29.5 ⚕ 29.5 **FUD** 090 J A2 50 ▭
AMA: 2018,Jan,8; 2017,Jan,8; 2016,Jan,13

69642 with ossicular chain reconstruction
38.0 ⚕ 38.0 **FUD** 090 J A2 50 ▭
AMA: 2018,Jan,8; 2017,Jan,8; 2016,Jan,13

69643 with intact or reconstructed wall, without ossicular chain reconstruction
34.7 ⚕ 34.7 **FUD** 090 J A2 50 ▭
AMA: 2018,Jan,8; 2017,Jan,8; 2016,Jan,13

69644 with intact or reconstructed canal wall, with ossicular chain reconstruction
42.0 ⚕ 42.0 **FUD** 090 J A2 50 ▭
AMA: 2018,Jan,8; 2017,Jan,8; 2016,Jan,13

69645 radical or complete, without ossicular chain reconstruction
41.4 ⚕ 41.4 **FUD** 090 J A2 50 ▭
AMA: 2018,Jan,8; 2017,Jan,8; 2016,Jan,13

69646 radical or complete, with ossicular chain reconstruction
44.1 ⚕ 44.1 **FUD** 090 J A2 80 50 ▭
AMA: 2018,Jan,8; 2017,Jan,8; 2016,Jan,13

69650-69662 Stapes Procedures

69650 Stapes mobilization
22.7 ⚕ 22.7 **FUD** 090 J A2 50 ▭
AMA: 2014,Jan,11; 1999,Oct,10

69660 Stapedectomy or stapedotomy with reestablishment of ossicular continuity, with or without use of foreign material;
26.2 ⚕ 26.2 **FUD** 090 J A2 50 ▭
AMA: 2014,Jan,11; 1999,Oct,10

69661 with footplate drill out
34.3 ⚕ 34.3 **FUD** 090 J A2 80 50 ▭
AMA: 2014,Jan,11; 1999,Oct,10

69662 Revision of stapedectomy or stapedotomy
32.7 ⚕ 32.7 **FUD** 090 J A2 50 ▭
AMA: 2014,Jan,11; 1999,Oct,10

69666-69706 [69714, 69716, 69717, 69719, 69726, 69727] Other Inner Ear Procedures

69666 Repair oval window fistula
22.9 ⚕ 22.9 **FUD** 090 J A2 80 50 ▭
AMA: 2014,Jan,11; 1999,Oct,10

69667 Repair round window fistula
22.9 ⚕ 22.9 **FUD** 090 J A2 80 50 ▭
AMA: 2014,Jan,11; 1999,Oct,10

69670 Mastoid obliteration (separate procedure)
26.8 ⚕ 26.8 **FUD** 090 J A2 80 50 ▭
AMA: 2014,Jan,11; 1999,Oct,10

69676 Tympanic neurectomy
23.6 ⚕ 23.6 **FUD** 090 J A2 50 ▭
AMA: 2014,Jan,11; 1999,Oct,10

▲ # **69714** Implantation, osseointegrated implant, skull; with percutaneous attachment to external speech processor
30.4 ⚕ 30.4 **FUD** 090 J J8 50 ▭
AMA: 2018,Jan,8; 2017,Jan,8; 2016,Jan,13

● # **69716** with magnetic transcutaneous attachment to external speech processor
0.00 ⚕ 0.00 **FUD** 000

▲ # **69717** Revision or replacement (including removal of existing device), osseointegrated implant, skull; with percutaneous attachment to external speech processor
31.9 ⚕ 31.9 **FUD** 090 J J8 50 ▭
AMA: 2014,Jan,11; 1999,Oct,10

● # **69719** with magnetic transcutaneous attachment to external speech processor
0.00 ⚕ 0.00 **FUD** 000

● # **69726** Removal, osseointegrated implant, skull; with percutaneous attachment to external speech processor
0.00 ⚕ 0.00 **FUD** 000

● # **69727** with magnetic transcutaneous attachment to external speech processor
0.00 ⚕ 0.00 **FUD** 000

69700 Closure postauricular fistula, mastoid (separate procedure)
19.1 ⚕ 19.1 **FUD** 090 T A2 50 ▭
AMA: 2014,Jan,11; 1999,Oct,10

69705 Nasopharyngoscopy, surgical, with dilation of eustachian tube (ie, balloon dilation); unilateral
EXCLUDES Nasal endoscopy, diagnostic (31231)
Nasopharyngoscopy with endoscope (92511)
5.06 ⚕ 89.2 **FUD** 000 J8 80 ▭

69706 bilateral
EXCLUDES Nasal endoscopy, diagnostic (31231)
Nasopharyngoscopy with endoscope (92511)
7.04 ⚕ 91.8 **FUD** 000 J8 80 ▭

69710-69719 [69714, 69716, 69717, 69719] Procedures Related to Hearing Aids/Auditory Implants

69710 Implantation or replacement of electromagnetic bone conduction hearing device in temporal bone
INCLUDES Removal existing device when performing replacement procedure
0.00 ⚕ 0.00 **FUD** XXX E ▭
AMA: 2014,Jan,11; 1999,Oct,10

69711 Removal or repair of electromagnetic bone conduction hearing device in temporal bone
24.0 ⚕ 24.0 **FUD** 090 J A2 80 50 ▭
AMA: 2014,Jan,11; 1999,Oct,10

69714 Resequenced code. See code following 69676.

~~**69715** with mastoidectomy~~
To report, see (69501-69530, 69535-69554, 69601-69604, 69610-69646, 69650-69662, 69666-69676)

69716	Resequenced code. See code following 69676.
69717	Resequenced code. See code following 69676.
69718	**with mastoidectomy**

To report, see (69501-69530, 69535-69554, 69601-69604, 69610-69646, 69650-69662, 69666-69676)

| 69719 | Resequenced code. See code following 69676. |

69720-69799 [69726, 69727] Procedures of the Facial Nerve

EXCLUDES *Extracranial suture facial nerve (64864)*

69720 **Decompression facial nerve, intratemporal; lateral to geniculate ganglion**
🔧 34.1 ✂ 34.1 **FUD** 090 J A2 80 50 ▭
AMA: 2014,Jan,11; 1999,Oct,10

69725 **including medial to geniculate ganglion**
🔧 53.5 ✂ 53.5 **FUD** 090 J 62 80 50 ▭
AMA: 2014,Jan,11; 1999,Oct,10

| 69726 | Resequenced code. See code following 69676. |
| 69727 | Resequenced code. See code following 69676. |

69740 **Suture facial nerve, intratemporal, with or without graft or decompression; lateral to geniculate ganglion**
🔧 33.2 ✂ 33.2 **FUD** 090 J A2 80 50 ▭
AMA: 2014,Jan,11; 1999,Oct,10

69745 **including medial to geniculate ganglion**
🔧 35.3 ✂ 35.3 **FUD** 090 J A2 80 50 ▭
AMA: 2014,Jan,11; 1999,Oct,10

69799 **Unlisted procedure, middle ear**
🔧 0.00 ✂ 0.00 **FUD** YYY T 80 50 ▭
AMA: 2019,Jan,14; 2018,Jan,8; 2017,Jan,8; 2016,Jan,13

69801-69915 Procedures of the Labyrinth

69801 **Labyrinthotomy, with perfusion of vestibuloactive drug(s), transcanal**

EXCLUDES *Myringotomy, tympanostomy on same ear (69420-69421, 69433, 69436)*
Procedure performed more than one time per day
🔧 3.58 ✂ 5.83 **FUD** 000 T P3 80 50 ▭
AMA: 2018,Jan,8; 2017,Jan,8; 2016,Jan,13

69805 **Endolymphatic sac operation; without shunt**
🔧 29.8 ✂ 29.8 **FUD** 090 J A2 80 50 ▭
AMA: 2014,Jan,11; 1999,Oct,10

69806 **with shunt**
🔧 26.6 ✂ 26.6 **FUD** 090 J A2 50 ▭
AMA: 2014,Jan,11; 1999,Oct,10

69905 **Labyrinthectomy; transcanal**
🔧 26.0 ✂ 26.0 **FUD** 090 J A2 50 ▭
AMA: 2014,Jan,11; 1999,Oct,10

69910 **with mastoidectomy**
🔧 28.7 ✂ 28.7 **FUD** 090 J A2 80 50 ▭
AMA: 2014,Jan,11; 1999,Oct,10

69915 **Vestibular nerve section, translabyrinthine approach**

EXCLUDES *Transcranial approach (69950)*
🔧 43.6 ✂ 43.6 **FUD** 090 J A2 80 50 ▭
AMA: 2014,Jan,11; 1999,Oct,10

69930-69949 Cochlear Implantation

CMS: 100-02,16,100 Hearing Devices

69930 **Cochlear device implantation, with or without mastoidectomy**
🔧 34.8 ✂ 34.8 **FUD** 090 J J8 80 50 ▭
AMA: 2014,Jan,11; 1999,Oct,10

The internal coil is secured to the temporal bone and an electrode is fed through the round window into the cochlea

69949 **Unlisted procedure, inner ear**
🔧 0.00 ✂ 0.00 **FUD** YYY T 80 50 ▭
AMA: 2014,Jan,11; 1999,Oct,10

69950-69979 Inner Ear Procedures via Craniotomy

EXCLUDES *External approach (69535)*

69950 **Vestibular nerve section, transcranial approach**
🔧 50.6 ✂ 50.6 **FUD** 090 C 80 50 ▭
AMA: 2014,Jan,11; 1999,Oct,10

69955 **Total facial nerve decompression and/or repair (may include graft)**
🔧 56.2 ✂ 56.2 **FUD** 090 J 62 80 50 ▭
AMA: 2014,Jan,11; 1999,Oct,10

69960 **Decompression internal auditory canal**
🔧 54.2 ✂ 54.2 **FUD** 090 J 62 80 50 ▭
AMA: 2014,Jan,11; 1999,Oct,10

69970 **Removal of tumor, temporal bone**
🔧 61.0 ✂ 61.0 **FUD** 090 J 62 80 50 ▭
AMA: 2014,Jan,11; 1999,Oct,10

69979 **Unlisted procedure, temporal bone, middle fossa approach**
🔧 0.00 ✂ 0.00 **FUD** YYY T 80 50 ▭
AMA: 2018,Jan,8; 2017,Jan,8; 2016,Jan,13

69990 Operating Microscope

EXCLUDES *Magnifying loupes*
Reporting code with (15756-15758, 15842, 19364, 19368, 20955-20962, 20969-20973, 22551-22552, 22856-22857 [22858], 22861, 26551-26554, 26556, 31526, 31531, 31536, 31541-31546, 31561, 31571, 43116, 43180, 43496, 46601, 46607, 49906, 61548, 63075-63078, 64727, 64820-64823, 64912-64913, 65091-68850 [66987, 66988, 67810], 0184T, 0308T, 0402T, 0583T)

+ **69990** **Microsurgical techniques, requiring use of operating microscope (List separately in addition to code for primary procedure)**
Code first primary procedure
🔧 6.40 ✂ 6.40 **FUD** ZZZ N N1 80 ▭
AMA: 2018,Feb,11; 2018,Jan,8; 2017,Dec,12; 2017,Dec,13; 2017,Dec,14; 2017,Jan,8; 2016,Feb,12; 2016,Jan,13

70010-70015 Radiography: Neurodiagnostic

70010 **Myelography, posterior fossa, radiological supervision and interpretation**
  🔧 1.73   ⚕ 1.73   **FUD** XXX   `02` `N1` `80` 🖵
  AMA: 2018,Jan,8; 2017,Jan,8; 2016,Jan,13

70015 **Cisternography, positive contrast, radiological supervision and interpretation**
  🔧 4.60   ⚕ 4.60   **FUD** XXX   `02` `N1` `80` 🖵
  AMA: 2014,Jan,11; 2012,Feb,9-10

70030-70390 Radiography: Head, Neck, Orofacial Structures

INCLUDES Minimum number views or more views when needed to adequately complete study
  Radiographs repeated during encounter due to substandard quality; only one unit reported
EXCLUDES Obtaining more films after initial film review, based on radiologist discretion, order for test, and change in patient's condition

70030 **Radiologic examination, eye, for detection of foreign body**
  🔧 0.87   ⚕ 0.87   **FUD** XXX   `01` `N1` `80` 🖵
  AMA: 2014,Jan,11; 2012,Feb,9-10

70100 **Radiologic examination, mandible; partial, less than 4 views**
  🔧 1.03   ⚕ 1.03   **FUD** XXX   `01` `N1` `80` 🖵
  AMA: 2014,Jan,11; 2012,Feb,9-10

70110 **complete, minimum of 4 views**
  🔧 1.19   ⚕ 1.19   **FUD** XXX   `01` `N1` `80` 🖵
  AMA: 2014,Jan,11; 2012,Feb,9-10

70120 **Radiologic examination, mastoids; less than 3 views per side**
  🔧 0.97   ⚕ 0.97   **FUD** XXX   `01` `N1` `80` 🖵
  AMA: 2014,Jan,11; 2012,Feb,9-10

70130 **complete, minimum of 3 views per side**
  🔧 1.68   ⚕ 1.68   **FUD** XXX   `01` `N1` `80` 🖵
  AMA: 2014,Jan,11; 2012,Feb,9-10

70134 **Radiologic examination, internal auditory meati, complete**
  🔧 1.59   ⚕ 1.59   **FUD** XXX   `01` `N1` `80` 🖵
  AMA: 2014,Jan,11; 2012,Feb,9-10

70140 **Radiologic examination, facial bones; less than 3 views**
  🔧 0.88   ⚕ 0.88   **FUD** XXX   `01` `N1` `80` 🖵
  AMA: 2014,Jan,11; 2012,Feb,9-10

70150 **complete, minimum of 3 views**
  🔧 1.29   ⚕ 1.29   **FUD** XXX   `01` `N1` `80` 🖵
  AMA: 2014,Jan,11; 2012,Feb,9-10

70160 **Radiologic examination, nasal bones, complete, minimum of 3 views**
  🔧 1.02   ⚕ 1.02   **FUD** XXX   `01` `N1` `80` 🖵
  AMA: 2014,Jan,11; 2012,Feb,9-10

70170 **Dacryocystography, nasolacrimal duct, radiological supervision and interpretation**
  EXCLUDES Injection contrast (68850)
  🔧 0.00   ⚕ 0.00   **FUD** XXX   `02` `N1` `80` 🖵
  AMA: 2014,Jan,11; 2012,Feb,9-10

70190 **Radiologic examination; optic foramina**
  🔧 1.08   ⚕ 1.08   **FUD** XXX   `01` `N1` `80` 🖵
  AMA: 2014,Jan,11; 2012,Feb,9-10

70200 **orbits, complete, minimum of 4 views**
  🔧 1.31   ⚕ 1.31   **FUD** XXX   `01` `N1` `80` 🖵
  AMA: 2014,Jan,11; 2012,Feb,9-10

70210 **Radiologic examination, sinuses, paranasal, less than 3 views**
  🔧 0.87   ⚕ 0.87   **FUD** XXX   `01` `N1` `80` 🖵
  AMA: 2014,Jan,11; 2012,Feb,9-10

70220 **Radiologic examination, sinuses, paranasal, complete, minimum of 3 views**
  🔧 1.10   ⚕ 1.10   **FUD** XXX   `01` `N1` `80` 🖵
  AMA: 2014,Jan,11; 2012,Feb,9-10

70240 **Radiologic examination, sella turcica**
  🔧 0.94   ⚕ 0.94   **FUD** XXX   `01` `N1` `80` 🖵
  AMA: 2014,Jan,11; 2012,Feb,9-10

70250 **X-ray of skull, fewer than 4 views**
  🔧 1.00   ⚕ 1.00   **FUD** XXX   `01` `N1` `80` 🖵
  AMA: 2014,Jan,11; 2012,Feb,9-10

70260 **complete, minimum of 4 views**
  🔧 1.24   ⚕ 1.24   **FUD** XXX   `01` `N1` `80` 🖵
  AMA: 2014,Jan,11; 2012,Feb,9-10

70300 **Radiologic examination, teeth; single view**
  🔧 0.39   ⚕ 0.39   **FUD** XXX   `01` `N1` `80` 🖵
  AMA: 2014,Jan,11; 2012,Feb,9-10

Section of incisor   Section of molar

70310 **partial examination, less than full mouth**
  🔧 1.06   ⚕ 1.06   **FUD** XXX   `01` `N1` `80` 🖵
  AMA: 2014,Jan,11; 2012,Feb,9-10

70320 **complete, full mouth**
  🔧 1.53   ⚕ 1.53   **FUD** XXX   `01` `N1` `80` 🖵
  AMA: 2014,Jan,11; 2012,Feb,9-10

70010 — 70320

Radiology

70328 Radiologic examination, temporomandibular joint, open and closed mouth; unilateral
  0.94   0.94   **FUD** XXX   01 N1 80 🔲
  AMA: 2014,Jan,11; 2012,Feb,9-10

70330 bilateral
  1.45   1.45   **FUD** XXX   01 N1 80 🔲
  AMA: 2018,Jan,8; 2017,Jan,8; 2016,Jan,13

70332 Temporomandibular joint arthrography, radiological supervision and interpretation
  INCLUDES   Fluoroscopic guidance (77002)
  2.15   2.15   **FUD** XXX   02 N1 80 🔲
  AMA: 2018,Jan,8; 2017,Jan,8; 2016,Jan,13

70336 Magnetic resonance (eg, proton) imaging, temporomandibular joint(s)
  8.68   8.68   **FUD** XXX   03 Z2 80 🔲
  AMA: 2018,Jan,8; 2017,Jan,8; 2016,Jan,13

70350 Cephalogram, orthodontic
  0.49   0.49   **FUD** XXX   01 N1 80 🔲
  AMA: 2018,Jan,8; 2017,Jan,8; 2016,Jan,13

70355 Orthopantogram (eg, panoramic x-ray)
  0.54   0.54   **FUD** XXX   01 N1 80 🔲
  AMA: 2014,Jan,11; 2012,Feb,9-10

70360 Radiologic examination; neck, soft tissue
  0.86   0.86   **FUD** XXX   01 N1 80 🔲
  AMA: 2014,Jan,11; 2012,Feb,9-10

70370 pharynx or larynx, including fluoroscopy and/or magnification technique
  2.49   2.49   **FUD** XXX   01 N1 80 🔲
  AMA: 2014,Jan,11; 2012,Feb,9-10

70371 Complex dynamic pharyngeal and speech evaluation by cine or video recording
  EXCLUDES   Laryngeal computed tomography (70490-70492)
  3.03   3.03   **FUD** XXX   01 N1 80 🔲
  AMA: 2018,Jan,8; 2017,Jan,8; 2016,Jan,13

70380 Radiologic examination, salivary gland for calculus
  1.01   1.01   **FUD** XXX   01 N1 80 🔲
  AMA: 2014,Jan,11; 2012,Feb,9-10

70390 Sialography, radiological supervision and interpretation
  3.16   3.16   **FUD** XXX   02 N1 80 🔲
  AMA: 2014,Jan,11; 2012,Feb,9-10

70450-70492 Computerized Tomography: Head, Neck, Face
CMS: 100-04,4,250.16 Multiple Procedure Payment Reduction: Certain Diagnostic Imaging Procedures Rendered by Physicians
  INCLUDES   Imaging using tomographic technique enhanced by computer imaging to create cross-sectional body plane view
  EXCLUDES   3D rendering (76376-76377)

70450 Computed tomography, head or brain; without contrast material
  3.25   3.25   **FUD** XXX   03 Z2 80 🔲
  AMA: 2018,Jan,8; 2017,Jan,8; 2016,Jan,13

70460 with contrast material(s)
  4.61   4.61   **FUD** XXX   03 Z2 80 🔲
  AMA: 2018,Jan,8; 2017,Jan,8; 2016,Jan,13

70470 without contrast material, followed by contrast material(s) and further sections
  5.38   5.38   **FUD** XXX   03 Z2 80 🔲
  AMA: 2018,Jan,8; 2017,Jan,8; 2016,Jan,13

70480 Computed tomography, orbit, sella, or posterior fossa or outer, middle, or inner ear; without contrast material
  5.64   5.64   **FUD** XXX   03 Z2 80 🔲
  AMA: 2018,Jan,8; 2017,Jan,8; 2016,Jan,13

70481 with contrast material(s)
  6.29   6.29   **FUD** XXX   03 Z2 80 🔲
  AMA: 2018,Jan,8; 2017,Jan,8; 2016,Jan,13

70482 without contrast material, followed by contrast material(s) and further sections
  6.97   6.97   **FUD** XXX   03 Z2 80 🔲
  AMA: 2014,Jan,11; 2012,Feb,9-10

70486 Computed tomography, maxillofacial area; without contrast material
  3.92   3.92   **FUD** XXX   03 Z2 80 🔲
  AMA: 2018,Jan,8; 2017,Jan,8; 2016,Jan,13

70487 with contrast material(s)
  4.70   4.70   **FUD** XXX   03 Z2 80 🔲
  AMA: 2014,Jan,11; 2012,Feb,9-10

70488 without contrast material, followed by contrast material(s) and further sections
  5.73   5.73   **FUD** XXX   03 Z2 80 🔲
  AMA: 2014,Jan,11; 2012,Feb,9-10

70490 Computed tomography, soft tissue neck; without contrast material
  EXCLUDES   CT cervical spine (72125)
  4.63   4.63   **FUD** XXX   03 Z2 80 🔲
  AMA: 2014,Jan,11; 2012,Feb,9-10

70491 with contrast material(s)
  EXCLUDES   CT cervical spine (72125)
  5.70   5.70   **FUD** XXX   03 Z2 80 🔲
  AMA: 2014,Jan,11; 2012,Feb,9-10

70492 without contrast material followed by contrast material(s) and further sections
  EXCLUDES   CT cervical spine (72125)
  6.89   6.89   **FUD** XXX   03 Z2 80 🔲
  AMA: 2014,Jan,11; 2012,Feb,9-10

70496-70498 Computerized Tomographic Angiography: Head and Neck
CMS: 100-04,4,250.16 Multiple Procedure Payment Reduction: Certain Diagnostic Imaging Procedures Rendered by Physicians
  INCLUDES   Computed tomography to visualize arterial and venous vessels
  EXCLUDES   Noninvasive arterial plaque analysis non-coronary computerized tomography angiography (0710T-0713T)

70496 Computed tomographic angiography, head, with contrast material(s), including noncontrast images, if performed, and image postprocessing
  8.35   8.35   **FUD** XXX   03 Z2 80 🔲
  AMA: 2018,Jan,8; 2017,Jan,8; 2016,Jan,13

70498 Computed tomographic angiography, neck, with contrast material(s), including noncontrast images, if performed, and image postprocessing
  8.34   8.34   **FUD** XXX   03 Z2 80 🔲
  AMA: 2018,Jan,8; 2017,Jan,8; 2016,Jan,13

70540-70543 Magnetic Resonance Imaging: Face, Neck, Orbits
CMS: 100-04,4,250.16 Multiple Procedure Payment Reduction: Certain Diagnostic Imaging Procedures Rendered by Physicians
  INCLUDES   Three-dimensional imaging that measures response oatomic nuclei in soft tissues to high-frequency radio waves when strong magnetic field applied
  EXCLUDES   Magnetic resonance angiography head/neck (70544-70549)
              Procedure performed more than one time per session

70540 Magnetic resonance (eg, proton) imaging, orbit, face, and/or neck; without contrast material(s)
  7.34   7.34   **FUD** XXX   03 Z2 80 🔲
  AMA: 2018,Jan,8; 2017,Jan,8; 2016,Jan,13

70542 with contrast material(s)
  8.72   8.72   **FUD** XXX   03 Z2 80 🔲
  AMA: 2018,Jan,8; 2017,Jan,8; 2016,Jan,13

70543 without contrast material(s), followed by contrast material(s) and further sequences
  11.1   11.1   **FUD** XXX   03 Z2 80 🔲
  AMA: 2018,Jan,8; 2017,Jan,8; 2016,Jan,13

70544-70549 Magnetic Resonance Angiography: Head and Neck

CMS: 100-04,13,40.1.1 Magnetic Resonance Angiography; 100-04,13,40.1.2 HCPCS Coding Requirements; 100-04,4,250.16 Multiple Procedure Payment Reduction: Certain Diagnostic Imaging Procedures Rendered by Physicians

> **INCLUDES** Magnetic fields and radio waves to produce detailed cross-sectional internal body structure images
> **EXCLUDES** *Reporting code with following unless separate diagnostic MRI performed (70551-70553)*

70544 **Magnetic resonance angiography, head; without contrast material(s)**
> 6.90   6.90   **FUD** XXX   Q3 Z2 80 ▭
> **AMA:** 2018,Jan,8; 2017,Jan,8; 2016,Jan,13

70545 **with contrast material(s)**
> 7.21   7.21   **FUD** XXX   Q3 Z2 80 ▭
> **AMA:** 2018,Jan,8; 2017,Jan,8; 2016,Jan,13

70546 **without contrast material(s), followed by contrast material(s) and further sequences**
> 10.4   10.4   **FUD** XXX   Q3 Z2 80 ▭
> **AMA:** 2018,Jan,8; 2017,Jan,8; 2016,Jan,13

70547 **Magnetic resonance angiography, neck; without contrast material(s)**
> 6.93   6.93   **FUD** XXX   Q3 Z2 80 ▭
> **AMA:** 2018,Jan,8; 2017,Jan,8; 2016,Jan,13

70548 **with contrast material(s)**
> 7.74   7.74   **FUD** XXX   Q3 Z2 80 ▭
> **AMA:** 2018,Jan,8; 2017,Jan,8; 2016,Jan,13

70549 **without contrast material(s), followed by contrast material(s) and further sequences**
> 10.9   10.9   **FUD** XXX   Q3 Z2 80 ▭
> **AMA:** 2018,Jan,8; 2017,Jan,8; 2016,Jan,13

70551-70553 Magnetic Resonance Imaging: Brain and Brain Stem

CMS: 100-04,4,200.3.2 Multi-Source Photon Stereotactic RadiosurgeryPlanning and Delivery; 100-04,4,250.16 Multiple Procedure Payment Reduction: Certain Diagnostic Imaging Procedures Rendered by Physicians

> **INCLUDES** Three-dimensional imaging that measures response oatomic nuclei in soft tissues to high-frequency radio waves when strong magnetic field applied
> **EXCLUDES** *Magnetic spectroscopy (76390)*

70551 **Magnetic resonance (eg, proton) imaging, brain (including brain stem); without contrast material**
> 6.28   6.28   **FUD** XXX   Q3 Z2 80 ▭
> **AMA:** 2018,Jan,8; 2017,Jan,8; 2016,Jan,13

70552 **with contrast material(s)**
> 8.69   8.69   **FUD** XXX   Q3 Z2 80 ▭
> **AMA:** 2018,Jan,8; 2017,Jan,8; 2016,Jan,13

70553 **without contrast material, followed by contrast material(s) and further sequences**
> 10.2   10.2   **FUD** XXX   Q3 Z2 80 ▭
> **AMA:** 2018,Jan,8; 2017,Jan,8; 2016,Jan,13

70554-70555 Magnetic Resonance Imaging: Brain Mapping

> **INCLUDES** Neuroimaging technique using MRI to identify and map signals related to brain activity
> **EXCLUDES** *Reporting code with following unless separate diagnostic MRI performed (70551-70553)*

70554 **Magnetic resonance imaging, brain, functional MRI; including test selection and administration of repetitive body part movement and/or visual stimulation, not requiring physician or psychologist administration**
> **EXCLUDES** *Functional brain mapping (96020)*
> *Testing performed by physician or psychologist (70555)*
> 12.1   12.1   **FUD** XXX   Q3 Z2 80 ▭
> **AMA:** 2018,Jan,8; 2017,Jan,8; 2016,Jan,13

70555 **requiring physician or psychologist administration of entire neurofunctional testing**
> **EXCLUDES** *Testing performed by technologist, nonphysician, or nonpsychologist (70554)*
> Code also (96020)
> 0.00   0.00   **FUD** XXX   S Z2 80 ▭
> **AMA:** 2018,Jan,8; 2017,Jan,8; 2016,Jan,13

70557-70559 Magnetic Resonance Imaging: Intraoperative

> **EXCLUDES** *Intracranial lesion stereotaxic biopsy with magnetic resonance guidance (61751, 77021-77022)*
> *Procedures performed more than one time per surgical encounter*
> *Reporting codes unless separate report generated*
> Code also stereotactic biopsy, aspiration, or excision, when performed with MRI (61751)

70557 **Magnetic resonance (eg, proton) imaging, brain (including brain stem and skull base), during open intracranial procedure (eg, to assess for residual tumor or residual vascular malformation); without contrast material**
> 0.00   0.00   **FUD** XXX   S Z2 80 ▭
> **AMA:** 2014,Jan,11; 2012,Feb,9-10

70558 **with contrast material(s)**
> 0.00   0.00   **FUD** XXX   S Z2 80 ▭
> **AMA:** 2014,Jan,11; 2012,Feb,9-10

70559 **without contrast material(s), followed by contrast material(s) and further sequences**
> 0.00   0.00   **FUD** XXX   S Z2 80 ▭
> **AMA:** 2014,Jan,11; 2012,Feb,9-10

71045-71130 Radiography: Thorax

71045 **Radiologic examination, chest; single view**
> **EXCLUDES** *Acute abdomen series, complete (2 or more views) including chest view (74022)*
> *Remotely performed CAD (0175T)*
> Code also concurrent computer-aided detection (CAD) (0174T)
> 0.72   0.72   **FUD** XXX   Q3 Z3 80 ▭
> **AMA:** 2019,Aug,8; 2019,May,10; 2019,Mar,10; 2018,Apr,7

71046 **2 views**
> **EXCLUDES** *Acute abdomen series, complete (2 or more views) including chest view (74022)*
> *Remotely performed CAD (0175T)*
> Code also concurrent computer-aided detection (CAD) (0174T)
> 0.89   0.89   **FUD** XXX   Q3 Z3 80 ▭
> **AMA:** 2019,Aug,8; 2019,Mar,10; 2018,Apr,7

71047 **3 views**
> **EXCLUDES** *Acute abdomen series, complete (2 or more views) including chest view (74022)*
> *Remotely performed CAD (0175T)*
> Code also concurrent computer-aided detection (CAD) (0174T)
> 1.16   1.16   **FUD** XXX   01 N1 80 ▭
> **AMA:** 2019,Mar,10; 2018,Apr,7

71048 **4 or more views**
> **EXCLUDES** *Acute abdomen series, complete (2 or more views) including chest view (74022)*
> *Remotely performed CAD (0175T)*
> Code also concurrent computer-aided detection (CAD) (0174T)
> 1.21   1.21   **FUD** XXX   01 N1 80 ▭
> **AMA:** 2019,Mar,10; 2018,Apr,7

● New Code   ▲ Revised Code   ○ Reinstated   ● New Web Release   ▲ Revised Web Release   + Add-on   Unlisted   Not Covered   # Resequenced
50 Optum Mod 50 Exempt   Ⓢ AMA Mod 51 Exempt   51 Optum Mod 51 Exempt   63 Mod 63 Exempt   ⩘ Non-FDA Drug   ★ Telemedicine   M Maternity   A Age Edit

Radiology

71100 **Radiologic examination, ribs, unilateral; 2 views**
🚑 1.00   ✂ 1.00   **FUD** XXX   `01` `N1` `80` `▢`
AMA: 2014,Jan,11; 2012,Feb,9-10

Hyoid bone
Manubrium of sternum
Trachea
Sternum
Xiphoid process

71101 including posteroanterior chest, minimum of 3 views
🚑 1.15   ✂ 1.15   **FUD** XXX   `01` `N1` `80` `▢`
AMA: 2014,Jan,11; 2012,Feb,9-10

71110 **Radiologic examination, ribs, bilateral; 3 views**
🚑 1.21   ✂ 1.21   **FUD** XXX   `01` `N1` `80` `▢`
AMA: 2014,Jan,11; 2012,Feb,9-10

71111 including posteroanterior chest, minimum of 4 views
🚑 1.44   ✂ 1.44   **FUD** XXX   `01` `N1` `80` `▢`
AMA: 2014,Jan,11; 2012,Feb,9-10

71120 **Radiologic examination; sternum, minimum of 2 views**
🚑 0.92   ✂ 0.92   **FUD** XXX   `01` `N1` `80` `▢`
AMA: 2014,Jan,11; 2012,Feb,9-10

71130 sternoclavicular joint or joints, minimum of 3 views
🚑 1.12   ✂ 1.12   **FUD** XXX   `01` `N1` `80` `▢`
AMA: 2014,Jan,11; 2012,Feb,9-10

71250-71271 Computerized Tomography: Thorax

INCLUDES   Imaging using tomographic technique enhanced by computer imaging to create cross-sectional body plane view
EXCLUDES   3D rendering (76376-76377)
CT breast (0633T-0638T)
CT heart (75571-75574)

71250 **Computed tomography, thorax, diagnostic; without contrast material**
EXCLUDES   CT thorax with contrast (71260-71270)
EXCLUDES   CT thorax for lung cancer screening (71271)
🚑 4.45   ✂ 4.45   **FUD** XXX   `03` `Z2` `80` `▢`
AMA: 2020,Sep,11; 2018,Jan,8; 2017,Jan,8; 2016,Jan,13

71260 with contrast material(s)
EXCLUDES   CT thorax for lung cancer screening (71271)
CT thorax without contrast (71250, 71270)
🚑 5.52   ✂ 5.52   **FUD** XXX   `03` `Z2` `80` `▢`
AMA: 2020,Sep,11; 2018,Jan,8; 2017,Jan,8; 2016,Jan,13

71270 without contrast material, followed by contrast material(s) and further sections
EXCLUDES   CT thorax for lung cancer screening (71271)
CT thorax with or without contrast only (71250, 71260)
🚑 6.53   ✂ 6.53   **FUD** XXX   `03` `Z2` `80` `▢`
AMA: 2020,Sep,11; 2018,Jan,8; 2017,Jan,8; 2016,Jan,13

71271 **Computed tomography, thorax, low dose for lung cancer screening, without contrast material(s)**
EXCLUDES   CT thorax not for lung cancer screening (71250, 71260, 71270)
🚑 4.32   ✂ 4.32   **FUD** XXX   `80` `▢`

71275 Computerized Tomographic Angiography: Thorax

CMS: 100-04,4,250.16 Multiple Procedure Payment Reduction: Certain Diagnostic Imaging Procedures Rendered by Physicians
INCLUDES   Multiple rapid thin section CT scans to create cross-sectional bone, organ, and tissue images
EXCLUDES   CT angiography coronary arteries including calcification score and/or cardiac morphology (75574)

71275 **Computed tomographic angiography, chest (noncoronary), with contrast material(s), including noncontrast images, if performed, and image postprocessing**
🚑 8.53   ✂ 8.53   **FUD** XXX   `03` `Z2` `80` `▢`
AMA: 2020,Sep,11; 2018,Jan,8; 2017,Jan,8; 2016,Jan,13

71550-71552 Magnetic Resonance Imaging: Thorax

CMS: 100-04,4,250.16 Multiple Procedure Payment Reduction: Certain Diagnostic Imaging Procedures Rendered by Physicians
INCLUDES   Three-dimensional imaging that measures response atomic nuclei in soft tissues to high-frequency radio waves when strong magnetic field applied
EXCLUDES   MRI of the breast (77046-77049)

71550 **Magnetic resonance (eg, proton) imaging, chest (eg, for evaluation of hilar and mediastinal lymphadenopathy); without contrast material(s)**
🚑 11.4   ✂ 11.4   **FUD** XXX   `03` `Z2` `80` `▢`
AMA: 2018,Jan,8; 2017,Jan,8; 2016,Jan,13

71551 with contrast material(s)
🚑 12.3   ✂ 12.3   **FUD** XXX   `03` `Z3` `80` `▢`
AMA: 2018,Jan,8; 2017,Jan,8; 2016,Jan,13

71552 without contrast material(s), followed by contrast material(s) and further sequences
🚑 15.9   ✂ 15.9   **FUD** XXX   `03` `Z2` `80` `▢`
AMA: 2018,Jan,8; 2017,Jan,8; 2016,Jan,13

71555 Magnetic Resonance Angiography: Thorax

CMS: 100-04,13,40.1.1 Magnetic Resonance Angiography; 100-04,13,40.1.2 HCPCS Coding Requirements; 100-04,4,250.16 Multiple Procedure Payment Reduction: Certain Diagnostic Imaging Procedures Rendered by Physicians

71555 **Magnetic resonance angiography, chest (excluding myocardium), with or without contrast material(s)**
🚑 10.8   ✂ 10.8   **FUD** XXX   `B` `80` `▢`
AMA: 2018,Jan,8; 2017,Jan,8; 2016,Jan,13

72020-72120 Radiography: Spine

INCLUDES   Minimum number views or more views when needed to adequately complete study
Radiographs repeated during encounter due to substandard quality; only one unit reported
EXCLUDES   Obtaining more films after initial film review, based on the radiologist discretion, an order for the test, and change in patient's condition

72020 **Radiologic examination, spine, single view, specify level**
EXCLUDES   Single view entire thoracic and lumbar spine (72081)
🚑 0.68   ✂ 0.68   **FUD** XXX   `01` `N1` `80` `▢`
AMA: 2018,Jan,8; 2017,Jan,8; 2016,Sep,4; 2016,Jan,13

72040 **Radiologic examination, spine, cervical; 2 or 3 views**
📷 1.07　👁 1.07　**FUD** XXX　　01 N1 80 ▣
AMA: 2018,Aug,10; 2018,Jan,8; 2017,Jan,8; 2016,Jan,13

Cervical
spine
C1–C4

Cervical
spine
C5–C7

Thoracic
spine
T1–T12

Detail of top two vertebrae

Odontoid
process

Atlas

Axis

Spinous
process

An x-ray of the cervical spine is performed

72050 **4 or 5 views**
📷 1.42　👁 1.42　**FUD** XXX　　01 N1 80 ▣
AMA: 2014,Jan,11; 2012,Feb,9-10

72052 **6 or more views**
📷 1.67　👁 1.67　**FUD** XXX　　01 N1 80 ▣
AMA: 2014,Jan,11; 2012,Feb,9-10

72070 **Radiologic examination, spine; thoracic, 2 views**
📷 0.96　👁 0.96　**FUD** XXX　　01 N1 80 ▣
AMA: 2018,Jan,8; 2017,Jan,8; 2016,Jan,13

72072 **thoracic, 3 views**
📷 1.08　👁 1.08　**FUD** XXX　　01 N1 80 ▣
AMA: 2018,Jan,8; 2017,Jan,8; 2016,Jan,13

72074 **thoracic, minimum of 4 views**
📷 1.21　👁 1.21　**FUD** XXX　　01 N1 80 ▣
AMA: 2018,Jan,8; 2017,Jan,8; 2016,Jan,13

72080 **thoracolumbar junction, minimum of 2 views**
EXCLUDES *Single view thoracolumbar junction (72020)*
📷 0.96　👁 0.96　**FUD** XXX　　01 N1 80 ▣
AMA: 2018,Jan,8; 2017,Jan,8; 2016,Sep,4; 2016,Jan,13

72081 **Radiologic examination, spine, entire thoracic and lumbar, including skull, cervical and sacral spine if performed (eg, scoliosis evaluation); one view**
📷 1.17　👁 1.17　**FUD** XXX　　01 N1 ▣
AMA: 2018,Jan,8; 2017,Jan,8; 2016,Sep,4

72082 **2 or 3 views**
📷 1.90　👁 1.90　**FUD** XXX　　01 N1 80 ▣
AMA: 2018,Jan,8; 2017,Jan,8; 2016,Sep,4

72083 **4 or 5 views**
📷 2.16　👁 2.16　**FUD** XXX　　S Z2 80 ▣
AMA: 2018,Jan,8; 2017,Jan,8; 2016,Sep,4

72084 **minimum of 6 views**
📷 2.52　👁 2.52　**FUD** XXX　　S Z2 80 ▣
AMA: 2018,Jan,8; 2017,Jan,8; 2016,Sep,4

72100 **Radiologic examination, spine, lumbosacral; 2 or 3 views**
📷 1.07　👁 1.07　**FUD** XXX　　01 N1 80 ▣
AMA: 2018,Jan,8; 2017,Jan,8; 2016,Jan,13

72110 **minimum of 4 views**
📷 1.36　👁 1.36　**FUD** XXX　　01 N1 80 ▣
AMA: 2018,Jan,8; 2017,Jan,8; 2016,Jan,13

72114 **complete, including bending views, minimum of 6 views**
📷 1.64　👁 1.64　**FUD** XXX　　01 N1 80 ▣
AMA: 2014,Jan,11; 2012,Feb,9-10

72120 **bending views only, 2 or 3 views**
📷 1.11　👁 1.11　**FUD** XXX　　01 N1 80 ▣
AMA: 2018,Jan,8; 2017,Jan,8; 2016,Aug,7

72125-72133 Computerized Tomography: Spine

CMS: 100-04,12,20.4.7 Services Not Meeting National Electrical Manufacturers Association (NEMA) Standard; 100-04,4,20.6.12 Use of HCPCS Modifier – CT; 100-04,4,250.16 Multiple Procedure Payment Reduction: Certain Diagnostic Imaging Procedures Rendered by Physicians

INCLUDES　Imaging using tomographic technique enhanced by computer imaging to create cross-sectional body plane view

EXCLUDES　*3D rendering (76376-76377)*

Code also intrathecal injection procedure when performed (61055, 62284)

72125 **Computed tomography, cervical spine; without contrast material**
📷 4.38　👁 4.38　**FUD** XXX　　03 Z2 80 ▣
AMA: 2020,Sep,11

72126 **with contrast material**
📷 6.40　👁 6.40　**FUD** XXX　　03 Z3 80 ▣
AMA: 2020,Sep,11; 2018,Jan,8; 2017,Jan,8; 2016,Jan,13

72127 **without contrast material, followed by contrast material(s) and further sections**
📷 6.48　👁 6.48　**FUD** XXX　　03 Z2 80 ▣
AMA: 2020,Sep,11

72128 **Computed tomography, thoracic spine; without contrast material**
📷 5.08　👁 5.08　**FUD** XXX　　03 Z2 80 ▣
AMA: 2020,Sep,11

72129 **with contrast material**
📷 5.54　👁 5.54　**FUD** XXX　　03 Z2 80 ▣
AMA: 2020,Sep,11; 2019,Jan,14; 2018,Jan,8; 2017,Jan,8; 2016,Jan,13

72130 **without contrast material, followed by contrast material(s) and further sections**
📷 6.49　👁 6.49　**FUD** XXX　　03 Z2 80 ▣
AMA: 2020,Sep,11

72131 **Computed tomography, lumbar spine; without contrast material**
📷 4.36　👁 4.36　**FUD** XXX　　03 Z2 80 ▣
AMA: 2020,Sep,11

72132 **with contrast material**
📷 5.51　👁 5.51　**FUD** XXX　　03 Z3 80 ▣
AMA: 2020,Sep,11; 2019,Jan,14; 2018,Jan,8; 2017,Jan,8; 2016,Jan,13

72133 **without contrast material, followed by contrast material(s) and further sections**
📷 6.45　👁 6.45　**FUD** XXX　　03 Z2 80 ▣
AMA: 2020,Sep,11

72141-72158 Magnetic Resonance Imaging: Spine

CMS: 100-04,4,250.16 Multiple Procedure Payment Reduction: Certain Diagnostic Imaging Procedures Rendered by Physicians

INCLUDES　Three-dimensional imaging that measures response atomic nuclei in soft tissues to high-frequency radio waves when strong magnetic field applied

EXCLUDES　*MR spectroscopy (0609T-0610T)*

Code also intrathecal injection procedure when performed (61055, 62284)

72141 **Magnetic resonance (eg, proton) imaging, spinal canal and contents, cervical; without contrast material**
📷 6.11　👁 6.11　**FUD** XXX　　03 Z2 80 ▣
AMA: 2018,Jan,8; 2017,Jan,8; 2016,Jan,13

72142 **with contrast material(s)**
EXCLUDES　*MRI cervical spinal canal performed without contrast followed by repeating study with contrast (72156)*
📷 8.88　👁 8.88　**FUD** XXX　　03 Z2 80 ▣
AMA: 2018,Jan,8; 2017,Jan,8; 2016,Jan,13

● New Code　▲ Revised Code　○ Reinstated　● New Web Release　▲ Revised Web Release　+ Add-on　Unlisted　Not Covered　# Resequenced
50 Optum Mod 50 Exempt　🚫 AMA Mod 51 Exempt　51 Optum Mod 51 Exempt　63 Mod 63 Exempt　✗ Non-FDA Drug　★ Telemedicine　M Maternity　A Age Edit

72146 Magnetic resonance (eg, proton) imaging, spinal canal and contents, thoracic; without contrast material
  6.11   6.11   **FUD** XXX   03 Z2 80 ▣
  AMA: 2018,Jan,8; 2017,Jan,8; 2016,Jan,13

72147 with contrast material(s)
  EXCLUDES   *MRI thoracic spinal canal performed without contrast followed by repeating study with contrast (72157)*
  8.82   8.82   **FUD** XXX   03 Z2 80 ▣
  AMA: 2018,Jan,8; 2017,Jan,8; 2016,Jan,13

72148 Magnetic resonance (eg, proton) imaging, spinal canal and contents, lumbar; without contrast material
  6.12   6.12   **FUD** XXX   03 Z2 80 ▣
  AMA: 2018,Jan,8; 2017,Jan,8; 2016,Jan,13

72149 with contrast material(s)
  EXCLUDES   *MRI lumbar spinal canal performed without contrast followed by repeating study with contrast (72158)*
  8.74   8.74   **FUD** XXX   03 Z2 80 ▣
  AMA: 2014,Jan,11; 2012,Feb,9-10

72156 Magnetic resonance (eg, proton) imaging, spinal canal and contents, without contrast material, followed by contrast material(s) and further sequences; cervical
  10.3   10.3   **FUD** XXX   03 Z2 80 ▣
  AMA: 2014,Jan,11; 2012,Feb,9-10

72157 thoracic
  10.5   10.5   **FUD** XXX   03 Z2 80 ▣
  AMA: 2014,Jan,11; 2012,Feb,9-10

72158 lumbar
  10.5   10.5   **FUD** XXX   03 Z2 80 ▣
  AMA: 2014,Jan,11; 2012,Feb,9-10

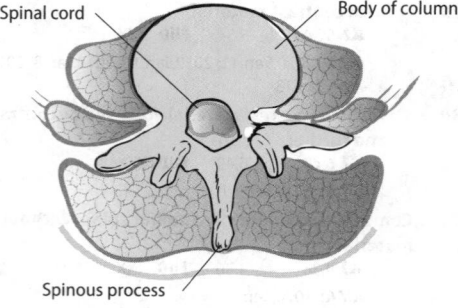

Superior view of thoracic spine and surrounding paraspinal muscles

Spinal cord — *Body of column* — *Spinous process*

72159 Magnetic Resonance Angiography: Spine

CMS: 100-04,13,40.1.1 Magnetic Resonance Angiography; 100-04,13,40.1.2 HCPCS Coding Requirements; 100-04,4,250.16 Multiple Procedure Payment Reduction: Certain Diagnostic Imaging Procedures Rendered by Physicians

72159 Magnetic resonance angiography, spinal canal and contents, with or without contrast material(s)
  11.2   11.2   **FUD** XXX   B 80 ▣
  AMA: 2018,Jan,8; 2017,Jan,8; 2016,Jan,13

72170-72190 Radiography: Pelvis

INCLUDES   Minimum number views or more views when needed to adequately complete study
  Radiographs repeated during encounter due to substandard quality; only one unit reported
EXCLUDES   *Combined CT or CT angiography abdomen and pelvis (74174, 74176-74178)*
  Obtaining more films after initial film review, based on radiologist discretion, order for test, and change in patient's condition
  Pelvimetry (74710)
  Second interpretation by requesting physician (included in E/M service)

72170 Radiologic examination, pelvis; 1 or 2 views
  0.80   0.80   **FUD** XXX   01 N1 80 ▣
  AMA: 2018,Jan,8; 2017,Jan,8; 2016,Aug,7; 2016,Jun,5; 2016,Jan,13

72190 complete, minimum of 3 views
  1.14   1.14   **FUD** XXX   01 N1 80 ▣
  AMA: 2016,Jun,5

72191 Computerized Tomographic Angiography: Pelvis

CMS: 100-04,4,250.16 Multiple Procedure Payment Reduction: Certain Diagnostic Imaging Procedures Rendered by Physicians

EXCLUDES   *Computed tomographic angiography (73706, 74174-74175, 75635)*
  Noninvasive arterial plaque analysis non-coronary computerized tomography angiography (0710T-0713T)

72191 Computed tomographic angiography, pelvis, with contrast material(s), including noncontrast images, if performed, and image postprocessing
  9.08   9.08   **FUD** XXX   03 Z2 80 ▣
  AMA: 2020,Sep,11; 2018,Jan,8; 2017,Jan,8; 2016,Jan,13

72192-72194 Computerized Tomography: Pelvis

CMS: 100-04,4,250.16 Multiple Procedure Payment Reduction: Certain Diagnostic Imaging Procedures Rendered by Physicians

EXCLUDES   *3D rendering (76376-76377)*
  Combined CT abdomen and pelvis (74176-74178)
  CT colonography, diagnostic (74261-74262)
  CT colonography, screening (74263)

72192 Computed tomography, pelvis; without contrast material
  4.09   4.09   **FUD** XXX   03 Z2 80 ▣
  AMA: 2020,Sep,11; 2018,Jan,8; 2017,Jan,8; 2016,Jan,13

72193 with contrast material(s)
  6.81   6.81   **FUD** XXX   03 Z2 80 ▣
  AMA: 2020,Sep,11; 2018,Jan,8; 2017,Jan,8; 2016,Jan,13

72194 without contrast material, followed by contrast material(s) and further sections
  7.66   7.66   **FUD** XXX   03 Z2 80 ▣
  AMA: 2020,Sep,11; 2018,Jan,8; 2017,Jan,8; 2016,Jan,13

72195-72197 Magnetic Resonance Imaging: Pelvis

CMS: 100-04,4,250.16 Multiple Procedure Payment Reduction: Certain Diagnostic Imaging Procedures Rendered by Physicians

INCLUDES   Three-dimensional imaging that measures response atomic nuclei in soft tissues to high-frequency radio waves when strong magnetic field applied
EXCLUDES   *MRI fetus(es) (74712-74713)*

72195 Magnetic resonance (eg, proton) imaging, pelvis; without contrast material(s)
  7.49   7.49   **FUD** XXX   03 Z2 80 ▣
  AMA: 2018,Jul,11; 2018,Jan,8; 2017,Jan,8; 2016,Jun,5; 2016,Jan,13

72196 with contrast material(s)
  8.74   8.74   **FUD** XXX   03 Z2 80 ▣
  AMA: 2018,Jul,11; 2018,Jan,8; 2017,Jan,8; 2016,Jun,5; 2016,Jan,13

72197 without contrast material(s), followed by contrast material(s) and further sequences
  10.9   10.9   **FUD** XXX   03 Z2 80 ▣
  AMA: 2018,Jul,11; 2018,Jan,8; 2017,Jan,8; 2016,Jun,5; 2016,Jan,13

72198 Magnetic Resonance Angiography: Pelvis

CMS: 100-04,13,40.1.1 Magnetic Resonance Angiography; 100-04,13,40.1.2 HCPCS Coding Requirements; 100-04,4,250.16 Multiple Procedure Payment Reduction: Certain Diagnostic Imaging Procedures Rendered by Physicians

INCLUDES   Magnetic fields and radio waves to produce detailed cross-sectional images arteries and veins

72198 Magnetic resonance angiography, pelvis, with or without contrast material(s)
  11.0   11.0   **FUD** XXX   B 80 ▣
  AMA: 2018,Jan,8; 2017,Jan,8; 2016,Jan,13

72200-72220 Radiography: Pelvisacral

INCLUDES Minimum number views or more views when needed to adequately complete study
Radiographs repeated during encounter due to substandard quality; only one unit reported

EXCLUDES *Obtaining more films after initial film review, based on radiologist discretion, order for, and change in patient's condition*
Second interpretation by requesting physician (included in E/M service)

72200 **Radiologic examination, sacroiliac joints; less than 3 views**
📷 0.90   ⚕ 0.90   **FUD** XXX   [01] [N1] [80] [▭]
AMA: 2014,Jan,11; 2012,Feb,9-10

72202 **3 or more views**
📷 1.07   ⚕ 1.07   **FUD** XXX   [01] [N1] [80] [▭]
AMA: 2014,Jan,11; 2012,Feb,9-10

72220 **Radiologic examination, sacrum and coccyx, minimum of 2 views**
📷 0.88   ⚕ 0.88   **FUD** XXX   [01] [N1] [80] [▭]
AMA: 2014,Jan,11; 2012,Feb,9-10

72240-72270 Myelography with Contrast: Spinal Cord

CMS: 100-04,13,30.1.3.1 Payment for Low Osmolar Contrast Material
EXCLUDES *Injection procedure for myelography (62284)*
Myelography (62302-62305)
Code also injection at C1-C2 for complete myelography (61055)

72240 **Myelography, cervical, radiological supervision and interpretation**
📷 3.14   ⚕ 3.14   **FUD** XXX   [02] [N1] [80] [▭]
AMA: 2018,Jan,8; 2017,Jan,8; 2016,Jan,13

72255 **Myelography, thoracic, radiological supervision and interpretation**
📷 2.99   ⚕ 2.99   **FUD** XXX   [02] [N1] [80] [▭]
AMA: 2018,Jan,8; 2017,Jan,8; 2016,Jan,13

72265 **Myelography, lumbosacral, radiological supervision and interpretation**
📷 2.90   ⚕ 2.90   **FUD** XXX   [02] [N1] [80] [▭]
AMA: 2018,Jan,8; 2017,Jan,8; 2016,Jan,13

72270 **Myelography, 2 or more regions (eg, lumbar/thoracic, cervical/thoracic, lumbar/cervical, lumbar/thoracic/cervical), radiological supervision and interpretation**
📷 4.00   ⚕ 4.00   **FUD** XXX   [02] [N1] [80] [▭]
AMA: 2018,Jan,8; 2017,Jan,8; 2016,Jan,13

72275 Radiography: Epidural Space

72275 ~~Epidurography, radiological supervision and interpretation~~
To report, see (62281-62282, 62321, 62323, 62325, 62327, 64479, 64480, 64483-64484)

72285 Radiography: Intervertebral Disc (Cervical/Thoracic)

CMS: 100-04,13,30.1.3.1 Payment for Low Osmolar Contrast Material
Code also discography injection procedure (62291)

72285 **Discography, cervical or thoracic, radiological supervision and interpretation**
📷 3.45   ⚕ 3.45   **FUD** XXX   [02] [N1] [80] [▭]
AMA: 2018,Jan,8; 2017,Jan,8; 2016,Jan,13

72295 Radiography: Intervertebral Disc (Lumbar)

CMS: 100-04,13,30.1.3.1 Payment for Low Osmolar Contrast Material
Code also discography injection procedure (62290)

72295 **Discography, lumbar, radiological supervision and interpretation**
📷 3.02   ⚕ 3.02   **FUD** XXX   [02] [N1] [80] [▭]
AMA: 2018,Jan,8; 2017,Feb,12; 2017,Jan,8; 2016,Jan,13

73000-73085 Radiography: Shoulder and Upper Arm

INCLUDES Minimum number views or more views when needed to adequately complete study
Radiographs repeated during encounter due to substandard quality; only one unit reported

EXCLUDES *Obtaining more films after initial film review, based on radiologist discretion, order for test, and change in patient's condition*
Second interpretation by requesting physician (included in E/M service)
Stress views upper body joint(s), when performed (77071)

73000 **Radiologic examination; clavicle, complete**
📷 0.88   ⚕ 0.88   **FUD** XXX   [01] [N1] [80] [▭]
AMA: 2014,Jan,11; 2012,Feb,9-10

Radiograph

Gold wedding band absorbs all x-rays (white)
Air allows all rays to reach film (black)
Soft tissues absorb part of rays and will vary in gray intensity
Calcium in bone absorbs most of rays and is nearly white
X-ray beam
Film

Posterioranterior (PA) chest study; lateral views also common

73010 **scapula, complete**
📷 0.78   ⚕ 0.78   **FUD** XXX   [01] [N1] [80] [▭]
AMA: 2014,Jan,11; 2012,Feb,9-10

73020 **Radiologic examination, shoulder; 1 view**
📷 0.60   ⚕ 0.60   **FUD** XXX   [01] [N1] [80] [▭]
AMA: 2014,Jan,11; 2012,Feb,9-10

73030 **complete, minimum of 2 views**
📷 0.93   ⚕ 0.93   **FUD** XXX   [01] [N1] [80] [▭]
AMA: 2014,Jan,11; 2012,Feb,9-10

73040 **Radiologic examination, shoulder, arthrography, radiological supervision and interpretation**
INCLUDES Fluoroscopic guidance (77002)
Code also arthrography injection procedure (23350)
📷 3.39   ⚕ 3.39   **FUD** XXX   [02] [N1] [80] [▭]
AMA: 2018,Jan,8; 2017,Jan,8; 2016,Jan,13

73050 **Radiologic examination; acromioclavicular joints, bilateral, with or without weighted distraction**
📷 0.88   ⚕ 0.88   **FUD** XXX   [01] [N1] [80] [▭]
AMA: 2014,Jan,11; 2012,Feb,9-10

73060 **humerus, minimum of 2 views**
📷 0.88   ⚕ 0.88   **FUD** XXX   [01] [N1] [80] [▭]
AMA: 2014,Jan,11; 2012,Feb,9-10

73070 **Radiologic examination, elbow; 2 views**
📷 0.80   ⚕ 0.80   **FUD** XXX   [01] [N1] [80] [▭]
AMA: 2018,Jan,8; 2017,Jan,8; 2016,Jan,13

73080 **complete, minimum of 3 views**
📷 0.87   ⚕ 0.87   **FUD** XXX   [01] [N1] [80] [▭]
AMA: 2014,Jan,11; 2012,Feb,9-10

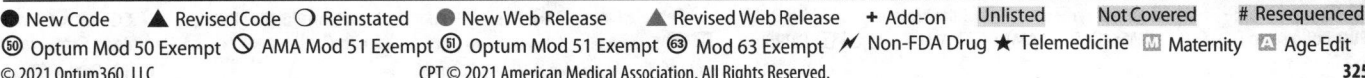

Radiology

73085 — 73502

73085 Radiologic examination, elbow, arthrography, radiological supervision and interpretation

> INCLUDES   Fluoroscopic guidance (77002)
> Code also arthrography injection procedure (24220)
> 🔳 3.18   ⅄ 3.18   **FUD** XXX   02 N1 80 ▭
>
> AMA: 2018,Jan,8; 2017,Jan,8; 2016,Jan,13

73090-73140 Radiography: Forearm and Hand

> INCLUDES   Minimum number views or more views when needed to adequately complete study
> Radiographs repeated during encounter due to substandard quality; only one unit reported
> EXCLUDES   *Obtaining more films after initial film review, based on radiologist discretion, order for test, and change in patient's condition*
> *Second interpretation by requesting physician (included in E/M service)*
> *Stress views upper body joint(s), when performed (77071)*

73090 Radiologic examination; forearm, 2 views

> 🔳 0.81   ⅄ 0.81   **FUD** XXX   01 N1 80 ▭
>
> AMA: 2018,Jan,8; 2017,Jan,8; 2016,Jan,13

73092 upper extremity, infant, minimum of 2 views   A

> 🔳 0.85   ⅄ 0.85   **FUD** XXX   01 N1 80 ▭
>
> AMA: 2014,Jan,11; 2012,Feb,9-10

73100 Radiologic examination, wrist; 2 views

> 🔳 0.92   ⅄ 0.92   **FUD** XXX   01 N1 80 ▭
>
> AMA: 2018,Oct,11; 2018,Jan,8; 2017,Jan,8; 2016,Jan,13

73110 complete, minimum of 3 views

> 🔳 1.09   ⅄ 1.09   **FUD** XXX   01 N1 80 ▭
>
> AMA: 2018,Oct,11; 2018,Jan,8; 2017,Jan,8; 2016,Jan,13

73115 Radiologic examination, wrist, arthrography, radiological supervision and interpretation

> INCLUDES   Fluoroscopic guidance (77002)
> Code also arthrography injection procedure (25246)
> 🔳 3.56   ⅄ 3.56   **FUD** XXX   02 N1 80 ▭
>
> AMA: 2018,Jan,8; 2017,Jan,8; 2016,Jan,13

73120 Radiologic examination, hand; 2 views

> 🔳 0.85   ⅄ 0.85   **FUD** XXX   01 N1 80 ▭
>
> AMA: 2018,Oct,11

73130 minimum of 3 views

> 🔳 0.94   ⅄ 0.94   **FUD** XXX   01 N1 80 ▭
>
> AMA: 2014,Jan,11; 2012,Feb,9-10

73140 Radiologic examination, finger(s), minimum of 2 views

> 🔳 1.00   ⅄ 1.00   **FUD** XXX   01 N1 80 ▭
>
> AMA: 2018,Jan,8; 2017,Jan,8; 2016,Jan,13

73200-73202 Computerized Tomography: Shoulder, Arm, Hand

CMS: 100-04,4,250.16 Multiple Procedure Payment Reduction: Certain Diagnostic Imaging Procedures Rendered by Physicians

> INCLUDES   Imaging using tomographic technique enhanced by computer imaging to create cross-sectional body plane view
> Intravascular, intrathecal, or intra-articular contrast materials when noted in code descriptor
> EXCLUDES   *3D rendering (76376-76377)*

73200 Computed tomography, upper extremity; without contrast material

> 🔳 5.03   ⅄ 5.03   **FUD** XXX   03 Z2 80 ▭
>
> AMA: 2018,Jan,8; 2017,Jan,8; 2016,Jan,13

73201 with contrast material(s)

> 🔳 6.28   ⅄ 6.28   **FUD** XXX   03 Z3 80 ▭
>
> AMA: 2018,Jan,8; 2017,Jan,8; 2016,Jan,13

73202 without contrast material, followed by contrast material(s) and further sections

> 🔳 7.82   ⅄ 7.82   **FUD** XXX   03 Z2 80 ▭
>
> AMA: 2014,Jan,11; 2012,Feb,9-10

73206 Computerized Tomographic Angiography: Shoulder, Arm, and Hand

CMS: 100-04,4,250.16 Multiple Procedure Payment Reduction: Certain Diagnostic Imaging Procedures Rendered by Physicians

> INCLUDES   Intravascular, intrathecal, or intra-articular contrast materials when noted in code descriptor
> Multiple rapid thin section CT scans to create cross-sectional images arteries and veins

73206 Computed tomographic angiography, upper extremity, with contrast material(s), including noncontrast images, if performed, and image postprocessing

> 🔳 9.24   ⅄ 9.24   **FUD** XXX   03 Z2 80 ▭
>
> AMA: 2018,Jan,8; 2017,Jan,8; 2016,Jan,13

73218-73223 Magnetic Resonance Imaging: Shoulder, Arm, Hand

CMS: 100-04,4,250.16 Multiple Procedure Payment Reduction: Certain Diagnostic Imaging Procedures Rendered by Physicians

> INCLUDES   Intravascular, intrathecal, or intra-articular contrast materials when noted in code descriptor
> Three-dimensional imaging that measures response atomic nuclei in soft tissues to high-frequency radio waves when strong magnetic field applied

73218 Magnetic resonance (eg, proton) imaging, upper extremity, other than joint; without contrast material(s)

> 🔳 10.1   ⅄ 10.1   **FUD** XXX   03 Z2 80 ▭
>
> AMA: 2018,Jan,8; 2017,Jan,8; 2016,Jan,13

73219 with contrast material(s)

> 🔳 10.9   ⅄ 10.9   **FUD** XXX   03 Z2 80 ▭
>
> AMA: 2018,Jan,8; 2017,Jan,8; 2016,Jan,13

73220 without contrast material(s), followed by contrast material(s) and further sequences

> 🔳 13.4   ⅄ 13.4   **FUD** XXX   03 Z2 80 ▭
>
> AMA: 2018,Jan,8; 2017,Jan,8; 2016,Jan,13

73221 Magnetic resonance (eg, proton) imaging, any joint of upper extremity; without contrast material(s)

> 🔳 6.47   ⅄ 6.47   **FUD** XXX   03 Z2 80 ▭
>
> AMA: 2018,Jan,8; 2017,Jan,8; 2016,Jan,13

73222 with contrast material(s)

> 🔳 10.2   ⅄ 10.2   **FUD** XXX   03 Z3 80 ▭
>
> AMA: 2018,Jan,8; 2017,Jan,8; 2016,Jan,13

73223 without contrast material(s), followed by contrast material(s) and further sequences

> 🔳 12.7   ⅄ 12.7   **FUD** XXX   03 Z2 80 ▭
>
> AMA: 2018,Jan,8; 2017,Jan,8; 2016,Jan,13

73225 Magnetic Resonance Angiography: Shoulder, Arm, Hand

CMS: 100-04,13,40.1.1 Magnetic Resonance Angiography; 100-04,4,250.16 Multiple Procedure Payment Reduction: Certain Diagnostic Imaging Procedures Rendered by Physicians

> INCLUDES   Intravascular, intrathecal, or intra-articular contrast materials when noted in code descriptor
> Magnetic fields and radio waves to produce detailed cross-sectional images arteries and veins

73225 Magnetic resonance angiography, upper extremity, with or without contrast material(s)

> 🔳 11.1   ⅄ 11.1   **FUD** XXX   B 80 ▭
>
> AMA: 2018,Jan,8; 2017,Jan,8; 2016,Jan,13

73501-73552 Radiography: Pelvic Region and Thigh

> EXCLUDES   *Stress views lower body joint(s), when performed (77071)*

73501 Radiologic examination, hip, unilateral, with pelvis when performed; 1 view

> 🔳 0.89   ⅄ 0.89   **FUD** XXX   01 N1 80 ▭
>
> AMA: 2018,Jan,8; 2017,Jan,8; 2016,Aug,7; 2016,Jun,8; 2016,Jan,13

73502 2-3 views

> 🔳 1.27   ⅄ 1.27   **FUD** XXX   01 N1 80 ▭
>
> AMA: 2018,Jan,8; 2017,Jan,8; 2016,Aug,7; 2016,Jun,8; 2016,Jan,13

| 26/TC PC/TC Only | A2-Z3 ASC Payment | 50 Bilateral | ♂ Male Only | ♀ Female Only | 🔳 Facility RVU | ⅄ Non-Facility RVU | ▭ CCI | ✖ CLIA |
| **FUD** Follow-up Days | **CMS:** IOM | **AMA:** CPT Asst | A-Y OPPSI | 80/80 Surg Assist Allowed / w/Doc | | ◩ Lab Crosswalk | | ✚ Radiology Crosswalk |

326   CPT © 2021 American Medical Association. All Rights Reserved.   © 2021 Optum360, LLC

73503 minimum of 4 views
1.57   1.57   **FUD** XXX   [01] [N1] [80] [▣]
AMA: 2018,Jan,8; 2017,Jan,8; 2016,Aug,7; 2016,Jun,8; 2016,Jan,13

73521 Radiologic examination, hips, bilateral, with pelvis when performed; 2 views
1.12   1.12   **FUD** XXX   [01] [N1] [80] [▣]
AMA: 2018,Jan,8; 2017,Jan,8; 2016,Aug,7; 2016,Jun,8; 2016,Jan,13

73522 3-4 views
1.46   1.46   **FUD** XXX   [01] [N1] [80] [▣]
AMA: 2018,Jan,8; 2017,Jan,8; 2016,Aug,7; 2016,Jun,8; 2016,Jan,13

73523 minimum of 5 views
1.65   1.65   **FUD** XXX   [S] [N1] [80] [▣]
AMA: 2018,Jan,8; 2017,Jan,8; 2016,Aug,7; 2016,Jun,8; 2016,Jan,13

73525 Radiologic examination, hip, arthrography, radiological supervision and interpretation
INCLUDES Fluoroscopic guidance (77002)
3.47   3.47   **FUD** XXX   [02] [N1] [80] [▣]
AMA: 2018,Jan,8; 2017,Jan,8; 2016,Nov,10; 2016,Aug,7; 2016,Jan,13

73551 Radiologic examination, femur; 1 view
0.82   0.82   **FUD** XXX   [01] [N1] [80] [▣]
AMA: 2018,Jan,8; 2017,Jan,8; 2016,Aug,7

73552 minimum 2 views
0.97   0.97   **FUD** XXX   [01] [N1] [80] [▣]
AMA: 2018,Jan,8; 2017,Nov,10; 2017,Jan,8; 2016,Aug,7

73560-73660 Radiography: Lower Leg, Ankle, and Foot

EXCLUDES Stress views lower body joint(s), when performed (77071)

73560 Radiologic examination, knee; 1 or 2 views
0.94   0.94   **FUD** XXX   [01] [N1] [80] [▣]
AMA: 2018,Jan,8; 2017,Jan,8; 2016,Jan,13

73562 3 views
1.10   1.10   **FUD** XXX   [01] [N1] [80] [▣]
AMA: 2014,Jan,11; 2012,Feb,9-10

73564 complete, 4 or more views
1.23   1.23   **FUD** XXX   [01] [N1] [80] [▣]
AMA: 2018,Jan,8; 2017,Jan,8; 2016,Jan,13

73565 both knees, standing, anteroposterior
1.09   1.09   **FUD** XXX   [01] [N1] [80] [▣]
AMA: 2018,Jan,8; 2017,Jan,8; 2016,Jan,13

73580 Radiologic examination, knee, arthrography, radiological supervision and interpretation
INCLUDES Fluoroscopic guidance (77002)
3.84   3.84   **FUD** XXX   [02] [N1] [80] [▣]
AMA: 2019,Aug,7; 2018,Jan,8; 2017,Jan,8; 2016,Jan,13

73590 Radiologic examination; tibia and fibula, 2 views
0.86   0.86   **FUD** XXX   [01] [N1] [80] [▣]
AMA: 2018,Jan,8; 2017,Nov,10; 2017,Jan,8; 2016,Jan,13

73592 lower extremity, infant, minimum of 2 views
0.85   0.85   **FUD** XXX   [A]
AMA: 2018,Jan,8; 2017,Nov,10

73600 Radiologic examination, ankle; 2 views
0.87   0.87   **FUD** XXX   [01] [N1] [80] [▣]
AMA: 2018,Jan,8; 2017,Jan,8; 2016,Jan,13

73610 complete, minimum of 3 views
0.98   0.98   **FUD** XXX   [01] [N1] [80] [▣]
AMA: 2018,Jan,8; 2017,Jan,8; 2016,Jan,13

73615 Radiologic examination, ankle, arthrography, radiological supervision and interpretation
INCLUDES Fluoroscopic guidance (77002)
3.61   3.61   **FUD** XXX   [02] [N1] [80] [▣]
AMA: 2018,Jan,8; 2017,Jan,8; 2016,Jan,13

73620 Radiologic examination, foot; 2 views
0.78   0.78   **FUD** XXX   [01] [N1] [80] [▣]
AMA: 2018,Jan,8; 2017,Jan,8; 2016,Jan,13

73630 complete, minimum of 3 views
0.92   0.92   **FUD** XXX   [01] [N1] [80] [▣]
AMA: 2014,Jan,11; 2012,Feb,9-10

73650 Radiologic examination; calcaneus, minimum of 2 views
0.79   0.79   **FUD** XXX   [01] [N1] [80] [▣]
AMA: 2014,Jan,11; 2012,Feb,9-10

73660 toe(s), minimum of 2 views
0.79   0.79   **FUD** XXX   [01] [N1] [80] [▣]
AMA: 2014,Jan,11; 2012,Feb,9-10

73700-73702 Computerized Tomography: Leg, Ankle, and Foot

CMS: 100-04,4,250.16 Multiple Procedure Payment Reduction: Certain Diagnostic Imaging Procedures Rendered by Physicians

EXCLUDES 3D rendering (76376-76377)

73700 Computed tomography, lower extremity; without contrast material
5.06   5.06   **FUD** XXX   [Q3] [Z2] [80] [▣]
AMA: 2018,Jan,8; 2017,Jan,8; 2016,Jan,13

73701 with contrast material(s)
5.45   5.45   **FUD** XXX   [Q3] [Z2] [80] [▣]
AMA: 2019,Aug,7; 2018,Jan,8; 2017,Jan,8; 2016,Jan,13

73702 without contrast material, followed by contrast material(s) and further sections
6.56   6.56   **FUD** XXX   [Q3] [Z2] [80] [▣]
AMA: 2019,Aug,7; 2018,Jan,8; 2017,Jan,8; 2016,Jan,13

73706 Computerized Tomographic Angiography: Leg, Ankle, and Foot

CMS: 100-04,4,250.16 Multiple Procedure Payment Reduction: Certain Diagnostic Imaging Procedures Rendered by Physicians

EXCLUDES CT angiography for aorto-iliofemoral runoff (75635)
Noninvasive arterial plaque analysis non-coronary computerized tomography angiography (0710T-0713T)

73706 Computed tomographic angiography, lower extremity, with contrast material(s), including noncontrast images, if performed, and image postprocessing
10.0   10.0   **FUD** XXX   [Q3] [Z2] [80] [▣]
AMA: 2018,Jan,8; 2017,Jan,8; 2016,Jan,13

73718-73723 Magnetic Resonance Imaging: Leg, Ankle, and Foot

CMS: 100-04,4,250.16 Multiple Procedure Payment Reduction: Certain Diagnostic Imaging Procedures Rendered by Physicians

73718 Magnetic resonance (eg, proton) imaging, lower extremity other than joint; without contrast material(s)
7.25   7.25   **FUD** XXX   [Q3] [Z2] [80] [▣]
AMA: 2018,Jan,8; 2017,Jan,8; 2016,Jan,13

73719 with contrast material(s)
8.58   8.58   **FUD** XXX   [Q3] [Z2] [80] [▣]
AMA: 2019,Aug,7; 2018,Jan,8; 2017,Jan,8; 2016,Jan,13

73720 without contrast material(s), followed by contrast material(s) and further sequences
10.9   10.9   **FUD** XXX   [Q3] [Z2] [80] [▣]
AMA: 2019,Aug,7; 2018,Jan,8; 2017,Jan,8; 2016,Jan,13

73721 Magnetic resonance (eg, proton) imaging, any joint of lower extremity; without contrast material
6.44   6.44   **FUD** XXX   [Q3] [Z2] [80] [▣]
AMA: 2018,Jan,8; 2017,Jan,8; 2016,Jan,13

73722 with contrast material(s)
10.3   10.3   **FUD** XXX   [Q3] [Z3] [80] [▣]
AMA: 2019,Aug,7; 2018,Jan,8; 2017,Jan,8; 2016,Jan,13

Radiology

73723 — 74183

73723	without contrast material(s), followed by contrast material(s) and further sequences

🎫 12.7 🔍 12.7 **FUD** XXX [03] [Z2] [80] 🖃

AMA: 2019,Aug,7; 2018,Jan,8; 2017,Jan,8; 2016,Jan,13

73725 Magnetic Resonance Angiography: Leg, Ankle, and Foot

CMS: 100-04,13,40.1.2 HCPCS Coding Requirements; 100-04,4,250.16 Multiple Procedure Payment Reduction: Certain Diagnostic Imaging Procedures Rendered by Physicians

73725	Magnetic resonance angiography, lower extremity, with or without contrast material(s)

🎫 10.8 🔍 10.8 **FUD** XXX [B] [80] 🖃

AMA: 2018,Jan,8; 2017,Jan,8; 2016,Jan,13

74018-74022 Radiography: Abdomen--General

74018	Radiologic examination, abdomen; 1 view

🎫 0.80 🔍 0.80 **FUD** XXX [01] [N1] [80] 🖃

AMA: 2020,Apr,10; 2019,May,10; 2018,Apr,7

74019	2 views

🎫 1.01 🔍 1.01 **FUD** XXX [01] [N1] [80] 🖃

AMA: 2018,Apr,7

74021	3 or more views

🎫 1.17 🔍 1.17 **FUD** XXX [01] [N1] [80] 🖃

AMA: 2018,Apr,7

74022	Radiologic examination, complete acute abdomen series, including 2 or more views of the abdomen (eg, supine, erect, decubitus), and a single view chest

🎫 1.36 🔍 1.36 **FUD** XXX [01] [N1] [80] 🖃

AMA: 2019,May,10; 2018,Apr,7; 2016,Jun,5

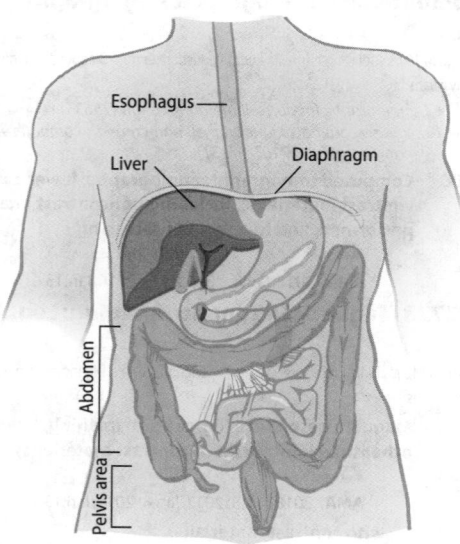

Esophagus
Liver
Diaphragm
Abdomen
Pelvis area

74150-74170 Computerized Tomography: Abdomen—General

CMS: 100-04,4,250.16 Multiple Procedure Payment Reduction: Certain Diagnostic Imaging Procedures Rendered by Physicians

EXCLUDES 3D rendering (76376-76377)
Combined CT abdomen and pelvis (74176-74178)
CT colonography, diagnostic (74261-74262)
CT colonography, screening (74263)

74150	Computed tomography, abdomen; without contrast material

🎫 4.20 🔍 4.20 **FUD** XXX [03] [Z2] [80] 🖃

AMA: 2020,Sep,11; 2018,Jan,8; 2017,Jan,8; 2016,Jun,5; 2016,Jan,13

74160	with contrast material(s)

🎫 6.96 🔍 6.96 **FUD** XXX [03] [Z2] [80] 🖃

AMA: 2020,Sep,11; 2018,Jan,8; 2017,Jan,8; 2016,Jun,5; 2016,Jan,13

74170	without contrast material, followed by contrast material(s) and further sections

🎫 7.85 🔍 7.85 **FUD** XXX [03] [Z2] [80] 🖃

AMA: 2020,Sep,11; 2018,Jan,8; 2017,Jan,8; 2016,Jun,5; 2016,Jan,13

74174-74175 Computerized Tomographic Angiography: Abdomen and Pelvis

CMS: 100-04,4,250.16 Multiple Procedure Payment Reduction: Certain Diagnostic Imaging Procedures Rendered by Physicians

EXCLUDES CT angiography for aorto-iliofemoral runoff (75635)
CT angiography, lower extremity (73706)
CT angiography, pelvis (72191)
Noninvasive arterial plaque analysis non-coronary computerized tomography angiography (0710T-0713T)

74174	Computed tomographic angiography, abdomen and pelvis, with contrast material(s), including noncontrast images, if performed, and image postprocessing

EXCLUDES 3D rendering (76376-76377)
CT angiography abdomen (74175)

🎫 11.4 🔍 11.4 **FUD** XXX [S] [Z2] [80] 🖃

AMA: 2020,Sep,11

74175	Computed tomographic angiography, abdomen, with contrast material(s), including noncontrast images, if performed, and image postprocessing

🎫 9.10 🔍 9.10 **FUD** XXX [03] [Z2] [80] 🖃

AMA: 2020,Sep,11; 2018,Jan,8; 2017,Jan,8; 2016,Jan,13

74176-74178 Computerized Tomography: Abdomen and Pelvis

CMS: 100-04,4,250.16 Multiple Procedure Payment Reduction: Certain Diagnostic Imaging Procedures Rendered by Physicians

EXCLUDES CT abdomen or pelvis alone (72192-72194, 74150-74170)
Procedure performed more than one time for each combined abdomen and pelvis examination

74176	Computed tomography, abdomen and pelvis; without contrast material

🎫 5.63 🔍 5.63 **FUD** XXX [03] [Z3] 🖃

AMA: 2020,Sep,11; 2018,Jan,8; 2017,Jan,8; 2016,Jan,13

74177	with contrast material(s)

🎫 9.21 🔍 9.21 **FUD** XXX [03] [Z2] 🖃

AMA: 2020,Sep,11; 2018,Jan,8; 2017,Jan,8; 2016,Jan,13

74178	without contrast material in one or both body regions, followed by contrast material(s) and further sections in one or both body regions

🎫 10.3 🔍 10.3 **FUD** XXX [03] [Z2] 🖃

AMA: 2020,Sep,11; 2018,Jan,8; 2017,Jan,8; 2016,Jan,13

74181-74183 Magnetic Resonance Imaging: Abdomen–General

CMS: 100-04,4,250.16 Multiple Procedure Payment Reduction: Certain Diagnostic Imaging Procedures Rendered by Physicians

74181	Magnetic resonance (eg, proton) imaging, abdomen; without contrast material(s)

🎫 6.34 🔍 6.34 **FUD** XXX [03] [Z2] [80] 🖃

AMA: 2018,Mar,11; 2018,Jan,8; 2017,Jan,8; 2016,Jan,13

74182	with contrast material(s)

🎫 9.90 🔍 9.90 **FUD** XXX [03] [Z2] [80] 🖃

AMA: 2018,Mar,11; 2018,Jan,8; 2017,Jan,8; 2016,Jan,13

74183	without contrast material(s), followed by with contrast material(s) and further sequences

🎫 11.0 🔍 11.0 **FUD** XXX [03] [Z2] [80] 🖃

AMA: 2018,Mar,11; 2018,Jan,8; 2017,Jan,8; 2016,Jan,13

26/TC PC/TC Only A2-Z3 ASC Payment 50 Bilateral ♂ Male Only ♀ Female Only 🎫 Facility RVU 🔍 Non-Facility RVU 🖃 CCI ❌ CLIA
FUD Follow-up Days CMS: IOM AMA: CPT Asst A-Y OPPSI 80/80 Surg Assist Allowed / w/Doc 🔲 Lab Crosswalk 🔳 Radiology Crosswalk

328
CPT © 2021 American Medical Association. All Rights Reserved.
© 2021 Optum360, LLC

74185 Magnetic Resonance Angiography: Abdomen–General

CMS: 100-04,13,40.1.1 Magnetic Resonance Angiography; 100-04,13,40.1.2 HCPCS Coding Requirements; 100-04,4,250.16 Multiple Procedure Payment Reduction: Certain Diagnostic Imaging Procedures Rendered by Physicians

74185 **Magnetic resonance angiography, abdomen, with or without contrast material(s)**
10.9   10.9   **FUD** XXX   B 80
AMA: 2018,Jan,8; 2017,Jan,8; 2016,Jan,13

74190 Peritoneography

74190 **Peritoneogram (eg, after injection of air or contrast), radiological supervision and interpretation**
EXCLUDES   *CT pelvis or abdomen (72192, 74150)*
Code also injection procedure (49400)
0.00   0.00   **FUD** XXX   02 N1 80
AMA: 2018,Jan,8; 2017,Jan,8; 2016,Jan,13

74210-74235 Radiography: Throat and Esophagus

EXCLUDES   *Percutaneous placement gastrostomy tube, endoscopic (43246)*
Percutaneous placement gastrostomy tube, fluoroscopic guidance (49440)

74210 **Radiologic examination, pharynx and/or cervical esophagus, including scout neck radiograph(s) and delayed image(s), when performed, contrast (eg, barium) study**
2.66   2.66   **FUD** XXX   01 N1 80
AMA: 2020,Aug,9

74220 **Radiologic examination, esophagus, including scout chest radiograph(s) and delayed image(s), when performed; single-contrast (eg, barium) study**
EXCLUDES   *Double-contrast study (74221)*
Small bowel follow-through (74248)
Upper GI tract studies (74240-74246)
2.73   2.73   **FUD** XXX   01 N1 80
AMA: 2020,Aug,9

74221 **double-contrast (eg, high-density barium and effervescent agent) study**
EXCLUDES   *Single-contrast study (74220)*
Small bowel follow-through (74248)
Upper GI tract studies (74240-74246)
3.06   3.06   **FUD** XXX   80
AMA: 2020,Aug,9

74230 **Radiologic examination, swallowing function, with cineradiography/videoradiography, including scout neck radiograph(s) and delayed image(s), when performed, contrast (eg, barium) study**
EXCLUDES   *Swallowing function motion fluoroscopic examination (92611)*
3.64   3.64   **FUD** XXX   01 Z2 80
AMA: 2020,Aug,9; 2018,Jan,8; 2017,Jan,8; 2016,Jan,13

74235 **Removal of foreign body(s), esophageal, with use of balloon catheter, radiological supervision and interpretation**
Code also procedure (43499)
0.00   0.00   **FUD** XXX   N N1 80
AMA: 2014,Jan,11; 2012,Feb,9-10

74240-74283 Radiography: Intestines

EXCLUDES   *Percutaneous placement gastrostomy tube, endoscopic (43246)*
Percutaneous placement gastrostomy tube, fluoroscopic guidance (49440)

74240 **Radiologic examination, upper gastrointestinal tract, including scout abdominal radiograph(s) and delayed image(s), when performed; single-contrast (eg, barium) study**
INCLUDES   Upper GI with KUB
EXCLUDES   *Double-contrast study (74246)*
Esophagus studies (74220-74221)
Code also small bowel follow-through when performed (74248)
3.39   3.39   **FUD** XXX   01 Z3 80
AMA: 2020,Aug,9; 2018,Jan,8; 2017,Jan,8; 2016,Sep,7

74246 **double-contrast (eg, high-density barium and effervescent agent) study, including glucagon, when administered**
INCLUDES   Upper GI with KUB
EXCLUDES   *Esophagus studies (74220-74221)*
Single-contrast study (74240)
3.90   3.90   **FUD** XXX   01 Z2 80
AMA: 2020,Aug,9; 2018,Jan,8; 2017,Jan,8; 2016,Sep,7

+ **74248** **Radiologic small intestine follow-through study, including multiple serial images (List separately in addition to code for primary procedure for upper GI radiologic examination)**
EXCLUDES   *Single- or double-contrast small intestine studies (74250-74251)*
Code first (74240, 74246)
2.32   2.32   **FUD** ZZZ   80
AMA: 2020,Aug,9

74250 **Radiologic examination, small intestine, including multiple serial images and scout abdominal radiograph(s), when performed; single-contrast (eg, barium) study**
EXCLUDES   *Double-contrast study (74251)*
Small bowel follow-through (74248)
3.18   3.18   **FUD** XXX   01 Z3 80
AMA: 2020,Aug,9; 2018,Jan,8; 2017,Jan,8; 2016,Sep,7

74251 **double-contrast (eg, high-density barium and air via enteroclysis tube) study, including glucagon, when administered**
EXCLUDES   *Single-contrast study (74250)*
Small bowel follow-through (74248)
Code also insertion long gastrointestinal tube (44500, 74340)
11.3   11.3   **FUD** XXX   S Z2 80
AMA: 2020,Aug,9; 2018,Jan,8; 2017,Jan,8; 2016,Sep,7

74261 **Computed tomographic (CT) colonography, diagnostic, including image postprocessing; without contrast material**
EXCLUDES   *3D rendering (76376-76377)*
CT abdomen or pelvis alone (72192-72194, 74150-74170)
Screening CT colonography (74263)
13.4   13.4   **FUD** XXX   03 Z2 80
AMA: 2020,Sep,11; 2020,Feb,13; 2018,Jan,8; 2017,Jan,8; 2016,Jan,13

74262 **with contrast material(s) including non-contrast images, if performed**
EXCLUDES   *3D rendering (76376-76377)*
CT abdomen or pelvis alone (72192-72194, 74150-74170)
Screening CT colonography (74263)
15.1   15.1   **FUD** XXX   03 Z2 80
AMA: 2020,Sep,11; 2020,Feb,13; 2018,Jan,8; 2017,Jan,8; 2016,Jan,13

74263 **Computed tomographic (CT) colonography, screening, including image postprocessing**
EXCLUDES   *3D rendering (76376-76377)*
CT abdomen or pelvis alone (72192-72194, 74150-74170)
CT colonography (74261-74262)
21.1   21.1   **FUD** XXX   E
AMA: 2020,Sep,11; 2020,Feb,13; 2018,Jan,8; 2017,Jan,8; 2016,Jan,13

74270 **Radiologic examination, colon, including scout abdominal radiograph(s) and delayed image(s), when performed; single-contrast (eg, barium) study**
EXCLUDES   *Double-contrast study (74280)*
4.34   4.34   **FUD** XXX   01 N1 80
AMA: 2020,Aug,9; 2018,Jan,8; 2017,Jan,8; 2016,Jan,13

74280 **double-contrast (eg, high density barium and air) study, including glucagon, when administered**
EXCLUDES   *Single-contrast study (74270)*
6.24   6.24   **FUD** XXX   S N1 80
AMA: 2020,Aug,9

● New Code   ▲ Revised Code   ○ Reinstated   ● New Web Release   ▲ Revised Web Release   + Add-on   Unlisted   Not Covered   # Resequenced
50 Optum Mod 50 Exempt   ⊘ AMA Mod 51 Exempt   51 Optum Mod 51 Exempt   63 Mod 63 Exempt   ✗ Non-FDA Drug   ★ Telemedicine   M Maternity   A Age Edit

Radiology

74283 — 74440

74283　　**Therapeutic enema, contrast or air, for reduction of intussusception or other intraluminal obstruction (eg, meconium ileus)**
　　　　　📠 7.00　　♋ 7.00　　**FUD** XXX　　　　　S Z2 80 ▭
　　　　　AMA: 2014,Jan,11; 2012,Feb,9-10

74290-74330 Radiography: Biliary Tract

74290　　**Cholecystography, oral contrast**
　　　　　📠 2.15　　♋ 2.15　　**FUD** XXX　　　　　01 N1 80 ▭
　　　　　AMA: 2014,Jan,11; 2012,Feb,9-10

74300　　**Cholangiography and/or pancreatography; intraoperative, radiological supervision and interpretation**
　　　　　📠 0.00　　♋ 0.00　　**FUD** XXX　　　　　N N1 80 ▭
　　　　　AMA: 2018,Jan,8; 2017,Jan,8; 2016,Jan,13

+ 74301　　**additional set intraoperative, radiological supervision and interpretation (List separately in addition to code for primary procedure)**
　　　　　Code first (74300)
　　　　　📠 0.00　　♋ 0.00　　**FUD** ZZZ　　　　　N N1 80 ▭
　　　　　AMA: 2015,Dec,3; 2014,Jan,11

74328　　**Endoscopic catheterization of the biliary ductal system, radiological supervision and interpretation**
　　　　　Code also ERCP (43261-43265, 43274-43278 [43274, 43275, 43276, 43277, 43278])
　　　　　📠 0.00　　♋ 0.00　　**FUD** XXX　　　　　N N1 80 ▭
　　　　　AMA: 2018,Jan,8; 2017,Jan,8; 2016,Jan,13

74329　　**Endoscopic catheterization of the pancreatic ductal system, radiological supervision and interpretation**
　　　　　Code also ERCP (43261-43265, 43274-43278 [43274, 43275, 43276, 43277, 43278])
　　　　　📠 0.00　　♋ 0.00　　**FUD** XXX　　　　　N N1 80 ▭
　　　　　AMA: 2014,Jan,11; 2012,Feb,9-10

74330　　**Combined endoscopic catheterization of the biliary and pancreatic ductal systems, radiological supervision and interpretation**
　　　　　Code also ERCP (43261-43265, 43274-43278 [43274, 43275, 43276, 43277, 43278])
　　　　　📠 0.00　　♋ 0.00　　**FUD** XXX　　　　　N N1 80 ▭
　　　　　AMA: 2014,Jan,11; 2012,Feb,9-10

74340-74363 Radiography: Bilidigestive Intubation

EXCLUDES　*Percutaneous placement gastrostomy tube, endoscopic (43246)*
　　　　　Percutaneous placement gastrotomy tube, fluoroscopic guidance (49440)

74340　　**Introduction of long gastrointestinal tube (eg, Miller-Abbott), including multiple fluoroscopies and images, radiological supervision and interpretation**
　　　　　Code also placement tube (44500)
　　　　　📠 0.00　　♋ 0.00　　**FUD** XXX　　　　　N N1 80 ▭
　　　　　AMA: 2020,Aug,9; 2018,Jan,8; 2017,Jan,8; 2016,Sep,9

74355　　**Percutaneous placement of enteroclysis tube, radiological supervision and interpretation**
　　　　　INCLUDES　Fluoroscopic guidance (77002)
　　　　　📠 0.00　　♋ 0.00　　**FUD** XXX　　　　　N N1 80 ▭
　　　　　AMA: 2018,Jan,8; 2017,Jan,8; 2016,Jan,13

74360　　**Intraluminal dilation of strictures and/or obstructions (eg, esophagus), radiological supervision and interpretation**
　　　　　EXCLUDES　*Esophagogastroduodenoscopy, flexible, transoral; with dilation esophagus (43233)*
　　　　　　　　　　Esophagoscopy, flexible, transoral; with dilation esophagus (43213-43214)
　　　　　📠 0.00　　♋ 0.00　　**FUD** XXX　　　　　N N1 80 ▭
　　　　　AMA: 2018,Jan,8; 2017,Jan,8; 2016,Jan,13

74363　　**Percutaneous transhepatic dilation of biliary duct stricture with or without placement of stent, radiological supervision and interpretation**
　　　　　EXCLUDES　*Surgical procedure (47555-47556)*
　　　　　📠 0.00　　♋ 0.00　　**FUD** XXX　　　　　N N1 80 ▭
　　　　　AMA: 2014,Jan,11; 2012,Feb,9-10

74400-74775 Radiography: Urogenital

74400　　**Urography (pyelography), intravenous, with or without KUB, with or without tomography**
　　　　　📠 3.60　　♋ 3.60　　**FUD** XXX　　　　　S Z2 80 ▭
　　　　　AMA: 2014,Jan,11; 2012,Feb,9-10

74410　　**Urography, infusion, drip technique and/or bolus technique;**
　　　　　📠 3.66　　♋ 3.66　　**FUD** XXX　　　　　S Z2 80 ▭
　　　　　AMA: 2014,Jan,11; 2012,Feb,9-10

74415　　**with nephrotomography**
　　　　　📠 4.28　　♋ 4.28　　**FUD** XXX　　　　　S Z2 80 ▭
　　　　　AMA: 2014,Jan,11; 2012,Feb,9-10

74420　　**Urography, retrograde, with or without KUB**
　　　　　📠 2.08　　♋ 2.08　　**FUD** XXX　　　　　S Z2 80 ▭
　　　　　AMA: 2018,Jan,8; 2017,Jan,8; 2016,Jan,13

74425　　**Urography, antegrade, radiological supervision and interpretation**
　　　　　EXCLUDES　*Injection for antegrade nephrostogram and/or ureterogram ([50430, 50431, 50432, 50433, 50434, 50435])*
　　　　　　　　　　Ureteral stent placement (50693-50695)
　　　　　Code also aspiration/injection renal cyst or pelvis, percutaneous (50390)
　　　　　Code also injection procedure:
　　　　　　ureterography or ureteropyelography (50684)
　　　　　　visualization ileal conduit/ureteropyelography (50690)
　　　　　Code also manometric study through nephrostomy or pyelostomy tube (50396)
　　　　　📠 3.66　　♋ 3.66　　**FUD** XXX　　　　　02 N1 80 ▭
　　　　　AMA: 2018,Jan,8; 2017,Jan,8; 2016,Jan,13; 2016,Jan,3

Nephrostomy catheter
Syringe with contrast
Ureter
Bladder
Contrast in urinary system
Contrast in urinary system
Nephrostogram

74430　　**Cystography, minimum of 3 views, radiological supervision and interpretation**
　　　　　📠 1.13　　♋ 1.13　　**FUD** XXX　　　　　02 N1 80 ▭
　　　　　AMA: 2014,Jan,11; 2012,Feb,9-10

74440　　**Vasography, vesiculography, or epididymography, radiological supervision and interpretation**　　　♂
　　　　　📠 2.59　　♋ 2.59　　**FUD** XXX　　　　　02 N1 80 ▭
　　　　　AMA: 2014,Jan,11; 2012,Feb,9-10

74445 Corpora cavernosography, radiological supervision and interpretation ♂

> INCLUDES Needle placement with fluoroscopic guidance (77002)
> 🔧 0.00   ⚖ 0.00   **FUD** XXX   02 N1 80 ▣
> **AMA:** 2018,Jan,8; 2017,Jan,8; 2016,Jan,13

74450 Urethrocystography, retrograde, radiological supervision and interpretation

> 🔧 0.00   ⚖ 0.00   **FUD** XXX   02 N1 80 ▣
> **AMA:** 2019,Oct,10

74455 Urethrocystography, voiding, radiological supervision and interpretation

> 🔧 2.55   ⚖ 2.55   **FUD** XXX   02 N1 80 ▣
> **AMA:** 2019,Oct,10

74470 Radiologic examination, renal cyst study, translumbar, contrast visualization, radiological supervision and interpretation

> INCLUDES Needle placement with fluoroscopic guidance (77002)
> 🔧 0.00   ⚖ 0.00   **FUD** XXX   02 N1 80 ▣
> **AMA:** 2018,Jan,8; 2017,Jan,8; 2016,Jan,13

74485 Dilation of ureter(s) or urethra, radiological supervision and interpretation

> EXCLUDES Change pyelostomy/nephrostomy tube ([50435])
> Nephrostomy tract dilation for procedure ([50436, 50437])
> Ureter dilation without radiologic guidance (52341, 52344)
> 🔧 3.19   ⚖ 3.19   **FUD** XXX   02 N1 80 ▣
> **AMA:** 2018,Jan,8; 2017,Jan,8; 2016,Jan,13; 2016,Jan,3

74710 Pelvimetry, with or without placental localization ♀

> EXCLUDES Imaging procedures on abdomen and pelvis (72170-72190, 74018-74019, 74021-74022, 74150-74170)
> 🔧 1.12   ⚖ 1.12   **FUD** XXX   01 N1 80 ▣
> **AMA:** 2014,Jan,11; 2012,Feb,9-10

74712 Magnetic resonance (eg, proton) imaging, fetal, including placental and maternal pelvic imaging when performed; single or first gestation ♀

> EXCLUDES Imaging maternal pelvis or placenta without fetal imaging (72195-72197)
> 🔧 13.3   ⚖ 13.3   **FUD** XXX   S Z2 80 ▣
> **AMA:** 2018,Jan,8; 2017,Jan,8; 2016,Jun,5

+ **74713** each additional gestation (List separately in addition to code for primary procedure) ♀

> EXCLUDES Imaging maternal pelvis or placenta without fetal imaging (72195-72197)
> Code first (74712)
> 🔧 6.46   ⚖ 6.46   **FUD** ZZZ   N N1 80 ▣
> **AMA:** 2018,Jan,8; 2017,Jan,8; 2016,Jun,5

74740 Hysterosalpingography, radiological supervision and interpretation ♀

> EXCLUDES Imaging procedures abdomen and pelvis (72170-72190, 74018-74019, 74021-74022, 74150-74170)
> Code also injection saline/contrast (58340)
> 🔧 2.54   ⚖ 2.54   **FUD** XXX   02 N1 80 ▣
> **AMA:** 2018,Jan,8; 2017,Jan,8; 2016,Jan,13

Tube
Ovary
Delivery apparatus
Uterus
Cervix
Vaginal canal

Hysterosalpingography (imaging of the uterus and tubes) is performed. Report for radiological supervision and interpretation

74742 Transcervical catheterization of fallopian tube, radiological supervision and interpretation ♀

> EXCLUDES Imaging procedures abdomen and pelvis (72170-72190, 74018-74019, 74021-74022, 74150-74170)
> Code also transcervical fallopian tube catheter (58345)
> 🔧 0.00   ⚖ 0.00   **FUD** XXX   N N1 80 ▣
> **AMA:** 2018,Jan,8; 2017,Jan,8; 2016,Jan,13

74775 Perineogram (eg, vaginogram, for sex determination or extent of anomalies) Ⓜ ♀

> EXCLUDES Imaging procedures abdomen and pelvis (72170-72190, 74018-74019, 74021-74022, 74150-74170)
> 🔧 0.00   ⚖ 0.00   **FUD** XXX   S Z2 80 ▣
> **AMA:** 2014,Jan,11; 2012,Feb,9-10

75557-75565 Magnetic Resonance Imaging: Heart Structure and Physiology

> INCLUDES Physiologic evaluation cardiac function
> EXCLUDES 3D rendering (76376-76377)
> Cardiac catheterization procedures (93451-93572)
> Reporting more than one code in this group per session
> Code also separate vascular injection (36000-36299)

75557 Cardiac magnetic resonance imaging for morphology and function without contrast material;

> 🔧 9.01   ⚖ 9.01   **FUD** XXX   03 Z2 80 ▣
> **AMA:** 2018,Jan,8; 2017,Jan,8; 2016,Jan,13

75559 with stress imaging

> INCLUDES Pharmacologic wall motion stress evaluation without contrast
> Code also stress testing when performed (93015-93018)
> 🔧 12.5   ⚖ 12.5   **FUD** XXX   03 Z2 80 ▣
> **AMA:** 2018,Jan,8; 2017,Jan,8; 2016,Jan,13

75561 Cardiac magnetic resonance imaging for morphology and function without contrast material(s), followed by contrast material(s) and further sequences;

> 🔧 11.8   ⚖ 11.8   **FUD** XXX   03 Z2 80 ▣
> **AMA:** 2018,Jan,8; 2017,Jan,8; 2016,Jan,13

75563 **with stress imaging**

INCLUDES Pharmacologic perfusion stress evaluation with contrast

Code also stress testing when performed (93015-93018)

🖐 14.0   ⚬ 14.0   **FUD** XXX   03 Z3 80 ▢

AMA: 2018,Jan,8; 2017,Jan,8; 2016,Jan,13

+ 75565 **Cardiac magnetic resonance imaging for velocity flow mapping (List separately in addition to code for primary procedure)**

Code first (75557, 75559, 75561, 75563)

🖐 1.51   ⚬ 1.51   **FUD** ZZZ   N N1 80 ▢

AMA: 2018,Jan,8; 2017,Jan,8; 2016,Jan,13

75571-75574 Computed Tomographic Imaging: Heart

CMS: 100-04,12,20.4.7 Services Not Meeting National Electrical Manufacturers Association (NEMA) Standard; 100-04,4,20.6.12 Use of HCPCS Modifier – CT; 100-04,4,250.16 Multiple Procedure Payment Reduction: Certain Diagnostic Imaging Procedures Rendered by Physicians

EXCLUDES 3D rendering (76376-76377)

Automated quantification/characterization coronary atherosclerotic plaque ([0623T, 0624T, 0625T, 0626T])

Fractional flow reserve (FFR) from coronary CT angiography data (0501T-0504T)

Reporting more than one code in this group per session

75571 **Computed tomography, heart, without contrast material, with quantitative evaluation of coronary calcium**

🖐 2.95   ⚬ 2.95   **FUD** XXX   Q1 N1 80 ▢

AMA: 2020,Sep,11; 2020,Jul,5; 2018,Jan,8; 2017,Jan,8; 2016,Jan,13

75572 **Computed tomography, heart, with contrast material, for evaluation of cardiac structure and morphology (including 3D image postprocessing, assessment of cardiac function, and evaluation of venous structures, if performed)**

INCLUDES Quantitative assessment(s) such as quantification coronary percentage stenosis, ejection fraction, stroke volume, ventricular volume, when performed

🖐 7.52   ⚬ 7.52   **FUD** XXX   S Z2 80 ▢

AMA: 2020,Sep,11; 2018,Jan,8; 2017,Jan,8; 2016,Jan,13

▲ **75573** **Computed tomography, heart, with contrast material, for evaluation of cardiac structure and morphology in the setting of congenital heart disease (including 3D image postprocessing, assessment of left ventricular [LV] cardiac function, right ventricular [RV] structure and function and evaluation of vascular structures, if performed)**

INCLUDES Quantitative assessment(s) such as quantification coronary percentage stenosis, ejection fraction, stroke volume, ventricular volume, when performed

🖐 10.1   ⚬ 10.1   **FUD** XXX   S Z2 80 ▢

AMA: 2020,Sep,11; 2018,Jan,8; 2017,Jan,8; 2016,Jan,13

75574 **Computed tomographic angiography, heart, coronary arteries and bypass grafts (when present), with contrast material, including 3D image postprocessing (including evaluation of cardiac structure and morphology, assessment of cardiac function, and evaluation of venous structures, if performed)**

INCLUDES Quantitative assessment(s) such as quantification coronary percentage stenosis, ejection fraction, stroke volume, ventricular volume, when performed

Code also:

Automated data analysis separately from CTA, when performed ([0623T, 0624T, 0625T, 0626T])

Noninvasive estimated coronary fractional flow reserve separately from CTA, when performed (0501T, 0502T, 0503T, 0504T)

🖐 10.1   ⚬ 10.1   **FUD** XXX   S Z2 80 ▢

AMA: 2020,Sep,11; 2018,Jan,8; 2017,Jan,8; 2016,Jan,13

75600-75774 Radiography: Arterial

INCLUDES Diagnostic angiography specifically included in interventional code description

Diagnostic procedures with interventional supervision and interpretation:
Angiography
Contrast injection
Fluoroscopic guidance for intervention
Post-angioplasty/atherectomy/stent angiography
Roadmapping
Vessel measurement

EXCLUDES Catheterization codes for diagnostic angiography lower extremity when access site other than site used for therapy required

Diagnostic angiogram during separate encounter from interventional procedure

Diagnostic angiography with interventional procedure if:
1. No previous catheter-based angiogram accessible and complete diagnostic procedure performed, and decision to proceed with interventional procedure based on diagnostic service, OR
2. Previous diagnostic angiogram accessible but documentation in medical record specifies that:
A. patient's condition has changed
B. insufficient imaging patient's anatomy and/or disease, OR
C. clinical change during procedure that necessitates new examination away from intervention site
3. Modifier 59 appended to code(s) for diagnostic radiological supervision and interpretation service to indicate guidelines were met

Intra-arterial procedures (36100-36248)

Intravenous procedures (36000, 36005-36015)

75600 **Aortography, thoracic, without serialography, radiological supervision and interpretation**

EXCLUDES Supravalvular aortography (93567)

🖐 5.65   ⚬ 5.65   **FUD** XXX   Q2 N1 80 ▢

AMA: 2014,Jan,11; 2012,Feb,9-10

75605 **Aortography, thoracic, by serialography, radiological supervision and interpretation**

EXCLUDES Supravalvular aortography (93567)

🖐 3.67   ⚬ 3.67   **FUD** XXX   Q2 N1 80 ▢

AMA: 2018,Jan,8; 2017,Jan,8; 2016,Jan,13

75625 **Aortography, abdominal, by serialography, radiological supervision and interpretation**

EXCLUDES Supravalvular aortography (93567)

🖐 3.92   ⚬ 3.92   **FUD** XXX   Q2 N1 80 ▢

AMA: 2020,Sep,14; 2018,Jan,8; 2017,Jan,8; 2016,Jan,13

75630 **Aortography, abdominal plus bilateral iliofemoral lower extremity, catheter, by serialography, radiological supervision and interpretation**

EXCLUDES Supravalvular aortography (93567)

🖐 4.81   ⚬ 4.81   **FUD** XXX   Q2 N1 80 ▢

AMA: 2020,Sep,14; 2018,Jan,8; 2017,Jan,8; 2016,Jan,13

75635 **Computed tomographic angiography, abdominal aorta and bilateral iliofemoral lower extremity runoff, with contrast material(s), including noncontrast images, if performed, and image postprocessing**

EXCLUDES 3D rendering (76376-76377)

CT angiography, abdomen, lower extremity, pelvis (72191, 73706, 74174-74175)

Noninvasive arterial plaque analysis non-coronary computerized tomography angiography (0710T-0713T)

🖐 12.4   ⚬ 12.4   **FUD** XXX   Q2 N1 80 ▢

AMA: 2020,Sep,11; 2018,Jan,8; 2017,Jan,8; 2016,Jan,13

75705 **Angiography, spinal, selective, radiological supervision and interpretation**

🖐 7.13   ⚬ 7.13   **FUD** XXX   Q2 N1 80 ▢

AMA: 2014,Jan,11; 2012,Feb,9-10

75710 **Angiography, extremity, unilateral, radiological supervision and interpretation**

🖐 4.73   ⚬ 4.73   **FUD** XXX   Q2 N1 80 ▢

AMA: 2018,Jan,8; 2017,Mar,3; 2017,Jan,8; 2016,Jan,13

26/TC PC/TC Only   A2-Z3 ASC Payment   50 Bilateral   ♂ Male Only   ♀ Female Only   🖐 Facility RVU   ⚬ Non-Facility RVU   ▢ CCI   ✖ CLIA
FUD Follow-up Days   **CMS:** IOM   **AMA:** CPT Asst   A-Y OPPSI   80/80 Surg Assist Allowed / w/Doc   Lab Crosswalk   Radiology Crosswalk

332   CPT © 2021 American Medical Association. All Rights Reserved.   © 2021 Optum360, LLC

75716 Angiography, extremity, bilateral, radiological supervision and interpretation
📷 4.94 ✂ 4.94 **FUD** XXX
02 N1 80 🖥
AMA: 2020,Sep,14; 2018,Jan,8; 2017,Jan,8; 2016,Jan,13

75726 Angiography, visceral, selective or supraselective (with or without flush aortogram), radiological supervision and interpretation
EXCLUDES Selective angiography, each additional visceral vessel examined after basic examination (75774)
📷 4.08 ✂ 4.08 **FUD** XXX
02 N1 80 🖥
AMA: 2014,Jan,11; 2012,Feb,9-10

75731 Angiography, adrenal, unilateral, selective, radiological supervision and interpretation
📷 4.60 ✂ 4.60 **FUD** XXX
02 Z3 80 🖥
AMA: 2014,Jan,11; 2012,Feb,9-10

75733 Angiography, adrenal, bilateral, selective, radiological supervision and interpretation
📷 4.97 ✂ 4.97 **FUD** XXX
02 N1 80 🖥
AMA: 2014,Jan,11; 2012,Feb,9-10

75736 Angiography, pelvic, selective or supraselective, radiological supervision and interpretation
📷 4.25 ✂ 4.25 **FUD** XXX
02 N1 80 🖥
AMA: 2014,Jan,11; 2012,Feb,9-10

75741 Angiography, pulmonary, unilateral, selective, radiological supervision and interpretation
📷 4.03 ✂ 4.03 **FUD** XXX
02 N1 80 🖥
AMA: 2019,Jun,3; 2018,Jan,8; 2017,Jan,8; 2016,Jan,13

75743 Angiography, pulmonary, bilateral, selective, radiological supervision and interpretation
📷 4.55 ✂ 4.55 **FUD** XXX
02 N1 80 🖥
AMA: 2019,Jun,3; 2018,Jan,8; 2017,Jan,8; 2016,Jan,13

75746 Angiography, pulmonary, by nonselective catheter or venous injection, radiological supervision and interpretation
EXCLUDES Nonselective injection procedure or catheter introduction with cardiac cath (93568)
📷 4.07 ✂ 4.07 **FUD** XXX
02 Z3 80 🖥
AMA: 2019,Jun,3

75756 Angiography, internal mammary, radiological supervision and interpretation
EXCLUDES Internal mammary angiography with cardiac cath (93455, 93457, 93459, 93461, 93564)
📷 4.62 ✂ 4.62 **FUD** XXX
02 N1 80 🖥
AMA: 2018,Jan,8; 2017,Jan,8; 2016,Jan,13

+ 75774 Angiography, selective, each additional vessel studied after basic examination, radiological supervision and interpretation (List separately in addition to code for primary procedure)
EXCLUDES Angiography (75600-75756)
Cardiac cath procedures (93452-93462, 93563-93568, 93593-93597)
Catheterizations (36215-36248)
Dialysis circuit angiography (current access), report modifier 52 with (36901)
Nonselective catheter placement, thoracic aorta (36221-36228)
Code also diagnostic angiography upper extremities and other vascular beds (except cervicocerebral vessels), when appropriate
Code first initial vessel
📷 3.04 ✂ 3.04 **FUD** ZZZ
N N1 80 🖥
AMA: 2020,Sep,14; 2018,Jan,8; 2017,Jan,8; 2016,Jan,13

75801-75893 Radiography: Lymphatic and Venous

INCLUDES Diagnostic venography specifically included in interventional code description
Diagnostic procedures with interventional supervision and interpretation:
Contrast injection
Fluoroscopic guidance for intervention
Post-angioplasty/venography
Roadmapping
Venography
Vessel measurement

EXCLUDES Diagnostic venogram during separate encounter from interventional procedure
Diagnostic venography with interventional procedure if:
1. No previous catheter-based venogram accessible and complete diagnostic procedure performed and decision to proceed with interventional procedure based on diagnostic service, OR
2. Previous diagnostic venogram accessible but documentation in medical record specifies that:
A. patient's condition has changed
B. insufficient imaging patient's anatomy and/or disease, OR
C. clinical change during procedure that necessitates new examination away from intervention site
Intravenous procedures (36000-36015, 36400-36510 [36465, 36466, 36482, 36483])
Lymphatic injection procedures (38790)

75801 Lymphangiography, extremity only, unilateral, radiological supervision and interpretation
📷 0.00 ✂ 0.00 **FUD** XXX
02 N1 80 🖥
AMA: 2014,Jan,11; 2012,Feb,9-10

75803 Lymphangiography, extremity only, bilateral, radiological supervision and interpretation
📷 0.00 ✂ 0.00 **FUD** XXX
02 Z2 80 🖥
AMA: 2014,Jan,11; 2012,Feb,9-10

75805 Lymphangiography, pelvic/abdominal, unilateral, radiological supervision and interpretation
📷 0.00 ✂ 0.00 **FUD** XXX
02 Z2 80 🖥
AMA: 2014,Jan,11; 2012,Feb,9-10

75807 Lymphangiography, pelvic/abdominal, bilateral, radiological supervision and interpretation
📷 0.00 ✂ 0.00 **FUD** XXX
02 N1 80 🖥
AMA: 2014,Jan,11; 2012,Feb,9-10

75809 Shuntogram for investigation of previously placed indwelling nonvascular shunt (eg, LeVeen shunt, ventriculoperitoneal shunt, indwelling infusion pump), radiological supervision and interpretation
Code also surgical procedure (49427, 61070)
📷 2.57 ✂ 2.57 **FUD** XXX
02 N1 80 🖥
AMA: 2018,Jan,8; 2017,Jan,8; 2016,Jan,13

75810 Splenoportography, radiological supervision and interpretation
📷 0.00 ✂ 0.00 **FUD** XXX
02 Z2 80 🖥
AMA: 2018,Jan,8; 2017,Jan,8; 2016,Jan,13

75820 Venography, extremity, unilateral, radiological supervision and interpretation
📷 3.04 ✂ 3.04 **FUD** XXX
02 N1 80 🖥
AMA: 2019,Mar,6; 2018,Jan,8; 2017,Jan,8; 2016,May,5; 2016,Jan,13

75822 Venography, extremity, bilateral, radiological supervision and interpretation
📷 3.56 ✂ 3.56 **FUD** XXX
02 Z3 80 🖥
AMA: 2014,Jan,11; 2012,Feb,9-10

75825 Venography, caval, inferior, with serialography, radiological supervision and interpretation
📷 3.55 ✂ 3.55 **FUD** XXX
02 N1 80 🖥
AMA: 2018,Jan,8; 2017,Feb,14; 2017,Jan,8; 2016,Jan,13

75827 Venography, caval, superior, with serialography, radiological supervision and interpretation
📷 3.69 ✂ 3.69 **FUD** XXX
02 N1 80 🖥
AMA: 2018,Jan,8; 2017,Jan,8; 2016,Jan,13

75831 Venography, renal, unilateral, selective, radiological supervision and interpretation
    🖪 3.84   ⅍ 3.84   **FUD** XXX   `02` `N1` `80` `▢`
    AMA: 2014,Jan,11; 2012,Feb,9-10

75833 Venography, renal, bilateral, selective, radiological supervision and interpretation
    🖪 4.45   ⅍ 4.45   **FUD** XXX   `02` `N1` `80` `▢`
    AMA: 2014,Jan,11; 2012,Feb,9-10

75840 Venography, adrenal, unilateral, selective, radiological supervision and interpretation
    🖪 3.97   ⅍ 3.97   **FUD** XXX   `02` `N1` `80` `▢`
    AMA: 2014,Jan,11; 2012,Feb,9-10

75842 Venography, adrenal, bilateral, selective, radiological supervision and interpretation
    🖪 4.84   ⅍ 4.84   **FUD** XXX   `02` `N1` `80` `▢`
    AMA: 2014,Jan,11; 2012,Feb,9-10

75860 Venography, venous sinus (eg, petrosal and inferior sagittal) or jugular, catheter, radiological supervision and interpretation
    🖪 3.89   ⅍ 3.89   **FUD** XXX   `02` `N1` `80` `▢`
    AMA: 2014,Jan,11; 2012,Feb,9-10

75870 Venography, superior sagittal sinus, radiological supervision and interpretation
    🖪 5.30   ⅍ 5.30   **FUD** XXX   `02` `Z3` `80` `▢`
    AMA: 2014,Jan,11; 2012,Feb,9-10

75872 Venography, epidural, radiological supervision and interpretation
    🖪 3.97   ⅍ 3.97   **FUD** XXX   `02` `N1` `80` `▢`
    AMA: 2014,Jan,11; 2012,Feb,9-10

75880 Venography, orbital, radiological supervision and interpretation
    🖪 3.44   ⅍ 3.44   **FUD** XXX   `02` `N1` `80` `▢`
    AMA: 2014,Jan,11; 2012,Feb,9-10

75885 Percutaneous transhepatic portography with hemodynamic evaluation, radiological supervision and interpretation
    🖪 4.29   ⅍ 4.29   **FUD** XXX   `02` `N1` `80` `▢`
    AMA: 2018,Jan,8; 2017,Jan,8; 2016,Jan,13

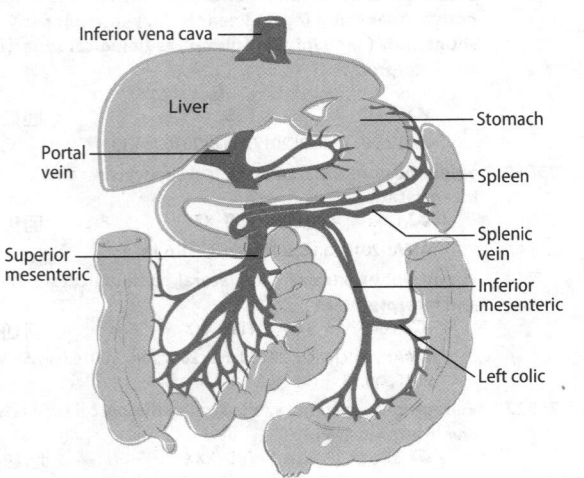

Schematic showing the portal vein

75887 Percutaneous transhepatic portography without hemodynamic evaluation, radiological supervision and interpretation
    🖪 4.24   ⅍ 4.24   **FUD** XXX   `02` `Z3` `80` `▢`
    AMA: 2018,Jan,8; 2017,Jan,8; 2016,Jan,13

75889 Hepatic venography, wedged or free, with hemodynamic evaluation, radiological supervision and interpretation
    🖪 3.81   ⅍ 3.81   **FUD** XXX   `02` `N1` `80` `▢`
    AMA: 2014,Jan,11; 2012,Feb,9-10

75891 Hepatic venography, wedged or free, without hemodynamic evaluation, radiological supervision and interpretation
    🖪 3.87   ⅍ 3.87   **FUD** XXX   `02` `N1` `80` `▢`
    AMA: 2014,Jan,11; 2012,Feb,9-10

75893 Venous sampling through catheter, with or without angiography (eg, for parathyroid hormone, renin), radiological supervision and interpretation
    Code also surgical procedure (36500)
    🖪 3.25   ⅍ 3.25   **FUD** XXX   `02` `N1` `80` `▢`
    AMA: 2014,Jan,11; 2012,Feb,9-10

75894-75902 Transcatheter Procedures

`INCLUDES` Diagnostic procedures with interventional supervision and interpretation:
    Angiography/venography
    Completion angiography/venography except for those services allowed by (75898)
    Contrast injection
    Fluoroscopic guidance for intervention
    Roadmapping
    Vessel measurement

`EXCLUDES` *Diagnostic angiography/venography performed same session as transcatheter therapy unless specifically included in code descriptor or excluded in venography/angiography notes (75600-75893)*

75894 Transcatheter therapy, embolization, any method, radiological supervision and interpretation
    `EXCLUDES` *Endovenous ablation therapy incompetent vein (36478-36479)*
        Transluminal balloon angioplasty (36475-36476)
        Vascular embolization or occlusion (37241-37244)
    🖪 0.00   ⅍ 0.00   **FUD** XXX   `N` `N1` `80` `▢`
    AMA: 2018,Mar,3; 2018,Jan,8; 2017,Jan,8; 2016,Nov,3; 2016,Jan,13

75898 Angiography through existing catheter for follow-up study for transcatheter therapy, embolization or infusion, other than for thrombolysis
    `EXCLUDES` *Percutaneous arterial transluminal mechanical thrombectomy (61645)*
        Prolonged endovascular intracranial administration pharmacologic agent(s) (61650-61651)
        Transcatheter therapy, arterial infusion for thrombolysis (37211-37214)
        Vascular embolization or occlusion (37241-37244)
    🖪 0.00   ⅍ 0.00   **FUD** XXX   `02` `Z2` `80` `▢`
    AMA: 2019,Sep,6; 2018,Jan,8; 2017,Jan,8; 2016,Jan,13

75901 Mechanical removal of pericatheter obstructive material (eg, fibrin sheath) from central venous device via separate venous access, radiologic supervision and interpretation
    `EXCLUDES` *Venous catheterization (36010-36012)*
    Code also surgical procedure (36595)
    🖪 6.15   ⅍ 6.15   **FUD** XXX   `N` `N1` `80` `▢`
    AMA: 2018,Jan,8; 2017,Jan,8; 2016,Jan,13

75902 Mechanical removal of intraluminal (intracatheter) obstructive material from central venous device through device lumen, radiologic supervision and interpretation
    `EXCLUDES` *Venous catheterization (36010-36012)*
    Code also surgical procedure (36596)
    🖪 2.40   ⅍ 2.40   **FUD** XXX   `N` `N1` `80` `▢`
    AMA: 2018,Jan,8; 2017,Jan,8; 2016,Jan,13

75956-75959 Endovascular Aneurysm Repair

INCLUDES Diagnostic procedures with interventional supervision and interpretation:
Angiography/venography
Completion angiography/venography except for those services allowed by (75898)
Contrast injection
Fluoroscopic guidance for intervention
Injection procedure only for transcatheter therapy or biopsy (36100-36299)
Percutaneous needle biopsy;
Pancreas (48102)
Retroperitoneal lymph node/mass (49180)
Roadmapping
Vessel measurement

EXCLUDES *Diagnostic angiography/venography performed same session as transcatheter therapy unless specifically included in code descriptor (75600-75893)*
Radiological supervision and interpretation for transluminal angioplasty in:
Femoral/popliteal arteries (37224-37227)
Iliac artery (37220-37223)
Tibial/peroneal artery (37228-37235)

75956 **Endovascular repair of descending thoracic aorta (eg, aneurysm, pseudoaneurysm, dissection, penetrating ulcer, intramural hematoma, or traumatic disruption); involving coverage of left subclavian artery origin, initial endoprosthesis plus descending thoracic aortic extension(s), if required, to level of celiac artery origin, radiological supervision and interpretation**

> Code also endovascular graft implantation (33880)
> 🔧 0.00   ⚕ 0.00   **FUD** XXX   C 80 ▢
> **AMA:** 2018,Jan,8; 2017,Jan,8; 2016,Jan,13

75957 **not involving coverage of left subclavian artery origin, initial endoprosthesis plus descending thoracic aortic extension(s), if required, to level of celiac artery origin, radiological supervision and interpretation**

> Code also endovascular graft implantation (33881)
> 🔧 0.00   ⚕ 0.00   **FUD** XXX   C 80 ▢
> **AMA:** 2018,Jan,8; 2017,Jan,8; 2016,Jan,13

75958 **Placement of proximal extension prosthesis for endovascular repair of descending thoracic aorta (eg, aneurysm, pseudoaneurysm, dissection, penetrating ulcer, intramural hematoma, or traumatic disruption), radiological supervision and interpretation**

> Code also:
> Placement each additional proximal extension(s) (75958)
> Proximal endovascular extension implantation (33883-33884)
> 🔧 0.00   ⚕ 0.00   **FUD** XXX   C 80 ▢
> **AMA:** 2018,Jan,8; 2017,Jan,8; 2016,Jan,13

75959 **Placement of distal extension prosthesis(s) (delayed) after endovascular repair of descending thoracic aorta, as needed, to level of celiac origin, radiological supervision and interpretation**

> INCLUDES Corresponding services for placement distal thoracic endovascular extension(s) placed during procedure following principal procedure
> EXCLUDES *Endovascular repair descending thoracic aorta (75956-75957)*
> *Reporting code more than one time no matter how many modules are deployed*
> Code also placement distal endovascular extension (33886)
> 🔧 0.00   ⚕ 0.00   **FUD** XXX   C 80 ▢
> **AMA:** 2018,Jan,8; 2017,Jan,8; 2016,Jan,13

75970 Percutaneous Transluminal Angioplasty

INCLUDES Diagnostic procedures with interventional supervision and interpretation:
Angiography/venography
Completion angiography/venography except for those services allowed by (75898)
Contrast injection
Fluoroscopic guidance for intervention
Roadmapping
Vessel measurement

EXCLUDES *Diagnostic angiography/venography performed same session as transcatheter therapy unless specifically included in code descriptor (75600-75893)*
Injection procedure only for transcatheter therapy or biopsy (36100-36299)
Percutaneous needle biopsy (48102)
Pancreas (48102)
Radiological supervision and interpretation for transluminal balloon angioplasty in:
Femoral/popliteal arteries (37224-37227)
Iliac artery (37220-37223)
Tibial/peroneal artery (37228-37235)
Retroperitoneal lymph node/mass (49180)
Transcatheter renal/ureteral biopsy (52007)

75970 **Transcatheter biopsy, radiological supervision and interpretation**

> 🔧 0.00   ⚕ 0.00   **FUD** XXX   N N1 80 ▢
> **AMA:** 2018,Jan,8

75984-75989 Percutaneous Drainage

75984 **Change of percutaneous tube or drainage catheter with contrast monitoring (eg, genitourinary system, abscess), radiological supervision and interpretation**

> EXCLUDES *Change only nephrostomy/pyelostomy tube ([50435])*
> *Cholecystostomy, percutaneous (47490)*
> *Introduction procedure only for percutaneous biliary drainage (47531-47544)*
> *Nephrostolithotomy/pyelostolithotomy, percutaneous (50080-50081)*
> *Percutaneous replacement gastrointestinal tube using fluoroscopic guidance (49450-49452)*
> *Removal and/or replacement internal ureteral stent using transurethral approach (50385-50386)*
> 🔧 2.79   ⚕ 2.79   **FUD** XXX   N N1 80 ▢
> **AMA:** 2014,Jan,11; 2012,Feb,9-10

75989 **Radiological guidance (ie, fluoroscopy, ultrasound, or computed tomography), for percutaneous drainage (eg, abscess, specimen collection), with placement of catheter, radiological supervision and interpretation**

> INCLUDES Imaging guidance
> EXCLUDES *Cholecystostomy (47490)*
> *Image-guided fluid collection drainage by catheter (10030, 49405-49407)*
> *Pericardial drainage (33017-33019)*
> *Thoracentesis (32554-32557)*
> 🔧 3.42   ⚕ 3.42   **FUD** XXX   N N1 80 ▢
> **AMA:** 2020,Jan,7; 2018,Jan,8; 2017,Jan,8; 2016,Jan,13

Radiology

76000-76145 Miscellaneous Techniques

EXCLUDES Arthrography:
Ankle (73615)
Elbow (73085)
Hip (73525)
Knee (73580)
Shoulder (73040)
Wrist (73115)
CT cerebral perfusion test (0042T)

76000 Fluoroscopy (separate procedure), up to 1 hour physician or other qualified health care professional time

EXCLUDES Extracorporeal membrane oxygenation (ECMO)/extracorporeal life support (ECLS) (33957-33959, [33962, 33963, 33964])
Insertion/removal/replacement wireless cardiac stimulator (0515T-0520T)
Insertion/replacement/removal leadless pacemaker ([33274, 33275])

📋 1.18   🔪 1.18   **FUD** XXX   S Z3 80 ▭

AMA: 2019,Sep,10; 2019,Sep,5; 2019,Jun,3; 2019,Mar,6; 2018,Apr,7; 2018,Mar,3; 2018,Jan,8; 2017,Jan,8; 2016,Nov,3; 2016,Aug,5; 2016,May,5; 2016,May,13; 2016,Mar,5; 2016,Jan,11; 2016,Jan,13

76010 Radiologic examination from nose to rectum for foreign body, single view, child   A

📋 0.81   🔪 0.81   **FUD** XXX   01 N1 60 ▭

AMA: 2018,Jan,8; 2017,Jan,8; 2016,Jan,13

76080 Radiologic examination, abscess, fistula or sinus tract study, radiological supervision and interpretation

EXCLUDES Contrast injections, radiology evaluation, and guidance via fluoroscopy for gastrostomy, duodenostomy, jejunostomy, gastro-jejunostomy, or cecostomy tube (49465)

📋 1.67   🔪 1.67   **FUD** XXX   02 N1 80 ▭

AMA: 2018,Jan,8; 2017,Jan,8; 2016,Jan,13

76098 Radiological examination, surgical specimen

EXCLUDES Breast biopsy with placement breast localization device(s) (19081-19086)
3D volumetric imaging/reconstruction breast or axillary lymph node tissue (0694T)

📋 1.21   🔪 1.21   **FUD** XXX   02 N1 80 ▭

AMA: 2012,Feb,9-10; 1997,Nov,1

76100 Radiologic examination, single plane body section (eg, tomography), other than with urography

EXCLUDES Nephrotomography (74415)
Panoramic x-ray (70355)

📋 2.75   🔪 2.75   **FUD** XXX   01 N1 80 ▭

AMA: 2012,Feb,9-10; 1997,Nov,1

~~76101 Radiologic examination, complex motion (ie, hypercycloidal) body section (eg, mastoid polytomography), other than with urography; unilateral~~

~~76102 bilateral~~

76120 Cineradiography/videoradiography, except where specifically included

📋 3.06   🔪 3.06   **FUD** XXX   01 N1 80 ▭

AMA: 2018,Jan,8; 2017,Jan,8; 2016,Jan,13

+ **76125 Cineradiography/videoradiography to complement routine examination (List separately in addition to code for primary procedure)**

Code first primary procedure
📋 0.00   🔪 0.00   **FUD** ZZZ   N N1 80 ▭

AMA: 2018,Jan,8; 2017,Jan,8; 2016,Jan,13

76140 Consultation on X-ray examination made elsewhere, written report

📋 0.00   🔪 0.00   **FUD** XXX   E ▭

AMA: 2018,Jan,8; 2017,Jan,8; 2016,Jan,13

76145 Medical physics dose evaluation for radiation exposure that exceeds institutional review threshold, including report

📋 24.3   🔪 24.3   **FUD** XXX   Z2 80 ▭

76376-76377 Three-dimensional Manipulation

INCLUDES 3D manipulation volumetric data set
Concurrent physician supervision image postprocessing
Rendering image

EXCLUDES 3D echocardiographic imaging/postprocessing during transesophageal echocardiography or transthoracic echocardiography for congenital cardiac anomalies ([93319])
Anatomic guide 3D-printed and designed from image data set (0561T-0562T)
Anatomic model 3D-printed from image data set (0559T-0560T)
Arthrography:
Ankle (73615)
Elbow (73085)
Hip (73525)
Knee (73580)
Shoulder (73040)
Wrist (73115)
Automated quantification/characterization coronary atherosclerotic plaque ([0623T, 0624T, 0625T, 0626T])
Cardiac MRI (75557, 75559, 75561, 75563, 75565)
Computer-aided detection MRI data for lesion, breast MRI (77046-77049)
CT angiography (70496, 70498, 71275, 72191, 73206, 73706, 74174-74175, 74261-74263, 75571-75574, 75635)
CT breast (0633T-0638T)
CT cerebral perfusion test (0042T)
Digital breast tomosynthesis (77061-77063)
Echocardiography, transesophageal (TEE) for guidance (93355)
Intraprocedural coronary fractional flow reserve (FFR) ([0523T])
Magnetic resonance angiography (70544-70549, 71555, 72159, 72198, 73225, 73725, 74185)
Noninvasive arterial plaque analysis non-coronary computerized tomography angiography (0710T-0713T)
Nuclear radiology procedures (78012-78999 [78429, 78430, 78431, 78432, 78433, 78434, 78804, 78830, 78831, 78832, 78835])
Physician planning patient-specific fenestrated visceral aortic endograft (34839)
Code also base imaging procedure(s)

76376 3D rendering with interpretation and reporting of computed tomography, magnetic resonance imaging, ultrasound, or other tomographic modality with image postprocessing under concurrent supervision; not requiring image postprocessing on an independent workstation

EXCLUDES 3D rendering (76377)
Bronchoscopy, with computer-assisted, image-guided navigation (31627)

📋 0.65   🔪 0.65   **FUD** XXX   N N1 80 ▭

AMA: 2019,Oct,10; 2019,Sep,10; 2019,Aug,5; 2018,Jul,11; 2018,Jan,8; 2017,Jan,8; 2016,Apr,8; 2016,Jan,13

76377 requiring image postprocessing on an independent workstation

EXCLUDES 3D rendering (76376)

📋 2.01   🔪 2.01   **FUD** XXX   N N1 80 ▭

AMA: 2019,Oct,10; 2019,Sep,10; 2019,Aug,5; 2018,Jul,11; 2018,Jan,8; 2017,Jan,8; 2016,Apr,8; 2016,Jan,13

76380 Computerized Tomography: Delimited

EXCLUDES Arthrography:
Ankle (73615)
Elbow (73085)
Hip (73525)
Knee (73580)
Shoulder (73040)
Wrist (73115)
CT cerebral perfusion test (0042T)

76380 Computed tomography, limited or localized follow-up study

📋 4.07   🔪 4.07   **FUD** XXX   01 N1 80 ▭

AMA: 2019,Mar,10; 2018,Jan,8; 2017,Jan,8; 2016,Jan,13

26/TC PC/TC Only   A2-Z3 ASC Payment   50 Bilateral   ♂ Male Only   ♀ Female Only   📋 Facility RVU   🔪 Non-Facility RVU   ▭ CCI   ✖ CLIA
FUD Follow-up Days   CMS: IOM   AMA: CPT Asst   A-Y OPPSI   80/80 Surg Assist Allowed / w/Doc   ◆ Lab Crosswalk   ✖ Radiology Crosswalk

336   CPT © 2021 American Medical Association. All Rights Reserved.   © 2021 Optum360, LLC

76390-76391 Magnetic Resonance Spectroscopy

EXCLUDES Arthrography:
Ankle (73615)
Elbow (73085)
Hip (73525)
Knee (73580)
Shoulder (73040)
Wrist (73115)
CT cerebral perfusion test (0042T)

76390 **Magnetic resonance spectroscopy**

EXCLUDES MRI
MR spectroscopy for discogenic pain (0609T-0610T)

11.9 11.9 **FUD** XXX E Z2

AMA: 2012,Feb,9-10; 1997,Nov,1

76391 **Magnetic resonance (eg, vibration) elastography**

6.54 6.54 **FUD** XXX Z2 80

AMA: 2019,Aug,3

76496-76499 Unlisted Radiology Procedures

76496 **Unlisted fluoroscopic procedure (eg, diagnostic, interventional)**

0.00 0.00 **FUD** XXX Q1 N1 80

AMA: 2012,Feb,9-10; 1997,Nov,1

76497 **Unlisted computed tomography procedure (eg, diagnostic, interventional)**

0.00 0.00 **FUD** XXX Q1 N1 80

AMA: 2018,Sep,10; 2018,Jan,8; 2017,Jan,8; 2016,Jan,13

76498 **Unlisted magnetic resonance procedure (eg, diagnostic, interventional)**

0.00 0.00 **FUD** XXX S Z2 80

AMA: 2019,Aug,5; 2018,Jul,11; 2018,Jan,8; 2017,Jan,8; 2016,Jan,13

76499 **Unlisted diagnostic radiographic procedure**

0.00 0.00 **FUD** XXX Q1 N1 80

AMA: 2018,Jan,8; 2017,Jan,8; 2016,Dec,15; 2016,Jul,8; 2016,Jan,13

76506 Ultrasound: Brain

INCLUDES Required permanent documentation ultrasound images except when diagnostic purpose is biometric measurement
Written documentation

EXCLUDES Noninvasive vascular studies, diagnostic (93880-93990)
Ultrasound not including thorough assessment organ or site, recorded image, and written report

76506 **Echoencephalography, real time with image documentation (gray scale) (for determination of ventricular size, delineation of cerebral contents, and detection of fluid masses or other intracranial abnormalities), including A-mode encephalography as secondary component where indicated**

3.25 3.25 **FUD** XXX Q1 N1 80

AMA: 2018,Jan,8; 2017,Jan,8; 2016,Jan,13

76510-76529 Ultrasound: Eyes

INCLUDES Required permanent documentation ultrasound images except when diagnostic purpose is biometric measurement
Written documentation

76510 **Ophthalmic ultrasound, diagnostic; B-scan and quantitative A-scan performed during the same patient encounter**

2.56 2.56 **FUD** XXX Q1 N1 80

AMA: 2018,Jan,8; 2017,Jan,8; 2016,Jan,13

76511 **quantitative A-scan only**

1.75 1.75 **FUD** XXX Q1 N1 80

AMA: 2019,Jan,12; 2018,Jan,8; 2017,Jan,8; 2016,Jan,13

76512 **B-scan (with or without superimposed non-quantitative A-scan)**

1.49 1.49 **FUD** XXX Q1 N1 80

AMA: 2019,Jan,12; 2018,Jan,8; 2017,Jan,8; 2016,Jan,13

76513 **anterior segment ultrasound, immersion (water bath) B-scan or high resolution biomicroscopy, unilateral or bilateral**

EXCLUDES Computerized ophthalmic testing other than by ultrasound (92132-92134)

2.81 2.81 **FUD** XXX Q1 N1 80

AMA: 2019,Jan,12; 2018,Jan,8; 2017,Jan,8; 2016,Jan,13

76514 **corneal pachymetry, unilateral or bilateral (determination of corneal thickness)**

INCLUDES Biometric measurement for which permanent image documentation not required

EXCLUDES Collagen cross-linking cornea (0402T)

0.34 0.34 **FUD** XXX Q1 N1 80

AMA: 2019,Jan,12; 2018,Jan,8; 2017,Jan,8; 2016,Feb,12; 2016,Jan,13

76516 **Ophthalmic biometry by ultrasound echography, A-scan;**

INCLUDES Biometric measurement for which permanent image documentation not required

1.36 1.36 **FUD** XXX Q1 N1 80

AMA: 2019,Jan,12; 2018,Jan,8; 2017,Jan,8; 2016,Jan,13

76519 **with intraocular lens power calculation**

INCLUDES Biometric measurement for which permanent image documentation not required
Written prescription that satisfies requirement for written report

EXCLUDES Partial coherence interferometry (92136)

1.88 1.88 **FUD** XXX Q1 N1 80

AMA: 2019,Jan,12; 2018,Jan,8; 2017,Jan,8; 2016,Jan,13

76529 **Ophthalmic ultrasonic foreign body localization**

2.35 2.35 **FUD** XXX Q1 N1 80

AMA: 2019,Jan,12; 2018,Jan,8; 2017,Jan,8; 2016,Jan,13

76536-76800 Ultrasound: Neck, Thorax, Abdomen, and Spine

INCLUDES Required permanent documentation ultrasound images except when diagnostic purpose is biometric measurement
Written documentation

EXCLUDES Focused ultrasound ablation uterine leiomyomata (0071T-0072T)
Ultrasound exam not including thorough assessment organ or site, recorded image, and written report

76536 **Ultrasound, soft tissues of head and neck (eg, thyroid, parathyroid, parotid), real time with image documentation**

3.27 3.27 **FUD** XXX Q1 N1 80

AMA: 2018,Jan,8; 2017,Oct,9; 2017,Jan,8; 2016,Jan,13

76604 **Ultrasound, chest (includes mediastinum), real time with image documentation**

2.51 2.51 **FUD** XXX Q1 N1 80

AMA: 2018,Jan,8; 2017,Oct,9; 2017,Jan,8; 2016,Jan,13

76641 **Ultrasound, breast, unilateral, real time with image documentation, including axilla when performed; complete**

INCLUDES Complete examination all four quadrants, retroareolar region, and axilla when performed

EXCLUDES Procedure performed more than one time per breast per session

3.02 3.02 **FUD** XXX Q1 N1 80 50

AMA: 2018,Jan,8; 2017,Oct,9; 2017,Jan,8; 2016,Jan,13

76642 **limited**

INCLUDES Examination not including all complete examination elements

EXCLUDES Procedure performed more than one time per breast per session

2.47 2.47 **FUD** XXX Q1 N1 80 50

AMA: 2018,Jan,8; 2017,Oct,9

76700 Ultrasound, abdominal, real time with image documentation; complete

> INCLUDES Real time scans:
> Common bile duct
> Gallbladder
> Inferior vena cava
> Kidneys
> Liver
> Pancreas
> Spleen
> Upper abdominal aorta

🔲 3.47   ⚖ 3.47   **FUD** XXX   [03] [Z2] [80] [▭]

AMA: 2018,Jan,8; 2017,Oct,9; 2017,Jan,8; 2016,Jan,13

76705 limited (eg, single organ, quadrant, follow-up)

🔲 2.57   ⚖ 2.57   **FUD** XXX   [03] [Z2] [80] [▭]

AMA: 2018,Jan,8; 2017,Oct,9; 2017,Jan,8; 2016,Jan,13

76706 Ultrasound, abdominal aorta, real time with image documentation, screening study for abdominal aortic aneurysm (AAA)

> EXCLUDES Diagnostic ultrasound aorta (76770-76775)
> Duplex scan aorta (93978-93979)

🔲 3.21   ⚖ 3.21   **FUD** XXX   [S] [80] [▭]

AMA: 2018,Jan,8; 2017,Sep,11

76770 Ultrasound, retroperitoneal (eg, renal, aorta, nodes), real time with image documentation; complete

> INCLUDES Complete assessment kidneys and bladder when history indicates urinary pathology
> Real time scans:
> Abdominal aorta
> Common iliac artery origins
> Inferior vena cava
> Kidneys

🔲 3.19   ⚖ 3.19   **FUD** XXX   [03] [Z2] [80] [▭]

AMA: 2018,Jan,8; 2017,Oct,9; 2017,Jan,8; 2016,Jan,13

76775 limited

🔲 1.66   ⚖ 1.66   **FUD** XXX   [01] [N1] [80] [▭]

AMA: 2018,Jan,8; 2017,Oct,9; 2017,Jan,8; 2016,Jan,13

76776 Ultrasound, transplanted kidney, real time and duplex Doppler with image documentation

> EXCLUDES Abdominal/pelvic/scrotal contents/retroperitoneal duplex scan (93975-93976)
> Transplanted kidney ultrasound without duplex doppler (76775)

🔲 4.41   ⚖ 4.41   **FUD** XXX   [03] [Z2] [80] [▭]

AMA: 2018,Jan,8; 2017,Jan,8; 2016,Jan,13

76800 Ultrasound, spinal canal and contents

🔲 4.04   ⚖ 4.04   **FUD** XXX   [01] [N1] [80] [▭]

AMA: 2018,Jan,8; 2017,Jan,8; 2016,Jan,13

76801-76802 Ultrasound: Pregnancy Less Than 14 Weeks

> INCLUDES Determination number gestational sacs and fetuses
> Gestational sac/fetal measurement appropriate for gestational age (younger than 14 weeks 0 days)
> Inspection maternal uterus and adnexa
> Quality analysis amniotic fluid volume/gestational sac shape
> Visualization fetal and placental anatomic formation
> Written documentation each exam component

> EXCLUDES Focused ultrasound ablation uterine leiomyomata (0071T-0072T)
> Ultrasound exam not including thorough assessment organ or site, recorded image, and written report

76801 Ultrasound, pregnant uterus, real time with image documentation, fetal and maternal evaluation, first trimester (< 14 weeks 0 days), transabdominal approach; single or first gestation   [M] ♀

> EXCLUDES Fetal nuchal translucency measurement, first trimester (76813)

🔲 3.45   ⚖ 3.45   **FUD** XXX   [S] [Z2] [80] [▭]

AMA: 2018,Jan,8; 2017,Jan,8; 2016,Jan,13

+ **76802** each additional gestation (List separately in addition to code for primary procedure)   [M] ♀

> EXCLUDES Fetal nuchal translucency measurement, first trimester (76814)

Code first (76801)

🔲 1.78   ⚖ 1.78   **FUD** ZZZ   [N] [N1] [80] [▭]

AMA: 2018,Jan,8; 2017,Jan,8; 2016,Jan,13

76805-76810 Ultrasound: Pregnancy of 14 Weeks or More

> INCLUDES Determination number gestational/chorionic sacs and fetuses
> Evaluation:
> Amniotic fluid
> Four chambered heart
> Intracranial, spinal, abdominal anatomy
> Placenta location
> Umbilical cord insertion site
> Examination maternal adnexa if visible
> Gestational sac/fetal measurement appropriate for gestational age (older than or equal to 14 weeks 0 days)
> Written documentation each exam component

> EXCLUDES Focused ultrasound ablation uterine leiomyomata (0071T-0072T)
> Ultrasound exam not including thorough assessment organ or site, recorded image, and written report

76805 Ultrasound, pregnant uterus, real time with image documentation, fetal and maternal evaluation, after first trimester (> or = 14 weeks 0 days), transabdominal approach; single or first gestation   [M] ♀

🔲 3.95   ⚖ 3.95   **FUD** XXX   [S] [Z2] [80] [▭]

AMA: 2018,Jan,8; 2017,Jan,8; 2016,Jan,13

+ **76810** each additional gestation (List separately in addition to code for primary procedure)   [M] ♀

Code first (76805)

🔲 2.59   ⚖ 2.59   **FUD** ZZZ   [N] [N1] [80] [▭]

AMA: 2018,Jan,8; 2017,Jan,8; 2016,Jan,13

76811-76812 Ultrasound: Pregnancy, with Additional Studies of Fetus

> INCLUDES Determination number gestational/chorionic sacs and fetuses
> Evaluation:
> Amniotic fluid
> Examination maternal adnexa if visible
> Focused ultrasound ablation uterine leiomyomata (0071T-0072T)
> Four-chambered heart
> Gestational sac/fetal measurement appropriate for gestational age (older than or equal to 14 weeks 0 days)
> Intracranial, spinal, abdominal anatomy
> Placenta location
> Ultrasound exam not including thorough assessment organ or site, recorded image, and written report
> Umbilical cord insertion site
> Written documentation each exam component
> Examination of maternal adnexa if visible
> Gestational sac/fetal measurement appropriate for gestational age (older than or equal to 14 weeks 0 days)
> Written documentation of each component of exam, including reason for nonvisualization, when applicable

> EXCLUDES Focused ultrasound ablation of uterine leiomyomata (0071T-0072T)
> Ultrasound exam that does not include thorough assessment organ or site, recorded image, and written report

76811 Ultrasound, pregnant uterus, real time with image documentation, fetal and maternal evaluation plus detailed fetal anatomic examination, transabdominal approach; single or first gestation   [M] ♀

🔲 5.01   ⚖ 5.01   **FUD** XXX   [S] [Z3] [80] [▭]

AMA: 2018,Jan,8; 2017,Jan,8; 2016,Jan,13

+ **76812** each additional gestation (List separately in addition to code for primary procedure)   [M] ♀

Code first (76811)

🔲 5.61   ⚖ 5.61   **FUD** ZZZ   [N] [N1] [80] [▭]

AMA: 2018,Jan,8; 2017,Jan,8; 2016,Jan,13

[26]/[TC] PC/TC Only   [A2]-[Z8] ASC Payment   [50] Bilateral   ♂ Male Only   ♀ Female Only   🔲 Facility RVU   ⚖ Non-Facility RVU   [▭] CCI   [✕] CLIA
FUD Follow-up Days   **CMS:** IOM   **AMA:** CPT Asst   [A]-[Y] OPPSI   [80]/[80] Surg Assist Allowed / w/Doc   [▨] Lab Crosswalk   [✚] Radiology Crosswalk

338   CPT © 2021 American Medical Association. All Rights Reserved.   © 2021 Optum360, LLC

76813-76828 Ultrasound: Other Fetal Evaluations

INCLUDES Required permanent documentation ultrasound images except when diagnostic purpose is biometric measurement
Written documentation

EXCLUDES *Focused ultrasound ablation uterine leiomyomata (0071T-0072T)*
Ultrasound exam not including thorough assessment organ or site, recorded image, and written report

76813 **Ultrasound, pregnant uterus, real time with image documentation, first trimester fetal nuchal translucency measurement, transabdominal or transvaginal approach; single or first gestation** M ♀
📷 3.42   ⚕ 3.42   **FUD** XXX   [01] [N1] [80] [▭]
AMA: 2018,Jan,8; 2017,Jan,8; 2016,Jan,13

+ **76814** **each additional gestation (List separately in addition to code for primary procedure)** M ♀
Code first (76813)
📷 2.22   ⚕ 2.22   **FUD** XXX   [N] [N1] [80] [▭]
AMA: 2018,Jan,8; 2017,Jan,8; 2016,Jan,13

76815 **Ultrasound, pregnant uterus, real time with image documentation, limited (eg, fetal heart beat, placental location, fetal position and/or qualitative amniotic fluid volume), 1 or more fetuses** M ♀
INCLUDES Exam concentrating on one or more elements
Reporting only one time per exam, not per element
EXCLUDES *Fetal nuchal translucency measurement, first trimester (76813-76814)*
📷 2.37   ⚕ 2.37   **FUD** XXX   [01] [N1] [80] [▭]
AMA: 2018,Jan,8; 2017,Jan,8; 2016,Jan,13

76816 **Ultrasound, pregnant uterus, real time with image documentation, follow-up (eg, re-evaluation of fetal size by measuring standard growth parameters and amniotic fluid volume, re-evaluation of organ system(s) suspected or confirmed to be abnormal on a previous scan), transabdominal approach, per fetus** M ♀
INCLUDES Re-evaluation fetal size, interval growth, or aberrancies noted on prior ultrasound
Code also modifier 59 for examination each additional fetus
📷 3.19   ⚕ 3.19   **FUD** XXX   [01] [N1] [80] [▭]
AMA: 2018,Jan,8; 2017,Jan,8; 2016,Jan,13

76817 **Ultrasound, pregnant uterus, real time with image documentation, transvaginal** M ♀
EXCLUDES *Transvaginal ultrasound, non-obstetrical (76830)*
Code also transabdominal obstetrical ultrasound, when performed
📷 2.73   ⚕ 2.73   **FUD** XXX   [01] [N1] [80] [▭]
AMA: 2018,Jan,8; 2017,Jan,8; 2016,Jan,13

76818 **Fetal biophysical profile; with non-stress testing** M ♀
Code also modifier 59 for each additional fetus
📷 3.44   ⚕ 3.44   **FUD** XXX   [S] [Z2] [80] [▭]
AMA: 2018,Jan,8; 2017,Jan,8; 2016,Jan,13

76819 **without non-stress testing** M ♀
EXCLUDES *Amniotic fluid index without non-stress test (76815)*
Code also modifier 59 for each additional fetus
📷 2.52   ⚕ 2.52   **FUD** XXX   [S] [Z3] [80] [▭]
AMA: 2018,Jan,8; 2017,Jan,8; 2016,Jan,13

76820 **Doppler velocimetry, fetal; umbilical artery** M
📷 1.35   ⚕ 1.35   **FUD** XXX   [01] [N1] [80] [▭]
AMA: 2018,Jan,8; 2017,Jan,8; 2016,Jul,8; 2016,Jan,13

76821 **middle cerebral artery** M
📷 2.61   ⚕ 2.61   **FUD** XXX   [01] [N1] [80] [▭]
AMA: 2018,Jan,8; 2017,Jan,8; 2016,Jan,13

76825 **Echocardiography, fetal, cardiovascular system, real time with image documentation (2D), with or without M-mode recording;** M ♀
📷 7.71   ⚕ 7.71   **FUD** XXX   [S] [Z3] [80] [▭]
AMA: 2018,Jan,8; 2017,Sep,14; 2017,Jan,8; 2016,Jan,13

76826 **follow-up or repeat study** M ♀
📷 4.58   ⚕ 4.58   **FUD** XXX   [S] [Z2] [80] [▭]
AMA: 2018,Jan,8; 2017,Sep,14

76827 **Doppler echocardiography, fetal, pulsed wave and/or continuous wave with spectral display; complete** M ♀
📷 2.07   ⚕ 2.07   **FUD** XXX   [01] [N1] [80] [▭]
AMA: 2018,Jan,8; 2017,Jan,8; 2016,Jan,13

76828 **follow-up or repeat study** M ♀
EXCLUDES *Color mapping (93325)*
📷 1.47   ⚕ 1.47   **FUD** XXX   [01] [N1] [80] [▭]
AMA: 2018,Jan,8; 2017,Jan,8; 2016,Jan,13

76830-76873 Ultrasound: Male and Female Genitalia

INCLUDES Required permanent documentation ultrasound images except when diagnostic purpose is biometric measurement
Written documentation

EXCLUDES *Focused ultrasound ablation uterine leiomyomata (0071T-0072T)*
Ultrasound exam not including thorough assessment organ or site, recorded image, and written report

76830 **Ultrasound, transvaginal** ♀
EXCLUDES *Transvaginal ultrasound, obstetric (76817)*
Code also transabdominal nonobstetrical ultrasound, when performed
📷 3.47   ⚕ 3.47   **FUD** XXX   [S] [Z2] [80] [▭]
AMA: 2018,Jan,8; 2017,Oct,9; 2017,Jan,8; 2016,Jan,13

Bladder   Pubic bone
Uterus
Ovary   Transducer
Rectum   Monitor

Ultrasound is performed in real time with image documentation by a transvaginal approach

76831 **Saline infusion sonohysterography (SIS), including color flow Doppler, when performed** ♀
Code also saline introduction for saline infusion sonohysterography (58340)
📷 3.36   ⚕ 3.36   **FUD** XXX   [03] [Z3] [80] [▭]
AMA: 2018,Jan,8; 2017,Jan,8; 2016,Jan,13

76856 **Ultrasound, pelvic (nonobstetric), real time with image documentation; complete**
INCLUDES Total examination female pelvic anatomy including:
Bladder measurement
Description and measurement uterus and adnexa
Description any pelvic pathology
Measurement, endometrium
Total examination male pelvis including:
Bladder measurement
Description any pelvic pathology
Evaluation prostate and seminal vesicles
📷 3.09   ⚕ 3.09   **FUD** XXX   [03] [Z2] [80] [▭]
AMA: 2018,Jan,8; 2017,Oct,9; 2017,Jan,8; 2016,Aug,9; 2016,Jan,13

76857   **limited or follow-up (eg, for follicles)**

> INCLUDES   Focused evaluation limited to:
>> Evaluation one or more elements listed in 76856 and/or
>> Re-evaluation one or more pelvic aberrancies noted on prior ultrasound
>> Urinary bladder alone
>
> EXCLUDES   *Bladder volume or post-voided residual measurement without bladder imaging (51798)*
>> *Urinary bladder and kidneys (76770)*

    🎫 1.37   🔨 1.37   **FUD** XXX   03 Z3 80 🖵

AMA: 2018,Jan,8; 2017,Oct,9; 2017,Jan,8; 2016,Jan,13

76870   **Ultrasound, scrotum and contents**   ♂

    🎫 2.96   🔨 2.96   **FUD** XXX   01 N1 80 🖵

AMA: 2018,Jan,8; 2017,Oct,9

76872   **Ultrasound, transrectal;**

> EXCLUDES   *Colonoscopy (45391-45392)*
>> *Cystourethroscopy with transurethral anterior prostate commissurotomy/drug dellivery (0619T)*
>> *Hemorrhoidectomy by transanal hemorrhoidal dearterialization ([46948])*
>> *Sigmoidoscopy (45341-45342)*
>> *Transurethral prostate ablation (0421T)*

    🎫 3.62   🔨 3.62   **FUD** XXX   S Z2 80 🖵

AMA: 2020,Feb,11; 2018,Nov,10; 2018,Jul,11; 2018,Jan,8; 2017,Oct,9; 2017,Jan,8; 2016,Jan,13

76873   **prostate volume study for brachytherapy treatment planning (separate procedure)**   ♂

    🎫 4.96   🔨 4.96   **FUD** XXX   S Z2 80 🖵

AMA: 2018,Jan,8; 2017,Jan,8; 2016,Jan,13

76881-76886 Ultrasound: Extremities

> EXCLUDES   *Doppler studies extremities (93925-93926, 93930-93931, 93970-93971)*

76881   **Ultrasound, complete joint (ie, joint space and peri-articular soft tissue structures) real-time with image documentation**

> INCLUDES   Real-time scans specific joint including assessment:
>> Joint space
>> Muscles
>> Other soft tissue
>> Tendons
>> Required permanent image documentation
>> Stress manipulations and dynamic imaging when performed
>> Written documentation including explanation any joint components not visualized

    🎫 2.19   🔨 2.19   **FUD** XXX   S Z3 80 🖵

AMA: 2018,Jan,8; 2017,Oct,9; 2017,Jan,8; 2016,Sep,9

76882   **Ultrasound, limited, joint or other nonvascular extremity structure(s) (eg, joint space, peri-articular tendon[s], muscle[s], nerve[s], other soft tissue structure[s], or soft tissue mass[es]), real-time with image documentation**

> INCLUDES   Limited joint examination or evaluation due to mass or other abnormality not requiring all complete joint evaluation components (76881)
>> Real-time scans specific joint including assessment:
>> Joint space
>> Muscles
>> Other soft tissue
>> Tendons
>> Required permanent image documentation
>> Written documentation including explanation any joint components not visualized

    🎫 1.62   🔨 1.62   **FUD** XXX   01 N1 80 🖵

AMA: 2018,Jan,8; 2017,Oct,9; 2017,Jan,8; 2016,Sep,9

76885   **Ultrasound, infant hips, real time with imaging documentation; dynamic (requiring physician or other qualified health care professional manipulation)**   A

    🎫 4.05   🔨 4.05   **FUD** XXX   01 N1 80 🖵

AMA: 2012,Feb,9-10; 2002,May,7

76886   **limited, static (not requiring physician or other qualified health care professional manipulation)**   A

    🎫 2.97   🔨 2.97   **FUD** XXX   01 N1 80 🖵

AMA: 2012,Feb,9-10; 2002,May,7

76932-76965 Imaging Guidance: Ultrasound

> INCLUDES   Required permanent documentation ultrasound images except when diagnostic purpose is biometric measurement
>> Written documentation
>
> EXCLUDES   *Focused ultrasound ablation uterine leiomyomata (0071T-0072T)*
>> *Ultrasound exam not including thorough assessment organ or site, recorded image, and written report*

76932   **Ultrasonic guidance for endomyocardial biopsy, imaging supervision and interpretation**

    🎫 0.00   🔨 0.00   **FUD** YYY   N N1 80 🖵

AMA: 2012,Feb,9-10; 2001,Sep,4

76936   **Ultrasound guided compression repair of arterial pseudoaneurysm or arteriovenous fistulae (includes diagnostic ultrasound evaluation, compression of lesion and imaging)**

    🎫 7.60   🔨 7.60   **FUD** XXX   S Z2 80 🖵

AMA: 2012,Feb,9-10; 2002,May,7

+ **76937**   **Ultrasound guidance for vascular access requiring ultrasound evaluation of potential access sites, documentation of selected vessel patency, concurrent realtime ultrasound visualization of vascular needle entry, with permanent recording and reporting (List separately in addition to code for primary procedure)**

> INCLUDES   Ultrasound guidance, needle placement (76942)
>
> EXCLUDES   *Endovascular venous arterialization, tibial or peroneal vein ([0620T])*
>> *Endovenous femoral-popliteal arterial revascularization (0505T)*
>> *Extremity venous noninvasive vascular diagnostic study performed separately from venous access guidance (93970-93971)*
>> *Insertion or replacement peripherally inserted central venous catheter (36568-36569, [36572, 36573], 36584)*
>> *Insertion, removal, or replacement permanent leadless pacemaker ([33274, 33275])*
>> *Insertion, removal, or repositioning vena cava filter (37191-37193)*
>> *Ligation perforator veins (37760-37761)*
>
> Code first primary procedure

    🎫 1.03   🔨 1.03   **FUD** ZZZ   N N1 80 🖵

AMA: 2019,May,3; 2019,Mar,6; 2018,Mar,3; 2018,Jan,8; 2017,Dec,3; 2017,Aug,10; 2017,Jul,3; 2017,Mar,3; 2017,Jan,8; 2016,Nov,3; 2016,Jul,6; 2016,Jan,13

76940   **Ultrasound guidance for, and monitoring of, parenchymal tissue ablation**

> EXCLUDES   *Ablation (20982-20983, [32994], 32998, 47370-47383, 50250, 50542, 50592-50593, 0582T, 0600T-0601T)*
>> *Ultrasound guidance:*
>>> *Intraoperative (76998)*
>>> *Needle placement (76942)*

    🎫 0.00   🔨 0.00   **FUD** YYY   N N1 80 🖵

AMA: 2018,Jan,8; 2017,Nov,8; 2017,Jan,8; 2016,Jan,13

76941   **Ultrasonic guidance for intrauterine fetal transfusion or cordocentesis, imaging supervision and interpretation**   M ♀

> Code also surgical procedure (36460, 59012)

    🎫 0.00   🔨 0.00   **FUD** XXX   N N1 80 🖵

AMA: 2012,Feb,9-10; 2001,Sep,4

26/TC PC/TC Only   A2-Z3 ASC Payment   50 Bilateral   ♂ Male Only   ♀ Female Only   🎫 Facility RVU   🔨 Non-Facility RVU   🖵 CCI   ❌ CLIA
FUD Follow-up Days   CMS: IOM   AMA: CPT Asst   A-Y OPPSI   80/80 Surg Assist Allowed / w/Doc   🔲 Lab Crosswalk   🔳 Radiology Crosswalk

340   CPT © 2021 American Medical Association. All Rights Reserved.   © 2021 Optum360, LLC

76942 Ultrasonic guidance for needle placement (eg, biopsy, aspiration, injection, localization device), imaging supervision and interpretation

> *EXCLUDES* *Arthrocentesis (20604, 20606, 20611)*
> *Autologous WBC injection (0481T)*
> *Breast biopsy with placement localization device(s) (19083)*
> *Core needle biopsy, lung or mediastinum (32408)*
> *Esophagogastroduodenoscopy (43237, 43242)*
> *Esophagoscopy (43232)*
> *Fine needle aspiration biopsy ([10004, 10005, 10006], 10021)*
> *Gastrointestinal endoscopic ultrasound (76975)*
> *Hemorrhoidectomy by transanal hemorrhoidal dearterialization ([46948])*
> *Image-guided fluid collection drainage by catheter (10030)*
> *Injection procedures (27096, 64479-64484, 0232T)*
> *Ligation (37760-37761)*
> *Paravertebral facet joint injections (64490-64491, 64493-64495, 0213T-0218T)*
> *Placement breast localization device(s) (19285)*
> *Sigmoidoscopy (45341-45342)*
> *Thoracentesis (32554-32557)*
> *Transperineal placement, periprostatic biodegradable material (55874)*
> *Transurethral ablation, malignant prostate tissue (0582T)*

> 🔧 1.61 ⚕ 1.61 **FUD** XXX   N N1 80 🖵

> **AMA:** 2020,Jun,10; 2020,Feb,11; 2020,Feb,9; 2020,Jan,7; 2019,Aug,10; 2019,Apr,4; 2019,Feb,8; 2018,Jul,11; 2018,Mar,3; 2018,Jan,8; 2017,Dec,13; 2017,Sep,6; 2017,Jun,10; 2017,Jan,8; 2016,Nov,3; 2016,Jun,3; 2016,Jan,13; 2016,Jan,9

76945 Ultrasonic guidance for chorionic villus sampling, imaging supervision and interpretation   M ♀

> Code also surgical procedure (59015)
> 🔧 0.00 ⚕ 0.00 **FUD** XXX   N N1 80 🖵

> **AMA:** 2012,Feb,9-10; 2001,Sep,4

76946 Ultrasonic guidance for amniocentesis, imaging supervision and interpretation   M ♀

> 🔧 0.91 ⚕ 0.91 **FUD** XXX   N N1 80 🖵

> **AMA:** 2012,Feb,9-10; 2001,Sep,4

76948 Ultrasonic guidance for aspiration of ova, imaging supervision and interpretation   M ♀

> 🔧 2.15 ⚕ 2.15 **FUD** XXX   N N1 80 🖵

> **AMA:** 2012,Feb,9-10; 2001,Sep,4

76965 Ultrasonic guidance for interstitial radioelement application

> 🔧 2.64 ⚕ 2.64 **FUD** XXX   N N1 80 🖵

> **AMA:** 2012,Feb,9-10; 1997,Nov,1

76975 Endoscopic Ultrasound

> *INCLUDES* Required permanent documentation ultrasound images except when diagnostic purpose is biometric measurement
> Written documentation
> *EXCLUDES* *Focused ultrasound ablation uterine leiomyomata (0071T-0072T)*
> *Ultrasound exam not including thorough assessment organ or site, recorded image, and written report*

76975 Gastrointestinal endoscopic ultrasound, supervision and interpretation

> *INCLUDES* Ultrasonic guidance (76942)
> *EXCLUDES* *Colonoscopy (44406-44407, 45391-45392)*
> *Esophagogastroduodenoscopy (43237-43238, 43240, 43242, 43259)*
> *Esophagoscopy (43231-43232)*
> *Sigmoidoscopy (45341-45342)*

> 🔧 0.00 ⚕ 0.00 **FUD** XXX   Q2 N1 80 🖵

> **AMA:** 2018,Jan,8; 2017,Jan,8; 2016,Jan,13

76977 Bone Density Measurements: Ultrasound

CMS: 100-02,15,80.5.5 Frequency Standards

> *INCLUDES* Required permanent documentation ultrasound images except when diagnostic purpose is biometric measurement
> Written documentation
> *EXCLUDES* *Ultrasound exam not including thorough assessment organ or site, recorded image, and written report*

76977 Ultrasound bone density measurement and interpretation, peripheral site(s), any method

> 🔧 0.20 ⚕ 0.20 **FUD** XXX   S Z3 80 🖵

> **AMA:** 2012,Feb,9-10; 1998,Nov,1

76978-76979 Targeted Dynamic Microbubble Sonographic Contrast Characterization: Ultrasound

> *INCLUDES* Intravenous injection (96374)

76978 Ultrasound, targeted dynamic microbubble sonographic contrast characterization (non-cardiac); initial lesion

> 🔧 9.21 ⚕ 9.21 **FUD** XXX   Z2 80 🖵

> **AMA:** 2019,Jun,9

+ 76979 each additional lesion with separate injection (List separately in addition to code for primary procedure)

> Code first (76978)
> 🔧 6.23 ⚕ 6.23 **FUD** ZZZ   N1 80 🖵

> **AMA:** 2019,Jun,9

76981-76983 Elastography: Ultrasound

> *EXCLUDES* *Quantitative ultrasound tissue characterization (0689T)*
> *Shear wave liver elastography (91200)*

76981 Ultrasound, elastography; parenchyma (eg, organ)

> *EXCLUDES* *Reporting code more than one time each session for same parenchymal organ and/or parenchymal organ and lesion*

> 🔧 3.04 ⚕ 3.04 **FUD** XXX   Z2 80 🖵

> **AMA:** 2019,Aug,3

76982 first target lesion

> 🔧 2.71 ⚕ 2.71 **FUD** XXX   Z2 80 🖵

> **AMA:** 2019,Aug,3

+ 76983 each additional target lesion (List separately in addition to code for primary procedure)

> *EXCLUDES* *Reporting code more than one time each session for same parenchymal organ and/or parenchymal organ and lesion*

> Code first (76982)
> 🔧 1.67 ⚕ 1.67 **FUD** ZZZ   N1 80 🖵

> **AMA:** 2019,Aug,3

76998-76999 Imaging Guidance During Surgery: Ultrasound

> *INCLUDES* Required permanent documentation ultrasound images except when diagnostic purpose is biometric measurement
> Written documentation
> *EXCLUDES* *Focused ultrasound ablation uterine leiomyomata (0071T-0072T)*
> *Ultrasound exam not including thorough assessment organ or site, recorded image, and written report*

76998 Ultrasonic guidance, intraoperative

> *EXCLUDES* *Ablation (47370-47371, 47380-47382)*
> *Endovenous ablation therapy incompetent vein (36475, 36479)*
> *Hemorrhoidectomy by transanal hemorrhoidal dearterialization ([46948])*
> *Ligation (37760-37761)*
> *Wireless cardiac stimulator (0515T-0520T)*

> 🔧 0.00 ⚕ 0.00 **FUD** XXX   N N1 80 🖵

> **AMA:** 2020,Feb,11; 2018,Mar,3; 2018,Jan,8; 2017,Apr,7; 2017,Jan,8; 2016,Nov,3; 2016,Jan,13

76999 Unlisted ultrasound procedure (eg, diagnostic, interventional)

> 🔧 0.00 ⚕ 0.00 **FUD** XXX   Q1 N1 80 🖵

> **AMA:** 2019,Dec,8; 2018,Jul,11; 2018,Jan,8; 2017,Jan,8; 2016,Jan,13

● New Code ▲ Revised Code ○ Reinstated ● New Web Release ▲ Revised Web Release + Add-on Unlisted Not Covered # Resequenced
🔟 Optum Mod 50 Exempt ⊘ AMA Mod 51 Exempt 51 Optum Mod 51 Exempt 63 Mod 63 Exempt ✎ Non-FDA Drug ★ Telemedicine M Maternity A Age Edit

77001-77022 Imaging Guidance Techniques

EXCLUDES *Imaging guidance, breast localization device(s) (19081, 19281, 19283)*

+ 77001 Fluoroscopic guidance for central venous access device placement, replacement (catheter only or complete), or removal (includes fluoroscopic guidance for vascular access and catheter manipulation, any necessary contrast injections through access site or catheter with related venography radiologic supervision and interpretation, and radiographic documentation of final catheter position) (List separately in addition to code for primary procedure)

INCLUDES Fluoroscopic guidance for needle placement (77002)

EXCLUDES *Any procedure codes that include fluoroscopic guidance in code descriptor*

Extracorporeal membrane oxygenation (ECMO)/extracorporeal life support (ECLS) (33957-33959, [33962, 33963, 33964])

Formal extremity venography performed separately from venous access and interpreted separately (36005, 75820, 75822, 75825, 75827)

Insertion peripherally inserted central venous catheter (PICC) (36568-36569, [36572, 36573])

Replacement peripherally inserted central venous catheter (PICC) (36584)

Code first primary procedure

🔹 2.71   ⚕ 2.71   **FUD** ZZZ   N NI 80 ▣

AMA: 2019,May,3; 2018,Jan,8; 2017,Jan,8; 2016,Jan,13

+ 77002 Fluoroscopic guidance for needle placement (eg, biopsy, aspiration, injection, localization device) (List separately in addition to code for primary procedure)

EXCLUDES *Ablation therapy (20982-20983)*

Any procedure codes that include fluoroscopic guidance in code descriptor:

Radiological guidance for percutaneous drainage by catheter (75989)

Transhepatic portography (75885, 75887)

Arthrography procedure(s) (70332, 73040, 73085, 73115, 73525, 73580, 73615)

Biopsy, breast, with placement breast localization device(s) (19081-19086)

Image-guided fluid collection drainage by catheter (10030)

Placement breast localization device(s) (19281-19288)

Platelet rich plasma injection(s) (0232T)

Thoracentesis (32554-32557)

Code first surgical procedure (10160, 20206, 20220, 20225, 20520, 20525-20526, 20550, 20551, 20552, 20553, 20555, 20600, 20605, 20610, 20612, 20615, 21116, 21550, 23350, 24220, 25246, 27093-27095, 27369, 27648, 32400, 32553, 36002, 38220-38222, 38505, 38794, 41019, 42400-42405, 47000-47001, 48102, 49180, 49411, 50200, 50390, 51100-51102, 55700, 55876, 60100, 62268-62269, 64400-64448, 64450, 64455, 64505, 64600-64605)

🔹 3.05   ⚕ 3.05   **FUD** ZZZ   N NI 80 ▣

AMA: 2020,Feb,9; 2020,Jan,7; 2019,Dec,8; 2019,Dec,12; 2019,Aug,7; 2019,Mar,6; 2019,Apr,4; 2019,Feb,8; 2018,Dec,10; 2018,Dec,10; 2018,Jan,8; 2017,Jun,10; 2017,Jan,8; 2016,Sep,9; 2016,Aug,7; 2016,Jun,3; 2016,Jan,9; 2016,Jan,13

+ 77003 Fluoroscopic guidance and localization of needle or catheter tip for spine or paraspinous diagnostic or therapeutic injection procedures (epidural or subarachnoid) (List separately in addition to code for primary procedure)

EXCLUDES *Any procedure codes that include fluoroscopic guidance in code descriptor*

Arthrodesis (22586)

Image-guided fluid collection drainage by catheter (10030)

Injection allogenic cellular and/or tissue-based product, intervertebral disc (0627T-0628T)

Injection medication (subarachnoid/interlaminar epidural) (62320-62327)

Spinal puncture (62270, [62328], 62272, [62329])

Code first (61050-61055, 62267, 62273, 62280-62284, 64449, 64510, 64517, 64520, 64610, 96450)

🔹 2.85   ⚕ 2.85   **FUD** ZZZ   N NI 80 ▣

AMA: 2020,Jun,10; 2019,Dec,8; 2018,Jan,8; 2017,Dec,13; 2017,Sep,6; 2017,Feb,9; 2017,Feb,12; 2017,Jan,8; 2016,Jan,11; 2016,Jan,9; 2016,Jan,13

77011 Computed tomography guidance for stereotactic localization

EXCLUDES *Arthrodesis (22586)*

🔹 6.57   ⚕ 6.57   **FUD** XXX   N NI ▣

AMA: 2018,Jan,8; 2017,Jan,8; 2016,Jan,13

77012 Computed tomography guidance for needle placement (eg, biopsy, aspiration, injection, localization device), radiological supervision and interpretation

EXCLUDES *Arthrodesis (22586)*

Autologous white blood cell concentrate (0481T)

Core needle biopsy, lung or mediastinum (32408)

Destruction paravertebral facet joint nerve by neurolysis ([64633, 64634, 64635, 64636])

Fine needle aspiration biopsy using CT guidance ([10009, 10010])

Image-guided fluid collection drainage by catheter (10030)

Injection allogenic cellular and/or tissue-based product, intervertebral disc (0629T-0630T)

Injection, paravertebral facet joint (64490-64495)

Platelet rich plasma injection(s) (0232T)

Sacroiliac joint arthrography (27096)

Spinal puncture (62270, [62328], 62272, [62329])

Thoracentesis (32554-32557)

Transforaminal epidural needle placement/injection (64479-64480, 64483-64484)

🔹 4.26   ⚕ 4.26   **FUD** XXX   N NI ▣

AMA: 2020,Jun,10; 2020,Jan,7; 2019,Dec,8; 2019,Apr,4; 2019,Feb,8; 2018,Jan,8; 2017,Sep,6; 2017,Feb,12; 2017,Jan,8; 2016,Jun,3; 2016,Jan,13

77013 Computed tomography guidance for, and monitoring of, parenchymal tissue ablation

EXCLUDES *Ablation therapy (20982-20983, [32994], 32998, 47382-47383, 50592-50593)*

Ablation, irreversible electroporation (0600T)

🔹 0.00   ⚕ 0.00   **FUD** XXX   N NI 80 ▣

AMA: 2018,Jan,8; 2017,Nov,8; 2017,Jan,8; 2016,Jan,13

77014 Computed tomography guidance for placement of radiation therapy fields

Code also placement interstitial device(s) for radiation therapy guidance (31627, 32553, 49411, 55876)

🔹 3.45   ⚕ 3.45   **FUD** XXX   N NI ▣

AMA: 2018,Jan,8; 2017,Jan,8; 2016,Feb,3; 2016,Jan,13

77021 Magnetic resonance imaging guidance for needle placement (eg, for biopsy, needle aspiration, injection, or placement of localization device) radiological supervision and interpretation

> EXCLUDES Autologous white blood cell concentrate (0481T)
> Biopsy, breast, with placement breast localization device(s) (19085)
> Core needle biopsy, lung or mediastinum (32408)
> Fine needle aspiration biopsy using MR guidance ([10011, 10012])
> Image-guided fluid collection drainage by catheter (10030)
> Placement breast localization device(s) (19287)
> Platelet rich plasma injection(s) (0232T)
> Surgical procedure
> Thoracentesis (32554-32557)

> 13.1   13.1   **FUD** XXX   N N1 ▢

> **AMA:** 2020,Jun,10; 2020,Feb,9; 2020,Jan,7; 2019,Apr,4; 2019,Feb,8; 2018,Jul,11; 2018,Jan,8; 2017,Jun,10; 2017,Jan,8; 2016,Jun,3; 2016,Jan,13

77022 Magnetic resonance imaging guidance for, and monitoring of, parenchymal tissue ablation

> EXCLUDES Ablation:
> Irreversible electroporation (0600T)
> Percutaneous radiofrequency ([32994], 32998, 47383-47383, 50592-50593)
> Reduction or eradication one or more bone tumors (20982-20983)
> Uterine leiomyomata by focused ablation (0071T-0072T)

> 0.00   0.00   **FUD** XXX   N N1 80 ▢

> **AMA:** 2019,Sep,10; 2018,Mar,3; 2018,Jan,8; 2017,Nov,8; 2017,Jan,8; 2016,Nov,3; 2016,Jan,13

77046-77067 Radiography: Breast

77046 Magnetic resonance imaging, breast, without contrast material; unilateral

> 7.02   7.02   **FUD** XXX   Z2 80 ▢

> **AMA:** 2019,Aug,5

77047 bilateral

> 7.08   7.08   **FUD** XXX   Z2 80 ▢

> **AMA:** 2019,Aug,5

77048 Magnetic resonance imaging, breast, without and with contrast material(s), including computer-aided detection (CAD real-time lesion detection, characterization and pharmacokinetic analysis), when performed; unilateral

> 11.1   11.1   **FUD** XXX   80 ▢

> **AMA:** 2019,Dec,14; 2019,Aug,5

77049 bilateral

> 11.1   11.1   **FUD** XXX   80 ▢

> **AMA:** 2019,Dec,14; 2019,Aug,5

77053 Mammary ductogram or galactogram, single duct, radiological supervision and interpretation

> Code also injection procedure (19030)

> 1.60   1.60   **FUD** XXX   Q2 N1 ▢

> **AMA:** 2018,Jan,8; 2017,Jan,8; 2016,Jan,13

77054 Mammary ductogram or galactogram, multiple ducts, radiological supervision and interpretation

> 2.07   2.07   **FUD** XXX   Q2 N1 ▢

> **AMA:** 2018,Jan,8; 2017,Jan,8; 2016,Jan,13

77061 Diagnostic digital breast tomosynthesis; unilateral

> EXCLUDES 3D rendering (76376-76377)
> Screening mammography (77067)

> 0.00   0.00   **FUD** XXX   E ▢

> **AMA:** 2020,Sep,14; 2018,Jan,8

77062 bilateral

> EXCLUDES 3D rendering (76376-76377)
> Screening mammography (77067)

> 0.00   0.00   **FUD** XXX   E ▢

> **AMA:** 2020,Sep,14; 2018,Jan,8; 2017,Jan,8; 2016,Dec,15

+ 77063 Screening digital breast tomosynthesis, bilateral (List separately in addition to code for primary procedure)

> EXCLUDES 3D rendering (76376-76377)
> Diagnostic mammography (77065-77066)

> Code first (77067)

> 1.55   1.55   **FUD** ZZZ   A ▢

> **AMA:** 2020,Sep,14; 2018,Jan,8; 2017,Jan,8; 2016,Dec,15

77065 Diagnostic mammography, including computer-aided detection (CAD) when performed; unilateral

> 3.78   3.78   **FUD** XXX   A 80 ▢

> **AMA:** 2020,Sep,14; 2019,Aug,5; 2018,Jan,8; 2017,Jan,8; 2016,Dec,15

77066 bilateral

> 4.76   4.76   **FUD** XXX   A 80 ▢

> **AMA:** 2020,Sep,14; 2019,Aug,5; 2018,Jan,8; 2017,Jan,8; 2016,Dec,15

77067 Screening mammography, bilateral (2-view study of each breast), including computer-aided detection (CAD) when performed

> EXCLUDES Breast scan, electrical impedance (76499)

> 3.86   3.86   **FUD** XXX   A 80 ▢

> **AMA:** 2020,Sep,14; 2019,Aug,5; 2018,Jan,8; 2017,Jan,8; 2016,Dec,15

77071-77092 [77085, 77086] Additional Evaluations of Bones and Joints

77071 Manual application of stress performed by physician or other qualified health care professional for joint radiography, including contralateral joint if indicated

> Code also interpretation stressed images according to anatomical site and number of views

> 1.50   1.50   **FUD** XXX   Q1 N1 80 26 ▢

> **AMA:** 2018,Jan,8; 2017,Jan,8; 2016,Jan,13

77072 Bone age studies

> 0.71   0.71   **FUD** XXX   Q1 N1 80 ▢

> **AMA:** 2018,Jan,8; 2017,Jan,8; 2016,Jan,13

77073 Bone length studies (orthoroentgenogram, scanogram)

> 1.24   1.24   **FUD** XXX   Q1 N1 80 ▢

> **AMA:** 2018,Jan,8; 2017,Jan,8; 2016,Jan,13

77074 Radiologic examination, osseous survey; limited (eg, for metastases)

> 1.78   1.78   **FUD** XXX   Q1 N1 80 ▢

> **AMA:** 2018,Jan,8; 2017,Jan,8; 2016,Jan,13

77075 complete (axial and appendicular skeleton)

> 2.68   2.68   **FUD** XXX   Q1 N1 80 ▢

> **AMA:** 2018,Jan,8; 2017,Jan,8; 2016,Jan,13

77076 Radiologic examination, osseous survey, infant

> 2.90   2.90   **FUD** XXX   Q1 N1 80 ▢

> **AMA:** 2018,Jan,8; 2017,Jan,8; 2016,Jan,13

77077 Joint survey, single view, 2 or more joints (specify)

> 1.29   1.29   **FUD** XXX   Q1 N1 80 ▢

> **AMA:** 2018,Jan,8; 2017,Jan,8; 2016,Jan,13

77078 Computed tomography, bone mineral density study, 1 or more sites, axial skeleton (eg, hips, pelvis, spine)

> 3.22   3.22   **FUD** XXX   S Z2 80 ▢

> **AMA:** 2018,Jan,8; 2017,Jan,8; 2016,Jan,13

77080 Dual-energy X-ray absorptiometry (DXA), bone density study, 1 or more sites; axial skeleton (eg, hips, pelvis, spine)

> EXCLUDES Dual-energy x-ray absorptiometry (DXA), bone density study ([77085])
> Vertebral fracture assessment via dual-energy x-ray absorptiometry (DXA) ([77086])

> 1.11   1.11   **FUD** XXX   S Z3 80 ▢

> **AMA:** 2018,Jan,8; 2017,Jan,8; 2016,Jan,13

77081 appendicular skeleton (peripheral) (eg, radius, wrist, heel)

> 0.91   0.91   **FUD** XXX   S Z3 80 ▢

> **AMA:** 2018,Jan,8; 2017,Jan,8; 2016,Jan,13

Radiology

77085 — 77306

77085 axial skeleton (eg, hips, pelvis, spine), including vertebral fracture assessment

EXCLUDES Dual-energy x-ray absorptiometry (DXA), bone density study (77080)
Vertebral fracture assessment via dual-energy x-ray absorptiometry (DXA) ([77086])

🖧 1.50   𝄜 1.50   **FUD** XXX   01 N1 80 ▭

77086 Vertebral fracture assessment via dual-energy X-ray absorptiometry (DXA)

EXCLUDES Dual-energy x-ray absorptiometry (DXA), bone density study (77080)
Therapy performed more than one time for treatment to specific area
Vertebral fracture assessment via dual-energy X-ray absorptiometry (DXA) ([77085])

🖧 0.99   𝄜 0.99   **FUD** XXX   01 N1 80 ▭

77084 Magnetic resonance (eg, proton) imaging, bone marrow blood supply

🖧 10.4   𝄜 10.4   **FUD** XXX   S Z2 80 ▭

AMA: 2018,Jan,8; 2017,Jan,8; 2016,Jan,13

77085 Resequenced code. See code following 77081.

77086 Resequenced code. See code before 77084.

● 77089 Trabecular bone score (TBS), structural condition of the bone microarchitecture; using dual X-ray absorptiometry (DXA) or other imaging data on gray-scale variogram, calculation, with interpretation and report on fracture-risk

EXCLUDES Interpretation and report only by other qualified health care professional (QHCP) (77092)
Technical calculation only (77091)
Technical preparation and data transmission to be performed elsewhere (77090)

● 77090 technical preparation and transmission of data for analysis to be performed elsewhere

EXCLUDES Trabecular bone score (TBS), complete (77089)

● 77091 technical calculation only

EXCLUDES Trabecular bone score (TBS), complete (77089)

● 77092 interpretation and report on fracture-risk only by other qualified health care professional

EXCLUDES Trabecular bone score (TBS), complete (77089)

77261-77263 Therapeutic Radiology: Treatment Planning

INCLUDES Determination:
  Appropriate treatment devices
  Number and size treatment ports
  Treatment method
  Treatment time/dosage
  Treatment volume
Interpretation special testing
Tumor localization
EXCLUDES Brachytherapy (0394T-0395T)
Radiation treatment delivery, superficial (77401)

77261 Therapeutic radiology treatment planning; simple

INCLUDES Planning for single treatment area included in single port or single parallel opposed ports with simple or no blocking

🖧 2.03   𝄜 2.03   **FUD** XXX   B 80 26 ▭

AMA: 2018,Jan,8; 2017,Jan,8; 2016,Feb,3; 2016,Jan,13

77262 intermediate

INCLUDES Planning for three or more converging ports, two separate treatment sites, multiple blocks, or special time dose constraints

🖧 3.06   𝄜 3.06   **FUD** XXX   B 80 26 ▭

AMA: 2018,Jan,8; 2017,Jan,8; 2016,Feb,3; 2016,Jan,13

77263 complex

INCLUDES Planning for very complex blocking, custom shielding blocks, tangential ports, special wedges or compensators, three or more separate treatment areas, rotational or special beam considerations, treatment modality combinations

🖧 4.78   𝄜 4.78   **FUD** XXX   B 80 26 ▭

AMA: 2018,Jan,8; 2017,Jan,8; 2016,Feb,3; 2016,Jan,13

77280-77299 [77295] Radiation Therapy Simulation

77280 Therapeutic radiology simulation-aided field setting; simple

INCLUDES Simulation single treatment site

🖧 7.85   𝄜 7.85   **FUD** XXX   S Z2 80 ▭

AMA: 2018,Jan,8; 2017,Jan,8; 2016,Jan,13

77285 intermediate

INCLUDES Two different treatment sites

🖧 13.1   𝄜 13.1   **FUD** XXX   S Z2 80 ▭

AMA: 2018,Jan,8; 2017,Jan,8; 2016,Jan,13

77290 complex

INCLUDES Brachytherapy
Complex blocking
Contrast material
Custom shielding blocks
Hyperthermia probe verification
Rotation, arc or particle therapy
Simulation to ≥ 3 treatment sites

🖧 14.0   𝄜 14.0   **FUD** XXX   S Z2 80 ▭

AMA: 2018,Jan,8; 2017,Jan,8; 2016,Sep,9; 2016,Jan,13

\+ 77293 Respiratory motion management simulation (List separately in addition to code for primary procedure)

Code first (77295, 77301)

🖧 12.7   𝄜 12.7   **FUD** ZZZ   N N1 80 ▭

AMA: 2018,Jan,8; 2017,Jan,8; 2016,Jan,13

77295 Resequenced code. See code before 77300.

77299 Unlisted procedure, therapeutic radiology clinical treatment planning

🖧 0.00   𝄜 0.00   **FUD** XXX   S Z2 80 ▭

AMA: 2018,Jan,8; 2017,Jan,8; 2016,Jan,13

77295-77370 [77295] Radiation Physics Services

77295 3-dimensional radiotherapy plan, including dose-volume histograms

🖧 13.8   𝄜 13.8   **FUD** XXX   S Z3 80 ▭

AMA: 2018,Jan,8; 2017,Jan,8; 2016,Jan,13

77300 Basic radiation dosimetry calculation, central axis depth dose calculation, TDF, NSD, gap calculation, off axis factor, tissue inhomogeneity factors, calculation of non-ionizing radiation surface and depth dose, as required during course of treatment, only when prescribed by the treating physician

EXCLUDES Brachytherapy (77316-77318, 77767-77772, 0394T-0395T)
Teletherapy plan (77306-77307, 77321)

🖧 1.88   𝄜 1.88   **FUD** XXX   S Z3 80 ▭

AMA: 2018,Jan,8; 2017,Jan,8; 2016,Jan,13

77301 Intensity modulated radiotherapy plan, including dose-volume histograms for target and critical structure partial tolerance specifications

🖧 54.0   𝄜 54.0   **FUD** XXX   S Z2 80 ▭

AMA: 2018,Jan,8; 2017,Jan,8; 2016,Jan,13

77306 Teletherapy isodose plan; simple (1 or 2 unmodified ports directed to a single area of interest), includes basic dosimetry calculation(s)

EXCLUDES Brachytherapy (0394T-0395T)
Radiation dosimetry calculation (77300)
Radiation treatment delivery (77401)
Therapy performed more than one time for treatment to specific area

🖧 4.23   𝄜 4.23   **FUD** XXX   S Z3 80 ▭

AMA: 2018,Jan,8; 2017,Jan,8; 2016,Feb,3

26/TC PC/TC Only   A2-Z3 ASC Payment   50 Bilateral   ♂ Male Only   ♀ Female Only   🖧 Facility RVU   𝄜 Non-Facility RVU   ▭ CCI   ✖ CLIA
FUD Follow-up Days   CMS: IOM   AMA: CPT Asst   A-Y OPPSI   80/80 Surg Assist Allowed / w/Doc   ▤ Lab Crosswalk   ⊞ Radiology Crosswalk

344   CPT © 2021 American Medical Association. All Rights Reserved.   © 2021 Optum360, LLC

77307 complex (multiple treatment areas, tangential ports, the use of wedges, blocking, rotational beam, or special beam considerations), includes basic dosimetry calculation(s)

> EXCLUDES Brachytherapy (0394T-0395T)
> Radiation dosimetry calculation (77300)
> Radiation treatment delivery (77401)
> Therapy performed more than one time for treatment to specific area

8.20   8.20   **FUD** XXX   [S] [Z3] [80] [▭]

AMA: 2018,Jan,8; 2017,Jan,8; 2016,Feb,3

77316 Brachytherapy isodose plan; simple (calculation[s] made from 1 to 4 sources, or remote afterloading brachytherapy, 1 channel), includes basic dosimetry calculation(s)

> EXCLUDES Brachytherapy (0394T-0395T)
> Radiation dosimetry calculation (77300)
> Radiation treatment delivery (77401)

6.17   6.17   **FUD** XXX   [S] [Z3] [80] [▭]

AMA: 2018,Jan,8; 2017,Jan,8; 2016,Feb,3

77317 intermediate (calculation[s] made from 5 to 10 sources, or remote afterloading brachytherapy, 2-12 channels), includes basic dosimetry calculation(s)

> EXCLUDES Brachytherapy (0394T-0395T)
> Radiation dosimetry calculation (77300)
> Radiation treatment delivery (77401)

8.09   8.09   **FUD** XXX   [S] [Z2] [80] [▭]

AMA: 2018,Jan,8; 2017,Jan,8

77318 complex (calculation[s] made from over 10 sources, or remote afterloading brachytherapy, over 12 channels), includes basic dosimetry calculation(s)

> EXCLUDES Brachytherapy (0394T-0395T)
> Radiation dosimetry calculation (77300)
> Radiation treatment delivery (77401)

11.5   11.5   **FUD** XXX   [S] [Z2] [80] [▭]

AMA: 2018,Jan,8; 2017,Jan,8; 2016,Feb,3

77321 Special teletherapy port plan, particles, hemibody, total body

2.68   2.68   **FUD** XXX   [S] [Z3] [80] [▭]

AMA: 2018,Jan,8; 2017,Jan,8; 2016,Jan,13

77331 Special dosimetry (eg, TLD, microdosimetry) (specify), only when prescribed by the treating physician

1.84   1.84   **FUD** XXX   [S] [Z3] [80] [▭]

AMA: 2018,Jan,8; 2017,Jan,8; 2016,Jan,13

77332 Treatment devices, design and construction; simple (simple block, simple bolus)

> EXCLUDES Brachytherapy (0394T-0395T)
> Radiation treatment delivery (77401)

1.34   1.34   **FUD** XXX   [S] [Z3] [80] [▭]

AMA: 2018,Jan,8; 2017,Jan,8; 2016,Feb,3; 2016,Jan,13

77333 intermediate (multiple blocks, stents, bite blocks, special bolus)

> EXCLUDES Brachytherapy (0394T-0395T)
> Radiation treatment delivery (77401)

3.41   3.41   **FUD** XXX   [S] [Z2] [80] [▭]

AMA: 2018,Jan,8; 2017,Jan,8; 2016,Feb,3; 2016,Jan,13

77334 complex (irregular blocks, special shields, compensators, wedges, molds or casts)

> EXCLUDES Brachytherapy (0394T-0395T)
> Radiation treatment delivery (77401)

3.61   3.61   **FUD** XXX   [S] [Z3] [80] [▭]

AMA: 2018,Jan,8; 2017,Jan,8; 2016,Sep,9; 2016,Feb,3; 2016,Jan,13

77336 Continuing medical physics consultation, including assessment of treatment parameters, quality assurance of dose delivery, and review of patient treatment documentation in support of the radiation oncologist, reported per week of therapy

> EXCLUDES Brachytherapy (0394T-0395T)
> Radiation treatment delivery (77401)

2.26   2.26   **FUD** XXX   [S] [Z2] [80] [TC] [▭]

AMA: 2018,Jan,8; 2017,Jan,8; 2016,Feb,3; 2016,Jan,13

77338 Multi-leaf collimator (MLC) device(s) for intensity modulated radiation therapy (IMRT), design and construction per IMRT plan

> EXCLUDES Immobilization in IMRT treatment (77332-77334)
> Intensity modulated radiation treatment delivery (IMRT) (77385)
> Reporting code more than one time per IMRT plan

14.1   14.1   **FUD** XXX   [S] [Z2] [80] [▭]

AMA: 2018,Jan,8; 2017,Jan,8; 2016,Jan,13

77370 Special medical radiation physics consultation

3.52   3.52   **FUD** XXX   [S] [Z2] [80] [TC] [▭]

AMA: 2018,Jan,8; 2017,Jan,8; 2016,Feb,3; 2016,Jan,13

77371-77399 [77385, 77386, 77387] Stereotactic Radiosurgery (SRS) Planning and Delivery

77371 Radiation treatment delivery, stereotactic radiosurgery (SRS), complete course of treatment of cranial lesion(s) consisting of 1 session; multi-source Cobalt 60 based

> EXCLUDES Guidance with computed tomography for radiation therapy field placement (77014)

0.00   0.00   **FUD** XXX   [J] [80] [TC] [▭]

AMA: 2018,Jan,8; 2017,Jan,8; 2016,Jan,13

77372 linear accelerator based

> EXCLUDES Guidance with computed tomography for radiation therapy field placement (77014)
> Radiation treatment supervision (77432)

30.2   30.2   **FUD** XXX   [J] [80] [TC] [▭]

AMA: 2018,Jan,8; 2017,Jan,8; 2016,Jan,13

77373 Stereotactic body radiation therapy, treatment delivery, per fraction to 1 or more lesions, including image guidance, entire course not to exceed 5 fractions

> EXCLUDES Guidance with computed tomography for radiation therapy field placement (77014)
> Intensity modulated radiation treatment delivery (IMRT) (77385-77386)
> Radiation treatment delivery (77401-77402, 77407, 77412)
> Single fraction cranial lesion(s) (77371-77372)

36.6   36.6   **FUD** XXX   [S] [80] [TC] [▭]

AMA: 2018,Jan,8; 2017,Jan,8; 2016,Jan,13

77385 Resequenced code. See code following 77417.

77386 Resequenced code. See code following 77417.

77387 Resequenced code. See code following 77417.

77399 Unlisted procedure, medical radiation physics, dosimetry and treatment devices, and special services

0.00   0.00   **FUD** XXX   [S] [Z2] [80] [▭]

AMA: 2018,Jan,8; 2017,Jan,8; 2016,Jan,13

● New Code ▲ Revised Code ○ Reinstated ● New Web Release ▲ Revised Web Release + Add-on Unlisted Not Covered # Resequenced
⑤⓪ Optum Mod 50 Exempt ⌀ AMA Mod 51 Exempt ⑤ⓘ Optum Mod 51 Exempt ⑥③ Mod 63 Exempt ✗ Non-FDA Drug ★ Telemedicine Ⓜ Maternity 🅐 Age Edit

77401-77425 [77385, 77386, 77387, 77424, 77425] Radiation Treatment

INCLUDES Technical component and assorted energy levels

77401 Radiation treatment delivery, superficial and/or ortho voltage, per day

EXCLUDES Continuing medical physics consultation (77336)
Isodose plan:
  Brachytherapy (77316-77318)
  Teletherapy (77306-77307)
Management:
  Intraoperative radiation treatment (77469-77470)
  Radiation therapy (77431-77432)
  Radiation treatment (77427)
  Stereotactic body radiation therapy (77435)
  Stereotactic body radiation therapy, treatment delivery (77373)
  Unlisted procedure, therapeutic radiology treatment management (77499)
Therapeutic radiology treatment planning (77261-77263)
Treatment devices, design and construction (77332-77334)
Code also E/M services when performed alone, as appropriate
🏥 0.70 👤 0.70 **FUD** XXX S Z3 80 TC 🖵
AMA: 2018,Jan,8; 2017,Jan,8; 2016,Feb,3; 2016,Jan,13

77402 Radiation treatment delivery, ≥1 MeV; simple
EXCLUDES Stereotactic body radiation therapy, treatment delivery (77373)
🏥 0.00 👤 0.00 **FUD** XXX S Z2 80 TC 🖵
AMA: 2018,Jan,8; 2017,Jan,8; 2016,Jun,9; 2016,Mar,7; 2016,Feb,3; 2016,Jan,13

77407 intermediate
EXCLUDES Stereotactic body radiation therapy, treatment delivery (77373)
🏥 0.00 👤 0.00 **FUD** XXX S Z2 80 TC 🖵
AMA: 2018,Jan,8; 2017,Jan,8; 2016,Jun,9; 2016,Mar,7; 2016,Feb,3; 2016,Jan,13

77412 complex
🏥 0.00 👤 0.00 **FUD** XXX S Z2 80 TC 🖵
AMA: 2018,Jan,8; 2017,Jan,8; 2016,Jun,9; 2016,Mar,7; 2016,Feb,3; 2016,Jan,13

77417 Therapeutic radiology port image(s)
🏥 0.32 👤 0.32 **FUD** XXX N N1 80 TC 🖵
AMA: 2018,Jan,8; 2017,Dec,14; 2017,Jan,8; 2016,Jan,13

\# **77385 Intensity modulated radiation treatment delivery (IMRT), includes guidance and tracking, when performed; simple**
🏥 0.00 👤 0.00 **FUD** XXX S Z2 80 TC 🖵
AMA: 2018,Jan,8; 2017,Jan,8; 2016,Feb,3

\# **77386 complex**
🏥 0.00 👤 0.00 **FUD** XXX S Z2 80 TC 🖵
AMA: 2018,Jan,8; 2017,Jan,8; 2016,Feb,3

\# **77387 Guidance for localization of target volume for delivery of radiation treatment, includes intrafraction tracking, when performed**
🏥 0.00 👤 0.00 **FUD** XXX N N1 80 🖵
AMA: 2018,Jan,8; 2017,Jan,8; 2016,Feb,3; 2016,Jan,13

\# **77424 Intraoperative radiation treatment delivery, x-ray, single treatment session**
🏥 0.00 👤 0.00 **FUD** XXX J Z2 🖵
AMA: 2018,Jan,8; 2017,Jan,8; 2016,Jan,13

\# **77425 Intraoperative radiation treatment delivery, electrons, single treatment session**
🏥 0.00 👤 0.00 **FUD** XXX J Z2 🖵
AMA: 2018,Jan,8; 2017,Jan,8; 2016,Jan,13

77423-77425 [77424, 77425] Neutron Therapy

77423 High energy neutron radiation treatment delivery, 1 or more isocenter(s) with coplanar or non-coplanar geometry with blocking and/or wedge, and/or compensator(s)
🏥 0.00 👤 0.00 **FUD** XXX S Z3 80 TC 🖵
AMA: 2018,Jan,8; 2017,Jan,8; 2016,Jan,13

77424 Resequenced code. See code following 77417.

77425 Resequenced code. See code following 77417.

77427-77499 Radiation Therapy Management

INCLUDES Assessment patient for medical evaluation and management (at least one per treatment management service) including:
  Coordination care/treatment
  Evaluation patient's response to treatment
Review:
  Dose delivery
  Dosimetry
  Lab tests
  Patient treatment set-up
  Port film
  Treatment parameters
  X-rays
Five fractions or treatment sessions regardless of time. Two or more fractions performed same day can be reported separately provided a distinct break in service exists between sessions and fractions are usually furnished on different days

EXCLUDES High dose rate electronic brachytherapy (0394T-0395T)
Radiation treatment delivery (77401)

77427 Radiation treatment management, 5 treatments
🏥 5.44 👤 5.44 **FUD** XXX B 26 🖵
AMA: 2018,Jan,8; 2017,Jan,8; 2016,Feb,3; 2016,Jan,13

77431 Radiation therapy management with complete course of therapy consisting of 1 or 2 fractions only
🏥 2.96 👤 2.96 **FUD** XXX B 80 26 🖵
AMA: 2018,Jan,8; 2017,Jan,8; 2016,Feb,3; 2016,Jan,13

77432 Stereotactic radiation treatment management of cranial lesion(s) (complete course of treatment consisting of 1 session)
🏥 12.1 👤 12.1 **FUD** XXX B 80 26 🖵
AMA: 2018,Jan,8; 2017,Jan,8; 2016,Feb,3; 2016,Jan,13

77435 Stereotactic body radiation therapy, treatment management, per treatment course, to 1 or more lesions, including image guidance, entire course not to exceed 5 fractions
🏥 18.1 👤 18.1 **FUD** XXX N N1 80 26 🖵
AMA: 2018,Jan,8; 2017,Jan,8; 2016,Feb,3; 2016,Jan,13

77469 Intraoperative radiation treatment management
🏥 9.00 👤 9.00 **FUD** XXX B 80 🖵
AMA: 2018,Jan,8; 2017,Jan,8; 2016,Feb,3

77470 Special treatment procedure (eg, total body irradiation, hemibody radiation, per oral or endocavitary irradiation)
🏥 3.79 👤 3.79 **FUD** XXX S Z3 80 🖵
AMA: 2018,Jan,8; 2017,Jan,8; 2016,Feb,3; 2016,Jan,13

77499 Unlisted procedure, therapeutic radiology treatment management
🏥 0.00 👤 0.00 **FUD** XXX B 80 🖵
AMA: 2018,Jan,8; 2017,Jan,8; 2016,Feb,3; 2016,Jan,13

77520-77525 Proton Therapy

EXCLUDES High dose rate electronic brachytherapy, per fraction (0394T-0395T)

77520 Proton treatment delivery; simple, without compensation
🏥 0.00 👤 0.00 **FUD** XXX S Z2 80 TC 🖵
AMA: 2018,Jan,8; 2017,Jan,8; 2016,Jan,13

77522 simple, with compensation
🏥 0.00 👤 0.00 **FUD** XXX S Z2 80 TC 🖵
AMA: 2012,Feb,9-10; 2010,Oct,3-4

77523 intermediate
🏥 0.00 👤 0.00 **FUD** XXX S Z2 80 TC 🖵
AMA: 2018,Jan,8; 2017,Jan,8; 2016,Jan,13

77525	complex

🚑 0.00 ⚕ 0.00 **FUD** XXX   [S] [Z2] [80] [TC] [▭]

AMA: 2012,Feb,9-10; 2010,Oct,3-4

77600-77620 Hyperthermia Treatment

CMS: 100-03,110.1 Hyperthermia for Treatment of Cancer

INCLUDES Heat generating devices
Interstitial insertion temperature sensors
Management during course therapy
Normal follow-up care for three months after completion
Physics planning

EXCLUDES *Initial E/M service*
Radiation therapy treatment (77371-77373, 77401-77412, 77423)

77600 **Hyperthermia, externally generated; superficial (ie, heating to a depth of 4 cm or less)**

🚑 12.7 ⚕ 12.7 **FUD** XXX   [S] [Z2] [80] [▭]

AMA: 2018,Jan,8; 2017,Jan,8; 2016,Jan,13

77605 **deep (ie, heating to depths greater than 4 cm)**

🚑 22.0 ⚕ 22.0 **FUD** XXX   [S] [Z2] [80] [▭]

AMA: 2018,Jan,8; 2017,Jan,8; 2016,Jan,13

77610 **Hyperthermia generated by interstitial probe(s); 5 or fewer interstitial applicators**

🚑 19.2 ⚕ 19.2 **FUD** XXX   [S] [Z2] [80] [▭]

AMA: 2018,Jan,8; 2017,Jan,8; 2016,Jan,13

77615 **more than 5 interstitial applicators**

🚑 30.1 ⚕ 30.1 **FUD** XXX   [S] [Z2] [80] [▭]

AMA: 2018,Jan,8; 2017,Jan,8; 2016,Jan,13

77620 **Hyperthermia generated by intracavitary probe(s)**

🚑 17.3 ⚕ 17.3 **FUD** XXX   [S] [Z2] [80] [▭]

AMA: 2018,Jan,8; 2017,Jan,8; 2016,Jan,13

77750-77799 Brachytherapy

CMS: 100-04,13,70.4 Clinical Brachytherapy; 100-04,13,70.5 Radiation Physics Services; 100-04,4,61.4.4 Billing for Brachytherapy Source Supervision, Handling and Loading Costs

INCLUDES Hospital admission and daily visits

EXCLUDES *Placement:*
Heyman capsules (58346)
Ovoids and tandems (57155)

77750 **Infusion or instillation of radioelement solution (includes 3-month follow-up care)**

🚑 10.9 ⚕ 10.9 **FUD** 090   [S] [Z2] [80] [▭]

AMA: 2018,Jan,8; 2017,Jan,8; 2016,Jan,13

77761 **Intracavitary radiation source application; simple**

🚑 11.4 ⚕ 11.4 **FUD** 090   [S] [Z3] [80] [▭]

AMA: 2018,Jan,8; 2017,Jan,8; 2016,Jan,13

77762 **intermediate**

🚑 15.1 ⚕ 15.1 **FUD** 090   [S] [Z3] [80] [▭]

AMA: 2018,Jan,8; 2017,Jan,8; 2016,Jan,13

77763 **complex**

🚑 21.4 ⚕ 21.4 **FUD** 090   [S] [Z3] [80] [▭]

AMA: 2018,Jan,8; 2017,Jan,8; 2016,Jan,13

77767 **Remote afterloading high dose rate radionuclide skin surface brachytherapy, includes basic dosimetry, when performed; lesion diameter up to 2.0 cm or 1 channel**

🚑 6.78 ⚕ 6.78 **FUD** XXX   [S] [Z2] [80] [▭]

77768 **lesion diameter over 2.0 cm and 2 or more channels, or multiple lesions**

🚑 10.1 ⚕ 10.1 **FUD** XXX   [S] [Z2] [80] [▭]

77770 **Remote afterloading high dose rate radionuclide interstitial or intracavitary brachytherapy, includes basic dosimetry, when performed; 1 channel**

🚑 9.51 ⚕ 9.51 **FUD** XXX   [S] [Z3] [80] [▭]

77771 **2-12 channels**

🚑 16.9 ⚕ 16.9 **FUD** XXX   [S] [Z2] [80] [▭]

77772 **over 12 channels**

🚑 25.5 ⚕ 25.5 **FUD** XXX   [S] [Z2] [80] [▭]

77778 **Interstitial radiation source application, complex, includes supervision, handling, loading of radiation source, when performed**

🚑 24.5 ⚕ 24.5 **FUD** 000   [S] [Z2] [80] [▭]

AMA: 2018,Jan,8; 2017,Jan,8; 2016,Jan,13

77789 **Surface application of low dose rate radionuclide source**

🚑 3.63 ⚕ 3.63 **FUD** 000   [S] [Z2] [60] [▭]

AMA: 2018,Jan,8; 2017,Jan,8; 2016,Jan,13

77790 **Supervision, handling, loading of radiation source**

🚑 0.43 ⚕ 0.43 **FUD** XXX   [N] [N1] [80] [TC] [▭]

AMA: 2018,Jan,8; 2017,Jan,8; 2016,Jan,13

77799 **Unlisted procedure, clinical brachytherapy**

🚑 0.00 ⚕ 0.00 **FUD** XXX   [S] [Z2] [80] [▭]

AMA: 2018,Jan,8; 2017,Jan,8; 2016,Jan,13

78012-78099 Nuclear Radiology: Thyroid, Parathyroid, Adrenal

EXCLUDES *Diagnostic services (see appropriate sections)*
Follow-up care (see appropriate section)
Code also radiopharmaceutical(s) and/or drug(s) supplied

78012 **Thyroid uptake, single or multiple quantitative measurement(s) (including stimulation, suppression, or discharge, when performed)**

🚑 2.34 ⚕ 2.34 **FUD** XXX   [S] [Z2] [80] [▭]

AMA: 2018,Jan,8; 2017,Jan,8; 2016,Jan,13

78013 **Thyroid imaging (including vascular flow, when performed);**

🚑 5.54 ⚕ 5.54 **FUD** XXX   [S] [Z2] [80] [▭]

AMA: 2018,Jan,8; 2017,Jan,8; 2016,Jan,13

78014 **with single or multiple uptake(s) quantitative measurement(s) (including stimulation, suppression, or discharge, when performed)**

🚑 6.86 ⚕ 6.86 **FUD** XXX   [S] [Z2] [80] [▭]

AMA: 2018,Jan,8; 2017,Jan,8; 2016,Jan,13

78015 **Thyroid carcinoma metastases imaging; limited area (eg, neck and chest only)**

🚑 6.43 ⚕ 6.43 **FUD** XXX   [S] [Z2] [80] [▭]

AMA: 2018,Jan,8; 2017,Jan,8; 2016,Jan,13

78016 **with additional studies (eg, urinary recovery)**

🚑 8.12 ⚕ 8.12 **FUD** XXX   [S] [Z2] [80] [▭]

AMA: 2018,Jan,8; 2017,Jan,8; 2016,Jan,13

78018 **whole body**

🚑 8.96 ⚕ 8.96 **FUD** XXX   [S] [Z2] [60] [▭]

AMA: 2018,Jan,8; 2017,Jan,8; 2016,Jan,13

+ 78020 **Thyroid carcinoma metastases uptake (List separately in addition to code for primary procedure)**

Code first (78018)

🚑 2.37 ⚕ 2.37 **FUD** ZZZ   [N] [N1] [80] [▭]

AMA: 2018,Jan,8; 2017,Jan,8; 2016,Jan,13

78070 **Parathyroid planar imaging (including subtraction, when performed);**

EXCLUDES *Distribution radiopharmaceutical agents or tumor localization (78800-78802, [78804], 78803)*
Radiopharmaceutical quantification measurements ([78835])
SPECT with concurrently acquired CT transmission scan ([78830, 78831, 78832])

🚑 8.48 ⚕ 8.48 **FUD** XXX   [S] [Z2] [80] [▭]

AMA: 2020,Oct,3; 2018,Jan,8; 2017,Jan,8; 2016,Dec,9; 2016,Dec,16; 2016,Jan,13

78071   **with tomographic (SPECT)**

> EXCLUDES   *Distribution radiopharmaceutical agents or tumor localization (78800-78802, [78804], 78803)*
> *Radiopharmaceutical quantification measurements ([78835])*
> *SPECT with concurrently acquired CT transmission scan ([78830, 78831, 78832])*

🚗 10.1   ⚖ 10.1   **FUD** XXX   S Z2 80 ▢

AMA: 2020,Oct,3; 2018,Jan,8; 2017,Jan,8; 2016,Dec,16; 2016,Dec,9

78072   **with tomographic (SPECT), and concurrently acquired computed tomography (CT) for anatomical localization**

> EXCLUDES   *Distribution radiopharmaceutical agents or tumor localization (78800-78802, [78804], 78803)*
> *Radiopharmaceutical quantification measurements ([78835])*
> *SPECT with concurrently acquired CT transmission scan ([78830, 78831, 78832])*

🚗 12.7   ⚖ 12.7   **FUD** XXX   S Z2 80 ▢

AMA: 2020,Oct,3; 2018,Jan,8; 2017,Jan,8; 2016,Dec,16; 2016,Dec,9

78075   **Adrenal imaging, cortex and/or medulla**

🚗 13.0   ⚖ 13.0   **FUD** XXX   S Z2 80 ▢

AMA: 2018,Jan,8; 2017,Jan,8; 2016,Jan,13

78099   **Unlisted endocrine procedure, diagnostic nuclear medicine**

🚗 0.00   ⚖ 0.00   **FUD** XXX   S Z2 80 ▢

AMA: 2018,Jan,8; 2017,Jan,8; 2016,Dec,9; 2016,Jan,13

Lateral view

Anterior view

Thyroglossal duct (dotted line)
Hyoid bone
Thyroid cartilage
Cricoid cartilage
Cricothyroid muscle
Thyroid gland
Trachea
Esophagus

Epiglottis
Hyoid bone
Pyramid lobe
Thyroid cartilage
Cricoid cartilage
Thyroid gland
Isthmus

78102-78199 Nuclear Radiology: Blood Forming Organs

> EXCLUDES   *Diagnostic services (see appropriate sections)*
> *Follow-up care (see appropriate section)*
> *Radioimmunoassays (82009-84999 [82042, 82652])*
> Code also radiopharmaceutical(s) and/or drug(s) supplied

78102   **Bone marrow imaging; limited area**

🚗 4.89   ⚖ 4.89   **FUD** XXX   S Z2 80 ▢

AMA: 2018,Jan,8; 2017,Jan,8; 2016,Jan,13

78103   **multiple areas**

🚗 6.27   ⚖ 6.27   **FUD** XXX   S Z2 80 ▢

AMA: 2012,Feb,9-10; 2007,Jan,28-31

78104   **whole body**

🚗 7.14   ⚖ 7.14   **FUD** XXX   S Z2 80 ▢

AMA: 2012,Feb,9-10; 2007,Jan,28-31

78110   **Plasma volume, radiopharmaceutical volume-dilution technique (separate procedure); single sampling**

🚗 1.99   ⚖ 1.99   **FUD** XXX   S Z2 80 ▢

AMA: 2012,Feb,9-10; 2007,Jan,28-31

78111   **multiple samplings**

🚗 2.11   ⚖ 2.11   **FUD** XXX   S Z2 80 ▢

AMA: 2012,Feb,9-10; 2007,Jan,28-31

78120   **Red cell volume determination (separate procedure); single sampling**

🚗 2.04   ⚖ 2.04   **FUD** XXX   S Z2 80 ▢

AMA: 2012,Feb,9-10; 2007,Jan,28-31

78121   **multiple samplings**

🚗 2.23   ⚖ 2.23   **FUD** XXX   S Z2 80 ▢

AMA: 2012,Feb,9-10; 2007,Jan,28-31

78122   **Whole blood volume determination, including separate measurement of plasma volume and red cell volume (radiopharmaceutical volume-dilution technique)**

🚗 2.75   ⚖ 2.75   **FUD** XXX   S Z2 80 ▢

AMA: 2012,Feb,9-10; 2007,Jan,28-31

78130   **Red cell survival study**

🚗 3.56   ⚖ 3.56   **FUD** XXX   S Z2 80 ▢

AMA: 2012,Feb,9-10; 2007,Jan,28-31

78140   **Labeled red cell sequestration, differential organ/tissue (eg, splenic and/or hepatic)**

🚗 3.19   ⚖ 3.19   **FUD** XXX   S Z2 80 ▢

AMA: 2012,Feb,9-10; 2007,Jan,28-31

78185   **Spleen imaging only, with or without vascular flow**

> EXCLUDES   *Liver imaging (78215-78216)*

🚗 4.88   ⚖ 4.88   **FUD** XXX   S Z2 80 ▢

AMA: 2012,Feb,9-10; 2007,Jan,28-31

78191   **Platelet survival study**

🚗 3.59   ⚖ 3.59   **FUD** XXX   S Z2 80 ▢

AMA: 2012,Feb,9-10; 2007,Jan,28-31

78195   **Lymphatics and lymph nodes imaging**

> EXCLUDES   *Sentinel node identification without scintigraphy (38792)*
> *Sentinel node removal (38500-38542)*

🚗 10.1   ⚖ 10.1   **FUD** XXX   S Z2 80 ▢

AMA: 2018,Jan,8; 2017,Jan,8; 2016,Jan,13

78199   **Unlisted hematopoietic, reticuloendothelial and lymphatic procedure, diagnostic nuclear medicine**

🚗 0.00   ⚖ 0.00   **FUD** XXX   S Z2 80 ▢

AMA: 2018,Jan,8; 2017,Jan,8; 2016,Jan,13

78201-78299 Nuclear Radiology: Digestive System

> EXCLUDES   *Diagnostic services (see appropriate sections)*
> *Follow-up care (see appropriate section)*
> Code also radiopharmaceutical(s) and/or drug(s) supplied

78201   **Liver imaging; static only**

> EXCLUDES   *Spleen imaging only (78185)*

🚗 5.46   ⚖ 5.46   **FUD** XXX   S Z2 80 ▢

AMA: 2018,Jan,8; 2017,Jan,8; 2016,Jan,13

78202   **with vascular flow**

> EXCLUDES   *Spleen imaging only (78185)*

🚗 5.88   ⚖ 5.88   **FUD** XXX   S Z2 80 ▢

AMA: 2012,Feb,9-10; 2007,Jan,28-31

78215   **Liver and spleen imaging; static only**

🚗 5.59   ⚖ 5.59   **FUD** XXX   S Z2 80 ▢

AMA: 2012,Feb,9-10; 2007,Jan,28-31

78216   **with vascular flow**

🚗 3.69   ⚖ 3.69   **FUD** XXX   S Z2 80 ▢

AMA: 2012,Feb,9-10; 2007,Jan,28-31

78226   **Hepatobiliary system imaging, including gallbladder when present;**

🚗 9.38   ⚖ 9.38   **FUD** XXX   S Z2 80 ▢

AMA: 2012,Feb,9-10

2B/TB PC/TC Only   A2-Z3 ASC Payment   50 Bilateral   ♂ Male Only   ♀ Female Only   🚗 Facility RVU   ⚖ Non-Facility RVU   ▢ CCI   ✖ CLIA
FUD Follow-up Days   **CMS:** IOM   **AMA:** CPT Asst   A-Y OPPSI   80/80 Surg Assist Allowed / w/Doc   ▤ Lab Crosswalk   ▣ Radiology Crosswalk

348   CPT © 2021 American Medical Association. All Rights Reserved.   © 2021 Optum360, LLC

78227 with pharmacologic intervention, including quantitative measurement(s) when performed
🔪 12.6   ⚖ 12.6   **FUD** XXX
S Z2 80 ▱
AMA: 2012,Feb,9-10

78230 Salivary gland imaging;
🔪 5.03   ⚖ 5.03   **FUD** XXX
S Z2 80 ▱
AMA: 2012,Feb,9-10; 2007,Jan,28-31

78231 with serial images
🔪 3.02   ⚖ 3.02   **FUD** XXX
S Z2 80 ▱
AMA: 2012,Feb,9-10; 2007,Jan,28-31

78232 Salivary gland function study
🔪 2.96   ⚖ 2.96   **FUD** XXX
S Z2 80 ▱
AMA: 2012,Feb,9-10; 2007,Jan,28-31

78258 Esophageal motility
🔪 6.19   ⚖ 6.19   **FUD** XXX
S Z2 80 ▱
AMA: 2012,Feb,9-10; 2007,Jan,28-31

78261 Gastric mucosa imaging
🔪 5.84   ⚖ 5.84   **FUD** XXX
S Z2 80 ▱
AMA: 2012,Feb,9-10; 2007,Jan,28-31

78262 Gastroesophageal reflux study
🔪 6.86   ⚖ 6.86   **FUD** XXX
S Z2 80 ▱
AMA: 2018,Jan,8; 2017,Jan,8; 2016,Jan,13

78264 Gastric emptying imaging study (eg, solid, liquid, or both);
EXCLUDES *Procedure performed more than one time per study*
🔪 9.52   ⚖ 9.52   **FUD** XXX
S Z2 80 ▱
AMA: 2018,Jan,8; 2017,Jan,8; 2016,Jan,13

78265 with small bowel transit
EXCLUDES *Procedure performed more than one time per study*
🔪 11.2   ⚖ 11.2   **FUD** XXX
S Z2 80 ▱
AMA: 2018,Jan,8; 2017,Jan,8

78266 with small bowel and colon transit, multiple days
EXCLUDES *Procedure performed more than one time per study*
🔪 12.3   ⚖ 12.3   **FUD** XXX
S Z2 80 ▱
AMA: 2018,Jan,8; 2017,Jan,8

78267 Urea breath test, C-14 (isotopic); acquisition for analysis
EXCLUDES *Breath hydrogen/methane test (91065)*
🔪 0.00   ⚖ 0.00   **FUD** XXX
A ▱
AMA: 2020,OctSE,1; 2020,OctSE,1; 2018,Jan,8; 2017,Jan,8; 2016,Jan,13

78268 analysis
EXCLUDES *Breath hydrogen/methane test (91065)*
🔪 0.00   ⚖ 0.00   **FUD** XXX
A ▱
AMA: 2020,OctSE,1; 2020,OctSE,1; 2018,Jan,8; 2017,Jan,8; 2016,Jan,13

78278 Acute gastrointestinal blood loss imaging
🔪 9.97   ⚖ 9.97   **FUD** XXX
S Z2 80 ▱
AMA: 2012,Feb,9-10; 2007,Jan,28-31

78282 Gastrointestinal protein loss
🔪 0.00   ⚖ 0.00   **FUD** XXX
S Z2 80 ▱
AMA: 2018,Jul,14

78290 Intestine imaging (eg, ectopic gastric mucosa, Meckel's localization, volvulus)
🔪 9.44   ⚖ 9.44   **FUD** XXX
S Z2 80 ▱
AMA: 2012,Feb,9-10; 2007,Jan,28-31

78291 Peritoneal-venous shunt patency test (eg, for LeVeen, Denver shunt)
Code also (49427)
🔪 7.30   ⚖ 7.30   **FUD** XXX
S Z2 80 ▱
AMA: 2012,Feb,9-10; 2007,Jan,28-31

78299 Unlisted gastrointestinal procedure, diagnostic nuclear medicine
🔪 0.00   ⚖ 0.00   **FUD** XXX
S Z2 80 ▱
AMA: 2018,Jan,8; 2017,Jan,8; 2016,Jan,13

78300-78399 Nuclear Radiology: Bones and Joints

EXCLUDES *Diagnostic services (see appropriate sections)*
Follow-up care (see appropriate section)
Code also radiopharmaceutical(s) and/or drug(s) supplied

78300 Bone and/or joint imaging; limited area
🔪 6.56   ⚖ 6.56   **FUD** XXX
S Z2 80 ▱
AMA: 2020,Oct,3; 2018,Jan,8; 2017,Jan,8; 2016,Jan,13

78305 multiple areas
🔪 8.08   ⚖ 8.08   **FUD** XXX
S Z2 80 ▱
AMA: 2020,Oct,3; 2018,Jan,8; 2017,Jan,8; 2016,Jan,13

78306 whole body
🔪 8.71   ⚖ 8.71   **FUD** XXX
S Z2 80 ▱
AMA: 2020,Oct,3; 2018,Jan,8; 2017,Jan,8; 2016,Jan,13

78315 3 phase study
🔪 9.91   ⚖ 9.91   **FUD** XXX
S Z2 80 ▱
AMA: 2020,Oct,3; 2018,Jan,8; 2017,Jan,8; 2016,Jan,13

78350 Bone density (bone mineral content) study, 1 or more sites; single photon absorptiometry
🔪 0.91   ⚖ 0.91   **FUD** XXX
E ▱
AMA: 2012,Feb,9-10; 2007,Jan,28-31

78351 dual photon absorptiometry, 1 or more sites
🔪 0.44   ⚖ 0.44   **FUD** XXX
E ▱
AMA: 2012,Feb,9-10; 2007,Jan,28-31

78399 Unlisted musculoskeletal procedure, diagnostic nuclear medicine
🔪 0.00   ⚖ 0.00   **FUD** XXX
S Z2 80 ▱
AMA: 2018,Jan,8; 2017,Jan,8; 2016,Jan,13

78414-78499 [78429, 78430, 78431, 78432, 78433, 78434] Nuclear Radiology: Heart and Vascular

EXCLUDES *Diagnostic services (see appropriate sections)*
Follow-up care (see appropriate section)
Code also radiopharmaceutical(s) and/or drug(s) supplied

78414 Determination of central c-v hemodynamics (non-imaging) (eg, ejection fraction with probe technique) with or without pharmacologic intervention or exercise, single or multiple determinations
🔪 0.00   ⚖ 0.00   **FUD** XXX
S Z2 80 ▱
AMA: 2018,Jan,8; 2017,Jan,8; 2016,Jan,13

78428 Cardiac shunt detection
🔪 5.30   ⚖ 5.30   **FUD** XXX
S Z2 80 ▱
AMA: 2018,Jan,8; 2017,Jan,8; 2016,Jan,13

78429 Resequenced code. See code following 78459.

78430 Resequenced code. See code following 78491.

78431 Resequenced code. See code following 78492.

78432 Resequenced code. See code following 78492.

78433 Resequenced code. See code following 78492.

78434 Resequenced code. See code following 78492.

78445 Non-cardiac vascular flow imaging (ie, angiography, venography)
🔪 5.60   ⚖ 5.60   **FUD** XXX
S Z2 80 ▱
AMA: 2018,Jan,8; 2017,Jan,8; 2016,Jan,13

78451 Myocardial perfusion imaging, tomographic (SPECT) (including attenuation correction, qualitative or quantitative wall motion, ejection fraction by first pass or gated technique, additional quantification, when performed); single study, at rest or stress (exercise or pharmacologic)
EXCLUDES *Distribution radiopharmaceutical agents or tumor localization (78800-78802, [78804], 78803)*
Radiopharmaceutical quantification measurements ([78835])
SPECT with concurrently acquired CT transmission scan ([78830, 78831, 78832])
Code also stress testing when performed (93015-93018)
🔪 9.63   ⚖ 9.63   **FUD** XXX
S Z2 80 ▱
AMA: 2020,Oct,3; 2020,Jul,5; 2018,Jan,8; 2017,Jan,8; 2016,Jan,13

Radiology

78452 — 78492

78452 multiple studies, at rest and/or stress (exercise or pharmacologic) and/or redistribution and/or rest reinjection

> EXCLUDES   Distribution radiopharmaceutical agents or tumor localization (78800-78802, [78804], 78803)
> Radiopharmaceutical quantification measurements ([78835])
> SPECT with concurrently acquired CT transmission scan ([78830, 78831, 78832])
> Code also stress testing when performed (93015-93018)
> 🚑 13.4   ⚕ 13.4   **FUD** XXX   S Z2 80 ▭

> **AMA:** 2020,Oct,3; 2020,Jul,5; 2018,Jan,8; 2017,Jan,8; 2016,Jan,13

78453 Myocardial perfusion imaging, planar (including qualitative or quantitative wall motion, ejection fraction by first pass or gated technique, additional quantification, when performed); single study, at rest or stress (exercise or pharmacologic)

> Code also stress testing when performed (93015-93018)
> 🚑 8.78   ⚕ 8.78   **FUD** XXX   S Z2 80 ▭

> **AMA:** 2020,Jul,5; 2018,Jan,8; 2017,Jan,8; 2016,Jan,13

78454 multiple studies, at rest and/or stress (exercise or pharmacologic) and/or redistribution and/or rest reinjection

> Code also stress testing when performed (93015-93018)
> 🚑 12.4   ⚕ 12.4   **FUD** XXX   S Z2 80 ▭

> **AMA:** 2020,Jul,5; 2018,Jan,8; 2017,Jan,8; 2016,Jan,13

78456 Acute venous thrombosis imaging, peptide
> 🚑 8.82   ⚕ 8.82   **FUD** XXX   S Z2 ▭

> **AMA:** 2018,Jan,8; 2017,Jan,8; 2016,Jan,13

78457 Venous thrombosis imaging, venogram; unilateral
> 🚑 5.02   ⚕ 5.02   **FUD** XXX   S Z2 80 ▭

> **AMA:** 2018,Jan,8; 2017,Jan,8; 2016,Jan,13

78458 bilateral
> 🚑 5.88   ⚕ 5.88   **FUD** XXX   S Z2 80 ▭

> **AMA:** 2018,Jan,8; 2017,Jan,8; 2016,Jan,13

78459 Myocardial imaging, positron emission tomography (PET), metabolic evaluation study (including ventricular wall motion[s] and/or ejection fraction[s], when performed), single study;

> INCLUDES   Examination CT transmission images for field of view anatomy review
> EXCLUDES   CT coronary calcium scoring (75571)
> CT for other than attenuation correction/anatomical localization; report site-specific CT code with modifier 59
> Myocardial perfusion studies (78491-78492)
> 🚑 0.00   ⚕ 0.00   **FUD** XXX   S Z2 80 ▭

> **AMA:** 2020,Jul,5; 2018,Jan,8; 2017,Jan,8; 2016,Jan,13

\#   **78429** with concurrently acquired computed tomography transmission scan

> INCLUDES   Examination CT transmission images for field of view anatomy review
> EXCLUDES   CT coronary calcium scoring (75571)
> CT for other than attenuation correction/anatomical localization; report site-specific CT code with modifier 59
> 🚑 0.00   ⚕ 0.00   **FUD** XXX   Z2 80 ▭

> **AMA:** 2020,Jul,5

78466 Myocardial imaging, infarct avid, planar; qualitative or quantitative
> 🚑 5.67   ⚕ 5.67   **FUD** XXX   S Z2 80 ▭

> **AMA:** 2012,Feb,9-10; 2010,May,5-6

78468 with ejection fraction by first pass technique
> 🚑 5.51   ⚕ 5.51   **FUD** XXX   S Z2 80 ▭

> **AMA:** 2018,Jan,8; 2017,Jan,8; 2016,Jan,13

78469 tomographic SPECT with or without quantification

> EXCLUDES   Distribution radiopharmaceutical agents or tumor localization (78800-78802, [78804], 78803)
> Myocardial sympathetic innervation imaging (0331T-0332T)
> Radiopharmaceutical quantification measurements ([78835])
> SPECT with concurrently acquired CT transmission scan ([78830, 78831, 78832])
> 🚑 6.39   ⚕ 6.39   **FUD** XXX   S Z2 80 ▭

> **AMA:** 2020,Oct,3; 2018,Nov,11; 2018,Jan,8; 2017,Jan,8; 2016,Jan,13

78472 Cardiac blood pool imaging, gated equilibrium; planar, single study at rest or stress (exercise and/or pharmacologic), wall motion study plus ejection fraction, with or without additional quantitative processing

> EXCLUDES   Cardiac blood pool imaging (78481, 78483, 78494)
> Myocardial perfusion imaging (78451-78454)
> Right ventricular ejection fraction by first pass technique (78496)
> Code also stress testing when performed (93015-93018)
> 🚑 6.51   ⚕ 6.51   **FUD** XXX   S Z2 80 ▭

> **AMA:** 2018,Jan,8; 2017,Jan,8; 2016,Jan,13

78473 multiple studies, wall motion study plus ejection fraction, at rest and stress (exercise and/or pharmacologic), with or without additional quantification

> EXCLUDES   Cardiac blood pool imaging (78481, 78483, 78494)
> Myocardial perfusion imaging (78451-78454)
> Code also stress testing when performed (93015-93018)
> 🚑 8.26   ⚕ 8.26   **FUD** XXX   S Z2 80 ▭

> **AMA:** 2018,Jan,8; 2017,Jan,8; 2016,Jan,13

78481 Cardiac blood pool imaging (planar), first pass technique; single study, at rest or with stress (exercise and/or pharmacologic), wall motion study plus ejection fraction, with or without quantification

> EXCLUDES   Myocardial perfusion imaging (78451-78454)
> Code also stress testing when performed (93015-93018)
> 🚑 5.03   ⚕ 5.03   **FUD** XXX   S Z2 80 ▭

> **AMA:** 2018,Jan,8; 2017,Jan,8; 2016,Jan,13

78483 multiple studies, at rest and with stress (exercise and/or pharmacologic), wall motion study plus ejection fraction, with or without quantification

> EXCLUDES   Blood flow studies brain (78610)
> Myocardial perfusion imaging (78451-78454)
> Code also stress testing when performed (93015-93018)
> 🚑 6.89   ⚕ 6.89   **FUD** XXX   S Z2 80 ▭

> **AMA:** 2018,Jan,8; 2017,Jan,8; 2016,Jan,13

78491 Myocardial imaging, positron emission tomography (PET), perfusion study (including ventricular wall motion[s] and/or ejection fraction[s], when performed); single study, at rest or stress (exercise or pharmacologic)

> Code also stress testing when performed (93015-93018)
> 🚑 0.00   ⚕ 0.00   **FUD** XXX   S Z2 80 ▭

> **AMA:** 2020,Jul,5; 2018,Jan,8; 2017,Jan,8; 2016,Jan,13

\#   **78430** single study, at rest or stress (exercise or pharmacologic), with concurrently acquired computed tomography transmission scan

> INCLUDES   Examination CT transmission images for field of view anatomy review
> Code also stress testing when performed (93015-93018)
> 🚑 0.00   ⚕ 0.00   **FUD** XXX   Z2 80 ▭

> **AMA:** 2020,Jul,5

78492 multiple studies at rest and stress (exercise or pharmacologic)

> Code also stress testing when performed (93015-93018)
> 🚑 0.00   ⚕ 0.00   **FUD** XXX   S Z2 80 ▭

> **AMA:** 2020,Jul,5; 2018,Jan,8; 2017,Jan,8; 2016,Jan,13

| 26/TC PC/TC Only | A2-Z3 ASC Payment | 50 Bilateral | ♂ Male Only | ♀ Female Only | 🚑 Facility RVU | ⚕ Non-Facility RVU | ▭ CCI | ✖ CLIA |
| FUD Follow-up Days | CMS: IOM | AMA: CPT Asst | A-Y OPPSI | 80/80 Surg Assist Allowed / w/Doc | 🔬 Lab Crosswalk | | 🔀 Radiology Crosswalk | |

350   CPT © 2021 American Medical Association. All Rights Reserved.   © 2021 Optum360, LLC

78431 multiple studies at rest and stress (exercise or pharmacologic), with concurrently acquired computed tomography transmission scan

INCLUDES Examination CT transmission images for field of view anatomy review

Code also stress testing when performed (93015-93018)

📷 2.62   🔍 2.62   **FUD** XXX   Z2 80 ▣

AMA: 2020,Jul,5

78432 Myocardial imaging, positron emission tomography (PET), combined perfusion with metabolic evaluation study (including ventricular wall motion[s] and/or ejection fraction[s], when performed), dual radiotracer (eg, myocardial viability);

Code also stress testing when performed (93015-93018)

📷 0.00   🔍 0.00   **FUD** XXX   Z2 80 ▣

AMA: 2020,Jul,5

78433 with concurrently acquired computed tomography transmission scan

INCLUDES Examination CT transmission images for field of view anatomy review

EXCLUDES CT for other than attenuation correction/anatomical localization; use site-specific CT code with modifier 59

Code also stress testing when performed (93015-93018)

📷 0.00   🔍 0.00   **FUD** XXX   Z2 80 ▣

AMA: 2020,Jul,5

+ # 78434 Absolute quantitation of myocardial blood flow (AQMBF), positron emission tomography (PET), rest and pharmacologic stress (List separately in addition to code for primary procedure)

EXCLUDES CT coronary calcium scoring (75571)
Myocardial imaging by planar or SPECT (78451-78454)

Code first ([78431], 78492)

📷 0.00   🔍 0.00   **FUD** ZZZ   N1 80 ▣

AMA: 2020,Jul,5

78494 Cardiac blood pool imaging, gated equilibrium, SPECT, at rest, wall motion study plus ejection fraction, with or without quantitative processing

EXCLUDES Distribution radiopharmaceutical agents or tumor localization (78800-78802, [78804], 78803)
Radiopharmaceutical quantification measurements ([78835])
SPECT with concurrently acquired CT transmission scan ([78830, 78831, 78832])

📷 6.47   🔍 6.47   **FUD** XXX   S Z2 80 ▣

AMA: 2020,Oct,3; 2018,Jan,8; 2017,Jan,8; 2016,Jan,13

+ 78496 Cardiac blood pool imaging, gated equilibrium, single study, at rest, with right ventricular ejection fraction by first pass technique (List separately in addition to code for primary procedure)

Code first (78472)

📷 1.23   🔍 1.23   **FUD** ZZZ   N N1 80 ▣

AMA: 2018,Jan,8; 2017,Jan,8; 2016,Jan,13

78499 Unlisted cardiovascular procedure, diagnostic nuclear medicine

📷 0.00   🔍 0.00   **FUD** XXX   S Z2 80 ▣

AMA: 2018,Jan,8; 2017,Jan,8; 2016,Jan,13

78579-78599 Nuclear Radiology: Lungs

EXCLUDES Diagnostic services (see appropriate sections)
Follow-up care (see appropriate sections)

Code also radiopharmaceutical(s) and/or drug(s) supplied

78579 Pulmonary ventilation imaging (eg, aerosol or gas)

EXCLUDES Procedure performed more than one time per imaging session

📷 5.36   🔍 5.36   **FUD** XXX   S Z2 80 ▣

AMA: 2012,Feb,9-10

78580 Pulmonary perfusion imaging (eg, particulate)

EXCLUDES Myocardial perfusion imaging (78451-78454)
Procedure performed more than one time per imaging session

📷 6.77   🔍 6.77   **FUD** XXX   S Z2 80 ▣

AMA: 2018,Jan,8; 2017,Jan,8; 2016,Jan,13

78582 Pulmonary ventilation (eg, aerosol or gas) and perfusion imaging

EXCLUDES Myocardial perfusion imaging (78451-78454)
Procedure performed more than one time per imaging session

📷 9.54   🔍 9.54   **FUD** XXX   S Z2 80 ▣

AMA: 2012,Feb,9-10

78597 Quantitative differential pulmonary perfusion, including imaging when performed

EXCLUDES Myocardial perfusion imaging (78451-78454)
Procedure performed more than one time per imaging session

📷 5.74   🔍 5.74   **FUD** XXX   S Z2 80 ▣

AMA: 2012,Feb,9-10

78598 Quantitative differential pulmonary perfusion and ventilation (eg, aerosol or gas), including imaging when performed

EXCLUDES Myocardial perfusion imaging (78451-78454)
Procedure performed more than one time per imaging session

📷 8.70   🔍 8.70   **FUD** XXX   S Z2 80 ▣

AMA: 2012,Feb,9-10

78599 Unlisted respiratory procedure, diagnostic nuclear medicine

📷 0.00   🔍 0.00   **FUD** XXX   S Z2 80 ▣

AMA: 2018,Jan,8; 2017,Jan,8; 2016,Jan,13

78600-78650 Nuclear Radiology: Brain/Cerebrospinal Fluid

EXCLUDES Diagnostic services (see appropriate sections)
Follow-up care (see appropriate section)

Code also radiopharmaceutical(s) and/or drug(s) supplied

78600 Brain imaging, less than 4 static views;

📷 5.26   🔍 5.26   **FUD** XXX   S Z2 80 ▣

AMA: 2018,Jan,8; 2017,Jan,8; 2016,Jan,13

X-ray beam

Linear focal plane

Schematic of frontal coronal CT section of skull

78601 with vascular flow

📷 6.20   🔍 6.20   **FUD** XXX   S Z2 80 ▣

AMA: 2012,Feb,9-10; 2007,Jan,28-31

78605 Brain imaging, minimum 4 static views;

📷 5.71   🔍 5.71   **FUD** XXX   S Z2 80 ▣

AMA: 2012,Feb,9-10; 2007,Jan,28-31

78606 with vascular flow

📷 9.50   🔍 9.50   **FUD** XXX   S Z2 80 ▣

AMA: 2012,Feb,9-10; 2007,Jan,28-31

Radiology

78608 — 78830

78608   **Brain imaging, positron emission tomography (PET); metabolic evaluation**
   🖪 0.00   ⚕ 0.00   **FUD** XXX   [S] [Z2] [80] [▣]
   AMA: 2012,Feb,9-10; 2007,Jan,28-31

78609   **perfusion evaluation**
   🖪 2.16   ⚕ 2.16   **FUD** XXX   [E] [▣]
   AMA: 2012,Feb,9-10; 2007,Jan,28-31

78610   **Brain imaging, vascular flow only**
   🖪 4.97   ⚕ 4.97   **FUD** XXX   [S] [Z2] [80] [▣]
   AMA: 2012,Feb,9-10; 2007,Jan,28-31

78630   **Cerebrospinal fluid flow, imaging (not including introduction of material); cisternography**
   Code also injection procedure (61000-61070, 62270-62327)
   🖪 9.66   ⚕ 9.66   **FUD** XXX   [S] [Z2] [80] [▣]
   AMA: 2018,Jan,8

78635   **ventriculography**
   Code also injection procedure (61000-61070, 62270-62294)
   🖪 9.77   ⚕ 9.77   **FUD** XXX   [S] [Z2] [80] [▣]
   AMA: 2012,Feb,9-10; 2007,Jan,28-31

78645   **shunt evaluation**
   Code also injection procedure (61000-61070, 62270-62294)
   🖪 9.28   ⚕ 9.28   **FUD** XXX   [S] [Z2] [80] [▣]
   AMA: 2012,Feb,9-10; 2007,Jan,28-31

78650   **Cerebrospinal fluid leakage detection and localization**
   Code also injection procedure (61000-61070, 62270-62294)
   🖪 7.89   ⚕ 7.89   **FUD** XXX   [S] [Z2] [80] [▣]
   AMA: 2012,Feb,9-10; 2007,Jan,28-31

78660-78699 Nuclear Radiology: Lacrimal Duct System

Code also radiopharmaceutical(s) and/or drug(s) supplied

78660   **Radiopharmaceutical dacryocystography**
   🖪 5.27   ⚕ 5.27   **FUD** XXX   [S] [Z2] [80] [▣]
   AMA: 2012,Feb,9-10; 2007,Jan,28-31

78699   **Unlisted nervous system procedure, diagnostic nuclear medicine**
   🖪 0.00   ⚕ 0.00   **FUD** XXX   [S] [Z2] [80] [▣]
   AMA: 2018,Jan,8; 2017,Jan,8; 2016,Jan,13

78700-78725 Nuclear Radiology: Renal Anatomy and Function

EXCLUDES   *Diagnostic services (see appropriate sections)*
Follow-up care (see appropriate section)
Renal endoscopy with insertion radioactive substances (77778)
Code also radiopharmaceutical(s) and/or drug(s) supplied

78700   **Kidney imaging morphology;**
   🖪 4.89   ⚕ 4.89   **FUD** XXX   [S] [Z2] [80] [▣]
   AMA: 2018,Jan,8; 2017,Jan,8; 2016,Jan,13

78701   **with vascular flow**
   🖪 6.25   ⚕ 6.25   **FUD** XXX   [S] [Z2] [80] [▣]
   AMA: 2012,Feb,9-10; 2007,Mar,7-8

78707   **with vascular flow and function, single study without pharmacological intervention**
   🖪 6.66   ⚕ 6.66   **FUD** XXX   [S] [Z2] [80] [▣]
   AMA: 2018,Jan,8; 2017,Jan,8; 2016,Jan,13

78708   **with vascular flow and function, single study, with pharmacological intervention (eg, angiotensin converting enzyme inhibitor and/or diuretic)**
   🖪 5.06   ⚕ 5.06   **FUD** XXX   [S] [Z2] [80] [▣]
   AMA: 2018,Jan,8; 2017,Jan,8; 2016,Jan,13

78709   **with vascular flow and function, multiple studies, with and without pharmacological intervention (eg, angiotensin converting enzyme inhibitor and/or diuretic)**
   🖪 10.5   ⚕ 10.5   **FUD** XXX   [S] [Z2] [80] [▣]
   AMA: 2018,Jan,8; 2017,Jan,8; 2016,Jan,13

78725   **Kidney function study, non-imaging radioisotopic study**
   🖪 3.10   ⚕ 3.10   **FUD** XXX   [S] [Z2] [80] [▣]
   AMA: 2012,Feb,9-10; 2007,Jan,28-31

78730-78799 Nuclear Radiology: Urogenital

EXCLUDES   *Diagnostic services (see appropriate sections)*
Follow-up care (see appropriate section)
Code also radiopharmaceutical(s) and/or drug(s) supplied

+   **78730**   **Urinary bladder residual study (List separately in addition to code for primary procedure)**
   EXCLUDES   *Measurement postvoid residual urine and /or bladder capacity using ultrasound (51798)*
Ultrasound imaging bladder only with measurement postvoid residual urine (76857)
   Code first (78740)
   🖪 2.17   ⚕ 2.17   **FUD** ZZZ   [N] [N1] [80] [▣]
   AMA: 2018,Jan,8; 2017,Jan,8; 2016,Jan,13

78740   **Ureteral reflux study (radiopharmaceutical voiding cystogram)**
   EXCLUDES   *Catheterization (51701-51703)*
   Code also urinary bladder residual study (78730)
   🖪 6.21   ⚕ 6.21   **FUD** XXX   [S] [Z2] [80] [▣]
   AMA: 2012,Feb,9-10; 2007,Jan,28-31

78761   **Testicular imaging with vascular flow**   ♂
   🖪 6.06   ⚕ 6.06   **FUD** XXX   [S] [Z2] [80] [▣]
   AMA: 2018,Jan,8; 2017,Jan,8; 2016,Jan,13

78799   **Unlisted genitourinary procedure, diagnostic nuclear medicine**
   🖪 0.00   ⚕ 0.00   **FUD** XXX   [S] [Z2] [80] [▣]
   AMA: 2018,Jan,8; 2017,Jan,8; 2016,Jan,13

78800-78835 [78804, 78830, 78831, 78832, 78835] Nuclear Radiology: Tumor Localization

EXCLUDES   *CSF studies requiring injection procedure (61055, 61070, 62320-62323)*
Code also radiopharmaceutical(s) and/or drug(s) supplied

78800   **Radiopharmaceutical localization of tumor, inflammatory process or distribution of radiopharmaceutical agent(s) (includes vascular flow and blood pool imaging, when performed); planar, single area (eg, head, neck, chest, pelvis), single day imaging**
   INCLUDES   Ocular radiophosphorus tumor identification
   EXCLUDES   *Specific organ (see appropriate site)*
   🖪 7.40   ⚕ 7.40   **FUD** XXX   [S] [Z2] [80] [▣]
   AMA: 2020,Oct,3; 2018,Nov,11; 2018,Jan,8; 2017,Jan,8; 2016,Jan,13

78801   **planar, 2 or more areas (eg, abdomen and pelvis, head and chest), 1 or more days imaging or single area imaging over 2 or more days**
   🖪 8.13   ⚕ 8.13   **FUD** XXX   [S] [Z2] [80] [▣]
   AMA: 2020,Oct,3; 2018,Jan,8; 2017,Jan,8; 2016,Jan,13

78802   **planar, whole body, single day imaging**
   🖪 8.93   ⚕ 8.93   **FUD** XXX   [S] [Z2] [80] [▣]
   AMA: 2020,Oct,3

\#   **78804**   **planar, whole body, requiring 2 or more days imaging**
   🖪 18.8   ⚕ 18.8   **FUD** XXX   [S] [Z2] [80] [▣]
   AMA: 2020,Oct,3

78803   **tomographic (SPECT), single area (eg, head, neck, chest, pelvis), single day imaging**
   🖪 11.1   ⚕ 11.1   **FUD** XXX   [S] [Z2] [80] [▣]
   AMA: 2020,Oct,3; 2020,Oct,14; 2018,Nov,11; 2018,Jan,8; 2017,Jan,8; 2016,Dec,9; 2016,Dec,16; 2016,Jan,13

78804   **Resequenced code. See code following 78802.**

\#   **78830**   **tomographic (SPECT) with concurrently acquired computed tomography (CT) transmission scan for anatomical review, localization and determination/detection of pathology, single area (eg, head, neck, chest, pelvis), single day imaging**
   🖪 14.0   ⚕ 14.0   **FUD** XXX   [Z2] [80] [▣]
   AMA: 2020,Oct,3

| 26/TC PC/TC Only | A2-Z3 ASC Payment | 50 Bilateral | ♂ Male Only | ♀ Female Only | 🖪 Facility RVU | ⚕ Non-Facility RVU | ▣ CCI | ✖ CLIA |
| **FUD** Follow-up Days | **CMS:** IOM | **AMA:** CPT Asst | A-Y OPPSI | 80/80 Surg Assist Allowed / w/Doc | | Lab Crosswalk | Radiology Crosswalk |

352   CPT © 2021 American Medical Association. All Rights Reserved.   © 2021 Optum360, LLC

\# **78831** tomographic (SPECT), minimum 2 areas (eg, pelvis and knees, abdomen and pelvis), single day imaging, or single area imaging over 2 or more days

🚑 20.3   ⚖ 20.3   **FUD** XXX   ⓩ² 80 ▭

AMA: 2020,Oct,3

\# **78832** tomographic (SPECT) with concurrently acquired computed tomography (CT) transmission scan for anatomical review, localization and determination/detection of pathology, minimum 2 areas (eg, pelvis and knees, abdomen and pelvis), single day imaging, or single area imaging over 2 or more days

🚑 26.4   ⚖ 26.4   **FUD** XXX   ⓩ² 80 ▭

AMA: 2020,Oct,3

+ \# **78835** Radiopharmaceutical quantification measurement(s) single area (List separately in addition to code for primary procedure)

Code first ([78830], [78832])

🚑 2.95   ⚖ 2.95   **FUD** ZZZ   80

AMA: 2020,Oct,3

78808 Intravenous Injection for Radiopharmaceutical Localization

Code also radiopharmaceutical(s) and/or drug(s) supplied

78808 Injection procedure for radiopharmaceutical localization by non-imaging probe study, intravenous (eg, parathyroid adenoma)

🚑 1.14   ⚖ 1.14   **FUD** XXX   01 N1 80 ▭

AMA: 2018,Jan,8; 2017,Jan,8; 2016,Dec,9

78811-78999 [78830, 78831, 78832, 78835] Nuclear Radiology: Diagnosis, Staging, Restaging or Monitoring Cancer

CMS: 100-03,220.6.17 Positron Emission Tomography (FDG) for Oncologic Conditions; 100-03,220.6.19 NaF-18 PET to Identify Bone Metastasis of Cancer; 100-03,220.6.9 FDG PET for Refractory Seizures; 100-04,13,60 Positron Emission Tomography (PET) Scans - General Information; 100-04,13,60.13 Billing for PET Scans for Specific Indications of Cervical Cancer; 100-04,13,60.15 Billing for CMS-Approved Clinical Trials for PET Scans; 100-04,13,60.16 Billing and Coverage for PET Scans; 100-04,13,60.17 Billing and Coverage Changes for PET Scans for Cervical Cancer; 100-04,13,60.2 Use of Gamma Cameras, Full and Partial Ring PET Scanners; 100-04,13,60.3 PET Scan Qualifying Conditions; 100-04,13,60.3.2 Tracer Codes Required for Positron Emission Tomography (PET) Scans

EXCLUDES *CT scan performed for other than attenuation correction and anatomical localization (report with appropriate site-specific CT code and modifier 59)*
Ocular radiophosphorus tumor identification (78800)
PET brain scan (78608-78609)
PET myocardial imaging (78459, 78491-78492)
Procedure performed more than one time per imaging session

Code also radiopharmaceutical(s) and/or drug(s) supplied

78811 Positron emission tomography (PET) imaging; limited area (eg, chest, head/neck)

🚑 0.00   ⚖ 0.00   **FUD** XXX   S ⓩ² 80 ▭

AMA: 2018,Jan,8; 2017,Jan,8; 2016,Jan,13

78812 skull base to mid-thigh

🚑 0.00   ⚖ 0.00   **FUD** XXX   S ⓩ² 80 ▭

AMA: 2018,Jan,8; 2017,Jan,8; 2016,Jan,13

78813 whole body

🚑 0.00   ⚖ 0.00   **FUD** XXX   S ⓩ² 80 ▭

AMA: 2018,Jan,8; 2017,Jan,8; 2016,Jan,13

78814 Positron emission tomography (PET) with concurrently acquired computed tomography (CT) for attenuation correction and anatomical localization imaging; limited area (eg, chest, head/neck)

🚑 0.00   ⚖ 0.00   **FUD** XXX   S ⓩ² 80 ▭

AMA: 2018,Jan,8; 2017,Jan,8; 2016,Jan,13

78815 skull base to mid-thigh

🚑 0.00   ⚖ 0.00   **FUD** XXX   S ⓩ² 80 ▭

AMA: 2018,Jan,8; 2017,Jan,8; 2016,Jan,13

78816 whole body

🚑 0.00   ⚖ 0.00   **FUD** XXX   S ⓩ² 80 ▭

AMA: 2020,Sep,11; 2018,Jan,8; 2017,Jan,8; 2016,Jan,13

78830 Resequenced code. See code following numeric code 78804.

78831 Resequenced code. See code following numeric code 78804.

78832 Resequenced code. See code following numeric code 78804.

78835 Resequenced code. See code following numeric code 78804.

78999 Unlisted miscellaneous procedure, diagnostic nuclear medicine

🚑 0.00   ⚖ 0.00   **FUD** XXX   S ⓩ² 80 ▭

AMA: 2018,Jan,8; 2017,Jan,8; 2016,Dec,9; 2016,Dec,16; 2016,Jan,13

79005-79999 Systemic Radiopharmaceutical Therapy

EXCLUDES *Imaging guidance*
Injection into artery, body cavity, or joint (see appropriate injection codes)
Radiological supervision and interpretation

79005 Radiopharmaceutical therapy, by oral administration

EXCLUDES *Monoclonal antibody treatment (79403)*

🚑 3.92   ⚖ 3.92   **FUD** XXX   S ⓩ³ 80 ▭

AMA: 2018,Jan,8; 2017,Jan,8; 2016,Jan,13

79101 Radiopharmaceutical therapy, by intravenous administration

EXCLUDES *Administration nonantibody radioelement solution including follow-up care (77750)*
Hydration infusion (96360)
Intravenous injection, IV push (96374-96375, 96409)
Radiolabeled monoclonal antibody IV infusion (79403)
Venipuncture (36400, 36410)

🚑 4.23   ⚖ 4.23   **FUD** XXX   S ⓩ³ 80 ▭

AMA: 2018,Jan,8; 2017,Jan,8; 2016,Jan,13

79200 Radiopharmaceutical therapy, by intracavitary administration

🚑 3.86   ⚖ 3.86   **FUD** XXX   S ⓩ³ 80 ▭

AMA: 2018,Jan,8; 2017,Jan,8; 2016,Jan,13

79300 Radiopharmaceutical therapy, by interstitial radioactive colloid administration

🚑 0.00   ⚖ 0.00   **FUD** XXX   S ⓩ² 80 ▭

AMA: 2018,Jan,8; 2017,Jan,8; 2016,Jan,13

79403 Radiopharmaceutical therapy, radiolabeled monoclonal antibody by intravenous infusion

EXCLUDES *Intravenous radiopharmaceutical therapy (79101)*

🚑 5.39   ⚖ 5.39   **FUD** XXX   S ⓩ³ 80 ▭

AMA: 2018,Jan,8; 2017,Jan,8; 2016,Jan,13

79440 Radiopharmaceutical therapy, by intra-articular administration

🚑 3.48   ⚖ 3.48   **FUD** XXX   S ⓩ³ 80 ▭

AMA: 2018,Jan,8; 2017,Jan,8; 2016,Jan,13

79445 Radiopharmaceutical therapy, by intra-arterial particulate administration

EXCLUDES *Intra-arterial injections (96373, 96420)*
Procedural and radiological supervision and interpretation for angiographic and interventional procedures before intra-arterial radiopharmaceutical therapy

🚑 0.00   ⚖ 0.00   **FUD** XXX   S ⓩ² 80 ▭

AMA: 2018,Jan,8; 2017,Jan,8; 2016,Jan,13

79999 Radiopharmaceutical therapy, unlisted procedure

🚑 0.00   ⚖ 0.00   **FUD** XXX   S ⓩ² 80 ▭

AMA: 2018,Jan,8; 2017,Jan,8; 2016,Jan,13

Medical Decision Making Table for Pathology Clinical Consultations

Medical Decision Making

Pathology clinical consultation services may be based on either the total time for consultation services performed on the date of consultation **or** the level of medical decision making as defined for each service.

The Medical Decision Making (MDM) Table for Pathology Clinical Consultations is a guide to assist in selecting the level of MDM for reporting pathology clinical consultation services. The table includes the levels of MDM (i.e., low, limited, moderate, high, extensive) and the three elements of MDM (i.e., number and complexity of problems addressed at the encounter, amount and/or complexity of data reviewed and analyzed, and risk of complications and/or morbidity or mortality of patient management). To qualify for a particular level of MDM, two of the three elements for that level of MDM must be met or exceeded. See Table 1: Medical Decision Making (MDM) Table for Pathology Clinical Consultations below.

Table 1: Medical Decision Making (MDM) Table for Pathology Clinical Consultations

Code	Level of MDM (based on 2 out of 3 elements of MDM)	Elements of Medical Decision Making		
		Number and Complexity of Problems Addressed	Amount and/or Complexity of Data to be Reviewed and Analyzed	Risk of Complications and/or Morbidity or Mortality of Patient Management

80503	Low	**Low**
		• **1** to **2** laboratory or pathology findings;
		or
		• **2** or more self-limited problems
			Limited
			(Must meet the requirements of at least 1 of the 2 categories)
			Category 1: Tests and documents
			• **Any combination of 2 from the following:**
			  - Review of prior note(s) from each unique source*;
			  - Review of result(s) of each unique test*;
			  - Ordering or recommending additional or follow-up testing*
			or
			Category 2: Assessment requiring an independent historian(s)
			(For the categories of independent interpretation of tests and discussion of management or test interpretation, see moderate or high)
				Low risk of morbidity from additional diagnostic testing or treatment

80504	Moderate	**Moderate** • **3** to **4** laboratory or pathology findings; or • **1** or more chronic illnesses with exacerbation, progression, or side effects of treatment; or • **2** or more stable chronic illnesses; or • **1** undiagnosed new problem with uncertain prognosis; or • **1** acute illness with systemic symptoms	**Moderate** *(Must meet the requirements of at least 1 out of 3 categories)* **Category 1: Tests, documents, or independent historian(s)** **Any combination of 3 from the following:** • Review of prior note(s) from each unique source*; • Review of the result(s) of each unique test*; • Ordering or recommending additional or follow-up testing* • Assessment requiring an independent historian(s) **or** **Category 2: Independent interpretation of tests** • Independent interpretation of a test performed by another physician/other qualified health care professional (not separately reported); **or** **Category 3: Discussion of management or test interpretation** • Discussion of management or test interpretation with external physician/other qualified health care professional/appropriate source (not separately reported)	**Moderate risk of morbidity from additional diagnostic testing or treatment** *Examples only:* Prescription drug management • Decision regarding minor surgery with identified patient or procedure risk factors • Decision regarding elective major surgery without identified patient or procedure risk factors • Diagnosis or treatment significantly limited by social determinants of health

Each unique test, order, or document contributes to the combination of 2 or combination of 3 in Category 1.

		Elements of Medical Decision Making		
Code	Level of MDM (based on 2 out of 3 elements of MDM)	Number and Complexity of Problems Addressed	Amount and/or Complexity of Data to be Reviewed and Analyzed	Risk of Complications and/or Morbidity or Mortality of Patient Management
80505	High	**High** • **5** or more laboratory or pathology findings; **or** • **1** or more chronic illnesses with severe exacerbation, progression, or side effects of treatment; **or** • **1** acute or chronic illness or injury that poses a threat to life or bodily function	**Extensive** *(Must meet the requirements of at least 2 out of 3 categories)* **Category 1: Tests, documents, or independent historian(s)** **Any combination of 3 from the following:** • Review of prior note(s) from each unique source*; • Review of the result(s) of each unique test*; • Ordering or recommending additional or follow-up testing* • Assessment requiring an independent historian(s) **or** **Category 2: Independent interpretation of tests** • Independent interpretation of a test performed by another physician/other qualified health care professional (not separately reported); **or** **Category 3: Discussion of management or test interpretation** • Discussion of management or test interpretation with external physician/other qualified health care professional/appropriate source (not separately reported)	**High risk of morbidity from additional diagnostic testing or treatment** *Examples only:* • Drug therapy requiring intensive monitoring for toxicity • Decision regarding elective major surgery with identified patient or procedure risk factors • Decision regarding emergency major surgery • Decision regarding hospitalization

Each unique test, order, or document contributes to the combination of 2 or combination of 3 in Category 1.

Medical Decision Making Table for Pathology Clinical Consultations

80047-80081 [80081] Multi-test Laboratory Panels

INCLUDES Specified test groups that may be reported in a panel

EXCLUDES *Reporting two or more panel codes including same tests; report panel with most tests in common to meet panel code definition*

Code also individual tests not part included in panel, when appropriate

80047   Basic metabolic panel (Calcium, ionized)

INCLUDES Calcium, ionized (82330)
Carbon dioxide (bicarbonate) (82374)
Chloride (82435)
Creatinine (82565)
Glucose (82947)
Potassium (84132)
Sodium (84295)
Urea nitrogen (BUN) (84520)

🖾 0.00   **FUD** XXX

AMA: 2020,Dec,3; 2020,Jun,3; 2018,Jan,8; 2017,Jan,8; 2016,Jan,13

80048   Basic metabolic panel (Calcium, total)

INCLUDES Calcium, total (82310)
Carbon dioxide (bicarbonate) (82374)
Chloride (82435)
Creatinine (82565)
Glucose (82947)
Potassium (84132)
Sodium (84295)
Urea nitrogen (BUN) (84520)

🖾 0.00   ✂ 0.00   **FUD** XXX

AMA: 2020,Dec,3; 2018,Jan,8; 2017,Jan,8; 2016,Jan,13

80050   General health panel

INCLUDES Complete blood count (CBC), automated, with:
Manual differential WBC count
Blood smear with manual differential AND complete (CBC), automated (85007, 85027)
Manual differential WBC count, buffy coat AND complete (CBC), automated (85009, 85027)
OR
Automated differential WBC count
Automated differential WBC count AND complete (CBC), automated/automated differential WBC count (85004, 85025)
Automated differential WBC count AND complete (CBC), automated (85004, 85027)
Comprehensive metabolic profile (80053)
Thyroid stimulating hormone (84443)

🖾 0.00   ✂ 0.00   **FUD** XXX

AMA: 2020,Dec,3; 2018,Jan,8; 2017,Jan,8; 2016,Jan,13

80051   Electrolyte panel

INCLUDES Carbon dioxide (bicarbonate) (82374)
Chloride (82435)
Potassium (84132)
Sodium (84295)

🖾 0.00   ✂ 0.00   **FUD** XXX

AMA: 2020,Dec,3; 2018,Jan,8; 2017,Jan,8; 2016,Jan,13

80053   Comprehensive metabolic panel

INCLUDES Albumin (82040)
Bilirubin, total (82247)
Calcium, total (82310)
Carbon dioxide (bicarbonate) (82374)
Chloride (82435)
Creatinine (82565)
Glucose (82947)
Phosphatase, alkaline (84075)
Potassium (84132)
Protein, total (84155)
Sodium (84295)
Transferase, alanine amino (ALT) (SGPT) (84460)
Transferase, aspartate amino (AST) (SGOT) (84450)
Urea nitrogen (BUN) (84520)

🖾 0.00   ✂ 0.00   **FUD** XXX

AMA: 2020,Dec,3; 2018,Jan,8; 2017,Jan,8; 2016,Jan,13

80055   Obstetric panel   M ♀

INCLUDES Complete blood count (CBC), automated, with:
Manual differential WBC count
Blood smear with manual differential AND complete (CBC), automated (85007, 85027)
Manual differential WBC count, buffy coat AND complete (CBC), automated (85009, 85027)
OR
Automated differential WBC count
Automated differential WBC count AND complete (CBC), automated/automated differential WBC count (85004, 85025)
Automated differential WBC count AND complete (CBC), automated (85004, 85027)
Blood typing, ABO and Rh (86900-86901)
Hepatitis B surface antigen (HBsAg) (87340)
RBC antibody screen, each serum technique (86850)
Rubella antibody (86762)
Syphilis test, non-treponemal antibody qualitative (86592)

EXCLUDES *Reporting code when syphilis screening provided using treponemal antibody approach. Instead, assign individual codes for tests performed in OB panel (86780)*

🖾 0.00   ✂ 0.00   **FUD** XXX

AMA: 2020,Dec,3; 2018,Jan,8; 2017,Jan,8; 2016,Jan,13

\# **80081   Obstetric panel (includes HIV testing)**   M ♀

INCLUDES Complete blood count (CBC), automated, with:
Manual differential WBC count
Blood smear with manual differential AND complete (CBC), automated (85007, 85027)
Manual differential WBC count, buffy count AND complete (CBC), automated (85009, 85027)
OR
Automated differential WBC count
Automated differential WBC count AND complete (CBC), automated/automated differential WBC count (85004, 85025)
Automated differential WBC count AND complete (CBC), automated (85004, 85027)
Blood typing, ABO and Rh (86900-86901)
Hepatitis B surface antigen (HBsAg) (87340)
HIV-1 antigens, with HIV-1 and HIV-2 antibodies, single result (87389)
RBC antibody screen, each serum technique (86850)
Rubella antibody (86762)
Syphilis test, non-treponemal antibody qualitative (86592)

EXCLUDES *Reporting code when syphilis screening provided using treponemal antibody approach. Instead, assign individual codes for tests performed in OB panel (86780)*

🖾 0.00   ✂ 0.00   **FUD** XXX

AMA: 2020,Dec,3; 2018,Jan,8; 2017,Jan,8; 2016,Jan,13

80061   Lipid panel

INCLUDES Cholesterol, serum, total (82465)
Lipoprotein, direct measurement, high density cholesterol (HDL cholesterol) (83718)
Triglycerides (84478)

🖾 0.00   ✂ 0.00   **FUD** XXX

AMA: 2020,Dec,3; 2018,Jan,8; 2017,Sep,11; 2017,Jan,8; 2016,Jan,13

80069   Renal function panel

INCLUDES Albumin (82040)
Calcium, total (82310)
Carbon dioxide (bicarbonate) (82374)
Chloride (82435)
Creatinine (82565)
Glucose (82947)
Phosphorus inorganic (phosphate) (84100)
Potassium (84132)
Sodium (84295)
Urea nitrogen (BUN) (84520)

🖾 0.00   ✂ 0.00   **FUD** XXX

AMA: 2020,Dec,3; 2018,Jan,8; 2017,Jan,8; 2016,Jan,13

80074 Acute hepatitis panel

INCLUDES Hepatitis A antibody (HAAb) IgM (86709)
Hepatitis B core antibody (HBcAb), IgM (86705)
Hepatitis B surface antigen (HBsAg) (87340)
Hepatitis C antibody (86803)

🚑 0.00   ⚕ 0.00   **FUD** XXX   Ⓠ ▭

AMA: 2020,Dec,3; 2018,Jan,8; 2017,Jan,8; 2016,Jan,13

80076 Hepatic function panel

INCLUDES Albumin (82040)
Bilirubin, direct (82248)
Bilirubin, total (82247)
Phosphatase, alkaline (84075)
Protein, total (84155)
Transferase, alanine amino (ALT) (SGPT) (84460)
Transferase, aspartate amino (AST) (SGOT) (84450)

🚑 0.00   ⚕ 0.00   **FUD** XXX   Ⓠ ▭

AMA: 2020,Dec,3; 2018,Jan,8; 2017,Jan,8; 2016,Jan,13

80081 Resequenced code. See code following 80055.

80305-80307 [80305, 80306, 80307] Nonspecific Drug Screening

INCLUDES All class testing procedures performed per modality
Validation testing

EXCLUDES *Confirmatory drug testing ([80320, 80321, 80322, 80323, 80324, 80325, 80326, 80327, 80328, 80329, 80330, 80331, 80332, 80333, 80334, 80335, 80336, 80337, 80338, 80339, 80340, 80341, 80342, 80343, 80344, 80345, 80346, 80347, 80348, 80349, 80350, 80351, 80352, 80353, 80354, 80355, 80356, 80357, 80358, 80359, 80360, 80361, 80362, 80363, 80364, 80365, 80366, 80367, 80368, 80369, 80370, 80371, 80372, 80373, 80374, 80375, 80376, 80377, 83992], [83992])*

\# **80305 Drug test(s), presumptive, any number of drug classes, any number of devices or procedures; capable of being read by direct optical observation only (eg, utilizing immunoassay [eg, dipsticks, cups, cards, or cartridges]), includes sample validation when performed, per date of service**

🚑 0.00   ⚕ 0.00   **FUD** XXX   ✖ Ⓠ ▭

AMA: 2020,Dec,3; 2018,Jul,14; 2018,Jan,8; 2017,Mar,6

\# **80306 read by instrument assisted direct optical observation (eg, utilizing immunoassay [eg, dipsticks, cups, cards, or cartridges]), includes sample validation when performed, per date of service**

🚑 0.00   ⚕ 0.00   **FUD** XXX   Ⓠ ▭

AMA: 2020,Dec,3; 2018,Jan,8; 2017,Mar,6

\# **80307 by instrument chemistry analyzers (eg, utilizing immunoassay [eg, EIA, ELISA, EMIT, FPIA, IA, KIMS, RIA]), chromatography (eg, GC, HPLC), and mass spectrometry either with or without chromatography, (eg, DART, DESI, GC-MS, GC-MS/MS, LC-MS, LC-MS/MS, LDTD, MALDI, TOF) includes sample validation when performed, per date of service**

🚑 0.00   ⚕ 0.00   **FUD** XXX   Ⓠ ▭

AMA: 2020,Dec,3; 2018,Jan,8; 2017,Mar,6

80320-80377 [80320, 80321, 80322, 80323, 80324, 80325, 80326, 80327, 80328, 80329, 80330, 80331, 80332, 80333, 80334, 80335, 80336, 80337, 80338, 80339, 80340, 80341, 80342, 80343, 80344, 80345, 80346, 80347, 80348, 80349, 80350, 80351, 80352, 80353, 80354, 80355, 80356, 80357, 80358, 80359, 80360, 80361, 80362, 80363, 80364, 80365, 80366, 80367, 80368, 80369, 80370, 80371, 80372, 80373, 80374, 80375, 80376, 80377, 83992] Confirmatory Drug Testing

INCLUDES Antihistamine drug tests ([80375, 80376, 80377])
Detection specific drugs using methods other than immunoassay or enzymatic technique

EXCLUDES *Definitive drug testing for any drug class not specified; report with NOS codes ([80375, 80376, 80377])*
Metabolites separate from code for drug except when distinct code available

\# **80320 Alcohols**

EXCLUDES *Alcohol (ethanol) therapeutic drug assay (82077)*

🚑 0.00   ⚕ 0.00   **FUD** XXX   Ⓑ ▭

AMA: 2020,Dec,3; 2018,Jan,8; 2017,Jan,8; 2016,Jan,13

\# **80321 Alcohol biomarkers; 1 or 2**

🚑 0.00   ⚕ 0.00   **FUD** XXX   Ⓑ ▭

AMA: 2020,Dec,3

\# **80322 3 or more**

🚑 0.00   ⚕ 0.00   **FUD** XXX   Ⓑ ▭

AMA: 2020,Dec,3

\# **80323 Alkaloids, not otherwise specified**

🚑 0.00   ⚕ 0.00   **FUD** XXX   Ⓑ ▭

AMA: 2020,Dec,3

\# **80324 Amphetamines; 1 or 2**

🚑 0.00   ⚕ 0.00   **FUD** XXX   Ⓑ ▭

AMA: 2020,Dec,3

\# **80325 3 or 4**

🚑 0.00   ⚕ 0.00   **FUD** XXX   Ⓑ ▭

AMA: 2020,Dec,3

\# **80326 5 or more**

🚑 0.00   ⚕ 0.00   **FUD** XXX   Ⓑ ▭

AMA: 2020,Dec,3

\# **80327 Anabolic steroids; 1 or 2**

🚑 0.00   ⚕ 0.00   **FUD** XXX   Ⓑ ▭

AMA: 2020,Dec,3

\# **80328 3 or more**

EXCLUDES *Analysis dihydrotestosterone for monitoring, endogenous levels of hormone (82642)*

🚑 0.00   ⚕ 0.00   **FUD** XXX   Ⓑ ▭

AMA: 2020,Dec,3

\# **80329 Analgesics, non-opioid; 1 or 2**

EXCLUDES *Acetaminophen therapeutic drug assay (80143)*
Salicylate therapeutic drug assay ([80179])

🚑 0.00   ⚕ 0.00   **FUD** XXX   Ⓑ ▭

AMA: 2020,Dec,3

\# **80330 3-5**

EXCLUDES *Acetaminophen therapeutic drug assay (80143)*
Salicylate therapeutic drug assay ([80179])

🚑 0.00   ⚕ 0.00   **FUD** XXX   Ⓑ ▭

AMA: 2020,Dec,3

\# **80331 6 or more**

EXCLUDES *Acetaminophen therapeutic drug assay (80143)*
Salicylate therapeutic drug assay ([80179])

🚑 0.00   ⚕ 0.00   **FUD** XXX   Ⓑ ▭

AMA: 2020,Dec,3

\# **80332 Antidepressants, serotonergic class; 1 or 2**

🚑 0.00   ⚕ 0.00   **FUD** XXX   Ⓑ ▭

AMA: 2020,Dec,3

#	80333	**3-5**					B ▣
		� 0.00	⚖ 0.00	**FUD** XXX			
		AMA: 2020,Dec,3					

#	80334	**6 or more**					B ▣
		� 0.00	⚖ 0.00	**FUD** XXX			
		AMA: 2020,Dec,3					

#	80335	**Antidepressants, tricyclic and other cyclicals; 1 or 2**					B ▣
		� 0.00	⚖ 0.00	**FUD** XXX			
		AMA: 2020,Dec,3					

#	80336	**3-5**					B ▣
		� 0.00	⚖ 0.00	**FUD** XXX			
		AMA: 2020,Dec,3					

#	80337	**6 or more**					B ▣
		� 0.00	⚖ 0.00	**FUD** XXX			
		AMA: 2020,Dec,3					

#	80338	**Antidepressants, not otherwise specified**					B ▣
		� 0.00	⚖ 0.00	**FUD** XXX			
		AMA: 2020,Dec,3					

#	80339	**Antiepileptics, not otherwise specified; 1-3**					B ▣
		� 0.00	⚖ 0.00	**FUD** XXX			
		AMA: 2020,Dec,3					

#	80340	**4-6**					B ▣
		� 0.00	⚖ 0.00	**FUD** XXX			
		AMA: 2020,Dec,3					

#	80341	**7 or more**					

EXCLUDES *Carbamazepine therapeutic drug assay (80156, 80157, [80161])*
Definitive drug testing for antihistamines ([80375, 80376, 80377])

🚓 0.00 ⚖ 0.00 **FUD** XXX — B ▣
AMA: 2020,Dec,3

#	80342	**Antipsychotics, not otherwise specified; 1-3**					B ▣
		🚓 0.00	⚖ 0.00	**FUD** XXX			
		AMA: 2020,Dec,3					

#	80343	**4-6**					B ▣
		🚓 0.00	⚖ 0.00	**FUD** XXX			
		AMA: 2020,Dec,3					

#	80344	**7 or more**					B ▣
		🚓 0.00	⚖ 0.00	**FUD** XXX			
		AMA: 2020,Dec,3					

#	80345	**Barbiturates**					B ▣
		🚓 0.00	⚖ 0.00	**FUD** XXX			
		AMA: 2020,Dec,3					

#	80346	**Benzodiazepines; 1-12**					B ▣
		🚓 0.00	⚖ 0.00	**FUD** XXX			
		AMA: 2020,Dec,3					

#	80347	**13 or more**					B ▣
		🚓 0.00	⚖ 0.00	**FUD** XXX			
		AMA: 2020,Dec,3					

#	80348	**Buprenorphine**					B ▣
		🚓 0.00	⚖ 0.00	**FUD** XXX			
		AMA: 2020,Dec,3					

#	80349	**Cannabinoids, natural**					B ▣
		🚓 0.00	⚖ 0.00	**FUD** XXX			
		AMA: 2020,Dec,3					

#	80350	**Cannabinoids, synthetic; 1-3**					B ▣
		🚓 0.00	⚖ 0.00	**FUD** XXX			
		AMA: 2020,Dec,3					

#	80351	**4-6**					B ▣
		🚓 0.00	⚖ 0.00	**FUD** XXX			
		AMA: 2020,Dec,3					

#	80352	**7 or more**					B ▣
		🚓 0.00	⚖ 0.00	**FUD** XXX			
		AMA: 2020,Dec,3					

#	80353	**Cocaine**					B ▣
		🚓 0.00	⚖ 0.00	**FUD** XXX			
		AMA: 2020,Dec,3					

#	80354	**Fentanyl**					B ▣
		🚓 0.00	⚖ 0.00	**FUD** XXX			
		AMA: 2020,Dec,3					

#	80355	**Gabapentin, non-blood**					

EXCLUDES *Therapeutic drug assay ([80171])*
🚓 0.00 ⚖ 0.00 **FUD** XXX — B ▣
AMA: 2020,Dec,3; 2018,Jan,8; 2017,Jan,8; 2016,Jan,13

#	80356	**Heroin metabolite**					B ▣
		🚓 0.00	⚖ 0.00	**FUD** XXX			
		AMA: 2020,Dec,3					

#	80357	**Ketamine and norketamine**					B ▣
		🚓 0.00	⚖ 0.00	**FUD** XXX			
		AMA: 2020,Dec,3					

#	80358	**Methadone**					B ▣
		🚓 0.00	⚖ 0.00	**FUD** XXX			
		AMA: 2020,Dec,3					

#	80359	**Methylenedioxyamphetamines (MDA, MDEA, MDMA)**					B ▣
		🚓 0.00	⚖ 0.00	**FUD** XXX			
		AMA: 2020,Dec,3					

#	80360	**Methylphenidate**					B ▣
		🚓 0.00	⚖ 0.00	**FUD** XXX			
		AMA: 2020,Dec,3					

#	80361	**Opiates, 1 or more**					B ▣
		🚓 0.00	⚖ 0.00	**FUD** XXX			
		AMA: 2020,Dec,3					

#	80362	**Opioids and opiate analogs; 1 or 2**					B ▣
		🚓 0.00	⚖ 0.00	**FUD** XXX			
		AMA: 2020,Dec,3					

#	80363	**3 or 4**					B ▣
		🚓 0.00	⚖ 0.00	**FUD** XXX			
		AMA: 2020,Dec,3					

#	80364	**5 or more**					B ▣
		🚓 0.00	⚖ 0.00	**FUD** XXX			
		AMA: 2020,Dec,3					

#	80365	**Oxycodone**					B ▣
		🚓 0.00	⚖ 0.00	**FUD** XXX			
		AMA: 2020,Dec,3					

#	83992	**Phencyclidine (PCP)**					E ▣
		🚓 0.00	⚖ 0.00	**FUD** XXX			
		AMA: 2020,Dec,3; 2018,Jan,8; 2017,Jan,8; 2016,Jan,13					

#	80366	**Pregabalin**					B ▣
		🚓 0.00	⚖ 0.00	**FUD** XXX			
		AMA: 2020,Dec,3					

#	80367	**Propoxyphene**					B ▣
		🚓 0.00	⚖ 0.00	**FUD** XXX			
		AMA: 2020,Dec,3					

#	80368	**Sedative hypnotics (non-benzodiazepines)**					B ▣
		🚓 0.00	⚖ 0.00	**FUD** XXX			
		AMA: 2020,Dec,3					

#	80369	**Skeletal muscle relaxants; 1 or 2**					B ▣
		🚓 0.00	⚖ 0.00	**FUD** XXX			
		AMA: 2020,Dec,3					

#	80370	**3 or more**					B ▣
		🚓 0.00	⚖ 0.00	**FUD** XXX			
		AMA: 2020,Dec,3					

● New Code ▲ Revised Code ○ Reinstated ● New Web Release ▲ Revised Web Release + Add-on Unlisted Not Covered # Resequenced
㊿ Optum Mod 50 Exempt Ⓝ AMA Mod 51 Exempt �51 Optum Mod 51 Exempt �63 Mod 63 Exempt ✗ Non-FDA Drug ★ Telemedicine Ⓜ Maternity Ⓐ Age Edit

#	80371	**Stimulants, synthetic**			
		0.00	0.00	**FUD** XXX	B 🖵
		AMA: 2020,Dec,3			

#	80372	**Tapentadol**			
		0.00	0.00	**FUD** XXX	B 🖵
		AMA: 2020,Dec,3			

#	80373	**Tramadol**			
		0.00	0.00	**FUD** XXX	B 🖵
		AMA: 2020,Dec,3			

#	80374	**Stereoisomer (enantiomer) analysis, single drug class**			
		Code also index drug analysis when appropriate			
		0.00	0.00	**FUD** XXX	B 🖵
		AMA: 2020,Dec,3			

#	80375	**Drug(s) or substance(s), definitive, qualitative or quantitative, not otherwise specified; 1-3**			
		0.00	0.00	**FUD** XXX	B 🖵
		AMA: 2020,Dec,3; 2018,Jan,8; 2017,Jan,8; 2016,Jan,13			

#	80376	**4-6**			
		0.00	0.00	**FUD** XXX	B 🖵
		AMA: 2020,Dec,3; 2018,Jan,8; 2017,Jan,8; 2016,Jan,13			

#	80377	**7 or more**			
		EXCLUDES Definitive drug testing for antihistamines ([80375, 80376, 80377])			
		0.00	0.00	**FUD** XXX	🖵
		AMA: 2020,Dec,3; 2018,Jan,8; 2017,Jan,8; 2016,Jan,13			

80143-80377 [80161, 80164, 80165, 80167, 80171, 80176, 80179, 80181, 80189, 80193, 80204, 80210, 80220, 80230, 80235, 80280, 80285, 80305, 80306, 80307, 80320, 80321, 80322, 80323, 80324, 80325, 80326, 80327, 80328, 80329, 80330, 80331, 80332, 80333, 80334, 80335, 80336, 80337, 80338, 80339, 80340, 80341, 80342, 80343, 80344, 80345, 80346, 80347, 80348, 80349, 80350, 80351, 80352, 80353, 80354, 80355, 80356, 80357, 80358, 80359, 80360, 80361, 80362, 80363, 80364, 80365, 80366, 80367, 80368, 80369, 80370, 80371, 80372, 80373, 80374, 80375, 80376, 80377]

Therapeutic Drug Levels

INCLUDES Monitoring known, prescribed or over-the-counter medication levels
Testing drug and metabolite(s) in primary code
Tests on specimens from blood, blood components, and spinal fluid

	80143	**Acetaminophen**			
		EXCLUDES Acetaminophen confirmatory drug testing ([80329, 80330, 80331])			
		0.00	0.00	**FUD** XXX	🖵
		AMA: 2020,Dec,3			

	80145	**Adalimumab**			
		0.00	0.00	**FUD** XXX	
		AMA: 2020,Dec,3			

	80150	**Amikacin**			
		0.00	0.00	**FUD** XXX	Q 🖵
		AMA: 2020,Dec,3; 2018,Jan,8; 2017,Jan,8; 2016,Jan,13			

	80151	**Amiodarone**			
		0.00	0.00	**FUD** XXX	🖵
		AMA: 2020,Dec,3			

	80155	**Caffeine**			
		0.00	0.00	**FUD** XXX	Q 🖵
		AMA: 2020,Dec,3			

	80156	**Carbamazepine; total**			
		0.00	0.00	**FUD** XXX	Q 🖵
		AMA: 2020,Dec,3; 2018,Jan,8; 2017,Jan,8; 2016,Jan,13			

	80157	**free**			
		0.00	0.00	**FUD** XXX	Q 🖵
		AMA: 2020,Dec,3; 2018,Jan,8; 2017,Jan,8; 2016,Jan,13			

#	80161	**-10,11-epoxide**			
		0.00	0.00	**FUD** XXX	🖵
		AMA: 2020,Dec,3			

	80158	**Cyclosporine**			
		0.00	0.00	**FUD** XXX	Q 🖵
		AMA: 2020,Dec,3; 2018,Jan,8; 2017,Jan,8; 2016,Jan,13			

	80159	**Clozapine**			
		0.00	0.00	**FUD** XXX	Q 🖵
		AMA: 2020,Dec,3			

80161	*Resequenced code. See code following 80157.*

	80162	**Digoxin; total**			
		0.00	0.00	**FUD** XXX	Q 🖵
		AMA: 2020,Dec,3; 2018,Jan,8; 2017,Jan,8; 2016,Jan,13			

	80163	**free**			
		0.00	0.00	**FUD** XXX	Q 🖵
		AMA: 2020,Dec,3; 2018,Jan,8; 2017,Jan,8; 2016,Jan,13			

80164	*Resequenced code. See code following 80201.*
80165	*Resequenced code. See code following 80201.*
80167	*Resequenced code. See code following 80169.*

	80168	**Ethosuximide**			
		0.00	0.00	**FUD** XXX	Q 🖵
		AMA: 2020,Dec,3; 2018,Jan,8; 2017,Jan,8; 2016,Jan,13			

	80169	**Everolimus**			
		0.00	0.00	**FUD** XXX	Q 🖵
		AMA: 2020,Dec,3			

#	80167	**Felbamate**			
		0.00	0.00	**FUD** XXX	🖵
		AMA: 2020,Dec,3			

#	80181	**Flecainide**			
		0.00	0.00	**FUD** XXX	🖵
		AMA: 2020,Dec,3			

#	80171	**Gabapentin, whole blood, serum, or plasma**			
		0.00	0.00	**FUD** XXX	Q 🖵
		AMA: 2020,Dec,3; 2018,Jan,8; 2017,Jan,8; 2016,Jan,13			

	80170	**Gentamicin**			
		0.00	0.00	**FUD** XXX	Q 🖵
		AMA: 2020,Dec,3; 2018,Jan,8; 2017,Jan,8; 2016,Jan,13			

80171	*Resequenced code. See code before 80170.*

	80173	**Haloperidol**			
		0.00	0.00	**FUD** XXX	Q 🖵
		AMA: 2020,Dec,3; 2018,Jan,8; 2017,Jan,8; 2016,Jan,13			

● #	80220	**Hydroxychloroquine**			
		0.00	0.00	**FUD** 000	

#	80230	**Infliximab**			
		0.00	0.00	**FUD** XXX	
		AMA: 2020,Dec,3			

#	80189	**Itraconazole**			
		0.00	0.00	**FUD** XXX	🖵
		AMA: 2020,Dec,3			

#	80235	**Lacosamide**			
		0.00	0.00	**FUD** XXX	
		AMA: 2020,Dec,3			

	80175	**Lamotrigine**			
		0.00	0.00	**FUD** XXX	Q 🖵
		AMA: 2020,Dec,3			

80176	*Resequenced code. See code following 80177.*

#	80193	**Leflunomide**			
		0.00	0.00	**FUD** XXX	🖵
		AMA: 2020,Dec,3			

	80177	**Levetiracetam**			
		0.00	0.00	**FUD** XXX	Q 🖵
		AMA: 2020,Dec,3			

26/TC PC/TC Only   A2-Z3 ASC Payment   50 Bilateral   ♂ Male Only   ♀ Female Only   Facility RVU   Non-Facility RVU   🖵 CCI   ☒ CLIA
FUD Follow-up Days   CMS: IOM   AMA: CPT Asst   A-Y OPPSI   80/80 Surg Assist Allowed / w/Doc   Lab Crosswalk   Radiology Crosswalk

360   CPT © 2021 American Medical Association. All Rights Reserved.   © 2021 Optum360, LLC

80176 — 80338

Pathology and Laboratory

#	**80176**	**Lidocaine**
		🔧 0.00 ⚕ 0.00 **FUD** XXX
		AMA: 2020,Dec,3; 2018,Jan,8; 2017,Jan,8; 2016,Jan,13
	80178	**Lithium**
		🔧 0.00 ⚕ 0.00 **FUD** XXX ☒
		AMA: 2020,Dec,3; 2018,Jan,8; 2017,Jan,8; 2016,Jan,13
#	**80204**	**Methotrexate**
		🔧 0.00 ⚕ 0.00 **FUD** XXX
		AMA: 2020,Dec,3
	80179	Resequenced code. See code before 80195.
	80180	**Mycophenolate (mycophenolic acid)**
		🔧 0.00 ⚕ 0.00 **FUD** XXX
		AMA: 2020,Dec,3
	80181	Resequenced code. See code following resequenced code 80167.
	80183	**Oxcarbazepine**
		🔧 0.00 ⚕ 0.00 **FUD** XXX
		AMA: 2020,Dec,3
	80184	**Phenobarbital**
		🔧 0.00 ⚕ 0.00 **FUD** XXX
		AMA: 2020,Dec,3; 2018,Jan,8; 2017,Jan,8; 2016,Jan,13
	80185	**Phenytoin; total**
		🔧 0.00 ⚕ 0.00 **FUD** XXX
		AMA: 2020,Dec,3; 2018,Jan,8; 2017,Jan,8; 2016,Jan,13
	80186	**free**
		🔧 0.00 ⚕ 0.00 **FUD** XXX
		AMA: 2020,Dec,3; 2018,Jan,8; 2017,Jan,8; 2016,Jan,13
	80187	**Posaconazole**
		🔧 0.00 ⚕ 0.00 **FUD** XXX
		AMA: 2020,Dec,3
	80188	**Primidone**
		🔧 0.00 ⚕ 0.00 **FUD** XXX
		AMA: 2020,Dec,3; 2018,Jan,8; 2017,Jan,8; 2016,Jan,13
	80189	Resequenced code. See code following resequenced code 80230.
	80190	**Procainamide;**
		🔧 0.00 ⚕ 0.00 **FUD** XXX
		AMA: 2020,Dec,3; 2018,Jan,8; 2017,Jan,8; 2016,Jan,13
	80192	**with metabolites (eg, n-acetyl procainamide)**
		🔧 0.00 ⚕ 0.00 **FUD** XXX
		AMA: 2020,Dec,3; 2018,Jan,8; 2017,Jan,8; 2016,Jan,13
	80193	Resequenced code. See code before 80177.
	80194	**Quinidine**
		🔧 0.00 ⚕ 0.00 **FUD** XXX
		AMA: 2020,Dec,3; 2018,Jan,8; 2017,Jan,8; 2016,Jan,13
#	**80210**	**Rufinamide**
		🔧 0.00 ⚕ 0.00 **FUD** XXX
		AMA: 2020,Dec,3
#	**80179**	**Salicylate**
		EXCLUDES *Salicylate confirmatory drug testing ([80329, 80330, 80331])*
		🔧 0.00 ⚕ 0.00 **FUD** XXX
		AMA: 2020,Dec,3
	80195	**Sirolimus**
		🔧 0.00 ⚕ 0.00 **FUD** XXX
		AMA: 2020,Dec,3; 2018,Jan,8; 2017,Jan,8; 2016,Jan,13
	80197	**Tacrolimus**
		🔧 0.00 ⚕ 0.00 **FUD** XXX
		AMA: 2020,Dec,3; 2018,Jan,8; 2017,Jan,8; 2016,Jan,13
	80198	**Theophylline**
		🔧 0.00 ⚕ 0.00 **FUD** XXX
		AMA: 2020,Dec,3; 2018,Jan,8; 2017,Jan,8; 2016,Jan,13

	80199	**Tiagabine**
		🔧 0.00 ⚕ 0.00 **FUD** XXX
		AMA: 2020,Dec,3
	80200	**Tobramycin**
		🔧 0.00 ⚕ 0.00 **FUD** XXX
		AMA: 2020,Dec,3; 2018,Jan,8; 2017,Jan,8; 2016,Jan,13
	80201	**Topiramate**
		🔧 0.00 ⚕ 0.00 **FUD** XXX
		AMA: 2020,Dec,3; 2018,Jan,8; 2017,Jan,8; 2016,Jan,13
#	**80164**	**Valproic acid (dipropylacetic acid); total**
		🔧 0.00 ⚕ 0.00 **FUD** XXX
		AMA: 2020,Dec,3; 2018,Jan,8; 2017,Jan,8; 2016,Jan,13
#	**80165**	**free**
		🔧 0.00 ⚕ 0.00 **FUD** XXX
		AMA: 2020,Dec,3; 2018,Jan,8; 2017,Jan,8; 2016,Jan,13
	80202	**Vancomycin**
		🔧 0.00 ⚕ 0.00 **FUD** XXX
		AMA: 2020,Dec,3; 2018,Jan,8; 2017,Jan,8; 2016,Jan,13
#	**80280**	**Vedolizumab**
		🔧 0.00 ⚕ 0.00 **FUD** XXX
		AMA: 2020,Dec,3
#	**80285**	**Voriconazole**
		🔧 0.00 ⚕ 0.00 **FUD** XXX
		AMA: 2020,Dec,3
	80203	**Zonisamide**
		🔧 0.00 ⚕ 0.00 **FUD** XXX
		AMA: 2020,Dec,3
	80204	Resequenced code. See code following 80178.
	80210	Resequenced code. See code following 80194.
	80220	Resequenced code. See code following 80173.
	80230	Resequenced code. See code following 80173.
	80235	Resequenced code. See code before 80175.
	80280	Resequenced code. See code following 80202.
	80285	Resequenced code. See code before 80203.
	80299	**Quantitation of therapeutic drug, not elsewhere specified**
		🔧 0.00 ⚕ 0.00 **FUD** XXX
		AMA: 2020,Dec,3; 2018,Jan,8; 2017,Jan,8; 2016,Jan,13
	80305	Resequenced code. See code before 80143.
	80306	Resequenced code. See code before 80143.
	80307	Resequenced code. See code before 80143.
	80320	Resequenced code. See code before 80143.
	80321	Resequenced code. See code before 80143.
	80322	Resequenced code. See code before 80143.
	80323	Resequenced code. See code before 80143.
	80324	Resequenced code. See code before 80143.
	80325	Resequenced code. See code before 80143.
	80326	Resequenced code. See code before 80143.
	80327	Resequenced code. See code before 80143.
	80328	Resequenced code. See code before 80143.
	80329	Resequenced code. See code before 80143.
	80330	Resequenced code. See code before 80143.
	80331	Resequenced code. See code before 80143.
	80332	Resequenced code. See code before 80143.
	80333	Resequenced code. See code before 80143.
	80334	Resequenced code. See code before 80143.
	80335	Resequenced code. See code before 80143.
	80336	Resequenced code. See code before 80143.
	80337	Resequenced code. See code before 80143.
	80338	Resequenced code. See code before 80143.

80339	Resequenced code. See code before 80143.
80340	Resequenced code. See code following resequenced code 80339.
80341	Resequenced code. See code before 80143.
80342	Resequenced code. See code before 80143.
80343	Resequenced code. See code before 80143.
80344	Resequenced code. See code before 80143.
80345	Resequenced code. See code before 80143.
80346	Resequenced code. See code before 80143.
80347	Resequenced code. See code before 80143.
80348	Resequenced code. See code before 80143.
80349	Resequenced code. See code before 80143.
80350	Resequenced code. See code before 80143.
80351	Resequenced code. See code before 80143.
80352	Resequenced code. See code before 80143.
80353	Resequenced code. See code before 80143.
80354	Resequenced code. See code before 80143.
80355	Resequenced code. See code before 80143.
80356	Resequenced code. See code before 80143.
80357	Resequenced code. See code before 80143.
80358	Resequenced code. See code before 80143.
80359	Resequenced code. See code before 80143.
80360	Resequenced code. See code before 80143.
80361	Resequenced code. See code before 80143.
80362	Resequenced code. See code before 80143.
80363	Resequenced code. See code before 80143.
80364	Resequenced code. See code before 80143.
80365	Resequenced code. See code before 80143.
80366	Resequenced code. See code before 80143.
80367	Resequenced code. See code before 80143.
80368	Resequenced code. See code before 80143.
80369	Resequenced code. See code before 80143.
80370	Resequenced code. See code before 80143.
80371	Resequenced code. See code before 80143.
80372	Resequenced code. See code before 80143.
80373	Resequenced code. See code before 80143.
80374	Resequenced code. See code before 80143.
80375	Resequenced code. See code before 80143.
80376	Resequenced code. See code before 80143.
80377	Resequenced code. See code before 80143.

80400-80439 Stimulation and Suppression Test Panels

EXCLUDES Administration evocative or suppressive material (96365-96368, 96372, 96374-96376, C8957)
Evocative or suppression test substances, when applicable
Physician monitoring and attendance during test (see E/M services)

80400   **ACTH stimulation panel; for adrenal insufficiency**
INCLUDES   Cortisol x 2 (82533)
🚑 0.00   ⚗ 0.00   **FUD** XXX   ⊡⊡
AMA: 2020,Dec,3; 2018,Jan,8; 2017,Jan,8; 2016,Jan,13

80402   **for 21 hydroxylase deficiency**
INCLUDES   17 hydroxyprogesterone X 2 (83498)
Cortisol x 2 (82533)
🚑 0.00   ⚗ 0.00   **FUD** XXX   ⊡⊡
AMA: 2020,Dec,3

80406   **for 3 beta-hydroxydehydrogenase deficiency**
INCLUDES   17 hydroxypregnenolone x 2 (84143)
Cortisol x 2 (82533)
🚑 0.00   ⚗ 0.00   **FUD** XXX   ⊡⊡
AMA: 2020,Dec,3

80408   **Aldosterone suppression evaluation panel (eg, saline infusion)**
INCLUDES   Aldosterone x 2 (82088)
Renin x 2 (84244)
🚑 0.00   ⚗ 0.00   **FUD** XXX   ⊡⊡
AMA: 2020,Dec,3

80410   **Calcitonin stimulation panel (eg, calcium, pentagastrin)**
INCLUDES   Calcitonin x 3 (82308)
🚑 0.00   ⚗ 0.00   **FUD** XXX   ⊡⊡
AMA: 2020,Dec,3

80412   **Corticotropic releasing hormone (CRH) stimulation panel**
INCLUDES   Adrenocorticotropic hormone (ACTH) x 6 (82024)
Cortisol x 6 (82533)
🚑 0.00   ⚗ 0.00   **FUD** XXX   ⊡⊡
AMA: 2020,Dec,3

80414   **Chorionic gonadotropin stimulation panel; testosterone response**
INCLUDES   Testosterone x 2 on three pooled blood samples (84403)
🚑 0.00   ⚗ 0.00   **FUD** XXX   ⊡⊡
AMA: 2020,Dec,3

80415   **estradiol response**
INCLUDES   Estradiol x 2 on three pooled blood samples (82670)
🚑 0.00   ⚗ 0.00   **FUD** XXX   ⊡⊡
AMA: 2020,Dec,3

80416   **Renal vein renin stimulation panel (eg, captopril)**
INCLUDES   Renin x 6 (84244)
🚑 0.00   ⚗ 0.00   **FUD** XXX   ⊡⊡
AMA: 2020,Dec,3

80417   **Peripheral vein renin stimulation panel (eg, captopril)**
INCLUDES   Renin x 2 (84244)
🚑 0.00   ⚗ 0.00   **FUD** XXX   ⊡⊡
AMA: 2020,Dec,3

80418   **Combined rapid anterior pituitary evaluation panel**
INCLUDES   Adrenocorticotropic hormone (ACTH) x 4 (82024)
Cortisol x 4 (82533)
Follicle stimulating hormone (FSH) x 4 (83001)
Human growth hormone x 4 (83003)
Luteinizing hormone (LH) x 4 (83002)
Prolactin x 4 (84146)
Thyroid stimulating hormone (TSH) x 4 (84443)
🚑 0.00   ⚗ 0.00   **FUD** XXX   ⊡⊡
AMA: 2020,Dec,3

80420   **Dexamethasone suppression panel, 48 hour**
INCLUDES   Cortisol x 2 (82533)
Free cortisol, urine x 2 (82530)
Volume measurement for timed collection x 2 (81050)
EXCLUDES   Single dose dexamethasone (82533)
🚑 0.00   ⚗ 0.00   **FUD** XXX   ⊡⊡
AMA: 2020,Dec,3

80422   **Glucagon tolerance panel; for insulinoma**
INCLUDES   Glucose x 3 (82947)
Insulin x 3 (83525)
🚑 0.00   ⚗ 0.00   **FUD** XXX   ⊡⊡
AMA: 2020,Dec,3

80424   **for pheochromocytoma**
INCLUDES   Catecholamines, fractionated x 2 (82384)
🚑 0.00   ⚗ 0.00   **FUD** XXX   ⊡⊡
AMA: 2020,Dec,3

80426 Gonadotropin releasing hormone stimulation panel

INCLUDES Follicle stimulating hormone (FSH) x 4 (83001)
Luteinizing hormone (LH) x 4 (83002)
⚕ 0.00 ⚗ 0.00 **FUD** XXX

AMA: 2020,Dec,3

80428 Growth hormone stimulation panel (eg, arginine infusion, l-dopa administration)

INCLUDES Human growth hormone (HGH) x 4 (83003)
⚕ 0.00 ⚗ 0.00 **FUD** XXX

AMA: 2020,Dec,3

80430 Growth hormone suppression panel (glucose administration)

INCLUDES Glucose x 3 (82947)
Human growth hormone (HGH) x 4 (83003)
⚕ 0.00 ⚗ 0.00 **FUD** XXX

AMA: 2020,Dec,3

80432 Insulin-induced C-peptide suppression panel

INCLUDES C-peptide x 5 (84681)
Glucose x 5 (82947)
Insulin (83525)
⚕ 0.00 ⚗ 0.00 **FUD** XXX

AMA: 2020,Dec,3

80434 Insulin tolerance panel; for ACTH insufficiency

INCLUDES Cortisol x 5 (82533)
Glucose x 5 (82947)
⚕ 0.00 ⚗ 0.00 **FUD** XXX

AMA: 2020,Dec,3

80435 for growth hormone deficiency

INCLUDES Glucose x 5 (82947)
Human growth hormone (HGH) x 5 (83003)
⚕ 0.00 ⚗ 0.00 **FUD** XXX

AMA: 2020,Dec,3

80436 Metyrapone panel

INCLUDES 11 deoxycortisol x 2 (82634)
Cortisol x 2 (82533)
⚕ 0.00 ⚗ 0.00 **FUD** XXX

AMA: 2020,Dec,3

80438 Thyrotropin releasing hormone (TRH) stimulation panel; 1 hour

INCLUDES Thyroid stimulating hormone (TSH) x 3 (84443)
⚕ 0.00 ⚗ 0.00 **FUD** XXX

AMA: 2020,Dec,3

80439 2 hour

INCLUDES Thyroid stimulating hormone (TSH) x 4 (84443)
⚕ 0.00 ⚗ 0.00 **FUD** XXX

AMA: 2020,Dec,3

80500-80506 Consultation By Clinical Pathologist

See also: Table 1: Medical Decision Making (MDM) Table for Pathology Clinical Consultations at beginning of Pathology chapter.

INCLUDES Appropriate consultation level selection based on total time for consultation services performed on date of service OR level of medical decision making
Clinical assessment, evaluation pathology/laboratory findings, other relevant clinical/diagnostic information requiring additional medical interpretative judgement
Consult rendered at request of physician, other qualified healt care professional (QHCP), or when mandated by federal or state regulation (i.e., Clinical Laboratory Improvement Amendments [CLIA])
Consultant time includes, when performed:
  Arriving at tentative conclusion/differential diagnosis
  Clinical consultation report documented in electronic or other health record
  Communicating with/referring to other health care professionals
  Ordering/recommending additional or follow up testing
  Reviewing complete medical history
  Reviewing test results, including all relevant past/current laboratory, pathology, radiology reports and images, and clinical testing/findings
  Total time spent on day of consultation personally spent by consultant, not clinical staff

EXCLUDES *Communicating laboratory/pathology results to patient, family, or caregiver (See appropriate E/M service level, if appropriate)*
Consultation, comprehensive, with records/specimen review and report, referred material (88325)
Consultation/report on referred material or slide prepared elsewhere (88321, 88323)
Reporting laboratory/pathology finding or other relevant clinical diagnostic information without medical interpretative judgement

80500 ~~Clinical pathology consultation; limited, without review of patient's history and medical records~~

To report, see (80503-80506)

80502 ~~comprehensive, for a complex diagnostic problem, with review of patient's history and medical records~~

To report, see (80503-80506)

● **80503** Pathology clinical consultation; for a clinical problem, with limited review of patient's history and medical records and straightforward medical decision making

EXCLUDES *Consultations including patient examination/evaluation (99241-99245, 99251-99255)*

● **80504** for a moderately complex clinical problem, with review of patient's history and medical records and moderate level of medical decision making

● **80505** for a highly complex clinical problem, with comprehensive review of patient's history and medical records and high level of medical decision making

● + **80506** prolonged service, each additional 30 minutes (List separately in addition to code for primary procedure)

EXCLUDES *Prolonged consultation time less than 15 additional minutes*
Code first (80505)
⚕ 0.00 ⚗ 0.00 **FUD** 000

81000-81099 Urine Tests

81000 Urinalysis, by dip stick or tablet reagent for bilirubin, glucose, hemoglobin, ketones, leukocytes, nitrite, pH, protein, specific gravity, urobilinogen, any number of these constituents; non-automated, with microscopy

⚕ 0.00 ⚗ 0.00 **FUD** XXX

AMA: 2020,Dec,3; 2018,Jul,14; 2018,Jan,8; 2017,Jan,8; 2016,Jan,13

81001 automated, with microscopy

⚕ 0.00 ⚗ 0.00 **FUD** XXX

AMA: 2020,Dec,3

81002 non-automated, without microscopy

INCLUDES Mosenthal test
⚕ 0.00 ⚗ 0.00 **FUD** XXX ☒

AMA: 2020,Dec,3; 2018,Jan,8; 2017,Jan,8; 2016,Jan,13

81003 automated, without microscopy
🔳 0.00 ⚖ 0.00 **FUD** XXX ❌ 🔲 🖵
AMA: 2020,Dec,3; 2018,Jan,8; 2017,Jan,8; 2016,Jan,13

81005 Urinalysis; qualitative or semiquantitative, except immunoassays
INCLUDES Benedict test for dextrose
EXCLUDES *Immunoassay, qualitative or semiquantitative (83518)*
Microalbumin (82043-82044)
Nonimmunoassay reagent strip analysis (81000, 81002)
🔳 0.00 ⚖ 0.00 **FUD** XXX 🔲 🖵
AMA: 2020,Dec,3; 2018,Jan,8; 2017,Jan,8; 2016,Jan,13

81007 bacteriuria screen, except by culture or dipstick
EXCLUDES *Culture (87086-87088)*
Dipstick (81000, 81002)
🔳 0.00 ⚖ 0.00 **FUD** XXX ❌ 🔲 🖵
AMA: 2020,Dec,3

81015 microscopic only
EXCLUDES *Sperm evaluation for retrograde ejaculation (89331)*
🔳 0.00 ⚖ 0.00 **FUD** XXX 🔲 🖵
AMA: 2020,Dec,3; 2018,Jan,8; 2017,Nov,10

81020 2 or 3 glass test
INCLUDES Valentine's test
🔳 0.00 ⚖ 0.00 **FUD** XXX 🔲 🖵
AMA: 2020,Dec,3

81025 Urine pregnancy test, by visual color comparison methods Ⓜ ♀
🔳 0.00 ⚖ 0.00 **FUD** XXX ❌ 🔲 🖵
AMA: 2020,Dec,3; 2018,Jan,8; 2017,Jan,8; 2016,Jan,13

81050 Volume measurement for timed collection, each
🔳 0.00 ⚖ 0.00 **FUD** XXX 🔲 🖵
AMA: 2020,Dec,3

81099 Unlisted urinalysis procedure
🔳 0.00 ⚖ 0.00 **FUD** XXX 🔲 🖵
AMA: 2020,Dec,3; 2018,Jan,8; 2017,Jan,8; 2016,Jan,13

81105-81364 [81105, 81106, 81107, 81108, 81109, 81110, 81111, 81112, 81120, 81121, 81161, 81162, 81163, 81164, 81165, 81166, 81167, 81168, 81173, 81174, 81184, 81185, 81186, 81187, 81188, 81189, 81190, 81191, 81192, 81193, 81194, 81200, 81201, 81202, 81203, 81204, 81205, 81206, 81207, 81208, 81209, 81210, 81219, 81227, 81230, 81231, 81233, 81234, 81238, 81239, 81245, 81246, 81250, 81257, 81258, 81259, 81261, 81262, 81263, 81264, 81265, 81266, 81267, 81268, 81269, 81271, 81274, 81277, 81278, 81279, 81283, 81284, 81285, 81286, 81287, 81288, 81289, 81291, 81292, 81293, 81294, 81295, 81301, 81302, 81303, 81304, 81306, 81307, 81308, 81309, 81312, 81320, 81324, 81325, 81326, 81332, 81334, 81336, 81337, 81338, 81339, 81343, 81344, 81345, 81347, 81348, 81349, 81351, 81352, 81353, 81357, 81361, 81362, 81363, 81364] Gene Analysis: Tier 1 Procedures

INCLUDES All analytical procedures in evaluation:
Amplification
Cell lysis
Detection
Digestion
Extraction
Nucleic acid stabilization
Code selection based on specific gene being reviewed
Evaluation constitutional or somatic gene variations
Evaluation gene variant presence using common gene variant name
Gene specific and genomic testing
Generally, all listed gene variants in code description (lists not all inclusive)
Genes described using Human Genome Organization (HUGO) approved names
Protein or disease examples in code description not all inclusive
Qualitative results unless otherwise stated
Tier 1 molecular pathology codes (81105-81254 [81161, 81162, 81163, 81164, 81165, 81166, 81167, 81173, 81174, 81184, 81185, 81186, 81187, 81188, 81189, 81190, 81200, 81201, 81202, 81203, 81204, 81205, 81206, 81207, 81208, 81209, 81210, 81219, 81227, 81230, 81231, 81233, 81234, 81238, 81239, 81245, 81246, 81250, 81257, 81258, 81259, 81265, 81266, 81267, 81268, 81269, 81284, 81285, 81286, 81289, 81361, 81362, 81363, 81364])

EXCLUDES *Full gene sequencing using separate gene variant assessment codes unless specifically stated in code description*
In situ hybridization analyses (88271-88275, 88365-88368 [88364, 88373, 88374])
Microbial identification (87149-87153, 87471-87801 [87623, 87624, 87625], 87900-87904 [87906, 87910, 87912])
Other related gene variants not listed in code description
Tier 1 molecular pathology codes (81370-81383)
Tier 2 codes (81400-81408)
Unlisted molecular pathology procedures ([81479])
Code also:
Modifier 26 when only interpretation and report performed
Services required before cell lysis

81105 Resequenced code. See code before 81260.

81106 Resequenced code. See code before 81260.

81107 Resequenced code. See code before 81260.

81108 Resequenced code. See code before 81260.

81109 Resequenced code. See code before 81260.

81110 Resequenced code. See code before 81260.

81111 Resequenced code. See code before 81260.

81112 Resequenced code. See code before 81260.

81120 Resequenced code. See code before 81260.

81121 Resequenced code. See code before 81260.

81161 Resequenced code. See code following numeric code 81231.

81162 Resequenced code. See code following resequenced code 81210.

81163 Resequenced code. See code following resequenced code 81210.

81164 Resequenced code. See code before 81212.

| 26/TC PC/TC Only | A2-Z3 ASC Payment | 50 Bilateral | ♂ Male Only | ♀ Female Only | 🔳 Facility RVU | ⚖ Non-Facility RVU | 🖵 CCI | ❌ CLIA |
| FUD Follow-up Days | CMS: IOM | AMA: CPT Asst | A-Y OPPSI | 80/80 Surg Assist Allowed / w/Doc | 🔲 Lab Crosswalk | 🔲 Radiology Crosswalk |

364
CPT © 2021 American Medical Association. All Rights Reserved.
© 2021 Optum360, LLC

81165	Resequenced code. See code following 81212.	
81166	Resequenced code. See code following 81212.	
81167	Resequenced code. See code following 81216.	
81168	Resequenced code. See code before 81218.	

81170 *ABL1 (ABL proto-oncogene 1, non-receptor tyrosine kinase)* (eg, acquired imatinib tyrosine kinase inhibitor resistance), gene analysis, variants in the kinase domain
   🔧 0.00   ✄ 0.00   **FUD** XXX   Ⓐ ▱
   AMA: 2020,Dec,3; 2018,Jan,8; 2017,Jan,8; 2016,Aug,9

81171 *AFF2 (AF4/FMR2 family, member 2 [FMR2])* (eg, fragile X mental retardation 2 [FRAXE]) gene analysis; evaluation to detect abnormal (eg, expanded) alleles
   🔧 0.00   ✄ 0.00   **FUD** XXX   ▱
   AMA: 2020,Dec,3

81172   characterization of alleles (eg, expanded size and methylation status)
   🔧 0.00   ✄ 0.00   **FUD** XXX   ▱
   AMA: 2020,Dec,3

81173	Resequenced code. See code following resequenced code 81204.	
81174	Resequenced code. See code following resequenced code 81204.	

\# **81201** *APC (adenomatous polyposis coli)* (eg, familial adenomatosis polyposis [FAP], attenuated FAP) gene analysis; full gene sequence
   🔧 0.00   ✄ 0.00   **FUD** XXX   Ⓐ ▱
   AMA: 2020,Dec,3; 2020,OctSE,1; 2020,OctSE,1; 2018,Nov,9; 2018,Jan,8; 2017,Jan,8; 2016,Aug,9; 2016,Jan,13

\# **81202**   known familial variants
   🔧 0.00   ✄ 0.00   **FUD** XXX   Ⓐ ▱
   AMA: 2020,Dec,3; 2020,OctSE,1; 2020,OctSE,1; 2018,Nov,9; 2018,Jan,8; 2017,Jan,8; 2016,Aug,9; 2016,Jan,13

\# **81203**   duplication/deletion variants
   🔧 0.00   ✄ 0.00   **FUD** XXX   Ⓐ ▱
   AMA: 2020,Dec,3; 2020,OctSE,1; 2020,OctSE,1; 2018,Nov,9; 2018,Jan,8; 2017,Jan,8; 2016,Aug,9; 2016,Jan,13

\# **81204** *AR (androgen receptor)* (eg, spinal and bulbar muscular atrophy, Kennedy disease, X chromosome inactivation) gene analysis; characterization of alleles (eg, expanded size or methylation status)
   🔧 0.00   ✄ 0.00   **FUD** XXX   ▱
   AMA: 2020,Dec,3; 2020,OctSE,1; 2020,OctSE,1; 2018,Nov,9

\# **81173**   full gene sequence
   🔧 0.00   ✄ 0.00   **FUD** XXX   ▱
   AMA: 2020,Dec,3

\# **81174**   known familial variant
   🔧 0.00   ✄ 0.00   **FUD** XXX   ▱
   AMA: 2020,Dec,3

\# **81200** *ASPA (aspartoacylase)* (eg, Canavan disease) gene analysis, common variants (eg, E285A, Y231X)
   🔧 0.00   ✄ 0.00   **FUD** XXX   Ⓐ ▱
   AMA: 2020,Dec,3; 2020,OctSE,1; 2020,OctSE,1; 2018,Nov,9; 2018,Jan,8; 2017,Jan,8; 2016,Aug,9; 2016,Jan,13

81175 *ASXL1 (additional sex combs like 1, transcriptional regulator)* (eg, myelodysplastic syndrome, myeloproliferative neoplasms, chronic myelomonocytic leukemia), gene analysis; full gene sequence
   🔧 0.00   ✄ 0.00   **FUD** XXX   Ⓐ ▱
   AMA: 2020,Dec,3

81176   targeted sequence analysis (eg, exon 12)
   🔧 0.00   ✄ 0.00   **FUD** XXX   Ⓐ ▱
   AMA: 2020,Dec,3

81177 *ATN1 (atrophin 1)* (eg, dentatorubral-pallidoluysian atrophy) gene analysis, evaluation to detect abnormal (eg, expanded) alleles
   🔧 0.00   ✄ 0.00   **FUD** XXX   ▱
   AMA: 2020,Dec,3

81178 *ATXN1 (ataxin 1)* (eg, spinocerebellar ataxia) gene analysis, evaluation to detect abnormal (eg, expanded) alleles
   🔧 0.00   ✄ 0.00   **FUD** XXX   ▱
   AMA: 2020,Dec,3; 2019,Sep,7

81179 *ATXN2 (ataxin 2)* (eg, spinocerebellar ataxia) gene analysis, evaluation to detect abnormal (eg, expanded) alleles
   🔧 0.00   ✄ 0.00   **FUD** XXX   ▱
   AMA: 2020,Dec,3; 2019,Sep,7

81180 *ATXN3 (ataxin 3)* (eg, spinocerebellar ataxia, Machado-Joseph disease) gene analysis, evaluation to detect abnormal (eg, expanded) alleles
   🔧 0.00   ✄ 0.00   **FUD** XXX   ▱
   AMA: 2020,Dec,3; 2019,Sep,7

81181 *ATXN7 (ataxin 7)* (eg, spinocerebellar ataxia) gene analysis, evaluation to detect abnormal (eg, expanded) alleles
   🔧 0.00   ✄ 0.00   **FUD** XXX   ▱
   AMA: 2020,Dec,3; 2019,Sep,7

81182 *ATXN8OS (ATXN8 opposite strand [non-protein coding])* (eg, spinocerebellar ataxia) gene analysis, evaluation to detect abnormal (eg, expanded) alleles
   🔧 0.00   ✄ 0.00   **FUD** XXX   ▱
   AMA: 2020,Dec,3; 2019,Sep,7

81183 *ATXN10 (ataxin 10)* (eg, spinocerebellar ataxia) gene analysis, evaluation to detect abnormal (eg, expanded) alleles
   🔧 0.00   ✄ 0.00   **FUD** XXX   ▱
   AMA: 2020,Dec,3; 2019,Sep,7

81184	Resequenced code. See code following resequenced code 81233.
81185	Resequenced code. See code following resequenced code 81233.
81186	Resequenced code. See code following resequenced code 81233.
81187	Resequenced code. See code following resequenced code 81268.
81188	Resequenced code. See code following resequenced code 81266.
81189	Resequenced code. See code following resequenced code 81266.
81190	Resequenced code. See code following resequenced code 81266.
81191	Resequenced code. See code following numeric code 81312.
81192	Resequenced code. See code following numeric code 81312.
81193	Resequenced code. See code following numeric code 81312.
81194	Resequenced code. See code following numeric code 81312.
81200	Resequenced code. See code before 81175.
81201	Resequenced code. See code following numeric code 81174.
81202	Resequenced code. See code following numeric code 81174.
81203	Resequenced code. See code following numeric code 81174.
81204	Resequenced code. See code following numeric code 81174.
81205	Resequenced code. See code following numeric code 81210.
81206	Resequenced code. See code following numeric code 81210.
81207	Resequenced code. See code following numeric code 81210.
81208	Resequenced code. See code following numeric code 81210.

● New Code   ▲ Revised Code   ○ Reinstated   ● New Web Release   ▲ Revised Web Release   + Add-on   Unlisted   Not Covered   # Resequenced
㊿ Optum Mod 50 Exempt   ⊘ AMA Mod 51 Exempt   ⑤¹ Optum Mod 51 Exempt   ㊿ Mod 63 Exempt   ✗ Non-FDA Drug   ★ Telemedicine   Ⓜ Maternity   Ⓐ Age Edit

© 2021 Optum360, LLC   CPT © 2021 American Medical Association. All Rights Reserved.   **365**

 # 81209 Resequenced code. See code following numeric code 81210.

 # 81210 Resequenced code. See code following resequenced code 81209.

 # 81205 *BCKDHB (branched-chain keto acid dehydrogenase E1, beta polypeptide) (eg, maple syrup urine disease) gene analysis, common variants (eg, R183P, G278S, E422X)*

🗲 0.00   ⚖ 0.00   **FUD** XXX   A ▯

AMA: 2020,Dec,3; 2020,OctSE,1; 2020,OctSE,1; 2018,Nov,9; 2018,Jan,8; 2017,Jan,8; 2016,Aug,9; 2016,Jan,13

 # 81206 *BCR/ABL1 (t(9;22)) (eg, chronic myelogenous leukemia) translocation analysis; major breakpoint, qualitative or quantitative*

🗲 0.00   ⚖ 0.00   **FUD** XXX   A ▯

AMA: 2020,Dec,3; 2020,OctSE,1; 2020,OctSE,1; 2018,Nov,9; 2018,Jan,8; 2017,Jan,8; 2016,Aug,9; 2016,Jan,13

 # 81207 minor breakpoint, qualitative or quantitative

🗲 0.00   ⚖ 0.00   **FUD** XXX   A ▯

AMA: 2020,Dec,3; 2020,OctSE,1; 2020,OctSE,1; 2018,Nov,9; 2018,Jan,8; 2017,Jan,8; 2016,Aug,9; 2016,Jan,13

 # 81208 other breakpoint, qualitative or quantitative

🗲 0.00   ⚖ 0.00   **FUD** XXX   A ▯

AMA: 2020,Dec,3; 2020,OctSE,1; 2020,OctSE,1; 2018,Nov,9; 2018,Jan,8; 2017,Jan,8; 2016,Aug,9; 2016,Jan,13

 # 81209 *BLM (Bloom syndrome, RecQ helicase-like) (eg, Bloom syndrome) gene analysis, 2281del6ins7 variant*

🗲 0.00   ⚖ 0.00   **FUD** XXX   A ▯

AMA: 2020,Dec,3; 2020,OctSE,1; 2020,OctSE,1; 2018,Nov,9; 2018,Jan,8; 2017,Jan,8; 2016,Aug,9; 2016,Jan,13

 # 81210 *BRAF (B-Raf proto-oncogene, serine/threonine kinase) (eg, colon cancer, melanoma), gene analysis, V600 variant(s)*

🗲 0.00   ⚖ 0.00   **FUD** XXX   A ▯

AMA: 2020,Dec,3; 2020,OctSE,1; 2020,OctSE,1; 2018,Nov,9; 2018,Jan,8; 2017,Jan,8; 2016,Aug,9; 2016,Jan,13

 # 81162 *BRCA1 (BRCA1, DNA repair associated), BRCA2 (BRCA2, DNA repair associated) (eg, hereditary breast and ovarian cancer) gene analysis; full sequence analysis and full duplication/deletion analysis (ie, detection of large gene rearrangements)*

EXCLUDES   *BRCA1 common duplication/deletion variant ([81479])*
BRCA1, BRCA2 full duplication/deletion analysis only (81164, 81166-81167, 81216)
BRCA1, BRCA2 full sequence analysis only (81163, 81165)
BRCA1, BRCA2 known familial variant only (81215, 81217)
Hereditary breast cancer genomic sequence analysis panel (81432)

🗲 0.00   ⚖ 0.00   **FUD** XXX   A ▯

AMA: 2020,Dec,3; 2019,May,5; 2018,Jan,8; 2017,Jan,8; 2016,Aug,9

 # 81163 full sequence analysis

EXCLUDES   *BRCA1 common duplication/deletion variant ([81479])*
BRCA1, BRCA2 full duplication/deletion analysis only (81164, 81216)
BRCA1, BRCA2 full sequence analysis and full duplication/deletion analysis (81162)
BRCA1, BRCA2 full sequence analysis only (81165)
Hereditary breast cancer genomic sequence analysis panel (81432)

🗲 0.00   ⚖ 0.00   **FUD** XXX   ▯

AMA: 2020,Dec,3; 2019,May,5

 # 81164 full duplication/deletion analysis (ie, detection of large gene rearrangements)

EXCLUDES   *BRCA1 common duplication/deletion variant ([81479])*
BRCA1, BRCA2 full sequence analysis and full duplication/deletion analysis (81162)
BRCA1, BRCA2 full sequence analysis only (81163)
BRCA1, BRCA2 full duplication/deletion analysis only (81166-81167)
BRCA1, BRCA2 known familial variant only (81217)

🗲 0.00   ⚖ 0.00   **FUD** XXX   ▯

AMA: 2020,Dec,3; 2019,May,5

81212 185delAG, 5385insC, 6174delT variants

🗲 0.00   ⚖ 0.00   **FUD** XXX   A ▯

AMA: 2020,Dec,3; 2020,OctSE,1; 2020,OctSE,1; 2019,May,5; 2018,Nov,9; 2018,Jan,8; 2017,Jan,8; 2016,Aug,9; 2016,Jan,13

 # 81165 *BRCA1 (BRCA1, DNA repair associated) (eg, hereditary breast and ovarian cancer) gene analysis; full sequence analysis*

EXCLUDES   *BRCA1 common duplication/deletion variant ([81479])*
BRCA1, BRCA2 full sequence analysis and full duplication/deletion analysis (81162)
BRCA1, BRCA2 full sequence analysis only (81163)
Hereditary breast cancer genomic sequence analysis panel (81432)

🗲 0.00   ⚖ 0.00   **FUD** XXX   ▯

AMA: 2020,Dec,3; 2019,May,5

 # 81166 full duplication/deletion analysis (ie, detection of large gene rearrangements)

EXCLUDES   *BRCA1 common duplication/deletion variant ([81479])*
BRCA1, BRCA2 full duplication/deletion analysis only (81164)
BRCA1, BRCA2 full sequence analysis and full duplication/deletion analysis (81162)

🗲 0.00   ⚖ 0.00   **FUD** XXX   ▯

AMA: 2020,Dec,3; 2019,May,5

81215 known familial variant

EXCLUDES   *BRCA1 common duplication/deletion variant ([81479])*

🗲 0.00   ⚖ 0.00   **FUD** XXX   A ▯

AMA: 2020,Dec,3; 2020,OctSE,1; 2020,OctSE,1; 2019,May,5; 2018,Nov,9; 2018,Jan,8; 2017,Jan,8; 2016,Aug,9; 2016,Jan,13

81216 *BRCA2 (BRCA2, DNA repair associated) (eg, hereditary breast and ovarian cancer) gene analysis; full sequence analysis*

EXCLUDES   *BRCA1, BRCA2 full sequence analysis only (81163)*
BRCA1, BRCA2 full sequence analysis and full duplication/deletion analysis (81162)
Hereditary breast cancer genomic sequence analysis panel (81432)

🗲 0.00   ⚖ 0.00   **FUD** XXX   A ▯

AMA: 2020,Dec,3; 2020,OctSE,1; 2020,OctSE,1; 2019,May,5; 2018,Nov,9; 2018,Jan,8; 2017,Jan,8; 2016,Aug,9; 2016,Jan,13

 # 81167 full duplication/deletion analysis (ie, detection of large gene rearrangements)

EXCLUDES   *BRCA1, BRCA2 full duplication/deletion analysis only (81164, 81167)*
BRCA1, BRCA2 full sequence analysis and full duplication/deletion analysis (81162)

🗲 0.00   ⚖ 0.00   **FUD** XXX   ▯

AMA: 2020,Dec,3; 2019,May,5

81217 known familial variant

EXCLUDES   *BRCA1, BRCA2 full duplication/deletion analysis only (81164, 81167)*
BRCA1, BRCA2 full sequence analysis and full duplication/deletion analysis (81162)

🗲 0.00   ⚖ 0.00   **FUD** XXX   A ▯

AMA: 2020,Dec,3; 2020,OctSE,1; 2020,OctSE,1; 2019,May,5; 2018,Nov,9; 2018,Jan,8; 2017,Jan,8; 2016,Aug,9; 2016,Jan,13

 # 81233 *BTK (Bruton's tyrosine kinase) (eg, chronic lymphocytic leukemia) gene analysis, common variants (eg, C481S, C481R, C481F)*

🗲 0.00   ⚖ 0.00   **FUD** XXX   ▯

AMA: 2020,Dec,3; 2020,OctSE,1; 2020,OctSE,1; 2018,Nov,9

26/TC PC/TC Only   A2-Z3 ASC Payment   50 Bilateral   ♂ Male Only   ♀ Female Only   🗲 Facility RVU   ⚖ Non-Facility RVU   ▯ CCI   ✖ CLIA
FUD Follow-up Days   CMS: IOM   AMA: CPT Asst   A-Y OPPSI   80/80 Surg Assist Allowed / w/Doc   ▯ Lab Crosswalk   ▯ Radiology Crosswalk

366   CPT © 2021 American Medical Association. All Rights Reserved.   © 2021 Optum360, LLC

\# 81184 **CACNA1A (calcium voltage-gated channel subunit alpha1 A) (eg, spinocerebellar ataxia) gene analysis; evaluation to detect abnormal (eg, expanded) alleles**
📋 0.00 ✂ 0.00 **FUD** XXX 🖵
AMA: 2020,Dec,3

\# 81185 **full gene sequence**
📋 0.00 ✂ 0.00 **FUD** XXX 🖵
AMA: 2020,Dec,3

\# 81186 **known familial variant**
📋 0.00 ✂ 0.00 **FUD** XXX 🖵
AMA: 2020,Dec,3

\# 81219 **CALR (calreticulin) (eg, myeloproliferative disorders), gene analysis, common variants in exon 9**
📋 0.00 ✂ 0.00 **FUD** XXX 🅐🖵
AMA: 2020,Dec,3; 2020,OctSE,1; 2020,OctSE,1; 2018,Nov,9; 2018,Jan,8; 2017,Jan,8; 2016,Aug,9

\# 81168 **CCND1/IGH (t(11;14)) (eg, mantle cell lymphoma) translocation analysis, major breakpoint, qualitative and quantitative, if performed**
📋 0.00 ✂ 0.00 **FUD** XXX 🖵
AMA: 2020,Dec,3

81218 **CEBPA (CCAAT/enhancer binding protein [C/EBP], alpha) (eg, acute myeloid leukemia), gene analysis, full gene sequence**
📋 0.00 ✂ 0.00 **FUD** XXX 🅐🖵
AMA: 2020,Dec,3; 2020,OctSE,1; 2020,OctSE,1; 2018,Nov,9; 2018,Jan,8; 2017,Jan,8; 2016,Aug,9

81219 **Resequenced code. See code before 81218.**

81220 **CFTR (cystic fibrosis transmembrane conductance regulator) (eg, cystic fibrosis) gene analysis; common variants (eg, ACMG/ACOG guidelines)**
EXCLUDES *Excludes Intron 8 poly-T analysis performed in conjunction with 81220 in R117H positive patient*
📋 0.00 ✂ 0.00 **FUD** XXX 🅐🖵
AMA: 2020,Dec,3; 2020,OctSE,1; 2020,OctSE,1; 2018,Nov,9; 2018,Jan,8; 2017,Jan,8; 2016,Aug,9; 2016,Jan,13

81221 **known familial variants**
📋 0.00 ✂ 0.00 **FUD** XXX 🅐🖵
AMA: 2020,Dec,3; 2020,OctSE,1; 2020,OctSE,1; 2018,Nov,9; 2018,Jan,8; 2017,Jan,8; 2016,Aug,9; 2016,Jan,13

81222 **duplication/deletion variants**
📋 0.00 ✂ 0.00 **FUD** XXX 🅐🖵
AMA: 2020,Dec,3; 2020,OctSE,1; 2020,OctSE,1; 2018,Nov,9; 2018,Jan,8; 2017,Jan,8; 2016,Aug,9; 2016,Jan,13

81223 **full gene sequence**
📋 0.00 ✂ 0.00 **FUD** XXX 🅐🖵
AMA: 2020,Dec,3; 2020,OctSE,1; 2020,OctSE,1; 2018,Nov,9; 2018,Jan,8; 2017,Jan,8; 2016,Aug,9; 2016,Jan,13

81224 **intron 8 poly-T analysis (eg, male infertility)**
📋 0.00 ✂ 0.00 **FUD** XXX 🅐🖵
AMA: 2020,Dec,3; 2020,OctSE,1; 2020,OctSE,1; 2018,Nov,9; 2018,Jan,8; 2017,Jan,8; 2016,Aug,9; 2016,Jan,13

\# 81267 **Chimerism (engraftment) analysis, post transplantation specimen (eg, hematopoietic stem cell), includes comparison to previously performed baseline analyses; without cell selection**
📋 0.00 ✂ 0.00 **FUD** XXX 🅐🖵
AMA: 2020,Dec,3; 2020,OctSE,1; 2020,OctSE,1; 2018,Nov,9; 2018,Jan,8; 2017,Jan,8; 2016,Aug,9; 2016,Jan,13

\# 81268 **with cell selection (eg, CD3, CD33), each cell type**
📋 0.00 ✂ 0.00 **FUD** XXX 🅐🖵
AMA: 2020,Dec,3; 2020,OctSE,1; 2020,OctSE,1; 2018,Nov,9; 2018,Jan,8; 2017,Jan,8; 2016,Aug,9; 2016,Jan,13

\# 81187 **CNBP (CCHC-type zinc finger nucleic acid binding protein) (eg, myotonic dystrophy type 2) gene analysis, evaluation to detect abnormal (eg, expanded) alleles**
📋 0.00 ✂ 0.00 **FUD** XXX 🖵
AMA: 2020,Dec,3

\# 81265 **Comparative analysis using Short Tandem Repeat (STR) markers; patient and comparative specimen (eg, pre-transplant recipient and donor germline testing, post-transplant non-hematopoietic recipient germline [eg, buccal swab or other germline tissue sample] and donor testing, twin zygosity testing, or maternal cell contamination of fetal cells)**
📋 0.00 ✂ 0.00 **FUD** XXX 🅐🖵
AMA: 2020,Dec,3; 2020,OctSE,1; 2020,OctSE,1; 2018,Nov,9; 2018,Jan,8; 2017,Jan,8; 2016,Aug,9; 2016,Jan,13

+ \# 81266 **each additional specimen (eg, additional cord blood donor, additional fetal samples from different cultures, or additional zygosity in multiple birth pregnancies) (List separately in addition to code for primary procedure)**
Code first ([81265])
📋 0.00 ✂ 0.00 **FUD** XXX 🅐🖵
AMA: 2020,Dec,3; 2020,OctSE,1; 2020,OctSE,1; 2018,Nov,9; 2018,Jan,8; 2017,Jan,8; 2016,Aug,9; 2016,Jan,13

\# 81188 **CSTB (cystatin B) (eg, Unverricht-Lundborg disease) gene analysis; evaluation to detect abnormal (eg, expanded) alleles**
📋 0.00 ✂ 0.00 **FUD** XXX 🖵
AMA: 2020,Dec,3

\# 81189 **full gene sequence**
📋 0.00 ✂ 0.00 **FUD** XXX 🖵
AMA: 2020,Dec,3

\# 81190 **known familial variant(s)**
📋 0.00 ✂ 0.00 **FUD** XXX 🖵
AMA: 2020,Dec,3

\# 81227 **CYP2C9 (cytochrome P450, family 2, subfamily C, polypeptide 9) (eg, drug metabolism), gene analysis, common variants (eg, *2, *3, *5, *6)**
📋 0.00 ✂ 0.00 **FUD** XXX 🅐🖵
AMA: 2020,Dec,3; 2020,OctSE,1; 2020,OctSE,1; 2018,Nov,9; 2018,Jan,8; 2017,Jan,8; 2016,Aug,9; 2016,Jan,13

81225 **CYP2C19 (cytochrome P450, family 2, subfamily C, polypeptide 19) (eg, drug metabolism), gene analysis, common variants (eg, *2, *3, *4, *8, *17)**
📋 0.00 ✂ 0.00 **FUD** XXX 🅐🖵
AMA: 2020,Dec,3; 2020,OctSE,1; 2020,OctSE,1; 2018,Nov,9; 2018,Jan,8; 2017,Jan,8; 2016,Aug,9; 2016,Jan,13

81226 **CYP2D6 (cytochrome P450, family 2, subfamily D, polypeptide 6) (eg, drug metabolism), gene analysis, common variants (eg, *2, *3, *4, *5, *6, *9, *10, *17, *19, *29, *35, *41, *1XN, *2XN, *4XN)**
📋 0.00 ✂ 0.00 **FUD** XXX 🅐🖵
AMA: 2020,Dec,3; 2020,OctSE,1; 2020,OctSE,1; 2018,Nov,9; 2018,Jan,8; 2017,Jan,8; 2016,Aug,9; 2016,Jan,13

81227 **Resequenced code. See code before 81225.**

\# 81230 **CYP3A4 (cytochrome P450 family 3 subfamily A member 4) (eg, drug metabolism), gene analysis, common variant(s) (eg, *2, *22)**
📋 0.00 ✂ 0.00 **FUD** XXX 🅐🖵
AMA: 2020,Dec,3; 2020,OctSE,1; 2020,OctSE,1; 2018,Nov,9

\# 81231 **CYP3A5 (cytochrome P450 family 3 subfamily A member 5) (eg, drug metabolism), gene analysis, common variants (eg, *2, *3, *4, *5, *6, *7)**
📋 0.00 ✂ 0.00 **FUD** XXX 🅐🖵
AMA: 2020,Dec,3; 2020,OctSE,1; 2020,OctSE,1; 2018,Nov,9

▲ **81228** **Cytogenomic (genome-wide) analysis for constitutional chromosomal abnormalities; interrogation of genomic regions for copy number variants, comparative genomic hybridization [CGH] microarray analysis**

EXCLUDES *Analyte-specific molecular pathology procedures included in microarray analysis*
When performed in conjunction with:
Cytogenomic (genome-wide) analysis for constitutional chromosomal abnormalities ([81349])
Single nucleotide polymorphism interrogation (81229)

🛏 0.00   ✂ 0.00   **FUD** XXX   Ⓐ 🖬

AMA: 2020,Dec,3; 2020,OctSE,1; 2020,OctSE,1; 2018,Nov,9; 2018,Jan,8; 2017,Apr,3; 2017,Jan,8; 2016,Aug,9; 2016,Jan,13

▲ **81229** **interrogation of genomic regions for copy number and single nucleotide polymorphism (SNP) variants, comparative genomic hybridization (CGH) microarray analysis**

EXCLUDES *Analyte-specific molecular pathology procedures included in microarray analysis*
Copy number variant detection using oligonucleotide interrogation only (81228)
Cytogenomic (genome-wide) analysis for constitutional chromosomal abnormalities ([81349])
Fetal genomic sequencing or other molecular multianalyte assays using circulating cell-free DNA in maternal blood ([81479], 81420, 81422)
Molecular cytogenetics; DNA probe (88271)

🛏 0.00   ✂ 0.00   **FUD** XXX   Ⓐ 🖬

AMA: 2020,Dec,3; 2020,OctSE,1; 2020,OctSE,1; 2018,Nov,9; 2018,Jan,8; 2017,Apr,3; 2017,Jan,8; 2016,Aug,9; 2016,Jan,13

● # **81349** **interrogation of genomic regions for copy number and loss-of-heterozygosity variants, low-pass sequencing analysis**

EXCLUDES *Analyte-specific molecular pathology procedures included in microarray analysis*
Chromosomal abnormalities by sequence analysis (81425-81426)
Chromosomal abnormalities not genome-wide, report instead code for targeted analyis or unlisted code ([81479])
Cytogenomic (genome-wide) analysis for constitutional chromosomal abnormalities (81228-81229)

🛏 0.00   ✂ 0.00   **FUD** 000

81277 **Cytogenomic neoplasia (genome-wide) microarray analysis, interrogation of genomic regions for copy number and loss-of-heterozygosity variants for chromosomal abnormalities**

EXCLUDES *Analyte-specific molecular pathology procedures included in microarray analysis for neoplasia*
Molecular cytogenetics; DNA probe (88271)

🛏 0.00   ✂ 0.00   **FUD** XXX

AMA: 2020,Dec,3; 2020,OctSE,1; 2020,OctSE,1; 2020,Feb,10

81230 **Resequenced code. See code following numeric code 81227.**

81231 **Resequenced code. See code following numeric code 81227.**

81161 **DMD (dystrophin) (eg, Duchenne/Becker muscular dystrophy) deletion analysis, and duplication analysis, if performed**

🛏 0.00   ✂ 0.00   **FUD** XXX   Ⓐ 🖬

AMA: 2020,Dec,3; 2020,OctSE,1; 2020,OctSE,1; 2018,Nov,9; 2018,Jan,8; 2017,Jan,8; 2016,Aug,9

81234 **DMPK (DM1 protein kinase) (eg, myotonic dystrophy type 1) gene analysis; evaluation to detect abnormal (expanded) alleles**

🛏 0.00   ✂ 0.00   **FUD** XXX   🖬

AMA: 2020,Dec,3; 2020,OctSE,1; 2020,OctSE,1; 2018,Nov,9

81239 **characterization of alleles (eg, expanded size)**

🛏 0.00   ✂ 0.00   **FUD** XXX   🖬

AMA: 2020,Dec,3; 2020,OctSE,1; 2020,OctSE,1; 2018,Nov,9

81232 **DPYD (dihydropyrimidine dehydrogenase) (eg, 5-fluorouracil/5-FU and capecitabine drug metabolism), gene analysis, common variant(s) (eg, *2A, *4, *5, *6)**

🛏 0.00   ✂ 0.00   **FUD** XXX   Ⓐ 🖬

AMA: 2020,Dec,3; 2020,OctSE,1; 2020,OctSE,1; 2018,Nov,9

81233 **Resequenced code. See code following 81217.**

81234 **Resequenced code. See code following numeric code 81231.**

81235 **EGFR (epidermal growth factor receptor) (eg, non-small cell lung cancer) gene analysis, common variants (eg, exon 19 LREA deletion, L858R, T790M, G719A, G719S, L861Q)**

🛏 0.00   ✂ 0.00   **FUD** XXX   Ⓐ 🖬

AMA: 2020,Dec,3; 2020,OctSE,1; 2020,OctSE,1; 2018,Nov,9; 2018,Jan,8; 2017,Jan,8; 2016,Aug,9; 2016,Jan,13

81236 **EZH2 (enhancer of zeste 2 polycomb repressive complex 2 subunit) (eg, myelodysplastic syndrome, myeloproliferative neoplasms) gene analysis, full gene sequence**

🛏 0.00   ✂ 0.00   **FUD** XXX   🖬

AMA: 2020,Dec,3; 2020,OctSE,1; 2020,OctSE,1; 2019,Jul,3; 2018,Nov,9

81237 **EZH2 (enhancer of zeste 2 polycomb repressive complex 2 subunit) (eg, diffuse large B-cell lymphoma) gene analysis, common variant(s) (eg, codon 646)**

🛏 0.00   ✂ 0.00   **FUD** XXX   🖬

AMA: 2020,Dec,3; 2020,OctSE,1; 2020,OctSE,1; 2019,Jul,3; 2018,Nov,9

81238 **Resequenced code. See code following 81241.**

81239 **Resequenced code. See code before 81232.**

81240 **F2 (prothrombin, coagulation factor II) (eg, hereditary hypercoagulability) gene analysis, 20210G>A variant**

🛏 0.00   ✂ 0.00   **FUD** XXX   Ⓐ 🖬

AMA: 2020,Dec,3; 2020,OctSE,1; 2020,OctSE,1; 2018,Nov,9; 2018,Jan,8; 2017,Jan,8; 2016,Aug,9; 2016,Jan,13

81241 **F5 (coagulation factor V) (eg, hereditary hypercoagulability) gene analysis, Leiden variant**

🛏 0.00   ✂ 0.00   **FUD** XXX   Ⓐ 🖬

AMA: 2020,Dec,3; 2020,OctSE,1; 2020,OctSE,1; 2018,Nov,9; 2018,Jan,8; 2017,Jan,8; 2016,Aug,9; 2016,Jan,13

81238 **F9 (coagulation factor IX) (eg, hemophilia B), full gene sequence**

🛏 0.00   ✂ 0.00   **FUD** XXX   Ⓐ 🖬

AMA: 2020,Dec,3; 2020,OctSE,1; 2020,OctSE,1; 2018,Nov,9

81242 **FANCC (Fanconi anemia, complementation group C) (eg, Fanconi anemia, type C) gene analysis, common variant (eg, IVS4+4A>T)**

🛏 0.00   ✂ 0.00   **FUD** XXX   Ⓐ 🖬

AMA: 2020,Dec,3; 2020,OctSE,1; 2020,OctSE,1; 2018,Nov,9; 2018,Jan,8; 2017,Jan,8; 2016,Aug,9; 2016,Jan,13

81245 **FLT3 (fms-related tyrosine kinase 3) (eg, acute myeloid leukemia), gene analysis; internal tandem duplication (ITD) variants (ie, exons 14, 15)**

🛏 0.00   ✂ 0.00   **FUD** XXX   Ⓐ 🖬

AMA: 2020,Dec,3; 2020,OctSE,1; 2020,OctSE,1; 2018,Nov,9; 2018,Jan,8; 2017,Jan,8; 2016,Aug,9; 2016,Jan,13

81246 **tyrosine kinase domain (TKD) variants (eg, D835, I836)**

🛏 0.00   ✂ 0.00   **FUD** XXX   Ⓐ 🖬

AMA: 2020,Dec,3; 2020,OctSE,1; 2020,OctSE,1; 2018,Nov,9; 2018,Jan,8; 2017,Jan,8; 2016,Aug,9; 2016,Jan,13

81243 **FMR1 (fragile X mental retardation 1) (eg, fragile X mental retardation) gene analysis; evaluation to detect abnormal (eg, expanded) alleles**

INCLUDES *Evaluation to detect and characterize abnormal alleles using single assay [i.e., PCR]*

EXCLUDES *Evaluation to detect and characterize abnormal alleles (81244)*

🛏 0.00   ✂ 0.00   **FUD** XXX   Ⓐ 🖬

AMA: 2020,Dec,3; 2020,OctSE,1; 2020,OctSE,1; 2019,Jul,3; 2018,Nov,9; 2018,Jan,8; 2017,Jan,8; 2016,Aug,9; 2016,Jan,13

26/TC PC/TC Only   A2-Z3 ASC Payment   50 Bilateral   ♂ Male Only   ♀ Female Only   🛏 Facility RVU   ✂ Non-Facility RVU   🖬 CCI   ☒ CLIA
FUD Follow-up Days   **CMS:** IOM   **AMA:** CPT Asst   Ⓐ-Ⓨ OPPSI   80/80 Surg Assist Allowed / w/Doc   ◼ Lab Crosswalk   ◼ Radiology Crosswalk

368   CPT © 2021 American Medical Association. All Rights Reserved.   © 2021 Optum360, LLC

81244 characterization of alleles (eg, expanded size and promoter methylation status)

EXCLUDES *Evaluation to detect and characterize abnormal alleles using single assay [i.e., PCR] (81243)*

🔲 0.00   ⚕   **FUD** XXX   Ⓐ 🔲

AMA: 2020,Dec,3; 2020,OctSE,1; 2020,OctSE,1; 2019,Jul,3; 2018,Nov,9; 2018,Jan,8; 2017,Jan,8; 2016,Aug,9; 2016,Jan,13

81245 **Resequenced code. See code following 81242.**

81246 **Resequenced code. See code following 81242.**

\# **81284** *FXN (frataxin)* (eg, Friedreich ataxia) gene analysis; evaluation to detect abnormal (expanded) alleles

🔲 0.00   ⚕   **FUD** XXX   🔲

AMA: 2020,Dec,3; 2020,OctSE,1; 2020,OctSE,1; 2018,Nov,9

\# **81285** characterization of alleles (eg, expanded size)

🔲 0.00   ⚕   **FUD** XXX   🔲

AMA: 2020,Dec,3; 2020,OctSE,1; 2020,OctSE,1; 2018,Nov,9

\# **81286** full gene sequence

🔲 0.00   ⚕   **FUD** XXX   🔲

AMA: 2020,Dec,3; 2020,OctSE,1; 2020,OctSE,1; 2018,Nov,9

\# **81289** known familial variant(s)

🔲 0.00   ⚕   **FUD** XXX   🔲

AMA: 2020,Dec,3; 2020,OctSE,1; 2020,OctSE,1; 2018,Nov,9

\# **81250** *G6PC (glucose-6-phosphatase, catalytic subunit)* (eg, Glycogen storage disease, type 1a, von Gierke disease) gene analysis, common variants (eg, R83C, Q347X)

🔲 0.00   ⚕   **FUD** XXX   Ⓐ 🔲

AMA: 2020,Dec,3; 2020,OctSE,1; 2020,OctSE,1; 2018,Nov,9; 2018,Jan,8; 2017,Jan,8; 2016,Aug,9; 2016,Jan,13

81247 *G6PD (glucose-6-phosphate dehydrogenase)* (eg, hemolytic anemia, jaundice), gene analysis; common variant(s) (eg, A, A-)

🔲 0.00   ⚕ 0.00   **FUD** XXX   Ⓐ 🔲

AMA: 2020,Dec,3; 2020,OctSE,1; 2020,OctSE,1; 2018,Nov,9

81248 known familial variant(s)

🔲 0.00   ⚕ 0.00   **FUD** XXX   Ⓐ 🔲

AMA: 2020,Dec,3; 2020,OctSE,1; 2020,OctSE,1; 2018,Nov,9

81249 full gene sequence

🔲 0.00   ⚕ 0.00   **FUD** XXX   Ⓐ 🔲

AMA: 2020,Dec,3; 2020,OctSE,1; 2020,OctSE,1; 2018,Nov,9

81250 **Resequenced code. See code before 81247.**

81251 *GBA (glucosidase, beta, acid)* (eg, Gaucher disease) gene analysis, common variants (eg, N370S, 84GG, L444P, IVS2+1G>A)

🔲 0.00   ⚕ 0.00   **FUD** XXX   Ⓐ 🔲

AMA: 2020,Dec,3; 2020,OctSE,1; 2020,OctSE,1; 2018,Nov,9; 2018,Jan,8; 2017,Jan,8; 2016,Aug,9; 2016,Jan,13

81252 *GJB2 (gap junction protein, beta 2, 26kDa, connexin 26)* (eg, nonsyndromic hearing loss) gene analysis; full gene sequence

🔲 0.00   ⚕ 0.00   **FUD** XXX   Ⓐ 🔲

AMA: 2020,Dec,3; 2020,OctSE,1; 2020,OctSE,1; 2018,Nov,9; 2018,Jan,8; 2017,Jan,8; 2016,Aug,9; 2016,Jan,13

81253 known familial variants

🔲 0.00   ⚕ 0.00   **FUD** XXX   Ⓐ 🔲

AMA: 2020,Dec,3; 2020,OctSE,1; 2020,OctSE,1; 2018,Nov,9; 2018,Jan,8; 2017,Jan,8; 2016,Aug,9; 2016,Jan,13

81254 *GJB6 (gap junction protein, beta 6, 30kDa, connexin 30)* (eg, nonsyndromic hearing loss) gene analysis, common variants (eg, 309kb [del(GJB6-D13S1830)] and 232kb [del(GJB6-D13S1854)])

🔲 0.00   ⚕ 0.00   **FUD** XXX   Ⓐ 🔲

AMA: 2020,Dec,3; 2020,OctSE,1; 2020,OctSE,1; 2018,Nov,9; 2018,Jan,8; 2017,Jan,8; 2016,Aug,9; 2016,Jan,13

\# **81257** *HBA1/HBA2 (alpha globin 1 and alpha globin 2)* (eg, alpha thalassemia, Hb Bart hydrops fetalis syndrome, HbH disease), gene analysis; common deletions or variant (eg, Southeast Asian, Thai, Filipino, Mediterranean, alpha3.7, alpha4.2, alpha20.5, Constant Spring)

🔲 0.00   ⚕   **FUD** XXX   Ⓐ 🔲

AMA: 2020,Dec,3; 2020,OctSE,1; 2020,OctSE,1; 2018,Nov,9; 2018,Jan,8; 2017,Jan,8; 2016,Aug,9; 2016,Jan,13

\# **81258** known familial variant

🔲 0.00   ⚕   **FUD** XXX   Ⓐ 🔲

AMA: 2020,Dec,3; 2020,OctSE,1; 2020,OctSE,1; 2018,Nov,9

\# **81259** full gene sequence

🔲 0.00   ⚕   **FUD** XXX   Ⓐ 🔲

AMA: 2020,Dec,3; 2020,OctSE,1; 2020,OctSE,1; 2018,Nov,9

\# **81269** duplication/deletion variants

🔲 0.00   ⚕   **FUD** XXX   Ⓐ 🔲

AMA: 2020,Dec,3; 2020,OctSE,1; 2020,OctSE,1; 2018,Nov,9

\# **81361** *HBB (hemoglobin, subunit beta)* (eg, sickle cell anemia, beta thalassemia, hemoglobinopathy); common variant(s) (eg, HbS, HbC, HbE)

🔲 0.00   ⚕   **FUD** XXX   Ⓐ 🔲

AMA: 2020,Dec,3; 2020,OctSE,1; 2020,OctSE,1; 2018,Nov,9

\# **81362** known familial variant(s)

🔲 0.00   ⚕   **FUD** XXX   Ⓐ 🔲

AMA: 2020,Dec,3; 2020,OctSE,1; 2020,OctSE,1; 2018,Nov,9

\# **81363** duplication/deletion variant(s)

🔲 0.00   ⚕   **FUD** XXX   Ⓐ 🔲

AMA: 2020,Dec,3; 2020,OctSE,1; 2020,OctSE,1; 2018,Nov,9; 2018,Sep,14

\# **81364** full gene sequence

🔲 0.00   ⚕   **FUD** XXX   Ⓐ 🔲

AMA: 2020,Dec,3; 2020,OctSE,1; 2020,OctSE,1; 2018,Nov,9; 2018,Sep,14

81255 *HEXA (hexosaminidase A [alpha polypeptide])* (eg, Tay-Sachs disease) gene analysis, common variants (eg, 1278insTATC, 1421+1G>C, G269S)

🔲 0.00   ⚕   **FUD** XXX   Ⓐ 🔲

AMA: 2020,Dec,3; 2020,OctSE,1; 2020,OctSE,1; 2018,Nov,9; 2018,Jan,8; 2017,Jan,8; 2016,Aug,9; 2016,Jan,13

81256 *HFE (hemochromatosis)* (eg, hereditary hemochromatosis) gene analysis, common variants (eg, C282Y, H63D)

🔲 0.00   ⚕ 0.00   **FUD** XXX   Ⓐ 🔲

AMA: 2020,Dec,3; 2020,OctSE,1; 2020,OctSE,1; 2018,Nov,9; 2018,Jan,8; 2017,Jan,8; 2016,Aug,9; 2016,Jan,13

81257 **Resequenced code. See code following 81254.**

81258 **Resequenced code. See code following 81254.**

81259 **Resequenced code. See code following 81254.**

\# **81271** *HTT (huntingtin)* (eg, Huntington disease) gene analysis; evaluation to detect abnormal (eg, expanded) alleles

🔲 0.00   ⚕ 0.00   **FUD** XXX   🔲

AMA: 2020,Dec,3; 2020,OctSE,1; 2020,OctSE,1; 2018,Nov,9

\# **81274** characterization of alleles (eg, expanded size)

🔲 0.00   ⚕ 0.00   **FUD** XXX   🔲

AMA: 2020,Dec,3; 2020,OctSE,1; 2020,OctSE,1; 2018,Nov,9

\# **81105** *Human Platelet Antigen 1 genotyping (HPA-1), ITGB3 (integrin, beta 3 [platelet glycoprotein IIIa], antigen CD61 [GPIIIa])* (eg, neonatal alloimmune thrombocytopenia [NAIT], post-transfusion purpura), gene analysis, common variant, HPA-1a/b (L33P)

🔲 0.00   ⚕ 0.00   **FUD** XXX   Ⓐ 🔲

AMA: 2020,Dec,3

● New Code   ▲ Revised Code   ○ Reinstated   ● New Web Release   ▲ Revised Web Release   + Add-on   Unlisted   Not Covered   \# Resequenced
⑤⓪ Optum Mod 50 Exempt   ⊘ AMA Mod 51 Exempt   ⑤① Optum Mod 51 Exempt   ⑥③ Mod 63 Exempt   ⚕ Non-FDA Drug   ★ Telemedicine   Ⓜ Maternity   Ⓐ Age Edit

\# 81106 **Human Platelet Antigen 2 genotyping (HPA-2), GP1BA (glycoprotein Ib [platelet], alpha polypeptide [GPIba]) (eg, neonatal alloimmune thrombocytopenia [NAIT], post-transfusion purpura), gene analysis, common variant, HPA-2a/b (T145M)**
🔲 0.00   ⚕ 0.00   **FUD** XXX   Ⓐ 🔲
AMA: 2020,Dec,3

\# 81107 **Human Platelet Antigen 3 genotyping (HPA-3), ITGA2B (integrin, alpha 2b [platelet glycoprotein IIb of IIb/IIIa complex], antigen CD41 [GPIIb]) (eg, neonatal alloimmune thrombocytopenia [NAIT], post-transfusion purpura), gene analysis, common variant, HPA-3a/b (I843S)**
🔲 0.00   ⚕ 0.00   **FUD** XXX   Ⓐ 🔲
AMA: 2020,Dec,3

\# 81108 **Human Platelet Antigen 4 genotyping (HPA-4), ITGB3 (integrin, beta 3 [platelet glycoprotein IIIa], antigen CD61 [GPIIIa]) (eg, neonatal alloimmune thrombocytopenia [NAIT], post-transfusion purpura), gene analysis, common variant, HPA-4a/b (R143Q)**
🔲 0.00   ⚕ 0.00   **FUD** XXX   Ⓐ 🔲
AMA: 2020,Dec,3

\# 81109 **Human Platelet Antigen 5 genotyping (HPA-5), ITGA2 (integrin, alpha 2 [CD49B, alpha 2 subunit of VLA-2 receptor] [GPIa]) (eg, neonatal alloimmune thrombocytopenia [NAIT], post-transfusion purpura), gene analysis, common variant (eg, HPA-5a/b (K505E))**
🔲 0.00   ⚕ 0.00   **FUD** XXX   Ⓐ 🔲
AMA: 2020,Dec,3

\# 81110 **Human Platelet Antigen 6 genotyping (HPA-6w), ITGB3 (integrin, beta 3 [platelet glycoprotein IIIa, antigen CD61] [GPIIIa]) (eg, neonatal alloimmune thrombocytopenia [NAIT], post-transfusion purpura), gene analysis, common variant, HPA-6a/b (R489Q)**
🔲 0.00   ⚕ 0.00   **FUD** XXX   Ⓐ 🔲
AMA: 2020,Dec,3

\# 81111 **Human Platelet Antigen 9 genotyping (HPA-9w), ITGA2B (integrin, alpha 2b [platelet glycoprotein IIb of IIb/IIIa complex, antigen CD41] [GPIIb]) (eg, neonatal alloimmune thrombocytopenia [NAIT], post-transfusion purpura), gene analysis, common variant, HPA-9a/b (V837M)**
🔲 0.00   ⚕ 0.00   **FUD** XXX   Ⓐ 🔲
AMA: 2020,Dec,3

\# 81112 **Human Platelet Antigen 15 genotyping (HPA-15), CD109 (CD109 molecule) (eg, neonatal alloimmune thrombocytopenia [NAIT], post-transfusion purpura), gene analysis, common variant, HPA-15a/b (S682Y)**
🔲 0.00   ⚕ 0.00   **FUD** XXX   Ⓐ 🔲
AMA: 2020,Dec,3

\# 81120 **IDH1 (isocitrate dehydrogenase 1 [NADP+], soluble) (eg, glioma), common variants (eg, R132H, R132C)**
🔲 0.00   ⚕ 0.00   **FUD** XXX   Ⓐ 🔲
AMA: 2020,Dec,3

\# 81121 **IDH2 (isocitrate dehydrogenase 2 [NADP+], mitochondrial) (eg, glioma), common variants (eg, R140W, R172M)**
🔲 0.00   ⚕ 0.00   **FUD** XXX   Ⓐ 🔲
AMA: 2020,Dec,3

\# 81283 **IFNL3 (interferon, lambda 3) (eg, drug response), gene analysis, rs12979860 variant**
🔲 0.00   ⚕ 0.00   **FUD** XXX   Ⓐ 🔲
AMA: 2020,Dec,3; 2020,OctSE,1; 2020,OctSE,1; 2018,Nov,9

\# 81261 **IGH@ (Immunoglobulin heavy chain locus) (eg, leukemias and lymphomas, B-cell), gene rearrangement analysis to detect abnormal clonal population(s); amplified methodology (eg, polymerase chain reaction)**
🔲 0.00   ⚕ 0.00   **FUD** XXX   Ⓐ 🔲
AMA: 2020,Dec,3; 2020,OctSE,1; 2020,OctSE,1; 2018,Nov,9; 2018,Jan,8; 2017,Jan,8; 2016,Aug,9; 2016,Jan,13

\# 81262 **direct probe methodology (eg, Southern blot)**
🔲 0.00   ⚕ 0.00   **FUD** XXX   Ⓐ 🔲
AMA: 2020,Dec,3; 2020,OctSE,1; 2020,OctSE,1; 2018,Nov,9; 2018,Jan,8; 2017,Jan,8; 2016,Aug,9; 2016,Jan,13

\# 81263 **IGH@ (Immunoglobulin heavy chain locus) (eg, leukemia and lymphoma, B-cell), variable region somatic mutation analysis**
🔲 0.00   ⚕ 0.00   **FUD** XXX   Ⓐ 🔲
AMA: 2020,Dec,3; 2020,OctSE,1; 2020,OctSE,1; 2018,Nov,9; 2018,Jan,8; 2017,Jan,8; 2016,Aug,9; 2016,Jan,13

\# 81278 **IGH@/BCL2 (t(14;18)) (eg, follicular lymphoma) translocation analysis, major breakpoint region (MBR) and minor cluster region (mcr) breakpoints, qualitative or quantitative**
🔲 0.00   ⚕ 0.00   **FUD** XXX   🔲
AMA: 2020,Dec,3; 2020,OctSE,1

\# 81264 **IGK@ (Immunoglobulin kappa light chain locus) (eg, leukemia and lymphoma, B-cell), gene rearrangement analysis, evaluation to detect abnormal clonal population(s)**
🔲 0.00   ⚕ 0.00   **FUD** XXX   Ⓐ 🔲
AMA: 2020,Dec,3; 2020,OctSE,1; 2020,OctSE,1; 2018,Nov,9; 2018,Jan,8; 2017,Jan,8; 2016,Aug,9; 2016,Jan,13

81260 **IKBKAP (inhibitor of kappa light polypeptide gene enhancer in B-cells, kinase complex-associated protein) (eg, familial dysautonomia) gene analysis, common variants (eg, 2507+6T>C, R696P)**
🔲 0.00   ⚕ 0.00   **FUD** XXX   Ⓐ 🔲
AMA: 2020,Dec,3; 2020,OctSE,1; 2020,OctSE,1; 2018,Nov,9; 2018,Jan,8; 2017,Jan,8; 2016,Aug,9; 2016,Jan,13

81261 *Resequenced code. See code before 81260.*

81262 *Resequenced code. See code before 81260.*

81263 *Resequenced code. See code before 81260.*

81264 *Resequenced code. See code before 81260.*

81265 *Resequenced code. See code following resequenced code 81187.*

81266 *Resequenced code. See code following resequenced code 81265.*

81267 *Resequenced code. See code following 81224.*

81268 *Resequenced code. See code following 81224.*

81269 *Resequenced code. See code following resequenced code 81259.*

81270 **JAK2 (Janus kinase 2) (eg, myeloproliferative disorder) gene analysis, p.Val617Phe (V617F) variant**
🔲 0.00   ⚕ 0.00   **FUD** XXX   Ⓐ 🔲
AMA: 2020,Dec,3; 2020,OctSE,1; 2020,OctSE,1; 2018,Nov,9; 2018,Jan,8; 2017,Jan,8; 2016,Aug,9; 2016,Jan,13

\# 81279 **JAK2 (Janus kinase 2) (eg, myeloproliferative disorder) targeted sequence analysis (eg, exons 12 and 13)**
🔲 0.00   ⚕ 0.00   **FUD** XXX   🔲
AMA: 2020,Dec,3; 2020,OctSE,1

81271 *Resequenced code. See code following numeric code 81259.*

81272 **KIT (v-kit Hardy-Zuckerman 4 feline sarcoma viral oncogene homolog) (eg, gastrointestinal stromal tumor [GIST], acute myeloid leukemia, melanoma), gene analysis, targeted sequence analysis (eg, exons 8, 11, 13, 17, 18)**
🔲 0.00   ⚕ 0.00   **FUD** XXX   Ⓐ 🔲
AMA: 2020,Dec,3; 2020,OctSE,1; 2020,OctSE,1; 2018,Nov,9; 2018,Jan,8; 2017,Jan,8; 2016,Aug,9

81273 **KIT (v-kit Hardy-Zuckerman 4 feline sarcoma viral oncogene homolog) (eg, mastocytosis), gene analysis, D816 variant**
🔲 0.00   ⚕ 0.00   **FUD** XXX   Ⓐ 🔲
AMA: 2020,Dec,3; 2020,OctSE,1; 2020,OctSE,1; 2018,Nov,9; 2018,Jan,8; 2017,Jan,8; 2016,Aug,9

81274 *Resequenced code. See code following resequenced code 81271.*

81275 **KRAS (Kirsten rat sarcoma viral oncogene homolog) (eg, carcinoma) gene analysis; variants in exon 2 (eg, codons 12 and 13)**
🔧 0.00 👤 0.00 **FUD** XXX Ⓐ▢
AMA: 2020,Dec,3; 2020,OctSE,1; 2020,OctSE,1; 2018,Nov,9; 2018,Jan,8; 2017,Jan,8; 2016,Aug,9; 2016,Jan,13

81276 **additional variant(s) (eg, codon 61, codon 146)**
🔧 0.00 👤 0.00 **FUD** XXX Ⓐ▢
AMA: 2020,Dec,3; 2020,OctSE,1; 2020,OctSE,1; 2018,Nov,9; 2018,Jan,8; 2017,Jan,8; 2016,Aug,9

81277 Resequenced code. See code following 81229.

81278 Resequenced code. See code following resequenced code 81263.

81279 Resequenced code. See code following 81270.

81283 Resequenced code. See code following resequenced code 81121.

81284 Resequenced code. See code following numeric code 81246.

81285 Resequenced code. See code following numeric code 81246.

81286 Resequenced code. See code following numeric code 81246.

81287 Resequenced code. See code following resequenced code 81304.

81288 Resequenced code. See code following resequenced code 81292.

81289 Resequenced code. See code following numeric code 81246.

81290 **MCOLN1 (mucolipin 1) (eg, Mucolipidosis, type IV) gene analysis, common variants (eg, IVS3-2A>G, del6.4kb)**
🔧 0.00 👤 0.00 **FUD** XXX Ⓐ▢
AMA: 2020,Dec,3; 2020,OctSE,1; 2020,OctSE,1; 2018,Nov,9; 2018,Jan,8; 2017,Jan,8; 2016,Aug,9; 2016,Jan,13

\# 81302 **MECP2 (methyl CpG binding protein 2) (eg, Rett syndrome) gene analysis; full sequence analysis**
🔧 0.00 👤 0.00 **FUD** XXX Ⓐ▢
AMA: 2020,Dec,3; 2020,OctSE,1; 2020,OctSE,1; 2018,Nov,9; 2018,Jan,8; 2017,Jan,8; 2016,Aug,9; 2016,Jan,13

\# 81303 **known familial variant**
🔧 0.00 👤 0.00 **FUD** XXX Ⓐ▢
AMA: 2020,Dec,3; 2020,OctSE,1; 2020,OctSE,1; 2018,Nov,9; 2018,Jan,8; 2017,Jan,8; 2016,Aug,9; 2016,Jan,13

\# 81304 **duplication/deletion variants**
🔧 0.00 👤 0.00 **FUD** XXX Ⓐ▢
AMA: 2020,Dec,3; 2020,OctSE,1; 2020,OctSE,1; 2018,Nov,9; 2018,Jan,8; 2017,Jan,8; 2016,Aug,9; 2016,Jan,13

\# 81287 **MGMT (O-6-methylguanine-DNA methyltransferase) (eg, glioblastoma multiforme), promoter methylation analysis**
🔧 0.00 👤 0.00 **FUD** XXX Ⓐ▢
AMA: 2020,Dec,3; 2020,OctSE,1; 2020,OctSE,1; 2019,Jul,3; 2018,Dec,10; 2018,Dec,10; 2018,Nov,9; 2018,Jan,8; 2017,Jan,8; 2016,Aug,9

\# 81301 **Microsatellite instability analysis (eg, hereditary non-polyposis colorectal cancer, Lynch syndrome) of markers for mismatch repair deficiency (eg, BAT25, BAT26), includes comparison of neoplastic and normal tissue, if performed**
🔧 0.00 👤 0.00 **FUD** XXX ▢
AMA: 2020,Dec,3; 2020,OctSE,1; 2020,OctSE,1; 2018,Nov,9; 2018,Jan,8; 2017,Jan,8; 2016,Aug,9; 2016,Jan,13

\# 81292 **MLH1 (mutL homolog 1, colon cancer, nonpolyposis type 2) (eg, hereditary non-polyposis colorectal cancer, Lynch syndrome) gene analysis; full sequence analysis**
🔧 0.00 👤 0.00 **FUD** XXX Ⓐ▢
AMA: 2020,Dec,3; 2020,OctSE,1; 2020,OctSE,1; 2018,Nov,9; 2018,Jan,8; 2017,Jan,8; 2016,Aug,9; 2016,Jan,13

\# 81288 **promoter methylation analysis**
🔧 0.00 👤 0.00 **FUD** XXX Ⓐ▢
AMA: 2020,Dec,3; 2020,OctSE,1; 2020,OctSE,1; 2018,Nov,9; 2018,Jan,8; 2017,Jan,8; 2016,Aug,9; 2016,Jan,13

\# 81293 **known familial variants**
🔧 0.00 👤 0.00 **FUD** XXX Ⓐ▢
AMA: 2020,Dec,3; 2020,OctSE,1; 2020,OctSE,1; 2018,Nov,9; 2018,Jan,8; 2017,Jan,8; 2016,Aug,9; 2016,Jan,13

\# 81294 **duplication/deletion variants**
🔧 0.00 👤 0.00 **FUD** XXX Ⓐ▢
AMA: 2020,Dec,3; 2020,OctSE,1; 2020,OctSE,1; 2018,Nov,9; 2018,Jan,8; 2017,Jan,8; 2016,Aug,9; 2016,Jan,13

\# 81338 **MPL (MPL proto-oncogene, thrombopoietin receptor) (eg, myeloproliferative disorder) gene analysis; common variants (eg, W515A, W515K, W515L, W515R)**
🔧 0.00 👤 0.00 **FUD** XXX ▢
AMA: 2020,Dec,3; 2020,OctSE,1

\# 81339 **sequence analysis, exon 10**
🔧 0.00 👤 0.00 **FUD** XXX ▢
AMA: 2020,Dec,3; 2020,OctSE,1

\# 81295 **MSH2 (mutS homolog 2, colon cancer, nonpolyposis type 1) (eg, hereditary non-polyposis colorectal cancer, Lynch syndrome) gene analysis; full sequence analysis**
🔧 0.00 👤 0.00 **FUD** XXX Ⓐ▢
AMA: 2020,Dec,3; 2020,OctSE,1; 2020,OctSE,1; 2018,Nov,9; 2018,Jan,8; 2017,Jan,8; 2016,Aug,9; 2016,Jan,13

81291 Resequenced code. See code before 81305.

81292 Resequenced code. See code before numeric code 81291.

81293 Resequenced code. See code before numeric code 81291.

81294 Resequenced code. See code before numeric code 81291.

81295 Resequenced code. See code before numeric code 81291.

81296 **known familial variants**
🔧 0.00 👤 0.00 **FUD** XXX Ⓐ▢
AMA: 2020,Dec,3; 2020,OctSE,1; 2020,OctSE,1; 2018,Nov,9; 2018,Jan,8; 2017,Jan,8; 2016,Aug,9; 2016,Jan,13

81297 **duplication/deletion variants**
🔧 0.00 👤 0.00 **FUD** XXX Ⓐ▢
AMA: 2020,Dec,3; 2020,OctSE,1; 2020,OctSE,1; 2018,Nov,9; 2018,Jan,8; 2017,Jan,8; 2016,Aug,9; 2016,Jan,13

81298 **MSH6 (mutS homolog 6 [E. coli]) (eg, hereditary non-polyposis colorectal cancer, Lynch syndrome) gene analysis; full sequence analysis**
🔧 0.00 👤 0.00 **FUD** XXX Ⓐ▢
AMA: 2020,Dec,3; 2020,OctSE,1; 2020,OctSE,1; 2018,Nov,9; 2018,Jan,8; 2017,Jan,8; 2016,Aug,9; 2016,Jan,13

81299 **known familial variants**
🔧 0.00 👤 0.00 **FUD** XXX Ⓐ▢
AMA: 2020,Dec,3; 2020,OctSE,1; 2020,OctSE,1; 2018,Nov,9; 2018,Jan,8; 2017,Jan,8; 2016,Aug,9; 2016,Jan,13

81300 **duplication/deletion variants**
🔧 0.00 👤 0.00 **FUD** XXX Ⓐ▢
AMA: 2020,Dec,3; 2020,OctSE,1; 2020,OctSE,1; 2018,Nov,9; 2018,Jan,8; 2017,Jan,8; 2016,Aug,9; 2016,Jan,13

81301 Resequenced code. See code following resequenced code 81287.

81302 Resequenced code. See code following 81290.

81303 Resequenced code. See code following 81290.

81304 Resequenced code. See code following 81290.

\# 81291 **MTHFR (5,10-methylenetetrahydrofolate reductase) (eg, hereditary hypercoagulability) gene analysis, common variants (eg, 677T, 1298C)**
🔧 0.00 👤 0.00 **FUD** XXX Ⓐ▢
AMA: 2020,Dec,3; 2020,OctSE,1; 2020,OctSE,1; 2018,Nov,9; 2018,Jan,8; 2017,Jan,8; 2016,Aug,9; 2016,Jan,13

81305 MYD88 (myeloid differentiation primary response 88) (eg, Waldenstrom's macroglobulinemia, lymphoplasmacytic leukemia) gene analysis, p.Leu265Pro (L265P) variant

⚙ 0.00   ⚙ 0.00   **FUD** XXX   🖵

AMA: 2020,Dec,3; 2020,OctSE,1; 2020,OctSE,1; 2019,Jul,3; 2018,Nov,9

81306 Resequenced code. See code before resequenced code 81312.

81307 Resequenced code. See code before 81313.

81308 Resequenced code. See code before 81313.

81309 Resequenced code. See code following 81314.

81310 NPM1 (nucleophosmin) (eg, acute myeloid leukemia) gene analysis, exon 12 variants

⚙ 0.00   ⚙ 0.00   **FUD** XXX   Ⓐ🖵

AMA: 2020,Dec,3; 2020,OctSE,1; 2020,OctSE,1; 2018,Nov,9; 2018,Jan,8; 2017,Jan,8; 2016,Aug,9; 2016,Jan,13

81311 NRAS (neuroblastoma RAS viral [v-ras] oncogene homolog) (eg, colorectal carcinoma), gene analysis, variants in exon 2 (eg, codons 12 and 13) and exon 3 (eg, codon 61)

⚙ 0.00   ⚙ 0.00   **FUD** XXX   Ⓐ🖵

AMA: 2020,Dec,3; 2020,OctSE,1; 2020,OctSE,1; 2018,Nov,9; 2018,Jan,8; 2017,Jan,8; 2016,Aug,9

81312 Resequenced code. See code before resequenced code 81307.

\# **81191** NTRK1 (neurotrophic receptor tyrosine kinase 1) (eg, solid tumors) translocation analysis

⚙ 0.00   ⚙ 0.00   **FUD** XXX   🖵

AMA: 2020,Dec,3

\# **81192** NTRK2 (neurotrophic receptor tyrosine kinase 2) (eg, solid tumors) translocation analysis

⚙ 0.00   ⚙ 0.00   **FUD** XXX   🖵

AMA: 2020,Dec,3

\# **81193** NTRK3 (neurotrophic receptor tyrosine kinase 3) (eg, solid tumors) translocation analysis

⚙ 0.00   ⚙ 0.00   **FUD** XXX   🖵

AMA: 2020,Dec,3

\# **81194** NTRK (neurotrophic receptor tyrosine kinase 1, 2, and 3) (eg, solid tumors) translocation analysis

[INCLUDES] Analysis NTRK1, NTRK2, and NTRK3 by single assay

⚙ 0.00   ⚙ 0.00   **FUD** XXX   🖵

AMA: 2020,Dec,3

\# **81306** NUDT15 (nudix hydrolase 15) (eg, drug metabolism) gene analysis, common variant(s) (eg, *2, *3, *4, *5, *6)

⚙ 0.00   ⚙ 0.00   **FUD** XXX

AMA: 2020,Dec,3; 2020,OctSE,1; 2020,OctSE,1; 2019,Jul,3; 2018,Nov,9

\# **81312** PABPN1 (poly[A] binding protein nuclear 1) (eg, oculopharyngeal muscular dystrophy) gene analysis, evaluation to detect abnormal (eg, expanded) alleles

⚙ 0.00   ⚙ 0.00   **FUD** XXX   🖵

AMA: 2020,Dec,3; 2020,OctSE,1; 2020,OctSE,1; 2018,Nov,9

\# **81307** PALB2 (partner and localizer of BRCA2) (eg, breast and pancreatic cancer) gene analysis; full gene sequence

⚙ 0.00   ⚙ 0.00   **FUD** XXX   🖵

AMA: 2020,Dec,3; 2020,OctSE,1; 2020,OctSE,1

\# **81308**   known familial variant

⚙ 0.00   ⚙ 0.00   **FUD** XXX   🖵

AMA: 2020,Dec,3; 2020,OctSE,1; 2020,OctSE,1

81313 PCA3/KLK3 (prostate cancer antigen 3 [non-protein coding]/kallikrein-related peptidase 3 [prostate specific antigen]) ratio (eg, prostate cancer)

⚙ 0.00   ⚙ 0.00   **FUD** XXX   Ⓐ🖵

AMA: 2020,Dec,3; 2020,OctSE,1; 2020,OctSE,1; 2018,Nov,9; 2018,Jan,8; 2017,Jan,8; 2016,Aug,9; 2016,Jan,13

81314 PDGFRA (platelet-derived growth factor receptor, alpha polypeptide) (eg, gastrointestinal stromal tumor [GIST]), gene analysis, targeted sequence analysis (eg, exons 12, 18)

⚙ 0.00   ⚙ 0.00   **FUD** XXX   Ⓐ🖵

AMA: 2020,Dec,3; 2020,OctSE,1; 2020,OctSE,1; 2018,Nov,9; 2018,Jan,8; 2017,Jan,8; 2016,Aug,9

\# **81309** PIK3CA (phosphatidylinositol-4, 5-biphosphate 3-kinase, catalytic subunit alpha) (eg, colorectal and breast cancer) gene analysis, targeted sequence analysis (eg, exons 7, 9, 20)

⚙ 0.00   ⚙ 0.00   **FUD** XXX   🖵

AMA: 2020,Dec,3; 2020,OctSE,1; 2020,OctSE,1; 2020,Apr,10

\# **81320** PLCG2 (phospholipase C gamma 2) (eg, chronic lymphocytic leukemia) gene analysis, common variants (eg, R665W, S707F, L845F)

⚙ 0.00   ⚙ 0.00   **FUD** XXX   🖵

AMA: 2020,Dec,3; 2020,OctSE,1; 2020,OctSE,1; 2019,Jul,3; 2018,Nov,9

81315 PML/RARalpha, (t(15;17)), (promyelocytic leukemia/retinoic acid receptor alpha) (eg, promyelocytic leukemia) translocation analysis; common breakpoints (eg, intron 3 and intron 6), qualitative or quantitative

⚙ 0.00   ⚙ 0.00   **FUD** XXX   Ⓐ🖵

AMA: 2020,Dec,3; 2020,OctSE,1; 2020,OctSE,1; 2018,Nov,9; 2018,Jan,8; 2017,Jan,8; 2016,Aug,9; 2016,Jan,13

81316   single breakpoint (eg, intron 3, intron 6 or exon 6), qualitative or quantitative

⚙ 0.00   ⚙ 0.00   **FUD** XXX   Ⓐ🖵

AMA: 2020,Dec,3; 2020,OctSE,1; 2020,OctSE,1; 2018,Nov,9; 2018,Jan,8; 2017,Jan,8; 2016,Aug,9; 2016,Jan,13

\# **81324** PMP22 (peripheral myelin protein 22) (eg, Charcot-Marie-Tooth, hereditary neuropathy with liability to pressure palsies) gene analysis; duplication/deletion analysis

⚙ 0.00   ⚙ 0.00   **FUD** XXX   Ⓐ🖵

AMA: 2020,Dec,3; 2020,OctSE,1; 2020,OctSE,1; 2018,Nov,9; 2018,Jan,8; 2017,Jan,8; 2016,Aug,9; 2016,Jan,13

\# **81325**   full sequence analysis

⚙ 0.00   ⚙ 0.00   **FUD** XXX   Ⓐ🖵

AMA: 2020,Dec,3; 2020,OctSE,1; 2020,OctSE,1; 2018,Nov,9; 2018,May,6; 2018,Jan,8; 2017,Jan,8; 2016,Aug,9; 2016,Jan,13

\# **81326**   known familial variant

⚙ 0.00   ⚙ 0.00   **FUD** XXX   Ⓐ🖵

AMA: 2020,Dec,3; 2020,OctSE,1; 2020,OctSE,1; 2018,Nov,9; 2018,Jan,8; 2017,Jan,8; 2016,Aug,9; 2016,Jan,13

81317 PMS2 (postmeiotic segregation increased 2 [S. cerevisiae]) (eg, hereditary non-polyposis colorectal cancer, Lynch syndrome) gene analysis; full sequence analysis

⚙ 0.00   ⚙ 0.00   **FUD** XXX   Ⓐ🖵

AMA: 2020,Dec,3; 2020,OctSE,1; 2020,OctSE,1; 2018,Nov,9; 2018,Jan,8; 2017,Jan,8; 2016,Aug,9; 2016,Jan,13

81318   known familial variants

⚙ 0.00   ⚙ 0.00   **FUD** XXX   Ⓐ🖵

AMA: 2020,Dec,3; 2020,OctSE,1; 2020,OctSE,1; 2018,Nov,9; 2018,Jan,8; 2017,Jan,8; 2016,Aug,9; 2016,Jan,13

81319   duplication/deletion variants

⚙ 0.00   ⚙ 0.00   **FUD** XXX   Ⓐ🖵

AMA: 2020,Dec,3; 2020,OctSE,1; 2020,OctSE,1; 2018,Nov,9; 2018,Jan,8; 2017,Jan,8; 2016,Aug,9; 2016,Jan,13

81320 Resequenced code. See code before 81315.

\# **81343** PPP2R2B (protein phosphatase 2 regulatory subunit Bbeta) (eg, spinocerebellar ataxia) gene analysis, evaluation to detect abnormal (eg, expanded) alleles

⚙ 0.00   ⚙ 0.00   **FUD** XXX   🖵

AMA: 2020,Dec,3; 2020,OctSE,1; 2020,OctSE,1; 2018,Nov,9

26/TC PC/TC Only   A2-Z3 ASC Payment   50 Bilateral   ♂ Male Only   ♀ Female Only   ⚙ Facility RVU   ⚙ Non-Facility RVU   🖵 CCI   ❎ CLIA
FUD Follow-up Days   CMS: IOM   AMA: CPT Asst   A-Y OPPSI   80/80 Surg Assist Allowed / w/Doc   🔻 Lab Crosswalk   🔻 Radiology Crosswalk

372   CPT © 2021 American Medical Association. All Rights Reserved.   © 2021 Optum360, LLC

81321   *PTEN (phosphatase and tensin homolog) (eg, Cowden syndrome, PTEN hamartoma tumor syndrome) gene analysis;* **full sequence analysis**

💭 0.00   ⚖ 0.00   **FUD** XXX   Ⓐ 🔲

AMA: 2020,Dec,3; 2020,OctSE,1; 2020,OctSE,1; 2018,Nov,9; 2018,Jan,8; 2017,Jan,8; 2016,Aug,9; 2016,Jan,13

81322   **known familial variant**

💭 0.00   ⚖ 0.00   **FUD** XXX   Ⓐ 🔲

AMA: 2020,Dec,3; 2020,OctSE,1; 2020,OctSE,1; 2018,Nov,9; 2018,Jan,8; 2017,Jan,8; 2016,Aug,9; 2016,Jan,13

81323   **duplication/deletion variant**

💭 0.00   ⚖ 0.00   **FUD** XXX   Ⓐ 🔲

AMA: 2020,Dec,3; 2020,OctSE,1; 2020,OctSE,1; 2018,Nov,9; 2018,Jan,8; 2017,Jan,8; 2016,Aug,9; 2016,Jan,13

81324   **Resequenced code. See code following 81316.**

81325   **Resequenced code. See code following 81316.**

81326   **Resequenced code. See code following 81316.**

\#   **81334**   *RUNX1 (runt related transcription factor 1) (eg, acute myeloid leukemia, familial platelet disorder with associated myeloid malignancy), gene analysis, targeted sequence analysis (eg, exons 3-8)*

💭 0.00   ⚖ 0.00   **FUD** XXX   Ⓐ 🔲

AMA: 2020,Dec,3; 2020,OctSE,1; 2020,OctSE,1; 2018,Nov,9

81327   *SEPT9 (Septin9) (eg, colorectal cancer) promoter methylation analysis*

💭 0.00   ⚖ 0.00   **FUD** XXX   Ⓐ 🔲

AMA: 2020,Dec,3; 2020,OctSE,1; 2020,OctSE,1; 2019,Jul,3; 2018,Nov,9

\#   **81332**   *SERPINA1 (serpin peptidase inhibitor, clade A, alpha-1 antiproteinase, antitrypsin, member 1) (eg, alpha-1-antitrypsin deficiency), gene analysis, common variants (eg, *S and *Z)*

💭 0.00   ⚖ 0.00   **FUD** XXX   Ⓐ 🔲

AMA: 2020,Dec,3; 2020,OctSE,1; 2020,OctSE,1; 2018,Nov,9; 2018,Jan,8; 2017,Jan,8; 2016,Aug,9; 2016,Jan,13

\#   **81347**   *SF3B1 (splicing factor [3b] subunit B1) (eg, myelodysplastic syndrome/acute myeloid leukemia) gene analysis, common variants (eg, A672T, E622D, L833F, R625C, R625L)*

💭 0.00   ⚖ 0.00   **FUD** XXX   🔲

AMA: 2020,Dec,3; 2020,OctSE,1

81328   *SLCO1B1 (solute carrier organic anion transporter family, member 1B1) (eg, adverse drug reaction), gene analysis, common variant(s) (eg, *5)*

💭 0.00   ⚖ 0.00   **FUD** XXX   Ⓐ 🔲

AMA: 2020,Dec,3; 2020,OctSE,1; 2020,OctSE,1; 2018,Nov,9

81329   *SMN1 (survival of motor neuron 1, telomeric) (eg, spinal muscular atrophy) gene analysis; dosage/deletion analysis (eg, carrier testing), includes SMN2 (survival of motor neuron 2, centromeric) analysis, if performed*

💭 0.00   ⚖ 0.00   **FUD** XXX   🔲

AMA: 2020,Dec,3; 2020,OctSE,1; 2020,OctSE,1; 2019,Jul,3; 2018,Nov,9

\#   **81336**   **full gene sequence**

💭 0.00   ⚖ 0.00   **FUD** XXX   🔲

AMA: 2020,Dec,3; 2020,OctSE,1; 2020,OctSE,1; 2019,Jul,3; 2018,Nov,9

\#   **81337**   **known familial sequence variant(s)**

💭 0.00   ⚖ 0.00   **FUD** XXX   🔲

AMA: 2020,Dec,3; 2020,OctSE,1; 2020,OctSE,1; 2019,Jul,3; 2018,Nov,9

81330   *SMPD1(sphingomyelin phosphodiesterase 1, acid lysosomal) (eg, Niemann-Pick disease, Type A) gene analysis, common variants (eg, R496L, L302P, fsP330)*

💭 0.00   ⚖ 0.00   **FUD** XXX   Ⓐ 🔲

AMA: 2020,Dec,3; 2020,OctSE,1; 2020,OctSE,1; 2018,Nov,9; 2018,Jan,8; 2017,Jan,8; 2016,Aug,9; 2016,Jan,13

81331   *SNRPN/UBE3A (small nuclear ribonucleoprotein polypeptide N and ubiquitin protein ligase E3A) (eg, Prader-Willi syndrome and/or Angelman syndrome), methylation analysis*

💭 0.00   ⚖ 0.00   **FUD** XXX   Ⓐ 🔲

AMA: 2020,Dec,3; 2020,OctSE,1; 2020,OctSE,1; 2018,Nov,9; 2018,Jan,8; 2017,Jan,8; 2016,Aug,9; 2016,Jan,13

81332   **Resequenced code. See code following 81327.**

\#   **81348**   *SRSF2 (serine and arginine-rich splicing factor 2) (eg, myelodysplastic syndrome, acute myeloid leukemia) gene analysis, common variants (eg, P95H, P95L)*

💭 0.00   ⚖ 0.00   **FUD** XXX   🔲

AMA: 2020,Dec,3; 2020,OctSE,1

\#   **81344**   *TBP (TATA box binding protein) (eg, spinocerebellar ataxia) gene analysis, evaluation to detect abnormal (eg, expanded) alleles*

💭 0.00   ⚖ 0.00   **FUD** XXX   🔲

AMA: 2020,Dec,3; 2020,OctSE,1; 2020,OctSE,1; 2018,Nov,9

\#   **81345**   *TERT (telomerase reverse transcriptase) (eg, thyroid carcinoma, glioblastoma multiforme) gene analysis, targeted sequence analysis (eg, promoter region)*

💭 0.00   ⚖ 0.00   **FUD** XXX   🔲

AMA: 2020,Dec,3; 2020,OctSE,1; 2020,OctSE,1; 2019,Jul,3; 2018,Nov,9

81333   *TGFBI (transforming growth factor beta-induced) (eg, corneal dystrophy) gene analysis, common variants (eg, R124H, R124C, R124L, R555W, R555Q)*

💭 0.00   ⚖ 0.00   **FUD** XXX   🔲

AMA: 2020,Dec,3; 2020,OctSE,1; 2020,OctSE,1; 2019,Jul,3; 2018,Nov,9

81334   **Resequenced code. See code following numeric code 81326.**

\#   **81351**   *TP53 (tumor protein 53) (eg, Li-Fraumeni syndrome) gene analysis; full gene sequence*

💭 0.00   ⚖ 0.00   **FUD** XXX   🔲

AMA: 2020,Dec,3; 2020,OctSE,1

\#   **81352**   **targeted sequence analysis (eg, 4 oncology)**

💭 0.00   ⚖ 0.00   **FUD** XXX   🔲

AMA: 2020,Dec,3; 2020,OctSE,1

\#   **81353**   **known familial variant**

💭 0.00   ⚖ 0.00   **FUD** XXX   🔲

AMA: 2020,Dec,3; 2020,OctSE,1

81335   *TPMT (thiopurine S-methyltransferase) (eg, drug metabolism), gene analysis, common variants (eg, *2, *3)*

💭 0.00   ⚖ 0.00   **FUD** XXX   Ⓐ 🔲

AMA: 2020,Dec,3; 2020,OctSE,1; 2020,OctSE,1; 2018,Nov,9

81336   **Resequenced code. See code following 81329.**

81337   **Resequenced code. See code following 81329.**

81338   **Resequenced code. See code following resequenced code 81294.**

81339   **Resequenced code. See code before resequenced code 81295.**

81340   *TRB@ (T cell antigen receptor, beta) (eg, leukemia and lymphoma), gene rearrangement analysis to detect abnormal clonal population(s); using amplification methodology (eg, polymerase chain reaction)*

💭 0.00   ⚖ 0.00   **FUD** XXX   Ⓐ 🔲

AMA: 2020,Dec,3; 2020,OctSE,1; 2020,OctSE,1; 2018,Nov,9; 2018,Jan,8; 2017,Jan,8; 2016,Aug,9; 2016,Jan,13

81341   **using direct probe methodology (eg, Southern blot)**

💭 0.00   ⚖ 0.00   **FUD** XXX   Ⓐ 🔲

AMA: 2020,Dec,3; 2020,OctSE,1; 2020,OctSE,1; 2018,Nov,9; 2018,Jan,8; 2017,Jan,8; 2016,Aug,9; 2016,Jan,13

81342 *TRG@ (T cell antigen receptor, gamma)* (eg, leukemia and lymphoma), gene rearrangement analysis, evaluation to detect abnormal clonal population(s)

    🗂 0.00   ⚕ 0.00   **FUD** XXX   A ▨

    AMA: 2020,Dec,3; 2020,OctSE,1; 2020,OctSE,1; 2018,Nov,9; 2018,Jan,8; 2017,Jan,8; 2016,Aug,9; 2016,Jan,13

81343 Resequenced code. See code following numeric code 81320.

81344 Resequenced code. See code following numeric code 81332.

81345 Resequenced code. See code following numeric code 81332.

81346 *TYMS (thymidylate synthetase)* (eg, 5-fluorouracil/5-FU drug metabolism), gene analysis, common variant(s) (eg, tandem repeat variant)

    🗂 0.00   ⚕ 0.00   **FUD** XXX   A ▨

    AMA: 2020,Dec,3; 2020,OctSE,1; 2020,OctSE,1; 2018,Nov,9

81347 Resequenced code. See code before 81328.

81348 Resequenced code. See code following numeric code 81332.

 # 81357 *U2AF1 (U2 small nuclear RNA auxiliary factor 1)* (eg, myelodysplastic syndrome, acute myeloid leukemia) gene analysis, common variants (eg, S34F, S34Y, Q157R, Q157P)

    🗂 0.00   ⚕ 0.00   **FUD** XXX   ▨

    AMA: 2020,Dec,3; 2020,OctSE,1

81349 Resequenced code. See code following 81229.

81350 *UGT1A1 (UDP glucuronosyltransferase 1 family, polypeptide A1)* (eg, drug metabolism, hereditary unconjugated hyperbilirubinemia [Gilbert syndrome]) gene analysis, common variants (eg, *28, *36, *37)

    🗂 0.00   ⚕ 0.00   **FUD** XXX   A ▨

    AMA: 2020,Dec,3; 2020,OctSE,1; 2020,OctSE,1; 2020,Apr,9; 2018,Nov,9; 2018,Jan,8; 2017,Jan,8; 2016,Aug,9; 2016,Jan,13

81351 Resequenced code. See code following 81333.

81352 Resequenced code. See code following 81333.

81353 Resequenced code. See code following 81333.

81355 *VKORC1 (vitamin K epoxide reductase complex, subunit 1)* (eg, warfarin metabolism), gene analysis, common variant(s) (eg, -1639G>A, c.173+1000C>T)

    🗂 0.00   ⚕ 0.00   **FUD** XXX   A ▨

    AMA: 2020,Dec,3; 2020,OctSE,1; 2020,OctSE,1; 2018,Nov,9; 2018,Jan,8; 2017,Jan,8; 2016,Aug,9; 2016,Jan,13

81357 Resequenced code. See code following 81346.

81360 *ZRSR2 (zinc finger CCCH-type, RNA binding motif and serine/arginine-rich 2)* (eg, myelodysplastic syndrome, acute myeloid leukemia) gene analysis, common variant(s) (eg, E65fs, E122fs, R448fs)

    🗂 0.00   ⚕ 0.00   **FUD** XXX   ▨

    AMA: 2020,Dec,3; 2020,OctSE,1

81361 Resequenced code. See code following resequenced code 81269.

81362 Resequenced code. See code following resequenced code 81269.

81363 Resequenced code. See code following resequenced code 81269.

81364 Resequenced code. See code following resequenced code 81269.

81370-81383 Human Leukocyte Antigen (HLA) Testing

INCLUDES Additional testing performed to resolve ambiguous allele combinations for high-resolution typing

All analytical procedures in evaluation:
    Amplification
    Cell lysis
    Detection
    Digestion
    Extraction
    Nucleic acid stabilization

Analysis to identify human leukocyte antigen (HLA) alleles and allele groups connected to specific diseases and individual response to drug therapy in addition to other clinical uses

Code selection based on specific gene being reviewed

Evaluation gene variant presence using common gene variant name

Generally, all listed gene variants in code description tested (lists not all inclusive)

Genes described using Human Genome Organization (HUGO) approved names

High-resolution typing resolves common well-defined (CWD) alleles usually identified by at least four-digits. Some instances when high-resolution typing may include ambiguities for rare alleles may be reported as string of alleles or National Marrow Donor Program (NMDP) code

Histocompatibility antigen testing

Intermediate resolution HLA testing identified by string of alleles or NMDP code

Low and intermediate resolution considered low resolution for code assignment

Low-resolution HLA type reporting identified by two-digit HLA name

Multiple variant alleles or allele groups identified by typing

One or more HLA genes in specific clinical circumstances

Protein or disease examples in code description not all inclusive

Qualitative results unless otherwise stated

Typing performed to determine recipient compatibility and potential donors undergoing solid organ or hematopoietic stem cell pretransplantation testing

EXCLUDES *Full gene sequencing using separate gene variant assessment codes unless specifically stated in code description*

HLA antigen typing by nonmolecular pathology methods (86812-86821)

In situ hybridization analyses (88271-88275, 88368-88375 [88377])

Microbial identification (87149-87153, 87471-87801 [87623, 87624, 87625], 87900-87904 [87906, 87910, 87912])

Other related gene variants not listed in code description

Tier 1 molecular pathology codes (81105-81254 [81161, 81162, 81163, 81164, 81165, 81166, 81167, 81173, 81174, 81184, 81185, 81186, 81187, 81188, 81189, 81190, 81200, 81201, 81202, 81203, 81204, 81205, 81206, 81207, 81208, 81209, 81210, 81219, 81227, 81230, 81231, 81233, 81234, 81238, 81239, 81245, 81246, 81250, 81257, 81258, 81259, 81265, 81266, 81267, 81268, 81269, 81284, 81285, 81286, 81289, 81361, 81362, 81363, 81364])

Tier 2 and unlisted molecular pathology procedures (81400-81408, [81479])

Code also:
    Modifier 26 when only interpretation and report performed
    Services required before cell lysis

81370 HLA Class I and II typing, low resolution (eg, antigen equivalents); *HLA-A, -B, -C, -DRB1/3/4/5, and -DQB1*

    🗂 0.00   ⚕ 0.00   **FUD** XXX   A ▨

    AMA: 2020,Dec,3; 2020,OctSE,1; 2020,OctSE,1; 2018,Nov,9; 2018,Jan,8; 2017,Jan,8; 2016,Aug,9; 2016,Jan,13

81371 *HLA-A, -B, and -DRB1* (eg, verification typing)

    🗂 0.00   ⚕ 0.00   **FUD** XXX   A ▨

    AMA: 2020,Dec,3; 2020,OctSE,1; 2020,OctSE,1; 2018,Nov,9; 2018,Jan,8; 2017,Jan,8; 2016,Aug,9; 2016,Jan,13

81372 HLA Class I typing, low resolution (eg, antigen equivalents); complete *(ie, HLA-A, -B, and -C)*

    EXCLUDES *Class I and II low-resolution HLA typing for HLA-A, -B, -C, -DRB1/3/4/5, and -DQB1 (81370)*

    🗂 0.00   ⚕ 0.00   **FUD** XXX   A ▨

    AMA: 2020,Dec,3; 2020,OctSE,1; 2020,OctSE,1; 2018,Nov,9; 2018,Jan,8; 2017,Jan,8; 2016,Aug,9; 2016,Jan,13

81373 one locus *(eg, HLA-A, -B, or -C)*, each

    EXCLUDES *Complete Class 1 (HLA-A, -B, and -C) low-resolution typing (81372)*

    Reporting presence or absence single antigen equivalent using low-resolution methodology (81374)

    🗂 0.00   ⚕ 0.00   **FUD** XXX   A ▨

    AMA: 2020,Dec,3; 2020,OctSE,1; 2020,OctSE,1; 2018,Nov,9; 2018,Jan,8; 2017,Jan,8; 2016,Aug,9; 2016,Jan,13

26/TC PC/TC Only   A2-Z3 ASC Payment   50 Bilateral   ♂ Male Only   ♀ Female Only   🗂 Facility RVU   ⚕ Non-Facility RVU   ▨ CCI   ✖ CLIA
FUD Follow-up Days   CMS: IOM   AMA: CPT Asst   A-Y OPPSI   80/80 Surg Assist Allowed / w/Doc   ◨ Lab Crosswalk   ▣ Radiology Crosswalk

374   CPT © 2021 American Medical Association. All Rights Reserved.   © 2021 Optum360, LLC

81374 **one antigen equivalent** *(eg, B*27), each*

> EXCLUDES *Testing for presence or absence more than two antigen equivalents at locus, report for each locus test (81373)*

🔧 0.00   ✂ 0.00   **FUD** XXX   A 🔲

AMA: 2020,Dec,3; 2020,OctSE,1; 2020,OctSE,1; 2018,Nov,9; 2018,Jan,8; 2017,Jan,8; 2016,Aug,9; 2016,Jan,13

81375 **HLA Class II typing, low resolution (eg, antigen equivalents); HLA-DRB1/3/4/5 and -DQB1**

> EXCLUDES *Class I and II low-resolution HLA typing for HLA-A, -B, -C, -DRB 1/3/4/5, and DQB1 (81370)*

🔧 0.00   ✂ 0.00   **FUD** XXX   A 🔲

AMA: 2020,Dec,3; 2020,OctSE,1; 2020,OctSE,1; 2018,Nov,9; 2018,Jan,8; 2017,Jan,8; 2016,Aug,9; 2016,Jan,13

81376 **one locus** *(eg, HLA-DRB1, -DRB3/4/5, -DQB1, -DQA1, -DPB1, or -DPA1), each*

> INCLUDES Low-resolution typing, HLA-DRB1/3/4/5 reported as single locus
> EXCLUDES *Low-resolution typing for HLA-DRB1/3/4/5 and -DQB1 (81375)*

🔧 0.00   ✂ 0.00   **FUD** XXX   A 🔲

AMA: 2020,Dec,3; 2020,OctSE,1; 2020,OctSE,1; 2018,Nov,9; 2018,Jan,8; 2017,Jan,8; 2016,Aug,9; 2016,Jan,13

81377 **one antigen equivalent, each**

> EXCLUDES *Testing for presence or absence more than two antigen equivalents at locus (81376)*

🔧 0.00   ✂ 0.00   **FUD** XXX   A 🔲

AMA: 2020,Dec,3; 2020,OctSE,1; 2020,OctSE,1; 2018,Nov,9; 2018,Jan,8; 2017,Jan,8; 2016,Aug,9; 2016,Jan,13

81378 **HLA Class I and II typing, high resolution (ie, alleles or allele groups), HLA-A, -B, -C, and -DRB1**

🔧 0.00   ✂ 0.00   **FUD** XXX   A 🔲

AMA: 2020,Dec,3; 2020,OctSE,1; 2020,OctSE,1; 2018,Nov,9; 2018,Jan,8; 2017,Jan,8; 2016,Aug,9; 2016,Jan,13

81379 **HLA Class I typing, high resolution (ie, alleles or allele groups); complete (ie, HLA-A, -B, and -C)**

🔧 0.00   ✂ 0.00   **FUD** XXX   A 🔲

AMA: 2020,Dec,3; 2020,OctSE,1; 2020,OctSE,1; 2018,Nov,9; 2018,Jan,8; 2017,Jan,8; 2016,Aug,9; 2016,Jan,13

81380 **one locus (eg, HLA-A, -B, or -C), each**

> EXCLUDES *Complete Class I high-resolution typing for HLA-A, -B, and -C (81379)*
> *Testing for presence or absence single allele or allele group using high-resolution methodology (81381)*

🔧 0.00   ✂ 0.00   **FUD** XXX   A 🔲

AMA: 2020,Dec,3; 2020,OctSE,1; 2020,OctSE,1; 2018,Nov,9; 2018,Jan,8; 2017,Jan,8; 2016,Aug,9; 2016,Jan,13

81381 **one allele or allele group (eg, B*57:01P), each**

> EXCLUDES *Testing for presence or absence more than two alleles or allele groups at locus, report for each locus (81380)*

🔧 0.00   ✂ 0.00   **FUD** XXX   A 🔲

AMA: 2020,Dec,3; 2020,OctSE,1; 2020,OctSE,1; 2018,Nov,9; 2018,Jan,8; 2017,Jan,8; 2016,Aug,9; 2016,Jan,13

81382 **HLA Class II typing, high resolution (ie, alleles or allele groups); one locus (eg, HLA-DRB1, -DRB3/4/5, -DQB1, -DQA1, -DPB1, or -DPA1), each**

> INCLUDES Typing one or all DRB3/4/5 genes regarded as one locus
> EXCLUDES *Testing for just presence or absence single allele or allele group using high-resolution methodology (81383)*

🔧 0.00   ✂ 0.00   **FUD** XXX   A 🔲

AMA: 2020,Dec,3; 2020,OctSE,1; 2020,OctSE,1; 2018,Nov,9; 2018,Jan,8; 2017,Jan,8; 2016,Jan,13

81383 **one allele or allele group (eg, HLA-DQB1*06:02P), each**

> EXCLUDES *Testing for presence or absence more than two alleles or allele groups at locus (81382)*

🔧 0.00   ✂ 0.00   **FUD** XXX   A 🔲

AMA: 2020,Dec,3; 2020,OctSE,1; 2020,OctSE,1; 2018,Nov,9; 2018,Jan,8; 2017,Jan,8; 2016,Jan,13

81400-81479 [81479] Molecular Pathology Tier 2 Procedures

> INCLUDES All analytical procedures in evaluation:
> Amplification
> Cell lysis
> Detection
> Digestion
> Extraction
> Nucleic acid stabilization
> Code selection based on specific gene being reviewed
> Codes arranged by technical resource level and work involved
> Evaluation gene variant presence using common gene variant name
> Generally, all listed gene variants in code description tested (lists not all inclusive)
> Genes described using Human Genome Organization (HUGO) approved names
> Histocompatibility testing
> Protein or disease examples in code description (lists not all inclusive)
> Qualitative results unless otherwise stated
> Specific analytes listed after code description for selecting appropriate molecular pathology procedure
> Targeted genomic testing (81410-81471 [81448])
> Testing for more rare diseases
> EXCLUDES *Full gene sequencing using separate gene variant assessment codes unless specifically stated in code description*
> *In situ hybridization analyses (88271-88275, 88365-88368 [88364, 88373, 88374])*
> *Microbial identification (87149-87153, 87471-87801 [87623, 87624, 87625], 87900-87904 [87906, 87910, 87912])*
> *Other related gene variants not listed in code description*
> *Tier 1 molecular pathology (81105-81254 [81161, 81162, 81163, 81164, 81165, 81166, 81167, 81173, 81174, 81184, 81185, 81186, 81187, 81188, 81189, 81190, 81200, 81201, 81202, 81203, 81204, 81205, 81206, 81207, 81208, 81209, 81210, 81219, 81227, 81230, 81231, 81233, 81234, 81238, 81239, 81245, 81246, 81250, 81257, 81258, 81259, 81265, 81266, 81267, 81268, 81269, 81284, 81285, 81286, 81289, 81361, 81362, 81363, 81364])*
> *Unlisted molecular pathology procedures ([81479])*

Code also:
   Services required before cell lysis
   Modifier 26 when only interpretation and report performed

81400 **Molecular pathology procedure, Level 1 (eg, identification of single germline variant [eg, SNP] by techniques such as restriction enzyme digestion or melt curve analysis)**

ACADM (acyl-CoA dehydrogenase, C-4 to C-12 straight chain, MCAD) (eg, medium chain acyl dehydrogenase deficiency), K304E variant

ACE (angiotensin converting enzyme) (eg, hereditary blood pressure regulation), insertion/deletion variant

AGTR1 (angiotensin II receptor, type 1) (eg, essential hypertension), 1166A>C variant

BCKDHA (branched chain keto acid dehydrogenase E1, alpha polypeptide) (eg, maple syrup urine disease, type 1A), Y438N variant

CCR5 (chemokine C-C motif receptor 5) (eg, HIV resistance), 32-bp deletion mutation/794 825del32 deletion

CLRN1 (clarin 1) (eg, Usher syndrome, type 3), N48K variant

F2 (coagulation factor 2) (eg, hereditary hypercoagulability), 1199G>A variant

F5 (coagulation factor V) (eg, hereditary hypercoagulability), HR2 variant

F7 (coagulation factor VII [serum prothrombin conversion accelerator]) (eg, hereditary hypercoagulability), R353Q variant

F13B (coagulation factor XIII, B polypeptide) (eg, hereditary hypercoagulability), V34L variant

FGB (fibrinogen beta chain) (eg, hereditary ischemic heart disease), -455G>A variant

FGFR1 (fibroblast growth factor receptor 1) (eg, Pfeiffer syndrome type 1, craniosynostosis), P252R variant

FGFR3 (fibroblast growth factor receptor 3) (eg, Muenke syndrome), P250R variant

FKTN (fukutin) (eg, Fukuyama congenital muscular dystrophy), retrotransposon insertion variant

GNE (glucosamine [UDP-N-acetyl]-2 -epimerase/N-acetylmannosamine kinase) (eg, inclusion body myopathy 2 [IBM2], Nonaka myopathy), M712T variant

IVD (isovaleryl-CoA dehydrogenase) (eg, isovaleric acidemia), A282V variant

LCT (lactase-phlorizin hydrolase) (eg, lactose intolerance), 13910 C>T variant

NEB (nebulin) (eg, nemaline myopathy 2), exon 55 deletion variant

PCDH15 (protocadherin-related 15) (eg, Usher syndrome type 1F), R245X variant

SERPINE1 (serpine peptidase inhibitor clade E, member 1, plasminogen activator inhibitor -1, PAI-1) (eg, thrombophilia), 4G variant

SHOC2 (soc-2 suppressor of clear homolog) (eg, Noonan-like syndrome with loose anagen hair), S2G variant

SRY (sex determining region Y) (eg, 46,XX testicular disorder of sex development, gonadal dysgenesis), gene analysis

TOR1A (torsin family 1, member A [torsin A]) (eg, early-onset primary dystonia [DYT1]), 907_909delGAG (904_906delGAG) variant

    🔧 0.00   ⚖ 0.00   **FUD** XXX   Ⓐ 🖨

    AMA: 2020,Dec,3; 2020,OctSE,1; 2020,OctSE,1; 2019,Jul,3; 2018,Nov,9; 2018,Jan,8; 2017,Jan,8; 2016,Aug,9; 2016,Jan,13

81401   **Molecular pathology procedure, Level 2 (eg, 2-10 SNPs, 1 methylated variant, or 1 somatic variant [typically using nonsequencing target variant analysis], or detection of a dynamic mutation disorder/triplet repeat)**

ABCC8 (ATP-binding cassette, sub-family C [CFTR/MRP], member 8) (eg, familial hyperinsulinism), common variants (eg, c.3898-9G>A [c.3992-9G>A], F1388del)

ABL1 (ABL proto oncogene 1, non-receptor tyrosine kinase) (eg, acquired imatinib resistance), T315I variant

ACADM (acyl-CoA dehydrogenase, C-4 to C-12 straight chain, MCAD) (eg, medium chain acyl dehydrogenase deficiency), common variants (eg, K304E, Y42H)

ADRB2 (adrenergic beta-2 receptor surface) (eg, drug metabolism), common variants (eg, G16R, Q27E)

APOB (apolipoprotein B) (eg, familial hypercholesterolemia type B), common variants (eg, R3500Q, R3500W)

APOE (apolipoprotein E) (eg, hyperlipoproteinemia type III, cardiovascular disease, Alzheimer disease), common variants (eg, *2, *3, *4)

CBFB/MYH11 (inv(16)) (eg, acute myeloid leukemia), qualitative, and quantitative, if performed

CBS (cystathionine-beta-synthase) (eg, homocystinuria, cystathionine beta-synthase deficiency), common variants (eg, I278T, G307S)

CFH/ARMS2 (complement factor H/age-related maculopathy susceptibility 2) (eg, macular degeneration), common variants (eg, Y402H [CFH], A69S [ARMS2])

DEK/NUP214 (t(6;9))(eg, acute myeloid leukemia), translocation analysis, qualitative, and quantitative, if performed

E2A/PBX1 (t(1;19)) (eg, acute lymphocytic leukemia), translocation analysis, qualitative, and quantitative, if performed

EML4/ALK (inv(2)) (eg, non-small cell lung cancer), translocation or inversion analysis

ETV6/RUNX1 (t(12;21)) (eg, acute lymphocytic leukemia), translocation analysis, qualitative and quantitative, if performed

EWSR1/ATF1 (t(12;22)) (eg, clear cell sarcoma), translocation analysis, qualitative, and quantitative, if performed

EWSR1/ERG (t(21;22)) (eg, Ewing sarcoma/peripheral neuroectodermal tumor), translocation analysis, qualitative and quantitative, if performed

EWSR1/FLI1 (t(11;22)) (eg, Ewing sarcoma/peripheral neuroectodermal tumor), translocation analysis, qualitative and quantitative, if performed

EWSR1/WT1 (t(11;22)) (eg, desmoplastic small round cell tumor), translocation analysis, qualitative and quantitative, if performed

F11 (coagulation factor XI) (eg, coagulation disorder), common variants (eg, E117X [Type II], F283L [Type III], IVS14del14, and IVS14+1G>A [Type I])

FGFR3 (fibroblast growth factor receptor 3) (eg, achondroplasia, hypochondroplasia), common variants (eg, 1138G>A, 1138G>C, 1620C>A, 1620C>G)

FIP1L1/PDGFRA (del[4q12]) (eg, imatinib-sensitive chronic eosinophilic leukemia), qualitative and quantitative, if performed

FLG (filaggrin) (eg, ichthyosis vulgaris), common variants (eg, R501X, 2282del4, R2447X, S3247X, 3702delG)

FOXO1/PAX3 (t(2;13)) (eg, alveolar rhabdomyosarcoma), translocation analysis, qualitative and quantitative, if performed

FOXO1/PAX7 (t(1;13)) (eg, alveolar rhabdomyosarcoma), translocation analysis, qualitative and quantitative, if performed

FUS/DDIT3 (t(12;16)) (eg, myxoid liposarcoma), translocation analysis, qualitative, and quantitative, if performed

GALC (galactosylceramidase) (eg, Krabbe disease), common variants (eg, c.857G>A, 30-kb deletion)

GALT (galactose-1-phosphate uridylyltransferase) (eg, galactosemia), common variants (eg, Q188R, S135L, K285N, T138M, L195P, Y209C, IVS2-2A>G, P171S, del5kb, N314D, L218L/N314D)

H19 (imprinted maternally expressed transcript [non-protein coding]) (eg, Beckwith-Wiedemann syndrome), methylation analysis

IGH@/BCL2 (t(14;18)) (eg, follicular lymphoma), translocation and analysis; single breakpoint (eg) major breakpoint region [MBR] or minor cluster region [mcr]), qualitative or quantitative

(When both MBR and mcr breakpoints are performed, report [81278])

KCNQ1OT1 (KCNQ1 overlapping transcript 1 [non-protein coding]) (e.g, Beckwith-Wiedemann syndrome), methylation analysis

LINC00518 (long intergenic non-protein coding RNA 518) (eg, melanoma), expression analysis

LRRK2 (leucine-rich repeat kinase 2) (eg, Parkinson disease), common variants (eg, R1441G, G2019S, I2020T)

MED12 (mediator complex subunit 12) (eg, FG syndrome type 1, Lujan syndrome), common variants (eg, R961W, N1007S)

MEG3/DLK1 (maternally expressed 3 [non-protein coding]/delta-like 1 homolog [Drosophila]) (eg, intrauterine growth retardation), methylation analysis

MLL/AFF1 (t(4;11)) (eg acute lymphoblastic leukemia), translocation analysis, qualitative and quantitative, if performed

MLL/MLLT3 (t(9;11)) (eg, acute myeloid leukemia) translocation analysis, qualitative and quantitative, if performed

MT-RNR1 (mitochondrially encoded 12S RNA) (eg, nonsyndromic hearing loss), common variants (eg, m.1555>G, m1494C>T)

MUTYH (mutY homolog [E.coli]) (eg, MYH-associated polyposis), common variants (eg, Y165C, G382D)

MT-ATP6 (mitochondrially encoded ATP synthase 6) (eg, neuropathy with ataxia and retinitis pigmentosa [NARP], Leigh syndrome), common variants (eg, m.8993T>G, m.8993T>C)

MT-ND4, MT-ND6 (mitochondrially encoded NADH dehydrogenase 4, mitochondrially encoded NADH dehydrogenase 6) (eg, Leber hereditary optic neuropathy [LHON]), common variants (eg m.11778G>A, m3460G>A, m14484T>C)

MT-ND5 (mitochondrially encoded tRNA leucine 1 [UUA/G], mitochondrially encoded NADH dehydrogenase 5) (eg, mitochondrial encephalopathy with lactic acidosis and stroke-like episodes [MELAS]), common variants (eg, m.3243A>G, m.3271T>C, m.3252A>G, m.13513G>A)

MT-TK (mitochondrially encoded tRNA lysine) (eg, myoclonic epilepsy with ragged-red fibers [MERRF]), common variants (eg, m8344A>G, m.8356T>C)

26/TC PC/TC Only   A2-Z3 ASC Payment   50 Bilateral   ♂ Male Only   ♀ Female Only   🔧 Facility RVU   ⚖ Non-Facility RVU   □ CCI   ✖ CLIA
FUD Follow-up Days   **CMS:** IOM   **AMA:** CPT Asst   Ⓐ-Ⓨ OPPSI   80/80 Surg Assist Allowed / w/Doc   Lab Crosswalk   Radiology Crosswalk

376   CPT © 2021 American Medical Association. All Rights Reserved.   © 2021 Optum360, LLC

MT-TL1 (mitochondrially encoded tRNA leucine 1[UUA/G]) (eg, diabetes and hearing loss), common variants (eg, m.3243A>G, m.14709 T>C) MT-TL1

MT-TS1, MT-RNR1 (mitochondrially encoded tRNA serine 1 [UCN], mitochondrially encoded 12S RNA) (eg, nonsyndromic sensorineural deafness [including aminoglycoside-induced nonsyndromic deafness]) common variants (eg, m.7445A>G, m.1555A>G)

NOD2 (nucleotide-binding oligomerization domain containing 2) (eg, Crohn's disease, Blau syndrome), common variants (eg, SNP 8, SNP 12, SNP 13)

NPM/ALK (t(2;5)) (eg, anaplastic large cell lymphoma), translocation analysis

PAX8/PPARG (t(2;3) (q13;p25)) (eg, follicular thyroid carcinoma), translocation analysis

PRAME (preferentially expressed antigen in melanoma)(eg, melanoma), expression analysis

PRSS1 (protease, serine, 1 [trypsin 1]) (eg, hereditary pancreatitis), common variants (eg, N29I, A16V, R122H)

PYGM (phosphorylase, glycogen, muscle) (eg, glycogen storage disease type V, McArdle disease), common variants (eg, R50X, G205S)

RUNX1/RUNX1T1 (t(8;21)) (eg, acute myeloid leukemia) translocation analysis, qualitative and quantitative, if performed

SS18/SSX1 (t(X;18)) (eg, synovial sarcoma), translocation analysis, qualitative and quantitative, if performed

SS18/SSX2 (t(X;18)) (eg, synovial sarcoma), translocation analysis, qualitative and quantitative, if performed

VWF (von Willebrand factor) (eg, von Willebrand disease type 2N), common variants (eg, T791M, R816W, R854Q)

    📷 0.00   ✂ 0.00   **FUD** XXX   Ⓐ ▢

    AMA: 2020,Dec,3; 2020,OctSE,1; 2020,OctSE,1; 2019,Sep,7; 2019,Jul,3; 2018,Nov,9; 2018,Jan,8; 2017,Jan,8; 2016,Aug,9; 2016,Jan,13

81402   Molecular pathology procedure, Level 3 (eg, >10 SNPs, 2-10 methylated variants, or 2-10 somatic variants [typically using non-sequencing target variant analysis], immunoglobulin and T-cell receptor gene rearrangements, duplication/deletion variants of 1 exon, loss of heterozygosity [LOH], uniparental disomy [UPD])

Chromosome 1p-/19q- (eg, glial tumors), deletion analysis

Chromosome 18q- (eg, D18S55, D18S58, D18S61, D18S64, and D18S69) (eg, colon cancer), allelic imbalance assessment (ie, loss of heterozygosity)

COL1A1/PDGFB (t(17;22)) (eg, dermatofibrosarcoma protuberans), translocation analysis, multiple breakpoints, qualitative, and quantitative, if performed

CYP21A2 (cytochrome P450, family 21, subfamily A, polypeptide 2) (eg, congenital adrenal hyperplasia, 21-hydroxylase deficiency), common variants (eg, IVS2-13G, P30L, I172N, exon 6 mutation cluster [I235N, V236E, M238K], V281L, L307FfsX6, Q318X, R356W, P453S, G110VfsX21, 30-kb deletion variant)

ESR1/PGR (receptor 1/progesterone receptor) ratio (eg, breast cancer)

MEFV (Mediterranean fever) (eg, familial Mediterranean fever), common variants (eg, E148Q, P369S, F479L, M680I, I692del, M694V, M694I, K695R, V726A, A744S, R761H)

TRD@ (T cell antigen receptor, delta) (eg, leukemia and lymphoma), gene rearrangement analysis, evaluation to detect abnormal clonal population

Uniparental disomy (UPD) (eg, Russell-Silver syndrome, Prader-Willi/Angelman syndrome), short tandem repeat (STR) analysis

    📷 0.00   ✂ 0.00   **FUD** XXX   Ⓐ ▢

    AMA: 2020,Dec,3; 2020,OctSE,1; 2020,OctSE,1; 2018,Nov,9; 2018,Jan,8; 2017,Jan,8; 2016,Aug,9; 2016,Jan,13

81403   Molecular pathology procedure, Level 4 (eg, analysis of single exon by DNA sequence analysis, analysis of >10 amplicons

using multiplex PCR in 2 or more independent reactions, mutation scanning or duplication/deletion variants of 2-5 exons)

ANG (angiogenin, ribonuclease, RNase A family, 5) (eg, amyotrophic lateral sclerosis), full gene sequence

ARX (aristaless-related homeobox) (eg, X-linked lissencephaly with ambiguous genitalia, X-linked mental retardation), duplication/deletion analysis

CEL (carboxyl ester lipase [bile salt-stimulated lipase]) (eg, maturity-onset diabetes of the young [MODY]), targeted sequence analysis of exon 11 (eg, c.1785delC, c.1686delT)

CTNNB1 (catenin [cadherin-associated protein], beta 1, 88kDa) (eg, desmoid tumors), targeted sequence analysis (eg, exon 3)

DAZ/SRY (deleted in azoospermia and sex determining region Y) (eg, male infertility), common deletions (eg, AZFa, AZFb, AZFc, AZFd)

DNMT3A (DNA [cytosine-5-]-methyltransferase 3 alpha) (eg, acute myeloid leukemia), targeted sequence analysis (eg, exon 23)

EPCAM (epithelial cell adhesion molecule) (eg, Lynch syndrome), duplication/deletion analysis

F8 (coagulation factor VIII) (eg, hemophilia A), inversion analysis, intron 1 and intron 22A

F12 (coagulation factor XII [Hageman factor]) (eg, angioedema, hereditary, type III; factor XII deficiency), targeted sequence analysis of exon 9

FGFR3 (fibroblast growth factor receptor 3) (eg, isolated craniosynostosis), targeted sequence analysis (eg, exon 7)

(For targeted sequence analysis of multiple FGFR3 exons, use 81404) (81404)

GJB1 (gap junction protein, beta 1) (eg, Charcot-Marie-Tooth X-linked), full gene sequence

GNAQ (guanine nucleotide-binding protein G[q] subunit alpha) (eg, uveal melanoma), common variants (eg, R183, Q209)

HRAS (v-Ha-ras Harvey rat sarcoma viral oncogene homolog) (eg, Costello syndrome), exon 2 sequence

Human erythrocyte antigen gene analyses (eg, SLC14A1 [Kidd blood group], BCAM [Lutheran blood group], ICAM4 [Landsteiner-Wiener blood group], SLC4A1 [Diego blood group], AQP1 [Colton blood group], ERMAP [Scianna blood group], RHCE [Rh blood group, CcEe antigens], KEL [Kell blood group], DARC [Duffy blood group], GYPA, GYPB, GYPE [MNS blood group], ART4 [Dombrock blood group]) (eg, sickle-cell disease, thalassemia, hemolytic transfusion reactions, hemolytic disease of the fetus or newborn), common variants

KCNC3 (potassium voltage-gated channel, Shaw-related subfamily, member 3) (eg, spinocerebellar ataxia), targeted sequence analysis (eg, exon 2)

KCNJ2 (potassium inwardly-rectifying channel, subfamily J, member 2) (eg, Andersen-Tawil syndrome), full gene sequence

KCNJ11 (potassium inwardly-rectifying channel, subfamily J, member 11) (eg, familial hyperinsulinism), full gene sequence

Killer cell immunoglobulin-like receptor (KIR) gene family (eg, hematopoietic stem cell transplantation), genotyping of KIR family genes

Known familial variant, not otherwise specified, for gene listed in Tier 1 or Tier 2, or identified during a genomic sequencing procedure, DNA sequence analysis, each variant exon

(For a known familial variant that is considered a common variant, use specific common variant Tier 1 or Tier 2 code)

MC4R (melanocortin 4 receptor) (eg, obesity), full gene sequence

*MICA (MHC class I polypeptide-related sequence A) (eg, solid organ transplantation), common variants (eg, *001, *002)*

MT-RNR1 (mitochondrially encoded 12S RNA) (eg, nonsyndromic hearing loss), full gene sequence

---

● New Code ▲ Revised Code ○ Reinstated ● New Web Release ▲ Revised Web Release + Add-on Unlisted Not Covered # Resequenced

㊿ Optum Mod 50 Exempt ⊘ AMA Mod 51 Exempt �51 Optum Mod 51 Exempt �63 Mod 63 Exempt ⚕ Non-FDA Drug ★ Telemedicine Ⓜ Maternity Ⓐ Age Edit

MT-TS1 (mitochondrially encoded tRNA serine 1) (eg, nonsyndromic hearing loss), full gene sequence

NDP (Norrie disease [pseudoglioma]) (eg, Norrie disease), duplication/deletion analysis

NHLRC1 (NHL repeat containing 1) (eg, progressive myoclonus epilepsy), full gene sequence

PHOX2B (paired-like homeobox 2b) (eg, congenital central hypoventilation syndrome), duplication/deletion analysis

PLN (phospholamban) (eg, dilated cardiomyopathy, hypertrophic cardiomyopathy), full gene sequence

RHD (Rh blood group, D antigen) (eg, hemolytic disease of the fetus and newborn, Rh maternal/fetal compatibility), deletion analysis (eg, exons 4, 5, and 7, pseudogene)

RHD (Rh blood group, D antigen) (eg, hemolytic disease of the fetus and newborn, Rh maternal/fetal compatibility), deletion analysis (eg, exons 4, 5, and 7, pseudogene), performed on cell-free fetal DNA in maternal blood

(For human erythrocyte gene analysis of RHD, use a separate unit of 81403)

SH2D1A (SH2 domain containing 1A) (eg, X-linked lymphoproliferative syndrome), duplication/deletion analysis

TWIST1 (twist homolog 1 [Drosophila]) (eg, Saethre-Chotzen syndrome), duplication/deletion analysis

UBA1 (ubiquitin-like modifier activating enzyme 1) (eg, spinal muscular atrophy, X-linked), targeted sequence analysis (eg, exon 15)

VHL (von Hippel-Lindau tumor suppressor) (eg, von Hippel-Lindau familial cancer syndrome), deletion/duplication analysis

VWF (von Willebrand factor) (eg, von Willebrand disease types 2A, 2B, 2M), targeted sequence analysis (eg, exon 28)

    📷 0.00   🔲 0.00   **FUD** XXX   A ▢

AMA: 2020,Dec,3; 2020,OctSE,1; 2020,OctSE,1; 2019,Jul,3; 2018,Nov,9; 2018,May,6; 2018,Jan,8; 2017,Jan,8; 2016,Aug,9; 2016,Jan,13

81404   **Molecular pathology procedure, Level 5 (eg, analysis of 2-5 exons by DNA sequence analysis, mutation scanning or duplication/deletion variants of 6-10 exons, or characterization of a dynamic mutation disorder/triplet repeat by Southern blot analysis)**

ACADS (acyl-CoA dehydrogenase, C-2 to C-3 short chain) (eg, short chain acyl-CoA dehydrogenase deficiency), targeted sequence analysis (eg, exons 5 and 6)

AQP2 (aquaporin 2 [collecting duct]) (eg, nephrogenic diabetes insipidus), full gene sequence

ARX (aristaless related homeobox) (eg, X-linked lissencephaly with ambiguous genitalia, X-linked mental retardation), full gene sequence

AVPR2 (arginine vasopressin receptor 2) (eg, nephrogenic diabetes insipidus), full gene sequence

BBS10 (Bardet-Biedl syndrome 10) (eg, Bardet-Biedl syndrome), full gene sequence

BTD (biotinidase) (eg, biotinidase deficiency), full gene sequence

C10orf2 (chromosome 10 open reading frame 2) (eg, mitochondrial DNA depletion syndrome), full gene sequence

CAV3 (caveolin 3) (eg, CAV3-related distal myopathy, limb-girdle muscular dystrophy type 1C), full gene sequence

CD40LG (CD40 ligand) (eg, X-linked hyper IgM syndrome), full gene sequence

CDKN2A (cyclin-dependent kinase inhibitor 2A) (eg, CDKN2A-related cutaneous malignant melanoma, familial atypical mole-malignant melanoma syndrome), full gene sequence

CLRN1 (clarin 1) (eg, Usher syndrome, type 3), full gene sequence

COX6B1 (cytochrome c oxidase subunit VIb polypeptide 1) (eg, mitochondrial respiratory chain complex IV deficiency), full gene sequence

CPT2 (carnitine palmitoyltransferase 2) (eg, carnitine palmitoyltransferase II deficiency), full gene sequence

CRX (cone-rod homeobox) (eg, cone-rod dystrophy 2, Leber congenital amaurosis), full gene sequence

CYP1B1 (cytochrome P450, family 1, subfamily B, polypeptide 1) (eg, primary congenital glaucoma), full gene sequence

EGR2 (early growth response 2) (eg, Charcot-Marie-Tooth), full gene sequence

EMD (emerin) (eg, Emery-Dreifuss muscular dystrophy), duplication/deletion analysis

EPM2A (epilepsy, progressive myoclonus type 2A, Lafora disease [laforin]) (eg, progressive myoclonus epilepsy), full gene sequence

FGF23 (fibroblast growth factor 23) (eg, hypophosphatemic rickets), full gene sequence

FGFR2 (fibroblast growth factor receptor 2) (eg, craniosynostosis, Apert syndrome, Crouzon syndrome), targeted sequence analysis (eg, exons 8, 10)

FGFR3 (fibroblast growth factor receptor 3) (eg, achondroplasia, hypochondroplasia), targeted sequence analysis (eg, exons 8, 11, 12, 13)

FHL1 (four and a half LIM domains 1) (eg, Emery-Dreifuss muscular dystrophy), full gene sequence

FKRP (Fukutin related protein) (eg, congenital muscular dystrophy type 1C [MDC1C], limb-girdle muscular dystrophy [LGMD] type 2I), full gene sequence

FOXG1 (forkhead box G1) (eg, Rett syndrome), full gene sequence

FSHMD1A (facioscapulohumeral muscular dystrophy 1A) (eg, facioscapulohumeral muscular dystrophy), evaluation to detect abnormal (eg, deleted) alleles

FSHMD1A (facioscapulohumeral muscular dystrophy 1A) (eg, facioscapulohumeral muscular dystrophy), characterization of haplotype(s) (ie, chromosome 4A and 4B haplotypes)

GH1 (growth hormone 1) (eg, growth hormone deficiency), full gene sequence

GP1BB (glycoprotein Ib [platelet], beta polypeptide) (eg, Bernard-Soulier syndrome type B), full gene sequence

(For common deletion variants of alpha globin 1 and alpha globin 2 genes, use 81257)

HNF1B (HNF1 homeobox B) (eg, maturity-onset diabetes of the young [MODY]), duplication/deletion analysis

HRAS (v-Ha-ras Harvey rat sarcoma viral oncogene homolog) (eg, Costello syndrome), full gene sequence

HSD3B2 (hydroxy-delta-5-steroid dehydrogenase, 3 beta- and steroid delta-isomerase 2) (eg, 3-beta-hydroxysteroid dehydrogenase type II deficiency), full gene sequence

HSD11B2 (hydroxysteroid [11-beta] dehydrogenase 2) (eg, mineralocorticoid excess syndrome), full gene sequence

HSPB1 (heat shock 27kDa protein 1) (eg, Charcot-Marie-Tooth disease), full gene sequence

INS (insulin) (eg, diabetes mellitus), full gene sequence

KCNJ1 (potassium inwardly-rectifying channel, subfamily J, member 1) (eg, Bartter syndrome), full gene sequence

KCNJ10 (potassium inwardly-rectifying channel, subfamily J, member 10) (eg, SeSAME syndrome, EAST syndrome, sensorineural hearing loss), full gene sequence

LITAF (lipopolysaccharide-induced TNF factor) (eg, Charcot-Marie-Tooth), full gene sequence

MEFV (Mediterranean fever) (eg, familial Mediterranean fever), full gene sequence

26/TC PC/TC Only   A2-Z3 ASC Payment   50 Bilateral   ♂ Male Only   ♀ Female Only   📷 Facility RVU   🔲 Non-Facility RVU   ▢ CCI   ❌ CLIA
FUD Follow-up Days   **CMS:** IOM   **AMA:** CPT Asst   A-Y OPPSI   80/80 Surg Assist Allowed / w/Doc   ❎ Lab Crosswalk   ❎ Radiology Crosswalk

378   CPT © 2021 American Medical Association. All Rights Reserved.   © 2021 Optum360, LLC

MEN1 (multiple endocrine neoplasia I) (eg, multiple endocrine neoplasia type 1, Wermer syndrome), duplication/deletion analysis

MMACHC (methylmalonic aciduria [cobalamin deficiency] cblC type, with homocystinuria) (eg, methylmalonic acidemia and homocystinuria), full gene sequence

MPV17 (MpV17 mitochondrial inner membrane protein) (eg, mitochondrial DNA depletion syndrome), duplication/deletion analysis

NDP (Norrie disease [pseudoglioma]) (eg, Norrie disease), full gene sequence

NDUFA1 (NADH dehydrogenase [ubiquinone] 1 alpha subcomplex, 1, 7.5kDa) (eg, Leigh syndrome, mitochondrial complex I deficiency), full gene sequence

NDUFAF2 (NADH dehydrogenase [ubiquinone] 1 alpha subcomplex, assembly factor 2) (eg, Leigh syndrome, mitochondrial complex I deficiency), full gene sequence

NDUFS4 (NADH dehydrogenase [ubiquinone] Fe-S protein 4, 18kDa [NADH-coenzyme Q reductase]) (eg, Leigh syndrome, mitochondrial complex I deficiency), full gene sequence

NIPA1 (non-imprinted in Prader-Willi/Angelman syndrome 1) (eg, spastic paraplegia), full gene sequence

NLGN4X (neuroligin 4, X-linked) (eg, autism spectrum disorders), duplication/deletion analysis

NPC2 (Niemann-Pick disease, type C2 [epididymal secretory protein E1]) (eg, Niemann-Pick disease type C2), full gene sequence

NR0B1 (nuclear receptor subfamily 0, group B, member 1) (eg, congenital adrenal hypoplasia), full gene sequence

PDX1 (pancreatic and duodenal homeobox 1) (eg, maturity-onset diabetes of the young [MODY]), full gene sequence

PHOX2B (paired-like homeobox 2b) (eg, congenital central hypoventilation syndrome), full gene sequence

PIK3CA (phosphatidylinositol-4,5-bisphosphate 3-kinase, catalytic subunit alpha) (eg, colorectal cancer), targeted sequence analysis (eg, exons 9 and 20)

PLP1 (proteolipid protein 1) (eg, Pelizaeus-Merzbacher disease, spastic paraplegia), duplication/deletion analysis

PQBP1 (polyglutamine binding protein 1) (eg, Renpenning syndrome), duplication/deletion analysis

PRNP (prion protein) (eg, genetic prion disease), full gene sequence

PROP1 (PROP paired-like homeobox 1) (eg, combined pituitary hormone deficiency), full gene sequence

PRPH2 (peripherin 2 [retinal degeneration, slow]) (eg, retinitis pigmentosa), full gene sequence

PRSS1 (protease, serine, 1 [trypsin 1]) (eg, hereditary pancreatitis), full gene sequence

RAF1 (v-raf-1 murine leukemia viral oncogene homolog 1) (eg, LEOPARD syndrome), targeted sequence analysis (eg, exons 7, 12, 14, 17)

RET (ret proto-oncogene) (eg, multiple endocrine neoplasia, type 2B and familial medullary thyroid carcinoma), common variants (eg, M918T, 2647_2648delinsTT, A883F)

RHO (rhodopsin) (eg, retinitis pigmentosa), full gene sequence

RP1 (retinitis pigmentosa 1) (eg, retinitis pigmentosa), full gene sequence

SCN1B (sodium channel, voltage-gated, type I, beta) (eg, Brugada syndrome), full gene sequence

SCO2 (SCO cytochrome oxidase deficient homolog 2 [SCO1L]) (eg, mitochondrial respiratory chain complex IV deficiency), full gene sequence

SDHC (succinate dehydrogenase complex, subunit C, integral membrane protein, 15kDa) (eg, hereditary paraganglioma-pheochromocytoma syndrome), duplication/deletion analysis

SDHD (succinate dehydrogenase complex, subunit D, integral membrane protein) (eg, hereditary paraganglioma), full gene sequence

SGCG (sarcoglycan, gamma [35kDa dystrophin-associated glycoprotein]) (eg, limb-girdle muscular dystrophy), duplication/deletion analysis

SH2D1A (SH2 domain containing 1A) (eg, X-linked lymphoproliferative syndrome), full gene sequence

SLC16A2 (solute carrier family 16, member 2 [thyroid hormone transporter]) (eg, specific thyroid hormone cell transporter deficiency, Allan-Herndon-Dudley syndrome), duplication/deletion analysis

SLC25A20 (solute carrier family 25 [carnitine/acylcarnitine translocase], member 20) (eg, carnitine-acylcarnitine translocase deficiency), duplication/deletion analysis

SLC25A4 (solute carrier family 25 [mitochondrial carrier; adenine nucleotide translocation], member 4) (eg, progressive external ophthalmoplegia), full gene sequence

SOD1 (superoxide dismutase 1, soluble) (eg, amyotrophic lateral sclerosis), full gene sequence

SPINK1 (serine peptidase inhibitor, Kazal type 1) (eg, hereditary pancreatitis), full gene sequence

STK11 (serine/threonine kinase 11) (eg, Peutz-Jeghers syndrome), duplication/deletion analysis

TACO1 (translational activator of mitochondrial encoded cytochrome c oxidase I) (eg, mitochondrial respiratory chain complex IV deficiency), full gene sequence

THAP1 (THAP domain containing, apoptosis associated protein 1) (eg, torsion dystonia), full gene sequence

TOR1A (torsin family 1, member A [torsin A]) (eg, torsion dystonia), full gene sequence

TTPA (tocopherol [alpha] transfer protein) (eg, ataxia), full gene sequence

TTR (transthyretin) (eg, familial transthyretin amyloidosis), full gene sequence

TWIST1 (twist homolog 1 [Drosophila]) (eg, Saethre-Chotzen syndrome), full gene sequence

TYR (tyrosinase [oculocutaneous albinism IA]) (eg, oculocutaneous albinism IA), full gene sequence

UGT1A1 (UDP glucuronosyltransferase 1 family, polypeptide A1) (eg, hereditary unconjugated hyperbilirubinemia [Crigler-Najjar syndrome]) full gene sequence

USH1G (Usher syndrome 1G [autosomal recessive]) (eg, Usher syndrome, type 1), full gene sequence

VWF (von Willebrand factor) (eg, von Willebrand disease type 1C), targeted sequence analysis (eg, exons 26, 27, 37)

VHL (von Hippel-Lindau tumor suppressor) (eg, von Hippel-Lindau familial cancer syndrome), full gene sequence

ZEB2 (zinc finger E-box binding homeobox 2) (eg, Mowat-Wilson syndrome), duplication/deletion analysis

ZNF41 (zinc finger protein 41) (eg, X-linked mental retardation 89), full gene sequence

    📷 0.00   ⚖ 0.00   **FUD** XXX   🅰 ⬚

AMA: 2020,Dec,3; 2020,OctSE,1; 2020,OctSE,1; 2020,Apr,9; 2019,Jul,3; 2018,Nov,9; 2018,May,6; 2018,Jan,8; 2017,Jan,8; 2016,Aug,9; 2016,Jan,13

▲ **81405** **Molecular pathology procedure, Level 6 (eg, analysis of 6-10 exons by DNA sequence analysis, mutation scanning or duplication/deletion variants of 11-25 exons, regionally targeted cytogenomic array analysis)**

ABCD1 (ATP-binding cassette, sub-family D [ALD], member 1) (eg, adrenoleukodystrophy), full gene sequence

ACADS (acyl-CoA dehydrogenase, C-2 to C-3 short chain) (eg, short chain acyl-CoA dehydrogenase deficiency), full gene sequence

● New Code   ▲ Revised Code   ○ Reinstated   ● New Web Release   ▲ Revised Web Release   + Add-on   Unlisted   Not Covered   # Resequenced
50 Optum Mod 50 Exempt   Ⓢ AMA Mod 51 Exempt   51 Optum Mod 51 Exempt   63 Mod 63 Exempt   ✕ Non-FDA Drug   ★ Telemedicine   Ⓜ Maternity   🅰 Age Edit

© 2021 Optum360, LLC   CPT © 2021 American Medical Association. All Rights Reserved.   **379**

ACTA2 (actin, alpha 2, smooth muscle, aorta) (eg, thoracic aortic aneurysms and aortic dissections), full gene sequence

ACTC1 (actin, alpha, cardiac muscle 1) (eg, familial hypertrophic cardiomyopathy), full gene sequence

ANKRD1 (ankyrin repeat domain 1) (eg, dilated cardiomyopathy), full gene sequence

APTX (aprataxin) (eg, ataxia with oculomotor apraxia 1), full gene sequence

ARSA (arylsulfatase A) (eg, arylsulfatase A deficiency), full gene sequence

BCKDHA (branched chain keto acid dehydrogenase E1, alpha polypeptide) (eg, maple syrup urine disease, type 1A), full gene sequence

BCS1L (BCS1-like [S. cerevisiae]) (eg, Leigh syndrome, mitochondrial complex III deficiency, GRACILE syndrome), full gene sequence

BMPR2 (bone morphogenetic protein receptor, type II [serine/threonine kinase]) (eg, heritable pulmonary arterial hypertension), duplication/deletion analysis

CASQ2 (calsequestrin 2 [cardiac muscle]) (eg, catecholaminergic polymorphic ventricular tachycardia), full gene sequence

CASR (calcium-sensing receptor) (eg, hypocalcemia), full gene sequence

CDKL5 (cyclin-dependent kinase-like 5) (eg, early infantile epileptic encephalopathy), duplication/deletion analysis

CHRNA4 (cholinergic receptor, nicotinic, alpha 4) (eg, nocturnal frontal lobe epilepsy), full gene sequence

CHRNB2 (cholinergic receptor, nicotinic, beta 2 [neuronal]) (eg, nocturnal frontal lobe epilepsy), full gene sequence

COX10 (COX10 homolog, cytochrome c oxidase assembly protein) (eg, mitochondrial respiratory chain complex IV deficiency), full gene sequence

COX15 (COX15 homolog, cytochrome c oxidase assembly protein) (eg, mitochondrial respiratory chain complex IV deficiency), full gene sequence

CPOX (coproporphyrinogen oxidase) (eg, hereditary coproporphyria), full gene sequence

CTRC (chymotrypsin C) (eg, hereditary pancreatitis), full gene sequence

CYP11B1 (cytochrome P450, family 11, subfamily B, polypeptide 1) (eg, congenital adrenal hyperplasia), full gene sequence

CYP17A1 (cytochrome P450, family 17, subfamily A, polypeptide 1) (eg, congenital adrenal hyperplasia), full gene sequence

CYP21A2 (cytochrome P450, family 21, subfamily A, polypeptide2) (eg, steroid 21-hydroxylase isoform, congenital adrenal hyperplasia), full gene sequence

Cytogenomic constitutional targeted microarray analysis of chromosome 22q13 by interrogation of genomic regions for copy number and single nucleotide polymorphism (SNP) variants for chromosomal abnormalities

(When performing cytogenomic [genome-wide] analysis for constitutional chromosomal abnormalities, see 81228, 81229, 81349)

(Do not report analyte-specific molecular pathology procedures separately when the specific analytes are included as part of the microarray analysis of chromosome 22q13)

(Do not report 88271 when performing cytogenomic microarray analysis)

DBT (dihydrolipoamide branched chain transacylase E2) (eg, maple syrup urine disease, type 2), duplication/deletion analysis

DCX (doublecortin) (eg, X-linked lissencephaly), full gene sequence

DES (desmin) (eg, myofibrillar myopathy), full gene sequence

DFNB59 (deafness, autosomal recessive 59) (eg, autosomal recessive nonsyndromic hearing impairment), full gene sequence

DGUOK (deoxyguanosine kinase) (eg, hepatocerebral mitochondrial DNA depletion syndrome), full gene sequence

DHCR7 (7-dehydrocholesterol reductase) (eg, Smith-Lemli-Opitz syndrome), full gene sequence

EIF2B2 (eukaryotic translation initiation factor 2B, subunit 2 beta, 39kDa) (eg, leukoencephalopathy with vanishing white matter), full gene sequence

EMD (emerin) (eg, Emery-Dreifuss muscular dystrophy), full gene sequence

ENG (endoglin) (eg, hereditary hemorrhagic telangiectasia, type 1), duplication/deletion analysis

EYA1 (eyes absent homolog 1 [Drosophila]) (eg, branchio-oto-renal [BOR] spectrum disorders), duplication/deletion analysis

FGFR1 (fibroblast growth factor receptor 1) (eg, Kallmann syndrome 2), full gene sequence

FH (fumarate hydratase) (eg, fumarate hydratase deficiency, hereditary leiomyomatosis with renal cell cancer), full gene sequence

FKTN (fukutin) (eg, limb-girdle muscular dystrophy [LGMD] type 2M or 2L), full gene sequence

FTSJ1 (FtsJ RNA methyltransferase homolog 1 [E. coli]) (eg, X-linked mental retardation 9), duplication/deletion analysis

GABRG2 (gamma-aminobutyric acid [GABA] A receptor, gamma 2) (eg, generalized epilepsy with febrile seizures), full gene sequence

GCH1 (GTP cyclohydrolase 1) (eg, autosomal dominant dopa-responsive dystonia), full gene sequence

GDAP1 (ganglioside-induced differentiation-associated protein 1) (eg, Charcot-Marie-Tooth disease), full gene sequence

GFAP (glial fibrillary acidic protein) (eg, Alexander disease), full gene sequence

GHR (growth hormone receptor) (eg, Laron syndrome), full gene sequence

GHRHR (growth hormone releasing hormone receptor) (eg, growth hormone deficiency), full gene sequence

GLA (galactosidase, alpha) (eg, Fabry disease), full gene sequence

HNF1A (HNF1 homeobox A) (eg, maturity-onset diabetes of the young [MODY]), full gene sequence

HNF1B (HNF1 homeobox B) (eg, maturity-onset diabetes of the young [MODY]), full gene sequence

HTRA1 (HtrA serine peptidase 1) (eg, macular degeneration), full gene sequence

IDS (iduronate 2-sulfatase) (eg, mucopolysaccharidosis, type II), full gene sequence

IL2RG (interleukin 2 receptor, gamma) (eg, X-linked severe combined immunodeficiency), full gene sequence

ISPD (isoprenoid synthase domain containing) (eg, muscle-eye-brain disease, Walker-Warburg syndrome), full gene sequence

KRAS (Kirsten rat sarcoma viral oncogene homolog) (eg, Noonan syndrome), full gene sequence

LAMP2 (lysosomal-associated membrane protein 2) (eg, Danon disease), full gene sequence

LDLR (low density lipoprotein receptor) (eg, familial hypercholesterolemia), duplication/deletion analysis

MEN1 (multiple endocrine neoplasia I) (eg, multiple endocrine neoplasia type 1, Wermer syndrome), full gene sequence

MMAA (methylmalonic aciduria [cobalamine deficiency] type A) (eg, MMAA-related methylmalonic acidemia), full gene sequence

MMAB (methylmalonic aciduria [cobalamine deficiency] type B) (eg, MMAA-related methylmalonic acidemia), full gene sequence

MPI (mannose phosphate isomerase) (eg, congenital disorder of glycosylation 1b), full gene sequence

MPV17 (MpV17 mitochondrial inner membrane protein) (eg, mitochondrial DNA depletion syndrome), full gene sequence

MPZ (myelin protein zero) (eg, Charcot-Marie-Tooth), full gene sequence

MTM1 (myotubularin 1) (eg, X-linked centronuclear myopathy), duplication/deletion analysis

MYL2 (myosin, light chain 2, regulatory, cardiac, slow) (eg, familial hypertrophic cardiomyopathy), full gene sequence

MYL3 (myosin, light chain 3, alkali, ventricular, skeletal, slow) (eg, familial hypertrophic cardiomyopathy), full gene sequence

MYOT (myotilin) (eg, limb-girdle muscular dystrophy), full gene sequence

NDUFS7 (NADH dehydrogenase [ubiquinone] Fe-S protein 7, 20kDa [NADH-coenzyme Q reductase]) (eg, Leigh syndrome, mitochondrial complex I deficiency), full gene sequence

NDUFS8 (NADH dehydrogenase [ubiquinone] Fe-S protein 8, 23kDa [NADH-coenzyme Q reductase]) (eg, Leigh syndrome, mitochondrial complex I deficiency), full gene sequence

NDUFV1 (NADH dehydrogenase [ubiquinone] flavoprotein 1, 51kDa) (eg, Leigh syndrome, mitochondrial complex I deficiency), full gene sequence

NEFL (neurofilament, light polypeptide) (eg, Charcot-Marie-Tooth), full gene sequence

NF2 (neurofibromin 2 [merlin]) (eg, neurofibromatosis, type 2), duplication/deletion analysis

NLGN3 (neuroligin 3) (eg, autism spectrum disorders), full gene sequence

NLGN4X (neuroligin 4, X-linked) (eg, autism spectrum disorders), full gene sequence

NPHP1 (nephronophthisis 1 [juvenile]) (eg, Joubert syndrome), deletion analysis, and duplication analysis, if performed

NPHS2 (nephrosis 2, idiopathic, steroid-resistant [podocin]) (eg, steroid-resistant nephrotic syndrome), full gene sequence

NSD1 (nuclear receptor binding SET domain protein 1) (eg, Sotos syndrome), duplication/deletion analysis

OTC (ornithine carbamoyltransferase) (eg, ornithine transcarbamylase deficiency), full gene sequence

PAFAH1B1 (platelet-activating factor acetylhydrolase 1b, regulatory subunit 1 [45kDa]) (eg, lissencephaly, Miller-Dieker syndrome), duplication/deletion analysis

PARK2 (Parkinson protein 2, E3 ubiquitin protein ligase [parkin]) (eg, Parkinson disease), duplication/deletion analysis

PCCA (propionyl CoA carboxylase, alpha polypeptide) (eg, propionic acidemia, type 1), duplication/deletion analysis

PCDH19 (protocadherin 19) (eg, epileptic encephalopathy), full gene sequence

PDHA1 (pyruvate dehydrogenase [lipoamide] alpha 1) (eg, lactic acidosis), duplication/deletion analysis

PDHB (pyruvate dehydrogenase [lipoamide] beta) (eg, lactic acidosis), full gene sequence

PINK1 (PTEN induced putative kinase 1) (eg, Parkinson disease), full gene sequence

PKLR (pyruvate kinase, liver and RBC) (eg, pyruvate kinase deficiency), full gene sequence

PLP1 (proteolipid protein 1) (eg, Pelizaeus-Merzbacher disease, spastic paraplegia), full gene sequence

POU1F1 (POU class 1 homeobox 1) (eg, combined pituitary hormone deficiency), full gene sequence

PQBP1 (polyglutamine binding protein 1) (eg, Renpenning syndrome), full gene sequence

PRX (periaxin) (eg, Charcot-Marie-Tooth disease), full gene sequence

PSEN1 (presenilin 1) (eg, Alzheimer's disease), full gene sequence

RAB7A (RAB7A, member RAS oncogene family) (eg, Charcot-Marie-Tooth disease), full gene sequence

RAI1 (retinoic acid induced 1) (eg, Smith-Magenis syndrome), full gene sequence

REEP1 (receptor accessory protein 1) (eg, spastic paraplegia), full gene sequence

RET (ret proto-oncogene) (eg, multiple endocrine neoplasia, type 2A and familial medullary thyroid carcinoma), targeted sequence analysis (eg, exons 10, 11, 13-16)

RPS19 (ribosomal protein S19) (eg, Diamond-Blackfan anemia), full gene sequence

RRM2B (ribonucleotide reductase M2 B [TP53 inducible]) (eg, mitochondrial DNA depletion), full gene sequence

SCO1 (SCO cytochrome oxidase deficient homolog 1) (eg, mitochondrial respiratory chain complex IV deficiency), full gene sequence

SDHB (succinate dehydrogenase complex, subunit B, iron sulfur) (eg, hereditary paraganglioma), full gene sequence

SDHC (succinate dehydrogenase complex, subunit C, integral membrane protein, 15kDa) (eg, hereditary paraganglioma-pheochromocytoma syndrome), full gene sequence

SGCA (sarcoglycan, alpha [50kDa dystrophin-associated glycoprotein]) (eg, limb-girdle muscular dystrophy), full gene sequence

SGCB (sarcoglycan, beta [43kDa dystrophin-associated glycoprotein]) (eg, limb-girdle muscular dystrophy), full gene sequence

SGCD (sarcoglycan, delta [35kDa dystrophin-associated glycoprotein]) (eg, limb-girdle muscular dystrophy), full gene sequence

SGCE (sarcoglycan, epsilon) (eg, myoclonic dystonia), duplication/deletion analysis

SGCG (sarcoglycan, gamma [35kDa dystrophin-associated glycoprotein]) (eg, limb-girdle muscular dystrophy), full gene sequence

SHOC2 (soc-2 suppressor of clear homolog) (eg, Noonan-like syndrome with loose anagen hair), full gene sequence

SHOX (short stature homeobox) (eg, Langer mesomelic dysplasia), full gene sequence

SIL1 (SIL1 homolog, endoplasmic reticulum chaperone [S. cerevisiae]) (eg, ataxia), full gene sequence

SLC2A1 (solute carrier family 2 [facilitated glucose transporter], member 1) (eg, glucose transporter type 1 [GLUT 1] deficiency syndrome), full gene sequence

SLC16A2 (solute carrier family 16, member 2 [thyroid hormone transporter]) (eg, specific thyroid hormone cell transporter deficiency, Allan-Herndon-Dudley syndrome), full gene sequence

SLC22A5 (solute carrier family 22 [organic cation/carnitine transporter], member 5) (eg, systemic primary carnitine deficiency), full gene sequence

SLC25A20 (solute carrier family 25 [carnitine/acylcarnitine translocase], member 20) (eg, carnitine-acylcarnitine translocase deficiency), full gene sequence

SMAD4 (SMAD family member 4) (eg, hemorrhagic telangiectasia syndrome, juvenile polyposis), duplication/deletion analysis

SPAST (spastin) (eg, spastic paraplegia), duplication/deletion analysis

SPG7 (spastic paraplegia 7 [pure and complicated autosomal recessive]) (eg, spastic paraplegia), duplication/deletion analysis

SPRED1 (sprouty-related, EVH1 domain containing 1) (eg, Legius syndrome), full gene sequence

STAT3 (signal transducer and activator of transcription 3 [acute-phase response factor]) (eg, autosomal dominant hyper-IgE syndrome), targeted sequence analysis (eg, exons 12, 13, 14, 16, 17, 20, 21)

STK11 (serine/threonine kinase 11) (eg, Peutz-Jeghers syndrome), full gene sequence

SURF1 (surfeit 1) (eg, mitochondrial respiratory chain complex IV deficiency), full gene sequence

TARDBP (TAR DNA binding protein) (eg, amyotrophic lateral sclerosis), full gene sequence

TBX5 (T-box 5) (eg, Holt-Oram syndrome), full gene sequence

TCF4 (transcription factor 4) (eg, Pitt-Hopkins syndrome), duplication/deletion analysis

TGFBR1 (transforming growth factor, beta receptor 1) (eg, Marfan syndrome), full gene sequence

TGFBR2 (transforming growth factor, beta receptor 2) (eg, Marfan syndrome), full gene sequence

THRB (thyroid hormone receptor, beta) (eg, thyroid hormone resistance, thyroid hormone beta receptor deficiency), full gene sequence or targeted sequence analysis of >5 exons

TK2 (thymidine kinase 2, mitochondrial) (eg, mitochondrial DNA depletion syndrome), full gene sequence

TNNC1 (troponin C type 1 [slow]) (eg, hypertrophic cardiomyopathy or dilated cardiomyopathy), full gene sequence

TNNI3 (troponin 1, type 3 [cardiac]) (eg, familial hypertrophic cardiomyopathy), full gene sequence

TPM1 (tropomyosin 1 [alpha]) (eg, familial hypertrophic cardiomyopathy), full gene sequence

TSC1 (tuberous sclerosis 1) (eg, tuberous sclerosis), duplication/deletion analysis

TYMP (thymidine phosphorylase) (eg, mitochondrial DNA depletion syndrome), full gene sequence

VWF (von Willebrand factor) (eg, von Willebrand disease type 2N), targeted sequence analysis (eg, exons 18-20, 23-25)

WT1 (Wilms tumor 1) (eg, Denys-Drash syndrome, familial Wilms tumor), full gene sequence

ZEB2 (zinc finger E-box binding homeobox 2) (eg, Mowat-Wilson syndrome), full gene sequence

🔾 0.00   🔾 0.00   **FUD** XXX   🅐 ▣

AMA: 2020,Dec,3; 2020,OctSE,1; 2020,OctSE,1; 2019,Jul,3; 2018,Nov,9; 2018,Sep,14; 2018,May,6; 2018,Jan,8; 2017,Jan,8; 2016,Aug,9; 2016,Jan,13

81406 **Molecular pathology procedure, Level 7 (eg, analysis of 11-25 exons by DNA sequence analysis, mutation scanning or duplication/deletion variants of 26-50 exons)**

ACADVL (acyl-CoA dehydrogenase, very long chain) (eg, very long chain acyl-coenzyme A dehydrogenase deficiency), full gene sequence

ACTN4 (actinin, alpha 4) (eg, focal segmental glomerulosclerosis), full gene sequence

AFG3L2 (AFG3 ATPase family gene 3-like 2 [S. cerevisiae]) (eg, spinocerebellar ataxia), full gene sequence

AIRE (autoimmune regulator) (eg, autoimmune polyendocrinopathy syndrome type 1), full gene sequence

ALDH7A1 (aldehyde dehydrogenase 7 family, member A1) (eg, pyridoxine-dependent epilepsy), full gene sequence

ANO5 (anoctamin 5) (eg, limb-girdle muscular dystrophy), full gene sequence

ANOS1 (anosim-1) (eg, Kallmann syndrome 1), full gene sequence

APP (amyloid beta [A4] precursor protein) (eg, Alzheimer's disease), full gene sequence

ASS1 (argininosuccinate synthase 1) (eg, citrullinemia type I), full gene sequence

ATL1 (atlastin GTPase 1) (eg, spastic paraplegia), full gene sequence

ATP1A2 (ATPase, Na+/K+ transporting, alpha 2 polypeptide) (eg, familial hemiplegic migraine), full gene sequence

ATP7B (ATPase, Cu++ transporting, beta polypeptide) (eg, Wilson disease), full gene sequence

BBS1 (Bardet-Biedl syndrome 1) (eg, Bardet-Biedl syndrome), full gene sequence

BBS2 (Bardet-Biedl syndrome 2) (eg, Bardet-Biedl syndrome), full gene sequence

BCKDHB (branched-chain keto acid dehydrogenase E1, beta polypeptide) (eg, maple syrup urine disease, type 1B), full gene sequence

BEST1 (bestrophin 1) (eg, vitelliform macular dystrophy), full gene sequence

BMPR2 (bone morphogenetic protein receptor, type II [serine/threonine kinase]) (eg, heritable pulmonary arterial hypertension), full gene sequence

BRAF (B-Raf proto-oncogene, serine/threonine kinase) (eg, Noonan syndrome), full gene sequence

BSCL2 (Berardinelli-Seip congenital lipodystrophy 2 [seipin]) (eg, Berardinelli-Seip congenital lipodystrophy), full gene sequence

BTK (Bruton agammaglobulinemia tyrosine kinase) (eg, X-linked agammaglobulinemia), full gene sequence

CACNB2 (calcium channel, voltage-dependent, beta 2 subunit) (eg, Brugada syndrome), full gene sequence

CAPN3 (calpain 3) (eg, limb-girdle muscular dystrophy [LGMD] type 2A, calpainopathy), full gene sequence

CBS (cystathionine-beta-synthase) (eg, homocystinuria, cystathionine beta-synthase deficiency), full gene sequence

CDH1 (cadherin 1, type 1, E-cadherin [epithelial]) (eg, hereditary diffuse gastric cancer), full gene sequence

CDKL5 (cyclin-dependent kinase-like 5) (eg, early infantile epileptic encephalopathy), full gene sequence

CLCN1 (chloride channel 1, skeletal muscle) (eg, myotonia congenita), full gene sequence

CLCNKB (chloride channel, voltage-sensitive Kb) (eg, Bartter syndrome 3 and 4b), full gene sequence

CNTNAP2 (contactin-associated protein-like 2) (eg, Pitt-Hopkins-like syndrome 1), full gene sequence

COL6A2 (collagen, type VI, alpha 2) (eg, collagen type VI-related disorders), duplication/deletion analysis

CPT1A (carnitine palmitoyltransferase 1A [liver]) (eg, carnitine palmitoyltransferase 1A [CPT1A] deficiency), full gene sequence

CRB1 (crumbs homolog 1 [Drosophila]) (eg, Leber congenital amaurosis), full gene sequence

CREBBP (CREB binding protein) (eg, Rubinstein-Taybi syndrome), duplication/deletion analysis

DBT (dihydrolipoamide branched chain transacylase E2) (eg, maple syrup urine disease, type 2), full gene sequence

DLAT (dihydrolipoamide S-acetyltransferase) (eg, pyruvate dehydrogenase E2 deficiency), full gene sequence

DLD (dihydrolipoamide dehydrogenase) (eg, maple syrup urine disease, type III), full gene sequence

DSC2 (desmocollin) (eg, arrhythmogenic right ventricular dysplasia/cardiomyopathy 11), full gene sequence

DSG2 (desmoglein 2) (eg, arrhythmogenic right ventricular dysplasia/cardiomyopathy 10), full gene sequence

DSP (desmoplakin) (eg, arrhythmogenic right ventricular dysplasia/cardiomyopathy 8), full gene sequence

EFHC1 (EF-hand domain [C-terminal] containing 1) (eg, juvenile myoclonic epilepsy), full gene sequence

EIF2B3 (eukaryotic translation initiation factor 2B, subunit 3 gamma, 58kDa) (eg, leukoencephalopathy with vanishing white matter), full gene sequence

EIF2B4 (eukaryotic translation initiation factor 2B, subunit 4 delta, 67kDa) (eg, leukoencephalopathy with vanishing white matter), full gene sequence

EIF2B5 (eukaryotic translation initiation factor 2B, subunit 5 epsilon, 82kDa) (eg, childhood ataxia with central nervous system hypomyelination/vanishing white matter), full gene sequence

ENG (endoglin) (eg, hereditary hemorrhagic telangiectasia, type 1), full gene sequence

EYA1 (eyes absent homolog 1 [Drosophila]) (eg, branchio-oto-renal [BOR] spectrum disorders), full gene sequence

F8 (coagulation factor VIII) (eg, hemophilia A), duplication/deletion analysis

FAH (fumarylacetoacetate hydrolase [fumarylacetoacetase]) (eg, tyrosinemia, type 1), full gene sequence

FASTKD2 (FAST kinase domains 2) (eg, mitochondrial respiratory chain complex IV deficiency), full gene sequence

FIG4 (FIG4 homolog, SAC1 lipid phosphatase domain containing [S. cerevisiae]) (eg, Charcot-Marie-Tooth disease), full gene sequence

FTSJ1 (FtsJ RNA methyltransferase homolog 1 [E. coli]) (eg, X-linked mental retardation 9), full gene sequence

FUS (fused in sarcoma) (eg, amyotrophic lateral sclerosis), full gene sequence

GAA (glucosidase, alpha; acid) (eg, glycogen storage disease type II [Pompe disease]), full gene sequence

GALC (galactosylceramidase) (eg, Krabbe disease), full gene sequence

GALT (galactose-1-phosphate uridylyltransferase) (eg, galactosemia), full gene sequence

GARS (glycyl-tRNA synthetase) (eg, Charcot-Marie-Tooth disease), full gene sequence

GCDH (glutaryl-CoA dehydrogenase) (eg, glutaricacidemia type 1), full gene sequence

GCK (glucokinase [hexokinase 4]) (eg, maturity-onset diabetes of the young [MODY]), full gene sequence

GLUD1 (glutamate dehydrogenase 1) (eg, familial hyperinsulinism), full gene sequence

GNE (glucosamine [UDP-N-acetyl]-2-epimerase/N-acetylmannosamine kinase) (eg, inclusion body myopathy 2 [IBM2], Nonaka myopathy), full gene sequence

GRN (granulin) (eg, frontotemporal dementia), full gene sequence

HADHA (hydroxyacyl-CoA dehydrogenase/3-ketoacyl-CoA thiolase/enoyl-CoA hydratase [trifunctional protein] alpha subunit) (eg, long chain acyl-coenzyme A dehydrogenase deficiency), full gene sequence

HADHB (hydroxyacyl-CoA dehydrogenase/3-ketoacyl-CoA thiolase/enoyl-CoA hydratase [trifunctional protein], beta subunit) (eg, trifunctional protein deficiency), full gene sequence

HEXA (hexosaminidase A, alpha polypeptide) (eg, Tay-Sachs disease), full gene sequence

HLCS (HLCS holocarboxylase synthetase) (eg, holocarboxylase synthetase deficiency), full gene sequence

HMBS (hydroxymethylbilane synthase) (eg, acute intermittent porphyria), full gene sequence

HNF4A (hepatocyte nuclear factor 4, alpha) (eg, maturity-onset diabetes of the young [MODY]), full gene sequence

IDUA (iduronidase, alpha-L-) (eg, mucopolysaccharidosis type I), full gene sequence

INF2 (inverted formin, FH2 and WH2 domain containing) (eg, focal segmental glomerulosclerosis), full gene sequence

IVD (isovaleryl-CoA dehydrogenase) (eg, isovaleric acidemia), full gene sequence

JAG1 (jagged 1) (eg, Alagille syndrome), duplication/deletion analysis

JUP (junction plakoglobin) (eg, arrhythmogenic right ventricular dysplasia/cardiomyopathy 11), full gene sequence

KCNH2 (potassium voltage-gated channel, subfamily H [eag-related], member 2) (eg, short QT syndrome, long QT syndrome), full gene sequence

KCNQ1 (potassium voltage-gated channel, KQT-like subfamily, member 1) (eg, short QT syndrome, long QT syndrome), full gene sequence

KCNQ2 (potassium voltage-gated channel, KQT-like subfamily, member 2) (eg, epileptic encephalopathy), full gene sequence

LDB3 (LIM domain binding 3) (eg, familial dilated cardiomyopathy, myofibrillar myopathy), full gene sequence

LDLR (low density lipoprotein receptor) (eg, familial hypercholesterolemia), full gene sequence

LEPR (leptin receptor(eg, obesity with hypogonadism), full gene sequence

LHCGR (luteinizing hormone/choriogonadotropin receptor) (eg, precocious male puberty), full gene sequence

LMNA (lamin A/C) (eg, Emery-Dreifuss muscular dystrophy [EDMD1, 2 and 3] limb-girdle muscular dystrophy [LGMD] type 1B, dilated cardiomyopathy [CMD1A], familial partial lipodystrophy [FPLD2]), full gene sequence

LRP5 (low density lipoprotein receptor-related protein 5) (eg, osteopetrosis), full gene sequence

MAP2K1 (mitogen-activated protein kinase 1) (eg, cardiofaciocutaneous syndrome), full gene sequence

MAP2K2 (mitogen-activated protein kinase 2) (eg, cardiofaciocutaneous syndrome), full gene sequence

MAPT (microtubule-associated protein tau) (eg, frontotemporal dementia), full gene sequence

MCCC1 (methylcrotonoyl-CoA carboxylase 1 [alpha]) (eg, 3-methylcrotonyl-CoA carboxylase deficiency), full gene sequence

MCCC2 (methylcrotonoyl-CoA carboxylase 2 [beta]) (eg, 3-methylcrotonyl carboxylase deficiency), full gene sequence

MFN2 (mitofusin 2) (eg, Charcot-Marie-Tooth disease), full gene sequence

MTM1 (myotubularin 1) (eg, X-linked centronuclear myopathy), full gene sequence

MUT (methylmalonyl CoA mutase) (eg, methylmalonic acidemia), full gene sequence

MUTYH (mutY homolog [E. coli]) (eg, MYH-associated polyposis), full gene sequence

NDUFS1 (NADH dehydrogenase [ubiquinone] Fe-S protein 1, 75kDa [NADH-coenzyme Q reductase]) (eg, Leigh syndrome, mitochondrial complex I deficiency), full gene sequence

NF2 (neurofibromin 2 [merlin]) (eg, neurofibromatosis, type 2), full gene sequence

NOTCH3 (notch 3) (eg, cerebral autosomal dominant arteriopathy with subcortical infarcts and leukoencephalopathy [CADASIL]), targeted sequence analysis (eg, exons 1-23)

NPC1 (Niemann-Pick disease, type C1) (eg, Niemann-Pick disease), full gene sequence

NPHP1 (nephronophthisis 1 [juvenile]) (eg, Joubert syndrome), full gene sequence

NSD1 (nuclear receptor binding SET domain protein 1) (eg, Sotos syndrome), full gene sequence

OPA1 (optic atrophy 1) (eg, optic atrophy), duplication/deletion analysis

OPTN (optineurin) (eg, amyotrophic lateral sclerosis), full gene sequence

PAFAH1B1 (platelet-activating factor acetylhydrolase 1b, regulatory subunit 1 [45kDa]) (eg, lissencephaly, Miller-Dieker syndrome), full gene sequence

---

PAH (phenylalanine hydroxylase) (eg, phenylketonuria), full gene sequence

PALB2 (partner and localizer of BRCA2) (eg, breast and pancreatic cancer), full gene sequence

PARK2 (Parkinson protein 2, E3 ubiquitin protein ligase [parkin]) (eg, Parkinson disease), full gene sequence

PAX2 (paired box 2) (eg, renal coloboma syndrome), full gene sequence

PC (pyruvate carboxylase) (eg, pyruvate carboxylase deficiency), full gene sequence

PCCA (propionyl CoA carboxylase, alpha polypeptide) (eg, propionic acidemia, type 1), full gene sequence

PCCB (propionyl CoA carboxylase, beta polypeptide) (eg, propionic acidemia), full gene sequence

PCDH15 (protocadherin-related 15) (eg, Usher syndrome type 1F), duplication/deletion analysis

PCSK9 (proprotein convertase subtilisin/kexin type 9) (eg familial hypercholesterolemia), full gene sequence

PDHA1 (pyruvate dehydrogenase [lipoamide] alpha 1) (eg, lactic acidosis), full gene sequence

PDHX (pyruvate dehydrogenase complex, component X) (eg, lactic acidosis), full gene sequence

PHEX (phosphate-regulating endopeptidase homolog, X-linked) (eg, hypophosphatemic rickets), full gene sequence

PKD2 (polycystic kidney disease 2 [autosomal dominant]) (eg, polycystic kidney disease), full gene sequence

PKP2 (plakophilin 2) (eg, arrhythmogenic right ventricular dysplasia/cardiomyopathy 9), full gene sequence

PNKD (eg, paroxysmal nonkinesigenic dyskinesia), full gene sequence

POLG (polymerase [DNA directed], gamma) (eg, Alpers-Huttenlocher syndrome, autosomal dominant progressive external ophthalmoplegia), full gene sequence

POMGNT1 (protein O-linked mannose beta1, 2-N acetylglucosaminyltransferase) (eg, muscle-eye-brain disease, Walker-Warburg syndrome), full gene sequence

POMT1 (protein-O-mannosyltransferase 1) (eg, limb-girdle muscular dystrophy [LGMD] type 2K, Walker-Warburg syndrome), full gene sequence

POMT2 (protein-O-mannosyltransferase 2) (eg, limb-girdle muscular dystrophy [LGMD] type 2N, Walker-Warburg syndrome), full gene sequence

PPOX (protoporphyrinogen oxidase) (eg, variegate porphyria), full gene sequence

PRKAG2 (protein kinase, AMP-activated, gamma 2 non-catalytic subunit) (eg, familial hypertrophic cardiomyopathy with Wolff-Parkinson-White syndrome, lethal congenital glycogen storage disease of heart), full gene sequence

PRKCG (protein kinase C, gamma) (eg, spinocerebellar ataxia), full gene sequence

PSEN2 (presenilin 2[Alzheimer's disease 4]) (eg, Alzheimer's disease), full gene sequence

PTPN11 (protein tyrosine phosphatase, non-receptor type 11) (eg, Noonan syndrome, LEOPARD syndrome), full gene sequence

PYGM (phosphorylase, glycogen, muscle) (eg, glycogen storage disease type V, McArdle disease), full gene sequence

RAF1 (v-raf-1 murine leukemia viral oncogene homolog 1) (eg, LEOPARD syndrome), full gene sequence

RET (ret proto-oncogene) (eg, Hirschsprung disease), full gene sequence

RPE65 (retinal pigment epithelium-specific protein 65kDa) (eg, retinitis pigmentosa, Leber congenital amaurosis), full gene sequence

RYR1 (ryanodine receptor 1, skeletal) (eg, malignant hyperthermia), targeted sequence analysis of exons with functionally-confirmed mutations

SCN4A (sodium channel, voltage-gated, type IV, alpha subunit) (eg, hyperkalemic periodic paralysis), full gene sequence

SCNN1A (sodium channel, nonvoltage-gated 1 alpha) (eg, pseudohypoaldosteronism), full gene sequence

SCNN1B (sodium channel, nonvoltage-gated 1, beta) (eg, Liddle syndrome, pseudohypoaldosteronism), full gene sequence

SCNN1G (sodium channel, nonvoltage-gated 1, gamma) (eg, Liddle syndrome, pseudohypoaldosteronism), full gene sequence

SDHA (succinate dehydrogenase complex, subunit A, flavoprotein [Fp]) (eg, Leigh syndrome, mitochondrial complex II deficiency), full gene sequence

SETX (senataxin) (eg, ataxia), full gene sequence

SGCE (sarcoglycan, epsilon) (eg, myoclonic dystonia), full gene sequence

SH3TC2 (SH3 domain and tetratricopeptide repeats 2) (eg, Charcot-Marie-Tooth disease), full gene sequence

SLC9A6 (solute carrier family 9 [sodium/hydrogen exchanger], member 6) (eg, Christianson syndrome), full gene sequence

SLC26A4 (solute carrier family 26, member 4) (eg, Pendred syndrome), full gene sequence

SLC37A4 (solute carrier family 37 [glucose-6-phosphate transporter], member 4) (eg, glycogen storage disease type Ib), full gene sequence

SMAD4 (SMAD family member 4) (eg, hemorrhagic telangiectasia syndrome, juvenile polyposis), full gene sequence

SOS1 (son of sevenless homolog 1) (eg, Noonan syndrome, gingival fibromatosis), full gene sequence

SPAST (spastin) (eg, spastic paraplegia), full gene sequence

SPG7 (spastic paraplegia 7 [pure and complicated autosomal recessive]) (eg, spastic paraplegia), full gene sequence

STXBP1 (syntaxin-binding protein 1) (eg, epileptic encephalopathy), full gene sequence

TAZ (tafazzin) (eg, methylglutaconic aciduria type 2, Barth syndrome), full gene sequence

TCF4 (transcription factor 4) (eg, Pitt-Hopkins syndrome), full gene sequence

TH (tyrosine hydroxylase) (eg, Segawa syndrome), full gene sequence

TMEM43 (transmembrane protein 43) (eg, arrhythmogenic right ventricular cardiomyopathy), full gene sequence

TNNT2 (troponin T, type 2 [cardiac]) (eg, familial hypertrophic cardiomyopathy), full gene sequence

TRPC6 (transient receptor potential cation channel, subfamily C, member 6) (eg, focal segmental glomerulosclerosis), full gene sequence

TSC1 (tuberous sclerosis 1) (eg, tuberous sclerosis), full gene sequence

TSC2 (tuberous sclerosis 2) (eg, tuberous sclerosis), duplication/deletion analysis

UBE3A (ubiquitin protein ligase E3A) (eg, Angelman syndrome) full gene sequence

UMOD (uromodulin) (eg, glomerulocystic kidney disease with hyperuricemia and isosthenuria), full gene sequence

VWF (von Willebrand factor) (von Willebrand disease type 2A), extended targeted sequence analysis (eg, exons 11-16, 24-26, 51, 52)

WAS (Wiskott-Aldrich syndrome [eczema-thrombocytopenia]) (eg, Wiskott-Aldrich syndrome), full gene sequence

📷 0.00   ⚖ 0.00   **FUD** XXX   Ⓐ 🖼

AMA: 2020,Dec,3; 2020,OctSE,1; 2020,OctSE,1; 2020,Feb,10; 2018,Nov,9; 2018,May,6; 2018,Jan,8; 2017,Apr,9; 2017,Jan,8; 2016,Aug,9; 2016,Jan,13

26/**TC** PC/TC Only   **A2**-**Z3** ASC Payment   **50** Bilateral   ♂ Male Only   ♀ Female Only   📷 Facility RVU   ⚖ Non-Facility RVU   ☐ CCI   ☒ CLIA
FUD Follow-up Days   **CMS:** IOM   **AMA:** CPT Asst   **A**-**Y** OPPSI   **80**/**80** Surg Assist Allowed / w/Doc   🔲 Lab Crosswalk   🔲 Radiology Crosswalk

384   CPT © 2021 American Medical Association. All Rights Reserved.   © 2021 Optum360, LLC

81407 Molecular pathology procedure, Level 8 (eg, analysis of 26-50 exons by DNA sequence analysis, mutation scanning or duplication/deletion variants of >50 exons, sequence analysis of multiple genes on one platform)

ABCC8 (ATP-binding cassette, sub-family C [CFTR/MRP], member 8) (eg, familial hyperinsulinism), full gene sequence

AGL (amylo-alpha-1, 6-glucosidase, 4-alpha-glucanotransferase) (eg, glycogen storage disease type III), full gene sequence

AHI1 (Abelson helper integration site 1) (eg, Joubert syndrome), full gene sequence

APOB (apolipoprotein B) (eg, familial hypercholesterolemia type B) full gene sequence

ASPM (asp [abnormal spindle] homolog, microcephaly associated [Drosophila]) (eg, primary microcephaly), full gene sequence

CHD7 (chromodomain helicase DNA binding protein 7) (eg, CHARGE syndrome), full gene sequence

COL4A4 (collagen, type IV, alpha 4) (eg, Alport syndrome), full gene sequence

COL4A5 (collagen, type IV, alpha 5) (eg, Alport syndrome), duplication/deletion analysis

COL6A1 (collagen, type VI, alpha 1) (eg, collagen type VI-related disorders), full gene sequence

COL6A2 (collagen, type VI, alpha 2) (eg, collagen type VI-related disorders), full gene sequence

COL6A3 (collagen, type VI, alpha 3) (eg, collagen type VI-related disorders), full gene sequence

CREBBP (CREB binding protein) (eg, Rubinstein-Taybi syndrome), full gene sequence

F8 (coagulation factor VIII) (eg, hemophilia A), full gene sequence

JAG1 (jagged 1) (eg, Alagille syndrome), full gene sequence

KDM5C (lysine [K]-specific demethylase 5C) (eg, X-linked mental retardation), full gene sequence

KIAA0196 (KIAA0196) (eg, spastic paraplegia), full gene sequence

L1CAM (L1 cell adhesion molecule) (eg, MASA syndrome, X-linked hydrocephaly), full gene sequence

LAMB2 (laminin, beta 2 [laminin S]) (eg, Pierson syndrome), full gene sequence

MYBPC3 (myosin binding protein C, cardiac) (eg, familial hypertrophic cardiomyopathy), full gene sequence

MYH6 (myosin, heavy chain 6, cardiac muscle, alpha) (eg, familial dilated cardiomyopathy), full gene sequence

MYH7 (myosin, heavy chain 7, cardiac muscle, beta) (eg, familial hypertrophic cardiomyopathy, Liang distal myopathy), full gene sequence

MYO7A (myosin VIIA) (eg, Usher syndrome, type 1), full gene sequence

NOTCH1 (notch 1) (eg, aortic valve disease), full gene sequence

NPHS1 (nephrosis 1, congenital, Finnish type [nephrin]) (eg, congenital Finnish nephrosis), full gene sequence

OPA1 (optic atrophy 1) (eg, optic atrophy), full gene sequence

PCDH15 (protocadherin-related 15) (eg, Usher syndrome, type 1), full gene sequence

PKD1 (polycystic kidney disease 1 [autosomal dominant]) (eg, polycystic kidney disease), full gene sequence

PLCE1 (phospholipase C, epsilon 1) (eg, nephrotic syndrome type 3), full gene sequence

SCN1A (sodium channel, voltage-gated, type 1, alpha subunit) (eg, generalized epilepsy with febrile seizures), full gene sequence

SCN5A (sodium channel, voltage-gated, type V, alpha subunit) (eg, familial dilated cardiomyopathy), full gene sequence

SLC12A1 (solute carrier family 12 [sodium/potassium/chloride transporters], member 1) (eg, Bartter syndrome), full gene sequence

SLC12A3 (solute carrier family 12 [sodium/chloride transporters], member 3) (eg, Gitelman syndrome), full gene sequence

SPG11 (spastic paraplegia 11 [autosomal recessive]) (eg, spastic paraplegia), full gene sequence

SPTBN2 (spectrin, beta, non-erythrocytic 2) (eg, spinocerebellar ataxia), full gene sequence

TMEM67 (transmembrane protein 67) (eg, Joubert syndrome), full gene sequence

TSC2 (tuberous sclerosis 2) (eg, tuberous sclerosis), full gene sequence

USH1C (Usher syndrome 1C [autosomal recessive, severe]) (eg, Usher syndrome, type 1), full gene sequence

VPS13B (vacuolar protein sorting 13 homolog B [yeast]) (eg, Cohen syndrome), duplication/deletion analysis

WDR62 (WD repeat domain 62) (eg, primary autosomal recessive microcephaly), full gene sequence

   📷 0.00   ✂ 0.00   **FUD** XXX   🅰 🖼

   AMA: 2020,Dec,3; 2020,OctSE,1; 2020,OctSE,1; 2019,Jul,3; 2018,Nov,9; 2018,May,6; 2018,Jan,8; 2017,Jan,8; 2016,Aug,9; 2016,Jan,13

81408 Molecular pathology procedure, Level 9 (eg, analysis of >50 exons in a single gene by DNA sequence analysis)

ABCA4 (ATP-binding cassette, sub-family A [ABC1], member 4) (eg, Stargardt disease, age-related macular degeneration), full gene sequence

ATM (ataxia telangiectasia mutated) (eg, ataxia telangiectasia), full gene sequence

CDH23 (cadherin-related 23) (eg, Usher syndrome, type 1), full gene sequence

CEP290 (centrosomal protein 290kDa) (eg, Joubert syndrome), full gene sequence

COL1A1 (collagen, type I, alpha 1) (eg, osteogenesis imperfecta, type I), full gene sequence

COL1A2 (collagen, type I, alpha 2) (eg, osteogenesis imperfecta, type I), full gene sequence

COL4A1 (collagen, type IV, alpha 1) (eg, brain small-vessel disease with hemorrhage), full gene sequence

COL4A3 (collagen, type IV, alpha 3 [Goodpasture antigen]) (eg, Alport syndrome), full gene sequence

COL4A5 (collagen, type IV, alpha 5) (eg, Alport syndrome), full gene sequence

DMD (dystrophin) (eg, Duchenne/Becker muscular dystrophy), full gene sequence

DYSF (dysferlin, limb girdle muscular dystrophy 2B [autosomal recessive]) (eg, limb-girdle muscular dystrophy), full gene sequence

FBN1 (fibrillin 1) (eg, Marfan syndrome), full gene sequence

ITPR1 (inositol 1,4,5-trisphosphate receptor, type 1) (eg, spinocerebellar ataxia), full gene sequence

LAMA2 (laminin, alpha 2) (eg, congenital muscular dystrophy), full gene sequence

LRRK2 (leucine-rich repeat kinase 2) (eg, Parkinson disease), full gene sequence

MYH11 (myosin, heavy chain 11, smooth muscle) (eg, thoracic aortic aneurysms and aortic dissections), full gene sequence

NEB (nebulin) (eg, nemaline myopathy 2), full gene sequence

NF1 (neurofibromin 1) (eg, neurofibromatosis, type 1), full gene sequence

PKHD1 (polycystic kidney and hepatic disease 1) (eg, autosomal recessive polycystic kidney disease), full gene sequence

RYR1 (ryanodine receptor 1, skeletal) (eg, malignant hyperthermia), full gene sequence

RYR2 (ryanodine receptor 2 [cardiac]) (eg, catecholaminergic polymorphic ventricular tachycardia, arrhythmogenic right ventricular dysplasia), full gene sequence or targeted sequence analysis of > 50 exons

USH2A (Usher syndrome 2A [autosomal recessive, mild]) (eg, Usher syndrome, type 2), full gene sequence

VPS13B (vacuolar protein sorting 13 homolog B [yeast]) (eg, Cohen syndrome), full gene sequence

VWF (von Willebrand factor) (eg, von Willebrand disease types 1 and 3), full gene sequence

🖩 0.00   🔧 0.00   **FUD** XXX   Ⓐ🖵

AMA: 2020,Dec,3; 2020,OctSE,1; 2020,OctSE,1; 2018,Nov,9; 2018,May,6; 2018,Jan,8; 2017,Jan,8; 2016,Aug,9; 2016,Jan,13

\# **81479** **Unlisted molecular pathology procedure**

🖩 0.00   🔧 0.00   **FUD** XXX   Ⓐ🖵

AMA: 2020,Dec,13; 2020,Dec,3; 2020,Oct,8; 2019,Jun,11; 2019,May,5; 2018,Dec,10; 2018,Dec,10; 2018,Nov,9; 2018,Sep,14; 2018,Jun,8; 2018,May,6; 2018,Jan,8; 2017,Apr,9; 2017,Jan,8; 2016,Sep,9; 2016,Aug,9; 2016,Apr,4; 2016,Jan,13

81410-81479 [81419, 81443, 81448, 81479] Genomic Sequencing

EXCLUDES Cytogenomic (genome-wide) analysis for constitutional chromosomal abnormalities (81228-81229, [81349], 81405-81406)
In situ hybridization analyses (88271-88275, 88365-88368 [88364, 88373, 88374])
Microbial identification (87149-87153, 87471-87801 [87623, 87624, 87625], 87900-87904 [87906, 87910, 87912])

81410 **Aortic dysfunction or dilation (eg, Marfan syndrome, Loeys Dietz syndrome, Ehler Danlos syndrome type IV, arterial tortuosity syndrome); genomic sequence analysis panel, must include sequencing of at least 9 genes, including *FBN1, TGFBR1, TGFBR2, COL3A1, MYH11, ACTA2, SLC2A10, SMAD3,* and *MYLK***

🖩 0.00   🔧 0.00   **FUD** XXX   Ⓐ🖵

AMA: 2020,Dec,3; 2018,Jan,8; 2017,Jan,8; 2016,Jan,13

81411 **duplication/deletion analysis panel, must include analyses for *TGFBR1, TGFBR2, MYH11,* and *COL3A1***

🖩 0.00   🔧 0.00   **FUD** XXX   Ⓐ🖵

AMA: 2020,Dec,3; 2018,Jan,8; 2017,Jan,8; 2016,Jan,13

81412 **Ashkenazi Jewish associated disorders (eg, Bloom syndrome, Canavan disease, cystic fibrosis, familial dysautonomia, Fanconi anemia group C, Gaucher disease, Tay-Sachs disease), genomic sequence analysis panel, must include sequencing of at least 9 genes, including *ASPA, BLM, CFTR, FANCC, GBA, HEXA, IKBKAP, MCOLN1,* and *SMPD1***

🖩 0.00   🔧 0.00   **FUD** XXX   Ⓐ🖵

AMA: 2020,Dec,3; 2018,Nov,9; 2018,Jan,8; 2017,Jan,8; 2016,Apr,4

81413 **Cardiac ion channelopathies (eg, Brugada syndrome, long QT syndrome, short QT syndrome, catecholaminergic polymorphic ventricular tachycardia); genomic sequence analysis panel, must include sequencing of at least 10 genes, including ANK2, CASQ2, CAV3, KCNE1, KCNE2, KCNH2, KCNJ2, KCNQ1, RYR2, and SCN5A**

EXCLUDES Evaluation cardiomyopathy (81439)

🖩 0.00   🔧 0.00   **FUD** XXX   Ⓐ🖵

AMA: 2020,Dec,3; 2018,Jan,8; 2017,Apr,3

81414 **duplication/deletion gene analysis panel, must include analysis of at least 2 genes, including KCNH2 and KCNQ1**

EXCLUDES Evaluation cardiomyopathy (81439)

🖩 0.00   🔧 0.00   **FUD** XXX   Ⓐ🖵

AMA: 2020,Dec,3; 2018,Jan,8; 2017,Apr,3

\# **81419** **Epilepsy genomic sequence analysis panel, must include analyses for *ALDH7A1, CACNA1A, CDKL5, CHD2, GABRG2, GRIN2A, KCNQ2, MECP2, PCDH19, POLG, PRRT2, SCN1A, SCN1B, SCN2A, SCN8A, SLC2A1, SLC9A6, STXBP1, SYNGAP1, TCF4, TPP1, TSC1, TSC2,* and *ZEB2***

🖩 0.00   🔧 0.00   **FUD** XXX   🖵

AMA: 2020,Dec,3

81415 **Exome (eg, unexplained constitutional or heritable disorder or syndrome); sequence analysis**

INCLUDES Chromosomal abnormality sequence analysis ([81349])

🖩 0.00   🔧 0.00   **FUD** XXX   Ⓐ🖵

AMA: 2020,Dec,3; 2018,Jan,8; 2017,Jan,8; 2016,Jan,13

\+ **81416** **sequence analysis, each comparator exome (eg, parents, siblings) (List separately in addition to code for primary procedure)**

INCLUDES Chromosomal abnormality sequence analysis ([81349])

Code first (81415)

🖩 0.00   🔧 0.00   **FUD** XXX   Ⓐ🖵

AMA: 2020,Dec,3; 2018,Jan,8; 2017,Jan,8; 2016,Jan,13

81417 **re-evaluation of previously obtained exome sequence (eg, updated knowledge or unrelated condition/syndrome)**

INCLUDES Chromosomal abnormality sequence analysis ([81349])

EXCLUDES Incidental results

🖩 0.00   🔧 0.00   **FUD** XXX   Ⓐ🖵

AMA: 2020,Dec,3; 2018,Jan,8; 2017,Jan,8; 2016,Jan,13

81419 **Resequenced code. See code following 81414.**

81420 **Fetal chromosomal aneuploidy (eg, trisomy 21, monosomy X) genomic sequence analysis panel, circulating cell-free fetal DNA in maternal blood, must include analysis of chromosomes 13, 18, and 21** Ⓜ

EXCLUDES Molecular cytogenetics (88271)

🖩 0.00   🔧 0.00   **FUD** XXX   Ⓐ🖵

AMA: 2020,Dec,3; 2018,Apr,10; 2018,Jan,8; 2017,Jan,8; 2016,Jan,13

81422 **Fetal chromosomal microdeletion(s) genomic sequence analysis (eg, DiGeorge syndrome, Cri-du-chat syndrome), circulating cell-free fetal DNA in maternal blood**

EXCLUDES Molecular cytogenetics (88271)

🖩 0.00   🔧 0.00   **FUD** XXX   Ⓐ🖵

AMA: 2020,Dec,3; 2018,Jan,8; 2017,Apr,3

\# **81443** **Genetic testing for severe inherited conditions (eg, cystic fibrosis, Ashkenazi Jewish-associated disorders [eg, Bloom syndrome, Canavan disease, Fanconi anemia type C, mucolipidosis type VI, Gaucher disease, Tay-Sachs disease], beta hemoglobinopathies, phenylketonuria, galactosemia), genomic sequence analysis panel, must include sequencing of at least 15 genes (eg, *ACADM, ARSA, ASPA, ATP7B, BCKDHA, BCKDHB, BLM, CFTR, DHCR7, FANCC, G6PC, GAA, GALT, GBA, GBE1, HBB, HEXA, IKBKAP, MCOLN1, PAH*)**

EXCLUDES When performed separately:
Ashkenazi Jewish-associated disorder analysis only (81412)
Fragile X mental retardation (FMR1) analysis (81243)
Hemoglobin A testing ([81257])
Spinal muscular atrophy (SMN1) analysis (81329)

🖩 0.00   🔧 0.00   **FUD** XXX   🖵

AMA: 2020,Dec,3; 2019,Jul,3; 2018,Nov,9

81425 **Genome (eg, unexplained constitutional or heritable disorder or syndrome); sequence analysis**

INCLUDES Chromosomal abnormality sequence analysis ([81349])

🖩 0.00   🔧 0.00   **FUD** XXX   Ⓐ🖵

AMA: 2020,Dec,3; 2018,Jan,8; 2017,Jan,8; 2016,Jan,13

\+ **81426** **sequence analysis, each comparator genome (eg, parents, siblings) (List separately in addition to code for primary procedure)**

INCLUDES Chromosomal abnormality sequence analysis ([81349])

Code first (81425)

🖩 0.00   🔧 0.00   **FUD** XXX   Ⓐ🖵

AMA: 2020,Dec,3; 2018,Jan,8; 2017,Jan,8; 2016,Jan,13

26/TC PC/TC Only	A2-Z3 ASC Payment	50 Bilateral	♂ Male Only	♀ Female Only	🖩 Facility RVU	🔧 Non-Facility RVU	🖵 CCI	☒ CLIA
FUD Follow-up Days	CMS: IOM	AMA: CPT Asst	A-Y OPPSI	80/80 Surg Assist Allowed / w/Doc	🔲 Lab Crosswalk	🔲 Radiology Crosswalk		

386

81427   re-evaluation of previously obtained genome sequence (eg, updated knowledge or unrelated condition/syndrome)

EXCLUDES   *Incidental results*

📋 0.00   ⚗ 0.00   **FUD** XXX   🅰 🖵

AMA: 2020,Dec,3; 2018,Jan,8; 2017,Jan,8; 2016,Jan,13

81430   Hearing loss (eg, nonsyndromic hearing loss, Usher syndrome, Pendred syndrome); genomic sequence analysis panel, must include sequencing of at least 60 genes, including *CDH23, CLRN1, GJB2, GPR98, MTRNR1, MYO7A, MYO15A, PCDH15, OTOF, SLC26A4, TMC1, TMPRSS3, USH1C, USH1G, USH2A,* and *WFS1*

📋 0.00   ⚗ 0.00   **FUD** XXX   🅰 🖵

AMA: 2020,Dec,3; 2018,Jan,8; 2017,Jan,8; 2016,Jan,13

81431   duplication/deletion analysis panel, must include copy number analyses for *STRC* and *DFNB1* deletions in *GJB2* and *GJB6* genes

📋 0.00   ⚗ 0.00   **FUD** XXX   🅰 🖵

AMA: 2020,Dec,3; 2018,Jan,8; 2017,Jan,8; 2016,Jan,13

81432   Hereditary breast cancer-related disorders (eg, hereditary breast cancer, hereditary ovarian cancer, hereditary endometrial cancer); genomic sequence analysis panel, must include sequencing of at least 10 genes, always including *BRCA1, BRCA2, CDH1, MLH1, MSH2, MSH6, PALB2, PTEN, STK11,* and *TP53*

📋 0.00   ⚗ 0.00   **FUD** XXX   🅰 🖵

AMA: 2020,Dec,3; 2019,May,5; 2018,Jan,8; 2017,Jan,8; 2016,Apr,4

81433   duplication/deletion analysis panel, must include analyses for *BRCA1, BRCA2, MLH1, MSH2,* and *STK11*

📋 0.00   ⚗ 0.00   **FUD** XXX   🅰 🖵

AMA: 2020,Dec,3; 2018,Jan,8; 2017,Jan,8; 2016,Apr,4

81434   Hereditary retinal disorders (eg, retinitis pigmentosa, Leber congenital amaurosis, cone-rod dystrophy), genomic sequence analysis panel, must include sequencing of at least 15 genes, including *ABCA4, CNGA1, CRB1, EYS, PDE6A, PDE6B, PRPF31, PRPH2, RDH12, RHO, RP1, RP2, RPE65, RPGR,* and *USH2A*

📋 0.00   ⚗ 0.00   **FUD** XXX   🅰 🖵

AMA: 2020,Dec,3; 2018,Jan,8; 2017,Jan,8; 2016,Apr,4

81435   Hereditary colon cancer disorders (eg, Lynch syndrome, PTEN hamartoma syndrome, Cowden syndrome, familial adenomatosis polyposis); genomic sequence analysis panel, must include sequencing of at least 10 genes, including *APC, BMPR1A, CDH1, MLH1, MSH2, MSH6, MUTYH, PTEN, SMAD4,* and *STK11*

📋 0.00   ⚗ 0.00   **FUD** XXX   🅰 🖵

AMA: 2020,Dec,3; 2018,Jan,8; 2017,Jan,8; 2016,Apr,4; 2016,Jan,13

81436   duplication/deletion analysis panel, must include analysis of at least 5 genes, including *MLH1, MSH2, EPCAM, SMAD4,* and *STK11*

📋 0.00   ⚗ 0.00   **FUD** XXX   🅰 🖵

AMA: 2020,Dec,3; 2018,Jan,8; 2017,Jan,8; 2016,Apr,4; 2016,Jan,13

81437   Hereditary neuroendocrine tumor disorders (eg, medullary thyroid carcinoma, parathyroid carcinoma, malignant pheochromocytoma or paraganglioma); genomic sequence analysis panel, must include sequencing of at least 6 genes, including *MAX, SDHB, SDHC, SDHD, TMEM127,* and *VHL*

📋 0.00   ⚗ 0.00   **FUD** XXX   🅰 🖵

AMA: 2020,Dec,3; 2018,Jan,8; 2017,Jan,8; 2016,Apr,4

81438   duplication/deletion analysis panel, must include analyses for *SDHB, SDHC, SDHD,* and *VHL*

📋 0.00   ⚗ 0.00   **FUD** XXX   🅰 🖵

AMA: 2020,Dec,3; 2018,Jan,8; 2017,Jan,8; 2016,Apr,4

81448   Hereditary peripheral neuropathies (eg, Charcot-Marie-Tooth, spastic paraplegia), genomic sequence analysis panel, must include sequencing of at least 5 peripheral neuropathy-related genes (eg, *BSCL2, GJB1, MFN2, MPZ, REEP1, SPAST, SPG11, SPTLC1*)

📋 0.00   ⚗ 0.00   **FUD** XXX   🅰 🖵

AMA: 2020,Dec,3; 2018,May,6

81439   Hereditary cardiomyopathy (eg, hypertrophic cardiomyopathy, dilated cardiomyopathy, arrhythmogenic right ventricular cardiomyopathy), genomic sequence analysis panel, must include sequencing of at least 5 cardiomyopathy-related genes (eg, *DSG2, MYBPC3, MYH7, PKP2, TTN*)

EXCLUDES   *Genetic sequencing for cardiac ion channelopathies (81413-81414)*

📋 0.00   ⚗ 0.00   **FUD** XXX   🅰 🖵

AMA: 2020,Dec,3; 2020,Dec,13; 2018,Sep,14; 2018,Jan,8; 2017,Apr,3

81440   Nuclear encoded mitochondrial genes (eg, neurologic or myopathic phenotypes), genomic sequence panel, must include analysis of at least 100 genes, including *BCS1L, C10orf2, COQ2, COX10, DGUOK, MPV17, OPA1, PDSS2, POLG, POLG2, RRM2B, SCO1, SCO2, SLC25A4, SUCLA2, SUCLG1, TAZ, TK2,* and *TYMP*

📋 0.00   ⚗ 0.00   **FUD** XXX   🅰 🖵

AMA: 2020,Dec,3; 2018,Jan,8; 2017,Jan,8; 2016,Jan,13

81442   Noonan spectrum disorders (eg, Noonan syndrome, cardio-facio-cutaneous syndrome, Costello syndrome, LEOPARD syndrome, Noonan-like syndrome), genomic sequence analysis panel, must include sequencing of at least 12 genes, including *BRAF, CBL, HRAS, KRAS, MAP2K1, MAP2K2, NRAS, PTPN11, RAF1, RIT1, SHOC2,* and *SOS1*

📋 0.00   ⚗ 0.00   **FUD** XXX   🅰 🖵

AMA: 2020,Dec,3; 2018,Jan,8; 2017,Jan,8; 2016,Apr,4

81443   **Resequenced code. See code following 81422.**

81445   Targeted genomic sequence analysis panel, solid organ neoplasm, DNA analysis, and RNA analysis when performed, 5-50 genes (eg, *ALK, BRAF, CDKN2A, EGFR, ERBB2, KIT, KRAS, NRAS, MET, PDGFRA, PDGFRB, PGR, PIK3CA, PTEN, RET*), interrogation for sequence variants and copy number variants or rearrangements, if performed

📋 0.00   ⚗ 0.00   **FUD** XXX   🅰 🖵

AMA: 2020,Dec,3; 2018,Jan,8; 2017,Jan,8; 2016,Apr,4; 2016,Jan,13

81448   **Resequenced code. See code following 81438.**

81450   Targeted genomic sequence analysis panel, hematolymphoid neoplasm or disorder, DNA analysis, and RNA analysis when performed, 5-50 genes (eg, *BRAF, CEBPA, DNMT3A, EZH2, FLT3, IDH1, IDH2, JAK2, KRAS, KIT, MLL, NRAS, NPM1, NOTCH1*), interrogation for sequence variants, and copy number variants or rearrangements, or isoform expression or mRNA expression levels, if performed

📋 0.00   ⚗ 0.00   **FUD** XXX   🅰 🖵

AMA: 2020,Dec,3; 2018,Jan,8; 2017,Jan,8; 2016,Apr,4; 2016,Jan,13

81455   Targeted genomic sequence analysis panel, solid organ or hematolymphoid neoplasm, DNA analysis, and RNA analysis when performed, 51 or greater genes (eg, *ALK, BRAF, CDKN2A, CEBPA, DNMT3A, EGFR, ERBB2, EZH2, FLT3, IDH1, IDH2, JAK2, KIT, KRAS, MLL, NPM1, NRAS, MET, NOTCH1, PDGFRA, PDGFRB, PGR, PIK3CA, PTEN, RET*), interrogation for sequence variants and copy number variants or rearrangements, if performed

📋 0.00   ⚗ 0.00   **FUD** XXX   🅰 🖵

AMA: 2020,Dec,3; 2018,Jan,8; 2017,Jan,8; 2016,Apr,4; 2016,Jan,13

81460 Whole mitochondrial genome (eg, Leigh syndrome, mitochondrial encephalomyopathy, lactic acidosis, and stroke-like episodes [MELAS], myoclonic epilepsy with ragged-red fibers [MERFF], neuropathy, ataxia, and retinitis pigmentosa [NARP], Leber hereditary optic neuropathy [LHON]), genomic sequence, must include sequence analysis of entire mitochondrial genome with heteroplasmy detection

🚑 0.00 ✂ 0.00 **FUD** XXX Ⓐ ▢

AMA: 2020,Dec,3; 2018,Jan,8; 2017,Jan,8; 2016,Jan,13

81465 Whole mitochondrial genome large deletion analysis panel (eg, Kearns-Sayre syndrome, chronic progressive external ophthalmoplegia), including heteroplasmy detection, if performed

🚑 0.00 ✂ 0.00 **FUD** XXX Ⓐ ▢

AMA: 2020,Dec,3; 2018,Jan,8; 2017,Jan,8; 2016,Jan,13

81470 X-linked intellectual disability (XLID) (eg, syndromic and non-syndromic XLID); genomic sequence analysis panel, must include sequencing of at least 60 genes, including *ARX, ATRX, CDKL5, FGD1, FMR1, HUWE1, IL1RAPL, KDM5C, L1CAM, MECP2, MED12, MID1, OCRL, RPS6KA3,* and *SLC16A2*

🚑 0.00 ✂ 0.00 **FUD** XXX Ⓐ ▢

AMA: 2020,Dec,3; 2018,Jan,8; 2017,Jan,8; 2016,Jan,13

81471 duplication/deletion gene analysis, must include analysis of at least 60 genes, including *ARX, ATRX, CDKL5, FGD1, FMR1, HUWE1, IL1RAPL, KDM5C, L1CAM, MECP2, MED12, MID1, OCRL, RPS6KA3,* and *SLC16A2*

🚑 0.00 ✂ 0.00 **FUD** XXX Ⓐ ▢

AMA: 2020,Dec,3; 2018,Jan,8; 2017,Jan,8; 2016,Jan,13

81479 **Resequenced code. See code following 81408.**

81490-81599 [81500, 81503, 81504, 81522, 81540, 81546, 81595, 81596] Multianalyte Assays

INCLUDES Procedures using multiple assay panel results (eg, molecular pathology, fluorescent in situ hybridization, non-nucleic acid-based) and other patient information to perform algorithmic analysis
Required analytical services (eg, amplification, cell lysis, detection, digestion, extraction, hybridization, nucleic acid stabilization) and algorithmic analysis

EXCLUDES *Genomic resequencing tests (81410-81471 [81448])*
In situ hybridization analyses (88271-88275, 88365-88368 [88364, 88373, 88374])
Microbial identification (87149-87153, 87471-87801 [87623, 87624, 87625], 87900-87904 [87906, 87910, 87912])
Multianalyte assays with algorithmic analyses without a Category I code (0002M-0007M, 0011M-0013M)
Code also procedures performed prior to cell lysis (eg, microdissection) (88380-88381)

81490 Autoimmune (rheumatoid arthritis), analysis of 12 biomarkers using immunoassays, utilizing serum, prognostic algorithm reported as a disease activity score

EXCLUDES *C-reactive protein (86140)*

🚑 0.00 ✂ 0.00 **FUD** XXX Ⓠ ▢

AMA: 2020,Dec,3

\# **81595** Cardiology (heart transplant), mRNA, gene expression profiling by real-time quantitative PCR of 20 genes (11 content and 9 housekeeping), utilizing subfraction of peripheral blood, algorithm reported as a rejection risk score

🚑 0.00 ✂ 0.00 **FUD** XXX Ⓐ ▢

AMA: 2020,Dec,3; 2019,Jun,11

81493 Coronary artery disease, mRNA, gene expression profiling by real-time RT-PCR of 23 genes, utilizing whole peripheral blood, algorithm reported as a risk score

🚑 0.00 ✂ 0.00 **FUD** XXX Ⓐ ▢

AMA: 2020,Dec,3

81500 **Resequenced code. See code following 81538.**

81503 **Resequenced code. See code before 81539.**

81504 **Resequenced code. See code following resequenced code 81546.**

81506 Endocrinology (type 2 diabetes), biochemical assays of seven analytes (glucose, HbA1c, insulin, hs-CRP, adiponectin, ferritin, interleukin 2-receptor alpha), utilizing serum or plasma, algorithm reporting a risk score

EXCLUDES *C-reactive protein; high sensitivity (hsCRP) (86141)*
Ferritin (82728)
Glucose (82947)
Hemoglobin; glycosylated (A1C) (83036)
Immunoassay for analyte other than infectious agent antibody or infectious agent antigen (83520)
Insulin; total (83525)
Unlisted chemistry procedure (84999)

🚑 0.00 ✂ 0.00 **FUD** XXX Ⓔ ▢

AMA: 2020,Dec,3; 2019,Jun,11

81507 Fetal aneuploidy (trisomy 21, 18, and 13) DNA sequence analysis of selected regions using maternal plasma, algorithm reported as a risk score for each trisomy ♀

EXCLUDES *Genome-wide microarray analysis (81228-81229)*
Low-pass sequencing analysis ([81349])
Molecular cytogenetics (88271)

🚑 0.00 ✂ 0.00 **FUD** XXX Ⓐ ▢

AMA: 2020,Dec,3; 2019,Jun,11; 2018,Apr,10

81508 Fetal congenital abnormalities, biochemical assays of two proteins (PAPP-A, hCG [any form]), utilizing maternal serum, algorithm reported as a risk score ♀

EXCLUDES *Gonadotropin, chorionic (hCG) (84702)*
Pregnancy-associated plasma protein-A (PAPP-A) (84163)

🚑 0.00 ✂ 0.00 **FUD** XXX Ⓔ ▢

AMA: 2020,Dec,3; 2019,Jun,11

81509 Fetal congenital abnormalities, biochemical assays of three proteins (PAPP-A, hCG [any form], DIA), utilizing maternal serum, algorithm reported as a risk score ♀

EXCLUDES *Gonadotropin, chorionic (hCG) (84702)*
Inhibin A (86336)
Pregnancy-associated plasma protein-A (PAPP-A) (84163)

🚑 0.00 ✂ 0.00 **FUD** XXX Ⓔ ▢

AMA: 2020,Dec,3; 2019,Jun,11

81510 Fetal congenital abnormalities, biochemical assays of three analytes (AFP, uE3, hCG [any form]), utilizing maternal serum, algorithm reported as a risk score ♀

EXCLUDES *Alpha-fetoprotein (AFP) (82105)*
Estriol (82677)
Gonadotropin, chorionic (hCG) (84702)

🚑 0.00 ✂ 0.00 **FUD** XXX Ⓔ ▢

AMA: 2020,Dec,3; 2019,Jun,11

81511 Fetal congenital abnormalities, biochemical assays of four analytes (AFP, uE3, hCG [any form], DIA) utilizing maternal serum, algorithm reported as a risk score (may include additional results from previous biochemical testing) ♀

EXCLUDES *Alpha-fetoprotein (AFP) (82105)*
Estriol (82677)
Gonadotropin, chorionic (hCG) (84702)
Inhibin A (86336)

🚑 0.00 ✂ 0.00 **FUD** XXX Ⓔ ▢

AMA: 2020,Dec,3; 2019,Jun,11

81512 Fetal congenital abnormalities, biochemical assays of five analytes (AFP, uE3, total hCG, hyperglycosylated hCG, DIA) utilizing maternal serum, algorithm reported as a risk score ♀

EXCLUDES *Alpha-fetoprotein (AFP) (82105)*
Estriol (82677)
Gonadotropin, chorionic (hCG) (84702)
Inhibin A (86336)

🚑 0.00 ✂ 0.00 **FUD** XXX Ⓔ ▢

AMA: 2020,Dec,3; 2019,Jun,11

| 26/TC PC/TC Only | A2-Z3 ASC Payment | 50 Bilateral | ♂ Male Only | ♀ Female Only | 🚑 Facility RVU | ✂ Non-Facility RVU | ▢ CCI | ✖ CLIA |
| **FUD** Follow-up Days | **CMS:** IOM | **AMA:** CPT Asst | Ⓐ-Ⓨ OPPSI | 80/80 Surg Assist Allowed / w/Doc | ▨ Lab Crosswalk | ▨ Radiology Crosswalk |

388 CPT © 2021 American Medical Association. All Rights Reserved. © 2021 Optum360, LLC

81513 Infectious disease, bacterial vaginosis, quantitative real-time amplification of RNA markers for Atopobium vaginae, Gardnerella vaginalis, and Lactobacillus species, utilizing vaginal-fluid specimens, algorithm reported as a positive or negative result for bacterial vaginosis ♀

🔧 0.00 ⚕ 0.00 **FUD** XXX 🖵

AMA: 2020,Dec,3

81514 Infectious disease, bacterial vaginosis and vaginitis, quantitative real-time amplification of DNA markers for Gardnerella vaginalis, Atopobium vaginae, Megasphaera type 1, Bacterial Vaginosis Associated Bacteria-2 (BVAB-2), and Lactobacillus species (L. crispatus and L. jensenii), utilizing vaginal-fluid specimens, algorithm reported as a positive or negative for high likelihood of bacterial vaginosis, includes separate detection of Trichomonas vaginalis and/or Candida species (C. albicans, C. tropicalis, C. parapsilosis, C. dubliniensis), Candida glabrata, Candida krusei, when reported ♀

EXCLUDES *Candida (87480-87482)*
Gardnerella vaginalis (87510-87512)
Trichomonas vaginalis (87660-87661)

🔧 0.00 ⚕ 0.00 **FUD** XXX 🖵

AMA: 2020,Dec,3

\# **81596** Infectious disease, chronic hepatitis C virus (HCV) infection, six biochemical assays (ALT, A2-macroglobulin, apolipoprotein A-1, total bilirubin, GGT, and haptoglobin) utilizing serum, prognostic algorithm reported as scores for fibrosis and necroinflammatory activity in liver

🔧 0.00 ⚕ 0.00 **FUD** XXX 🖵

AMA: 2020,Dec,3; 2019,Jun,11; 2019,Jul,3

81518 Oncology (breast), mRNA, gene expression profiling by real-time RT-PCR of 11 genes (7 content and 4 housekeeping), utilizing formalin-fixed paraffin-embedded tissue, algorithms reported as percentage risk for metastatic recurrence and likelihood of benefit from extended endocrine therapy

🔧 0.00 ⚕ 0.00 **FUD** XXX 🖵

AMA: 2020,Dec,3; 2019,Jun,11; 2019,Jul,3

\# **81522** Oncology (breast), mRNA, gene expression profiling by RT-PCR of 12 genes (8 content and 4 housekeeping), utilizing formalin-fixed paraffin-embedded tissue, algorithm reported as recurrence risk score

🔧 0.00 ⚕ 0.00 **FUD** XXX 🖵

AMA: 2020,Dec,3

81519 Oncology (breast), mRNA, gene expression profiling by real-time RT-PCR of 21 genes, utilizing formalin-fixed paraffin embedded tissue, algorithm reported as recurrence score

🔧 0.00 ⚕ 0.00 **FUD** XXX A 🖵

AMA: 2020,Dec,3; 2019,Jun,11; 2018,Jan,8; 2017,Jan,8; 2016,Jan,13

81520 Oncology (breast), mRNA gene expression profiling by hybrid capture of 58 genes (50 content and 8 housekeeping), utilizing formalin-fixed paraffin-embedded tissue, algorithm reported as a recurrence risk score

🔧 0.00 ⚕ 0.00 **FUD** XXX A 🖵

AMA: 2020,Dec,3; 2019,Jun,11; 2018,Jun,8

81521 Oncology (breast), mRNA, microarray gene expression profiling of 70 content genes and 465 housekeeping genes, utilizing fresh frozen or formalin-fixed paraffin-embedded tissue, algorithm reported as index related to risk of distant metastasis

EXCLUDES *Oncology (breast), mRNA, next-generation sequencing gene expression profiling, when performed on same specimen (81523)*

🔧 0.00 ⚕ 0.00 **FUD** XXX A 🖵

AMA: 2020,Dec,3; 2019,Jun,11; 2018,Jun,8

81522 Resequenced code. See code following 81518.

● **81523** Oncology (breast), mRNA, next-generation sequencing gene expression profiling of 70 content genes and 31 housekeeping genes, utilizing formalin-fixed paraffin-embedded tissue, algorithm reported as index related to risk to distant metastasis

EXCLUDES *Oncology (breast), mRNA, microarray gene expression profiling, when performed on same specimen (81521)*

81525 Oncology (colon), mRNA, gene expression profiling by real-time RT-PCR of 12 genes (7 content and 5 housekeeping), utilizing formalin-fixed paraffin-embedded tissue, algorithm reported as a recurrence score

🔧 0.00 ⚕ 0.00 **FUD** XXX A 🖵

AMA: 2020,Dec,3; 2019,Jun,11

81528 Oncology (colorectal) screening, quantitative real-time target and signal amplification of 10 DNA markers (*KRAS* mutations, promoter methylation of *NDRG4* and *BMP3*) and fecal hemoglobin, utilizing stool, algorithm reported as a positive or negative result

EXCLUDES *Blood, occult, by fecal hemoglobin (82274)*
KRAS (Kirsten rat sarcoma viral oncogene homolog) (81275)

🔧 0.00 ⚕ 0.00 **FUD** XXX A 🖵

AMA: 2020,Dec,3; 2019,Jun,11

81529 Oncology (cutaneous melanoma), mRNA, gene expression profiling by real-time RT-PCR of 31 genes (28 content and 3 housekeeping), utilizing formalin-fixed paraffin-embedded tissue, algorithm reported as recurrence risk, including likelihood of sentinel lymph node metastasis

🔧 0.00 ⚕ 0.00 **FUD** XXX 🖵

AMA: 2020,Dec,3

81535 Oncology (gynecologic), live tumor cell culture and chemotherapeutic response by DAPI stain and morphology, predictive algorithm reported as a drug response score; first single drug or drug combination

🔧 0.00 ⚕ 0.00 **FUD** XXX Q 🖵

AMA: 2020,Dec,3; 2019,Jun,11

\+ **81536** each additional single drug or drug combination (List separately in addition to code for primary procedure)

Code first (81535)

🔧 0.00 ⚕ 0.00 **FUD** XXX Q 🖵

AMA: 2020,Dec,3; 2019,Jun,11

81538 Oncology (lung), mass spectrometric 8-protein signature, including amyloid A, utilizing serum, prognostic and predictive algorithm reported as good versus poor overall survival

🔧 0.00 ⚕ 0.00 **FUD** XXX Q 🖵

AMA: 2020,Dec,3; 2019,Jun,11

\# **81500** Oncology (ovarian), biochemical assays of two proteins (CA-125 and HE4), utilizing serum, with menopausal status, algorithm reported as a risk score ♀

EXCLUDES *Human epididymis protein 4 (HE4) (86305)*
Immunoassay for tumor antigen, quantitative; CA 125 (86304)

🔧 0.00 ⚕ 0.00 **FUD** XXX E 🖵

AMA: 2020,Dec,3; 2019,Jun,11

\# **81503** Oncology (ovarian), biochemical assays of five proteins (CA-125, apolipoprotein A1, beta-2 microglobulin, transferrin, and pre-albumin), utilizing serum, algorithm reported as a risk score ♀

EXCLUDES *Apolipoprotein (82172)*
Beta-2 microglobulin (82232)
Immunoassay for tumor antigen, quantitative; CA 125 (86304)
Prealbumin (84134)
Transferrin (84466)

🔧 0.00 ⚕ 0.00 **FUD** XXX Q 🖵

AMA: 2020,Dec,3; 2019,Jun,11

81539 Oncology (high-grade prostate cancer), biochemical assay of four proteins (Total PSA, Free PSA, Intact PSA, and human kallikrein-2 [hK2]), utilizing plasma or serum, prognostic algorithm reported as a probability score ♂
  🚑 0.00 ⚕ 0.00 **FUD** XXX [Q] [▭]
  AMA: 2020,Dec,3; 2019,Jun,11; 2018,Jan,8; 2017,Apr,3

81540 Resequenced code. See code before 81552.

81541 Oncology (prostate), mRNA gene expression profiling by real-time RT-PCR of 46 genes (31 content and 15 housekeeping), utilizing formalin-fixed paraffin-embedded tissue, algorithm reported as a disease-specific mortality risk score
  🚑 0.00 ⚕ 0.00 **FUD** XXX [A] [▭]
  AMA: 2020,Dec,3; 2019,Jun,11; 2018,Aug,8

81542 Oncology (prostate), mRNA, microarray gene expression profiling of 22 content genes, utilizing formalin-fixed paraffin-embedded tissue, algorithm reported as metastasis risk score ♂
  🚑 0.00 ⚕ 0.00 **FUD** XXX
  AMA: 2020,Dec,3; 2020,Oct,8

81546 Resequenced code. See code following 81551.

81551 Oncology (prostate), promoter methylation profiling by real-time PCR of 3 genes (*GSTP1, APC, RASSF1*), utilizing formalin-fixed paraffin-embedded tissue, algorithm reported as a likelihood of prostate cancer detection on repeat biopsy
  🚑 0.00 ⚕ 0.00 **FUD** XXX [A] [▭]
  AMA: 2020,Dec,3; 2019,Jun,11; 2018,Aug,8

\# **81546** Oncology (thyroid), mRNA, gene expression analysis of 10,196 genes, utilizing fine needle aspirate, algorithm reported as a categorical result (eg, benign or suspicious)
  🚑 0.00 ⚕ 0.00 **FUD** XXX [▭]
  AMA: 2020,Dec,3

\# **81504** Oncology (tissue of origin), microarray gene expression profiling of > 2000 genes, utilizing formalin-fixed paraffin-embedded tissue, algorithm reported as tissue similarity scores
  🚑 0.00 ⚕ 0.00 **FUD** XXX [A] [▭]
  AMA: 2020,Dec,3; 2019,Jun,11

\# **81540** Oncology (tumor of unknown origin), mRNA, gene expression profiling by real-time RT-PCR of 92 genes (87 content and 5 housekeeping) to classify tumor into main cancer type and subtype, utilizing formalin-fixed paraffin-embedded tissue, algorithm reported as a probability of a predicted main cancer type and subtype
  🚑 0.00 ⚕ 0.00 **FUD** XXX [A] [▭]
  AMA: 2020,Dec,3; 2019,Jun,11

81552 Oncology (uveal melanoma), mRNA, gene expression profiling by real-time RT-PCR of 15 genes (12 content and 3 housekeeping), utilizing fine needle aspirate or formalin-fixed paraffin-embedded tissue, algorithm reported as risk of metastasis
  🚑 0.00 ⚕ 0.00 **FUD** XXX [▭]
  AMA: 2020,Dec,3; 2020,Jan,10

81554 Pulmonary disease (idiopathic pulmonary fibrosis [IPF]), mRNA, gene expression analysis of 190 genes, utilizing transbronchial biopsies, diagnostic algorithm reported as categorical result (eg, positive or negative for high probability of usual interstitial pneumonia [UIP])
  🚑 0.00 ⚕ 0.00 **FUD** XXX [▭]
  AMA: 2020,Dec,3

● **81560** Transplantation medicine (allograft rejection, pediatric liver and small bowel), measurement of donor and third-party-induced CD154+T-cytotoxic memory cells, utilizing whole peripheral blood, algorithm reported as a rejection risk score
  EXCLUDES Blood count (85032)
    Cryopreservation (88240)
    Flow cytometry (88184-88185, 88187)
    HLA typing (86821)
    Lymphocyte transformation, mitogen, antigen induced blastogenesis (86353)
    Thawing, expansion frozen cells (88241)
    Tissue cultures, non-neoplastic disorders (88230)

81595 Resequenced code. See code following 81490.

81596 Resequenced code. See code following 81514.

81599 Unlisted multianalyte assay with algorithmic analysis
  🚑 0.00 ⚕ 0.00 **FUD** XXX [E] [▭]
  AMA: 2020,Dec,3; 2019,Jun,11; 2018,Jun,8; 2018,Apr,10

82009-82030 Chemistry: Acetaldehyde—Adenosine

INCLUDES Clinical information not requested by ordering physician
  Mathematically calculated results
  Quantitative analysis unless otherwise specified
  Specimens from any source unless otherwise specified

EXCLUDES Analytes from nonrequested laboratory analysis
  Calculated results representing score or probability derived by algorithm
  Drug testing ([80305, 80306, 80307], [80324, 80325, 80326, 80327, 80328, 80329, 80330, 80331, 80332, 80333, 80334, 80335, 80336, 80337, 80338, 80339, 80340, 80341, 80342, 80343, 80344, 80345, 80346, 80347, 80348, 80349, 80350, 80351, 80352, 80353, 80354, 80355, 80356, 80357, 80358, 80359, 80360, 80361, 80362, 80363, 80364, 80365, 80366, 80367, 80368, 80369, 80370, 80371, 80372, 80373, 80374, 80375, 80376, 80377, 83992])
  Organ or disease panels (80048-80076 [80081])
  Therapeutic drug assays (80150-80299 [80164, 80165, 80171])

82009 Ketone body(s) (eg, acetone, acetoacetic acid, beta-hydroxybutyrate); qualitative
  🚑 0.00 ⚕ 0.00 **FUD** XXX [Q] [▭]
  AMA: 2020,Dec,3; 2018,Jan,8; 2017,Jan,8; 2016,Jan,13

82010 quantitative
  🚑 0.00 ⚕ 0.00 **FUD** XXX [X] [Q] [▭]
  AMA: 2020,Dec,3; 2018,Jan,8; 2017,Jan,8; 2016,Jan,13

82013 Acetylcholinesterase
  EXCLUDES Acid phosphatase (84060-84066)
    Gastric acid analysis (82930)
  🚑 0.00 ⚕ 0.00 **FUD** XXX [Q] [▭]
  AMA: 2020,Dec,3

82016 Acylcarnitines; qualitative, each specimen
  🚑 0.00 ⚕ 0.00 **FUD** XXX [Q] [▭]
  AMA: 2020,Dec,3

82017 quantitative, each specimen
  EXCLUDES Carnitine (82379)
  🚑 0.00 ⚕ 0.00 **FUD** XXX [Q] [▭]
  AMA: 2020,Dec,3

82024 Adrenocorticotropic hormone (ACTH)
  🚑 0.00 ⚕ 0.00 **FUD** XXX [Q] [▭]
  AMA: 2020,Dec,3

82030 Adenosine, 5-monophosphate, cyclic (cyclic AMP)
  🚑 0.00 ⚕ 0.00 **FUD** XXX [Q] [▭]
  AMA: 2020,Dec,3

82040-82042 [82042] Chemistry: Albumin

INCLUDES Clinical information not requested by ordering physician
Mathematically calculated results
Quantitative analysis unless otherwise specified
Specimens from any other sources unless otherwise specified

EXCLUDES *Analytes from nonrequested laboratory analysis*
Calculated results representing score or probability derived by algorithm
Drug testing ([80305, 80306, 80307], [80324, 80325, 80326, 80327, 80328, 80329, 80330, 80331, 80332, 80333, 80334, 80335, 80336, 80337, 80338, 80339, 80340, 80341, 80342, 80343, 80344, 80345, 80346, 80347, 80348, 80349, 80350, 80351, 80352, 80353, 80354, 80355, 80356, 80357, 80358, 80359, 80360, 80361, 80362, 80363, 80364, 80365, 80366, 80367, 80368, 80369, 80370, 80371, 80372, 80373, 80374, 80375, 80376, 80377, 83992])
Organ or disease panels (80048-80076 [80081])
Therapeutic drug assays (80150-80299 [80164, 80165, 80171])

82040 **Albumin; serum, plasma or whole blood**
0.00 0.00 **FUD** XXX
AMA: 2020,Dec,3; 2018,Jan,8; 2017,Jan,8; 2016,Jan,13

82042 **Resequenced code. See code following 82045.**

82043 **urine (eg, microalbumin), quantitative**
0.00 0.00 **FUD** XXX
AMA: 2020,Dec,3; 2018,Jan,8; 2017,Jan,8; 2016,Jan,13

82044 **urine (eg, microalbumin), semiquantitative (eg, reagent strip assay)**
EXCLUDES *Prealbumin (84134)*
0.00 0.00 **FUD** XXX
AMA: 2020,Dec,3; 2018,Jan,8; 2017,Jan,8; 2016,Jan,13

82045 **ischemia modified**
0.00 0.00 **FUD** XXX
AMA: 2020,Dec,3

\# **82042** **other source, quantitative, each specimen**
EXCLUDES *Total protein (84155-84157, 84160)*
0.00 0.00 **FUD** XXX
AMA: 2020,Dec,3

82075-82107 Chemistry: Alcohol—Alpha-fetoprotein (AFP)

INCLUDES Clinical information not requested by ordering physician
Mathematically calculated results
Quantitative analysis unless otherwise specified
Specimens from any source unless otherwise specified

EXCLUDES *Analytes from nonrequested laboratory analysis*
Calculated results representing score or probability derived by algorithm
Drug testing ([80305, 80306, 80307], [80324, 80325, 80326, 80327, 80328, 80329, 80330, 80331, 80332, 80333, 80334, 80335, 80336, 80337, 80338, 80339, 80340, 80341, 80342, 80343, 80344, 80345, 80346, 80347, 80348, 80349, 80350, 80351, 80352, 80353, 80354, 80355, 80356, 80357, 80358, 80359, 80360, 80361, 80362, 80363, 80364, 80365, 80366, 80367, 80368, 80369, 80370, 80371, 80372, 80373, 80374, 80375, 80376, 80377, 83992])
Organ or disease panels (80048-80076 [80081])
Therapeutic drug assays (80150-80299 [80164, 80165, 80171])

82075 **Alcohol (ethanol); breath**
0.00 0.00 **FUD** XXX
AMA: 2020,Dec,3

82077 **any specimen except urine and breath, immunoassay (eg, IA, EIA, ELISA, RIA, EMIT, FPIA) and enzymatic methods (eg, alcohol dehydrogenase)**
EXCLUDES *Alcohol (ethanol) confirmatory drug testing ([80320])*
0.00 0.00 **FUD** XXX
AMA: 2020,Dec,3

82085 **Aldolase**
0.00 0.00 **FUD** XXX
AMA: 2020,Dec,3

82088 **Aldosterone**
EXCLUDES *Alkaline phosphatase (84075, 84080)*
Alphaketoglutarate (82009-82010)
Alphatocopherol (VitaminE) (84446)
0.00 0.00 **FUD** XXX
AMA: 2020,Dec,3

82103 **Alpha-1-antitrypsin; total**
0.00 0.00 **FUD** XXX
AMA: 2020,Dec,3

82104 **phenotype**
0.00 0.00 **FUD** XXX
AMA: 2020,Dec,3

82105 **Alpha-fetoprotein (AFP); serum**
0.00 0.00 **FUD** XXX
AMA: 2020,Dec,3

82106 **amniotic fluid**
0.00 0.00 **FUD** XXX
AMA: 2020,Dec,3

82107 **AFP-L3 fraction isoform and total AFP (including ratio)**
0.00 0.00 **FUD** XXX
AMA: 2020,Dec,3

82108 Chemistry: Aluminum

CMS: 100-02,11,20.2 ESRD Laboratory Services

INCLUDES Clinical information not requested by ordering physician
Mathematically calculated results
Quantitative analysis unless otherwise specified
Specimens from any source unless otherwise specified

EXCLUDES *Analytes from nonrequested laboratory analysis*
Calculated results representing score or probability derived by algorithm
Drug testing ([80305, 80306, 80307], [80324, 80325, 80326, 80327, 80328, 80329, 80330, 80331, 80332, 80333, 80334, 80335, 80336, 80337, 80338, 80339, 80340, 80341, 80342, 80343, 80344, 80345, 80346, 80347, 80348, 80349, 80350, 80351, 80352, 80353, 80354, 80355, 80356, 80357, 80358, 80359, 80360, 80361, 80362, 80363, 80364, 80365, 80366, 80367, 80368, 80369, 80370, 80371, 80372, 80373, 80374, 80375, 80376, 80377, 83992])
Organ or disease panels (80048-80076 [80081])
Therapeutic drug assays (80150-80299 [80164, 80165, 80171])

82108 **Aluminum**
0.00 0.00 **FUD** XXX
AMA: 2020,Dec,3

82120-82261 Chemistry: Amines—Biotinidase

INCLUDES Clinical information not requested by ordering physician
Mathematically calculated results
Quantitative analysis unless otherwise specified
Specimens from any source unless otherwise specified

EXCLUDES *Analytes from nonrequested laboratory analysis*
Calculated results representing score or probability derived by algorithm
Drug testing ([80305, 80306, 80307], [80324, 80325, 80326, 80327, 80328, 80329, 80330, 80331, 80332, 80333, 80334, 80335, 80336, 80337, 80338, 80339, 80340, 80341, 80342, 80343, 80344, 80345, 80346, 80347, 80348, 80349, 80350, 80351, 80352, 80353, 80354, 80355, 80356, 80357, 80358, 80359, 80360, 80361, 80362, 80363, 80364, 80365, 80366, 80367, 80368, 80369, 80370, 80371, 80372, 80373, 80374, 80375, 80376, 80377, 83992])
Organ or disease panels (80048-80076 [80081])
Therapeutic drug assays (80150-80299 [80164, 80165, 80171])

82120 **Amines, vaginal fluid, qualitative**
EXCLUDES *Combined pH and amines test for vaginitis (82120, 83986)*
0.00 0.00 **FUD** XXX
AMA: 2020,Dec,3; 2018,Jan,8; 2017,Jan,8; 2016,Jan,13

82127 **Amino acids; single, qualitative, each specimen**
0.00 0.00 **FUD** XXX
AMA: 2020,Dec,3

82128 **multiple, qualitative, each specimen**
0.00 0.00 **FUD** XXX
AMA: 2020,Dec,3

82131 **single, quantitative, each specimen**
INCLUDES Van Slyke method
0.00 0.00 **FUD** XXX
AMA: 2020,Dec,3; 2018,Jan,8; 2017,Jan,8; 2016,Jan,13

82135 **Aminolevulinic acid, delta (ALA)**
0.00 0.00 **FUD** XXX
AMA: 2020,Dec,3

82136 **Amino acids, 2 to 5 amino acids, quantitative, each specimen**
0.00 0.00 **FUD** XXX
AMA: 2020,Dec,3

● New Code ▲ Revised Code ○ Reinstated ● New Web Release ▲ Revised Web Release + Add-on Unlisted Not Covered \# Resequenced
⑤⓪ Optum Mod 50 Exempt ⦰ AMA Mod 51 Exempt ⑤① Optum Mod 51 Exempt ⑥③ Mod 63 Exempt ⁄ Non-FDA Drug ★ Telemedicine Ⓜ Maternity Ⓐ Age Edit

CPT © 2021 American Medical Association. All Rights Reserved.

82139 Amino acids, 6 or more amino acids, quantitative, each specimen
🚑 0.00   ⅗ 0.00   **FUD** XXX   ⓠ▱
AMA: 2020,Dec,3

82140 Ammonia
🚑 0.00   ⅗ 0.00   **FUD** XXX   ⓠ▱
AMA: 2020,Dec,3

82143 Amniotic fluid scan (spectrophotometric)   Ⓜ ♀
EXCLUDES Amobarbital ([80345])
L/S ratio (83661)
🚑 0.00   ⅗ 0.00   **FUD** XXX   ⓠ▱
AMA: 2020,Dec,3

82150 Amylase
🚑 0.00   ⅗ 0.00   **FUD** XXX   ⌧ⓠ▱
AMA: 2020,Dec,3

82154 Androstanediol glucuronide
🚑 0.00   ⅗ 0.00   **FUD** XXX   ⓠ▱
AMA: 2020,Dec,3; 2018,Jan,8; 2017,Jan,8; 2016,Jan,13

82157 Androstenedione
🚑 0.00   ⅗ 0.00   **FUD** XXX   ⓠ▱
AMA: 2020,Dec,3

82160 Androsterone
🚑 0.00   ⅗ 0.00   **FUD** XXX   ⓠ▱
AMA: 2020,Dec,3

82163 Angiotensin II
🚑 0.00   ⅗ 0.00   **FUD** XXX   ⓠ▱
AMA: 2020,Dec,3

82164 Angiotensin I - converting enzyme (ACE)
EXCLUDES Antidiuretic hormone (ADH) (84588)
Antimony (83015)
Antitrypsin, alpha-1- (82103-82104)
🚑 0.00   ⅗ 0.00   **FUD** XXX   ⓠ▱
AMA: 2020,Dec,3

82172 Apolipoprotein, each
🚑 0.00   ⅗ 0.00   **FUD** XXX   ⓠ▱
AMA: 2020,Dec,3

82175 Arsenic
EXCLUDES Heavy metal screening (83015)
🚑 0.00   ⅗ 0.00   **FUD** XXX   ⓠ▱
AMA: 2020,Dec,3

82180 Ascorbic acid (Vitamin C), blood
EXCLUDES Aspirin (acetylsalicylic acid) ([80329, 80330, 80331])
Atherogenic index, blood, ultracentrifugation, quantitative (83701)
Salicylate therapeutic drug assay ([80179])
🚑 0.00   ⅗ 0.00   **FUD** XXX   ⓠ▱
AMA: 2020,Dec,3

82190 Atomic absorption spectroscopy, each analyte
🚑 0.00   ⅗ 0.00   **FUD** XXX   ⓠ▱
AMA: 2020,Dec,3

82232 Beta-2 microglobulin
🚑 0.00   ⅗ 0.00   **FUD** XXX   ⓠ▱
AMA: 2020,Dec,3

82239 Bile acids; total
🚑 0.00   ⅗ 0.00   **FUD** XXX   ⓠ▱
AMA: 2020,Dec,3

82240 cholylglycine
EXCLUDES Bile pigments, urine (81000-81005)
🚑 0.00   ⅗ 0.00   **FUD** XXX   ⓠ▱
AMA: 2020,Dec,3

82247 Bilirubin; total
INCLUDES Van Den Bergh test
🚑 0.00   ⅗ 0.00   **FUD** XXX   ⌧ⓠ▱
AMA: 2020,Dec,3; 2018,Jan,8; 2017,Jan,8; 2016,Jan,13

82248 direct
🚑 0.00   ⅗ 0.00   **FUD** XXX   ⓠ▱
AMA: 2020,Dec,3; 2018,Jan,8; 2017,Jan,8; 2016,Jan,13

82252 feces, qualitative
🚑 0.00   ⅗ 0.00   **FUD** XXX   ⓠ▱
AMA: 2020,Dec,3

82261 Biotinidase, each specimen
🚑 0.00   ⅗ 0.00   **FUD** XXX   ⓠ▱
AMA: 2020,Dec,3

82270-82274 Chemistry: Occult Blood

CMS: 100-04,16,70.8 CLIA Waived Tests; 100-04,18,60 Colorectal Cancer Screening
INCLUDES Clinical information not requested by ordering physician
Mathematically calculated results
Quantitative analysis unless otherwise specified
Specimens from any source unless otherwise specified
EXCLUDES Analytes from nonrequested laboratory analysis
Calculated results representing score or probability derived by algorithm
Drug testing ([80305, 80306, 80307], [80324, 80325, 80326, 80327, 80328, 80329, 80330, 80331, 80332, 80333, 80334, 80335, 80336, 80337, 80338, 80339, 80340, 80341, 80342, 80343, 80344, 80345, 80346, 80347, 80348, 80349, 80350, 80351, 80352, 80353, 80354, 80355, 80356, 80357, 80358, 80359, 80360, 80361, 80362, 80363, 80364, 80365, 80366, 80367, 80368, 80369, 80370, 80371, 80372, 80373, 80374, 80375, 80376, 80377, 83992])
Organ or disease panels (80048-80076 [80081])
Therapeutic drug assays (80150-80299 [80164, 80165, 80171])

82270 Blood, occult, by peroxidase activity (eg, guaiac), qualitative; feces, consecutive collected specimens with single determination, for colorectal neoplasm screening (ie, patient was provided 3 cards or single triple card for consecutive collection)
INCLUDES Day test
🚑 0.00   ⅗ 0.00   **FUD** XXX   ⌧Ⓐ▱
AMA: 2020,Dec,3; 2018,Jan,8; 2017,Jan,8; 2016,Jan,13

82271 other sources
🚑 0.00   ⅗ 0.00   **FUD** XXX   ⌧ⓠ▱
AMA: 2020,Dec,3

82272 Blood, occult, by peroxidase activity (eg, guaiac), qualitative, feces, 1-3 simultaneous determinations, performed for other than colorectal neoplasm screening
🚑 0.00   ⅗ 0.00   **FUD** XXX   ⌧ⓠ▱
AMA: 2020,Dec,3; 2018,Jan,8; 2017,Jan,8; 2016,Jan,13

82274 Blood, occult, by fecal hemoglobin determination by immunoassay, qualitative, feces, 1-3 simultaneous determinations
🚑 0.00   ⅗ 0.00   **FUD** XXX   ⌧ⓠ▱
AMA: 2020,Dec,3

82286-82308 [82652] Chemistry: Bradykinin—Calcitonin

INCLUDES Clinical information not requested by ordering physician
Mathematically calculated results
Quantitative analysis unless otherwise specified
Specimens from any source unless otherwise specified
EXCLUDES Analytes from nonrequested laboratory analysis
Calculated results representing score or probability derived by algorithm
Drug testing ([80305, 80306, 80307], [80324, 80325, 80326, 80327, 80328, 80329, 80330, 80331, 80332, 80333, 80334, 80335, 80336, 80337, 80338, 80339, 80340, 80341, 80342, 80343, 80344, 80345, 80346, 80347, 80348, 80349, 80350, 80351, 80352, 80353, 80354, 80355, 80356, 80357, 80358, 80359, 80360, 80361, 80362, 80363, 80364, 80365, 80366, 80367, 80368, 80369, 80370, 80371, 80372, 80373, 80374, 80375, 80376, 80377, 83992])
Organ or disease panels (80048-80076 [80081])
Therapeutic drug assays (80150-80299 [80164, 80165, 80171])

82286 Bradykinin
🚑 0.00   ⅗ 0.00   **FUD** XXX   ⓠ▱
AMA: 2020,Dec,3

82300 Cadmium
🚑 0.00   ⅗ 0.00   **FUD** XXX   ⓠ▱
AMA: 2020,Dec,3

82306 Vitamin D; 25 hydroxy, includes fraction(s), if performed
🚑 0.00   ⅗ 0.00   **FUD** XXX   ⓠ▱
AMA: 2020,Dec,3

| # | 82652 | 1, 25 dihydroxy, includes fraction(s), if performed

**82652** **1, 25 dihydroxy, includes fraction(s), if performed**
🚑 0.00 ✂ 0.00 **FUD** XXX
AMA: 2020,Dec,3

82308 **Calcitonin**
🚑 0.00 ✂ 0.00 **FUD** XXX
AMA: 2020,Dec,3

82310-82373 Chemistry: Calcium, total; Carbohydrate Deficient Transferrin

INCLUDES Clinical information not requested by ordering physician
Mathematically calculated results
Quantitative analysis unless otherwise specified
Specimens from any source unless otherwise specified
EXCLUDES *Analytes from nonrequested laboratory analysis*
Calculated results representing score or probability derived by algorithm
Drug testing ([80305, 80306, 80307], [80324, 80325, 80326, 80327, 80328, 80329, 80330, 80331, 80332, 80333, 80334, 80335, 80336, 80337, 80338, 80339, 80340, 80341, 80342, 80343, 80344, 80345, 80346, 80347, 80348, 80349, 80350, 80351, 80352, 80353, 80354, 80355, 80356, 80357, 80358, 80359, 80360, 80361, 80362, 80363, 80364, 80365, 80366, 80367, 80368, 80369, 80370, 80371, 80372, 80373, 80374, 80375, 80376, 80377, 83992])
Organ or disease panels (80048-80076 [80081])
Therapeutic drug assays (80150-80299 [80164, 80165, 80171])

82310 **Calcium; total**
🚑 0.00 ✂ 0.00 **FUD** XXX
AMA: 2020,Dec,3; 2018,Jan,8; 2017,Jan,8; 2016,Jan,13

82330 **ionized**
🚑 0.00 ✂ 0.00 **FUD** XXX
AMA: 2020,Dec,3; 2018,Jan,8; 2017,Jan,8; 2016,Jan,13

82331 **after calcium infusion test**
🚑 0.00 ✂ 0.00 **FUD** XXX
AMA: 2020,Dec,3

82340 **urine quantitative, timed specimen**
🚑 0.00 ✂ 0.00 **FUD** XXX
AMA: 2020,Dec,3

82355 **Calculus; qualitative analysis**
🚑 0.00 ✂ 0.00 **FUD** XXX
AMA: 2020,Dec,3

82360 **quantitative analysis, chemical**
🚑 0.00 ✂ 0.00 **FUD** XXX
AMA: 2020,Dec,3

82365 **infrared spectroscopy**
🚑 0.00 ✂ 0.00 **FUD** XXX
AMA: 2020,Dec,3

82370 **X-ray diffraction**
🚑 0.00 ✂ 0.00 **FUD** XXX
AMA: 2020,Dec,3

82373 **Carbohydrate deficient transferrin**
🚑 0.00 ✂ 0.00 **FUD** XXX
AMA: 2020,Dec,3

82374 Chemistry: Carbon Dioxide

CMS: 100-02,11,20.2 ESRD Laboratory Services; 100-02,11,30.2.2 Automated Multi-Channel Chemistry (AMCC) Tests; 100-04,16,40.6.1 Automated Multi-Channel Chemistry (AMCC) Tests for ESRD Beneficiaries; 100-04,16,70.8 CLIA Waived Tests; 100-04,16,90.2 Organ or Disease Oriented Panels

INCLUDES Clinical information not requested by ordering physician
Mathematically calculated results
Quantitative analysis unless otherwise specified
Specimens from any source unless otherwise specified
EXCLUDES *Analytes from nonrequested laboratory analysis*
Calculated results representing score or probability derived by algorithm
Drug testing ([80305, 80306, 80307], [80324, 80325, 80326, 80327, 80328, 80329, 80330, 80331, 80332, 80333, 80334, 80335, 80336, 80337, 80338, 80339, 80340, 80341, 80342, 80343, 80344, 80345, 80346, 80347, 80348, 80349, 80350, 80351, 80352, 80353, 80354, 80355, 80356, 80357, 80358, 80359, 80360, 80361, 80362, 80363, 80364, 80365, 80366, 80367, 80368, 80369, 80370, 80371, 80372, 80373, 80374, 80375, 80376, 80377, 83992])
Organ or disease panels (80048-80076 [80081])
Therapeutic drug assays (80150-80299 [80164, 80165, 80171])

82374 **Carbon dioxide (bicarbonate)**
EXCLUDES *Blood gases (82803)*
🚑 0.00 ✂ 0.00 **FUD** XXX
AMA: 2020,Dec,3; 2018,Jan,8; 2017,Jan,8; 2016,Jan,13

82375-82376 Chemistry: Carboxyhemoglobin (Carbon Monoxide)

INCLUDES Clinical information not requested by ordering physician
Mathematically calculated results
Specimens from any source unless otherwise specified
EXCLUDES *Analytes from nonrequested laboratory analysis*
Calculated results representing score or probability derived by algorithm
Drug testing ([80305, 80306, 80307], [80324, 80325, 80326, 80327, 80328, 80329, 80330, 80331, 80332, 80333, 80334, 80335, 80336, 80337, 80338, 80339, 80340, 80341, 80342, 80343, 80344, 80345, 80346, 80347, 80348, 80349, 80350, 80351, 80352, 80353, 80354, 80355, 80356, 80357, 80358, 80359, 80360, 80361, 80362, 80363, 80364, 80365, 80366, 80367, 80368, 80369, 80370, 80371, 80372, 80373, 80374, 80375, 80376, 80377, 83992])
Organ or disease panels (80048-80076 [80081])
Transcutaneous measurement of carboxyhemoglobin (88740)

82375 **Carboxyhemoglobin; quantitative**
🚑 0.00 ✂ 0.00 **FUD** XXX
AMA: 2020,Dec,3; 2018,Jan,8; 2017,Jan,8; 2016,Jan,13

82376 **qualitative**
🚑 0.00 ✂ 0.00 **FUD** XXX
AMA: 2020,Dec,3

82378 Chemistry: Carcinoembryonic Antigen (CEA)

CMS: 100-03,190.26 Carcinoembryonic Antigen (CEA)
INCLUDES Clinical information not requested by ordering physician
EXCLUDES *Analytes from nonrequested laboratory analysis*
Calculated results representing score or probability derived by algorithm

82378 **Carcinoembryonic antigen (CEA)**
🚑 0.00 ✂ 0.00 **FUD** XXX
AMA: 2020,Dec,3; 2018,Jan,8; 2017,Jan,8; 2016,Jan,13

82379-82415 Chemistry: Carnitine—Chloramphenicol

INCLUDES Clinical information not requested by ordering physician
Mathematically calculated results
Quantitative analysis unless otherwise specified
Specimens from any source unless otherwise specified
EXCLUDES *Analytes from nonrequested laboratory analysis*
Calculated results representing score or probability derived by algorithm
Drug testing ([80305, 80306, 80307], [80324, 80325, 80326, 80327, 80328, 80329, 80330, 80331, 80332, 80333, 80334, 80335, 80336, 80337, 80338, 80339, 80340, 80341, 80342, 80343, 80344, 80345, 80346, 80347, 80348, 80349, 80350, 80351, 80352, 80353, 80354, 80355, 80356, 80357, 80358, 80359, 80360, 80361, 80362, 80363, 80364, 80365, 80366, 80367, 80368, 80369, 80370, 80371, 80372, 80373, 80374, 80375, 80376, 80377, 83992])
Organ or disease panels (80048-80076 [80081])
Therapeutic drug assays (80150-80299 [80164, 80165, 80171])

82379 **Carnitine (total and free), quantitative, each specimen**
EXCLUDES *Acylcarnitine (82016-82017)*
🚑 0.00 ✂ 0.00 **FUD** XXX
AMA: 2020,Dec,3

82380 **Carotene**
🚑 0.00 ✂ 0.00 **FUD** XXX
AMA: 2020,Dec,3

Pathology and Laboratory

82382	**Catecholamines; total urine**
	🚑 0.00 ⚕ 0.00 **FUD** XXX Q ▫
	AMA: 2020,Dec,3
82383	**blood**
	🚑 0.00 ⚕ 0.00 **FUD** XXX Q ▫
	AMA: 2020,Dec,3
82384	**fractionated**
	EXCLUDES *Urine metabolites (83835, 84585)*
	🚑 0.00 ⚕ 0.00 **FUD** XXX Q ▫
	AMA: 2020,Dec,3
82387	**Cathepsin-D**
	🚑 0.00 ⚕ 0.00 **FUD** XXX Q ▫
	AMA: 2020,Dec,3
82390	**Ceruloplasmin**
	🚑 0.00 ⚕ 0.00 **FUD** XXX Q ▫
	AMA: 2020,Dec,3
82397	**Chemiluminescent assay**
	🚑 0.00 ⚕ 0.00 **FUD** XXX Q ▫
	AMA: 2020,Dec,3; 2018,Jan,8; 2017,Jan,8; 2016,Jan,13
82415	**Chloramphenicol**
	🚑 0.00 ⚕ 0.00 **FUD** XXX Q ▫
	AMA: 2020,Dec,3

82435-82438 Chemistry: Chloride

INCLUDES Clinical information not requested by ordering physician
Mathematically calculated results
Quantitative analysis unless otherwise specified
Specimens from any source unless otherwise specified

EXCLUDES *Analytes from nonrequested laboratory analysis*
Calculated results representing score or probability derived by algorithm
Organ or disease panels (80048-80076 [80081])
Therapeutic drug assays (80150-80299 [80164, 80165, 80171])

82435	**Chloride; blood**
	🚑 0.00 ⚕ 0.00 **FUD** XXX ✗ Q ▫
	AMA: 2020,Dec,3; 2018,Jan,8; 2017,Jan,8; 2016,Jan,13
82436	**urine**
	🚑 0.00 ⚕ 0.00 **FUD** XXX Q ▫
	AMA: 2020,Dec,3
82438	**other source**
	EXCLUDES *Sweat collections by iontophoresis (89230)*
	🚑 0.00 ⚕ 0.00 **FUD** XXX Q ▫
	AMA: 2020,Dec,3; 2018,Jan,8; 2017,Jan,8; 2016,Jan,13

82441 Chemistry: Chlorinated Hydrocarbons

INCLUDES Clinical information not requested by ordering physician
Mathematically calculated results
Quantitative analysis unless otherwise specified
Specimens from any source unless otherwise specified

EXCLUDES *Analytes from nonrequested laboratory analysis*
Calculated results representing a score or probability derived by algorithm

82441	**Chlorinated hydrocarbons, screen**
	EXCLUDES *Cholecalciferol (Vitamin D) (82306)*
	🚑 0.00 ⚕ 0.00 **FUD** XXX Q ▫
	AMA: 2020,Dec,3

82465 Chemistry: Cholesterol, Total

CMS: 100-03,190.23 Lipid Testing; 100-04,16,40.6.1 Automated Multi-Channel Chemistry (AMCC) Tests for ESRD Beneficiaries; 100-04,16,70.8 CLIA Waived Tests; 100-04,16,90.2 Organ or Disease Oriented Panels

INCLUDES Clinical information not requested by ordering physician
Mathematically calculated results
Quantitative analysis unless otherwise specified

EXCLUDES *Analytes from nonrequested laboratory analysis*
Calculated results representing score or probability derived by algorithm
Organ or disease panels (80048-80076 [80081])

82465	**Cholesterol, serum or whole blood, total**
	EXCLUDES *High density lipoprotein (HDL) (83718)*
	🚑 0.00 ⚕ 0.00 **FUD** XXX ✗ A ▫
	AMA: 2020,Dec,3; 2018,Jan,8; 2017,Jan,8; 2016,Jan,13

82480-82507 Chemistry: Cholinesterase—Citrate

INCLUDES Clinical information not requested by ordering physician
Mathematically calculated results
Quantitative analysis unless otherwise specified
Specimens from any source unless otherwise specified

EXCLUDES *Analytes from nonrequested laboratory analysis*
Calculated results representing score or probability derived by algorithm
Drug testing ([80305, 80306, 80307], [80324, 80325, 80326, 80327, 80328, 80329, 80330, 80331, 80332, 80333, 80334, 80335, 80336, 80337, 80338, 80339, 80340, 80341, 80342, 80343, 80344, 80345, 80346, 80347, 80348, 80349, 80350, 80351, 80352, 80353, 80354, 80355, 80356, 80357, 80358, 80359, 80360, 80361, 80362, 80363, 80364, 80365, 80366, 80367, 80368, 80369, 80370, 80371, 80372, 80373, 80374, 80375, 80376, 80377, 83992])
Organ or disease panels (80048-80076 [80081])
Therapeutic drug assays (80150-80299 [80164, 80165, 80171])

82480	**Cholinesterase; serum**
	🚑 0.00 ⚕ 0.00 **FUD** XXX Q ▫
	AMA: 2020,Dec,3
82482	**RBC**
	🚑 0.00 ⚕ 0.00 **FUD** XXX Q ▫
	AMA: 2020,Dec,3
82485	**Chondroitin B sulfate, quantitative**
	EXCLUDES *Chorionic gonadotropin (84702-84703)*
	🚑 0.00 ⚕ 0.00 **FUD** XXX Q ▫
	AMA: 2020,Dec,3
82495	**Chromium**
	🚑 0.00 ⚕ 0.00 **FUD** XXX Q ▫
	AMA: 2020,Dec,3
82507	**Citrate**
	EXCLUDES *Cocaine, qualitative analysis ([80353])*
	Codeine, qualitative analysis ([80361])
	Complement (86160-86162)
	🚑 0.00 ⚕ 0.00 **FUD** XXX Q ▫
	AMA: 2020,Dec,3

82523 Chemistry: Collagen Crosslinks, Any Method

CMS: 100-03,190.19 NCD for Collagen Crosslinks, Any Method; 100-04,16,70.8 CLIA Waived Tests

INCLUDES Clinical information not requested by ordering physician
Mathematically calculated results
Quantitative analysis unless otherwise specified
Specimens from any source unless otherwise specified

EXCLUDES *Analytes from nonrequested laboratory analysis*
Calculated results representing score or probability derived by algorithm
Organ or disease panels (80048-80076 [80081])
Therapeutic drug assays (80150-80299 [80164, 80165, 80171])

82523	**Collagen cross links, any method**
	🚑 0.00 ⚕ 0.00 **FUD** XXX ✗ Q ▫
	AMA: 2020,Dec,3

82525-82735 [82652, 82653, 82681] Chemistry: Copper—Fluoride

INCLUDES Clinical information not requested by ordering physician
Mathematically calculated results
Quantitative analysis unless otherwise specified
Specimens from any source unless otherwise specified

EXCLUDES *Analytes from nonrequested laboratory analysis*
Calculated results representing score or probability derived by algorithm
Drug testing ([80305, 80306, 80307], [80324, 80325, 80326, 80327, 80328, 80329, 80330, 80331, 80332, 80333, 80334, 80335, 80336, 80337, 80338, 80339, 80340, 80341, 80342, 80343, 80344, 80345, 80346, 80347, 80348, 80349, 80350, 80351, 80352, 80353, 80354, 80355, 80356, 80357, 80358, 80359, 80360, 80361, 80362, 80363, 80364, 80365, 80366, 80367, 80368, 80369, 80370, 80371, 80372, 80373, 80374, 80375, 80376, 80377, 83992])
Organ or disease panels (80048-80076 [80081])
Therapeutic drug assays (80150-80299 [80164, 80165, 80171])

82525	**Copper**
	EXCLUDES *Coproporphyrin (84119-84120)*
	Corticosteroids (83491)
	🚑 0.00 ⚕ 0.00 **FUD** XXX Q ▫
	AMA: 2020,Dec,3

26/TC PC/TC Only   A2-Z3 ASC Payment   50 Bilateral   ♂ Male Only   ♀ Female Only   🚑 Facility RVU   ⚕ Non-Facility RVU   ▫ CCI   ✗ CLIA
FUD Follow-up Days   CMS: IOM   AMA: CPT Asst   A-Y OPPSI   80/80 Surg Assist Allowed / w/Doc   ▫ Lab Crosswalk   ▫ Radiology Crosswalk

394   CPT © 2021 American Medical Association. All Rights Reserved.   © 2021 Optum360, LLC

82528 **Corticosterone**
INCLUDES Porter-Silber test
🚑 0.00   ⚕ 0.00   **FUD** XXX   Q ▯
AMA: 2020,Dec,3

82530 **Cortisol; free**
🚑 0.00   ⚕ 0.00   **FUD** XXX   Q ▯
AMA: 2020,Dec,3; 2018,Jan,8; 2017,Jan,8; 2016,Jan,13

82533   **total**
🚑 0.00   ⚕ 0.00   **FUD** XXX   Q ▯
AMA: 2020,Dec,3; 2018,Jan,8; 2017,Jan,8; 2016,Jan,13

82540 **Creatine**
🚑 0.00   ⚕ 0.00   **FUD** XXX   Q ▯
AMA: 2020,Dec,3

82542 **Column chromatography, includes mass spectrometry, if performed (eg, HPLC, LC, LC/MS, LC/MS-MS, GC, GC/MS-MS, GC/MS, HPLC/MS), non-drug analyte(s) not elsewhere specified, qualitative or quantitative, each specimen**
EXCLUDES *Column chromatography/mass spectrometry drugs/substances ([80305, 80306, 80307], [80320, 80321, 80322, 80323, 80324, 80325, 80326, 80327, 80328, 80329, 80330, 80331, 80332, 80333, 80334, 80335, 80336, 80337, 80338, 80339, 80340, 80341, 80342, 80343, 80344, 80345, 80346, 80347, 80348, 80349, 80350, 80351, 80352, 80353, 80354, 80355, 80356, 80357, 80358, 80359, 80360, 80361, 80362, 80363, 80364, 80365, 80366, 80367, 80368, 80369, 80370, 80371, 80372, 80373, 80374, 80375, 80376, 80377, 83992])*
Procedure performed more than one time per specimen
🚑 0.00   ⚕ 0.00   **FUD** XXX   Q ▯
AMA: 2020,Dec,3; 2018,Jan,8; 2017,Jan,8; 2016,Jan,13

82550 **Creatine kinase (CK), (CPK); total**
🚑 0.00   ⚕ 0.00   **FUD** XXX   ✗ Q ▯
AMA: 2020,Dec,3; 2018,Jan,8; 2017,Jan,8; 2016,Jan,13

82552   **isoenzymes**
🚑 0.00   ⚕ 0.00   **FUD** XXX   Q ▯
AMA: 2020,Dec,3; 2018,Jan,8; 2017,Jan,8; 2016,Jan,13

82553   **MB fraction only**
🚑 0.00   ⚕ 0.00   **FUD** XXX   Q ▯
AMA: 2020,Dec,3; 2018,Jan,8; 2017,Jan,8; 2016,Jan,13

82554   **isoforms**
🚑 0.00   ⚕ 0.00   **FUD** XXX   Q ▯
AMA: 2020,Dec,3; 2018,Jan,8; 2017,Jan,8; 2016,Jan,13

82565 **Creatinine; blood**
🚑 0.00   ⚕ 0.00   **FUD** XXX   ✗ Q ▯
AMA: 2020,Dec,3; 2018,Jan,8; 2017,Jan,8; 2016,Jan,13

82570   **other source**
🚑 0.00   ⚕ 0.00   **FUD** XXX   ✗ Q ▯
AMA: 2020,Dec,3

82575   **clearance**
INCLUDES Holten test
🚑 0.00   ⚕ 0.00   **FUD** XXX   Q ▯
AMA: 2020,Dec,3

82585 **Cryofibrinogen**
🚑 0.00   ⚕ 0.00   **FUD** XXX   Q ▯
AMA: 2020,Dec,3

82595 **Cryoglobulin, qualitative or semi-quantitative (eg, cryocrit)**
EXCLUDES *Crystals, pyrophosphate vs urate (89060)*
Quantitative, cryoglobulin (82784-82785)
🚑 0.00   ⚕ 0.00   **FUD** XXX   Q ▯
AMA: 2020,Dec,3

82600 **Cyanide**
🚑 0.00   ⚕ 0.00   **FUD** XXX   Q ▯
AMA: 2020,Dec,3

82607 **Cyanocobalamin (Vitamin B-12);**
EXCLUDES *Cyclic AMP (82030)*
Cyclosporine (80158)
🚑 0.00   ⚕ 0.00   **FUD** XXX   Q ▯
AMA: 2020,Dec,3

82608   **unsaturated binding capacity**
EXCLUDES *Cyclic AMP (82030)*
Cyclosporine (80158)
🚑 0.00   ⚕ 0.00   **FUD** XXX   Q ▯
AMA: 2020,Dec,3

82610 **Cystatin C**
🚑 0.00   ⚕ 0.00   **FUD** XXX   Q ▯
AMA: 2020,Dec,3; 2018,Jan,8; 2017,Jan,8; 2016,Jan,13

82615 **Cystine and homocystine, urine, qualitative**
🚑 0.00   ⚕ 0.00   **FUD** XXX   Q ▯
AMA: 2020,Dec,3

82626 **Dehydroepiandrosterone (DHEA)**
EXCLUDES *Anabolic steroids ([80327, 80328])*
🚑 0.00   ⚕ 0.00   **FUD** XXX   Q ▯
AMA: 2020,Dec,3; 2018,Jan,8; 2017,Jan,8; 2016,Jan,13

82627 **Dehydroepiandrosterone-sulfate (DHEA-S)**
EXCLUDES *Delta-aminolevulinicacid (ALA) (82135)*
🚑 0.00   ⚕ 0.00   **FUD** XXX   Q ▯
AMA: 2020,Dec,3; 2018,Jan,8; 2017,Jan,8; 2016,Jan,13

82633 **Desoxycorticosterone, 11-**
🚑 0.00   ⚕ 0.00   **FUD** XXX   Q ▯
AMA: 2020,Dec,3

82634 **Deoxycortisol, 11-**
EXCLUDES *Dexamethasone suppression test (80420)*
Diastase, urine (82150)
🚑 0.00   ⚕ 0.00   **FUD** XXX   Q ▯
AMA: 2020,Dec,3

82638 **Dibucaine number**
EXCLUDES *Dichloroethane (82441)*
Dichloromethane (82441)
Diethylether (84600)
🚑 0.00   ⚕ 0.00   **FUD** XXX   Q ▯
AMA: 2020,Dec,3

82642 **Dihydrotestosterone (DHT)**
EXCLUDES *Anabolic drug testing analysis dihydrotestosterone ([80327, 80328])*
Dipropylaceticacid ([80164])
Dopamine (82382)
Duodenal contents, individual enzymes for intubation and collection (43756-43757)
🚑 0.00   ⚕ 0.00   **FUD** XXX   ▯
AMA: 2020,Dec,3

82652 **Resequenced code. See code following 82306.**

82653 **Resequnced code. See code following 82656.**

▲ **82656** **Elastase, pancreatic (EL-1), fecal; qualitative or semi-quantitative**
🚑 0.00   ⚕ 0.00   **FUD** XXX   Q ▯
AMA: 2020,Dec,3; 2018,Jan,8; 2017,Jan,8; 2016,Jan,13

● # **82653**   **quantitative**
🚑 0.00   ⚕ 0.00   **FUD** 000

82657 **Enzyme activity in blood cells, cultured cells, or tissue, not elsewhere specified; nonradioactive substrate, each specimen**
🚑 0.00   ⚕ 0.00   **FUD** XXX   Q ▯
AMA: 2020,Dec,3

82658   **radioactive substrate, each specimen**
🚑 0.00   ⚕ 0.00   **FUD** XXX   Q ▯
AMA: 2020,Dec,3

82664	**Electrophoretic technique, not elsewhere specified**	
	EXCLUDES *Endocrine receptor assays (84233-84235)*	
	📋 0.00 ⚕ 0.00 **FUD** XXX	Q 🖳
	AMA: 2020,Dec,3	

82668	**Erythropoietin**	
	📋 0.00 ⚕ 0.00 **FUD** XXX	Q 🖳
	AMA: 2020,Dec,3	

82670	**Estradiol; total**	
	📋 0.00 ⚕ 0.00 **FUD** XXX	Q 🖳
	AMA: 2020,Dec,3	

# 82681	**free, direct measurement (eg, equilibrium dialysis)**	
	📋 0.00 ⚕ 0.00 **FUD** XXX	
	AMA: 2020,Dec,3	

82671	**Estrogens; fractionated**	
	EXCLUDES *Estrogen receptor assay (84233)*	
	📋 0.00 ⚕ 0.00 **FUD** XXX	Q 🖳
	AMA: 2020,Dec,3	

82672	**total**	
	EXCLUDES *Estrogen receptor assay (84233)*	
	📋 0.00 ⚕ 0.00 **FUD** XXX	Q 🖳
	AMA: 2020,Dec,3	

82677	**Estriol**	
	📋 0.00 ⚕ 0.00 **FUD** XXX	Q 🖳
	AMA: 2020,Dec,3	

82679	**Estrone**	
	EXCLUDES *Alcohol (ethanol) definitive drug testing ([80320])*	
	Alcohol (ethanol) therapeutic drug assay (82077)	
	📋 0.00 ⚕ 0.00 **FUD** XXX	✖ Q 🖳
	AMA: 2020,Dec,3	

82681	**Resequenced code. See code following 82670.**

82693	**Ethylene glycol**	
	📋 0.00 ⚕ 0.00 **FUD** XXX	Q 🖳
	AMA: 2020,Dec,3	

82696	**Etiocholanolone**	
	EXCLUDES *Fractionation ketosteroids (83593)*	
	📋 0.00 ⚕ 0.00 **FUD** XXX	Q 🖳
	AMA: 2020,Dec,3	

82705	**Fat or lipids, feces; qualitative**	
	📋 0.00 ⚕ 0.00 **FUD** XXX	Q 🖳
	AMA: 2020,Dec,3	

82710	**quantitative**	
	📋 0.00 ⚕ 0.00 **FUD** XXX	Q 🖳
	AMA: 2020,Dec,3	

82715	**Fat differential, feces, quantitative**	
	📋 0.00 ⚕ 0.00 **FUD** XXX	Q 🖳
	AMA: 2020,Dec,3	

82725	**Fatty acids, nonesterified**	
	📋 0.00 ⚕ 0.00 **FUD** XXX	Q 🖳
	AMA: 2020,Dec,3	

82726	**Very long chain fatty acids**	
	EXCLUDES *Long-chain (C20-22) omega-3 fatty acids in red blood cell (RBC) membranes (84999)*	
	📋 0.00 ⚕ 0.00 **FUD** XXX	Q 🖳
	AMA: 2020,Dec,3	

82728	**Ferritin**	
	EXCLUDES *Fetal hemoglobin (83030, 83033, 85460)*	
	Fetoprotein, alpha-1 (82105-82106)	
	📋 0.00 ⚕ 0.00 **FUD** XXX	Q 🖳
	AMA: 2020,Dec,3	

82731	**Fetal fibronectin, cervicovaginal secretions, semi-quantitative**	
		M ♀
	📋 0.00 ⚕ 0.00 **FUD** XXX	Q 🖳
	AMA: 2020,Dec,3	

82735	**Fluoride**	
	EXCLUDES *Foam stability test (83662)*	
	📋 0.00 ⚕ 0.00 **FUD** XXX	Q 🖳
	AMA: 2020,Dec,3	

82746-82941 Chemistry: Folic Acid—Gastrin

INCLUDES Clinical information not requested by ordering physician
Mathematically calculated results
Quantitative analysis unless otherwise specified
Specimens from any source unless otherwise specified

EXCLUDES *Analytes from nonrequested laboratory analysis*
Calculated results representing score or probability derived by algorithm
Drug testing ([80305, 80306, 80307], [80324, 80325, 80326, 80327, 80328, 80329, 80330, 80331, 80332, 80333, 80334, 80335, 80336, 80337, 80338, 80339, 80340, 80341, 80342, 80343, 80344, 80345, 80346, 80347, 80348, 80349, 80350, 80351, 80352, 80353, 80354, 80355, 80356, 80357, 80358, 80359, 80360, 80361, 80362, 80363, 80364, 80365, 80366, 80367, 80368, 80369, 80370, 80371, 80372, 80373, 80374, 80375, 80376, 80377, 83992])
Organ or disease panels (80048-80076 [80081])
Therapeutic drug assays (80150-80299 [80164, 80165, 80171])

82746	**Folic acid; serum**	
	📋 0.00 ⚕ 0.00 **FUD** XXX	Q 🖳
	AMA: 2020,Dec,3	

82747	**RBC**	
	EXCLUDES *Follicle stimulating hormone (FSH) (83001)*	
	📋 0.00 ⚕ 0.00 **FUD** XXX	Q 🖳
	AMA: 2020,Dec,3	

82757	**Fructose, semen**	
	EXCLUDES *Fructosamine (82985)*	
	Fructose, TLC screen (84375)	
	📋 0.00 ⚕ 0.00 **FUD** XXX	Q 🖳
	AMA: 2020,Dec,3	

82759	**Galactokinase, RBC**	
	📋 0.00 ⚕ 0.00 **FUD** XXX	Q 🖳
	AMA: 2020,Dec,3	

82760	**Galactose**	
	📋 0.00 ⚕ 0.00 **FUD** XXX	Q 🖳
	AMA: 2020,Dec,3	

82775	**Galactose-1-phosphate uridyl transferase; quantitative**	
	📋 0.00 ⚕ 0.00 **FUD** XXX	Q 🖳
	AMA: 2020,Dec,3	

82776	**screen**	
	📋 0.00 ⚕ 0.00 **FUD** XXX	Q 🖳
	AMA: 2020,Dec,3	

82777	**Galectin-3**	
	📋 0.00 ⚕ 0.00 **FUD** XXX	Q 🖳
	AMA: 2020,Dec,3	

82784	**Gammaglobulin (immunoglobulin); IgA, IgD, IgG, IgM, each**	
	INCLUDES Farr test	
	📋 0.00 ⚕ 0.00 **FUD** XXX	Q 🖳
	AMA: 2020,Dec,3; 2018,Jan,8; 2017,Jan,8; 2016,Jan,13	

82785	**IgE**	
	INCLUDES Farr test	
	EXCLUDES *Allergen specific, IgE (86003, 86005)*	
	📋 0.00 ⚕ 0.00 **FUD** XXX	Q 🖳
	AMA: 2020,Dec,3; 2018,Jan,8; 2017,Jan,8; 2016,Jan,13	

82787	**immunoglobulin subclasses (eg, IgG1, 2, 3, or 4), each**	
	EXCLUDES *Gamma-glutamyltransferase (GGT) (82977)*	
	📋 0.00 ⚕ 0.00 **FUD** XXX	Q 🖳
	AMA: 2020,Dec,3	

82800	**Gases, blood, pH only**	
	📋 0.00 ⚕ 0.00 **FUD** XXX	Q 🖳
	AMA: 2020,Dec,3	

82803	**Gases, blood, any combination of pH, pCO2, pO2, CO2, HCO3 (including calculated O2 saturation);**	
	INCLUDES Two or more listed analytes	
	📋 0.00 ⚕ 0.00 **FUD** XXX	Q 🖳
	AMA: 2020,Dec,3	

26/TC PC/TC Only	A2-Z3 ASC Payment	50 Bilateral	♂ Male Only	♀ Female Only	📋 Facility RVU	⚕ Non-Facility RVU	🖳 CCI	✖ CLIA
FUD Follow-up Days	**CMS:** IOM	**AMA:** CPT Asst	A-Y OPPSI	80/80 Surg Assist Allowed / w/Doc		🗎 Lab Crosswalk	🗎 Radiology Crosswalk	

396   CPT © 2021 American Medical Association. All Rights Reserved.   © 2021 Optum360, LLC

82805 with O2 saturation, by direct measurement, except pulse oximetry
  💰 0.00   🔬 0.00   **FUD** XXX   🔲 🔲
  AMA: 2020,Dec,3

82810 Gases, blood, O2 saturation only, by direct measurement, except pulse oximetry
  EXCLUDES Pulse oximetry (94760)
  💰 0.00   🔬 0.00   **FUD** XXX   🔲 🔲
  AMA: 2020,Dec,3

82820 Hemoglobin-oxygen affinity (pO2 for 50% hemoglobin saturation with oxygen)
  EXCLUDES Gastric acid analysis (82930)
  💰 0.00   🔬 0.00   **FUD** XXX   🔲 🔲
  AMA: 2020,Dec,3

82930 Gastric acid analysis, includes pH if performed, each specimen
  💰 0.00   🔬 0.00   **FUD** XXX   🔲 🔲
  AMA: 2020,Dec,3; 2018,Jan,8; 2017,Jan,8; 2016,Jan,13

82938 Gastrin after secretin stimulation
  💰 0.00   🔬 0.00   **FUD** XXX   🔲 🔲
  AMA: 2020,Dec,3

82941 Gastrin
  EXCLUDES Gentamicin (80170)
      GGT (82977)
      Qualitative column chromatography report specific analyte or (82542)
  💰 0.00   🔬 0.00   **FUD** XXX   🔲 🔲
  AMA: 2020,Dec,3

82943-82962 Chemistry: Glucagon—Glucose Testing

CMS: 100-03,190.20 Blood Glucose Testing

INCLUDES Clinical information not requested by ordering physician
    Mathematically calculated results
    Quantitative analysis unless otherwise specified
    Specimens from any source unless otherwise specified
EXCLUDES Analytes from nonrequested laboratory analysis
    Calculated results representing score or probability derived by algorithm
    Organ or disease panels (80048-80076 [80081])
    Therapeutic drug assays (80150-80299 [80164, 80165, 80171])
Code also glucose administration injection (96374)

82943 Glucagon
  💰 0.00   🔬 0.00   **FUD** XXX   🔲 🔲
  AMA: 2020,Dec,3

82945 Glucose, body fluid, other than blood
  💰 0.00   🔬 0.00   **FUD** XXX   🔲 🔲
  AMA: 2020,Dec,3

82946 Glucagon tolerance test
  💰 0.00   🔬 0.00   **FUD** XXX   🔲 🔲
  AMA: 2020,Dec,3

82947 Glucose; quantitative, blood (except reagent strip)
  💰 0.00   🔬 0.00   **FUD** XXX   ❌ 🅰 🔲
  AMA: 2020,Dec,3; 2018,Jan,8; 2017,Jan,8; 2016,Jan,13

82948 blood, reagent strip
  💰 0.00   🔬 0.00   **FUD** XXX   🔲 🔲
  AMA: 2020,Dec,3; 2018,Jan,8; 2017,Jan,8; 2016,Jan,13

82950 post glucose dose (includes glucose)
  💰 0.00   🔬 0.00   **FUD** XXX   ❌ 🅰 🔲
  AMA: 2020,Dec,3; 2018,Jan,8; 2017,Jan,8; 2016,Jan,13

82951 tolerance test (GTT), 3 specimens (includes glucose)
  💰 0.00   🔬 0.00   **FUD** XXX   ❌ 🅰 🔲
  AMA: 2020,Dec,3; 2018,Jan,8; 2017,Jan,8; 2016,Jan,13

+ 82952 tolerance test, each additional beyond 3 specimens (List separately in addition to code for primary procedure)
  EXCLUDES Insulin tolerance test (80434-80435)
      Leucine tolerance test (80428)
      Semiquantitative urine glucose (81000, 81002, 81005, 81099)
  Code first (82951)
  💰 0.00   🔬 0.00   **FUD** XXX   ❌ 🔲 🔲
  AMA: 2020,Dec,3; 2018,Jan,8; 2017,Jan,8; 2016,Jan,13

82955 Glucose-6-phosphate dehydrogenase (G6PD); quantitative
  Code also glucose tolerance test with medication, when performed (96374)
  💰 0.00   🔬 0.00   **FUD** XXX   🔲 🔲
  AMA: 2020,Dec,3

82960 screen
  Code also glucose tolerance test with medication, when performed (96374)
  💰 0.00   🔬 0.00   **FUD** XXX   🔲 🔲
  AMA: 2020,Dec,3

82962 Glucose, blood by glucose monitoring device(s) cleared by the FDA specifically for home use
  💰 0.00   🔬 0.00   **FUD** XXX   ❌ 🔲 🔲
  AMA: 2020,Dec,3; 2018,Jan,8; 2017,Jan,8; 2016,Jan,13

82963-83690 [83529] Chemistry: Glucosidase—Lipase

INCLUDES Clinical information not requested by ordering physician
    Mathematically calculated results
    Quantitative analysis unless otherwise specified
    Specimens from any source unless otherwise specified
EXCLUDES Analytes from nonrequested laboratory analysis
    Calculated results representing score or probability derived by algorithm
    Drug testing ([80305, 80306, 80307], [80324, 80325, 80326, 80327, 80328, 80329, 80330, 80331, 80332, 80333, 80334, 80335, 80336, 80337, 80338, 80339, 80340, 80341, 80342, 80343, 80344, 80345, 80346, 80347, 80348, 80349, 80350, 80351, 80352, 80353, 80354, 80355, 80356, 80357, 80358, 80359, 80360, 80361, 80362, 80363, 80364, 80365, 80366, 80367, 80368, 80369, 80370, 80371, 80372, 80373, 80374, 80375, 80376, 80377, 83992])
    Organ or disease panels (80048-80076 [80081])
    Therapeutic drug assays (80150-80299 [80164, 80165, 80171])

82963 Glucosidase, beta
  💰 0.00   🔬 0.00   **FUD** XXX   🔲 🔲
  AMA: 2020,Dec,3

82965 Glutamate dehydrogenase
  💰 0.00   🔬 0.00   **FUD** XXX   🔲 🔲
  AMA: 2020,Dec,3

82977 Glutamyltransferase, gamma (GGT)
  💰 0.00   🔬 0.00   **FUD** XXX   ❌ 🔲 🔲
  AMA: 2020,Dec,3; 2018,Jan,8; 2017,Jan,8; 2016,Jan,13

82978 Glutathione
  💰 0.00   🔬 0.00   **FUD** XXX   🔲 🔲
  AMA: 2020,Dec,3

82979 Glutathione reductase, RBC
  EXCLUDES Glycohemoglobin (83036)
  💰 0.00   🔬 0.00   **FUD** XXX   🔲 🔲
  AMA: 2020,Dec,3

82985 Glycated protein
  EXCLUDES Gonadotropin chorionic (hCG) (84702-84703)
  💰 0.00   🔬 0.00   **FUD** XXX   ❌ 🔲 🔲
  AMA: 2020,Dec,3; 2018,Jan,8; 2017,Jan,8; 2016,Jan,13

83001 Gonadotropin; follicle stimulating hormone (FSH)
  💰 0.00   🔬 0.00   **FUD** XXX   ❌ 🔲 🔲
  AMA: 2020,Dec,3

83002 luteinizing hormone (LH)
  EXCLUDES Luteinizing releasing factor (LRH) (83727)
  💰 0.00   🔬 0.00   **FUD** XXX   ❌ 🔲 🔲
  AMA: 2020,Dec,3

83003 Growth hormone, human (HGH) (somatotropin)
  EXCLUDES Antibody to human growth hormone (86277)
  💰 0.00   🔬 0.00   **FUD** XXX   🔲 🔲
  AMA: 2020,Dec,3

83006 Growth stimulation expressed gene 2 (ST2, Interleukin 1 receptor like-1)
 ⚙ 0.00 ⚕ 0.00 **FUD** XXX 🔲🖵
 AMA: 2020,Dec,3

83009 Helicobacter pylori, blood test analysis for urease activity, non-radioactive isotope (eg, C-13)
 EXCLUDES *H. pylori, breath test analysis for urease activity (83013-83014)*
 ⚙ 0.00 ⚕ 0.00 **FUD** XXX 🔲🖵
 AMA: 2020,Dec,3

83010 Haptoglobin; quantitative
 ⚙ 0.00 ⚕ 0.00 **FUD** XXX 🔲🖵
 AMA: 2020,Dec,3

83012 phenotypes
 ⚙ 0.00 ⚕ 0.00 **FUD** XXX 🔲🖵
 AMA: 2020,Dec,3

83013 Helicobacter pylori; breath test analysis for urease activity, non-radioactive isotope (eg, C-13)
 ⚙ 0.00 ⚕ 0.00 **FUD** XXX 🔲🖵
 AMA: 2020,Dec,3; 2020,OctSE,1; 2020,OctSE,1; 2018,Jan,8; 2017,Jan,8; 2016,Jan,13

83014 drug administration
 EXCLUDES *H. pylori:*
   Blood test analysis for urease activity (83009)
   Enzyme immunoassay (87339)
   Liquid scintillation counter (78267-78268)
   Stool (87338)
 ⚙ 0.00 ⚕ 0.00 **FUD** XXX 🔲🖵
 AMA: 2020,Dec,3; 2020,OctSE,1; 2020,OctSE,1; 2018,Jan,8; 2017,Jan,8; 2016,Jan,13

83015 Heavy metal (eg, arsenic, barium, beryllium, bismuth, antimony, mercury); qualitative, any number of analytes
 INCLUDES Reinsch test
 ⚙ 0.00 ⚕ 0.00 **FUD** XXX 🔲🖵
 AMA: 2020,Dec,3

83018 quantitative, each, not elsewhere specified
 EXCLUDES *Evaluation known heavy metal with specific code*
 ⚙ 0.00 ⚕ 0.00 **FUD** XXX 🔲🖵
 AMA: 2020,Dec,3

83020 Hemoglobin fractionation and quantitation; electrophoresis (eg, A2, S, C, and/or F)
 ⚙ 0.00 ⚕ 0.00 **FUD** XXX 🔲 80 🖵
 AMA: 2020,Dec,3

83021 chromatography (eg, A2, S, C, and/or F)
 EXCLUDES *Analysis glycosylated (A1c) hemoglobin by chromatography or electrophoresis without identified hemoglobin variant (83036)*
 ⚙ 0.00 ⚕ 0.00 **FUD** XXX 🔲🖵
 AMA: 2020,Dec,3; 2018,Jan,8; 2017,Jan,8; 2016,Jan,13

83026 Hemoglobin; by copper sulfate method, non-automated
 ⚙ 0.00 ⚕ 0.00 **FUD** XXX ❌🔲🖵
 AMA: 2020,Dec,3

83030 F (fetal), chemical
 ⚙ 0.00 ⚕ 0.00 **FUD** XXX 🔲🖵
 AMA: 2020,Dec,3

83033 F (fetal), qualitative
 ⚙ 0.00 ⚕ 0.00 **FUD** XXX 🔲🖵
 AMA: 2020,Dec,3

83036 glycosylated (A1C)
 EXCLUDES *Analysis glycosylated (A1c) hemoglobin by chromatography or electrophoresis without identified hemoglobin variant (83020-83021)*
   Detection hemoglobin, fecal, by immunoassay (82274)
 ⚙ 0.00 ⚕ 0.00 **FUD** XXX ❌🔲🖵
 AMA: 2020,Dec,3; 2018,Jan,8; 2017,Jan,8; 2016,Jan,13

83037 glycosylated (A1C) by device cleared by FDA for home use
 ⚙ 0.00 ⚕ 0.00 **FUD** XXX ❌🔲🖵
 AMA: 2020,Dec,3; 2018,Jan,8; 2017,Jan,8; 2016,Jan,13

83045 methemoglobin, qualitative
 ⚙ 0.00 ⚕ 0.00 **FUD** XXX 🔲🖵
 AMA: 2020,Dec,3

83050 methemoglobin, quantitative
 EXCLUDES *Transcutaneous methemoglobin test (88741)*
 ⚙ 0.00 ⚕ 0.00 **FUD** XXX 🔲🖵
 AMA: 2020,Dec,3; 2018,Jan,8; 2017,Jan,8; 2016,Jan,13

83051 plasma
 ⚙ 0.00 ⚕ 0.00 **FUD** XXX 🔲🖵
 AMA: 2020,Dec,3

83060 sulfhemoglobin, quantitative
 ⚙ 0.00 ⚕ 0.00 **FUD** XXX 🔲🖵
 AMA: 2020,Dec,3

83065 thermolabile
 ⚙ 0.00 ⚕ 0.00 **FUD** XXX 🔲🖵
 AMA: 2020,Dec,3

83068 unstable, screen
 ⚙ 0.00 ⚕ 0.00 **FUD** XXX 🔲🖵
 AMA: 2020,Dec,3

83069 urine
 ⚙ 0.00 ⚕ 0.00 **FUD** XXX 🔲🖵
 AMA: 2020,Dec,3

83070 Hemosiderin, qualitative
 EXCLUDES *HIAA (83497)*
   Qualitative column chromatography report specific analyte or (82542)
 ⚙ 0.00 ⚕ 0.00 **FUD** XXX 🔲🖵
 AMA: 2020,Dec,3

83080 b-Hexosaminidase, each assay
 ⚙ 0.00 ⚕ 0.00 **FUD** XXX 🔲🖵
 AMA: 2020,Dec,3

83088 Histamine
 EXCLUDES *Hollander test (43754-43755)*
 ⚙ 0.00 ⚕ 0.00 **FUD** XXX 🔲🖵
 AMA: 2020,Dec,3

83090 Homocysteine
 ⚙ 0.00 ⚕ 0.00 **FUD** XXX 🔲🖵
 AMA: 2020,Dec,3; 2018,Jan,8; 2017,Jan,8; 2016,Jan,13

83150 Homovanillic acid (HVA)
 EXCLUDES *Hormone testing report from alphabetic list in Chemistry section*
   Hydrogen/methane breath test (91065)
 ⚙ 0.00 ⚕ 0.00 **FUD** XXX 🔲🖵
 AMA: 2020,Dec,3

83491 Hydroxycorticosteroids, 17- (17-OHCS)
 EXCLUDES *Cortisol (82530, 82533)*
   Deoxycortisol (82634)
 ⚙ 0.00 ⚕ 0.00 **FUD** XXX 🔲🖵
 AMA: 2020,Dec,3

83497 Hydroxyindolacetic acid, 5-(HIAA)
 EXCLUDES *5-Hydroxytryptamine (84260)*
   Urine qualitative test (81005)
 ⚙ 0.00 ⚕ 0.00 **FUD** XXX 🔲🖵
 AMA: 2020,Dec,3

83498 Hydroxyprogesterone, 17-d
 ⚙ 0.00 ⚕ 0.00 **FUD** XXX 🔲🖵
 AMA: 2020,Dec,3

83500 Hydroxyproline; free
 ⚙ 0.00 ⚕ 0.00 **FUD** XXX 🔲🖵
 AMA: 2020,Dec,3

26/TC PC/TC Only	A2-Z3 ASC Payment	50 Bilateral	♂ Male Only	♀ Female Only	⚙ Facility RVU	⚕ Non-Facility RVU	🖵 CCI	❌ CLIA
FUD Follow-up Days	**CMS:** IOM	**AMA:** CPT Asst	A-Y OPPSI	80/80 Surg Assist Allowed / w/Doc	🖵 Lab Crosswalk		🖵 Radiology Crosswalk	

83505 **total**
🚑 0.00 ⚕ 0.00 **FUD** XXX ⊠🔲🔲
AMA: 2020,Dec,3

83516 **Immunoassay for analyte other than infectious agent antibody or infectious agent antigen; qualitative or semiquantitative, multiple step method**
🚑 0.00 ⚕ 0.00 **FUD** XXX ⊠🔲🔲
AMA: 2020,Dec,3; 2020,OctSE,1; 2020,OctSE,1; 2020,AugSE,1; 2020,AugSE,1; 2020,AugSE,1

83518 **qualitative or semiquantitative, single step method (eg, reagent strip)**
🚑 0.00 ⚕ 0.00 **FUD** XXX 🔲🔲
AMA: 2020,Dec,3; 2020,OctSE,1; 2020,OctSE,1

83519 **quantitative, by radioimmunoassay (eg, RIA)**
🚑 0.00 ⚕ 0.00 **FUD** XXX 🔲🔲
AMA: 2020,Dec,3; 2020,OctSE,1; 2020,OctSE,1; 2018,Jan,8; 2017,Jan,8; 2016,Jan,13

83520 **quantitative, not otherwise specified**
> **EXCLUDES** Immunoassays for antibodies to infectious agent antigen report specific analyte/method from Immunology
> Immunoassay of tumor antigens not elsewhere specified (86316)
> Immunoglobulins (82784, 82785)

🚑 0.00 ⚕ 0.00 **FUD** XXX 🔲🔲
AMA: 2020,Dec,3; 2020,OctSE,1; 2020,OctSE,1

● **83521** **Immunoglobulin light chains (ie, kappa, lambda), free, each**

83525 **Insulin; total**
> **EXCLUDES** Proinsulin (84206)

🚑 0.00 ⚕ 0.00 **FUD** XXX 🔲🔲
AMA: 2020,Dec,3

83527 **free**
🚑 0.00 ⚕ 0.00 **FUD** XXX 🔲🔲
AMA: 2020,Dec,3; 2018,Jan,8; 2017,Jan,8; 2016,Jan,13

● # **83529** **Interleukin-6 (IL-6)**
🚑 0.00 ⚕ 0.00 **FUD** 000
AMA: 2020,Dec,3

83528 **Intrinsic factor**
> **EXCLUDES** Intrinsic factor antibodies (86340)

🚑 0.00 ⚕ 0.00 **FUD** XXX 🔲🔲
AMA: 2020,Dec,3

83529 **Resequnced code. See code following 83527.**

83540 **Iron**
🚑 0.00 ⚕ 0.00 **FUD** XXX 🔲🔲
AMA: 2020,Dec,3; 2018,Jan,8; 2017,Jan,8; 2016,Jan,13

83550 **Iron binding capacity**
🚑 0.00 ⚕ 0.00 **FUD** XXX 🔲🔲
AMA: 2020,Dec,3

83570 **Isocitric dehydrogenase (IDH)**
> **EXCLUDES** Isonicotinic acid hydrazide, INH, report specific method
> Isopropyl alcohol ([80320])

🚑 0.00 ⚕ 0.00 **FUD** XXX 🔲🔲
AMA: 2020,Dec,3

83582 **Ketogenic steroids, fractionation**
> **EXCLUDES** Ketone bodies:
> Serum (82009, 82010)
> Urine (81000-81003)

🚑 0.00 ⚕ 0.00 **FUD** XXX 🔲🔲
AMA: 2020,Dec,3

83586 **Ketosteroids, 17- (17-KS); total**
🚑 0.00 ⚕ 0.00 **FUD** XXX 🔲🔲
AMA: 2020,Dec,3

83593 **fractionation**
🚑 0.00 ⚕ 0.00 **FUD** XXX 🔲🔲
AMA: 2020,Dec,3

83605 **Lactate (lactic acid)**
🚑 0.00 ⚕ 0.00 **FUD** XXX ⊠🔲🔲
AMA: 2020,Dec,3

83615 **Lactate dehydrogenase (LD), (LDH);**
🚑 0.00 ⚕ 0.00 **FUD** XXX 🔲🔲
AMA: 2020,Dec,3; 2018,Jan,8; 2017,Jan,8; 2016,Jan,13

83625 **isoenzymes, separation and quantitation**
🚑 0.00 ⚕ 0.00 **FUD** XXX 🔲🔲
AMA: 2020,Dec,3; 2018,Jan,8; 2017,Jan,8; 2016,Jan,13

83630 **Lactoferrin, fecal; qualitative**
🚑 0.00 ⚕ 0.00 **FUD** XXX 🔲🔲
AMA: 2020,Dec,3; 2018,Jan,8; 2017,Jan,8; 2016,Jan,13

83631 **quantitative**
🚑 0.00 ⚕ 0.00 **FUD** XXX 🔲🔲
AMA: 2020,Dec,3; 2018,Jan,8; 2017,Jan,8; 2016,Jan,13

83632 **Lactogen, human placental (HPL) human chorionic somatomammotropin** Ⓜ
🚑 0.00 ⚕ 0.00 **FUD** XXX 🔲🔲
AMA: 2020,Dec,3

83633 **Lactose, urine, qualitative**
> **EXCLUDES** Lactase deficiency breath hydrogen/methane test (91065)
> Lactose tolerance test (82951, 82952)

🚑 0.00 ⚕ 0.00 **FUD** XXX 🔲🔲
AMA: 2020,Dec,3

83655 **Lead**
🚑 0.00 ⚕ 0.00 **FUD** XXX ⊠🔲🔲
AMA: 2020,Dec,3

83661 **Fetal lung maturity assessment; lecithin sphingomyelin (L/S) ratio** Ⓜ
🚑 0.00 ⚕ 0.00 **FUD** XXX 🔲🔲
AMA: 2020,Dec,3; 2018,Jan,8; 2017,Jan,8; 2016,Jan,13

83662 **foam stability test** Ⓜ
🚑 0.00 ⚕ 0.00 **FUD** XXX 🔲🔲
AMA: 2020,Dec,3

83663 **fluorescence polarization** Ⓜ
🚑 0.00 ⚕ 0.00 **FUD** XXX 🔲🔲
AMA: 2020,Dec,3

83664 **lamellar body density** Ⓜ
> **EXCLUDES** Phosphatidylglycerol (84081)

🚑 0.00 ⚕ 0.00 **FUD** XXX 🔲🔲
AMA: 2020,Dec,3

83670 **Leucine aminopeptidase (LAP)**
🚑 0.00 ⚕ 0.00 **FUD** XXX 🔲🔲
AMA: 2020,Dec,3

83690 **Lipase**
🚑 0.00 ⚕ 0.00 **FUD** XXX 🔲🔲
AMA: 2020,Dec,3

83695-83727 Chemistry: Lipoprotein—Luteinizing Releasing Factor

> **INCLUDES** Clinical information not requested by ordering physician
> Mathematically calculated results
> Quantitative analysis unless otherwise specified
> Specimens from any source unless otherwise specified

> **EXCLUDES** Analytes from nonrequested laboratory analysis
> Calculated results representing score or probability derived by algorithm
> Organ or disease panels (80048-80076 [80081])
> Therapeutic drug assays (80150-80299 [80164, 80165, 80171])

83695 **Lipoprotein (a)**
🚑 0.00 ⚕ 0.00 **FUD** XXX 🔲🔲
AMA: 2020,Dec,3; 2018,Jan,8; 2017,Jan,8; 2016,Jan,13

83698 **Lipoprotein-associated phospholipase A2 (Lp-PLA2)**
🚑 0.00 ⚕ 0.00 **FUD** XXX 🔲🔲
AMA: 2020,Dec,3

83700 Lipoprotein, blood; electrophoretic separation and quantitation
🔧 0.00   ⚖ 0.00   **FUD** XXX   ▣ ▢
AMA: 2020,Dec,3; 2018,Jan,8; 2017,Jan,8; 2016,Jan,13

83701 high resolution fractionation and quantitation of lipoproteins including lipoprotein subclasses when performed (eg, electrophoresis, ultracentrifugation)
🔧 0.00   ⚖ 0.00   **FUD** XXX   ▣ ▢
AMA: 2020,Dec,3; 2018,Jan,8; 2017,Jan,8; 2016,Jan,13

83704 quantitation of lipoprotein particle number(s) (eg, by nuclear magnetic resonance spectroscopy), includes lipoprotein particle subclass(es), when performed
🔧 0.00   ⚖ 0.00   **FUD** XXX   ▣ ▢
AMA: 2020,Dec,3; 2018,Jan,8; 2017,Jan,8; 2016,Jan,13

83718 Lipoprotein, direct measurement; high density cholesterol (HDL cholesterol)
🔧 0.00   ⚖ 0.00   **FUD** XXX   ☒ Ⓐ ▢
AMA: 2020,Dec,3; 2018,Jan,8; 2017,Jan,8; 2016,Jan,13

83719 VLDL cholesterol
🔧 0.00   ⚖ 0.00   **FUD** XXX   ▣ ▢
AMA: 2020,Dec,3; 2018,Jan,8; 2017,Jan,8; 2016,Jan,13

83721 LDL cholesterol
EXCLUDES   Fractionation by high resolution electrophoresis or ultracentrifugation (83701)
Lipoprotein particle numbers and subclasses analysis by nuclear magnetic resonance spectroscopy (83704)
🔧 0.00   ⚖ 0.00   **FUD** XXX   ☒ ▣ ▢
AMA: 2020,Dec,3; 2018,Jan,8; 2017,Jan,8; 2016,Jan,13

83722 small dense LDL cholesterol
EXCLUDES   Fractionation by high resolution electrophoresis or ultracentrifugation (83701)
Lipoprotein particle numbers/subclass analysis by nuclear magnetic resonance spectroscopy (83704)
🔧 0.00   ⚖ 0.00   **FUD** XXX   ▢
AMA: 2020,Dec,3

83727 Luteinizing releasing factor (LRH)
EXCLUDES   alpha-2-Macroglobulin (86329)
Luteinizing hormone (LH) (83002)
🔧 0.00   ⚖ 0.00   **FUD** XXX   ▣ ▢
AMA: 2020,Dec,3

83735-83885 Chemistry: Magnesium—Nickel

INCLUDES   Clinical information not requested by the ordering physician
Mathematically calculated results
Quantitative analysis unless otherwise specified
Specimens from any source unless otherwise specified
EXCLUDES   Analytes from nonrequested laboratory analysis
Calculated results representing a score or probability derived by algorithm
Organ or disease panels (80048-80076 [80081])
Therapeutic drug assays (80150-80299 [80164, 80165, 80171])

83735 Magnesium
🔧 0.00   ⚖ 0.00   **FUD** XXX   ▣ ▢
AMA: 2020,Dec,3

83775 Malate dehydrogenase
EXCLUDES   Maltose tolerance (82951, 82952)
Mammotropin (84146)
🔧 0.00   ⚖ 0.00   **FUD** XXX   ▣ ▢
AMA: 2020,Dec,3

83785 Manganese
🔧 0.00   ⚖ 0.00   **FUD** XXX   ▣ ▢
AMA: 2020,Dec,3

83789 Mass spectrometry and tandem mass spectrometry (eg, MS, MS/MS, MALDI, MS-TOF, QTOF), non-drug analyte(s) not elsewhere specified, qualitative or quantitative, each specimen
EXCLUDES   Column chromatography/mass spectrometry drugs or substances ([80305], [80306], [80307], [80320, 80321, 80322, 80323, 80324, 80325, 80326, 80327, 80328, 80329, 80330, 80331, 80332, 80333, 80334, 80335, 80336, 80337, 80338, 80339, 80340, 80341, 80342, 80343, 80344, 80345, 80346, 80347, 80348, 80349, 80350, 80351, 80352, 80353, 80354, 80355, 80356, 80357, 80358, 80359, 80360, 80361, 80362, 80363, 80364, 80365, 80366, 80367, 80368, 80369, 80370, 80371, 80372, 80373, 80374, 80375, 80376, 80377, 83992])
Procedure performed more than one time per specimen
Report specific analyte testing with code(s) from Chemistry section
🔧 0.00   ⚖ 0.00   **FUD** XXX   ▣ ▢
AMA: 2020,Dec,3

83825 Mercury, quantitative
EXCLUDES   Mercury screen (83015)
🔧 0.00   ⚖ 0.00   **FUD** XXX   ▣ ▢
AMA: 2020,Dec,3

83835 Metanephrines
EXCLUDES   Catecholamines (82382-82384)
Methamphetamine ([80324], [80325], [80326])
Methane breath test (91065)
🔧 0.00   ⚖ 0.00   **FUD** XXX   ▣ ▢
AMA: 2020,Dec,3

83857 Methemalbumin
EXCLUDES   Methemoglobin (83045, 83050)
Methyl alcohol ([80320])
Microalbumin
Quantitative (82043)
Semiquantitative (82044)
🔧 0.00   ⚖ 0.00   **FUD** XXX   ▣ ▢
AMA: 2020,Dec,3

83861 Microfluidic analysis utilizing an integrated collection and analysis device, tear osmolarity
EXCLUDES   beta-2 Microglobulin (82232)
Code also when performed on both eyes 83861 X 2
🔧 0.00   ⚖ 0.00   **FUD** XXX   ☒ ▣ ▢
AMA: 2020,Dec,3

83864 Mucopolysaccharides, acid, quantitative
🔧 0.00   ⚖ 0.00   **FUD** XXX   ▣ ▢
AMA: 2020,Dec,3

83872 Mucin, synovial fluid (Ropes test)
🔧 0.00   ⚖ 0.00   **FUD** XXX   ▣ ▢
AMA: 2020,Dec,3

83873 Myelin basic protein, cerebrospinal fluid
EXCLUDES   Oligoclonal bands (83916)
🔧 0.00   ⚖ 0.00   **FUD** XXX   ▣ ▢
AMA: 2020,Dec,3

83874 Myoglobin
🔧 0.00   ⚖ 0.00   **FUD** XXX   ▣ ▢
AMA: 2020,Dec,3; 2018,Jan,8; 2017,Jan,8; 2016,Jan,13

83876 Myeloperoxidase (MPO)
🔧 0.00   ⚖ 0.00   **FUD** XXX   ▣ ▢
AMA: 2020,Dec,3

83880 Natriuretic peptide
🔧 0.00   ⚖ 0.00   **FUD** XXX   ☒ ▣ ▢
AMA: 2020,Dec,3; 2018,Jan,8; 2017,Jan,8; 2016,Jan,13

83883 Nephelometry, each analyte not elsewhere specified
🔧 0.00   ⚖ 0.00   **FUD** XXX   ▣ ▢
AMA: 2020,Dec,3

83885 Nickel
🔧 0.00   ⚖ 0.00   **FUD** XXX   ▣ ▢
AMA: 2020,Dec,3

83915-84066 [83992] Chemistry: Nucleotidase 5'-—Phosphatase (Acid)

INCLUDES Clinical information not requested by ordering physician
Mathematically calculated results
Quantitative analysis unless otherwise specified
Specimens from any source unless otherwise specified

EXCLUDES Analytes from nonrequested laboratory analysis
Calculated results representing score or probability derived by algorithm
Drug testing ([80305, 80306, 80307], [80324, 80325, 80326, 80327, 80328, 80329, 80330, 80331, 80332, 80333, 80334, 80335, 80336, 80337, 80338, 80339, 80340, 80341, 80342, 80343, 80344, 80345, 80346, 80347, 80348, 80349, 80350, 80351, 80352, 80353, 80354, 80355, 80356, 80357, 80358, 80359, 80360, 80361, 80362, 80363, 80364, 80365, 80366, 80367, 80368, 80369, 80370, 80371, 80372, 80373, 80374, 80375, 80376, 80377, 83992])
Organ or disease panels (80048-80076 [80081])
Therapeutic drug assays (80150-80299 [80164, 80165, 80171])

83915 **Nucleotidase 5'-**
🔧 0.00   ✂ 0.00   **FUD** XXX
AMA: 2020,Dec,3

83916 **Oligoclonal immune (oligoclonal bands)**
🔧 0.00   ✂ 0.00   **FUD** XXX
AMA: 2020,Dec,3

83918 **Organic acids; total, quantitative, each specimen**
🔧 0.00   ✂ 0.00   **FUD** XXX
AMA: 2020,Dec,3; 2018,Jan,8; 2017,Jan,8; 2016,Jan,13

83919 **qualitative, each specimen**
🔧 0.00   ✂ 0.00   **FUD** XXX
AMA: 2020,Dec,3

83921 **Organic acid, single, quantitative**
🔧 0.00   ✂ 0.00   **FUD** XXX
AMA: 2020,Dec,3

83930 **Osmolality; blood**
EXCLUDES Tear osmolarity (83861)
🔧 0.00   ✂ 0.00   **FUD** XXX
AMA: 2020,Dec,3

83935 **urine**
EXCLUDES Tear osmolarity (83861)
🔧 0.00   ✂ 0.00   **FUD** XXX
AMA: 2020,Dec,3

83937 **Osteocalcin (bone g1a protein)**
🔧 0.00   ✂ 0.00   **FUD** XXX
AMA: 2020,Dec,3; 2018,Jan,8; 2017,Jan,8; 2016,Jan,13

83945 **Oxalate**
🔧 0.00   ✂ 0.00   **FUD** XXX
AMA: 2020,Dec,3

83950 **Oncoprotein; HER-2/neu**
EXCLUDES Tissue (88342, 88365)
🔧 0.00   ✂ 0.00   **FUD** XXX
AMA: 2020,Dec,3

83951 **des-gamma-carboxy-prothrombin (DCP)**
🔧 0.00   ✂ 0.00   **FUD** XXX
AMA: 2020,Dec,3

83970 **Parathormone (parathyroid hormone)**
EXCLUDES Chlorinated hydrocarbon screen (82441)
Quantitative pesticide report code for specific method
🔧 0.00   ✂ 0.00   **FUD** XXX
AMA: 2020,Dec,3

83986 **pH; body fluid, not otherwise specified**
EXCLUDES Blood pH (82800, 82803)
🔧 0.00   ✂ 0.00   **FUD** XXX ☒
AMA: 2020,Dec,3; 2018,Jan,8; 2017,Jan,8; 2016,May,13; 2016,Jan,13

83987 **exhaled breath condensate**
EXCLUDES Blood pH (82800, 82803)
Phenobarbital ([80345])
🔧 0.00   ✂ 0.00   **FUD** XXX
AMA: 2020,Dec,3

83992 **Resequenced code. See code following resequenced code 80365.**

83993 **Calprotectin, fecal**
🔧 0.00   ✂ 0.00   **FUD** XXX
AMA: 2020,Dec,3; 2018,Jan,8; 2017,Jan,8; 2016,Jan,13

84030 **Phenylalanine (PKU), blood**
INCLUDES Guthrie test
EXCLUDES Phenylalanine-tyrosine ratio (84030, 84510)
🔧 0.00   ✂ 0.00   **FUD** XXX
AMA: 2020,Dec,3

84035 **Phenylketones, qualitative**
🔧 0.00   ✂ 0.00   **FUD** XXX
AMA: 2020,Dec,3

84060 **Phosphatase, acid; total**
🔧 0.00   ✂ 0.00   **FUD** XXX
AMA: 2020,Dec,3

84066 **prostatic**
🔧 0.00   ✂ 0.00   **FUD** XXX
AMA: 2020,Dec,3

84075-84080 Chemistry: Phosphatase (Alkaline)

CMS: 100-03,160.17 Payment for L-Dopa /Associated Inpatient Hospital Services

INCLUDES Clinical information not requested by ordering physician
Mathematically calculated results
Quantitative analysis unless otherwise specified
Specimens from any source unless otherwise specified

EXCLUDES Analytes from nonrequested laboratory analysis
Calculated results representing score or probability derived by algorithm
Organ or disease panels (80048-80076 [80081])

84075 **Phosphatase, alkaline;**
🔧 0.00   ✂ 0.00   **FUD** XXX ☒
AMA: 2020,Dec,3; 2018,Jan,8; 2017,Jan,8; 2016,Jan,13

84078 **heat stable (total not included)**
🔧 0.00   ✂ 0.00   **FUD** XXX
AMA: 2020,Dec,3

84080 **isoenzymes**
🔧 0.00   ✂ 0.00   **FUD** XXX
AMA: 2020,Dec,3

84081-84150 Chemistry: Phosphatidylglycerol—Prostaglandin

INCLUDES Clinical information not requested by ordering physician
Mathematically calculated results
Quantitative analysis unless otherwise specified
Specimens from any source unless otherwise specified

EXCLUDES Analytes from nonrequested laboratory analysis
Calculated results representing score or probability derived by algorithm
Organ or disease panels (80048-80076 [80081])
Therapeutic drug assays (80150-80299 [80164, 80165, 80171])

84081 **Phosphatidylglycerol**
EXCLUDES Cholinesterase (82480, 82482)
Inorganic phosphates (84100)
Organic phosphates, report code for specific method
🔧 0.00   ✂ 0.00   **FUD** XXX
AMA: 2020,Dec,3

84085 **Phosphogluconate, 6-, dehydrogenase, RBC**
🔧 0.00   ✂ 0.00   **FUD** XXX
AMA: 2020,Dec,3

84087 **Phosphohexose isomerase**
🔧 0.00   ✂ 0.00   **FUD** XXX
AMA: 2020,Dec,3

84100 **Phosphorus inorganic (phosphate);**
🔧 0.00   ✂ 0.00   **FUD** XXX
AMA: 2020,Dec,3; 2018,Jan,8; 2017,Jan,8; 2016,Jan,13

84105 **urine**
EXCLUDES Pituitary gonadotropins (83001-83002)
PKU (84030, 84035)
🔧 0.00   ✂ 0.00   **FUD** XXX
AMA: 2020,Dec,3

84106 **Porphobilinogen, urine; qualitative**
🔧 0.00 🔬 0.00 **FUD** XXX   Q 🖳
AMA: 2020,Dec,3

84110 **quantitative**
🔧 0.00 🔬 0.00 **FUD** XXX   Q 🖳
AMA: 2020,Dec,3

84112 **Evaluation of cervicovaginal fluid for specific amniotic fluid protein(s) (eg, placental alpha microglobulin-1 [PAMG-1], placental protein 12 [PP12], alpha-fetoprotein), qualitative, each specimen** ♀
🔧 0.00 🔬 0.00 **FUD** XXX   Q 🖳
AMA: 2020,Dec,3

84119 **Porphyrins, urine; qualitative**
🔧 0.00 🔬 0.00 **FUD** XXX   Q 🖳
AMA: 2020,Dec,3

84120 **quantitation and fractionation**
🔧 0.00 🔬 0.00 **FUD** XXX   Q 🖳
AMA: 2020,Dec,3

84126 **Porphyrins, feces, quantitative**
EXCLUDES Porphyrin precursors (82135, 84106, 84110)
Protoporphyrin, RBC (84202, 84203)
🔧 0.00 🔬 0.00 **FUD** XXX   Q 🖳
AMA: 2020,Dec,3

84132 **Potassium; serum, plasma or whole blood**
🔧 0.00 🔬 0.00 **FUD** XXX   ✖ Q 🖳
AMA: 2020,Dec,3; 2018,Jan,8; 2017,Jan,8; 2016,Jan,13

84133 **urine**
🔧 0.00 🔬 0.00 **FUD** XXX   Q 🖳
AMA: 2020,Dec,3

84134 **Prealbumin**
EXCLUDES Microalbumin (82043-82044)
🔧 0.00 🔬 0.00 **FUD** XXX   Q 🖳
AMA: 2020,Dec,3

84135 **Pregnanediol** ♀
🔧 0.00 🔬 0.00 **FUD** XXX   Q 🖳
AMA: 2020,Dec,3

84138 **Pregnanetriol** ♀
🔧 0.00 🔬 0.00 **FUD** XXX   Q 🖳
AMA: 2020,Dec,3

84140 **Pregnenolone**
🔧 0.00 🔬 0.00 **FUD** XXX   Q 🖳
AMA: 2020,Dec,3; 2018,Jan,8; 2017,Jan,8; 2016,Jan,13

84143 **17-hydroxypregnenolone**
🔧 0.00 🔬 0.00 **FUD** XXX   Q 🖳
AMA: 2020,Dec,3; 2018,Jan,8; 2017,Jan,8; 2016,Jan,13

84144 **Progesterone**
EXCLUDES Progesterone receptor assay (84234)
Proinsulin (84206)
🔧 0.00 🔬 0.00 **FUD** XXX   Q 🖳
AMA: 2020,Dec,3

84145 **Procalcitonin (PCT)**
🔧 0.00 🔬 0.00 **FUD** XXX   Q 🖳
AMA: 2020,Dec,3

84146 **Prolactin**
🔧 0.00 🔬 0.00 **FUD** XXX   Q 🖳
AMA: 2020,Dec,3

84150 **Prostaglandin, each**
🔧 0.00 🔬 0.00 **FUD** XXX   Q 🖳
AMA: 2020,Dec,3

84152-84154 Chemistry: Prostate Specific Antigen
CMS: 100-03,190.31 Prostate Specific Antigen (PSA); 100-03,210.1 Prostate Cancer Screening Tests
INCLUDES Clinical information not requested by ordering physician
Mathematically calculated results
Quantitative analysis unless otherwise specified
EXCLUDES Analytes from nonrequested laboratory analysis
Calculated results representing score or probability derived by algorithm

84152 **Prostate specific antigen (PSA); complexed (direct measurement)** ♂
🔧 0.00 🔬 0.00 **FUD** XXX   Q 🖳
AMA: 2020,Dec,3

84153 **total** ♂
🔧 0.00 🔬 0.00 **FUD** XXX   Q 🖳
AMA: 2020,Dec,3; 2018,Jan,8; 2017,Jan,8; 2016,Jan,13

84154 **free** ♂
🔧 0.00 🔬 0.00 **FUD** XXX   Q 🖳
AMA: 2020,Dec,3; 2018,Jan,8; 2017,Jan,8; 2016,Jan,13

84155-84157 Chemistry: Protein, Total (Not by Refractometry)
INCLUDES Clinical information not requested by ordering physician
Mathematically calculated results
EXCLUDES Analytes from nonrequested laboratory analysis
Calculated results representing score or probability derived by algorithm
Organ or disease panels (80048-80076 [80081])

84155 **Protein, total, except by refractometry; serum, plasma or whole blood**
🔧 0.00 🔬 0.00 **FUD** XXX   ✖ Q 🖳
AMA: 2020,Dec,3; 2018,Jan,8; 2017,Jan,8; 2016,Jan,13

84156 **urine**
🔧 0.00 🔬 0.00 **FUD** XXX   Q 🖳
AMA: 2020,Dec,3

84157 **other source (eg, synovial fluid, cerebrospinal fluid)**
🔧 0.00 🔬 0.00 **FUD** XXX   Q 🖳
AMA: 2020,Dec,3

84160-84432 Chemistry: Protein, Total (Refractometry)—Thyroglobulin
INCLUDES Clinical information not requested by ordering physician
Mathematically calculated results
Quantitative analysis unless otherwise specified
Specimens from any source unless otherwise specified
EXCLUDES Analytes from nonrequested laboratory analysis
Calculated results representing score or probability derived by algorithm
Drug testing ([80305, 80306, 80307], [80324, 80325, 80326, 80327, 80328, 80329, 80330, 80331, 80332, 80333, 80334, 80335, 80336, 80337, 80338, 80339, 80340, 80341, 80342, 80343, 80344, 80345, 80346, 80347, 80348, 80349, 80350, 80351, 80352, 80353, 80354, 80355, 80356, 80357, 80358, 80359, 80360, 80361, 80362, 80363, 80364, 80365, 80366, 80367, 80368, 80369, 80370, 80371, 80372, 80373, 80374, 80375, 80376, 80377, 83992])
Organ or disease panels (80048-80076 [80081])
Therapeutic drug assays (80150-80299 [80164, 80165, 80171])

84160 **Protein, total, by refractometry, any source**
EXCLUDES Urine total protein, dipstick method (81000-81003)
🔧 0.00 🔬 0.00 **FUD** XXX   Q 🖳
AMA: 2020,Dec,3

84163 **Pregnancy-associated plasma protein-A (PAPP-A)** ♀
🔧 0.00 🔬 0.00 **FUD** XXX   Q 🖳
AMA: 2020,Dec,3

84165 **Protein; electrophoretic fractionation and quantitation, serum**
🔧 0.00 🔬 0.00 **FUD** XXX   Q 80 🖳
AMA: 2020,Dec,3

84166 **electrophoretic fractionation and quantitation, other fluids with concentration (eg, urine, CSF)**
🔧 0.00 🔬 0.00 **FUD** XXX   Q 80 🖳
AMA: 2020,Dec,3

84181 **Western Blot, with interpretation and report, blood or other body fluid**
🔧 0.00 🔬 0.00 **FUD** XXX Q 80 ▭
AMA: 2020,Dec,3

84182 **Western Blot, with interpretation and report, blood or other body fluid, immunological probe for band identification, each**
EXCLUDES *Western Blot tissue analysis (88371)*
🔧 0.00 🔬 0.00 **FUD** XXX Q 80 ▭
AMA: 2020,Dec,3

84202 **Protoporphyrin, RBC; quantitative**
🔧 0.00 🔬 0.00 **FUD** XXX Q ▭
AMA: 2020,Dec,3

84203 **screen**
🔧 0.00 🔬 0.00 **FUD** XXX Q ▭
AMA: 2020,Dec,3

84206 **Proinsulin**
EXCLUDES *Pseudocholinesterase (82480)*
🔧 0.00 🔬 0.00 **FUD** XXX Q ▭
AMA: 2020,Dec,3

84207 **Pyridoxal phosphate (Vitamin B-6)**
🔧 0.00 🔬 0.00 **FUD** XXX Q ▭
AMA: 2020,Dec,3

84210 **Pyruvate**
🔧 0.00 🔬 0.00 **FUD** XXX Q ▭
AMA: 2020,Dec,3

84220 **Pyruvate kinase**
🔧 0.00 🔬 0.00 **FUD** XXX Q ▭
AMA: 2020,Dec,3

84228 **Quinine**
🔧 0.00 🔬 0.00 **FUD** XXX Q ▭
AMA: 2020,Dec,3; 2018,Jan,8; 2017,Jan,8; 2016,Jan,13

84233 **Receptor assay; estrogen**
🔧 0.00 🔬 0.00 **FUD** XXX Q ▭
AMA: 2020,Dec,3

84234 **progesterone**
🔧 0.00 🔬 0.00 **FUD** XXX Q ▭
AMA: 2020,Dec,3

84235 **endocrine, other than estrogen or progesterone (specify hormone)**
🔧 0.00 🔬 0.00 **FUD** XXX Q ▭
AMA: 2020,Dec,3

84238 **non-endocrine (specify receptor)**
🔧 0.00 🔬 0.00 **FUD** XXX Q ▭
AMA: 2020,Dec,3; 2018,Jan,8; 2017,Jan,8; 2016,Jan,13

84244 **Renin**
🔧 0.00 🔬 0.00 **FUD** XXX Q ▭
AMA: 2020,Dec,3

84252 **Riboflavin (Vitamin B-2)**
EXCLUDES *Salicylates ([80329], [80330], [80331])*
Salicylate therapeutic drug assay ([80179])
Secretin test reported with appropriate analyses (43756, 43757, 99070)
🔧 0.00 🔬 0.00 **FUD** XXX Q ▭
AMA: 2020,Dec,3

84255 **Selenium**
🔧 0.00 🔬 0.00 **FUD** XXX Q ▭
AMA: 2020,Dec,3

84260 **Serotonin**
EXCLUDES *Urine metabolites (HIAA) (83497)*
🔧 0.00 🔬 0.00 **FUD** XXX Q ▭
AMA: 2020,Dec,3

84270 **Sex hormone binding globulin (SHBG)**
🔧 0.00 🔬 0.00 **FUD** XXX Q ▭
AMA: 2020,Dec,3; 2018,Jan,8; 2017,Jan,8; 2016,Jan,13

84275 **Sialic acid**
EXCLUDES *Sickle hemoglobin (85660)*
🔧 0.00 🔬 0.00 **FUD** XXX Q ▭
AMA: 2020,Dec,3

84285 **Silica**
🔧 0.00 🔬 0.00 **FUD** XXX Q ▭
AMA: 2020,Dec,3

84295 **Sodium; serum, plasma or whole blood**
🔧 0.00 🔬 0.00 **FUD** XXX ✕ Q ▭
AMA: 2020,Dec,3; 2018,Jan,8; 2017,Jan,8; 2016,Jan,13

84300 **urine**
🔧 0.00 🔬 0.00 **FUD** XXX Q ▭
AMA: 2020,Dec,3

84302 **other source**
EXCLUDES *Somatomammotropin (83632)*
Somatotropin (83003)
🔧 0.00 🔬 0.00 **FUD** XXX Q ▭
AMA: 2020,Dec,3; 2018,Jan,8; 2017,Jan,8; 2016,Jan,13

84305 **Somatomedin**
🔧 0.00 🔬 0.00 **FUD** XXX Q ▭
AMA: 2020,Dec,3; 2018,Jan,8; 2017,Jan,8; 2016,Jan,13

84307 **Somatostatin**
🔧 0.00 🔬 0.00 **FUD** XXX Q ▭
AMA: 2020,Dec,3; 2018,Jan,8; 2017,Jan,8; 2016,Jan,13

84311 **Spectrophotometry, analyte not elsewhere specified**
🔧 0.00 🔬 0.00 **FUD** XXX Q ▭
AMA: 2020,Dec,3

84315 **Specific gravity (except urine)**
EXCLUDES *Stone analysis (82355-82370)*
Suppression of growth stimulation expressed gene 2 [ST2] testing (83006)
Urine specific gravity (81000-81003)
🔧 0.00 🔬 0.00 **FUD** XXX Q ▭
AMA: 2020,Dec,3

84375 **Sugars, chromatographic, TLC or paper chromatography**
🔧 0.00 🔬 0.00 **FUD** XXX Q ▭
AMA: 2020,Dec,3

84376 **Sugars (mono-, di-, and oligosaccharides); single qualitative, each specimen**
🔧 0.00 🔬 0.00 **FUD** XXX Q ▭
AMA: 2020,Dec,3; 2018,Jan,8; 2017,Jan,8; 2016,Jan,13

84377 **multiple qualitative, each specimen**
🔧 0.00 🔬 0.00 **FUD** XXX Q ▭
AMA: 2020,Dec,3; 2018,Jan,8; 2017,Jan,8; 2016,Jan,13

84378 **single quantitative, each specimen**
🔧 0.00 🔬 0.00 **FUD** XXX Q ▭
AMA: 2020,Dec,3

84379 **multiple quantitative, each specimen**
🔧 0.00 🔬 0.00 **FUD** XXX Q ▭
AMA: 2020,Dec,3; 2018,Jan,8; 2017,Jan,8; 2016,Jan,13

84392 **Sulfate, urine**
EXCLUDES *Sulfhemoglobin (83060)*
T-3 (84479-84481)
T-4 (84436-84439)
🔧 0.00 🔬 0.00 **FUD** XXX Q ▭
AMA: 2020,Dec,3

84402 **Testosterone; free**
EXCLUDES *Anabolic steroids ([80327, 80328])*
🔧 0.00 🔬 0.00 **FUD** XXX Q ▭
AMA: 2020,Dec,3

84403 **total**
EXCLUDES *Anabolic steroids ([80327, 80328])*
🔧 0.00 🔬 0.00 **FUD** XXX Q ▭
AMA: 2020,Dec,3

84410 bioavailable, direct measurement (eg, differential precipitation)
⚕ 0.00 ⚕ 0.00 **FUD** XXX 🔲 🔲
AMA: 2020,Dec,3

84425 Thiamine (Vitamin B-1)
⚕ 0.00 ⚕ 0.00 **FUD** XXX 🔲 🔲
AMA: 2020,Dec,3

84430 Thiocyanate
⚕ 0.00 ⚕ 0.00 **FUD** XXX 🔲 🔲
AMA: 2020,Dec,3

84431 Thromboxane metabolite(s), including thromboxane if performed, urine
Code also determination concurrent urine creatinine (82570)
⚕ 0.00 ⚕ 0.00 **FUD** XXX 🔲 🔲
AMA: 2020,Dec,3

84432 Thyroglobulin
EXCLUDES *Thyroglobulin antibody (86800)*
Thyrotropin releasing hormone (TRH) (80438, 80439)
⚕ 0.00 ⚕ 0.00 **FUD** XXX 🔲 🔲
AMA: 2020,Dec,3; 2018,Jan,8; 2017,Jan,8; 2016,Jan,13

84436-84445 Chemistry: Thyroid Tests
CMS: 100-03,190.22 Thyroid Testing
INCLUDES Clinical information not requested by the ordering physician
Mathematically calculated results
Quantitative analysis unless otherwise specified
Specimens from any source unless otherwise specified
EXCLUDES *Analytes from nonrequested laboratory analysis*
Calculated results representing a score or probability derived by algorithm
Organ or disease panels (80048-80076 [80081])
Therapeutic drug assays (80150-80299 [80164, 80165, 80171])

84436 Thyroxine; total
⚕ 0.00 ⚕ 0.00 **FUD** XXX 🔲 🔲
AMA: 2020,Dec,3; 2018,Jan,8; 2017,Jan,8; 2016,Jan,13

84437 requiring elution (eg, neonatal)
⚕ 0.00 ⚕ 0.00 **FUD** XXX 🔲 🔲
AMA: 2020,Dec,3

84439 free
⚕ 0.00 ⚕ 0.00 **FUD** XXX 🔲 🔲
AMA: 2020,Dec,3

84442 Thyroxine binding globulin (TBG)
⚕ 0.00 ⚕ 0.00 **FUD** XXX 🔲 🔲
AMA: 2020,Dec,3

84443 Thyroid stimulating hormone (TSH)
⚕ 0.00 ⚕ 0.00 **FUD** XXX ❌ 🔲 🔲
AMA: 2020,Dec,3

84445 Thyroid stimulating immune globulins (TSI)
EXCLUDES *Tobramycin (80200)*
⚕ 0.00 ⚕ 0.00 **FUD** XXX 🔲 🔲
AMA: 2020,Dec,3; 2018,Jan,8; 2017,Jan,8; 2016,Jan,13

84446-84449 Chemistry: Tocopherol Alpha—Transcortin
INCLUDES Clinical information not requested by ordering physician
Mathematically calculated results
Quantitative analysis unless otherwise specified
Specimens from any source unless otherwise specified
EXCLUDES *Analytes from nonrequested laboratory analysis*
Calculated results representing a score or probability derived by algorithm
Organ or disease panels (80048-80076 [80081])
Therapeutic drug assays (80150-80299 [80164, 80165, 80171])

84446 Tocopherol alpha (Vitamin E)
⚕ 0.00 ⚕ 0.00 **FUD** XXX 🔲 🔲
AMA: 2020,Dec,3

84449 Transcortin (cortisol binding globulin)
⚕ 0.00 ⚕ 0.00 **FUD** XXX 🔲 🔲
AMA: 2020,Dec,3; 2018,Jan,8; 2017,Jan,8; 2016,Jan,13

84450-84460 Chemistry: Transferase
CMS: 100-02,11,30.2.2 Automated Multi-Channel Chemistry (AMCC) Tests; 100-03,160.17 Payment for L-Dopa /Associated Inpatient Hospital Services; 100-04,16,40.6.1 Automated Multi-Channel Chemistry (AMCC) Tests for ESRD Beneficiaries; 100-04,16,70.8 CLIA Waived Tests
INCLUDES Clinical information not requested by ordering physician
Mathematically calculated results
Quantitative analysis unless otherwise specified
EXCLUDES *Analytes from nonrequested laboratory analysis*
Calculated results representing score or probability derived by algorithm

84450 Transferase; aspartate amino (AST) (SGOT)
⚕ 0.00 ⚕ 0.00 **FUD** XXX ❌ 🔲 🔲
AMA: 2020,Dec,3; 2018,Jan,8; 2017,Jan,8; 2016,Jan,13

84460 alanine amino (ALT) (SGPT)
⚕ 0.00 ⚕ 0.00 **FUD** XXX ❌ 🔲 🔲
AMA: 2020,Dec,3; 2018,Jan,8; 2017,Jan,8; 2016,Jan,13

84466 Chemistry: Transferrin
CMS: 100-02,11,20.2 ESRD Laboratory Services; 100-03,190.18 Serum Iron Studies
INCLUDES Clinical information not requested by ordering physician
Mathematically calculated results
Quantitative analysis unless otherwise specified
EXCLUDES *Analytes from nonrequested laboratory analysis*
Calculated results representing score or probability derived by algorithm

84466 Transferrin
EXCLUDES *Iron binding capacity (83550)*
⚕ 0.00 ⚕ 0.00 **FUD** XXX 🔲 🔲
AMA: 2020,Dec,3; 2018,Jan,8; 2017,Jan,8; 2016,Jan,13

84478 Chemistry: Triglycerides
CMS: 100-02,11,30.2.2 Automated Multi-Channel Chemistry (AMCC) Tests; 100-03,190.23 Lipid Testing; 100-04,16,70.8 CLIA Waived Tests; 100-04,16,90.2 Organ or Disease Oriented Panels
INCLUDES Clinical information not requested by ordering physician
Mathematically calculated results
EXCLUDES *Analytes from nonrequested laboratory analysis*
Calculated results representing score or probability derived by algorithm
Organ or disease panels (80048-80076 [80081])

84478 Triglycerides
⚕ 0.00 ⚕ 0.00 **FUD** XXX ❌ 🅰 🔲
AMA: 2020,Dec,3; 2018,Jan,8; 2017,Jan,8; 2016,Jan,13

84479-84482 Chemistry: Thyroid Hormone—Triiodothyronine
CMS: 100-03,190.22 Thyroid Testing
INCLUDES Clinical information not requested by ordering physician
Mathematically calculated results
Quantitative analysis unless otherwise specified
Specimens from any source unless otherwise specified
EXCLUDES *Analytes from nonrequested laboratory analysis*
Calculated results representing score or probability derived by algorithm
Organ or disease panels (80048-80076 [80081])

84479 Thyroid hormone (T3 or T4) uptake or thyroid hormone binding ratio (THBR)
⚕ 0.00 ⚕ 0.00 **FUD** XXX 🔲 🔲
AMA: 2020,Dec,3; 2018,Jan,8; 2017,Jan,8; 2016,Jan,13

84480 Triiodothyronine T3; total (TT-3)
⚕ 0.00 ⚕ 0.00 **FUD** XXX 🔲 🔲
AMA: 2020,Dec,3

84481 free
⚕ 0.00 ⚕ 0.00 **FUD** XXX 🔲 🔲
AMA: 2020,Dec,3

84482 reverse
⚕ 0.00 ⚕ 0.00 **FUD** XXX 🔲 🔲
AMA: 2020,Dec,3; 2018,Jan,8; 2017,Jan,8; 2016,Jan,13

84484-84512 Chemistry: Troponin (Quantitative)—Troponin (Qualitative)

INCLUDES   Clinical information not requested by ordering physician
Mathematically calculated results
Specimens from any source unless otherwise specified

EXCLUDES   *Analytes from nonrequested laboratory analysis*
Calculated results representing score or probability derived by algorithm
Organ or disease panels

84484   **Troponin, quantitative**

EXCLUDES   *Qualitative troponin assay (84512)*

🛠 0.00   ⚖ 0.00   **FUD** XXX   🔲🖥

AMA: 2020,Dec,3; 2018,Jan,8; 2017,Jan,8; 2016,Jan,13

84485   **Trypsin; duodenal fluid**

🛠 0.00   ⚖ 0.00   **FUD** XXX   🔲🖥

AMA: 2020,Dec,3

84488   **feces, qualitative**

🛠 0.00   ⚖ 0.00   **FUD** XXX   🔲🖥

AMA: 2020,Dec,3

84490   **feces, quantitative, 24-hour collection**

🛠 0.00   ⚖ 0.00   **FUD** XXX   🔲🖥

AMA: 2020,Dec,3

84510   **Tyrosine**

EXCLUDES   *Urate crystal identification (89060)*

🛠 0.00   ⚖ 0.00   **FUD** XXX   🔲🖥

AMA: 2020,Dec,3

84512   **Troponin, qualitative**

EXCLUDES   *Quantitative troponin assay (84484)*

🛠 0.00   ⚖ 0.00   **FUD** XXX   🔲🖥

AMA: 2020,Dec,3; 2018,Jan,8; 2017,Jan,8; 2016,Jan,13

84520-84525 Chemistry: Urea Nitrogen (Blood)

CMS: 100-03,160.17 Payment for L-Dopa /Associated Inpatient Hospital Services

INCLUDES   Clinical information not requested by ordering physician
Mathematically calculated results

EXCLUDES   *Analytes from nonrequested laboratory analysis*
Calculated results representing score or probability derived by algorithm
Organ or disease panels (80048-80076 [80081])

84520   **Urea nitrogen; quantitative**

🛠 0.00   ⚖ 0.00   **FUD** XXX   ❌🔲🖥

AMA: 2020,Dec,3; 2018,Jan,8; 2017,Jan,8; 2016,Jan,13

84525   **semiquantitative (eg, reagent strip test)**

INCLUDES   Patterson's test

🛠 0.00   ⚖ 0.00   **FUD** XXX   🔲🖥

AMA: 2020,Dec,3; 2018,Jan,8; 2017,Jan,8; 2016,Jan,13

84540-84630 Chemistry: Urea Nitrogen (Urine)—Zinc

INCLUDES   Clinical information not requested by ordering physician
Mathematically calculated results
Quantitative analysis unless otherwise specified
Specimens from any source unless otherwise specified

EXCLUDES   *Analytes from nonrequested laboratory analysis*
Calculated results representing score or probability derived by algorithm
Organ or disease panels (80048-80076 [80081])
Therapeutic drug assays (80150-80299 [80164, 80165, 80171])

84540   **Urea nitrogen, urine**

🛠 0.00   ⚖ 0.00   **FUD** XXX   🔲🖥

AMA: 2020,Dec,3

84545   **Urea nitrogen, clearance**

🛠 0.00   ⚖ 0.00   **FUD** XXX   🔲🖥

AMA: 2020,Dec,3

84550   **Uric acid; blood**

🛠 0.00   ⚖ 0.00   **FUD** XXX   ❌🔲🖥

AMA: 2020,Dec,3; 2018,Jan,8; 2017,Jan,8; 2016,Jan,13

84560   **other source**

🛠 0.00   ⚖ 0.00   **FUD** XXX   🔲🖥

AMA: 2020,Dec,3

84577   **Urobilinogen, feces, quantitative**

🛠 0.00   ⚖ 0.00   **FUD** XXX   🔲🖥

AMA: 2020,Dec,3

84578   **Urobilinogen, urine; qualitative**

🛠 0.00   ⚖ 0.00   **FUD** XXX   🔲🖥

AMA: 2020,Dec,3

84580   **quantitative, timed specimen**

🛠 0.00   ⚖ 0.00   **FUD** XXX   🔲🖥

AMA: 2020,Dec,3

84583   **semiquantitative**

EXCLUDES   *Uroporphyrins (84120)*
Valproic acid (dipropylacetic acid) ([80164])

🛠 0.00   ⚖ 0.00   **FUD** XXX   🔲🖥

AMA: 2020,Dec,3

84585   **Vanillylmandelic acid (VMA), urine**

🛠 0.00   ⚖ 0.00   **FUD** XXX   🔲🖥

AMA: 2020,Dec,3

84586   **Vasoactive intestinal peptide (VIP)**

🛠 0.00   ⚖ 0.00   **FUD** XXX   🔲🖥

AMA: 2020,Dec,3; 2018,Jan,8; 2017,Jan,8; 2016,Jan,13

84588   **Vasopressin (antidiuretic hormone, ADH)**

🛠 0.00   ⚖ 0.00   **FUD** XXX   🔲🖥

AMA: 2020,Dec,3; 2018,Jan,7

84590   **Vitamin A**

EXCLUDES   *Vitamin B-1 (84425)*
Vitamin B-2 (84252)
Vitamin B-6 (84207)
Vitamin B-12 (82607)
Vitamin C (82180)
Vitamin D (82306, [82652])
Vitamin E (84446)

🛠 0.00   ⚖ 0.00   **FUD** XXX   🔲🖥

AMA: 2020,Dec,3

84591   **Vitamin, not otherwise specified**

🛠 0.00   ⚖ 0.00   **FUD** XXX   🔲🖥

AMA: 2020,Dec,3

84597   **Vitamin K**

EXCLUDES   *Vanillylmandelic acid (VMA) (84585)*

🛠 0.00   ⚖ 0.00   **FUD** XXX   🔲🖥

AMA: 2020,Dec,3

84600   **Volatiles (eg, acetic anhydride, diethylether)**

EXCLUDES   *Carbon tetrachloride, dichloroethane, dichloromethane (82441)*
Isopropyl alcohol and methanol ([80320])
Volume, blood, RISA, or Cr-51 (78110, 78111)

🛠 0.00   ⚖ 0.00   **FUD** XXX   🔲🖥

AMA: 2020,Dec,3

84620   **Xylose absorption test, blood and/or urine**

EXCLUDES   *Administration (99070)*

🛠 0.00   ⚖ 0.00   **FUD** XXX   🔲🖥

AMA: 2020,Dec,3

84630   **Zinc**

🛠 0.00   ⚖ 0.00   **FUD** XXX   🔲🖥

AMA: 2020,Dec,3

84681-84999 Other and Unlisted Chemistry Tests

INCLUDES   Clinical information not requested by ordering physician
Mathematically calculated results
Quantitative analysis unless otherwise specified
Specimens from any source unless otherwise specified

EXCLUDES   *Analytes from nonrequested laboratory analysis*
Calculated results representing score or probability derived by algorithm
Confirmational testing, not otherwise specified drug ([80375, 80376, 80377], 80299)
Organ or disease panels (80048-80076 [80081])

84681   **C-peptide**

🛠 0.00   ⚖ 0.00   **FUD** XXX   🔲🖥

AMA: 2020,Dec,3

84702   **Gonadotropin, chorionic (hCG); quantitative**

🛠 0.00   ⚖ 0.00   **FUD** XXX   🔲🖥

AMA: 2020,Dec,3

● New Code   ▲ Revised Code   ○ Reinstated   ⬤ New Web Release   ▲ Revised Web Release   + Add-on   Unlisted   Not Covered   # Resequenced
⑤⓪ Optum Mod 50 Exempt   Ⓢ AMA Mod 51 Exempt   ⑤① Optum Mod 51 Exempt   ⑥③ Mod 63 Exempt   ✗ Non-FDA Drug   ★ Telemedicine   Ⓜ Maternity   Ⓐ Age Edit

84703   **qualitative**
> EXCLUDES   *Urine pregnancy test by visual color comparison (81025)*
> 🔧 0.00   ⚕ 0.00   **FUD** XXX   ☒ 🔲 🖳
> AMA: 2020,Dec,3

84704   **free beta chain**
> 🔧 0.00   ⚕ 0.00   **FUD** XXX   🔲 🖳
> AMA: 2020,Dec,3; 2018,Jan,8; 2017,Jan,8; 2016,Jan,13

84830   **Ovulation tests, by visual color comparison methods for human luteinizing hormone**   ♀
> 🔧 0.00   ⚕ 0.00   **FUD** XXX   ☒ 🔲
> AMA: 2020,Dec,3; 2018,Jan,8; 2017,Jan,8; 2016,Jan,13

84999   **Unlisted chemistry procedure**
> EXCLUDES   *Definitive drug testing, not otherwise specified ([80375], [80376], [80377], 80299)*
> 🔧 0.00   ⚕ 0.00   **FUD** XXX   🔲 🖳
> AMA: 2020,Dec,3; 2018,Jan,8; 2017,Jan,8; 2016,Jan,13

85002 Bleeding Time Test

> EXCLUDES   *Agglutinins (86000, 86156, 86157)*
> *Antiplasmin (85410)*
> *Antithrombin III (85300, 85301)*
> *Blood banking procedures (86077-86079)*

85002   **Bleeding time**
> 🔧 0.00   ⚕ 0.00   **FUD** XXX   🔲 🖳
> AMA: 2020,Dec,3; 2018,Jan,8; 2017,Jan,8; 2016,Jan,13

85004-85049 Blood Counts

CMS: 100-03,190.15 Blood Counts
> EXCLUDES   *Agglutinins (86000, 86156-86157)*
> *Antiplasmin (85410)*
> *Antithrombin III (85300-85301)*
> *Blood banking procedures (86850-86999)*

85004   **Blood count; automated differential WBC count**
> 🔧 0.00   ⚕ 0.00   **FUD** XXX   🔲 🖳
> AMA: 2020,Dec,3; 2018,Jan,8; 2017,Jan,8; 2016,Jan,13

85007   **blood smear, microscopic examination with manual differential WBC count**
> 🔧 0.00   ⚕ 0.00   **FUD** XXX   🔲 🖳
> AMA: 2020,Dec,3; 2018,Jan,8; 2017,Jan,8; 2016,Jan,13

85008   **blood smear, microscopic examination without manual differential WBC count**
> EXCLUDES   *Cell count other fluids (eg, CSF) (89050-89051)*
> 🔧 0.00   ⚕ 0.00   **FUD** XXX   🔲 🖳
> AMA: 2020,Dec,3; 2018,Jan,8; 2017,Jan,8; 2016,Jan,13

85009   **manual differential WBC count, buffy coat**
> EXCLUDES   *Eosinophils, nasal smear (89190)*
> 🔧 0.00   ⚕ 0.00   **FUD** XXX   🔲 🖳
> AMA: 2020,Dec,3; 2018,Jan,8; 2017,Jan,8; 2016,Jan,13

85013   **spun microhematocrit**
> 🔧 0.00   ⚕ 0.00   **FUD** XXX   ☒ 🔲 🖳
> AMA: 2020,Dec,3

85014   **hematocrit (Hct)**
> 🔧 0.00   ⚕ 0.00   **FUD** XXX   ☒ 🔲 🖳
> AMA: 2020,Dec,3; 2018,Jan,8; 2017,Jan,8; 2016,Jan,13

85018   **hemoglobin (Hgb)**
> EXCLUDES   *Immunoassay, hemoglobin, fecal (82274)*
> *Other hemoglobin determination (83020-83069)*
> *Transcutaneous hemoglobin measurement (88738)*
> 🔧 0.00   ⚕ 0.00   **FUD** XXX   🔲 🖳
> AMA: 2020,Dec,3; 2018,Jan,8; 2017,Jan,8; 2016,Jan,13

85025   **complete (CBC), automated (Hgb, Hct, RBC, WBC and platelet count) and automated differential WBC count**
> 🔧 0.00   ⚕ 0.00   **FUD** XXX   ☒ 🔲 🖳
> AMA: 2020,Dec,3; 2018,Jan,8; 2017,Jan,8; 2016,Jan,13

85027   **complete (CBC), automated (Hgb, Hct, RBC, WBC and platelet count)**
> 🔧 0.00   ⚕ 0.00   **FUD** XXX   🔲 🖳
> AMA: 2020,Dec,3; 2018,Jan,8; 2017,Jan,8; 2016,Jan,13

85032   **manual cell count (erythrocyte, leukocyte, or platelet) each**
> 🔧 0.00   ⚕ 0.00   **FUD** XXX   🔲 🖳
> AMA: 2020,Dec,3; 2018,Jan,8; 2017,Jan,8; 2016,Jan,13

85041   **red blood cell (RBC), automated**
> EXCLUDES   *Complete blood count (85025, 85027)*
> 🔧 0.00   ⚕ 0.00   **FUD** XXX   🔲 🖳
> AMA: 2020,Dec,3; 2018,Jan,8; 2017,Jan,8; 2016,Jan,13

85044   **reticulocyte, manual**
> 🔧 0.00   ⚕ 0.00   **FUD** XXX   🔲 🖳
> AMA: 2020,Dec,3; 2018,Jan,8; 2017,Jan,8; 2016,Jan,13

85045   **reticulocyte, automated**
> 🔧 0.00   ⚕ 0.00   **FUD** XXX   🔲 🖳
> AMA: 2020,Dec,3; 2018,Jan,8; 2017,Jan,8; 2016,Jan,13

85046   **reticulocytes, automated, including 1 or more cellular parameters (eg, reticulocyte hemoglobin content [CHr], immature reticulocyte fraction [IRF], reticulocyte volume [MRV], RNA content), direct measurement**
> 🔧 0.00   ⚕ 0.00   **FUD** XXX   🔲 🖳
> AMA: 2020,Dec,3

85048   **leukocyte (WBC), automated**
> 🔧 0.00   ⚕ 0.00   **FUD** XXX   🔲 🖳
> AMA: 2020,Dec,3; 2018,Jan,8; 2017,Jan,8; 2016,Jan,13

85049   **platelet, automated**
> 🔧 0.00   ⚕ 0.00   **FUD** XXX   🔲 🖳
> AMA: 2020,Dec,3

85055-85705 Coagulopathy Testing

> EXCLUDES   *Agglutinins (86000, 86156-86157)*
> *Antiplasmin (85410)*
> *Antithrombin III (85300-85301)*
> *Blood banking procedures (86850-86999)*

85055   **Reticulated platelet assay**
> 🔧 0.00   ⚕ 0.00   **FUD** XXX   🔲 🖳
> AMA: 2020,Dec,3

85060   **Blood smear, peripheral, interpretation by physician with written report**
> 🔧 0.70   ⚕ 0.70   **FUD** XXX   Ⓑ 80 🖳
> AMA: 2020,Dec,3

85097   **Bone marrow, smear interpretation**
> EXCLUDES   *Bone biopsy (20220, 20225, 20240, 20245, 20250-20251)*
> *Special stains (88312-88313)*
> 🔧 1.42   ⚕ 2.11   **FUD** XXX   02 80 🖳
> AMA: 2020,Dec,3; 2018,Jan,8; 2017,Jan,8; 2016,Jan,13

85130   **Chromogenic substrate assay**
> EXCLUDES   *Circulating anticoagulant screen (mixing studies) (85611, 85732)*
> 🔧 0.00   ⚕ 0.00   **FUD** XXX   🔲 🖳
> AMA: 2020,Dec,3

85170   **Clot retraction**
> 🔧 0.00   ⚕ 0.00   **FUD** XXX   🔲 🖳
> AMA: 2020,Dec,3

85175   **Clot lysis time, whole blood dilution**
> EXCLUDES   *Clotting factor I (fibrinogen) (85384, 85385)*
> 🔧 0.00   ⚕ 0.00   **FUD** XXX   🔲 🖳
> AMA: 2020,Dec,3

85210   **Clotting; factor II, prothrombin, specific**
> EXCLUDES   *Prothrombin time (85610-85611)*
> *Russell viper venom time (85612-85613)*
> 🔧 0.00   ⚕ 0.00   **FUD** XXX   🔲 🖳
> AMA: 2020,Dec,3

85220   **factor V (AcG or proaccelerin), labile factor**
> 🔧 0.00   ⚕ 0.00   **FUD** XXX   🔲 🖳
> AMA: 2020,Dec,3

85230   **factor VII (proconvertin, stable factor)**
> 🔧 0.00   ⚕ 0.00   **FUD** XXX   🔲 🖳
> AMA: 2020,Dec,3

26/TC PC/TC Only   A2-Z3 ASC Payment   50 Bilateral   ♂ Male Only   ♀ Female Only   🔧 Facility RVU   ⚕ Non-Facility RVU   🖳 CCI   ☒ CLIA
FUD Follow-up Days   **CMS:** IOM   **AMA:** CPT Asst   A-Y OPPSI   80/80 Surg Assist Allowed / w/Doc   🔲 Lab Crosswalk   ⊞ Radiology Crosswalk

406   CPT © 2021 American Medical Association. All Rights Reserved.   © 2021 Optum360, LLC

85240   factor VIII (AHG), 1-stage
        0.00   0.00   FUD XXX
        AMA: 2020,Dec,3

85244   factor VIII related antigen
        0.00   0.00   FUD XXX
        AMA: 2020,Dec,3

85245   factor VIII, VW factor, ristocetin cofactor
        0.00   0.00   FUD XXX
        AMA: 2020,Dec,3

85246   factor VIII, VW factor antigen
        0.00   0.00   FUD XXX
        AMA: 2020,Dec,3

85247   factor VIII, von Willebrand factor, multimetric analysis
        0.00   0.00   FUD XXX
        AMA: 2020,Dec,3

85250   factor IX (PTC or Christmas)
        0.00   0.00   FUD XXX
        AMA: 2020,Dec,3

85260   factor X (Stuart-Prower)
        0.00   0.00   FUD XXX
        AMA: 2020,Dec,3

85270   factor XI (PTA)
        0.00   0.00   FUD XXX
        AMA: 2020,Dec,3

85280   factor XII (Hageman)
        0.00   0.00   FUD XXX
        AMA: 2020,Dec,3

85290   factor XIII (fibrin stabilizing)
        0.00   0.00   FUD XXX
        AMA: 2020,Dec,3

85291   factor XIII (fibrin stabilizing), screen solubility
        0.00   0.00   FUD XXX
        AMA: 2020,Dec,3

85292   prekallikrein assay (Fletcher factor assay)
        0.00   0.00   FUD XXX
        AMA: 2020,Dec,3

85293   high molecular weight kininogen assay (Fitzgerald factor assay)
        0.00   0.00   FUD XXX
        AMA: 2020,Dec,3

85300   Clotting inhibitors or anticoagulants; antithrombin III, activity
        0.00   0.00   FUD XXX
        AMA: 2020,Dec,3

85301   antithrombin III, antigen assay
        0.00   0.00   FUD XXX
        AMA: 2020,Dec,3

85302   protein C, antigen
        0.00   0.00   FUD XXX
        AMA: 2020,Dec,3

85303   protein C, activity
        0.00   0.00   FUD XXX
        AMA: 2020,Dec,3

85305   protein S, total
        0.00   0.00   FUD XXX
        AMA: 2020,Dec,3

85306   protein S, free
        0.00   0.00   FUD XXX
        AMA: 2020,Dec,3

85307   Activated Protein C (APC) resistance assay
        0.00   0.00   FUD XXX
        AMA: 2020,Dec,3

85335   Factor inhibitor test
        0.00   0.00   FUD XXX
        AMA: 2020,Dec,3

85337   Thrombomodulin
        EXCLUDES   Mixing studies for inhibitors (85732)
        0.00   0.00   FUD XXX
        AMA: 2020,Dec,3

85345   Coagulation time; Lee and White
        0.00   0.00   FUD XXX
        AMA: 2020,Dec,3

85347   activated
        0.00   0.00   FUD XXX
        AMA: 2020,Dec,3; 2019,Apr,10

85348   other methods
        EXCLUDES   Differential count (85007-85009, 85025)
                   Duke bleeding time (85002)
                   Eosinophils, nasal smear (89190)
        0.00   0.00   FUD XXX
        AMA: 2020,Dec,3

85360   Euglobulin lysis
        EXCLUDES   Fetal hemoglobin (83030, 83033, 85460)
        0.00   0.00   FUD XXX
        AMA: 2020,Dec,3

85362   Fibrin(ogen) degradation (split) products (FDP) (FSP); agglutination slide, semiquantitative
        EXCLUDES   Immunoelectrophoresis (86320)
        0.00   0.00   FUD XXX
        AMA: 2020,Dec,3

85366   paracoagulation
        0.00   0.00   FUD XXX
        AMA: 2020,Dec,3

85370   quantitative
        0.00   0.00   FUD XXX
        AMA: 2020,Dec,3

85378   Fibrin degradation products, D-dimer; qualitative or semiquantitative
        0.00   0.00   FUD XXX
        AMA: 2020,Dec,3; 2018,Jan,8; 2017,Jan,8; 2016,Jan,13

85379   quantitative
        INCLUDES   Ultrasensitive and standard sensitivity quantitative D-dimer (85379)
        0.00   0.00   FUD XXX
        AMA: 2020,Dec,3

85380   ultrasensitive (eg, for evaluation for venous thromboembolism), qualitative or semiquantitative
        0.00   0.00   FUD XXX
        AMA: 2020,Dec,3; 2018,Jan,8; 2017,Jan,8; 2016,Jan,13

85384   Fibrinogen; activity
        0.00   0.00   FUD XXX
        AMA: 2020,Dec,3; 2019,Apr,10

85385   antigen
        0.00   0.00   FUD XXX
        AMA: 2020,Dec,3

85390   Fibrinolysins or coagulopathy screen, interpretation and report
        0.00   0.00   FUD XXX
        AMA: 2020,Dec,3; 2019,Apr,10

85396   Coagulation/fibrinolysis assay, whole blood (eg, viscoelastic clot assessment), including use of any pharmacologic additive(s), as indicated, including interpretation and written report, per day
        0.58   0.58   FUD XXX
        AMA: 2020,Dec,3; 2019,Apr,10

85397   Coagulation and fibrinolysis, functional activity, not otherwise specified (eg, ADAMTS-13), each analyte
        0.00   0.00   FUD XXX
        AMA: 2020,Dec,3

85400	**Fibrinolytic factors and inhibitors; plasmin**

🖸 0.00 ⚕ 0.00 **FUD** XXX Q 🖵
AMA: 2020,Dec,3

85410 alpha-2 antiplasmin
🖸 0.00 ⚕ 0.00 **FUD** XXX Q 🖵
AMA: 2020,Dec,3

85415 plasminogen activator
🖸 0.00 ⚕ 0.00 **FUD** XXX Q 🖵
AMA: 2020,Dec,3

85420 plasminogen, except antigenic assay
🖸 0.00 ⚕ 0.00 **FUD** XXX Q 🖵
AMA: 2020,Dec,3

85421 plasminogen, antigenic assay
EXCLUDES Fragility, red blood cell (85547, 85555-85557)
🖸 0.00 ⚕ 0.00 **FUD** XXX Q 🖵
AMA: 2020,Dec,3

85441 Heinz bodies; direct
🖸 0.00 ⚕ 0.00 **FUD** XXX Q 🖵
AMA: 2020,Dec,3

85445 induced, acetyl phenylhydrazine
EXCLUDES Hematocrit (PCV) (85014, 85025, 85027)
Hemoglobin (83020-83068, 85018, 85025, 85027)
🖸 0.00 ⚕ 0.00 **FUD** XXX Q 🖵
AMA: 2020,Dec,3

85460 Hemoglobin or RBCs, fetal, for fetomaternal hemorrhage; differential lysis (Kleihauer-Betke) M ♀
EXCLUDES Hemoglobin F (83030, 83033)
Hemolysins (86940-86941)
🖸 0.00 ⚕ 0.00 **FUD** XXX Q 🖵
AMA: 2020,Dec,3; 2018,Jan,8; 2017,Jan,8; 2016,Jan,13

85461 rosette M ♀
🖸 0.00 ⚕ 0.00 **FUD** XXX Q 🖵
AMA: 2020,Dec,3

85475 Hemolysin, acid
INCLUDES Ham test
EXCLUDES Hemolysins and agglutinins (86940-86941)
🖸 0.00 ⚕ 0.00 **FUD** XXX Q 🖵
AMA: 2020,Dec,3

85520 Heparin assay
🖸 0.00 ⚕ 0.00 **FUD** XXX Q 🖵
AMA: 2020,Dec,3

85525 Heparin neutralization
🖸 0.00 ⚕ 0.00 **FUD** XXX Q 🖵
AMA: 2020,Dec,3; 2018,Jan,8; 2017,Aug,9

85530 Heparin-protamine tolerance test
🖸 0.00 ⚕ 0.00 **FUD** XXX Q 🖵
AMA: 2020,Dec,3

85536 Iron stain, peripheral blood
EXCLUDES Iron stains on bone marrow or other tissues with physician evaluation (88313)
🖸 0.00 ⚕ 0.00 **FUD** XXX Q 🖵
AMA: 2020,Dec,3

85540 Leukocyte alkaline phosphatase with count
🖸 0.00 ⚕ 0.00 **FUD** XXX Q 🖵
AMA: 2020,Dec,3

85547 Mechanical fragility, RBC
🖸 0.00 ⚕ 0.00 **FUD** XXX Q 🖵
AMA: 2020,Dec,3

85549 Muramidase
EXCLUDES Nitroblue tetrazolium dye test (86384)
🖸 0.00 ⚕ 0.00 **FUD** XXX Q 🖵
AMA: 2020,Dec,3

85555 Osmotic fragility, RBC; unincubated
🖸 0.00 ⚕ 0.00 **FUD** XXX Q 🖵
AMA: 2020,Dec,3

85557 incubated
EXCLUDES Packed cell volume (85013)
Parasites, blood (eg, malaria smears) (87207)
Partial thromboplastin time (85730, 85732)
Plasmin (85400)
Plasminogen (85420)
Plasminogen activator (85415)
🖸 0.00 ⚕ 0.00 **FUD** XXX Q 🖵
AMA: 2020,Dec,3

85576 Platelet, aggregation (in vitro), each agent
EXCLUDES Thromboxane metabolite(s), including thromboxane, when performed, in urine (84431)
🖸 0.00 ⚕ 0.00 **FUD** XXX ✖ Q 80 🖵
AMA: 2020,Dec,3; 2019,Apr,10; 2018,Jan,8; 2017,Jan,8; 2016,Jan,13

85597 Phospholipid neutralization; platelet
🖸 0.00 ⚕ 0.00 **FUD** XXX Q 🖵
AMA: 2020,Dec,3; 2018,Jan,8; 2017,Jan,8; 2016,Jan,13

85598 hexagonal phospholipid
🖸 0.00 ⚕ 0.00 **FUD** XXX Q 🖵
AMA: 2020,Dec,3; 2018,Jan,8; 2017,Jan,8; 2016,Jan,13

85610 Prothrombin time;
🖸 0.00 ⚕ 0.00 **FUD** XXX ✖ Q 🖵
AMA: 2020,Dec,3

85611 substitution, plasma fractions, each
🖸 0.00 ⚕ 0.00 **FUD** XXX Q 🖵
AMA: 2020,Dec,3

85612 Russell viper venom time (includes venom); undiluted
🖸 0.00 ⚕ 0.00 **FUD** XXX Q 🖵
AMA: 2020,Dec,3

85613 diluted
EXCLUDES Red blood cell count (85025, 85027, 85041)
🖸 0.00 ⚕ 0.00 **FUD** XXX Q 🖵
AMA: 2020,Dec,3

85635 Reptilase test
EXCLUDES Reticulocyte count (85044-85045)
🖸 0.00 ⚕ 0.00 **FUD** XXX Q 🖵
AMA: 2020,Dec,3

85651 Sedimentation rate, erythrocyte; non-automated
🖸 0.00 ⚕ 0.00 **FUD** XXX ✖ Q 🖵
AMA: 2020,Dec,3

85652 automated
INCLUDES Westergren test
🖸 0.00 ⚕ 0.00 **FUD** XXX Q 🖵
AMA: 2020,Dec,3

85660 Sickling of RBC, reduction
EXCLUDES Hemoglobin electrophoresis (83020)
Smears (87207)
🖸 0.00 ⚕ 0.00 **FUD** XXX Q 🖵
AMA: 2020,Dec,3

85670 Thrombin time; plasma
🖸 0.00 ⚕ 0.00 **FUD** XXX Q 🖵
AMA: 2020,Dec,3

85675 titer
🖸 0.00 ⚕ 0.00 **FUD** XXX Q 🖵
AMA: 2020,Dec,3

85705 Thromboplastin inhibition, tissue
EXCLUDES Individual clotting factors (85245-85247)
🖸 0.00 ⚕ 0.00 **FUD** XXX Q 🖵
AMA: 2020,Dec,3

85730-85732 Partial Thromboplastin Time (PTT)

EXCLUDES *Agglutinins (86000, 86156-86157)*
Antiplasmin (85410)
Antithrombin III (85300-85301)
Blood banking procedures (86850-86999)

85730 **Thromboplastin time, partial (PTT); plasma or whole blood**

INCLUDES Hicks-Pitney test
🚑 0.00 ⚕ 0.00 **FUD** XXX 🔲 🔲
AMA: 2020,Dec,3

85732 **substitution, plasma fractions, each**
🚑 0.00 ⚕ 0.00 **FUD** XXX 🔲 🔲
AMA: 2020,Dec,3; 2018,Jan,8; 2017,Jan,8; 2016,Jan,13

85810-85999 Blood Viscosity and Unlisted Hematology Procedures

85810 **Viscosity**

EXCLUDES *von Willebrand factor assay (85245-85247)*
WBC count (85025, 85027, 85048, 89050)
🚑 0.00 ⚕ 0.00 **FUD** XXX 🔲
AMA: 2020,Dec,3; 2018,Jan,8; 2017,Jan,8; 2016,Jan,13

85999 **Unlisted hematology and coagulation procedure**
🚑 0.00 ⚕ 0.00 **FUD** XXX 🔲 🔲
AMA: 2020,Dec,3; 2018,Jan,8; 2017,Aug,9; 2017,Jan,8; 2016,Jan,13

86015-86053 [86015, 86051, 86052, 86053] Antibody Testing

● # **86015** **Actin (smooth muscle) antibody (ASMA), each**

EXCLUDES *Antibodies:*
Actinomyces (86602)
Adrenal cortex (86255-86256)
🚑 0.00 ⚕ 0.00 **FUD** 000

86000 **Agglutinins, febrile (eg, Brucella, Francisella, Murine typhus, Q fever, Rocky Mountain spotted fever, scrub typhus), each antigen**

EXCLUDES *Infectious agent antibodies (86602-86804)*
🚑 0.00 ⚕ 0.00 **FUD** XXX 🔲 🔲
AMA: 2020,Dec,3; 2018,Jan,8; 2017,Jan,8; 2016,Jan,13

86001 **Allergen specific IgG quantitative or semiquantitative, each allergen**

EXCLUDES *Agglutinins and autohemolysins (86940-86941)*
🚑 0.00 ⚕ 0.00 **FUD** XXX 🔲 🔲
AMA: 2020,Dec,3

86003 **Allergen specific IgE; quantitative or semiquantitative, crude allergen extract, each**

EXCLUDES *Total quantitative IgE (82785)*
🚑 0.00 ⚕ 0.00 **FUD** XXX 🔲 🔲
AMA: 2020,Dec,3; 2018,Jan,8; 2017,Jan,8; 2016,Jan,13

86005 **qualitative, multiallergen screen (eg, disk, sponge, card)**

EXCLUDES *Total qualitative IgE (83518)*
🚑 0.00 ⚕ 0.00 **FUD** XXX 🔲 🔲
AMA: 2020,Dec,3; 2018,Jan,8; 2017,Jan,8; 2016,Jan,13

86008 **quantitative or semiquantitative, recombinant or purified component, each**

EXCLUDES *Alpha-1 antitrypsin (82103, 82104)*
Alpha-1 feto-protein (82105, 82106)
Anti-AChR (acetylcholine receptor) antibody titer (86255, 86256)
Anticardiolipin antibody (86147)
Anti-deoxyribonuclease titer (86215)
Anti-DNA (86225)
🚑 0.00 ⚕ 0.00 **FUD** XXX 🔲 🔲
AMA: 2020,Dec,3

86015 **Resequenced code. See code before 86000.**

86021 **Antibody identification; leukocyte antibodies**
🚑 0.00 ⚕ 0.00 **FUD** XXX 🔲 🔲
AMA: 2020,Dec,3; 2020,AugSE,1; 2020,AugSE,1; 2020,AugSE,1

86022 **platelet antibodies**
🚑 0.00 ⚕ 0.00 **FUD** XXX 🔲 🔲
AMA: 2020,Dec,3; 2020,AugSE,1; 2020,AugSE,1; 2020,AugSE,1

86023 **platelet associated immunoglobulin assay**
🚑 0.00 ⚕ 0.00 **FUD** XXX 🔲 🔲
AMA: 2020,Dec,3; 2020,AugSE,1; 2020,AugSE,1; 2020,AugSE,1

● **86036** **Antineutrophil cytoplasmic antibody (ANCA); screen, each antibody**

● **86037** **titer, each antibody**

86038 **Antinuclear antibodies (ANA);**
🚑 0.00 ⚕ 0.00 **FUD** XXX 🔲 🔲
AMA: 2020,Dec,3

86039 **titer**

EXCLUDES *Antistreptococcal antibody, ie, anti-DNAse (86215)*
Antistreptokinase titer (86590)
🚑 0.00 ⚕ 0.00 **FUD** XXX 🔲 🔲
AMA: 2020,Dec,3

86051 **Resequenced code. See code following 86063.**
86052 **Resequenced code. See code following 86063.**
86053 **Resequenced code. See code following 86063.**

86060 **Antistreptolysin 0; titer**

EXCLUDES *Antibodies, infectious agents (86602-86804)*
🚑 0.00 ⚕ 0.00 **FUD** XXX 🔲 🔲
AMA: 2020,Dec,3

86063 **screen**

EXCLUDES *Antibodies to blastomyces (86612)*
Antibodies, infectious agents (86602-86804)
🚑 0.00 ⚕ 0.00 **FUD** XXX 🔲 🔲
AMA: 2020,Dec,3

● # **86051** **Aquaporin-4 (neuromyelitis optica [NMO]) antibody; enzyme-linked immunosorbent immunoassay (ELISA)**
🚑 0.00 ⚕ 0.00 **FUD** 000

● # **86052** **cell-based immunofluorescence assay (CBA), each**
🚑 0.00 ⚕ 0.00 **FUD** 000

● # **86053** **flow cytometry (ie, fluorescence-activated cell sorting [FACS]), each**
🚑 0.00 ⚕ 0.00 **FUD** 000

86077-86079 Blood Bank Services

86077 **Blood bank physician services; difficult cross match and/or evaluation of irregular antibody(s), interpretation and written report**
🚑 1.46 ⚕ 1.57 **FUD** XXX 🔲 🔲 🔲
AMA: 2020,Dec,3

86078 **investigation of transfusion reaction including suspicion of transmissible disease, interpretation and written report**
🚑 1.46 ⚕ 1.57 **FUD** XXX 🔲 🔲 🔲
AMA: 2020,Dec,3

86079 **authorization for deviation from standard blood banking procedures (eg, use of outdated blood, transfusion of Rh incompatible units), with written report**

EXCLUDES *Brucella antibodies (86622)*
Candida antibodies (86628)
Candida skin test (86485)
🚑 1.46 ⚕ 1.56 **FUD** XXX 🔲 🔲 🔲
AMA: 2020,Dec,3

86140-86344 [86152, 86153, 86328] Diagnostic Immunology Testing

86140 **C-reactive protein;**

EXCLUDES *Candidiasis (86628)*
🚑 0.00 ⚕ 0.00 **FUD** XXX 🔲 🔲
AMA: 2020,Dec,3

86141   **high sensitivity (hsCRP)**
⚙ 0.00   ⚖ 0.00   **FUD** XXX   Q ▢
AMA: 2020,Dec,3

86146   **Beta 2 Glycoprotein I antibody, each**
⚙ 0.00   ⚖ 0.00   **FUD** XXX   Q ▢
AMA: 2020,Dec,3

86147   **Cardiolipin (phospholipid) antibody, each Ig class**
⚙ 0.00   ⚖ 0.00   **FUD** XXX   Q ▢
AMA: 2020,Dec,3

86152   **Cell enumeration using immunologic selection and identification in fluid specimen (eg, circulating tumor cells in blood);**
EXCLUDES   Flow cytometric immunophenotyping (88184-88189)
            Flow cytometric quantitation (86355-86357,
               86359-86361, 86367)
Code also physician interpretation/report when performed
([86153])
⚙ 0.00   ⚖ 0.00   **FUD** XXX   Q ▢
AMA: 2020,Dec,3

86153   **physician interpretation and report, when required**
EXCLUDES   Flow cytometric immunophenotyping (88184-88189)
            Flow cytometric quantitation (86355-86357,
               86359-86361, 86367)
Code first cell enumeration, when performed ([86152])
⚙ 0.00   ⚖ 0.00   **FUD** 000   B 80 ▢
AMA: 2020,Dec,3

86148   **Anti-phosphatidylserine (phospholipid) antibody**
EXCLUDES   Antiprothrombin (phospholipid cofactor) antibody
               (86849)
⚙ 0.00   ⚖ 0.00   **FUD** XXX   Q ▢
AMA: 2020,Dec,3; 2018,Jan,8; 2017,Jan,8; 2016,Jan,13

86152   Resequenced code. See code following 86147.

86153   Resequenced code. See code before 86148.

86155   **Chemotaxis assay, specify method**
EXCLUDES   Antibodies, coccidioides (86635)
            Clostridium difficile toxin (87230)
            Skin test, coccidioides (86490)
⚙ 0.00   ⚖ 0.00   **FUD** XXX   Q ▢
AMA: 2020,Dec,3

86156   **Cold agglutinin; screen**
⚙ 0.00   ⚖ 0.00   **FUD** XXX   ▢
AMA: 2020,Dec,3

86157   **titer**
⚙ 0.00   ⚖ 0.00   **FUD** XXX   Q ▢
AMA: 2020,Dec,3

86160   **Complement; antigen, each component**
⚙ 0.00   ⚖ 0.00   **FUD** XXX   Q ▢
AMA: 2020,Dec,3

86161   **functional activity, each component**
⚙ 0.00   ⚖ 0.00   **FUD** XXX   Q ▢
AMA: 2020,Dec,3

86162   **total hemolytic (CH50)**
⚙ 0.00   ⚖ 0.00   **FUD** XXX   Q ▢
AMA: 2020,Dec,3

86171   **Complement fixation tests, each antigen**
EXCLUDES   Coombs test
⚙ 0.00   ⚖ 0.00   **FUD** XXX   Q ▢
AMA: 2020,Dec,3

86200   **Cyclic citrullinated peptide (CCP), antibody**
⚙ 0.00   ⚖ 0.00   **FUD** XXX   Q ▢
AMA: 2020,Dec,3; 2018,Jan,8; 2017,Jan,8; 2016,Jan,13

86215   **Deoxyribonuclease, antibody**
⚙ 0.00   ⚖ 0.00   **FUD** XXX   Q ▢
AMA: 2020,Dec,3

86225   **Deoxyribonucleic acid (DNA) antibody; native or double stranded**
EXCLUDES   Echinococcus antibodies, report code for specific method
            HIV antibody tests (86701-86703)
⚙ 0.00   ⚖ 0.00   **FUD** XXX   Q ▢
AMA: 2020,Dec,3

86226   **single stranded**
EXCLUDES   Anti-D.S, DNA, IFA, eg, using C. Lucilae (86255-86256)
⚙ 0.00   ⚖ 0.00   **FUD** XXX   Q ▢
AMA: 2020,Dec,3

● **86231**   **Endomysial antibody (EMA), each immunoglobulin (Ig) class**

86235   **Extractable nuclear antigen, antibody to, any method (eg, nRNP, SS-A, SS-B, Sm, RNP, Sc170, J01), each antibody**
⚙ 0.00   ⚖ 0.00   **FUD** XXX   Q ▢
AMA: 2020,Dec,3

86255   **Fluorescent noninfectious agent antibody; screen, each antibody**
⚙ 0.00   ⚖ 0.00   **FUD** XXX   Q 80 ▢
AMA: 2020,Dec,3; 2020,AugSE,1; 2020,AugSE,1; 2020,AugSE,1

86256   **titer, each antibody**
EXCLUDES   Fluorescent technique for antigen identification in tissue
               (88346, [88350])
            FTA (86780)
            Gel (agar) diffusion tests (86331)
            Indirect fluorescence (88346, [88350])
⚙ 0.00   ⚖ 0.00   **FUD** XXX   Q 80 ▢
AMA: 2020,Dec,3; 2020,AugSE,1; 2020,AugSE,1; 2020,AugSE,1

● **86258**   **Gliadin (deamidated) (DGP) antibody, each immunoglobulin (Ig) class**

86277   **Growth hormone, human (HGH), antibody**
⚙ 0.00   ⚖ 0.00   **FUD** XXX   Q ▢
AMA: 2020,Dec,3

86280   **Hemagglutination inhibition test (HAI)**
EXCLUDES   Antibodies to infectious agents (86602-86804)
            Rubella (86762)
⚙ 0.00   ⚖ 0.00   **FUD** XXX   Q ▢
AMA: 2020,Dec,3

86294   **Immunoassay for tumor antigen, qualitative or semiquantitative (eg, bladder tumor antigen)**
EXCLUDES   Qualitative NMP22 protein (86386)
⚙ 0.00   ⚖ 0.00   **FUD** XXX   ☒ Q ▢
AMA: 2020,Dec,3

86300   **Immunoassay for tumor antigen, quantitative; CA 15-3 (27.29)**
⚙ 0.00   ⚖ 0.00   **FUD** XXX   Q ▢
AMA: 2020,Dec,3

86301   **CA 19-9**
⚙ 0.00   ⚖ 0.00   **FUD** XXX   Q ▢
AMA: 2020,Dec,3

86304   **CA 125**
EXCLUDES   Antibody, hepatitis delta agent (86692)
            Measurement serum HER-2/neu oncoprotein (83950)
⚙ 0.00   ⚖ 0.00   **FUD** XXX   Q ▢
AMA: 2020,Dec,3

86305   **Human epididymis protein 4 (HE4)**
⚙ 0.00   ⚖ 0.00   **FUD** XXX   Q ▢
AMA: 2020,Dec,3

86308   **Heterophile antibodies; screening**
EXCLUDES   Antibodies, infectious agents (86602-86804)
⚙ 0.00   ⚖ 0.00   **FUD** XXX   ☒ Q ▢
AMA: 2020,Dec,3

86309   **titer**
EXCLUDES   Antibodies, infectious agents (86602-86804)
⚙ 0.00   ⚖ 0.00   **FUD** XXX   Q ▢
AMA: 2020,Dec,3

86310   titers after absorption with beef cells and guinea pig kidney

> EXCLUDES   *Antibodies, infectious agents (86602-86804)*
> *Histoplasma antibodies (86698)*
> *Histoplasmosis skin test (86510)*
> *Human growth hormone antibody (86277)*

🚑 0.00   ⚕ 0.00   **FUD** XXX   Q 💬

AMA: 2020,Dec,3

86316   Immunoassay for tumor antigen, other antigen, quantitative (eg, CA 50, 72-4, 549), each

🚑 0.00   ⚕ 0.00   **FUD** XXX   Q 💬

AMA: 2020,Dec,3; 2018,Jan,8; 2017,Jan,8; 2016,Jan,13

86317   Immunoassay for infectious agent antibody, quantitative, not otherwise specified

> EXCLUDES   *Immunoassay techniques for infectious antigens (87301-87451)*
> *Immunoassay techniques for noninfectious antigens (83516, 83518-83520)*
> *Immunoassay techniques with direct/visual observation for infectious antigens (87802-87899 [87806, 87811])*
> *Particle agglutination test (86403)*

🚑 0.00   ⚕ 0.00   **FUD** XXX   Q 💬

AMA: 2020,Dec,3; 2020,OctSE,1; 2020,OctSE,1

86318   Immunoassay for infectious agent antibody(ies), qualitative or semiquantitative, single-step method (eg, reagent strip);

🚑 0.00   ⚕ 0.00   **FUD** XXX   X Q 💬

AMA: 2020,Dec,3; 2020,AugSE,1; 2020,AugSE,1; 2020,AugSE,1; 2018,Jan,8; 2017,Jan,8; 2016,Jan,13

**86328**   severe acute respiratory syndrome coronavirus 2 (SARS-CoV-2) (Coronavirus disease [COVID-19])

> INCLUDES   Testing for antibodies only
> EXCLUDES   *Severe acute respiratory syndrome coronavirus 2 [SARS-CoV-2] [coronavirus disease [COVID-19]] testing via multiple-step method (86769)*
> *Testing for presence neutralizing antibodies that block cell infection ([86408, 86409])*

🚑 0.00   ⚕ 0.00   **FUD** XXX   💬

AMA: 2020,Dec,3; 2020,SepSE,1; 2020,AugSE,1; 2020,SepSE,1; 2020,AugSE,1; 2020,AugSE,1

86320   Immunoelectrophoresis; serum

🚑 0.00   ⚕ 0.00   **FUD** XXX   Q 80 💬

AMA: 2020,Dec,3

86325   other fluids (eg, urine, cerebrospinal fluid) with concentration

🚑 0.00   ⚕ 0.00   **FUD** XXX   Q 80 💬

AMA: 2020,Dec,3

86327   crossed (2-dimensional assay)

🚑 0.00   ⚕ 0.00   **FUD** XXX   Q 80 💬

AMA: 2020,Dec,3

86328   **Resequenced code. See code following 86318.**

86329   Immunodiffusion; not elsewhere specified

🚑 0.00   ⚕ 0.00   **FUD** XXX   Q 💬

AMA: 2020,Dec,3; 2018,Jan,8; 2017,Jan,8; 2016,Jan,13

86331   gel diffusion, qualitative (Ouchterlony), each antigen or antibody

🚑 0.00   ⚕ 0.00   **FUD** XXX   Q 💬

AMA: 2020,Dec,3

86332   Immune complex assay

🚑 0.00   ⚕ 0.00   **FUD** XXX   Q 💬

AMA: 2020,Dec,3

86334   Immunofixation electrophoresis; serum

🚑 0.00   ⚕ 0.00   **FUD** XXX   Q 80 💬

AMA: 2020,Dec,3

86335   other fluids with concentration (eg, urine, CSF)

🚑 0.00   ⚕ 0.00   **FUD** XXX   Q 80 💬

AMA: 2020,Dec,3

86336   Inhibin A

🚑 0.00   ⚕ 0.00   **FUD** XXX   Q 💬

AMA: 2020,Dec,3

86337   Insulin antibodies

🚑 0.00   ⚕ 0.00   **FUD** XXX   Q 💬

AMA: 2020,Dec,3

86340   Intrinsic factor antibodies

> EXCLUDES   *Antibodies, leptospira (86720)*
> *Leukoagglutinins (86021)*

🚑 0.00   ⚕ 0.00   **FUD** XXX   Q 💬

AMA: 2020,Dec,3

86341   Islet cell antibody

🚑 0.00   ⚕ 0.00   **FUD** XXX   Q 💬

AMA: 2020,Dec,3; 2018,Jan,8; 2017,Jan,8; 2016,Jan,13

86343   Leukocyte histamine release test (LHR)

🚑 0.00   ⚕ 0.00   **FUD** XXX   Q 💬

AMA: 2020,Dec,3

86344   Leukocyte phagocytosis

🚑 0.00   ⚕ 0.00   **FUD** XXX   Q 💬

AMA: 2020,Dec,3

86352 Assay Cellular Function

86352   Cellular function assay involving stimulation (eg, mitogen or antigen) and detection of biomarker (eg, ATP)

🚑 0.00   ⚕ 0.00   **FUD** XXX   Q 💬

AMA: 2020,Dec,3

86353 Lymphocyte Mitogen Response Assay

CMS: 100-03,190.8 Lymphocyte Mitogen Response Assays

86353   Lymphocyte transformation, mitogen (phytomitogen) or antigen induced blastogenesis

> EXCLUDES   *Cellular function assay with stimulation and biomarker detection (86352)*
> *Malaria antibodies (86750)*

🚑 0.00   ⚕ 0.00   **FUD** XXX   Q 💬

AMA: 2020,Dec,3

86355-86596 [86362, 86363, 86364, 86408, 86409, 86413] Additional Diagnostic Immunology Testing

86355   B cells, total count

> EXCLUDES   *Flow cytometry interpretation (88187-88189)*

🚑 0.00   ⚕ 0.00   **FUD** XXX   Q 💬

AMA: 2020,Dec,3; 2018,Jan,8; 2017,Jan,8; 2016,Jan,13

86356   Mononuclear cell antigen, quantitative (eg, flow cytometry), not otherwise specified, each antigen

> EXCLUDES   *Flow cytometry interpretation (88187-88189)*

🚑 0.00   ⚕ 0.00   **FUD** XXX   Q 💬

AMA: 2020,Dec,3; 2018,Jan,8; 2017,Jan,8; 2016,Jan,13

● **#**   **86362**   Myelin oligodendrocyte glycoprotein (MOG-IgG1) antibody; cell-based immunofluorescence assay (CBA), each

🚑 0.00   ⚕ 0.00   **FUD** 000

● **#**   **86363**   flow cytometry (ie, fluorescence-activated cell sorting [FACS]), each

🚑 0.00   ⚕ 0.00   **FUD** 000

86357   Natural killer (NK) cells, total count

> EXCLUDES   *Flow cytometry interpretation (88187-88189)*

🚑 0.00   ⚕ 0.00   **FUD** XXX   Q 💬

AMA: 2020,Dec,3; 2018,Jan,8; 2017,Jan,8; 2016,Jan,13

● **#**   **86364**   Tissue transglutaminase, each immunoglobulin (Ig) class

🚑 0.00   ⚕ 0.00   **FUD** 000

86359   T cells; total count

> EXCLUDES   *Flow cytometry interpretation (88187-88189)*

🚑 0.00   ⚕ 0.00   **FUD** XXX   Q 💬

AMA: 2020,Dec,3; 2018,Jan,8; 2017,Jan,8; 2016,Jan,13

● New Code   ▲ Revised Code   ○ Reinstated   ● New Web Release   ▲ Revised Web Release   + Add-on   Unlisted   Not Covered   # Resequenced

⑤⓪ Optum Mod 50 Exempt   ⊘ AMA Mod 51 Exempt   ⑤① Optum Mod 51 Exempt   ⑥③ Mod 63 Exempt   ✏ Non-FDA Drug   ★ Telemedicine   Ⓜ Maternity   Ⓐ Age Edit

86360 absolute CD4 and CD8 count, including ratio
> EXCLUDES *Flow cytometry interpretation (88187-88189)*
> 🚗 0.00   ⚗ 0.00   **FUD** XXX   Q ▣
>
> AMA: 2020,Dec,3; 2018,Jan,8; 2017,Jan,8; 2016,Jan,13

86361 absolute CD4 count
> EXCLUDES *Flow cytometry interpretation (88187-88189)*
> 🚗 0.00   ⚗ 0.00   **FUD** XXX   Q ▣
>
> AMA: 2020,Dec,3; 2018,Jan,8; 2017,Jan,8; 2016,Jan,13

86362 Resequenced code. See code following 86356.

86363 Resequenced code. See code following 86356.

86364 Resequenced code. See code following 86357.

86367 Stem cells (ie, CD34), total count
> EXCLUDES *Flow cytometric immunophenotyping, potential hematolymphoid neoplasia assessment (88184-88189)*
> *Flow cytometry interpretation (88187-88189)*
> 🚗 0.00   ⚗ 0.00   **FUD** XXX   Q ▣
>
> AMA: 2020,Dec,3; 2018,Jan,8; 2017,Jan,8; 2016,Jan,13

86376 Microsomal antibodies (eg, thyroid or liver-kidney), each
> 🚗 0.00   ⚗ 0.00   **FUD** XXX   Q ▣
>
> AMA: 2020,Dec,3; 2020,AugSE,1; 2020,AugSE,1; 2020,AugSE,1

● **86381** Mitochondrial antibody (eg, M2), each

86382 Neutralization test, viral
> 🚗 0.00   ⚗ 0.00   **FUD** XXX   Q ▣
>
> AMA: 2020,Dec,3

● # **86408** Neutralizing antibody, severe acute respiratory syndrome coronavirus 2 (SARS-CoV-2) (Coronavirus disease [COVID-19]); screen
> INCLUDES Testing for presence neutralizing antibodies that block cell infection
> EXCLUDES *Testing for presence antibodies only ([86328])*
> 🚗 0.00   ⚗ 0.00   **FUD** XXX
>
> AMA: 2020,Dec,3; 2020,AugSE,1

● # **86409** titer
> INCLUDES Testing for presence neutralizing antibodies that block cell infection
> EXCLUDES *Testing for presence antibodies only ([86328])*
> 🚗 0.00   ⚗ 0.00   **FUD** XXX
>
> AMA: 2020,Dec,3; 2020,AugSE,1

● # **86413** Severe acute respiratory syndrome coronavirus 2 (SARS-CoV-2) (Coronavirus disease [COVID-19]) antibody, quantitative
> INCLUDES Testing for presence and adaptive immune response to SARS-CoV-2
> 🚗 0.00   ⚗ 0.00   **FUD** XXX
>
> AMA: 2020,Dec,3; 2020,SepSE,1

86384 Nitroblue tetrazolium dye test (NTD)
> 🚗 0.00   ⚗ 0.00   **FUD** XXX   Q ▣
>
> AMA: 2020,Dec,3

86386 Nuclear Matrix Protein 22 (NMP22), qualitative
> EXCLUDES *Ouchterlony diffusion (86331)*
> *Platelet antibodies (86022, 86023)*
> 🚗 0.00   ⚗ 0.00   **FUD** XXX   ✖ Q ▣
>
> AMA: 2020,Dec,3

86403 Particle agglutination; screen, each antibody
> 🚗 0.00   ⚗ 0.00   **FUD** XXX   Q ▣
>
> AMA: 2020,Dec,3; 2020,OctSE,1; 2020,OctSE,1

86406 titer, each antibody
> EXCLUDES *Pregnancy test (84702, 84703)*
> *Rapid plasma reagin test (RPR) (86592, 86593)*
> 🚗 0.00   ⚗ 0.00   **FUD** XXX   Q ▣
>
> AMA: 2020,Dec,3

86408 Resequenced code. See code following 86382.

86409 Resequenced code. See code following 86382.

86413 Resequenced code. See code following resequenced code 86409.

86430 Rheumatoid factor; qualitative
> 🚗 0.00   ⚗ 0.00   **FUD** XXX   Q ▣
>
> AMA: 2020,Dec,3

86431 quantitative
> EXCLUDES *Serologic syphilis testing (86592, 86593)*
> 🚗 0.00   ⚗ 0.00   **FUD** XXX   Q ▣
>
> AMA: 2020,Dec,3

86480 Tuberculosis test, cell mediated immunity antigen response measurement; gamma interferon
> 🚗 0.00   ⚗ 0.00   **FUD** XXX   Q ▣
>
> AMA: 2020,Dec,3; 2019,Dec,12; 2018,Jan,8; 2017,Jan,8; 2016,Jan,13

86481 enumeration of gamma interferon-producing T-cells in cell suspension
> 🚗 0.00   ⚗ 0.00   **FUD** XXX   Q ▣
>
> AMA: 2020,Dec,3; 2019,Dec,12

86485 Skin test; candida
> EXCLUDES *Candida antibody (86628)*
> 🚗 0.00   ⚗ 0.00   **FUD** XXX   Q1 80 TC ▣
>
> AMA: 2020,Dec,3

86486 unlisted antigen, each
> 🚗 0.15   ⚗ 0.15   **FUD** XXX   Q1 80 TC ▣
>
> AMA: 2020,Dec,3

86490 coccidioidomycosis
> 🚗 2.49   ⚗ 2.49   **FUD** XXX   Q1 80 TC ▣
>
> AMA: 2020,Dec,3

86510 histoplasmosis
> EXCLUDES *Histoplasma antibody (86698)*
> 🚗 0.19   ⚗ 0.19   **FUD** XXX   Q1 80 TC ▣
>
> AMA: 2020,Dec,3

86580 tuberculosis, intradermal
> INCLUDES Heaf test
> Intradermal Mantoux test
> EXCLUDES *Antibodies to sporothrix, report code for specific method*
> *Skin test for allergy (95012-95199)*
> *Smooth muscle antibody ([86015])*
> *Tuberculosis test, cell mediated immunity measurement gamma interferon antigen response (86480)*
> 🚗 0.26   ⚗ 0.26   **FUD** XXX   Q1 80 TC ▣
>
> AMA: 2020,Dec,3

86590 Streptokinase, antibody
> EXCLUDES *Antibodies, infectious agents (86602-86804)*
> *Streptolysin O antibody, antistreptolysin O (86060, 86063)*
> 🚗 0.00   ⚗ 0.00   **FUD** XXX   Q ▣
>
> AMA: 2020,Dec,3

86592 Syphilis test, non-treponemal antibody; qualitative (eg, VDRL, RPR, ART)
> INCLUDES Wasserman test
> EXCLUDES *Antibodies to infectious agents (86602-86804)*
> 🚗 0.00   ⚗ 0.00   **FUD** XXX   A ▣
>
> AMA: 2020,Dec,3

86593 quantitative
> EXCLUDES *Antibodies, infectious agents (86602-86804)*
> *Tetanus antibody (86774)*
> *Thyroglobulin (84432)*
> *Thyroglobulin antibody (86800)*
> *Thyroid microsomal antibody (86376)*
> *Toxoplasma antibody (86777-86778)*
> 🚗 0.00   ⚗ 0.00   **FUD** XXX   A ▣
>
> AMA: 2020,Dec,3

● **86596** Voltage-gated calcium channel antibody, each

| 26/TC PC/TC Only | A2-Z3 ASC Payment | 50 Bilateral | ♂ Male Only | ♀ Female Only | 🚗 Facility RVU | ⚗ Non-Facility RVU | ▣ CCI | ✖ CLIA |
| **FUD** Follow-up Days | **CMS:** IOM | **AMA:** CPT Asst | A-Y OPPSI | 80/80 Surg Assist Allowed / w/Doc | 🔲 Lab Crosswalk | 🔲 Radiology Crosswalk |

412   CPT © 2021 American Medical Association. All Rights Reserved.   © 2021 Optum360, LLC

86602-86698 Testing for Antibodies to Infectious Agents: Actinomyces—Histoplasma

INCLUDES Qualitative or semiquantitative immunoassays performed by multiple-step methods for detection, antibodies to infectious agents

EXCLUDES Detection:

Antibodies other than those to infectious agents, see specific antibody or method

Infectious agent/antigen (87260-87899 [87623, 87624, 87625, 87806])

Immunoassays by single-step method (86318, [86328])

86602 **Antibody; actinomyces**
🚑 0.00   ✂ 0.00   **FUD** XXX   🔲🖼
AMA: 2020,Dec,3; 2020,OctSE,1; 2020,OctSE,1; 2020,AugSE,1; 2020,AugSE,1; 2020,AugSE,1; 2018,Jan,8; 2017,Jan,8; 2016,Jan,13

86603 **adenovirus**
🚑 0.00   ✂ 0.00   **FUD** XXX   🔲🖼
AMA: 2020,Dec,3; 2020,OctSE,1; 2020,OctSE,1; 2020,AugSE,1; 2020,AugSE,1; 2020,AugSE,1

86606 **Aspergillus**
🚑 0.00   ✂ 0.00   **FUD** XXX   🔲🖼
AMA: 2020,Dec,3; 2020,OctSE,1; 2020,OctSE,1; 2020,AugSE,1; 2020,AugSE,1; 2020,AugSE,1

86609 **bacterium, not elsewhere specified**
🚑 0.00   ✂ 0.00   **FUD** XXX   🔲🖼
AMA: 2020,Dec,3; 2020,OctSE,1; 2020,OctSE,1; 2020,AugSE,1; 2020,AugSE,1; 2020,AugSE,1

86611 **Bartonella**
🚑 0.00   ✂ 0.00   **FUD** XXX   🔲🖼
AMA: 2020,Dec,3; 2020,OctSE,1; 2020,OctSE,1; 2020,AugSE,1; 2020,AugSE,1; 2020,AugSE,1

86612 **Blastomyces**
🚑 0.00   ✂ 0.00   **FUD** XXX   🔲🖼
AMA: 2020,Dec,3; 2020,OctSE,1; 2020,OctSE,1; 2020,AugSE,1; 2020,AugSE,1; 2020,AugSE,1

86615 **Bordetella**
🚑 0.00   ✂ 0.00   **FUD** XXX   🔲🖼
AMA: 2020,Dec,3; 2020,OctSE,1; 2020,OctSE,1; 2020,AugSE,1; 2020,AugSE,1; 2020,AugSE,1

86617 **Borrelia burgdorferi (Lyme disease) confirmatory test (eg, Western Blot or immunoblot)**
🚑 0.00   ✂ 0.00   **FUD** XXX   🔲🖼
AMA: 2020,Dec,3; 2020,OctSE,1; 2020,OctSE,1; 2020,AugSE,1; 2020,AugSE,1; 2020,AugSE,1

86618 **Borrelia burgdorferi (Lyme disease)**
🚑 0.00   ✂ 0.00   **FUD** XXX   ❌🔲🖼
AMA: 2020,Dec,3; 2020,OctSE,1; 2020,OctSE,1; 2020,AugSE,1; 2020,AugSE,1; 2020,AugSE,1

86619 **Borrelia (relapsing fever)**
🚑 0.00   ✂ 0.00   **FUD** XXX   🔲🖼
AMA: 2020,Dec,3; 2020,OctSE,1; 2020,OctSE,1; 2020,AugSE,1; 2020,AugSE,1; 2020,AugSE,1

86622 **Brucella**
🚑 0.00   ✂ 0.00   **FUD** XXX   🔲🖼
AMA: 2020,Dec,3; 2020,OctSE,1; 2020,OctSE,1; 2020,AugSE,1; 2020,AugSE,1; 2020,AugSE,1

86625 **Campylobacter**
🚑 0.00   ✂ 0.00   **FUD** XXX   🔲🖼
AMA: 2020,Dec,3; 2020,OctSE,1; 2020,OctSE,1; 2020,AugSE,1; 2020,AugSE,1; 2020,AugSE,1

86628 **Candida**
EXCLUDES Candida skin test (86485)
🚑 0.00   ✂ 0.00   **FUD** XXX   🔲🖼
AMA: 2020,Dec,3; 2020,OctSE,1; 2020,OctSE,1; 2020,AugSE,1; 2020,AugSE,1; 2020,AugSE,1

86631 **Chlamydia**
🚑 0.00   ✂ 0.00   **FUD** XXX   🅰🖼
AMA: 2020,Dec,3; 2020,OctSE,1; 2020,OctSE,1; 2020,AugSE,1; 2020,AugSE,1; 2020,AugSE,1

86632 **Chlamydia, IgM**
EXCLUDES Chlamydia antigen (87270, 87320)
Fluorescent antibody technique (86255-86256)
🚑 0.00   ✂ 0.00   **FUD** XXX   🅰🖼
AMA: 2020,Dec,3; 2020,OctSE,1; 2020,OctSE,1; 2020,AugSE,1; 2020,AugSE,1; 2020,AugSE,1

86635 **Coccidioides**
EXCLUDES Severe Acute Respiratory Syndrome Coronavirus 2 [SARS-CoV-2] [Coronavirus disease {COVID-19}] antibody testing ([86328], 86769)
🚑 0.00   ✂ 0.00   **FUD** XXX   🔲🖼
AMA: 2020,Dec,3; 2020,OctSE,1; 2020,OctSE,1; 2020,AugSE,1; 2020,AugSE,1; 2020,AugSE,1

86638 **Coxiella burnetii (Q fever)**
🚑 0.00   ✂ 0.00   **FUD** XXX   🔲🖼
AMA: 2020,Dec,3; 2020,OctSE,1; 2020,OctSE,1; 2020,AugSE,1; 2020,AugSE,1; 2020,AugSE,1

86641 **Cryptococcus**
🚑 0.00   ✂ 0.00   **FUD** XXX   🔲🖼
AMA: 2020,Dec,3; 2020,OctSE,1; 2020,OctSE,1; 2020,AugSE,1; 2020,AugSE,1; 2020,AugSE,1

86644 **cytomegalovirus (CMV)**
🚑 0.00   ✂ 0.00   **FUD** XXX   🔲🖼
AMA: 2020,Dec,3; 2020,OctSE,1; 2020,OctSE,1; 2020,AugSE,1; 2020,AugSE,1; 2020,AugSE,1

86645 **cytomegalovirus (CMV), IgM**
🚑 0.00   ✂ 0.00   **FUD** XXX   🔲🖼
AMA: 2020,Dec,3; 2020,OctSE,1; 2020,OctSE,1; 2020,AugSE,1; 2020,AugSE,1; 2020,AugSE,1; 2018,Jan,8; 2017,Jan,8; 2016,Jan,13

86648 **Diphtheria**
🚑 0.00   ✂ 0.00   **FUD** XXX   🔲🖼
AMA: 2020,Dec,3; 2020,OctSE,1; 2020,OctSE,1; 2020,AugSE,1; 2020,AugSE,1; 2020,AugSE,1

86651 **encephalitis, California (La Crosse)**
🚑 0.00   ✂ 0.00   **FUD** XXX   🔲🖼
AMA: 2020,Dec,3; 2020,OctSE,1; 2020,OctSE,1; 2020,AugSE,1; 2020,AugSE,1; 2020,AugSE,1

86652 **encephalitis, Eastern equine**
🚑 0.00   ✂ 0.00   **FUD** XXX   🔲🖼
AMA: 2020,Dec,3; 2020,OctSE,1; 2020,OctSE,1; 2020,AugSE,1; 2020,AugSE,1; 2020,AugSE,1

86653 **encephalitis, St. Louis**
🚑 0.00   ✂ 0.00   **FUD** XXX   🔲🖼
AMA: 2020,Dec,3; 2020,OctSE,1; 2020,OctSE,1; 2020,AugSE,1; 2020,AugSE,1; 2020,AugSE,1

86654 **encephalitis, Western equine**
🚑 0.00   ✂ 0.00   **FUD** XXX   🔲🖼
AMA: 2020,Dec,3; 2020,OctSE,1; 2020,OctSE,1; 2020,AugSE,1; 2020,AugSE,1; 2020,AugSE,1

86658 **enterovirus (eg, coxsackie, echo, polio)**
EXCLUDES Antibodies to:
Trichinella (86784)
Trypanosoma—see code for specific methodology
Tuberculosis (86580)
Viral—see code for specific methodology
🚑 0.00   ✂ 0.00   **FUD** XXX   🔲🖼
AMA: 2020,Dec,3; 2020,OctSE,1; 2020,OctSE,1; 2020,AugSE,1; 2020,AugSE,1; 2020,AugSE,1

86663 **Epstein-Barr (EB) virus, early antigen (EA)**
🚑 0.00   ✂ 0.00   **FUD** XXX   🔲🖼
AMA: 2020,Dec,3; 2020,OctSE,1; 2020,OctSE,1; 2020,AugSE,1; 2020,AugSE,1; 2020,AugSE,1

86664 **Epstein-Barr (EB) virus, nuclear antigen (EBNA)**
🚑 0.00   ✂ 0.00   **FUD** XXX   🔲🖼
AMA: 2020,Dec,3; 2020,OctSE,1; 2020,OctSE,1; 2020,AugSE,1; 2020,AugSE,1; 2020,AugSE,1

86665 Epstein-Barr (EB) virus, viral capsid (VCA)
🔲 0.00 ⚖ 0.00 **FUD** XXX   🔲🔲
AMA: 2020,Dec,3; 2020,OctSE,1; 2020,OctSE,1; 2020,AugSE,1; 2020,AugSE,1; 2020,AugSE,1

86666 Ehrlichia
🔲 0.00 ⚖ 0.00 **FUD** XXX   🔲🔲
AMA: 2020,Dec,3; 2020,OctSE,1; 2020,OctSE,1; 2020,AugSE,1; 2020,AugSE,1; 2020,AugSE,1

86668 Francisella tularensis
🔲 0.00 ⚖ 0.00 **FUD** XXX   🔲🔲
AMA: 2020,Dec,3; 2020,OctSE,1; 2020,OctSE,1; 2020,AugSE,1; 2020,AugSE,1; 2020,AugSE,1

86671 fungus, not elsewhere specified
🔲 0.00 ⚖ 0.00 **FUD** XXX   🔲🔲
AMA: 2020,Dec,3; 2020,OctSE,1; 2020,OctSE,1; 2020,AugSE,1; 2020,AugSE,1; 2020,AugSE,1

86674 Giardia lamblia
🔲 0.00 ⚖ 0.00 **FUD** XXX   🔲🔲
AMA: 2020,Dec,3; 2020,OctSE,1; 2020,OctSE,1; 2020,AugSE,1; 2020,AugSE,1; 2020,AugSE,1

86677 Helicobacter pylori
🔲 0.00 ⚖ 0.00 **FUD** XXX   🔲🔲
AMA: 2020,Dec,3; 2020,OctSE,1; 2020,OctSE,1; 2020,AugSE,1; 2020,AugSE,1; 2020,AugSE,1; 2018,Jan,8; 2017,Jan,8; 2016,Jan,13

86682 helminth, not elsewhere specified
🔲 0.00 ⚖ 0.00 **FUD** XXX   🔲🔲
AMA: 2020,Dec,3; 2020,OctSE,1; 2020,OctSE,1; 2020,AugSE,1; 2020,AugSE,1; 2020,AugSE,1

86684 Haemophilus influenza
🔲 0.00 ⚖ 0.00 **FUD** XXX   🔲🔲
AMA: 2020,Dec,3; 2020,OctSE,1; 2020,OctSE,1; 2020,AugSE,1; 2020,AugSE,1; 2020,AugSE,1

86687 HTLV-I
🔲 0.00 ⚖ 0.00 **FUD** XXX   🔲🔲
AMA: 2020,Dec,3; 2020,OctSE,1; 2020,OctSE,1; 2020,AugSE,1; 2020,AugSE,1; 2020,AugSE,1

86688 HTLV-II
🔲 0.00 ⚖ 0.00 **FUD** XXX   🔲🔲
AMA: 2020,Dec,3; 2020,OctSE,1; 2020,OctSE,1; 2020,AugSE,1; 2020,AugSE,1; 2020,AugSE,1

86689 HTLV or HIV antibody, confirmatory test (eg, Western Blot)
🔲 0.00 ⚖ 0.00 **FUD** XXX   🔲🔲
AMA: 2020,Dec,3; 2020,OctSE,1; 2020,OctSE,1; 2020,AugSE,1; 2020,AugSE,1; 2020,AugSE,1; 2018,Jan,8; 2017,Jan,8; 2016,Jan,13

86692 hepatitis, delta agent
> *EXCLUDES* Hepatitis delta agent, antigen (87380)

🔲 0.00 ⚖ 0.00 **FUD** XXX   🔲🔲
AMA: 2020,Dec,3; 2020,OctSE,1; 2020,OctSE,1; 2020,AugSE,1; 2020,AugSE,1; 2020,AugSE,1

86694 herpes simplex, non-specific type test
🔲 0.00 ⚖ 0.00 **FUD** XXX   🔲🔲
AMA: 2020,Dec,3; 2020,OctSE,1; 2020,OctSE,1; 2020,AugSE,1; 2020,AugSE,1; 2020,AugSE,1

86695 herpes simplex, type 1
🔲 0.00 ⚖ 0.00 **FUD** XXX   🔲🔲
AMA: 2020,Dec,3; 2020,OctSE,1; 2020,OctSE,1; 2020,AugSE,1; 2020,AugSE,1; 2020,AugSE,1; 2018,Jan,8; 2017,Jan,8; 2016,Jan,13

86696 herpes simplex, type 2
🔲 0.00 ⚖ 0.00 **FUD** XXX   🔲🔲
AMA: 2020,Dec,3; 2020,OctSE,1; 2020,OctSE,1; 2020,AugSE,1; 2020,AugSE,1; 2020,AugSE,1

86698 histoplasma
🔲 0.00 ⚖ 0.00 **FUD** XXX   🔲🔲
AMA: 2020,Dec,3; 2020,OctSE,1; 2020,OctSE,1; 2020,AugSE,1; 2020,AugSE,1; 2020,AugSE,1

86701-86703 Testing for HIV Antibodies
CMS: 100-03,190.14 Human Immunodeficiency Virus Testing (Diagnosis); 100-03,190.9 Serologic Testing for Acquired Immunodeficiency Syndrome (AIDS)

> *INCLUDES* Qualitative or semiquantitative immunoassays performed by multiple-step methods for detection, antibodies to infectious agents
> *EXCLUDES* Confirmatory test for HIV antibody (86689)
> HIV-1 antigen (87390)
> HIV-1 antigen(s) with HIV 1 and 2 antibodies, single result (87389)
> HIV-2 antigen (87391)
> Immunoassays by single-step method (86318)

Code also modifier 92 for test performed using kit or transportable instrument comprising (all or part) single-use, disposable analytical chamber

86701 Antibody; HIV-1
🔲 0.00 ⚖ 0.00 **FUD** XXX   ❌🔲🔲
AMA: 2020,Dec,3; 2020,OctSE,1; 2020,OctSE,1; 2020,AugSE,1; 2020,AugSE,1; 2020,AugSE,1; 2018,Jan,8; 2017,Jan,8; 2016,Jan,13

86702 HIV-2
🔲 0.00 ⚖ 0.00 **FUD** XXX   🔲🔲
AMA: 2020,Dec,3; 2020,OctSE,1; 2020,OctSE,1; 2020,AugSE,1; 2020,AugSE,1; 2020,AugSE,1; 2018,Jan,8; 2017,Jan,8; 2016,Jan,13

86703 HIV-1 and HIV-2, single result
🔲 0.00 ⚖ 0.00 **FUD** XXX   🔲🔲
AMA: 2020,Dec,3; 2020,OctSE,1; 2020,OctSE,1; 2020,AugSE,1; 2020,AugSE,1; 2020,AugSE,1; 2018,Jan,8; 2017,Jan,8; 2016,Jan,13

86704-86804 Testing for Infectious Disease Antibodies: Hepatitis—Yersinia
> *INCLUDES* Qualitative or semiquantitative immunoassays performed by multiple-step methods for detection, antibodies to infectious agents
> *EXCLUDES* Detection of:
> Antibodies other than those to infectious agents, see specific antibody or method
> Infectious agent/antigen (87260-87899 [87623, 87624, 87625, 87806])
> Immunoassays by single-step method (86318)

86704 Hepatitis B core antibody (HBcAb); total
🔲 0.00 ⚖ 0.00 **FUD** XXX   🔲🔲
AMA: 2020,Dec,3; 2020,OctSE,1; 2020,OctSE,1; 2020,AugSE,1; 2020,AugSE,1; 2018,Jan,8; 2017,Jan,8; 2016,Jan,13

86705 IgM antibody
🔲 0.00 ⚖ 0.00 **FUD** XXX   🔲🔲
AMA: 2020,Dec,3; 2020,OctSE,1; 2020,OctSE,1; 2020,AugSE,1; 2020,AugSE,1; 2018,Jan,8; 2017,Jan,8; 2016,Jan,13

86706 Hepatitis B surface antibody (HBsAb)
🔲 0.00 ⚖ 0.00 **FUD** XXX   🔲🔲
AMA: 2020,Dec,3; 2020,OctSE,1; 2020,OctSE,1; 2020,AugSE,1; 2020,AugSE,1

86707 Hepatitis Be antibody (HBeAb)
🔲 0.00 ⚖ 0.00 **FUD** XXX   🔲🔲
AMA: 2020,Dec,3; 2020,OctSE,1; 2020,OctSE,1; 2020,AugSE,1; 2020,AugSE,1

86708 Hepatitis A antibody (HAAb)
🔲 0.00 ⚖ 0.00 **FUD** XXX   🔲🔲
AMA: 2020,Dec,3; 2020,OctSE,1; 2020,OctSE,1; 2020,AugSE,1; 2020,AugSE,1; 2018,Jan,8; 2017,Jan,8; 2016,Jan,13

86709 Hepatitis A antibody (HAAb), IgM antibody
🔲 0.00 ⚖ 0.00 **FUD** XXX   🔲🔲
AMA: 2020,Dec,3; 2020,OctSE,1; 2020,OctSE,1; 2020,AugSE,1; 2020,AugSE,1; 2018,Jan,8; 2017,Jan,8; 2016,Jan,13

86710 Antibody; influenza virus
🔲 0.00 ⚖ 0.00 **FUD** XXX   🔲🔲
AMA: 2020,Dec,3; 2020,OctSE,1; 2020,OctSE,1; 2020,AugSE,1; 2020,AugSE,1; 2018,Jan,8; 2017,Jan,8; 2016,Jan,13

86711 JC (John Cunningham) virus
🔲 0.00 ⚖ 0.00 **FUD** XXX   🔲🔲
AMA: 2020,Dec,3; 2020,OctSE,1; 2020,OctSE,1; 2020,AugSE,1; 2020,AugSE,1

86713 Legionella
🔲 0.00 ⚖ 0.00 **FUD** XXX   🔲🔲
AMA: 2020,Dec,3; 2020,OctSE,1; 2020,OctSE,1; 2020,AugSE,1; 2020,AugSE,1

26/TC PC/TC Only   A2-Z3 ASC Payment   50 Bilateral   ♂ Male Only   ♀ Female Only   Facility RVU   Non-Facility RVU   CCI   CLIA
FUD Follow-up Days   **CMS:** IOM   **AMA:** CPT Asst   A-Y OPPSI   80/80 Surg Assist Allowed / w/Doc   Lab Crosswalk   Radiology Crosswalk

414   CPT © 2021 American Medical Association. All Rights Reserved.   © 2021 Optum360, LLC

86717	**Leishmania**

🔧 0.00   ⚕ 0.00   **FUD** XXX   ▣ ▢

AMA: 2020,Dec,3; 2020,OctSE,1; 2020,OctSE,1; 2020,AugSE,1; 2020,AugSE,1; 2020,AugSE,1

86720	**Leptospira**

🔧 0.00   ⚕ 0.00   **FUD** XXX   ▣ ▢

AMA: 2020,Dec,3; 2020,OctSE,1; 2020,OctSE,1; 2020,AugSE,1; 2020,AugSE,1; 2020,AugSE,1

86723	**Listeria monocytogenes**

🔧 0.00   ⚕ 0.00   **FUD** XXX   ▣ ▢

AMA: 2020,Dec,3; 2020,OctSE,1; 2020,OctSE,1; 2020,AugSE,1; 2020,AugSE,1; 2020,AugSE,1

86727	**lymphocytic choriomeningitis**

🔧 0.00   ⚕ 0.00   **FUD** XXX   ▣ ▢

AMA: 2020,Dec,3; 2020,OctSE,1; 2020,OctSE,1; 2020,AugSE,1; 2020,AugSE,1; 2020,AugSE,1

86732	**mucormycosis**

🔧 0.00   ⚕ 0.00   **FUD** XXX   ▣ ▢

AMA: 2020,Dec,3; 2020,OctSE,1; 2020,OctSE,1; 2020,AugSE,1; 2020,AugSE,1; 2020,AugSE,1

86735	**mumps**

🔧 0.00   ⚕ 0.00   **FUD** XXX   ▣ ▢

AMA: 2020,Dec,3; 2020,OctSE,1; 2020,OctSE,1; 2020,AugSE,1; 2020,AugSE,1; 2020,AugSE,1; 2018,Jan,8; 2017,Jan,8; 2016,Jan,13

86738	**mycoplasma**

🔧 0.00   ⚕ 0.00   **FUD** XXX   ▣ ▢

AMA: 2020,Dec,3; 2020,OctSE,1; 2020,OctSE,1; 2020,AugSE,1; 2020,AugSE,1

86741	**Neisseria meningitidis**

🔧 0.00   ⚕ 0.00   **FUD** XXX   ▣ ▢

AMA: 2020,Dec,3; 2020,OctSE,1; 2020,OctSE,1; 2020,AugSE,1; 2020,AugSE,1

86744	**Nocardia**

🔧 0.00   ⚕ 0.00   **FUD** XXX   ▣ ▢

AMA: 2020,Dec,3; 2020,OctSE,1; 2020,OctSE,1; 2020,AugSE,1; 2020,AugSE,1

86747	**parvovirus**

🔧 0.00   ⚕ 0.00   **FUD** XXX   ▣ ▢

AMA: 2020,Dec,3; 2020,OctSE,1; 2020,OctSE,1; 2020,AugSE,1; 2020,AugSE,1

86750	**Plasmodium (malaria)**

🔧 0.00   ⚕ 0.00   **FUD** XXX   ▣ ▢

AMA: 2020,Dec,3; 2020,OctSE,1; 2020,OctSE,1; 2020,AugSE,1; 2020,AugSE,1

86753	**protozoa, not elsewhere specified**

🔧 0.00   ⚕ 0.00   **FUD** XXX   ▣ ▢

AMA: 2020,Dec,3; 2020,OctSE,1; 2020,OctSE,1; 2020,AugSE,1; 2020,AugSE,1

86756	**respiratory syncytial virus**

🔧 0.00   ⚕ 0.00   **FUD** XXX   ▣ ▢

AMA: 2020,Dec,3; 2020,OctSE,1; 2020,OctSE,1; 2020,AugSE,1; 2020,AugSE,1

86757	**Rickettsia**

🔧 0.00   ⚕ 0.00   **FUD** XXX   ▣ ▢

AMA: 2020,Dec,3; 2020,OctSE,1; 2020,OctSE,1; 2020,AugSE,1; 2020,AugSE,1

86759	**rotavirus**

🔧 0.00   ⚕ 0.00   **FUD** XXX   ▣ ▢

AMA: 2020,Dec,3; 2020,OctSE,1; 2020,OctSE,1; 2020,AugSE,1; 2020,AugSE,1

86762	**rubella**

🔧 0.00   ⚕ 0.00   **FUD** XXX   ▣ ▢

AMA: 2020,Dec,3; 2020,OctSE,1; 2020,OctSE,1; 2020,AugSE,1; 2020,AugSE,1

86765	**rubeola**

🔧 0.00   ⚕ 0.00   **FUD** XXX   ▣ ▢

AMA: 2020,Dec,3; 2020,OctSE,1; 2020,OctSE,1; 2020,AugSE,1; 2020,AugSE,1; 2020,AugSE,1

86768	**Salmonella**

🔧 0.00   ⚕ 0.00   **FUD** XXX   ▣ ▢

AMA: 2020,Dec,3; 2020,OctSE,1; 2020,OctSE,1; 2020,AugSE,1; 2020,AugSE,1; 2020,AugSE,1

86769	**severe acute respiratory syndrome coronavirus 2 (SARS-CoV-2) (Coronavirus disease [COVID-19])**

EXCLUDES *Antibody, severe acute respiratory syndrome coronavirus 2 (SARS-CoV-2) (coronavirus disease [COVID-19]), includes titer(s) (0224U)*
Severe acute respiratory syndrome coronavirus 2 (SARS-CoV-2) (coronavirus disease [COVID-19]) antibody testing via single-step method ([86328])

🔧 0.00   ⚕ 0.00   **FUD** XXX   ▢

AMA: 2020,Dec,3; 2020,OctSE,1; 2020,SepSE,1; 2020,OctSE,1; 2020,AugSE,1; 2020,SepSE,1; 2020,AugSE,1; 2020,AugSE,1; 2020,May,3; 2020,JuneSE,1

86771	**Shigella**

🔧 0.00   ⚕ 0.00   **FUD** XXX   ▣ ▢

AMA: 2020,Dec,3; 2020,OctSE,1; 2020,OctSE,1; 2020,AugSE,1; 2020,AugSE,1

86774	**tetanus**

🔧 0.00   ⚕ 0.00   **FUD** XXX   ▣ ▢

AMA: 2020,Dec,3; 2020,OctSE,1; 2020,OctSE,1; 2020,AugSE,1; 2020,AugSE,1

86777	**Toxoplasma**

🔧 0.00   ⚕ 0.00   **FUD** XXX   ▣ ▢

AMA: 2020,Dec,3; 2020,OctSE,1; 2020,OctSE,1; 2020,AugSE,1; 2020,AugSE,1

86778	**Toxoplasma, IgM**

🔧 0.00   ⚕ 0.00   **FUD** XXX   ▣ ▢

AMA: 2020,Dec,3; 2020,OctSE,1; 2020,OctSE,1; 2020,AugSE,1; 2020,AugSE,1

86780	**Treponema pallidum**

EXCLUDES *Nontreponemal antibody analysis syphilis testing (86592-86593)*

🔧 0.00   ⚕ 0.00   **FUD** XXX   ✖ Ⓐ ▢

AMA: 2020,Dec,3; 2020,OctSE,1; 2020,OctSE,1; 2020,AugSE,1; 2020,AugSE,1

86784	**Trichinella**

🔧 0.00   ⚕ 0.00   **FUD** XXX   ▣ ▢

AMA: 2020,Dec,3; 2020,OctSE,1; 2020,OctSE,1; 2020,AugSE,1; 2020,AugSE,1

86787	**varicella-zoster**

🔧 0.00   ⚕ 0.00   **FUD** XXX   ▣ ▢

AMA: 2020,Dec,3; 2020,OctSE,1; 2020,OctSE,1; 2020,AugSE,1; 2020,AugSE,1

86788	**West Nile virus, IgM**

🔧 0.00   ⚕ 0.00   **FUD** XXX   ▣ ▢

AMA: 2020,Dec,3; 2020,OctSE,1; 2020,OctSE,1; 2020,AugSE,1; 2020,AugSE,1

86789	**West Nile virus**

🔧 0.00   ⚕ 0.00   **FUD** XXX   ▣ ▢

AMA: 2020,Dec,3; 2020,OctSE,1; 2020,OctSE,1; 2020,AugSE,1; 2020,AugSE,1

86790	**virus, not elsewhere specified**

🔧 0.00   ⚕ 0.00   **FUD** XXX   ▣ ▢

AMA: 2020,Dec,3; 2020,OctSE,1; 2020,OctSE,1; 2020,AugSE,1; 2020,AugSE,1

86793	**Yersinia**

🔧 0.00   ⚕ 0.00   **FUD** XXX   ▣ ▢

AMA: 2020,Dec,3; 2020,OctSE,1; 2020,OctSE,1; 2020,AugSE,1; 2020,AugSE,1

● New Code   ▲ Revised Code   ○ Reinstated   ● New Web Release   ▲ Revised Web Release   + Add-on   Unlisted   Not Covered   # Resequenced
㊿ Optum Mod 50 Exempt   ⊘ AMA Mod 51 Exempt   ㊿ Optum Mod 51 Exempt   ㊿ Mod 63 Exempt   ⚡ Non-FDA Drug   ★ Telemedicine   Ⓜ Maternity   Ⓐ Age Edit

© 2021 Optum360, LLC   CPT © 2021 American Medical Association. All Rights Reserved.   415

86794   **Zika virus, IgM**
    0.00   0.00   **FUD** XXX
    AMA: 2020,Dec,3; 2020,OctSE,1; 2020,OctSE,1; 2020,AugSE,1; 2020,AugSE,1; 2020,AugSE,1

86800   **Thyroglobulin antibody**
    EXCLUDES   *Thyroglobulin (84432)*
    0.00   0.00   **FUD** XXX
    AMA: 2020,Dec,3; 2020,OctSE,1; 2020,OctSE,1; 2020,AugSE,1; 2020,AugSE,1; 2020,AugSE,1

86803   **Hepatitis C antibody;**
    0.00   0.00   **FUD** XXX
    AMA: 2020,Dec,3; 2020,OctSE,1; 2020,OctSE,1; 2020,AugSE,1; 2020,AugSE,1; 2020,AugSE,1

86804   **confirmatory test (eg, immunoblot)**
    0.00   0.00   **FUD** XXX
    AMA: 2020,Dec,3; 2020,OctSE,1; 2020,OctSE,1; 2020,AugSE,1; 2020,AugSE,1; 2020,AugSE,1; 2018,Jan,8; 2017,Jan,8; 2016,Jan,13

86805-86808 Pre-Transplant Antibody Cross Matching

86805   **Lymphocytotoxicity assay, visual crossmatch; with titration**
    0.00   0.00   **FUD** XXX
    AMA: 2020,Dec,3; 2018,Jan,8; 2017,Jan,8; 2016,Jan,13

86806   **without titration**
    0.00   0.00   **FUD** XXX
    AMA: 2020,Dec,3

86807   **Serum screening for cytotoxic percent reactive antibody (PRA); standard method**
    0.00   0.00   **FUD** XXX
    AMA: 2020,Dec,3; 2018,Jan,8; 2017,Jan,8; 2016,Jan,13

86808   **quick method**
    0.00   0.00   **FUD** XXX
    AMA: 2020,Dec,3; 2018,Jan,8; 2017,Jan,8; 2016,Jan,13

86812-86826 Histocompatibility Testing

CMS: 100-03,110.23 Stem Cell Transplantation; 100-03,190.1 Histocompatibility Testing; 100-04,3,90.3 Stem Cell Transplantation; 100-04,3,90.3.1 Allogeneic Stem Cell Transplantation; 100-04,3,90.3.3 Billing for Allogeneic Stem Cell Transplants; 100-04,32,90 Billing for Stem Cell Transplantation; 100-04,4,231.11 Billing for Allogeneic Stem Cell Transplants

    EXCLUDES   *HLA typing by molecular pathology techniques (81370-81383)*

86812   **HLA typing; A, B, or C (eg, A10, B7, B27), single antigen**
    0.00   0.00   **FUD** XXX
    AMA: 2020,Dec,3; 2018,Jan,8; 2017,Jan,8; 2016,Jan,13

86813   **A, B, or C, multiple antigens**
    0.00   0.00   **FUD** XXX
    AMA: 2020,Dec,3; 2018,Jan,8; 2017,Jan,8; 2016,Jan,13

86816   **DR/DQ, single antigen**
    0.00   0.00   **FUD** XXX
    AMA: 2020,Dec,3; 2018,Jan,8; 2017,Jan,8; 2016,Jan,13

86817   **DR/DQ, multiple antigens**
    0.00   0.00   **FUD** XXX
    AMA: 2020,Dec,3; 2018,Jan,8; 2017,Jan,8; 2016,Jan,13

86821   **lymphocyte culture, mixed (MLC)**
    0.00   0.00   **FUD** XXX
    AMA: 2020,Dec,3; 2018,Jan,8; 2017,Jan,8; 2016,Jan,13

86825   **Human leukocyte antigen (HLA) crossmatch, non-cytotoxic (eg, using flow cytometry); first serum sample or dilution**
    INCLUDES   *Autologous HLA crossmatch*
    EXCLUDES   *B cells (86355)*
             Flow cytometry (88184-88189)
             Lymphocytotoxicity visual crossmatch (86805-86806)
             T cells (86359)
    0.00   0.00   **FUD** XXX
    AMA: 2020,Dec,3; 2020,Aug,14

+ 86826   **each additional serum sample or sample dilution (List separately in addition to primary procedure)**
    INCLUDES   *Autologous HLA crossmatch*
    EXCLUDES   *B cells (86355)*
             Flow cytometry (88184-88189)
             Lymphocytotoxicity visual crossmatch (86805-86806)
             T cells (86359)
    Code first (86825)
    0.00   0.00   **FUD** XXX
    AMA: 2020,Dec,3; 2020,Aug,14

86828-86849 HLA Antibodies

86828   **Antibody to human leukocyte antigens (HLA), solid phase assays (eg, microspheres or beads, ELISA, flow cytometry); qualitative assessment of the presence or absence of antibody(ies) to HLA Class I and Class II HLA antigens**
    Code also solid phase testing, untreated and treated specimens, either class of HLA after treatment (86828-86833)
    0.00   0.00   **FUD** XXX
    AMA: 2020,Dec,3

86829   **qualitative assessment of the presence or absence of antibody(ies) to HLA Class I or Class II HLA antigens**
    Code also solid phase testing, untreated and treated specimens, either class of HLA after treatment (86828-86833)
    0.00   0.00   **FUD** XXX
    AMA: 2020,Dec,3

86830   **antibody identification by qualitative panel using complete HLA phenotypes, HLA Class I**
    Code also solid phase testing, untreated and treated specimens, either class of HLA after treatment (86828-86833)
    0.00   0.00   **FUD** XXX
    AMA: 2020,Dec,3

86831   **antibody identification by qualitative panel using complete HLA phenotypes, HLA Class II**
    Code also solid phase testing, untreated and treated specimens, either class of HLA after treatment (86828-86833)
    0.00   0.00   **FUD** XXX
    AMA: 2020,Dec,3

86832   **high definition qualitative panel for identification of antibody specificities (eg, individual antigen per bead methodology), HLA Class I**
    Code also solid phase testing, untreated and treated specimens, either class of HLA after treatment (86828-86833)
    0.00   0.00   **FUD** XXX
    AMA: 2020,Dec,3

86833   **high definition qualitative panel for identification of antibody specificities (eg, individual antigen per bead methodology), HLA Class II**
    Code also solid phase testing, untreated and treated specimens, either class of HLA after treatment (86828-86833)
    0.00   0.00   **FUD** XXX
    AMA: 2020,Dec,3

86834   **semi-quantitative panel (eg, titer), HLA Class I**
    0.00   0.00   **FUD** XXX
    AMA: 2020,Dec,3

86835   **semi-quantitative panel (eg, titer), HLA Class II**
    0.00   0.00   **FUD** XXX
    AMA: 2020,Dec,3

86849   **Unlisted immunology procedure**
    0.00   0.00   **FUD** XXX
    AMA: 2020,Dec,3; 2019,Dec,12; 2018,Jan,8; 2017,Jan,8; 2016,Jan,13

86850-86999 Transfusion Services

    EXCLUDES   *Apheresis (36511-36512)*
             Therapeutic phlebotomy (99195)

86850   **Antibody screen, RBC, each serum technique**
    0.00   0.00   **FUD** XXX
    AMA: 2020,Dec,3; 2020,AugSE,1; 2020,AugSE,1; 2020,AugSE,1; 2018,Jan,8; 2017,Jan,8; 2016,Jan,13

86860 Antibody elution (RBC), each elution
    🔪 0.00   ⚖ 0.00   **FUD** XXX   01 ▭
    AMA: 2020,Dec,3; 2020,AugSE,1; 2020,AugSE,1; 2020,AugSE,1

86870 Antibody identification, RBC antibodies, each panel for each serum technique
    🔪 0.00   ⚖ 0.00   **FUD** XXX   02 ▭
    AMA: 2020,Dec,3; 2020,AugSE,1; 2020,AugSE,1; 2020,AugSE,1; 2018,Jan,8; 2017,Jan,8; 2016,Jan,13

86880 Antihuman globulin test (Coombs test); direct, each antiserum
    🔪 0.00   ⚖ 0.00   **FUD** XXX   01 ▭
    AMA: 2020,Dec,3

86885 indirect, qualitative, each reagent red cell
    🔪 0.00   ⚖ 0.00   **FUD** XXX   01 ▭
    AMA: 2020,Dec,3; 2018,Jan,8; 2017,Jan,8; 2016,Jan,13

86886 indirect, each antibody titer
    EXCLUDES   *Indirect antihuman globulin (Coombs) test for RBC antibody identification using reagent red cell panels (86870)*
    Indirect antihuman globulin (Coombs) test for RBC antibody screening (86850)
    🔪 0.00   ⚖ 0.00   **FUD** XXX   01 ▭
    AMA: 2020,Dec,3; 2018,Jan,8; 2017,Jan,8; 2016,Jan,13

86890 Autologous blood or component, collection processing and storage; predeposited
    🔪 0.00   ⚖ 0.00   **FUD** XXX   01 ▭
    AMA: 2020,Dec,3; 2018,Jan,8; 2017,Jan,8; 2016,Jan,13

86891 intra- or postoperative salvage
    🔪 0.00   ⚖ 0.00   **FUD** XXX   01 ▭
    AMA: 2020,Dec,3

86900 Blood typing, serologic; ABO
    🔪 0.00   ⚖ 0.00   **FUD** XXX   01 ▭
    AMA: 2020,Dec,3

86901 Rh (D)
    🔪 0.00   ⚖ 0.00   **FUD** XXX   01 ▭
    AMA: 2020,Dec,3; 2018,Jan,8; 2017,Jan,8; 2016,Jan,13

86902 antigen testing of donor blood using reagent serum, each antigen test
    Code also one time for each antigen, each unit blood, when multiple units tested for same antigen
    🔪 0.00   ⚖ 0.00   **FUD** XXX   01 ▭
    AMA: 2020,Dec,3

86904 antigen screening for compatible unit using patient serum, per unit screened
    🔪 0.00   ⚖ 0.00   **FUD** XXX   01 ▭
    AMA: 2020,Dec,3

86905 RBC antigens, other than ABO or Rh (D), each
    🔪 0.00   ⚖ 0.00   **FUD** XXX   01 ▭
    AMA: 2020,Dec,3

86906 Rh phenotyping, complete
    EXCLUDES   *Reporting molecular pathology procedures for human erythrocyte antigen typing (81403)*
    🔪 0.00   ⚖ 0.00   **FUD** XXX   01 ▭
    AMA: 2020,Dec,3

86910 Blood typing, for paternity testing, per individual; ABO, Rh and MN
    🔪 0.00   ⚖ 0.00   **FUD** XXX   E ▭
    AMA: 2020,Dec,3

86911 each additional antigen system
    🔪 0.00   ⚖ 0.00   **FUD** XXX   E ▭
    AMA: 2020,Dec,3

86920 Compatibility test each unit; immediate spin technique
    🔪 0.00   ⚖ 0.00   **FUD** XXX   01 ▭
    AMA: 2020,Dec,3; 2018,Jan,8; 2017,Jan,8; 2016,Jan,13

86921 incubation technique
    🔪 0.00   ⚖ 0.00   **FUD** XXX   01 ▭
    AMA: 2020,Dec,3; 2018,Jan,8; 2017,Jan,8; 2016,Jan,13

86922 antiglobulin technique
    🔪 0.00   ⚖ 0.00   **FUD** XXX   01 ▭
    AMA: 2020,Dec,3; 2018,Jan,8; 2017,Jan,8; 2016,Jan,13

86923 electronic
    EXCLUDES   *Other compatibility test techniques (86920-86922)*
    🔪 0.00   ⚖ 0.00   **FUD** XXX   01 ▭
    AMA: 2020,Dec,3; 2018,Jan,8; 2017,Jan,8; 2016,Jan,13

86927 Fresh frozen plasma, thawing, each unit
    🔪 0.00   ⚖ 0.00   **FUD** XXX   S ▭
    AMA: 2020,Dec,3

86930 Frozen blood, each unit; freezing (includes preparation)
    🔪 0.00   ⚖ 0.00   **FUD** XXX   01 ▭
    AMA: 2020,Dec,3; 2018,Jan,8; 2017,Jan,8; 2016,Jan,13

86931 thawing
    🔪 0.00   ⚖ 0.00   **FUD** XXX   01 ▭
    AMA: 2020,Dec,3; 2018,Jan,8; 2017,Jan,8; 2016,Jan,13

86932 freezing (includes preparation) and thawing
    🔪 0.00   ⚖ 0.00   **FUD** XXX   01 ▭
    AMA: 2020,Dec,3; 2018,Jan,8; 2017,Jan,8; 2016,Jan,13

86940 Hemolysins and agglutinins; auto, screen, each
    🔪 0.00   ⚖ 0.00   **FUD** XXX   Q ▭
    AMA: 2020,Dec,3

86941 incubated
    🔪 0.00   ⚖ 0.00   **FUD** XXX   Q ▭
    AMA: 2020,Dec,3

86945 Irradiation of blood product, each unit
    🔪 0.00   ⚖ 0.00   **FUD** XXX   01 ▭
    AMA: 2020,Dec,3; 2018,Jan,8; 2017,Jan,8; 2016,Jan,13

86950 Leukocyte transfusion
    EXCLUDES   *Infusion allogeneic lymphocytes (38242)*
    Leukapheresis (36511)
    🔪 0.00   ⚖ 0.00   **FUD** XXX   01 ▭
    AMA: 2020,Dec,3; 2018,Jan,8; 2017,Jan,8; 2016,Jan,13

86960 Volume reduction of blood or blood product (eg, red blood cells or platelets), each unit
    🔪 0.00   ⚖ 0.00   **FUD** XXX   01 ▭
    AMA: 2020,Dec,3; 2018,Jan,8; 2017,Jan,8; 2016,Jan,13

86965 Pooling of platelets or other blood products
    EXCLUDES   *Autologous WBC injection (0481T)*
    Injection platelet rich plasma (0232T)
    🔪 0.00   ⚖ 0.00   **FUD** XXX   01 ▭
    AMA: 2020,Dec,3; 2018,Jan,8; 2017,Jan,8; 2016,Jan,13

86970 Pretreatment of RBCs for use in RBC antibody detection, identification, and/or compatibility testing; incubation with chemical agents or drugs, each
    🔪 0.00   ⚖ 0.00   **FUD** XXX   01 ▭
    AMA: 2020,Dec,3

86971 incubation with enzymes, each
    🔪 0.00   ⚖ 0.00   **FUD** XXX   01 ▭
    AMA: 2020,Dec,3

86972 by density gradient separation
    🔪 0.00   ⚖ 0.00   **FUD** XXX   01 ▭
    AMA: 2020,Dec,3

86975 Pretreatment of serum for use in RBC antibody identification; incubation with drugs, each
    🔪 0.00   ⚖ 0.00   **FUD** XXX   01 ▭
    AMA: 2020,Dec,3

86976 by dilution
    🔪 0.00   ⚖ 0.00   **FUD** XXX   01 ▭
    AMA: 2020,Dec,3

86977 incubation with inhibitors, each
    🔪 0.00   ⚖ 0.00   **FUD** XXX   01 ▭
    AMA: 2020,Dec,3

86978 by differential red cell absorption using patient RBCs or RBCs of known phenotype, each absorption
🔧 0.00 ⚖ 0.00 **FUD** XXX
AMA: 2020,Dec,3

86985 Splitting of blood or blood products, each unit
🔧 0.00 ⚖ 0.00 **FUD** XXX
AMA: 2020,Dec,3; 2018,Jan,8; 2017,Jan,8; 2016,Jan,13

86999 Unlisted transfusion medicine procedure
🔧 0.00 ⚖ 0.00 **FUD** XXX
AMA: 2020,Dec,3; 2018,Jan,8; 2017,Jan,8; 2016,Jan,13

87003-87118 Identification of Microorganisms

INCLUDES Bacteriology, mycology, parasitology, and virology
EXCLUDES Additional tests using molecular probes, chromatography, nucleic acid resequencing, or immunologic techniques (87140-87158)
Code also:
Modifier 59 for multiple specimens or sites
Modifier 91 for repeat procedures performed on same day

87003 Animal inoculation, small animal, with observation and dissection
🔧 0.00 ⚖ 0.00 **FUD** XXX
AMA: 2020,Dec,3

87015 Concentration (any type), for infectious agents
EXCLUDES Direct smear for ova and parasites (87177)
🔧 0.00 ⚖ 0.00 **FUD** XXX
AMA: 2020,Dec,3

87040 Culture, bacterial; blood, aerobic, with isolation and presumptive identification of isolates (includes anaerobic culture, if appropriate)
🔧 0.00 ⚖ 0.00 **FUD** XXX
AMA: 2020,Dec,3; 2018,Jan,8; 2017,Jan,8; 2016,Jan,13

87045 stool, aerobic, with isolation and preliminary examination (eg, KIA, LIA), Salmonella and Shigella species
🔧 0.00 ⚖ 0.00 **FUD** XXX
AMA: 2020,Dec,3

87046 stool, aerobic, additional pathogens, isolation and presumptive identification of isolates, each plate
🔧 0.00 ⚖ 0.00 **FUD** XXX
AMA: 2020,Dec,3; 2018,Jan,8; 2017,Jan,8; 2016,Jan,13

87070 any other source except urine, blood or stool, aerobic, with isolation and presumptive identification of isolates
EXCLUDES Urine (87088)
🔧 0.00 ⚖ 0.00 **FUD** XXX
AMA: 2020,Dec,3; 2018,Jan,8; 2017,Jan,8; 2016,Jan,13

87071 quantitative, aerobic with isolation and presumptive identification of isolates, any source except urine, blood or stool
EXCLUDES Urine (87088)
🔧 0.00 ⚖ 0.00 **FUD** XXX
AMA: 2020,Dec,3; 2018,Jan,8; 2017,Jan,8; 2016,Jan,13

87073 quantitative, anaerobic with isolation and presumptive identification of isolates, any source except urine, blood or stool
EXCLUDES Definitive identification isolates (87076, 87077)
Typing isolates (87140-87158)
🔧 0.00 ⚖ 0.00 **FUD** XXX
AMA: 2020,Dec,3; 2018,Jan,8; 2017,Jan,8; 2016,Jan,13

87075 any source, except blood, anaerobic with isolation and presumptive identification of isolates
🔧 0.00 ⚖ 0.00 **FUD** XXX
AMA: 2020,Dec,3

87076 anaerobic isolate, additional methods required for definitive identification, each isolate
🔧 0.00 ⚖ 0.00 **FUD** XXX
AMA: 2020,Dec,3; 2018,Jan,8; 2017,Jan,8; 2016,Jan,13

87077 aerobic isolate, additional methods required for definitive identification, each isolate
🔧 0.00 ⚖ 0.00 **FUD** XXX
AMA: 2020,Dec,3; 2018,Jan,8; 2017,Jan,8; 2016,Jan,13

87081 Culture, presumptive, pathogenic organisms, screening only;
🔧 0.00 ⚖ 0.00 **FUD** XXX
AMA: 2020,Dec,3; 2018,Jan,8; 2017,Jan,8; 2016,Jan,13

87084 with colony estimation from density chart
🔧 0.00 ⚖ 0.00 **FUD** XXX
AMA: 2020,Dec,3

87086 Culture, bacterial; quantitative colony count, urine
🔧 0.00 ⚖ 0.00 **FUD** XXX
AMA: 2020,Dec,3; 2018,Jan,8; 2017,Jan,8; 2016,Jan,13

87088 with isolation and presumptive identification of each isolate, urine
🔧 0.00 ⚖ 0.00 **FUD** XXX
AMA: 2020,Dec,3; 2018,Jan,8; 2017,Jan,8; 2016,Jan,13

87101 Culture, fungi (mold or yeast) isolation, with presumptive identification of isolates; skin, hair, or nail
🔧 0.00 ⚖ 0.00 **FUD** XXX
AMA: 2020,Dec,3; 2018,Jan,8; 2017,Jan,8; 2016,Jan,13

87102 other source (except blood)
🔧 0.00 ⚖ 0.00 **FUD** XXX
AMA: 2020,Dec,3

87103 blood
🔧 0.00 ⚖ 0.00 **FUD** XXX
AMA: 2020,Dec,3

87106 Culture, fungi, definitive identification, each organism; yeast
🔧 0.00 ⚖ 0.00 **FUD** XXX
AMA: 2020,Dec,3

87107 mold
🔧 0.00 ⚖ 0.00 **FUD** XXX
AMA: 2020,Dec,3

87109 Culture, mycoplasma, any source
🔧 0.00 ⚖ 0.00 **FUD** XXX
AMA: 2020,Dec,3

87110 Culture, chlamydia, any source
EXCLUDES Immunofluorescence staining shell vials (87140)
🔧 0.00 ⚖ 0.00 **FUD** XXX
AMA: 2020,Dec,3

87116 Culture, tubercle or other acid-fast bacilli (eg, TB, AFB, mycobacteria) any source, with isolation and presumptive identification of isolates
EXCLUDES Concentration (87015)
🔧 0.00 ⚖ 0.00 **FUD** XXX
AMA: 2020,Dec,3

87118 Culture, mycobacterial, definitive identification, each isolate
🔧 0.00 ⚖ 0.00 **FUD** XXX
AMA: 2020,Dec,3

87140-87158 [87154] Additional Culture Typing Techniques

INCLUDES Bacteriology, mycology, parasitology, and virology
EXCLUDES Reporting molecular procedure codes as substitute for codes in this range (81105-81183 [81173, 81174, 81200, 81201, 81202, 81203, 81204], 81400-81408, [81479])
Code also:
Definitive identification
Modifier 59 for multiple specimens or sites
Modifier 91 for repeat procedures performed on same day

87140 Culture, typing; immunofluorescent method, each antiserum
🔧 0.00 ⚖ 0.00 **FUD** XXX
AMA: 2020,Dec,3; 2020,OctSE,1; 2020,OctSE,1; 2018,Jan,8; 2017,Jan,8; 2016,Jan,13

87143 gas liquid chromatography (GLC) or high pressure liquid chromatography (HPLC) method
🔧 0.00   ⚖ 0.00   **FUD** XXX   🔲🖰
AMA: 2020,Dec,3; 2020,OctSE,1; 2020,OctSE,1

87147 immunologic method, other than immunofluorescence (eg, agglutination grouping), per antiserum
🔧 0.00   ⚖ 0.00   **FUD** XXX   🔲🖰
AMA: 2020,Dec,3; 2020,OctSE,1; 2020,OctSE,1; 2018,Jan,8; 2017,Jan,8; 2016,Jan,13

87149 identification by nucleic acid (DNA or RNA) probe, direct probe technique, per culture or isolate, each organism probed
🔧 0.00   ⚖ 0.00   **FUD** XXX   🔲🖰
AMA: 2020,Dec,3; 2020,OctSE,1; 2020,OctSE,1; 2018,Jan,8; 2017,Jan,8; 2016,Jan,13

87150 identification by nucleic acid (DNA or RNA) probe, amplified probe technique, per culture or isolate, each organism probed
🔧 0.00   ⚖ 0.00   **FUD** XXX   🔲🖰
AMA: 2020,Dec,3; 2020,OctSE,1; 2020,OctSE,1; 2018,Jan,8; 2017,Jan,8; 2016,Jan,13

● # **87154** identification of blood pathogen and resistance typing, when performed, by nucleic acid (DNA or RNA) probe, multiplexed amplified probe technique including multiplex reverse transcription, when performed, per culture or isolate, 6 or more targets
🔧 0.00   ⚖ 0.00   **FUD** 000

87152 identification by pulse field gel typing
🔧 0.00   ⚖ 0.00   **FUD** XXX   🔲🖰
AMA: 2020,Dec,3; 2020,OctSE,1; 2020,OctSE,1; 2018,Jan,8; 2017,Jan,8; 2016,Jan,13

87153 identification by nucleic acid sequencing method, each isolate (eg, sequencing of the 16S rRNA gene)
🔧 0.00   ⚖ 0.00   **FUD** XXX   🔲🖰
AMA: 2020,Dec,3; 2020,OctSE,1; 2020,OctSE,1; 2018,Jan,8; 2017,Jan,8; 2016,Jan,13

87154 **Resequenced code. See code following 87150.**

87158 other methods
🔧 0.00   ⚖ 0.00   **FUD** XXX   🔲🖰
AMA: 2020,Dec,3; 2020,OctSE,1; 2020,OctSE,1; 2018,Jan,8; 2017,Jan,8; 2016,Jan,13

87164-87255 Identification of Organism from Primary Source and Sensitivity Studies

INCLUDES Bacteriology, mycology, parasitology, and virology
EXCLUDES *Additional tests using molecular probes, chromatography, or immunologic techniques (87140-87158)*
Code also:
Modifier 59 for multiple specimens or sites
Modifier 91 for repeat procedures performed on same day

87164 Dark field examination, any source (eg, penile, vaginal, oral, skin); includes specimen collection
🔧 0.00   ⚖ 0.00   **FUD** XXX   🔲⑧⓪🖰
AMA: 2020,Dec,3

87166 without collection
🔧 0.00   ⚖ 0.00   **FUD** XXX   🔲🖰
AMA: 2020,Dec,3

87168 Macroscopic examination; arthropod
🔧 0.00   ⚖ 0.00   **FUD** XXX   🔲🖰
AMA: 2020,Dec,3

87169 parasite
🔧 0.00   ⚖ 0.00   **FUD** XXX   🔲🖰
AMA: 2020,Dec,3

87172 Pinworm exam (eg, cellophane tape prep)
🔧 0.00   ⚖ 0.00   **FUD** XXX   🔲🖰
AMA: 2020,Dec,3

87176 Homogenization, tissue, for culture
🔧 0.00   ⚖ 0.00   **FUD** XXX   🔲🖰
AMA: 2020,Dec,3

87177 Ova and parasites, direct smears, concentration and identification
EXCLUDES *Coccidia or microsporidia exam (87207)*
Complex special stain (trichrome, iron hematoxylin) (87209)
Concentration for infectious agents (87015)
Direct smears from primary source (87207)
Nucleic acid probes in cytologic material (88365)
🔧 0.00   ⚖ 0.00   **FUD** XXX   🔲🖰
AMA: 2020,Dec,3; 2018,Jan,8; 2017,Jan,8; 2016,Jan,13

87181 Susceptibility studies, antimicrobial agent; agar dilution method, per agent (eg, antibiotic gradient strip)
🔧 0.00   ⚖ 0.00   **FUD** XXX   🔲🖰
AMA: 2020,Dec,3; 2018,Jan,8; 2017,Jan,8; 2016,Jan,13

87184 disk method, per plate (12 or fewer agents)
🔧 0.00   ⚖ 0.00   **FUD** XXX   🔲🖰
AMA: 2020,Dec,3; 2018,Jan,8; 2017,Jan,8; 2016,Jan,13

87185 enzyme detection (eg, beta lactamase), per enzyme
🔧 0.00   ⚖ 0.00   **FUD** XXX   🔲🖰
AMA: 2020,Dec,3; 2018,Jan,8; 2017,Jan,8; 2016,Jan,13

87186 microdilution or agar dilution (minimum inhibitory concentration [MIC] or breakpoint), each multi-antimicrobial, per plate
🔧 0.00   ⚖ 0.00   **FUD** XXX   🔲🖰
AMA: 2020,Dec,3; 2018,Jan,8; 2017,Jan,8; 2016,Jan,13

+ **87187** microdilution or agar dilution, minimum lethal concentration (MLC), each plate (List separately in addition to code for primary procedure)
Code first (87186, 87188)
🔧 0.00   ⚖ 0.00   **FUD** XXX   🔲🖰
AMA: 2020,Dec,3; 2018,Jan,8; 2017,Jan,8; 2016,Jan,13

87188 macrobroth dilution method, each agent
🔧 0.00   ⚖ 0.00   **FUD** XXX   🔲🖰
AMA: 2020,Dec,3; 2018,Jan,8; 2017,Jan,8; 2016,Jan,13

87190 mycobacteria, proportion method, each agent
EXCLUDES *Other mycobacterial susceptibility studies (87181, 87184, 87186, 87188)*
🔧 0.00   ⚖ 0.00   **FUD** XXX   🔲🖰
AMA: 2020,Dec,3

87197 Serum bactericidal titer (Schlichter test)
🔧 0.00   ⚖ 0.00   **FUD** XXX   🔲🖰
AMA: 2020,Dec,3

87205 Smear, primary source with interpretation; Gram or Giemsa stain for bacteria, fungi, or cell types
🔧 0.00   ⚖ 0.00   **FUD** XXX   🔲🖰
AMA: 2020,Dec,3; 2018,Jan,8; 2017,Jan,8; 2016,Jan,13

87206 fluorescent and/or acid fast stain for bacteria, fungi, parasites, viruses or cell types
🔧 0.00   ⚖ 0.00   **FUD** XXX   🔲🖰
AMA: 2020,Dec,3

87207 special stain for inclusion bodies or parasites (eg, malaria, coccidia, microsporidia, trypanosomes, herpes viruses)
EXCLUDES *Direct smears with concentration and identification (87177)*
Fat, fibers, meat, nasal eosinophils, starch (89049-89240)
Thick smear preparation (87015)
🔧 0.00   ⚖ 0.00   **FUD** XXX   🔲⑧⓪🖰
AMA: 2020,Dec,3; 2018,Jan,8; 2017,Jan,8; 2016,Jan,13

87209 complex special stain (eg, trichrome, iron hemotoxylin) for ova and parasites
🔧 0.00   ⚖ 0.00   **FUD** XXX   🔲🖰
AMA: 2020,Dec,3; 2018,Jan,8; 2017,Jan,8; 2016,Jan,13

87210	**wet mount for infectious agents (eg, saline, India ink, KOH preps)**

> **EXCLUDES** *KOH evaluation skin, hair, or nails (87220)*

🔳 0.00 ✂ 0.00 **FUD** XXX ❌ Ⓠ 🖵

AMA: 2020,Dec,3; 2018,Jan,8; 2017,Jan,8; 2016,May,13

87220	**Tissue examination by KOH slide of samples from skin, hair, or nails for fungi or ectoparasite ova or mites (eg, scabies)**

🔳 0.00 ✂ 0.00 **FUD** XXX Ⓠ 🖵

AMA: 2020,Dec,3

87230	**Toxin or antitoxin assay, tissue culture (eg, Clostridium difficile toxin)**

🔳 0.00 ✂ 0.00 **FUD** XXX Ⓠ 🖵

AMA: 2020,Dec,3

87250	**Virus isolation; inoculation of embryonated eggs, or small animal, includes observation and dissection**

🔳 0.00 ✂ 0.00 **FUD** XXX Ⓠ 🖵

AMA: 2020,Dec,3; 2020,OctSE,1; 2020,OctSE,1

87252	**tissue culture inoculation, observation, and presumptive identification by cytopathic effect**

🔳 0.00 ✂ 0.00 **FUD** XXX Ⓠ 🖵

AMA: 2020,Dec,3

87253	**tissue culture, additional studies or definitive identification (eg, hemabsorption, neutralization, immunofluorescence stain), each isolate**

> **EXCLUDES** *Electron microscopy (88348)*
> *Inclusion bodies in:*
> *Fluids (88106)*
> *Smears (87207-87210)*
> *Tissue sections (88304-88309)*

🔳 0.00 ✂ 0.00 **FUD** XXX Ⓠ 🖵

AMA: 2020,Dec,3

87254	**centrifuge enhanced (shell vial) technique, includes identification with immunofluorescence stain, each virus**

Code also (87252)

🔳 0.00 ✂ 0.00 **FUD** XXX Ⓠ 🖵

AMA: 2020,Dec,3; 2018,Jan,8; 2017,Jan,8; 2016,Jan,13

87255	**including identification by non-immunologic method, other than by cytopathic effect (eg, virus specific enzymatic activity)**

🔳 0.00 ✂ 0.00 **FUD** XXX Ⓠ 🖵

AMA: 2020,Dec,3; 2020,OctSE,1; 2020,OctSE,1; 2018,Jan,8; 2017,Jan,8; 2016,Jan,13

87260-87300 Fluorescence Microscopy by Organism

INCLUDES Primary source only

EXCLUDES *Comparable tests on culture material (87140-87158)*
Identification antibodies (86602-86804)
Immunoassay techniques with direct/visual observation for infectious antigens (87260-87300)
Microscopic identification infectious agents via direct/indirect immunofluorescent assay (IFA) techniques (87301-87451, 87802-87899 [87806, 87811])
Nonspecific agent detection (87299, 87449, 87797-87799, 87899)
Code also modifier 59 for different species or strains reported by same code

87260	**Infectious agent antigen detection by immunofluorescent technique; adenovirus**

🔳 0.00 ✂ 0.00 **FUD** XXX Ⓠ 🖵

AMA: 2020,Dec,3; 2020,OctSE,1; 2020,OctSE,1; 2020,AugSE,1; 2020,AugSE,1; 2020,AugSE,1

87265	**Bordetella pertussis/parapertussis**

🔳 0.00 ✂ 0.00 **FUD** XXX Ⓠ 🖵

AMA: 2020,Dec,3; 2020,OctSE,1; 2020,OctSE,1; 2020,AugSE,1; 2020,AugSE,1; 2020,AugSE,1

87267	**Enterovirus, direct fluorescent antibody (DFA)**

🔳 0.00 ✂ 0.00 **FUD** XXX Ⓠ 🖵

AMA: 2020,Dec,3; 2020,OctSE,1; 2020,OctSE,1; 2020,AugSE,1; 2020,AugSE,1; 2018,Jan,8; 2017,Jan,8; 2016,Jan,13

87269	**giardia**

🔳 0.00 ✂ 0.00 **FUD** XXX Ⓠ 🖵

AMA: 2020,Dec,3; 2020,OctSE,1; 2020,OctSE,1; 2020,AugSE,1; 2020,AugSE,1; 2020,AugSE,1

87270	**Chlamydia trachomatis**

🔳 0.00 ✂ 0.00 **FUD** XXX Ⓐ 🖵

AMA: 2020,Dec,3; 2020,OctSE,1; 2020,OctSE,1; 2020,AugSE,1; 2020,AugSE,1; 2020,AugSE,1

87271	**Cytomegalovirus, direct fluorescent antibody (DFA)**

🔳 0.00 ✂ 0.00 **FUD** XXX Ⓠ 🖵

AMA: 2020,Dec,3; 2020,OctSE,1; 2020,OctSE,1; 2020,AugSE,1; 2020,AugSE,1; 2018,Jan,8; 2017,Jan,8; 2016,Jan,13

87272	**cryptosporidium**

🔳 0.00 ✂ 0.00 **FUD** XXX Ⓠ 🖵

AMA: 2020,Dec,3; 2020,OctSE,1; 2020,OctSE,1; 2020,AugSE,1; 2020,AugSE,1; 2020,AugSE,1

87273	**Herpes simplex virus type 2**

🔳 0.00 ✂ 0.00 **FUD** XXX Ⓠ 🖵

AMA: 2020,Dec,3; 2020,OctSE,1; 2020,OctSE,1; 2020,AugSE,1; 2020,AugSE,1; 2020,AugSE,1

87274	**Herpes simplex virus type 1**

🔳 0.00 ✂ 0.00 **FUD** XXX Ⓠ 🖵

AMA: 2020,Dec,3; 2020,OctSE,1; 2020,OctSE,1; 2020,AugSE,1; 2020,AugSE,1; 2020,AugSE,1

87275	**influenza B virus**

🔳 0.00 ✂ 0.00 **FUD** XXX Ⓠ 🖵

AMA: 2020,Dec,3; 2020,OctSE,1; 2020,OctSE,1; 2020,AugSE,1; 2020,AugSE,1; 2020,AugSE,1; 2018,Jan,8; 2017,Jan,8; 2016,Jan,13

87276	**influenza A virus**

🔳 0.00 ✂ 0.00 **FUD** XXX Ⓠ 🖵

AMA: 2020,Dec,3; 2020,OctSE,1; 2020,OctSE,1; 2020,AugSE,1; 2020,AugSE,1; 2020,AugSE,1; 2018,Jan,8; 2017,Jan,8; 2016,Jan,13

87278	**Legionella pneumophila**

🔳 0.00 ✂ 0.00 **FUD** XXX Ⓠ 🖵

AMA: 2020,Dec,3; 2020,OctSE,1; 2020,OctSE,1; 2020,AugSE,1; 2020,AugSE,1; 2020,AugSE,1

87279	**Parainfluenza virus, each type**

🔳 0.00 ✂ 0.00 **FUD** XXX Ⓠ 🖵

AMA: 2020,Dec,3; 2020,OctSE,1; 2020,OctSE,1; 2020,AugSE,1; 2020,AugSE,1; 2020,AugSE,1

87280	**respiratory syncytial virus**

🔳 0.00 ✂ 0.00 **FUD** XXX Ⓠ 🖵

AMA: 2020,Dec,3; 2020,OctSE,1; 2020,OctSE,1; 2020,AugSE,1; 2020,AugSE,1; 2020,AugSE,1

87281	**Pneumocystis carinii**

🔳 0.00 ✂ 0.00 **FUD** XXX Ⓠ 🖵

AMA: 2020,Dec,3; 2020,OctSE,1; 2020,OctSE,1; 2020,AugSE,1; 2020,AugSE,1; 2020,AugSE,1

87283	**Rubeola**

🔳 0.00 ✂ 0.00 **FUD** XXX Ⓠ 🖵

AMA: 2020,Dec,3; 2020,OctSE,1; 2020,OctSE,1; 2020,AugSE,1; 2020,AugSE,1; 2020,AugSE,1

87285	**Treponema pallidum**

🔳 0.00 ✂ 0.00 **FUD** XXX Ⓠ 🖵

AMA: 2020,Dec,3; 2020,OctSE,1; 2020,OctSE,1; 2020,AugSE,1; 2020,AugSE,1; 2020,AugSE,1

87290	**Varicella zoster virus**

🔳 0.00 ✂ 0.00 **FUD** XXX Ⓠ 🖵

AMA: 2020,Dec,3; 2020,OctSE,1; 2020,OctSE,1; 2020,AugSE,1; 2020,AugSE,1; 2020,AugSE,1

87299	**not otherwise specified, each organism**

🔳 0.00 ✂ 0.00 **FUD** XXX Ⓠ 🖵

AMA: 2020,Dec,3; 2020,OctSE,1; 2020,OctSE,1; 2020,AugSE,1; 2020,AugSE,1; 2020,AugSE,1; 2018,Jan,8; 2017,Jan,8; 2016,Jan,13

87300 Infectious agent antigen detection by immunofluorescent technique, polyvalent for multiple organisms, each polyvalent antiserum

> EXCLUDES Physician evaluation infectious disease agents by immunofluorescence (88346)

🚗 0.00 ⚕ 0.00 **FUD** XXX 🔲🔲

AMA: 2020,Dec,3; 2020,OctSE,1; 2020,OctSE,1; 2020,AugSE,1; 2020,AugSE,1; 2020,AugSE,1

87301-87451 [87428] Enzyme Immunoassay Technique by Organism

INCLUDES Primary source only
EXCLUDES Comparable tests on culture material (87140-87158)
Identification antibodies (86602-86804)
Nonspecific agent detection (87449, 87797-87799, 87899)
Code also modifier 59 for different species or strains reported by same code

▲ **87301** Infectious agent antigen detection by immunoassay technique, (eg, enzyme immunoassay [EIA], enzyme-linked immunosorbent assay [ELISA], fluorescence immunoassay [FIA], immunochemiluminometric assay [IMCA]) qualitative or semiquantitative; adenovirus enteric types 40/41

🚗 0.00 ⚕ 0.00 **FUD** XXX 🔲🔲

AMA: 2020,Dec,3; 2020,OctSE,1; 2020,NovSE,1; 2020,OctSE,1; 2020,AugSE,1; 2020,AugSE,1; 2020,AugSE,1; 2020,May,3; 2020,JuneSE,1; 2018,Jan,8; 2017,Jan,8; 2016,Jan,13

▲ **87305** Aspergillus

🚗 0.00 ⚕ 0.00 **FUD** XXX 🔲🔲

AMA: 2020,Dec,3; 2020,OctSE,1; 2020,OctSE,1; 2020,AugSE,1; 2020,AugSE,1; 2020,AugSE,1

▲ **87320** Chlamydia trachomatis

🚗 0.00 ⚕ 0.00 **FUD** XXX 🔲🔲

AMA: 2020,Dec,3; 2020,OctSE,1; 2020,OctSE,1; 2020,AugSE,1; 2020,AugSE,1; 2020,AugSE,1

▲ **87324** Clostridium difficile toxin(s)

🚗 0.00 ⚕ 0.00 **FUD** XXX 🔲🔲

AMA: 2020,Dec,3; 2020,OctSE,1; 2020,OctSE,1; 2020,AugSE,1; 2020,AugSE,1; 2020,AugSE,1

▲ **87327** Cryptococcus neoformans

> EXCLUDES Cryptococcus latex agglutination (86403)

🚗 0.00 ⚕ 0.00 **FUD** XXX 🔲🔲

AMA: 2020,Dec,3; 2020,OctSE,1; 2020,OctSE,1; 2020,AugSE,1; 2020,AugSE,1; 2020,AugSE,1

▲ **87328** cryptosporidium

🚗 0.00 ⚕ 0.00 **FUD** XXX 🔲🔲

AMA: 2020,Dec,3; 2020,OctSE,1; 2020,OctSE,1; 2020,AugSE,1; 2020,AugSE,1; 2020,AugSE,1

▲ **87329** giardia

🚗 0.00 ⚕ 0.00 **FUD** XXX 🔲🔲

AMA: 2020,Dec,3; 2020,OctSE,1; 2020,OctSE,1; 2020,AugSE,1; 2020,AugSE,1; 2020,AugSE,1

▲ **87332** cytomegalovirus

🚗 0.00 ⚕ 0.00 **FUD** XXX 🔲🔲

AMA: 2020,Dec,3; 2020,OctSE,1; 2020,OctSE,1; 2020,AugSE,1; 2020,AugSE,1; 2020,AugSE,1

▲ **87335** Escherichia coli O157

> EXCLUDES Giardia antigen (87329)

🚗 0.00 ⚕ 0.00 **FUD** XXX 🔲🔲

AMA: 2020,Dec,3; 2020,OctSE,1; 2020,OctSE,1; 2020,AugSE,1; 2020,AugSE,1

▲ **87336** Entamoeba histolytica dispar group

🚗 0.00 ⚕ 0.00 **FUD** XXX 🔲🔲

AMA: 2020,Dec,3; 2020,OctSE,1; 2020,OctSE,1; 2020,AugSE,1; 2020,AugSE,1

▲ **87337** Entamoeba histolytica group

🚗 0.00 ⚕ 0.00 **FUD** XXX 🔲🔲

AMA: 2020,Dec,3; 2020,OctSE,1; 2020,OctSE,1; 2020,AugSE,1; 2020,AugSE,1

▲ **87338** Helicobacter pylori, stool

🚗 0.00 ⚕ 0.00 **FUD** XXX ❌🔲🔲

AMA: 2020,Dec,3; 2020,OctSE,1; 2020,OctSE,1; 2020,AugSE,1; 2020,AugSE,1; 2020,AugSE,1; 2018,Jan,8; 2017,Jan,8; 2016,Jan,13

▲ **87339** Helicobacter pylori

> EXCLUDES H. pylori:
> Breath and blood by mass spectrometry (83013-83014)
> Liquid scintillation counter (78267-78268)
> Stool (87338)

🚗 0.00 ⚕ 0.00 **FUD** XXX 🔲🔲

AMA: 2020,Dec,3; 2020,OctSE,1; 2020,OctSE,1; 2020,AugSE,1; 2020,AugSE,1; 2020,AugSE,1

▲ **87340** hepatitis B surface antigen (HBsAg)

🚗 0.00 ⚕ 0.00 **FUD** XXX 🔲🔲

AMA: 2020,Dec,3; 2020,OctSE,1; 2020,OctSE,1; 2020,AugSE,1; 2020,AugSE,1; 2020,AugSE,1; 2018,Jan,8; 2017,Jan,8; 2016,Jan,13

▲ **87341** hepatitis B surface antigen (HBsAg) neutralization

🚗 0.00 ⚕ 0.00 **FUD** XXX 🅰🔲

AMA: 2020,Dec,3; 2020,OctSE,1; 2020,OctSE,1; 2020,AugSE,1; 2020,AugSE,1

▲ **87350** hepatitis Be antigen (HBeAg)

🚗 0.00 ⚕ 0.00 **FUD** XXX 🔲🔲

AMA: 2020,Dec,3; 2020,OctSE,1; 2020,OctSE,1; 2020,AugSE,1; 2020,AugSE,1

▲ **87380** hepatitis, delta agent

🚗 0.00 ⚕ 0.00 **FUD** XXX 🔲🔲

AMA: 2020,Dec,3; 2020,OctSE,1; 2020,OctSE,1; 2020,AugSE,1; 2020,AugSE,1

▲ **87385** Histoplasma capsulatum

🚗 0.00 ⚕ 0.00 **FUD** XXX 🔲🔲

AMA: 2020,Dec,3; 2020,OctSE,1; 2020,OctSE,1; 2020,AugSE,1; 2020,AugSE,1

▲ **87389** HIV-1 antigen(s), with HIV-1 and HIV-2 antibodies, single result

Code also modifier 92 for test performed using kit or transportable instrument comprising (all or part) single-use, disposable analytical chamber

🚗 0.00 ⚕ 0.00 **FUD** XXX ❌🔲🔲

AMA: 2020,Dec,3; 2020,OctSE,1; 2020,OctSE,1; 2020,AugSE,1; 2020,AugSE,1

▲ **87390** HIV-1

🚗 0.00 ⚕ 0.00 **FUD** XXX 🔲🔲

AMA: 2020,Dec,3; 2020,OctSE,1; 2020,OctSE,1; 2020,AugSE,1; 2020,AugSE,1

▲ **87391** HIV-2

🚗 0.00 ⚕ 0.00 **FUD** XXX 🔲🔲

AMA: 2020,Dec,3; 2020,OctSE,1; 2020,OctSE,1; 2020,AugSE,1; 2020,AugSE,1

▲ **87400** Influenza, A or B, each

🚗 0.00 ⚕ 0.00 **FUD** XXX 🔲🔲

AMA: 2020,Dec,3; 2020,OctSE,1; 2020,NovSE,1; 2020,OctSE,1; 2020,AugSE,1; 2020,AugSE,1; 2020,AugSE,1; 2018,Jan,8; 2017,Jan,8; 2016,Jan,13

▲ **87420** respiratory syncytial virus

🚗 0.00 ⚕ 0.00 **FUD** XXX 🔲🔲

AMA: 2020,Dec,3; 2020,OctSE,1; 2020,OctSE,1; 2020,AugSE,1; 2020,AugSE,1

▲ **87425** rotavirus

🚗 0.00 ⚕ 0.00 **FUD** XXX 🔲🔲

AMA: 2020,Dec,3; 2020,OctSE,1; 2020,OctSE,1; 2020,AugSE,1; 2020,AugSE,1

▲ **87426** severe acute respiratory syndrome coronavirus (eg, SARS-CoV, SARS-CoV-2 [COVID-19])

AMA: 2020,Dec,3; 2020,OctSE,1; 2020,NovSE,1; 2020,OctSE,1; 2020,AugSE,1; 2020,AugSE,1; 2020,AugSE,1

● # **87428** **severe acute respiratory syndrome coronavirus (eg, SARS-CoV, SARS-CoV-2 [COVID-19]) and influenza virus types A and B**
🐘 0.00 ⚕ 0.00 **FUD** XXX ▫
AMA: 2020,Dec,3; 2020,OctSE,1

▲ **87427** **Shiga-like toxin**
🐘 0.00 ⚕ 0.00 **FUD** XXX ▫▫
AMA: 2020,Dec,3; 2020,OctSE,1; 2020,OctSE,1; 2020,AugSE,1; 2020,AugSE,1; 2020,AugSE,1

87428 Resequenced code. See code following 87426.

▲ **87430** **Streptococcus, group A**
🐘 0.00 ⚕ 0.00 **FUD** XXX ▫▫
AMA: 2020,Dec,3; 2020,OctSE,1; 2020,OctSE,1; 2020,AugSE,1; 2020,AugSE,1; 2020,AugSE,1; 2018,Jan,8; 2017,Jan,8; 2016,Jan,13

▲ **87449** **not otherwise specified, each organism**
🐘 0.00 ⚕ 0.00 **FUD** XXX ✖▫▫
AMA: 2020,Dec,3; 2020,OctSE,1; 2020,OctSE,1; 2020,AugSE,1; 2020,AugSE,1; 2020,AugSE,1; 2018,Jan,8; 2017,Jan,8; 2016,Jan,13

87450 **single step method, not otherwise specified, each organism**
To report, see (87301-87451 [87428], 87802-87899 [87806, 87811])

▲ **87451** **polyvalent for multiple organisms, each polyvalent antiserum**
🐘 0.00 ⚕ 0.00 **FUD** XXX ▫▫
AMA: 2020,Dec,3; 2020,OctSE,1; 2020,OctSE,1; 2020,AugSE,1; 2020,AugSE,1; 2020,AugSE,1

87471-87801 [87623, 87624, 87625] Detection Infectious Agent by Probe Techniques

INCLUDES Primary source only
EXCLUDES *Comparable tests on culture material (87140-87158)*
Identification antibodies (86602-86804)
Nonspecific agent detection (87299, 87449, 87797-87799, 87899)
Reporting molecular procedure codes as substitute for codes in this range (81161-81408 [81105, 81106, 81107, 81108, 81109, 81110, 81111, 81112, 81120, 81121, 81161, 81162, 81230, 81231, 81238, 81269, 81283, 81287, 81288, 81334])
Code also modifier 59 for different species or strains reported by same code

87471 **Infectious agent detection by nucleic acid (DNA or RNA); Bartonella henselae and Bartonella quintana, amplified probe technique**
🐘 0.00 ⚕ 0.00 **FUD** XXX ▫▫
AMA: 2020,Dec,3; 2020,OctSE,1; 2020,Oct,11; 2020,OctSE,1; 2020,AugSE,1; 2020,AugSE,1; 2018,Jan,8; 2017,Jan,8; 2016,Jan,13

87472 **Bartonella henselae and Bartonella quintana, quantification**
🐘 0.00 ⚕ 0.00 **FUD** XXX ▫▫
AMA: 2020,Dec,3; 2020,OctSE,1; 2020,OctSE,1; 2020,AugSE,1; 2020,AugSE,1; 2020,AugSE,1; 2018,Jan,8; 2017,Jan,8; 2016,Jan,13

87475 **Borrelia burgdorferi, direct probe technique**
🐘 0.00 ⚕ 0.00 **FUD** XXX ▫▫
AMA: 2020,Dec,3; 2020,OctSE,1; 2020,OctSE,1; 2020,AugSE,1; 2020,AugSE,1; 2020,AugSE,1; 2018,Jan,8; 2017,Jan,8; 2016,Jan,13

87476 **Borrelia burgdorferi, amplified probe technique**
🐘 0.00 ⚕ 0.00 **FUD** XXX ▫▫
AMA: 2020,Dec,3; 2020,OctSE,1; 2020,OctSE,1; 2020,AugSE,1; 2020,AugSE,1; 2020,AugSE,1; 2018,Jan,8; 2017,Jan,8; 2016,Jan,13

87480 **Candida species, direct probe technique**
🐘 0.00 ⚕ 0.00 **FUD** XXX ▫▫
AMA: 2020,Dec,3; 2020,OctSE,1; 2020,OctSE,1; 2020,AugSE,1; 2020,AugSE,1; 2020,AugSE,1; 2018,Jan,8; 2017,Jan,8; 2016,Jan,13

87481 **Candida species, amplified probe technique**
🐘 0.00 ⚕ 0.00 **FUD** XXX ▫▫
AMA: 2020,Dec,3; 2020,OctSE,1; 2020,OctSE,1; 2020,AugSE,1; 2020,AugSE,1; 2020,AugSE,1; 2018,Jan,8; 2017,Jan,8; 2016,Jan,13

87482 **Candida species, quantification**
🐘 0.00 ⚕ 0.00 **FUD** XXX ▫▫
AMA: 2020,Dec,3; 2020,OctSE,1; 2020,OctSE,1; 2020,AugSE,1; 2020,AugSE,1; 2020,AugSE,1; 2018,Jan,8; 2017,Jan,8; 2016,Jan,13

87483 **central nervous system pathogen (eg, Neisseria meningitidis, Streptococcus pneumoniae, Listeria, Haemophilus influenzae, E. coli, Streptococcus agalactiae, enterovirus, human parechovirus, herpes simplex virus type 1 and 2, human herpesvirus 6, cytomegalovirus, varicella zoster virus, Cryptococcus), includes multiplex reverse transcription, when performed, and multiplex amplified probe technique, multiple types or subtypes, 12-25 targets**
🐘 0.00 ⚕ 0.00 **FUD** XXX ▫▫
AMA: 2020,Dec,3; 2020,OctSE,1; 2020,OctSE,1; 2020,AugSE,1; 2020,AugSE,1; 2020,AugSE,1

87485 **Chlamydia pneumoniae, direct probe technique**
🐘 0.00 ⚕ 0.00 **FUD** XXX ▫▫
AMA: 2020,Dec,3; 2020,OctSE,1; 2020,OctSE,1; 2020,AugSE,1; 2020,AugSE,1; 2018,Jan,8; 2017,Jan,8; 2016,Jan,13

87486 **Chlamydia pneumoniae, amplified probe technique**
🐘 0.00 ⚕ 0.00 **FUD** XXX ▫▫
AMA: 2020,Dec,3; 2020,OctSE,1; 2020,OctSE,1; 2020,AugSE,1; 2020,AugSE,1; 2018,Jan,8; 2017,Jan,8; 2016,Jan,13

87487 **Chlamydia pneumoniae, quantification**
🐘 0.00 ⚕ 0.00 **FUD** XXX ▫▫
AMA: 2020,Dec,3; 2020,OctSE,1; 2020,OctSE,1; 2020,AugSE,1; 2020,AugSE,1; 2018,Jan,8; 2017,Jan,8; 2016,Jan,13

87490 **Chlamydia trachomatis, direct probe technique**
🐘 0.00 ⚕ 0.00 **FUD** XXX Ⓐ▫
AMA: 2020,Dec,3; 2020,OctSE,1; 2020,OctSE,1; 2020,AugSE,1; 2020,AugSE,1; 2018,Jan,8; 2017,Jan,8; 2016,Jan,13

87491 **Chlamydia trachomatis, amplified probe technique**
🐘 0.00 ⚕ 0.00 **FUD** XXX Ⓐ▫
AMA: 2020,Dec,3; 2020,OctSE,1; 2020,OctSE,1; 2020,AugSE,1; 2020,AugSE,1; 2018,Jan,8; 2017,Jan,8; 2016,Jan,13

87492 **Chlamydia trachomatis, quantification**
🐘 0.00 ⚕ 0.00 **FUD** XXX ▫▫
AMA: 2020,Dec,3; 2020,OctSE,1; 2020,OctSE,1; 2020,AugSE,1; 2020,AugSE,1; 2018,Jan,8; 2017,Jan,8; 2016,Jan,13

87493 **Clostridium difficile, toxin gene(s), amplified probe technique**
🐘 0.00 ⚕ 0.00 **FUD** XXX ▫▫
AMA: 2020,Dec,3; 2020,OctSE,1; 2020,OctSE,1; 2020,AugSE,1; 2020,AugSE,1; 2018,Jan,8; 2017,Jan,8; 2016,Jan,13

87495 **cytomegalovirus, direct probe technique**
🐘 0.00 ⚕ 0.00 **FUD** XXX ▫▫
AMA: 2020,Dec,3; 2020,OctSE,1; 2020,OctSE,1; 2020,AugSE,1; 2020,AugSE,1; 2018,Jan,8; 2017,Jan,8; 2016,Jan,13

87496 **cytomegalovirus, amplified probe technique**
🐘 0.00 ⚕ 0.00 **FUD** XXX ▫▫
AMA: 2020,Dec,3; 2020,OctSE,1; 2020,OctSE,1; 2020,AugSE,1; 2020,AugSE,1; 2018,Jan,8; 2017,Jan,8; 2016,Jan,13

87497 **cytomegalovirus, quantification**
🐘 0.00 ⚕ 0.00 **FUD** XXX ▫▫
AMA: 2020,Dec,3; 2020,OctSE,1; 2020,OctSE,1; 2020,AugSE,1; 2020,AugSE,1; 2018,Jan,8; 2017,Jan,8; 2016,Jan,13

87498 **enterovirus, amplified probe technique, includes reverse transcription when performed**
🐘 0.00 ⚕ 0.00 **FUD** XXX ▫▫
AMA: 2020,Dec,3; 2020,OctSE,1; 2020,OctSE,1; 2020,AugSE,1; 2020,AugSE,1; 2018,Jan,8; 2017,Jan,8; 2016,Jan,13

87500 **vancomycin resistance (eg, enterococcus species van A, van B), amplified probe technique**
🐘 0.00 ⚕ 0.00 **FUD** XXX ▫▫
AMA: 2020,Dec,3; 2020,OctSE,1; 2020,OctSE,1; 2020,AugSE,1; 2020,AugSE,1; 2018,Jan,8; 2017,Jan,8; 2016,Jan,13

87501 influenza virus, includes reverse transcription, when performed, and amplified probe technique, each type or subtype

    0.00   0.00   **FUD** XXX

AMA: 2020,Dec,3; 2020,OctSE,1; 2020,OctSE,1; 2020,AugSE,1; 2020,AugSE,1; 2020,AugSE,1; 2018,Jan,8; 2017,Jan,8; 2016,Jan,13

87502 influenza virus, for multiple types or sub-types, includes multiplex reverse transcription, when performed, and multiplex amplified probe technique, first 2 types or sub-types

    0.00   0.00   **FUD** XXX

AMA: 2020,Dec,3; 2020,OctSE,1; 2020,OctSE,1; 2020,AugSE,1; 2020,AugSE,1; 2020,AugSE,1; 2018,Jan,8; 2017,Jan,8; 2016,Jan,13

+ 87503 influenza virus, for multiple types or sub-types, includes multiplex reverse transcription, when performed, and multiplex amplified probe technique, each additional influenza virus type or sub-type beyond 2 (List separately in addition to code for primary procedure)

Code first (87502)

    0.00   0.00   **FUD** XXX

AMA: 2020,Dec,3; 2020,OctSE,1; 2020,OctSE,1; 2020,AugSE,1; 2020,AugSE,1; 2020,AugSE,1; 2018,Jan,8; 2017,Jan,8; 2016,Jan,13

87505 gastrointestinal pathogen (eg, Clostridium difficile, E. coli, Salmonella, Shigella, norovirus, Giardia), includes multiplex reverse transcription, when performed, and multiplex amplified probe technique, multiple types or subtypes, 3-5 targets

    0.00   0.00   **FUD** XXX

AMA: 2020,Dec,3; 2020,OctSE,1; 2020,OctSE,1; 2020,AugSE,1; 2020,AugSE,1; 2020,AugSE,1

87506 gastrointestinal pathogen (eg, Clostridium difficile, E. coli, Salmonella, Shigella, norovirus, Giardia), includes multiplex reverse transcription, when performed, and multiplex amplified probe technique, multiple types or subtypes, 6-11 targets

    0.00   0.00   **FUD** XXX

AMA: 2020,Dec,3; 2020,OctSE,1; 2020,OctSE,1; 2020,AugSE,1; 2020,AugSE,1; 2020,AugSE,1

87507 gastrointestinal pathogen (eg, Clostridium difficile, E. coli, Salmonella, Shigella, norovirus, Giardia), includes multiplex reverse transcription, when performed, and multiplex amplified probe technique, multiple types or subtypes, 12-25 targets

    0.00   0.00   **FUD** XXX

AMA: 2020,Dec,3; 2020,OctSE,1; 2020,OctSE,1; 2020,AugSE,1; 2020,AugSE,1; 2020,AugSE,1

87510 Gardnerella vaginalis, direct probe technique

    0.00   0.00   **FUD** XXX

AMA: 2020,Dec,3; 2020,OctSE,1; 2020,OctSE,1; 2020,AugSE,1; 2020,AugSE,1; 2020,AugSE,1; 2018,Jan,8; 2017,Jan,8; 2016,Jan,13

87511 Gardnerella vaginalis, amplified probe technique

    0.00   0.00   **FUD** XXX

AMA: 2020,Dec,3; 2020,OctSE,1; 2020,OctSE,1; 2020,AugSE,1; 2020,AugSE,1; 2020,AugSE,1; 2018,Jan,8; 2017,Jan,8; 2016,Jan,13

87512 Gardnerella vaginalis, quantification

    0.00   0.00   **FUD** XXX

AMA: 2020,Dec,3; 2020,OctSE,1; 2020,OctSE,1; 2020,AugSE,1; 2020,AugSE,1; 2020,AugSE,1; 2018,Jan,8; 2017,Jan,8; 2016,Jan,13

87516 hepatitis B virus, amplified probe technique

    0.00   0.00   **FUD** XXX

AMA: 2020,Dec,3; 2020,OctSE,1; 2020,OctSE,1; 2020,AugSE,1; 2020,AugSE,1; 2020,AugSE,1; 2018,Jan,8; 2017,Jan,8; 2016,Jan,13

87517 hepatitis B virus, quantification

    0.00   0.00   **FUD** XXX

AMA: 2020,Dec,3; 2020,OctSE,1; 2020,OctSE,1; 2020,AugSE,1; 2020,AugSE,1; 2020,AugSE,1; 2018,Jan,8; 2017,Jan,8; 2016,Jan,13

87520 hepatitis C, direct probe technique

    0.00   0.00   **FUD** XXX

AMA: 2020,Dec,3; 2020,OctSE,1; 2020,OctSE,1; 2020,AugSE,1; 2020,AugSE,1; 2020,AugSE,1; 2018,Jan,8; 2017,Jan,8; 2016,Jan,13

87521 hepatitis C, amplified probe technique, includes reverse transcription when performed

    0.00   0.00   **FUD** XXX

AMA: 2020,Dec,3; 2020,OctSE,1; 2020,OctSE,1; 2020,AugSE,1; 2020,AugSE,1; 2020,AugSE,1; 2018,Jan,8; 2017,Jan,8; 2016,Jan,13

87522 hepatitis C, quantification, includes reverse transcription when performed

    0.00   0.00   **FUD** XXX

AMA: 2020,Dec,3; 2020,OctSE,1; 2020,OctSE,1; 2020,AugSE,1; 2020,AugSE,1; 2020,AugSE,1; 2018,Jan,8; 2017,Jan,8; 2016,Jan,13

87525 hepatitis G, direct probe technique

    0.00   0.00   **FUD** XXX

AMA: 2020,Dec,3; 2020,OctSE,1; 2020,OctSE,1; 2020,AugSE,1; 2020,AugSE,1; 2020,AugSE,1; 2018,Jan,8; 2017,Jan,8; 2016,Jan,13

87526 hepatitis G, amplified probe technique

    0.00   0.00   **FUD** XXX

AMA: 2020,Dec,3; 2020,OctSE,1; 2020,OctSE,1; 2020,AugSE,1; 2020,AugSE,1; 2020,AugSE,1; 2018,Jan,8; 2017,Jan,8; 2016,Jan,13

87527 hepatitis G, quantification

    0.00   0.00   **FUD** XXX

AMA: 2020,Dec,3; 2020,OctSE,1; 2020,OctSE,1; 2020,AugSE,1; 2020,AugSE,1; 2020,AugSE,1; 2018,Jan,8; 2017,Jan,8; 2016,Jan,13

87528 Herpes simplex virus, direct probe technique

    0.00   0.00   **FUD** XXX

AMA: 2020,Dec,3; 2020,OctSE,1; 2020,OctSE,1; 2020,AugSE,1; 2020,AugSE,1; 2020,AugSE,1; 2018,Jan,8; 2017,Jan,8; 2016,Jan,13

87529 Herpes simplex virus, amplified probe technique

    0.00   0.00   **FUD** XXX

AMA: 2020,Dec,3; 2020,OctSE,1; 2020,OctSE,1; 2020,AugSE,1; 2020,AugSE,1; 2020,AugSE,1; 2018,Jan,8; 2017,Jan,8; 2016,Jan,13

87530 Herpes simplex virus, quantification

    0.00   0.00   **FUD** XXX

AMA: 2020,Dec,3; 2020,OctSE,1; 2020,OctSE,1; 2020,AugSE,1; 2020,AugSE,1; 2020,AugSE,1; 2018,Jan,8; 2017,Jan,8; 2016,Jan,13

87531 Herpes virus-6, direct probe technique

    0.00   0.00   **FUD** XXX

AMA: 2020,Dec,3; 2020,OctSE,1; 2020,OctSE,1; 2020,AugSE,1; 2020,AugSE,1; 2020,AugSE,1; 2018,Jan,8; 2017,Jan,8; 2016,Jan,13

87532 Herpes virus-6, amplified probe technique

    0.00   0.00   **FUD** XXX

AMA: 2020,Dec,3; 2020,OctSE,1; 2020,OctSE,1; 2020,AugSE,1; 2020,AugSE,1; 2020,AugSE,1; 2018,Jan,8; 2017,Jan,8; 2016,Jan,13

87533 Herpes virus-6, quantification

    0.00   0.00   **FUD** XXX

AMA: 2020,Dec,3; 2020,OctSE,1; 2020,OctSE,1; 2020,AugSE,1; 2020,AugSE,1; 2020,AugSE,1; 2018,Jan,8; 2017,Jan,8; 2016,Jan,13

87534 HIV-1, direct probe technique

    0.00   0.00   **FUD** XXX

AMA: 2020,Dec,3; 2020,OctSE,1; 2020,OctSE,1; 2020,AugSE,1; 2020,AugSE,1; 2020,AugSE,1; 2018,Jan,8; 2017,Jan,8; 2016,Jan,13

87535 HIV-1, amplified probe technique, includes reverse transcription when performed

    0.00   0.00   **FUD** XXX

AMA: 2020,Dec,3; 2020,OctSE,1; 2020,OctSE,1; 2020,AugSE,1; 2020,AugSE,1; 2020,AugSE,1; 2018,Jan,8; 2017,Jan,8; 2016,Jan,13

87536 HIV-1, quantification, includes reverse transcription when performed

    0.00   0.00   **FUD** XXX

AMA: 2020,Dec,3; 2020,OctSE,1; 2020,OctSE,1; 2020,AugSE,1; 2020,AugSE,1; 2020,AugSE,1; 2018,Jan,8; 2017,Jan,8; 2016,Jan,13

87537 HIV-2, direct probe technique

    0.00   0.00   **FUD** XXX

AMA: 2020,Dec,3; 2020,OctSE,1; 2020,OctSE,1; 2020,AugSE,1; 2020,AugSE,1; 2020,AugSE,1; 2018,Jan,8; 2017,Jan,8; 2016,Jan,13

87538 HIV-2, amplified probe technique, includes reverse transcription when performed
🖵 0.00 ⚕ 0.00 **FUD** XXX   ⒬ ▣
AMA: 2020,Dec,3; 2020,OctSE,1; 2020,OctSE,1; 2020,AugSE,1; 2020,AugSE,1; 2020,AugSE,1; 2018,Jan,8; 2017,Jan,8; 2016,Jan,13

87539 HIV-2, quantification, includes reverse transcription when performed
🖵 0.00 ⚕ 0.00 **FUD** XXX   ⒬ ▣
AMA: 2020,Dec,3; 2020,OctSE,1; 2020,OctSE,1; 2020,AugSE,1; 2020,AugSE,1; 2020,AugSE,1; 2018,Jan,8; 2017,Jan,8; 2016,Jan,13

\# **87623** Human Papillomavirus (HPV), low-risk types (eg, 6, 11, 42, 43, 44)
🖵 0.00 ⚕ 0.00 **FUD** XXX   ⒬ ▣
AMA: 2020,Dec,3; 2020,OctSE,1; 2020,OctSE,1; 2020,AugSE,1; 2020,AugSE,1; 2020,AugSE,1

\# **87624** Human Papillomavirus (HPV), high-risk types (eg, 16, 18, 31, 33, 35, 39, 45, 51, 52, 56, 58, 59, 68)
INCLUDES Low- and high-risk types in one assay
🖵 0.00 ⚕ 0.00 **FUD** XXX   ⒬ ▣
AMA: 2020,Dec,3; 2020,OctSE,1; 2020,OctSE,1; 2020,AugSE,1; 2020,AugSE,1; 2020,AugSE,1; 2018,Jan,8; 2017,Jan,8; 2016,Jan,13

\# **87625** Human Papillomavirus (HPV), types 16 and 18 only, includes type 45, if performed
EXCLUDES *HPV detection (genotyping) (0500T)*
🖵 0.00 ⚕ 0.00 **FUD** XXX   ⒬ ▣
AMA: 2020,Dec,3; 2020,OctSE,1; 2020,OctSE,1; 2020,AugSE,1; 2020,AugSE,1; 2020,AugSE,1; 2018,Jan,8; 2017,Jan,8; 2016,Jan,13

87540 Legionella pneumophila, direct probe technique
🖵 0.00 ⚕ 0.00 **FUD** XXX   ⒬ ▣
AMA: 2020,Dec,3; 2020,OctSE,1; 2020,OctSE,1; 2020,AugSE,1; 2020,AugSE,1; 2020,AugSE,1; 2018,Jan,8; 2017,Jan,8; 2016,Jan,13

87541 Legionella pneumophila, amplified probe technique
🖵 0.00 ⚕ 0.00 **FUD** XXX   ⒬ ▣
AMA: 2020,Dec,3; 2020,OctSE,1; 2020,OctSE,1; 2020,AugSE,1; 2020,AugSE,1; 2020,AugSE,1; 2018,Jan,8; 2017,Jan,8; 2016,Jan,13

87542 Legionella pneumophila, quantification
🖵 0.00 ⚕ 0.00 **FUD** XXX   ⒬ ▣
AMA: 2020,Dec,3; 2020,OctSE,1; 2020,OctSE,1; 2020,AugSE,1; 2020,AugSE,1; 2020,AugSE,1; 2018,Jan,8; 2017,Jan,8; 2016,Jan,13

87550 Mycobacteria species, direct probe technique
🖵 0.00 ⚕ 0.00 **FUD** XXX   ⒬ ▣
AMA: 2020,Dec,3; 2020,OctSE,1; 2020,OctSE,1; 2020,AugSE,1; 2020,AugSE,1; 2020,AugSE,1; 2018,Jan,8; 2017,Jan,8; 2016,Jan,13

87551 Mycobacteria species, amplified probe technique
🖵 0.00 ⚕ 0.00 **FUD** XXX   ⒬ ▣
AMA: 2020,Dec,3; 2020,OctSE,1; 2020,OctSE,1; 2020,AugSE,1; 2020,AugSE,1; 2020,AugSE,1; 2018,Jan,8; 2017,Jan,8; 2016,Jan,13

87552 Mycobacteria species, quantification
🖵 0.00 ⚕ 0.00 **FUD** XXX   ⒬ ▣
AMA: 2020,Dec,3; 2020,OctSE,1; 2020,OctSE,1; 2020,AugSE,1; 2020,AugSE,1; 2020,AugSE,1; 2018,Jan,8; 2017,Jan,8; 2016,Jan,13

87555 Mycobacteria tuberculosis, direct probe technique
🖵 0.00 ⚕ 0.00 **FUD** XXX   ⒬ ▣
AMA: 2020,Dec,3; 2020,OctSE,1; 2020,OctSE,1; 2020,AugSE,1; 2020,AugSE,1; 2020,AugSE,1; 2018,Jan,8; 2017,Jan,8; 2016,Jan,13

87556 Mycobacteria tuberculosis, amplified probe technique
🖵 0.00 ⚕ 0.00 **FUD** XXX   ⒬ ▣
AMA: 2020,Dec,3; 2020,OctSE,1; 2020,OctSE,1; 2020,AugSE,1; 2020,AugSE,1; 2020,AugSE,1; 2018,Jan,8; 2017,Jan,8; 2016,Jan,13

87557 Mycobacteria tuberculosis, quantification
🖵 0.00 ⚕ 0.00 **FUD** XXX   ⒬ ▣
AMA: 2020,Dec,3; 2020,OctSE,1; 2020,OctSE,1; 2020,AugSE,1; 2020,AugSE,1; 2020,AugSE,1; 2018,Jan,8; 2017,Jan,8; 2016,Jan,13

87560 Mycobacteria avium-intracellulare, direct probe technique
🖵 0.00 ⚕ 0.00 **FUD** XXX   ⒬ ▣
AMA: 2020,Dec,3; 2020,OctSE,1; 2020,OctSE,1; 2020,AugSE,1; 2020,AugSE,1; 2020,AugSE,1; 2018,Jan,8; 2017,Jan,8; 2016,Jan,13

87561 Mycobacteria avium-intracellulare, amplified probe technique
🖵 0.00 ⚕ 0.00 **FUD** XXX   ⒬ ▣
AMA: 2020,Dec,3; 2020,OctSE,1; 2020,OctSE,1; 2020,AugSE,1; 2020,AugSE,1; 2020,AugSE,1; 2018,Jan,8; 2017,Jan,8; 2016,Jan,13

87562 Mycobacteria avium-intracellulare, quantification
🖵 0.00 ⚕ 0.00 **FUD** XXX   ⒬ ▣
AMA: 2020,Dec,3; 2020,OctSE,1; 2020,OctSE,1; 2020,AugSE,1; 2020,AugSE,1; 2020,AugSE,1; 2018,Jan,8; 2017,Jan,8; 2016,Jan,13

87563 Mycoplasma genitalium, amplified probe technique
AMA: 2020,Dec,3; 2020,OctSE,1; 2020,Oct,11; 2020,OctSE,1; 2020,AugSE,1; 2020,AugSE,1; 2020,AugSE,1

87580 Mycoplasma pneumoniae, direct probe technique
🖵 0.00 ⚕ 0.00 **FUD** XXX   ⒬ ▣
AMA: 2020,Dec,3; 2020,OctSE,1; 2020,OctSE,1; 2020,AugSE,1; 2020,AugSE,1; 2020,AugSE,1; 2018,Jan,8; 2017,Jan,8; 2016,Jan,13

87581 Mycoplasma pneumoniae, amplified probe technique
🖵 0.00 ⚕ 0.00 **FUD** XXX   ⒬ ▣
AMA: 2020,Dec,3; 2020,OctSE,1; 2020,OctSE,1; 2020,AugSE,1; 2020,AugSE,1; 2020,AugSE,1; 2018,Jan,8; 2017,Jan,8; 2016,Jan,13

87582 Mycoplasma pneumoniae, quantification
🖵 0.00 ⚕ 0.00 **FUD** XXX   ⒬ ▣
AMA: 2020,Dec,3; 2020,OctSE,1; 2020,OctSE,1; 2020,AugSE,1; 2020,AugSE,1; 2020,AugSE,1; 2018,Jan,8; 2017,Jan,8; 2016,Jan,13

87590 Neisseria gonorrhoeae, direct probe technique
🖵 0.00 ⚕ 0.00 **FUD** XXX   Ⓐ ▣
AMA: 2020,Dec,3; 2020,OctSE,1; 2020,OctSE,1; 2020,AugSE,1; 2020,AugSE,1; 2020,AugSE,1; 2018,Jan,8; 2017,Jan,8; 2016,Jan,13

87591 Neisseria gonorrhoeae, amplified probe technique
🖵 0.00 ⚕ 0.00 **FUD** XXX   Ⓐ ▣
AMA: 2020,Dec,3; 2020,OctSE,1; 2020,OctSE,1; 2020,AugSE,1; 2020,AugSE,1; 2020,AugSE,1; 2018,Jan,8; 2017,Jan,8; 2016,Jan,13

87592 Neisseria gonorrhoeae, quantification
🖵 0.00 ⚕ 0.00 **FUD** XXX   ⒬ ▣
AMA: 2020,Dec,3; 2020,OctSE,1; 2020,OctSE,1; 2020,AugSE,1; 2020,AugSE,1; 2020,AugSE,1; 2018,Jan,8; 2017,Jan,8; 2016,Jan,13

87623 **Resequenced code. See code following 87539.**

87624 **Resequenced code. See code following 87539.**

87625 **Resequenced code. See code before 87540.**

87631 respiratory virus (eg, adenovirus, influenza virus, coronavirus, metapneumovirus, parainfluenza virus, respiratory syncytial virus, rhinovirus), includes multiplex reverse transcription, when performed, and multiplex amplified probe technique, multiple types or subtypes, 3-5 targets
INCLUDES Detection multiple respiratory viruses with one test
EXCLUDES *Assay for severe acute respiratory syndrome coronavirus 2 (SARS-CoV-2) (Coronavirus disease) (COVID-19) (87635)*
Assays for typing or subtyping influenza viruses only (87501-87503)
Single test for detection multiple infectious organisms (87800-87801)
🖵 0.00 ⚕ 0.00 **FUD** XXX   ✖ ⒬ ▣
AMA: 2020,Dec,3; 2020,OctSE,1; 2020,OctSE,1; 2020,AugSE,1; 2020,AugSE,1; 2020,AugSE,1; 2020,Apr,3; 2020,Mar,3; 2018,Jan,8; 2017,Jan,8; 2016,Jan,13

26/TC PC/TC Only	A2-Z3 ASC Payment	50 Bilateral	♂ Male Only	♀ Female Only	🖵 Facility RVU	⚕ Non-Facility RVU	▣ CCI	✖ CLIA
FUD Follow-up Days	CMS: IOM	AMA: CPT Asst	A-Y OPPSI	80/80 Surg Assist Allowed / w/Doc	▣ Lab Crosswalk	▣ Radiology Crosswalk

424
CPT © 2021 American Medical Association. All Rights Reserved.
© 2021 Optum360, LLC

87632 respiratory virus (eg, adenovirus, influenza virus, coronavirus, metapneumovirus, parainfluenza virus, respiratory syncytial virus, rhinovirus), includes multiplex reverse transcription, when performed, and multiplex amplified probe technique, multiple types or subtypes, 6-11 targets

INCLUDES Detection multiple respiratory viruses with one test

EXCLUDES Assay for severe acute respiratory syndrome coronavirus 2 (SARS-CoV-2) (Coronavirus disease) (COVID-19) (87635)

Assays for typing or subtyping influenza viruses only (87501-87503)

Single test to detect multiple infectious organisms (87800-87801)

🚗 0.00   ⚖ 0.00   **FUD** XXX   🔲 🖵

AMA: 2020,Dec,3; 2020,OctSE,1; 2020,OctSE,1; 2020,AugSE,1; 2020,AugSE,1; 2020,AugSE,1; 2020,Apr,3; 2020,Mar,3; 2018,Jan,8; 2017,Jan,8; 2016,Jan,13

87633 respiratory virus (eg, adenovirus, influenza virus, coronavirus, metapneumovirus, parainfluenza virus, respiratory syncytial virus, rhinovirus), includes multiplex reverse transcription, when performed, and multiplex amplified probe technique, multiple types or subtypes, 12-25 targets

INCLUDES Detection multiple respiratory viruses with one test

EXCLUDES Assay for severe acute respiratory syndrome coronavirus 2 (SARS-CoV-2) (Coronavirus disease) (COVID-19) (87635)

Assays for typing or subtyping influenza viruses only (87501-87503)

Single test to detect multiple infectious organisms (87800-87801)

🚗 0.00   ⚖ 0.00   **FUD** XXX   ❌ 🔲 🖵

AMA: 2020,Dec,3; 2020,OctSE,1; 2020,OctSE,1; 2020,AugSE,1; 2020,AugSE,1; 2020,Apr,3; 2020,Mar,3; 2018,Jan,8; 2017,Jan,8; 2016,Jan,13

87634 respiratory syncytial virus, amplified probe technique

EXCLUDES Assays for RSV with other respiratory viruses (87631-87633)

🚗 0.00   ⚖ 0.00   **FUD** XXX   ❌ 🔲 🖵

AMA: 2020,Dec,3; 2020,OctSE,1; 2020,OctSE,1; 2020,AugSE,1; 2020,AugSE,1; 2020,AugSE,1

87635 severe acute respiratory syndrome coronavirus 2 (SARS-CoV-2) (Coronavirus disease [COVID-19]), amplified probe technique

EXCLUDES HCPCS codes for reporting coronavirus testing (U0001-U0002)

Single procedure nucleic acid assays to detect multiple respiratory viruses by multiplex reaction (87631-87633)

Code also code 87635, with modifier 59, for assays performed on specimens from different anatomic locations, when performed

🚗 0.00   ⚖ 0.00   **FUD** XXX   🖵

AMA: 2020,Dec,3; 2020,OctSE,1; 2020,OctSE,1; 2020,AugSE,1; 2020,AugSE,1; 2020,AugSE,1; 2020,Apr,3; 2020,Mar,3

● **87636** severe acute respiratory syndrome coronavirus 2 (SARS-CoV-2) (Coronavirus disease [COVID-19]) and influenza virus types A and B, multiplex amplified probe technique

EXCLUDES Nucleic acid detection multiple respiratory infectious agents (87631-87633):

Including severe acute respiratory syndrome coronavirus 2 (SARS-CoV-2) (Coronavirus disease) (COVID-19) with additional agents beyond influenza A and B and respiratory syncytial virus

Not including severe acute respiratory syndrome coronavirus 2 (SARS-CoV-2) (Coronavirus disease) (COVID-19)

🚗 0.00   ⚖ 0.00   **FUD** XXX   🖵

AMA: 2020,Dec,3; 2020,OctSE,1; 2020,NovSE,1

● **87637** severe acute respiratory syndrome coronavirus 2 (SARS-CoV-2) (Coronavirus disease [COVID-19]), influenza virus types A and B, and respiratory syncytial virus, multiplex amplified probe technique

EXCLUDES Nucleic acid detection multiple respiratory infectious agents (87631-87633):

Including severe acute respiratory syndrome coronavirus 2 (SARS-CoV-2) (coronavirus disease) (COVID-19) with additional agents beyond influenza A and B and respiratory syncytial virus

Not including severe acute respiratory syndrome coronavirus 2 (SARS-CoV-2) (coronavirus disease) (COVID-19)

🚗 0.00   ⚖ 0.00   **FUD** XXX   🖵

AMA: 2020,Dec,3; 2020,OctSE,1; 2020,NovSE,1

87640 Staphylococcus aureus, amplified probe technique

🚗 0.00   ⚖ 0.00   **FUD** XXX   🔲 🖵

AMA: 2020,Dec,3; 2020,OctSE,1; 2020,OctSE,1; 2020,AugSE,1; 2020,AugSE,1; 2020,AugSE,1; 2018,Jan,8; 2017,Jan,8; 2016,Jan,13

87641 Staphylococcus aureus, methicillin resistant, amplified probe technique

EXCLUDES Assays that detect methicillin resistance and identify Staphylococcus aureus using single nucleic acid sequence (87641)

🚗 0.00   ⚖ 0.00   **FUD** XXX   🔲 🖵

AMA: 2020,Dec,3; 2020,OctSE,1; 2020,OctSE,1; 2020,AugSE,1; 2020,AugSE,1; 2020,AugSE,1; 2018,Jan,8; 2017,Jan,8; 2016,Jan,13

87650 Streptococcus, group A, direct probe technique

🚗 0.00   ⚖ 0.00   **FUD** XXX   🔲 🖵

AMA: 2020,Dec,3; 2020,OctSE,1; 2020,OctSE,1; 2020,AugSE,1; 2020,AugSE,1; 2020,AugSE,1; 2018,Jan,8; 2017,Jan,8; 2016,Jan,13

87651 Streptococcus, group A, amplified probe technique

🚗 0.00   ⚖ 0.00   **FUD** XXX   ❌ 🔲 🖵

AMA: 2020,Dec,3; 2020,OctSE,1; 2020,OctSE,1; 2020,AugSE,1; 2020,AugSE,1; 2020,AugSE,1; 2018,Jan,8; 2017,Jan,8; 2016,Jan,13

87652 Streptococcus, group A, quantification

🚗 0.00   ⚖ 0.00   **FUD** XXX   🔲 🖵

AMA: 2020,Dec,3; 2020,OctSE,1; 2020,OctSE,1; 2020,AugSE,1; 2020,AugSE,1; 2020,AugSE,1; 2018,Jan,8; 2017,Jan,8; 2016,Jan,13

87653 Streptococcus, group B, amplified probe technique

🚗 0.00   ⚖ 0.00   **FUD** XXX   🔲 🖵

AMA: 2020,Dec,3; 2020,OctSE,1; 2020,OctSE,1; 2020,AugSE,1; 2020,AugSE,1; 2020,AugSE,1; 2018,Jan,8; 2017,Jan,8; 2016,Jan,13

87660 Trichomonas vaginalis, direct probe technique

🚗 0.00   ⚖ 0.00   **FUD** XXX   🔲 🖵

AMA: 2020,Dec,3; 2020,OctSE,1; 2020,OctSE,1; 2020,AugSE,1; 2020,AugSE,1; 2020,AugSE,1; 2018,Jan,8; 2017,Jan,8; 2016,Jan,13

87661 Trichomonas vaginalis, amplified probe technique

🚗 0.00   ⚖ 0.00   **FUD** XXX

AMA: 2020,Dec,3; 2020,OctSE,1; 2020,OctSE,1; 2020,AugSE,1; 2020,AugSE,1; 2020,AugSE,1

87662 Zika virus, amplified probe technique

🚗 0.00   ⚖ 0.00   **FUD** XXX   🔲 🖵

AMA: 2020,Dec,3; 2020,OctSE,1; 2020,OctSE,1; 2020,AugSE,1; 2020,AugSE,1; 2020,AugSE,1

87797 Infectious agent detection by nucleic acid (DNA or RNA), not otherwise specified; direct probe technique, each organism

🚗 0.00   ⚖ 0.00   **FUD** XXX   🔲 🖵

AMA: 2020,Dec,3; 2020,OctSE,1; 2020,OctSE,1; 2020,AugSE,1; 2020,AugSE,1; 2020,AugSE,1; 2018,Jan,8; 2017,Jan,8; 2016,Aug,9; 2016,Jan,13

87798 amplified probe technique, each organism

🚗 0.00   ⚖ 0.00   **FUD** XXX   🔲 🖵

AMA: 2020,Dec,3; 2020,Oct,11; 2020,OctSE,1; 2020,OctSE,1; 2020,AugSE,1; 2020,AugSE,1; 2020,AugSE,1; 2018,Jan,8; 2017,Jan,8; 2016,Jan,13

● New Code   ▲ Revised Code   ○ Reinstated   ● New Web Release   ▲ Revised Web Release   + Add-on   Unlisted   Not Covered   # Resequenced
⑤⓪ Optum Mod 50 Exempt   Ⓢ AMA Mod 51 Exempt   ㊿ Optum Mod 51 Exempt   ㊿ Mod 63 Exempt   ∕ Non-FDA Drug   ★ Telemedicine   Ⓜ Maternity   🅰 Age Edit

Pathology and Laboratory

87799 — 87910

87799   **quantification, each organism**
🏥 0.00   🔬 0.00   **FUD** XXX   Q ▢
AMA: 2020,Dec,3; 2020,OctSE,1; 2020,OctSE,1; 2020,AugSE,1; 2020,AugSE,1; 2020,AugSE,1; 2018,Jan,8; 2017,Jan,8; 2016,Jan,13

87800   **Infectious agent detection by nucleic acid (DNA or RNA), multiple organisms; direct probe(s) technique**
INCLUDES   Single test to detect multiple infectious organisms
EXCLUDES   *Detection specific infectious agents not otherwise specified (87797-87799)*
     Each specific organism nucleic acid detection from primary source (87471-87660 [87623, 87624, 87625])
🏥 0.00   🔬 0.00   **FUD** XXX   A ▢
AMA: 2020,Dec,3; 2020,OctSE,1; 2020,OctSE,1; 2020,AugSE,1; 2020,AugSE,1; 2020,AugSE,1; 2018,Jan,8; 2017,Jan,8; 2016,Aug,9; 2016,Jan,13

87801   **amplified probe(s) technique**
INCLUDES   Single test to detect multiple infectious organisms
EXCLUDES   *Detection multiple respiratory viruses with one test (87631-87633)*
     Detection specific infectious agents not otherwise specified (87797-87799)
     Each specific organism nucleic acid detection from primary source (87471-87660 [87623, 87624, 87625])
🏥 0.00   🔬 0.00   **FUD** XXX   Q ▢
AMA: 2020,Dec,3; 2020,OctSE,1; 2020,OctSE,1; 2020,AugSE,1; 2020,AugSE,1; 2020,AugSE,1; 2018,Jan,8; 2017,Jan,8; 2016,Jan,13

87802-87899 [87806, 87811] Detection Infectious Agent by Immunoassay with Direct Optical Observation

▲ 87802   **Infectious agent antigen detection by immunoassay with direct optical (ie, visual) observation; Streptococcus, group B**
🏥 0.00   🔬 0.00   **FUD** XXX   Q ▢
AMA: 2020,Dec,3; 2020,OctSE,1; 2020,OctSE,1; 2020,AugSE,1; 2020,AugSE,1; 2020,AugSE,1

▲ 87803   **Clostridium difficile toxin A**
🏥 0.00   🔬 0.00   **FUD** XXX   Q ▢
AMA: 2020,Dec,3; 2020,OctSE,1; 2020,OctSE,1; 2020,AugSE,1; 2020,AugSE,1

▲ # 87806   **HIV-1 antigen(s), with HIV-1 and HIV-2 antibodies**
🏥 0.00   🔬 0.00   **FUD** XXX   ✖ Q ▢
AMA: 2020,Dec,3; 2020,OctSE,1; 2020,OctSE,1; 2020,AugSE,1; 2020,AugSE,1

87806   Resequenced code. See code following 87803.

▲ 87807   **respiratory syncytial virus**
🏥 0.00   🔬 0.00   **FUD** XXX   ✖ Q ▢
AMA: 2020,Dec,3; 2020,OctSE,1; 2020,OctSE,1; 2020,AugSE,1; 2020,AugSE,1

● # 87811   **severe acute respiratory syndrome coronavirus 2 (SARS-CoV-2) (Coronavirus disease [COVID-19])**
🏥 0.00   🔬 0.00   **FUD** XXX
AMA: 2020,Dec,3; 2020,OctSE,1

▲ 87808   **Trichomonas vaginalis**
🏥 0.00   🔬 0.00   **FUD** XXX   ✖ Q ▢
AMA: 2020,Dec,3; 2020,OctSE,1; 2020,OctSE,1; 2020,AugSE,1; 2020,AugSE,1

▲ 87809   **adenovirus**
🏥 0.00   🔬 0.00   **FUD** XXX   ✖ Q ▢
AMA: 2020,Dec,3; 2020,OctSE,1; 2020,OctSE,1; 2020,AugSE,1; 2020,AugSE,1; 2018,Jan,8; 2017,Jan,8; 2016,Jan,13

▲ 87810   **Chlamydia trachomatis**
🏥 0.00   🔬 0.00   **FUD** XXX   A ▢
AMA: 2020,Dec,3; 2020,OctSE,1; 2020,OctSE,1; 2020,AugSE,1; 2020,AugSE,1; 2020,AugSE,1; 2018,Jan,8; 2017,Jan,8; 2016,Jan,13

87811   Resequenced code. See code following 87807.

▲ 87850   **Neisseria gonorrhoeae**
🏥 0.00   🔬 0.00   **FUD** XXX   A ▢
AMA: 2020,Dec,3; 2020,OctSE,1; 2020,OctSE,1; 2020,AugSE,1; 2020,AugSE,1; 2020,AugSE,1; 2018,Jan,8; 2017,Jan,8; 2016,Jan,13

▲ 87880   **Streptococcus, group A**
🏥 0.00   🔬 0.00   **FUD** XXX   ✖ Q ▢
AMA: 2020,Dec,3; 2020,OctSE,1; 2020,OctSE,1; 2020,AugSE,1; 2020,AugSE,1; 2020,AugSE,1; 2018,Jan,8; 2017,Jan,8; 2016,Jan,13

▲ 87899   **not otherwise specified**
🏥 0.00   🔬 0.00   **FUD** XXX   ✖ Q ▢
AMA: 2020,Dec,3; 2020,OctSE,1; 2020,OctSE,1; 2020,AugSE,1; 2020,AugSE,1; 2020,AugSE,1; 2018,Jan,8; 2017,Jan,8; 2016,Jan,13

87900-87999 [87906, 87910, 87912] Drug Sensitivity Genotype/Phenotype

87900   **Infectious agent drug susceptibility phenotype prediction using regularly updated genotypic bioinformatics**
🏥 0.00   🔬 0.00   **FUD** XXX   Q ▢
AMA: 2020,Dec,3; 2020,OctSE,1; 2020,OctSE,1; 2018,Jan,8; 2017,Jan,8; 2016,Jan,13

87910   **Infectious agent genotype analysis by nucleic acid (DNA or RNA); cytomegalovirus**
EXCLUDES   *HPV detection (genotyping) (0500T)*
     HIV-1 infectious agent phenotype prediction (87900)
🏥 0.00   🔬 0.00   **FUD** XXX   Q ▢
AMA: 2020,Dec,3; 2018,Jan,8; 2017,Jan,8; 2016,Jan,13

87901   **HIV-1, reverse transcriptase and protease regions**
EXCLUDES   *Infectious agent drug susceptibility phenotype prediction for HIV-1 (87900)*
🏥 0.00   🔬 0.00   **FUD** XXX   Q ▢
AMA: 2020,Dec,3; 2020,OctSE,1; 2020,OctSE,1; 2018,Jan,8; 2017,Jan,8; 2016,Jan,13

87906   **HIV-1, other region (eg, integrase, fusion)**
EXCLUDES   *HIV-1 infectious agent phenotype prediction (87900)*
🏥 0.00   🔬 0.00   **FUD** XXX   Q ▢
AMA: 2020,Dec,3; 2018,Jan,8; 2017,Jan,8; 2016,Jan,13

87912   **Hepatitis B virus**
🏥 0.00   🔬 0.00   **FUD** XXX   Q ▢
AMA: 2020,Dec,3; 2018,Jan,8; 2017,Jan,8; 2016,Jan,13

87902   **Hepatitis C virus**
🏥 0.00   🔬 0.00   **FUD** XXX   Q ▢
AMA: 2020,Dec,3; 2020,OctSE,1; 2020,OctSE,1; 2018,Jan,8; 2017,Jan,8; 2016,Jan,13

87903   **Infectious agent phenotype analysis by nucleic acid (DNA or RNA) with drug resistance tissue culture analysis, HIV 1; first through 10 drugs tested**
🏥 0.00   🔬 0.00   **FUD** XXX   Q ▢
AMA: 2020,Dec,3; 2020,OctSE,1; 2020,OctSE,1; 2018,Jan,8; 2017,Jan,8; 2016,Jan,13

+ 87904   **each additional drug tested (List separately in addition to code for primary procedure)**
Code first (87903)
🏥 0.00   🔬 0.00   **FUD** XXX   Q ▢
AMA: 2020,Dec,3; 2018,Jan,8; 2017,Jan,8; 2016,Jan,13

87905   **Infectious agent enzymatic activity other than virus (eg, sialidase activity in vaginal fluid)**
EXCLUDES   *Virus isolation identified by nonimmunologic method, and by noncytopathic effect (87255)*
🏥 0.00   🔬 0.00   **FUD** XXX   ✖ Q ▢
AMA: 2020,Dec,3

87906   Resequenced code. See code following 87901.

87910   Resequenced code. See code following 87900.

| *87912* | Resequenced code. See code before 87902. |

87999   Unlisted microbiology procedure
🔲 0.00   ⚘ 0.00   **FUD** XXX   N 🔲
AMA: 2020,Dec,3; 2018,Jan,8; 2017,Jan,8; 2016,Jan,13

88000-88099 Autopsy Services
CMS: 100-02,15,80.1 Payment for Clinical Laboratory Services
INCLUDES   Services for physicians only

88000   Necropsy (autopsy), gross examination only; without CNS
🔲 0.00   ⚘ 0.00   **FUD** XXX   E 🔲
AMA: 2020,Dec,3; 2018,Jan,8; 2017,Jan,8; 2016,Jan,13

88005   with brain
🔲 0.00   ⚘ 0.00   **FUD** XXX   E 🔲
AMA: 2020,Dec,3

88007   with brain and spinal cord
🔲 0.00   ⚘ 0.00   **FUD** XXX   E 🔲
AMA: 2020,Dec,3

88012   infant with brain   A
🔲 0.00   ⚘ 0.00   **FUD** XXX   E 🔲
AMA: 2020,Dec,3

88014   stillborn or newborn with brain   A
🔲 0.00   ⚘ 0.00   **FUD** XXX   E 🔲
AMA: 2020,Dec,3

88016   macerated stillborn   A
🔲 0.00   ⚘ 0.00   **FUD** XXX   E 🔲
AMA: 2020,Dec,3

88020   Necropsy (autopsy), gross and microscopic; without CNS
🔲 0.00   ⚘ 0.00   **FUD** XXX   E 🔲
AMA: 2020,Dec,3

88025   with brain
🔲 0.00   ⚘ 0.00   **FUD** XXX   E 🔲
AMA: 2020,Dec,3

88027   with brain and spinal cord
🔲 0.00   ⚘ 0.00   **FUD** XXX   E 🔲
AMA: 2020,Dec,3

88028   infant with brain   A
🔲 0.00   ⚘ 0.00   **FUD** XXX   E 🔲
AMA: 2020,Dec,3

88029   stillborn or newborn with brain   A
🔲 0.00   ⚘ 0.00   **FUD** XXX   E 🔲
AMA: 2020,Dec,3

88036   Necropsy (autopsy), limited, gross and/or microscopic; regional
🔲 0.00   ⚘ 0.00   **FUD** XXX   E 🔲
AMA: 2020,Dec,3

88037   single organ
🔲 0.00   ⚘ 0.00   **FUD** XXX   E 🔲
AMA: 2020,Dec,3

88040   Necropsy (autopsy); forensic examination
🔲 0.00   ⚘ 0.00   **FUD** XXX   E 🔲
AMA: 2020,Dec,3

88045   coroner's call
🔲 0.00   ⚘ 0.00   **FUD** XXX   E 🔲
AMA: 2020,Dec,3

88099   Unlisted necropsy (autopsy) procedure
🔲 0.00   ⚘ 0.00   **FUD** XXX   E 🔲
AMA: 2020,Dec,3; 2018,Jan,8; 2017,Jan,8; 2016,Jan,13

88104-88140 Cytopathology: Other Than Cervical/Vaginal

88104   Cytopathology, fluids, washings or brushings, except cervical or vaginal; smears with interpretation
🔲 1.93   ⚘ 1.93   **FUD** XXX   Q1 80 🔲
AMA: 2020,Dec,3; 2018,Jan,8; 2017,Jan,8; 2016,Jan,13

88106   simple filter method with interpretation
EXCLUDES   *Cytopathology smears with interpretation (88104)*
    Selective cellular enhancement (nongynecological)
        including filter transfer techniques (88112)
🔲 1.81   ⚘ ___   **FUD** XXX   Q1 80 🔲
AMA: 2020,Dec,3; 2018,Jan,8; 2017,Jan,8; 2016,Jan,13

88108   Cytopathology, concentration technique, smears and interpretation (eg, Saccomanno technique)
EXCLUDES   *Cervical or vaginal smears (88150-88155)*
    Gastric intubation with lavage (43754-43755)
📷 (74340)
🔲 1.75   ⚘ 1.75   **FUD** XXX   Q1 80 🔲
AMA: 2020,Dec,3; 2018,Jan,8; 2017,Jan,8; 2016,Jan,13

88112   Cytopathology, selective cellular enhancement technique with interpretation (eg, liquid based slide preparation method), except cervical or vaginal
EXCLUDES   *Cytopathology cellular enhancement technique (88108)*
🔲 1.90   ⚘ 1.90   **FUD** XXX   Q1 80 🔲
AMA: 2020,Dec,3

88120   Cytopathology, in situ hybridization (eg, FISH), urinary tract specimen with morphometric analysis, 3-5 molecular probes, each specimen; manual
EXCLUDES   *More than five probes (88399)*
    Morphometric in situ hybridization on specimens other
        than urinary tract (88367-88368 [88373, 88374])
🔲 16.3   ⚘ 16.3   **FUD** XXX   Q2 80 🔲
AMA: 2020,Dec,3

88121   using computer-assisted technology
EXCLUDES   *More than five probes (88399)*
    Morphometric in situ hybridization on specimens other
        than urinary tract (88367-88368 [88373, 88374])
🔲 12.4   ⚘ 12.4   **FUD** XXX   Q1 80 🔲
AMA: 2020,Dec,3

88125   Cytopathology, forensic (eg, sperm)
🔲 0.75   ⚘ 0.75   **FUD** XXX   Q1 80 🔲
AMA: 2020,Dec,3

88130   Sex chromatin identification; Barr bodies
🔲 0.00   ⚘ 0.00   **FUD** XXX   Q 🔲
AMA: 2020,Dec,3

88140   peripheral blood smear, polymorphonuclear drumsticks
EXCLUDES   *Guard stain (88313)*
🔲 0.00   ⚘ 0.00   **FUD** XXX   Q 🔲
AMA: 2020,Dec,3; 2018,Jan,8; 2017,Jan,8; 2016,Jan,13

88141-88155 Pap Smears
CMS: 100-03,210.2 Screening Pap Smears/Pelvic Examinations for Early Cancer Detection
EXCLUDES   *Non-Bethesda method (88150-88153)*

88141   Cytopathology, cervical or vaginal (any reporting system), requiring interpretation by physician   ♀
Code also (88142-88153, 88164-88167, 88174-88175)
🔲 0.90   ⚘ 0.90   **FUD** XXX   N 80 26 🔲
AMA: 2020,Dec,3; 2018,Jan,8; 2017,Jan,8; 2016,Jan,13

88142   Cytopathology, cervical or vaginal (any reporting system), collected in preservative fluid, automated thin layer preparation; manual screening under physician supervision   ♀
INCLUDES   Bethesda or non-Bethesda method
🔲 0.00   ⚘ 0.00   **FUD** XXX   Q 🔲
AMA: 2020,Dec,3; 2018,Jan,8; 2017,Jan,8; 2016,Jan,13

88143   with manual screening and rescreening under physician supervision   ♀
INCLUDES   Bethesda or non-Bethesda method
EXCLUDES   *Automated screening automated thin layer preparation*
        (88174-88175)
🔲 0.00   ⚘ 0.00   **FUD** XXX   Q 🔲
AMA: 2020,Dec,3; 2018,Jan,8; 2017,Jan,8; 2016,Jan,13

88147   Cytopathology smears, cervical or vaginal; screening by automated system under physician supervision ♀
   🔧 0.00   ⚗ 0.00   **FUD** XXX   [Q] [CCI]
   AMA: 2020,Dec,3; 2018,Jan,8; 2017,Jan,8; 2016,Jan,13

88148   screening by automated system with manual rescreening under physician supervision ♀
   🔧 0.00   ⚗ 0.00   **FUD** XXX   [Q] [CCI]
   AMA: 2020,Dec,3; 2018,Jan,8; 2017,Jan,8; 2016,Jan,13

88150   Cytopathology, slides, cervical or vaginal; manual screening under physician supervision ♀
   EXCLUDES   *Bethesda method Pap smears (88164-88167)*
   🔧 0.00   ⚗ 0.00   **FUD** XXX   [Q] [CCI]
   AMA: 2020,Dec,3; 2018,Jan,8; 2017,Jan,8; 2016,Jan,13

88152   with manual screening and computer-assisted rescreening under physician supervision
   EXCLUDES   *Bethesda method Pap smears (88164-88167)*
   🔧 0.00   ⚗ 0.00   **FUD** XXX   [Q] [CCI]
   AMA: 2020,Dec,3; 2018,Jan,8; 2017,Jan,8; 2016,Jan,13

88153   with manual screening and rescreening under physician supervision ♀
   EXCLUDES   *Bethesda method Pap smears (88164-88167)*
   🔧 0.00   ⚗ 0.00   **FUD** XXX   [Q] [CCI]
   AMA: 2020,Dec,3; 2018,Jan,8; 2017,Jan,8; 2016,Jan,13

+ 88155   Cytopathology, slides, cervical or vaginal, definitive hormonal evaluation (eg, maturation index, karyopyknotic index, estrogenic index) (List separately in addition to code[s] for other technical and interpretation services) ♀
   Code first (88142-88153, 88164-88167, 88174-88175)
   🔧 0.00   ⚗ 0.00   **FUD** XXX   [Q] [CCI]
   AMA: 2020,Dec,3; 2018,Jan,8; 2017,Jan,8; 2016,Jan,13

88160-88162 Cytopathology Smears (Other Than Pap)

88160   Cytopathology, smears, any other source; screening and interpretation
   🔧 2.01   ⚗ 2.01   **FUD** XXX   [Q1] [80] [CCI]
   AMA: 2020,Dec,3

88161   preparation, screening and interpretation
   🔧 1.93   ⚗ 1.93   **FUD** XXX   [Q1] [80] [CCI]
   AMA: 2020,Dec,3; 2018,Jan,8; 2017,Jan,8; 2016,Jan,13

88162   extended study involving over 5 slides and/or multiple stains
   EXCLUDES   *Aerosol collection sputum (89220)*
             Special stains (88312-88314)
   🔧 2.80   ⚗ 2.80   **FUD** XXX   [Q1] [80] [CCI]
   AMA: 2020,Dec,3

88164-88167 Pap Smears: Bethesda System

CMS: 100-03,210.2 Screening Pap Smears/Pelvic Examinations for Early Cancer Detection
   EXCLUDES   *Non-Bethesda method (88150-88153)*

88164   Cytopathology, slides, cervical or vaginal (the Bethesda System); manual screening under physician supervision ♀
   🔧 0.00   ⚗ 0.00   **FUD** XXX   [Q] [CCI]
   AMA: 2020,Dec,3; 2018,Jan,8; 2017,Jan,8; 2016,Jan,13

88165   with manual screening and rescreening under physician supervision ♀
   🔧 0.00   ⚗ 0.00   **FUD** XXX   [Q] [CCI]
   AMA: 2020,Dec,3; 2018,Jan,8; 2017,Jan,8; 2016,Jan,13

88166   with manual screening and computer-assisted rescreening under physician supervision ♀
   🔧 0.00   ⚗ 0.00   **FUD** XXX   [Q] [CCI]
   AMA: 2020,Dec,3; 2018,Jan,8; 2017,Jan,8; 2016,Jan,13

88167   with manual screening and computer-assisted rescreening using cell selection and review under physician supervision ♀
   EXCLUDES   *Fine needle aspiration ([10004, 10005, 10006, 10007, 10008, 10009, 10010, 10011, 10012])*
   🔧 0.00   ⚗ 0.00   **FUD** XXX   [Q] [CCI]
   AMA: 2020,Dec,3; 2018,Jan,8; 2017,Jan,8; 2016,Jan,13

88172-88177 [88177] Cytopathology of Needle Biopsy

EXCLUDES   *Fine needle aspiration (10021, [10004, 10005, 10006, 10007, 10008, 10009, 10010, 10011, 10012])*

88172   Cytopathology, evaluation of fine needle aspirate; immediate cytohistologic study to determine adequacy for diagnosis, first evaluation episode, each site
   INCLUDES   Submission complete set cytologic material for evaluation no matter how many needle passes performed or slides prepared from each site
   EXCLUDES   *Cytologic examination during intraoperative pathology consultation (88333-88334)*
   🔧 1.58   ⚗ 1.58   **FUD** XXX   [Q1] [80] [CCI]
   AMA: 2020,Dec,3; 2019,Feb,8; 2019,Apr,4; 2018,Jan,8; 2017,Jan,8; 2016,Jan,13; 2016,Jan,11

88173   interpretation and report
   INCLUDES   Interpretation and report from each anatomical site no matter how many passes or evaluation episodes performed during aspiration
   EXCLUDES   *Cytologic examination during intraoperative pathology consultation (88333-88334)*
   🔧 4.36   ⚗ 4.36   **FUD** XXX   [Q1] [80] [CCI]
   AMA: 2020,Dec,3; 2019,Apr,4; 2019,Feb,8; 2018,Jan,8; 2017,Jan,8; 2016,Jan,13

+ # 88177   immediate cytohistologic study to determine adequacy for diagnosis, each separate additional evaluation episode, same site (List separately in addition to code for primary procedure)
   Code also each additional immediate repeat evaluation episode(s) required from same site (i.e., previous sample inadequate)
   Code first (88172)
   🔧 0.84   ⚗ 0.84   **FUD** ZZZ   [N] [80] [CCI]
   AMA: 2020,Dec,3; 2019,Apr,4; 2018,Jan,8; 2017,Jan,8; 2016,Jan,11

88174-88177 [88177] Pap Smears: Automated Screening

EXCLUDES   *Non-Bethesda method (88150-88153)*

88174   Cytopathology, cervical or vaginal (any reporting system), collected in preservative fluid, automated thin layer preparation; screening by automated system, under physician supervision ♀
   INCLUDES   Bethesda or non-Bethesda method
   🔧 0.00   ⚗ 0.00   **FUD** XXX   [Q] [CCI]
   AMA: 2020,Dec,3; 2018,Jan,8; 2017,Jan,8; 2016,Jan,13

88175   with screening by automated system and manual rescreening or review, under physician supervision ♀
   INCLUDES   Bethesda or non-Bethesda method
   EXCLUDES   *Manual screening (88142-88143)*
   🔧 0.00   ⚗ 0.00   **FUD** XXX   [Q] [CCI]
   AMA: 2020,Dec,3; 2018,Jan,8; 2017,Jan,8; 2016,Jan,13

88177   **Resequenced code. See code following 88173.**

88182-88199 Cytopathology Using the Fluorescence-Activated Cell Sorter

88182   Flow cytometry, cell cycle or DNA analysis
   EXCLUDES   *DNA ploidy analysis by morphometric technique (88358)*
   🔧 3.89   ⚗ 3.89   **FUD** XXX   [Q2] [80] [CCI]
   AMA: 2020,Dec,3; 2018,Jan,8; 2017,Jan,8; 2016,Jan,13

88184   Flow cytometry, cell surface, cytoplasmic, or nuclear marker, technical component only; first marker
   🔧 1.88   ⚗ 1.88   **FUD** XXX   [Q2] [80] [TC] [CCI]
   AMA: 2020,Dec,3; 2018,Jan,8; 2017,Jan,8; 2016,Jan,13

| 26/TC PC/TC Only | A2-Z3 ASC Payment | 50 Bilateral | ♂ Male Only | ♀ Female Only | 🔧 Facility RVU | ⚗ Non-Facility RVU | CCI | ☒ CLIA |
| FUD Follow-up Days | CMS: IOM | AMA: CPT Asst | A-Y OPPSI | 80/80 Surg Assist Allowed / w/Doc | Lab Crosswalk | Radiology Crosswalk |

428   CPT © 2021 American Medical Association. All Rights Reserved.   © 2021 Optum360, LLC

+	**88185**	**each additional marker (List separately in addition to code for first marker)**

Code first (88184)

0.69   0.69   **FUD** ZZZ   N 80 TC

AMA: 2020,Dec,3; 2018,Jan,8; 2017,Jan,8; 2016,Jan,13

88187   **Flow cytometry, interpretation; 2 to 8 markers**

EXCLUDES   *Antibody assessment by flow cytometry (83516-83520, 86000-86849 [86152, 86153])*
Cell enumeration by immunologic selection and identification ([86152, 86153])
Interpretation (86355-86357, 86359-86361, 86367)

1.08   1.08   **FUD** XXX   B 80 26

AMA: 2020,Dec,3; 2018,Jan,8; 2017,Jan,8; 2016,Jan,13

88188   **9 to 15 markers**

EXCLUDES   *Antibody assessment by flow cytometry (83516-83520, 86000-86849 [86152, 86153])*
Cell enumeration by immunologic selection and identification ([86152, 86153])
Interpretation (86355-86357, 86359-86361, 86367)

1.83   1.83   **FUD** XXX   B 80 26

AMA: 2020,Dec,3; 2018,Jan,8; 2017,Jan,8; 2016,Jan,13

88189   **16 or more markers**

EXCLUDES   *Antibody assessment by flow cytometry (83516-83520, 86000-86849 [86152, 86153])*
Cell enumeration using immunologic selection and identification in fluid sample ([86152, 86153])
Interpretation (86355-86357, 86359-86361, 86367)

2.45   2.45   **FUD** XXX   B 80 26

AMA: 2020,Dec,3; 2018,Jan,8; 2017,Jan,8; 2016,Jan,13

88199   **Unlisted cytopathology procedure**

EXCLUDES   *Electron microscopy (88348)*

0.00   0.00   **FUD** XXX   01 80

AMA: 2020,Dec,3; 2018,Jan,8; 2017,Jan,8; 2016,Jan,13

88230-88299 Cytogenic Studies

CMS: 100-03,190.3 Cytogenic Studies

EXCLUDES   *Acetylcholinesterase (82013)*
Alpha-fetoprotein (amniotic fluid or serum) (82105-82106)
Microdissection (88380)
Molecular pathology codes (81105-81383 [81105, 81106, 81107, 81108, 81109, 81110, 81111, 81112, 81120, 81121, 81161, 81162, 81163, 81164, 81165, 81166, 81167, 81173, 81174, 81184, 81185, 81186, 81187, 81188, 81189, 81190, 81200, 81201, 81202, 81203, 81204, 81205, 81206, 81207, 81208, 81209, 81210, 81219, 81227, 81230, 81231, 81233, 81234, 81238, 81239, 81245, 81246, 81250, 81257, 81258, 81259, 81261, 81262, 81263, 81264, 81265, 81266, 81267, 81268, 81269, 81271, 81274, 81283, 81284, 81285, 81286, 81287, 81288, 81289, 81291, 81292, 81293, 81294, 81295, 81301, 81302, 81303, 81304, 81306, 81312, 81320, 81324, 81325, 81326, 81332, 81334, 81336, 81337, 81343, 81344, 81345, 81361, 81362, 81363, 81364], 81400-81408, [81479], 81410-81471 [81448], 81500-81512, 81599)

88230   **Tissue culture for non-neoplastic disorders; lymphocyte**

0.00   0.00   **FUD** XXX   Q

AMA: 2020,Dec,3; 2018,Jan,8; 2017,Jan,8; 2016,Jan,13

88233   **skin or other solid tissue biopsy**

0.00   0.00   **FUD** XXX   Q

AMA: 2020,Dec,3; 2018,Jan,8; 2017,Jan,8; 2016,Jan,13

88235   **amniotic fluid or chorionic villus cells**   M

0.00   0.00   **FUD** XXX   Q

AMA: 2020,Dec,3; 2018,Jan,8; 2017,Jan,8; 2016,Jan,13

88237   **Tissue culture for neoplastic disorders; bone marrow, blood cells**

0.00   0.00   **FUD** XXX   Q

AMA: 2020,Dec,3; 2018,Jan,8; 2017,Jan,8; 2016,Jan,13

88239   **solid tumor**

0.00   0.00   **FUD** XXX   Q

AMA: 2020,Dec,3; 2018,Jan,8; 2017,Jan,8; 2016,Jan,13

88240   **Cryopreservation, freezing and storage of cells, each cell line**

EXCLUDES   *Therapeutic cryopreservation and storage (38207)*

0.00   0.00   **FUD** XXX   Q

AMA: 2020,Dec,3; 2018,Jan,8; 2017,Jan,8; 2016,Jan,13

88241   **Thawing and expansion of frozen cells, each aliquot**

EXCLUDES   *Therapeutic thawing of prior harvest (38208)*

0.00   0.00   **FUD** XXX   Q

AMA: 2020,Dec,3; 2018,Jan,8; 2017,Jan,8; 2016,Jan,13

88245   **Chromosome analysis for breakage syndromes; baseline Sister Chromatid Exchange (SCE), 20-25 cells**

0.00   0.00   **FUD** XXX   Q

AMA: 2020,Dec,3; 2018,Jan,8; 2017,Jan,8; 2016,Jan,13

88248   **baseline breakage, score 50-100 cells, count 20 cells, 2 karyotypes (eg, for ataxia telangiectasia, Fanconi anemia, fragile X)**

0.00   0.00   **FUD** XXX   Q

AMA: 2020,Dec,3; 2018,Jan,8; 2017,Jan,8; 2016,Jan,13

88249   **score 100 cells, clastogen stress (eg, diepoxybutane, mitomycin C, ionizing radiation, UV radiation)**

0.00   0.00   **FUD** XXX   Q

AMA: 2020,Dec,3; 2018,Jan,8; 2017,Jan,8; 2016,Jan,13

88261   **Chromosome analysis; count 5 cells, 1 karyotype, with banding**

0.00   0.00   **FUD** XXX   Q

AMA: 2020,Dec,3; 2018,Jan,8; 2017,Jan,8; 2016,Jan,13

88262   **count 15-20 cells, 2 karyotypes, with banding**

0.00   0.00   **FUD** XXX   Q

AMA: 2020,Dec,3; 2019,Aug,10; 2018,Jan,8; 2017,Jan,8; 2016,Jan,13

88263   **count 45 cells for mosaicism, 2 karyotypes, with banding**

0.00   0.00   **FUD** XXX   Q

AMA: 2020,Dec,3; 2018,Jan,8; 2017,Jan,8; 2016,Jan,13

88264   **analyze 20-25 cells**

0.00   0.00   **FUD** XXX   Q

AMA: 2020,Dec,3; 2019,Aug,10; 2018,Jan,8; 2017,Jan,8; 2016,Jan,13

88267   **Chromosome analysis, amniotic fluid or chorionic villus, count 15 cells, 1 karyotype, with banding**   M ♀

0.00   0.00   **FUD** XXX   Q

AMA: 2020,Dec,3; 2018,Jan,8; 2017,Jan,8; 2016,Jan,13

88269   **Chromosome analysis, in situ for amniotic fluid cells, count cells from 6-12 colonies, 1 karyotype, with banding**   M ♀

0.00   0.00   **FUD** XXX   Q

AMA: 2020,Dec,3; 2018,Jan,8; 2017,Jan,8; 2016,Jan,13

88271   **Molecular cytogenetics; DNA probe, each (eg, FISH)**

EXCLUDES   *Cytogenomic microarray analysis (81228-81229, [81349], 81405-81406, [81479])*
Fetal chromosome analysis using maternal blood (81420-81422)

0.00   0.00   **FUD** XXX   Q

AMA: 2020,Dec,3; 2020,Feb,10; 2018,Jan,8; 2017,Apr,3; 2017,Jan,8; 2016,Jan,13

88272   **chromosomal in situ hybridization, analyze 3-5 cells (eg, for derivatives and markers)**

0.00   0.00   **FUD** XXX   Q

AMA: 2020,Dec,3; 2018,Jan,8; 2017,Jan,8; 2016,Jan,13

88273   **chromosomal in situ hybridization, analyze 10-30 cells (eg, for microdeletions)**

0.00   0.00   **FUD** XXX   Q

AMA: 2020,Dec,3; 2018,Jan,8; 2017,Jan,8; 2016,Jan,13

88274   **interphase in situ hybridization, analyze 25-99 cells**

0.00   0.00   **FUD** XXX   Q

AMA: 2020,Dec,3; 2018,Jan,8; 2017,Jan,8; 2016,Jan,13

88275   **interphase in situ hybridization, analyze 100-300 cells**

0.00   0.00   **FUD** XXX   Q

AMA: 2020,Dec,3; 2018,Jan,8; 2017,Jan,8; 2016,Jan,13

88280   **Chromosome analysis; additional karyotypes, each study**

0.00   0.00   **FUD** XXX   Q

AMA: 2020,Dec,3; 2018,Jan,8; 2017,Jan,8; 2016,Jan,13

88283   additional specialized banding technique (eg, NOR, C-banding)

     🚑 0.00   ⚗ 0.00   **FUD** XXX   [Q] [▭]

     AMA: 2020,Dec,3; 2018,Jan,8; 2017,Jan,8; 2016,Jan,13

88285   additional cells counted, each study

     🚑 0.00   ⚗ 0.00   **FUD** XXX   [Q] [▭]

     AMA: 2020,Dec,3; 2018,Jan,8; 2017,Jan,8; 2016,Jan,13

88289   additional high resolution study

     🚑 0.00   ⚗ 0.00   **FUD** XXX   [Q] [▭]

     AMA: 2020,Dec,3; 2018,Jan,8; 2017,Jan,8; 2016,Jan,13

88291   Cytogenetics and molecular cytogenetics, interpretation and report

     🚑 0.94   ⚗ 0.94   **FUD** XXX   [M] [80] [26] [▭]

     AMA: 2020,Dec,3; 2018,Jan,8; 2017,Jan,8; 2016,Jan,13

88299   Unlisted cytogenetic study

     🚑 0.00   ⚗ 0.00   **FUD** XXX   [Q1] [80] [▭]

     AMA: 2020,Dec,3; 2018,Jan,8; 2017,Jan,8; 2016,Jan,13

88300 Evaluation of Surgical Specimen: Gross Anatomy

CMS: 100-02,15,80.1 Payment for Clinical Laboratory Services

   [INCLUDES]   Attainment, examination, and reporting
           Unit of service is the specimen
   [EXCLUDES]   *Additional procedures (88311-88365 [88341, 88350], 88399)*
           Microscopic exam (88302-88309)

88300   Level I - Surgical pathology, gross examination only

     🚑 0.44   ⚗ 0.44   **FUD** XXX   [Q1] [80] [▭]

     AMA: 2020,Dec,3; 2018,Jan,8; 2017,Jan,8; 2016,Jan,13

88302-88309 Evaluation of Surgical Specimens: Gross and Microscopic Anatomy

CMS: 100-02,15,80.1 Payment for Clinical Laboratory Services

   [INCLUDES]   Attainment, examination, and reporting
           Unit of service is the specimen
   [EXCLUDES]   *Additional procedures (88311-88365 [88341, 88350], 88399)*
           Mohs surgery (17311-17315)

88302   Level II - Surgical pathology, gross and microscopic examination

       [INCLUDES]   Confirming identification and disease absence:
            Appendix, incidental
            Fallopian tube, sterilization
            Fingers or toes traumatic amputation
            Foreskin, newborn
            Hernia sac, any site
            Hydrocele sac
            Nerve
            Skin, plastic repair
            Sympathetic ganglion
            Testis, castration
            Vaginal mucosa, incidental
            Vas deferens, sterilization

     🚑 0.87   ⚗ 0.87   **FUD** XXX   [Q1] [80] [▭]

     AMA: 2020,Dec,3; 2018,Jan,8; 2017,Jan,8; 2016,Jan,13

88304   Level III - Surgical pathology, gross and microscopic examination

       [INCLUDES]   Abortion, induced
            Abscess
            Anal tag
            Aneurysm-atrial/ventricular
            Appendix, other than incidental
            Artery, atheromatous plaque
            Bartholin's gland cyst
            Bone fragment(s), other than pathologic fracture
            Bursa/ synovial cyst
            Carpal tunnel tissue
            Cartilage, shavings
            Cholesteatoma
            Colon, colostomy stoma
            Conjunctiva-biopsy/pterygium
            Cornea
            Diverticulum-esophagus/small intestine
            Dupuytren's contracture tissue
            Femoral head, other than fracture
            Fissure/fistula
            Foreskin, other than newborn
            Gallbladder
            Ganglion cyst
            Hematoma
            Hemorrhoids
            Hydatid of Morgagni
            Intervertebral disc
            Joint, loose body
            Meniscus
            Mucocele, salivary
            Neuroma-Morton's/traumatic
            Pilonidal cyst/sinus
            Polyps, inflammatory-nasal/sinusoidal
            Skin-cyst/tag/debridement
            Soft tissue, debridement
            Soft tissue, lipoma
            Spermatocele
            Tendon/tendon sheath
            Testicular appendage
            Thrombus or embolus
            Tonsil and/or adenoids
            Varicocele
            Vas deferens, other than sterilization
            Vein, varicosity

     🚑 1.16   ⚗ 1.16   **FUD** XXX   [Q1] [80] [▭]

     AMA: 2020,Dec,3; 2018,Jan,8; 2017,Jan,8; 2016,Jan,13

88305   Level IV - Surgical pathology, gross and microscopic examination

       [INCLUDES]   Abortion, spontaneous/missed
            Artery, biopsy
            Bone exostosis
            Bone marrow, biopsy
            Brain/meninges, other than for tumor resection
            Breast biopsy without microscopic assessment of surgical margin
            Breast reduction mammoplasty
            Bronchus, biopsy
            Cell block, any source
            Cervix, biopsy
            Colon, biopsy
            Duodenum, biopsy
            Endocervix, curettings/biopsy
            Endometrium, curettings/biopsy
            Esophagus, biopsy
            Extremity, amputation, traumatic
            Fallopian tube, biopsy
            Fallopian tube, ectopic pregnancy
            Femoral head, fracture
            Finger/toes, amputation, nontraumatic
            Gingiva/oral mucosa, biopsy
            Heart valve
            Joint resection
            Kidney biopsy
            Larynx biopsy

Leiomyoma(s), uterine myomectomy-without uterus
Lip, biopsy/wedge resection
Lung, transbronchial biopsy
Lymph node, biopsy
Muscle, biopsy
Nasal mucosa, biopsy
Nasopharynx/oropharynx, biopsy
Nerve biopsy
Odontogenic/dental cyst
Omentum, biopsy
Ovary, biopsy/wedge resection
Ovary with or without tube, nonneoplastic
Parathyroid gland
Peritoneum, biopsy
Pituitary tumor
Placenta, other than third trimester
Pleura/pericardium-biopsy/tissue
Polyp:
    Cervical/endometrial
    Colorectal
    Stomach/small intestine
Prostate:
    Needle biopsy
    TUR
Salivary gland, biopsy
Sinus, paranasal biopsy
Skin, other than cyst/tag/debridement/plastic repair
Small intestine, biopsy
Soft tissue, other than
        tumor/mas/lipoma/debridement
Spleen
Stomach biopsy
Synovium
Testis, other than tumor/biopsy, castration
Thyroglossal duct/brachial cleft cyst
Tongue, biopsy
Tonsil, biopsy
Trachea biopsy
Ureter, biopsy
Urethra, biopsy
Urinary bladder, biopsy
Uterus, with or without tubes and ovaries, for
        prolapse
Vagina biopsy
Vulva/labial biopsy

🔲 1.95   🔲 1.95   **FUD** XXX   [01] [80] 🔲

AMA: 2020,Dec,3; 2018,May,3; 2018,Jan,8; 2017,Jan,8;
2016,Jan,13

88307 **Level V - Surgical pathology, gross and microscopic examination**

[INCLUDES] Adrenal resection
Bone, biopsy/curettings
Bone fragment(s), pathologic fractures
Brain, biopsy
Brain meninges, tumor resection
Breast, excision of lesion, requiring microscopic
        evaluation of surgical margins
Breast, mastectomy-partial/simple
Cervix, conization
Colon, segmental resection, other than for tumor
Extremity, amputation, nontraumatic
Eye, enucleation
Kidney, partial/total nephrectomy
Larynx, partial/total resection
Liver
    Biopsy, needle/wedge
    Partial resection
Lung, wedge biopsy
Lymph nodes, regional resection
Mediastinum, mass
Myocardium, biopsy
Odontogenic tumor
Ovary with or without tube, neoplastic
Pancreas, biopsy
Placenta, third trimester
Prostate, except radical resection
Salivary gland
Sentinel lymph node
Small intestine, resection, other than for tumor
Soft tissue mass (except lipoma)-biopsy/simple
        excision
Stomach-subtotal/total resection, other than for
        tumor
Testis, biopsy
Thymus, tumor
Thyroid, total/lobe
Ureter, resection
Urinary bladder, TUR
Uterus, with or without tubes and ovaries, other than
        neoplastic/prolapse

🔲 7.80   🔲 7.80   **FUD** XXX   [02] [80] 🔲

AMA: 2020,Dec,3; 2018,Jan,8; 2017,Jan,8; 2016,Jan,13

88309 **Level VI - Surgical pathology, gross and microscopic examination**

[INCLUDES] Bone resection
Breast, mastectomy-with regional lymph nodes
Colon:
    Segmental resection for tumor
    Total resection
Esophagus, partial/total resection
Extremity, disarticulation
Fetus, with dissection
Larynx, partial/total resection-with regional lymph
        nodes
Lung-total/lobe/segment resection
Pancreas, total/subtotal resection
Prostate, radical resection
Small intestine, resection for tumor
Soft tissue tumor, extensive resection
Stomach, subtotal/total resection for tumor
Testis, tumor
Tongue/tonsil, resection for tumor
Urinary bladder, partial/total resection
Uterus, with or without tubes and ovaries, neoplastic
Vulva, total/subtotal resection

[EXCLUDES] *Evaluation fine needle aspirate (88172-88173)*
*Fine needle aspiration (10021, [10004, 10005, 10006,
        10007, 10008, 10009, 10010, 10011, 10012])*

🔲 11.8   🔲 11.8   **FUD** XXX   [02] [80] 🔲

AMA: 2020,Dec,3; 2018,Jan,8; 2017,Jan,8; 2016,Jan,13

Pathology and Laboratory *(side tab)*

88311 — 88348 *(side tab)*

88311-88399 [88341, 88350, 88364, 88373, 88374, 88377]
Additional Surgical Pathology Services
CMS: 100-02,15,80.1 Payment for Clinical Laboratory Services

+ 88311 **Decalcification procedure (List separately in addition to code for surgical pathology examination)**
> Code first surgical pathology exam (88302-88309)
> 🏥 0.61   ⚕ 0.61   **FUD** XXX   N 80 ▱
> **AMA:** 2020,Dec,3; 2018,Jan,8; 2017,Jan,8; 2016,Jan,13

88312 **Special stain including interpretation and report; Group I for microorganisms (eg, acid fast, methenamine silver)**
> INCLUDES   Reporting one unit for each special stain performed on surgical pathology block, cytologic sample, or hematologic smear
> 🏥 2.97   ⚕ 2.97   **FUD** XXX   Q1 80 ▱
> **AMA:** 2020,Dec,3; 2018,Jan,8; 2017,Jan,8; 2016,Jan,13

88313 **Group II, all other (eg, iron, trichrome), except stain for microorganisms, stains for enzyme constituents, or immunocytochemistry and immunohistochemistry**
> INCLUDES   Reporting one unit for each special stain performed on surgical pathology block, cytologic sample, or hematologic smear
> EXCLUDES   Immunocytochemistry and immunohistochemistry (88342)
> 🏥 2.14   ⚕ 2.14   **FUD** XXX   Q1 80 ▱
> **AMA:** 2020,Dec,3; 2018,Jan,8; 2017,Jan,8; 2016,Jan,13

+ 88314 **histochemical stain on frozen tissue block (List separately in addition to code for primary procedure)**
> INCLUDES   Reporting one unit for each special stain on each frozen surgical pathology block
> EXCLUDES   Routine frozen section stain during Mohs surgery (17311-17315)
>   Special stain performed on frozen tissue section specimen to identify enzyme constituents (88319)
> Code also modifier 59 for nonroutine histochemical stain on frozen section during Mohs surgery
> Code first (17311-17315, 88302-88309, 88331-88332)
> 🏥 2.60   ⚕ 2.60   **FUD** XXX   N 80 ▱
> **AMA:** 2020,Dec,3; 2018,Jan,8; 2017,Jan,8; 2016,Jan,13

88319 **Group III, for enzyme constituents**
> INCLUDES   Reporting one unit for each special stain on each frozen surgical pathology block
> EXCLUDES   Detection of enzyme constituents by immunohistochemical or immunocytochemical methodology (88342)
> 🏥 3.15   ⚕ 3.15   **FUD** XXX   Q2 80 ▱
> **AMA:** 2020,Dec,3; 2018,Jan,8; 2017,Jan,8; 2016,Jan,13

88321 **Consultation and report on referred slides prepared elsewhere**
> 🏥 2.42   ⚕ 2.85   **FUD** XXX   Q1 80 ▱
> **AMA:** 2020,Dec,3; 2018,Jan,8; 2017,Jan,8; 2016,Jan,13

88323 **Consultation and report on referred material requiring preparation of slides**
> 🏥 3.26   ⚕ 3.26   **FUD** XXX   Q1 80 ▱
> **AMA:** 2020,Dec,3; 2018,Jan,8; 2017,Jan,8; 2016,Jan,13

88325 **Consultation, comprehensive, with review of records and specimens, with report on referred material**
> 🏥 4.18   ⚕ 4.96   **FUD** XXX   Q1 80 ▱
> **AMA:** 2020,Dec,3; 2018,Jan,8; 2017,Jan,8; 2016,Jan,13

88329 **Pathology consultation during surgery;**
> 🏥 1.04   ⚕ 1.47   **FUD** XXX   Q1 80 ▱
> **AMA:** 2020,Dec,3; 2018,Jan,8; 2017,Jan,8; 2016,Jan,13

88331 **first tissue block, with frozen section(s), single specimen**
> Code also cytologic evaluation performed at same time (88334)
> 🏥 2.78   ⚕ 2.78   **FUD** XXX   Q1 80 ▱
> **AMA:** 2020,Dec,3; 2018,Jan,8; 2017,Jan,8; 2016,Jan,13

+ 88332 **each additional tissue block with frozen section(s) (List separately in addition to code for primary procedure)**
> Code first (88331)
> 🏥 1.51   ⚕ 1.51   **FUD** XXX   N 80 ▱
> **AMA:** 2020,Dec,3; 2018,Jan,8; 2017,Jan,8; 2016,Jan,13

88333 **cytologic examination (eg, touch prep, squash prep), initial site**
> EXCLUDES   Intraprocedural cytologic evaluation fine needle aspirate (88172)
>   Nonintraoperative cytologic examination (88160-88162)
> 🏥 2.55   ⚕ 2.55   **FUD** XXX   Q2 80 ▱
> **AMA:** 2020,Dec,3; 2018,Jan,8; 2017,Jan,8; 2016,Jan,13

+ 88334 **cytologic examination (eg, touch prep, squash prep), each additional site (List separately in addition to code for primary procedure)**
> EXCLUDES   Intraprocedural cytologic evaluation fine needle aspirate (88172)
>   Nonintraoperative cytologic examination (88160-88162)
>   Percutaneous needle biopsy requiring intraprocedural cytologic examination (88333)
> Code first (88331, 88333)
> 🏥 1.60   ⚕ 1.60   **FUD** ZZZ   N 80 ▱
> **AMA:** 2020,Dec,3; 2018,Jan,8; 2017,Jan,8; 2016,Jan,13

88341   **Resequenced code. See code following 88342.**

88342 **Immunohistochemistry or immunocytochemistry, per specimen; initial single antibody stain procedure**
> EXCLUDES   Morphometric analysis, tumor immunohistochemistry, on same antibody (88360-88361)
>   Multiplex antibody stain (88344)
>   Reporting code more than one time for each specific antibody
> 🏥 2.97   ⚕ 2.97   **FUD** XXX   Q2 80 ▱
> **AMA:** 2020,Dec,3; 2018,Jan,8; 2017,Jan,8; 2016,Jan,13

+ # 88341 **each additional single antibody stain procedure (List separately in addition to code for primary procedure)**
> EXCLUDES   Morphometric analysis (88360-88361)
>   Multiplex antibody stain (88344)
>   Reporting code more than one time for each specific antibody
> Code first (88342)
> 🏥 2.61   ⚕ 2.61   **FUD** ZZZ   N 80 ▱
> **AMA:** 2020,Dec,3; 2018,Jan,8; 2017,Jan,8; 2016,Jan,13

88344 **each multiplex antibody stain procedure**
> INCLUDES   Staining with multiple antibodies on same slide
> EXCLUDES   Morphometric analysis, tumor immunohistochemistry, on same antibody (88360-88361)
>   Reporting code more than one time for each specific antibody
> 🏥 4.86   ⚕ 4.86   **FUD** XXX   Q1 80 ▱
> **AMA:** 2020,Dec,3; 2018,Jan,8; 2017,Jan,8; 2016,Jan,13

88346 **Immunofluorescence, per specimen; initial single antibody stain procedure**
> EXCLUDES   Fluorescent in situ hybridization studies (88364-88369 [88364, 88373, 88374, 88377])
>   Multiple immunofluorescence analysis (88399)
> 🏥 3.56   ⚕ 3.56   **FUD** XXX   Q2 80 ▱
> **AMA:** 2020,Dec,3; 2018,Jan,8; 2017,Jan,8; 2016,Jan,13

+ # 88350 **each additional single antibody stain procedure (List separately in addition to code for primary procedure)**
> EXCLUDES   Fluorescent in situ hybridization studies (88364-88369 [88364, 88373, 88374, 88377])
>   Multiple immunofluorescence analysis (88399)
> Code first (88346)
> 🏥 2.18   ⚕ 2.18   **FUD** ZZZ   N 80 ▱
> **AMA:** 2020,Dec,3

88348 **Electron microscopy, diagnostic**
> 🏥 10.1   ⚕ 10.1   **FUD** XXX   Q2 80 ▱
> **AMA:** 2020,Dec,3

| 26/TC PC/TC Only | A2-Z3 ASC Payment | 50 Bilateral | ♂ Male Only | ♀ Female Only | 🏥 Facility RVU | ⚕ Non-Facility RVU | ▱ CCI | ▨ CLIA |
| **FUD** Follow-up Days | **CMS:** IOM | **AMA:** CPT Asst | A-Y OPPSI | 80/80 Surg Assist Allowed / w/Doc | ▨ Lab Crosswalk | ▨ Radiology Crosswalk | | |

432   CPT © 2021 American Medical Association. All Rights Reserved.   © 2021 Optum360, LLC

88350 Resequenced code. See code following 88346.

88355 Morphometric analysis; skeletal muscle
 3.88 3.88 **FUD** XXX
AMA: 2020,Dec,3; 2018,Jan,8; 2017,Jan,8; 2016,Jan,13

88356 nerve
 6.66 6.66 **FUD** XXX
AMA: 2020,Dec,3; 2018,Jan,8; 2017,Jan,8; 2016,Jan,13

88358 tumor (eg, DNA ploidy)
EXCLUDES *Special stain, Group II (88313)*
 3.77 3.77 **FUD** XXX
AMA: 2020,Dec,3; 2018,Jan,8; 2017,Jan,8; 2016,Jan,13

88360 Morphometric analysis, tumor immunohistochemistry (eg, Her-2/neu, estrogen receptor/progesterone receptor), quantitative or semiquantitative, per specimen, each single antibody stain procedure; manual
EXCLUDES *Additional stain procedures unless each test for different antibody (88341, 88342, 88344)*
Morphometric analysis using in situ hybridization techniques (88367-88368 [88373, 88374])
 3.53 3.53 **FUD** XXX
AMA: 2020,Dec,3; 2018,Jan,8; 2017,Jan,8; 2016,Jan,13

88361 using computer-assisted technology
EXCLUDES *Additional stain procedures unless each test for different antibody (88341, 88342, 88344)*
Morphometric analysis using in situ hybridization techniques (88367-88368 [88373, 88374])
 3.58 3.58 **FUD** XXX
AMA: 2020,Dec,3; 2018,Jan,8; 2017,Jan,8; 2016,Jan,13

88362 Nerve teasing preparations
 6.44 6.44 **FUD** XXX
AMA: 2020,Dec,3; 2018,Jan,8; 2017,Jan,8; 2016,Jan,13

88363 Examination and selection of retrieved archival (ie, previously diagnosed) tissue(s) for molecular analysis (eg, KRAS mutational analysis)
INCLUDES *Archival retrieval only*
 0.57 0.67 **FUD** XXX
AMA: 2020,Dec,3; 2018,Jan,8; 2017,Jan,8; 2016,Jan,13

88364 Resequenced code. See code following 88365.

88365 In situ hybridization (eg, FISH), per specimen; initial single probe stain procedure
EXCLUDES *Morphometric analysis probe stain procedures with same probe (88367, [88374], 88368, [88377])*
 4.99 4.99 **FUD** XXX
AMA: 2020,Dec,3; 2018,Nov,11; 2018,Jan,8; 2017,Jan,8; 2016,Jan,13

+ # **88364** each additional single probe stain procedure (List separately in addition to code for primary procedure)
Code first (88365)
 3.89 3.89 **FUD** ZZZ
AMA: 2020,Dec,3

88366 each multiplex probe stain procedure
EXCLUDES *Morphometric analysis probe stain procedures (88367, [88374], 88368, [88377])*
 7.80 7.80 **FUD** XXX
AMA: 2020,Dec,3

88367 Morphometric analysis, in situ hybridization (quantitative or semi-quantitative), using computer-assisted technology, per specimen; initial single probe stain procedure
EXCLUDES *In situ hybridization probe stain procedures for same probe (88365, 88366, 88368, [88377])*
Morphometric in situ hybridization evaluation urinary tract cytologic specimens (88120-88121)
 3.19 3.19 **FUD** XXX
AMA: 2020,Dec,3; 2018,Jan,8; 2017,Jan,8; 2016,Jan,13

+ # **88373** each additional single probe stain procedure (List separately in addition to code for primary procedure)
Code first (88367)
 2.08 2.08 **FUD** ZZZ
AMA: 2020,Dec,3

88374 each multiplex probe stain procedure
EXCLUDES *In situ hybridization probe stain procedures for same probe (88365, 88366, 88368, [88377])*
 9.65 9.65 **FUD** XXX
AMA: 2020,Dec,3

88368 Morphometric analysis, in situ hybridization (quantitative or semi-quantitative), manual, per specimen; initial single probe stain procedure
EXCLUDES *In situ hybridization probe stain procedures for same probe (88365, 88366-88367, [88374])*
Morphometric in situ hybridization evaluation urinary tract cytologic specimens (88120-88121)
 3.71 3.71 **FUD** XXX
AMA: 2020,Dec,3; 2018,Jan,8; 2017,Jan,8; 2016,Jan,13

+ **88369** each additional single probe stain procedure (List separately in addition to code for primary procedure)
Code first (88368)
 3.23 3.23 **FUD** ZZZ
AMA: 2020,Dec,3

88377 each multiplex probe stain procedure
EXCLUDES *In situ hybridization probe stain procedures for same probe (88365, 88366-88367, [88374])*
Morphometric in situ hybridization evaluation, urinary tract cytologic specimens (88120-88121)
 11.4 11.4 **FUD** XXX
AMA: 2020,Dec,3

88371 Protein analysis of tissue by Western Blot, with interpretation and report;
 0.00 0.00 **FUD** XXX
AMA: 2020,Dec,3; 2018,Jan,8; 2017,Jan,8; 2016,Jan,13

88372 immunological probe for band identification, each
 0.00 0.00 **FUD** XXX
AMA: 2020,Dec,3; 2018,Jan,8; 2017,Jan,8; 2016,Jan,13

88373 Resequenced code. See code following 88367.

88374 Resequenced code. See code following 88367.

88375 Optical endomicroscopic image(s), interpretation and report, real-time or referred, each endoscopic session
EXCLUDES *Endoscopic procedures that include optical endomicroscopy (43206, 43252, 0397T)*
 1.42 1.42 **FUD** XXX
AMA: 2020,Dec,3; 2018,Jan,8; 2017,Jan,8; 2016,Jan,13

88377 Resequenced code. See code following 88369.

88380 Microdissection (ie, sample preparation of microscopically identified target); laser capture
EXCLUDES *Microdissection, manual procedure (88381)*
 3.82 3.82 **FUD** XXX
AMA: 2020,Dec,3; 2018,Aug,3; 2018,Jan,8; 2017,Jan,8; 2016,Jan,13

88381 manual
EXCLUDES *Microdissection, laser capture procedure (88380)*
 5.07 5.07 **FUD** XXX
AMA: 2020,Dec,3; 2018,Aug,3; 2018,Jan,8; 2017,Jan,8; 2016,Jan,13

88387 Macroscopic examination, dissection, and preparation of tissue for non-microscopic analytical studies (eg, nucleic acid-based molecular studies); each tissue preparation (eg, a single lymph node)
EXCLUDES *Pathology consultation during surgery (88329-88334, 88388)*
Tissue preparation for microbiologic cultures or flow cytometric studies
 1.00 1.00 **FUD** XXX
AMA: 2020,Dec,3; 2018,Jan,8; 2017,Jan,8; 2016,Jan,13

+   88388   in conjunction with a touch imprint, intraoperative consultation, or frozen section, each tissue preparation (eg, a single lymph node) (List separately in addition to code for primary procedure)

> EXCLUDES   Tissue preparation for microbiologic cultures or flow cytometric studies

Code first (88329-88334)
🔧 1.04   ⚕ 1.04   **FUD** XXX   N 80 ▭

AMA: 2020,Dec,3; 2018,Jan,8; 2017,Jan,8; 2016,Jan,13

88399   **Unlisted surgical pathology procedure**
🔧 0.00   ⚕ 0.00   **FUD** XXX   Q1 80 ▭

AMA: 2020,Dec,3; 2018,Jan,8; 2017,Jan,8; 2016,Jan,13

88720-88749 Transcutaneous Procedures

> EXCLUDES   Transcutaneous oxyhemoglobin measurement (0493T)
> Wavelength fluorescent spectroscopy advanced glycation end products (skin) (88749)

88720   **Bilirubin, total, transcutaneous**

> EXCLUDES   Transdermal oxygen saturation testing (94760-94762)

🔧 0.00   ⚕ 0.00   **FUD** XXX   Q ▭

AMA: 2020,Dec,3; 2020,May,13; 2018,Jan,8; 2017,Jan,8; 2016,Jan,13

88738   **Hemoglobin (Hgb), quantitative, transcutaneous**

> EXCLUDES   In vitro hemoglobin measurement (85018)

🔧 0.00   ⚕ 0.00   **FUD** XXX   Q ▭

AMA: 2020,Dec,3; 2018,Jan,8; 2017,Jan,8; 2016,Jan,13

88740   **Hemoglobin, quantitative, transcutaneous, per day; carboxyhemoglobin**

> EXCLUDES   In vitro carboxyhemoglobin measurement (82375)

🔧 0.00   ⚕ 0.00   **FUD** XXX   Q ▭

AMA: 2020,Dec,3; 2018,Jan,8; 2017,Jan,8; 2016,Jan,13

88741   **methemoglobin**

> EXCLUDES   In vitro quantitative methemoglobin measurement (83050)

🔧 0.00   ⚕ 0.00   **FUD** XXX   Q ▭

AMA: 2020,Dec,3; 2018,Jan,8; 2017,Jan,8; 2016,Jan,13

88749   **Unlisted in vivo (eg, transcutaneous) laboratory service**

> INCLUDES   All in vivo measurements not specifically listed

🔧 0.00   ⚕ 0.00   **FUD** XXX   Q ▭

AMA: 2020,Dec,3

89049-89240 Other Pathology Services

89049   **Caffeine halothane contracture test (CHCT) for malignant hyperthermia susceptibility, including interpretation and report**
🔧 1.75   ⚕ 7.13   **FUD** XXX   Q1 80 ▭

AMA: 2020,Dec,3; 2018,Jan,8; 2017,Jan,8; 2016,Jan,13

89050   **Cell count, miscellaneous body fluids (eg, cerebrospinal fluid, joint fluid), except blood;**
🔧 0.00   ⚕ 0.00   **FUD** XXX   Q ▭

AMA: 2020,Dec,3; 2018,Jan,8; 2017,Jan,8; 2016,Jan,13

89051   **with differential count**
🔧 0.00   ⚕ 0.00   **FUD** XXX   Q ▭

AMA: 2020,Dec,3; 2018,Jan,8; 2017,Jan,8; 2016,Jan,13

89055   **Leukocyte assessment, fecal, qualitative or semiquantitative**
🔧 0.00   ⚕ 0.00   **FUD** XXX   Q ▭

AMA: 2020,Dec,3; 2018,Jan,8; 2017,Jan,8; 2016,Jan,13

89060   **Crystal identification by light microscopy with or without polarizing lens analysis, tissue or any body fluid (except urine)**

> EXCLUDES   Crystal identification on paraffin embedded tissue

🔧 0.00   ⚕ 0.00   **FUD** XXX   Q 80 ▭

AMA: 2020,Dec,3; 2018,Jan,8; 2017,Jan,8; 2016,Jan,13

89125   **Fat stain, feces, urine, or respiratory secretions**
🔧 0.00   ⚕ 0.00   **FUD** XXX   Q ▭

AMA: 2020,Dec,3; 2018,Jan,8; 2017,Jan,8; 2016,Jan,13

89160   **Meat fibers, feces**
🔧 0.00   ⚕ 0.00   **FUD** XXX   Q ▭

AMA: 2020,Dec,3; 2018,Jan,8; 2017,Jan,8; 2016,Jan,13

89190   **Nasal smear for eosinophils**

> EXCLUDES   Occult blood feces (82270)
> Paternity tests (86910)

🔧 0.00   ⚕ 0.00   **FUD** XXX   Q ▭

AMA: 2020,Dec,3; 2018,Jan,8; 2017,Jan,8; 2016,Jan,13

89220   **Sputum, obtaining specimen, aerosol induced technique (separate procedure)**
🔧 0.46   ⚕ 0.46   **FUD** XXX   Q1 80 TC ▭

AMA: 2020,Dec,3; 2018,Jan,8; 2017,Jan,8; 2016,Jan,13

89230   **Sweat collection by iontophoresis**
🔧 0.08   ⚕ 0.08   **FUD** XXX   Q1 80 TC ▭

AMA: 2020,Dec,3; 2018,Jan,8; 2017,Jan,8; 2016,Jan,13

89240   **Unlisted miscellaneous pathology test**
🔧 0.00   ⚕ 0.00   **FUD** XXX   Q1 80 ▭

AMA: 2020,Dec,3; 2018,Jan,8; 2017,Jan,8; 2016,Jan,13

89250-89398 Infertility Treatment Services

CMS: 100-02,1,100 Treatment for Infertility

89250   **Culture of oocyte(s)/embryo(s), less than 4 days;**
🔧 0.00   ⚕ 0.00   **FUD** XXX   Q1 ▭

AMA: 2020,Dec,3; 2018,Jan,8; 2017,Jan,8; 2016,Jan,13

89251   **with co-culture of oocyte(s)/embryos**

> EXCLUDES   Extended culture oocyte(s)/embryo(s) (89272)

🔧 0.00   ⚕ 0.00   **FUD** XXX   Q2 ▭

AMA: 2020,Dec,3; 2018,Jan,8; 2017,Jan,8; 2016,Jan,13

89253   **Assisted embryo hatching, microtechniques (any method)**
🔧 0.00   ⚕ 0.00   **FUD** XXX   Q1 ▭

AMA: 2020,Dec,3; 2018,Jan,8; 2017,Jan,8; 2016,Jan,13

89254   **Oocyte identification from follicular fluid**
🔧 0.00   ⚕ 0.00   **FUD** XXX   Q1 ▭

AMA: 2020,Dec,3; 2018,Jan,8; 2017,Jan,8; 2016,Jan,13

89255   **Preparation of embryo for transfer (any method)**
🔧 0.00   ⚕ 0.00   **FUD** XXX   Q1 ▭

AMA: 2020,Dec,3; 2018,Jan,8; 2017,Jan,8; 2016,Jan,13

89257   **Sperm identification from aspiration (other than seminal fluid)**

> EXCLUDES   Semen analysis (89300-89320)
> Sperm identification from testis tissue (89264)

🔧 0.00   ⚕ 0.00   **FUD** XXX   Q1 ▭

AMA: 2020,Dec,3; 2018,Jan,8; 2017,Jan,8; 2016,Jan,13

89258   **Cryopreservation; embryo(s)**
🔧 0.00   ⚕ 0.00   **FUD** XXX   Q2 ▭

AMA: 2020,Dec,3; 2018,Jan,8; 2017,Jan,8; 2016,Jan,13

89259   **sperm**

> EXCLUDES   Cryopreservation testicular reproductive tissue (89335)

🔧 0.00   ⚕ 0.00   **FUD** XXX   Q1 ▭

AMA: 2020,Dec,3; 2018,Jan,8; 2017,Jan,8; 2016,Jan,13

89260   **Sperm isolation; simple prep (eg, sperm wash and swim-up) for insemination or diagnosis with semen analysis**
🔧 0.00   ⚕ 0.00   **FUD** XXX   Q1 ▭

AMA: 2020,Dec,3; 2018,Jan,8; 2017,Jan,8; 2016,Jan,13

89261   **complex prep (eg, Percoll gradient, albumin gradient) for insemination or diagnosis with semen analysis**

> EXCLUDES   Semen analysis without sperm wash or swim-up (89320)

🔧 0.00   ⚕ 0.00   **FUD** XXX   Q1 ▭

AMA: 2020,Dec,3; 2018,Jan,8; 2017,Jan,8; 2016,Jan,13

89264   **Sperm identification from testis tissue, fresh or cryopreserved**   ♂

> EXCLUDES   Biopsy testis (54500, 54505)
> Semen analysis (89300-89320)
> Sperm identification from aspiration (89257)

🔧 0.00   ⚕ 0.00   **FUD** XXX   Q1 ▭

AMA: 2020,Dec,3; 2018,Jan,8; 2017,Jan,8; 2016,Jan,13

26/TC PC/TC Only	A2-Z3 ASC Payment	50 Bilateral	♂ Male Only	♀ Female Only	🔧 Facility RVU	⚕ Non-Facility RVU	▭ CCI	⊠ CLIA
FUD Follow-up Days	**CMS:** IOM	**AMA:** CPT Asst	A-Y OPPSI	80/80 Surg Assist Allowed / w/Doc		◼ Lab Crosswalk		⊞ Radiology Crosswalk

89268 Insemination of oocytes
🔧 0.00 ⚕ 0.00 **FUD** XXX 〔Q1〕🖵
AMA: 2020,Dec,3; 2018,Jan,8; 2017,Jan,8; 2016,Jan,13

89272 Extended culture of oocyte(s)/embryo(s), 4-7 days
🔧 0.00 ⚕ 0.00 **FUD** XXX 〔Q2〕🖵
AMA: 2020,Dec,3; 2018,Jan,8; 2017,Jan,8; 2016,Jan,13

89280 Assisted oocyte fertilization, microtechnique; less than or equal to 10 oocytes
🔧 0.00 ⚕ 0.00 **FUD** XXX 〔Q2〕🖵
AMA: 2020,Dec,3; 2018,Jan,8; 2017,Jan,8; 2016,Jan,13

89281 greater than 10 oocytes
🔧 0.00 ⚕ 0.00 **FUD** XXX 〔Q1〕🖵
AMA: 2020,Dec,3; 2018,Jan,8; 2017,Jan,8; 2016,Jan,13

89290 Biopsy, oocyte polar body or embryo blastomere, microtechnique (for pre-implantation genetic diagnosis); less than or equal to 5 embryos
🔧 0.00 ⚕ 0.00 **FUD** XXX 〔Q1〕🖵
AMA: 2020,Dec,3; 2018,Jan,8; 2017,Jan,8; 2016,Jan,13

89291 greater than 5 embryos
🔧 0.00 ⚕ 0.00 **FUD** XXX 〔Q1〕🖵
AMA: 2020,Dec,3; 2018,Jan,8; 2017,Jan,8; 2016,Jan,13

89300 Semen analysis; presence and/or motility of sperm including Huhner test (post coital)
🔧 0.00 ⚕ 0.00 **FUD** XXX ✖〔Q〕🖵
AMA: 2020,Dec,3; 2018,Jan,8; 2017,Jan,8; 2016,Jan,13

89310 motility and count (not including Huhner test) ♂
🔧 0.00 ⚕ 0.00 **FUD** XXX 〔Q〕🖵
AMA: 2020,Dec,3; 2018,Jan,8; 2017,Jan,8; 2016,Jan,13

89320 volume, count, motility, and differential ♂
  EXCLUDES *Skin testing (86485-86580, 95012-95199)*
🔧 0.00 ⚕ 0.00 **FUD** XXX 〔Q〕🖵
AMA: 2020,Dec,3; 2018,Jan,8; 2017,Jan,8; 2016,Jan,13

89321 sperm presence and motility of sperm, if performed ♂
  EXCLUDES *Hyaluronan binding assay (HBA) (89398)*
🔧 0.00 ⚕ 0.00 **FUD** XXX ✖〔Q〕🖵
AMA: 2020,Dec,3; 2018,Jan,8; 2017,Jan,8; 2016,Jan,13

89322 volume, count, motility, and differential using strict morphologic criteria (eg, Kruger) ♂
🔧 0.00 ⚕ 0.00 **FUD** XXX 〔Q〕🖵
AMA: 2020,Dec,3; 2018,Jan,8; 2017,Jan,8; 2016,Jan,13

89325 Sperm antibodies ♂
  EXCLUDES *Medicolegal identification sperm (88125)*
🔧 0.00 ⚕ 0.00 **FUD** XXX 〔Q〕🖵
AMA: 2020,Dec,3; 2018,Jan,8; 2017,Jan,8; 2016,Jan,13

89329 Sperm evaluation; hamster penetration test ♂
🔧 0.00 ⚕ 0.00 **FUD** XXX 〔Q〕🖵
AMA: 2020,Dec,3; 2018,Jan,8; 2017,Jan,8; 2016,Jan,13

89330 cervical mucus penetration test, with or without spinnbarkeit test ♂
🔧 0.00 ⚕ 0.00 **FUD** XXX 〔Q〕🖵
AMA: 2020,Dec,3; 2018,Jan,8; 2017,Jan,8; 2016,Jan,13

89331 Sperm evaluation, for retrograde ejaculation, urine (sperm concentration, motility, and morphology, as indicated) ♂
  EXCLUDES *Detection sperm in urine (81015)*
  Code also semen analysis on concurrent sperm specimen (89300-89322)
🔧 0.00 ⚕ 0.00 **FUD** XXX 〔Q〕🖵
AMA: 2020,Dec,3; 2018,Jan,8; 2017,Jan,8; 2016,Jan,13

89335 Cryopreservation, reproductive tissue, testicular
  EXCLUDES *Cryopreservation:*
    Embryo(s) (89258)
    Immature oocyte(s) (89398)
    Mature oocytes (89337)
    Ovarian reproductive tissue (89398)
    Sperm (89259)
🔧 0.00 ⚕ 0.00 **FUD** XXX 〔Q1〕🖵
AMA: 2020,Dec,3; 2018,Jan,8; 2017,Jan,8; 2016,Jan,13

89337 Cryopreservation, mature oocyte(s) ♀
  EXCLUDES *Cryopreservation immature oocyte[s] (89398)*
🔧 0.00 ⚕ 0.00 **FUD** XXX 〔Q1〕🖵
AMA: 2020,Dec,3; 2018,Jan,8; 2017,Jan,8; 2016,Jan,13

89342 Storage (per year); embryo(s)
🔧 0.00 ⚕ 0.00 **FUD** XXX 〔Q1〕🖵
AMA: 2020,Dec,3; 2018,Jan,8; 2017,Jan,8; 2016,Jan,13

89343 sperm/semen
🔧 0.00 ⚕ 0.00 **FUD** XXX 〔Q1〕🖵
AMA: 2020,Dec,3; 2018,Jan,8; 2017,Jan,8; 2016,Jan,13

89344 reproductive tissue, testicular/ovarian
🔧 0.00 ⚕ 0.00 **FUD** XXX 〔Q1〕🖵
AMA: 2020,Dec,3; 2018,Jan,8; 2017,Jan,8; 2016,Jan,13

89346 oocyte(s)
🔧 0.00 ⚕ 0.00 **FUD** XXX 〔Q2〕🖵
AMA: 2020,Dec,3; 2018,Jan,8; 2017,Jan,8; 2016,Jan,13

89352 Thawing of cryopreserved; embryo(s)
🔧 0.00 ⚕ 0.00 **FUD** XXX 〔Q1〕🖵
AMA: 2020,Dec,3; 2018,Jan,8; 2017,Jan,8; 2016,Jan,13

89353 sperm/semen, each aliquot
🔧 0.00 ⚕ 0.00 **FUD** XXX 〔Q1〕🖵
AMA: 2020,Dec,3; 2018,Jan,8; 2017,Jan,8; 2016,Jan,13

89354 reproductive tissue, testicular/ovarian
🔧 0.00 ⚕ 0.00 **FUD** XXX 〔Q1〕🖵
AMA: 2020,Dec,3; 2018,Jan,8; 2017,Jan,8; 2016,Jan,13

89356 oocytes, each aliquot
🔧 0.00 ⚕ 0.00 **FUD** XXX 〔Q1〕🖵
AMA: 2020,Dec,3; 2018,Jan,8; 2017,Jan,8; 2016,Jan,13

89398 Unlisted reproductive medicine laboratory procedure
  INCLUDES Cryopreservation:
    Immature oocytes
    Ovarian reproductive tissue
    Hyaluronan binding assay (HBA)
🔧 0.00 ⚕ 0.00 **FUD** XXX 〔Q1〕🖵
AMA: 2020,Dec,3

0001U-0305U Proprietary Laboratory Analysis (PLA)

In response to the Protecting Access to Medicare Act of 2014 (PAMA), which focuses on payment and coding of clinical laboratory studies paid for under the Medicare Clinical Laboratory Fee Schedule (CLFS), the AMA has developed a new category of CPT codes known as Proprietary Laboratory Analyses (PLA), which are released on a quarterly basis. These alphanumeric codes appear at the end of the Pathology and Laboratory chapter of the CPT book and include a wide range of tests. Codes in this section can also be found in Appendix L along with the procedure's proprietary name and clinical laboratory or manufacturer. When multiple codes have identical code descriptors and can only be distinguished by a proprietary test name, instructional notes are provided to help ensure accurate code assignment.

  INCLUDES All necessary investigative services
    PLA codes take priority over other CPT codes
  EXCLUDES *Additional procedures necessary before cell lysis (88380-88381)*

0001U Red blood cell antigen typing, DNA, human erythrocyte antigen gene analysis of 35 antigens from 11 blood groups, utilizing whole blood, common RBC alleles reported
  INCLUDES PreciseType® HEA Test, Immucor, Inc
🔧 0.00 ⚕ 0.00 **FUD** 000 〔A〕🖵
AMA: 2019,Jun,11

0002U Oncology (colorectal), quantitative assessment of three urine metabolites (ascorbic acid, succinic acid and carnitine) by liquid chromatography with tandem mass spectrometry (LC-MS/MS) using multiple reaction monitoring acquisition, algorithm reported as likelihood of adenomatous polyps

INCLUDES PolypDX™, Atlantic Diagnostic Laboratories, LLC, Metabolomic Technologies Inc

🚗 0.00   **FUD** 000   Q ▣

AMA: 2018,Aug,3

0003U Oncology (ovarian) biochemical assays of five proteins (apolipoprotein A-1, CA 125 II, follicle stimulating hormone, human epididymis protein 4, transferrin), utilizing serum, algorithm reported as a likelihood score

INCLUDES Overa (OVA1 Next Generation), Aspira Labs, Inc, Vermillion, Inc

🚗 0.00   ⚕ 0.00   **FUD** 000   Q ▣

0005U Oncology (prostate) gene expression profile by real-time RT-PCR of 3 genes (*ERG, PCA3,* and *SPDEF*), urine, algorithm reported as risk score

INCLUDES ExosomeDx® Prostate (IntelliScore), Exosome Diagnostics, Inc, Exosome Diagnostics, Inc

🚗 0.00   ⚕ 0.00   **FUD** 000   Q ▣

0007U Drug test(s), presumptive, with definitive confirmation of positive results, any number of drug classes, urine, includes specimen verification including DNA authentication in comparison to buccal DNA, per date of service

INCLUDES ToxProtect, Genotox Laboratories LTD

🚗 0.00   ⚕ 0.00   **FUD** 000   Q ▣

AMA: 2018,Jan,6

0008U Helicobacter pylori detection and antibiotic resistance, DNA, 16S and 23S rRNA, gyrA, pbp1, rdxA and rpoB, next-generation sequencing, formalin-fixed paraffin-embedded or fresh tissue or fecal sample, predictive, reported as positive or negative for resistance to clarithromycin, fluoroquinolones, metronidazole, amoxicillin, tetracycline, and rifabutin

INCLUDES AmHPR® H. pylori Antibiotic Resistance Panel, American Molecular Laboratories, Inc

🚗 0.00   ⚕ 0.00   **FUD** 000   A ▣

0009U Oncology (breast cancer), ERBB2 (HER2) copy number by FISH, tumor cells from formalin fixed paraffin embedded tissue isolated using image-based dielectrophoresis (DEP) sorting, reported as ERBB2 gene amplified or non-amplified

INCLUDES DEPArray™ HER2, PacificDx

🚗 0.00   **FUD** 000   Q ▣

0010U Infectious disease (bacterial), strain typing by whole genome sequencing, phylogenetic-based report of strain relatedness, per submitted isolate

INCLUDES Bacterial Typing by Whole Genome Sequencing, Mayo Clinic

🚗 0.00   ⚕ 0.00   **FUD** 000   A ▣

0011U Prescription drug monitoring, evaluation of drugs present by LC-MS/MS, using oral fluid, reported as a comparison to an estimated steady-state range, per date of service including all drug compounds and metabolites

INCLUDES Cordant CORE™, Cordant Health Solutions

🚗 0.00   ⚕ 0.00   **FUD** 000   Q ▣

0012U Germline disorders, gene rearrangement detection by whole genome next-generation sequencing, DNA, whole blood, report of specific gene rearrangement(s)

INCLUDES MatePair Targeted Rearrangements, Congenital, Mayo Clinic

🚗 0.00   ⚕ 0.00   **FUD** 000   A ▣

0013U Oncology (solid organ neoplasia), gene rearrangement detection by whole genome next-generation sequencing, DNA, fresh or frozen tissue or cells, report of specific gene rearrangement(s)

INCLUDES MatePair Targeted Rearrangements, Oncology, Mayo Clinic

🚗 0.00   ⚕ 0.00   **FUD** 000   A ▣

0014U Hematology (hematolymphoid neoplasia), gene rearrangement detection by whole genome next-generation sequencing, DNA, whole blood or bone marrow, report of specific gene rearrangement(s)

INCLUDES MatePair Targeted Rearrangements, Hematologic, Mayo Clinic

🚗 0.00   ⚕ 0.00   **FUD** 000   A ▣

0016U Oncology (hematolymphoid neoplasia), RNA, *BCR/ABL1* major and minor breakpoint fusion transcripts, quantitative PCR amplification, blood or bone marrow, report of fusion not detected or detected with quantitation

INCLUDES BCR-ABL1 major and minor breakpoint fusion transcripts, University of Iowa, Department of Pathology, Asuragen

🚗 0.00   ⚕ 0.00   **FUD** 000   A ▣

0017U Oncology (hematolymphoid neoplasia), *JAK2* mutation, DNA, PCR amplification of exons 12-14 and sequence analysis, blood or bone marrow, report of *JAK2* mutation not detected or detected

INCLUDES *JAK2* Mutation, University of Iowa, Department of Pathology

🚗 0.00   ⚕ 0.00   **FUD** 000   A ▣

0018U Oncology (thyroid), microRNA profiling by RT-PCR of 10 microRNA sequences, utilizing fine needle aspirate, algorithm reported as a positive or negative result for moderate to high risk of malignancy

INCLUDES ThyraMIR™, Interpace Diagnostics

🚗 0.00   ⚕ 0.00   **FUD** 000   A ▣

0019U Oncology, RNA, gene expression by whole transcriptome sequencing, formalin-fixed paraffin embedded tissue or fresh frozen tissue, predictive algorithm reported as potential targets for therapeutic agents

INCLUDES OncoTarget/OncoTreat, Columbia University Department of Pathology and Cell Biology, Darwin Health

🚗 0.00   ⚕ 0.00   **FUD** 000   A ▣

0021U Oncology (prostate), detection of 8 autoantibodies (ARF 6, NKX3-1, 5'-UTR-BMI1, CEP 164, 3'-UTR-Ropporin, Desmocollin, AURKAIP-1, CSNK2A2), multiplexed immunoassay and flow cytometry serum, algorithm reported as risk score

INCLUDES Apifiny®, Armune BioScience, Inc

🚗 0.00   ⚕ 0.00   **FUD** 000   Q ▣

0022U Targeted genomic sequence analysis panel, non-small cell lung neoplasia, DNA and RNA analysis, 23 genes, interrogation for sequence variants and rearrangements, reported as presence/absence of variants and associated therapy(ies) to consider

INCLUDES Oncomine™ Dx Target Test, Thermo Fisher Scientific

🚗 0.00   ⚕ 0.00   **FUD** 000   ▣

0023U Oncology (acute myelogenous leukemia), DNA, genotyping of internal tandem duplication, p.D835, p.I836, using mononuclear cells, reported as detection or non-detection of *FLT3* mutation and indication for or against the use of midostaurin

INCLUDES LeukoStrat® CDx *FLT3* Mutation Assay, LabPMM LLC, an Invivoscribe Technologies, Inc Company, Invivoscribe Technologies, Inc

🚗 0.00   ⚕ 0.00   **FUD** 000   A ▣

0024U Glycosylated acute phase proteins (GlycA), nuclear magnetic resonance spectroscopy, quantitative

INCLUDES GlycA, Laboratory Corporation of America, Laboratory Corporation of America

🚗 0.00   ⚕ 0.00   **FUD** 000   Q ▣

0025U Tenofovir, by liquid chromatography with tandem mass spectrometry (LC-MS/MS), urine, quantitative

INCLUDES UrSure Tenofovir Quantification Test, Synergy Medical Laboratories, UrSure Inc

🚗 0.00   ⚕ 0.00   **FUD** 000   Q ▣

0026U Oncology (thyroid), DNA and mRNA of 112 genes, next-generation sequencing, fine needle aspirate of thyroid nodule, algorithmic analysis reported as a categorical result ("Positive, high probability of malignancy" or "Negative, low probability of malignancy")

INCLUDES Thyroseq Genomic Classifier, CBLPath, Inc, University of Pittsburgh Medical Center

🚚 0.00 ⚕ 0.00 **FUD** 000 A▣

0027U *JAK2 (Janus kinase 2)* (eg, myeloproliferative disorder) gene analysis, targeted sequence analysis exons 12-15

INCLUDES *JAK2* Exons 12 to 15 Sequencing, Mayo Clinic, Mayo Clinic

🚚 0.00 ⚕ 0.00 **FUD** 000 A▣

0029U Drug metabolism (adverse drug reactions and drug response), targeted sequence analysis (ie, *CYP1A2, CYP2C19, CYP2C9, CYP2D6, CYP3A4, CYP3A5, CYP4F2, SLCO1B1, VKORC1* and rs12777823)

INCLUDES Focused Pharmacogenomics Panel, Mayo Clinic, Mayo Clinic

🚚 0.00 ⚕ 0.00 **FUD** 000 A▣

0030U Drug metabolism (warfarin drug response), targeted sequence analysis (ie, *CYP2C9, CYP4F2, VKORC1*, rs12777823)

INCLUDES Warfarin Response Genotype, Mayo Clinic, Mayo Clinic

🚚 0.00 ⚕ 0.00 **FUD** 000 A▣

0031U *CYP1A2 (cytochrome P450 family 1, subfamily A, member 2)* (eg, drug metabolism) gene analysis, common variants (ie, *1F, *1K, *6, *7)

INCLUDES Cytochrome P450 1A2 Genotype, Mayo Clinic, Mayo Clinic

🚚 0.00 ⚕ 0.00 **FUD** 000 A▣

0032U *COMT (catechol-O-methyltransferase)(drug metabolism)* gene analysis, c.472G>A (rs4680) variant

INCLUDES Catechol-O-Methyltransferase (*COMT*) Genotype, Mayo Clinic, Mayo Clinic

🚚 0.00 ⚕ 0.00 **FUD** 000 A▣

0033U *HTR2A (5-hydroxytryptamine receptor 2A), HTR2C (5-hydroxytryptamine receptor 2C)* (eg, citalopram metabolism) gene analysis, common variants (ie, *HTR2A* rs7997012 [c.614-2211T>C], *HTR2C* rs3813929 [c.-759C>T] and rs1414334 [c.551-3008C>G])

INCLUDES Serotonin Receptor Genotype (*HTR2A* and *HTR2C*), Mayo Clinic, Mayo Clinic

🚚 0.00 ⚕ 0.00 **FUD** 000 A▣

0034U *TPMT (thiopurine S-methyltransferase), NUDT15 (nudix hydroxylase 15)(eg, thiopurine metabolism)*, gene analysis, common variants (ie, *TPMT *2, *3A, *3B, *3C, *4, *5, *6, *8, *12; NUDT15 *3, *4, *5)

INCLUDES Thiopurine Methyltransferase (*TPMT*) and Nudix Hydrolase (*NUDT15*) Genotyping, Mayo Clinic, Mayo Clinic

🚚 0.00 ⚕ 0.00 **FUD** 000 A▣

0035U Neurology (prion disease), cerebrospinal fluid, detection of prion protein by quaking-induced conformational conversion, qualitative

INCLUDES Real-time quaking-induced conversion for prion detection (RT-QuIC), National Prion Disease Pathology Surveillance Center

🚚 0.00 ⚕ 0.00 **FUD** 000 ▣

0036U Exome (ie, somatic mutations), paired formalin-fixed paraffin-embedded tumor tissue and normal specimen, sequence analyses

INCLUDES EXaCT-1 Whole Exome Testing, Lab of Oncology-Molecular Detection, Weill Cornell Medicine-Clinical Genomics Laboratory

🚚 0.00 ⚕ 0.00 **FUD** 000 ▣

0037U Targeted genomic sequence analysis, solid organ neoplasm, DNA analysis of 324 genes, interrogation for sequence variants, gene copy number amplifications, gene rearrangements, microsatellite instability and tumor mutational burden

INCLUDES FoundationOne CDx™ (F1CDx), Foundation Medicine, Inc, Foundation Medicine, Inc

🚚 0.00 ⚕ 0.00 **FUD** 000 ▣

0038U Vitamin D, 25 hydroxy D2 and D3, by LC-MS/MS, serum microsample, quantitative

INCLUDES Sensieva™ Droplet 25OH Vitamin D2/D3 Microvolume LC/MS Assay, InSource Diagnostics, InSource Diagnostics

🚚 0.00 ⚕ 0.00 **FUD** 000 ▣

0039U Deoxyribonucleic acid (DNA) antibody, double stranded, high avidity

INCLUDES Anti-dsDNA, High Salt/Avidity, University of Washington, Department of Laboratory Medicine, Bio-Rad

🚚 0.00 ⚕ 0.00 **FUD** 000 ▣

0040U *BCR/ABL1 (t(9;22))* (eg, chronic myelogenous leukemia) translocation analysis, major breakpoint, quantitative

INCLUDES MRDx BCR-ABL Test, MolecularMD, MolecularMD

🚚 0.00 ⚕ 0.00 **FUD** 000 ▣

0041U Borrelia burgdorferi, antibody detection of 5 recombinant protein groups, by immunoblot, IgM

INCLUDES Lyme ImmunoBlot IgM, IGeneX Inc, ID-FISH Technology Inc. (ASR) (Lyme ImmunoBlot IgM Strips Only)

🚚 0.00 ⚕ 0.00 **FUD** 000 ▣

0042U Borrelia burgdorferi, antibody detection of 12 recombinant protein groups, by immunoblot, IgG

INCLUDES Lyme ImmunoBlot IgG, IGeneX Inc, ID-FISH Technology Inc (ASR) (Lyme ImmunoBlot IgG Strips Only)

🚚 0.00 ⚕ 0.00 **FUD** 000 ▣

0043U Tick-borne relapsing fever Borrelia group, antibody detection to 4 recombinant protein groups, by immunoblot, IgM

INCLUDES Tick-Borne Relapsing Fever (TBRF) Borrelia ImmunoBlots IgM Test, IGeneX Inc, ID-FISH Technology Inc (Provides TBRF ImmunoBlot IgM Strips)

🚚 0.00 ⚕ 0.00 **FUD** 000 ▣

0044U Tick-borne relapsing fever Borrelia group, antibody detection to 4 recombinant protein groups, by immunoblot, IgG

INCLUDES Tick-Borne Relapsing Fever (TBRF) Borrelia ImmunoBlots IgG Test, IGeneX Inc, ID-FISH Technology Inc (Provides TBRF ImmunoBlot IgG Strips)

🚚 0.00 ⚕ 0.00 **FUD** 000 ▣

0045U Oncology (breast ductal carcinoma in situ), mRNA, gene expression profiling by real-time RT-PCR of 12 genes (7 content and 5 housekeeping), utilizing formalin-fixed paraffin-embedded tissue, algorithm reported as recurrence score

INCLUDES The Oncotype DX® Breast DCIS Score™ Test, Genomic Health, Inc, Genomic Health, Inc

🚚 0.00 ⚕ 0.00 **FUD** 000 ▣

0046U *FLT3 (fms-related tyrosine kinase 3)* (eg, acute myeloid leukemia) internal tandem duplication (ITD) variants, quantitative

INCLUDES FLT3 ITD MRD by NGS, LabPMM LLC, an Invivoscribe Technologies, Inc Company

🚚 0.00 ⚕ 0.00 **FUD** 000 ▣

0047U Oncology (prostate), mRNA, gene expression profiling by real-time RT-PCR of 17 genes (12 content and 5 housekeeping), utilizing formalin-fixed paraffin-embedded tissue, algorithm reported as a risk score

INCLUDES Oncotype DX Genomic Prostate Score, Genomic Health, Inc, Genomic Health, Inc

🚗 0.00   ⚖ 0.00   **FUD** 000   ▯

0048U Oncology (solid organ neoplasia), DNA, targeted sequencing of protein-coding exons of 468 cancer-associated genes, including interrogation for somatic mutations and microsatellite instability, matched with normal specimens, utilizing formalin-fixed paraffin-embedded tumor tissue, report of clinically significant mutation(s)

INCLUDES MSK-IMPACT (Integrated Mutation Profiling of Actionable Cancer Targets), Memorial Sloan Kettering Cancer Center

🚗 0.00   ⚖ 0.00   **FUD** 000   ▯

0049U NPM1 (nucleophosmin) (eg, acute myeloid leukemia) gene analysis, quantitative

INCLUDES *NPM1* MRD by NGS, LabPMM LLC, an Invivoscribe Technologies, Inc Company

🚗 0.00   ⚖ 0.00   **FUD** 000   ▯

0050U Targeted genomic sequence analysis panel, acute myelogenous leukemia, DNA analysis, 194 genes, interrogation for sequence variants, copy number variants or rearrangements

INCLUDES MyAML NGS Panel, LabPMM LLC, an Invivoscribe Technologies, Inc Company

🚗 0.00   ⚖ 0.00   **FUD** 000   ▯

▲ **0051U** Prescription drug monitoring, evaluation of drugs present by liquid chromatography tandem mass spectrommetry (LC-MS/MS), urine or blood, 31 drug panel, reported as quantitative results, detected or not detected, per date of service

INCLUDES UCompliDx, Elite Medical Laboratory Solutions, LLC, Elite Medical Laboratory Solutions, LLC (LDT)

🚗 0.00   ⚖ 0.00   **FUD** 000   ▯

0052U Lipoprotein, blood, high resolution fractionation and quantitation of lipoproteins, including all five major lipoprotein classes and subclasses of HDL, LDL, and VLDL by vertical auto profile ultracentrifugation

INCLUDES VAP Cholesterol Test, VAP Diagnostics Laboratory, Inc, VAP Diagnostics Laboratory, Inc

🚗 0.00   ⚖ 0.00   **FUD** 000   ▯

0053U Oncology (prostate cancer), FISH analysis of 4 genes (*ASAP1, HDAC9, CHD1* and *PTEN*), needle biopsy specimen, algorithm reported as probability of higher tumor grade

INCLUDES Prostate Cancer Risk Panel, Mayo Clinic, Laboratory Developed Test

🚗 0.00   ⚖ 0.00   **FUD** 000   ▯

0054U Prescription drug monitoring, 14 or more classes of drugs and substances, definitive tandem mass spectrometry with chromatography, capillary blood, quantitative report with therapeutic and toxic ranges, including steady-state range for the prescribed dose when detected, per date of service

INCLUDES AssuranceRx Micro Serum, Firstox Laboratories, LLC, Firstox Laboratories, LLC

🚗 0.00   ⚖ 0.00   **FUD** 000   ▯

0055U Cardiology (heart transplant), cell-free DNA, PCR assay of 96 DNA target sequences (94 single nucleotide polymorphism targets and two control targets), plasma

INCLUDES myTAIHEART, TAI Diagnostics, Inc, TAI Diagnostics, Inc

🚗 0.00   ⚖ 0.00   **FUD** 000   ▯

0056U Hematology (acute myelogenous leukemia), DNA, whole genome next-generation sequencing to detect gene rearrangement(s), blood or bone marrow, report of specific gene rearrangement(s)

INCLUDES MatePair Acute Myeloid Leukemia Panel, Mayo Clinic, Laboratory Developed Test

🚗 0.00   ⚖ 0.00   **FUD** 000   ▯

0058U Oncology (Merkel cell carcinoma), detection of antibodies to the Merkel cell polyoma virus oncoprotein (small T antigen), serum, quantitative

INCLUDES Merkel SmT Oncoprotein Antibody Titer, University of Washington, Department of Laboratory Medicine

🚗 0.00   ⚖ 0.00   **FUD** 000   ▯

0059U Oncology (Merkel cell carcinoma), detection of antibodies to the Merkel cell polyoma virus capsid protein (VP1), serum, reported as positive or negative

INCLUDES Merkel Virus VP1 Capsid Antibody, University of Washington, Department of Laboratory Medicine

🚗 0.00   ⚖ 0.00   **FUD** 000   ▯

0060U Twin zygosity, genomic targeted sequence analysis of chromosome 2, using circulating cell-free fetal DNA in maternal blood

INCLUDES Twins Zygosity PLA, Natera, Inc, Natera, Inc

🚗 0.00   ⚖ 0.00   **FUD** 000   ▯

0061U Transcutaneous measurement of five biomarkers (tissue oxygenation [StO2], oxyhemoglobin [ctHbO2], deoxyhemoglobin [ctHbR], papillary and reticular dermal hemoglobin concentrations [ctHb1 and ctHb2]), using spatial frequency domain imaging (SFDI) and multi-spectral analysis

INCLUDES Transcutaneous multispectral measurement of tissue oxygenation and hemoglobin using spatial frequency domain imaging (SFDI), Modulated Imaging, Inc, Modulated Imaging, Inc

🚗 0.00   ⚖ 0.00   **FUD** 000   ▯

0062U Autoimmune (systemic lupus erythematosus), IgG and IgM analysis of 80 biomarkers, utilizing serum, algorithm reported with a risk score

INCLUDES SLE-key® Rule Out, Veracis Inc, Veracis Inc

🚗 0.00   ⚖ 0.00   **FUD** 000   ▯

0063U Neurology (autism), 32 amines by LC-MS/MS, using plasma, algorithm reported as metabolic signature associated with autism spectrum disorder

INCLUDES NPDX ASD ADM Panel I, Stemina Biomarker Discovery, Inc, Stemina Biomarker Discovery, Inc d/b/a NeuroPointDX

🚗 0.00   ⚖ 0.00   **FUD** 000   ▯

0064U Antibody, Treponema pallidum, total and rapid plasma reagin (RPR), immunoassay, qualitative

INCLUDES BioPlex 2200 Syphilis Total & RPR Assay, Bio-Rad Laboratories, Bio-Rad Laboratories

🚗 0.00   ⚖ 0.00   **FUD** 000   ▯

0065U Syphilis test, non-treponemal antibody, immunoassay, qualitative (RPR)

INCLUDES BioPlex 2200 RPR Assay, Bio-Rad Laboratories, Bio-Rad Laboratories

🚗 0.00   ⚖ 0.00   **FUD** 000   ▯

0066U Placental alpha-micro globulin-1 (PAMG-1), immunoassay with direct optical observation, cervico-vaginal fluid, each specimen

INCLUDES PartoSure™ Test, Parsagen Diagnostics, Inc, Parsagen Diagnostics, Inc, a QIAGEN Company

🚗 0.00   ⚖ 0.00   **FUD** 000   ▯

26/TC PC/TC Only   A2-Z3 ASC Payment   50 Bilateral   ♂ Male Only   ♀ Female Only   🚗 Facility RVU   ⚖ Non-Facility RVU   ▯ CCI   ✕ CLIA
FUD Follow-up Days   **CMS:** IOM   **AMA:** CPT Asst   A-Y OPPSI   80/80 Surg Assist Allowed / w/Doc   ▯ Lab Crosswalk   ▯ Radiology Crosswalk

0067U Oncology (breast), immunohistochemistry, protein expression profiling of 4 biomarkers (matrix metalloproteinase-1 [MMP-1], carcinoembryonic antigen-related cell adhesion molecule 6 [CEACAM6], hyaluronoglucosaminidase [HYAL1], highly expressed in cancer protein [HEC1]), formalin-fixed paraffin-embedded precancerous breast tissue, algorithm reported as carcinoma risk score

INCLUDES BBDRisk Dx™, Silbiotech, Inc, Silbiotech, Inc

0.00   0.00   **FUD** 000

0068U Candida species panel (*C. albicans, C. glabrata, C. parapsilosis, C. kruseii, C tropicalis, and C. auris*), amplified probe technique with qualitative report of the presence or absence of each species

INCLUDES MYCODART-PCR™ Dual Amplification Real Time PCR Panel for 6 Candida species, RealTime Laboratories, Inc/MycoDART, Inc, RealTime Laboratories, Inc

0.00   0.00   **FUD** 000

0069U Oncology (colorectal), microRNA, RT-PCR expression profiling of miR-31-3p, formalin-fixed paraffin-embedded tissue, algorithm reported as an expression score

INCLUDES miR-31now™, GoPath Laboratories, GoPath Laboratories

0.00   0.00   **FUD** 000

0070U *CYP2D6 (cytochrome P450, family 2, subfamily D, polypeptide 6) (eg, drug metabolism) gene analysis, common and select rare variants (ie, *2, *3, *4, *4N, *5, *6, *7, *8, *9, *10, *11, *12, *13, *14A, *14B, *15, *17, *29, *35, *36, *41, *57, *61, *63, *68, *83, *xN)*

INCLUDES *CYP2D6* Common Variants and Copy Number, Mayo Clinic, Laboratory Developed Test

0.00   0.00   **FUD** 000

+ 0071U *CYP2D6 (cytochrome P450, family 2, subfamily D, polypeptide 6) (eg, drug metabolism) gene analysis, full gene sequence (List separately in addition to code for primary procedure)*

INCLUDES *CYP2D6* Full Gene Sequencing, Mayo Clinic, Laboratory Developed Test

Code first (0070U)

0.00   0.00   **FUD** 000

+ 0072U *CYP2D6 (cytochrome P450, family 2, subfamily D, polypeptide 6) (eg, drug metabolism) gene analysis, targeted sequence analysis (ie, CYP2D6-2D7 hybrid gene) (List separately in addition to code for primary procedure)*

INCLUDES *CYP2D6-2D7* Hybrid Gene Targeted Sequence Analysis, Mayo Clinic, Laboratory Developed Test

Code first (0070U)

0.00   0.00   **FUD** 000

+ 0073U *CYP2D6 (cytochrome P450, family 2, subfamily D, polypeptide 6) (eg, drug metabolism) gene analysis, targeted sequence analysis (ie, CYP2D7-2D6 hybrid gene) (List separately in addition to code for primary procedure)*

INCLUDES *CYP2D7-2D6* Hybrid Gene Targeted Sequence Analysis, Mayo Clinic, Laboratory Developed Test

Code first (0070U)

0.00   0.00   **FUD** 000

+ 0074U *CYP2D6 (cytochrome P450, family 2, subfamily D, polypeptide 6) (eg, drug metabolism) gene analysis, targeted sequence analysis (ie, non-duplicated gene when duplication/multiplication is trans) (List separately in addition to code for primary procedure)*

INCLUDES *CYP2D6* trans-duplication/multiplication non-duplicated gene targeted sequence analysis, Mayo Clinic, Laboratory Developed Test

Code first (0070U)

0.00   0.00   **FUD** 000

+ 0075U *CYP2D6 (cytochrome P450, family 2, subfamily D, polypeptide 6) (eg, drug metabolism) gene analysis, targeted sequence analysis (ie, 5' gene duplication/multiplication) (List separately in addition to code for primary procedure)*

INCLUDES *CYP2D6* 5' gene duplication/multiplication targeted sequence analysis, Mayo Clinic, Laboratory Developed Test

Code first (0070U)

0.00   0.00   **FUD** 000

+ 0076U *CYP2D6 (cytochrome P450, family 2, subfamily D, polypeptide 6) (eg, drug metabolism) gene analysis, targeted sequence analysis (ie, 3' gene duplication/ multiplication) (List separately in addition to code for primary procedure)*

INCLUDES *CYP2D6* 3' gene duplication/multiplication targeted sequence analysis, Mayo Clinic, Laboratory Developed Test

Code first (0070U)

0.00   0.00   **FUD** 000

0077U Immunoglobulin paraprotein (M-protein), qualitative, immunoprecipitation and mass spectrometry, blood or urine, including isotype

INCLUDES M-Protein Detection and Isotyping by MALDI-TOF Mass Spectrometry, Mayo Clinic, Laboratory Developed Test

0.00   0.00   **FUD** 000

0078U Pain management (opioid-use disorder) genotyping panel, 16 common variants (ie, ABCB1, COMT, DAT1, DBH, DOR, DRD1, DRD2, DRD4, GABA, GAL, HTR2A, HTTLPR, MTHFR, MUOR, OPRK1, OPRM1), buccal swab or other germline tissue sample, algorithm reported as positive or negative risk of opioid-use disorder

INCLUDES INFINITI® Neural Response Panel, PersonalizeDx Labs, AutoGenomics Inc

0.00   0.00   **FUD** 000

0079U Comparative DNA analysis using multiple selected single-nucleotide polymorphisms (SNPs), urine and buccal DNA, for specimen identity verification

INCLUDES ToxLok™, InSource Diagnostics, InSource Diagnostics

0.00   0.00   **FUD** 000

0080U Oncology (lung), mass spectrometric analysis of galectin-3-binding protein and scavenger receptor cysteine-rich type 1 protein M130, with five clinical risk factors (age, smoking status, nodule diameter, nodule-spiculation status and nodule location), utilizing plasma, algorithm reported as a categorical probability of malignancy

INCLUDES BDX-XL2, Biodesix®, Inc, Biodesix®, Inc

0.00   0.00   **FUD** 000

0082U Drug test(s), definitive, 90 or more drugs or substances, definitive chromatography with mass spectrometry, and presumptive, any number of drug classes, by instrument chemistry analyzer (utilizing immunoassay), urine, report of presence or absence of each drug, drug metabolite or substance with description and severity of significant interactions per date of service

INCLUDES NextGen Precision™ Testing, Precision Diagnostics, Precision Diagnostics LBN Precision Toxicology, LLC

0.00   0.00   **FUD** 000

0083U Oncology, response to chemotherapy drugs using motility contrast tomography, fresh or frozen tissue, reported as likelihood of sensitivity or resistance to drugs or drug combinations

INCLUDES Onco4D™, Animated Dynamics, Inc, Animated Dynamics, Inc

0.00   0.00   **FUD** 000

● New Code   ▲ Revised Code   ○ Reinstated   ● New Web Release   ▲ Revised Web Release   + Add-on   Unlisted   Not Covered   # Resequenced
🔟 Optum Mod 50 Exempt   ⬨ AMA Mod 51 Exempt   🔟 Optum Mod 51 Exempt   ⑥③ Mod 63 Exempt   ✗ Non-FDA Drug   ★ Telemedicine   Ⓜ Maternity   Ⓐ Age Edit

0084U Red blood cell antigen typing, DNA, genotyping of 10 blood groups with phenotype prediction of 37 red blood cell antigens

INCLUDES BLOODchip® ID CORE XT™, Grifols Diagnostic Solutions Inc

🔧 0.00 ⚕ 0.00 **FUD** 000 ▣

0086U Infectious disease (bacterial and fungal), organism identification, blood culture, using rRNA FISH, 6 or more organism targets, reported as positive or negative with phenotypic minimum inhibitory concentration (MIC)-based antimicrobial susceptibility

INCLUDES Accelerate PhenoTest™ BC kit, Accelerate Diagnostics, Inc

🔧 0.00 ⚕ 0.00 **FUD** 000 ▣

0087U Cardiology (heart transplant), mRNA gene expression profiling by microarray of 1283 genes, transplant biopsy tissue, allograft rejection and injury algorithm reported as a probability score

INCLUDES Molecular Microscope® MMDx—Heart, Kashi Clinical Laboratories

🔧 0.00 ⚕ 0.00 **FUD** 000 ▣

0088U Transplantation medicine (kidney allograft rejection), microarray gene expression profiling of 1494 genes, utilizing transplant biopsy tissue, algorithm reported as a probability score for rejection

INCLUDES Molecular Microscope® MMDx—Kidney, Kashi Clinical Laboratories

🔧 0.00 ⚕ 0.00 **FUD** 000 ▣

0089U Oncology (melanoma), gene expression profiling by RTqPCR, *PRAME* and *LINC00518*, superficial collection using adhesive patch(es)

INCLUDES Pigmented Lesion Assay (PLA), DermTech

🔧 0.00 ⚕ 0.00 **FUD** 000 ▣

▲ **0090U** Oncology (cutaneous melanoma), mRNA gene expression profiling by RT-PCR of 23 genes (14 content and 9 housekeeping), utilizing formalin-fixed paraffin-embedded (FFPE) tissue, algorithm reported as a categorical result (ie, benign, intermediate, malignant)

INCLUDES myPath® Melanoma, Castle Biosciences, Inc

🔧 0.00 ⚕ 0.00 **FUD** 000 ▣

0091U Oncology (colorectal) screening, cell enumeration of circulating tumor cells, utilizing whole blood, algorithm, for the presence of adenoma or cancer, reported as a positive or negative result

INCLUDES FirstSightCRC™, CellMax Life

🔧 0.00 ⚕ 0.00 **FUD** 000 ▣

0092U Oncology (lung), three protein biomarkers, immunoassay using magnetic nanosensor technology, plasma, algorithm reported as risk score for likelihood of malignancy

INCLUDES REVEAL Lung Nodule Characterization, MagArray, Inc

🔧 0.00 ⚕ 0.00 **FUD** 000 ▣

0093U Prescription drug monitoring, evaluation of 65 common drugs by LC-MS/MS, urine, each drug reported detected or not detected

INCLUDES ComplyRX, Claro Labs

🔧 0.00 ⚕ 0.00 **FUD** 000 ▣

0094U Genome (eg, unexplained constitutional or heritable disorder or syndrome), rapid sequence analysis

INCLUDES RCIGM Rapid Whole Genome Sequencing, Rady Children's Institute for Genomic Medicine (RCIGM)

🔧 0.00 ⚕ 0.00 **FUD** 000

0095U Inflammation (eosinophilic esophagitis), ELISA analysis of eotaxin-3 *(CCL26 [C-C motif chemokine ligand 26])* and major basic protein *(PRG2 [proteoglycan 2, pro eosinophil major basic protein])*, specimen obtained by swallowed nylon string, algorithm reported as predictive probability index for active eosinophilic esophagitis

INCLUDES Esophageal String Test™ (EST), Cambridge Biomedical, Inc

🔧 0.00 ⚕ 0.00 **FUD** 000

0096U Human papillomavirus (HPV), high-risk types (ie, 16, 18, 31, 33, 35, 39, 45, 51, 52, 56, 58, 59, 66, 68), male urine

INCLUDES HPV, High-Risk, Male Urine, Molecular Testing Labs

🔧 0.00 ⚕ 0.00 **FUD** 000

0097U Gastrointestinal pathogen, multiplex reverse transcription and multiplex amplified probe technique, multiple types or subtypes, 22 targets (Campylobacter [C. jejuni/C. coli/C. upsaliensis], Clostridium difficile [C. difficile] toxin A/B, Plesiomonas shigelloides, Salmonella, Vibrio [V. parahaemolyticus/V. vulnificus/V. cholerae], including specific identification of Vibrio cholerae, Yersinia enterocolitica, Enteroaggregative Escherichia coli [EAEC], Enteropathogenic Escherichia coli [EPEC], Enterotoxigenic Escherichia coli [ETEC] lt/st, Shiga-like toxin-producing Escherichia coli [STEC] stx1/stx2 [including specific identification of the E. coli O157 serogroup within STEC], Shigella/Enteroinvasive Escherichia coli [EIEC], Cryptosporidium, Cyclospora cayetanensis, Entamoeba histolytica, Giardia lamblia [also known as G. intestinalis and G. duodenalis], adenovirus F 40/41, astrovirus, norovirus GI/GII, rotavirus A, sapovirus [Genogroups I, II, IV, and V])

INCLUDES BioFire® FilmArray® Gastrointestinal (GI) Panel, BioFire® Diagnostics

🔧 0.00 ⚕ 0.00 **FUD** 000

~~0098U~~ ~~Respiratory pathogen, multiplex reverse transcription and multiplex amplified probe technique, multiple types or subtypes, 14 targets (adenovirus, coronavirus, human metapneumovirus, influenza A, influenza A subtype H1, influenza A subtype H3, influenza A subtype H1-2009, influenza B, parainfluenza virus, human rhinovirus/enterovirus, respiratory syncytial virus, Bordetella pertussis, Chlamydophila pneumoniae, Mycoplasma pneumoniae)~~

~~0099U~~ ~~Respiratory pathogen, multiplex reverse transcription and multiplex amplified probe technique, multiple types or subtypes, 20 targets (adenovirus, coronavirus 229E, coronavirus HKU1, coronavirus, coronavirus OC43, human metapneumovirus, influenza A, influenza A subtype, influenza A subtype H3, influenza A subtype H1-2009, influenza, parainfluenza virus, parainfluenza virus 2, parainfluenza virus 3, parainfluenza virus 4, human rhinovirus/enterovirus, respiratory syncytial virus, Bordetella pertussis, Chlamydophila pneumonia, Mycoplasma pneumoniae)~~

~~0100U~~ ~~Respiratory pathogen, multiplex reverse transcription and multiplex amplified probe technique, multiple types or subtypes, 21 targets (adenovirus, coronavirus 229E, coronavirus HKU1, coronavirus NL63, coronavirus OC43, human metapneumovirus, human rhinovirus/enterovirus, influenza A, including subtypes H1, H1-2009, and H3, influenza B, parainfluenza virus 1, parainfluenza virus 2, parainfluenza virus 3, parainfluenza virus 4, respiratory syncytial virus, Bordetella parapertussis [IS1001], Bordetella pertussis [ptxP], Chlamydia pneumoniae, Mycoplasma pneumoniae)~~

26/TC PC/TC Only 42-23 ASC Payment 50 Bilateral ♂ Male Only ♀ Female Only 🔧 Facility RVU ⚕ Non-Facility RVU ▣ CCI ✕ CLIA
FUD Follow-up Days CMS: IOM AMA: CPT Asst A-Y OPPSI 80/80 Surg Assist Allowed / w/Doc ▤ Lab Crosswalk ▦ Radiology Crosswalk

440 CPT © 2021 American Medical Association. All Rights Reserved. © 2021 Optum360, LLC

0101U Hereditary colon cancer disorders (eg, Lynch syndrome, *PTEN* hamartoma syndrome, Cowden syndrome, familial adenomatosis polyposis), genomic sequence analysis panel utilizing a combination of NGS, Sanger, MLPA, and array CGH, with MRNA analytics to resolve variants of unknown significance when indicated (15 genes [sequencing and deletion/duplication], *EPCAM* and *GREM1* [deletion/duplication only])

INCLUDES ColoNext®, Ambry Genetics®, Ambry Genetics®
🚗 0.00   🩺 0.00   **FUD** 000

0102U Hereditary breast cancer-related disorders (eg, hereditary breast cancer, hereditary ovarian cancer, hereditary endometrial cancer), genomic sequence analysis panel utilizing a combination of NGS, Sanger, MLPA, and array CGH, with mRNA analytics to resolve variants of unknown significance when indicated (17 genes [sequencing and deletion/duplication])

INCLUDES BreastNext®, Ambry Genetics®, Ambry Genetics®
🚗 0.00   🩺 0.00   **FUD** 000

0103U Hereditary ovarian cancer (eg, hereditary ovarian cancer, hereditary endometrial cancer), genomic sequence analysis panel utilizing a combination of NGS, Sanger, MLPA, and array CGH, with MRNA analytics to resolve variants of unknown significance when indicated (24 genes [sequencing and deletion/duplication], *EPCAM* [deletion/duplication only])

INCLUDES OvaNext®, Ambry Genetics®, Ambry Genetics®
🚗 0.00   🩺 0.00   **FUD** 000

0105U Nephrology (chronic kidney disease), multiplex electrochemiluminescent immunoassay (ECLIA) of tumor necrosis factor receptor 1A, receptor superfamily 2 *(TNFR1, TNFR2)*, and kidney injury molecule-1 (KIM-1) combined with longitudinal clinical data, including *APOL1* genotype if available, and plasma (isolated fresh or frozen), algorithm reported as probability score for rapid kidney function decline (RKFD)

INCLUDES KidneyIntelX™, RenalytixAI, RenalytixAI
🚗 0.00   🩺 0.00   **FUD** 000

0106U Gastric emptying, serial collection of 7 timed breath specimens, non-radioisotope carbon-13 (^{13}C) spirulina substrate, analysis of each specimen by gas isotope ratio mass spectrometry, reported as rate of $^{13}CO_2$ excretion

INCLUDES 13C-Spirulina Gastric Emptying Breath Test (GEBT), Cairn Diagnostics d/b/a Advanced Breath Diagnostics, LLC, Cairn Diagnostics d/b/a Advanced Breath Diagnostics, LLC
🚗 0.00   🩺 0.00   **FUD** 000

0107U Clostridium difficile toxin(s) antigen detection by immunoassay technique, stool, qualitative, multiple-step method

INCLUDES Singulex Clarity C. diff toxins A/B assay, Singulex
🚗 0.00   🩺 0.00   **FUD** 000

0108U Gastroenterology (Barrett's esophagus), whole slide-digital imaging, including morphometric analysis, computer-assisted quantitative immunolabeling of 9 protein biomarkers (p16, AMACR, p53, CD68, COX-2, CD45RO, HIF1a, HER-2, K20) and morphology, formalin-fixed paraffin-embedded tissue, algorithm reported as risk of progression to high-grade dysplasia or cancer

INCLUDES TissueCypher® Barrett's Esophagus Assay, Cernostics, Cernostics
🚗 0.00   🩺 0.00   **FUD** 000

0109U Infectious disease (Aspergillus species), real-time PCR for detection of DNA from 4 species (*A. fumigatus, A. terreus, A. niger,* and *A. flavus)*, blood, lavage fluid, or tissue, qualitative reporting of presence or absence of each species

INCLUDES MYCODART-PCR™ Dual Amplification Real Time PCR Panel for 4 Aspergillus species, RealTime Laboratories, Inc/MycoDART, Inc
🚗 0.00   🩺 0.00   **FUD** 000

0110U Prescription drug monitoring, one or more oral oncology drug(s) and substances, definitive tandem mass spectrometry with chromatography, serum or plasma from capillary blood or venous blood, quantitative report with steady-state range for the prescribed drug(s) when detected

INCLUDES Oral OncolyticAssuranceRX, Firstox Laboratories, LLC, Firstox Laboratories, LLC
🚗 0.00   🩺 0.00   **FUD** 000

0111U Oncology (colon cancer), targeted *KRAS* (codons 12, 13, and 61) and *NRAS* (codons 12, 13, and 61) gene analysis utilizing formalin-fixed paraffin-embedded tissue

INCLUDES Praxis(™) Extended RAS Panel, Illumina, Illumina
🚗 0.00   🩺 0.00   **FUD** 000

0112U Infectious agent detection and identification, targeted sequence analysis (16S and 18S rRNA genes) with drug-resistance gene

INCLUDES MicroGenDX qPCR & NGS For Infection, MicroGenDX, MicroGenDX

0113U Oncology (prostate), measurement of *PCA3* and *TMPRSS2-ERG* in urine and PSA in serum following prostatic massage, by RNA amplification and fluorescence-based detection, algorithm reported as risk score

INCLUDES MiPS (Mi-Prostate Score), MLabs, Mlabs
🚗 0.00   🩺 0.00   **FUD** 000

0114U Gastroenterology (Barrett's esophagus), *VIM* and *CCNA1* methylation analysis, esophageal cells, algorithm reported as likelihood for Barrett's esophagus

INCLUDES EsoGuard™, Lucid Diagnostics, Lucid Diagnostics
🚗 0.00   🩺 0.00   **FUD** 000

0115U Respiratory infectious agent detection by nucleic acid (DNA and RNA), 18 viral types and subtypes and 2 bacterial targets, amplified probe technique, including multiplex reverse transcription for RNA targets, each analyte reported as detected or not detected

INCLUDES ePlex Respiratory Pathogen (RP) Panel, GenMark Diagnostics, Inc, GenMark Diagnostics, Inc
🚗 0.00   🩺 0.00   **FUD** 000
AMA: 2020,Apr,3

0116U Prescription drug monitoring, enzyme immunoassay of 35 or more drugs confirmed with LC-MS/MS, oral fluid, algorithm results reported as a patient-compliance measurement with risk of drug to drug interactions for prescribed medications

INCLUDES Snapshot Oral Fluid Compliance, Ethos Laboratories
🚗 0.00   🩺 0.00   **FUD** 000

0117U Pain management, analysis of 11 endogenous analytes (methylmalonic acid, xanthurenic acid, homocysteine, pyroglutamic acid, vanilmandelate, 5-hydroxyindoleacetic acid, hydroxymethylglutarate, ethylmalonate, 3-hydroxypropyl mercapturic acid (3-HPMA), quinolinic acid, kynurenic acid), LC-MS/MS, urine, algorithm reported as a pain-index score with likelihood of atypical biochemical function associated with pain

INCLUDES Foundation PI^{SM}, Ethos Laboratories
🚗 0.00   🩺 0.00   **FUD** 000

Pathology and Laboratory

0118U — 0140U

0118U Transplantation medicine, quantification of donor-derived cell-free DNA using whole genome next-generation sequencing, plasma, reported as percentage of donor-derived cell-free DNA in the total cell-free DNA

INCLUDES Viracor TRAC™ dd-cfDNA, Viracor Eurofins, Viracor Eurofins

🔧 0.00   ⚖ 0.00   **FUD** 000   ▫

0119U Cardiology, ceramides by liquid chromatography-tandem mass spectrometry, plasma, quantitative report with risk score for major cardiovascular events

INCLUDES MI-HEART Ceramides, Plasma, Mayo Clinic, Laboratory Developed Test

🔧 0.00   ⚖ 0.00   **FUD** 000   ▫

0120U Oncology (B-cell lymphoma classification), mRNA, gene expression profiling by fluorescent probe hybridization of 58 genes (45 content and 13 housekeeping genes), formalin-fixed paraffin-embedded tissue, algorithm reported as likelihood for primary mediastinal B-cell lymphoma (PMBCL) and diffuse large B-cell lymphoma (DLBCL) with cell of origin subtyping in the latter

INCLUDES Lymph3Cx Lymphoma Molecular Subtyping Assay, Mayo Clinic, Laboratory Developed Test

EXCLUDES *Oncology (diffuse large B-cell lymphoma [DLBCL]), mRNA, gene expression profiling by fluorescent probe hybridization of 20 genes (0017M)*

🔧 0.00   ⚖ 0.00   **FUD** 000   ▫

0121U Sickle cell disease, microfluidic flow adhesion (VCAM-1), whole blood

INCLUDES Flow Adhesion of Whole Blood on VCAM-1 (FAB-V), Functional Fluidics, Functional Fluidics

🔧 0.00   ⚖ 0.00   **FUD** 000   ▫

0122U Sickle cell disease, microfluidic flow adhesion (P-Selectin), whole blood

INCLUDES Flow Adhesion of Whole Blood to P-SELECTIN (WB-PSEL), Functional Fluidics, Functional Fluidics

🔧 0.00   ⚖ 0.00   **FUD** 000   ▫

0123U Mechanical fragility, RBC, shear stress and spectral analysis profiling

INCLUDES Mechanical Fragility, RBC by shear stress profiling and spectral analysis, Functional Fluidics, Functional Fluidics

🔧 0.00   ⚖ 0.00   **FUD** 000   ▫

0129U Hereditary breast cancer-related disorders (eg, hereditary breast cancer, hereditary ovarian cancer, hereditary endometrial cancer), genomic sequence analysis and deletion/duplication analysis panel *(ATM, BRCA1, BRCA2, CDH1, CHEK2, PALB2, PTEN,* and *TP53)*

INCLUDES BRCAplus, Ambry Genetics

🔧 0.00   ⚖ 0.00   **FUD** 000   ▫

+ 0130U Hereditary colon cancer disorders (eg, Lynch syndrome, PTEN hamartoma syndrome, Cowden syndrome, familial adenomatosis polyposis), targeted mRNA sequence analysis panel *(APC, CDH1, CHEK2, MLH1, MSH2, MSH6, MUTYH, PMS2, PTEN,* and *TP53)* (List separately in addition to code for primary procedure)

INCLUDES +RNAinsight™ for ColoNext®, Ambry Genetics

Code first (81435, 0101U)

🔧 0.00   ⚖ 0.00   **FUD** 000   ▫

+ 0131U Hereditary breast cancer-related disorders (eg, hereditary breast cancer, hereditary ovarian cancer, hereditary endometrial cancer), targeted mRNA sequence analysis panel (13 genes) (List separately in addition to code for primary procedure)

INCLUDES +RNAinsight™ for BreastNext®, Ambry Genetics

Code first ([81162], 81432, 0102U)

🔧 0.00   ⚖ 0.00   **FUD** 000   ▫

+ 0132U Hereditary ovarian cancer-related disorders (eg, hereditary breast cancer, hereditary ovarian cancer, hereditary endometrial cancer), targeted mRNA sequence analysis panel (17 genes) (List separately in addition to code for primary procedure)

INCLUDES +RNAinsight™ for OvaNext®, Ambry Genetics

Code first ([81162], 81432, 0103U)

🔧 0.00   ⚖ 0.00   **FUD** 000   ▫

+ 0133U Hereditary prostate cancer-related disorders, targeted mRNA sequence analysis panel (11 genes) (List separately in addition to code for primary procedure)

INCLUDES +RNAinsight™ for ProstateNext®, Ambry Genetics

Code first ([81162])

🔧 0.00   ⚖ 0.00   **FUD** 000   ▫

+ 0134U Hereditary pan cancer (eg, hereditary breast and ovarian cancer, hereditary endometrial cancer, hereditary colorectal cancer), targeted mRNA sequence analysis panel (18 genes) (List separately in addition to code for primary procedure)

INCLUDES +RNAinsight™ for CancerNext®, Ambry Genetics

Code first ([81162], 81432, 81435)

🔧 0.00   ⚖ 0.00   **FUD** 000   ▫

+ 0135U Hereditary gynecological cancer (eg, hereditary breast and ovarian cancer, hereditary endometrial cancer, hereditary colorectal cancer), targeted mRNA sequence analysis panel (12 genes) (List separately in addition to code for primary procedure)

INCLUDES +RNAinsight™ for GYNPlus®, Ambry Genetics

Code first ([81162])

🔧 0.00   ⚖ 0.00   **FUD** 000   ▫

+ 0136U *ATM (ataxia telangiectasia mutated)* (eg, ataxia telangiectasia) mRNA sequence analysis (List separately in addition to code for primary procedure)

INCLUDES +RNAinsight™ for *ATM*, Ambry Genetics

Code first (81408)

🔧 0.00   ⚖ 0.00   **FUD** 000   ▫

+ 0137U *PALB2 (partner and localizer of BRCA2)* (eg, breast and pancreatic cancer) mRNA sequence analysis (List separately in addition to code for ...

INCLUDES +RNAinsight™ for *PALB2*, Ambry Genetics

Code first (81406)

🔧 0.00   ⚖ 0.00   **FUD** 000   ▫

+ 0138U *BRCA1 (BRCA1, DNA repair associated), BRCA2 (BRCA2, DNA repair associated)* (eg, hereditary breast and ovarian cancer) mRNA sequence analysis (List separately in addition to code for primary procedure)

INCLUDES +RNAinsight™ for *BRCA1/2*, Ambry Genetics

Code first ([81162])

🔧 0.00   ⚖ 0.00   **FUD** 000   ▫

0139U ~~Neurology (autism spectrum disorder [ASD]), quantitative measurements of 6 central carbon metabolites (ie, a-ketoglutarate, alanine, lactate, phenylalanine, pyruvate, and succinate), LC-MS/MS, plasma, algorithmic analysis with result reported as negative or positive (with metabolic subtypes of ASD)~~

0140U Infectious disease (fungi), fungal pathogen identification, DNA (15 fungal targets), blood culture, amplified probe technique, each target reported as detected or not detected

INCLUDES ePlex® BCID Fungal Pathogens Panel, GenMark Diagnostics, Inc, GenMark Diagnostics, Inc

🔧 0.00   ⚖ 0.00   **FUD** 000   ▫

| 26/TC PC/TC Only | A2-Z3 ASC Payment | 50 Bilateral | ♂ Male Only | ♀ Female Only | 🔧 Facility RVU | ⚖ Non-Facility RVU | ▫ CCI | ❌ CLIA |
| **FUD** Follow-up Days | **CMS:** IOM | **AMA:** CPT Asst | A-Y OPPSI | 80/80 Surg Assist Allowed / w/Doc | ◤ Lab Crosswalk | ◤ Radiology Crosswalk |

442   CPT © 2021 American Medical Association. All Rights Reserved.   © 2021 Optum360, LLC

0141U Infectious disease (bacteria and fungi), gram-positive organism identification and drug resistance element detection, DNA (20 gram-positive bacterial targets, 4 resistance genes, 1 pan gram-negative bacterial target, 1 pan Candida target), blood culture, amplified probe technique, each target reported as detected or not detected

INCLUDES ePlex® BCID Gram-Positive Panel, GenMark Diagnostics, Inc, GenMark Diagnostics, Inc

🚗 0.00 👤 0.00 **FUD** 000

0142U Infectious disease (bacteria and fungi), gram-negative bacterial identification and drug resistance element detection, DNA (21 gram-negative bacterial targets, 6 resistance genes, 1 pan gram-positive bacterial target, 1 pan Candida target), amplified probe technique, each target reported as detected or not detected

INCLUDES ePlex® BCID Gram-Negative Panel, GenMark Diagnostics, Inc, GenMark Diagnostics, Inc

🚗 0.00 👤 0.00 **FUD** 000

0143U Drug assay, definitive, 120 or more drugs or metabolites, urine, quantitative liquid chromatography with tandem mass spectrometry (LC-MS/MS) using multiple reaction monitoring (MRM), with drug or metabolite description, comments including sample validation, per date of service

INCLUDES CareViewRx, Newstar Medical Laboratories, LLC, Newstar Medical Laboratories, LLC

EXCLUDES *PsychViewRx Plus analysis by Newstar Medical Laboratories, LLC. To report, see (0150U)*

🚗 0.00 👤 0.00 **FUD** 000

0144U Drug assay, definitive, 160 or more drugs or metabolites, urine, quantitative liquid chromatography with tandem mass spectrometry (LC-MS/MS) using multiple reaction monitoring (MRM), with drug or metabolite description, comments including sample validation, per date of service

INCLUDES CareViewRx Plus, Newstar Medical Laboratories, LLC, Newstar Medical Laboratories, LLC

🚗 0.00 👤 0.00 **FUD** 000

0145U Drug assay, definitive, 65 or more drugs or metabolites, urine, quantitative liquid chromatography with tandem mass spectrometry (LC-MS/MS) using multiple reaction monitoring (MRM), with drug or metabolite description, comments including sample validation, per date of service

INCLUDES PainViewRx, Newstar Medical Laboratories, LLC, Newstar Medical Laboratories, LLC

🚗 0.00 👤 0.00 **FUD** 000

0146U Drug assay, definitive, 80 or more drugs or metabolites, urine, by quantitative liquid chromatography with tandem mass spectrometry (LC-MS/MS) using multiple reaction monitoring (MRM), with drug or metabolite description, comments including sample validation, per date of service

INCLUDES PainViewRx Plus, Newstar Medical Laboratories, LLC, Newstar Medical Laboratories, LLC

🚗 0.00 👤 0.00 **FUD** 000

0147U Drug assay, definitive, 85 or more drugs or metabolites, urine, quantitative liquid chromatography with tandem mass spectrometry (LC-MS/MS) using multiple reaction monitoring (MRM), with drug or metabolite description, comments including sample validation, per date of service

INCLUDES RiskViewRx, Newstar Medical Laboratories, LLC, Newstar Medical Laboratories, LLC

🚗 0.00 👤 0.00 **FUD** 000

0148U Drug assay, definitive, 100 or more drugs or metabolites, urine, quantitative liquid chromatography with tandem mass spectrometry (LC-MS/MS) using multiple reaction monitoring (MRM), with drug or metabolite description, comments including sample validation, per date of service

INCLUDES RiskViewRx Plus, Newstar Medical Laboratories, LLC, Newstar Medical Laboratories, LLC

🚗 0.00 👤 0.00 **FUD** 000

0149U Drug assay, definitive, 60 or more drugs or metabolites, urine, quantitative liquid chromatography with tandem mass spectrometry (LC-MS/MS) using multiple reaction monitoring (MRM), with drug or metabolite description, comments including sample validation, per date of service

INCLUDES PsychViewRx, Newstar Medical Laboratories, LLC, Newstar Medical Laboratories, LLC

🚗 0.00 👤 0.00 **FUD** 000

0150U Drug assay, definitive, 120 or more drugs or metabolites, urine, quantitative liquid chromatography with tandem mass spectrometry (LC-MS/MS) using multiple reaction monitoring (MRM), with drug or metabolite description, comments including sample validation, per date of service

INCLUDES PsychViewRx Plus, Newstar Medical Laboratories, LLC, Newstar Medical Laboratories, LLC

EXCLUDES *CareViewRx analysis by Newstar Medical Laboratories, LLC. To report, see (0143U)*

🚗 0.00 👤 0.00 **FUD** 000

0151U Infectious disease (bacterial or viral respiratory tract infection), pathogen specific nucleic acid (DNA or RNA), 33 targets, real-time semi-quantitative PCR, bronchoalveolar lavage, sputum, or endotracheal aspirate, detection of 33 organismal and antibiotic resistance genes with limited semi-quantitative results

INCLUDES BioFire® FilmArray® Pneumonia Panel, BioFire® Diagnostics, BioFire® Diagnostics

🚗 0.00 👤 0.00 **FUD** 000

AMA: 2020,Apr,3

▲ **0152U** Infectious disease (bacteria, fungi, parasites, and DNA viruses), microbial cell-free DNA, plasma, untargeted next-generation sequencing, report for significant positive pathogens

INCLUDES Karius® Test, Karius Inc, Karius Inc

0153U Oncology (breast), mRNA, gene expression profiling by next-generation sequencing of 101 genes, utilizing formalin-fixed paraffin-embedded tissue, algorithm reported as a triple negative breast cancer clinical subtype(s) with information on immune cell involvement

INCLUDES Insight TNBCtype™, Insight Molecular Labs

🚗 0.00 👤 0.00 **FUD** 000

0154U Oncology (urothelial cancer), RNA, analysis by real-time RT-PCR of the *FGFR3 (fibroblast growth factor receptor3)* gene analysis (ie, p.R248C [c.742C>T], p.S249C [c.746C>G], p.G370C [c.1108G>T], p.Y373C [c.1118A>G], FGFR3-TACC3v1, and FGFR3-TACC3v3) utilizing formalin-fixed paraffin-embedded urothelial cancer tumor tissue, reported as *FGFR* gene alteration status

INCLUDES therascreen® *FGFR* RGQ RT-PCR Kit, QIAGEN, QIAGEN GmbH

🚗 0.00 👤 0.00 **FUD** 000

AMA: 2020,Jun,11

0155U Oncology (breast cancer), DNA, *PIK3CA (phosphatidylinositol-4,5-bisphosphate 3-kinase, catalytic subunit alpha)* (eg, breast cancer) gene analysis (ie, p.C420R, p.E542K, p.E545A, p.E545D [g.1635G>T only], p.E545G, p.E545K, p.Q546E, p.Q546R, p.H1047L, p.H1047R, p.H1047Y), utilizing formalin-fixed paraffin-embedded breast tumor tissue, reported as *PIK3CA* gene mutation status

INCLUDES therascreen® *PIK3CA* RGQ PCR Kit, QIAGEN, QIAGEN GmbH

🚗 0.00 👤 0.00 **FUD** 000

AMA: 2020,Jun,11

0156U Copy number (eg, intellectual disability, dysmorphology), sequence analysis

INCLUDES SMASH™, New York Genome Center, Marvel Genomics™

🚗 0.00 👤 0.00 **FUD** 000

● New Code ▲ Revised Code ○ Reinstated ● New Web Release ▲ Revised Web Release + Add-on Unlisted Not Covered # Resequenced

㊿ Optum Mod 50 Exempt 👤 AMA Mod 51 Exempt �51 Optum Mod 51 Exempt �63 Mod 63 Exempt ✎ Non-FDA Drug ★ Telemedicine Ⓜ Maternity Ⓐ Age Edit

+ **0157U** *APC (APC regulator of WNT signaling pathway)* (eg, familial adenomatosis polyposis [FAP]) mRNA sequence analysis (List separately in addition to code for primary procedure)

     INCLUDES   CustomNext + RNA: APC, Ambry Genetics®, Ambry Genetics®

     Code first ([81201])

     🔧 0.00   🔨 0.00   **FUD** 000   🖻

+ **0158U** *MLH1 (mutL homolog 1)* (eg, hereditary non-polyposis colorectal cancer, Lynch syndrome) mRNA sequence analysis (List separately in addition to code for primary procedure)

     INCLUDES   CustomNext + RNA: MLH1, Ambry Genetics®, Ambry Genetics®

     Code first ([81292])

     🔧 0.00   🔨 0.00   **FUD** 000   🖻

+ **0159U** *MSH2 (mutS homolog 2)* (eg, hereditary colon cancer, Lynch syndrome) mRNA sequence analysis (List separately in addition to code for primary procedure)

     INCLUDES   CustomNext + RNA: MSH2, Ambry Genetics®, Ambry Genetics®

     Code first ([81295])

     🔧 0.00   🔨 0.00   **FUD** 000   🖻

+ **0160U** *MSH6 (mutS homolog 6)* (eg, hereditary colon cancer, Lynch syndrome) mRNA sequence analysis (List separately in addition to code for primary procedure)

     INCLUDES   CustomNext + RNA: MSH6, Ambry Genetics®, Ambry Genetics®

     Code first (81298)

     🔧 0.00   🔨 0.00   **FUD** 000   🖻

+ **0161U** *PMS2 (PMS1 homolog 2, mismatch repair system component)* (eg, hereditary non-polyposis colorectal cancer, Lynch syndrome) mRNA sequence analysis (List separately in addition to code for primary procedure)

     INCLUDES   CustomNext + RNA: PMS2, Ambry Genetics®, Ambry Genetics®

     Code first (81317)

     🔧 0.00   🔨 0.00   **FUD** 000   🖻

+ **0162U** Hereditary colon cancer (Lynch syndrome), targeted mRNA sequence analysis panel *(MLH1, MSH2, MSH6, PMS2)* (List separately in addition to code for primary procedure)

     INCLUDES   CustomNext + RNA: Lynch (MLH1, MSH2, MSH6, PMS2), Ambry Genetics®, Ambry Genetics®

     Code first ([81292], [81295], 81298, 81317, 81435)

     🔧 0.00   🔨 0.00   **FUD** 000   🖻

0163U Oncology (colorectal) screening, biochemical enzyme-linked immunosorbent assay (ELISA) of 3 plasma or serum proteins (teratocarcinoma derived growth factor-1 [TDGF-1, Cripto-1], carcinoembryonic antigen [CEA], extracellular matrix protein [ECM]), with demographic data (age, gender, CRC-screening compliance) using a proprietary algorithm and reported as likelihood of CRC or advanced adenomas

     INCLUDES   BeScreened™-CRC, Beacon Biomedical Inc, Beacon Biomedical Inc

     🔧 0.00   🔨 0.00   **FUD** 000   🖻

     AMA: 2020,Jun,11

0164U Gastroenterology (irritable bowel syndrome [IBS]), immunoassay for anti-CdtB and anti-vinculin antibodies, utilizing plasma, algorithm for elevated or not elevated qualitative results

     INCLUDES   ibs-smart™, Gemelli Biotech, Gemelli Biotech

     🔧 0.00   🔨 0.00   **FUD** 000   🖻

     AMA: 2020,Jun,11

0165U Peanut allergen-specific quantitative assessment of multiple epitopes using enzyme-linked immunosorbent assay (ELISA), blood, individual epitope results and probability of peanut allergy

     INCLUDES   VeriMAP™ Peanut Dx – Bead-based Epitope Assay, AllerGenis™ Clinical Laboratory, AllerGenis™ LLC

     🔧 0.00   🔨 0.00   **FUD** 000

     AMA: 2020,Jun,11

0166U Liver disease, 10 biochemical assays (α2-macroglobulin, haptoglobin, apolipoprotein A1, bilirubin, GGT, ALT, AST, triglycerides, cholesterol, fasting glucose) and biometric and demographic data, utilizing serum, algorithm reported as scores for fibrosis, necroinflammatory activity, and steatosis with a summary interpretation

     INCLUDES   LiverFASt™, Fibronostics, Fibronostics

     🔧 0.00   🔨 0.00   **FUD** 000   🖻

     AMA: 2020,Jun,11

0167U Gonadotropin, chorionic (hCG), immunoassay with direct optical observation, blood

     INCLUDES   ADEXUSDx hCG Test, NOWDiagnostics, NOWDiagnostics

     🔧 0.00   🔨 0.00   **FUD** 000   🖻

     AMA: 2020,Jun,11

~~**0168U** Fetal aneuploidy (trisomy 21, 18, and 13) DNA sequence analysis of selected regions using maternal plasma without fetal fraction cutoff, algorithm reported as a risk score for each trisomy~~

0169U *NUDT15 (nudix hydrolase 15)* and *TPMT (thiopurine S-methyltransferase)* (eg, drug metabolism) gene analysis, common variants

     INCLUDES   NT (NUDT15 and TPMT) genotyping panel, RPRD Diagnostics

     🔧 0.00   🔨 0.00   **FUD** 000   🖻

     AMA: 2020,Jun,11

0170U Neurology (autism spectrum disorder [ASD]), RNA, next-generation sequencing, saliva, algorithmic analysis, and results reported as predictive probability of ASD diagnosis

     INCLUDES   Clarifi™, Quadrant Biosciences, Inc, Quadrant Biosciences, Inc

     🔧 0.00   🔨 0.00   **FUD** 000   🖻

     AMA: 2020,Jun,11

0171U Targeted genomic sequence analysis panel, acute myeloid leukemia, myelodysplastic syndrome, and myeloproliferative neoplasms, DNA analysis, 23 genes, interrogation for sequence variants, rearrangements and minimal residual disease, reported as presence/absence

     INCLUDES   MyMRD® NGS Panel, Laboratory for Personalized Molecular Medicine, Laboratory for Personalized Molecular Medicine

     🔧 0.00   🔨 0.00   **FUD** 000   🖻

     AMA: 2020,Jun,11

0172U Oncology (solid tumor as indicated by the label), somatic mutation analysis of *BRCA1 (BRCA1, DNA repair associated)*, *BRCA2 (BRCA2, DNA repair associated)* and analysis of homologous recombination deficiency pathways, DNA, formalin-fixed paraffin-embedded tissue, algorithm quantifying tumor genomic instability score

     INCLUDES   myChoice® CDx, Myriad Genetics Laboratories, Inc, Myriad Genetics Laboratories, Inc

     🔧 0.00   🔨 0.00   **FUD** 000   🖻

0173U Psychiatry (ie, depression, anxiety), genomic analysis panel, includes variant analysis of 14 genes

     INCLUDES   Psych HealthPGx Panel, RPRD Diagnostics, RPRD Diagnostics

     🔧 0.00   🔨 0.00   **FUD** 000   🖻

0174U Oncology (solid tumor), mass spectrometric 30 protein targets, formalin-fixed paraffin-embedded tissue, prognostic and predictive algorithm reported as likely, unlikely, or uncertain benefit of 39 chemotherapy and targeted therapeutic oncology agents

     INCLUDES   LC-MS/MS Targeted Proteomic Assay, OncoOmicDx Laboratory, LDT

     🔧 0.00   🔨 0.00   **FUD** 000   🖻

26/TC PC/TC Only   A2-Z3 ASC Payment   50 Bilateral   ♂ Male Only   ♀ Female Only   🔧 Facility RVU   🔨 Non-Facility RVU   🖻 CCI   ❌ CLIA

FUD Follow-up Days   **CMS:** IOM   **AMA:** CPT Asst   A-Y OPPSI   80/80 Surg Assist Allowed / w/Doc   🖥 Lab Crosswalk   🖥 Radiology Crosswalk

444   CPT © 2021 American Medical Association. All Rights Reserved.   © 2021 Optum360, LLC

0175U **Psychiatry (eg, depression, anxiety), genomic analysis panel, variant analysis of 15 genes**

INCLUDES Genomind® Professional PGx Express™ CORE, Genomind, Inc, Genomind, Inc

🚗 0.00 ⚖ 0.00 **FUD** 000

0176U **Cytolethal distending toxin B (CdtB) and vinculin IgG antibodies by immunoassay (ie, ELISA)**

INCLUDES IBSSchek®, Commonwealth Diagnostics International, Inc, Commonwealth Diagnostics International, Inc

🚗 0.00 ⚖ 0.00 **FUD** 000

0177U **Oncology (breast cancer), DNA, *PIK3CA (phosphatidylinositol-4,5-bisphosphate 3-kinase catalytic subunit alpha)* gene analysis of 11 gene variants utilizing plasma, reported as *PIK3CA* gene mutation status**

INCLUDES therascreen® *PIK3CA* RGQ PCR Kit, QIAGEN, QIAGEN GmbH

🚗 0.00 ⚖ 0.00 **FUD** 000 ▱

0178U **Peanut allergen-specific quantitative assessment of multiple epitopes using enzyme-linked immunosorbent assay (ELISA), blood, report of minimum eliciting exposure for a clinical reaction**

INCLUDES VeriMAP™ Peanut Reactivity Threshold - Bead Based Epitope Assay, AllerGenis™ Clinical Laboratory, AllerGenis™ LLC

🚗 0.00 ⚖ 0.00 **FUD** 000

0179U **Oncology (non-small cell lung cancer), cell-free DNA, targeted sequence analysis of 23 genes (single nucleotide variations, insertions and deletions, fusions without prior knowledge of partner/breakpoint, copy number variations), with report of significant mutation(s)**

INCLUDES Resolution ctDx Lung™, Resolution Bioscience, Resolution Bioscience, Inc

🚗 0.00 ⚖ 0.00 **FUD** 000

0180U **Red cell antigen (ABO blood group) genotyping (ABO), gene analysis Sanger/chain termination/conventional sequencing, *ABO (ABO, alpha 1-3-N-acetylgalactosaminyltransferase and alpha 1-3-galactosyltransferase)* gene, including subtyping, 7 exons**

INCLUDES Navigator ABO Sequencing, Grifols Immunohematology Center, Grifols Immunohematology Center

🚗 0.00 ⚖ 0.00 **FUD** 000

0181U **Red cell antigen (Colton blood group) genotyping (CO), gene analysis, *AQP1 (aquaporin 1 [Colton blood group])* exon 1**

INCLUDES Navigator CO Sequencing, Grifols Immunohematology Center, Grifols Immunohematology Center

🚗 0.00 ⚖ 0.00 **FUD** 000

0182U **Red cell antigen (Cromer blood group) genotyping (CROM), gene analysis, *CD55 (CD55 molecule [Cromer blood group])* exons 1-10**

INCLUDES Navigator CROM Sequencing, Grifols Immunohematology Center, Grifols Immunohematology Center

🚗 0.00 ⚖ 0.00 **FUD** 000

0183U **Red cell antigen (Diego blood group) genotyping (DI), gene analysis, *SLC4A1 (solute carrier family 4 member 1 [Diego blood group])* exon 19**

INCLUDES Navigator DI Sequencing, Grifols Immunohematology Center, Grifols Immunohematology Center

🚗 0.00 ⚖ 0.00 **FUD** 000

0184U **Red cell antigen (Dombrock blood group) genotyping (DO), gene analysis, *ART4 (ADP-ribosyltransferase 4 [Dombrock blood group])* exon 2**

INCLUDES Navigator DO Sequencing, Grifols Immunohematology Center, Grifols Immunohematology Center

🚗 0.00 ⚖ 0.00 **FUD** 000

0185U **Red cell antigen (H blood group) genotyping (FUT1), gene analysis, *FUT1 (fucosyltransferase 1 [H blood group])* exon 4**

INCLUDES Navigator FUT1 Sequencing, Grifols Immunohematology Center, Grifols Immunohematology Center

🚗 0.00 ⚖ 0.00 **FUD** 000

0186U **Red cell antigen (H blood group) genotyping (FUT2), gene analysis, *FUT2 (fucosyltransferase 2)* exon 2**

INCLUDES Navigator FUT2 Sequencing, Grifols Immunohematology Center, Grifols Immunohematology Center

🚗 0.00 ⚖ 0.00 **FUD** 000

0187U **Red cell antigen (Duffy blood group) genotyping (FY), gene analysis, *ACKR1 (atypical chemokine receptor 1 [Duffy blood group])* exons 1-2**

INCLUDES Navigator FY Sequencing, Grifols Immunohematology Center, Grifols Immunohematology Center

🚗 0.00 ⚖ 0.00 **FUD** 000

0188U **Red cell antigen (Gerbich blood group) genotyping (GE), gene analysis, *GYPC (glycophorin C [Gerbich blood group])* exons 1-4**

INCLUDES Navigator GE Sequencing, Grifols Immunohematology Center, Grifols Immunohematology Center

🚗 0.00 ⚖ 0.00 **FUD** 000

0189U **Red cell antigen (MNS blood group) genotyping (GYPA), gene analysis, *GYPA (glycophorin A [MNS blood group])* introns 1, 5, exon 2**

INCLUDES Navigator GYPA Sequencing, Grifols Immunohematology Center, Grifols Immunohematology Center

🚗 0.00 ⚖ 0.00 **FUD** 000

0190U **Red cell antigen (MNS blood group) genotyping (GYPB), gene analysis, *GYPB (glycophorin B [MNS blood group])* introns 1, 5, pseudoexon 3**

INCLUDES Navigator GYPB Sequencing, Grifols Immunohematology Center, Grifols Immunohematology Center

🚗 0.00 ⚖ 0.00 **FUD** 000

0191U **Red cell antigen (Indian blood group) genotyping (IN), gene analysis, *CD44 (CD44 molecule [Indian blood group])* exons 2, 3, 6**

INCLUDES Navigator IN Sequencing, Grifols Immunohematology Center, Grifols Immunohematology Center

🚗 0.00 ⚖ 0.00 **FUD** 000

0192U **Red cell antigen (Kidd blood group) genotyping (JK), gene analysis, *SLC14A1 (solute carrier family 14 member 1 [Kidd blood group])* gene promoter, exon 9**

INCLUDES Navigator JK Sequencing, Grifols Immunohematology Center, Grifols Immunohematology Center

🚗 0.00 ⚖ 0.00 **FUD** 000

0193U **Red cell antigen (JR blood group) genotyping (JR), gene analysis, *ABCG2 (ATP binding cassette subfamily G member 2 [Junior blood group])* exons 2-26**

INCLUDES Navigator JR Sequencing, Grifols Immunohematology Center, Grifols Immunohematology Center

🚗 0.00 ⚖ 0.00 **FUD** 000

0194U **Red cell antigen (Kell blood group) genotyping (KEL), gene analysis, *KEL (Kell metallo-endopeptidase [Kell blood group])* exon 8**

INCLUDES Navigator KEL Sequencing, Grifols Immunohematology Center, Grifols Immunohematology Center

🚗 0.00 ⚖ 0.00 **FUD** 000

0195U ***KLF1 (Kruppel-like factor 1)*, targeted sequencing (ie, exon 13)**

INCLUDES Navigator *KLF1* Sequencing, Grifols Immunohematology Center, Grifols Immunohematology Center

🚗 0.00 ⚖ 0.00 **FUD** 000

0196U Red cell antigen (Lutheran blood group) genotyping (LU), gene analysis, *BCAM (basal cell adhesion molecule [Lutheran blood group])* exon 3

INCLUDES Navigator LU Sequencing, Grifols Immunohematology Center, Grifols Immunohematology Center
0.00 0.00 **FUD** 000

0197U Red cell antigen (Landsteiner-Wiener blood group) genotyping (LW), gene analysis, *ICAM4 (intercellular adhesion molecule 4 [Landsteiner-Wiener blood group])* exon 1

INCLUDES Navigator LW Sequencing, Grifols Immunohematology Center, Grifols Immunohematology Center
0.00 0.00 **FUD** 000

0198U Red cell antigen (RH blood group) genotyping (RHD and RHCE), gene analysis Sanger/chain termination/conventional sequencing, *RHD (Rh blood group D antigen) exons 1-10 and RHCE (Rh blood group CcEe antigens) exon 5*

INCLUDES Navigator RHD/CE Sequencing, Grifols Immunohematology Center, Grifols Immunohematology Center
0.00 0.00 **FUD** 000

0199U Red cell antigen (Scianna blood group) genotyping (SC), gene analysis, *ERMAP (erythroblast membrane associated protein [Scianna blood group])* exons 4, 12

INCLUDES Navigator SC Sequencing, Grifols Immunohematology Center, Grifols Immunohematology Center
0.00 0.00 **FUD** 000

0200U Red cell antigen (Kx blood group) genotyping (XK), gene analysis, *XK (X-linked Kx blood group)* exons 1-3

INCLUDES Navigator XK Sequencing, Grifols Immunohematology Center, Grifols Immunohematology Center
0.00 0.00 **FUD** 000

0201U Red cell antigen (Yt blood group) genotyping (YT), gene analysis, *ACHE (acetylcholinesterase [Cartwright blood group])* exon 2

INCLUDES Navigator YT Sequencing, Grifols Immunohematology Center, Grifols Immunohematology Center
0.00 0.00 **FUD** 000

0202U Infectious disease (bacterial or viral respiratory tract infection), pathogen-specific nucleic acid (DNA or RNA), 22 targets including severe acute respiratory syndrome coronavirus 2 (SARS-CoV-2), qualitative RT-PCR, nasopharyngeal swab, each pathogen reported as detected or not detected

INCLUDES BioFire® Respiratory Panel 2.1 (RP2.1), BioFire® Diagnostics, BioFire® Diagnostics, LLC
EXCLUDES *QIAstat-Dx Respiratory SARS CoV-2 Panel, QIAGEN Sciences, QIAGEN GmbH. To report, see (0223U)*
0.00 0.00 **FUD** 000
AMA: 2020,AugSE,1; 2020,AugSE,1; 2020,AugSE,1; 2020,MaySE,1; 2020,May,3; 2020,JuneSE,1

0203U Autoimmune (inflammatory bowel disease), mRNA, gene expression profiling by quantitative RT-PCR, 17 genes (15 target and 2 reference genes), whole blood, reported as a continuous risk score and classification of inflammatory bowel disease aggressiveness

INCLUDES PredictSURE IBD™ Test, KSL Diagnostics, PredictImmune Ltd
0.00 0.00 **FUD** 000

0204U Oncology (thyroid), mRNA, gene expression analysis of 593 genes (including *BRAF, RAS, RET, PAX8,* and *NTRK*) for sequence variants and rearrangements, utilizing fine needle aspirate, reported as detected or not detected

INCLUDES Afirma Xpression Atlas, Veracyte, Inc, Veracyte, Inc
0.00 0.00 **FUD** 000

0205U Ophthalmology (age-related macular degeneration), analysis of 3 gene variants (2 *CFH* gene, 1 *ARMS2* gene), using PCR and MALDI-TOF, buccal swab, reported as positive or negative for neovascular age-related macular-degeneration risk associated with zinc supplements

INCLUDES Vita Risk®, Arctic Medical Laboratories, Arctic Medical Laboratories
0.00 0.00 **FUD** 000

0206U Neurology (Alzheimer disease); cell aggregation using morphometric imaging and protein kinase C-epsilon (PKCe) concentration in response to amylospheroid treatment by ELISA, cultured skin fibroblasts, each reported as positive or negative for Alzheimer disease

INCLUDES DISCERN™, NeuroDiagnostics, NeuroDiagnostics
0.00 0.00 **FUD** 000

+ **0207U** quantitative imaging of phosphorylated *ERK1* and *ERK2* in response to bradykinin treatment by in situ immunofluorescence, using cultured skin fibroblasts, reported as a probability index for Alzheimer disease (List separately in addition to code for primary procedure)

INCLUDES DISCERN™, NeuroDiagnostics, NeuroDiagnostics
Code first (0206U)
0.00 0.00 **FUD** 000

0208U ~~Oncology (medullary thyroid carcinoma), mRNA, gene expression analysis of 108 genes, utilizing fine needle aspirate, algorithm reported as positive or negative for medullary thyroid carcinoma~~

0209U Cytogenomic constitutional (genome-wide) analysis, interrogation of genomic regions for copy number, structural changes and areas of homozygosity for chromosomal abnormalities

INCLUDES CNGnome™, PerkinElmer Genomics, PerkinElmer Genomics
0.00 0.00 **FUD** 000

0210U Syphilis test, non-treponemal antibody, immunoassay, quantitative (RPR)

INCLUDES BioPlex 2200 RPR Assay - Quantitative, Bio-Rad Laboratories, Bio-Rad Laboratories
0.00 0.00 **FUD** 000

0211U Oncology (pan-tumor), DNA and RNA by next-generation sequencing, utilizing formalin-fixed paraffin-embedded tissue, interpretative report for single nucleotide variants, copy number alterations, tumor mutational burden, and microsatellite instability, with therapy association

INCLUDES MI Cancer Seek™ - NGS Analysis, Caris MPI d/b/a Caris Life Sciences, Caris MPI d/b/a Caris Life Sciences
0.00 0.00 **FUD** 000

0212U Rare diseases (constitutional/heritable disorders), whole genome and mitochondrial DNA sequence analysis, including small sequence changes, deletions, duplications, short tandem repeat gene expansions, and variants in non-uniquely mappable regions, blood or saliva, identification and categorization of genetic variants, proband

INCLUDES Genomic Unity® Whole Genome Analysis – Proband, Variantyx Inc, Variantyx Inc
EXCLUDES *Genome (e.g., unexplained constitutional or heritable disorder or syndrome); sequence analysis (81425)*
0.00 0.00 **FUD** 000

0213U Rare diseases (constitutional/heritable disorders), whole genome and mitochondrial DNA sequence analysis, including small sequence changes, deletions, duplications, short tandem repeat gene expansions, and variants in non-uniquely mappable regions, blood or saliva, identification and categorization of genetic variants, each comparator genome (eg, parent, sibling)

> INCLUDES   Genomic Unity® Whole Genome Analysis - Comparator, Variantyx Inc, Variantyx Inc
>
> EXCLUDES   Genome (e.g., unexplained constitutional or heritable disorder or syndrome); sequence analysis, each comparator genome (e.g., parents, siblings) (81426)

📋 0.00   ⚕ 0.00   **FUD** 000

0214U Rare diseases (constitutional/heritable disorders), whole exome and mitochondrial DNA sequence analysis, including small sequence changes, deletions, duplications, short tandem repeat gene expansions, and variants in non-uniquely mappable regions, blood or saliva, identification and categorization of genetic variants, proband

> INCLUDES   Genomic Unity® Exome Plus Analysis - Proband, Variantyx Inc, Variantyx Inc
>
> EXCLUDES   Exome (e.g., unexplained constitutional or heritable disorder or syndrome); sequence analysis (81415)

📋 0.00   ⚕ 0.00   **FUD** 000

0215U Rare diseases (constitutional/heritable disorders), whole exome and mitochondrial DNA sequence analysis, including small sequence changes, deletions, duplications, short tandem repeat gene expansions, and variants in non-uniquely mappable regions, blood or saliva, identification and categorization of genetic variants, each comparator exome (eg, parent, sibling)

> INCLUDES   Genomic Unity® Exome Plus Analysis - Comparator, Variantyx Inc, Variantyx Inc
>
> EXCLUDES   Exome (e.g., unexplained constitutional or heritable disorder or syndrome); sequence analysis, each comparator exome (e.g., parents, siblings) (81416)

📋 0.00   ⚕ 0.00   **FUD** 000

0216U Neurology (inherited ataxias), genomic DNA sequence analysis of 12 common genes including small sequence changes, deletions, duplications, short tandem repeat gene expansions, and variants in non-uniquely mappable regions, blood or saliva, identification and categorization of genetic variants

> INCLUDES   Genomic Unity® Ataxia Repeat Expansion and Sequence Analysis, Variantyx Inc, Variantyx Inc

📋 0.00   ⚕ 0.00   **FUD** 000

0217U Neurology (inherited ataxias), genomic DNA sequence analysis of 51 genes including small sequence changes, deletions, duplications, short tandem repeat gene expansions, and variants in non-uniquely mappable regions, blood or saliva, identification and categorization of genetic variants

> INCLUDES   Genomic Unity® Comprehensive Ataxia Repeat Expansion and Sequence Analysis, Variantyx Inc, Variantyx Inc

📋 0.00   ⚕ 0.00   **FUD** 000

0218U Neurology (muscular dystrophy), *DMD* gene sequence analysis, including small sequence changes, deletions, duplications, and variants in non-uniquely mappable regions, blood or saliva, identification and characterization of genetic variants

> INCLUDES   Genomic Unity® DMD Analysis, Variantyx Inc, Variantyx Inc

📋 0.00   ⚕ 0.00   **FUD** 000

0219U Infectious agent (human immunodeficiency virus), targeted viral next-generation sequence analysis (ie, protease [PR], reverse transcriptase [RT], integrase [INT]), algorithm reported as prediction of antiviral drug susceptibility

> INCLUDES   Sentosa® SQ HIV-1 Genotyping Assay, Vela Diagnostics USA, Inc, Vela Operations Singapore Pte Ltd

📋 0.00   ⚕ 0.00   **FUD** 000

0220U Oncology (breast cancer), image analysis with artificial intelligence assessment of 12 histologic and immunohistochemical features, reported as a recurrence score

> INCLUDES   PreciseDx™ Breast Cancer Test, PreciseDx, PreciseDx

📋 0.00   ⚕ 0.00   **FUD** 000

0221U Red cell antigen (ABO blood group) genotyping (ABO), gene analysis, next-generation sequencing, *ABO (ABO, alpha 1-3-N-acetylgalactosaminyltransferase and alpha 1-3-galactosyltransferase)* gene

> INCLUDES   Navigator ABO Blood Group NGS, Grifols Immunohematology Center, Grifols Immunohematology Center

📋 0.00   ⚕ 0.00   **FUD** 000

0222U Red cell antigen (RH blood group) genotyping (RHD and RHCE), gene analysis, next-generation sequencing, RH proximal promoter, exons 1-10, portions of introns 2-3

> INCLUDES   Navigator Rh Blood Group NGS, Grifols Immunohematology Center, Grifols Immunohematology Center

📋 0.00   ⚕ 0.00   **FUD** 000

● **0223U** Infectious disease (bacterial or viral respiratory tract infection), pathogen-specific nucleic acid (DNA or RNA), 22 targets including severe acute respiratory syndrome coronavirus 2 (SARS-CoV-2), qualitative RT-PCR, nasopharyngeal swab, each pathogen reported as detected or not detected

> INCLUDES   QIAstat-Dx Respiratory SARS CoV-2 Panel, QIAGEN Sciences, QIAGEN GmbH
>
> EXCLUDES   BioFire® Respiratory Panel 2.1 (RP2.1), BioFire® Diagnostics, BioFire® Diagnostics, LLC. To report, see (0202U)

AMA: 2020,AugSE,1; 2020,AugSE,1; 2020,AugSE,1

● **0224U** Antibody, severe acute respiratory syndrome coronavirus 2 (SARS-CoV-2) (coronavirus disease [COVID-19]), includes titer(s), when performed

> INCLUDES   COVID-19 Antibody Test, Mt Sinai, Mount Sinai Laboratory
>
> EXCLUDES   Antibody; severe acute respiratory syndrome coronavirus 2 (SARS-CoV-2) (coronavirus disease [COVID-19]) (86769)

AMA: 2020,AugSE,1; 2020,AugSE,1; 2020,AugSE,1

● **0225U** Infectious disease (bacterial or viral respiratory tract infection) pathogen-specific DNA and RNA, 21 targets, including severe acute respiratory syndrome coronavirus 2 (SARS-CoV-2), amplified probe technique, including multiplex reverse transcription for RNA targets, each analyte reported as detected or not detected

> INCLUDES   ePlex® Respiratory Pathogen Panel 2, GenMark Dx, GenMark Diagnostics, Inc

AMA: 2020,AugSE,1

● **0226U** Surrogate viral neutralization test (sVNT), severe acute respiratory syndrome coronavirus 2 (SARS-CoV-2) (coronavirus disease [COVID-19]), ELISA, plasma, serum

> INCLUDES   Tru-Immune™, Ethos Laboratories, GenScript® USA Inc

AMA: 2020,AugSE,1

● **0227U** Drug assay, presumptive, 30 or more drugs or metabolites, urine, liquid chromatography with tandem mass spectrometry (LC-MS/MS) using multiple reaction monitoring (MRM), with drug or metabolite description, includes sample validation

> INCLUDES   Comprehensive Screen, Aspenti Health

📋 0.00   ⚕ 0.00   **FUD** 000

● New Code   ▲ Revised Code   ○ Reinstated   ● New Web Release   ▲ Revised Web Release   + Add-on   Unlisted   Not Covered   # Resequenced
⑤⓪ Optum Mod 50 Exempt   Ⓝ AMA Mod 51 Exempt   ⑤① Optum Mod 51 Exempt   ⑥③ Mod 63 Exempt   ✗ Non-FDA Drug   ★ Telemedicine   Ⓜ Maternity   Ⓐ Age Edit

CPT © 2021 American Medical Association. All Rights Reserved.

0228U Oncology (prostate), multianalyte molecular profile by photometric detection of macromolecules adsorbed on nanosponge array slides with machine learning, utilizing first morning voided urine, algorithm reported as likelihood of prostate cancer

INCLUDES PanGIA Prostate, Genetics Institute of America, Entopsis, LLC

0229U *BCAT1 (Branched chain amino acid transaminase 1)* or *IKZF1 (IKAROS family zinc finger 1)* (eg, colorectal cancer) promoter methylation analysis

INCLUDES Colvera®, Clinical Genomics Pathology Inc

0230U *AR (androgen receptor)* (eg, spinal and bulbar muscular atrophy, Kennedy disease, X chromosome inactivation), full sequence analysis, including small sequence changes in exonic and intronic regions, deletions, duplications, short tandem repeat (STR) expansions, mobile element insertions, and variants in non-uniquely mappable regions

INCLUDES Genomic Unity® AR Analysis, Variantyx Inc, Variantyx Inc

0231U *CACNA1A (calcium voltage-gated channel subunit alpha 1A)* (eg, spinocerebellar ataxia), full gene analysis, including small sequence changes in exonic and intronic regions, deletions, duplications, short tandem repeat (STR) gene expansions, mobile element insertions, and variants in non-uniquely mappable regions

INCLUDES Genomic Unity® CACNA1A Analysis, Variantyx Inc, Variantyx Inc

0232U *CSTB (cystatin B)* (eg, progressive myoclonic epilepsy type 1A, Unverricht-Lundborg disease), full gene analysis, including small sequence changes in exonic and intronic regions, deletions, duplications, short tandem repeat (STR) expansions, mobile element insertions, and variants in non-uniquely mappable regions

INCLUDES Genomic Unity® CSTB Analysis, Variantyx Inc, Variantyx Inc

0233U *FXN (frataxin)* (eg, Friedreich ataxia), gene analysis, including small sequence changes in exonic and intronic regions, deletions, duplications, short tandem repeat (STR) expansions, mobile element insertions, and variants in non-uniquely mappable regions

INCLUDES Genomic Unity® FXN Analysis, Variantyx Inc, Variantyx Inc

0234U *MECP2 (methyl CpG binding protein 2)* (eg, Rett syndrome), full gene analysis, including small sequence changes in exonic and intronic regions, deletions, duplications, mobile element insertions, and variants in non-uniquely mappable regions

INCLUDES Genomic Unity® MECP2 Analysis, Variantyx Inc, Variantyx Inc

0235U *PTEN (phosphatase and tensin homolog)* (eg, Cowden syndrome, PTEN hamartoma tumor syndrome), full gene analysis, including small sequence changes in exonic and intronic regions, deletions, duplications, mobile element insertions, and variants in non-uniquely mappable regions

INCLUDES Genomic Unity® PTEN Analysis, Variantyx Inc, Variantyx Inc

0236U *SMN1 (survival of motor neuron 1, telomeric)* and *SMN2 (survival of motor neuron 2, centromeric)* (eg, spinal muscular atrophy) full gene analysis, including small sequence changes in exonic and intronic regions, duplications, deletions, and mobile element insertions

INCLUDES Genomic Unity® SMN1/2 Analysis, Variantyx Inc, Variantyx Inc

0237U Cardiac ion channelopathies (eg, Brugada syndrome, long QT syndrome, short QT syndrome, catecholaminergic polymorphic ventricular tachycardia), genomic sequence analysis panel including *ANK2, CASQ2, CAV3, KCNE1, KCNE2, KCNH2, KCNJ2, KCNQ1, RYR2,* and *SCN5A,* including small sequence changes in exonic and intronic regions, deletions, duplications, mobile element insertions, and variants in non-uniquely mappable regions

INCLUDES Genomic Unity® Cardiac Ion Channelopathies Analysis, Variantyx Inc, Variantyx Inc

0238U Oncology (Lynch syndrome), genomic DNA sequence analysis of *MLH1, MSH2, MSH6, PMS2,* and *EPCAM,* including small sequence changes in exonic and intronic regions, deletions, duplications, mobile element insertions, and variants in non-uniquely mappable regions

INCLUDES Genomic Unity® Lynch Syndrome Analysis, Variantyx Inc, Variantyx Inc

0239U Targeted genomic sequence analysis panel, solid organ neoplasm, cell-free DNA, analysis of 311 or more genes, interrogation for sequence variants, including substitutions, insertions, deletions, select rearrangements, and copy number variations

INCLUDES FoundationOne® Liquid CDx, Foundation Medicine, Inc, Foundation Medicine, Inc

0240U Infectious disease (viral respiratory tract infection), pathogen-specific RNA, 3 targets (severe acute respiratory syndrome coronavirus 2 [SARS-CoV-2], influenza A, influenza B), upper respiratory specimen, each pathogen reported as detected or not detected

INCLUDES Xpert® Xpress SARS-CoV-2/Flu/RSV (SARS-CoV-2 & Flu targets only), Cepheid

🚑 0.00 ⚕ 0.00 **FUD** 000 ▣

AMA: 2020,OctSE,1

0241U Infectious disease (viral respiratory tract infection), pathogen-specific RNA, 4 targets (severe acute respiratory syndrome coronavirus 2 [SARS-CoV-2], influenza A, influenza B, respiratory syncytial virus [RSV]), upper respiratory specimen, each pathogen reported as detected or not detected

INCLUDES Xpert® Xpress SARS-CoV-2/Flu/RSV (all targets), Cepheid

🚑 0.00 ⚕ 0.00 **FUD** 000 ▣

AMA: 2020,OctSE,1

0242U Targeted genomic sequence analysis panel, solid organ neoplasm, cell-free circulating DNA analysis of 55-74 genes, interrogation for sequence variants, gene copy number amplifications, and gene rearrangements

INCLUDES Guardant360® CDx, Guardant Health Inc, Guardant Health Inc

0243U Obstetrics (preeclampsia), biochemical assay of placental-growth factor, time-resolved fluorescence immunoassay, maternal serum, predictive algorithm reported as a risk score for preeclampsia ♀

INCLUDES PIGF Preeclampsia Screen, PerkinElmer Genetics, PerkinElmer Genetics, Inc

🚑 0.00 ⚕ 0.00 **FUD** 000

0244U Oncology (solid organ), DNA, comprehensive genomic profiling, 257 genes, interrogation for single-nucleotide variants, insertions/deletions, copy number alterations, gene rearrangements, tumor-mutational burden and microsatellite instability, utilizing formalin-fixed paraffin-embedded tumor tissue

INCLUDES Oncotype MAP™ Pan-Cancer Tissue Test, Paradigm Diagnostics, Inc, Paradigm Diagnostics, Inc

26/TC PC/TC Only A2-Z3 ASC Payment 50 Bilateral ♂ Male Only ♀ Female Only 🚑 Facility RVU ⚕ Non-Facility RVU ▣ CCI ▣ CLIA
FUD Follow-up Days **CMS:** IOM **AMA:** CPT Asst A-Y OPPSI 80/80 Surg Assist Allowed / w/Doc ▣ Lab Crosswalk ▣ Radiology Crosswalk

448   CPT © 2021 American Medical Association. All Rights Reserved.   © 2021 Optum360, LLC

● **0245U** Oncology (thyroid), mutation analysis of 10 genes and 37 RNA fusions and expression of 4 mRNA markers using next-generation sequencing, fine needle aspirate, report includes associated risk of malignancy expressed as a percentage

INCLUDES ThyGeNEXT® Thyroid Oncogene Panel, Interpace Diagnostics, Interpace Diagnostics

● **0246U** Red blood cell antigen typing, DNA, genotyping of at least 16 blood groups with phenotype prediction of at least 51 red blood cell antigens

INCLUDES PrecisionBlood™, San Diego Blood Bank, San Diego Blood Bank

● **0247U** Obstetrics (preterm birth), insulin-like growth factor-binding protein 4 (IBP4), sex hormone-binding globulin (SHBG), quantitative measurement by LC-MS/MS, utilizing maternal serum, combined with clinical data, reported as predictive-risk stratification for spontaneous preterm birth

INCLUDES PreTRM®, Sera Prognostics, Sera Prognostics, Inc®

● **0248U** Oncology (brain), spheroid cell culture in a 3D microenvironment, 12 drug panel, tumor-response prediction for each drug

INCLUDES 3D Predict Glioma, KIYATEC®, Inc

● **0249U** Oncology (breast), semiquantitative analysis of 32 phosphoproteins and protein analytes, includes laser capture microdissection, with algorithmic analysis and interpretative report

INCLUDES Theralink® Reverse Phase Protein Array (RPPA), Theralink® Technologies, Inc, Theralink® Technologies, Inc

● **0250U** Oncology (solid organ neoplasm), targeted genomic sequence DNA analysis of 505 genes, interrogation for somatic alterations (SNVs [single nucleotide variant], small insertions and deletions, one amplification, and four translocations), microsatellite instability and tumor-mutation burden

INCLUDES PGDx elio™ tissue complete, Personal Genome Diagnostics, Inc, Personal Genome Diagnostics, Inc

● **0251U** Hepcidin-25, enzyme-linked immunosorbent assay (ELISA), serum or plasma

INCLUDES Intrinsic Hepcidin IDx™ Test, IntrinsicDx, Intrinsic LifeSciences™ LLC

● **0252U** Fetal aneuploidy short tandem–repeat comparative analysis, fetal DNA from products of conception, reported as normal (euploidy), monosomy, trisomy, or partial deletion/duplication, mosaicism, and segmental aneuploidy

INCLUDES POC (Products of Conception), Igenomix®, Igenomix® USA

● **0253U** Reproductive medicine (endometrial receptivity analysis), RNA gene expression profile, 238 genes by next-generation sequencing, endometrial tissue, predictive algorithm reported as endometrial window of implantation (eg, pre-receptive, receptive, post-receptive) ♀

INCLUDES ERA® (Endometrial Receptivity Analysis), Igenomix®, Igenomix® USA

🔲 0.00 ⚬ 0.00 **FUD** 000

● **0254U** Reproductive medicine (preimplantation genetic assessment), analysis of 24 chromosomes using embryonic DNA genomic sequence analysis for aneuploidy, and a mitochondrial DNA score in euploid embryos, results reported as normal (euploidy), monosomy, trisomy, or partial deletion/duplication, mosaicism, and segmental aneuploidy, per embryo tested

INCLUDES SMART PGT-A (Pre-implantation Genetic Testing - Aneuploidy), Igenomix®, Igenomix® USA

● **0255U** Andrology (infertility), sperm-capacitation assessment of ganglioside GM1 distribution patterns, fluorescence microscopy, fresh or frozen specimen, reported as percentage of capacitated sperm and probability of generating a pregnancy score

INCLUDES Cap-Score™ Test, Androvia LifeSciences, Avantor Clinical Services (previously known as Therapak)

● **0256U** Trimethylamine/trimethylamine N-oxide (TMA/TMAO) profile, tandem mass spectrometry (MS/MS), urine, with algorithmic analysis and interpretive report

INCLUDES Trimethylamine (TMA) and TMA N-Oxide, Children's Hospital Colorado Laboratory

● **0257U** Very long chain acyl-coenzyme A (CoA) dehydrogenase (VLCAD), leukocyte enzyme activity, whole blood

INCLUDES Very-Long Chain Acyl-CoA Dehydrogenase (VLCAD) Enzyme Activity, Children's Hospital Colorado Laboratory

● **0258U** Autoimmune (psoriasis), mRNA, next-generation sequencing, gene expression profiling of 50-100 genes, skin-surface collection using adhesive patch, algorithm reported as likelihood of response to psoriasis biologics

INCLUDES Mind.Px, Mindera, Mindera Corporation

● **0259U** Nephrology (chronic kidney disease), nuclear magnetic resonance spectroscopy measurement of myo-inositol, valine, and creatinine, algorithmically combined with cystatin C (by immunoassay) and demographic data to determine estimated glomerular filtration rate (GFR), serum, quantitative

INCLUDES GFR by NMR, Labtech™ Diagnostics

● **0260U** Rare diseases (constitutional/heritable disorders), identification of copy number variations, inversions, insertions, translocations, and other structural variants by optical genome mapping

INCLUDES Augusta Optical Genome Mapping, Georgia Esoteric and Molecular (GEM) Laboratory, LLC, Bionano Genomics Inc

EXCLUDES *Praxis Optical Genome Mapping, Praxis Genomics LLC (0264U)*

● **0261U** Oncology (colorectal cancer), image analysis with artificial intelligence assessment of 4 histologic and immunohistochemical features (CD3 and CD8 within tumor-stroma border and tumor core), tissue, reported as immune response and recurrence-risk score

INCLUDES Immunoscore®, HalioDx, HalioDx

● **0262U** Oncology (solid tumor), gene expression profiling by real-time RT-PCR of 7 gene pathways (*ER, AR, PI3K, MAPK, HH, TGFB, Notch*), formalin-fixed paraffin-embedded (FFPE), algorithm reported as gene pathway activity score

INCLUDES OncoSignal 7 Pathway Signal, Protean BioDiagnostics, Philips Electronics Nederland BV

● **0263U** Neurology (autism spectrum disorder [ASD]), quantitative measurements of 16 central carbon metabolites (ie, α-ketoglutarate, alanine, lactate, phenylalanine, pyruvate, succinate, carnitine, citrate, fumarate, hypoxanthine, inosine, malate, S-sulfocysteine, taurine, urate, and xanthine), liquid chromatography tandem mass spectrometry (LC-MS/MS), plasma, algorithmic analysis with result reported as negative or positive (with metabolic subtypes of ASD)

INCLUDES NPDX ASD and Central Carbon Energy Metabolism, Stemina Biomarker Discovery, Inc, Stemina Biomarker Discovery, Inc

● **0264U** Rare diseases (constitutional/heritable disorders), identification of copy number variations, inversions, insertions, translocations, and other structural variants by optical genome mapping

INCLUDES Praxis Optical Genome Mapping, Praxis Genomics LLC

EXCLUDES *Augusta Optical Genome Mapping, Georgia Esoteric and Molecular (GEM) Laboratory, LLC, Bionano Genomics Inc (0260U)*

● **0265U** Rare constitutional and other heritable disorders, whole genome and mitochondrial DNA sequence analysis, blood, frozen and formalin-fixed paraffin-embedded (FFPE) tissue, saliva, buccal swabs or cell lines, identification of single nucleotide and copy number variants

INCLUDES Praxis Whole Genome Sequencing, Praxis Genomics LLC

● **0266U** Unexplained constitutional or other heritable disorders or syndromes, tissue-specific gene expression by whole-transcriptome and next-generation sequencing, blood, formalin-fixed paraffin-embedded (FFPE) tissue or fresh frozen tissue, reported as presence or absence of splicing or expression changes

INCLUDES Praxis Transcriptome, Praxis Genomics LLC

● **0267U** Rare constitutional and other heritable disorders, identification of copy number variations, inversions, insertions, translocations, and other structural variants by optical genome mapping and whole genome sequencing

INCLUDES Praxis Combined Whole Genome Sequencing and Optical Genome Mapping, Praxis Genomics LLC

● **0268U** Hematology (atypical hemolytic uremic syndrome [aHUS]), genomic sequence analysis of 15 genes, blood, buccal swab, or amniotic fluid

INCLUDES Versiti™ aHUS Genetic Evaluation, Versiti™ Diagnostic Laboratories, Versiti™

● **0269U** Hematology (autosomal dominant congenital thrombocytopenia), genomic sequence analysis of 14 genes, blood, buccal swab, or amniotic fluid

INCLUDES Versiti™ Autosomal Dominant Thrombocytopenia Panel, Versiti™ Diagnostic Laboratories, Versiti™

● **0270U** Hematology (congenital coagulation disorders), genomic sequence analysis of 20 genes, blood, buccal swab, or amniotic fluid

INCLUDES Versiti™ Coagulation Disorder Panel, Versiti™ Diagnostic Laboratories, Versiti™

● **0271U** Hematology (congenital neutropenia), genomic sequence analysis of 23 genes, blood, buccal swab, or amniotic fluid

INCLUDES Versiti™ Congenital Neutropenia Panel, Versiti™ Diagnostic Laboratories, Versiti™

● **0272U** Hematology (genetic bleeding disorders), genomic sequence analysis of 51 genes, blood, buccal swab, or amniotic fluid, comprehensive

INCLUDES Versiti™ Comprehensive Bleeding Disorder Panel, Versiti™ Diagnostic Laboratories, Versiti™

● **0273U** Hematology (genetic hyperfibrinolysis, delayed bleeding), genomic sequence analysis of 8 genes (*F13A1, F13B, FGA, FGB, FGG, SERPINA1, SERPINE1, SERPINF2, PLAU*), blood, buccal swab, or amniotic fluid

INCLUDES Versiti™ Fibrinolytic Disorder Panel, Versiti™ Diagnostic Laboratories, Versiti™

● **0274U** Hematology (genetic platelet disorders), genomic sequence analysis of 43 genes, blood, buccal swab, or amniotic fluid

INCLUDES Versiti™ Comprehensive Platelet Disorder Panel, Versiti™ Diagnostic Laboratories, Versiti™

● **0275U** Hematology (heparin-induced thrombocytopenia), platelet antibody reactivity by flow cytometry, serum

INCLUDES Versiti™ Heparin-Induced Thrombocytopenia Evaluation – PEA, Versiti™ Diagnostic Laboratories, Versiti™

● **0276U** Hematology (inherited thrombocytopenia), genomic sequence analysis of 23 genes, blood, buccal swab, or amniotic fluid

INCLUDES Versiti™ Inherited Thrombocytopenia Panel, Versiti™ Diagnostic Laboratories, Versiti™

● **0277U** Hematology (genetic platelet function disorder), genomic sequence analysis of 31 genes, blood, buccal swab, or amniotic fluid

INCLUDES Versiti™ Platelet Function Disorder Panel, Versiti™ Diagnostic Laboratories, Versiti™

● **0278U** Hematology (genetic thrombosis), genomic sequence analysis of 12 genes, blood, buccal swab, or amniotic fluid

INCLUDES Versiti™ Thrombosis Panel, Versiti™ Diagnostic Laboratories, Versiti™

● **0279U** Hematology (von Willebrand disease [VWD]), von Willebrand factor (VWF) and collagen III binding by enzyme-linked immunosorbent assays (ELISA), plasma, report of collagen III binding

INCLUDES Versiti™ VWF Collagen III Binding, Versiti™ Diagnostic Laboratories, Versiti™

● **0280U** Hematology (von Willebrand disease [VWD]), von Willebrand factor (VWF) and collagen IV binding by enzyme-linked immunosorbent assays (ELISA), plasma, report of collagen IV binding

INCLUDES Versiti™ VWF Collagen IV Binding, Versiti™ Diagnostic Laboratories, Versiti™

● **0281U** Hematology (von Willebrand disease [VWD]), von Willebrand propeptide, enzyme-linked immunosorbent assays (ELISA), plasma, diagnostic report of von Willebrand factor (VWF) propeptide antigen level

INCLUDES Versiti™ VWF Propeptide Antigen, Versiti™ Diagnostic Laboratories, Versiti™

● **0282U** Red blood cell antigen typing, DNA, genotyping of 12 blood group system genes to predict 44 red blood cell antigen phenotypes

INCLUDES Versiti™ Red Cell Genotyping Panel, Versiti™ Diagnostic Laboratories, Versiti™

● **0283U** von Willebrand factor (VWF), type 2B, platelet-binding evaluation, radioimmunoassay, plasma

INCLUDES Versiti™ VWD Type 2B Evaluation, Versiti™ Diagnostic Laboratories, Versiti™

● **0284U** von Willebrand factor (VWF), type 2N, factor VIII and VWF binding evaluation, enzyme-linked immunosorbent assays (ELISA), plasma

INCLUDES Versiti™ VWD Type 2N Binding, Versiti™ Diagnostic Laboratories, Versiti™

● **0285U** Oncology, response to radiation, cell-free DNA, quantitative branched chain DNA amplification, plasma, reported as a radiation toxicity score

INCLUDES RadTox™ cfDNA test, DiaCarta Clinical Lab, DiaCarta Inc

● **0286U** *CEP72 (centrosomal protein, 72-KDa), NUDT15 (nudix hydrolase 15)* and *TPMT (thiopurine S-methyltransferase)* (eg, drug metabolism) gene analysis, common variants

INCLUDES CNT *(CEP72, TPMT and NUDT15)* genotyping panel, RPRD Diagnostics

● **0287U** Oncology (thyroid), DNA and mRNA, next-generation sequencing analysis of 112 genes, fine needle aspirate or formalin-fixed paraffin-embedded (FFPE) tissue, algorithmic prediction of cancer recurrence, reported as a categorical risk result (low, intermediate, high)

INCLUDES ThyroSeq® CRC, CBLPath, Inc, University of Pittsburgh Medical Center

● **0288U** Oncology (lung), mRNA, quantitative PCR analysis of 11 genes (*BAG1, BRCA1, CDC6, CDK2AP1, ERBB3, FUT3, IL11, LCK, RND3, SH3BGR, WNT3A*) and 3 reference genes (*ESD, TBP, YAP1*), formalin-fixed paraffin-embedded (FFPE) tumor tissue, algorithmic interpretation reported as a recurrence risk score

INCLUDES DetermaRx™, Oncocyte Corporation

| 26/TC PC/TC Only | A2-Z3 ASC Payment | 50 Bilateral | ♂ Male Only | ♀ Female Only | 🖪 Facility RVU | Non-Facility RVU | CCI | ☒ CLIA |
| FUD Follow-up Days | CMS: IOM | AMA: CPT Asst | A-Y OPPSI | 80/80 Surg Assist Allowed / w/Doc | Lab Crosswalk | Radiology Crosswalk |

450   CPT © 2021 American Medical Association. All Rights Reserved.   © 2021 Optum360, LLC

● **0289U** Neurology (Alzheimer disease), mRNA, gene expression profiling by RNA sequencing of 24 genes, whole blood, algorithm reported as predictive risk score
INCLUDES MindX Blood Test™ - Memory/Alzheimer's, MindX Sciences™ Laboratory, MindX Sciences™ Inc

● **0290U** Pain management, mRNA, gene expression profiling by RNA sequencing of 36 genes, whole blood, algorithm reported as predictive risk score
INCLUDES MindX Blood Test™ - Pain, MindX Sciences™ Laboratory, MindX Sciences™ Inc

● **0291U** Psychiatry (mood disorders), mRNA, gene expression profiling by RNA sequencing of 144 genes, whole blood, algorithm reported as predictive risk score
INCLUDES MindX Blood Test™ - Mood, MindX Sciences™ Laboratory, MindX Sciences™ Inc

● **0292U** Psychiatry (stress disorders), mRNA, gene expression profiling by RNA sequencing of 72 genes, whole blood, algorithm reported as predictive risk score
INCLUDES MindX Blood Test™ - Stress, MindX Sciences™ Laboratory, MindX Sciences™ Inc

● **0293U** Psychiatry (suicidal ideation), mRNA, gene expression profiling by RNA sequencing of 54 genes, whole blood, algorithm reported as predictive risk score
INCLUDES MindX Blood Test™ - Suicidality, MindX Sciences™ Laboratory, MindX Sciences™ Inc

● **0294U** Longevity and mortality risk, mRNA, gene expression profiling by RNA sequencing of 18 genes, whole blood, algorithm reported as predictive risk score
INCLUDES MindX Blood Test™ - Longevity, MindX Sciences™ Laboratory, MindX Sciences™ Inc

● **0295U** Oncology (breast ductal carcinoma in situ), protein expression profiling by immunohistochemistry of 7 proteins (COX2, FOXA1, HER2, Ki-67, p16, PR, SIAH2), with 4 clinicopathologic factors (size, age, margin status, palpability), utilizing formalin-fixed paraffin-embedded (FFPE) tissue, algorithm reported as a recurrence risk score
INCLUDES DCISionRT®, PreludeDx™, Prelude Corporation

● **0296U** Oncology (oral and/or oropharyngeal cancer), gene expression profiling by RNA sequencing at least 20 molecular features (eg, human and/or microbial mRNA), saliva, algorithm reported as positive or negative for signature associated with malignancy
INCLUDES mRNA CancerDetect™, Viome Life Sciences, Inc, Viome Life Sciences, Inc

● **0297U** Oncology (pan tumor), whole genome sequencing of paired malignant and normal DNA specimens, fresh or formalin-fixed paraffin-embedded (FFPE) tissue, blood or bone marrow, comparative sequence analyses and variant identification
INCLUDES Praxis Somatic Whole Genome Sequencing, Praxis Genomics LLC

● **0298U** Oncology (pan tumor), whole transcriptome sequencing of paired malignant and normal RNA specimens, fresh or formalin-fixed paraffin-embedded (FFPE) tissue, blood or bone marrow, comparative sequence analyses and expression level and chimeric transcript identification
INCLUDES Praxis Somatic Transcriptome, Praxis Genomics LLC

● **0299U** Oncology (pan tumor), whole genome optical genome mapping of paired malignant and normal DNA specimens, fresh frozen tissue, blood, or bone marrow, comparative structural variant identification
INCLUDES Praxis Somatic Optical Genome Mapping, Praxis Genomics LLC

● **0300U** Oncology (pan tumor), whole genome sequencing and optical genome mapping of paired malignant and normal DNA specimens, fresh tissue, blood, or bone marrow, comparative sequence analyses and variant identification
INCLUDES Praxis Somatic Combined Whole Genome Sequencing and Optical Genome Mapping, Praxis Genomics LLC

● **0301U** Infectious agent detection by nucleic acid (DNA or RNA), Bartonella henselae and Bartonella quintana, droplet digital PCR (ddPCR);
INCLUDES Bartonella ddPCR, Galaxy Diagnostics Inc

● **0302U** following liquid enhancement
INCLUDES Bartonella Digital ePCR™, Galaxy Diagnostics Inc

● **0303U** Hematology, red blood cell (RBC) adhesion to endothelial/subendothelial adhesion molecules, functional assessment, whole blood, with algorithmic analysis and result reported as an RBC adhesion index; hypoxic
INCLUDES Hypoxic BioChip Adhesion, BioChip Labs™, BioChip Labs™

● **0304U** normoxic
INCLUDES Normoxic BioChip Adhesion, BioChip Labs™, BioChip Labs™

● **0305U** Hematology, red blood cell (RBC) functionality and deformity as a function of shear stress, whole blood, reported as a maximum elongation index
INCLUDES Ektacytometry, BioChip Labs™, BioChip Labs™

90281-90399 Immunoglobulin Products

INCLUDES Immune globulin product only
    Anti-infectives
    Antitoxins
    Isoantibodies
    Monoclonal antibodies
Code also (96365-96372, 96374-96375)

90281 **Immune globulin (Ig), human, for intramuscular use**
INCLUDES Gamastan
0.00   0.00   **FUD** XXX
AMA: 2020,NovSE,1; 2020,Jan,11; 2018,Jan,8; 2017,Jan,8; 2016,Jan,13

90283 **Immune globulin (IgIV), human, for intravenous use**
0.00   0.00   **FUD** XXX
AMA: 2020,NovSE,1; 2020,Jan,11; 2018,Jan,8; 2017,Jan,8; 2016,Jan,13

90284 **Immune globulin (SCIg), human, for use in subcutaneous infusions, 100 mg, each**
0.00   0.00   **FUD** XXX
AMA: 2020,NovSE,1; 2020,Jan,11; 2018,Jan,8; 2017,Jan,8; 2016,Jan,13

90287 **Botulinum antitoxin, equine, any route**
0.00   0.00   **FUD** XXX
AMA: 2020,NovSE,1; 2020,Jan,11; 2018,Jan,8; 2017,Jan,8; 2016,Jan,13

90288 **Botulism immune globulin, human, for intravenous use**
0.00   0.00   **FUD** XXX
AMA: 2020,NovSE,1; 2020,Jan,11; 2018,Jan,8; 2017,Jan,8; 2016,Jan,13

90291 **Cytomegalovirus immune globulin (CMV-IgIV), human, for intravenous use**
INCLUDES Cytogram
0.00   0.00   **FUD** XXX
AMA: 2020,NovSE,1; 2020,Jan,11; 2018,Jan,8; 2017,Jan,8; 2016,Jan,13

90296 **Diphtheria antitoxin, equine, any route**
0.00   0.00   **FUD** XXX
AMA: 2020,NovSE,1; 2020,Jan,11; 2018,Jan,8; 2017,Jan,8; 2016,Jan,13

90371 **Hepatitis B immune globulin (HBIg), human, for intramuscular use**
INCLUDES HBIG
0.00   0.00   **FUD** XXX
AMA: 2020,NovSE,1; 2020,Jan,11; 2018,Jan,8; 2017,Jan,8; 2016,Jan,13

90375 **Rabies immune globulin (RIg), human, for intramuscular and/or subcutaneous use**
INCLUDES HyperRAB
0.00   0.00   **FUD** XXX
AMA: 2020,NovSE,1; 2020,Jan,11; 2018,Jan,8; 2017,Jan,8; 2016,Jan,13

90376 **Rabies immune globulin, heat-treated (RIg-HT), human, for intramuscular and/or subcutaneous use**
0.00   0.00   **FUD** XXX
AMA: 2020,NovSE,1; 2020,Jan,11; 2018,Jan,8; 2017,Jan,8; 2016,Jan,13

90377 **Rabies immune globulin, heat- and solvent/detergent-treated (RIg-HT S/D), human, for intramuscular and/or subcutaneous use**
0.00   0.00   **FUD** XXX

90378 **Respiratory syncytial virus, monoclonal antibody, recombinant, for intramuscular use, 50 mg, each**
INCLUDES Synagis
0.00   0.00   **FUD** XXX
AMA: 2020,NovSE,1; 2020,Jan,11; 2018,Jan,8; 2017,Jan,8; 2016,Jan,13

90384 **Rho(D) immune globulin (RhIg), human, full-dose, for intramuscular use**
0.00   0.00   **FUD** XXX
AMA: 2020,NovSE,1; 2020,Jan,11; 2018,Jan,8; 2017,Jan,8; 2016,Jan,13

90385 **Rho(D) immune globulin (RhIg), human, mini-dose, for intramuscular use**
0.00   0.00   **FUD** XXX
AMA: 2020,NovSE,1; 2020,Jan,11; 2018,Jan,8; 2017,Jan,8; 2016,Jan,13

90386 **Rho(D) immune globulin (RhIgIV), human, for intravenous use**
0.00   0.00   **FUD** XXX
AMA: 2020,NovSE,1; 2020,Jan,11; 2018,Jan,8; 2017,Jan,8; 2016,Jan,13

90389 **Tetanus immune globulin (TIg), human, for intramuscular use**
INCLUDES HyperTET S/D (Tetanus Immune Globulin)
0.00   0.00   **FUD** XXX
AMA: 2020,NovSE,1; 2020,Jan,11; 2018,Jan,8; 2017,Jan,8; 2016,Jan,13

90393 **Vaccinia immune globulin, human, for intramuscular use**
0.00   0.00   **FUD** XXX
AMA: 2020,NovSE,1; 2020,Jan,11; 2018,Jan,8; 2017,Jan,8; 2016,Jan,13

90396 **Varicella-zoster immune globulin, human, for intramuscular use**
INCLUDES VariZIG
0.00   0.00   **FUD** XXX
AMA: 2020,NovSE,1; 2020,Jan,11; 2018,Jan,8; 2017,Jan,8; 2016,Jan,13

90399 **Unlisted immune globulin**
0.00   0.00   **FUD** XXX
AMA: 2020,NovSE,1; 2020,Jan,11; 2018,Jan,8; 2017,Jan,8; 2016,Jan,13

90460-90461 Injections Provided with Counseling

INCLUDES All components influenza vaccine, report one time only
Combination vaccines which comprise multiple vaccine components
Components (all antigens) in vaccines to prevent disease due to specific organisms
Counseling by physician or other qualified health care professional
Multivalent antigens or multiple antigen serotypes against single organisms considered one component
Patient/family face-to-face counseling by doctor or qualified health care professional for patients age 18 years and younger
EXCLUDES Administration influenza and pneumococcal vaccine for Medicare patients (G0008-G0009)
Allergy testing (95004-95028)
Bacterial/viral/fungal skin tests (86485-86580)
Diagnostic or therapeutic injections (96365-96371, 96372-96379)
Reporting with severe acute respiratory syndrome coronavirus 2 (SARS-CoV-2) (coronavirus disease [COVID-19]) vaccine when not administered with separately identifiable vaccine/toxoid ([91300, 91301, 91302, 91303, 91304, 91305, 91306, 91307])
Vaccines provided without face-to-face counseling from physician or qualified health care professional or to patients age 18 years and older (90471-90474)
Code also:
Significant, separately identifiable E/M service when appropriate
Toxoid/vaccine (90476-90749 [90619, 90620, 90621, 90625, 90630, 90644, 90672, 90673, 90674, 90750, 90756])

90460 **Immunization administration through 18 years of age via any route of administration, with counseling by physician or other qualified health care professional; first or only component of each vaccine or toxoid administered**
Code also each additional component in vaccine (e.g., 5-year-old receives DtaP-IPV IM administration, and MMR/Varicella vaccines SQ administration. Report initial component two times, and additional components six times)
0.47   0.47   **FUD** XXX
AMA: 2020,DecSE,1; 2020,DecSE,1; 2020,NovBULL,2; 2020,NovSE,1; 2020,Jul,11; 2020,Jan,11; 2018,Nov,7; 2018,Jan,8; 2017,Jan,8; 2016,Oct,6; 2016,Jan,13

+ 90461 each additional vaccine or toxoid component administered (List separately in addition to code for primary procedure) Ⓐ

Code also each additional component in vaccine (e.g., 5-year-old receives DtaP-IPV IM administration, and MMR/Varicella vaccines SQ administration. Report initial component two times, and additional components six times)

Code first initial component in each vaccine provided (90460)

🔲 0.36   ⚖ 0.36   **FUD** ZZZ

Ⓑ ⑧⓪ ▭

AMA: 2020,DecSE,1; 2020,DecSE,1; 2020,NovSE,1; 2020,Jul,11; 2020,Jan,11; 2018,Nov,7; 2018,Jan,8; 2017,Jan,8; 2016,Oct,6; 2016,Jan,13

90471-0104A [0001A, 0002A, 0003A, 0004A, 0011A, 0012A, 0013A, 0014A, 0021A, 0022A, 0023A, 0024A, 0031A, 0032A, 0033A, 0034A, 0041A, 0042A, 0043A, 0044A, 0051A, 0052A, 0053A, 0054A, 0061A, 0062A, 0063A, 0064A, 0071A, 0072A, 0073A, 0074A, 0081A, 0082A, 0083A, 0084A, 0091A, 0092A, 0093A, 0094A, 0101A, 0102A, 0103A, 0104A] Injections and Other Routes of Administration Without Physician Counseling

EXCLUDES Administration influenza and pneumococcal vaccine for Medicare patients (G0008-G0009)
Administration vaccine with counseling (90460-90461)
Allergy testing (95004-95028)
Bacterial/viral/fungal skin tests (86485-86580)
Diagnostic or therapeutic injections (96365-96371, 96374)
Patient/family face-to-face counseling
Reporting with severe acute respiratory syndrome coronavirus 2 (SARS-CoV-2) (Coronavirus disease [COVID-19]) vaccine when not administered with separately identifiable vaccine/toxoid ([91300, 91301, 91302, 91303, 91304, 91305, 91306, 91307])

Code also:
Significant, separately identifiable E/M service when appropriate
Toxoid/vaccine (90476-90749 [90619, 90620, 90621, 90625, 90630, 90644, 90672, 90673, 90674, 90750, 90756])

90471 Immunization administration (includes percutaneous, intradermal, subcutaneous, or intramuscular injections); 1 vaccine (single or combination vaccine/toxoid)

EXCLUDES Intranasal/oral administration (90473)

🔲 0.47   ⚖ 0.47   **FUD** XXX

⓪① ⑧⓪ ▭

AMA: 2020,NovSE,1; 2020,Jul,11; 2020,Jan,11; 2019,Jun,11; 2018,Nov,7; 2018,Jan,8; 2017,Jan,8; 2016,Oct,6; 2016,Jan,13

+ 90472 each additional vaccine (single or combination vaccine/toxoid) (List separately in addition to code for primary procedure)

EXCLUDES BCG vaccine, intravesical administration (51720, 90586)
Immune globulin administration (96365-96371, 96374)
Immune globulin product (90281-90399)

Code first initial vaccine (90460, 90471, 90473)

🔲 0.36   ⚖ 0.36   **FUD** ZZZ

Ⓝ ⑧⓪ ▭

AMA: 2020,NovSE,1; 2020,Jul,11; 2020,Jan,11; 2018,Nov,7; 2018,Jan,8; 2017,Jan,8; 2016,Oct,6; 2016,Jan,13

90473 Immunization administration by intranasal or oral route; 1 vaccine (single or combination vaccine/toxoid)

EXCLUDES Administration by injection (90471)

🔲 0.47   ⚖ 0.47   **FUD** XXX

⓪① ⑧⓪ ▭

AMA: 2020,NovSE,1; 2020,Jan,11; 2018,Nov,7; 2018,Jan,8; 2017,Jan,8; 2016,Jan,13

+ 90474 each additional vaccine (single or combination vaccine/toxoid) (List separately in addition to code for primary procedure)

Code first initial vaccine (90460, 90471, 90473)

🔲 0.36   ⚖ 0.36   **FUD** ZZZ

Ⓝ ⑧⓪ ▭

AMA: 2020,NovSE,1; 2018,Nov,7; 2018,Jan,8; 2017,Jan,8; 2016,Jan,13

● **0001A Immunization administration by intramuscular injection of severe acute respiratory syndrome coronavirus 2 (SARS-CoV-2) (coronavirus disease [COVID-19]) vaccine, mRNA-LNP, spike protein, preservative free, 30 mcg/0.3mL dosage, diluent reconstituted; first dose**

INCLUDES Pfizer-BioNTech COVID-19 vaccine, Comirnaty

Code also vaccine ([91300])

🔲 0.00   ⚖ 0.00   **FUD** XXX

● **0002A second dose**

INCLUDES Pfizer-BioNTech COVID-19 vaccine, Comirnaty

Code also vaccine ([91300])

🔲 0.00   ⚖ 0.00   **FUD** XXX

● **0003A third dose**

INCLUDES Pfizer-BioNTech COVID-19 vaccine, Comirnaty

Code also vaccine ([91300])

🔲 0.00   ⚖ 0.00   **FUD** 000

● **0004A booster dose**

INCLUDES Pfizer-BioNTech COVID-19 vaccine, Comirnaty

Code also vaccine ([91300])

🔲 0.00   ⚖ 0.00   **FUD** 000

● # **0051A Immunization administration by intramuscular injection of severe acute respiratory syndrome coronavirus 2 (SARS-CoV-2) (coronavirus disease [COVID-19]) vaccine, mRNA-LNP, spike protein, preservative free, 30 mcg/0.3 mL dosage, tris-sucrose formulation; first dose**

INCLUDES Pfizer-BioNTech COVID-19 vaccine

Code also vaccine ([91305])

🔲 0.00   ⚖ 0.00   **FUD** 000

● # **0052A second dose**

INCLUDES Pfizer-BioNTech COVID-19 vaccine

Code also vaccine ([91305])

🔲 0.00   ⚖ 0.00   **FUD** 000

● # **0053A third dose**

INCLUDES Pfizer-BioNTech COVID-19 vaccine

Code also vaccine ([91305])

🔲 0.00   ⚖ 0.00   **FUD** 000

● # **0054A booster dose**

INCLUDES Pfizer-BioNTech COVID-19 vaccine

Code also vaccine ([91305])

🔲 0.00   ⚖ 0.00   **FUD** 000

● # **0071A Immunization administration by intramuscular injection of severe acute respiratory syndrome coronavirus 2 (SARS-CoV-2) (coronavirus disease [COVID-19]) vaccine, mRNA-LNP, spike protein, preservative free, 10 mcg/0.2 mL dosage, diluent reconstituted, tris-sucrose formulation; first dose**

INCLUDES Pfizer-BioNTech COVID-19 vaccine

Code also vaccine ([91307])

🔲 0.00   ⚖ 0.00   **FUD** 000

● # **0072A second dose**

INCLUDES Pfizer-BioNTech COVID-19 vaccine

Code also vaccine ([91307])

🔲 0.00   ⚖ 0.00   **FUD** 000

● **0011A Immunization administration by intramuscular injection of severe acute respiratory syndrome coronavirus 2 (SARS-CoV-2) (coronavirus disease [COVID-19]) vaccine, mRNA-LNP, spike protein, preservative free, 100 mcg/0.5mL dosage; first dose**

INCLUDES Moderna COVID-19 vaccine

Code also vaccine ([91301])

🔲 0.00   ⚖ 0.00   **FUD** XXX

● **0012A second dose**

INCLUDES Moderna COVID-19 vaccine

Code also vaccine ([91301])

🔲 0.00   ⚖ 0.00   **FUD** XXX

● **0013A** **third dose**

INCLUDES Moderna COVID-19 vaccine
Code also vaccine ([91301])
🚑 0.00 ⚕ 0.00 **FUD** 000

● # **0064A** **Immunization administration by intramuscular injection of severe acute respiratory syndrome coronavirus 2 (SARS-CoV-2) (coronavirus disease [COVID-19]) vaccine, mRNA-LNP, spike protein, preservative free, 50 mcg/0.25 mL dosage, booster dose**

INCLUDES Moderna COVID-19 vaccine
Code also vaccine ([91306])
🚑 0.00 ⚕ 0.00 **FUD** 000

● **0014A** **PLACEHOLDER ONLY**
🚑 0.00 ⚕ 0.00 **FUD** 000

● **0021A** **Immunization administration by intramuscular injection of severe acute respiratory syndrome coronavirus 2 (SARS-CoV-2) (coronavirus disease [COVID-19]) vaccine, DNA, spike protein, chimpanzee adenovirus Oxford 1 (ChAdOx1) vector, preservative free, $5x10^{10}$ viral particles/0.5mL dosage; first dose**

INCLUDES AstraZeneca COVID-19 vaccine
Code also vaccine [91302]
🚑 0.00 ⚕ 0.00 **FUD** 000

● **0022A** **second dose**

INCLUDES AstraZeneca COVID-19 vaccine
Code also vaccine [91302]
🚑 0.00 ⚕ 0.00 **FUD** 000

● **0023A** **PLACEHOLDER ONLY**
🚑 0.00 ⚕ 0.00 **FUD** 000

● **0024A** **PLACEHOLDER ONLY**
🚑 0.00 ⚕ 0.00 **FUD** 000

● **0031A** **Immunization administration by intramuscular injection of severe acute respiratory syndrome coronavirus 2 (SARS-CoV-2) (coronavirus disease [COVID-19]) vaccine, DNA, spike protein, adenovirus type 26 (Ad26) vector, preservative free, $5x10^{10}$ viral particles/0.5mL dosage; single dose**

INCLUDES Janssen COVID-19 vaccine
Code also vaccine ([91303])
🚑 0.00 ⚕ 0.00 **FUD** XXX

● **0034A** **booster dose**

INCLUDES Janssen COVID-19 vaccine
Code also vaccine ([91303])
🚑 0.00 ⚕ 0.00 **FUD** 000

● **0032A** **PLACEHOLDER ONLY**
🚑 0.00 ⚕ 0.00 **FUD** 000

● **0033A** **PLACEHOLDER ONLY**
🚑 0.00 ⚕ 0.00 **FUD** 000

● **0041A** **Immunization administration by intramuscular injection of severe acute respiratory syndrome coronavirus 2 (SARS-CoV-2) (coronavirus disease [COVID-19]) vaccine, recombinant spike protein nanoparticle, saponin-based adjuvant, preservative free, 5 mcg/0.5mL dosage; first dose**

INCLUDES Novavax COVID-19 vaccine
Code also vaccine ([91304])
🚑 0.00 ⚕ 0.00 **FUD** 000

● **0042A** **second dose**

INCLUDES Novavax COVID-19 vaccine
Code also vaccine ([91304])
🚑 0.00 ⚕ 0.00 **FUD** 000

● **0043A** **PLACEHOLDER ONLY**
🚑 0.00 ⚕ 0.00 **FUD** 000

● **0044A** **PLACEHOLDER ONLY**
🚑 0.00 ⚕ 0.00 **FUD** 000

● **0061A** **PLACEHOLDER ONLY**
🚑 0.00 ⚕ 0.00 **FUD** 000

● **0062A** **PLACEHOLDER ONLY**
🚑 0.00 ⚕ 0.00 **FUD** 000

● **0063A** **PLACEHOLDER ONLY**
🚑 0.00 ⚕ 0.00 **FUD** 000

● **0073A** **PLACEHOLDER ONLY**
🚑 0.00 ⚕ 0.00 **FUD** 000

● **0074A** **PLACEHOLDER ONLY**
🚑 0.00 ⚕ 0.00 **FUD** 000

● **0081A** **PLACEHOLDER ONLY**
🚑 0.00 ⚕ 0.00 **FUD** 000

● **0082A** **PLACEHOLDER ONLY**
🚑 0.00 ⚕ 0.00 **FUD** 000

● **0083A** **PLACEHOLDER ONLY**
🚑 0.00 ⚕ 0.00 **FUD** 000

● **0084A** **PLACEHOLDER ONLY**
🚑 0.00 ⚕ 0.00 **FUD** 000

● **0091A** **PLACEHOLDER ONLY**
🚑 0.00 ⚕ 0.00 **FUD** 000

● **0092A** **PLACEHOLDER ONLY**
🚑 0.00 ⚕ 0.00 **FUD** 000

● **0093A** **PLACEHOLDER ONLY**
🚑 0.00 ⚕ 0.00 **FUD** 000

● **0094A** **PLACEHOLDER ONLY**
🚑 0.00 ⚕ 0.00 **FUD** 000

● **0101A** **PLACEHOLDER ONLY**
🚑 0.00 ⚕ 0.00 **FUD** 000

● **0102A** **PLACEHOLDER ONLY**
🚑 0.00 ⚕ 0.00 **FUD** 000

● **0103A** **PLACEHOLDER ONLY**
🚑 0.00 ⚕ 0.00 **FUD** 000

● **0104A** **PLACEHOLDER ONLY**
🚑 0.00 ⚕ 0.00 **FUD** 000

91300-90759 [90619, 90620, 90621, 90625, 90626, 90627, 90630, 90644, 90672, 90673, 90674, 90677, 90694, 90750, 90756, 90758, 90759, 91300, 91301, 91302, 91303, 91304, 91305, 91306, 91307, 91308, 91309, 91310] Vaccination Products

INCLUDES Patient's age for reporting purposes, not for product license
Vaccine product only
EXCLUDES *Immune globulins and administration (90281-90399, 96365-96375)*
Reporting each combination vaccine component individually
Code also:
Administration vaccine (90460-90461, 90471-90474, [0001A, 0002A, 0003A, 0004A], [0011A, 0012A], [0013A], [0021A, 0022A], [0031A], [0034A], [0041A, 0042A], [0051A, 0052A, 0053A, 0054A], [0064A], [0071A, 0072A]
Significant separately identifiable E/M service when appropriate

● # **91300** **Severe acute respiratory syndrome coronavirus 2 (SARS-CoV-2) (coronavirus disease [COVID-19]) vaccine, mRNA-LNP, spike protein, preservative free, 30 mcg/0.3mL dosage, diluent reconstituted, for intramuscular use**

INCLUDES Pfizer-BioNTech COVID-19 vaccine, Comirnaty
Code also vaccine administration ([0001A], [0002A], [0003A], [0004A])
🚑 0.00 ⚕ 0.00 **FUD** XXX
AMA: 2020,DecSE,1; 2020,DecSE,1

Medicine

91305 — 90644

● # **91305** Severe acute respiratory syndrome coronavirus 2 (SARS-CoV-2) (coronavirus disease [COVID-19]) vaccine, mRNA-LNP, spike protein, preservative free, 30 mcg/0.3 mL dosage, tris-sucrose formulation, for intramuscular use
INCLUDES   Pfizer-BioNTech COVID-19 vaccine
Code also vaccine administration ([0051A], [0052A], [0053A], [0054A])
🚑 0.00   ⚕ 0.00   **FUD** 000   ✗

● # **91307** Severe acute respiratory syndrome coronavirus 2 (SARS-CoV-2) (coronavirus disease [COVID-19]) vaccine, mRNA-LNP, spike protein, preservative free, 10 mcg/0.2 mL dosage, diluent reconstituted, tris-sucrose formulation, for intramuscular use
INCLUDES   Pfizer-BioNTech COVID-19 vaccine
Code also vaccine administration ([0071A, 0072A])
🚑 0.00   ⚕ 0.00   **FUD** 000   ✗

● # **91301** Severe acute respiratory syndrome coronavirus 2 (SARS-CoV2) (coronavirus disease [COVID-19]) vaccine, mRNA-LNP, spike protein, preservative free, 100 mcg/0.5mL dosage, for intramuscular use
INCLUDES   Moderna COVID-19 vaccine
Code also vaccine administration ([0011A], [0012A], [0013A])
🚑 0.00   ⚕ 0.00   **FUD** XXX   ▭
AMA: 2020,DecSE,1; 2020,DecSE,1

● # **91306** Severe acute respiratory syndrome coronavirus 2 (SARS-CoV-2) (coronavirus disease [COVID-19]) vaccine, mRNA-LNP, spike protein, preservative free, 50 mcg/0.25 mL dosage, for intramuscular use
INCLUDES   Moderna COVID-19 vaccine
Code also vaccine administration ([0064A])
🚑 0.00   ⚕ 0.00   **FUD** 000

● # **91302** Severe acute respiratory syndrome coronavirus 2 (SARS-CoV-2) (coronavirus disease [COVID-19]) vaccine, DNA, spike protein, chimpanzee adenovirus Oxford 1 (ChAdOx1) vector, preservative free, 5×10^{10} viral particles/0.5mL dosage, for intramuscular use
INCLUDES   AstraZeneca COVID-19 vaccine
Code also vaccine administration ([0021A], [0022A])
🚑 0.00   ⚕ 0.00   **FUD** 000   ✗ ▭
AMA: 2020,DecSE,1; 2020,DecSE,1

● # **91303** Severe acute respiratory syndrome coronavirus 2 (SARSCoV-2) (coronavirus disease [COVID-19]) vaccine, DNA, spike protein, adenovirus type 26 (Ad26) vector, preservative free, 5×10^{10} viral particles/0.5mL dosage, for intramuscular use
INCLUDES   Janssen COVID-19 vaccine
Code also vaccine administration ([0031A], [0034A])
🚑 0.00   ⚕ 0.00   **FUD** XXX   U1 ▭

● # **91304** Severe acute respiratory syndrome coronavirus 2 (SARS-CoV-2) (coronavirus disease [COVID-19]) vaccine, recombinant spike protein nanoparticle, saponin-based adjuvant, preservative free, 5 mcg/0.5mL dosage, for intramuscular use
INCLUDES   Novavax COVID-19 vaccine
Code also vaccine administration ([0041A, 0042A])
🚑 0.00   ⚕ 0.00   **FUD** 000   ✗ ▭

● # **91308** PLACEHOLDER ONLY
🚑 0.00   ⚕ 0.00   **FUD** 000   ✗

● # **91309** PLACEHOLDER ONLY
🚑 0.00   ⚕ 0.00   **FUD** 000   ✗

● # **91310** PLACEHOLDER ONLY
🚑 0.00   ⚕ 0.00   **FUD** 000   ✗

90476 Adenovirus vaccine, type 4, live, for oral use
INCLUDES   Adeno-4
🚑 0.00   ⚕ 0.00   **FUD** XXX   SI N NI ▭
AMA: 2020,DecSE,1; 2020,DecSE,1; 2020,NovSE,1; 2018,Jan,8; 2017,Jan,8; 2016,Jan,13

90477 Adenovirus vaccine, type 7, live, for oral use
INCLUDES   Adeno-7
🚑 0.00   ⚕ 0.00   **FUD** XXX   SI M ▭
AMA: 2020,DecSE,1; 2020,DecSE,1; 2020,NovSE,1; 2018,Jan,8; 2017,Jan,8; 2016,Jan,13

90581 Anthrax vaccine, for subcutaneous or intramuscular use
INCLUDES   BioThrax
🚑 0.00   ⚕ 0.00   **FUD** XXX   SI E ▭
AMA: 2020,DecSE,1; 2020,DecSE,1; 2020,NovSE,1; 2018,Jan,8; 2017,Jan,8; 2016,Jan,13

90585 Bacillus Calmette-Guerin vaccine (BCG) for tuberculosis, live, for percutaneous use
INCLUDES   Mycobax
🚑 0.00   ⚕ 0.00   **FUD** XXX   SI M ▭
AMA: 2020,DecSE,1; 2020,DecSE,1; 2020,NovSE,1; 2018,Jan,8; 2017,Jan,8; 2016,Jan,13

90586 Bacillus Calmette-Guerin vaccine (BCG) for bladder cancer, live, for intravesical use
INCLUDES   TheraCys
            TICE BCG
🚑 0.00   ⚕ 0.00   **FUD** XXX   SI B ▭
AMA: 2020,DecSE,1; 2020,DecSE,1; 2020,NovSE,1; 2020,Jan,11; 2018,Jan,8; 2017,Jan,8; 2016,Jan,13

90587 Dengue vaccine, quadrivalent, live, 3 dose schedule, for subcutaneous use
🚑 0.00   ⚕ 0.00   **FUD** XXX   SI E ▭
AMA: 2020,DecSE,1; 2020,DecSE,1; 2020,NovSE,1; 2018,Nov,7; 2018,Jan,8

90619 Resequenced code. See code following 90734.

90620 Resequenced code. See code following 90734.

90621 Resequenced code. See code following 90734.

90625 Resequenced code. See code following 90723.

90626 Resequenced code. See code following 90715.

90627 Resequenced code. See code following 90715.

90630 Resequenced code. See code following 90654.

90632 Hepatitis A vaccine (HepA), adult dosage, for intramuscular use   A
INCLUDES   Havrix
            Vaqta
🚑 0.00   ⚕ 0.00   **FUD** XXX   SI N NI ▭
AMA: 2020,DecSE,1; 2020,DecSE,1; 2020,NovSE,1; 2018,Jan,8; 2017,Jan,8; 2016,Jan,13

90633 Hepatitis A vaccine (HepA), pediatric/adolescent dosage-2 dose schedule, for intramuscular use   A
INCLUDES   Havrix
            Vaqta
🚑 0.00   ⚕ 0.00   **FUD** XXX   SI N NI ▭
AMA: 2020,DecSE,1; 2020,DecSE,1; 2020,NovSE,1; 2018,Jan,8; 2017,Jan,8; 2016,Jan,13

90634 Hepatitis A vaccine (HepA), pediatric/adolescent dosage-3 dose schedule, for intramuscular use   A
INCLUDES   Havrix
🚑 0.00   ⚕ 0.00   **FUD** XXX   SI N NI ▭
AMA: 2020,DecSE,1; 2020,DecSE,1; 2020,NovSE,1; 2018,Jan,8; 2017,Jan,8; 2016,Jan,13

90636 Hepatitis A and hepatitis B vaccine (HepA-HepB), adult dosage, for intramuscular use   A
INCLUDES   Twinrix
🚑 0.00   ⚕ 0.00   **FUD** XXX   SI N NI ▭
AMA: 2020,DecSE,1; 2020,DecSE,1; 2020,NovSE,1; 2018,Jan,8; 2017,Jan,8; 2016,Jan,13

90644 Resequenced code. See code following 90732.

90647 Haemophilus influenzae type b vaccine (Hib), PRP-OMP conjugate, 3 dose schedule, for intramuscular use

INCLUDES PedvaxHIB

🚑 0.00   ⚕ 0.00   **FUD** XXX   50 N M1 🖼

AMA: 2020,DecSE,1; 2020,DecSE,1; 2020,NovSE,1; 2018,Jan,8; 2017,Jan,8; 2016,Jan,13

90648 Haemophilus influenzae type b vaccine (Hib), PRP-T conjugate, 4 dose schedule, for intramuscular use

INCLUDES ActHIB
Hiberix
OmniHIB

🚑 0.00   ⚕ 0.00   **FUD** XXX   50 N M1 🖼

AMA: 2020,DecSE,1; 2020,DecSE,1; 2020,NovSE,1; 2018,Jan,8; 2017,Jan,8; 2016,Jan,13

90649 Human Papillomavirus vaccine, types 6, 11, 16, 18, quadrivalent (4vHPV), 3 dose schedule, for intramuscular use

INCLUDES Gardasil

🚑 0.00   ⚕ 0.00   **FUD** XXX   50 M 🖼

AMA: 2020,DecSE,1; 2020,DecSE,1; 2020,NovSE,1; 2018,Jan,8; 2017,Jan,8; 2016,Jan,13

90650 Human Papillomavirus vaccine, types 16, 18, bivalent (2vHPV), 3 dose schedule, for intramuscular use

INCLUDES Cervarix

🚑 0.00   ⚕ 0.00   **FUD** XXX   50 M 🖼

AMA: 2020,DecSE,1; 2020,DecSE,1; 2020,NovSE,1; 2018,Jan,8; 2017,Jan,8; 2016,Jan,13

90651 Human Papillomavirus vaccine types 6, 11, 16, 18, 31, 33, 45, 52, 58, nonavalent (9vHPV), 2 or 3 dose schedule, for intramuscular use

INCLUDES GARDASIL 9

🚑 0.00   ⚕ 0.00   **FUD** XXX   50 M 🖼

AMA: 2020,DecSE,1; 2020,DecSE,1; 2020,NovSE,1; 2018,Nov,7; 2018,Jan,8; 2017,Jan,8; 2016,Jan,13

90653 Influenza vaccine, inactivated (IIV), subunit, adjuvanted, for intramuscular use

INCLUDES Fluad

🚑 0.00   ⚕ 0.00   **FUD** XXX   50 L L1 🖼

AMA: 2020,DecSE,1; 2020,DecSE,1; 2020,NovSE,1; 2019,Jun,11; 2018,Jan,8; 2017,Jan,8; 2016,Oct,6; 2016,Jan,13

90654 Influenza virus vaccine, trivalent (IIV3), split virus, preservative-free, for intradermal use

INCLUDES Fluzone intradermal

🚑 0.00   ⚕ 0.00   **FUD** XXX   50 L L1 🖼

AMA: 2020,DecSE,1; 2020,DecSE,1; 2020,NovSE,1; 2018,Jan,8; 2017,Jan,8; 2016,Jan,13

90630 Influenza virus vaccine, quadrivalent (IIV4), split virus, preservative free, for intradermal use

INCLUDES Fluzone Intradermal Quadrivalent

🚑 0.00   ⚕ 0.00   **FUD** XXX   50 L L1 🖼

AMA: 2020,DecSE,1; 2020,DecSE,1; 2020,NovSE,1; 2018,Jan,8; 2016,Jan,13

90655 Influenza virus vaccine, trivalent (IIV3), split virus, preservative free, 0.25 mL dosage, for intramuscular use   🅰

INCLUDES Afluria
Fluzone, no preservative, pediatric dose

🚑 0.00   ⚕ 0.00   **FUD** XXX   50 L L1 🖼

AMA: 2020,DecSE,1; 2020,DecSE,1; 2020,NovSE,1; 2018,Jan,8; 2017,Jan,8; 2016,Oct,6; 2016,May,9; 2016,Jan,13

90656 Influenza virus vaccine, trivalent (IIV3), split virus, preservative free, 0.5 mL dosage, for intramuscular use   🅰

INCLUDES Afluria

🚑 0.00   ⚕ 0.00   **FUD** XXX   50 L L1 🖼

AMA: 2020,DecSE,1; 2020,DecSE,1; 2020,NovSE,1; 2018,Jan,8; 2017,Jan,8; 2016,Oct,6; 2016,May,9; 2016,Jan,13

90657 Influenza virus vaccine, trivalent (IIV3), split virus, 0.25 mL dosage, for intramuscular use   🅰

INCLUDES Afluria
Flulaval
Fluvirin
Fluzone (5 ml vial [0.25ml dose])

🚑 0.00   ⚕ 0.00   **FUD** XXX   50 L L1 🖼

AMA: 2020,DecSE,1; 2020,DecSE,1; 2020,NovSE,1; 2018,Jan,8; 2017,Jan,8; 2016,Oct,6; 2016,May,9; 2016,Jan,13

90658 Influenza virus vaccine, trivalent (IIV3), split virus, 0.5 mL dosage, for intramuscular use   🅰

INCLUDES Afluria
Flulaval
Fluvirin
Fluzone

🚑 0.00   ⚕ 0.00   **FUD** XXX   50 E 🖼

AMA: 2020,DecSE,1; 2020,DecSE,1; 2020,NovSE,1; 2018,Jan,8; 2017,Jan,8; 2016,Oct,6; 2016,May,9; 2016,Jan,13

90660 Influenza virus vaccine, trivalent, live (LAIV3), for intranasal use

INCLUDES FluMist

🚑 0.00   ⚕ 0.00   **FUD** XXX   50 L L1 🖼

AMA: 2020,DecSE,1; 2020,DecSE,1; 2020,NovSE,1; 2018,Jan,8; 2017,Jan,8; 2016,Jan,13

90672 Influenza virus vaccine, quadrivalent, live (LAIV4), for intranasal use

INCLUDES FluMist Quadrivalent

🚑 0.00   ⚕ 0.00   **FUD** XXX   50 L L1 🖼

AMA: 2020,DecSE,1; 2020,DecSE,1; 2020,NovSE,1; 2018,Jan,8; 2017,Jan,8; 2016,Jan,13

90661 Influenza virus vaccine (ccIIV3), derived from cell cultures, subunit, preservative and antibiotic free, for intramuscular use

INCLUDES Flucelvax

🚑 0.00   ⚕ 0.00   **FUD** XXX   50 L L1 🖼

AMA: 2020,DecSE,1; 2020,DecSE,1; 2020,NovSE,1; 2018,Jan,8; 2017,Jan,8; 2016,Oct,6; 2016,Jan,13

90674 Influenza virus vaccine, quadrivalent (ccIIV4), derived from cell cultures, subunit, preservative and antibiotic free, 0.5 mL dosage, for intramuscular use

INCLUDES Flucelvax Quadrivalent

🚑 0.00   ⚕ 0.00   **FUD** XXX   50 L L1 🖼

AMA: 2020,DecSE,1; 2020,DecSE,1; 2020,NovSE,1; 2018,Jan,8; 2017,Jan,8; 2016,Oct,6

90756 Influenza virus vaccine, quadrivalent (ccIIV4), derived from cell cultures, subunit, antibiotic free, 0.5mL dosage, for intramuscular use

INCLUDES Flucelvax Quadrivalent

🚑 0.00   ⚕ 0.00   **FUD** XXX   50 L L1 🖼

AMA: 2018,Nov,7

90673 Influenza virus vaccine, trivalent (RIV3), derived from recombinant DNA, hemagglutinin (HA) protein only, preservative and antibiotic free, for intramuscular use

🚑 0.00   ⚕ 0.00   **FUD** XXX   50 L L1 🖼

AMA: 2020,DecSE,1; 2020,DecSE,1; 2020,NovSE,1; 2018,Jan,8; 2017,Jan,8; 2016,Jan,13

90662 Influenza virus vaccine (IIV), split virus, preservative free, enhanced immunogenicity via increased antigen content, for intramuscular use

INCLUDES Fluzone high-dose Quadrivalent

🚑 0.00   ⚕ 0.00   **FUD** XXX   50 L L1 🖼

AMA: 2020,DecSE,1; 2020,DecSE,1; 2020,NovSE,1; 2018,Jan,8; 2017,Jan,8; 2016,Jan,13

90664 Influenza virus vaccine, live (LAIV), pandemic formulation, for intranasal use

🚑 0.00   ⚕ 0.00   **FUD** XXX   50 E 🖼

AMA: 2020,DecSE,1; 2020,DecSE,1; 2020,NovSE,1; 2018,Jan,8; 2017,Jan,8; 2016,Jan,13

90666 Influenza virus vaccine (IIV), pandemic formulation, split virus, preservative free, for intramuscular use
    0.00   0.00   **FUD** XXX   ✔ Ⓢ Ⓔ ▭
 AMA: 2020,DecSE,1; 2020,DecSE,1; 2020,NovSE,1; 2018,Jan,8; 2017,Jan,8; 2016,Jan,13

90667 Influenza virus vaccine (IIV), pandemic formulation, split virus, adjuvanted, for intramuscular use
    0.00   0.00   **FUD** XXX   ✔ Ⓢ Ⓔ ▭
 AMA: 2020,DecSE,1; 2020,DecSE,1; 2020,NovSE,1; 2018,Jan,8; 2017,Jan,8; 2016,Jan,13

90668 Influenza virus vaccine (IIV), pandemic formulation, split virus, for intramuscular use
    0.00   0.00   **FUD** XXX   ✔ Ⓢ Ⓔ ▭
 AMA: 2020,DecSE,1; 2020,DecSE,1; 2020,NovSE,1; 2018,Jan,8; 2017,Jan,8; 2016,Jan,13

90670 Pneumococcal conjugate vaccine, 13 valent (PCV13), for intramuscular use
 INCLUDES   Prevnar 13
    0.00   0.00   **FUD** XXX   Ⓢ Ⓛ L1 ▭
 AMA: 2020,DecSE,1; 2020,DecSE,1; 2020,NovSE,1; 2018,Jan,8; 2017,Jan,8; 2016,Jan,13

● **90671** Pneumococcal conjugate vaccine, 15 valent (PCV15), for intramuscular use
    0.00   0.00   **FUD** XXX   ✔

● # **90677** Pneumococcal conjugate vaccine, 20 valent (PCV20), for intramuscular use
    0.00   0.00   **FUD** XXX   L1

90672 Resequenced code. See code following 90660.

90673 Resequenced code. See code before 90662.

90674 Resequenced code. See code following 90661.

90675 Rabies vaccine, for intramuscular use
 INCLUDES   Imovax
           RabAvert
    0.00   0.00   **FUD** XXX   Ⓢ Ⓚ K2 ▭
 AMA: 2020,DecSE,1; 2020,DecSE,1; 2020,NovSE,1; 2018,Jan,8; 2017,Jan,8; 2016,Jan,13

90676 Rabies vaccine, for intradermal use
    0.00   0.00   **FUD** XXX   Ⓢ Ⓚ K2 ▭
 AMA: 2020,DecSE,1; 2020,DecSE,1; 2020,NovSE,1; 2018,Jan,8; 2017,Jan,8; 2016,Jan,13

90677 Resequenced code. See code following 90671.

90680 Rotavirus vaccine, pentavalent (RV5), 3 dose schedule, live, for oral use
 INCLUDES   RotaTeq
    0.00   0.00   **FUD** XXX   Ⓢ Ⓝ N1 ▭
 AMA: 2020,DecSE,1; 2020,DecSE,1; 2020,NovSE,1; 2018,Jan,8; 2017,Jan,8; 2016,Jan,13

90681 Rotavirus vaccine, human, attenuated (RV1), 2 dose schedule, live, for oral use
 INCLUDES   Rotarix
    0.00   0.00   **FUD** XXX   Ⓢ Ⓜ ▭
 AMA: 2020,DecSE,1; 2020,DecSE,1; 2020,NovSE,1; 2018,Jan,8; 2017,Jan,8; 2016,Jan,13

90682 Influenza virus vaccine, quadrivalent (RIV4), derived from recombinant DNA, hemagglutinin (HA) protein only, preservative and antibiotic free, for intramuscular use
 INCLUDES   Flublok Quadrivalent
    0.00   0.00   **FUD** XXX   Ⓢ Ⓛ L1 ▭
 AMA: 2020,DecSE,1; 2020,DecSE,1; 2020,NovSE,1; 2018,Nov,7; 2018,Jan,8; 2017,Jan,8

90685 Influenza virus vaccine, quadrivalent (IIV4), split virus, preservative free, 0.25 mL, for intramuscular use   Ⓐ
 INCLUDES   Afluria Quadrivalent
    0.00   0.00   **FUD** XXX   Ⓢ Ⓛ L1 ▭
 AMA: 2020,DecSE,1; 2020,DecSE,1; 2020,NovSE,1; 2018,Jan,8; 2017,Jan,8; 2016,Oct,6; 2016,May,9; 2016,Jan,13

90686 Influenza virus vaccine, quadrivalent (IIV4), split virus, preservative free, 0.5 mL dosage, for intramuscular use   Ⓐ
 INCLUDES   Afluria Quadrivalent
           Fluarix Quadrivalent
           Flulaval Quadrivalent
           Fluzone Quadrivalent
    0.00   0.00   **FUD** XXX   Ⓢ Ⓛ L1 ▭
 AMA: 2020,DecSE,1; 2020,DecSE,1; 2020,NovSE,1; 2018,Jan,8; 2017,Jan,8; 2016,Oct,6; 2016,May,9; 2016,Jan,13

90687 Influenza virus vaccine, quadrivalent (IIV4), split virus, 0.25 mL dosage, for intramuscular use   Ⓐ
 INCLUDES   Afluria Quadrivalent
           Fluzone Quadrivalent
    0.00   0.00   **FUD** XXX   Ⓢ Ⓛ L1 ▭
 AMA: 2020,DecSE,1; 2020,DecSE,1; 2020,NovSE,1; 2018,Jan,8; 2017,Jan,8; 2016,Oct,6; 2016,May,9; 2016,Jan,13

90688 Influenza virus vaccine, quadrivalent (IIV4), split virus, 0.5 mL dosage, for intramuscular use   Ⓐ
 INCLUDES   Afluria Quadrivalent
           Fluzone Quadrivalent
    0.00   0.00   **FUD** XXX   Ⓢ Ⓛ L1 ▭
 AMA: 2020,DecSE,1; 2020,DecSE,1; 2020,NovSE,1; 2020,Jul,11; 2018,Jan,8; 2017,Jan,8; 2016,Oct,6; 2016,May,9; 2016,Jan,13

90689 Influenza virus vaccine quadrivalent (IIV4), inactivated, adjuvanted, preservative free, 0.25 mL dosage, for intramuscular use
    0.00   0.00   **FUD** XXX   Ⓢ L1 ▭
 AMA: 2020,DecSE,1; 2020,DecSE,1; 2020,NovSE,1; 2020,Jul,11; 2019,Jul,10; 2018,Nov,7

\# **90694** Influenza virus vaccine, quadrivalent (aIIV4), inactivated, adjuvanted, preservative free, 0.5 mL dosage, for intramuscular use
 INCLUDES   Fluad Quadrivalent
    0.00   0.00   **FUD** XXX   Ⓢ L1 ▭
 AMA: 2020,DecSE,1; 2020,DecSE,1; 2020,NovSE,1; 2020,Jul,11

90690 Typhoid vaccine, live, oral
 INCLUDES   Vivotif
    0.00   0.00   **FUD** XXX   Ⓢ Ⓝ N1 ▭
 AMA: 2020,DecSE,1; 2020,DecSE,1; 2020,NovSE,1; 2020,Jul,11; 2018,Jan,8; 2017,Jan,8; 2016,Jan,13

90691 Typhoid vaccine, Vi capsular polysaccharide (ViCPs), for intramuscular use
 INCLUDES   Typhim Vi
    0.00   0.00   **FUD** XXX   Ⓢ Ⓝ N1 ▭
 AMA: 2020,DecSE,1; 2020,DecSE,1; 2020,NovSE,1; 2020,Jul,11; 2018,Jan,8; 2017,Jan,8; 2016,Jan,13

90694 Resequenced code. See code following 90689.

90696 Diphtheria, tetanus toxoids, acellular pertussis vaccine and inactivated poliovirus vaccine (DTaP-IPV), when administered to children 4 through 6 years of age, for intramuscular use   Ⓐ
 INCLUDES   KINRIX
           Quadracel
    0.00   0.00   **FUD** XXX   Ⓢ Ⓝ N1 ▭
 AMA: 2020,DecSE,1; 2020,DecSE,1; 2020,NovSE,1; 2018,Jan,8; 2017,Jan,8; 2016,Jan,13

90697 Diphtheria, tetanus toxoids, acellular pertussis vaccine, inactivated poliovirus vaccine, Haemophilus influenzae type b PRP-OMP conjugate vaccine, and hepatitis B vaccine (DTaP-IPV-Hib-HepB), for intramuscular use
    0.00   0.00   **FUD** XXX   Ⓢ Ⓜ ▭
 AMA: 2020,DecSE,1; 2020,DecSE,1; 2020,NovSE,1; 2018,Jan,8; 2017,Jan,8; 2016,Jan,13

90698 Diphtheria, tetanus toxoids, acellular pertussis vaccine, Haemophilus influenzae type b, and inactivated poliovirus vaccine, (DTaP-IPV/Hib), for intramuscular use

INCLUDES Pentacel

🔧 0.00 ⚕ 0.00 **FUD** XXX ⑤ N NI ▭

AMA: 2020,DecSE,1; 2020,DecSE,1; 2020,NovSE,1; 2018,Jan,8; 2017,Jan,8; 2016,Jan,13

90700 Diphtheria, tetanus toxoids, and acellular pertussis vaccine (DTaP), when administered to individuals younger than 7 years, for intramuscular use ▣

INCLUDES Daptacel
Infanrix

🔧 0.00 ⚕ 0.00 **FUD** XXX ⑤ N ▭

AMA: 2020,DecSE,1; 2020,DecSE,1; 2020,NovSE,1; 2018,Jan,8; 2017,Jan,8; 2016,Jan,13

90702 Diphtheria and tetanus toxoids adsorbed (DT) when administered to individuals younger than 7 years, for intramuscular use ▣

INCLUDES Diphtheria and Tetanus Toxoids Adsorbed USP (For Pediatric Use)

🔧 0.00 ⚕ 0.00 **FUD** XXX ⑤ N ▭

AMA: 2020,DecSE,1; 2020,DecSE,1; 2020,NovSE,1; 2018,Jan,8; 2017,Jan,8; 2016,Jan,13

90707 Measles, mumps and rubella virus vaccine (MMR), live, for subcutaneous use

INCLUDES M-M-R II

🔧 0.00 ⚕ 0.00 **FUD** XXX ⑤ N ▭

AMA: 2020,DecSE,1; 2020,DecSE,1; 2020,NovSE,1; 2018,Jan,8; 2017,Jan,8; 2016,Jan,13

90710 Measles, mumps, rubella, and varicella vaccine (MMRV), live, for subcutaneous use

INCLUDES ProQuad

🔧 0.00 ⚕ 0.00 **FUD** XXX ⑤ N ▭

AMA: 2020,DecSE,1; 2020,DecSE,1; 2020,NovSE,1; 2018,Jan,8; 2017,Jan,8; 2016,Jan,13

90713 Poliovirus vaccine, inactivated (IPV), for subcutaneous or intramuscular use

INCLUDES IPOL

🔧 0.00 ⚕ 0.00 **FUD** XXX ⑤ N ▭

AMA: 2020,DecSE,1; 2020,DecSE,1; 2020,NovSE,1; 2018,Jan,8; 2017,Jan,8; 2016,Jan,13

90714 Tetanus and diphtheria toxoids adsorbed (Td), preservative free, when administered to individuals 7 years or older, for intramuscular use ▣

INCLUDES Tenivac
Tetanus-diphtheria toxoids absorbed

🔧 0.00 ⚕ 0.00 · **FUD** XXX ⑤ N ▭

AMA: 2020,DecSE,1; 2020,DecSE,1; 2020,NovSE,1; 2018,Jan,8; 2017,Jan,8; 2016,Jan,13

90715 Tetanus, diphtheria toxoids and acellular pertussis vaccine (Tdap), when administered to individuals 7 years or older, for intramuscular use ▣

INCLUDES Adacel
Boostrix

🔧 0.00 ⚕ 0.00 **FUD** XXX ⑤ N ▭

AMA: 2020,DecSE,1; 2020,DecSE,1; 2020,NovSE,1; 2018,Jan,8; 2017,Jan,8; 2016,Jan,13

● # **90626** Tick-borne encephalitis virus vaccine, inactivated; 0.25 mL dosage, for intramuscular use

INCLUDES TicoVac Junior®

🔧 0.00 ⚕ 0.00 **FUD** XXX ✎

● # **90627** 0.5 mL dosage, for intramuscular use

INCLUDES TicoVac®

🔧 0.00 ⚕ 0.00 **FUD** XXX ✎

90716 Varicella virus vaccine (VAR), live, for subcutaneous use

INCLUDES Varivax

🔧 0.00 ⚕ 0.00 **FUD** XXX ⑤ M ▭

AMA: 2020,DecSE,1; 2020,DecSE,1; 2020,NovSE,1; 2018,Jan,8; 2017,Jan,8; 2016,Jan,13

90717 Yellow fever vaccine, live, for subcutaneous use

INCLUDES YF-VAX

🔧 0.00 ⚕ 0.00 **FUD** XXX ⑤ N NI ▭

AMA: 2020,DecSE,1; 2020,DecSE,1; 2020,NovSE,1; 2018,Jan,8; 2017,Jan,8; 2016,Jan,13

90723 Diphtheria, tetanus toxoids, acellular pertussis vaccine, hepatitis B, and inactivated poliovirus vaccine (DTaP-HepB-IPV), for intramuscular use

INCLUDES PEDIARIX

🔧 0.00 ⚕ 0.00 **FUD** XXX ⑤ M ▭

AMA: 2020,DecSE,1; 2020,DecSE,1; 2020,NovSE,1; 2018,Jan,8; 2017,Jan,8; 2016,Jan,13

90625 Cholera vaccine, live, adult dosage, 1 dose schedule, for oral use ▣

🔧 0.00 ⚕ 0.00 **FUD** XXX ⑤ E ▭

AMA: 2020,DecSE,1; 2020,DecSE,1; 2020,NovSE,1; 2018,Jan,8; 2017,Jan,8; 2016,Oct,6; 2016,Jan,13

90732 Pneumococcal polysaccharide vaccine, 23-valent (PPSV23), adult or immunosuppressed patient dosage, when administered to individuals 2 years or older, for subcutaneous or intramuscular use ▣

INCLUDES Pneumovax 23

🔧 0.00 ⚕ 0.00 **FUD** XXX ⑤ L L1 ▭

AMA: 2020,DecSE,1; 2020,DecSE,1; 2020,NovSE,1; 2018,Jan,8; 2017,Jan,8; 2016,Jan,13

90644 Meningococcal conjugate vaccine, serogroups C & Y and Haemophilus influenzae type b vaccine (Hib-MenCY), 4 dose schedule, when administered to children 6 weeks-18 months of age, for intramuscular use ▣

INCLUDES MenHibrix

🔧 0.00 ⚕ 0.00 **FUD** XXX ⑤ M ▭

AMA: 2020,DecSE,1; 2020,DecSE,1; 2020,NovSE,1; 2018,Jan,8; 2017,Jan,8; 2016,Jan,13

90733 Meningococcal polysaccharide vaccine, serogroups A, C, Y, W-135, quadrivalent (MPSV4), for subcutaneous use

INCLUDES Menomune-A/C/Y/W-135

🔧 0.00 ⚕ 0.00 **FUD** XXX ⑤ M ▭

AMA: 2020,DecSE,1; 2020,DecSE,1; 2020,NovSE,1; 2018,Jan,8; 2017,Jan,8; 2016,Jan,13

90734 Meningococcal conjugate vaccine, serogroups A, C, W, Y, quadrivalent, diphtheria toxoid carrier (MenACWY-D) or CRM197 carrier (MenACWY-CRM), for intramuscular use

INCLUDES Menactra
Menveo

🔧 0.00 ⚕ 0.00 **FUD** XXX ⑤ M ▭

AMA: 2020,DecSE,1; 2020,DecSE,1; 2020,NovSE,1; 2020,Jan,11; 2018,Jan,8; 2017,Jan,8; 2016,Oct,6; 2016,Jan,13

90619 Meningococcal conjugate vaccine, serogroups A, C, W, Y, quadrivalent, tetanus toxoid carrier (MenACWY-TT), for intramuscular use

🔧 0.00 ⚕ 0.00 **FUD** XXX ⑤ ▭

AMA: 2020,DecSE,1; 2020,DecSE,1; 2020,NovSE,1; 2020,Jan,11

90620 Meningococcal recombinant protein and outer membrane vesicle vaccine, serogroup B (MenB-4C), 2 dose schedule, for intramuscular use

INCLUDES Bexsero

🔧 0.00 ⚕ 0.00 **FUD** XXX ⑤ M ▭

AMA: 2020,DecSE,1; 2020,DecSE,1; 2020,NovSE,1; 2018,Nov,7; 2018,Jan,8; 2017,Jan,8; 2016,Jan,13

\# **90621** **Meningococcal recombinant lipoprotein vaccine, serogroup B (MenB-FHbp), 2 or 3 dose schedule, for intramuscular use**

INCLUDES   Trumenba

🔧 0.00   ⚕ 0.00   **FUD** XXX   Ⓢ Ⓜ ▭

AMA: 2020,DecSE,1; 2020,DecSE,1; 2020,NovSE,1; 2018,Nov,7; 2018,Jan,8; 2017,Jan,8; 2016,Jan,13

90736 **Zoster (shingles) vaccine (HZV), live, for subcutaneous injection**

INCLUDES   Zostavax

🔧 0.00   ⚕ 0.00   **FUD** XXX   Ⓢ Ⓜ ▭

AMA: 2020,DecSE,1; 2020,DecSE,1; 2020,NovSE,1; 2018,Nov,7; 2018,Jan,8; 2017,Jan,8; 2016,Jan,13

\# **90750** **Zoster (shingles) vaccine (HZV), recombinant, subunit, adjuvanted, for intramuscular use**

🔧 0.00   ⚕ 0.00   **FUD** XXX   Ⓢ Ⓜ ▭

AMA: 2018,Nov,7

90738 **Japanese encephalitis virus vaccine, inactivated, for intramuscular use**

INCLUDES   Ixiaro

🔧 0.00   ⚕ 0.00   **FUD** XXX   Ⓢ Ⓜ ▭

AMA: 2020,DecSE,1; 2020,DecSE,1; 2020,NovSE,1; 2018,Jan,8; 2017,Jan,8; 2016,Jan,13

90739 **Hepatitis B vaccine (HepB), adult dosage, 2 dose schedule, for intramuscular use**

🔧 0.00   ⚕ 0.00   **FUD** XXX   Ⓢ Ⓔ ▭

AMA: 2020,DecSE,1; 2020,DecSE,1; 2020,NovSE,1; 2018,Nov,7; 2018,Jan,8; 2017,Jan,8; 2016,Jan,13

90740 **Hepatitis B vaccine (HepB), dialysis or immunosuppressed patient dosage, 3 dose schedule, for intramuscular use**

INCLUDES   Recombivax HB

🔧 0.00   ⚕ 0.00   **FUD** XXX   Ⓢ Ⓕ F4 ▭

AMA: 2020,DecSE,1; 2020,DecSE,1; 2020,NovSE,1; 2018,Jan,8; 2017,Jan,8; 2016,Jan,13

90743 **Hepatitis B vaccine (HepB), adolescent, 2 dose schedule, for intramuscular use**

INCLUDES   Energix-B
              Recombivax HB

🔧 0.00   ⚕ 0.00   **FUD** XXX   Ⓐ

                                            Ⓢ Ⓕ F4 ▭

AMA: 2020,DecSE,1; 2020,DecSE,1; 2020,NovSE,1; 2018,Jan,8; 2017,Jan,8; 2016,Jan,13

90744 **Hepatitis B vaccine (HepB), pediatric/adolescent dosage, 3 dose schedule, for intramuscular use**

INCLUDES   Energix-B
              Flucelvax Quadrivalent
              Recombivax HB

🔧 0.00   ⚕ 0.00   **FUD** XXX   Ⓐ   Ⓢ Ⓕ F4 ▭

AMA: 2020,DecSE,1; 2020,DecSE,1; 2020,NovSE,1; 2018,Jan,8; 2017,Jan,8; 2016,Jan,13

90746 **Hepatitis B vaccine (HepB), adult dosage, 3 dose schedule, for intramuscular use**

INCLUDES   Energix-B
              Recombivax HB

🔧 0.00   ⚕ 0.00   **FUD** XXX   Ⓢ Ⓕ F4 ▭

AMA: 2020,DecSE,1; 2020,DecSE,1; 2020,NovSE,1; 2018,Jan,8; 2017,Jan,8; 2016,Jan,13

● \# **90759** **Hepatitis B vaccine (HepB), 3-antigen (S, Pre-S1, Pre-S2), 10 mcg dosage, 3 dose schedule, for intramuscular use**

🔧 0.00   ⚕ 0.00   **FUD** 000   ✎

90747 **Hepatitis B vaccine (HepB), dialysis or immunosuppressed patient dosage, 4 dose schedule, for intramuscular use**

INCLUDES   Energix-B
              RECOMBIVAX dialysis

🔧 0.00   ⚕ 0.00   **FUD** XXX   Ⓢ Ⓕ F4 ▭

AMA: 2020,DecSE,1; 2020,DecSE,1; 2020,NovSE,1; 2018,Jan,8; 2017,Jan,8; 2016,Jan,13

90748 **Hepatitis B and Haemophilus influenzae type b vaccine (Hib-HepB), for intramuscular use**

INCLUDES   COMVAX

🔧 0.00   ⚕ 0.00   **FUD** XXX   Ⓢ Ⓔ ▭

AMA: 2020,DecSE,1; 2020,DecSE,1; 2020,NovSE,1; 2018,Jan,8; 2017,Jan,8; 2016,Jan,13

● \# **90758** **Zaire ebolavirus vaccine, live, for intramuscular use**

INCLUDES   Ervebo®

🔧 0.00   ⚕ 0.00   **FUD** XXX

90749 **Unlisted vaccine/toxoid**

🔧 0.00   ⚕ 0.00   **FUD** XXX   Ⓢ Ⓝ M1 ▭

AMA: 2020,DecSE,1; 2020,DecSE,1; 2020,NovSE,1; 2018,Jan,8; 2017,Jan,8; 2016,Jan,13

90750 **Resequenced code. See code following 90736.**

90756 **Resequenced code. See code following 90661.**

90758 **Resequenced code. See code following 90748.**

90759 **Resequenced code. See code following 90746.**

90785 Complex Interactive Encounter

CMS: 100-02,15,160 Clinical Psychologist Services; 100-02,15,170 Clinical Social Worker (CSW) Services; 100-03,10.3 Inpatient Pain Rehabilitation Programs; 100-03,10.4 Outpatient Hospital Pain Rehabilitation Programs; 100-03,130.1 Inpatient Stays for Alcoholism Treatment; 100-04,12,100 Teaching Physician Services; 100-04,4,260.1 Special Partial Hospitalization Billing Requirements forHospitals, Community Mental Health Centers, and Critical Access Hospitals; 100-04,4,260.1.1 Bill Review for Partial Hospitalization Services Provided in Community Mental Health Centers (CMHC)

INCLUDES   Complicated communication issues affecting psychiatric service
              Involved communication with:
                    Emotionally charged or dissonant family members
                    Patients wanting others present during visit (e.g., family member, translator)
                    Patients with impaired or undeveloped verbal skills
                    Patients with third parties responsible for their care (e.g., parents, guardians)
                    Third-party involvement (e.g., schools, probation and parole officers, child protective agencies)
              One or more following activity:
                    Discussion sentinel event demanding third-party involvement (i.e., abuse or neglect reported to state agency)
                    Interference by caregiver's behavior or emotional state to understand and assist in treatment plan
                    Managing discordant communication complicating care among participating members (e.g., arguing, reactivity)
                    Nonverbal communication methods (e.g., toys, other devices, or translator) to eliminate communication barriers

EXCLUDES   *Adaptive behavior assessment/treatment ([97151, 97152, 97153, 97154, 97155, 97156, 97157, 97158], 0362T, 0373T)*
              Crisis psychotherapy (90839-90840)
              Psychological or neuropsychological test administration (96136-96139, 96146)
              Psychological testing evaluation services (96130-96133)

\+ **90785** **Interactive complexity (List separately in addition to the code for primary procedure)**

Code first, when performed (90791-90792, 90832-90834, 90836-90838, 90853)

🔧 0.39   ⚕ 0.42   **FUD** ZZZ   ★ Ⓝ ▭

AMA: 2020,Aug,3; 2018,Nov,3; 2018,Jul,12; 2018,Apr,9; 2018,Jan,8; 2017,Jan,8; 2016,Dec,11; 2016,Jan,13

26/TC PC/TC Only   A2-Z3 ASC Payment   50 Bilateral   ♂ Male Only   ♀ Female Only   🔧 Facility RVU   ⚕ Non-Facility RVU   ▭ CCI   ✖ CLIA

FUD Follow-up Days   **CMS:** IOM   **AMA:** CPT Asst   A-Y OPPSI   80/80 Surg Assist Allowed / w/Doc   Lab Crosswalk   Radiology Crosswalk

460   CPT © 2021 American Medical Association. All Rights Reserved.   © 2021 Optum360, LLC

90791-90792 Psychiatric Evaluations

CMS: 100-02,15,170 Clinical Social Worker (CSW) Services; 100-03,10.3 Inpatient Pain Rehabilitation Programs; 100-03,130.1 Inpatient Stays for Alcoholism Treatment; 100-03,130.2 Outpatient Hospital Services for Alcoholism; 100-04,12,100 Teaching Physician Services; 100-04,12,190.3 List of Telehealth Services; 100-04,12,190.6 Payment Methodology for Physician/Practitioner at the Distant Site ; 100-04,12,190.6.1 Submission of Telehealth Claims for Distant Site Practitioners; 100-04,12,190.7 Contractor Editing of Telehealth Claims; 100-04,4,260.1 Special Partial Hospitalization Billing Requirements forHospitals, Community Mental Health Centers, and Critical Access Hospitals; 100-04,4,260.1.1 Bill Review for Partial Hospitalization Services Provided in Community Mental Health Centers (CMHC)

INCLUDES Diagnostic assessment or reassessment without psychotherapy services

EXCLUDES *Adaptive behavior assessment/treatment ([97151, 97152, 97153, 97154, 97155, 97156, 97157, 97158], 0362T, 0373T)*
Crisis psychotherapy (90839-90840)
E/M services (99202-99337 [99224, 99225, 99226], 99341-99350, 99366-99368, 99401-99443 [99415, 99416, 99417, 99421, 99422, 99423, 99439])
Code also interactive complexity services when applicable (90785)

90791 **Psychiatric diagnostic evaluation**
⏱ 3.54   ⚖ 3.89   **FUD** XXX   ★ 03 ▢

AMA: 2020,Oct,14; 2020,Aug,3; 2018,Nov,3; 2018,Jul,12; 2018,Apr,9; 2018,Jan,8; 2017,Nov,3; 2017,Jan,8; 2016,Jan,13

90792 **Psychiatric diagnostic evaluation with medical services**
⏱ 4.01   ⚖ 4.37   **FUD** XXX   ★ 03 ▢

AMA: 2020,Oct,14; 2020,Aug,3; 2019,Dec,14; 2018,Nov,3; 2018,Jul,12; 2018,Apr,9; 2018,Jan,8; 2017,Nov,3; 2017,Jan,8; 2016,Jan,13

90832-90838 Psychotherapy Services

CMS: 100-02,15,160 Clinical Psychologist Services; 100-02,15,170 Clinical Social Worker (CSW) Services; 100-03,130.1 Inpatient Stays for Alcoholism Treatment; 100-03,130.2 Outpatient Hospital Services for Alcoholism; 100-03,130.3 Chemical Aversion Therapy for Treatment of Alcoholism; 100-04,12,100 Teaching Physician Services; 100-04,12,160 Independent Psychologist Services; 100-04,12,170 Clinical Psychologist Services; 100-04,12,190.3 List of Telehealth Services; 100-04,12,190.6 Payment Methodology for Physician/Practitioner at the Distant Site ; 100-04,12,190.6.1 Submission of Telehealth Claims for Distant Site Practitioners; 100-04,12,190.7 Contractor Editing of Telehealth Claims

INCLUDES Face-to-face time with patient (family, other informers may also be present)
Pharmacologic management in time allocated to psychotherapy service codes
Psychotherapy only (90832, 90834, 90837)
Psychotherapy with separately identifiable medical E/M services includes add-on codes (90833, 90836, 90838)
Service times no less than 16 minutes
Services provided in all settings
Therapeutic communication to:
Ameliorate patient's mental and behavioral symptoms
Modify behavior
Support and encourage personality growth and development
Treatment for:
Behavior disturbances
Mental illness

EXCLUDES *Adaptive behavior assessment/treatment ([97151, 97152, 97153, 97154, 97155, 97156, 97157, 97158], 0362T, 0373T)*
Crisis psychotherapy (90839-90840)
Family psychotherapy (90846-90847)
Code also interactive complexity services with time provider spends performing service reflected in time for appropriate psychotherapy code (90785)

90832 **Psychotherapy, 30 minutes with patient**
⏱ 1.76   ⚖ 1.90   **FUD** XXX   ★ 03 ▢

AMA: 2020,Dec,13; 2020,Aug,3; 2018,Nov,3; 2018,Jul,12; 2018,Jan,8; 2017,Nov,3; 2017,Sep,11; 2017,Jan,8; 2016,Dec,11; 2016,Jan,13

+ 90833 **Psychotherapy, 30 minutes with patient when performed with an evaluation and management service (List separately in addition to the code for primary procedure)**
Code first (99202-99255 [99224, 99225, 99226], 99304-99337, 99341-99350)
⏱ 1.84   ⚖ 1.97   **FUD** ZZZ   ★ N ▢

AMA: 2020,Dec,13; 2020,Aug,3; 2018,Nov,3; 2018,Jul,12; 2018,Jan,8; 2017,Nov,3; 2017,Jan,8; 2016,Dec,11; 2016,Jan,13

90834 **Psychotherapy, 45 minutes with patient**
⏱ 2.35   ⚖ 2.53   **FUD** XXX   ★ 03 ▢

AMA: 2020,Dec,13; 2020,Aug,3; 2018,Nov,3; 2018,Jul,12; 2018,Jan,8; 2017,Nov,3; 2017,Jan,8; 2016,Dec,11; 2016,Jan,13

+ 90836 **Psychotherapy, 45 minutes with patient when performed with an evaluation and management service (List separately in addition to the code for primary procedure)**
Code first (99202-99255 [99224, 99225, 99226], 99304-99337, 99341-99350)
⏱ 2.33   ⚖ 2.49   **FUD** ZZZ   ★ N ▢

AMA: 2020,Dec,13; 2020,Aug,3; 2018,Nov,3; 2018,Jul,12; 2018,Jan,8; 2017,Nov,3; 2017,Jan,8; 2016,Dec,11; 2016,Jan,13

90837 **Psychotherapy, 60 minutes with patient**
Code also prolonged service for psychotherapy performed without E/M service face-to-face with patient lasting 90 minutes or longer (99354-99357)
⏱ 3.53   ⚖ 3.80   **FUD** XXX   ★ 03 ▢

AMA: 2020,Dec,13; 2020,Sep,3; 2020,Aug,3; 2018,Nov,3; 2018,Jul,12; 2018,Jan,8; 2017,Nov,3; 2017,Jan,8; 2016,Dec,11; 2016,Jan,13

+ 90838 **Psychotherapy, 60 minutes with patient when performed with an evaluation and management service (List separately in addition to the code for primary procedure)**
Code first (99202-99255 [99224, 99225, 99226], 99304-99337, 99341-99350)
⏱ 3.08   ⚖ 3.29   **FUD** ZZZ   ★ N ▢

AMA: 2020,Dec,13; 2020,Aug,3; 2018,Nov,3; 2018,Jul,12; 2018,Jan,8; 2017,Nov,3; 2017,Jan,8; 2016,Dec,11; 2016,Jan,13

90839-90840 Services for Patients in Crisis

CMS: 100-02,15,170 Clinical Social Worker (CSW) Services; 100-03,130.1 Inpatient Stays for Alcoholism Treatment; 100-03,130.3 Chemical Aversion Therapy for Treatment of Alcoholism; 100-04,12,100 Teaching Physician Services; 100-04,12,160 Independent Psychologist Services; 100-04,12,160.1 Payment of Independent Psychologist Services; 100-04,12,170 Clinical Psychologist Services

INCLUDES 30 minutes or more face-to-face time with patient (for all or part service) and/or family providing crisis psychotherapy
All time spent exclusively with patient (for all or part service) and/or family, even if time not continuous
Emergent care to patient in severe distress (e.g., life threatening or complex)
Institute interventions to minimize psychological trauma
Measures to ease crisis and reestablish safety
Psychotherapy

EXCLUDES *Adaptive behavior assessment/treatment ([97151, 97152, 97153, 97154, 97155, 97156, 97157, 97158], 0362T, 0373T)*
Other psychiatric services (90785-90899)

90839 **Psychotherapy for crisis; first 60 minutes**
INCLUDES First 30-74 minutes crisis psychotherapy per day
EXCLUDES *Reporting code more than one time per day, even when service not continuous on that date*
⏱ 3.69   ⚖ 3.96   **FUD** XXX   ★ 03 80 ▢

AMA: 2020,Aug,3; 2018,Nov,3; 2018,Jul,12; 2018,Jan,8; 2017,Nov,3; 2017,Jan,8; 2016,Jan,13

+ 90840 **each additional 30 minutes (List separately in addition to code for primary service)**
INCLUDES Up to 30 minutes time beyond initial 74 minutes
Code first (90839)
⏱ 1.76   ⚖ 1.90   **FUD** ZZZ   ★ N 80 ▢

AMA: 2020,Aug,3; 2018,Nov,3; 2018,Jul,12; 2018,Jan,8; 2017,Nov,3; 2017,Jan,8; 2016,Jan,13

90845-90863 Additional Psychotherapy Services

CMS: 100-02,15,170 Clinical Social Worker (CSW) Services; 100-03,10.3 Inpatient Pain Rehabilitation Programs; 100-03,10.4 Outpatient Hospital Pain Rehabilitation Programs

EXCLUDES *Adaptive behavior assessment/treatment ([97151, 97152, 97153, 97154, 97155, 97156, 97157, 97158], 0362T, 0373T)*
Analysis/programming neurostimulators for vagus nerve stimulation therapy (95970, 95976-95977)
Crisis psychotherapy (90839-90840)

90845 **Psychoanalysis**
⏱ 2.52   ⚖ 2.70   **FUD** XXX   ★ 03 80 ▢

AMA: 2020,Aug,3; 2018,Nov,3; 2018,Jul,12; 2018,Jan,8; 2017,Jan,8; 2016,Jan,13

Medicine (side tab)

90846 — 90882 (side tab)

90846 **Family psychotherapy (without the patient present), 50 minutes**

EXCLUDES *Service times less than 26 minutes*

⚕ 2.85   ⚕ 3.06   **FUD** XXX   ★ 03 80 ▭

AMA: 2020,Aug,3; 2018,Nov,3; 2018,Jul,12; 2018,Jan,8; 2017,Nov,3; 2017,Mar,10; 2017,Jan,8; 2016,Dec,11; 2016,Jan,13

90847 **Family psychotherapy (conjoint psychotherapy) (with patient present), 50 minutes**

EXCLUDES *Service times less than 26 minutes*
Service times more than 80 minutes, see prolonged services (99354-99357)

⚕ 2.96   ⚕ 3.18   **FUD** XXX   ★ 03 80 ▭

AMA: 2020,Sep,3; 2020,Aug,3; 2018,Nov,3; 2018,Jul,12; 2018,Jan,8; 2017,Nov,3; 2017,Jan,8; 2016,Dec,11; 2016,Jan,13

90849 **Multiple-family group psychotherapy**

⚕ 0.87   ⚕ 1.17   **FUD** XXX   03 80 ▭

AMA: 2020,Aug,3; 2018,Nov,3; 2018,Jul,12; 2018,Jan,8; 2017,Nov,3; 2017,Jan,8; 2016,Jan,13

90853 **Group psychotherapy (other than of a multiple-family group)**

Code also group psychotherapy with interactive complexity (90785)

⚕ 0.70   ⚕ 0.76   **FUD** XXX   03 80 ▭

AMA: 2020,Aug,3; 2018,Nov,3; 2018,Jul,12; 2018,Jan,8; 2017,Nov,3; 2017,Mar,10; 2017,Jan,8; 2016,Jan,13

+ **90863** **Pharmacologic management, including prescription and review of medication, when performed with psychotherapy services (List separately in addition to the code for primary procedure)**

INCLUDES *Pharmacologic management in time allocated to psychotherapy service codes*

Code first (90832, 90834, 90837)

⚕ 0.70   ⚕ 0.74   **FUD** XXX   ★ E ▭

AMA: 2020,Aug,3; 2018,Nov,3; 2018,Jul,12; 2018,Jan,8; 2017,Jan,8; 2016,Jan,13

90865-90870 Other Psychiatric Treatment

EXCLUDES *Adaptive behavior assessment/treatment ([97151, 97152, 97153, 97154, 97155, 97156, 97157, 97158], 0362T, 0373T)*
Analysis/programming neurostimulators for vagus nerve stimulation therapy (95970, 95976-95977)
Crisis psychotherapy (90839-90840)

90865 **Narcosynthesis for psychiatric diagnostic and therapeutic purposes (eg, sodium amobarbital (Amytal) interview)**

⚕ 3.61   ⚕ 4.80   **FUD** XXX   03 80 ▭

AMA: 2020,Aug,3; 2018,Nov,3; 2018,Jul,12; 2018,Jan,8; 2017,Jan,8; 2016,Jan,13

90867 **Therapeutic repetitive transcranial magnetic stimulation (TMS) treatment; initial, including cortical mapping, motor threshold determination, delivery and management**

INCLUDES *E/M services related directly to:*
  Cortical mapping
  Delivery and management TMS services
  Motor threshold determination

EXCLUDES *Electromyography (95860, 95870)*
Evoked potential studies (95928, 95929, [95939])
Medication management
Reporting code more than one time for each treatment course
Significant, separately identifiable E/M service
Significant, separately identifiable psychotherapy service
Subsequent transcranial magnetic stimulation (TMS) treatment:
  Delivery and management (90868)
  Motor threshold redetermination (90869)

⚕ 0.00   ⚕ 0.00   **FUD** 000   S ▭

AMA: 2020,Aug,3; 2018,Nov,3; 2018,Jul,12

90868 **subsequent delivery and management, per session**

INCLUDES *E/M services related directly to:*
  Cortical mapping
  Delivery and management TMS services
  Motor threshold determination

EXCLUDES *Medication management*
Significant, separately identifiable E/M service
Significant, separately identifiable psychotherapy service

⚕ 0.00   ⚕ 0.00   **FUD** 000   S ▭

AMA: 2020,Aug,3; 2018,Nov,3; 2018,Jul,12

90869 **subsequent motor threshold re-determination with delivery and management**

INCLUDES *E/M services related directly to:*
  Cortical mapping
  Delivery and management TMS services
  Motor threshold determination

EXCLUDES *Electromyography (95860, 95870)*
Evoked potential studies (95928-95929, [95939])
Medication management
Significant, separately identifiable E/M service
Significant, separately identifiable psychotherapy service
Transcranial magnetic stimulation (TMS) treatment:
  Initial (90867)
  Subsequent delivery and managment (90868)

⚕ 0.00   ⚕ 0.00   **FUD** 000   S ▭

AMA: 2020,Aug,3; 2018,Nov,3; 2018,Jul,12

90870 **Electroconvulsive therapy (includes necessary monitoring)**

⚕ 3.11   ⚕ 4.99   **FUD** 000   S 80 ▭

AMA: 2020,Aug,3; 2018,Nov,3; 2018,Jul,12; 2018,Jan,8; 2017,Jan,8; 2016,Jan,13

90875-90880 Psychiatric Therapy with Biofeedback or Hypnosis

CMS: 100-02,15,170 Clinical Social Worker (CSW) Services; 100-04,12,160 Independent Psychologist Services; 100-04,12,160.1 Payment of Independent Psychologist Services; 100-04,12,170 Clinical Psychologist Services

EXCLUDES *Adaptive behavior assessment/treatment ([97151, 97152, 97153, 97154, 97155, 97156, 97157, 97158], 0362T, 0373T)*
Analysis/programming neurostimulators for vagus nerve stimulation therapy (95970, 95976-95977)
Crisis psychotherapy (90839-90840)

90875 **Individual psychophysiological therapy incorporating biofeedback training by any modality (face-to-face with the patient), with psychotherapy (eg, insight oriented, behavior modifying or supportive psychotherapy); 30 minutes**

⚕ 1.73   ⚕ 1.80   **FUD** XXX   E ▭

AMA: 2020,Aug,3; 2018,Nov,3; 2018,Jul,12; 2018,Jan,8; 2017,Jan,8; 2016,Jan,13

90876 **45 minutes**

⚕ 2.74   ⚕ 3.05   **FUD** XXX   E ▭

AMA: 2020,Aug,3; 2018,Nov,3; 2018,Jul,12; 2018,Jan,8; 2017,Jan,8; 2016,Jan,13

90880 **Hypnotherapy**

⚕ 2.58   ⚕ 2.98   **FUD** XXX   03 80 ▭

AMA: 2020,Aug,3; 2018,Nov,3; 2018,Jul,12; 2018,Jan,8; 2017,Jan,8; 2016,Jan,13

90882-90899 Psychiatric Services without Patient Face-to-Face Contact

CMS: 100-04,12,160 Independent Psychologist Services; 100-04,12,160.1 Payment of Independent Psychologist Services

EXCLUDES *Analysis/programming neurostimulators for vagus nerve stimulation therapy (95970, 95976-95977)*
Crisis psychotherapy (90839-90840)

90882 **Environmental intervention for medical management purposes on a psychiatric patient's behalf with agencies, employers, or institutions**

⚕ 0.00   ⚕ 0.00   **FUD** XXX   E ▭

AMA: 2020,Aug,3; 2018,Nov,3; 2018,Jul,12; 2018,Jan,8; 2017,Jan,8; 2016,Jan,13

26/TC PC/TC Only   A2-Z3 ASC Payment   50 Bilateral   ♂ Male Only   ♀ Female Only   ⚕ Facility RVU   ⚕ Non-Facility RVU   ▭ CCI   ✖ CLIA
FUD Follow-up Days   CMS: IOM   AMA: CPT Asst   A-Y OPPSI   80/80 Surg Assist Allowed / w/Doc   ▧ Lab Crosswalk   ▨ Radiology Crosswalk

462   CPT © 2021 American Medical Association. All Rights Reserved.   © 2021 Optum360, LLC

90885 Psychiatric evaluation of hospital records, other psychiatric reports, psychometric and/or projective tests, and other accumulated data for medical diagnostic purposes

🔪 1.41   🖐 1.41   **FUD** XXX   N ▢

AMA: 2020,Dec,13; 2020,Aug,3; 2018,Nov,3; 2018,Jul,12; 2018,Jan,8; 2017,Jan,8; 2016,Jan,13

90887 Interpretation or explanation of results of psychiatric, other medical examinations and procedures, or other accumulated data to family or other responsible persons, or advising them how to assist patient

EXCLUDES   *Adaptive behavior assessment/treatment ([97151, 97152, 97153, 97154, 97155, 97156, 97157, 97158], 0362T, 0373T)*

🔪 2.14   🖐 2.48   **FUD** XXX   N ▢

AMA: 2020,Aug,3; 2018,Nov,3; 2018,Jul,12; 2018,Jan,8; 2017,Jan,8; 2016,Jan,13

90889 Preparation of report of patient's psychiatric status, history, treatment, or progress (other than for legal or consultative purposes) for other individuals, agencies, or insurance carriers

🔪 0.00   🖐 0.00   **FUD** XXX   N ▢

AMA: 2020,Aug,3; 2018,Nov,3; 2018,Jul,12; 2018,Jan,8; 2017,Jan,8; 2016,Jan,13

90899 Unlisted psychiatric service or procedure

🔪 0.00   🖐 0.00   **FUD** XXX   03 80 ▢

AMA: 2020,Aug,3; 2018,Nov,3; 2018,Jul,12; 2018,Jan,8; 2017,Jan,8; 2016,Jan,13

90901-90913 Biofeedback Therapy

EXCLUDES   *Psychophysiological therapy utilizing biofeedback training (90875-90876)*

90901 Biofeedback training by any modality

🔪 0.57   🖐 1.15   **FUD** 000   A 80 ▢

AMA: 2020,Jun,13; 2018,Jan,8; 2017,Jan,8; 2016,Jan,13

90912 Biofeedback training, perineal muscles, anorectal or urethral sphincter, including EMG and/or manometry, when performed; initial 15 minutes of one-on-one physician or other qualified health care professional contact with the patient

EXCLUDES   *Incontinence treatment using pulsed magnetic neuromodulation (53899)*
Testing rectal sensation, tone, and compliance (91120)

🔪 1.26   🖐 2.27   **FUD** 000   80 ▢

AMA: 2020,Jun,13

+ **90913** each additional 15 minutes of one-on-one physician or other qualified health care professional contact with the patient (List separately in addition to code for primary procedure)

EXCLUDES   *Incontinence treatment using pulsed magnetic neuromodulation (53899)*
Testing rectal sensation, tone, and compliance (91120)
Code first (90912)

🔪 0.70   🖐 0.92   **FUD** ZZZ   80 ▢

AMA: 2020,Jun,13

90935-90940 Hemodialysis Services: Inpatient ESRD and Outpatient Non-ESRD

CMS: 100-02,11,20 Renal Dialysis Items and Services ; 100-04,3,100.6 Inpatient Renal Services

EXCLUDES   *Attendance by physician or other qualified health care provider for prolonged period of time (99354-99360 [99415, 99416])*
Blood specimen collection from partial/complete implantable venous access device (36591)
Declotting cannula (36831, 36833, 36860-36861)
Hemodialysis home visit by non-physician health care professional (99512)
Therapeutic apheresis procedures (36511-36516)
Therapeutic ultrafiltration (0692T)
Thrombolytic agent declotting implanted vascular access device/catheter (36593)

Code also significant separately identifiable E/M service not related to dialysis procedure or renal failure with modifier 25 (99202-99215, 99217-99223 [99224, 99225, 99226], 99231-99239, 99241-99245, 99281-99285, 99291-99292, 99304-99318, 99324-99337, 99341-99350, 99466-99467, 99468-99472, 99475-99480)

90935 Hemodialysis procedure with single evaluation by a physician or other qualified health care professional

INCLUDES   All E/M services related to patient's renal disease rendered on day dialysis performed
Inpatient ESRD and non-ESRD procedures
Only one patient evaluation related to hemodialysis procedure
Outpatient non-ESRD dialysis

🔪 2.07   🖐 2.07   **FUD** 000   S 80 ▢

AMA: 2018,Jan,8; 2017,Jan,8; 2016,Jan,13

90937 Hemodialysis procedure requiring repeated evaluation(s) with or without substantial revision of dialysis prescription

INCLUDES   All E/M services related to patient's renal disease rendered on day dialysis performed
Inpatient ESRD and non-ESRD procedures
Outpatient non-ESRD dialysis
Re-evaluation patient during hemodialysis procedure

🔪 2.95   🖐 2.95   **FUD** 000   B 80 ▢

AMA: 2018,Jan,8; 2017,Jan,8; 2016,Jan,13

90940 Hemodialysis access flow study to determine blood flow in grafts and arteriovenous fistulae by an indicator method

EXCLUDES   *Hemodialysis access duplex scan (93990)*

🔪 0.00   🖐 0.00   **FUD** XXX   N ▢

AMA: 2018,Jan,8; 2017,Jan,8; 2016,Jan,13

90945-90947 Dialysis Techniques Other Than Hemodialysis

CMS: 100-04,12,40.3 Global Surgery Review; 100-04,3,100.6 Inpatient Renal Services

INCLUDES   All E/M services related to patient's renal disease rendered on day dialysis performed
Procedures other than hemodialysis:
    Continuous renal replacement therapies
    Hemofiltration
    Peritoneal dialysis

EXCLUDES   *Attendance by physician or other qualified health care provider for prolonged time period (99354-99360 [99415, 99416])*
Hemodialysis
Therapeutic ultrafiltration (0692T)
Tunneled intraperitoneal catheter insertion
    Open (49421)
    Percutaneous (49418)

Code also significant, separately identifiable E/M service not related to dialysis procedure or renal failure with modifier 25 (99202-99215, 99217-99223 [99224, 99225, 99226], 99231-99239, 99241-99245, 99281-99285, 99291-99292, 99304-99318, 99324-99337, 99341-99350, 99466-99467, 99468-99472, 99475-99480)

90945 Dialysis procedure other than hemodialysis (eg, peritoneal dialysis, hemofiltration, or other continuous renal replacement therapies), with single evaluation by a physician or other qualified health care professional

INCLUDES   Only one patient evaluation related to procedure
EXCLUDES   *Peritoneal dialysis home infusion (99601, 99602)*

🔪 2.42   🖐 2.42   **FUD** 000   V 80 ▢

AMA: 2018,Jan,8; 2017,Jan,8; 2016,Jan,13

90947   **Dialysis procedure other than hemodialysis (eg, peritoneal dialysis, hemofiltration, or other continuous renal replacement therapies) requiring repeated evaluations by a physician or other qualified health care professional, with or without substantial revision of dialysis prescription**

      EXCLUDES *Re-evaluation during procedure*

      3.51   3.51   **FUD** 000   B 80 ▭

      AMA: 2018,Jan,8; 2017,Jan,8; 2016,Jan,13

90951-90962 End-stage Renal Disease Monthly Outpatient Services

CMS: 100-02,11,20 Renal Dialysis Items and Services ; 100-04,12,190.3 List of Telehealth Services; 100-04,12,190.3.4 ESRD-Related Services as a Telehealth Service; 100-04,8,140.1 ESRD-Related Services Under the Monthly Capitation Payment

INCLUDES   Establishing dialyzing cycle
           Management dialysis visits
           Outpatient E/M dialysis visits
           Patient management during dialysis for month
           Telephone calls

EXCLUDES *ESRD/non-ESRD dialysis services performed in inpatient setting (90935-90937, 90945-90947)*
           Non-ESRD dialysis services performed in outpatient setting (90935-90937, 90945-90947)
           Non-ESRD related E/M services that cannot be performed during dialysis session
           Services provided in same month with:
             Chronic care management ([99437], [99439, 99490, 99491])
             Complex chronic care management (99487-99489)
             Principal care management services ([99424, 99425, 99426, 99427])
           Therapeutic ultrafiltration (0692T)

90951   **End-stage renal disease (ESRD) related services monthly, for patients younger than 2 years of age to include monitoring for the adequacy of nutrition, assessment of growth and development, and counseling of parents; with 4 or more face-to-face visits by a physician or other qualified health care professional per month** A

      26.6   26.6   **FUD** XXX   ★ M 80 ▭

      AMA: 2018,Feb,11; 2018,Jan,8; 2017,Jan,8; 2016,Jan,13

90952   **with 2-3 face-to-face visits by a physician or other qualified health care professional per month** A

      0.00   0.00   **FUD** XXX   ★ M 80 ▭

      AMA: 2018,Feb,11; 2018,Jan,8; 2017,Jan,8; 2016,Jan,13

90953   **with 1 face-to-face visit by a physician or other qualified health care professional per month** A

      0.00   0.00   **FUD** XXX   M 80 ▭

      AMA: 2018,Feb,11; 2018,Jan,8; 2017,Jan,8; 2016,Jan,13

90954   **End-stage renal disease (ESRD) related services monthly, for patients 2-11 years of age to include monitoring for the adequacy of nutrition, assessment of growth and development, and counseling of parents; with 4 or more face-to-face visits by a physician or other qualified health care professional per month** A

      23.0   23.0   **FUD** XXX   ★ M 80 ▭

      AMA: 2018,Feb,11; 2018,Jan,8; 2017,Jan,8; 2016,Jan,13

90955   **with 2-3 face-to-face visits by a physician or other qualified health care professional per month** A

      13.0   13.0   **FUD** XXX   ★ M 80 ▭

      AMA: 2018,Feb,11; 2018,Jan,8; 2017,Jan,8; 2016,Jan,13

90956   **with 1 face-to-face visit by a physician or other qualified health care professional per month** A

      9.05   9.05   **FUD** XXX   M 80 ▭

      AMA: 2018,Feb,11; 2018,Jan,8; 2017,Jan,8; 2016,Jan,13

90957   **End-stage renal disease (ESRD) related services monthly, for patients 12-19 years of age to include monitoring for the adequacy of nutrition, assessment of growth and development, and counseling of parents; with 4 or more face-to-face visits by a physician or other qualified health care professional per month** A

      18.3   18.3   **FUD** XXX   ★ M 80 ▭

      AMA: 2018,Feb,11; 2018,Jan,8; 2017,Jan,8; 2016,Jan,13

90958   **with 2-3 face-to-face visits by a physician or other qualified health care professional per month** A

      12.3   12.3   **FUD** XXX   ★ M 80 ▭

      AMA: 2018,Feb,11; 2018,Jan,8; 2017,Jan,8; 2016,Jan,13

90959   **with 1 face-to-face visit by a physician or other qualified health care professional per month** A

      8.40   8.40   **FUD** XXX   M 80 ▭

      AMA: 2018,Feb,11; 2018,Jan,8; 2017,Jan,8; 2016,Jan,13

90960   **End-stage renal disease (ESRD) related services monthly, for patients 20 years of age and older; with 4 or more face-to-face visits by a physician or other qualified health care professional per month** A

      8.02   8.02   **FUD** XXX   ★ M 80 ▭

      AMA: 2018,Feb,11; 2018,Jan,8; 2017,Jan,8; 2016,Jan,13

90961   **with 2-3 face-to-face visits by a physician or other qualified health care professional per month** A

      6.78   6.78   **FUD** XXX   ★ M 80 ▭

      AMA: 2018,Feb,11; 2018,Jan,8; 2017,Jan,8; 2016,Jan,13

90962   **with 1 face-to-face visit by a physician or other qualified health care professional per month** A

      5.23   5.23   **FUD** XXX   M 80 ▭

      AMA: 2018,Feb,11; 2018,Jan,8; 2017,Jan,8; 2016,Jan,13

90963-90966 End-stage Renal Disease Monthly Home Dialysis Services

CMS: 100-02,11,20 Renal Dialysis Items and Services ; 100-04,12,190.3.4 ESRD-Related Services as a Telehealth Service; 100-04,8,140.1 ESRD-Related Services Under the Monthly Capitation Payment; 100-04,8,140.1.1 Payment for Managing Patients on Home Dialysis

INCLUDES   ESRD services for home dialysis patients
           Services provided for full month

EXCLUDES *Services provided in same month with:*
           Chronic care management ([99437], [99439, 99490, 99491])
           Complex chronic care management (99487-99489)
           Principal care management services ([99424, 99425, 99426, 99427])
           Therapeutic ultrafiltration (0692T)

90963   **End-stage renal disease (ESRD) related services for home dialysis per full month, for patients younger than 2 years of age to include monitoring for the adequacy of nutrition, assessment of growth and development, and counseling of parents** A

      15.4   15.4   **FUD** XXX   ★ M 80 ▭

      AMA: 2018,Feb,11; 2018,Jan,8; 2017,Jan,8; 2016,Jan,13

90964   **End-stage renal disease (ESRD) related services for home dialysis per full month, for patients 2-11 years of age to include monitoring for the adequacy of nutrition, assessment of growth and development, and counseling of parents** A

      13.4   13.4   **FUD** XXX   ★ M 80 ▭

      AMA: 2018,Feb,11; 2018,Jan,8; 2017,Jan,8; 2016,Jan,13

90965   **End-stage renal disease (ESRD) related services for home dialysis per full month, for patients 12-19 years of age to include monitoring for the adequacy of nutrition, assessment of growth and development, and counseling of parents** A

      12.8   12.8   **FUD** XXX   ★ M 80 ▭

      AMA: 2018,Feb,11; 2018,Jan,8; 2017,Jan,8; 2016,Jan,13

90966   **End-stage renal disease (ESRD) related services for home dialysis per full month, for patients 20 years of age and older** A

      6.77   6.77   **FUD** XXX   ★ M 80 ▭

      AMA: 2018,Feb,11; 2018,Jan,8; 2017,Jan,8; 2016,Jan,13

26/TC PC/TC Only   A2-Z3 ASC Payment   50 Bilateral   ♂ Male Only   ♀ Female Only   Facility RVU   Non-Facility RVU   CCI   CLIA
FUD Follow-up Days   CMS: IOM   AMA: CPT Asst   A-Y OPPSI   80/80 Surg Assist Allowed / w/Doc   Lab Crosswalk   Radiology Crosswalk

464   CPT © 2021 American Medical Association. All Rights Reserved.   © 2021 Optum360, LLC

90967-90970 End-stage Renal Disease Services: Partial Month

CMS: 100-02,11,20 Renal Dialysis Items and Services

INCLUDES ESRD services for less than full month, such as:
Outpatient ESRD-related services initiated prior to assessment completion
Patient spending partial month as hospital inpatient
Patient who is transient, dies, recovers, or undergoes kidney transplant
Services reported on daily basis, less hospitalization days

EXCLUDES *Services provided in same month with:*
Chronic care management ([99437], [99439, 99490, 99491])
Complex chronic care management (99487-99489)
Principal care management services ([99424, 99425, 99426, 99427])
Therapeutic ultrafiltration (0692T)

90967 **End-stage renal disease (ESRD) related services for dialysis less than a full month of service, per day; for patients younger than 2 years of age** A
🔲 0.51   ⚕ 0.51   **FUD** XXX   ★ M 80 🖥
AMA: 2018,Feb,11; 2018,Jan,8; 2017,Jan,8; 2016,Jan,13

90968 **for patients 2-11 years of age** A
🔲 0.45   ⚕ 0.45   **FUD** XXX   ★ M 80 🖥
AMA: 2018,Feb,11; 2018,Jan,8; 2017,Jan,8; 2016,Jan,13

90969 **for patients 12-19 years of age** A
🔲 0.43   ⚕ 0.43   **FUD** XXX   ★ M 80 🖥
AMA: 2018,Feb,11; 2018,Jan,8; 2017,Jan,8; 2016,Jan,13

90970 **for patients 20 years of age and older** A
🔲 0.22   ⚕ 0.22   **FUD** XXX   ★ M 80 🖥
AMA: 2018,Feb,11; 2018,Jan,8; 2017,Jan,8; 2016,Jan,13

90989-90993 Dialysis Training Services

CMS: 100-04,3,100.6 Inpatient Renal Services

EXCLUDES *Therapeutic ultrafiltration (0692T)*

90989 **Dialysis training, patient, including helper where applicable, any mode, completed course**
🔲 0.00   ⚕ 0.00   **FUD** XXX   B 🖥
AMA: 2018,Feb,11; 2018,Jan,8; 2017,Jan,8; 2016,Jan,13

90993 **Dialysis training, patient, including helper where applicable, any mode, course not completed, per training session**
🔲 0.00   ⚕ 0.00   **FUD** XXX   B 🖥
AMA: 2018,Feb,11; 2018,Jan,8; 2017,Jan,8; 2016,Jan,13

90997-90999 Hemoperfusion and Unlisted Dialysis Procedures

CMS: 100-04,3,100.6 Inpatient Renal Services

EXCLUDES *Therapeutic ultrafiltration (0692T)*

90997 **Hemoperfusion (eg, with activated charcoal or resin)**
🔲 2.56   ⚕ 2.56   **FUD** 000   B 80 🖥
AMA: 2018,Feb,11

90999 **Unlisted dialysis procedure, inpatient or outpatient**
🔲 0.00   ⚕ 0.00   **FUD** XXX   B 80 🖥
AMA: 2018,Feb,11

91010-91022 Esophageal Manometry

91010 **Esophageal motility (manometric study of the esophagus and/or gastroesophageal junction) study with interpretation and report;**
EXCLUDES *Esophageal motility studies with high-resolution esophageal pressure topography (91299)*
Code also for esophageal motility studies with stimulant or perfusion (91013)
🔲 5.70   ⚕ 5.70   **FUD** 000   S 80 🖥
AMA: 2018,Feb,11

+ **91013** **with stimulation or perfusion (eg, stimulant, acid or alkali perfusion) (List separately in addition to code for primary procedure)**
EXCLUDES *Esophageal motility studies with high-resolution esophageal pressure topography (91299)*
Reporting code more than one time for each session
Code first (91010)
🔲 0.73   ⚕ 0.73   **FUD** ZZZ   N 80 🖥
AMA: 2018,Feb,11

91020 **Gastric motility (manometric) studies**
EXCLUDES *Gastrointestinal imaging by wireless capsule (91112)*
🔲 7.35   ⚕ 7.35   **FUD** 000   S 80 🖥
AMA: 2018,Feb,11; 2018,Jan,8; 2017,Jan,8; 2016,Jan,13

Liver
Stomach
Colon
Small intestine

Gastric pertains to the stomach; peptic is a term for ulcers caused by digestive juices in the stomach, duodenum or jejunum; duodenal ulcers are more common in young people, gastric in the elderly

Esophagus
Mucosal and muscle layers
Fundus
Rugae (folds lining the stomach)
Duodenum
Pyloric sphincter
Inner stomach (area where gastric ulcers occur)

91022 **Duodenal motility (manometric) study**
EXCLUDES *Fluoroscopy (76000)*
Gastric motility study (91020)
Gastrointestinal imaging by wireless capsule (91112)
🔲 4.79   ⚕ 4.79   **FUD** 000   S 80 🖥
AMA: 2018,Feb,11; 2018,Jan,8; 2017,Jan,8; 2016,Jan,13

91030-91040 Esophageal Reflux Tests

EXCLUDES *Duodenal intubation/aspiration (43756-43757)*
Esophagoscopy (43180-43233 [43211, 43212, 43213, 43214])
Insertion:
Esophageal tamponade tube (43460)
Insertion long gastrointestinal tube (44500)
Radiologic services, gastrointestinal (74210-74363)
Upper gastrointestinal endoscopy (43235-43259 [43233, 43266, 43270])

91030 **Esophagus, acid perfusion (Bernstein) test for esophagitis**
🔲 3.94   ⚕ 3.94   **FUD** 000   S 80 🖥
AMA: 2018,Feb,11

91034 **Esophagus, gastroesophageal reflux test; with nasal catheter pH electrode(s) placement, recording, analysis and interpretation**
🔲 5.41   ⚕ 5.41   **FUD** 000   S 80 🖥
AMA: 2018,Feb,11; 2018,Jan,8; 2017,Jan,8; 2016,Jan,13

91035 **with mucosal attached telemetry pH electrode placement, recording, analysis and interpretation**
INCLUDES Endoscopy only to place device
🔲 13.7   ⚕ 13.7   **FUD** 000   S 72 80 🖥
AMA: 2018,Feb,11; 2018,Jan,8; 2017,Jan,8; 2016,Jan,13

91037 **Esophageal function test, gastroesophageal reflux test with nasal catheter intraluminal impedance electrode(s) placement, recording, analysis and interpretation;**
🔲 4.71   ⚕ 4.71   **FUD** 000   S 80 🖥
AMA: 2018,Feb,11

91038 **prolonged (greater than 1 hour, up to 24 hours)**
🔲 12.4   ⚕ 12.4   **FUD** 000   S 80 🖥
AMA: 2018,Feb,11; 2018,Jan,8; 2017,Jan,8; 2016,Jan,13

91040   **Esophageal balloon distension study, diagnostic, with provocation when performed**

EXCLUDES *Reporting code more than one time for each session*
🛠 14.4   👐 14.4   **FUD** 000   S 80 ▭
AMA: 2018,Feb,11; 2018,Jan,8; 2017,Jan,6

91065 Breath Analysis

CMS: 100-03,100.5 Diagnostic Breath Analysis

EXCLUDES *H. pylori breath test analysis, radioactive (C-14) or nonradioactive (C-13) (78268, 83013)*
Code also each challenge administered

91065   **Breath hydrogen or methane test (eg, for detection of lactase deficiency, fructose intolerance, bacterial overgrowth, or oro-cecal gastrointestinal transit)**

🛠 2.26   👐 2.26   **FUD** 000   S 80 ▭
AMA: 2018,Feb,11; 2018,Jan,8; 2017,Jan,8; 2016,Jan,13

91110-91310 [91113, 91300, 91301, 91302, 91303, 91304, 91305, 91306, 91307, 91308, 91309, 91310] Additional Gastrointestinal Diagnostic/Therapeutic Procedures

EXCLUDES *Abdominal paracentesis (49082-49084)*
Abdominal paracentesis with medication administration (96440, 96446)
Anoscopy (46600-46615)
Colonoscopy (45378-45393 [45388, 45390, 45398])
Duodenal intubation/aspiration (43756-43757)
Esophagoscopy (43180-43233 [43211, 43212, 43213, 43214])
Proctosigmoidoscopy (45300-45327)
Radiologic services, gastrointestinal (74210-74363)
Sigmoidoscopy (45330-45350 [45346])
Small intestine/stomal endoscopy (44360-44408 [44381, 44401])
Upper gastrointestinal endoscopy (43235-43259 [43233, 43266, 43270])

91110   **Gastrointestinal tract imaging, intraluminal (eg, capsule endoscopy), esophagus through ileum, with interpretation and report**

INCLUDES *Incidental colon visualization*
EXCLUDES *Imaging esophagus (91111)*
Intraluminal capsule endoscopy GI tract ([91113])
Magnetically controlled capsule endoscopy (0651T)
Code also modifier 52 when ileum not visualized
🛠 24.3   👐 24.3   **FUD** XXX   T 80 ▭
AMA: 2018,Feb,11; 2018,Jan,8; 2017,Jan,8; 2016,Jan,13

91111   **Gastrointestinal tract imaging, intraluminal (eg, capsule endoscopy), esophagus with interpretation and report**

INCLUDES *Incidental colon, duodenum, esophagus, ileum, or stomach visualization*
EXCLUDES *Imaging esophagus through ileum (91110)*
Intraluminal capsule endoscopy GI tract ([91113])
Magnetically controlled capsule endoscopy (0651T)
Wireless capsule to measure transit times or pressure in gastrointestinal tract (91112)
🛠 22.8   👐 22.8   **FUD** XXX   T 80 ▭
AMA: 2018,Feb,11; 2018,Jan,8; 2017,Jan,8; 2016,Jan,13

● # **91113**   **Gastrointestinal tract imaging, intraluminal (eg, capsule endoscopy), colon, with interpretation and report**

INCLUDES *Incidental duodenum, esophagus, ileum, or stomach visualization*
EXCLUDES *Imaging esophagus or esophagus through ileum (91110, 91111)*
🛠 0.00   👐 0.00   **FUD** 000

91112   **Gastrointestinal transit and pressure measurement, stomach through colon, wireless capsule, with interpretation and report**

EXCLUDES *Colon motility study (91117)*
Duodenal motility study (91022)
Gastric motility studies (91020)
pH body fluid (83986)
🛠 40.9   👐 40.9   **FUD** XXX   T 80 ▭
AMA: 2018,Feb,11; 2018,Jan,8; 2017,Jan,8; 2016,Jan,13

91113   Resequenced code. See code following 91111.

91117   **Colon motility (manometric) study, minimum 6 hours continuous recording (including provocation tests, eg, meal, intracolonic balloon distension, pharmacologic agents, if performed), with interpretation and report**

EXCLUDES *Anal manometry (91122)*
Rectal sensation, tone and compliance testing (91120)
Reporting code more than one time no matter how many provocations
Wireless capsule to measure transit times or pressure in gastrointestinal tract (91112)
🛠 3.96   👐 3.96   **FUD** 000   T 80 ▭
AMA: 2018,Feb,11; 2018,Jan,8; 2017,Jan,8; 2016,Jan,13

91120   **Rectal sensation, tone, and compliance test (ie, response to graded balloon distension)**

EXCLUDES *Anorectal manometry (91122)*
Biofeedback training (90912, 90913)
Colon motility study (91117)
🛠 13.7   👐 13.7   **FUD** XXX   S 80 ▭
AMA: 2020,Jun,13; 2018,Feb,11; 2018,Jan,8; 2017,Jan,8; 2016,Jan,13

91122   **Anorectal manometry**

EXCLUDES *Colon motility study (91117)*
🛠 7.13   👐 7.13   **FUD** 000   T 80 ▭
AMA: 2018,Feb,11

91132   **Electrogastrography, diagnostic, transcutaneous;**

🛠 9.16   👐 9.16   **FUD** XXX   S 80 ▭
AMA: 2018,Feb,11

91133   **with provocative testing**

🛠 7.44   👐 7.44   **FUD** XXX   Q1 80 ▭
AMA: 2018,Feb,11

91200   **Liver elastography, mechanically induced shear wave (eg, vibration), without imaging, with interpretation and report**

EXCLUDES *Ultrasound elastography parenchyma (76981-76983)*
🛠 1.05   👐 1.05   **FUD** XXX   Q1 80 ▭
AMA: 2019,Aug,3; 2018,Feb,11; 2018,Jan,8; 2017,Oct,9

91299   **Unlisted diagnostic gastroenterology procedure**

🛠 0.00   👐 0.00   **FUD** XXX   S 80 ▭
AMA: 2018,Feb,11; 2018,Jan,8; 2017,Jan,8; 2016,Jan,13

91300   **Resequenced code. See code before 90476.**

91301   **Resequenced code. See code before 90476.**

91302   **Resequenced code. See code before 90476.**

91303   **Resequenced code. See code before 90476.**

91304   **Resequenced code. See code before 90476.**

91305   **Resequenced code. See code following resequenced code 91300.**

91306   **Resequenced code. See code following resequenced code 91301.**

91307   **Resequenced code. See code following resequenced code 91305.**

91308   **Resequenced code. See code before 90476.**

91309   **Resequenced code. See code before 90476.**

91310   **Resequenced code. See code before 90476.**

92002-92014 Ophthalmic Medical Services

CMS: 100-02,15,30.4 Optometrist's Services

INCLUDES Routine ophthalmoscopy
Services provided to established patients who have received professional services from physician or other qualified health care provider or another physician or other qualified health care professional within same group practice/exact same specialty and subspecialty within past three years
Services provided to new patients who have received no professional services from physician or other qualified health care provider or another physician or other qualified health care professional within same group practice/exact same specialty and subspecialty within past three years

EXCLUDES Retinal polarization scan (0469T)
Surgical procedures on eye/ocular adnexa (65091-68899 [66987, 66988, 67810])
Visual screening tests (99173-99174 [99177])

92002 **Ophthalmological services: medical examination and evaluation with initiation of diagnostic and treatment program; intermediate, new patient**

INCLUDES Evaluation new/existing condition complicated by new diagnostic or management problem
Integrated services where medical decision making cannot be separated from examination methods
Intermediate services:
External ocular/adnexal examination
General medical observation
History
Other diagnostic procedures:
Biomicroscopy
Mydriasis
Ophthalmoscopy
Tonometry
Problems not related to primary diagnosis

🚑 1.34 👥 2.37 **FUD** XXX V 80 🖵

AMA: 2018,Feb,11; 2018,Feb,3; 2018,Jan,8; 2017,Sep,14; 2017,Jan,8; 2016,Jan,13

92004 **comprehensive, new patient, 1 or more visits**

INCLUDES Comprehensive services:
Basic sensorimotor examination
Biomicroscopy
Dilation (cycloplegia)
External examinations
General medical observation
Gross visual fields
History
Initiation diagnostic/treatment programs
Mydriasis
Ophthalmoscopic examinations
Other diagnostic procedures
Prescription medication
Special diagnostic/treatment services
Tonometry
General evaluation complete visual system
Integrated services where medical decision making cannot be separated from examination methods
Single service that need not be performed at one session

🚑 2.81 👥 4.26 **FUD** XXX V 80 🖵

AMA: 2018,Feb,11; 2018,Feb,3; 2018,Jan,8; 2017,Sep,14; 2017,Jan,8; 2016,Nov,9; 2016,Jan,13

92012 **Ophthalmological services: medical examination and evaluation, with initiation or continuation of diagnostic and treatment program; intermediate, established patient**

INCLUDES Evaluation new/existing condition complicated by new diagnostic or management problem
Integrated services where medical decision making cannot be separated from examination methods
Problems not related to primary diagnosis
Intermediate services:
External ocular/adnexal examination
General medical observation
History
Other diagnostic procedures:
Biomicroscopy
Mydriasis
Ophthalmoscopy
Tonometry

🚑 1.49 👥 2.49 **FUD** XXX V 80 🖵

AMA: 2018,Feb,11; 2018,Feb,3; 2018,Jan,8; 2017,Sep,14; 2017,Jan,8; 2016,Jan,13

92014 **comprehensive, established patient, 1 or more visits**

INCLUDES General evaluation complete visual system
Integrated services where medical decision making cannot be separated from examination methods
Single service that need not be performed at one session
Comprehensive services:
Basic sensorimotor examination
Biomicroscopy
Dilation (cycloplegia)
External examinations
General medical observation
Gross visual fields
History
Initiation diagnostic/treatment programs
Mydriasis
Ophthalmoscopic examinations
Other diagnostic procedures
Prescription medication
Special diagnostic/treatment services
Tonometry

🚑 2.25 👥 3.57 **FUD** XXX V 80 🖵

AMA: 2018,Feb,11; 2018,Feb,3; 2018,Jan,8; 2017,Sep,14; 2017,Jan,8; 2016,Nov,9; 2016,Jan,13

92015-92145 Ophthalmic Special Services

INCLUDES Routine ophthalmoscopy
EXCLUDES Surgical procedures on eye/ocular adnexa (65091-68899 [66987, 66988, 67810])
Code also:
E/M services, when performed
General ophthalmological services, when performed (92002-92014)

92015 **Determination of refractive state**

INCLUDES Lens prescription:
Absorptive factor
Axis
Impact resistance
Lens power
Prism
Specification lens type:
Bifocal
Monofocal

EXCLUDES Ocular screening, instrument based (99173-99174 [99177])

🚑 0.55 👥 0.56 **FUD** XXX E 🖵

AMA: 2020,Dec,13; 2018,Feb,11; 2018,Jan,8; 2017,Jan,8; 2016,Mar,10; 2016,Jan,13

92018 **Ophthalmological examination and evaluation, under general anesthesia, with or without manipulation of globe for passive range of motion or other manipulation to facilitate diagnostic examination; complete**

🚑 4.06 👥 4.06 **FUD** XXX J 80 🖵

AMA: 2018,Feb,11; 2018,Jan,8; 2017,Jan,8; 2016,Jan,13

92019 limited

📠 2.05   ⚕ 2.05   **FUD** XXX   [J] [80] 🖵

AMA: 2018,Feb,11; 2018,Jan,8; 2017,Jan,8; 2016,Jan,13

92020 Gonioscopy (separate procedure)

EXCLUDES   *Gonioscopy under general anesthesia (92018)*
Laser trabeculostomy ab interno (0621T-0622T)

📠 0.60   ⚕ 0.78   **FUD** XXX   [01] [80] 🖵

AMA: 2018,Feb,11; 2018,Jan,8; 2017,Jan,8; 2016,Jan,13

92025 Computerized corneal topography, unilateral or bilateral, with interpretation and report

EXCLUDES   *Corneal transplant procedures (65710-65771)*
Manual keratoscopy

📠 1.04   ⚕ 1.04   **FUD** XXX   [01] [80] 🖵

AMA: 2018,Feb,11; 2018,Jan,8; 2017,Jan,8; 2016,Jan,13

92060 Sensorimotor examination with multiple measurements of ocular deviation (eg, restrictive or paretic muscle with diplopia) with interpretation and report (separate procedure)

📠 1.79   ⚕ 1.79   **FUD** XXX   [01] [80] 🖵

AMA: 2018,Feb,11; 2018,Jan,8; 2017,Jan,8; 2016,Jan,13

▲ 92065 Orthoptic training

📠 1.49   ⚕ 1.49   **FUD** XXX   [01] [80] 🖵

AMA: 2018,Feb,11; 2018,Jan,8; 2017,Jan,8; 2016,Jan,13

92071 Fitting of contact lens for treatment of ocular surface disease

EXCLUDES   *Contact lens service for keratoconus (92072)*
Code also lens supply with appropriate supply code or (99070)

📠 0.95   ⚕ 1.07   **FUD** XXX   [N] [80] [50] 🖵

AMA: 2018,Feb,11

92072 Fitting of contact lens for management of keratoconus, initial fitting

EXCLUDES   *Contact lens service for disease ocular surface (92071)*
Subsequent fittings (99211-99215, 92012-92014)
Code also lens supply with appropriate supply code or (99070)

📠 2.84   ⚕ 3.72   **FUD** XXX   [N] [80] 🖵

AMA: 2018,Feb,11; 2018,Jan,8; 2017,Sep,14; 2017,Jan,8; 2016,Jan,13

92081 Visual field examination, unilateral or bilateral, with interpretation and report; limited examination (eg, tangent screen, Autoplot, arc perimeter, or single stimulus level automated test, such as Octopus 3 or 7 equivalent)

INCLUDES   Gross visual testing/confrontation testing

📠 0.95   ⚕ 0.95   **FUD** XXX   [01] [80] 🖵

AMA: 2018,Feb,11; 2018,Jan,8; 2017,Jan,8; 2016,Jan,13

92082 intermediate examination (eg, at least 2 isopters on Goldmann perimeter, or semiquantitative, automated suprathreshold screening program, Humphrey suprathreshold automatic diagnostic test, Octopus program 33)

INCLUDES   Gross visual testing/confrontation testing

📠 1.34   ⚕ 1.34   **FUD** XXX   [01] [80] 🖵

AMA: 2018,Feb,11; 2018,Jan,8; 2017,Jan,8; 2016,Jan,13

92083 extended examination (eg, Goldmann visual fields with at least 3 isopters plotted and static determination within the central 30°, or quantitative, automated threshold perimetry, Octopus program G-1, 32 or 42, Humphrey visual field analyzer full threshold programs 30-2, 24-2, or 30/60-2)

INCLUDES   Gross visual field testing/confrontation testing
EXCLUDES   *Assessment visual field, by data transmission, by patient to surveillance center (0378T-0379T)*

📠 1.78   ⚕ 1.78   **FUD** XXX   [01] [80] 🖵

AMA: 2018,Feb,11; 2018,Jan,8; 2017,Jan,8; 2016,Jan,13

92100 Serial tonometry (separate procedure) with multiple measurements of intraocular pressure over an extended time period with interpretation and report, same day (eg, diurnal curve or medical treatment of acute elevation of intraocular pressure)

EXCLUDES   *Intraocular pressure monitoring for 24 hours or more (0329T)*
Ocular blood flow measurements (0198T)
Single-episode tonometry (99202-99215, 92002-92004)

📠 0.96   ⚕ 2.32   **FUD** XXX   [N] [80] 🖵

AMA: 2018,Feb,11; 2018,Jan,8; 2017,Jan,8; 2016,Jan,13

92132 Scanning computerized ophthalmic diagnostic imaging, anterior segment, with interpretation and report, unilateral or bilateral

EXCLUDES   *Imaging anterior segment with specular microscopy and endothelial cell analysis (92286)*
Scanning computerized ophthalmic diagnostic imaging optic nerve and retina (92133-92134)
Tear film imaging (0330T)

📠 0.89   ⚕ 0.89   **FUD** XXX   [01] [80] 🖵

AMA: 2018,Feb,11; 2018,Jan,8; 2017,Jan,8; 2016,Jan,13

92133 Scanning computerized ophthalmic diagnostic imaging, posterior segment, with interpretation and report, unilateral or bilateral; optic nerve

EXCLUDES   *Remote imaging for retinal disease (92227-92228)*
Scanning computerized ophthalmic imaging retina same visit (92134)

📠 1.05   ⚕ 1.05   **FUD** XXX   [01] [80] 🖵

AMA: 2018,Feb,11; 2018,Jan,8; 2017,Jan,8; 2016,Jan,13

92134 retina

EXCLUDES   *Remote imaging for retinal disease (92227-92228)*
Scanning computerized ophthalmic imaging retina same visit (92134)

📠 1.15   ⚕ 1.15   **FUD** XXX   [01] [80] 🖵

AMA: 2018,Feb,11; 2018,Jan,8; 2017,Jan,8; 2016,Jan,13

92136 Ophthalmic biometry by partial coherence interferometry with intraocular lens power calculation

EXCLUDES   *Tear film imaging (0330T)*

📠 1.76   ⚕ 1.76   **FUD** XXX   [01] [80] 🖵

AMA: 2018,Feb,11; 2018,Jan,8; 2017,Jan,8; 2016,Jan,13

92145 Corneal hysteresis determination, by air impulse stimulation, unilateral or bilateral, with interpretation and report

📠 0.42   ⚕ 0.42   **FUD** XXX   [01] [80] 🖵

AMA: 2018,Feb,11

92201-92287 Other Ophthalmology Services

EXCLUDES   *Ophthalmological exam under anesthesia (92018)*
Prescription, fitting, and/or medical supervision ocular prosthesis adaptation by physician (99202-99215, 99241-99245, 92002-92014)
Surgical procedures on eye/ocular adnexa (65091-68899 [66987, 66988, 67810])

92201 Ophthalmoscopy, extended; with retinal drawing and scleral depression of peripheral retinal disease (eg, for retinal tear, retinal detachment, retinal tumor) with interpretation and report, unilateral or bilateral

EXCLUDES   *Fundus photography with interpretation and report (92250)*

📠 0.65   ⚕ 0.71   **FUD** XXX   [80] 🖵

AMA: 2019,Dec,3

92202 with drawing of optic nerve or macula (eg, for glaucoma, macular pathology, tumor) with interpretation and report, unilateral or bilateral

EXCLUDES   *Fundus photography with interpretation and report (92250)*

📠 0.42   ⚕ 0.45   **FUD** XXX   [80] 🖵

AMA: 2019,Dec,3

| 26/TC PC/TC Only | A2-Z3 ASC Payment | 50 Bilateral | ♂ Male Only | ♀ Female Only | 📠 Facility RVU | ⚕ Non-Facility RVU | 🖵 CCI | ☒ CLIA |
| FUD Follow-up Days | CMS: IOM | AMA: CPT Asst | A-Y OPPSI | 80/80 Surg Assist Allowed / w/Doc | | 🖵 Lab Crosswalk | 🖵 Radiology Crosswalk | |

468   CPT © 2021 American Medical Association. All Rights Reserved.   © 2021 Optum360, LLC

Medicine

92019 — 92202

92227 Imaging of retina for detection or monitoring of disease; with remote clinical staff review and report, unilateral or bilateral

EXCLUDES *Fundus photography with interpretation and report (92250)*
Imaging for retinal disease:
Point of care automated analysis and report (92229)
Remote interpretation and report (92228)
Scanning computerized ophthalmic imaging:
Optic nerve (92133)
Retina (92134)

🔲 0.40 🔲 0.40 **FUD** XXX ★ 🔲 🔲 🔲 🔲

AMA: 2019,Aug,10; 2018,Feb,11; 2018,Jan,8; 2017,Jan,8; 2016,Jul,8; 2016,Jan,13

92228 with remote physician or other qualified health care professional interpretation and report, unilateral or bilateral

EXCLUDES *Fundus photography with interpretation and report (92250)*
Imaging for retinal disease:
Point of care automated analysis and report (92229)
Remote clinical staff review and report (92227)
Scanning computerized ophthalmic imaging:
Optic nerve (92133)
Retina (92134)

🔲 0.97 🔲 0.97 **FUD** XXX ★ 🔲 🔲 🔲

AMA: 2018,Feb,11; 2018,Jan,8; 2017,Jan,8; 2016,Jan,13

92229 point-of-care automated analysis and report, unilateral or bilateral

EXCLUDES *Fundus photography with interpretation and report (92250)*
Remote imaging for retinal disease (92227-92228)
Scanning computerized ophthalmic imaging:
Optic nerve (92133)
Retina (92134)

🔲 0.00 🔲 0.00 **FUD** XXX 🔲 🔲 🔲

92230 Fluorescein angioscopy with interpretation and report

🔲 0.95 🔲 1.83 **FUD** XXX 🔲 🔲 🔲

AMA: 2018,Feb,11; 2018,Jan,8; 2017,Jan,8; 2016,Jan,13

92235 Fluorescein angiography (includes multiframe imaging) with interpretation and report, unilateral or bilateral

EXCLUDES *Fluorescein and indocyanine-green angiography (92242)*

🔲 2.93 🔲 2.93 **FUD** XXX 🔲 🔲 🔲

AMA: 2018,Feb,11; 2018,Jan,8; 2017,Jun,8; 2017,Jan,8; 2016,Jan,13

92240 Indocyanine-green angiography (includes multiframe imaging) with interpretation and report, unilateral or bilateral

EXCLUDES *Fluorescein and indocyanine-green angiography (92242)*

🔲 5.69 🔲 5.69 **FUD** XXX 🔲 🔲 🔲

AMA: 2018,Feb,11; 2018,Jan,8; 2017,Jun,8; 2017,Jan,8; 2016,Jan,13

92242 Fluorescein angiography and indocyanine-green angiography (includes multiframe imaging) performed at the same patient encounter with interpretation and report, unilateral or bilateral

🔲 6.71 🔲 6.71 **FUD** XXX 🔲 🔲 🔲

AMA: 2018,Feb,11; 2018,Jan,8; 2017,Jun,8

92250 Fundus photography with interpretation and report

🔲 1.27 🔲 1.27 **FUD** XXX 🔲 🔲 🔲

AMA: 2019,Dec,3; 2018,Feb,11; 2018,Jan,8; 2017,Jan,8; 2016,Jul,8; 2016,Jan,13

92260 Ophthalmodynamometry

🔲 0.31 🔲 0.55 **FUD** XXX 🔲 🔲 🔲

AMA: 2018,Feb,11; 2018,Jan,8; 2017,Jan,8; 2016,Jan,13

92265 Needle oculoelectromyography, 1 or more extraocular muscles, 1 or both eyes, with interpretation and report

🔲 2.45 🔲 2.45 **FUD** XXX 🔲 🔲 🔲

AMA: 2018,Feb,11; 2018,Jan,8; 2017,Jan,8; 2016,Jan,13

92270 Electro-oculography with interpretation and report

EXCLUDES *Recording saccadic eye movement (92700)*
Vestibular function testing (92537-92538, 92540-92542, 92544-92549)

🔲 2.73 🔲 2.73 **FUD** XXX 🔲 🔲 🔲

AMA: 2020,Apr,7; 2018,Feb,11; 2018,Jan,8; 2017,Jan,8; 2016,Jan,13

92273 Electroretinography (ERG), with interpretation and report; full field (ie, ffERG, flash ERG, Ganzfeld ERG)

EXCLUDES *Pattern electroretinography (PERG) (0509T)*

🔲 3.78 🔲 3.78 **FUD** XXX 🔲 🔲

AMA: 2019,Jan,12

92274 multifocal (mfERG)

EXCLUDES *Pattern electroretinography (PERG) (0509T)*

🔲 2.56 🔲 2.56 **FUD** XXX 🔲 🔲

AMA: 2019,Jan,12

92283 Color vision examination, extended, eg, anomaloscope or equivalent

🔲 1.49 🔲 1.49 **FUD** XXX 🔲 🔲 🔲

AMA: 2018,Feb,11; 2018,Jan,8; 2017,Jan,8; 2016,Jan,13

92284 Dark adaptation examination with interpretation and report

🔲 1.68 🔲 1.68 **FUD** XXX 🔲 🔲 🔲

AMA: 2018,Feb,11; 2018,Jan,8; 2017,Jan,8; 2016,Jan,13

92285 External ocular photography with interpretation and report for documentation of medical progress (eg, close-up photography, slit lamp photography, goniophotography, stereo-photography)

🔲 0.62 🔲 0.62 **FUD** XXX 🔲 🔲 🔲

AMA: 2018,Feb,11; 2018,Jan,8; 2017,Jan,8; 2016,Jan,13

92286 Anterior segment imaging with interpretation and report; with specular microscopy and endothelial cell analysis

🔲 1.10 🔲 1.10 **FUD** XXX 🔲 🔲 🔲

AMA: 2018,Feb,11; 2018,Jan,8; 2017,Jan,8; 2016,Jan,13

92287 with fluorescein angiography

🔲 4.46 🔲 4.46 **FUD** XXX 🔲 🔲 🔲

AMA: 2018,Feb,11; 2018,Jan,8; 2017,Jan,8; 2016,Jan,13

92310-92326 Services Related to Contact Lenses

CMS: 100-02,15,30.4 Optometrist's Services

INCLUDES Incidental revision lens during training period
Patient training/instruction
Specification optical/physical characteristics:
Curvature
Flexibility
Gas-permeability
Power
Size

EXCLUDES *Extended wear lenses follow up (92012-92014)*
General ophthalmological services
Therapeutic/surgical use contact lens (68340, 92071-92072)

92310 Prescription of optical and physical characteristics of and fitting of contact lens, with medical supervision of adaptation; corneal lens, both eyes, except for aphakia

Code also modifier 52 for prescription and fitting only one eye

🔲 1.69 🔲 2.80 **FUD** XXX 🔲 🔲

AMA: 2018,Feb,11; 2018,Jan,8; 2017,Jan,8; 2016,Jan,13

92311 corneal lens for aphakia, 1 eye

🔲 1.57 🔲 2.94 **FUD** XXX 🔲 🔲 🔲

AMA: 2018,Feb,11; 2018,Jan,8; 2017,Jan,8; 2016,Jan,13

92312 corneal lens for aphakia, both eyes

🔲 1.81 🔲 3.40 **FUD** XXX 🔲 🔲 🔲

AMA: 2018,Feb,11; 2018,Jan,8; 2017,Jan,8; 2016,Jan,13

92313   **corneoscleral lens**
    🔧 1.31   📐 2.78   **FUD** XXX   `01` `80` 🖵
    AMA: 2018,Feb,11; 2018,Jan,8; 2017,Jan,8; 2016,Jan,13

92314   **Prescription of optical and physical characteristics of contact lens, with medical supervision of adaptation and direction of fitting by independent technician; corneal lens, both eyes except for aphakia**
    Code also modifier 52 for prescription and fitting only one eye
    🔧 1.00   📐 2.36   **FUD** XXX   `E` 🖵
    AMA: 2018,Feb,11; 2018,Jan,8; 2017,Jan,8; 2016,Jan,13

92315   **corneal lens for aphakia, 1 eye**
    🔧 0.62   📐 2.19   **FUD** XXX   `01` `80` 🖵
    AMA: 2018,Feb,11; 2018,Jan,8; 2017,Jan,8; 2016,Jan,13

92316   **corneal lens for aphakia, both eyes**
    🔧 0.92   📐 2.76   **FUD** XXX   `01` `80` 🖵
    AMA: 2018,Feb,11; 2018,Jan,8; 2017,Jan,8; 2016,Jan,13

92317   **corneoscleral lens**
    🔧 0.61   📐 2.32   **FUD** XXX   `01` `80` 🖵
    AMA: 2018,Feb,11; 2018,Jan,8; 2017,Jan,8; 2016,Jan,13

92325   **Modification of contact lens (separate procedure), with medical supervision of adaptation**
    🔧 1.24   📐 1.24   **FUD** XXX   `01` `80` 🖵
    AMA: 2018,Feb,11; 2018,Jan,8; 2017,Jan,8; 2016,Jan,13

92326   **Replacement of contact lens**
    🔧 1.06   📐 1.06   **FUD** XXX   `01` `80` 🖵
    AMA: 2018,Feb,11; 2018,Jan,8; 2017,Jan,8; 2016,Jan,13

92340-92499 Services Related to Eyeglasses

CMS: 100-02,15,30.4 Optometrist's Services
INCLUDES Anatomical facial characteristics measurement
Final adjustment of spectacles to visual axes/anatomical topography
Written laboratory specifications
EXCLUDES *Materials supply*

92340   **Fitting of spectacles, except for aphakia; monofocal**
    🔧 0.53   📐 0.99   **FUD** XXX   `E` 🖵
    AMA: 2018,Feb,11; 2018,Jan,8; 2017,Jan,8; 2016,Jan,13

92341   **bifocal**
    🔧 0.68   📐 1.14   **FUD** XXX   `E` 🖵
    AMA: 2018,Feb,11; 2018,Jan,8; 2017,Jan,8; 2016,Jan,13

92342   **multifocal, other than bifocal**
    🔧 0.78   📐 1.23   **FUD** XXX   `E` 🖵
    AMA: 2018,Feb,11; 2018,Jan,8; 2017,Jan,8; 2016,Jan,13

92352   **Fitting of spectacle prosthesis for aphakia; monofocal**
    🔧 0.53   📐 1.17   **FUD** XXX   `01` 🖵
    AMA: 2018,Feb,11; 2018,Jan,8; 2017,Jan,8; 2016,Jan,13

92353   **multifocal**
    🔧 0.72   📐 1.36   **FUD** XXX   `01` 🖵
    AMA: 2018,Feb,11; 2018,Jan,8; 2017,Jan,8; 2016,Jan,13

92354   **Fitting of spectacle mounted low vision aid; single element system**
    🔧 0.37   📐 0.37   **FUD** XXX   `01` 🖵
    AMA: 2018,Feb,11; 2018,Jan,8; 2017,Jan,8; 2016,Jan,13

92355   **telescopic or other compound lens system**
    🔧 0.59   📐 0.59   **FUD** XXX   `01` 🖵
    AMA: 2018,Feb,11; 2018,Jan,8; 2017,Jan,8; 2016,Jan,13

92358   **Prosthesis service for aphakia, temporary (disposable or loan, including materials)**
    🔧 0.31   📐 0.31   **FUD** XXX   `01` 🖵
    AMA: 2018,Feb,11; 2018,Jan,8; 2017,Jan,8; 2016,Jan,13

92370   **Repair and refitting spectacles; except for aphakia**
    🔧 0.46   📐 0.88   **FUD** XXX   `E` 🖵
    AMA: 2018,Feb,11; 2018,Jan,8; 2017,Jan,8; 2016,Jan,13

92371   **spectacle prosthesis for aphakia**
    🔧 0.33   📐 0.33   **FUD** XXX   `01` 🖵
    AMA: 2018,Feb,11; 2018,Jan,8; 2017,Jan,8; 2016,Jan,13

92499   **Unlisted ophthalmological service or procedure**
    🔧 0.00   📐 0.00   **FUD** XXX   `01` `80` 🖵
    AMA: 2020,Dec,13; 2020,Aug,14; 2019,Jan,12; 2018,Jul,3; 2018,Feb,11; 2018,Jan,8; 2017,Jan,8; 2016,Jan,13

92502-92526 [92517, 92518, 92519] Special Procedures of the Ears/Nose/Throat

INCLUDES Anterior rhinoscopy, tuning fork testing, otoscopy, or removal non-impacted cerumen
Diagnostic/treatment services not generally included in E/M service
EXCLUDES *Laryngoscopy with stroboscopy (31579)*

92502   **Otolaryngologic examination under general anesthesia**
    🔧 2.73   📐 2.73   **FUD** 000   `T` `80` 🖵
    AMA: 2018,Feb,11; 2018,Jan,8; 2017,Jan,8; 2016,Sep,6

92504   **Binocular microscopy (separate diagnostic procedure)**
    🔧 0.27   📐 0.83   **FUD** XXX   `N` `80` 🖵
    AMA: 2018,Feb,11; 2018,Jan,8; 2017,Jan,8; 2016,Sep,6; 2016,Jan,13

92507   **Treatment of speech, language, voice, communication, and/or auditory processing disorder; individual**
    EXCLUDES *Adaptive behavior treatment ([97153], [97155])*
    Auditory rehabilitation:
      Postlingual hearing loss (92633)
      Prelingual hearing loss (92630)
      Programming cochlear implant (92601-92604)
    🔧 2.23   📐 2.23   **FUD** XXX   `A` `80` 🖵
    AMA: 2018,Dec,7; 2018,Dec,7; 2018,Nov,3; 2018,Feb,11; 2018,Jan,8; 2017,Jan,8; 2016,Sep,6; 2016,Jan,13

92508   **group, 2 or more individuals**
    EXCLUDES *Adaptive behavior treatment ([97154], [97158])*
    Auditory rehabilitation:
      Postlingual hearing loss (92633)
      Prelingual hearing loss (92630)
      Programming cochlear implant (92601-92604)
    🔧 0.68   📐 0.68   **FUD** XXX   `A` `80` 🖵
    AMA: 2018,Nov,3; 2018,Feb,11; 2018,Jan,8; 2017,Jan,8; 2016,Sep,6; 2016,Jan,13

92511   **Nasopharyngoscopy with endoscope (separate procedure)**
    EXCLUDES *Diagnostic flexible laryngoscopy (31575)*
    Drug-induced sleep endoscopy (42975)
    Nasopharyngoscopic dilation eustachian tube (69705-69706)
    Transnasal esophagoscopy (43197-43198)
    🔧 1.08   📐 3.15   **FUD** 000   `T` `80` 🖵
    AMA: 2018,Feb,11; 2018,Jan,8; 2017,Jul,7; 2017,Jan,8; 2016,Dec,13; 2016,Sep,6

92512   **Nasal function studies (eg, rhinomanometry)**
    🔧 0.80   📐 1.68   **FUD** XXX   `S` `80` 🖵
    AMA: 2018,Feb,11; 2018,Jan,8; 2017,Jan,8; 2016,Sep,6

92516   **Facial nerve function studies (eg, electroneuronography)**
    🔧 0.65   📐 1.94   **FUD** XXX   `S` `80` 🖵
    AMA: 2018,Feb,11; 2018,Jan,8; 2017,Jan,8; 2016,Sep,6

92517   **Resequenced code. See code following 92549.**

92518   **Resequenced code. See code following 92549.**

92519   **Resequenced code. See code following 92549.**

92520   **Laryngeal function studies (ie, aerodynamic testing and acoustic testing)**
    EXCLUDES *Other laryngeal function testing (92700)*
    Swallowing/laryngeal sensory testing with flexible fiberoptic endoscope (92611-92617)
    Code also modifier 52 for single test
    🔧 1.15   📐 2.23   **FUD** XXX   `01` `80` 🖵
    AMA: 2018,Feb,11; 2018,Jan,8; 2017,Jan,8; 2016,Sep,6; 2016,Jan,13

`26`/`16` PC/TC Only   `A2`-`Z3` ASC Payment   `50` Bilateral   ♂ Male Only   ♀ Female Only   🔧 Facility RVU   📐 Non-Facility RVU   🖵 CCI   ✖ CLIA
FUD Follow-up Days   **CMS:** IOM   **AMA:** CPT Asst   `A`-`Y` OPPSI   `80`/`80` Surg Assist Allowed / w/Doc   Lab Crosswalk   Radiology Crosswalk

470   CPT © 2021 American Medical Association. All Rights Reserved.   © 2021 Optum360, LLC

92521 **Evaluation of speech fluency (eg, stuttering, cluttering)**

INCLUDES Ability to execute motor movements needed for speech

Comprehension written and verbal expression

Determination patient's ability to create and communicate expressive thought

Evaluation ability to produce speech sound

🚗 3.21 ⚖ 3.21 **FUD** XXX A 80 ▭

AMA: 2018,Feb,11; 2018,Jan,8; 2017,Jan,8; 2016,Sep,6; 2016,Jan,13

92522 **Evaluation of speech sound production (eg, articulation, phonological process, apraxia, dysarthria);**

INCLUDES Ability to execute motor movements needed for speech

Comprehension written and verbal expression

Determination patient's ability to create and communicate expressive thought

Evaluation ability to produce speech sound

🚗 2.60 ⚖ 2.60 **FUD** XXX A 80 ▭

AMA: 2018,Feb,11; 2018,Jan,8; 2017,Jan,8; 2016,Sep,6; 2016,Jan,13

92523 **with evaluation of language comprehension and expression (eg, receptive and expressive language)**

INCLUDES Ability to execute motor movements needed for speech

Comprehension written and verbal expression

Determination patient's ability to create and communicate expressive thought

Evaluation ability to produce speech sound

🚗 5.54 ⚖ 5.54 **FUD** XXX A 80 ▭

AMA: 2018,Feb,11; 2018,Jan,8; 2017,Jan,8; 2016,Sep,6; 2016,Jan,13

92524 **Behavioral and qualitative analysis of voice and resonance**

INCLUDES Ability to execute motor movements needed for speech

Comprehension written and verbal expression

Determination patient's ability to create and communicate expressive thought

Evaluation ability to produce speech sound

🚗 2.51 ⚖ 2.51 **FUD** XXX A 80 ▭

AMA: 2018,Feb,11; 2018,Jan,8; 2017,Jan,8; 2016,Sep,6; 2016,Jan,13

92526 **Treatment of swallowing dysfunction and/or oral function for feeding**

🚗 2.44 ⚖ 2.44 **FUD** XXX A 80 ▭

AMA: 2018,Feb,11; 2018,Jan,8; 2017,Jan,8; 2016,Sep,6

92531-92519 [92517, 92518, 92519] Vestibular Function Tests

92531 **Spontaneous nystagmus, including gaze**

EXCLUDES When performed with E/M services (99202-99215, 99218-99223 [99224, 99225, 99226], 99231-99236, 99241-99245, 99304-99318, 99324-99337)

🚗 0.00 ⚖ 0.00 **FUD** XXX N ▭

AMA: 2020,Aug,14; 2018,Feb,11

92532 **Positional nystagmus test**

EXCLUDES When performed with E/M services (99202-99215, 99218-99223 [99224, 99225, 99226], 99231-99236, 99241-99245, 99304-99318, 99324-99337)

🚗 0.00 ⚖ 0.00 **FUD** XXX N ▭

AMA: 2020,Aug,14; 2018,Feb,11

92533 **Caloric vestibular test, each irrigation (binaural, bithermal stimulation constitutes 4 tests)**

INCLUDES Barany caloric test

🚗 0.00 ⚖ 0.00 **FUD** XXX N ▭

AMA: 2020,Aug,14; 2018,Feb,11; 2018,Jan,8; 2017,Jan,8; 2016,Jan,13

92534 **Optokinetic nystagmus test**

🚗 0.00 ⚖ 0.00 **FUD** XXX N ▭

AMA: 2020,Aug,14; 2018,Feb,11

92537 **Caloric vestibular test with recording, bilateral; bithermal (ie, one warm and one cool irrigation in each ear for a total of four irrigations)**

EXCLUDES Electro-oculography (92270)

Monothermal caloric vestibular test (92538)

Code also modifier 52 when only three irrigations performed

🚗 1.18 ⚖ 1.18 **FUD** XXX S 80 ▭

AMA: 2020,Aug,14; 2018,Feb,11

92538 **monothermal (ie, one irrigation in each ear for a total of two irrigations)**

EXCLUDES Bithermal caloric vestibular test (92537)

Electro-oculography (92270)

Code also modifier 52 only one irrigation performed

🚗 0.64 ⚖ 0.64 **FUD** XXX S 80 ▭

AMA: 2020,Aug,14; 2018,Feb,11

92540 **Basic vestibular evaluation, includes spontaneous nystagmus test with eccentric gaze fixation nystagmus, with recording, positional nystagmus test, minimum of 4 positions, with recording, optokinetic nystagmus test, bidirectional foveal and peripheral stimulation, with recording, and oscillating tracking test, with recording**

EXCLUDES Vestibular function tests (92270, 92541-92542, 92544-92545)

🚗 3.04 ⚖ 3.04 **FUD** XXX S 80 ▭

AMA: 2020,Aug,14; 2018,Feb,11; 2018,Jan,8; 2017,Jan,8; 2016,Jan,13

92541 **Spontaneous nystagmus test, including gaze and fixation nystagmus, with recording**

EXCLUDES Vestibular function tests (92270, 92540, 92542, 92544-92545)

🚗 0.72 ⚖ 0.72 **FUD** XXX 01 80 ▭

AMA: 2020,Aug,14; 2019,Jan,12; 2018,Feb,11; 2018,Jan,8; 2017,Jan,8; 2016,Jan,13

92542 **Positional nystagmus test, minimum of 4 positions, with recording**

EXCLUDES Vestibular function tests (92270, 92540-92541, 92544-92545)

🚗 0.84 ⚖ 0.84 **FUD** XXX 01 80 ▭

AMA: 2020,Aug,14; 2018,Feb,11; 2018,Jan,8; 2017,Jan,8; 2016,Jan,13

92544 **Optokinetic nystagmus test, bidirectional, foveal or peripheral stimulation, with recording**

EXCLUDES Vestibular function tests (92270, 92540-92542, 92545)

🚗 0.50 ⚖ 0.50 **FUD** XXX S 80 ▭

AMA: 2020,Aug,14; 2018,Feb,11; 2018,Jan,8; 2017,Jan,8; 2016,Jan,13

92545 **Oscillating tracking test, with recording**

EXCLUDES Vestibular function tests (92270, 92540-92542, 92544)

🚗 0.47 ⚖ 0.47 **FUD** XXX S 80 ▭

AMA: 2020,Aug,14; 2018,Feb,11; 2018,Jan,8; 2017,Jan,8; 2016,Jan,13

92546 **Sinusoidal vertical axis rotational testing**

EXCLUDES Electro-oculography (92270)

🚗 3.15 ⚖ 3.15 **FUD** XXX S 80 ▭

AMA: 2020,Aug,14; 2018,Feb,11; 2018,Jan,8; 2017,Jan,8; 2016,Jan,13

+ 92547 **Use of vertical electrodes (List separately in addition to code for primary procedure)**

EXCLUDES Electro-oculography (92270)

Unlisted vestibular tests (92700)

Code first (92540-92546)

🚗 0.21 ⚖ 0.21 **FUD** ZZZ N 80 TC ▭

AMA: 2020,Aug,14; 2018,Feb,11; 2018,Jan,8; 2017,Jan,8; 2016,Jan,13

92548   Computerized dynamic posturography sensory organization test (CDP-SOT), 6 conditions (ie, eyes open, eyes closed, visual sway, platform sway, eyes closed platform sway, platform and visual sway), including interpretation and report;

     EXCLUDES   Electro-oculography (92270)

     🖥 1.41   🔧 1.41   **FUD** XXX   01 80 🔲

     AMA: 2020,Aug,14; 2020,Apr,7; 2018,Feb,11; 2018,Jan,8; 2017,Jan,8; 2016,Jan,13

92549   with motor control test (MCT) and adaptation test (ADT)

     EXCLUDES   Electro-oculography (92270)

     🖥 1.80   🔧 1.80   **FUD** XXX   80 🔲

     AMA: 2020,Aug,14; 2020,Apr,7

**92517**   Vestibular evoked myogenic potential (VEMP) testing, with interpretation and report; cervical (cVEMP)

     EXCLUDES   Electro-oculography (92270)
          Vestibular evoked myogenic potential testing:
            Cervical and ocular ([92519])
            Ocular ([92518])

     🖥 1.26   🔧 2.50   **FUD** XXX   80 🔲

**92518**   ocular (oVEMP)

     EXCLUDES   Electro-oculography (92270)
          Vestibular evoked myogenic potential testing:
            Cervical ([92517])
            Cervical and ocular ([92519])

     🖥 1.26   🔧 2.33   **FUD** XXX   80 🔲

**92519**   cervical (cVEMP) and ocular (oVEMP)

     EXCLUDES   Electro-oculography (92270)
          Vestibular evoked myogenic potential testing:
            Cervical only ([92517])
            Ocular only ([92518])

     🖥 1.89   🔧 3.88   **FUD** XXX   80 🔲

92550-92597 [92558, 92597, 92650, 92651, 92652, 92653]
Hearing and Speech Tests

   INCLUDES   Calibrated electronic equipment, recording results, and report with interpretation
          Diagnostic/treatment services not generally included in comprehensive otorhinolaryngologic evaluation or office visit
          Testing both ears
          Tuning fork and whisper tests
   EXCLUDES   Evaluation speech/language/hearing problems using performance observation/assessment (92521-92524)
   Code also modifier 52 for unilateral testing

92550   Tympanometry and reflex threshold measurements

     INCLUDES   Tympanometry, acoustic reflex testing individual codes (92567-92568)

     🖥 0.62   🔧 0.62   **FUD** XXX   01 80 🔲

     AMA: 2018,Feb,11; 2018,Jan,8; 2017,Jan,8; 2016,Jan,13

92551   Screening test, pure tone, air only

     🖥 0.33   🔧 0.33   **FUD** XXX   E 🔲

     AMA: 2018,Feb,11; 2018,Jan,8; 2017,Jan,8; 2016,Jan,13

92552   Pure tone audiometry (threshold); air only

     EXCLUDES   Automated test (0208T)

     🖥 0.89   🔧 0.89   **FUD** XXX   01 80 TC 🔲

     AMA: 2018,Feb,11; 2018,Jan,8; 2017,Jan,8; 2016,Jan,13

92553   air and bone

     EXCLUDES   Automated test (0209T)

     🖥 1.08   🔧 1.08   **FUD** XXX   01 80 TC 🔲

     AMA: 2018,Feb,11; 2018,Jan,8; 2017,Jan,8; 2016,Jan,13

92555   Speech audiometry threshold;

     EXCLUDES   Automated test (0210T)

     🖥 0.68   🔧 0.68   **FUD** XXX   01 80 TC 🔲

     AMA: 2018,Feb,11; 2018,Jan,8; 2017,Jan,8; 2016,Jan,13

92556   with speech recognition

     EXCLUDES   Automated test (0211T)

     🖥 1.07   🔧 1.07   **FUD** XXX   01 80 TC 🔲

     AMA: 2018,Feb,11; 2018,Jan,8; 2017,Jan,8; 2016,Jan,13

92557   Comprehensive audiometry threshold evaluation and speech recognition (92553 and 92556 combined)

     EXCLUDES   Automated test (0208T-0212T)
          Evaluation/selection hearing aid (92590-92595)

     🖥 0.93   🔧 1.08   **FUD** XXX   01 80 🔲

     AMA: 2018,Feb,11; 2018,Jan,8; 2017,Jan,8; 2016,Jan,13

92558   Resequenced code. See code before 92587.

92559   ~~Audiometric testing of groups~~

     To report, see (92700)

92560   ~~Bekesy audiometry; screening~~

     To report, see (92700)

92561   ~~diagnostic~~

     To report, see (92700)

92562   Loudness balance test, alternate binaural or monaural

     INCLUDES   ABLB test

     🖥 1.25   🔧 1.25   **FUD** XXX   01 80 TC 🔲

     AMA: 2018,Feb,11; 2018,Jan,8; 2017,Jan,8; 2016,Jan,13

92563   Tone decay test

     🖥 0.86   🔧 0.86   **FUD** XXX   01 80 TC 🔲

     AMA: 2018,Feb,11; 2018,Jan,8; 2017,Jan,8; 2016,Jan,13

92564   ~~Short increment sensitivity index (SISI)~~

     To report, see (92700)

92565   Stenger test, pure tone

     🖥 0.44   🔧 0.44   **FUD** XXX   01 80 TC 🔲

     AMA: 2018,Feb,11; 2018,Jan,8; 2017,Jan,8; 2016,Jan,13

92567   Tympanometry (impedance testing)

     🖥 0.31   🔧 0.45   **FUD** XXX   01 80 🔲

     AMA: 2018,Feb,11; 2018,Jan,8; 2017,Jan,8; 2016,Jan,13

92568   Acoustic reflex testing, threshold

     🖥 0.44   🔧 0.45   **FUD** XXX   01 80 🔲

     AMA: 2018,Feb,11; 2018,Jan,8; 2017,Jan,8; 2016,Jan,13

92570   Acoustic immittance testing, includes tympanometry (impedance testing), acoustic reflex threshold testing, and acoustic reflex decay testing

     INCLUDES   Tympanometry, acoustic reflex testing individual codes (92567-92568)

     🖥 0.85   🔧 0.92   **FUD** XXX   01 80 🔲

     AMA: 2018,Feb,11; 2018,Jan,8; 2017,Jan,8; 2016,Jan,13

92571   Filtered speech test

     🖥 0.76   🔧 0.76   **FUD** XXX   01 80 TC 🔲

     AMA: 2018,Feb,11; 2018,Jan,8; 2017,Jan,8; 2016,Jan,13

92572   Staggered spondaic word test

     🖥 1.21   🔧 1.21   **FUD** XXX   01 80 TC 🔲

     AMA: 2018,Feb,11; 2018,Jan,8; 2017,Jan,8; 2016,Jan,13

92575   Sensorineural acuity level test

     🖥 1.79   🔧 1.79   **FUD** XXX   01 80 TC 🔲

     AMA: 2018,Feb,11; 2018,Jan,8; 2017,Jan,8; 2016,Jan,13

92576   Synthetic sentence identification test

     🖥 1.03   🔧 1.03   **FUD** XXX   01 80 TC 🔲

     AMA: 2018,Feb,11; 2018,Jan,8; 2017,Jan,8; 2016,Jan,13

92577   Stenger test, speech

     🖥 0.39   🔧 0.39   **FUD** XXX   01 80 🔲

     AMA: 2018,Feb,11; 2018,Jan,8; 2017,Jan,8; 2016,Jan,13

92579   Visual reinforcement audiometry (VRA)

     🖥 1.09   🔧 1.32   **FUD** XXX   01 80 🔲

     AMA: 2018,Feb,11; 2018,Jan,8; 2017,Jan,8; 2016,Jan,13

92582   Conditioning play audiometry

     🖥 2.06   🔧 2.06   **FUD** XXX   01 80 TC 🔲

     AMA: 2018,Feb,11; 2018,Jan,8; 2017,Jan,8; 2016,Jan,13

92583   Select picture audiometry

     🖥 1.35   🔧 1.35   **FUD** XXX   01 80 TC 🔲

     AMA: 2018,Feb,11; 2018,Jan,8; 2017,Jan,8; 2016,Jan,13

92584   Electrocochleography

     🖥 2.09   🔧 2.09   **FUD** XXX   S 80 🔲

     AMA: 2018,Feb,11; 2018,Jan,8; 2017,Jan,8; 2016,Jan,13

26/TC PC/TC Only	A2-Z3 ASC Payment	50 Bilateral	♂ Male Only	♀ Female Only	🖥 Facility RVU	🔧 Non-Facility RVU	🔲 CCI	✖ CLIA
FUD Follow-up Days	CMS: IOM	AMA: CPT Asst	A-Y OPPSI	80/80 Surg Assist Allowed / w/Doc		🔲 Lab Crosswalk	🔲 Radiology Crosswalk	

472   CPT © 2021 American Medical Association. All Rights Reserved.   © 2021 Optum360, LLC

(left column)

**92650** **Auditory evoked potentials; screening of auditory potential with broadband stimuli, automated analysis**
🔧 0.83   ⚖ 0.83   **FUD** XXX   80 ▣
AMA: 2020,Oct,9

**92651** **for hearing status determination, broadband stimuli, with interpretation and report**
EXCLUDES *Auditory evoked potentials, neurodiagnostic ([92653])*
Threshold estimation ([92652])
🔧 2.62   ⚖ 2.62   **FUD** XXX   80 ▣
AMA: 2020,Oct,9

**92652** **for threshold estimation at multiple frequencies, with interpretation and report**
EXCLUDES *Hearing status determination ([92651])*
Auditory evoked potentials, neurodiagnostic ([92653])
🔧 3.43   ⚖ 3.43   **FUD** XXX   80 ▣
AMA: 2020,Oct,9

**92653** **neurodiagnostic, with interpretation and report**
EXCLUDES *Hearing status determination ([92651])*
Threshold estimation ([92652])
🔧 2.51   ⚖ 2.51   **FUD** XXX   80 ▣
AMA: 2020,Oct,9

**92558** **Evoked otoacoustic emissions, screening (qualitative measurement of distortion product or transient evoked otoacoustic emissions), automated analysis**
🔧 0.25   ⚖ 0.28   **FUD** XXX   E ▣
AMA: 2018,Feb,11; 2018,Jan,8; 2017,Jan,8; 2016,Jan,13

92587 **Distortion product evoked otoacoustic emissions; limited evaluation (to confirm the presence or absence of hearing disorder, 3-6 frequencies) or transient evoked otoacoustic emissions, with interpretation and report**
🔧 0.63   ⚖ 0.63   **FUD** XXX   S 80 ▣
AMA: 2018,Feb,11; 2018,Jan,8; 2017,Jan,8; 2016,Jan,13

92588 **comprehensive diagnostic evaluation (quantitative analysis of outer hair cell function by cochlear mapping, minimum of 12 frequencies), with interpretation and report**
EXCLUDES *Evaluation central auditory function (92620-92621)*
🔧 0.96   ⚖ 0.96   **FUD** XXX   S 80 ▣
AMA: 2018,Feb,11; 2018,Jan,8; 2017,Jan,8; 2016,Jan,13

92590 **Hearing aid examination and selection; monaural**
🔧 0.00   ⚖ 0.00   **FUD** XXX   E ▣
AMA: 2020,Jul,3; 2018,Feb,11; 2018,Jan,8; 2017,Jan,8; 2016,Jan,13

92591 **binaural**
🔧 0.00   ⚖ 0.00   **FUD** XXX   E ▣
AMA: 2020,Jul,3; 2018,Feb,11; 2018,Jan,8; 2017,Jan,8; 2016,Jan,13

92592 **Hearing aid check; monaural**
🔧 0.00   ⚖ 0.00   **FUD** XXX   E ▣
AMA: 2020,Jul,3; 2018,Feb,11; 2018,Jan,8; 2017,Jan,8; 2016,Jan,13

92593 **binaural**
🔧 0.00   ⚖ 0.00   **FUD** XXX   E ▣
AMA: 2020,Jul,3; 2018,Feb,11; 2018,Jan,8; 2017,Jan,8; 2016,Jan,13

92594 **Electroacoustic evaluation for hearing aid; monaural**
🔧 0.00   ⚖ 0.00   **FUD** XXX   E ▣
AMA: 2020,Jul,3; 2018,Feb,11; 2018,Jan,8; 2017,Jan,8; 2016,Jan,13

92595 **binaural**
🔧 0.00   ⚖ 0.00   **FUD** XXX   E ▣
AMA: 2020,Jul,3; 2018,Feb,11; 2018,Jan,8; 2017,Jan,8; 2016,Jan,13

92596 **Ear protector attenuation measurements**
🔧 1.84   ⚖ 1.84   **FUD** XXX   Q1 80 TC
AMA: 2018,Feb,11; 2018,Jan,8; 2017,Jan,8; 2016,Jan,13

92597 **Resequenced code. See code following 92604.**

92601-92609 [92597, 92618] Services Related to Hearing and Speech Devices

INCLUDES Diagnostic/treatment services not generally included in comprehensive otorhinolaryngologic evaluation or office visit

92601 **Diagnostic analysis of cochlear implant, patient younger than 7 years of age; with programming**   A
INCLUDES Connection to cochlear implant
Postoperative analysis/fitting previously placed external devices
Stimulator programming
EXCLUDES *Cochlear implant placement (69930)*
🔧 3.57   ⚖ 4.68   **FUD** XXX   S 80 ▣
AMA: 2020,Jul,3; 2018,Feb,11; 2018,Jan,8; 2017,Jan,8; 2016,Sep,6; 2016,Jan,13

92602 **subsequent reprogramming**   A
INCLUDES Internal stimulator re-programming
Subsequent sessions for external transmitter measurements/adjustment
EXCLUDES *Analysis with programming (92601)*
Aural rehabilitation services after cochlear implant (92626-92627, 92630-92633)
Cochlear implant placement (69930)
🔧 2.03   ⚖ 2.96   **FUD** XXX   S 80 ▣
AMA: 2020,Jul,3; 2018,Feb,11; 2018,Jan,8; 2017,Jan,8; 2016,Sep,6; 2016,Jan,13

92603 **Diagnostic analysis of cochlear implant, age 7 years or older; with programming**   A
INCLUDES Connection to cochlear implant
Postoperative analysis/fitting previously placed external devices
Stimulator programming
EXCLUDES *Cochlear implant placement (69930)*
🔧 3.47   ⚖ 4.37   **FUD** XXX   S 80 ▣
AMA: 2020,Jul,3; 2018,Feb,11; 2018,Jan,8; 2017,Jan,8; 2016,Sep,6; 2016,Jan,13

92604 **subsequent reprogramming**   A
INCLUDES Internal stimulator reprogramming
Subsequent sessions for external transmitter measurements/adjustment
EXCLUDES *Analysis with programming (92603)*
Cochlear implant placement (69930)
🔧 1.94   ⚖ 2.64   **FUD** XXX   S 80 ▣
AMA: 2020,Jul,3; 2018,Feb,11; 2018,Jan,8; 2017,Jan,8; 2016,Sep,6; 2016,Jan,13

**92597** **Evaluation for use and/or fitting of voice prosthetic device to supplement oral speech**
EXCLUDES *Augmentative or alternative communication device services (92605, [92618], 92607-92608)*
🔧 2.06   ⚖ 2.06   **FUD** XXX   A 80 ▣
AMA: 2018,Feb,11; 2018,Jan,8; 2017,Jan,8; 2016,Jan,13

92605 **Evaluation for prescription of non-speech-generating augmentative and alternative communication device, face-to-face with the patient; first hour**
EXCLUDES *Prosthetic voice device fitting or use evaluation (92597)*
🔧 2.53   ⚖ 2.65   **FUD** XXX   A ▣
AMA: 2018,Feb,11; 2018,Jan,8; 2017,Jan,8; 2016,Jan,13

+ # **92618** **each additional 30 minutes (List separately in addition to code for primary procedure)**
Code first (92605)
🔧 0.94   ⚖ 0.96   **FUD** ZZZ   A ▣
AMA: 2018,Feb,11

92606 **Therapeutic service(s) for the use of non-speech-generating device, including programming and modification**
🔧 2.05   ⚖ 2.39   **FUD** XXX   A ▣
AMA: 2018,Feb,11; 2018,Jan,8; 2017,Jan,8; 2016,Jan,13

Medicine

92607 — 92633

92607 Evaluation for prescription for speech-generating augmentative and alternative communication device, face-to-face with the patient; first hour
EXCLUDES Evaluation for prescription non-speech generating device (92605)
Evaluation for use/fitting voice prosthetic (92597)
🚗 3.66 ⚕ 3.66 **FUD** XXX [A] [80] ▭
AMA: 2018,Feb,11; 2018,Jan,8; 2017,Jan,8; 2016,Jan,13

+ 92608 each additional 30 minutes (List separately in addition to code for primary procedure)
Code first initial hour (92607)
🚗 1.47 ⚕ 1.47 **FUD** ZZZ [A] [80] ▭
AMA: 2018,Feb,11; 2018,Jan,8; 2017,Jan,8; 2016,Jan,13

92609 Therapeutic services for the use of speech-generating device, including programming and modification
EXCLUDES Therapeutic services for use non-speech generating device (92606)
🚗 3.08 ⚕ 3.08 **FUD** XXX [A] [80] ▭
AMA: 2018,Feb,11; 2018,Jan,8; 2017,Jan,8; 2016,Jan,13

92610-92618 [92618] Swallowing Evaluations

92610 Evaluation of oral and pharyngeal swallowing function
EXCLUDES Evaluation with flexible endoscope (92612-92617)
Motion fluoroscopic evaluation swallowing function (92611)
🚗 2.07 ⚕ 2.47 **FUD** XXX [A] [80] ▭
AMA: 2018,Feb,11; 2018,Jan,8; 2017,Apr,8; 2017,Jan,8; 2016,Jan,13

92611 Motion fluoroscopic evaluation of swallowing function by cine or video recording
EXCLUDES Diagnostic flexible laryngoscopy (31575)
Evaluation oral/pharyngeal swallowing function (92610)
📷 (74230)
🚗 2.55 ⚕ 2.55 **FUD** XXX [A] [80] ▭
AMA: 2020,Aug,9; 2018,Feb,11; 2018,Jan,8; 2017,Apr,8; 2017,Jan,8; 2016,Sep,6; 2016,Jan,13

92612 Flexible endoscopic evaluation of swallowing by cine or video recording;
EXCLUDES Diagnostic flexible fiberoptic laryngoscopy (31575)
Flexible endoscopic examination/testing without cine or video recording (92700)
🚗 1.94 ⚕ 5.42 **FUD** XXX [A] [80] ▭
AMA: 2018,Feb,11; 2018,Jan,8; 2017,Jul,7; 2017,Apr,8; 2017,Jan,8; 2016,Dec,13; 2016,Sep,6; 2016,Jan,13

92613 interpretation and report only
EXCLUDES Diagnostic flexible laryngoscopy (31575)
Oral/pharyngeal swallowing function examination (92610)
Swallowing function motion fluoroscopic examination (92611)
🚗 1.07 ⚕ 1.07 **FUD** XXX [B] [80] ▭
AMA: 2018,Feb,11; 2018,Jan,8; 2017,Jul,7; 2017,Apr,8; 2017,Jan,8; 2016,Dec,13; 2016,Sep,6; 2016,Jan,13

92614 Flexible endoscopic evaluation, laryngeal sensory testing by cine or video recording;
EXCLUDES Diagnostic flexible laryngoscopy (31575)
Flexible endoscopic examination/testing without cine or video recording (92700)
🚗 1.90 ⚕ 4.03 **FUD** XXX [A] [80] ▭
AMA: 2018,Feb,11; 2018,Jan,8; 2017,Jul,7; 2017,Apr,8; 2017,Jan,8; 2016,Dec,13; 2016,Sep,6; 2016,Jan,13

92615 interpretation and report only
EXCLUDES Diagnostic flexible laryngoscopy (31575)
🚗 0.95 ⚕ 0.95 **FUD** XXX [E] [80] ▭
AMA: 2018,Feb,11; 2018,Jan,8; 2017,Jul,7; 2017,Apr,8; 2017,Jan,8; 2016,Dec,13; 2016,Sep,6; 2016,Jan,13

92616 Flexible endoscopic evaluation of swallowing and laryngeal sensory testing by cine or video recording;
EXCLUDES Diagnostic flexible fiberoptic laryngoscopy (31575)
Flexible endoscopic examination/testing without cine or video recording (92700)
🚗 2.84 ⚕ 5.85 **FUD** XXX [A] [80] ▭
AMA: 2018,Feb,11; 2018,Jan,8; 2017,Jul,7; 2017,Apr,8; 2017,Jan,8; 2016,Dec,13; 2016,Sep,6; 2016,Jan,13

92617 interpretation and report only
EXCLUDES Diagnostic flexible laryngoscopy (31575)
🚗 1.18 ⚕ 1.18 **FUD** XXX [E] [80] ▭
AMA: 2018,Feb,11; 2018,Jan,8; 2017,Jul,7; 2017,Apr,8; 2017,Jan,8; 2016,Dec,13; 2016,Sep,6; 2016,Jan,13

92618 Resequenced code. See code following 92605.

92620-92700 [92650, 92651, 92652, 92653] Diagnostic Hearing Evaluations and Rehabilitation
INCLUDES Diagnostic/treatment services not generally included in comprehensive otorhinolaryngologic evaluation or office visit

92620 Evaluation of central auditory function, with report; initial 60 minutes
EXCLUDES Voice analysis (92521-92524)
🚗 2.33 ⚕ 2.67 **FUD** XXX [Q1] [80] ▭
AMA: 2018,Feb,11; 2018,Jan,8; 2017,Jan,8; 2016,Jan,13

+ 92621 each additional 15 minutes (List separately in addition to code for primary procedure)
EXCLUDES Voice analysis (92521-92524)
Code first (92620)
🚗 0.54 ⚕ 0.64 **FUD** ZZZ [N] [80] ▭
AMA: 2018,Feb,11; 2018,Jan,8; 2017,Jan,8; 2016,Jan,13

92625 Assessment of tinnitus (includes pitch, loudness matching, and masking)
EXCLUDES Loudness test (92562)
Code also modifier 52 for unilateral procedure
🚗 1.78 ⚕ 1.99 **FUD** XXX [Q1] [80] ▭
AMA: 2018,Feb,11; 2018,Jan,8; 2017,Jan,8; 2016,Jan,13

92626 Evaluation of auditory function for surgically implanted device(s) candidacy or postoperative status of a surgically implanted device(s); first hour
INCLUDES Assessment to determine patient's proficiency in remaining hearing to identify speech
Face-to-face time spent with patient or family
EXCLUDES Hearing aid evaluation, fitting, follow-up, or selection (92590-92591, 92592-92593, 92594-92595)
🚗 2.16 ⚕ 2.55 **FUD** XXX [Q1] [80] ▭
AMA: 2020,Jul,3; 2018,Feb,11; 2018,Jan,8; 2017,Jan,8; 2016,Sep,6; 2016,Jan,13

+ 92627 each additional 15 minutes (List separately in addition to code for primary procedure)
INCLUDES Assessment to determine patient's proficiency in remaining hearing to identify speech
Face-to-face time spent with patient or family
EXCLUDES Hearing aid evaluation, fitting, follow-up, or selection (92590-92591, 92592-92593, 92594-92595)
Code first initial hour (92626)
🚗 0.51 ⚕ 0.64 **FUD** ZZZ [N] [80] ▭
AMA: 2020,Jul,3; 2018,Feb,11; 2018,Jan,8; 2017,Jan,8; 2016,Sep,6; 2016,Jan,13

92630 Auditory rehabilitation; prelingual hearing loss
🚗 0.00 ⚕ 0.00 **FUD** XXX [E] ▭
AMA: 2018,Feb,11; 2018,Jan,8; 2017,Jan,8; 2016,Sep,6; 2016,Jan,13

92633 postlingual hearing loss
🚗 0.00 ⚕ 0.00 **FUD** XXX [E] ▭
AMA: 2018,Feb,11; 2018,Jan,8; 2017,Jan,8; 2016,Sep,6; 2016,Jan,13

92640   **Diagnostic analysis with programming of auditory brainstem implant, per hour**

> EXCLUDES   *Nonprogramming services (cardiac monitoring)*
> 🔧 2.74   ⚕ 3.24   **FUD** XXX   S 80 🖵
> **AMA:** 2018,Feb,11

92650   **Resequenced code. See code following 92584.**

92651   **Resequenced code. See code following 92584.**

92652   **Resequenced code. See code following 92584.**

92653   **Resequenced code. See code following 92584.**

92700   **Unlisted otorhinolaryngological service or procedure**

> INCLUDES   Lombard test
> 🔧 0.00   ⚕ 0.00   **FUD** XXX   Q1 80 🖵
> **AMA:** 2018,Feb,11; 2018,Jan,8; 2017,Apr,8; 2017,Jan,8; 2016,Sep,6; 2016,Jan,13

92920-92953 [92920, 92921, 92924, 92925, 92928, 92929, 92933, 92934, 92937, 92938, 92941, 92943, 92944] Emergency Cardiac Procedures

92920   **Resequenced code. See code following 92998.**

92921   **Resequenced code. See code following 92998.**

92924   **Resequenced code. See code following 92998.**

92925   **Resequenced code. See code following 92998.**

92928   **Resequenced code. See code following 92998.**

92929   **Resequenced code. See code following 92998.**

92933   **Resequenced code. See code following 92998.**

92934   **Resequenced code. See code following 92998.**

92937   **Resequenced code. See code following 92998.**

92938   **Resequenced code. See code following 92998.**

92941   **Resequenced code. See code following 92998.**

92943   **Resequenced code. See code following 92998.**

92944   **Resequenced code. See code following 92998.**

92950   **Cardiopulmonary resuscitation (eg, in cardiac arrest)**

> INCLUDES   Cardiac defibrillation
> EXCLUDES   *Critical care services (99291-99292)*
> 🔧 5.36   ⚕ 9.16   **FUD** 000   S 80 🖵
> **AMA:** 2018,Feb,11; 2018,Jan,8; 2017,Jan,8; 2016,Jan,13

92953   **Temporary transcutaneous pacing**

> EXCLUDES   *Direction ambulance/rescue personnel by physician or other qualified health care professional (99288)*
> 🔧 0.03   ⚕ 0.03   **FUD** 000   Q3 80 🖵
> **AMA:** 2019,Aug,8; 2018,Feb,11; 2018,Jan,8; 2017,Jan,8; 2016,Jan,13

92960-92961 Cardioversion

92960   **Cardioversion, elective, electrical conversion of arrhythmia; external**

> 🔧 3.13   ⚕ 4.51   **FUD** 000   S 80 🖵
> **AMA:** 2018,Feb,11; 2018,Jan,8; 2017,Jan,8; 2016,Jan,13

92961   **internal (separate procedure)**

> EXCLUDES   *Device evaluation for implantable defibrillator/multi-lead pacemaker system (93282-93284, 93287, 93289, 93295-93296)*
> *Electrophysiological studies (93618-93624, 93631, 93640-93642)*
> *Intracardiac ablation (93650-93657, 93662)*
> 🔧 7.17   ⚕ 7.17   **FUD** 000   S 🖵
> **AMA:** 2018,Feb,11; 2018,Jan,8; 2017,Jan,8; 2016,Jan,13

92970-92979 [92973, 92974, 92975, 92977, 92978, 92979] Circulatory Assist: External/Internal

> EXCLUDES   *Atrial septostomy, any method (33741)*
> *Catheter placement for use in circulatory assist devices (intra-aortic balloon pump) (33970)*

92970   **Cardioassist-method of circulatory assist; internal**

> 🔧 5.49   ⚕ 5.49   **FUD** 000   C 80 🖵
> **AMA:** 2018,Feb,11

92971   **external**

> 🔧 2.91   ⚕ 2.91   **FUD** 000   C 80 🖵
> **AMA:** 2018,Feb,11

92973   **Resequenced code. See code following 92998.**

92974   **Resequenced code. See code following 92998.**

92975   **Resequenced code. See code following 92998.**

92977   **Resequenced code. See code following 92998.**

92978   **Resequenced code. See code following 92998.**

92979   **Resequenced code. See code following 92998.**

92986-92990 Percutaneous Procedures of Heart Valves and Septum

> EXCLUDES   *Atrial septostomy, any method (33741)*

92986   **Percutaneous balloon valvuloplasty; aortic valve**

> 🔧 38.1   ⚕ 38.1   **FUD** 090   J 80 🖵
> **AMA:** 2018,Feb,11; 2018,Jan,8; 2017,Jan,8; 2016,Jan,13

92987   **mitral valve**

> 🔧 39.5   ⚕ 39.5   **FUD** 090   J 80 🖵
> **AMA:** 2018,Feb,11; 2018,Jan,8; 2017,Jan,8; 2016,Jan,13

92990   **pulmonary valve**

> 🔧 31.6   ⚕ 31.6   **FUD** 090   J 80 🖵
> **AMA:** 2018,Feb,11; 2018,Jan,8; 2017,Jan,8; 2016,Jan,13

92997-92998 Percutaneous Angioplasty: Pulmonary Artery

92997   **Percutaneous transluminal pulmonary artery balloon angioplasty; single vessel**

> 🔧 19.0   ⚕ 19.0   **FUD** 000   J 80 🖵
> **AMA:** 2018,Feb,11; 2018,Jan,8; 2017,Jul,3; 2017,Jan,8; 2016,Mar,5; 2016,Jan,13

+   92998   **each additional vessel (List separately in addition to code for primary procedure)**

> Code first single vessel (92997)
> 🔧 9.44   ⚕ 9.44   **FUD** ZZZ   N 80 🖵
> **AMA:** 2018,Feb,11; 2018,Jan,8; 2017,Jul,3; 2017,Jan,8; 2016,Mar,5; 2016,Jan,13

92920-92944 [92920, 92921, 92924, 92925, 92928, 92929, 92933, 92934, 92937, 92938, 92941, 92943, 92944]
Intravascular Coronary Procedures

INCLUDES
Accessing vessel
Additional procedures performed in third branch, major coronary artery
All procedures performed in all branch segments, coronary arteries
  Branches left anterior descending (diagonals), left circumflex (marginals), and right (posterior descending, posterolaterals)
  Distal, proximal, and mid segments
All procedures performed in all segments, major coronary arteries through native vessels:
  Distal, proximal, and mid segments
  Left main, left anterior descending, left circumflex, right, and ramus intermedius arteries
All procedures performed in major coronary arteries or recognized coronary artery branches through coronary artery bypass graft
  Sequential bypass graft with more than single distal anastomosis as one graft
  Branching bypass grafts (e.g., "Y" grafts) include coronary vessel for primary graft, with each branch off primary graft making up an additional coronary vessel
  Each coronary artery bypass graft denotes single coronary vessel
  Embolic protection devices when used
Arteriotomy closure through access sheath
Atherectomy (e.g., directional, laser, rotational)
Balloon angioplasty (e.g., cryoplasty, cutting balloon, wired balloons)
Cardiac catheterization and related procedures when included in coronary revascularization service (93454-93461, 93563-93564)
Imaging once procedure complete
Percutaneous coronary interventions (PCI) for coronary vessel disease, native and bypass grafts
Procedures in left main and ramus intermedius coronary artery branches as they are unrecognized for individual code assignment
Radiological supervision and interpretation intervention(s)
Reporting most comprehensive treatment in given vessel according to intensity hierarchy for base and add-on codes:
  Add-on codes: 92944 = 92938 > 92934 > 92925 > 92929 > 92921
  Base codes (report only one): 92943 = 92941 = 92933 > 92924 > 92937 = 92928 > 92920
Revascularization achieved with single procedure when single lesion continues from one target vessel (major artery, branch, or bypass graft) to another target vessel
Selective vessel catheterization
Stenting (e.g., balloon expandable, bare metal, covered, drug eluting, self-expanding)
Traversing lesion

EXCLUDES
Application intravascular radioelements (77770-77772)
Insertion device for coronary intravascular brachytherapy (92974)
Reduction septum (e.g., alcohol ablation) (93799)

Code also add-on codes for procedures performed during same session in additional recognized target vessel branches
Code also diagnostic angiography during interventional procedure when:
  No previous catheter-based coronary angiography study available, and full diagnostic study performed, with decision to perform intervention based on that study
  Previous study available, but documentation states patient's condition changed since previous study or target area visualization inadequate, or change occurs during procedure warranting additional evaluation outside current target area
Code also diagnostic angiography performed at session separate from interventional procedure
Code also individual base codes for treatment major native coronary artery segment and another segment same artery requiring treatment through bypass graft when performed at same time
Code also procedures for both vessels for bifurcation lesion
Code also procedures performed in second branch major coronary artery
Code also treatment arterial segment requiring access through bypass graft

---

 # 92920   **Percutaneous transluminal coronary angioplasty; single major coronary artery or branch**
    15.4   15.4   **FUD** 000   J J8 80
    AMA: 2018,Feb,11; 2018,Jan,8; 2017,Jul,3; 2017,Jan,8; 2016,Jan,13

Catheter is advanced to affected portion of coronary artery

A stent is placed

Aorta

Left coronary artery

Plaque

Inflated balloon

Right coronary artery

A balloon may be inflated or other intravascular therapy may accompany the procedure

+ # 92921   **each additional branch of a major coronary artery (List separately in addition to code for primary procedure)**
    Code first (92920, 92924, 92928, 92933, 92937, 92941, 92943)
    0.00   0.00   **FUD** ZZZ   N N1
    AMA: 2018,Feb,11; 2018,Jan,8; 2017,Jul,3; 2017,Jan,8; 2016,Jan,13

 # 92924   **Percutaneous transluminal coronary atherectomy, with coronary angioplasty when performed; single major coronary artery or branch**
    18.4   18.4   **FUD** 000   J 80
    AMA: 2018,Feb,11; 2018,Jan,8; 2017,Jul,3; 2017,Jan,8; 2016,Jan,13

+ # 92925   **each additional branch of a major coronary artery (List separately in addition to code for primary procedure)**
    Code first (92924, 92928, 92933, 92937, 92941, 92943)
    0.00   0.00   **FUD** ZZZ   N
    AMA: 2018,Feb,11; 2018,Jan,8; 2017,Jul,3; 2017,Jan,8; 2016,Jan,13

 # 92928   **Percutaneous transcatheter placement of intracoronary stent(s), with coronary angioplasty when performed; single major coronary artery or branch**
    17.2   17.2   **FUD** 000   J J8 80
    AMA: 2018,Feb,11; 2018,Jan,8; 2017,Jul,3; 2017,Feb,14; 2017,Jan,8; 2017,Jan,6; 2016,Jan,13

+ # 92929   **each additional branch of a major coronary artery (List separately in addition to code for primary procedure)**
    Code first (92928, 92933, 92937, 92941, 92943)
    0.00   0.00   **FUD** ZZZ   N N1
    AMA: 2018,Feb,11; 2018,Jan,8; 2017,Jul,3; 2017,Jan,8; 2017,Jan,6; 2016,Jan,13

 # 92933   **Percutaneous transluminal coronary atherectomy, with intracoronary stent, with coronary angioplasty when performed; single major coronary artery or branch**
    19.3   19.3   **FUD** 000   J 80
    AMA: 2018,Feb,11; 2018,Jan,8; 2017,Jul,3; 2017,Jan,8; 2016,Jan,13

26/ TC PC/TC Only   A2-Z3 ASC Payment   50 Bilateral   ♂ Male Only   ♀ Female Only   Facility RVU   Non-Facility RVU   CCI   CLIA
FUD Follow-up Days   **CMS:** IOM   **AMA:** CPT Asst   A-Y OPPSI   80/80 Surg Assist Allowed / w/Doc   Lab Crosswalk   Radiology Crosswalk

476   CPT © 2021 American Medical Association. All Rights Reserved.   © 2021 Optum360, LLC

+ # 92934 each additional branch of a major coronary artery (List separately in addition to code for primary procedure)

Code first (92933, 92937, 92941, 92943)

🔧 0.00   ☂ 0.00   **FUD** ZZZ   N 💬

AMA: 2018,Feb,11; 2018,Jan,8; 2017,Jul,3; 2017,Jan,8; 2016,Jan,13

 # 92937 Percutaneous transluminal revascularization of or through coronary artery bypass graft (internal mammary, free arterial, venous), any combination of intracoronary stent, atherectomy and angioplasty, including distal protection when performed; single vessel

🔧 17.2   ☂ 17.2   **FUD** 000   J 80 💬

AMA: 2018,Feb,11; 2018,Jan,8; 2017,Jul,3; 2017,Feb,14; 2017,Jan,8; 2016,Jan,13

+ # 92938 each additional branch subtended by the bypass graft (List separately in addition to code for primary procedure)

Code first (92937)

🔧 0.00   ☂ 0.00   **FUD** ZZZ   N 💬

AMA: 2018,Feb,11; 2018,Jan,8; 2017,Jul,3; 2017,Jan,8; 2016,Jan,13

 # 92941 Percutaneous transluminal revascularization of acute total/subtotal occlusion during acute myocardial infarction, coronary artery or coronary artery bypass graft, any combination of intracoronary stent, atherectomy and angioplasty, including aspiration thrombectomy when performed, single vessel

INCLUDES   Aspiration thrombectomy, when performed
Embolic protection
Rheolytic thrombectomy

EXCLUDES   *Transcatheter intracoronary infusion supersaturated oxygen therapy [SSO2] (0659T)*

Code also treatment additional vessels, when appropriate (92920-92938, 92943-92944)

🔧 19.3   ☂ 19.3   **FUD** 000   C 80 💬

AMA: 2020,Jul,13; 2018,Feb,11; 2018,Jan,8; 2017,Jul,3; 2017,Feb,14; 2017,Jan,8; 2016,Jan,13

 # 92943 Percutaneous transluminal revascularization of chronic total occlusion, coronary artery, coronary artery branch, or coronary artery bypass graft, any combination of intracoronary stent, atherectomy and angioplasty; single vessel

INCLUDES   Antegrade flow deficiency with angiography and clinical criteria indicating chronic total occlusion

🔧 19.3   ☂ 19.3   **FUD** 000   J 80 💬

AMA: 2018,Feb,11; 2018,Jan,8; 2017,Jul,3; 2017,Jan,8; 2016,Jan,13

+ # 92944 each additional coronary artery, coronary artery branch, or bypass graft (List separately in addition to code for primary procedure)

EXCLUDES   *Application intravascular radioelements (77770-77772)*

Code first (92924, 92928, 92933, 92937, 92941, 92943)

🔧 0.00   ☂ 0.00   **FUD** ZZZ   N 💬

AMA: 2018,Feb,11; 2018,Jan,8; 2017,Jul,3; 2017,Jan,8; 2016,Jan,13

92973-92979 [92973, 92974, 92975, 92977, 92978, 92979] Additional Coronary Artery Procedures

+ # 92973 Percutaneous transluminal coronary thrombectomy mechanical (List separately in addition to code for primary procedure)

EXCLUDES   *Aspiration thrombectomy*

Code first (92920, 92924, 92928, 92933, 92937, 92941, 92943, 92975, 93454-93461, 93563-93564)

🔧 5.12   ☂ 5.12   **FUD** ZZZ   N 80 💬

AMA: 2020,Jul,13; 2018,Feb,11; 2018,Jan,8; 2017,Feb,14; 2017,Jan,8; 2016,Jan,13

+ # 92974 Transcatheter placement of radiation delivery device for subsequent coronary intravascular brachytherapy (List separately in addition to code for primary procedure)

EXCLUDES   *Application intravascular radioelements (77770-77772)*

Code first (92920, 92924, 92928, 92933, 92937, 92941, 92943, 93454-93461)

🔧 4.72   ☂ 4.72   **FUD** ZZZ   N 80 💬

AMA: 2018,Feb,11; 2018,Jan,8; 2017,Feb,14; 2017,Jan,8; 2016,Jan,13

 # 92975 Thrombolysis, coronary; by intracoronary infusion, including selective coronary angiography

EXCLUDES   *Thrombolysis, cerebral (37195)*
Thrombolysis other than coronary ([37211, 37212, 37213, 37214])

🔧 10.9   ☂ 10.9   **FUD** 000   C 80 💬

AMA: 2018,Feb,11

 # 92977 by intravenous infusion

EXCLUDES   *Thrombolysis, cerebral (37195)*
Thrombolysis other than coronary ([37211, 37212, 37213, 37214])

🔧 1.51   ☂ 1.51   **FUD** XXX   T 80 💬

AMA: 2018,Feb,11

+ # 92978 Endoluminal imaging of coronary vessel or graft using intravascular ultrasound (IVUS) or optical coherence tomography (OCT) during diagnostic evaluation and/or therapeutic intervention including imaging supervision, interpretation and report; initial vessel (List separately in addition to code for primary procedure)

Code first primary procedure (92920, 92924, 92928, 92933, 92937, 92941, 92943, 92975, 93454-93461, 93563-93564)

🔧 0.00   ☂ 0.00   **FUD** ZZZ   N 80 💬

AMA: 2018,Feb,11; 2018,Jan,8; 2017,Jan,8; 2016,Jan,13

+ # 92979 each additional vessel (List separately in addition to code for primary procedure)

INCLUDES   Transducer manipulations/repositioning in vessel examined, before and after therapeutic intervention

EXCLUDES   *Intravascular spectroscopy (93799)*

Code first initial vessel (92978)

🔧 0.00   ☂ 0.00   **FUD** ZZZ   N 80 💬

AMA: 2018,Feb,11; 2018,Jan,8; 2017,Jan,8; 2016,Jan,13

93000-93010 Electrocardiographic Services

INCLUDES   Specific order for service, separate written and signed report, and documentation medical necessity

EXCLUDES   *Acoustic cardiography (93799)*
Echocardiography (93303-93350)
Intracardiac ischemia monitoring system (0525T-0532T)
Reporting codes for telemetry monitoring strip review

93000 Electrocardiogram, routine ECG with at least 12 leads; with interpretation and report

🔧 0.48   ☂ 0.48   **FUD** XXX   M 80 💬

AMA: 2020,Dec,3; 2018,Feb,11; 2018,Jan,8; 2017,Oct,3; 2017,Jan,8; 2016,Jan,13

93005 tracing only, without interpretation and report

🔧 0.24   ☂ 0.24   **FUD** XXX   01 80 TC 💬

AMA: 2020,Dec,3; 2018,Feb,11; 2018,Jan,8; 2017,Oct,3; 2017,Jan,8; 2016,Apr,8; 2016,Jan,13

93010 **interpretation and report only**
🔌 0.24   ⚗ 0.24   **FUD** XXX   B 80 26 ▢

AMA: 2020,Dec,3; 2018,Feb,11; 2018,Jan,8; 2017,Oct,3;
2017,Jan,8; 2016,Apr,8; 2016,Jan,13

Sinoatrial node
(pacemaker)

Internodal tracts:
  Anterior
  Middle
  Posterior

Atrioventricular
node

Common bundle
(of His)

Atrioventricular
block

Accessory
bundle (of Kent)

Right bundle
branch

Right bundle
branch block

Moderator band

Purkinje fibers

Bachmann's
bundle

Left bundle
branch block

Left bundle branch:
  Anterior fascicle
  Posterior fascicle

Left bundle
branch
hemiblock

Conduction system of the heart

93015-93018 Stress Test

93015 **Cardiovascular stress test using maximal or submaximal treadmill or bicycle exercise, continuous electrocardiographic monitoring, and/or pharmacological stress; with supervision, interpretation and report**
🔌 2.01   ⚗ 2.01   **FUD** XXX   B 80 ▢

AMA: 2020,Dec,3; 2020,Jul,5; 2018,Feb,11; 2018,Jan,8;
2017,Oct,3; 2017,Jan,8; 2016,Jan,13

93016 **supervision only, without interpretation and report**
🔌 0.63   ⚗ 0.63   **FUD** XXX   B 80 26 ▢

AMA: 2020,Dec,3; 2020,Jul,5; 2018,Feb,11; 2018,Jan,8;
2017,Oct,3; 2017,Jan,8; 2016,Jan,13

93017 **tracing only, without interpretation and report**
🔌 0.96   ⚗ 0.96   **FUD** XXX   Q1 80 TC ▢

AMA: 2020,Dec,3; 2020,Jul,5; 2018,Feb,11; 2018,Jan,8;
2017,Oct,3; 2017,Jan,8; 2016,Jan,13

93018 **interpretation and report only**
🔌 0.42   ⚗ 0.42   **FUD** XXX   B 80 26 ▢

AMA: 2020,Dec,3; 2020,Jul,5; 2018,Feb,11; 2018,Jan,8;
2017,Oct,3; 2017,Jan,8; 2016,Jan,13

93024 Provocation Test for Coronary Vasospasm

93024 **Ergonovine provocation test**
🔌 3.12   ⚗ 3.12   **FUD** XXX   Q1 80 ▢

AMA: 2018,Feb,11

93025 Microvolt T-Wave Alternans

CMS: 100-03,20.30 Microvolt T-Wave Alternans (MTWA); 100-04,32,370 Microvolt T-wave Alternans;
100-04,32,370.1 Coding and Claims Processing for MTWA; 100-04,32,370.2 Messaging for MTWA

INCLUDES   Specific order for service, separate written and signed report, and
documentation medical necessity

EXCLUDES   *Echocardiography (93303-93350)*
Reporting codes for telemetry monitoring strip review

93025 **Microvolt T-wave alternans for assessment of ventricular arrhythmias**
🔌 4.23   ⚗ 4.23   **FUD** XXX   S 80 ▢

AMA: 2018,Feb,11; 2018,Jan,8; 2017,Jan,8; 2016,Jan,13

93040-93042 Rhythm Strips

INCLUDES   Specific order for service, separate written and signed report, and
documentation medical necessity

EXCLUDES   *Device evaluation ([93261], 93279-93289 [93260], 93291-93296, 93298)*
Echocardiography (93303-93350)
Reporting codes for telemetry monitoring strip review

93040 **Rhythm ECG, 1-3 leads; with interpretation and report**
🔌 0.36   ⚗ 0.36   **FUD** XXX   B 80 ▢

AMA: 2020,Dec,3; 2020,Sep,7; 2018,Feb,11; 2018,Jan,8;
2017,Oct,3; 2017,Jan,8; 2016,Jan,13

93041 **tracing only without interpretation and report**
🔌 0.16   ⚗ 0.16   **FUD** XXX   Q1 80 TC ▢

AMA: 2020,Dec,3; 2018,Feb,11; 2018,Jan,8; 2017,Oct,3;
2017,Jan,8; 2016,Jan,13

93042 **interpretation and report only**
🔌 0.20   ⚗ 0.20   **FUD** XXX   B 80 26 ▢

AMA: 2020,Dec,3; 2018,Feb,11; 2018,Jan,8; 2017,Oct,3;
2017,Jan,8; 2016,Jan,13

93050 Arterial Waveform Analysis

EXCLUDES   *Reporting code with any intra-arterial diagnostic or interventional procedure*

93050 **Arterial pressure waveform analysis for assessment of central arterial pressures, includes obtaining waveform(s), digitization and application of nonlinear mathematical transformations to determine central arterial pressures and augmentation index, with interpretation and report, upper extremity artery, non-invasive**
🔌 0.46   ⚗ 0.46   **FUD** XXX   Q1 80 ▢

AMA: 2018,Feb,11

93224-93227 Holter Monitor

INCLUDES   Cardiac monitoring using in-person as well as remote technology for
electrocardiographic data assessment
Up to 48 hours recording on continuous basis

EXCLUDES   *Echocardiography (93303-93355 [93356])*
Implantable patient activated cardiac event recorders (93285, 93291, 93297-93298)
More than 48 hours monitoring ([93241, 93242, 93243, 93244, 93245, 93246, 93247, 93248])

Code also modifier 52 when less than 12 hours continuous recording provided

93224 **External electrocardiographic recording up to 48 hours by continuous rhythm recording and storage; includes recording, scanning analysis with report, review and interpretation by a physician or other qualified health care professional**
🔌 2.51   ⚗ 2.51   **FUD** XXX   M 80 ▢

AMA: 2020,Nov,10; 2018,Feb,11; 2018,Jan,8; 2017,Jan,8;
2016,Jan,13

93225 **recording (includes connection, recording, and disconnection)**
🔌 0.73   ⚗ 0.73   **FUD** XXX   Q1 80 TC ▢

AMA: 2020,Nov,10; 2018,Feb,11; 2018,Jan,8; 2017,Jan,8;
2016,Jan,13

93226 **scanning analysis with report**
🔌 1.03   ⚗ 1.03   **FUD** XXX   Q1 80 TC ▢

AMA: 2020,Nov,10; 2018,Feb,11; 2018,Jan,8; 2017,Jan,8;
2016,Jan,13

93227 **review and interpretation by a physician or other qualified health care professional**
🔌 0.75   ⚗ 0.75   **FUD** XXX   M 80 26 ▢

AMA: 2020,Nov,10; 2018,Mar,5; 2018,Feb,11; 2018,Jan,8;
2017,Jan,8; 2016,Jan,13

26/TC PC/TC Only   A2-Z3 ASC Payment   50 Bilateral   ♂ Male Only   ♀ Female Only   🔌 Facility RVU   ⚗ Non-Facility RVU   ▢ CCI   CLIA
FUD Follow-up Days   **CMS:** IOM   **AMA:** CPT Asst   A-Y OPPSI   80/80 Surg Assist Allowed / w/Doc   Lab Crosswalk   Radiology Crosswalk

478   CPT © 2021 American Medical Association. All Rights Reserved.   © 2021 Optum360, LLC

93241-93248 [93241, 93242, 93243, 93244, 93245, 93246, 93247, 93248] External Electrocardiographic Recording

INCLUDES Cardiac monitoring using in-person as well as remote technology for electrocardiographic data assessment

EXCLUDES During same monitoring period:
External ECG event recording up to 30 days (93268-93272)
External ECG event recording without 24 hour attended monitoring (0497T-0498T)
Remote physiological monitoring, collection and interpretation ([99453, 99454], [99091])
Echocardiography (93303-93355 [93356])
Implantable patient activated cardiac event recorders (93285, 93291, 93297-93298)
Less than 48 hours monitoring (93224-93227)

\# **93241** **External electrocardiographic recording for more than 48 hours up to 7 days by continuous rhythm recording and storage; includes recording, scanning analysis with report, review and interpretation**
　　EXCLUDES More than 7 days and up to 15 days monitoring ([93245, 93246, 93247, 93248])
　　🚗 0.00　⚕ 0.00　**FUD** XXX　　　　　80 ▢

\# **93242** **recording (includes connection and initial recording)**
　　EXCLUDES More than 7 days and up to 15 days monitoring ([93245, 93246, 93247, 93248])
　　🚗 0.44　⚕ 0.44　**FUD** XXX　　　　80 TC ▢

\# **93243** **scanning analysis with report**
　　EXCLUDES More than 7 days and up to 15 days monitoring ([93245, 93246, 93247, 93248])
　　🚗 0.00　⚕ 0.00　**FUD** XXX　　　　80 TC ▢

\# **93244** **review and interpretation**
　　EXCLUDES More than 7 days and up to 15 days monitoring ([93245, 93246, 93247, 93248])
　　🚗 0.71　⚕ 0.71　**FUD** XXX　　　　80 26 ▢

\# **93245** **External electrocardiographic recording for more than 7 days up to 15 days by continuous rhythm recording and storage; includes recording, scanning analysis with report, review and interpretation**
　　EXCLUDES More than 48 hours up to 7 days monitoring ([93241, 93242, 93243, 93244])
　　🚗 0.00　⚕ 0.00　**FUD** XXX　　　　　80 ▢

\# **93246** **recording (includes connection and initial recording)**
　　EXCLUDES More than 48 hours up to 7 days monitoring ([93241, 93242, 93243, 93244])
　　🚗 0.44　⚕ 0.44　**FUD** XXX　　　　80 TC ▢

\# **93247** **scanning analysis with report**
　　EXCLUDES More than 48 hours up to 7 days monitoring ([93241, 93242, 93243, 93244])
　　🚗 0.00　⚕ 0.00　**FUD** XXX　　　　80 TC ▢

\# **93248** **review and interpretation**
　　EXCLUDES More than 48 hours up to 7 days monitoring ([93241, 93242, 93243, 93244])
　　🚗 0.78　⚕ 0.78　**FUD** XXX　　　　80 26 ▢

93228-93248 [93241, 93242, 93243, 93244, 93245, 93246, 93247, 93248] Remote Cardiovascular Telemetry

INCLUDES Cardiac monitoring using in-person as well as remote technology for electrocardiographic data assessment
Mobile telemetry monitors with capacity to:
Detect arrhythmias
Real-time data analysis for signal quality evaluation quality
Records ECG rhythm on continuous basis using external electrodes on patient
Transmit tracing at any time
Transmit data to attended surveillance center where technician available to respond to device or rhythm alerts and contact physician or qualified health care professional when needed

EXCLUDES Reporting code more than one time in 30-day period

93228 **External mobile cardiovascular telemetry with electrocardiographic recording, concurrent computerized real time data analysis and greater than 24 hours of accessible ECG data storage (retrievable with query) with ECG triggered and patient selected events transmitted to a remote attended surveillance center for up to 30 days; review and interpretation with report by a physician or other qualified health care professional**
　　EXCLUDES Cardiovascular monitors that do not perform automatic ECG triggered transmissions to attended surveillance center (93224-93227, 93268-93272)
　　🚗 0.74　⚕ 0.74　**FUD** XXX　　★ M 80 26 ▢
　　AMA: 2020,Nov,10; 2018,Feb,11; 2018,Jan,8; 2017,Jan,8; 2016,Jan,13

93229 **technical support for connection and patient instructions for use, attended surveillance, analysis and transmission of daily and emergent data reports as prescribed by a physician or other qualified health care professional**
　　🚗 19.9　⚕ 19.9　**FUD** XXX　　★ S 80 TC ▢
　　AMA: 2020,Nov,10; 2018,Feb,11; 2018,Jan,8; 2017,Jan,8; 2016,Jan,13

93241 **Resequenced code. See code following 93227.**
93242 **Resequenced code. See code following 93227.**
93243 **Resequenced code. See code following 93227.**
93244 **Resequenced code. See code following 93227.**
93245 **Resequenced code. See code following 93227.**
93246 **Resequenced code. See code following 93227.**
93247 **Resequenced code. See code following 93227.**
93248 **Resequenced code. See code following 93227.**

93260-93272 [93260, 93261, 93264] Event Monitors

INCLUDES ECG rhythm derived elements, which differ from physiologic data and include heart rhythm, rate, ST analysis, heart rate variability, T-wave alternans, among others
Event monitors that:
Record ECGs in response to patient activation or automatic detection algorithm (or both)
Require attended surveillance
Transmit data upon request (although not immediately when activated)

EXCLUDES Monitoring cardiovascular devices (93279-93289 [93260], 93291-93296, 93298)

93260 **Resequenced code. See code following 93284.**
93261 **Resequenced code. See code following 93289.**
93264 **Resequenced code. See code before 93279.**

93268 **External patient and, when performed, auto activated electrocardiographic rhythm derived event recording with symptom-related memory loop with remote download capability up to 30 days, 24-hour attended monitoring; includes transmission, review and interpretation by a physician or other qualified health care professional**
　　EXCLUDES Implantable patient activated cardiac event recorders (93285, 93291, 93298)
　　Subcutaneous cardiac rhythm monitor (33285)
　　🚗 5.70　⚕ 5.70　**FUD** XXX　　★ M 80 ▢
　　AMA: 2020,Nov,10; 2018,Feb,11; 2018,Jan,8; 2017,Jan,8; 2016,Jan,13

93270 recording (includes connection, recording, and disconnection)

🔹 0.26　　🔸 0.26　　**FUD** XXX　　★ 01 80 TC ▢

AMA: 2020,Nov,10; 2018,Feb,11; 2018,Jan,8; 2017,Jan,8; 2016,Jan,13

93271 transmission and analysis

🔹 4.72　　🔸 4.72　　**FUD** XXX　　★ S 80 TC ▢

AMA: 2020,Nov,10; 2018,Feb,11; 2018,Jan,8; 2017,Jan,8; 2016,Jan,13

93272 review and interpretation by a physician or other qualified health care professional

EXCLUDES *Implantable patient activated cardiac event recorders (93285, 93291, 93298)*

Subcutaneous cardiac rhythm monitor (33285)

🔹 0.72　　🔸 0.72　　**FUD** XXX　　★ M 80 26 ▢

AMA: 2020,Nov,10; 2018,Mar,5; 2018,Feb,11; 2018,Jan,8; 2017,Jan,8; 2016,Jan,13

93278 Signal-averaged Electrocardiography

EXCLUDES *Echocardiography (93303-93355)*

Code also modifier 26 for interpretation and report only

93278 Signal-averaged electrocardiography (SAECG), with or without ECG

🔹 0.85　　🔸 0.85　　**FUD** XXX　　01 80 ▢

AMA: 2018,Feb,11; 2018,Jan,8; 2017,Jan,8; 2016,Jan,13

93264 [93264] Wireless Pulmonary Artery Pressure Sensor Monitoring

INCLUDES Data collection from internal sensor in pulmonary artery

Downloads, interpretation, analysis, and report that must occur at least one time per week

Transmission and storage of data

EXCLUDES *Reporting code wehn monitoring for less than 30-day period*

Reporting code more than one time in 30 days ·

\#　**93264** Remote monitoring of a wireless pulmonary artery pressure sensor for up to 30 days, including at least weekly downloads of pulmonary artery pressure recordings, interpretation(s), trend analysis, and report(s) by a physician or other qualified health care professional

🔹 1.03　　🔸 1.43　　**FUD** XXX　　80 ▢

AMA: 2020,Feb,7; 2019,Oct,3; 2019,Jun,3

93279-93298 [93260, 93261] Monitoring of Cardiovascular Devices

INCLUDES Implantable cardiovascular monitor (ICM) interrogation:

Analysis at least one recorded physiologic cardiovascular data element from either internal or external sensors

Programmed parameters

Implantable defibrillator interrogation:

Battery

Capture and sensing functions

Leads

Presence or absence therapy for ventricular tachyarrhythmias

Programmed parameters

Underlying heart rhythm

Implantable loop recorder (ILR) interrogation:

Heart rate and rhythm during recorded episodes from both patient-initiated and device detected events

Programmed parameters

In-person interrogation/device evaluation (93288)

In-person periprocedural device evaluation/programming device system parameters (93286)

Interrogation evaluation device

Pacemaker interrogation:

Battery

Capture and sensing functions

Heart rhythm

Leads

Programmed parameters

Time period established by initiation remote monitoring or 91st day implantable defibrillator/pacemaker monitoring or 31st day ILR monitoring and extending for succeeding 30- or 90-day period

EXCLUDES *Wearable device monitoring (93224-93272)*

93279 Programming device evaluation (in person) with iterative adjustment of the implantable device to test the function of the device and select optimal permanent programmed values with analysis, review and report by a physician or other qualified health care professional; single lead pacemaker system or leadless pacemaker system in one cardiac chamber

EXCLUDES *External ECG event recording up to 30 days (93268-93272)*

Peri-procedural and interrogation device evaluation (93286, 93288)

Rhythm strips (93040-93042)

Code also body surface-activation mapping, pacemaker or pacing cardioverter-defibrillator lead(s), for electrical synchrony optimization, when performed during same session (0696T)

🔹 1.72　　🔸 1.72　　**FUD** XXX　　01 80 ▢

AMA: 2019,Oct,3; 2019,Mar,6; 2018,Feb,11; 2018,Jan,8; 2017,Jan,8; 2016,Aug,5; 2016,May,5; 2016,Jan,13

93280 dual lead pacemaker system

EXCLUDES *External ECG event recording up to 30 days (93268-93272)*

Peri-procedural and interrogation device evaluation (93286, 93288) ·

Rhythm strips (93040-93042)

🔹 2.03　　🔸 2.03　　**FUD** XXX　　01 80 ▢

AMA: 2019,Oct,3; 2018,Feb,11; 2018,Jan,8; 2017,Jan,8; 2016,Aug,5; 2016,May,5; 2016,Jan,13

93281 multiple lead pacemaker system

EXCLUDES *External ECG event recording up to 30 days (93268-93272)*

Peri-procedural and interrogation device evaluation (93286, 93288)

Rhythm strips (93040-93042)

Code also body surface-activation mapping, pacemaker or pacing cardioverter-defibrillator lead(s), for electrical synchrony optimization, when performed during same session (0696T)

🔹 2.17　　🔸 2.17　　**FUD** XXX　　01 80 ▢

AMA: 2019,Oct,3; 2018,Feb,11; 2018,Jan,8; 2017,Jan,8; 2016,Aug,5; 2016,May,5; 2016,Jan,13

26/TC PC/TC Only　　A2-Z3 ASC Payment　　50 Bilateral　　♂ Male Only　　♀ Female Only　　🔹 Facility RVU　　🔸 Non-Facility RVU　　▢ CCI　　✖ CLIA

FUD Follow-up Days　　**CMS:** IOM　　**AMA:** CPT Asst　　A-Y OPPSI　　80/80 Surg Assist Allowed / w/Doc　　▢ Lab Crosswalk　　▢ Radiology Crosswalk

480　　CPT © 2021 American Medical Association. All Rights Reserved.　　© 2021 Optum360, LLC

93282 **single lead transvenous implantable defibrillator system**

EXCLUDES *Device evaluation subcutaneous lead defibrillator system (93260)*
External ECG event recording up to 30 days (93268-93272)
Peri-procedural and interrogation device evaluation (93287, 93289)
Rhythm strips (93040-93042)
Wearable cardio-defibrillator system services (93745)

2.08   2.08   **FUD** XXX   [01][80][💻]

AMA: 2019,Oct,3; 2018,Feb,11; 2018,Jan,8; 2017,Jan,8; 2016,Aug,5; 2016,Jan,13

93283 **dual lead transvenous implantable defibrillator system**

EXCLUDES *External ECG event recording up to 30 days (93268-93272)*
Peri-procedural and interrogation device evaluation (93287, 93289)
Rhythm strips (93040-93042)

2.60   2.60   **FUD** XXX   [01][80][💻]

AMA: 2019,Oct,3; 2018,Feb,11; 2018,Jan,8; 2017,Jan,8; 2016,Aug,5; 2016,Jan,13

93284 **multiple lead transvenous implantable defibrillator system**

EXCLUDES *External ECG event recording up to 30 days (93268-93272)*
Peri-procedural and interrogation device evaluation (93287, 93289)
Rhythm strips (93040-93042)

Code also body surface-activation mapping, pacemaker or pacing cardioverter-defibrillator lead(s), for electrical synchrony optimization, when performed during same session (0696T)

2.81   2.81   **FUD** XXX   [01][80][💻]

AMA: 2019,Oct,3; 2018,Feb,11; 2018,Jan,8; 2017,Jan,8; 2016,Aug,5; 2016,Jan,13

\# **93260** **implantable subcutaneous lead defibrillator system**

EXCLUDES *Device evaluation (93261, 93282, 93287)*
External ECG event recording up to 30 days (93268-93272)
Insertion/removal/replacement implantable defibrillator (33240, 33241, [33262], [33270, 33271, 33272, 33273])
Rhythm strips (93040-93042)

2.04   2.04   **FUD** XXX   [01][80][💻]

AMA: 2019,Oct,3; 2018,Feb,11; 2018,Jan,8; 2017,Jan,8; 2016,Aug,5; 2016,Jan,13

93285 **subcutaneous cardiac rhythm monitor system**

EXCLUDES *Device evaluation (93279-93284, 93291)*
External ECG event recording up to 30 days (93268-93272)
Insertion subcutaneous cardiac rhythm monitor (33285)
Remote programming device evaluation (0650T)
Rhythm strips (93040-93042)

1.52   1.52   **FUD** XXX   [01][80][💻]

AMA: 2019,Oct,3; 2019,Apr,3; 2018,Feb,11; 2018,Jan,8; 2017,Jan,8; 2016,Aug,5; 2016,Jan,13

93286 **Peri-procedural device evaluation (in person) and programming of device system parameters before or after a surgery, procedure, or test with analysis, review and report by a physician or other qualified health care professional; single, dual, or multiple lead pacemaker system, or leadless pacemaker system**

INCLUDES One evaluation and programming (if performed once before and once after, report as two units)

EXCLUDES *Device evaluation (93279-93281, 93288)*
External ECG event recording up to 30 days (93268-93272)
Rhythm strips (93040-93042)
Services related to cardiac contractility modulation systems (0408T-0411T, 0414T-0415T)
Subcutaneous implantable defibrillator peri-procedural device evaluation and programming (93260, 93261)

Code also body surface-activation mapping, pacemaker or pacing cardioverter-defibrillator lead(s), for electrical synchrony optimization, when performed during same session (0696T)

1.14   1.14   **FUD** XXX   [N][80][💻]

AMA: 2019,Oct,3; 2019,Mar,6; 2018,Feb,11; 2018,Jan,8; 2017,Jan,8; 2016,Aug,5; 2016,May,5; 2016,Jan,13

93287 **single, dual, or multiple lead implantable defibrillator system**

INCLUDES One evaluation and programming (if performed once before and once after, report as two units)

EXCLUDES *Device evaluation (93282-93284, 93289)*
External ECG event recording up to 30 days (93268-93272)
Rhythm strips (93040-93042)
Services related to cardiac contractility modulation systems (0408T-0411T, 0414T-0415T)
Subcutaneous implantable defibrillator peri-procedural device evaluation and programming (93260, 93261)

Code also body surface-activation mapping, pacemaker or pacing cardioverter-defibrillator lead(s), for electrical synchrony optimization, when performed during same session (0696T)

1.36   1.36   **FUD** XXX   [N][80][💻]

AMA: 2019,Oct,3; 2018,Feb,11; 2018,Jan,8; 2017,Jan,8; 2016,Aug,5; 2016,May,5; 2016,Jan,13

93288 **Interrogation device evaluation (in person) with analysis, review and report by a physician or other qualified health care professional, includes connection, recording and disconnection per patient encounter; single, dual, or multiple lead pacemaker system, or leadless pacemaker system**

EXCLUDES *Device evaluation (93279-93281, 93286, 93294-93295)*
External ECG event recording up to 30 days (93268-93272)
Rhythm strips (93040-93042)

Code also body surface-activation mapping, pacemaker or pacing cardioverter-defibrillator lead(s), for electrical synchrony optimization, when performed during same session (0696T)

1.39   1.39   **FUD** XXX   [01][80][💻]

AMA: 2019,Oct,3; 2019,Mar,6; 2018,Feb,11; 2018,Jan,8; 2017,Jan,8; 2016,Aug,5; 2016,May,5; 2016,Jan,13

93289 **single, dual, or multiple lead transvenous implantable defibrillator system, including analysis of heart rhythm derived data elements**

EXCLUDES *Monitoring physiologic cardiovascular data elements derived from implantable defibrillator (93290)*
Device evaluation (93261, 93282-93284, 93287, 93295-93296)
External ECG event recording up to 30 days (93268-93272)
Rhythm strips (93040-93042)

Code also body surface-activation mapping, pacemaker or pacing cardioverter-defibrillator lead(s), for electrical synchrony optimization, when performed during same session (0696T)

1.87   1.87   **FUD** XXX   [01][80][💻]

AMA: 2019,Oct,3; 2018,Feb,11; 2018,Jan,8; 2017,Jan,8; 2016,Aug,5; 2016,May,5; 2016,Jan,13

**93261** **implantable subcutaneous lead defibrillator system**

EXCLUDES Device evaluation (93260, 93287, 93289)
External ECG event recording up to 30 days
(93268-93272)
Insertion/removal/replacement implantable defibrillator
(33240, 33241, [33262], [33270, 33271, 33272,
33273])
Rhythm strips (93040-93042)

🔲 1.87 ⚖ 1.87 **FUD** XXX   🔲01 🔲80 🖵

AMA: 2019,Oct,3; 2018,Feb,11; 2018,Jan,8; 2017,Jan,8;
2016,Aug,5; 2016,Jan,13

93290 **implantable cardiovascular physiologic monitor system,
including analysis of 1 or more recorded physiologic
cardiovascular data elements from all internal and external
sensors**

EXCLUDES Device evaluation (93297)
Heart rhythm derived data (93289)

🔲 1.34 ⚖ 1.34 **FUD** XXX   🔲01 🔲80 🖵

AMA: 2020,Feb,7; 2019,Oct,3; 2018,Feb,11; 2018,Jan,8;
2017,Jan,8; 2016,Aug,5; 2016,Jan,13

93291 **subcutaneous cardiac rhythm monitor system, including
heart rhythm derived data analysis**

EXCLUDES Device evaluation (93288-93290 [93261], 93298)
External ECG event recording up to 30 days
(93268-93272)
Insertion subcutaneous cardiac rhythm monitor (33285)
Remote programming device evaluation subcutaneous
cardiac rhythm monitor system (0650T)
Rhythm strips (93040-93042)

🔲 1.22 ⚖ 1.22 **FUD** XXX   🔲01 🔲80 🖵

AMA: 2019,Oct,3; 2019,Apr,3; 2018,Feb,11; 2018,Jan,8;
2017,Jan,8; 2016,Aug,5; 2016,Jan,13

93292 **wearable defibrillator system**

EXCLUDES External ECG event recording up to 30 days
(93268-93272)
Rhythm strips (93040-93042)
Wearable cardioverter-defibrillator system (93745)

🔲 1.14 ⚖ 1.14 **FUD** XXX   🔲01 🔲80 🖵

AMA: 2019,Oct,3; 2018,Feb,11; 2018,Jan,8; 2017,Jan,8;
2016,Aug,5; 2016,Jan,13

93293 **Transtelephonic rhythm strip pacemaker evaluation(s) single,
dual, or multiple lead pacemaker system, includes recording
with and without magnet application with analysis, review
and report(s) by a physician or other qualified health care
professional, up to 90 days**

EXCLUDES Device evaluation (93294)
External ECG event recording up to 30 days
(93268-93272)
Rhythm strips (93040-93042)
Reporting code more than one time in 90-day period
Reporting code when monitoring period less than 30
days

🔲 1.46 ⚖ 1.46 **FUD** XXX   🔲01 🔲80 🖵

AMA: 2019,Oct,3; 2018,Feb,11; 2018,Jan,8; 2017,Jan,8;
2016,Aug,5; 2016,Jan,13

93294 **Interrogation device evaluation(s) (remote), up to 90 days;
single, dual, or multiple lead pacemaker system, or leadless
pacemaker system with interim analysis, review(s) and
report(s) by a physician or other qualified health care
professional**

EXCLUDES Device evaluation (93288, 93293)
External ECG event recording up to 30 days
(93268-93272)
Rhythm strips (93040-93042)
Reporting code more than one time in 90-day period
Reporting code when monitoring period less than 30
days

🔲 0.87 ⚖ 0.87 **FUD** XXX   🔲M 🔲80 🔲26 🖵

AMA: 2019,Oct,3; 2019,Mar,6; 2018,Feb,11; 2018,Jan,8;
2017,Jan,8; 2016,Aug,5; 2016,Jan,13

93295 **single, dual, or multiple lead implantable defibrillator
system with interim analysis, review(s) and report(s) by a
physician or other qualified health care professional**

EXCLUDES Device evaluation (93289)
External ECG event recording up to 30 days
(93268-93272)
Remote interrogation device evaluation implantable
cardioverter-defibrillator with substernal lead
(0578T, 0579T)
Remote monitoring physiological cardiovascular data
(93297)
Rhythm strips (93040-93042)
Reporting code more than one time in 90-day period
Reporting code when monitoring period less than 30
days

🔲 1.26 ⚖ 1.26 **FUD** XXX   🔲M 🔲80 🔲26 🖵

AMA: 2019,Oct,3; 2018,Feb,11; 2018,Jan,8; 2017,Jan,8;
2016,Aug,5; 2016,Jan,13

93296 **single, dual, or multiple lead pacemaker system, leadless
pacemaker system, or implantable defibrillator system,
remote data acquisition(s), receipt of transmissions and
technician review, technical support and distribution of
results**

EXCLUDES Device evaluation (93288-93289)
External ECG event recording up to 30 days
(93268-93272)
Remote interrogation device evaluation implantable
cardioverter-defibrillator with substernal lead
(0578T, 0579T)
Rhythm strips (93040-93042)
Reporting code more than one time in 90-day period
Reporting code when monitoring period less than 30
days

🔲 0.72 ⚖ 0.72 **FUD** XXX   🔲01 🔲80 🔲TC 🖵

AMA: 2019,Oct,3; 2019,Mar,6; 2019,Jan,6; 2018,Feb,11;
2018,Jan,8; 2017,Jan,8; 2016,Aug,5; 2016,Jan,13

93297 **Interrogation device evaluation(s), (remote) up to 30 days;
implantable cardiovascular physiologic monitor system,
including analysis of 1 or more recorded physiologic
cardiovascular data elements from all internal and external
sensors, analysis, review(s) and report(s) by a physician or
other qualified health care professional**

EXCLUDES Collection and interpretation physiologic data digitally
stored and/or transmitted ([99091])
Device evaluation (93290, 93298)
Heart rhythm derived data (93295)
Remote monitoring physiologic parameter(s) with daily
recording(s) or programmed alert(s) ([99454])
Remote monitoring wireless pulmonary artery pressure
sensor (93264)
Reporting code more than one time in 30-day period
Reporting code when monitoring period less than 10
days

Code also for technical component (G2066)

🔲 0.75 ⚖ 0.75 **FUD** XXX   🔲M 🔲80 🔲26 🖵

AMA: 2020,Feb,12; 2019,Oct,3; 2018,Feb,11; 2018,Jan,8;
2017,Jan,8; 2016,Aug,5; 2016,Jan,13

| 🔲26/🔲TC PC/TC Only | 🔲A2-🔲Z3 ASC Payment | 🔲50 Bilateral | ♂ Male Only | ♀ Female Only | 🔲 Facility RVU | ⚖ Non-Facility RVU | 🔲 CCI | ❌ CLIA |
| **FUD** Follow-up Days | **CMS:** IOM | **AMA:** CPT Asst | 🔲A-🔲Y OPPSI | 🔲80/🔲80 Surg Assist Allowed / w/Doc | 🔲 Lab Crosswalk | 🔲 Radiology Crosswalk |

482   CPT © 2021 American Medical Association. All Rights Reserved.   © 2021 Optum360, LLC

93298   **subcutaneous cardiac rhythm monitor system, including analysis of recorded heart rhythm data, analysis, review(s) and report(s) by a physician or other qualified health care professional**

> EXCLUDES   *Collection and interpretation physiologic data digitally stored and/or transmitted ([99091])*
> *Device evaluation (93291, 93297)*
> *External ECG event recording up to 30 days (93268-93272)*
> *Implantation patient-activated cardiac event recorder (33285)*
> *Remote monitoring physiologic parameter(s) with daily recording(s) or programmed alert(s) ([99454])*
> Code also for technical component (G2066)
> *Reporting code more than one time in 30-day period*
> *Reporting code when monitoring period less than 10 days*
> *Rhythm strips (93040-93042)*

🚗 0.75   ⚖ 0.75   **FUD** XXX   M 80 26 ▢

AMA: 2020,Feb,12; 2019,Oct,3; 2019,Apr,3; 2018,Feb,11; 2018,Jan,8; 2017,Jan,8; 2016,Aug,5; 2016,Jan,13

93303-93356 [93319, 93356] Echocardiography

INCLUDES   Interpretation and report
Obtaining ultrasonic signals from heart/great arteries
Report study including:
    Description recognized abnormalities
    Documentation all clinically relevant findings including obtained quantitative measurements
    Interpretation all information obtained
Two-dimensional image/doppler ultrasonic signal documentation
Ultrasound exam:
    Adjacent great vessels
    Cardiac chambers/valves
    Pericardium
EXCLUDES   *Contrast agents and/or drugs used for pharmacological stress*
Echocardiography, fetal (76825-76828)
Ultrasound with thorough examination organ(s) or anatomic region/documentation image/final written report

93303   **Transthoracic echocardiography for congenital cardiac anomalies; complete**

🚗 6.58   ⚖ 6.58   **FUD** XXX   S 80 ▢

AMA: 2020,Jul,12; 2020,Apr,10; 2020,Jan,7; 2018,Feb,11; 2018,Jan,8; 2017,Jan,8; 2016,Jan,13

93304   **follow-up or limited study**

🚗 4.52   ⚖ 4.52   **FUD** XXX   S 80 ▢

AMA: 2020,Jul,12; 2020,Jan,7; 2018,Feb,11; 2018,Jan,8; 2017,Jan,8; 2016,Jan,13

93306   **Echocardiography, transthoracic, real-time with image documentation (2D), includes M-mode recording, when performed, complete, with spectral Doppler echocardiography, and with color flow Doppler echocardiography**

> INCLUDES   Doppler and color flow
> Two-dimensional and M-mode
> EXCLUDES   *Transthoracic without spectral and color doppler (93307)*

🚗 5.86   ⚖ 5.86   **FUD** XXX   S 80 ▢

AMA: 2020,Jul,12; 2020,May,12; 2020,Jan,7; 2018,Dec,10; 2018,Dec,10; 2018,Feb,11; 2018,Jan,8; 2017,Jan,8; 2016,Apr,8; 2016,Jan,13

93307   **Echocardiography, transthoracic, real-time with image documentation (2D), includes M-mode recording, when performed, complete, without spectral or color Doppler echocardiography**

> INCLUDES   Additional structures that may be viewed such as pulmonary vein or artery, pulmonic valve, inferior vena cava
> Obtaining/recording appropriate measurements
> Two-dimensional/selected M-mode exam:
>   Adjacent portions aorta
>   Aortic/mitral/tricuspid valves
>   Left/right atria
>   Left/right ventricles
>   Pericardium
> Using multiple views as required to obtain complete functional/anatomic evaluation
> EXCLUDES   *Doppler echocardiography (93320-93321, 93325)*

🚗 3.97   ⚖ 3.97   **FUD** XXX   S 80 ▢

AMA: 2020,Jul,12; 2020,May,12; 2020,Jan,7; 2018,Feb,11; 2018,Jan,8; 2017,Jan,8; 2016,Apr,8; 2016,Jan,13

93308   **Echocardiography, transthoracic, real-time with image documentation (2D), includes M-mode recording, when performed, follow-up or limited study**

> INCLUDES   Exam that does not evaluate/document attempt to evaluate all structures comprising complete echocardiographic exam

🚗 2.79   ⚖ 2.79   **FUD** XXX   S 80 ▢

AMA: 2020,Jul,12; 2020,May,12; 2020,Jan,7; 2018,Dec,10; 2018,Dec,10; 2018,Feb,11; 2018,Jan,8; 2017,Jan,8; 2016,Apr,8; 2016,Jan,13

93312   **Echocardiography, transesophageal, real-time with image documentation (2D) (with or without M-mode recording); including probe placement, image acquisition, interpretation and report**

> EXCLUDES   *Transesophageal echocardiography (93355)*

🚗 6.96   ⚖ 6.96   **FUD** XXX   S 80 ▢

AMA: 2020,Jan,7; 2018,Feb,11; 2018,Jan,8; 2017,Jan,8; 2016,Jan,13

93313   **placement of transesophageal probe only**

> EXCLUDES   *Procedure when performed by same person performing transesophageal echocardiography (93355)*

🚗 0.33   ⚖ 0.33   **FUD** XXX   S 80 ▢

AMA: 2020,Jan,7; 2018,Feb,11; 2018,Jan,8; 2017,Jan,8; 2016,Jan,13

93314   **image acquisition, interpretation and report only**

> EXCLUDES   *Transesophageal echocardiography (93355)*

🚗 6.68   ⚖ 6.68   **FUD** XXX   N 80 ▢

AMA: 2020,Jan,7; 2018,Feb,11; 2018,Jan,8; 2017,Jan,8; 2016,Jan,13

93315   **Transesophageal echocardiography for congenital cardiac anomalies; including probe placement, image acquisition, interpretation and report**

> EXCLUDES   *Transesophageal echocardiography (93355)*

🚗 0.00   ⚖ 0.00   **FUD** XXX   S 80 ▢

AMA: 2020,Jan,7; 2018,Feb,11; 2018,Jan,8; 2017,Jan,8; 2016,Jan,13

93316   **placement of transesophageal probe only**

> EXCLUDES   *Transesophageal echocardiography (93355)*

🚗 0.79   ⚖ 0.79   **FUD** XXX   S 80 ▢

AMA: 2020,Jan,7; 2018,Feb,11; 2018,Jan,8; 2017,Jan,8; 2016,Jan,13

93317   **image acquisition, interpretation and report only**

> EXCLUDES   *Transesophageal echocardiography (93355)*

🚗 0.00   ⚖ 0.00   **FUD** XXX   N 80 ▢

AMA: 2020,Jan,7; 2018,Feb,11; 2018,Jan,8; 2017,Jan,8; 2016,Jan,13

● + # **93319** **3D echocardiographic imaging and postprocessing during transesophageal echocardiography, or during transthoracic echocardiography for congenital cardiac anomalies, for the assessment of cardiac structure(s) (eg, cardiac chambers and valves, left atrial appendage, interatrial septum, interventricular septum) and function, when performed (List separately in addition to code for echocardiographic imaging)**

> EXCLUDES *3D rendering (76376, 76377)*
> *Doppler echocardiography color flow velocity mapping (93325)*
> *Echocardiography, transesophageal (TEE) for guidance (93355)*
>
> Code first (93303-93304, 93312, 93314-93315, 93317)
>
> 🖫 0.00   ⚕ 0.00   **FUD** 000

93318 **Echocardiography, transesophageal (TEE) for monitoring purposes, including probe placement, real time 2-dimensional image acquisition and interpretation leading to ongoing (continuous) assessment of (dynamically changing) cardiac pumping function and to therapeutic measures on an immediate time basis**

> EXCLUDES *Transesophageal echocardiography (93355)*
>
> 🖫 0.00   ⚕ 0.00   **FUD** XXX   S 80 ▭
>
> **AMA:** 2020,Jan,7; 2018,Feb,11; 2018,Jan,8; 2017,Jan,8; 2016,Jan,13

93319 **Resequenced code. See code following 93317.**

+ **93320** **Doppler echocardiography, pulsed wave and/or continuous wave with spectral display (List separately in addition to codes for echocardiographic imaging); complete**

> EXCLUDES *Transesophageal echocardiography (93355)*
>
> Code first (93303-93304, 93312, 93314-93315, 93317, 93350-93351)
>
> 🖫 1.51   ⚕ 1.51   **FUD** ZZZ   N 80 ▭
>
> **AMA:** 2020,May,12; 2020,Jan,7; 2018,Feb,11; 2018,Jan,8; 2017,Jan,8; 2016,Jan,13

+ **93321** **follow-up or limited study (List separately in addition to codes for echocardiographic imaging)**

> EXCLUDES *Transesophageal echocardiography (93355)*
>
> Code first (93303-93304, 93308, 93312, 93314-93315, 93317, 93350-93351)
>
> 🖫 0.75   ⚕ 0.75   **FUD** ZZZ   N 80 ▭
>
> **AMA:** 2020,Jan,7; 2018,Feb,11; 2018,Jan,8; 2017,Jan,8; 2016,Jan,13

+ **93325** **Doppler echocardiography color flow velocity mapping (List separately in addition to codes for echocardiography)**

> EXCLUDES *Transesophageal echocardiography (93355)*
>
> Code first (76825-76828, 93303-93304, 93308, 93312, 93314-93315, 93317, 93350-93351)
>
> 🖫 0.70   ⚕ 0.70   **FUD** ZZZ   N 80 ▭
>
> **AMA:** 2020,May,12; 2020,Jan,7; 2018,Feb,11; 2018,Jan,8; 2017,Jan,8; 2016,Jul,8; 2016,Jan,13

93350 **Echocardiography, transthoracic, real-time with image documentation (2D), includes M-mode recording, when performed, during rest and cardiovascular stress test using treadmill, bicycle exercise and/or pharmacologically induced stress, with interpretation and report;**

> EXCLUDES *Cardiovascular stress test, complete procedure (93015)*
>
> Code also exercise stress testing (93016-93018)
>
> 🖫 5.31   ⚕ 5.31   **FUD** XXX   S 80 ▭
>
> **AMA:** 2020,Jul,12; 2018,Feb,11; 2018,Jan,8; 2017,Jan,8; 2016,Apr,8; 2016,Jan,13

93351 **including performance of continuous electrocardiographic monitoring, with supervision by a physician or other qualified health care professional**

> INCLUDES *Stress echocardiogram performed with complete cardiovascular stress test*
>
> EXCLUDES *Cardiovascular stress test (93015-93018)*
> *Echocardiography (93350)*
> *Professional only components complete stress test and stress echocardiogram performed in facility by same physician, append modifier 26*
> *Reporting code for professional component (modifier 26 appended) with (93016, 93018, 93350)*
>
> Code also components cardiovascular stress test when professional services not performed by same physician performing stress echocardiogram (93016-93018)
>
> 🖫 6.57   ⚕ 6.57   **FUD** XXX   S ▭
>
> **AMA:** 2020,Jul,12; 2018,Feb,11; 2018,Jan,8; 2017,Jan,8; 2016,Apr,8; 2016,Jan,13

+ # **93356** **Myocardial strain imaging using speckle tracking-derived assessment of myocardial mechanics (List separately in addition to codes for echocardiography imaging)**

> EXCLUDES *Reporting code more than one time for each session*
>
> Code first (93303-93304, 93306, 93307, 93308, 93350-93351)
>
> 🖫 0.34   ⚕ 1.13   **FUD** ZZZ   80 ▭
>
> **AMA:** 2020,Jul,12; 2020,Apr,10

+ **93352** **Use of echocardiographic contrast agent during stress echocardiography (List separately in addition to code for primary procedure)**

> EXCLUDES *Reporting code more than one time for each stress echocardiogram*
>
> Code first (93350, 93351)
>
> 🖫 0.95   ⚕ 0.95   **FUD** ZZZ   M 80 ▭
>
> **AMA:** 2018,Feb,11; 2018,Jan,8; 2017,Jan,8; 2016,Jan,13

93355 **Echocardiography, transesophageal (TEE) for guidance of a transcatheter intracardiac or great vessel(s) structural intervention(s) (eg, TAVR, transcatheter pulmonary valve replacement, mitral valve repair, paravalvular regurgitation repair, left atrial appendage occlusion/closure, ventricular septal defect closure) (peri-and intra-procedural), real-time image acquisition and documentation, guidance with quantitative measurements, probe manipulation, interpretation, and report, including diagnostic transesophageal echocardiography and, when performed, administration of ultrasound contrast, Doppler, color flow, and 3D**

> EXCLUDES *3D rendering (76376-76377)*
> *Doppler echocardiography (93320-93321, 93325)*
> *Transesophageal echocardiography (93312-93318)*
> *Transesophageal probe positioning by different provider (93313)*
>
> 🖫 6.49   ⚕ 6.49   **FUD** XXX   N 80 ▭
>
> **AMA:** 2018,Feb,11

93356 **Resequenced code. See code following 93351.**

93451-93505 Heart Catheterization

INCLUDES Access site imaging and placement closure device
Catheter insertion and positioning
Contrast injection (except as listed below)
Imaging and insertion closure device
Radiology supervision and interpretation
Roadmapping angiography

EXCLUDES *Congenital cardiac catheterization procedures (93593-93597)*

Code also separately identifiable:
Aortography (93567)
Noncardiac angiography (see radiology and vascular codes)
Pulmonary angiography (93568)
Right ventricular or atrial injection (93566)

93451 Right heart catheterization including measurement(s) of oxygen saturation and cardiac output, when performed

INCLUDES Cardiac output review
Insertion catheter into one or more right cardiac chambers or areas
Obtaining samples for blood gas

EXCLUDES *Catheterization procedures including right side heart (93453, 93456-93457, 93460-93461)*
Implantation wireless pulmonary artery pressure sensor (33289)
Indicator dilution studies (93598)
Percutaneous repair congenital interatrial defect (93580)
Swan-Ganz catheter insertion (93503)
Transcatheter implantation interatrial septal shunt device, percutaneous approach (0613T)
Transcatheter left ventricular restoration device implantation ([0643T])
Transcatheter ultrasound ablation nerves innervating pulmonary arteries, percutaneous approach (0632T)
Valve repair or annulus reconstruction (33418, 0345T, 0483T, 0484T, 0544T, 0545T)

Code also administration medication or exercise to repeat assessment hemodynamic measurement (93463-93464)

🖐 23.9 ✂ 23.9 **FUD** 000 [J] [G2] [80] [▢]

AMA: 2019,Jun,3; 2019,Mar,6; 2018,Dec,10; 2018,Dec,10; 2018,Feb,11; 2018,Jan,8; 2017,Dec,13; 2017,Jul,3; 2017,Jan,8; 2016,Mar,5; 2016,Jan,13

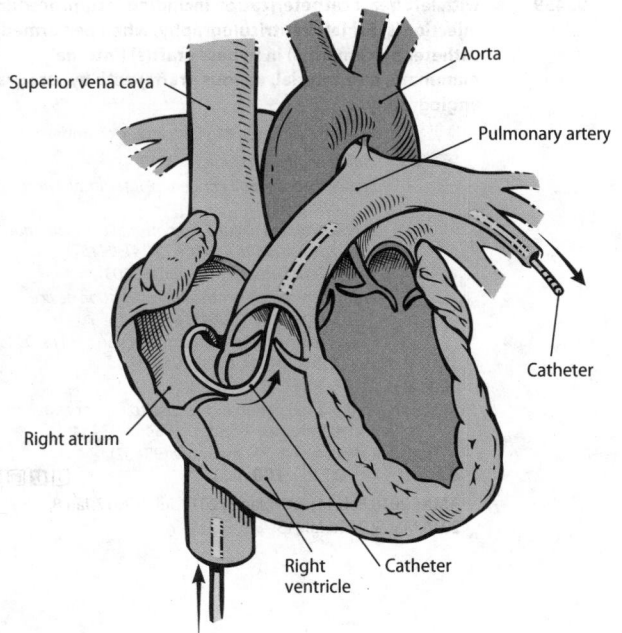

Superior vena cava
Aorta
Pulmonary artery
Catheter
Right atrium
Right ventricle
Catheter

93452 Left heart catheterization including intraprocedural injection(s) for left ventriculography, imaging supervision and interpretation, when performed

INCLUDES Insertion catheter into left cardiac chambers

EXCLUDES *Catheterization procedures including injections for left ventriculography (93453, 93458-93461)*
Indicator dilution studies (93598)
Percutaneous repair congenital interatrial defect (93580)
Services related to cardiac contractility modulation systems (0408T-0411T, 0414T-0415T)
Swan-Ganz catheter insertion (93503)
Transcatheter left ventricular restoration device implantation ([0643T])
Valve repair or annulus reconstruction (33418, 0345T, 0483T, 0484T, 0544T, 0545T)

Code also:
Administration medication or exercise to repeat assessment hemodynamic measurement (93463-93464)
Transapical or transseptal puncture (93462)

🖐 25.9 ✂ 25.9 **FUD** 000 [J] [62] [80] [▢]

AMA: 2018,Feb,11; 2018,Jan,8; 2017,Jul,3; 2017,Jan,8; 2016,Jan,13

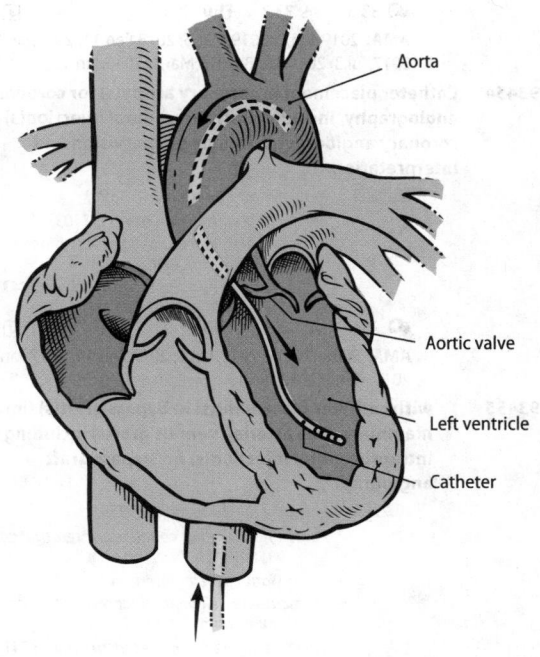

Aorta
Aortic valve
Left ventricle
Catheter

93453 **Combined right and left heart catheterization including intraprocedural injection(s) for left ventriculography, imaging supervision and interpretation, when performed**

INCLUDES Cardiac output review

Insertion catheter into left cardiac chambers

Insertion catheter into one or more right cardiac chambers or areas

Obtaining samples for blood gas

EXCLUDES *Catheterization procedures (93451-93452, 93456-93461)*

Indicator dilution studies (93598)

Percutaneous repair congenital interatrial defect (93580)

Services related to cardiac contractility modulation systems (0408T-0411T, 0414T-0415T)

Swan-Ganz catheter insertion (93503)

Transcatheter left ventricular restoration device implantation ([0643T])

Valve repair or annulus reconstruction (33418, 0345T, 0483T, 0484T, 0544T, 0545T)

Code also:

Administration medication or exercise to repeat assessment hemodynamic measurement (93463-93464)

Transapical or transseptal puncture (93462)

🔧 33.3   ⚕ 33.3   **FUD** 000   J 62 80 📭

AMA: 2019,Jun,3; 2019,Mar,6; 2018,Feb,11; 2018,Jan,8; 2017,Jul,3; 2017,Jan,8; 2016,Mar,5; 2016,Jan,13

93454 **Catheter placement in coronary artery(s) for coronary angiography, including intraprocedural injection(s) for coronary angiography, imaging supervision and interpretation;**

EXCLUDES *Indicator dilution studies (93598)*

Swan-Ganz catheter insertion (93503)

Transcatheter left ventricular restoration device implantation ([0643T])

Valve repair or annulus reconstruction (33418, 0345T, 0483T, 0484T, 0544T, 0545T)

🔧 25.9   ⚕ 25.9   **FUD** 000   J 62 80 📭

AMA: 2018,Feb,11; 2018,Jan,8; 2017,Feb,14; 2017,Jan,8; 2016,Mar,5; 2016,Jan,13

93455 **with catheter placement(s) in bypass graft(s) (internal mammary, free arterial, venous grafts) including intraprocedural injection(s) for bypass graft angiography**

EXCLUDES *Indicator dilution studies (93598)*

Percutaneous repair congenital interatrial defect (93580)

Swan-Ganz catheter insertion (93503)

Transcatheter left ventricular restoration device implantation ([0643T])

Valve repair or annulus reconstruction (33418, 0345T, 0483T, 0484T, 0544T, 0545T)

🔧 28.6   ⚕ 28.6   **FUD** 000   J 62 80 📭

AMA: 2018,Feb,11; 2018,Jan,8; 2017,Jan,8; 2016,Mar,5; 2016,Jan,13

93456 **with right heart catheterization**

INCLUDES Cardiac output review

Insertion catheter into one or more right cardiac chambers or areas

Obtaining samples for blood gas

EXCLUDES *Indicator dilution studies (93598)*

Percutaneous repair congenital interatrial defect (93580)

Swan-Ganz catheter insertion (93503)

Transcatheter left ventricular restoration device implantation ([0643T])

Valve repair or annulus reconstruction (33418, 0345T, 0483T, 0484T, 0544T, 0545T)

Code also administration medication or exercise to repeat assessment hemodynamic measurement (93463-93464)

🔧 32.8   ⚕ 32.8   **FUD** 000   J 62 80 📭

AMA: 2019,Jun,3; 2019,Mar,6; 2018,Feb,11; 2018,Jan,8; 2017,Jul,3; 2017,Jan,8; 2016,Mar,5; 2016,Jan,13

93457 **with catheter placement(s) in bypass graft(s) (internal mammary, free arterial, venous grafts) including intraprocedural injection(s) for bypass graft angiography and right heart catheterization**

INCLUDES Cardiac output review

Insertion catheter into one more right cardiac chambers or areas

Obtaining samples for blood gas

EXCLUDES *Indicator dilution studies (93598)*

Percutaneous repair congenital interatrial defect (93580)

Swan-Ganz catheter insertion (93503)

Transcatheter left ventricular restoration device implantation ([0643T])

Valve repair or annulus reconstruction (33418, 0345T, 0483T, 0484T, 0544T, 0545T)

Code also administration medication or exercise to repeat assessment hemodynamic measurement (93463-93464)

🔧 36.4   ⚕ 36.4   **FUD** 000   J 62 80 📭

AMA: 2019,Jun,3; 2019,Mar,6; 2018,Feb,11; 2018,Jan,8; 2017,Jan,8; 2016,Mar,5; 2016,Jan,13

93458 **with left heart catheterization including intraprocedural injection(s) for left ventriculography, when performed**

INCLUDES Insertion catheter into left cardiac chambers

EXCLUDES *Indicator dilution studies (93598)*

Percutaneous repair congenital interatrial defect (93580)

Services related to cardiac contractility modulation systems (0408T-0411T, 0414T-0415T)

Swan-Ganz catheter insertion (93503)

Transcatheter left ventricular restoration device implantation ([0643T])

Valve repair or annulus reconstruction (33418, 0345T, 0483T, 0484T, 0544T, 0545T)

Code also:

Administration medication or exercise to repeat assessment hemodynamic measurement (93463-93464)

Transapical or transseptal puncture (93462)

🔧 30.4   ⚕ 30.4   **FUD** 000   J 62 80 📭

AMA: 2018,Feb,11; 2018,Jan,8; 2017,Jul,3; 2017,Jan,8; 2016,Mar,5; 2016,Jan,13

93459 **with left heart catheterization including intraprocedural injection(s) for left ventriculography, when performed, catheter placement(s) in bypass graft(s) (internal mammary, free arterial, venous grafts) with bypass graft angiography**

INCLUDES Insertion catheter into left cardiac chambers

EXCLUDES *Indicator dilution studies (93598)*

Percutaneous repair congenital interatrial defect (93580)

Services related to cardiac contractility modulation systems (0408T-0411T, 0414T-0415T)

Swan-Ganz catheter insertion (93503)

Transcatheter left ventricular restoration device implantation ([0643T])

Valve repair or annulus reconstruction (33418, 0345T, 0483T, 0484T, 0544T, 0545T)

Code also:

Administration medication or exercise to repeat assessment hemodynamic measurement (93463-93464)

Transapical or transseptal puncture (93462)

🔧 33.1   ⚕ 33.1   **FUD** 000   J 62 80 📭

AMA: 2018,Feb,11; 2018,Jan,8; 2017,Jul,3; 2017,Jan,8; 2016,Mar,5; 2016,Jan,13

93460 **with right and left heart catheterization including intraprocedural injection(s) for left ventriculography, when performed**

INCLUDES Cardiac output review
Insertion catheter into left cardiac chambers
Insertion catheter into one or more right cardiac chambers or areas
Obtaining samples for blood gas

EXCLUDES *Indicator dilution studies (93598)*
Percutaneous repair congenital interatrial defect (93580)
Services related to cardiac contractility modulation systems (0408T-0411T, 0414T-0415T)
Swan-Ganz catheter insertion (93503)
Transcatheter left ventricular restoration device implantation ([0643T])
Valve repair or annulus reconstruction (33418, 0345T, 0483T, 0484T, 0544T, 0545T)

Code also:
Administration medication or exercise to repeat assessment hemodynamic measurement (93463-93464)
Transapical or transseptal puncture (93462)

🔧 36.6 ⚙ 36.6 **FUD** 000   J 62 80 ▭

AMA: 2019,Jun,3; 2019,Mar,6; 2018,Feb,11; 2018,Jan,8; 2017,Jul,3; 2017,Jan,8; 2016,Mar,5; 2016,Jan,13

93461 **with right and left heart catheterization including intraprocedural injection(s) for left ventriculography, when performed, catheter placement(s) in bypass graft(s) (internal mammary, free arterial, venous grafts) with bypass graft angiography**

INCLUDES Cardiac output review
Insertion catheter into left cardiac chambers
Insertion catheter into one or more right cardiac chambers or areas
Obtaining samples for blood gas

EXCLUDES *Indicator dilution studies (93598)*
Percutaneous repair congenital interatrial defect (93580)
Services related to cardiac contractility modulation systems (0408T-0411T, 0414T-0415T)
Swan-Ganz catheter insertion (93503)
Transcatheter left ventricular restoration device implantation ([0643T])
Valve repair or annulus reconstruction (33418, 0345T, 0483T, 0484T, 0544T, 0545T)

Code also:
Administration medication or exercise to repeat assessment hemodynamic measurement (93463-93464)
Transapical or transseptal puncture (93462)

🔧 41.0 ⚙ 41.0 **FUD** 000   J 62 80 ▭

AMA: 2019,Jun,3; 2019,Mar,6; 2018,Feb,11; 2018,Jan,8; 2017,Jul,3; 2017,Jan,8; 2016,Mar,5; 2016,Jan,13

+ 93462 **Left heart catheterization by transseptal puncture through intact septum or by transapical puncture (List separately in addition to code for primary procedure)**

INCLUDES Insertion catheter into left cardiac chambers

EXCLUDES *Comprehensive electrophysiologic evaluation (93656)*
Transseptal approach for percutaneous closure paravalvular leak (93590)
Valve repair or annulus reconstruction unless performed with transapical puncture (33418, 0345T, 0544T)

Code also, when performed:
Percutaneous closure paravalvular leak when transapical puncture (93590-93591)
Percutaneous closure ventricular septal defect (93581)
Code first (33477, 33741, 33745, 93452-93453, 93458-93461, 93582, 93595-93597, 93653-93654)

🔧 6.11 ⚙ 6.11 **FUD** ZZZ   N N1 80 ▭

AMA: 2020,Nov,7; 2018,Feb,11; 2018,Jan,8; 2017,Sep,3; 2017,Jul,3; 2017,Jan,8; 2016,Jan,13

+ 93463 **Pharmacologic agent administration (eg, inhaled nitric oxide, intravenous infusion of nitroprusside, dobutamine, milrinone, or other agent) including assessing hemodynamic measurements before, during, after and repeat pharmacologic agent administration, when performed (List separately in addition to code for primary procedure)**

EXCLUDES *Coronary interventional procedures (92920-92944, 92975, 92977)*
Reporting code more than one time per catheterization

Code first (33477, 93451-93453, 93456-93461, 93580-93582, 93593-93597)

🔧 2.82 ⚙ 2.82 **FUD** ZZZ   N 80 ▭

AMA: 2018,Feb,11; 2018,Jan,8; 2017,Jan,8; 2016,Jan,13

+ 93464 **Physiologic exercise study (eg, bicycle or arm ergometry) including assessing hemodynamic measurements before and after (List separately in addition to code for primary procedure)**

EXCLUDES *Administration of pharmacologic agent (93463)*
Reporting code more than one time per catheterization

Code first (33477, 93451-93453, 93456-93461, 93593-93597)

🔧 6.89 ⚙ 6.89 **FUD** ZZZ   N 80 ▭

AMA: 2018,Feb,11; 2018,Jan,8; 2017,Jan,8; 2016,Jan,13

93503 **Insertion and placement of flow directed catheter (eg, Swan-Ganz) for monitoring purposes**

EXCLUDES *Diagnostic cardiac catheterization (93451-93461, 93593-93594)*
Subsequent monitoring (99356-99357)
Transcatheter ultrasound ablation nerves innervating pulmonary arteries, percutaneous approach (0632T)

🔧 2.55 ⚙ 2.55 **FUD** 000   T 80 ▭

AMA: 2018,Feb,11; 2018,Jan,8; 2017,Jan,8; 2016,Jan,13

93505 **Endomyocardial biopsy**

EXCLUDES *Cardiac blood pool imaging (78472-78473, 78481)*
Transcatheter insertion brachytherapy delivery device (92974)

🔧 20.1 ⚙ 20.1 **FUD** 000   T 80 ▭

AMA: 2018,Feb,11; 2018,Jan,8; 2017,Dec,13; 2017,Jan,8; 2016,Jan,13

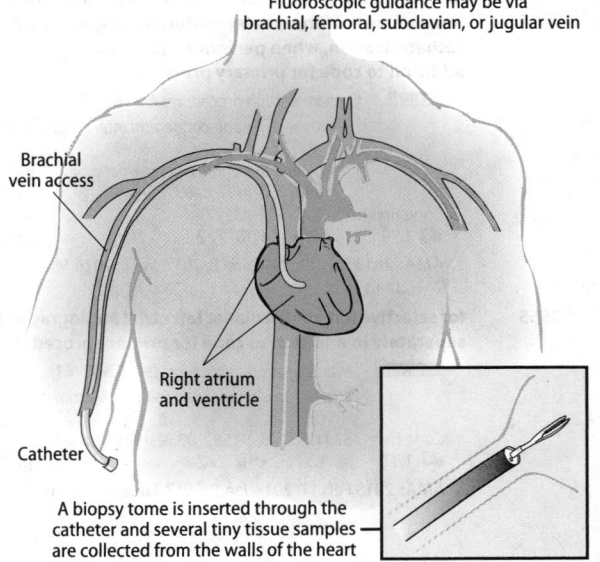

Fluoroscopic guidance may be via brachial, femoral, subclavian, or jugular vein

Brachial vein access

Right atrium and ventricle

Catheter

A biopsy tome is inserted through the catheter and several tiny tissue samples are collected from the walls of the heart

93530-93533 Congenital Heart Defect Catheterization

93530 ~~Right heart catheterization, for congenital cardiac anomalies~~

To report, see (93593-93594)

~~93531~~ ~~Combined right heart catheterization and retrograde left~~
~~heart catheterization, for congenital cardiac anomalies~~
To report, see (93462, 93596-93597)

~~93532~~ ~~Combined right heart catheterization and transseptal left~~
~~heart catheterization through intact septum with or without~~
~~retrograde left heart catheterization, for congenital cardiac~~
~~anomalies~~
To report, see (93462, 93596-93597)

~~93533~~ ~~Combined right heart catheterization and transseptal left~~
~~heart catheterization through existing septal opening, with~~
~~or without retrograde left heart catheterization, for~~
~~congenital cardiac anomalies~~
To report, see (93462, 93596-93597)

93561-93568 Injection Procedures

INCLUDES   Automatic power injector
Catheter repositioning
Radiology supervision and interpretation

~~93561~~ ~~Indicator dilution studies such as dye or thermodilution,~~
~~including arterial and/or venous catheterization; with cardiac~~
~~output measurement (separate procedure)~~
To report, see (93598)

~~93562~~ ~~subsequent measurement of cardiac output~~
To report, see (93598)

+ **93563** **Injection procedure during cardiac catheterization including**
imaging supervision, interpretation, and report; for selective
coronary angiography during congenital heart catheterization
(List separately in addition to code for primary procedure)

EXCLUDES   *Catheterization procedures (93452-93461)*
Valve repair or annulus reconstruction (33418, 0345T,
0483T, 0484T, 0544T, 0545T)
Code first (33741, 33745, 93582, 93593-93597)
🔧 1.69   ✂ 1.69   **FUD** ZZZ   N 80 💻

AMA: 2018,Feb,11; 2018,Jan,8; 2017,Jan,8; 2016,Mar,5;
2016,Jan,13

+ **93564** **for selective opacification of aortocoronary venous or**
arterial bypass graft(s) (eg, aortocoronary saphenous vein,
free radial artery, or free mammary artery graft) to one or
more coronary arteries and in situ arterial conduits (eg,
internal mammary), whether native or used for bypass to
one or more coronary arteries during congenital heart
catheterization, when performed (List separately in
addition to code for primary procedure)

EXCLUDES   *Catheterization procedures (93452-93461)*
Percutaneous repair congenital interatrial defect
(93580)
Valve repair or annulus reconstruction (33418, 0345T,
0483T, 0484T, 0544T, 0545T)
Code first (93582, 93593-93597)
🔧 1.79   ✂ 1.79   **FUD** ZZZ   N 80 💻

AMA: 2018,Feb,11; 2018,Jan,8; 2017,Jan,8; 2016,Mar,5;
2016,Jan,13

+ **93565** **for selective left ventricular or left atrial angiography (List**
separately in addition to code for primary procedure)

EXCLUDES   *Catheterization procedures (93452-93461)*
Percutaneous repair congenital interatrial defect
(93580)
Code first (33741, 33745, 93582, 93593-93597)
🔧 1.31   ✂ 1.31   **FUD** ZZZ   N 80 💻

AMA: 2018,Feb,11; 2018,Jan,8; 2017,Jan,8; 2016,Jan,13

+ **93566** **for selective right ventricular or right atrial angiography**
(List separately in addition to code for primary
procedure)

EXCLUDES   *Annulus reconstruction (0545T)*
Percutaneous repair congenital interatrial defect
(93580)
Right ventriculography when performed during
insertion leadless pacemaker ([33274])
Code first (33741, 33745, 93451, 93453, 93456-93457,
93460-93461, 93582, 93593-93597)
🔧 1.35   ✂ 4.38   **FUD** ZZZ   N NI 80 💻

AMA: 2019,Mar,6; 2018,Feb,11; 2018,Jan,8; 2017,Jan,8;
2016,Aug,5; 2016,May,5; 2016,Mar,5; 2016,Jan,13

+ **93567** **for supravalvular aortography (List separately in addition**
to code for primary procedure)

EXCLUDES   *Abdominal aortography or non-supravalvular thoracic*
aortography at same time as cardiac
catheterization (36221, 75600-75630)
Code first (33741, 33745, 93451-93461, 93593-93597)
🔧 1.53   ✂ 3.71   **FUD** ZZZ   N NI 80 💻

AMA: 2018,Feb,11; 2018,Jan,8; 2017,Jan,8; 2016,Mar,5;
2016,Jan,13

+ **93568** **for pulmonary angiography (List separately in addition to**
code for primary procedure)

EXCLUDES   *Transcatheter ultrasound ablation nerves innervating*
pulmonary arteries, percutaneous approach
(0632T)
Code first (33741, 33745, 93451, 93453, 93456-93457,
93460-93461, 93580-93583, 93593-93597)
🔧 1.38   ✂ 3.97   **FUD** ZZZ   N NI 80 💻

AMA: 2019,Jun,3; 2019,Apr,10; 2018,Feb,11; 2018,Jan,8;
2017,Jan,8; 2016,Mar,5; 2016,Jan,13

93571-93572 Coronary Artery Doppler Studies

INCLUDES   Doppler transducer manipulations/repositioning within vessel examined,
during coronary angiography/therapeutic intervention (angioplasty)
EXCLUDES   *Intraprocedural coronary fractional flow reserve (FFR) ([0523T])*

+ **93571** **Intravascular Doppler velocity and/or pressure derived**
coronary flow reserve measurement (coronary vessel or graft)
during coronary angiography including pharmacologically
induced stress; initial vessel (List separately in addition to
code for primary procedure)

Code first ([92920], [92924], [92928], [92933], [92937], [92941],
[92943], [92975], 93454-93461, 93563-93564, 93593-93597)
🔧 0.00   ✂ 0.00   **FUD** ZZZ   N NI 80 💻

AMA: 2018,Feb,11; 2018,Jan,8; 2017,Jan,8; 2016,Jan,13

+ **93572** **each additional vessel (List separately in addition to code**
for primary procedure)

Code first initial vessel (93571)
🔧 0.00   ✂ 0.00   **FUD** ZZZ   N NI 80 💻

AMA: 2018,Feb,11; 2018,Jan,8; 2017,Jan,8; 2016,Jan,13

93580-93583 Percutaneous Repair of Congenital Heart Defects

93580 **Percutaneous transcatheter closure of congenital interatrial**
communication (ie, Fontan fenestration, atrial septal defect)
with implant

INCLUDES   Injection contrast for atrial/ventricular angiograms
(93565-93566)
Right heart catheterization (93451, 93456-93457,
93593-93594)

EXCLUDES   *Left heart catheterization (93452, 93458-93459, 93595)*
Measurement cardiac output (93598)
Other contrast injections (93563-93564, 93567-93568)
Right and left heart catheterization (93453,
93460-93461, 93596-93597)
Code also echocardiography, when performed (93303-93317,
93662)
🔧 28.4   ✂ 28.4   **FUD** 000   J 80 💻

AMA: 2018,Feb,11; 2018,Jan,8; 2017,Jan,8; 2016,Jan,13

26/TC PC/TC Only   A2-Z3 ASC Payment   50 Bilateral   ♂ Male Only   ♀ Female Only   🔧 Facility RVU   ✂ Non-Facility RVU   💻 CCI   ❌ CLIA
FUD Follow-up Days   **CMS:** IOM   **AMA:** CPT Asst   A-Y OPPSI   80/80 Surg Assist Allowed / w/Doc   Lab Crosswalk   Radiology Crosswalk

488   CPT © 2021 American Medical Association. All Rights Reserved.   © 2021 Optum360, LLC

Medicine

93581 **Percutaneous transcatheter closure of a congenital ventricular septal defect with implant**

INCLUDES   Injection contrast for atrial/ventricular angiograms (93565-93566)
Right heart catheterization (93451, 93456-93457, 93593-93594)

EXCLUDES   *Left heart catheterization (93452, 93458-93459, 93595)*
Measurement cardiac output (93598)
Other contrast injections (93563-93564, 93567-93568)
Right and left heart catheterization (93453, 93460-93461, 93596-93597)

Code also echocardiography, when performed (93303-93317, 93662)

🚑 38.7   ✂ 38.7   **FUD** 000   J 80 🖥

AMA: 2018,Feb,11; 2018,Jan,8; 2017,Jan,8; 2016,Jan,13

93582 **Percutaneous transcatheter closure of patent ductus arteriosus**

INCLUDES   Aorta catheter placement (36200)
Aortography (75600-75605, 93567)
Heart catheterization (93451, 93453, 93456-93461, 93593-93598)

EXCLUDES   *Catheterization pulmonary artery (36013-36014)*
Intracardiac echocardiographic services (93662) ·
Ligation repair (33820, 33822, 33824)
Other cardiac angiographic procedures (93563-93566, 93568)
Other echocardiographic services by different provider (93315-93317)

🚑 19.4   ✂ 19.4   **FUD** 000   J 80 🖥

AMA: 2019,Apr,10; 2018,Feb,11; 2018,Jan,8; 2017,Jan,8; 2016,Jan,13

93583 **Percutaneous transcatheter septal reduction therapy (eg, alcohol septal ablation) including temporary pacemaker insertion when performed**

INCLUDES   Alcohol injection (93463)
Coronary angiography during procedure to roadmap, guide intervention, measure vessel, and complete angiography (93454-93461, 93563, 93563, 93565)
Left heart catheterization (93452-93453, 93458-93461, 93595-93597)
Temporary pacemaker insertion (33210-33211)

EXCLUDES   *Intracardiac echocardiographic services when performed (93662)*
Myectomy (surgical ventriculomyotomy) to treat idiopathic hypertrophic subaortic stenosis (33416)
Other echocardiographic services rendered by different provider (93312-93317)

Code also diagnostic cardiac catheterization procedures if patient's condition (clinical indication) changed since intervention or prior study, no available prior catheter-based diagnostic study in treatment zone, or prior study not adequate (93451, 93454-93457, 93563-93564, 93566-93568, 93593-93594, 93598)

🚑 21.6   ✂ 21.6   **FUD** 000   C 80 🖥

AMA: 2018,Feb,11

93590-93592 Percutaneous Repair Paravalvular Leak

INCLUDES   Access with insertion and positioning of device
Angiography
Fluoroscopy (76000)
Imaging guidance
Left heart catheterization (93452-93453, 93458-93461, 93565, 93595-93597)

Code also diagnostic cardiac catheterization procedures if patient's condition (clinical indication) changed since intervention or prior study, no available prior catheter-based diagnostic study in treatment zone, or prior study not adequate; append modifier 59 (93451, 93454-93457, 93563-93564, 93593-93594, 93598)

93590 **Percutaneous transcatheter closure of paravalvular leak; initial occlusion device, mitral valve**

INCLUDES   Transseptal puncture (93462)

Code also for transapical puncture/left heart catheterization, when performed (93462)

🚑 31.2   ✂ 31.2   **FUD** 000   J 80 🖥

AMA: 2018,Feb,11; 2018,Jan,8; 2017,Sep,3

93591 **initial occlusion device, aortic valve**

Code also for transapical puncture/left heart catheterization, when performed (93462)

🚑 25.7   ✂ 25.7   **FUD** 000   J 80 🖥

AMA: 2018,Feb,11; 2018,Jan,8; 2017,Sep,3

+ **93592** **each additional occlusion device (List separately in addition to code for primary procedure)**

Code first (93590-93591)

🚑 11.3   ✂ 11.3   **FUD** ZZZ   N 80 🖥

AMA: 2018,Feb,11; 2018,Jan,8; 2017,Sep,3

93593-93598 Cardiac Catheterization for Congenital Heart Defects

INCLUDES   Access site imaging and placement closure device
Cardiac output review
Evaluation anomalous coronary arteries arising from pulmonary arterial system
Insertion catheter into one or more right cardiac chambers or areas
Obtaining samples for blood gas
Radiologic supervision and interpretation
Roadmapping angiography

EXCLUDES   *Angiography/ventriculography (93565-93566)*
Angiography native coronary arteries/bypass arteries during same operative session (93563-93564)
Cardiac cath on noncongenital heart (93451-93453, 93456-93461)
Contrast injections (93563-93568)
Percutaneous repair congenital interarterial defect (93580)
Swan-Ganz catheter insertion (93503)

Code also, when performed:
Pharmacologic agent administration (93463)
Physiologic exercise study during procedure (93464)
Transapical or transseptal access (93462)

● **93593** **Right heart catheterization for congenital heart defect(s) including imaging guidance by the proceduralist to advance the catheter to the target zone; normal native connections**

● **93594** **abnormal native connections**

● **93595** **Left heart catheterization for congenital heart defect(s) including imaging guidance by the proceduralist to advance the catheter to the target zone, normal or abnormal native connections**

● **93596** **Right and left heart catheterization for congenital heart defect(s) including imaging guidance by the proceduralist to advance the catheter to the target zone(s); normal native connections**

● **93597** **abnormal native connections**

● + **93598** **Cardiac output measurement(s), thermodilution or other indicator dilution method, performed during cardiac catheterization for the evaluation of congenital heart defects (List separately in addition to code for primary procedure)**

Code first (93593-93597)

🚑 0.00   ✂ 0.00   **FUD** 000

93600-93603 Recording of Intracardiac Electrograms

INCLUDES   Unusual situations in which there may be recording/pacing/attempt at arrhythmia induction from only one side heart

EXCLUDES   *Comprehensive electrophysiological studies (93619-93620, 93653-93654, 93656)*

93600 **Bundle of His recording**

🚑 0.00   ✂ 0.00   **FUD** 000   ⊘ J 80 🖥

AMA: 2018,Feb,11; 2018,Jan,8; 2017,Jan,8; 2016,Jan,13

93602 **Intra-atrial recording**

🚑 0.00   ✂ 0.00   **FUD** 000   ⊘ J 80 🖥

AMA: 2018,Feb,11; 2018,Jan,8; 2017,Jan,8; 2016,Jan,13

93603 **Right ventricular recording**

🚑 0.00   ✂ 0.00   **FUD** 000   ⊘ J 80 🖥

AMA: 2018,Feb,11; 2018,Jan,8; 2017,Jan,8; 2016,Jan,13

93609-93613 Intracardiac Mapping and Pacing

+ 93609 **Intraventricular and/or intra-atrial mapping of tachycardia site(s) with catheter manipulation to record from multiple sites to identify origin of tachycardia (List separately in addition to code for primary procedure)**

> EXCLUDES *Intracardiac 3D mapping (93613)*
> *Intracardiac ablation with 3D mapping (93654)*
> Code first (93620, 93653, 93656)
> 📇 0.00 ⚖ 0.00 **FUD** ZZZ N 80 💻
> **AMA:** 2018,Feb,11; 2018,Jan,8; 2017,Jan,8; 2016,Jan,13

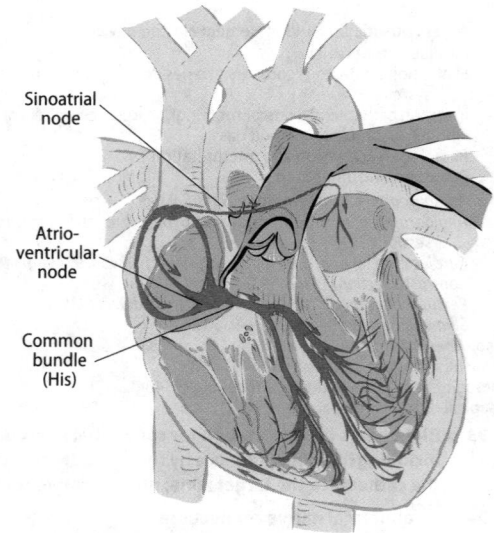

Sinoatrial node

Atrio-ventricular node

Common bundle (His)

Tachycardia is rapid heartbeat

93610 **Intra-atrial pacing**

> INCLUDES Unusual situations in which there may be recording/pacing/attempt at arrhythmia induction from only one side heart
> EXCLUDES *Comprehensive electrophysiological studies (93619-93620)*
> *Intracardiac ablation (93653-93654, 93656)*
> 📇 0.00 ⚖ 0.00 **FUD** 000 ⊘ J 80 💻
> **AMA:** 2018,Feb,11; 2018,Jan,8; 2017,Jan,8; 2016,Jan,13

93612 **Intraventricular pacing**

> INCLUDES Unusual situations in which there may be recording/pacing/attempt at arrhythmia induction from only one side heart
> EXCLUDES *Comprehensive electrophysiological studies (93619-93622)*
> *Intracardiac ablation (93653-93654, 93656)*
> 📇 0.00 ⚖ 0.00 **FUD** 000 ⊘ J 80 💻
> **AMA:** 2018,Feb,11; 2018,Jan,8; 2017,Jan,8; 2016,Jan,13

+ 93613 **Intracardiac electrophysiologic 3-dimensional mapping (List separately in addition to code for primary procedure)**

> EXCLUDES *Intracardiac ablation with 3D mapping (93654)*
> *Mapping tachycardia site (93609)*
> Code first (93620)
> 📇 8.63 ⚖ 8.63 **FUD** ZZZ N 80 💻
> **AMA:** 2018,Feb,11; 2018,Jan,8; 2017,Jan,8; 2016,Jan,13

93615-93616 Recording and Pacing via Esophagus

93615 **Esophageal recording of atrial electrogram with or without ventricular electrogram(s);**

> 📇 0.00 ⚖ 0.00 **FUD** 000 ⊘ J 80 💻
> **AMA:** 2018,Feb,11; 2018,Jan,8; 2017,Jan,8; 2016,Jan,13

93616 **with pacing**

> 📇 0.00 ⚖ 0.00 **FUD** 000 ⊘ J 80 💻
> **AMA:** 2018,Feb,11; 2018,Jan,8; 2017,Jan,8; 2016,Jan,13

93618 Pacing to Produce an Arrhythmia

CMS: 100-03,20.12 Diagnostic Endocardial Electrical Stimulation (Pacing)

> INCLUDES Unusual situations in which there may be recording/pacing/attempt at arrhythmia induction from only one side heart
> EXCLUDES *Comprehensive electrophysiological studies (93619-93622)*
> *Intracardiac ablation (93653-93656, 93656)*
> *Intracardiac phonocardiogram (93799)*

93618 **Induction of arrhythmia by electrical pacing**

> 📇 0.00 ⚖ 0.00 **FUD** 000 ⊘ J 80 💻
> **AMA:** 2018,Feb,11; 2018,Jan,8; 2017,Jan,8; 2016,Jan,13

93619-93623 Comprehensive Electrophysiological Studies

CMS: 100-03,20.12 Diagnostic Endocardial Electrical Stimulation (Pacing)

93619 **Comprehensive electrophysiologic evaluation with right atrial pacing and recording, right ventricular pacing and recording, His bundle recording, including insertion and repositioning of multiple electrode catheters, without induction or attempted induction of arrhythmia**

> INCLUDES Evaluation sinus node/atrioventricular node/His-Purkinje conduction system without arrhythmia induction
> EXCLUDES *Comprehensive electrophysiological studies (93620-93622)*
> *Intracardiac ablation (93653-93657)*
> *Intracardiac pacing (93610, 93612, 93618)*
> *Recording intracardiac electrograms (93600-93603)*
> 📇 0.00 ⚖ 0.00 **FUD** 000 J 80 💻
> **AMA:** 2018,Feb,11; 2018,Jan,8; 2017,Jan,8; 2016,Jan,13

93620 **Comprehensive electrophysiologic evaluation including insertion and repositioning of multiple electrode catheters with induction or attempted induction of arrhythmia; with right atrial pacing and recording, right ventricular pacing and recording, His bundle recording**

> INCLUDES Recording/pacing/attempted arrhythmia induction from one or more site(s) in heart
> EXCLUDES *Comprehensive electrophysiological study without induction/attempted induction arrhythmia (93619)*
> *Intracardiac ablation (93653-93657)*
> *Intracardiac pacing (93610, 93612, 93618)*
> *Recording intracardiac electrograms (93600-93603)*
> 📇 0.00 ⚖ 0.00 **FUD** 000 J 80 💻
> **AMA:** 2018,Feb,11; 2018,Jan,8; 2017,Jan,8; 2016,Jan,13

+ 93621 **with left atrial pacing and recording from coronary sinus or left atrium (List separately in addition to code for primary procedure)**

> INCLUDES Recording/pacing/attempted arrhythmia induction from one or more site(s) in heart
> EXCLUDES *Intracardiac ablation (93656)*
> Code first (93620)
> 📇 0.00 ⚖ 0.00 **FUD** ZZZ N 80 💻
> **AMA:** 2018,Feb,11; 2018,Jan,8; 2017,Jan,8; 2016,Jan,13

+ 93622 **with left ventricular pacing and recording (List separately in addition to code for primary procedure)**

> EXCLUDES *Intracardiac ablation (93654)*
> Code first (93620, 93653, 93656)
> 📇 0.00 ⚖ 0.00 **FUD** ZZZ N 80 💻
> **AMA:** 2018,Feb,11; 2018,Jan,8; 2017,Jan,8; 2016,Jan,13

+ 93623 **Programmed stimulation and pacing after intravenous drug infusion (List separately in addition to code for primary procedure)**

> INCLUDES Recording/pacing/attempted arrhythmia induction from one or more site(s) in heart
> EXCLUDES *Reporting code more than one time per day*
> Code first comprehensive electrophysiologic evaluation (93610, 93612, 93619-93620, 93653-93654, 93656)
> 📇 0.00 ⚖ 0.00 **FUD** ZZZ N 80 💻
> **AMA:** 2018,Feb,11; 2018,Jan,8; 2017,Jan,8; 2016,Jan,13

26/TC PC/TC Only A2-Z3 ASC Payment 50 Bilateral ♂ Male Only ♀ Female Only 📇 Facility RVU ⚖ Non-Facility RVU 💻 CCI ❌ CLIA
FUD Follow-up Days **CMS:** IOM **AMA:** CPT Asst A-Y OPPSI 80/80 Surg Assist Allowed / w/Doc Lab Crosswalk Radiology Crosswalk

490

CPT © 2021 American Medical Association. All Rights Reserved.

© 2021 Optum360, LLC

93624-93631 Followup and Intraoperative Electrophysiologic Studies

CMS: 100-03,20.12 Diagnostic Endocardial Electrical Stimulation (Pacing)

93624 Electrophysiologic follow-up study with pacing and recording to test effectiveness of therapy, including induction or attempted induction of arrhythmia

INCLUDES Recording/pacing/attempted arrhythmia induction from one or more site(s) in heart

🔧 0.00 ⚖ 0.00 **FUD** 000 J 80 ▢

AMA: 2018,Feb,11; 2018,Jan,8; 2017,Jan,8; 2016,Jan,13

93631 Intra-operative epicardial and endocardial pacing and mapping to localize the site of tachycardia or zone of slow conduction for surgical correction

EXCLUDES Operative ablation arrhythmogenic focus or pathway by separate provider (33250-33261)

🔧 0.00 ⚖ 0.00 **FUD** 000 N 80 ▢

AMA: 2018,Feb,11; 2018,Jan,8; 2017,Jan,8; 2016,Jan,13

93640-93644 Electrophysiologic Studies of Cardioverter-Defibrillators

INCLUDES Recording/pacing/attempted arrhythmia induction from one or more site(s) in heart

93640 Electrophysiologic evaluation of single or dual chamber pacing cardioverter-defibrillator leads including defibrillation threshold evaluation (induction of arrhythmia, evaluation of sensing and pacing for arrhythmia termination) at time of initial implantation or replacement;

🔧 0.00 ⚖ 0.00 **FUD** 000 N 80 ▢

AMA: 2018,Feb,11; 2018,Jan,8; 2017,Jan,8; 2016,Jan,13

93641 with testing of single or dual chamber pacing cardioverter-defibrillator pulse generator

EXCLUDES Single/dual chamber pacing cardioverter-defibrillators reprogramming/electronic analysis, subsequent/periodic (93282-93283, 93289, 93292, 93295, 93642)

🔧 0.00 ⚖ 0.00 **FUD** 000 N 80 ▢

AMA: 2018,Feb,11; 2018,Jan,8; 2017,Jan,8; 2016,Jan,13

93642 Electrophysiologic evaluation of single or dual chamber transvenous pacing cardioverter-defibrillator (includes defibrillation threshold evaluation, induction of arrhythmia, evaluation of sensing and pacing for arrhythmia termination, and programming or reprogramming of sensing or therapeutic parameters)

🔧 9.78 ⚖ 9.78 **FUD** 000 J 80 ▢

AMA: 2018,Feb,11; 2018,Jan,8; 2017,Jan,8; 2016,Jan,13

93644 Electrophysiologic evaluation of subcutaneous implantable defibrillator (includes defibrillation threshold evaluation, induction of arrhythmia, evaluation of sensing for arrhythmia termination, and programming or reprogramming of sensing or therapeutic parameters)

EXCLUDES Electrophysiological evaluation subcutaneous implantable defibrillator system with substernal electrode (0577T)
Insertion/replacement subcutaneous implantable defibrillator ([33270])
Subcutaneous cardioverter-defibrillator electrophysiologic evaluation, subsequent/periodic (93260-93261)

🔧 5.63 ⚖ 5.63 **FUD** 000 N 80 ▢

AMA: 2018,Feb,11

93650-93657 Intracardiac Ablation

INCLUDES Ablation services include selective delivery cryo-energy or radiofrequency to targeted tissue
Electrophysiologic studies performed in same session with ablation

93650 Intracardiac catheter ablation of atrioventricular node function, atrioventricular conduction for creation of complete heart block, with or without temporary pacemaker placement

🔧 17.2 ⚖ 17.2 **FUD** 000 J 80 ▢

AMA: 2018,Feb,11; 2018,Jan,8; 2017,Jan,8; 2016,Jan,13

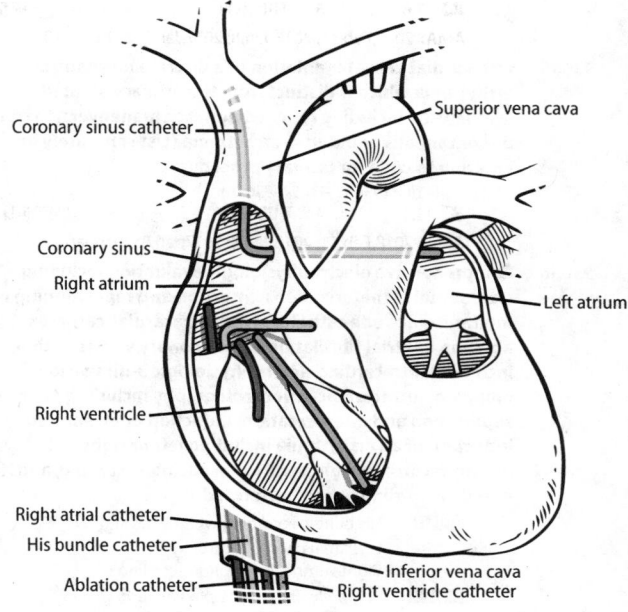

Coronary sinus catheter
Superior vena cava
Coronary sinus
Right atrium
Left atrium
Right ventricle
Right atrial catheter
His bundle catheter
Ablation catheter
Inferior vena cava
Right ventricle catheter

▲ **93653** Comprehensive electrophysiologic evaluation with insertion and repositioning of multiple electrode catheters, induction or attempted induction of an arrhythmia with right atrial pacing and recording and catheter ablation of arrhythmogenic focus, including intracardiac electrophysiologic 3-dimensional mapping, right ventricular pacing and recording, left atrial pacing and recording from coronary sinus or left atrium, and His bundle recording, when performed; with treatment of supraventricular tachycardia by ablation of fast or slow atrioventricular pathway, accessory atrioventricular connection, cavo-tricuspid isthmus or other single atrial focus or source of atrial re-entry

EXCLUDES Comprehensive electrophysiological studies (93619-93621)
Electrophysiologic evaluation pacing cardioverter defibrillator (93642)
Intracardiac ablation with transseptal catheterization (93656)
Intracardiac ablation with treatment ventricular arrhythmia (93654)
Intracardiac electrophysiologic 3D mapping (93613)
Intracardiac pacing (93610, 93612, 93618)
Recording intracardiac electrograms (93600-93603)

🔧 24.3 ⚖ 24.3 **FUD** 000 J 80 ▢

AMA: 2018,Feb,11; 2018,Jan,8; 2017,Jan,8; 2016,Jan,13

▲ 93654 with treatment of ventricular tachycardia or focus of ventricular ectopy including left ventricular pacing and recording, when performed

> EXCLUDES Comprehensive electrophysiological studies (93619-93620, 93622)
> Device evaluation (93279-93284, 93286-93289)
> Intracardiac ablation with transseptal catheterization (93656)
> Intracardiac ablation with treatment supraventricular tachycardia (93653)
> Intracardiac pacing (93609-93613, 93618)
> Recording intracardiac electrograms (93600-93603)

🔲 32.6 ⚖ 32.6 **FUD** 000   [J] [80] ▯

AMA: 2018,Feb,11; 2018,Jan,8; 2017,Jan,8; 2016,Jan,13

+ 93655 Intracardiac catheter ablation of a discrete mechanism of arrhythmia which is distinct from the primary ablated mechanism, including repeat diagnostic maneuvers, to treat a spontaneous or induced arrhythmia (List separately in addition to code for primary procedure)

> Code first (93653-93654, 93656)

🔲 12.4 ⚖ 12.4 **FUD** ZZZ   [N] [80] ▯

AMA: 2018,Feb,11; 2018,Jan,8; 2017,Jan,8; 2016,Jan,13

▲ 93656 Comprehensive electrophysiologic evaluation including transseptal catheterizations, insertion and repositioning of multiple electrode catheters with intracardiac catheter ablation of atrial fibrillation by pulmonary vein isolation, including intracardiac electrophysiologic 3-dimensional mapping, intracardiac echocardiography including imaging supervision and interpretation, induction or attempted induction of an arrhythmia including left or right atrial pacing/recording, right ventricular pacing/recording, and His bundle recording, when performed

> INCLUDES His bundle recording when indicated
> Left atrial pacing/recording
> Right ventricular pacing/recording
> EXCLUDES Comprehensive electrophysiological studies (93619-93621)
> Device evaluation (93279-93284, 93286-93289)
> Electrophysiologic evaluation with treatment ventricular tachycardia (93654)
> Intracardiac ablation with treatment supraventricular tachycardia (93653)
> Intracardiac echocardiography during diagnostic/therapeutic intervention (93662)
> Intracardiac electrophysiologic 3D mapping (93613)
> Intracardiac pacing (93610, 93612, 93618)
> Left heart catheterization by transseptal puncture (93462)
> Recording intracardiac electrograms (93600-93603)

🔲 32.7 ⚖ 32.7 **FUD** 000   [J] [80] ▯

AMA: 2020,Nov,12; 2019,Sep,10; 2018,Feb,11; 2018,Jan,8; 2017,Jan,8; 2016,Jan,13

+ 93657 Additional linear or focal intracardiac catheter ablation of the left or right atrium for treatment of atrial fibrillation remaining after completion of pulmonary vein isolation (List separately in addition to code for primary procedure)

> Code first (93656)

🔲 12.3 ⚖ 12.3 **FUD** ZZZ   [N] [80] ▯

AMA: 2020,Nov,12; 2019,Sep,10; 2018,Feb,11; 2018,Jan,8; 2017,Jan,8; 2016,Jan,13

93660-93662 Other Tests for Cardiac Function

93660 Evaluation of cardiovascular function with tilt table evaluation, with continuous ECG monitoring and intermittent blood pressure monitoring, with or without pharmacological intervention

> EXCLUDES Autonomic nervous system function testing (95921, 95924)

🔲 4.51 ⚖ 4.51 **FUD** 000   [S] [80] ▯

AMA: 2018,Feb,11; 2018,Jan,8; 2017,Jan,8; 2016,Jan,13

+ 93662 Intracardiac echocardiography during therapeutic/diagnostic intervention, including imaging supervision and interpretation (List separately in addition to code for primary procedure)

> EXCLUDES Internal cardioversion (92961)
> Transcatheter implantation interatrial septal shunt device, percutaneous approach (0613T)
> Transcatheter tricuspid valve repair with prosthesis, percutaneous approach (0569T-0570T)
> Code first (as appropriate) ([33274, 33275], 33340, 33361-33366, 33418, 33477, 33741, 33745, 92986-92987, 92990, 92997, 93451-93461, 93505, 93580-93583, 93590-93591, 93593-93597, 93620, 93653-93654, 93656, 0345T, 0483T-0484T, 0543T, 0544T, 0545T)

🔲 0.00 ⚖ 0.00 **FUD** ZZZ   [N] [80] ▯

AMA: 2018,Feb,11; 2018,Jan,8; 2017,Jan,8; 2016,Jan,13

93668 Rehabilitation Services: Peripheral Arterial Disease

CMS: 100-03,1,20.35 Supervised Exercise Therapy (SET) for Symptomatic Peripheral Artery Disease (PAD)(Effective May 25, 2017; 100-04,32,390 Supervised exercise therapy (SET) Symptomatic Peripheral Artery Disease; 100-04,32,390.1 General Billing Requirements for Supervised exercise therapy (SET) for PAD; 100-04,32,390.2 Coding Requirements for SET for PAD; 100-04,32,390.3 Special Billing Requirements for Professional Claims; 100-04,32,390.4 Special Billing Requirements for Institutional Claims; 100-04,32,390.5 Common Working File (CWF) Requirements; 100-04,32,390.6 Applicable Medicare Summary Notice (MSN), Remittance Advice Remark Codes (RARCs), and Claim Adjustment Reason Code (CARC) Messaging

> INCLUDES Monitoring:
> Other cardiovascular limitations for workload adjustment
> Patient's claudication threshold
> Motorized treadmill or track
> Sessions lasting 45-60 minutes
> Supervision by exercise physiologist/nurse
> Code also appropriate E/M service, when performed

93668 Peripheral arterial disease (PAD) rehabilitation, per session

🔲 0.50 ⚖ 0.50 **FUD** XXX   [S] [80] [TC] ▯

AMA: 2018,Feb,11

93701-93702 Thoracic Electrical Bioimpedance

> EXCLUDES Bioelectrical impedance analysis whole body (0358T)
> Indirect measurement left ventricular filling pressure by computerized calibration arterial waveform response to Valsalva (93799)

93701 Bioimpedance-derived physiologic cardiovascular analysis

🔲 0.71 ⚖ 0.71 **FUD** XXX   [Q1] [80] [TC] ▯

AMA: 2018,Feb,11; 2018,Jan,8; 2017,Jan,8; 2016,Jan,13

93702 Bioimpedance spectroscopy (BIS), extracellular fluid analysis for lymphedema assessment(s)

🔲 3.50 ⚖ 3.50 **FUD** XXX   [S] [80] [TC] ▯

AMA: 2018,Feb,11

93724 Electronic Analysis of Pacemaker Function

93724 Electronic analysis of antitachycardia pacemaker system (includes electrocardiographic recording, programming of device, induction and termination of tachycardia via implanted pacemaker, and interpretation of recordings)

🔲 8.04 ⚖ 8.04 **FUD** 000   [S] [80] ▯

AMA: 2018,Feb,11; 2018,Jan,8; 2017,Jan,8; 2016,Jan,13

93740 Temperature Gradient Assessment

93740 Temperature gradient studies

🔲 0.23 ⚖ 0.23 **FUD** XXX   [Q1] ▯

AMA: 2018,Feb,11

93745 Wearable Cardioverter-Defibrillator System Services

> EXCLUDES Device evaluation (93282, 93292)

93745 Initial set-up and programming by a physician or other qualified health care professional of wearable cardioverter-defibrillator includes initial programming of system, establishing baseline electronic ECG, transmission of data to data repository, patient instruction in wearing system and patient reporting of problems or events

🔲 0.00 ⚖ 0.00 **FUD** XXX   [S] [80] ▯

AMA: 2018,Feb,11

26/TC PC/TC Only   A2-Z3 ASC Payment   50 Bilateral   ♂ Male Only   ♀ Female Only   🔲 Facility RVU   ⚖ Non-Facility RVU   ▯ CCI   ✖ CLIA

FUD Follow-up Days   **CMS:** IOM   **AMA:** CPT Asst   A-Y OPPSI   80/80 Surg Assist Allowed / w/Doc   Lab Crosswalk   Radiology Crosswalk

93750 Ventricular Assist Device (VAD) Interrogation

CMS: 100-03,20.9 Artificial Hearts and Related Devices; 100-03,20.9.1 Ventricular Assist Devices; 100-04,32,320.1 Artificial Hearts Prior to May 1, 2008; 100-04,32,320.2 Coding for Artificial Hearts After May 1, 2008; 100-04,32,320.3 Ventricular Assist Devices; 100-04,32,320.3.1 Post-cardiotomy; 100-04,32,320.3.2 Bridge- to -Transplantation; 100-04,32,320.3.3 Other

> EXCLUDES *Insertion ventricular assist device (33975-33976, 33979)*
> *Removal/replacement ventricular assist device (33981-33983)*

93750 Interrogation of ventricular assist device (VAD), in person, with physician or other qualified health care professional analysis of device parameters (eg, drivelines, alarms, power surges), review of device function (eg, flow and volume status, septum status, recovery), with programming, if performed, and report

  🔲 1.32   ⚖ 1.58   **FUD** XXX   S 80 🖳

  AMA: 2018,Dec,10; 2018,Dec,10; 2018,Feb,11; 2018,Jan,8; 2017,Jan,8; 2016,Jan,13

93770 Peripheral Venous Blood Pressure Assessment

CMS: 100-03,20.19 Ambulatory Blood Pressure Monitoring (20.19)

> EXCLUDES *Cannulization, central venous (36500, 36555-36556)*

93770 Determination of venous pressure

  🔲 0.23   ⚖ 0.23   **FUD** XXX   N 🖳

  AMA: 2018,Feb,11

93784-93790 Ambulatory Blood Pressure Monitoring

CMS: 100-03,20.19 Ambulatory Blood Pressure Monitoring (20.19); 100-04,32,10.1 Ambulatory Blood Pressure Monitoring Billing Requirements

> EXCLUDES *Self-measured blood pressure monitoring ([99473, 99474])*

93784 Ambulatory blood pressure monitoring, utilizing report-generating software, automated, worn continuously for 24 hours or longer; including recording, scanning analysis, interpretation and report

  🔲 1.51   ⚖ 1.51   **FUD** XXX   B 80 🖳

  AMA: 2020,Apr,5; 2018,Feb,11

93786 recording only

  🔲 0.83   ⚖ 0.83   **FUD** XXX   Q1 80 TC 🖳

  AMA: 2020,Apr,5; 2018,Feb,11

93788 scanning analysis with report

  🔲 0.15   ⚖ 0.15   **FUD** XXX   Q1 80 TC 🖳

  AMA: 2020,Apr,5; 2018,Feb,11

93790 review with interpretation and report

  🔲 0.53   ⚖ 0.53   **FUD** XXX   M 80 26 🖳

  AMA: 2020,Apr,5; 2018,Feb,11

93792-93793 INR Monitoring

CMS: 100-03,190.11 Home PT/INR Monitoring for Anticoagulation Management

> EXCLUDES *Chronic care management services provided during same month ([99439, 99490, 99491])*
> *Complex chronic care management services provided during same month (99487-99489)*
> *Online digital assessment and management services by nonphysician healthcare professional (98970-98972)*
> *Online digital evaluation and management services by physician or other qualified health care professional ([99421, 99422, 99423])*
> *Telephone assessment and management service by nonphysician healthcare professional (98966-98968)*
> *Telephone evaluation and management service by physician or other qualified healthcare professional (99441-99443)*

93792 Patient/caregiver training for initiation of home international normalized ratio (INR) monitoring under the direction of a physician or other qualified health care professional, face-to-face, including use and care of the INR monitor, obtaining blood sample, instructions for reporting home INR test results, and documentation of patient's/caregiver's ability to perform testing and report results

  Code also:
    INR home monitoring equipment with appropriate supply code or (99070)
    Significantly separately identifiable E/M service on same date service; append modifier 25

  🔲 1.84   ⚖ 1.84   **FUD** XXX   B 80 TC 🖳

  AMA: 2018,Mar,7; 2018,Feb,11

93793 Anticoagulant management for a patient taking warfarin, must include review and interpretation of a new home, office, or lab international normalized ratio (INR) test result, patient instructions, dosage adjustment (as needed), and scheduling of additional test(s), when performed

> EXCLUDES *E/M services performed same date (99202-99215, 99241-99245)*
> *Reporting code more than one time per day*

  🔲 0.33   ⚖ 0.33   **FUD** XXX   B 80 26 🖳

  AMA: 2020,Feb,7; 2018,Mar,7; 2018,Feb,11; 2018,Jan,8; 2017,Nov,10

93797-93799 Cardiac Rehabilitation

CMS: 100-02,15,232 Cardiac Rehabilitation (CR) and Intensive Cardiac Rehabilitation (ICR) Services Furnished On or After January 1, 2010; 100-04,32,140.2 Cardiac Rehabilitation On or After January 1, 2010; 100-04,32,140.2.1 Coding Cardiac Rehabilitation Services On or After January 1, 2010; 100-04,32,140.2.2.2 Institutional Claims for CR and ICR Services; 100-04,32,140.2.2.4 CR Services Exceeding 36 Sessions; 100-04,32,140.3 Intensive Cardiac Rehabilitation On or After January 1, 2010; 100-08,15,4.2.8 Cardiac Rehabilitation (CR) and Intensive Cardiac Rehabilitation (ICR)

93797 Physician or other qualified health care professional services for outpatient cardiac rehabilitation; without continuous ECG monitoring (per session)

  🔲 0.25   ⚖ 0.46   **FUD** 000   S 80 🖳

  AMA: 2018,Feb,11

93798 with continuous ECG monitoring (per session)

  🔲 0.40   ⚖ 0.72   **FUD** 000   S 80 🖳

  AMA: 2018,Feb,11

93799 Unlisted cardiovascular service or procedure

  🔲 0.00   ⚖ 0.00   **FUD** XXX   S 80 🖳

  AMA: 2020,Nov,7; 2018,Dec,10; 2018,Dec,10; 2018,Sep,10; 2018,Aug,10; 2018,Feb,11; 2018,Jan,8; 2017,Jan,8; 2016,May,5; 2016,Jan,13

93880-93895 Noninvasive Tests Extracranial/Intracranial Arteries

> INCLUDES Patient care required to perform/supervise studies and interpret results
> EXCLUDES *Hand-held Dopplers that do not provide hard copy or vascular flow bidirectional analysis (see E/M codes)*

93880 Duplex scan of extracranial arteries; complete bilateral study

> EXCLUDES *Common carotid intima-media thickness (IMT) studies (93895)*

  🔲 5.70   ⚖ 5.70   **FUD** XXX   S 80 🖳

  AMA: 2018,Feb,11; 2018,Jan,8; 2017,Jan,8; 2016,Jan,13

93882 unilateral or limited study

> EXCLUDES *Common carotid intima-media thickness (IMT) studies (93895)*

  🔲 3.64   ⚖ 3.64   **FUD** XXX   S 80 🖳

  AMA: 2018,Feb,11; 2018,Jan,8; 2017,Jan,8; 2016,Jan,13

93886 Transcranial Doppler study of the intracranial arteries; complete study

> INCLUDES Complete transcranial doppler (TCD) study
> Ultrasound evaluation right/left anterior circulation territories and posterior circulation territory

  🔲 7.67   ⚖ 7.67   **FUD** XXX   S 80 🖳

  AMA: 2018,Feb,11; 2018,Jan,8; 2017,Jan,8; 2016,Jan,13

93888 limited study

> INCLUDES Limited TCD study
> Ultrasound examination two or fewer territories (right/left anterior circulation, posterior circulation)

  🔲 4.47   ⚖ 4.47   **FUD** XXX   S 80 🖳

  AMA: 2018,Feb,11; 2018,Jan,8; 2017,Jan,8; 2016,Jan,13

93890 vasoreactivity study

> EXCLUDES *Limited TCD study (93888)*

  🔲 7.82   ⚖ 7.82   **FUD** XXX   Q1 80 🖳

  AMA: 2018,Feb,11; 2018,Jan,8; 2017,Jan,8; 2016,Jan,13

93892 emboli detection without intravenous microbubble injection

EXCLUDES Limited TCD study (93888)

⚕ 8.81   ℥ 8.81   **FUD** XXX   01 80 ▢

AMA: 2018,Feb,11; 2018,Jan,8; 2017,Jan,8; 2016,Jan,13

93893 emboli detection with intravenous microbubble injection

EXCLUDES Limited TCD study (93888)

⚕ 10.1   ℥ 10.1   **FUD** XXX   01 80 ▢

AMA: 2018,Feb,11; 2018,Jan,8; 2017,Jan,8; 2016,Jan,13

93895 Quantitative carotid intima media thickness and carotid atheroma evaluation, bilateral

EXCLUDES Complete and limited duplex studies (93880, 93882)

⚕ 0.00   ℥ 0.00   **FUD** XXX   E 80 ▢

AMA: 2018,Feb,11

93922-93971 Noninvasive Vascular Studies: Extremities

CMS: 100-04,8,180 Noninvasive Studies for ESRD Patients

INCLUDES Patient care required to perform/supervise studies and interpret results

EXCLUDES Hand-held Dopplers that do not provide hard copy or vascular flow bidirectional analysis (see E/M codes)

93922 Limited bilateral noninvasive physiologic studies of upper or lower extremity arteries, (eg, for lower extremity: ankle/brachial indices at distal posterior tibial and anterior tibial/dorsalis pedis arteries plus bidirectional, Doppler waveform recording and analysis at 1-2 levels, or ankle/brachial indices at distal posterior tibial and anterior tibial/dorsalis pedis arteries plus volume plethysmography at 1-2 levels, or ankle/brachial indices at distal posterior tibial and anterior tibial/dorsalis pedis arteries with, transcutaneous oxygen tension measurement at 1-2 levels)

INCLUDES Evaluation:

Doppler analysis bidirectional blood flow

Nonimaging physiologic recordings pressure

Oxygen tension measurements and/or plethysmography

Lower extremity (potential levels include high thigh, low thigh, calf, ankle, metatarsal and toes) limited study includes either:

Ankle/brachial indices distal posterior tibial and anterior tibial/dorsalis pedis arteries plus bidirectional Doppler waveform recording and analysis 1-2 levels; OR

Ankle/brachial indices distal posterior tibial and anterior tibial/dorsalis pedis arteries plus volume plethysmography 1-2 levels; OR

Ankle/brachial indices distal posterior tibial and anterior tibial/dorsalis pedis arteries with transcutaneous oxygen tension measurements 1-2 levels

Unilateral provocative functional measurement

Unilateral study 3 or move levels

Upper extremity (potential levels include arm, forearm, wrist, and digits) limited study includes:

Doppler-determined systolic pressures and bidirectional waveform recording with analysis 1-2 levels; OR

Doppler-determined systolic pressures and transcutaneous oxygen tension measurements 1-2 levels; OR

Doppler-determined systolic pressures and volume plethysmography 1-2 levels

EXCLUDES Reporting code more than one time for lower extremity(ies)

Reporting code more than one time for upper extremity(ies)

Transcutaneous oxyhemoglobin, deoxyhemoglobin and tissue oxygenation measurement (0631T)

Transcutaneous oxyhemoglobin measurement (0493T)

Code also:

Modifier 52 for unilateral study 1-2 levels

Twice for upper and lower extremity study; append modifier 59 on second code

⚕ 2.40   ℥ 2.40   **FUD** XXX   01 80 ▢

AMA: 2019,Oct,8; 2018,Feb,11; 2018,Jan,8; 2017,Jan,8; 2016,Jan,13

26/TC PC/TC Only	A2-Z3 ASC Payment	50 Bilateral	♂ Male Only	♀ Female Only	⚕ Facility RVU	℥ Non-Facility RVU	▢ CCI	✖ CLIA
FUD Follow-up Days	**CMS:** IOM	**AMA:** CPT Asst	A-Y OPPSI	80/80 Surg Assist Allowed / w/Doc		▣ Lab Crosswalk	▣ Radiology Crosswalk	

494   CPT © 2021 American Medical Association. All Rights Reserved.   © 2021 Optum360, LLC

93923 Complete bilateral noninvasive physiologic studies of upper or lower extremity arteries, 3 or more levels (eg, for lower extremity: ankle/brachial indices at distal posterior tibial and anterior tibial/dorsalis pedis arteries plus segmental blood pressure measurements with bidirectional Doppler waveform recording and analysis, at 3 or more levels, or ankle/brachial indices at distal posterior tibial and anterior tibial/dorsalis pedis arteries plus segmental volume plethysmography at 3 or more levels, or ankle/brachial indices at distal posterior tibial and anterior tibial/dorsalis pedis arteries plus segmental transcutaneous oxygen tension measurements at 3 or more levels), or single level study with provocative functional maneuvers (eg, measurements with postural provocative tests, or measurements with reactive hyperemia)

INCLUDES Evaluation:
Doppler analysis bidirectional blood flow
Nonimaging physiologic recordings pressures
Oxygen tension measurements
Lower extremity:
Ankle/brachial indices distal posterior tibial and anterior tibial/dorsalis pedis arteries plus bidirectional Doppler waveform recording and analysis 3 or more levels; OR
Ankle/brachial indices distal posterior tibial and anterior tibial/dorsalis pedis arteries with transcutaneous oxygen tension measurements 3 or more levels; OR
Ankle/brachial indices distal posterior tibial and anterior tibial/dorsalis pedis arteries plus volume plethysmography 3 or more levels; OR
Provocative functional maneuvers and measurement single level
Upper extremity complete study:
Doppler-determined systolic pressures and bidirectional waveform recording with analysis 3 or more levels; OR
Doppler-determined systolic pressures and transcutaneous oxygen tension measurements 3 or more levels; OR
Doppler-determined systolic pressures and volume plethysmography 3 or more levels; OR
EXCLUDES Reporting code more than one time for lower extremity(ies)
Reporting coe more than one time for upper extremity(ies)
Transcutaneous oxyhemoglobin, deoxyhemoglobin and tissue oxygenation measurement (0631T)
Unilateral study 3 or more levels (93922)
Code also twice for upper and lower extremity study and append modifier 59
🚑 3.74 ⚕ 3.74 **FUD** XXX Ⓢ 80 🖵
AMA: 2020,Sep,14; 2019,Oct,8; 2018,Feb,11; 2018,Jan,8; 2017,Jan,8; 2016,Jan,13

93924 Noninvasive physiologic studies of lower extremity arteries, at rest and following treadmill stress testing, (ie, bidirectional Doppler waveform or volume plethysmography recording and analysis at rest with ankle/brachial indices immediately after and at timed intervals following performance of a standardized protocol on a motorized treadmill plus recording of time of onset of claudication or other symptoms, maximal walking time, and time to recovery) complete bilateral study

INCLUDES Evaluation:
Doppler analysis bidirectional blood flow
Nonimaging physiologic recordings pressures
Oxygen tension measurements
Plethysmography
EXCLUDES Noninvasive vascular studies extremities (93922-93923)
Other types exercise
🚑 4.67 ⚕ 4.67 **FUD** XXX Ⓢ 80 🖵
AMA: 2019,Oct,8; 2018,Feb,11; 2018,Jan,8; 2017,Jan,8; 2016,Jan,13

93925 Duplex scan of lower extremity arteries or arterial bypass grafts; complete bilateral study

EXCLUDES Preoperative arterial inflow and venous outflow duplex scan for creation hemodialysis access, same extremities (93985)
🚑 7.17 ⚕ 7.17 **FUD** XXX Ⓢ 80 🖵
AMA: 2019,Oct,8; 2018,Feb,11; 2018,Jan,8; 2017,Jan,8; 2016,Sep,9; 2016,Jan,13

93926 unilateral or limited study

EXCLUDES Preoperative arterial inflow and venous outflow duplex scan for creation hemodialysis access, same extremity (93986)
🚑 4.24 ⚕ 4.24 **FUD** XXX Ⓢ 80 🖵
AMA: 2019,Oct,8; 2018,Feb,11; 2018,Jan,8; 2017,Jan,8; 2016,Sep,9; 2016,Jan,13

93930 Duplex scan of upper extremity arteries or arterial bypass grafts; complete bilateral study

EXCLUDES Preoperative arterial inflow and venous outflow duplex scan for creation hemodialysis access, same extremity(ies) (93985-93986)
🚑 5.83 ⚕ 5.83 **FUD** XXX Ⓢ 80 🖵
AMA: 2019,Oct,8; 2018,Feb,11; 2018,Jan,8; 2017,Jan,8; 2016,Sep,9; 2016,Jan,13

93931 unilateral or limited study

EXCLUDES Preoperative arterial inflow and venous outflow duplex scan for creation hemodialysis access, same extremity (93985-93986)
🚑 3.64 ⚕ 3.64 **FUD** XXX Ⓢ 80 🖵
AMA: 2019,Oct,8; 2018,Feb,11; 2018,Jan,8; 2017,Jan,8; 2016,Sep,9; 2016,Jan,13

93970 Duplex scan of extremity veins including responses to compression and other maneuvers; complete bilateral study

EXCLUDES Endovenous ablation (36475-36476, 36478-36479)
Preoperative arterial inflow and venous outflow duplex scan for creation hemodialysis access, same extremity(ies) (93985-93986)
🚑 5.51 ⚕ 5.51 **FUD** XXX Ⓢ 80 🖵
AMA: 2019,Oct,8; 2018,Mar,3; 2018,Feb,11; 2018,Jan,8; 2017,Jan,8; 2016,Nov,3; 2016,Sep,9; 2016,Jan,13

93971 unilateral or limited study

EXCLUDES Endovenous ablation (36475-36476, 36478-36479)
Preoperative arterial inflow and venous outflow duplex scan for creation hemodialysis access, same extremity (93985-93986)
🚑 3.44 ⚕ 3.44 **FUD** XXX Ⓢ 80 🖵
AMA: 2019,Oct,8; 2018,Mar,3; 2018,Feb,11; 2018,Jan,8; 2017,Jan,8; 2016,Nov,3; 2016,Sep,9; 2016,Jan,13

93975-93981 Noninvasive Vascular Studies: Abdomen/Chest/Pelvis

93975 Duplex scan of arterial inflow and venous outflow of abdominal, pelvic, scrotal contents and/or retroperitoneal organs; complete study
🚑 7.88 ⚕ 7.88 **FUD** XXX Ⓢ 80 🖵
AMA: 2018,Feb,11; 2018,Jan,8; 2017,Jan,8; 2016,Aug,9; 2016,Jan,13

93976 limited study
🚑 4.64 ⚕ 4.64 **FUD** XXX Ⓢ 80 🖵
AMA: 2018,Feb,11; 2018,Jan,8; 2017,Jan,8; 2016,Aug,9; 2016,Jan,13

93978 Duplex scan of aorta, inferior vena cava, iliac vasculature, or bypass grafts; complete study
EXCLUDES Ultrasound screening for abdominal aortic aneurysm (76706)
🚑 5.32 ⚕ 5.32 **FUD** XXX Ⓢ 80 🖵
AMA: 2018,Feb,11; 2018,Jan,8; 2017,Jan,8; 2016,Jan,13

93979 unilateral or limited study

EXCLUDES　*Ultrasound screening for abdominal aortic aneurysm (76706)*

🚑 3.42　⚕ 3.42　**FUD** XXX　　　01 80 ▢

AMA: 2018,Feb,11; 2018,Jan,8; 2017,Jan,8; 2016,Jan,13

93980 Duplex scan of arterial inflow and venous outflow of penile vessels; complete study

🚑 3.46　⚕ 3.46　**FUD** XXX　　　S 80 ▢

AMA: 2018,Feb,11; 2018,Jan,8; 2017,Jan,8; 2016,Jan,13

93981 follow-up or limited study

🚑 2.08　⚕ 2.08　**FUD** XXX　　　S 80 ▢

AMA: 2018,Feb,11; 2018,Jan,8; 2017,Jan,8; 2016,Jan,13

93985-93998 Noninvasive Vascular Studies: Hemodialysis Access

93985 Duplex scan of arterial inflow and venous outflow for preoperative vessel assessment prior to creation of hemodialysis access; complete bilateral study

EXCLUDES　*Duplex scan extremity arteries only, same extremity(ies) (93925, 93930)*
Duplex scan extremity veins only, same extremity(ies) (93970)
Duplex scan hemodialysis access, arterial inflow, and venous outflow, same extremity(ies) (93990)
Physiologic arterial evaluation extremities (93922-93924)

🚑 7.53　⚕ 7.53　**FUD** XXX　　　P2 80 ▢

93986 complete unilateral study

EXCLUDES　*Duplex scan extremity arteries only, same extremity (93926, 93931)*
Duplex scan extremity veins only, same extremity (93971)
Duplex scan hemodialysis access, arterial inflow and venous outflow, same extremity (93990)
Physiologic arterial evaluation extremities (93922-93924)

🚑 4.37　⚕ 4.37　**FUD** XXX　　　P2 80 ▢

93990 Duplex scan of hemodialysis access (including arterial inflow, body of access and venous outflow)

EXCLUDES　*Hemodialysis access flow measurement by indicator method (90940)*

🚑 4.39　⚕ 4.39　**FUD** XXX　　　01 80 ▢

AMA: 2019,Oct,8; 2018,Feb,11; 2018,Jan,8; 2017,Jan,8; 2016,Jan,13

93998 Unlisted noninvasive vascular diagnostic study

🚑 0.00　⚕ 0.00　**FUD** XXX　　　01 80 ▢

AMA: 2018,Feb,11; 2018,Jan,8; 2017,Jan,8; 2016,Jan,13

94002-94005 Ventilator Management Services

94002 Ventilation assist and management, initiation of pressure or volume preset ventilators for assisted or controlled breathing; hospital inpatient/observation, initial day

EXCLUDES　*E/M services*

🚑 2.64　⚕ 2.64　**FUD** XXX　　　03 80 ▢

AMA: 2019,Aug,8; 2018,Feb,11; 2018,Jan,8; 2017,Jan,8; 2016,Jan,13

94003 hospital inpatient/observation, each subsequent day

EXCLUDES　*E/M services*

🚑 1.89　⚕ 1.89　**FUD** XXX　　　03 80 ▢

AMA: 2019,Aug,8; 2018,Feb,11; 2018,Jan,8; 2017,Jan,8; 2016,Jan,13

94004 nursing facility, per day

EXCLUDES　*E/M services*

🚑 1.40　⚕ 1.40　**FUD** XXX　　　B 80 ▢

AMA: 2019,Aug,8; 2018,Feb,11; 2018,Jan,8; 2017,Jan,8; 2016,Jan,13

94005 Home ventilator management care plan oversight of a patient (patient not present) in home, domiciliary or rest home (eg, assisted living) requiring review of status, review of laboratories and other studies and revision of orders and respiratory care plan (as appropriate), within a calendar month, 30 minutes or more

Code also when different provider reports care plan oversight in same 30 days (99339-99340, 99374-99378)

🚑 2.61　⚕ 2.61　**FUD** XXX　　　M ▢

AMA: 2018,Feb,11; 2018,Jan,8; 2017,Jan,8; 2016,Jan,13

94010-94799 [94619] Respiratory Services: Diagnostic and Therapeutic

INCLUDES　Laboratory procedure(s)
Test results interpretation
EXCLUDES　*Separately identifiable E/M service*

94010 Spirometry, including graphic record, total and timed vital capacity, expiratory flow rate measurement(s), with or without maximal voluntary ventilation

INCLUDES　Measurement expiratory airflow and volumes
EXCLUDES　*Diffusing capacity (94729)*
Other respiratory function services (94150, 94200, 94375, 94728)

🚑 1.00　⚕ 1.00　**FUD** XXX　　　01 80 ▢

AMA: 2020,Dec,3; 2019,May,10; 2019,Mar,10; 2019,Apr,10; 2018,Feb,11; 2018,Jan,8; 2017,Jan,8; 2016,Jan,13

94011 Measurement of spirometric forced expiratory flows in an infant or child through 2 years of age

🚑 2.48　⚕ 2.48　**FUD** XXX　　　01 80 ▢

AMA: 2020,Dec,3; 2019,Mar,10; 2018,Feb,11; 2018,Jan,8; 2017,Jan,8; 2016,Jan,13

94012 Measurement of spirometric forced expiratory flows, before and after bronchodilator, in an infant or child through 2 years of age

🚑 4.01　⚕ 4.01　**FUD** XXX　　　01 80 ▢

AMA: 2020,Dec,3; 2019,Mar,10; 2018,Feb,11; 2018,Jan,8; 2017,Jan,8; 2016,Jan,13

94013 Measurement of lung volumes (ie, functional residual capacity [FRC], forced vital capacity [FVC], and expiratory reserve volume [ERV]) in an infant or child through 2 years of age

🚑 0.55　⚕ 0.55　**FUD** XXX　　　S 80 ▢

AMA: 2020,Dec,3; 2019,Mar,10; 2018,Feb,11; 2018,Jan,8; 2017,Jan,8; 2016,Jan,13

94014 Patient-initiated spirometric recording per 30-day period of time; includes reinforced education, transmission of spirometric tracing, data capture, analysis of transmitted data, periodic recalibration and review and interpretation by a physician or other qualified health care professional

🚑 1.58　⚕ 1.58　**FUD** XXX　　　01 80 ▢

AMA: 2020,Dec,3; 2019,Mar,10; 2018,Feb,11; 2018,Jan,8; 2017,Jan,8; 2016,Jan,13

94015 recording (includes hook-up, reinforced education, data transmission, data capture, trend analysis, and periodic recalibration)

🚑 0.86　⚕ 0.86　**FUD** XXX　　　01 80 TC ▢

AMA: 2020,Dec,3; 2019,Mar,10; 2018,Feb,11; 2018,Jan,8; 2017,Jan,8; 2016,Jan,13

94016 review and interpretation only by a physician or other qualified health care professional

🚑 0.72　⚕ 0.72　**FUD** XXX　　　A 80 26 ▢

AMA: 2020,Dec,3; 2019,Mar,10; 2018,Feb,11; 2018,Jan,8; 2017,Jan,8; 2016,Jan,13

94060 **Bronchodilation responsiveness, spirometry as in 94010, pre- and post-bronchodilator administration**

> INCLUDES   Spirometry performed prior to and after bronchodilator has been administered
> EXCLUDES   *Bronchospasm prolonged exercise test with pre- and post-spirometry (94617, [94619])*
> *Diffusing capacity (94729)*
> *Other respiratory function services (94150, 94200, 94375, 94640, 94728)*
> Code also bronchodilator supply with appropriate supply code or (99070)

> 🚑 1.67   ⚕ 1.67   **FUD** XXX   Ⓢ 80 ▭

AMA: 2020,Dec,3; 2019,Mar,10; 2019,Apr,10; 2018,Feb,11; 2018,Jan,8; 2017,Jan,8; 2016,Jan,13

94070 **Bronchospasm provocation evaluation, multiple spirometric determinations as in 94010, with administered agents (eg, antigen[s], cold air, methacholine)**

> EXCLUDES   *Diffusing capacity (94729)*
> *Inhalation treatment (diagnostic or therapeutic) (94640)*
> Code also antigen(s) administration with appropriate supply code or (99070)

> 🚑 1.69   ⚕ 1.69   **FUD** XXX   Ⓢ 80 ▭

AMA: 2020,Dec,3; 2019,Mar,10; 2018,Feb,11; 2018,Jan,8; 2017,Jan,8; 2016,Jan,13

94150 **Vital capacity, total (separate procedure)**

> EXCLUDES   *Other respiratory function services (94010, 94060, 94728)*
> *Thoracic gas volumes (94726-94727)*

> 🚑 0.71   ⚕ 0.71   **FUD** XXX   01 ▭

AMA: 2020,Dec,3; 2019,Mar,10; 2018,Sep,14; 2018,Feb,11; 2018,Jan,8; 2017,Jan,8; 2016,Jan,13

94200 **Maximum breathing capacity, maximal voluntary ventilation**

> EXCLUDES   *Other respiratory function services (94010, 94060)*

> 🚑 0.63   ⚕ 0.63   **FUD** XXX   01 80 ▭

AMA: 2020,Dec,3; 2019,Mar,10; 2018,Feb,11; 2018,Jan,8; 2017,Jan,8; 2016,Jan,13

94375 **Respiratory flow volume loop**

> INCLUDES   Obstruction pattern identification in central or peripheral airways (inspiratory and/or expiratory)
> EXCLUDES   *Diffusing capacity (94729)*
> *Other respiratory function services (94010, 94060, 94728)*

> 🚑 1.10   ⚕ 1.10   **FUD** XXX   01 80 ▭

AMA: 2020,Dec,3; 2019,Mar,10; 2018,Feb,11; 2018,Jan,8; 2017,Jan,8; 2016,Jan,13

94450 **Breathing response to hypoxia (hypoxia response curve)**

> EXCLUDES   *HAST - high altitude simulation test (94452, 94453)*

> 🚑 1.88   ⚕ 1.88   **FUD** XXX   01 80 ▭

AMA: 2020,Dec,3; 2019,Mar,10; 2018,Feb,11; 2018,Jan,8; 2017,Jan,8; 2016,Jan,13

94452 **High altitude simulation test (HAST), with interpretation and report by a physician or other qualified health care professional;**

> EXCLUDES   *HAST test with supplemental oxygen titration (94453)*
> *Noninvasive pulse oximetry (94760-94761)*
> *Obtaining arterial blood gases (36600)*

> 🚑 1.48   ⚕ 1.48   **FUD** XXX   01 80 ▭

AMA: 2020,Dec,3; 2019,Mar,10; 2018,Feb,11; 2018,Jan,8; 2017,Jan,8; 2016,Jan,13

94453 **with supplemental oxygen titration**

> EXCLUDES   *HAST test without supplemental oxygen titration (94452)*
> *Noninvasive pulse oximetry (94760-94761)*
> *Obtaining arterial blood gases (36600)*

> 🚑 2.03   ⚕ 2.03   **FUD** XXX   01 80 ▭

AMA: 2020,Dec,3; 2019,Mar,10; 2018,Feb,11; 2018,Jan,8; 2017,Jan,8; 2016,Jan,13

94610 **Intrapulmonary surfactant administration by a physician or other qualified health care professional through endotracheal tube**

> INCLUDES   Reporting once per dosing episode
> EXCLUDES   *Intubation, endotracheal (31500)*
> *Neonatal critical care (99468-99472)*

> 🚑 1.59   ⚕ 1.59   **FUD** XXX   ⊘ 01 80 ▭

AMA: 2020,Dec,3; 2019,Mar,10; 2018,Feb,11; 2018,Jan,8; 2017,Jan,8; 2016,Jan,13

94617 **Exercise test for bronchospasm, including pre- and post-spirometry and pulse oximetry; with electrocardiographic recording(s)**

> EXCLUDES   *Cardiovascular stress test (93015-93018)*
> *ECG monitoring (93000-93010, 93040-93042)*
> *Pulse oximetry (94760-94761)*

> 🚑 2.58   ⚕ 2.58   **FUD** XXX   01 80 ▭

AMA: 2020,Dec,3; 2019,May,10; 2019,Mar,10; 2018,Feb,11; 2018,Jan,8; 2017,Oct,3

\# **94619** **without electrocardiographic recording(s)**

> EXCLUDES   *Cardiovascular stress test (93015-93018)*
> *ECG monitoring (93000-93010, 93040-93042)*
> *Pulse oximetry (94760-94761)*

> 🚑 2.16   ⚕ 2.16   **FUD** XXX   80 ▭

AMA: 2020,Dec,3

94618 **Pulmonary stress testing (eg, 6-minute walk test), including measurement of heart rate, oximetry, and oxygen titration, when performed**

> EXCLUDES   *Pulse oximetry (94760-94761)*

> 🚑 0.95   ⚕ 0.95   **FUD** XXX   01 80 ▭

AMA: 2020,Dec,3; 2019,May,10; 2019,Mar,10; 2018,Feb,11; 2018,Jan,8; 2017,Oct,3

94619 **Resequenced code. See code following 94617.**

94621 **Cardiopulmonary exercise testing, including measurements of minute ventilation, CO_2 production, O_2 uptake, and electrocardiographic recordings**

> EXCLUDES   *Cardiovascular stress test (93015-93018)*
> *ECG monitoring (93000-93010, 93040-93042)*
> *Oxygen uptake expired gas analysis (94680-94690)*
> *Pulse oximetry (94760-94761)*

> 🚑 4.50   ⚕ 4.50   **FUD** XXX   Ⓢ 80 ▭

AMA: 2020,Dec,3; 2019,May,10; 2019,Mar,10; 2018,Feb,11; 2018,Jan,8; 2017,Oct,3; 2017,Jan,8; 2016,Jan,13

● **94625** **Physician or other qualified health care professional services for outpatient pulmonary rehabilitation; without continuous oximetry monitoring (per session)**

> EXCLUDES   *Pulse oximetry, noninvasive (94760-94761)*

● **94626** **with continuous oximetry monitoring (per session)**

> EXCLUDES   *Pulse oximetry, noninvasive (94760-94761)*

94640 **Pressurized or nonpressurized inhalation treatment for acute airway obstruction for therapeutic purposes and/or for diagnostic purposes such as sputum induction with an aerosol generator, nebulizer, metered dose inhaler or intermittent positive pressure breathing (IPPB) device**

> EXCLUDES   *One hour or more continuous inhalation treatment (94644, 94645)*
> *Other respiratory function services (94060, 94070)*
> Code also modifier 76 when more than one inhalation treatment performed on same date

> 🚑 0.51   ⚕ 0.51   **FUD** XXX   01 80 ▭

AMA: 2020,Dec,3; 2019,Mar,10; 2018,Feb,11; 2018,Jan,8; 2017,Jan,8; 2016,Jan,13

94642 **Aerosol inhalation of pentamidine for pneumocystis carinii pneumonia treatment or prophylaxis**

> 🚑 0.00   ⚕ 0.00   **FUD** XXX   01 80 ▭

AMA: 2020,Dec,3; 2019,Mar,10; 2018,Feb,11; 2018,Jan,8; 2017,Jan,8; 2016,Jan,13

94644   Continuous inhalation treatment with aerosol medication for acute airway obstruction; first hour

      EXCLUDES   *Services less than one hour (94640)*

      🔧 1.40   🔨 1.40   **FUD** XXX   [Q1] [80] 🖳

      AMA: 2020,Dec,3; 2019,Mar,10; 2018,Feb,11; 2018,Jan,8; 2017,Jan,8; 2016,Jan,13

+ 94645   each additional hour (List separately in addition to code for primary procedure)

      Code first initial hour (94644)

      🔧 0.47   🔨 0.47   **FUD** XXX   [N] [80] 🖳

      AMA: 2020,Dec,3; 2019,Mar,10; 2018,Feb,11; 2018,Jan,8; 2017,Jan,8; 2016,Jan,13

94660   Continuous positive airway pressure ventilation (CPAP), initiation and management

      🔧 1.09   🔨 1.81   **FUD** XXX   [Q1] [80] 🖳

      AMA: 2020,Dec,3; 2019,Aug,8; 2019,Mar,10; 2018,Feb,11; 2018,Jan,8; 2017,Jan,8; 2016,Jan,13

94662   Continuous negative pressure ventilation (CNP), initiation and management

      🔧 1.03   🔨 1.03   **FUD** XXX   [Q3] [80] 🖳

      AMA: 2020,Dec,3; 2019,Aug,8; 2019,Mar,10; 2018,Feb,11; 2018,Jan,8; 2017,Jan,8; 2016,Jan,13

94664   Demonstration and/or evaluation of patient utilization of an aerosol generator, nebulizer, metered dose inhaler or IPPB device

      INCLUDES   Reporting only one time per day

      🔧 0.48   🔨 0.48   **FUD** XXX   [Q1] [80] 🖳

      AMA: 2020,Dec,3; 2019,Mar,10; 2018,Feb,11; 2018,Jan,8; 2017,Jan,8; 2016,Jan,13

94667   Manipulation chest wall, such as cupping, percussing, and vibration to facilitate lung function; initial demonstration and/or evaluation

      🔧 0.70   🔨 0.70   **FUD** XXX   [Q1] [80] 🖳

      AMA: 2020,Dec,3; 2019,Mar,10; 2018,Feb,11; 2018,Jan,8; 2017,Jan,8; 2016,Jan,13

94668   subsequent

      🔧 0.92   🔨 0.92   **FUD** XXX   [Q1] [80] 🖳

      AMA: 2020,Dec,3; 2019,Mar,10; 2018,Feb,11; 2018,Jan,8; 2017,Jan,8; 2016,Jan,13

94669   Mechanical chest wall oscillation to facilitate lung function, per session

      INCLUDES   Application external wrap or vest to provide mechanical oscillation

      🔧 0.90   🔨 0.90   **FUD** XXX   [Q1] [80] 🖳

      AMA: 2020,Dec,3; 2019,Mar,10; 2018,Feb,11; 2018,Jan,8; 2017,Jan,8; 2016,Jan,13

94680   Oxygen uptake, expired gas analysis; rest and exercise, direct, simple

      EXCLUDES   *Cardiopulmonary stress testing (94621)*

      🔧 1.51   🔨 1.51   **FUD** XXX   [Q1] [80] 🖳

      AMA: 2020,Dec,3; 2019,Mar,10; 2018,Feb,11; 2017,Oct,3; 2017,Jan,8; 2016,Jan,13

94681   including CO2 output, percentage oxygen extracted

      EXCLUDES   *Cardiopulmonary stress testing (94621)*

      🔧 1.49   🔨 1.49   **FUD** XXX   [Q1] [80] 🖳

      AMA: 2020,Dec,3; 2019,Mar,10; 2018,Feb,11; 2017,Oct,3; 2017,Jan,8; 2016,Jan,13

94690   rest, indirect (separate procedure)

      EXCLUDES   *Arterial puncture (36600)*
                   Cardiopulmonary stress testing (94621)

      🔧 1.43   🔨 1.43   **FUD** XXX   [Q1] [80] 🖳

      AMA: 2020,Dec,3; 2019,Mar,10; 2018,Feb,11; 2018,Jan,8; 2017,Oct,3; 2017,Jan,8; 2016,Jan,13

94726   Plethysmography for determination of lung volumes and, when performed, airway resistance

      INCLUDES   Airway resistance
                   Determination:
                      Functional residual capacity
                      Residual volume
                      Total lung capacity

      EXCLUDES   *Airway resistance by oscillometry (94728)*
                   Bronchial provocation (94070)
                   Diffusing capacity (94729)
                   Gas dilution or washout (94727)
                   Spirometry (94010, 94060)

      🔧 1.51   🔨 1.51   **FUD** XXX   [Q1] [80] 🖳

      AMA: 2020,Dec,3; 2019,Mar,10; 2018,Feb,11; 2018,Jan,8; 2017,Jan,8; 2016,Jan,13

94727   Gas dilution or washout for determination of lung volumes and, when performed, distribution of ventilation and closing volumes

      INCLUDES   Closing volume
                   Lung volume measurement
                   Ventilation distribution

      EXCLUDES   *Bronchial provocation (94070)*
                   Diffusing capacity (94729)
                   Plethysmography for lung volume/airway resistance (94726)
                   Spirometry (94010, 94060)

      🔧 1.23   🔨 1.23   **FUD** XXX   [Q1] [80] 🖳

      AMA: 2020,Dec,3; 2019,Mar,10; 2018,Feb,11; 2018,Jan,8; 2017,Jan,8; 2016,Jan,13

94728   Airway resistance by oscillometry

      EXCLUDES   *Diffusing capacity (94729)*
                   Gas dilution techniques
                   Other respiratory function services (94010, 94060, 94070, 94375, 94726)

      🔧 1.15   🔨 1.15   **FUD** XXX   [Q1] [80] 🖳

      AMA: 2020,Dec,3; 2019,Mar,10; 2018,Feb,11; 2018,Jan,8; 2017,Jan,8; 2016,Jan,13

+ 94729   Diffusing capacity (eg, carbon monoxide, membrane) (List separately in addition to code for primary procedure)

      Code first (94010, 94060, 94070, 94375, 94726-94728)

      🔧 1.59   🔨 1.59   **FUD** ZZZ   [N] [80] 🖳

      AMA: 2020,Dec,3; 2019,Mar,10; 2018,Feb,11; 2018,Jan,8; 2017,Jan,8; 2016,Jan,13

94760   Noninvasive ear or pulse oximetry for oxygen saturation; single determination

      EXCLUDES   *Blood gases (82803-82810)*
                   Cardiopulmonary stress testing (94621)
                   Exercise test for bronchospasm (94617)
                   Pulmonary stress testing (94618)

      🔧 0.07   🔨 0.07   **FUD** XXX   [N] [80] [TC] 🖳

      AMA: 2020,Dec,3; 2019,Aug,8; 2019,Mar,10; 2019,Jan,6; 2018,Feb,11; 2018,Jan,8; 2017,Oct,3; 2017,Jan,8; 2016,Jan,13

94761   multiple determinations (eg, during exercise)

      EXCLUDES   *Cardiopulmonary stress testing (94621)*
                   Exercise test for bronchospasm (94617, [94619])
                   Pulmonary stress testing (94618)

      🔧 0.12   🔨 0.12   **FUD** XXX   [N] [80] [TC] 🖳

      AMA: 2020,Dec,3; 2019,Aug,8; 2019,Mar,10; 2018,Feb,11; 2018,Jan,8; 2017,Oct,3; 2017,Jan,8; 2016,Jan,13

94762   by continuous overnight monitoring (separate procedure)

      🔧 0.71   🔨 0.71   **FUD** XXX   [Q3] [80] [TC] 🖳

      AMA: 2020,Dec,3; 2019,Aug,8; 2019,Mar,10; 2018,Feb,11; 2018,Jan,8; 2017,Jan,8; 2016,Jan,13

94772   Circadian respiratory pattern recording (pediatric pneumogram), 12-24 hour continuous recording, infant   [A]

      EXCLUDES   *Electromyograms/EEG/ECG/respiration recordings*

      🔧 0.00   🔨 0.00   **FUD**   [S] [80] 🖳

      AMA: 2020,Dec,3; 2019,Mar,10; 2018,Feb,11; 2018,Jan,8; 2017,Jan,8; 2016,Jan,13

26/TC PC/TC Only   [A2]-[Z3] ASC Payment   [50] Bilateral   ♂ Male Only   ♀ Female Only   🔧 Facility RVU   🔨 Non-Facility RVU   🖳 CCI   ❌ CLIA
FUD Follow-up Days   **CMS:** IOM   **AMA:** CPT Asst   [A]-[Y] OPPSI   80/80 Surg Assist Allowed / w/Doc   🖳 Lab Crosswalk   🖳 Radiology Crosswalk

94774 Pediatric home apnea monitoring event recording including respiratory rate, pattern and heart rate per 30-day period of time; includes monitor attachment, download of data, review, interpretation, and preparation of a report by a physician or other qualified health care professional `A`

INCLUDES Oxygen saturation monitoring
EXCLUDES *Event monitors (93268-93272)*
Holter monitor (93224-93227)
Pediatric home apnea services (94775-94777)
Remote cardiovascular telemetry (93228-93229)
Sleep testing (95805-95811 [95800, 95801])

0.00 0.00 **FUD** YYY `B` `80`
AMA: 2020,Dec,3; 2019,Mar,10; 2018,Feb,11; 2018,Jan,8; 2017,Jan,8; 2016,Jan,13

94775 monitor attachment only (includes hook-up, initiation of recording and disconnection) `A`

INCLUDES Oxygen saturation monitoring
EXCLUDES *Event monitors (93268-93272)*
Holter monitor (93224-93227)
Remote cardiovascular telemetry (93228-93229)
Sleep testing (95805-95811 [95800, 95801])

0.00 0.00 **FUD** YYY `S` `80` `TC`
AMA: 2020,Dec,3; 2019,Mar,10; 2018,Feb,11; 2018,Jan,8; 2017,Jan,8; 2016,Jan,13

94776 monitoring, download of information, receipt of transmission(s) and analyses by computer only `A`

INCLUDES Oxygen saturation monitoring
EXCLUDES *Event monitors (93268-93272)*
Holter monitor (93224-93227)
Remote cardiovascular telemetry (93228-93229)
Sleep testing (95805-95811 [95800, 95801])

0.00 0.00 **FUD** YYY `S` `80` `TC`
AMA: 2020,Dec,3; 2019,Mar,10; 2018,Feb,11; 2018,Jan,8; 2017,Jan,8; 2016,Jan,13

94777 review, interpretation and preparation of report only by a physician or other qualified health care professional `A`

INCLUDES Oxygen saturation monitoring
EXCLUDES *Event monitors (93268-93272)*
Holter monitor (93224-93227)
Remote cardiovascular telemetry (93228-93229)
Sleep testing (95805-95811 [95800, 95801])

0.00 0.00 **FUD** YYY `B` `80` `26`
AMA: 2020,Dec,3; 2019,Mar,10; 2018,Feb,11; 2018,Jan,8; 2017,Jan,8; 2016,Jan,13

94780 Car seat/bed testing for airway integrity, for infants through 12 months of age, with continual clinical staff observation and continuous recording of pulse oximetry, heart rate and respiratory rate, with interpretation and report; 60 minutes `A`

EXCLUDES *Pediatric and neonatal critical care services (99468-99476, 99477-99480)*
Pulse oximetry (94760-94761)
Reporting code for service less than 60 minutes
Rhythm strips (93040-93042)

0.68 1.45 **FUD** XXX `01`
AMA: 2020,Dec,3; 2019,Mar,10; 2018,Feb,11; 2018,Jan,8; 2017,Jan,8; 2016,Jan,13

+ **94781** each additional full 30 minutes (List separately in addition to code for primary procedure) `A`
Code first (94780)
0.24 0.57 **FUD** ZZZ `N`
AMA: 2020,Dec,3; 2019,Mar,10; 2018,Feb,11; 2018,Jan,8; 2017,Jan,8; 2016,Jan,13

94799 Unlisted pulmonary service or procedure
0.00 0.00 **FUD** XXX `01` `80`
AMA: 2020,Dec,3; 2019,Mar,10; 2018,Sep,14; 2018,Feb,11; 2018,Jan,8; 2017,Jan,8; 2016,Jan,13

95004-95070 Allergy Tests

EXCLUDES *Drugs administered for intractable/severe allergic reaction (eg, antihistamines, epinephrine, steroids) (96372)*
E/M services when reporting test interpretation/report
Laboratory tests for allergies (86000-86999 [86152, 86153])
Code also:
Medical conferences regarding equipment use (e.g., air filters, humidifiers, dehumidifiers), climate therapy, physical, occupational, and recreation therapy using appropriate E/M codes
Significant, separately identifiable E/M services appending modifier 25, when performed (99202-99215, 99217-99223 [99224, 99225, 99226], 99231-99233, 99241-99255, 99281-99285, 99304-99318, 99324-99337, 99341-99350, 99381-99429 [99415, 99416, 99417, 99421, 99422, 99423])

95004 Percutaneous tests (scratch, puncture, prick) with allergenic extracts, immediate type reaction, including test interpretation and report, specify number of tests
0.12 0.12 **FUD** XXX `01` `80`
AMA: 2018,Feb,11; 2018,Jan,8; 2017,Jan,8; 2016,Jan,13

95012 Nitric oxide expired gas determination
0.57 0.57 **FUD** XXX `01` `80`
AMA: 2018,Feb,11; 2018,Jan,8; 2017,Jan,8; 2016,Jan,13

95017 Allergy testing, any combination of percutaneous (scratch, puncture, prick) and intracutaneous (intradermal), sequential and incremental, with venoms, immediate type reaction, including test interpretation and report, specify number of tests
0.11 0.23 **FUD** XXX `01` `80`
AMA: 2018,Feb,11; 2018,Jan,8; 2017,Jan,8; 2016,Jan,13

95018 Allergy testing, any combination of percutaneous (scratch, puncture, prick) and intracutaneous (intradermal), sequential and incremental, with drugs or biologicals, immediate type reaction, including test interpretation and report, specify number of tests
0.21 0.61 **FUD** XXX `01` `80`
AMA: 2018,Feb,11; 2018,Jan,8; 2017,Jan,8; 2016,Jan,13

95024 Intracutaneous (intradermal) tests with allergenic extracts, immediate type reaction, including test interpretation and report, specify number of tests
0.03 0.23 **FUD** XXX `01` `80`
AMA: 2018,Feb,11; 2018,Jan,8; 2017,Jan,8; 2016,Jan,13

95027 Intracutaneous (intradermal) tests, sequential and incremental, with allergenic extracts for airborne allergens, immediate type reaction, including test interpretation and report, specify number of tests
0.13 0.13 **FUD** XXX `01` `80`
AMA: 2018,Feb,11; 2018,Jan,8; 2017,Jan,8; 2016,Jan,13

95028 Intracutaneous (intradermal) tests with allergenic extracts, delayed type reaction, including reading, specify number of tests
0.37 0.37 **FUD** XXX `01` `80` `TC`
AMA: 2018,Feb,11; 2018,Jan,8; 2017,Jan,8; 2016,Jan,13

95044 Patch or application test(s) (specify number of tests)
0.16 0.16 **FUD** XXX `01` `80`
AMA: 2018,Feb,11; 2018,Jan,8; 2017,Jan,8; 2016,Jan,13

95052 Photo patch test(s) (specify number of tests)
0.19 0.19 **FUD** XXX `01` `80`
AMA: 2018,Feb,11; 2018,Jan,8; 2017,Jan,8; 2016,Jan,13

95056 Photo tests
1.31 1.31 **FUD** XXX `01` `80`
AMA: 2018,Feb,11; 2018,Jan,8; 2017,Jan,8; 2016,Jan,13

95060 Ophthalmic mucous membrane tests
0.99 0.99 **FUD** XXX `01` `80` `TC`
AMA: 2018,Feb,11; 2018,Jan,8; 2017,Jan,8; 2016,Jan,13

95065 Direct nasal mucous membrane test
0.74 0.74 **FUD** XXX `01` `80` `TC`
AMA: 2018,Feb,11; 2018,Jan,8; 2017,Jan,8; 2016,Jan,13

95070	**Inhalation bronchial challenge testing (not including necessary pulmonary function tests), with histamine, methacholine, or similar compounds**

EXCLUDES *Pulmonary function tests (94060, 94070)*

🔧 0.90   ⚖ 0.90   **FUD** XXX   S 80 TC ▢

AMA: 2018,Feb,11; 2018,Jan,8; 2017,Jan,8; 2016,Jan,13

95076-95079 Challenge Ingestion Testing

CMS: 100-03,110.12 Challenge Ingestion Food Testing

INCLUDES   Assessment and monitoring for allergic reactions (eg, blood pressure, peak flow meter)
Testing time until test ends or to point E/M service needed

EXCLUDES *Reporting code for testing time less than 61 minutes, such as positive challenge resulting in ending test (report E/M codes as appropriate)*
Code also interventions when appropriate (eg, injection of epinephrine or steroid)

95076	**Ingestion challenge test (sequential and incremental ingestion of test items, eg, food, drug or other substance); initial 120 minutes of testing**

INCLUDES   First 120 minutes testing time (not face-to-face time with physician)

🔧 2.15   ⚖ 3.43   **FUD** XXX   S 80 ▢

AMA: 2018,Feb,11; 2018,Jan,8; 2017,Jan,8; 2016,Jan,13

+ 95079	**each additional 60 minutes of testing (List separately in addition to code for primary procedure)**

INCLUDES   Includes each 60 minutes additional testing time (not face-to-face time with physician)
Code first (95076)

🔧 1.97   ⚖ 2.42   **FUD** ZZZ   N 80 ▢

AMA: 2018,Feb,11; 2018,Jan,8; 2017,Jan,8; 2016,Jan,13

95115-95199 Allergy Immunotherapy

CMS: 100-03,110.9 Antigens Prepared for Sublingual Administration

INCLUDES   Allergen immunotherapy professional services

EXCLUDES *Bacterial/viral/fungal extracts skin testing (86485-86580, 95028)*
Procedures for testing: (see Pathology/Immunology section or code:) (95199)
    Leukocyte histamine release (LHR)
    Lymphocytic transformation test (LTT)
    Mast cell degranulation test (MCDT)
    Migration inhibitory factor test (MIF)
    Nitroblue tetrazolium dye test (NTD)
    Radioallergosorbent testing (RAST)
    Rat mast cell technique (RMCT)
    Transfer factor test (TFT)
Special reports for allergy patients (99080)
Code also significant separately identifiable E/M services, when performed

95115	**Professional services for allergen immunotherapy not including provision of allergenic extracts; single injection**

🔧 0.26   ⚖ 0.26   **FUD** XXX   01 80 ▢

AMA: 2020,Sep,14; 2019,Jun,14; 2018,Feb,11; 2018,Jan,8; 2017,Jan,8; 2016,Jan,13

95117	**2 or more injections**

🔧 0.30   ⚖ 0.30   **FUD** XXX   01 80 ▢

AMA: 2020,Sep,14; 2019,Jun,14; 2018,Feb,11; 2018,Jan,8; 2017,Jan,8; 2016,Jan,13

95120	**Professional services for allergen immunotherapy in the office or institution of the prescribing physician or other qualified health care professional, including provision of allergenic extract; single injection**

🔧 0.00   ⚖ 0.00   **FUD** XXX   E ▢

AMA: 2018,Feb,11; 2018,Jan,8; 2017,Jan,8; 2016,Jan,13

95125	**2 or more injections**

🔧 0.00   ⚖ 0.00   **FUD** XXX   E ▢

AMA: 2018,Feb,11; 2018,Jan,8; 2017,Jan,8; 2016,Jan,13

95130	**single stinging insect venom**

🔧 0.00   ⚖ 0.00   **FUD** XXX   E ▢

AMA: 2018,Feb,11; 2018,Jan,8; 2017,Jan,8; 2016,Jan,13

95131	**2 stinging insect venoms**

🔧 0.00   ⚖ 0.00   **FUD** XXX   E ▢

AMA: 2018,Feb,11; 2018,Jan,8; 2017,Jan,8; 2016,Jan,13

95132	**3 stinging insect venoms**

🔧 0.00   ⚖ 0.00   **FUD** XXX   E ▢

AMA: 2018,Feb,11; 2018,Jan,8; 2017,Jan,8; 2016,Jan,13

95133	**4 stinging insect venoms**

🔧 0.00   ⚖ 0.00   **FUD** XXX   E ▢

AMA: 2018,Feb,11; 2018,Jan,8; 2017,Jan,8; 2016,Jan,13

95134	**5 stinging insect venoms**

🔧 0.00   ⚖ 0.00   **FUD** XXX   E ▢

AMA: 2018,Feb,11; 2018,Jan,8; 2017,Jan,8; 2016,Jan,13

95144	**Professional services for the supervision of preparation and provision of antigens for allergen immunotherapy, single dose vial(s) (specify number of vials)**

INCLUDES   Single dose vial/single dose of antigen administered in one injection

🔧 0.09   ⚖ 0.41   **FUD** XXX   01 80 ▢

AMA: 2018,Feb,11; 2018,Jan,8; 2017,Jan,8; 2016,Jan,13

95145	**Professional services for the supervision of preparation and provision of antigens for allergen immunotherapy (specify number of doses); single stinging insect venom**

🔧 0.09   ⚖ 0.81   **FUD** XXX   01 80 ▢

AMA: 2018,Feb,11; 2018,Jan,8; 2017,Jan,8; 2016,Jan,13

95146	**2 single stinging insect venoms**

🔧 0.09   ⚖ 1.50   **FUD** XXX   01 80 ▢

AMA: 2018,Feb,11; 2018,Jan,8; 2017,Jan,8; 2016,Jan,13

95147	**3 single stinging insect venoms**

🔧 0.09   ⚖ 1.55   **FUD** XXX   01 80 ▢

AMA: 2018,Feb,11; 2018,Jan,8; 2017,Jan,8; 2016,Jan,13

95148	**4 single stinging insect venoms**

🔧 0.09   ⚖ 2.23   **FUD** XXX   01 80 ▢

AMA: 2018,Feb,11; 2018,Jan,8; 2017,Jan,8; 2016,Jan,13

95149	**5 single stinging insect venoms**

🔧 0.09   ⚖ 2.97   **FUD** XXX   01 80 ▢

AMA: 2018,Feb,11; 2018,Jan,8; 2017,Jan,8; 2016,Jan,13

95165	**Professional services for the supervision of preparation and provision of antigens for allergen immunotherapy; single or multiple antigens (specify number of doses)**

🔧 0.09   ⚖ 0.40   **FUD** XXX   01 80 ▢

AMA: 2018,Feb,11; 2018,Jan,8; 2017,Jan,8; 2016,Jan,13

95170	**whole body extract of biting insect or other arthropod (specify number of doses)**

INCLUDES   Dose which is amount of antigen(s) administered in single injection from multiple dose vial

🔧 0.09   ⚖ 0.30   **FUD** XXX   01 80 ▢

AMA: 2018,Feb,11; 2018,Jan,8; 2017,Jan,8; 2016,Jan,13

95180	**Rapid desensitization procedure, each hour (eg, insulin, penicillin, equine serum)**

🔧 2.96   ⚖ 3.92   **FUD** XXX   01 80 ▢

AMA: 2019,Jun,14; 2018,Feb,11; 2018,Jan,8; 2017,Jan,8; 2016,Jan,13

95199	**Unlisted allergy/clinical immunologic service or procedure**

🔧 0.00   ⚖ 0.00   **FUD** XXX   01 80 ▢

AMA: 2018,Feb,11; 2018,Jan,8; 2017,Jan,8; 2016,Jan,13

95249-95251 [95249] Glucose Monitoring By Subcutaneous Device

EXCLUDES *Physiologic data collection/interpretation (99091)*
Code also when data receiver owned by patient for sensor placement, hook-up, monitor calibration, training, and printout (95999)

95249	**Resequenced code. See code following 95250.**

95250	**Ambulatory continuous glucose monitoring of interstitial tissue fluid via a subcutaneous sensor for a minimum of 72 hours; physician or other qualified health care professional (office) provided equipment, sensor placement, hook-up, calibration of monitor, patient training, removal of sensor, and printout of recording**

EXCLUDES *Reporting code more than one time per month*
Subcutaneous pocket with insertion interstitial glucose monitor (0446T)

🔧 4.26   ⚖ 4.26   **FUD** XXX   V 80 TC ▢

AMA: 2019,Jan,6; 2018,Jun,6; 2018,Mar,5; 2018,Feb,11; 2018,Jan,8; 2017,Jan,8; 2016,Jan,13

2G/TC PC/TC Only   A2 -Z3 ASC Payment   50 Bilateral   ♂ Male Only   ♀ Female Only   🔧 Facility RVU   ⚖ Non-Facility RVU   ■ CCI   ✖ CLIA
FUD Follow-up Days   **CMS:** IOM   **AMA:** CPT Asst   A -Y OPPSI   80/80 Surg Assist Allowed / w/Doc   ▢ Lab Crosswalk   ▣ Radiology Crosswalk

 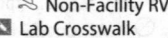

500   CPT © 2021 American Medical Association. All Rights Reserved.   © 2021 Optum360, LLC

\# **95249** **patient-provided equipment, sensor placement, hook-up, calibration of monitor, patient training, and printout of recording**

> INCLUDES Performing complete collection initial data in provider's office
>
> EXCLUDES *Reporting code more than one time during period patient owns data receiver*
> *Subcutaneous pocket with insertion interstitial glucose monitor (0446T)*
>
> 1.54 1.54 **FUD** XXX [S] [80] [TC] [□]
>
> **AMA:** 2018,Jun,6; 2018,Feb,11

95251 **analysis, interpretation and report**

> EXCLUDES *Reporting code more than one time per month*
>
> 1.02 1.02 **FUD** XXX [B] [80] [26] [□]
>
> **AMA:** 2018,Jun,6; 2018,Mar,5; 2018,Feb,11; 2018,Jan,8; 2017,Jan,8; 2016,Jan,13

95700-95783 [95700, 95705, 95706, 95707, 95708, 95709, 95710, 95711, 95712, 95713, 95714, 95715, 95716, 95717, 95718, 95719, 95720, 95721, 95722, 95723, 95724, 95725, 95726, 95782, 95783, 95800, 95801] Sleep Studies

> INCLUDES Assessment sleep disorders in adults and children
> Continuous and simultaneous monitoring and recording physiological sleep parameters six hours or more
> Evaluation patient's response to therapies
> Physician:
>   Interpretation
>   Recording
>   Report
> Portable and in-laboratory technology
> Recording sessions may be:
>   Attended studies that include technologist or qualified health care professional presence to respond to patient needs or technical issues at bedside
>   Remote without technologist or qualified health professional presence
>   Unattended without technologist or qualified health care professional presence
> Testing parameters include:
>   Actigraphy: Noninvasive portable device to record gross motor movements to approximate sleep and wakeful periods
>   Electrooculogram (EOG): Records electrical activity associated with eye movements
>   Maintenance of wakefulness test (MWT): Attended study to determine patient's ability to stay awake
>   Multiple sleep latency test (MSLT): Attended study to determine patient tendency to fall asleep
>   Peripheral arterial tonometry (PAT): Pulsatile volume changes in digit measured to determine activity in sympathetic nervous system for respiratory analysis
>   Polysomnography: Attended continuous, simultaneous recording physiological sleep parameters for at least six hours in sleep laboratory setting that also includes four or more:
>   1. Airflow-oral and/or nasal
>   2. Bilateral anterior tibialis EMG
>   3. Electrocardiogram (ECG)
>   4. Oxyhemoglobin saturation, SpO2
>   5. Respiratory effort
>   Positive airway pressure (PAP): Noninvasive devices to treat sleep-related disorders
>   Respiratory airflow (ventilation): Assessment air movement during inhalation and exhalation as measured by nasal pressure sensors and thermistor
>   Respiratory analysis: Assessment respiration components obtained by other methods such as airflow or peripheral arterial tone
>   Respiratory effort: Diaphragm and/or intercostal muscle contraction for airflow measured using transducers to estimate thoracic and abdominal motion
>   Respiratory movement: Measures chest and abdomen movement during respiration
>   Sleep latency: Pertains to time it takes to get to sleep
>   Sleep staging: Determining separate sleep levels according to physiological measurements
>   Total sleep time: Determined by actigraphy and other methods
>
> EXCLUDES *E/M services*

Code	Note
95700	**Resequenced code. See code following 95967.**
95705	**Resequenced code. See code following 95967.**
95706	**Resequenced code. See code following 95967.**
95707	**Resequenced code. See code following 95967.**
95708	**Resequenced code. See code following 95967.**
95709	**Resequenced code. See code following 95967.**
95710	**Resequenced code. See code following 95967.**
95711	**Resequenced code. See code following 95967.**
95712	**Resequenced code. See code following 95967.**
95713	**Resequenced code. See code following 95967.**
95714	**Resequenced code. See code following 95967.**
95715	**Resequenced code. See code following 95967.**
95716	**Resequenced code. See code following 95967.**
95717	**Resequenced code. See code following 95967.**
95718	**Resequenced code. See code following 95967.**
95719	**Resequenced code. See code following 95967.**
95720	**Resequenced code. See code following 95967.**
95721	**Resequenced code. See code following 95967.**
95722	**Resequenced code. See code following 95967.**
95723	**Resequenced code. See code following 95967.**
95724	**Resequenced code. See code following 95967.**
95725	**Resequenced code. See code following 95967.**
95726	**Resequenced code. See code following 95967.**
95782	**Resequenced code. See code following 95811.**
95783	**Resequenced code. See code following 95811.**
95800	**Resequenced code. See code following 95806.**
95801	**Resequenced code. See code following 95806.**

95803 **Actigraphy testing, recording, analysis, interpretation, and report (minimum of 72 hours to 14 consecutive days of recording)**

> EXCLUDES *Reporting code more than one time in 14-day period*
> *Sleep studies (95806-95811 [95800, 95801])*
>
> 4.22 4.22 **FUD** XXX [Q1] [80] [□]
>
> **AMA:** 2018,Feb,11; 2018,Jan,8; 2017,Jan,8; 2016,Jan,13

95805 **Multiple sleep latency or maintenance of wakefulness testing, recording, analysis and interpretation of physiological measurements of sleep during multiple trials to assess sleepiness**

> INCLUDES Physiological sleep parameters as measured by:
>   Frontal, central, and occipital EEG leads (three leads)
>   Left and right EOG
>   Submental EMG lead
>
> EXCLUDES *Polysomnography (95808-95811)*
> *Sleep study, not attended (95806)*
>
> Code also modifier 52 when less than four nap opportunities recorded
>
> 11.7 11.7 **FUD** XXX [S] [80] [□]
>
> **AMA:** 2018,Feb,11; 2018,Jan,8; 2017,Jan,8; 2016,Jan,13

95806 **Sleep study, unattended, simultaneous recording of, heart rate, oxygen saturation, respiratory airflow, and respiratory effort (eg, thoracoabdominal movement)**

> EXCLUDES *Arterial waveform analysis (93050)*
> *Event monitors (93268-93272)*
> *Holter monitor (93224-93227)*
> *Remote cardiovascular telemetry (93228-93229)*
> *Rhythm strips (93041-93042)*
> *Unattended sleep study with minimum heart rate, oxygen saturation, and respiratory analysis measurement ([95801])*
> *Unattended sleep study with heart rate, oxygen saturation, respiratory analysis, and sleep time measurement ([95800])*
>
> Code also modifier 52 for fewer than six hours recording
>
> 3.30 3.30 **FUD** XXX [S] [80] [□]
>
> **AMA:** 2018,Feb,11; 2018,Jan,8; 2017,Jan,8; 2016,Jan,13

Medicine

95800 — 95783

**95800** **Sleep study, unattended, simultaneous recording; heart rate, oxygen saturation, respiratory analysis (eg, by airflow or peripheral arterial tone), and sleep time**

> **EXCLUDES** *Actigraphy testing (95803)*
> *Arterial waveform analysis (93050)*
> *Event monitors (93268-93272)*
> *Holter monitor (93224-93227)*
> *Remote cardiovascular telemetry (93228-93229)*
> *Rhythm strips (93041-93042)*
> *Unattended sleep study with heart rate, oxygen saturation, respiratory airflow and respiratory effort measurement (95806)*
> *Unattended sleep study with minimum heart rate, oxygen saturation, and respiratory analysis measurement ([95801])*

Code also modifier 52 for fewer than 6 hours recording
🛏 4.68   ⚗ 4.68   **FUD** XXX   [S] [80] [▦]

AMA: 2018,Feb,11; 2018,Jan,8; 2017,Jan,8; 2016,Jan,13

**95801** **minimum of heart rate, oxygen saturation, and respiratory analysis (eg, by airflow or peripheral arterial tone)**

> **EXCLUDES** *Arterial waveform analysis (93050)*
> *Event monitors (93268-93272)*
> *Holter monitor (93224-93227)*
> *Remote cardiovascular telemetry (93228-93229)*
> *Rhythm strips (93041-93042)*
> *Unattended sleep study with heart rate, oxygen saturation, respiratory airflow and respiratory effort measurement (95806)*
> *Unattended sleep study with heart rate, oxygen saturation, respiratory analysis, and sleep time measurement ([95800])*

Code also modifier 52 for fewer than 6 hours recording
🛏 2.52   ⚗ 2.52   **FUD** XXX   [01] [80] [▦]

AMA: 2018,Feb,11; 2018,Jan,8; 2017,Jan,8; 2016,Jan,13

95807 **Sleep study, simultaneous recording of ventilation, respiratory effort, ECG or heart rate, and oxygen saturation, attended by a technologist**

> **EXCLUDES** *Polysomnography (95808-95811)*
> *Sleep study, not attended (95806)*

Code also modifier 52 for fewer than six hours recording
🛏 11.4   ⚗ 11.4   **FUD** XXX   [S] [80] [▦]

AMA: 2018,Feb,11; 2018,Jan,8; 2017,Jan,8; 2016,Jan,13

95808 **Polysomnography; any age, sleep staging with 1-3 additional parameters of sleep, attended by a technologist**

> **EXCLUDES** *Sleep study, not attended (95806)*

🛏 18.4   ⚗ 18.4   **FUD** XXX   [S] [80] [▦]

AMA: 2018,Feb,11; 2018,Jan,8; 2017,Jan,8; 2016,Jan,13

95810 **age 6 years or older, sleep staging with 4 or more additional parameters of sleep, attended by a technologist** [A]

> **EXCLUDES** *Sleep study, not attended (95806)*

Code also modifier 52 for fewer than six hours recording
🛏 17.2   ⚗ 17.2   **FUD** XXX   [S] [80] [▦]

AMA: 2018,Feb,11; 2018,Jan,8; 2017,Jan,8; 2016,Jan,13

95811 **age 6 years or older, sleep staging with 4 or more additional parameters of sleep, with initiation of continuous positive airway pressure therapy or bilevel ventilation, attended by a technologist** [A]

> **EXCLUDES** *Sleep study, not attended (95806)*

Code also modifier 52 for fewer than six hours recording
🛏 18.1   ⚗ 18.1   **FUD** XXX   [S] [80] [▦]

AMA: 2018,Feb,11; 2018,Jan,8; 2017,Jan,8; 2016,Jan,13

Core areas of monitoring for polysomnography

**95782** **younger than 6 years, sleep staging with 4 or more additional parameters of sleep, attended by a technologist** [A]

Code also modifier 52 for fewer than 7 hours recording
🛏 25.4   ⚗ 25.4   **FUD** XXX   [S] [80] [▦]

AMA: 2018,Feb,11; 2018,Jan,8; 2017,Jan,8; 2016,Jan,13

**95783** **younger than 6 years, sleep staging with 4 or more additional parameters of sleep, with initiation of continuous positive airway pressure therapy or bi-level ventilation, attended by a technologist** [A]

Code also modifier 52 for fewer than seven hours recording
🛏 27.1   ⚗ 27.1   **FUD** XXX   [S] [80] [▦]

AMA: 2018,Feb,11; 2018,Jan,8; 2017,Jan,8; 2016,Jan,13

95812-95830 [95829] Evaluation of Brain Activity by Electroencephalogram

INCLUDES Only time when time is recorded, data collected, and does not include set-up and take-down

EXCLUDES E/M services

95812 Electroencephalogram (EEG) extended monitoring; 41-60 minutes

INCLUDES
Hyperventilation
Photic stimulation
Physician interpretation
Recording 41-60 minutes
Report

EXCLUDES
EEG digital analysis (95957)
EEG during nonintracranial surgery (95955)
Long-term EEG (two hours or more) ([95700, 95705, 95706, 95707, 95708, 95709, 95710, 95711, 95712, 95713, 95714, 95715, 95716, 95717, 95718, 95719, 95720, 95721, 95722, 95723, 95724, 95725, 95726])
Wada test (95958)

Code also modifier 26 for physician interpretation only

🚑 9.19 ☟ 9.19 **FUD** XXX [S][80][▭]

AMA: 2018,Dec,3; 2018,Dec,3; 2018,Feb,11; 2018,Jan,8; 2017,Jan,8; 2016,Jan,13

95813 61-119 minutes

INCLUDES
Hyperventilation
Photic stimulation
Physician interpretation
Recording 61 minutes or more
Report

EXCLUDES
EEG digital analysis (95957)
EEG during nonintracranial surgery (95955)
Long-term EEG (two hours or more) ([95700, 95705, 95706, 95707, 95708, 95709, 95710, 95711, 95712, 95713, 95714, 95715, 95716, 95717, 95718, 95719, 95720, 95721, 95722, 95723, 95724, 95725, 95726])
Wada test (95958)

Code also modifier 26 for physician interpretation only

🚑 11.5 ☟ 11.5 **FUD** XXX [S][80][▭]

AMA: 2018,Dec,3; 2018,Dec,3; 2018,Feb,11; 2018,Jan,8; 2017,Jan,8; 2016,Jan,13

95816 Electroencephalogram (EEG); including recording awake and drowsy

INCLUDES
Photic stimulation
Physician interpretation
Recording 20-40 minutes
Report

EXCLUDES
EEG digital analysis (95957)
EEG during nonintracranial surgery (95955)
Long-term EEG (two hours or more) ([95700, 95705, 95706, 95707, 95708, 95709, 95710, 95711, 95712, 95713, 95714, 95715, 95716, 95717, 95718, 95719, 95720, 95721, 95722, 95723, 95724, 95725, 95726])
Wada test (95958)

Code also modifier 26 for physician interpretation only

🚑 10.3 ☟ 10.3 **FUD** XXX [S][80][▭]

AMA: 2018,Dec,3; 2018,Dec,3; 2018,Feb,11; 2018,Jan,8; 2017,Jan,8; 2016,Jan,13

95819 including recording awake and asleep

INCLUDES
Hyperventilation
Photic stimulation
Physician interpretation
Recording 20-40 minutes
Report

EXCLUDES
EEG digital analysis (95957)
EEG during nonintracranial surgery (95955)
Long-term EEG (two hours or more) ([95700, 95705, 95706, 95707, 95708, 95709, 95710, 95711, 95712, 95713, 95714, 95715, 95716, 95717, 95718, 95719, 95720, 95721, 95722, 95723, 95724, 95725, 95726])
Wada test (95958)

Code also modifier 26 for interpretation only

🚑 12.2 ☟ 12.2 **FUD** XXX [S][80][▭]

AMA: 2018,Dec,3; 2018,Dec,3; 2018,Feb,11; 2018,Jan,8; 2017,Jan,8; 2016,Jan,13

95822 recording in coma or sleep only

INCLUDES
Hyperventilation
Photic stimulation
Physician interpretation
Recording 20-40 minutes
Report

EXCLUDES
EEG digital analysis (95957)
EEG during nonintracranial surgery (95955)
Long-term EEG (two hours or more) ([95700, 95705, 95706, 95707, 95708, 95709, 95710, 95711, 95712, 95713, 95714, 95715, 95716, 95717, 95718, 95719, 95720, 95721, 95722, 95723, 95724, 95725, 95726])
Wada test (95958)

Code also modifier 26 for interpretation only

🚑 11.0 ☟ 11.0 **FUD** XXX [S][80][▭]

AMA: 2018,Dec,3; 2018,Dec,3; 2018,Feb,11; 2018,Jan,8; 2017,Jan,8; 2016,Jan,13

95824 cerebral death evaluation only

INCLUDES
Physician interpretation
Recording
Report

EXCLUDES
EEG digital analysis (95957)
EEG during nonintracranial surgery (95955)
Long-term EEG (two hours or more) ([95700, 95705, 95706, 95707, 95708, 95709, 95710, 95711, 95712, 95713, 95714, 95715, 95716, 95717, 95718, 95719, 95720, 95721, 95722, 95723, 95724, 95725, 95726])
Wada test (95958)

Code also modifier 26 for physician interpretation only

🚑 0.00 ☟ 0.00 **FUD** XXX [S][80][▭]

AMA: 2018,Feb,11

95829 Resequenced code. See code following 95830.

95830 Insertion by physician or other qualified health care professional of sphenoidal electrodes for electroencephalographic (EEG) recording

🚑 2.64 ☟ 10.9 **FUD** XXX [B][80][▭]

AMA: 2018,Feb,11

95829-95836 [95829, 95836] Evaluation of Brain Activity by Electrocorticography

\# **95829 Electrocorticogram at surgery (separate procedure)**

INCLUDES
EEG recording from electrodes placed in or on brain
Interpretation and review during surgical procedure

Code also modifier 26 for interpretation only

🚑 53.6 ☟ 53.6 **FUD** XXX [N][80][▭]

AMA: 2018,Dec,3; 2018,Dec,3; 2018,Feb,11

Medicine

95836 — 95885

#	95836	**Electrocorticogram from an implanted brain neurostimulator pulse generator/transmitter, including recording, with interpretation and written report, up to 30 days**

INCLUDES Intracranial recordings up to 30 days (unattended) with storage for later review

EXCLUDES EEG digital analysis (95957)

Programming neurostimulator during 30-day period ([95983, 95984])

Reporting code more than one time for documented 30-day period

🖙 3.19 ⚕ 3.19 **FUD** XXX   80 🖵

AMA: 2018,Dec,3; 2018,Dec,3

95836-95857 [95836] Evaluation of Muscles and Range of Motion

95836 **Resequenced code. See code following 95830.**

95851 **Range of motion measurements and report (separate procedure); each extremity (excluding hand) or each trunk section (spine)**

🖙 0.22 ⚕ 0.59 **FUD** XXX   A 80 🖵

AMA: 2018,Feb,11; 2018,Jan,8; 2017,Jan,8; 2016,Dec,16; 2016,Jan,13

95852 **hand, with or without comparison with normal side**

🖙 0.17 ⚕ 0.53 **FUD** XXX   A 80 🖵

AMA: 2018,Feb,11; 2018,Jan,8; 2017,Jan,8; 2016,Jan,13

95857 **Cholinesterase inhibitor challenge test for myasthenia gravis**

🖙 0.85 ⚕ 1.54 **FUD** XXX   S 80 🖵

AMA: 2018,Feb,11; 2018,Jan,8; 2017,Jan,8; 2016,Jan,13

95860-95887 [95885, 95886, 95887] Evaluation of Nerve and Muscle Function: EMGs with/without Nerve Conduction Studies

INCLUDES Physician interpretation
Recording
Report

EXCLUDES E/M services

95860 **Needle electromyography; 1 extremity with or without related paraspinal areas**

INCLUDES Testing five or more muscles per extremity

EXCLUDES Dynamic electromyography during motion analysis studies (96002-96003)

Guidance for chemodenervation (95873-95874)

🖙 3.40 ⚕ 3.40 **FUD** XXX   Q1 80 🖵

AMA: 2018,Feb,11; 2018,Jan,8; 2017,Jan,8; 2016,Jan,13

95861 **2 extremities with or without related paraspinal areas**

INCLUDES Testing five or more muscles per extremity

EXCLUDES Dynamic electromyography during motion analysis studies (96002-96003)

Guidance for chemodenervation (95873-95874)

🖙 4.87 ⚕ 4.87 **FUD** XXX   Q1 80 🖵

AMA: 2018,Feb,11; 2018,Jan,8; 2017,Jan,8; 2016,Jan,13

95863 **3 extremities with or without related paraspinal areas**

INCLUDES Testing five or more muscles per extremity

EXCLUDES Dynamic electromyography during motion analysis studies (96002-96003)

Guidance for chemodenervation (95873-95874)

🖙 6.02 ⚕ 6.02 **FUD** XXX   S 80 🖵

AMA: 2018,Feb,11; 2018,Jan,8; 2017,Jan,8; 2016,Jan,13

95864 **4 extremities with or without related paraspinal areas**

INCLUDES Testing five or more muscles per extremity

EXCLUDES Dynamic electromyography during motion analysis studies (96002-96003)

Guidance for chemodenervation (95873-95874)

🖙 7.07 ⚕ 7.07 **FUD** XXX   S 80 🖵

AMA: 2018,Feb,11; 2018,Jan,8; 2017,Jan,8; 2016,Jan,13

95865 **larynx**

EXCLUDES Dynamic electromyography during motion analysis studies (96002-96003)

Guidance for chemodenervation (95873-95874)

Code also modifier 52 for unilateral procedure

🖙 4.34 ⚕ 4.34 **FUD** XXX   Q1 80 🖵

AMA: 2018,Feb,11; 2018,Jan,8; 2017,Jan,8; 2016,Jan,13

95866 **hemidiaphragm**

EXCLUDES Dynamic electromyography during motion analysis studies (96002-96003)

Guidance for chemodenervation (95873-95874)

🖙 3.83 ⚕ 3.83 **FUD** XXX   Q1 80 🖵

AMA: 2018,Feb,11; 2018,Jan,8; 2017,Jan,8; 2016,Jan,13

95867 **cranial nerve supplied muscle(s), unilateral**

EXCLUDES Guidance for chemodenervation (95873-95874)

🖙 3.05 ⚕ 3.05 **FUD** XXX   S 80 🖵

AMA: 2018,Feb,11; 2018,Jan,8; 2017,Jan,8; 2016,Jan,13

95868 **cranial nerve supplied muscles, bilateral**

EXCLUDES Guidance for chemodenervation (95873-95874)

🖙 4.00 ⚕ 4.00 **FUD** XXX   S 80 🖵

AMA: 2018,Feb,11; 2018,Jan,8; 2017,Jan,8; 2016,Jan,13

95869 **thoracic paraspinal muscles (excluding T1 or T12)**

EXCLUDES Dynamic electromyography during motion analysis studies (96002-96003)

Guidance for chemodenervation (95873-95874)

🖙 2.71 ⚕ 2.71 **FUD** XXX   Q1 80 🖵

AMA: 2018,Feb,11; 2018,Jan,8; 2017,Jan,8; 2016,Jan,13

95870 **limited study of muscles in 1 extremity or non-limb (axial) muscles (unilateral or bilateral), other than thoracic paraspinal, cranial nerve supplied muscles, or sphincters**

INCLUDES Adson test

Testing four or less muscles per extremity

EXCLUDES Anal/urethral sphincter/detrusor/urethra/perineum musculature (51785-51792)

Complete study extremities (95860-95864)

Dynamic electromyography during motion analysis studies (96002-96003)

Eye muscles (92265)

Guidance for chemodenervation (95873-95874)

🖙 2.56 ⚕ 2.56 **FUD** XXX   Q1 80 🖵

AMA: 2018,Feb,11; 2018,Jan,8; 2017,Jan,8; 2016,Jan,13

95872 **Needle electromyography using single fiber electrode, with quantitative measurement of jitter, blocking and/or fiber density, any/all sites of each muscle studied**

EXCLUDES Dynamic electromyography during motion analysis studies (96002-96003)

🖙 5.66 ⚕ 5.66 **FUD** XXX   S 80 🖵

AMA: 2018,Feb,11; 2018,Jan,8; 2017,Jan,8; 2016,Jan,13

+ #	95885	**Needle electromyography, each extremity, with related paraspinal areas, when performed, done with nerve conduction, amplitude and latency/velocity study; limited (List separately in addition to code for primary procedure)**

INCLUDES Testing four or less muscles per extremity

EXCLUDES Dynamic electromyography during motion analysis studies (96002-96003)

Motor and sensory nerve conduction (95905)

Needle electromyography extremities (95860-95864, 95870)

Reporting code more than one time per extremity

Code also, when applicable, for combined maximum total four units per patient when all four extremities tested ([95886])

Code first nerve conduction tests (95907-95913)

🖙 1.77 ⚕ 1.77 **FUD** ZZZ   N 80 🖵

AMA: 2020,Nov,12; 2018,Feb,11; 2018,Jan,8; 2017,Jul,10; 2017,Jan,8; 2016,Jan,13

+ # **95886**   **complete, five or more muscles studied, innervated by three or more nerves or four or more spinal levels (List separately in addition to code for primary procedure)**

INCLUDES Testing five or more muscles per extremity

EXCLUDES *Dynamic electromyography during motion analysis studies (96002-96003)*
Motor and sensory nerve conduction (95905)
Needle electromyography extremities (95860-95864, 95870)
Reporting code more than one time per extremity

Code also, when applicable, for combined maximum total four units per patient when all four extremities tested ([95885])
Code first nerve conduction tests (95907-95913)

🔧 2.75   ✂ 2.75   **FUD** ZZZ   N 80 ▱

AMA: 2020,Nov,12; 2018,Feb,11; 2018,Jan,8; 2017,Jul,10; 2017,Jan,8; 2016,Jan,13

+ # **95887**   **Needle electromyography, non-extremity (cranial nerve supplied or axial) muscle(s) done with nerve conduction, amplitude and latency/velocity study (List separately in addition to code for primary procedure)**

INCLUDES Nerve study unilateral cranial nerve innervated muscles

EXCLUDES *Dynamic electromyography during motion analysis studies (96002-96003)*
Guidance for chemodenervation (95874)
Motor and sensory nerve conduction (95905)
Needle electromyography cranial nerve supplied muscles (95867-95868)
Needle electromyography except for thoracic paraspinal, cranial nerve supplied muscles, or sphincters (95870)
Nerve study extra-ocular or laryngeal nerves
Reporting code more than once per anatomic site

Code also twice when performed bilaterally
Code first nerve conduction tests (95907-95913)

🔧 2.40   ✂ 2.40   **FUD** ZZZ   N 80 ▱

AMA: 2018,Feb,11; 2018,Jan,8; 2017,Jul,10; 2017,Jan,8; 2016,Jan,13

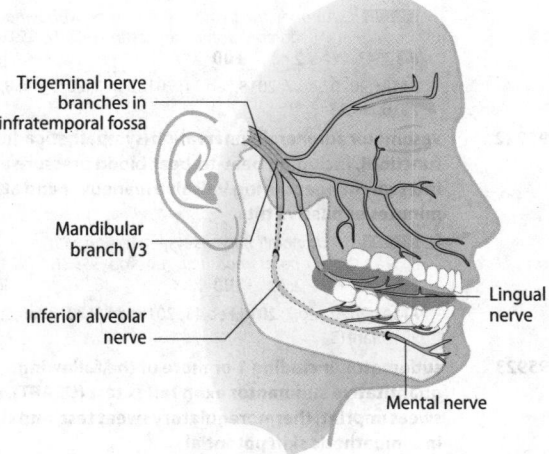

Trigeminal nerve branches in infratemporal fossa

Mandibular branch V3

Inferior alveolar nerve

Lingual nerve

Mental nerve

Cranial nerves: trigeminal branches of lower face and select facial nerves

Needle EMG is performed to determine conduction, amplitude, and latency/velocity

+   95873   **Electrical stimulation for guidance in conjunction with chemodenervation (List separately in addition to code for primary procedure)**

EXCLUDES *Chemodenervation larynx (64617)*
Injection anesthetic or steroid, sacroiliac joint (64451)
Needle electromyography (95860-95870)
Needle electromyography guidance for chemodenervation (95874)
Radiofrequency ablation, sacroiliac joint ([64625])
Reporting more than one guidance code for each chemodenervation code

Code first chemodenervation (64612, 64615-64616, 64642-64647)

🔧 2.17   ✂ 2.17   **FUD** ZZZ   N 80 ▱

AMA: 2019,Dec,8; 2019,Apr,9; 2018,Feb,11; 2018,Jan,8; 2017,Jan,8; 2016,Jan,13

+   95874   **Needle electromyography for guidance in conjunction with chemodenervation (List separately in addition to code for primary procedure)**

EXCLUDES *Chemodenervation larynx (64617)*
Injection anesthetic or steroid, sacroiliac joint (64451)
Needle electromyography (95860-95870)
Needle electromyography guidance for chemodenervation (95873)
Radiofrequency ablation, sacroiliac joint ([64625])
Reporting more than one guidance code for each chemodenervation code

Code first chemodenervation (64612, 64615-64616, 64642-64647)

🔧 2.23   ✂ 2.23   **FUD** ZZZ   N 80 ▱

AMA: 2020,Dec,13; 2019,Dec,8; 2019,Apr,9; 2018,Feb,11; 2018,Jan,8; 2017,Jan,8; 2016,Jan,13

     95875   **Ischemic limb exercise test with serial specimen(s) acquisition for muscle(s) metabolite(s)**

🔧 3.78   ✂ 3.78   **FUD** XXX   S 80 ▱

AMA: 2018,Feb,11; 2018,Jan,8; 2017,Jan,8; 2016,Jan,13

     95885   **Resequenced code. See code following 95872.**

     95886   **Resequenced code. See code following 95872.**

     95887   **Resequenced code. See code before 95873.**

95905-95913 Evaluation of Nerve Function: Nerve Conduction Studies

INCLUDES Conduction studies motor and sensory nerves
Reports from on-site examiner including interpretation results using established methodologies, calculations, comparisons to normal studies, and interpretation by physician or other qualified health care professional
Single conduction study comprising sensory and motor conduction test with/without F or H wave testing, and all orthodromic and antidromic impulses
Total number tests performed indicate appropriate code

EXCLUDES *Reporting code for more than one study when multiple sites on same nerve tested*

Code also electromyography performed with nerve conduction studies, as appropriate ([95885, 95886, 95887])

     95905   **Motor and/or sensory nerve conduction, using preconfigured electrode array(s), amplitude and latency/velocity study, each limb, includes F-wave study when performed, with interpretation and report**

INCLUDES Study with preconfigured electrodes that are customized to a specific body location

EXCLUDES *Needle electromyography ([95885, 95886])*
Nerve conduction studies (95907-95913)
Reporting code more than one time for each limb studied

🔧 1.53   ✂ 1.53   **FUD** XXX   ⊘ 01 80 ▱

AMA: 2018,Feb,11; 2018,Jan,8; 2017,Jan,8; 2016,Jan,13

     95907   **Nerve conduction studies; 1-2 studies**

🔧 2.71   ✂ 2.71   **FUD** XXX   S 80 ▱

AMA: 2018,Aug,10; 2018,Feb,11; 2018,Jan,8; 2017,Dec,14; 2017,Jan,8; 2016,Jan,13

Medicine

95908 — 95924

	95908	**3-4 studies**
		🔻 3.44 ⚸ 3.44 **FUD** XXX [S] [80] 🖵
		AMA: 2018,Aug,10; 2018,Feb,11; 2018,Jan,8; 2017,Jan,8; 2016,Jan,13
	95909	**5-6 studies**
		🔻 4.12 ⚸ 4.12 **FUD** XXX [S] [80] 🖵
		AMA: 2018,Aug,10; 2018,Feb,11; 2018,Jan,8; 2017,Jan,8; 2016,Jan,13
	95910	**7-8 studies**
		🔻 5.42 ⚸ 5.42 **FUD** XXX [S] [80] 🖵
		AMA: 2018,Aug,10; 2018,Feb,11; 2018,Jan,8; 2017,Jan,8; 2016,Jan,13
	95911	**9-10 studies**
		🔻 6.49 ⚸ 6.49 **FUD** XXX [S] [80] 🖵
		AMA: 2018,Aug,10; 2018,Feb,11; 2018,Jan,8; 2017,Jan,8; 2016,Jan,13
	95912	**11-12 studies**
		🔻 7.43 ⚸ 7.43 **FUD** XXX [S] [80] 🖵
		AMA: 2018,Aug,10; 2018,Feb,11; 2018,Jan,8; 2017,Jan,8; 2016,Jan,13
	95913	**13 or more studies**
		🔻 8.60 ⚸ 8.60 **FUD** XXX [S] [80] 🖵
		AMA: 2018,Aug,10; 2018,Feb,11; 2018,Jan,8; 2017,Jan,8; 2016,Jan,13

95940-95941 [95940, 95941] Intraoperative Neurophysiological Monitoring

INCLUDES   Monitoring, testing, and data evaluation during surgical procedures by monitoring professional dedicated only to performing necessary testing and monitoring
Monitoring services provided by anesthesiologist or surgeon separately

EXCLUDES   *Baseline neurophysiologic monitoring*
EEG during nonintracranial surgery (95955)
Electrocorticography ([95829])
Intraoperative cortical and subcortical mapping (95961-95962)
Neurostimulator programming/analysis (95971-95972, 95976-95977, [95983, 95984])
Time required for set-up, recording, interpretation, and electrode removal

Code also:
Baseline studies (eg, EMGs, NCVs), no more than one time per operative session
Services provided after midnight using date when monitoring started and total monitoring time
Standby time prior to procedure (99360)
Code first ([92653], 95822, 95860-95870, 95907-95913, 95925-95937 [95938, 95939])

+ #   95940   Continuous intraoperative neurophysiology monitoring in the operating room, one on one monitoring requiring personal attendance, each 15 minutes (List separately in addition to code for primary procedure)

INCLUDES   15 minute increments monitoring service
Based on time spent monitoring, despite number tests or parameters monitored
Continuous intraoperative neurophysiologic monitoring by dedicated monitoring professional in operating room providing one-on-one patient care
Monitoring time distinct from baseline neurophysiologic study time(s) or other services (e.g., mapping)
Monitoring time may begin prior to incision
Total all monitoring time for procedures overlapping midnight

EXCLUDES   *Time spent in executing or interpreting baseline neurophysiologic study or studies*

Code also monitoring from outside operative room, when applicable ([95941])

🔻 0.93   ⚸ 0.93   **FUD** XXX   [N] [80] 🖵

AMA: 2020,Oct,9; 2020,Oct,14; 2018,Feb,11; 2018,Jan,8; 2017,Aug,8; 2017,Jan,8; 2016,Jan,13

+ #   95941   Continuous intraoperative neurophysiology monitoring, from outside the operating room (remote or nearby) or for monitoring of more than one case while in the operating room, per hour (List separately in addition to code for primary procedure)

INCLUDES   Based on time spent monitoring, despite number tests or parameters monitored
Monitoring time distinct from baseline neurophysiologic study time(s) or other services (e.g., mapping)
One hour increments monitoring service

🔻 0.00   ⚸ 0.00   **FUD** XXX   [N] 🖵

AMA: 2020,Oct,9; 2020,Oct,14; 2018,Feb,11; 2018,Jan,8; 2017,Aug,8; 2017,Jan,8; 2016,Jan,13

95921-95924 Evaluation of Autonomic Nervous System

INCLUDES   Physician interpretation
Recording
Report
Testing for autonomic dysfunction including site and autonomic subsystems

| | 95921 | **Testing of autonomic nervous system function; cardiovagal innervation (parasympathetic function), including 2 or more of the following: heart rate response to deep breathing with recorded R-R interval, Valsalva ratio, and 30:15 ratio** |

INCLUDES   Data storage for waveform analysis
Display on monitor
Minimum two elements performed:
  Cardiovascular function indicated by 30:15 ration (R/R interval at beat 30)/(R-R interval at beat 15)
  Heart rate response to deep breathing obtained by visual quantitative recording analysis with patient taking five to six breaths per minute
  Valsalva ratio (at least two) obtained by dividing highest heart rate by lowest
Monitoring heart rate by electrocardiography; rate obtained from time between two successive R waves (R-R interval)
Testing most usually in prone position
Tilt table testing, when performed

EXCLUDES   *Autonomic nervous system testing with sympathetic adrenergic function testing (95922, 95924)*

🔻 2.43   ⚸ 2.43   **FUD** XXX   [S] [80] 🖵

AMA: 2020,Sep,7; 2018,Feb,11; 2018,Jan,8; 2017,Jan,8; 2016,Jan,13

95922   vasomotor adrenergic innervation (sympathetic adrenergic function), including beat-to-beat blood pressure and R-R interval changes during Valsalva maneuver and at least 5 minutes of passive tilt

EXCLUDES   *Autonomic nervous system testing with parasympathetic function (95921, 95924)*

🔻 2.70   ⚸ 2.70   **FUD** XXX   [Q1] [80] 🖵

AMA: 2020,Sep,7; 2018,Feb,11; 2018,Jan,8; 2017,Jan,8; 2016,Jan,13

95923   sudomotor, including 1 or more of the following: quantitative sudomotor axon reflex test (QSART), silastic sweat imprint, thermoregulatory sweat test, and changes in sympathetic skin potential

🔻 3.64   ⚸ 3.64   **FUD** XXX   [Q1] [80] 🖵

AMA: 2020,Sep,7; 2018,Feb,11; 2018,Jan,8; 2017,Jan,8; 2016,Jan,13

95924   combined parasympathetic and sympathetic adrenergic function testing with at least 5 minutes of passive tilt

INCLUDES   Tilt table testing adrenergic and parasympathetic function

EXCLUDES   *Autonomic nervous system testing with parasympathetic function (95921-95922)*

🔻 4.25   ⚸ 4.25   **FUD** XXX   [S] [80] 🖵

AMA: 2020,Sep,7; 2018,Feb,11; 2018,Jan,8; 2017,Jan,8; 2016,Jan,13

95925-95943 [95938, 95939, 95940, 95941]
Neurotransmission Studies

95925 Short-latency somatosensory evoked potential study, stimulation of any/all peripheral nerves or skin sites, recording from the central nervous system; in upper limbs

EXCLUDES *Auditory evoked potentials ([92653])*

Evoked potential study both upper and lower limbs ([95938])

Evoked potential study lower limbs (95926)

🔧 3.73   ⚕ 3.73   **FUD** XXX   S 80 ▢

AMA: 2018,Feb,11; 2018,Jan,8; 2017,Jan,8; 2016,Jan,13

95926 in lower limbs

EXCLUDES *Auditory evoked potentials ([92653])*

Evoked potential study both upper and lower limbs ([95938])

Evoked potential study upper limbs (95925)

🔧 3.76   ⚕ 3.76   **FUD** XXX   S 80 ▢

AMA: 2018,Feb,11; 2018,Jan,8; 2017,Jan,8; 2016,Jan,13

\# **95938** in upper and lower limbs

🔧 9.88   ⚕ 9.88   **FUD** XXX   S 80 ▢

AMA: 2018,Feb,11; 2018,Jan,8; 2017,Jan,8; 2016,Jan,13

95927 in the trunk or head

EXCLUDES *Auditory evoked potentials ([92653])*

Code also modifier 52 for unilateral test

🔧 3.75   ⚕ 3.75   **FUD** XXX   S 80 ▢

AMA: 2020,Oct,9; 2018,Feb,11; 2018,Jan,8; 2017,Jan,8; 2016,Jan,13

95928 Central motor evoked potential study (transcranial motor stimulation); upper limbs

EXCLUDES *Central motor evoked potential study lower limbs (95929)*

🔧 6.20   ⚕ 6.20   **FUD** XXX   S 80 ▢

AMA: 2018,Feb,11; 2018,Jan,8; 2017,Jan,8; 2016,Jan,13

95929 lower limbs

EXCLUDES *Central motor evoked potential study upper limbs (95928)*

🔧 6.57   ⚕ 6.57   **FUD** XXX   S 80 ▢

AMA: 2018,Feb,11; 2018,Jan,8; 2017,Jan,8; 2016,Jan,13

\# **95939** in upper and lower limbs

EXCLUDES *Central motor evoked potential study either lower or upper limbs (95928-95929)*

🔧 14.8   ⚕ 14.8   **FUD** XXX   S 80 ▢

AMA: 2018,Feb,11; 2018,Jan,8; 2017,Jan,8; 2016,Jan,13

95930 Visual evoked potential (VEP) checkerboard or flash testing, central nervous system except glaucoma, with interpretation and report

EXCLUDES *Visual acuity screening using automated visual evoked potential devices (0333T)*

Visual evoked glaucoma testing ([0464T])

🔧 1.88   ⚕ 1.88   **FUD** XXX   S 80 ▢

AMA: 2018,Feb,11; 2018,Feb,3; 2018,Jan,8; 2017,Jan,8; 2016,Jan,13

95933 Orbicularis oculi (blink) reflex, by electrodiagnostic testing

🔧 2.33   ⚕ 2.33   **FUD** XXX   01 80 ▢

AMA: 2018,Feb,11; 2018,Jan,8; 2017,Jul,10; 2017,Jan,8; 2016,Jan,13

95937 Neuromuscular junction testing (repetitive stimulation, paired stimuli), each nerve, any 1 method

🔧 2.48   ⚕ 2.48   **FUD** XXX   S 80 ▢

AMA: 2020,Aug,14; 2018,Feb,11; 2018,Jan,8; 2017,Jan,8; 2016,Feb,13; 2016,Jan,13

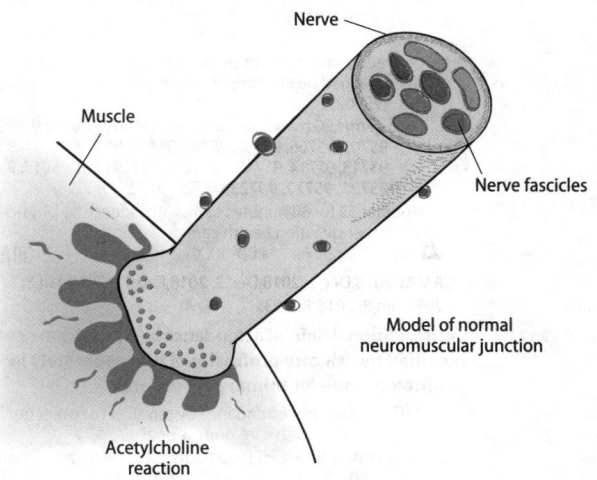

Model of normal neuromuscular junction

A selected neuromuscular junction is repeatedly stimulated. The test is useful to demonstrate reduced muscle action potential from fatigue

95938 Resequenced code. See code following 95926.

95939 Resequenced code. See code following 95929.

95940 Resequenced code. See code following 95913.

95941 Resequenced code. See code following 95913.

95943 ~~Simultaneous, independent, quantitative measures of both parasympathetic function and sympathetic function, based on time-frequency analysis of heart rate variability concurrent with time-frequency analysis of continuous respiratory activity, with mean heart rate and blood pressure measures, during rest, paced (deep) breathing, Valsalva maneuvers, and head-up postural change~~

To report, see (95999)

95954-95962 Electroencephalography For Seizure Monitoring/Intraoperative Use

EXCLUDES *E/M services*

95954 Pharmacological or physical activation requiring physician or other qualified health care professional attendance during EEG recording of activation phase (eg, thiopental activation test)

🔧 11.0   ⚕ 11.0   **FUD** XXX   S 80 ▢

AMA: 2018,Feb,11; 2018,Jan,8; 2017,Jan,8; 2016,Jan,13

95955 Electroencephalogram (EEG) during nonintracranial surgery (eg, carotid surgery)

🔧 5.94   ⚕ 5.94   **FUD** XXX   N 80 ▢

AMA: 2018,Feb,11; 2018,Jan,8; 2017,Jan,8; 2016,Jan,13

95957 Digital analysis of electroencephalogram (EEG) (eg, for epileptic spike analysis)

EXCLUDES *Use of automated spike and seizure detection/trending software, when performed ([95700, 95705, 95706, 95707, 95708, 95709, 95710, 95711, 95712, 95713, 95714, 95715, 95716, 95717, 95718, 95719, 95720, 95721, 95722, 95723, 95724, 95725, 95726])*

🔧 7.24   ⚕ 7.24   **FUD** XXX   N 80 ▢

AMA: 2018,Dec,3; 2018,Dec,3; 2018,Feb,11; 2018,Jan,8; 2017,Jan,8; 2016,Jan,13

95958 Wada activation test for hemispheric function, including electroencephalographic (EEG) monitoring

🔧 16.4   ⚕ 16.4   **FUD** XXX   S 80 ▢

AMA: 2018,Feb,11

Medicine

95961   Functional cortical and subcortical mapping by stimulation and/or recording of electrodes on brain surface, or of depth electrodes, to provoke seizures or identify vital brain structures; initial hour of attendance by a physician or other qualified health care professional

> **INCLUDES**   One hour attendance by physician or other qualified health care professional
>
> Code also:
>
> > Each additional hour attendance by physician or other qualified health care professional, when appropriate (95962)
> >
> > Long-term EEG (two hours or more), when performed ([95700, 95705, 95706, 95707, 95708, 95709, 95710, 95711, 95712, 95713, 95714, 95715, 95716, 95717, 95718, 95719, 95720, 95721, 95722, 95723, 95724, 95725, 95726])
> >
> > Modifier 52 for 30 minutes or less attendance by physician or other qualified health care professional
>
> 🖥 8.79   ✎ 8.79   **FUD** XXX   Ⓢ 80 ▢
>
> **AMA:** 2018,Dec,3; 2018,Dec,3; 2018,Feb,11; 2018,Jan,8; 2017,Jan,8; 2016,Jan,13

+ 95962   each additional hour of attendance by a physician or other qualified health care professional (List separately in addition to code for primary procedure)

> **INCLUDES**   One hour attendance by physician or other qualified health care professional
>
> Code also long-term EEG (two hours or more), when performed ([95700, 95705, 95706, 95707, 95708, 95709, 95710, 95711, 95712, 95713, 95714, 95715, 95716, 95717, 95718, 95719, 95720, 95721, 95722, 95723, 95724, 95725, 95726])
>
> Code first initial hour (95961)
>
> 🖥 7.44   ✎ 7.44   **FUD** ZZZ   Ⓝ 80 ▢
>
> **AMA:** 2018,Feb,11; 2018,Jan,8; 2017,Jan,8; 2016,Jan,13

95965-95967 Magnetoencephalography

> **INCLUDES**   Physician interpretation
> Recording
> Report
>
> **EXCLUDES**   *CT provided with magnetoencephalography (70450-70470, 70496)*
> *Electroencephalography provided with magnetoencephalography (95812-95824)*
> *E/M services*
> *MRI provided with magnetoencephalography (70551-70553)*
> *Somatosensory evoked potentials/auditory evoked potentials/visual evoked potentials provided with magnetic evoked field responses ([92653], 95925, 95926, 95930)*

95965   Magnetoencephalography (MEG), recording and analysis; for spontaneous brain magnetic activity (eg, epileptic cerebral cortex localization)

> 🖥 0.00   ✎ 0.00   **FUD** XXX   Ⓢ 80 ▢
>
> **AMA:** 2018,Feb,11

95966   for evoked magnetic fields, single modality (eg, sensory, motor, language, or visual cortex localization)

> 🖥 0.00   ✎ 0.00   **FUD** XXX   Ⓢ 80 ▢
>
> **AMA:** 2018,Feb,11

+ 95967   for evoked magnetic fields, each additional modality (eg, sensory, motor, language, or visual cortex localization) (List separately in addition to code for primary procedure)

> Code first single modality (95966)
>
> 🖥 0.00   ✎ 0.00   **FUD** ZZZ   Ⓝ 80 ▢
>
> **AMA:** 2020,Oct,9; 2018,Feb,11

95700-95726 [95700, 95705, 95706, 95707, 95708, 95709, 95710, 95711, 95712, 95713, 95714, 95715, 95716, 95717, 95718, 95719, 95720, 95721, 95722, 95723, 95724, 95725, 95726] Electronencephalogram (EEG)

> **INCLUDES**   Automated spike and seizure detection/trending software, when performed
> Determination:
>   Eligibility for epilepsy surgery
>   Location and type seizures
> Differentiation seizures from other conditions
> Monitoring:
>   Seizure treatment
>   Status epilepticus
>
> **EXCLUDES**   *Diagnostic EEG recording time less than two hours*
> *Routine EEG (95812-95813, 95816, 95819, 95822)*
>
> Code also cortical or subcortical mapping, when performed (95961-95962)

 # 95700   Electroencephalogram (EEG) continuous recording, with video when performed, setup, patient education, and takedown when performed, administered in person by EEG technologist, minimum of 8 channels

> **INCLUDES**   Technical component
>
> **EXCLUDES**   *EEG performed using patient-placed electrodes, performed by non-EEG technologist, or remote supervision by EEG technologist (95999)*
> *Reporting code more than one time each session*
>
> 🖥 0.00   ✎ 0.00   **FUD** XXX   80 ▢

 # 95705   Electroencephalogram (EEG), without video, review of data, technical description by EEG technologist, 2-12 hours; unmonitored

> **INCLUDES**   Technical component
>
> **EXCLUDES**   *Reporting code more than one time to capture complete long-term EEG session or final 2-12 hour segment past 26 hours*
>
> 🖥 0.00   ✎ 0.00   **FUD** XXX   80 ▢

 # 95706   with intermittent monitoring and maintenance

> **INCLUDES**   Technical component
>
> **EXCLUDES**   *Reporting code more than one time to capture complete long-term EEG session or final 2-12 hour segment past 26 hours*
>
> 🖥 0.00   ✎ 0.00   **FUD** XXX   80 ▢

 # 95707   with continuous, real-time monitoring and maintenance

> **INCLUDES**   Technical component
>
> **EXCLUDES**   *Reporting code more than one time to capture complete long-term EEG session or final 2-12 hour segment past 26 hours*
>
> 🖥 0.00   ✎ 0.00   **FUD** XXX   80 ▢

 # 95708   Electroencephalogram (EEG), without video, review of data, technical description by EEG technologist, each increment of 12-26 hours; unmonitored

> **INCLUDES**   Technical component
>
> 🖥 0.00   ✎ 0.00   **FUD** XXX   80 ▢

 # 95709   with intermittent monitoring and maintenance

> **INCLUDES**   Technical component
>
> 🖥 0.00   ✎ 0.00   **FUD** XXX   80 ▢

 # 95710   with continuous, real-time monitoring and maintenance

> **INCLUDES**   Technical component
>
> 🖥 0.00   ✎ 0.00   **FUD** XXX   80 ▢

 # 95711   Electroencephalogram with video (VEEG), review of data, technical description by EEG technologist, 2-12 hours; unmonitored

> **INCLUDES**   Technical component
>
> **EXCLUDES**   *Reporting code more than one time to capture complete long-term EEG session or final 2-12 hour segment past 26 hours*
>
> 🖥 0.00   ✎ 0.00   **FUD** XXX   80 ▢

95712 with intermittent monitoring and maintenance

INCLUDES Technical component

EXCLUDES *Reporting code more than one time to capture complete long-term EEG session or final 2-12 hour segment past 26 hours*

🚑 0.00   ⚕ 0.00   **FUD** XXX   80 ▱

95713 with continuous, real-time monitoring and maintenance

INCLUDES Technical component

EXCLUDES *Reporting code more than one time to capture complete long-term EEG session or final 2-12 hour segment past 26 hours*

🚑 0.00   ⚕ 0.00   **FUD** XXX   80 ▱

95714 Electroencephalogram with video (VEEG), review of data, technical description by EEG technologist, each increment of 12-26 hours; unmonitored

INCLUDES Technical component

🚑 0.00   ⚕ 0.00   **FUD** XXX   80 ▱

95715 with intermittent monitoring and maintenance

INCLUDES Technical component

🚑 0.00   ⚕ 0.00   **FUD** XXX   80 ▱

95716 with continuous, real-time monitoring and maintenance

INCLUDES Technical component

🚑 0.00   ⚕ 0.00   **FUD** XXX   80 ▱

95717 Electroencephalogram (EEG), continuous recording, physician or other qualified health care professional review of recorded events, analysis of spike and seizure detection, interpretation and report, 2-12 hours of EEG recording; without video

INCLUDES Professional component

EXCLUDES *Professional interpretation for recordings greater than 36 hours and for which entire professional report generated retroactively ([95721, 95722, 95723, 95724, 95725, 95726])*

Reporting code more than one time to capture complete long-term EEG session or final 2-12 hour segment past 24 hours

🚑 2.90   ⚕ 2.94   **FUD** XXX   80 ▱

95718 with video (VEEG)

INCLUDES Professional component

EXCLUDES *Professional interpretation for recordings greater than 36 hours and for which entire professional report generated retroactively ([95721, 95722, 95723, 95724, 95725, 95726])*

Reporting code more than one time to capture complete long-term EEG session or final 2-12 hour segment past 24 hours

🚑 3.81   ⚕ 3.87   **FUD** XXX   80 ▱

95719 Electroencephalogram (EEG), continuous recording, physician or other qualified health care professional review of recorded events, analysis of spike and seizure detection, each increment of greater than 12 hours, up to 26 hours of EEG recording, interpretation and report after each 24-hour period; without video

INCLUDES Professional component

Single report or multiple reports during 26-hour reporting period

EXCLUDES *Professional interpretation for recordings greater than 36 hours and for which entire professional report generated retroactively ([95721, 95722, 95723, 95724, 95725, 95726])*

Reporting code more than once for multiple day studies after each 24-hour period during extended EEG recording time ([95719, 95720])

Reporting code more than one time to capture between12-26 hours

Code also EEG, 2-12 hours for studies longer than 26 hours ([95717, 95718])

🚑 4.50   ⚕ 4.55   **FUD** XXX   80 ▱

95720 with video (VEEG)

INCLUDES Professional component

Single report or multiple reports during 26-hour reporting period

EXCLUDES *Professional interpretation for recordings greater than 36 hours and for which entire professional report generated retroactively ([95721, 95722, 95723, 95724, 95725, 95726])*

Reporting code more than one time to capture between 12-26 hours

Reporting code more than once for multiple day studies after each 24-hour period during extended EEG recording time ([95719, 95720])

Code also EEG, 2-12 hours for studies longer than 26 hours ([95717, 95718])

🚑 5.90   ⚕ 5.99   **FUD** XXX   80 ▱

95721 Electroencephalogram (EEG), continuous recording, physician or other qualified health care professional review of recorded events, analysis of spike and seizure detection, interpretation, and summary report, complete study; greater than 36 hours, up to 60 hours of EEG recording, without video

INCLUDES Professional interpretation for recordings greater than 36 hours and for which entire professional report generated retroactively

EXCLUDES *EEG, continuous recording, less than 36 hours ([95717, 95718, 95719, 95720])*

🚑 5.92   ⚕ 6.04   **FUD** XXX   80 ▱

95722 greater than 36 hours, up to 60 hours of EEG recording, with video (VEEG)

INCLUDES Professional interpretation for recordings greater than 36 hours and for which entire professional report generated retroactively

EXCLUDES *EEG, continuous recording, less than 36 hours ([95717, 95718, 95719, 95720])*

🚑 7.20   ⚕ 7.33   **FUD** XXX   80 ▱

95723 greater than 60 hours, up to 84 hours of EEG recording, without video

INCLUDES Professional interpretation for recordings greater than 36 hours and for which entire professional report generated retroactively

EXCLUDES *EEG, continuous recording, less than 36 hours ([95717, 95718, 95719, 95720])*

🚑 7.33   ⚕ 7.49   **FUD** XXX   80 ▱

95724 greater than 60 hours, up to 84 hours of EEG recording, with video (VEEG)

INCLUDES Professional interpretation for recordings greater than 36 hours and for which entire professional report generated retroactively

EXCLUDES *EEG, continuous recording, less than 36 hours ([95717, 95718, 95719, 95720])*

🚑 9.18   ⚕ 9.36   **FUD** XXX   80 ▱

95725 greater than 84 hours of EEG recording, without video

INCLUDES Professional interpretation for recordings greater than 36 hours and for which entire professional report generated retroactively

EXCLUDES *EEG, continuous recording, less than 36 hours ([95717, 95718, 95719, 95720])*

🚑 8.34   ⚕ 8.55   **FUD** XXX   80 ▱

AMA: 2011,Jan,11; 2009,Jan,11-31

95726 greater than 84 hours of EEG recording, with video (VEEG)

INCLUDES Professional interpretation for recordings greater than 36 hours and for which entire professional report generated retroactively

EXCLUDES *EEG, continuous recording, less than 36 hours ([95717, 95718, 95719, 95720])*

🚑 11.6   ⚕ 11.8   **FUD** XXX   80 ▱

● New Code   ▲ Revised Code   ○ Reinstated   ● New Web Release   ▲ Revised Web Release   + Add-on   Unlisted   Not Covered   # Resequenced

㊿ Optum Mod 50 Exempt   ⊘ AMA Mod 51 Exempt   ⑤ Optum Mod 51 Exempt   ㊿ Mod 63 Exempt   ✏ Non-FDA Drug   ★ Telemedicine   Ⓜ Maternity   Ⓐ Age Edit

© 2021 Optum360, LLC   CPT © 2021 American Medical Association. All Rights Reserved.   **509**

Medicine

95970 — 95992

95970-95984 [95983, 95984] Evaluation of Implanted Neurostimulator with/without Programming

INCLUDES   Documentation settings, electrode impedances system parameters before programming
Insertion electrode array(s) into target area (permanent or trial)
Multiple adjustments to parameters necessary during programming session
Neurostimulators distinguished by nervous system area stimulated:
  Brain: Deep brain stimulation or cortical stimulation (brain surface)
  Cranial nerves: Includes 12 pairs cranial nerves, branches, divisions, intracranial and extracranial segments
  Spinal cord and peripheral nerves: Nerves originating in spinal cord and nerves and ganglia outside spinal cord
  Parameters (vary by system) include:
    Amplitude
    Burst
    Cycling on/off
    Detection algorithms
    Dose lockout
    Frequency
    Pulse width
    Responsive neurostimulation

EXCLUDES   *Implantation/replacement neurostimulator electrodes (43647, 43881, 61850-61868, 63650-63655, 64553-64581)*
Neurostimulation system, posterior tibial nerve (0587T-0590T)
Neurostimulator pulse generator/receiver:
 Insertion (61885-61886, 63685, 64568, 64582, 64590)
 Revision/removal (61888, 63688, 64569, 64570, 64583-64584, 64595)
Revision/removal neurostimulator electrodes (43648, 43882, 61880, 63661-63664, 64569-64570, 64583-64585)

95970   **Electronic analysis of implanted neurostimulator pulse generator/transmitter (eg, contact group[s], interleaving, amplitude, pulse width, frequency [Hz], on/off cycling, burst, magnet mode, dose lockout, patient selectable parameters, responsive neurostimulation, detection algorithms, closed loop parameters, and passive parameters) by physician or other qualified health care professional; with brain, cranial nerve, spinal cord, peripheral nerve, or sacral nerve, neurostimulator pulse generator/transmitter, without programming**

  INCLUDES   Analysis implanted neurostimulator without programming
  EXCLUDES   *Programming with analysis (95971-95972, 95976-95977, [95983, 95984])*
  📠 0.53   ⚖ 0.54   **FUD** XXX   01 80 💻
  AMA: 2019,Feb,6; 2018,Oct,8; 2018,Feb,11; 2018,Jan,8; 2017,Jan,8; 2016,Jul,7; 2016,Jan,13

95971   **with simple spinal cord or peripheral nerve (eg, sacral nerve) neurostimulator pulse generator/transmitter programming by physician or other qualified health care professional**

  EXCLUDES   *Programming neurostimulator for complex spinal cord or peripheral nerve (95972)*
  📠 1.17   ⚖ 1.44   **FUD** XXX   S 80 💻
  AMA: 2019,Feb,6; 2018,Oct,8; 2018,Feb,11; 2018,Jan,8; 2017,Jan,8; 2016,Jul,7; 2016,Jan,13

95972   **with complex spinal cord or peripheral nerve (eg, sacral nerve) neurostimulator pulse generator/transmitter programming by physician or other qualified health care professional**

  📠 1.19   ⚖ 1.62   **FUD** XXX   S 80 💻
  AMA: 2019,Feb,6; 2018,Oct,8; 2018,Feb,11; 2018,Jan,8; 2017,Jan,8; 2016,Jul,7; 2016,Jan,13

95976   **with simple cranial nerve neurostimulator pulse generator/transmitter programming by physician or other qualified health care professional**

  EXCLUDES   *Programming neurostimulator for complex cranial nerve (95977)*
  📠 1.16   ⚖ 1.18   **FUD** XXX   80 💻
  AMA: 2019,Feb,6

95977   **with complex cranial nerve neurostimulator pulse generator/transmitter programming by physician or other qualified health care professional**

  📠 1.52   ⚖ 1.54   **FUD** XXX   80 💻
  AMA: 2019,Feb,6

 # 95983   **with brain neurostimulator pulse generator/transmitter programming, first 15 minutes face-to-face time with physician or other qualified health care professional**

  📠 1.44   ⚖ 1.46   **FUD** XXX   80 💻
  AMA: 2019,Feb,6; 2018,Dec,3; 2018,Dec,3

+ # 95984   **with brain neurostimulator pulse generator/transmitter programming, each additional 15 minutes face-to-face time with physician or other qualified health care professional (List separately in addition to code for primary procedure)**

  Code first ([95983])
  📠 1.26   ⚖ 1.27   **FUD** ZZZ   80 💻
  AMA: 2019,Feb,6; 2018,Dec,3; 2018,Dec,3

95980   **Electronic analysis of implanted neurostimulator pulse generator system (eg, rate, pulse amplitude and duration, configuration of wave form, battery status, electrode selectability, output modulation, cycling, impedance and patient measurements) gastric neurostimulator pulse generator/transmitter; intraoperative, with programming**

  INCLUDES   Gastric neurostimulator lesser curvature
  EXCLUDES   *Analysis, with programming when performed, vagus nerve trunk stimulator for morbid obesity (0312T, 0317T)*
  📠 1.32   ⚖ 1.32   **FUD** XXX   N 80 💻
  AMA: 2018,Feb,11; 2018,Jan,8; 2017,Jan,8; 2016,Jul,7; 2016,Jan,13

95981   **subsequent, without reprogramming**

  EXCLUDES   *Analysis, with programming when performed, vagus nerve trunk stimulator for morbid obesity (0312T, 0317T)*
  📠 0.51   ⚖ 0.97   **FUD** XXX   01 80 💻
  AMA: 2018,Feb,11; 2018,Jan,8; 2017,Jan,8; 2016,Jul,7; 2016,Jan,13

95982   **subsequent, with reprogramming**

  EXCLUDES   *Analysis, with programming when performed, vagus nerve trunk stimulator for morbid obesity (0312T, 0317T)*
  📠 1.04   ⚖ 1.55   **FUD** XXX   01 80 💻
  AMA: 2018,Feb,11; 2018,Jan,8; 2017,Jan,8; 2016,Jul,7; 2016,Jan,13

95983   Resequenced code. See code following 95977.

95984   Resequenced code. See code following 95977.

95990-95991 Refill/Upkeep of Implanted Drug Delivery Pump to Central Nervous System

EXCLUDES   *Analysis/reprogramming implanted pump for infusion (62367-62370)*
E/M services

95990   **Refilling and maintenance of implantable pump or reservoir for drug delivery, spinal (intrathecal, epidural) or brain (intraventricular), includes electronic analysis of pump, when performed;**

  📠 2.62   ⚖ 2.62   **FUD** XXX   S 80 💻
  AMA: 2018,Feb,11; 2018,Jan,8; 2017,Jan,8; 2016,Jan,13

95991   **requiring skill of a physician or other qualified health care professional**

  📠 1.14   ⚖ 3.30   **FUD** XXX   T 80 💻
  AMA: 2018,Feb,11; 2018,Jan,8; 2017,Jan,8; 2016,Jan,13

95992-95999 Other and Unlisted Neurological Procedures

95992   **Canalith repositioning procedure(s) (eg, Epley maneuver, Semont maneuver), per day**

  EXCLUDES   *Nystagmus testing (92531-92532)*
  📠 1.07   ⚖ 1.25   **FUD** XXX   A 80 💻
  AMA: 2018,Feb,11; 2018,Jan,8; 2017,Jan,8; 2016,Jan,13

| 95999 | Unlisted neurological or neuromuscular diagnostic procedure |

🔲 0.00   🔲 0.00   **FUD** XXX   [01] [80] 🖥

AMA: 2018,Aug,10; 2018,Feb,11; 2018,Jan,8; 2017,Jan,8; 2016,Jan,13

96000-96004 Motion Analysis Studies

CMS: 100-02,15,230.4 Services By a Physical/Occupational Therapist in Private Practice

INCLUDES Services provided as part major therapeutic/diagnostic decision making
Services provided in dedicated motion analysis department with these capabilities:
3D kinetics/dynamic electromyography
Computerized 3D kinematics
Videotaping from front/back/both sides

EXCLUDES *E/M services*
Gait training (97116)
Needle electromyography (95860-95872 [95885, 95886, 95887])

| 96000 | Comprehensive computer-based motion analysis by video-taping and 3D kinematics; |

🔲 2.72   🔲 2.72   **FUD** XXX   [S] [80] 🖥

AMA: 2018,Feb,11; 2018,Jan,8; 2017,Jan,8; 2016,Jan,13

| 96001 | with dynamic plantar pressure measurements during walking |

🔲 3.65   🔲 3.65   **FUD** XXX   [S] [80] 🖥

AMA: 2018,Feb,11; 2018,Jan,8; 2017,Jan,8; 2016,Jan,13

| 96002 | Dynamic surface electromyography, during walking or other functional activities, 1-12 muscles |

🔲 0.63   🔲 0.63   **FUD** XXX   [S] [80] 🖥

AMA: 2018,Feb,11; 2018,Jan,8; 2017,Jan,8; 2016,Jan,13

| 96003 | Dynamic fine wire electromyography, during walking or other functional activities, 1 muscle |

🔲 0.49   🔲 0.49   **FUD** XXX   [01] [80] 🖥

AMA: 2018,Feb,11; 2018,Jan,8; 2017,Jan,8; 2016,Jan,13

| 96004 | Review and interpretation by physician or other qualified health care professional of comprehensive computer-based motion analysis, dynamic plantar pressure measurements, dynamic surface electromyography during walking or other functional activities, and dynamic fine wire electromyography, with written report |

🔲 3.27   🔲 3.27   **FUD** XXX   [B] [80] [26] 🖥

AMA: 2018,Feb,11; 2018,Jan,8; 2017,Jan,8; 2016,Jan,13

96020 Neurofunctional Brain Testing

INCLUDES Selection/administration, testing:
Cognition
Determining validity neurofunctional testing relative to separately interpreted functional magnetic resonance images
Functional neuroimaging
Language
Memory
Monitoring performance of testing
Movement
Other neurological functions
Sensation

EXCLUDES *Clinical depression treatment by repetitive transcranial magnetic stimulation (90867-90868)*
Developmental test administration (96112-96113)
E/M services on same date
MRI brain (70554-70555)
Neurobehavioral status examination (96116, 96121)
Neuropsychological testing (96132-96133)
Psychological testing (96130-96131)

| 96020 | Neurofunctional testing selection and administration during noninvasive imaging functional brain mapping, with test administered entirely by a physician or other qualified health care professional (ie, psychologist), with review of test results and report |

🔲 0.00   🔲 0.00   **FUD** XXX   [N] [80] 🖥

AMA: 2018,Feb,11; 2018,Jan,8; 2017,Jan,8; 2016,Jan,13

96040 Genetic Counseling Services

INCLUDES Analysis for genetic risk assessment
Counseling patient/family
Counseling services
Face-to-face interviews
Obtaining structured family genetic history
Pedigree construction
Review medical data/family information
Services provided by trained genetic counselor
Services provided during one or more sessions
Thirty minutes face-to-face time, reported one time for each 16-30 minutes service

EXCLUDES *Education/genetic counseling by physician or other qualified health care provider to group (99078)*
Education/genetic counseling by physician or other qualified health care provider to individual; report appropriate E/M code
Education regarding genetic risks by nonphysician to group (98961, 98962)
Genetic counseling and/or risk factor reduction intervention from physician or other qualified health care provider provided to patients without symptoms/diagnosis (99401-99412)
Reporting code when 15 minutes or less face-to-face time provided

| 96040 | Medical genetics and genetic counseling services, each 30 minutes face-to-face with patient/family |

🔲 1.30   🔲 1.30   **FUD** XXX   ★ [B] 🖥

AMA: 2018,Feb,11; 2018,Jan,8; 2017,Jan,8; 2016,Jan,13

97151-97158 [97151, 97152, 97153, 97154, 97155, 97156, 97157, 97158] Adaptive Behavior Assessments and Treatments

INCLUDES Adaptive behavior deficits (e.g., impairment in social, communication, self care skills)
Assessment and treatment that focuses on:
Maladaptive behaviors (e.g., repetitive movements, risk harm to self, others, property)
Secondary functional impairment due to consequences deficient adaptive and maladaptive behaviors (e.g., communication, play, leisure, social interactions)
Treatment determined based on goals and targets identified in assessments

| # | 97151 | Behavior identification assessment, administered by a physician or other qualified health care professional, each 15 minutes of the physician's or other qualified health care professional's time face-to-face with patient and/or guardian(s)/caregiver(s) administering assessments and discussing findings and recommendations, and non-face-to-face analyzing past data, scoring/interpreting the assessment, and preparing the report/treatment plan |

EXCLUDES *Health and behavior assessment and intervention (96156, 96158-96159, [96164, 96165], [96167, 96168], [96170, 96171])*
Medical team conference (99366-99368)
Neurobehavioral status examination (96116, 96121)
Neuropsychological testing (96132-96133, 96136-96139, 96146)
Psychiatric diagnostic evaluation (90791-90792)
Speech evaluations (92521-92524)

Code also:
More than one time on same or different days until assessment complete
Supporting assessment depending on time patient spends face-to-face with one or more technicians (counting only time spent by one technician) ([97152], 0362T)

🔲 0.00   🔲 0.00   **FUD** XXX   [80] 🖥

AMA: 2018,Nov,3

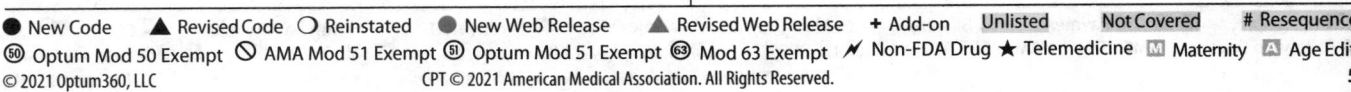

Medicine

97152 — 97157

97152 Behavior identification-supporting assessment, administered by one technician under the direction of a physician or other qualified health care professional, face-to-face with the patient, each 15 minutes

EXCLUDES *Health and behavior assessment and intervention (96156, 96158-96159, [96164, 96165], [96167, 96168], [96170, 96171])*
Medical team conference (99366-99368)
Neurobehavioral status examination (96116, 96121)
Neuropsychological testing (96132-96133, 96136-96139, 96146)
Psychiatric diagnostic evaluation (90791-90792)
Speech evaluations (92521-92524)

Code also:
  More than one time on same or different days until assessment complete
  Supporting assessment depending on time patient spends face-to-face with one or more technicians (counting only time spent by one technician) ([97152], 0362T)

🖐 0.00   🔧 0.00   **FUD** XXX   80 🖵

AMA: 2018,Nov,3

97153 Adaptive behavior treatment by protocol, administered by technician under the direction of a physician or other qualified health care professional, face-to-face with one patient, each 15 minutes

INCLUDES Face-to-face service with one patient only
Provided by technician under physician/other qualified healthcare professional direction

EXCLUDES *Aphasia and cognitive performance testing (96105, [96125])*
Behavioral/developmental screening/testing (96110-96113 [96127])
Health and behavior assessment and intervention (96156, 96158-96159, [96164, 96165], [96167, 96168], [96170, 96171])
Health risk assessment (96160-96161)
Neurobehavioral status examination (96116, 96121)
Psychiatric services (90785-90899)
Testing administration with scoring (96136-96139, 96146)
Testing evaluation (96130-96133)
Therapeutic procedure(s), individual patient (97129)
Treatment speech disorders (individual) (92507)

🖐 0.00   🔧 0.00   **FUD** XXX   80 🖵

AMA: 2020,Jul,10; 2018,Nov,3

97154 Group adaptive behavior treatment by protocol, administered by technician under the direction of a physician or other qualified health care professional, face-to-face with two or more patients, each 15 minutes

INCLUDES Face-to-face service with one patient only
Provided by technician under physician/other qualified healthcare professional direction

EXCLUDES *Aphasia and cognitive performance testing (96105, [96125])*
Behavioral/developmental screening/testing (96110-96113, [96127])
Health and behavior assessment and intervention (96156, 96158-96159, [96164, 96165], [96167, 96168], [96170, 96171])
Neurobehavioral status examination (96116, 96121)
Psychiatric services (90785-90899)
Testing administration with scoring (96136-96139, 96146)
Testing evaluation (96130-96133)
Therapeutic procedure(s) group, two or more patients (97150)
Treatment speech disorders (group) (92508)

🖐 0.00   🔧 0.00   **FUD** XXX   80 🖵

AMA: 2018,Nov,3

97155 Adaptive behavior treatment with protocol modification, administered by physician or other qualified health care professional, which may include simultaneous direction of technician, face-to-face with one patient, each 15 minutes

INCLUDES Face-to-face service with one patient only
Provided by technician under physician/other qualified healthcare professional direction

EXCLUDES *Aphasia and cognitive performance testing (96105, [96125])*
Behavioral/developmental screening/testing (96110-96113, [96127])
Health and behavior assessment and intervention (96156, 96158-96159, [96164, 96165], [96167, 96168], [96170, 96171])
Neurobehavioral status examination (96116, 96121)
Psychiatric services (90785-90899)
Testing administration with scoring (96136-96139, 96146)
Testing evaluation (96130-96133)
Therapeutic procedure(s), individual patient (97129)
Treatment speech disorders (individual) (92507)

🖐 0.00   🔧 0.00   **FUD** XXX   80 🖵

AMA: 2020,Jul,10; 2018,Nov,3

97156 Family adaptive behavior treatment guidance, administered by physician or other qualified health care professional (with or without the patient present), face-to-face with guardian(s)/caregiver(s), each 15 minutes

INCLUDES Provided by physician/other qualified healthcare professional
Without patient presence

EXCLUDES *Aphasia and cognitive performance testing (96105, [96125])*
Behavioral/developmental screening/testing (96110-96113 [96127])
Health and behavior assessment and intervention (96156, 96158-96159, [96164, 96165], [96167, 96168], [96170, 96171])
Neurobehavioral status examination (96116, 96121)
Psychiatric services (90785-90899)
Testing administration with scoring (96136-96139, 96146)
Testing evaluation (96130-96133)

🖐 0.00   🔧 0.00   **FUD** XXX   80 🖵

AMA: 2018,Nov,3

97157 Multiple-family group adaptive behavior treatment guidance, administered by physician or other qualified health care professional (without the patient present), face-to-face with multiple sets of guardians/caregivers, each 15 minutes

INCLUDES Provided by physician/other qualified healthcare professional
Without patient presence

EXCLUDES *Aphasia and cognitive performance testing (96105, [96125])*
Behavioral/developmental screening/testing (96110-96113 [96127])
Groups more than eight families
Health and behavior assessment and intervention (96156, 96158-96159, [96164, 96165], [96167, 96168], [96170, 96171])
Neurobehavioral status examination (96116, 96121)
Psychiatric services (90785-90899)
Testing administration with scoring (96136-96139, 96146)
Testing evaluation (96130-96133)

🖐 0.00   🔧 0.00   **FUD** XXX   80 🖵

AMA: 2018,Nov,3

26/TC PC/TC Only   A2-Z3 ASC Payment   50 Bilateral   ♂ Male Only   ♀ Female Only   🖐 Facility RVU   🔧 Non-Facility RVU   🖵 CCI   ✖ CLIA
FUD Follow-up Days   **CMS:** IOM   **AMA:** CPT Asst   A-Y OPPSI   80/80 Surg Assist Allowed / w/Doc   ◨ Lab Crosswalk   ◨ Radiology Crosswalk

512   CPT © 2021 American Medical Association. All Rights Reserved.   © 2021 Optum360, LLC

 # 97158 Group adaptive behavior treatment with protocol modification, administered by physician or other qualified health care professional, face-to-face with multiple patients, each 15 minutes

INCLUDES Face-to-face service with one patient only
Provided by technician under physician/other qualified healthcare professional direction

EXCLUDES *Aphasia and cognitive performance testing (96105, [96125])*
Behavioral/developmental screening/testing (96110-96113 [96127])
Groups more than eight families
Health and behavior assessment and intervention (96156, 96158-96159, [96164, 96165], [96167, 96168], [96170, 96171])
Neurobehavioral status examination (96116, 96121)
Psychiatric services (90785-90899)
Testing administration with scoring (96136-96139, 96146)
Testing evaluation (96130-96133)
Therapeutic procedure(s) group of two or more patients (97150)
Treatment speech disorders (group) (92508)

🔧 0.00 ⚕ 0.00 **FUD** XXX   80 💻

AMA: 2018,Nov,3

96105-96146 [96125, 96127] Testing Services

INCLUDES Interpretation and report when performed by qualified healthcare professional
Results when automatically generated

EXCLUDES *Adaptive behavior assessments and treatments ([97151, 97152, 97153, 97154, 97155, 97156, 97157, 97158], 0362T, 0373T)*
Cognitive skills development (97129, 97533)

96105 Assessment of aphasia (includes assessment of expressive and receptive speech and language function, language comprehension, speech production ability, reading, spelling, writing, eg, by Boston Diagnostic Aphasia Examination) with interpretation and report, per hour

EXCLUDES *Reporting code for less than 31 minutes*

🔧 2.96 ⚕ 2.96 **FUD** XXX   A 80 💻

AMA: 2018,Nov,3; 2018,Oct,5; 2018,Feb,11; 2018,Jan,8; 2017,Jan,8; 2016,Jan,13

 # 96125 Standardized cognitive performance testing (eg, Ross Information Processing Assessment) per hour of a qualified health care professional's time, both face-to-face time administering tests to the patient and time interpreting these test results and preparing the report

EXCLUDES *Neuropsychological testing (96132-96139, 96146)*

🔧 3.12 ⚕ 3.12 **FUD** XXX   A 80 💻

AMA: 2018,Nov,3; 2018,Oct,5; 2018,Feb,11; 2018,Jan,8; 2017,Jan,8; 2016,Jan,13

96110 Developmental screening (eg, developmental milestone survey, speech and language delay screen), with scoring and documentation, per standardized instrument

EXCLUDES *Emotional/behavioral assessment ([96127])*

🔧 0.28 ⚕ 0.28 **FUD** XXX   E 💻

AMA: 2018,Nov,3; 2018,Feb,11; 2018,Jan,8; 2017,Feb,14; 2017,Jan,8; 2016,Jan,13

96112 Developmental test administration (including assessment of fine and/or gross motor, language, cognitive level, social, memory and/or executive functions by standardized developmental instruments when performed), by physician or other qualified health care professional, with interpretation and report; first hour

EXCLUDES *Reporting code for less than 31 minutes*

🔧 3.61 ⚕ 3.83 **FUD** XXX   80 💻

AMA: 2018,Nov,3

+ 96113 each additional 30 minutes (List separately in addition to code for primary procedure)

EXCLUDES *Reporting code for less than 16 minutes*

🔧 1.65 ⚕ 1.74 **FUD** ZZZ   80 💻

AMA: 2018,Nov,3

 # 96127 Brief emotional/behavioral assessment (eg, depression inventory, attention-deficit/hyperactivity disorder [ADHD] scale), with scoring and documentation, per standardized instrument

🔧 0.15 ⚕ 0.15 **FUD** XXX   01 80 TC 💻

AMA: 2018,Nov,3; 2018,Oct,5; 2018,Apr,9; 2018,Feb,11; 2018,Jan,8; 2017,Feb,14; 2017,Jan,8; 2016,Jan,13

96116 Neurobehavioral status exam (clinical assessment of thinking, reasoning and judgment, [eg, acquired knowledge, attention, language, memory, planning and problem solving, and visual spatial abilities]), by physician or other qualified health care professional, both face-to-face time with the patient and time interpreting test results and preparing the report; first hour

EXCLUDES *Neuropsychological testing (96132-96139, 96146)*
Reporting code for less than 31 minutes

🔧 2.41 ⚕ 2.70 **FUD** XXX   ★ 03 80 💻

AMA: 2018,Nov,3; 2018,Oct,5; 2018,Feb,11; 2018,Jan,8; 2017,Jan,8; 2016,Jan,13

+ 96121 each additional hour (List separately in addition to code for primary procedure)

EXCLUDES *Reporting code for less than 31 minutes*
Code first (96116)

🔧 2.22 ⚕ 2.39 **FUD** ZZZ   80 💻

AMA: 2018,Nov,3

96125 Resequenced code. See code following 96105.

96127 Resequenced code. See code following 96113.

96130 Psychological testing evaluation services by physician or other qualified health care professional, including integration of patient data, interpretation of standardized test results and clinical data, clinical decision making, treatment planning and report, and interactive feedback to the patient, family member(s) or caregiver(s), when performed; first hour

EXCLUDES *Reporting code for less than 31 minutes*

🔧 3.08 ⚕ 3.38 **FUD** XXX   80 💻

AMA: 2019,Dec,14; 2019,Sep,10; 2018,Nov,3

+ 96131 each additional hour (List separately in addition to code for primary procedure)

EXCLUDES *Reporting code for less than 31 minutes*

🔧 2.37 ⚕ 2.60 **FUD** ZZZ   80 💻

AMA: 2019,Dec,14; 2019,Sep,10; 2018,Nov,3

96132 Neuropsychological testing evaluation services by physician or other qualified health care professional, including integration of patient data, interpretation of standardized test results and clinical data, clinical decision making, treatment planning and report, and interactive feedback to the patient, family member(s) or caregiver(s), when performed; first hour

EXCLUDES *Reporting code for less than 31 minutes*

🔧 3.04 ⚕ 3.78 **FUD** XXX   80 💻

AMA: 2019,Dec,14; 2019,Sep,10; 2018,Nov,3

+ 96133 each additional hour (List separately in addition to code for primary procedure)

EXCLUDES *Reporting code for less than 31 minutes*

🔧 2.34 ⚕ 2.84 **FUD** ZZZ   80 💻

AMA: 2019,Dec,14; 2019,Sep,10; 2018,Nov,3

96136 Psychological or neuropsychological test administration and scoring by physician or other qualified health care professional, two or more tests, any method; first 30 minutes

EXCLUDES *Reporting code for less than 16 minutes*
Code also testing evaluation on same or different days (96130-96133)

🔧 0.70 ⚕ 1.33 **FUD** XXX   80 💻

AMA: 2020,Aug,3; 2019,Dec,14; 2019,Sep,10; 2018,Nov,3

● New Code ▲ Revised Code ○ Reinstated ● New Web Release ▲ Revised Web Release + Add-on Unlisted Not Covered # Resequenced
50 Optum Mod 50 Exempt ⊘ AMA Mod 51 Exempt 51 Optum Mod 51 Exempt 63 Mod 63 Exempt ∥ Non-FDA Drug ★ Telemedicine M Maternity A Age Edit

CPT © 2021 American Medical Association. All Rights Reserved.

Medicine

96137 — 96171

+ 96137 each additional 30 minutes (List separately in addition to code for primary procedure)

> *EXCLUDES* *Reporting code for less than 16 minutes*
> Code also testing evaluation on same or different days (96130-96133)
> 🛢 0.55　⚕ 1.22　**FUD** ZZZ　　　　80 ▣
> **AMA:** 2020,Aug,3; 2019,Dec,14; 2019,Sep,10; 2018,Nov,3

96138 Psychological or neuropsychological test administration and scoring by technician, two or more tests, any method; first 30 minutes

> *EXCLUDES* *Reporting code for less than 16 minutes*
> Code also testing evaluation on same or different days (96130-96133)
> 🛢 1.07　⚕ 1.07　**FUD** XXX　　　　80 ▣
> **AMA:** 2018,Nov,3

+ 96139 each additional 30 minutes (List separately in addition to code for primary procedure)

> *EXCLUDES* *Reporting code for less than 16 minutes*
> Code also testing evaluation on same or different days (96130-96133)
> 🛢 1.07　⚕ 1.07　**FUD** ZZZ　　　　80 ▣
> **AMA:** 2018,Nov,3

96146 Psychological or neuropsychological test administration, with single automated, standardized instrument via electronic platform, with automated result only

> *EXCLUDES* *Testing provided by physician, other qualified healthcare professional, or technician ([96127], 96136-96139)*
> 🛢 0.06　⚕ 0.06　**FUD** XXX
> **AMA:** 2018,Nov,3

96156-96171 [96164, 96165, 96167, 96168, 96170, 96171] Biopsychosocial Assessment/Intervention

> *INCLUDES* Services for patients that have primary physical illnesses/diagnoses/symptoms who may benefit from assessments/interventions that focus on biopsychosocial factors related to patient's health status
> Services used to identify factors important to prevention/treatment/management physical health problems:
> Behavioral
> Cognitive
> Emotional
> Psychological
> Social

> *EXCLUDES* Adaptive behavior services ([97151, 97152, 97153, 97154, 97155, 97156, 97157, 97158], 0362T, 0373T)
> E/M services same date
> Health and behavior assessment and intervention (96156, 96158-96159)
> Preventive medicine counseling services (99401-99412)

96156 Health behavior assessment, or re-assessment (ie, health-focused clinical interview, behavioral observations, clinical decision making)

> *EXCLUDES* *Psychotherapy services (90785-90899)*
> 🛢 2.51　⚕ 2.77　**FUD** XXX　　　　80 ▣
> **AMA:** 2020,Aug,3; 2020,Jul,7

96158 Health behavior intervention, individual, face-to-face; initial 30 minutes

> *EXCLUDES* *Psychotherapy services (90785-90899)*
> 🛢 1.71　⚕ 1.89　**FUD** XXX　　　　80 ▣
> **AMA:** 2020,Aug,3; 2020,Jul,7

+ 96159 each additional 15 minutes (List separately in addition to code for primary service)

> *EXCLUDES* *Psychotherapy services (90785-90899)*
> Code first (96158)
> 🛢 0.59　⚕ 0.66　**FUD** ZZZ　　　　80 ▣
> **AMA:** 2020,Aug,3; 2020,Jul,7

 # 96164 Health behavior intervention, group (2 or more patients), face-to-face; initial 30 minutes

> *EXCLUDES* *Psychotherapy services (90785-90899)*
> 🛢 0.25　⚕ 0.28　**FUD** XXX　　　　80 ▣
> **AMA:** 2020,Aug,3; 2020,Jul,7

+ # 96165 each additional 15 minutes (List separately in addition to code for primary service)

> *EXCLUDES* *Psychotherapy services (90785-90899)*
> Code first ([96164])
> 🛢 0.11　⚕ 0.13　**FUD** ZZZ　　　　80 ▣
> **AMA:** 2020,Aug,3; 2020,Jul,7

 # 96167 Health behavior intervention, family (with the patient present), face-to-face; initial 30 minutes

> *EXCLUDES* *Psychotherapy services (90785-90899)*
> 🛢 1.83　⚕ 2.03　**FUD** XXX　　　　80 ▣
> **AMA:** 2020,Aug,3

+ # 96168 each additional 15 minutes (List separately in addition to code for primary service)

> *EXCLUDES* *Psychotherapy services (90785-90899)*
> Code first ([96167])
> 🛢 0.65　⚕ 0.72　**FUD** ZZZ　　　　80 ▣
> **AMA:** 2020,Aug,3

 # 96170 Health behavior intervention, family (without the patient present), face-to-face; initial 30 minutes

> *EXCLUDES* *Psychotherapy services (90785-90899)*
> 🛢 2.19　⚕ 2.30　**FUD** XXX　　　　▣
> **AMA:** 2020,Aug,3

+ # 96171 each additional 15 minutes (List separately in addition to code for primary service)

> *EXCLUDES* *Psychotherapy services (90785-90899)*
> Code first ([96170])
> 🛢 0.80　⚕ 0.84　**FUD** ZZZ　　　　▣
> **AMA:** 2020,Aug,3

96160-96171 [96164, 96165, 96167, 96168, 96170, 96171] Health Risk Assessments

96160 Administration of patient-focused health risk assessment instrument (eg, health hazard appraisal) with scoring and documentation, per standardized instrument

> 🛢 0.09　⚕ 0.09　**FUD** ZZZ　　　　★ Ⓢ ▣
> **AMA:** 2020,Aug,3; 2018,Feb,11; 2018,Jan,8; 2017,Feb,14; 2017,Jan,8; 2016,Nov,5

96161 Administration of caregiver-focused health risk assessment instrument (eg, depression inventory) for the benefit of the patient, with scoring and documentation, per standardized instrument

> 🛢 0.07　⚕ 0.07　**FUD** ZZZ　　　　★ Ⓢ ▣
> **AMA:** 2020,Aug,3; 2018,Feb,11; 2018,Jan,8; 2017,Feb,14; 2017,Jan,8; 2016,Nov,5

96164 Resequenced code. See code following 96159.

96165 Resequenced code. See code following 96159.

96167 Resequenced code. See code following 96159.

96168 Resequenced code. See code following 96159.

96170 Resequenced code. See code following 96159.

96171 Resequenced code. See code following 96159.

26/TC PC/TC Only　　A2-Z3 ASC Payment　　50 Bilateral　　♂ Male Only　　♀ Female Only　　🛢 Facility RVU　　⚕ Non-Facility RVU　　▣ CCI　　❌ CLIA
FUD Follow-up Days　　**CMS:** IOM　　**AMA:** CPT Asst　　A-Y OPPSI　　80/80 Surg Assist Allowed / w/Doc　　Lab Crosswalk　　Radiology Crosswalk

514　　　　　　　　　　　　　　CPT © 2021 American Medical Association. All Rights Reserved.　　　　　　　　　　© 2021 Optum360, LLC

96360-96361 Intravenous Fluid Infusion for Hydration (Nonchemotherapy)

CMS: 100-04,4,230.2 OPPS Drug Administration

INCLUDES Administration prepackaged fluids and electrolytes
Coding hierarchy rules for facility reporting only:
  Chemotherapy services primary to diagnostic, prophylactic, and therapeutic services
  Diagnostic, prophylactic, and therapeutic services primary to hydration services
  Infusions primary to pushes
  Pushes primary to injections
    Constant observance/attendance by person administering drug or substance
    Infusion 15 minutes or less
Direct supervision by physician or other qualified health care provider:
  Direction personnel
Minimal supervision for:
  Consent
  Safety oversight
  Supervision personnel
If done to facilitate injection/infusion:
  Flush at infusion end
  Indwelling IV, subcutaneous catheter/port access
  Local anesthesia
  Start IV
  Supplies/tubing/syringes
Report initial code for primary reason for visit despite order infusions or injections given
Treatment plan verification

EXCLUDES *Catheter/port declotting (36593)*
Drugs/other substances
Minimal infusion to keep vein open or during other therapeutic infusions
Reporting code for hydration infusion 31 minutes or less
Reporting code for second initial service on same date for accessing multilumen catheter, restarting IV, or when two IV lines are needed to meet infusion rate
Services provided by physicians or other qualified health care providers in facility settings
Significant separately identifiable E/M service, when performed

96360 **Intravenous infusion, hydration; initial, 31 minutes to 1 hour**

EXCLUDES *Reporting code when service performed as concurrent infusion*

1.07 1.07 **FUD** XXX S 80

AMA: 2019,Jun,5; 2018,Feb,11; 2018,Jan,8; 2017,Jan,8; 2016,Jan,13

+ 96361 **each additional hour (List separately in addition to code for primary procedure)**

INCLUDES Hydration infusion of more than 30 minutes beyond 1 hour
Hydration provided as secondary or subsequent service after different initial service via same IV access site

Code first (96360)

0.38 0.38 **FUD** ZZZ S 80

AMA: 2019,Jun,5; 2018,Feb,11; 2018,Jan,8; 2017,Jan,8; 2016,Jan,13

96365-96371 Infusions: Diagnostic/Preventive/Therapeutic

CMS: 100-04,4,230.2 OPPS Drug Administration

INCLUDES Administration fluid
Administration substances/drugs
Coding hierarchy rules for facility reporting:
  Chemotherapy services primary to diagnostic, prophylactic, and therapeutic services
  Diagnostic, prophylactic, and therapeutic services primary to hydration services
  Infusions primary to pushes
  Pushes primary to injections
Constant presence by health care professional administering substance/drug
Direct supervision by physician or other qualified health care provider:
  Consent
  Direction personnel
  Patient assessment
  Safety oversight
  Supervision personnel
If done to facilitate injection/infusion:
  Flush at infusion end
  Indwelling IV, subcutaneous catheter/port access
  Local anesthesia
  Start IV
  Supplies/tubing/syringes
Infusion 16 minutes or more
Training to assess patient and monitor vital signs
Training to prepare/dose/dispose
Treatment plan verification

EXCLUDES *Catheter/port declotting (36593)*
Mechanical scalp cooling (0662T-0663T)
Services provided by physicians or other qualified health care providers in facility settings
Significant separately identifiable E/M service, when performed
Reporting code for second initial service on same date for accessing multilumen catheter, restarting IV, or when two IV lines needed to meet infusion rate
Reporting code with other procedures where IV push or infusion is integral to procedure

Code also drugs/materials

96365 **Intravenous infusion, for therapy, prophylaxis, or diagnosis (specify substance or drug); initial, up to 1 hour**

Code also second initial service with modifier 59 when patient's condition or drug protocol mandates use of two IV lines

2.02 2.02 **FUD** XXX S 80

AMA: 2020,NovSE,1; 2020,Jan,11; 2018,Dec,8; 2018,Dec,8; 2018,Sep,14; 2018,May,10; 2018,Feb,11; 2018,Jan,8; 2017,Jan,8; 2016,Jan,13

+ 96366 **each additional hour (List separately in addition to code for primary procedure)**

INCLUDES Additional hours sequential infusion
Infusion intervals more than 30 minutes beyond one hour
Second and subsequent infusions same drug or substance

Code also additional infusion, when appropriate (96367)
Code first (96365)

0.61 0.61 **FUD** ZZZ S 80

AMA: 2020,NovSE,1; 2020,Jan,11; 2018,Sep,14; 2018,Feb,11; 2018,Jan,8; 2017,Jan,8; 2016,Jan,13

+ 96367 **additional sequential infusion of a new drug/substance, up to 1 hour (List separately in addition to code for primary procedure)**

INCLUDES Secondary or subsequent service with new drug or substance after different initial service via same IV access

EXCLUDES *Reporting code more than one time per sequential infusion same mix*

Code first (96365, 96374, 96409, 96413)

0.88 0.88 **FUD** ZZZ S 80

AMA: 2020,NovSE,1; 2020,Jan,11; 2018,Feb,11; 2018,Jan,8; 2017,Jan,8; 2016,Jan,13

+ 96368 concurrent infusion (List separately in addition to code for primary procedure)

> [EXCLUDES] *Reporting code more than one time per service date*
>
> Code first (96365, 96366, 96413, 96415, 96416)
>
> 🖥 0.59   ⚘ 0.59   **FUD** ZZZ   Ⓝ 80 ▭
>
> **AMA:** 2020,NovSE,1; 2020,Jan,11; 2018,Feb,11; 2018,Jan,8; 2017,Jan,8; 2016,Jan,13

96369 Subcutaneous infusion for therapy or prophylaxis (specify substance or drug); initial, up to 1 hour, including pump set-up and establishment of subcutaneous infusion site(s)

> [EXCLUDES] *Infusions 15 minutes or less (96372)*
>
> *Reporting code more than one time per encounter*
>
> 🖥 4.69   ⚘ 4.69   **FUD** XXX   Ⓢ 80 ▭
>
> **AMA:** 2020,NovSE,1; 2020,Jan,11; 2018,Feb,11; 2018,Jan,8; 2017,Jan,8; 2016,Jan,13

+ 96370 each additional hour (List separately in addition to code for primary procedure)

> [INCLUDES] Infusions more than 30 minutes beyond one hour
>
> Code first (96369)
>
> 🖥 0.44   ⚘ 0.44   **FUD** ZZZ   Ⓢ 80 ▭
>
> **AMA:** 2020,NovSE,1; 2020,Jan,11; 2018,Feb,11; 2018,Jan,8; 2017,Jan,8; 2016,Jan,13

+ 96371 additional pump set-up with establishment of new subcutaneous infusion site(s) (List separately in addition to code for primary procedure)

> [EXCLUDES] *Reporting code more than one time per encounter*
>
> Code first (96369)
>
> 🖥 1.84   ⚘ 1.84   **FUD** ZZZ   Ⓠ1 80 ▭
>
> **AMA:** 2020,NovSE,1; 2020,Jan,11; 2018,Feb,11; 2018,Jan,8; 2017,Jan,8; 2016,Jan,13

96372-96379 Injections: Diagnostic/Preventive/Therapeutic

CMS: 100-04,4,230.2 OPPS Drug Administration

[INCLUDES] Administration fluid
Administration substances/drugs
Coding hierarchy rules for facility reporting:
  Chemotherapy services primary to diagnostic, prophylactic, and therapeutic services
  Diagnostic, prophylactic, and therapeutic services primary to hydration services
  Infusions primary to pushes
  Pushes primary to injections
Constant presence by health care professional administering substance/drug
Direct supervision by physician or other qualified health care provider:
  Consent
  Direction personnel
  Patient assessment
  Safety oversight
  Supervision personnel
If done to facilitate injection/infusion:
  Flush at infusion end
  Indwelling IV, subcutaneous catheter/port access
  Local anesthesia
  Start IV
  Supplies/tubing/syringes
Infusion 15 minutes or less
Training to assess patient and monitor vital signs
Training to prepare/dose/dispose
Treatment plan verification

[EXCLUDES] *Catheter/port declotting (36593)*
Mechanical scalp cooling (0662T-0663T)
Reporting code for second initial service on same date for accessing multilumen catheter, restarting IV, or when two IV lines needed to meet infusion rate
Reporting code with other procedures where IV push or infusion is integral to procedure
Services provided by physicians or other qualified health care providers in facility settings
Significant separately identifiable E/M service, when performed
Code also drugs/materials

96372 Therapeutic, prophylactic, or diagnostic injection (specify substance or drug); subcutaneous or intramuscular

> [INCLUDES] Direct supervision by physician or other qualified health care provider when reported by physician/other qualified health care provider. When reported by hospital, physician/other qualified health care provider need not be present
>
> Hormonal therapy injections (non-antineoplastic) (96372)
>
> [EXCLUDES] *Administration vaccines/toxoids (90460-90461, 90471-90472, [0001A, 0002A, 0003A, 0004A], [0051A, 0052A, 0053A, 0054A], [0071A, 0072A], [0011A, 0012A, 0013A], [0064A], [0021A, 0022A], [0031A], [0034A], [0041A, 0042A])*
>
> *Allergen immunotherapy injections (95115-95117)*
> *Antineoplastic hormonal injections (96402)*
> *Antineoplastic nonhormonal injections (96401)*
> *Injections administered without direct supervision by physician or other qualified health care provider (99211)*
> *Intradermal cancer immunotherapy (0708T-0709T)*
>
> 🖥 0.47   ⚘ 0.47   **FUD** XXX   Ⓠ1 80 ▭
>
> **AMA:** 2018,Dec,10; 2018,Dec,10; 2018,Feb,11; 2018,Jan,8; 2017,Jan,8; 2016,Oct,9; 2016,Jan,13

96373 intra-arterial

> 🖥 0.53   ⚘ 0.53   **FUD** XXX   Ⓢ 80 ▭
>
> **AMA:** 2018,Feb,11; 2018,Jan,8; 2017,Jan,8; 2016,Jan,13

96374 intravenous push, single or initial substance/drug

> 🖥 1.10   ⚘ 1.10   **FUD** XXX   Ⓢ 80 ▭
>
> **AMA:** 2020,NovSE,1; 2020,Jan,11; 2019,Sep,5; 2019,Jun,9; 2018,Feb,11; 2018,Jan,8; 2017,Jan,8; 2016,Jan,13

26/TC PC/TC Only   A2-Z3 ASC Payment   50 Bilateral   ♂ Male Only   ♀ Female Only   🖥 Facility RVU   ⚘ Non-Facility RVU   ▭ CCI   ☒ CLIA
FUD Follow-up Days   CMS: IOM   AMA: CPT Asst   A-Y OPPSI   80/80 Surg Assist Allowed / w/Doc   ▭ Lab Crosswalk   Radiology Crosswalk

516   CPT © 2021 American Medical Association. All Rights Reserved.   © 2021 Optum360, LLC

+ **96375** **each additional sequential intravenous push of a new substance/drug (List separately in addition to code for primary procedure)**

INCLUDES IV push new substance/drug provided as secondary or subsequent service after different initial service via same IV access site

Code first (96365, 96374, 96409, 96413)

🔲 0.47   ⚖ 0.47   **FUD** ZZZ   ⑤ 80 🖾

AMA: 2019,Sep,5; 2018,Feb,11; 2018,Jan,8; 2017,Jan,8; 2016,Jan,13

+ **96376** **each additional sequential intravenous push of the same substance/drug provided in a facility (List separately in addition to code for primary procedure)**

INCLUDES Facilities only

EXCLUDES IV push performed within 30 minutes push same substance or drug
Services performed by any nonfacilty provider

Code first (96365, 96374, 96409, 96413)

🔲 0.00   ⚖ 0.00   **FUD** ZZZ   Ⓝ 🖾

AMA: 2018,Dec,8; 2018,Dec,8; 2018,Feb,11; 2018,Jan,8; 2017,Jan,8; 2016,Jan,13

96377 **Application of on-body injector (includes cannula insertion) for timed subcutaneous injection**

🔲 0.56   ⚖ 0.56   **FUD** XXX   ⑪ 80 🖾

AMA: 2018,Feb,11; 2018,Jan,8; 2017,Jan,8; 2016,Oct,9

96379 **Unlisted therapeutic, prophylactic, or diagnostic intravenous or intra-arterial injection or infusion**

🔲 0.00   ⚖ 0.00   **FUD** XXX   ⑪ 80 🖾

AMA: 2018,Feb,11; 2018,Jan,8; 2017,Jan,8; 2016,Jan,13

96401-96411 Chemotherapy and Other Complex Drugs, Biologicals: Injection and IV Push

CMS: 100-03,110.2 Certain Drugs Distributed by the National Cancer Institute; 100-03,110.6 Scalp Hypothermia During Chemotherapy, to Prevent Hair Loss; 100-04,4,230.2 OPPS Drug Administration

INCLUDES Highly complex services that require direct supervision for:
Consent
Patient assessment
Safety oversight
Supervision
More intense work and monitoring clinical staff by physician or other qualified health care provider due to greater risk severe patient reactions
Parenteral administration:
Anti-neoplastic agents for noncancer diagnoses
Monoclonal antibody agents
Nonradionuclide antineoplastic drugs
Other biologic response modifiers

EXCLUDES Reporting code for second initial service on same date for accessing multilumen catheter, restarting IV, or when two IV lines needed to meet infusion rate

96401 **Chemotherapy administration, subcutaneous or intramuscular; non-hormonal anti-neoplastic**

EXCLUDES Intradermal cancer immunotherapy (0708T-0709T)
Services performed by physicians or other qualified health care providers in facility settings

🔲 2.24   ⚖ 2.24   **FUD** XXX   ⑪ 80 🖾

AMA: 2018,Feb,11; 2018,Jan,8; 2017,Jan,8; 2016,Jan,13

96402 **hormonal anti-neoplastic**

EXCLUDES Services performed by physicians or other qualified health care providers in facility settings

🔲 0.87   ⚖ 0.87   **FUD** XXX   ⑪ 80 🖾

AMA: 2018,Feb,11; 2018,Jan,8; 2017,Jan,8; 2016,Jan,13

96405 **Chemotherapy administration; intralesional, up to and including 7 lesions**

🔲 0.84   ⚖ 2.31   **FUD** 000   ⑪ 🖾

AMA: 2018,Feb,11; 2018,Jan,8; 2017,Jan,8; 2016,Jan,13

96406 **intralesional, more than 7 lesions**

🔲 1.31   ⚖ 3.46   **FUD** 000   ⑤ 🖾

AMA: 2018,Feb,11; 2018,Jan,8; 2017,Jan,8; 2016,Jan,13

96409 **intravenous, push technique, single or initial substance/drug**

INCLUDES Push technique includes:
Administration injection directly into vessel or access line by health care professional; or
Infusion less than or equal to 15 minutes

EXCLUDES Insertion arterial and venous cannula(s) for extracorpororeal circulation (36823)
Services performed by physicians or other qualified health care providers in facility settings

🔲 3.05   ⚖ 3.05   **FUD** XXX   ⑤ 80 🖾

AMA: 2018,Feb,11; 2018,Jan,8; 2017,Jan,8; 2016,Jan,13

+ **96411** **intravenous, push technique, each additional substance/drug (List separately in addition to code for primary procedure)**

INCLUDES Push technique includes:
Administration injection directly into vessel or access line by health care professional; or
Infusion less than or equal to 15 minutes

EXCLUDES Insertion arterial and venous cannula(s) for extracorpororeal circulation (36823)
Services performed by physicians or other qualified health care providers in facility settings

Code first initial substance/drug (96409, 96413)

🔲 1.65   ⚖ 1.65   **FUD** ZZZ   ⑤ 80 🖾

AMA: 2018,Feb,11; 2018,Jan,8; 2017,Jan,8; 2016,Jan,13

96413-96417 Chemotherapy and Complex Drugs, Biologicals: Intravenous Infusion

CMS: 100-03,110.2 Certain Drugs Distributed by the National Cancer Institute; 100-03,110.6 Scalp Hypothermia During Chemotherapy, to Prevent Hair Loss; 100-04,4,230.2 OPPS Drug Administration

INCLUDES Administration:
  Access to IV/catheter/port
  Drug preparation
  Flushing at infusion completion
  Hydration fluid
  Local anesthesia
  Routine tubing/syringe/supplies
  Starting IV
Highly complex services that require direct supervision for:
  Consent
  Patient assessment
  Safety oversight
  Supervision
More intense work and monitoring clinical staff by physician or other
  qualified health care provider due to greater risk severe patient
  reactions
Parenteral administration:
  Antineoplastic agents for noncancer diagnoses
  Monoclonal antibody agents
  Nonradionuclide antineoplastic drugs
  Other biologic response modifiers

EXCLUDES *Administration nonchemotherapy agents such as
    antibiotics/steroids/analgesics*
Declotting catheter/port (36593)
Home infusion (99601-99602)
*Insertion arterial and venous cannula(s) for extracorpororeal circulation
    (36823)*
*Reporting code for second initial service on same date for accessing multilumen
    catheter, restarting IV, or when two IV lines needed to meet infusion rate*
*Services provided by physicians or other qualified health care providers in
    facility settings*

Code also:
  Drug or substance
  Significant separately identifiable E/M service, when performed

96413 Chemotherapy administration, intravenous infusion technique; up to 1 hour, single or initial substance/drug

INCLUDES Push technique includes:
    Administration injection directly into vessel or
      access line by health care professional; or
    Infusion less than or equal to 15 minutes

EXCLUDES *Hydration administered as secondary or subsequent
      service via same IV access site (96361)*
*Therapeutic/prophylactic/diagnostic drug
      infusion/injection through the same intravenous
      access (96366, 96367, 96375)*

Code also second initial service with modifier 59 when patient's
    condition or drug protocol mandates use of two IV lines

🖪 3.97   ⅀ 3.97   **FUD** XXX   S 80 ▯

AMA: 2018,Feb,11; 2018,Jan,8; 2017,Jan,8; 2016,Jan,13

+ 96415 each additional hour (List separately in addition to code for primary procedure)

INCLUDES Infusion intervals more than 30 minutes past 1-hour
      increments

Code first initial hour (96413)

🖪 0.86   ⅀ 0.86   **FUD** ZZZ   S 80 ▯

AMA: 2018,Feb,11; 2018,Jan,8; 2017,Jan,8; 2016,Jan,13

96416 initiation of prolonged chemotherapy infusion (more than 8 hours), requiring use of a portable or implantable pump

EXCLUDES *Portable or implantable infusion pump/reservoir
      refilling/maintenance for drug delivery
      (96521-96523)*

🖪 3.98   ⅀ 3.98   **FUD** XXX   S 80 ▯

AMA: 2018,Feb,11; 2018,Jan,8; 2017,Jan,8; 2016,Jan,13

+ 96417 each additional sequential infusion (different substance/drug), up to 1 hour (List separately in addition to code for primary procedure)

INCLUDES Push technique includes:
    Administration injection directly into vessel or
      access line by health care professional; or
    Infusion less than or equal to 15 minutes

EXCLUDES *Additional hour(s) sequential infusion (96415)*
*Reporting code more than one time per sequential
      infusion*

Code first initial substance/drug (96413)

🖪 1.92   ⅀ 1.92   **FUD** ZZZ   S 80 ▯

AMA: 2018,Feb,11; 2018,Jan,8; 2017,Jan,8; 2016,Jan,13

96420-96425 Chemotherapy and Complex Drugs, Biologicals: Intra-arterial

CMS: 100-03,110.2 Certain Drugs Distributed by the National Cancer Institute; 100-03,110.6 Scalp Hypothermia During Chemotherapy, to Prevent Hair Loss; 100-04,4,230.2 OPPS Drug Administration

INCLUDES Administration:
  Access to IV/catheter/port
  Drug preparation
  Flushing at infusion completion
  Hydration fluid
  Local anesthesia
  Routine tubing/syringe/supplies
  Starting IV
Highly complex services that require direct supervision for:
  Consent
  Patient assessment
  Safety oversight
  Supervision
More intense work and monitoring clinical staff by physician or other
  qualified health care provider due to greater risk severe patient
  reactions
Parenteral administration:
  Antineoplastic agents for noncancer diagnoses
  Monoclonal antibody agents
  Nonradionuclide antineoplastic drugs
  Other biologic response modifiers

EXCLUDES *Administration nonchemotherapy agents such as
    antibiotics/steroids/analgesics*
Declotting catheter/port (36593)
Home infusion (99601-99602)
*Reporting code for second initial service on same date for accessing multilumen
    catheter, restarting IV, or when two IV lines needed to meet an infusion
    rate*
*Services provided by physicians or other qualified health care providers in
    facility settings*

Code also:
  Significant separately identifiable E/M service, when performed
  Drug or substance

96420 Chemotherapy administration, intra-arterial; push technique

INCLUDES Push technique includes:
    Administration injection directly into vessel or
      access line by health care professional; or
    Infusion less than or equal to 15 minutes
  Regional chemotherapy perfusion

EXCLUDES *Insertion arterial and venous cannula(s) for
      extracorpororeal circulation (36823)*
Placement intra-arterial catheter

🖪 2.95   ⅀ 2.95   **FUD** XXX   S 80 ▯

AMA: 2018,Feb,11; 2018,Jan,8; 2017,Jan,8; 2016,Mar,3; 2016,Jan,13

96422 infusion technique, up to 1 hour

INCLUDES Push technique includes:
    Administration injection directly into vessel or
      access line by health care professional; or
    Infusion less than or equal to 15 minutes
  Regional chemotherapy perfusion

EXCLUDES *Insertion arterial and venous cannula(s) for
      extracorpororeal circulation (36823)*
Placement intra-arterial catheter

🖪 4.85   ⅀ 4.85   **FUD** XXX   S 80 ▯

AMA: 2018,Feb,11; 2018,Jan,8; 2017,Jan,8; 2016,Mar,3; 2016,Jan,13

26/TC PC/TC Only   A2-Z3 ASC Payment   50 Bilateral   ♂ Male Only   ♀ Female Only   🖪 Facility RVU   ⅀ Non-Facility RVU   ▯ CCI   ✖ CLIA
FUD Follow-up Days   **CMS:** IOM   **AMA:** CPT Asst   A-Y OPPSI   80/80 Surg Assist Allowed / w/Doc   Lab Crosswalk   Radiology Crosswalk

518   CPT © 2021 American Medical Association. All Rights Reserved.   © 2021 Optum360, LLC

+   96423   infusion technique, each additional hour (List separately in addition to code for primary procedure)

> INCLUDES   Infusion intervals more than 30 minutes past 1-hour increments
> Regional chemotherapy perfusion
> EXCLUDES   *Insertion arterial and venous cannula(s) for extracorpororeal circulation (36823)*
> *Placement intra-arterial catheter*
> Code first initial hour (96422)
> 🔲 2.24   ⚖ 2.24   **FUD** ZZZ   [S] [80] [▭]
>
> **AMA:** 2018,Feb,11; 2018,Jan,8; 2017,Jan,8; 2016,Mar,3; 2016,Jan,13

96425   infusion technique, initiation of prolonged infusion (more than 8 hours), requiring the use of a portable or implantable pump

> INCLUDES   Regional chemotherapy perfusion
> EXCLUDES   *Insertion arterial and venous cannula(s) for extracorpororeal circulation (36823)*
> *Placement intra-arterial catheter*
> *Portable or implantable infusion pump/reservoir refilling/maintenance for drug delivery (96521-96523)*
> 🔲 5.14   ⚖ 5.14   **FUD** XXX   [S] [80] [▭]
>
> **AMA:** 2018,Feb,11; 2018,Jan,8; 2017,Jan,8; 2016,Mar,3; 2016,Jan,13

96440-96450 Chemotherapy Administration: Intrathecal/Peritoneal Cavity/Pleural Cavity

CMS: 100-03,110.2 Certain Drugs Distributed by the National Cancer Institute; 100-04,4,230.2 OPPS Drug Administration

96440   Chemotherapy administration into pleural cavity, requiring and including thoracentesis

> 🔲 3.57   ⚖ 23.6   **FUD** 000   [S] [80] [▭]
>
> **AMA:** 2018,Feb,11; 2018,Jan,8; 2017,Jan,8; 2016,Jan,13

96446   Chemotherapy administration into the peritoneal cavity via indwelling port or catheter

> 🔲 0.79   ⚖ 5.78   **FUD** XXX   [S] [80] [▭]
>
> **AMA:** 2018,Feb,11; 2018,Jan,8; 2017,Jan,8; 2016,Jan,13

96450   Chemotherapy administration, into CNS (eg, intrathecal), requiring and including spinal puncture

> EXCLUDES   *Chemotherapy administration, intravesical/bladder (51720)*
> *Fluoroscopy (77003)*
> *Insertion catheter/reservoir:*
>   *Intraventricular (61210, 61215)*
>   *Subarachnoid (62350-62351, 62360-62362)*
> 🔲 2.27   ⚖ 5.13   **FUD** 000   [S] [80] [▭]
>
> **AMA:** 2018,Feb,11; 2018,Jan,8; 2017,Jan,8; 2016,Jan,13

96521-96523 Refill/Upkeep of Drug Delivery Device

CMS: 100-04,4,230.2 OPPS Drug Administration

> INCLUDES   Administration:
>   Access to IV/catheter/port
>   Drug preparation
>   Flushing at infusion completion
>   Hydration fluid
>   Local anesthesia
>   Routine tubing/syringe/supplies
>   Starting IV
> Highly complex services that require direct supervision for:
>   Consent
>   Patient assessment
>   Safety oversight
>   Supervision
> Parenteral administration:
>   Antineoplastic agents for noncancer diagnoses
>   Monoclonal antibody agents
>   Nonradionuclide antineoplastic drugs
>   Other biologic response modifiers
> Therapeutic drugs other than chemotherapy
> EXCLUDES   *Administration nonchemotherapy agents such as antibiotics/steroids/analgesics*
> *Blood specimen collection from completely implantable venous access device (36591)*
> *Declotting catheter/port (36593)*
> *Home infusion (99601-99602)*
> *Services provided by physicians or other qualified health care providers in facility settings*
> Code also:
>   Drug or substance
>   Significant separately identifiable E/M service, when performed

96521   Refilling and maintenance of portable pump

> 🔲 4.13   ⚖ 4.13   **FUD** XXX   [S] [80] [▭]
>
> **AMA:** 2018,Feb,11; 2018,Jan,8; 2017,Jan,8; 2016,Jan,13

96522   Refilling and maintenance of implantable pump or reservoir for drug delivery, systemic (eg, intravenous, intra-arterial)

> EXCLUDES   *Implantable infusion pump refilling/maintenance for spinal/brain drug delivery (95990-95991)*
> 🔲 3.39   ⚖ 3.39   **FUD** XXX   [S] [80] [▭]
>
> **AMA:** 2018,Feb,11; 2018,Jan,8; 2017,Jan,8; 2016,Jan,13

96523   Irrigation of implanted venous access device for drug delivery systems

> EXCLUDES   *Direct supervision by physician or other qualified health care provider in facility settings*
> *Reporting code with any other services on same service date*
> 🔲 0.77   ⚖ 0.77   **FUD** XXX   [Q1] [80] [▭]
>
> **AMA:** 2018,Feb,11; 2018,Jan,8; 2017,Jan,8; 2016,Jan,13

96542-96549 Chemotherapy Injection Into Brain

CMS: 100-04,4,230.2 OPPS Drug Administration

INCLUDES Administration:
  Access to IV/catheter/port
  Drug preparation
  Flushing at infusion completion
  Hydration fluid
  Local anesthesia
  Routine tubing/syringe/supplies
  Starting IV
Highly complex services that require direct supervision for:
  Consent
  Patient assessment
  Safety oversight
  Supervision
Parenteral administration:
  Antineoplastic agents for noncancer diagnoses
  Monoclonal antibody agents
  Nonradionuclide antineoplastic drugs
  Other biologic response modifiers

EXCLUDES *Administration nonchemotherapy agents such as antibiotics/steroids/analgesics*
Blood specimen collection from completely implantable venous access device (36591)
Declotting catheter/port (36593)
Home infusion (99601-99602)

Code also:
  Drug or substance
  Significant separately identifiable E/M service, when performed

96542 Chemotherapy injection, subarachnoid or intraventricular via subcutaneous reservoir, single or multiple agents

EXCLUDES *Oral radioactive isotope therapy (79005)*

🔹 1.19 　 ⚕ 3.77 　 **FUD** XXX 　 　 S 80 ▭

AMA: 2018,Feb,11; 2018,Jan,8; 2017,Jan,8; 2016,Jan,13

96549 Unlisted chemotherapy procedure

🔹 0.00 　 ⚕ 0.00 　 **FUD** XXX 　 　 01 80 ▭

AMA: 2018,Feb,11; 2018,Jan,8; 2017,Jan,8; 2016,Jan,13

96567-96574 Destruction of Lesions: Photodynamic Therapy

EXCLUDES *Ocular photodynamic therapy (67221)*

96567 Photodynamic therapy by external application of light to destroy premalignant lesions of the skin and adjacent mucosa with application and illumination/activation of photosensitive drug(s), per day

INCLUDES Services provided without direct participation by physician or other qualified healthcare professional

🔹 3.50 　 ⚕ 3.50 　 **FUD** XXX 　 　 01 80 ▭

AMA: 2018,Jul,14; 2018,Feb,10; 2018,Feb,11; 2018,Jan,8; 2017,Jan,8; 2016,Jan,13

+ 96570 Photodynamic therapy by endoscopic application of light to ablate abnormal tissue via activation of photosensitive drug(s); first 30 minutes (List separately in addition to code for endoscopy or bronchoscopy procedures of lung and gastrointestinal tract)

Code also:
  For 38-52 minutes (96571)
  Modifier 52 when services with report less than 23 minutes
Code first (31641, 43229)

🔹 1.48 　 ⚕ 1.48 　 **FUD** ZZZ 　 　 N ▭

AMA: 2018,Feb,11; 2018,Jan,8; 2017,Jan,8; 2016,Jan,13

+ 96571 each additional 15 minutes (List separately in addition to code for endoscopy or bronchoscopy procedures of lung and gastrointestinal tract)

EXCLUDES *23-37 minutes service (96570)*

Code first (96570)
Code first when appropriate (31641, 43229)

🔹 0.83 　 ⚕ 0.83 　 **FUD** ZZZ 　 　 N ▭

AMA: 2018,Feb,11; 2018,Jan,8; 2017,Jan,8; 2016,Jan,13

96573 Photodynamic therapy by external application of light to destroy premalignant lesions of the skin and adjacent mucosa with application and illumination/activation of photosensitizing drug(s) provided by a physician or other qualified health care professional, per day

INCLUDES Application photosensitizer to lesions at anatomical site
Debridement, when performed
Light to activate photosensitizer for destruction premalignant lesions

EXCLUDES *Debridement lesion with photodynamic therapy provided by physician or other qualified healthcare professional (96574)*
Photodynamic therapy by external application light to same anatomical site (96567)
Services provided to same area on same date as photodynamic therapy:
  Biopsy (11102-11107)
  Debridement (11000-11001, 11004-11005)
  Excision lesion (11400-11471)
  Shaving lesion (11300-11313)

🔹 6.03 　 ⚕ 6.03 　 **FUD** 000 　 　 01 80 ▭

AMA: 2018,Jul,14; 2018,Feb,11; 2018,Feb,10

96574 Debridement of premalignant hyperkeratotic lesion(s) (ie, targeted curettage, abrasion) followed with photodynamic therapy by external application of light to destroy premalignant lesions of the skin and adjacent mucosa with application and illumination/activation of photosensitizing drug(s) provided by a physician or other qualified health care professional, per day

INCLUDES Application photosensitizer to lesions at anatomical site
Debridement, when performed
Light to activate photosensitizer for destruction premalignant lesions

EXCLUDES *Photodynamic therapy by external application light for destruction premalignant lesions (96573)*
Photodynamic therapy by external application light to same anatomical site (96567)
Services provided to same area on same as photodynamic therapy:
  Biopsy (11102-11107)
  Debridement (11000-11001, 11004-11005)
  Excision lesion (11400-11471)
  Shaving lesion (11300-11313)

🔹 7.25 　 ⚕ 7.25 　 **FUD** 000 　 　 01 80 ▭

AMA: 2018,Feb,10; 2018,Feb,11

96900-96999 Diagnostic/Therapeutic Skin Procedures

EXCLUDES *E/M services*
Injection, intralesional (11900-11901)

96900 Actinotherapy (ultraviolet light)

EXCLUDES *Rhinophototherapy (30999)*

🔲 (88160-88161)

🔹 0.61 　 ⚕ 0.61 　 **FUD** XXX 　 　 01 80 ▭

AMA: 2018,Feb,11; 2018,Jan,8; 2017,Jan,8; 2016,Nov,9; 2016,Sep,3; 2016,Jan,13

96902 Microscopic examination of hairs plucked or clipped by the examiner (excluding hair collected by the patient) to determine telogen and anagen counts, or structural hair shaft abnormality

🔲 (88160-88161)

🔹 0.59 　 ⚕ 0.62 　 **FUD** XXX 　 　 N ▭

AMA: 2018,Feb,11

96904 Whole body integumentary photography, for monitoring of high risk patients with dysplastic nevus syndrome or a history of dysplastic nevi, or patients with a personal or familial history of melanoma

🔲 (88160-88161)

🔹 1.82 　 ⚕ 1.82 　 **FUD** XXX 　 　 N 80 ▭

AMA: 2018,Feb,11

26/TC PC/TC Only　 A2-Z3 ASC Payment　 50 Bilateral　 ♂ Male Only　 ♀ Female Only　 🔹 Facility RVU　 ⚕ Non-Facility RVU　 ▭ CCI　 🔲 CLIA
FUD Follow-up Days　 CMS: IOM　 AMA: CPT Asst　 A-Y OPPSI　 80/80 Surg Assist Allowed / w/Doc　 🔲 Lab Crosswalk　 Radiology Crosswalk

520 　 CPT © 2021 American Medical Association. All Rights Reserved. 　 © 2021 Optum360, LLC

96910 Photochemotherapy; tar and ultraviolet B (Goeckerman treatment) or petrolatum and ultraviolet B
    (88160-88161)
    3.24   3.24   **FUD** XXX   01 80
    AMA: 2018,Feb,11; 2018,Jan,8; 2017,Jan,8; 2016,Sep,3; 2016,Jan,13

96912 psoralens and ultraviolet A (PUVA)
    (88160-88161)
    2.75   2.75   **FUD** XXX   01 80
    AMA: 2018,Feb,11; 2018,Jan,8; 2017,Jan,8; 2016,Sep,3; 2016,Jan,13

96913 Photochemotherapy (Goeckerman and/or PUVA) for severe photoresponsive dermatoses requiring at least 4-8 hours of care under direct supervision of the physician (includes application of medication and dressings)
    (88160-88161)
    3.91   3.91   **FUD** XXX   T 80
    AMA: 2018,Feb,11; 2018,Jan,8; 2017,Jan,8; 2016,Sep,3

96920 Laser treatment for inflammatory skin disease (psoriasis); total area less than 250 sq cm
    EXCLUDES   *Destruction by laser:*
        Benign lesions (17110-17111)
        Cutaneous vascular proliferative lesions (17106-17108)
        Malignant lesions (17260-17286)
        Premalignant lesions (17000-17004)
    (88160-88161)
    1.90   4.64   **FUD** 000   01
    AMA: 2020,Jul,13; 2018,Feb,11; 2018,Jan,8; 2017,Jan,8; 2016,Sep,3; 2016,Jan,13

96921 250 sq cm to 500 sq cm
    EXCLUDES   *Destruction by laser:*
        Benign lesions (17110-17111)
        Cutaneous vascular proliferative lesions (17106-17108)
        Malignant lesions (17260-17286)
        Premalignant lesions (17000-17004)
    (88160-88161)
    2.14   5.09   **FUD** 000   01
    AMA: 2020,Jul,13; 2018,Feb,11; 2018,Jan,8; 2017,Jan,8; 2016,Sep,3; 2016,Jan,13

96922 over 500 sq cm
    EXCLUDES   *Destruction by laser:*
        Benign lesions (17110-17111)
        Cutaneous vascular proliferative lesions (17106-17108)
        Malignant lesions (17260-17286)
        Premalignant lesions (17000-17004)
    (88160-88161)
    3.43   6.91   **FUD** 000   01
    AMA: 2020,Jul,13; 2018,Feb,11; 2018,Jan,8; 2017,Jan,8; 2016,Sep,3; 2016,Jan,13

96931 Reflectance confocal microscopy (RCM) for cellular and sub-cellular imaging of skin; image acquisition and interpretation and report, first lesion
    EXCLUDES   *Optical coherence tomography for skin imaging (0470T-0471T)*
        Reflectance confocal microscopy examination without generated mosaic images (96999)
    4.83   4.83   **FUD** XXX   M 80
    AMA: 2018,Feb,11; 2018,Jan,8; 2017,Sep,9

96932 image acquisition only, first lesion
    EXCLUDES   *Optical coherence tomography for skin imaging (0470T-0471T)*
        Reflectance confocal microscopy examination without generated mosaic images (96999)
    3.51   3.51   **FUD** XXX   01 80 TC
    AMA: 2018,Feb,11; 2018,Jan,8; 2017,Sep,9

96933 interpretation and report only, first lesion
    EXCLUDES   *Optical coherence tomography for skin imaging (0470T-0471T)*
        Reflectance confocal microscopy examination without generated mosaic images (96999)
    1.16   1.16   **FUD** XXX   B 80 26
    AMA: 2018,Feb,11; 2018,Jan,8; 2017,Sep,9

+ 96934 image acquisition and interpretation and report, each additional lesion (List separately in addition to code for primary procedure)
    EXCLUDES   *Optical coherence tomography for skin imaging (0470T-0471T)*
        Reflectance confocal microscopy examination without generated mosaic images (96999)
    Code first (96931)
    2.74   2.74   **FUD** ZZZ   N 80
    AMA: 2018,Feb,11; 2018,Jan,8; 2017,Sep,9

+ 96935 image acquisition only, each additional lesion (List separately in addition to code for primary procedure)
    EXCLUDES   *Optical coherence tomography for skin imaging (0470T-0471T)*
        Reflectance confocal microscopy examination without generated mosaic images (96999)
    Code first (96932)
    1.26   1.26   **FUD** ZZZ   N 80 TC
    AMA: 2018,Feb,11; 2018,Jan,8; 2017,Sep,9

+ 96936 interpretation and report only, each additional lesion (List separately in addition to code for primary procedure)
    EXCLUDES   *Optical coherence tomography for skin imaging (0470T-0471T)*
        Reflectance confocal microscopy examination without generated mosaic images (96999)
    Code first (96933)
    1.26   1.26   **FUD** ZZZ   N 80 26
    AMA: 2018,Feb,11; 2018,Jan,8; 2017,Sep,9

96999 Unlisted special dermatological service or procedure
    0.00   0.00   **FUD** XXX   01 80
    AMA: 2020,Jul,13; 2018,Feb,11; 2018,Jan,8; 2017,Sep,9; 2017,Jan,8; 2016,Sep,3; 2016,Jan,13

97161-97164 [97161, 97162, 97163, 97164] Assessment: Physical Therapy

CMS: 100-02,15,220 Coverage of Outpatient Rehabilitation Therapy Services; 100-02,15,220.4 Functional Reporting; 100-02,15,230 Practice of Physical Therapy, Occupational Therapy, and Speech-Language Pathology; 100-02,15,230.1 Practice of Physical Therapy; 100-02,15,230.4 Services By a Physical/Occupational Therapist in Private Practice; 100-04,5,10.3.2 Therapy Cap Exceptions; 100-04,5,10.3.3 Use of the KX Modifier; 100-04,5,10.6 Functional Reporting; 100-04,5,20.2 Reporting Units of Service

    INCLUDES   Care plan creation
        Evaluation body systems as defined in 1997 E/M documentation guidelines:
        Cardiovascular system: Vital signs, edema extremities
        Integumentary system: Inspection for skin abnormalities
        Mental status: Orientation, judgment, thought processes
        Musculoskeletal system: Evaluation gait and station, motion range, muscle strength, height, and weight
        Neuromuscular evaluation: Balance, abnormal movements
    EXCLUDES   *Biofeedback traning via EMG (90901)*
        Joint motion range (95851-95852)
        Transcutaneous nerve stimulation (TENS) (97014, 97032)

 # 97161 Physical therapy evaluation: low complexity, requiring these components: A history with no personal factors and/or comorbidities that impact the plan of care; An examination of body system(s) using standardized tests and measures addressing 1-2 elements from any of the following: body structures and functions, activity limitations, and/or participation restrictions; A clinical presentation with stable and/or uncomplicated characteristics; and Clinical decision making of low complexity using standardized patient assessment instrument and/or measurable assessment of functional outcome. Typically, 20 minutes are spent face-to-face with the patient and/or family.
    2.40   2.40   **FUD** XXX   ★ 51 A 80
    AMA: 2018,May,5; 2018,Feb,11; 2018,Jan,8; 2017,Aug,3; 2017,Jun,6; 2017,Jan,8

**97162** Physical therapy evaluation: moderate complexity, requiring these components: A history of present problem with 1-2 personal factors and/or comorbidities that impact the plan of care; An examination of body systems using standardized tests and measures in addressing a total of 3 or more elements from any of the following: body structures and functions, activity limitations, and/or participation restrictions; An evolving clinical presentation with changing characteristics; and Clinical decision making of moderate complexity using standardized patient assessment instrument and/or measurable assessment of functional outcome. Typically, 30 minutes are spent face-to-face with the patient and/or family.

     2.40   2.40   **FUD** XXX   ★ ⑤ Ⓐ 80 ▱

AMA: 2018,May,5; 2018,Feb,11; 2018,Jan,8; 2017,Aug,3; 2017,Jun,6; 2017,Jan,8

**97163** Physical therapy evaluation: high complexity, requiring these components: A history of present problem with 3 or more personal factors and/or comorbidities that impact the plan of care; An examination of body systems using standardized tests and measures addressing a total of 4 or more elements from any of the following: body structures and functions, activity limitations, and/or participation restrictions; A clinical presentation with unstable and unpredictable characteristics; and Clinical decision making of high complexity using standardized patient assessment instrument and/or measurable assessment of functional outcome. Typically, 45 minutes are spent face-to-face with the patient and/or family.

     2.40   2.40   **FUD** XXX   ⑤ Ⓐ 80 ▱

AMA: 2018,May,5; 2018,Feb,11; 2018,Jan,8; 2017,Aug,3; 2017,Jun,6; 2017,Jan,8

**97164** Re-evaluation of physical therapy established plan of care, requiring these components: An examination including a review of history and use of standardized tests and measures is required; and Revised plan of care using a standardized patient assessment instrument and/or measurable assessment of functional outcome Typically, 20 minutes are spent face-to-face with the patient and/or family.

     1.63   1.63   **FUD** XXX   ⑤ Ⓐ 80 ▱

AMA: 2018,May,5; 2018,Feb,11; 2018,Jan,8; 2017,Aug,3; 2017,Jun,6; 2017,Jan,8

97165-97168 [97165, 97166, 97167, 97168] Assessment: Occupational Therapy

CMS: 100-02,15,220 Coverage of Outpatient Rehabilitation Therapy Services; 100-02,15,220.4 Functional Reporting; 100-02,15,230 Practice of Physical Therapy, Occupational Therapy, and Speech-Language Pathology; 100-02,15,230.1 Practice of Physical Therapy; 100-02,15,230.2 Practice of Occupational Therapy; 100-02,15,230.4 Services By a Physical/Occupational Therapist in Private Practice; 100-04,5,10.3.2 Therapy Cap Exceptions; 100-04,5,10.3.3 Use of the KX Modifier; 100-04,5,10.6 Functional Reporting; 100-04,5,20.2 Reporting Units of Service

INCLUDES Care plan creation
Evaluations as appropriate
Medical history
Occupational status
Past therapy history

**97165** Occupational therapy evaluation, low complexity, requiring these components: An occupational profile and medical and therapy history, which includes a brief history including review of medical and/or therapy records relating to the presenting problem; An assessment(s) that identifies 1-3 performance deficits (ie, relating to physical, cognitive, or psychosocial skills) that result in activity limitations and/or participation restrictions; and Clinical decision making of low complexity, which includes an analysis of the occupational profile, analysis of data from problem-focused assessment(s), and consideration of a limited number of treatment options. Patient presents with no comorbidities that affect occupational performance. Modification of tasks or assistance (eg, physical or verbal) with assessment(s) is not necessary to enable completion of evaluation component. Typically, 30 minutes are spent face-to-face with the patient and/or family.

     2.58   2.58   **FUD** XXX   ★ ⑤ Ⓐ 80 ▱

AMA: 2018,May,5; 2018,Feb,11; 2018,Jan,8; 2017,Jun,6; 2017,Feb,3; 2017,Jan,8

**97166** Occupational therapy evaluation, moderate complexity, requiring these components: An occupational profile and medical and therapy history, which includes an expanded review of medical and/or therapy records and additional review of physical, cognitive, or psychosocial history related to current functional performance; An assessment(s) that identifies 3-5 performance deficits (ie, relating to physical, cognitive, or psychosocial skills) that result in activity limitations and/or participation restrictions; and Clinical decision making of moderate analytic complexity, which includes an analysis of the occupational profile, analysis of data from detailed assessment(s), and consideration of several treatment options. Patient may present with comorbidities that affect occupational performance. Minimal to moderate modification of tasks or assistance (eg, physical or verbal) with assessment(s) is necessary to enable patient to complete evaluation component. Typically, 45 minutes are spent face-to-face with the patient and/or family.

     2.58   2.58   **FUD** XXX   ★ ⑤ Ⓐ 80 ▱

AMA: 2018,May,5; 2018,Feb,11; 2018,Jan,8; 2017,Jun,6; 2017,Feb,3; 2017,Jan,8

97167
Occupational therapy evaluation, high complexity, requiring these components: An occupational profile and medical and therapy history, which includes review of medical and/or therapy records and extensive additional review of physical, cognitive, or psychosocial history related to current functional performance; An assessment(s) that identifies 5 or more performance deficits (ie, relating to physical, cognitive, or psychosocial skills) that result in activity limitations and/or participation restrictions; and Clinical decision making of high analytic complexity, which includes an analysis of the patient profile, analysis of data from comprehensive assessment(s), and consideration of multiple treatment options. Patient presents with comorbidities that affect occupational performance. Significant modification of tasks or assistance (eg, physical or verbal) with assessment(s) is necessary to enable patient to complete evaluation component. Typically, 60 minutes are spent face-to-face with the patient and/or family.

🚑 2.58 ⚕ 2.58 **FUD** XXX

AMA: 2018,May,5; 2018,Feb,11; 2018,Jan,8; 2017,Jun,6; 2017,Feb,3; 2017,Jan,8

97168
Re-evaluation of occupational therapy established plan of care, requiring these components: An assessment of changes in patient functional or medical status with revised plan of care; An update to the initial occupational profile to reflect changes in condition or environment that affect future interventions and/or goals; and A revised plan of care. A formal reevaluation is performed when there is a documented change in functional status or a significant change to the plan of care is required. Typically, 30 minutes are spent face-to-face with the patient and/or family.

🚑 1.77 ⚕ 1.77 **FUD** XXX

AMA: 2018,May,5; 2018,Feb,11; 2018,Jan,8; 2017,Jun,6; 2017,Feb,3; 2017,Jan,8

97169-97172 [97169, 97170, 97171, 97172] Assessment: Athletic Training

CMS: 100-02,15,220 Coverage of Outpatient Rehabilitation Therapy Services; 100-02,15,230 Practice of Physical Therapy, Occupational Therapy, and Speech-Language Pathology; 100-02,15,230.1 Practice of Physical Therapy

INCLUDES Care plan creation
Evaluation body systems as defined in 1997 E/M documentation guidelines:
Cardiovascular system: Vital signs, edema extremities
Integumentary system: Inspection for skin abnormalities
Musculoskeletal system: Evaluation gait and station, motion range, muscle strength, height, and weight
Neuromuscular evaluation: Balance, abnormal movements

97169
Athletic training evaluation, low complexity, requiring these components: A history and physical activity profile with no comorbidities that affect physical activity; An examination of affected body area and other symptomatic or related systems addressing 1-2 elements from any of the following: body structures, physical activity, and/or participation deficiencies; and Clinical decision making of low complexity using standardized patient assessment instrument and/or measurable assessment of functional outcome. Typically, 15 minutes are spent face-to-face with the patient and/or family.

🚑 0.00 ⚕ 0.00 **FUD** XXX

AMA: 2018,May,5; 2018,Feb,11; 2018,Jan,8; 2017,Jun,6; 2017,Jan,8

97170
Athletic training evaluation, moderate complexity, requiring these components: A medical history and physical activity profile with 1-2 comorbidities that affect physical activity; An examination of affected body area and other symptomatic or related systems addressing a total of 3 or more elements from any of the following: body structures, physical activity, and/or participation deficiencies; and Clinical decision making of moderate complexity using standardized patient assessment instrument and/or measurable assessment of functional outcome. Typically, 30 minutes are spent face-to-face with the patient and/or family.

🚑 0.00 ⚕ 0.00 **FUD** XXX

AMA: 2018,May,5; 2018,Feb,11; 2018,Jan,8; 2017,Jun,6; 2017,Jan,8

97171
Athletic training evaluation, high complexity, requiring these components: A medical history and physical activity profile, with 3 or more comorbidities that affect physical activity; A comprehensive examination of body systems using standardized tests and measures addressing a total of 4 or more elements from any of the following: body structures, physical activity, and/or participation deficiencies; Clinical presentation with unstable and unpredictable characteristics; and Clinical decision making of high complexity using standardized patient assessment instrument and/or measurable assessment of functional outcome. Typically, 45 minutes are spent face-to-face with the patient and/or family.

🚑 0.00 ⚕ 0.00 **FUD** XXX

AMA: 2018,May,5; 2018,Feb,11; 2018,Jan,8; 2017,Jun,6; 2017,Jan,8

97172
Re-evaluation of athletic training established plan of care requiring these components: An assessment of patient's current functional status when there is a documented change; and A revised plan of care using a standardized patient assessment instrument and/or measurable assessment of functional outcome with an update in management options, goals, and interventions. Typically, 20 minutes are spent face-to-face with the patient and/or family.

🚑 0.00 ⚕ 0.00 **FUD** XXX

AMA: 2018,May,5; 2018,Feb,11; 2018,Jan,8; 2017,Jun,6; 2017,Jan,8

97010-97028 Physical Therapy Treatment Modalities: Supervised

CMS: 100-02,15,220 Coverage of Outpatient Rehabilitation Therapy Services; 100-02,15,220.4 Functional Reporting; 100-02,15,230 Practice of Physical Therapy, Occupational Therapy, and Speech-Language Pathology; 100-02,15,230.1 Practice of Physical Therapy; 100-02,15,230.2 Practice of Occupational Therapy; 100-02,15,230.4 Services By a Physical/Occupational Therapist in Private Practice; 100-03,10.3 Inpatient Pain Rehabilitation Programs; 100-03,10.4 Outpatient Hospital Pain Rehabilitation Programs; 100-03,160.17 Payment for L-Dopa /Associated Inpatient Hospital Services; 100-04,5,10 Part B Outpatient Rehabilitation and Comprehensive Outpatient Rehabilitation Facility (CORF) Services - General; 100-04,5,10.3.2 Therapy Cap Exceptions; 100-04,5,10.3.3 Use of the KX Modifier; 100-04,5,20.2 Reporting Units of Service

INCLUDES Adding incremental treatment time intervals for same visit to calculate total service time

EXCLUDES Direct patient contact by provider
Electromyography (95860-95872 [95885, 95886, 95887])
EMG biofeedback training (90901)
Muscle and motion range tests ([97161, 97162, 97163, 97164, 97165, 97166, 97167, 97168, 97169, 97170, 97171, 97172])
Nerve conduction studies (95905-95913)

97010
Application of a modality to 1 or more areas; hot or cold packs

🚑 0.18 ⚕ 0.18 **FUD** XXX

AMA: 2018,May,5; 2018,Feb,11; 2018,Jan,8; 2017,Jan,8; 2016,Jun,8; 2016,Jan,13

97012
traction, mechanical

🚑 0.42 ⚕ 0.42 **FUD** XXX

AMA: 2020,Jul,13; 2018,May,5; 2018,Feb,11; 2018,Jan,8; 2017,Jan,8; 2016,Jun,8; 2016,Jan,13

● New Code   ▲ Revised Code   ○ Reinstated   ● New Web Release   ▲ Revised Web Release   + Add-on   Unlisted   Not Covered   # Resequenced
⑤⓪ Optum Mod 50 Exempt   Ⓢ AMA Mod 51 Exempt   ⑤ Optum Mod 51 Exempt   ⑥③ Mod 63 Exempt   ✗ Non-FDA Drug   ★ Telemedicine   Ⓜ Maternity   Ⓐ Age Edit

97014 electrical stimulation (unattended)
EXCLUDES *Acupuncture with electrical stimulation (97813, 97814)*
🦵 0.42 ⚖ 0.42 **FUD** XXX ⑤ Ⓔ ▦
AMA: 2019,Jul,10; 2018,Oct,11; 2018,Oct,8; 2018,May,5; 2018,Feb,11; 2018,Jan,8; 2017,Jan,8; 2016,Jan,13

97016 vasopneumatic devices
🦵 0.36 ⚖ 0.36 **FUD** XXX ⑤ Ⓐ 80 ▦
AMA: 2018,May,5; 2018,Feb,11; 2018,Jan,8; 2017,Jan,8; 2016,Jan,13

97018 paraffin bath
🦵 0.20 ⚖ 0.20 **FUD** XXX ⑤ Ⓐ 80 ▦
AMA: 2018,May,5; 2018,Feb,11; 2018,Jan,8; 2017,Jan,8; 2016,Jan,13

97022 whirlpool
🦵 0.51 ⚖ 0.51 **FUD** XXX ⑤ Ⓐ 80 ▦
AMA: 2018,May,5; 2018,Feb,11; 2018,Jan,8; 2017,Jan,8; 2016,Jan,13

97024 diathermy (eg, microwave)
🦵 0.20 ⚖ 0.20 **FUD** XXX ⑤ Ⓐ 80 ▦
AMA: 2018,May,5; 2018,Feb,11; 2018,Jan,8; 2017,Jan,8; 2016,Jan,13

97026 infrared
🦵 0.18 ⚖ 0.18 **FUD** XXX ⑤ Ⓐ 80 ▦
AMA: 2018,May,5; 2018,Feb,11; 2018,Jan,8; 2017,Jan,8; 2016,Jan,13

97028 ultraviolet
🦵 0.23 ⚖ 0.23 **FUD** XXX ⑤ Ⓐ 80 ▦
AMA: 2018,May,5; 2018,Feb,11; 2018,Jan,8; 2017,Jan,8; 2016,Jan,13

97032-97039 Physical Therapy Treatment Modalities: Constant Attendance
CMS: 100-02,15,220 Coverage of Outpatient Rehabilitation Therapy Services; 100-02,15,220.4 Functional Reporting; 100-02,15,230 Practice of Physical Therapy, Occupational Therapy, and Speech-Language Pathology; 100-02,15,230.1 Practice of Physical Therapy; 100-02,15,230.2 Practice of Occupational Therapy; 100-02,15,230.4 Services By a Physical/Occupational Therapist in Private Practice; 100-03,10.3 Inpatient Pain Rehabilitation Programs; 100-03,10.4 Outpatient Hospital Pain Rehabilitation Programs; 100-03,160.17 Payment for L-Dopa /Associated Inpatient Hospital Services; 100-04,5,10 Part B Outpatient Rehabilitation and Comprehensive Outpatient Rehabilitation Facility (CORF) Services - General; 100-04,5,10.3.2 Therapy Cap Exceptions; 100-04,5,10.3.3 Use of the KX Modifier; 100-04,5,20.2 Reporting Units of Service
INCLUDES Adding incremental treatment time intervals for same visit to calculate total service time
Direct patient contact by provider
EXCLUDES *Electromyography (95860-95872 [95885, 95886, 95887])*
EMG biofeedback training (90901)
Muscle and motion range tests ([97161, 97162, 97163, 97164, 97165, 97166, 97167, 97168, 97169, 97170, 97171, 97172])
Nerve conduction studies (95905-95913)

97032 Application of a modality to 1 or more areas; electrical stimulation (manual), each 15 minutes
EXCLUDES *Transcutaneous electrical modulation pain reprocessing (TEMPR) (scrambler therapy) (0278T)*
🦵 0.42 ⚖ 0.42 **FUD** XXX ⑤ Ⓐ 80 ▦
AMA: 2019,Jul,10; 2018,Oct,11; 2018,Oct,8; 2018,May,5; 2018,Feb,11; 2018,Jan,8; 2017,Jan,8; 2016,Jan,13

97033 iontophoresis, each 15 minutes
🦵 0.59 ⚖ 0.59 **FUD** XXX ⑤ Ⓐ 80 ▦
AMA: 2018,May,5; 2018,Feb,11; 2018,Jan,8; 2017,Jan,8; 2016,Jan,13

97034 contrast baths, each 15 minutes
🦵 0.43 ⚖ 0.43 **FUD** XXX ⑤ Ⓐ 80 ▦
AMA: 2018,May,5; 2018,Feb,11; 2018,Jan,8; 2017,Jan,8; 2016,Jan,13

97035 ultrasound, each 15 minutes
🦵 0.39 ⚖ 0.39 **FUD** XXX ⑤ Ⓐ 80 ▦
AMA: 2018,May,5; 2018,Feb,11; 2018,Jan,8; 2017,Jan,8; 2016,Jan,13

97036 Hubbard tank, each 15 minutes
🦵 0.99 ⚖ 0.99 **FUD** XXX ⑤ Ⓐ 80 ▦
AMA: 2018,May,5; 2018,Feb,11; 2018,Jan,8; 2017,Jan,8; 2016,Jan,13

97039 Unlisted modality (specify type and time if constant attendance)
🦵 0.00 ⚖ 0.00 **FUD** XXX Ⓐ 80 ▦
AMA: 2020,Jul,13; 2018,May,5; 2018,Feb,11; 2018,Jan,8; 2017,Jan,8; 2016,Nov,9; 2016,Jun,8; 2016,Jan,13

97110-97546 [97151, 97152, 97153, 97154, 97155, 97156, 97157, 97158, 97161, 97162, 97163, 97164, 97165, 97166, 97167, 97168, 97169, 97170, 97171, 97172] Other Therapeutic Techniques With Direct Patient Contact
CMS: 100-02,15,220 Coverage of Outpatient Rehabilitation Therapy Services; 100-02,15,230 Practice of Physical Therapy, Occupational Therapy, and Speech-Language Pathology; 100-02,15,230.1 Practice of Physical Therapy; 100-02,15,230.2 Practice of Occupational Therapy; 100-02,15,230.4 Services By a Physical/Occupational Therapist in Private Practice; 100-03,10.3 Inpatient Pain Rehabilitation Programs; 100-03,10.4 Outpatient Hospital Pain Rehabilitation Programs; 100-04,5,10 Part B Outpatient Rehabilitation and Comprehensive Outpatient Rehabilitation Facility (CORF) Services - General; 100-04,5,20.2 Reporting Units of Service
INCLUDES Application clinical skills/services to improve function
Direct patient contact by provider
EXCLUDES *Electromyography (95860-95872 [95885, 95886, 95887])*
EMG biofeedback training (90901)
Muscle and motion range tests ([97161, 97162, 97163, 97164, 97165, 97166, 97167, 97168, 97169, 97170, 97171, 97172])
Nerve conduction studies (95905-95913)

97110 Therapeutic procedure, 1 or more areas, each 15 minutes; therapeutic exercises to develop strength and endurance, range of motion and flexibility
🦵 0.87 ⚖ 0.87 **FUD** XXX ★ ⑤ Ⓐ 80 ▦
AMA: 2019,Jun,14; 2018,Dec,7; 2018,Dec,7; 2018,May,5; 2018,Feb,11; 2018,Jan,8; 2017,Dec,14; 2017,Jan,8; 2016,Jun,8; 2016,Jan,13

97112 neuromuscular reeducation of movement, balance, coordination, kinesthetic sense, posture, and/or proprioception for sitting and/or standing activities
🦵 0.99 ⚖ 0.99 **FUD** XXX ★ ⑤ Ⓐ 80 ▦
AMA: 2018,May,5; 2018,Feb,11; 2018,Jan,8; 2017,Jan,8; 2016,Jan,13

97113 aquatic therapy with therapeutic exercises
🦵 1.10 ⚖ 1.10 **FUD** XXX ⑤ Ⓐ 80 ▦
AMA: 2018,May,5; 2018,Feb,11; 2018,Jan,8; 2017,Jan,8; 2016,Jan,13

97116 gait training (includes stair climbing)
EXCLUDES *Comprehensive gait/motion analysis (96000-96003)*
🦵 0.86 ⚖ 0.86 **FUD** XXX ★ Ⓐ 80 ▦
AMA: 2018,May,5; 2018,Feb,11; 2018,Jan,8; 2017,Jan,8; 2016,Jan,13

97124 massage, including effleurage, petrissage and/or tapotement (stroking, compression, percussion)
EXCLUDES *Myofascial release (97140)*
🦵 0.81 ⚖ 0.81 **FUD** XXX ⑤ Ⓐ 80 ▦
AMA: 2020,Jul,10; 2019,Jun,14; 2018,May,5; 2018,Feb,11; 2018,Jan,8; 2017,Jan,8; 2016,Jun,8; 2016,Jan,13

97129 Therapeutic interventions that focus on cognitive function (eg, attention, memory, reasoning, executive function, problem solving, and/or pragmatic functioning) and compensatory strategies to manage the performance of an activity (eg, managing time or schedules, initiating, organizing, and sequencing tasks), direct (one-on-one) patient contact; initial 15 minutes
EXCLUDES *Adaptive behavior treatment ([97153], [97155])*
Reporting code more than one time per day
🦵 0.67 ⚖ 0.68 **FUD** XXX ⑤ 80 ▦
AMA: 2020,Jul,10

| 26/TC PC/TC Only | 42-43 ASC Payment | 50 Bilateral | ♂ Male Only | ♀ Female Only | 🦵 Facility RVU | ⚖ Non-Facility RVU | CCI | ☒ CLIA |
| FUD Follow-up Days | CMS: IOM | AMA: CPT Asst | A-Y OPPSI | 80/80 Surg Assist Allowed / w/Doc | ▦ Lab Crosswalk | ☒ Radiology Crosswalk |

524

+ 97130 each additional 15 minutes (List separately in addition to code for primary procedure)

EXCLUDES *Adaptive behavior treatment ([97153], [97155])*
Code first (97129)

⏣ 0.65 ⚕ 0.65 **FUD** ZZZ ⑤⑧⓪☐

AMA: 2020,Jul,10

97139 Unlisted therapeutic procedure (specify)

⏣ 0.00 ⚕ 0.00 **FUD** XXX Ⓐ⑧⓪☐

AMA: 2018,May,5; 2018,Feb,11; 2018,Jan,8; 2017,Jan,8; 2016,Jan,13

97140 Manual therapy techniques (eg, mobilization/manipulation, manual lymphatic drainage, manual traction), 1 or more regions, each 15 minutes

EXCLUDES *Insertion needle without injection ([20560, 20561])*

⏣ 0.79 ⚕ 0.79 **FUD** XXX ⑤Ⓐ⑧⓪☐

AMA: 2020,Jul,10; 2020,Feb,9; 2019,Jun,14; 2018,May,5; 2018,Feb,11; 2018,Jan,8; 2017,Jan,8; 2016,Nov,9; 2016,Sep,9; 2016,Aug,3; 2016,Jan,13

97150 Therapeutic procedure(s), group (2 or more individuals)

INCLUDES Constant attendance by physician/therapist
Reporting this procedure for each group member

EXCLUDES *Adaptive behavior services ([97154], [97158])*
Osteopathic manipulative treatment (98925-98929)

⏣ 0.52 ⚕ 0.52 **FUD** XXX ⑤Ⓐ⑧⓪☐

AMA: 2020,Jul,7; 2018,Nov,3; 2018,May,5; 2018,Feb,11; 2018,Jan,8; 2017,Jan,8; 2016,Jan,13

97151 Resequenced code. See code following 96040.

97152 Resequenced code. See code following 96040.

97153 Resequenced code. See code following 96040.

97154 Resequenced code. See code following 96040.

97155 Resequenced code. See code following 96040.

97156 Resequenced code. See code following 96040.

97157 Resequenced code. See code following 96040.

97158 Resequenced code. See code following 96040.

97161 Resequenced code. See code before 97010.

97162 Resequenced code. See code before 97010.

97163 Resequenced code. See code before 97010.

97164 Resequenced code. See code before 97010.

97165 Resequenced code. See code before 97010.

97166 Resequenced code. See code before 97010.

97167 Resequenced code. See code before 97010.

97168 Resequenced code. See code before 97010.

97169 Resequenced code. See code before 97010.

97170 Resequenced code. See code before 97010.

97171 Resequenced code. See code before 97010.

97172 Resequenced code. See code before 97010.

97530 Therapeutic activities, direct (one-on-one) patient contact (use of dynamic activities to improve functional performance), each 15 minutes

⏣ 1.13 ⚕ 1.13 **FUD** XXX ★⑤Ⓐ⑧⓪☐

AMA: 2018,Dec,7; 2018,Dec,7; 2018,May,5; 2018,Feb,11; 2018,Jan,8; 2017,Jan,8; 2016,Jan,13

97533 Sensory integrative techniques to enhance sensory processing and promote adaptive responses to environmental demands, direct (one-on-one) patient contact, each 15 minutes

⏣ 1.21 ⚕ 1.21 **FUD** XXX ⑤Ⓐ⑧⓪☐

AMA: 2018,May,5; 2018,Feb,11; 2018,Jan,8; 2017,Jan,8; 2016,Jan,13

97535 Self-care/home management training (eg, activities of daily living (ADL) and compensatory training, meal preparation, safety procedures, and instructions in use of assistive technology devices/adaptive equipment) direct one-on-one contact, each 15 minutes

⏣ 0.97 ⚕ 0.97 **FUD** XXX ★⑤Ⓐ⑧⓪☐

AMA: 2018,May,5; 2018,Feb,11; 2018,Jan,8; 2017,Jan,8; 2016,Aug,3; 2016,Jan,13

97537 Community/work reintegration training (eg, shopping, transportation, money management, avocational activities and/or work environment/modification analysis, work task analysis, use of assistive technology device/adaptive equipment), direct one-on-one contact, each 15 minutes

EXCLUDES *Wheelchair management/propulsion training (97542)*

⏣ 0.93 ⚕ 0.93 **FUD** XXX ⑤Ⓐ⑧⓪☐

AMA: 2018,May,5; 2018,Feb,11; 2018,Jan,8; 2017,Jan,8; 2016,Jan,13

97542 Wheelchair management (eg, assessment, fitting, training), each 15 minutes

⏣ 0.94 ⚕ 0.94 **FUD** XXX ⑤Ⓐ⑧⓪☐

AMA: 2018,May,5; 2018,Feb,11; 2018,Jan,8; 2017,Jan,8; 2016,Jan,13

97545 Work hardening/conditioning; initial 2 hours

⏣ 0.00 ⚕ 0.00 **FUD** XXX ⑤Ⓐ⑧⓪☐

AMA: 2018,May,5; 2018,Feb,11; 2018,Jan,8; 2017,Jan,8; 2016,Jan,13

+ 97546 each additional hour (List separately in addition to code for primary procedure)

Code first initial two hours (97545)

⏣ 0.00 ⚕ 0.00 **FUD** ZZZ ⑤Ⓐ⑧⓪☐

AMA: 2018,May,5; 2018,Feb,11; 2018,Jan,8; 2017,Jan,8; 2016,Jan,13

97597-97610 Treatment of Wounds

CMS: 100-02,15,220.4 Functional Reporting; 100-02,15,230.4 Services By a Physical/Occupational Therapist in Private Practice; 100-03,270.3 Blood-derived Products for Chronic Nonhealing Wounds; 100-04,4,200.9 Billing for "Sometimes Therapy" Services that May be Paid as Non-Therapy Services; 100-04,5,10 Part B Outpatient Rehabilitation and Comprehensive Outpatient Rehabilitation Facility (CORF) Services - General; 100-04,5,10.3.2 Therapy Cap Exceptions; 100-04,5,10.3.3 Use of the KX Modifier

INCLUDES Direct patient contact
Removing devitalized/necrotic tissue and promoting healing
EXCLUDES Burn wound debridement (16020-16030)

97597 Debridement (eg, high pressure waterjet with/without suction, sharp selective debridement with scissors, scalpel and forceps), open wound, (eg, fibrin, devitalized epidermis and/or dermis, exudate, debris, biofilm), including topical application(s), wound assessment, use of a whirlpool, when performed and instruction(s) for ongoing care, per session, total wound(s) surface area; first 20 sq cm or less

INCLUDES Chemical cauterization (17250)
🚗 0.68 ✂ 2.52 **FUD** 000 ⑤ T 80 🖳
AMA: 2018,May,5; 2018,Feb,11; 2018,Jan,8; 2017,Jan,8; 2016,Oct,3; 2016,Aug,9; 2016,Jan,13

Wound may be washed, addressed with scissors, and/or tweezers and scalpel

+ **97598** each additional 20 sq cm, or part thereof (List separately in addition to code for primary procedure)

INCLUDES Chemical cauterization (17250)
Code first (97597)
🚗 0.32 ✂ 0.79 **FUD** ZZZ ⑤ N 80 🖳
AMA: 2018,May,5; 2018,Feb,11; 2018,Jan,8; 2017,Jan,8; 2016,Oct,3; 2016,Aug,9; 2016,Jan,13

97602 Removal of devitalized tissue from wound(s), non-selective debridement, without anesthesia (eg, wet-to-moist dressings, enzymatic, abrasion, larval therapy), including topical application(s), wound assessment, and instruction(s) for ongoing care, per session

INCLUDES Chemical cauterization (17250)
🚗 0.00 ✂ 0.00 **FUD** XXX ⑤ 01 🖳
AMA: 2018,May,5; 2018,Feb,11; 2018,Jan,8; 2017,Jan,8; 2016,Oct,3; 2016,Jan,13

97605 Negative pressure wound therapy (eg, vacuum assisted drainage collection), utilizing durable medical equipment (DME), including topical application(s), wound assessment, and instruction(s) for ongoing care, per session; total wound(s) surface area less than or equal to 50 square centimeters

EXCLUDES Negative pressure wound therapy using disposable medical equipment (97607-97608)
🚗 0.74 ✂ 1.24 **FUD** XXX ⑤ 01 80 🖳
AMA: 2018,May,5; 2018,Feb,11; 2018,Jan,8; 2017,Jan,8; 2016,Feb,13; 2016,Jan,13

97606 total wound(s) surface area greater than 50 square centimeters

EXCLUDES Negative pressure wound therapy using disposable medical equipment (97607-97608)
🚗 0.80 ✂ 1.46 **FUD** XXX ⑤ 01 80 🖳
AMA: 2018,May,5; 2018,Feb,11; 2018,Jan,8; 2017,Jan,8; 2016,Feb,13; 2016,Jan,13

97607 Negative pressure wound therapy, (eg, vacuum assisted drainage collection), utilizing disposable, non-durable medical equipment including provision of exudate management collection system, topical application(s), wound assessment, and instructions for ongoing care, per session; total wound(s) surface area less than or equal to 50 square centimeters

EXCLUDES Negative pressure wound therapy using durable medical equipment (97605-97606)
🚗 0.00 ✂ 0.00 **FUD** XXX ⑤ T 80 🖳
AMA: 2018,May,5; 2018,Feb,11; 2018,Jan,8; 2017,Jan,8; 2016,Jan,13

97608 total wound(s) surface area greater than 50 square centimeters

EXCLUDES Negative pressure wound therapy using durable medical equipment (97605-97606)
🚗 0.00 ✂ 0.00 **FUD** XXX ⑤ T 80 🖳
AMA: 2018,May,5; 2018,Feb,11; 2018,Jan,8; 2017,Jan,8; 2016,Jan,13

97610 Low frequency, non-contact, non-thermal ultrasound, including topical application(s), when performed, wound assessment, and instruction(s) for ongoing care, per day

🚗 0.48 ✂ 6.39 **FUD** XXX ⑤ 01 80 🖳
AMA: 2018,May,5; 2018,Feb,11; 2018,Jan,8; 2017,Jan,8; 2016,Jan,13

97750-97799 Assessments and Training

CMS: 100-02,15,220 Coverage of Outpatient Rehabilitation Therapy Services; 100-02,15,220.4 Functional Reporting; 100-02,15,230 Practice of Physical Therapy, Occupational Therapy, and Speech-Language Pathology; 100-02,15,230.1 Practice of Physical Therapy; 100-02,15,230.2 Practice of Occupational Therapy; 100-02,15,230.4 Services By a Physical/Occupational Therapist in Private Practice; 100-04,5,10 Part B Outpatient Rehabilitation and Comprehensive Outpatient Rehabilitation Facility (CORF) Services - General; 100-04,5,10.3.2 Exceptions Process; 100-04,5,10.3.3 Use of the KX Modifier

97750 Physical performance test or measurement (eg, musculoskeletal, functional capacity), with written report, each 15 minutes

INCLUDES Direct patient contact
EXCLUDES Electromyography (95860-95872, [95885, 95886, 95887])
Joint motion range (95851-95852)
Nerve velocity determination (95905, 95907-95913)
🚗 0.99 ✂ 0.99 **FUD** XXX ★⑤ A 80 🖳
AMA: 2018,May,5; 2018,Feb,11; 2018,Jan,8; 2017,Jan,8; 2016,Jan,13

97755 Assistive technology assessment (eg, to restore, augment or compensate for existing function, optimize functional tasks and/or maximize environmental accessibility), direct one-on-one contact, with written report, each 15 minutes

> INCLUDES Direct patient contact
> EXCLUDES *Augmentative/alternative communication device (92605, 92607)*
> *Electromyography (95860-95872, [95885, 95886, 95887])*
> *Joint motion range (95851-95852)*
> *Nerve velocity determination (95905, 95907-95913)*
>
> 1.08   1.08 **FUD** XXX ★ ⑤ A 80
>
> **AMA:** 2018,May,5; 2018,Feb,11

97760 Orthotic(s) management and training (including assessment and fitting when not otherwise reported), upper extremity(ies), lower extremity(ies) and/or trunk, initial orthotic(s) encounter, each 15 minutes

> EXCLUDES *Gait training, when performed on same extremity (97116)*
>
> 1.35   1.35 **FUD** XXX ★ ⑤ A 80
>
> **AMA:** 2018,May,5; 2018,Feb,11; 2018,Jan,8; 2017,Jan,8; 2016,Jan,13

97761 Prosthetic(s) training, upper and/or lower extremity(ies), initial prosthetic(s) encounter, each 15 minutes

> 1.16   1.16 **FUD** XXX ★ ⑤ A 80
>
> **AMA:** 2018,May,5; 2018,Feb,11; 2018,Jan,8; 2017,Jan,8; 2016,Jan,13

97763 Orthotic(s)/prosthetic(s) management and/or training, upper extremity(ies), lower extremity(ies), and/or trunk, subsequent orthotic(s)/prosthetic(s) encounter, each 15 minutes

> EXCLUDES *Initial encounter for orthotics and prosthetics management and training (97760-97761)*
>
> 1.50   1.50 **FUD** XXX ⑤ A 80
>
> **AMA:** 2018,May,5; 2018,Feb,11

97799 Unlisted physical medicine/rehabilitation service or procedure

> 0.00   0.00 **FUD** XXX A 80
>
> **AMA:** 2018,May,5; 2018,Feb,11; 2018,Jan,8; 2017,Jan,8; 2016,Nov,9; 2016,Jan,13

97802-97804 Medical Nutrition Therapy Services

CMS: 100-02,13,220 Preventive Health Services; 100-03,180.1 Medical Nutrition Therapy; 100-04,12,190.3 List of Telehealth Services; 100-04,12,190.6 Payment Methodology for Physician/Practitioner at the Distant Site; 100-04,12,190.6.1 Submission of Telehealth Claims for Distant Site Practitioners; 100-04,12,190.7 Contractor Editing of Telehealth Claims; 100-04,4,300 Medical Nutrition Therapy Services; 100-04,4,300.6 CWF Edits for MNT/DSMT

> EXCLUDES *Medical nutrition therapy assessment/intervention provided by physician or other qualified health care provider; report appropriate E/M codes*

97802 Medical nutrition therapy; initial assessment and intervention, individual, face-to-face with the patient, each 15 minutes

> 0.96   1.05 **FUD** XXX ★ A 80
>
> **AMA:** 2020,Jul,7; 2018,Feb,11; 2018,Jan,8; 2017,Jan,8; 2016,Jan,13

97803 re-assessment and intervention, individual, face-to-face with the patient, each 15 minutes

> 0.82   0.91 **FUD** XXX ★ A 80
>
> **AMA:** 2020,Jul,7; 2018,Feb,11; 2018,Jan,8; 2017,Jan,8; 2016,Jan,13

97804 group (2 or more individual(s)), each 30 minutes

> 0.45   0.48 **FUD** XXX ★ A 80
>
> **AMA:** 2020,Jul,7; 2018,Feb,11; 2018,Jan,8; 2017,Jan,8; 2016,Jan,13

97810-97814 Acupuncture

CMS: 100-03,10.3 Inpatient Pain Rehabilitation Programs; 100-03,10.4 Outpatient Hospital Pain Rehabilitation Programs; 100-03,30.3 Acupuncture; 100-03,30.3.1 Acupuncture for Fibromyalgia; 100-03,30.3.2 Acupuncture for Osteoarthritis; 100-04,32,410 Acupuncture for Chronic Low Back Pain (cLBP); 100-04,32,410.1 Coverage Requirements; 100-04,32,410.3 Institutional Claims Bill Type and Revenue Coding Information; 100-04,32,410.4 Messaging

> INCLUDES 15 minute increments face-to-face contact with patient
> Reporting only one code for each 15 minute increment
> EXCLUDES *Insertion needle without injection ([20560, 20561])*
> Code also significant separately identifiable E/M service with modifier 25, when performed

97810 Acupuncture, 1 or more needles; without electrical stimulation, initial 15 minutes of personal one-on-one contact with the patient

> EXCLUDES *Treatment with electrical stimulation (97813-97814)*
>
> 0.87   1.03 **FUD** XXX E
>
> **AMA:** 2020,Feb,9; 2018,Feb,11; 2018,Jan,8; 2017,Jan,8; 2016,Jan,13

+ 97811 without electrical stimulation, each additional 15 minutes of personal one-on-one contact with the patient, with re-insertion of needle(s) (List separately in addition to code for primary procedure)

> EXCLUDES *Treatment with electrical stimulation (97813-97814)*
> Code first initial 15 minutes (97810)
>
> 0.72   0.78 **FUD** ZZZ E
>
> **AMA:** 2020,Feb,9; 2018,Feb,11; 2018,Jan,8; 2017,Jan,8; 2016,Jan,13

97813 with electrical stimulation, initial 15 minutes of personal one-on-one contact with the patient

> EXCLUDES *Treatment without electrical stimulation (97813-97814)*
>
> 0.94   1.13 **FUD** XXX E
>
> **AMA:** 2020,Feb,9; 2018,Feb,11; 2018,Jan,8; 2017,Jan,8; 2016,Jan,13

+ 97814 with electrical stimulation, each additional 15 minutes of personal one-on-one contact with the patient, with re-insertion of needle(s) (List separately in addition to code for primary procedure)

> EXCLUDES *Treatment without electrical stimulation (97813-97814)*
> Code first initial 15 minutes (97813)
>
> 0.79   0.91 **FUD** ZZZ E
>
> **AMA:** 2020,Feb,9; 2018,Feb,11; 2018,Jan,8; 2017,Jan,8; 2016,Jan,13

98925-98929 Osteopathic Manipulation

CMS: 100-03,150.1 Manipulation

> INCLUDES Body regions:
> Abdomen/visceral region
> Cervical region
> Head region
> Lower extremities
> Lumbar region
> Pelvic region
> Rib cage region
> Sacral region
> Thoracic region
> Upper extremities
> Physician applied manual treatment done to eliminate/alleviate somatic dysfunction and related disorders with multiple techniques
> Code also significant separately identifiable E/M service with modifier 25, when performed

98925 Osteopathic manipulative treatment (OMT); 1-2 body regions involved

> 0.68   0.89 **FUD** 000 01 80
>
> **AMA:** 2018,Aug,9; 2018,Feb,11; 2018,Jan,8; 2017,Dec,14; 2017,Jan,8; 2016,Jan,13

98926 3-4 body regions involved

> 1.02   1.28 **FUD** 000 01 80
>
> **AMA:** 2018,Aug,9; 2018,Feb,11; 2018,Jan,8; 2017,Jan,8; 2016,Jan,13

● New Code ▲ Revised Code ○ Reinstated ● New Web Release ▲ Revised Web Release + Add-on Unlisted Not Covered # Resequenced

⑤⓪ Optum Mod 50 Exempt ⊘ AMA Mod 51 Exempt ⑤① Optum Mod 51 Exempt ⑥③ Mod 63 Exempt ✔ Non-FDA Drug ★ Telemedicine M Maternity A Age Edit

© 2021 Optum360, LLC   CPT © 2021 American Medical Association. All Rights Reserved.   **527**

Medicine

98927 — 98967

98927   5-6 body regions involved
📠 1.35   🔖 1.68   **FUD** 000   01 80 🖵

AMA: 2018,Aug,9; 2018,Feb,11; 2018,Jan,8; 2017,Jan,8; 2016,Jan,13

98928   7-8 body regions involved
📠 1.69   🔖 2.04   **FUD** 000   01 80 🖵

AMA: 2018,Aug,9; 2018,Feb,11; 2018,Jan,8; 2017,Jan,8; 2016,Jan,13

98929   9-10 body regions involved
📠 2.05   🔖 2.44   **FUD** 000   01 80 🖵

AMA: 2018,Aug,9; 2018,Feb,11; 2018,Jan,8; 2017,Jan,8; 2016,Jan,13

98940-98943 Chiropractic Manipulation

CMS: 100-01,5,70.6 Chiropractors; 100-02,15,240 Chiropractic Services - General; 100-02,15,240.1.3 Necessity for Treatment; 100-02,15,30.5 Chiropractor's Services; 100-03,150.1 Manipulation

INCLUDES   Five extraspinal regions:
    Abdomen
    Head, including temporomandibular joint, excluding atlanto-occipital region
    Lower extremities
    Rib cage, not including costotransverse/costovertebral joints
    Upper extremities
  Five spinal regions:
    Cervical region (atlanto-occipital joint)
    Lumbar region
    Pelvic region (sacro-iliac joint)
    Sacral region
    Thoracic region (costovertebral/costotransverse joints)
  Manual treatment performed to influence joint/neurophysical function
Code also significant separately identifible E/M service with modifier 25, when performed

98940   Chiropractic manipulative treatment (CMT); spinal, 1-2 regions
📠 0.64   🔖 0.80   **FUD** 000   01 80 🖵

AMA: 2018,Nov,11; 2018,Feb,11; 2018,Jan,8; 2017,Jan,8; 2016,Jan,13

98941   spinal, 3-4 regions
📠 0.98   🔖 1.16   **FUD** 000   01 80 🖵

AMA: 2018,Nov,11; 2018,Feb,11; 2018,Jan,8; 2017,Jan,8; 2016,Jan,13

98942   spinal, 5 regions
📠 1.33   🔖 1.50   **FUD** 000   01 80 🖵

AMA: 2018,Nov,11; 2018,Feb,11; 2018,Jan,8; 2017,Jan,8; 2016,Jan,13

98943   extraspinal, 1 or more regions
📠 0.67   🔖 0.77   **FUD** XXX   E 🖵

AMA: 2018,Nov,11; 2018,Feb,11; 2018,Jan,8; 2017,Jan,8; 2016,Jan,13

98960-98962 Self-Management Training

INCLUDES   Education/training services:
    Prescribed by physician or other qualified health care professional
    Provided by qualified nonphysician health care provider
  Standardized curriculum that may be modified as necessary for:
    Clinical needs
    Cultural norms
    Health literacy
  Teaching patient how to manage illness/delay comorbidity(s)

EXCLUDES   *Collection/interpretation physiologic data ([99091])*
Complex chronic care management (99487, 99489)
Counseling/education to group (99078)
Counseling/risk factor reduction without symptoms/established disease (99401-99412)
Genetic counseling education services (96040, 98961-98962)
Health and behavior assessment and intervention (96156, 96158-96159, [96164, 96165], [96167, 96168], [96170, 96171])
Medical nutrition therapy (97802-97804)
Physician supervision in home, domiciliary, or rest home (99339, 99340, 99374-99375, 99379-99380)
Services provided in which would be reported with other services
Services provided with cumulative time of less than 5 minutes
Supervision hospice patient (99377-99378)
Transitional care management (99495, 99496)

98960   Education and training for patient self-management by a qualified, nonphysician health care professional using a standardized curriculum, face-to-face with the patient (could include caregiver/family) each 30 minutes; individual patient
📠 0.77   🔖 0.77   **FUD** XXX   ★ E 🖵

AMA: 2020,Jul,7; 2018,Aug,6; 2018,Feb,11; 2018,Jan,8; 2017,Jan,8; 2016,Jan,13

98961   2-4 patients
INCLUDES   Group education regarding genetic risks
📠 0.38   🔖 0.38   **FUD** XXX   ★ E 🖵

AMA: 2020,Jul,7; 2018,Aug,6; 2018,Feb,11; 2018,Jan,8; 2017,Jan,8; 2016,Jan,13

98962   5-8 patients
INCLUDES   Group education regarding genetic risks
📠 0.28   🔖 0.28   **FUD** XXX   ★ E 🖵

AMA: 2020,Jul,7; 2018,Aug,6; 2018,Feb,11; 2018,Jan,8; 2017,Jan,8; 2016,Jan,13

98966-98968 Nonphysician Telephone Services

INCLUDES   Assessment and management services provided by telephone by qualified health care professional
  Care episodes initiated by established patient or his/her guardian

EXCLUDES   *Call initiated by qualified health care professional*
Calls during postoperative period
Decision to see patient at next available urgent care appointment
Decision to see patient within 24 hours from patient call
Monitoring INR (93792-93793)
Patient management services during same time frame as ([99439, 99490, 99491], 99487-99489)
Principal care management services during same time frame as ([99426], [99427])
Reporting codes when same codes billed within past seven days
Telephone services considered previous or subsequent service component
Telephone services provided by physician (99441-99443)

98966   Telephone assessment and management service provided by a qualified nonphysician health care professional to an established patient, parent, or guardian not originating from a related assessment and management service provided within the previous 7 days nor leading to an assessment and management service or procedure within the next 24 hours or soonest available appointment; 5-10 minutes of medical discussion
📠 0.36   🔖 0.39   **FUD** XXX   E 80 🖵

AMA: 2018,Mar,7; 2018,Feb,11; 2018,Jan,8; 2017,Jan,8; 2016,Jan,13

98967   11-20 minutes of medical discussion
📠 0.72   🔖 0.76   **FUD** XXX   E 80 🖵

AMA: 2018,Mar,7; 2018,Feb,11; 2018,Jan,8; 2017,Jan,8; 2016,Jan,13

 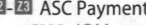

98968 **21-30 minutes of medical discussion**
🔲 1.08 ⚖ 1.12 **FUD** XXX   E 80 ▢
AMA: 2018,Mar,7; 2018,Feb,11; 2018,Jan,8; 2017,Jan,8; 2016,Jan,13

98970-98972 Nonphysician Online Service

INCLUDES Timely reply to patient as well as:
Ordering laboratory services
Permanent service record; either hard copy or electronic
Providing prescription
Related telephone calls
EXCLUDES *Monitoring INR (93792-93793)*
Online digital assessment and management service provided by qualified health care professional ([99421, 99422, 99423])
Online evaluation service:
Provided during postoperative period
Provided more than once in seven day period
Related to service provided in previous seven days
Provided with cumulative time less than 5 minutes
Where time would be reported as another service
Patient management services during same time frame as:
Chronic care management ([99437], [99439, 99490, 99491])
Collection/interpretation physiologic data ([99091])
Complex chronic care management (99487-99489)
Physician supervision in home, domiciliary, or rest home (99339-99340, 99374-99375, 99379-99380)
Principal care management services ([99426, 99427])
Supervision hospice patient (99377-99378)

98970 **Qualified nonphysician health care professional online digital assessment and management, for an established patient, for up to 7 days, cumulative time during the 7 days; 5-10 minutes**
🔲 0.00 ⚖ 0.00 **FUD** XXX   80 ▢
AMA: 2020,Jan,3

98971 **11-20 minutes**
🔲 0.00 ⚖ 0.00 **FUD** XXX   80 ▢
AMA: 2020,Jan,3

98972 **21 or more minutes**
🔲 0.00 ⚖ 0.00 **FUD** XXX   80 ▢
AMA: 2020,Jan,3

98975-98977 Remote Therapeutic Monitoring Services

INCLUDES Device:
Set-up and patient education
Supply
EXCLUDES *Physiological monitoring services ([99453], [99454])*
Pulse oximetry, noninvasive (94760)
Remote device interrogation (93296)
Remote physiologic monitoring treatment management services ([99457])
Reporting when monitoring less than 16 days
Self-measured blood pressure monitoring ([99473, 99474])
Therapeutic monitoring treatment management services (98980)

● **98975** **Remote therapeutic monitoring (eg, respiratory system status, musculoskeletal system status, therapy adherence, therapy response); initial set-up and patient education on use of equipment**
EXCLUDES *Reporting more than once per episode of care*

● **98976** **device(s) supply with scheduled (eg, daily) recording(s) and/or programmed alert(s) transmission to monitor respiratory system, each 30 days**

● **98977** **device(s) supply with scheduled (eg, daily) recording(s) and/or programmed alert(s) transmission to monitor musculoskeletal system, each 30 days**

98980-98981 Remote Therapeutic Monitoring Treatment Management Services

INCLUDES Patient management via remote therapeutic monitoring for specific treatment plan
EXCLUDES *Time counted during month of reporting for:*
E/M service(s) (99202-99205, 99211-99215, 99221-99223, 99231-99233, 99251-99255, 99324-99328, 99334-99337, 99341-99345, 99347-99350)
Other reported services

● **98980** **Remote therapeutic monitoring treatment management services, physician or other qualified health care professional time in a calendar month requiring at least one interactive communication with the patient or caregiver during the calendar month; first 20 minutes**
INCLUDES Reporting once each 30 days
EXCLUDES *Collection/interpretation physiologic data (99091)*
Remote monitoring wireless pulmonary artery sensor (93264)
Remote physiologic monitoring treatment management services (99457-99458)
Reporting services less than 20 minutes
Self-measured blood pressure monitoring ([99473, 99474])

● + **98981** **each additional 20 minutes (List separately in addition to code for primary procedure)**
EXCLUDES *Reporting services less than additional 20 minutes*
Code first (98980)
🔲 0.00 ⚖ 0.00 **FUD** 000

99000-99091 [99091] Supplemental Services and Supplies

INCLUDES Supplemental reporting for services adjunct to basic service provided

99000 **Handling and/or conveyance of specimen for transfer from the office to a laboratory**
🔲 0.00 ⚖ 0.00 **FUD** XXX   E ▢
AMA: 2018,Dec,10; 2018,Dec,10; 2018,Feb,11; 2018,Jan,8; 2017,Jan,8; 2016,Jan,13

99001 **Handling and/or conveyance of specimen for transfer from the patient in other than an office to a laboratory (distance may be indicated)**
🔲 0.00 ⚖ 0.00 **FUD** XXX   E ▢
AMA: 2018,Dec,10; 2018,Dec,10; 2018,Feb,11; 2018,Jan,8; 2017,Jan,8; 2016,Jan,13

99002 **Handling, conveyance, and/or any other service in connection with the implementation of an order involving devices (eg, designing, fitting, packaging, handling, delivery or mailing) when devices such as orthotics, protectives, prosthetics are fabricated by an outside laboratory or shop but which items have been designed, and are to be fitted and adjusted by the attending physician or other qualified health care professional**
EXCLUDES *Venous blood routine collection (36415)*
🔲 0.00 ⚖ 0.00 **FUD** XXX   B ▢
AMA: 2018,Dec,10; 2018,Dec,10; 2018,Feb,11; 2018,Jan,8; 2017,Jan,8; 2016,Jan,13

99024 **Postoperative follow-up visit, normally included in the surgical package, to indicate that an evaluation and management service was performed during a postoperative period for a reason(s) related to the original procedure**
🔲 0.00 ⚖ 0.00 **FUD** XXX   B ▢
AMA: 2018,Dec,10; 2018,Dec,10; 2018,Feb,11; 2018,Jan,8; 2017,Jul,9; 2017,Jan,3; 2017,Jan,8; 2016,Jan,13

99026 **Hospital mandated on call service; in-hospital, each hour**
EXCLUDES *Physician stand-by services with prolonged physician attendance (99360)*
Time spent providing procedures or services that may be separately reported
🔲 0.00 ⚖ 0.00 **FUD** XXX   E ▢
AMA: 2018,Dec,10; 2018,Dec,10; 2018,Feb,11; 2018,Jan,8; 2017,Jan,8; 2016,Jan,13

99027   **out-of-hospital, each hour**

> EXCLUDES *Physician stand-by services with prolonged physician attendance (99360)*
> *Time spent providing procedures or services that may be separately reported*

📓 0.00   ⚕ 0.00   **FUD** XXX   E 🖵

AMA: 2018,Dec,10; 2018,Dec,10; 2018,Feb,11; 2018,Jan,8; 2017,Jan,8; 2016,Jan,13

99050   **Services provided in the office at times other than regularly scheduled office hours, or days when the office is normally closed (eg, holidays, Saturday or Sunday), in addition to basic service**

> Code also more than one adjunct code per encounter when appropriate
> Code first basic service provided

📓 0.00   ⚕ 0.00   **FUD** XXX   S B 🖵

AMA: 2018,Dec,10; 2018,Dec,10; 2018,Feb,11; 2018,Jan,8; 2017,Jan,8; 2016,Jan,13

99051   **Service(s) provided in the office during regularly scheduled evening, weekend, or holiday office hours, in addition to basic service**

> Code also more than one adjunct code per encounter when appropriate
> Code first basic service provided

📓 0.00   ⚕ 0.00   **FUD** XXX   S B 🖵

AMA: 2018,Dec,10; 2018,Dec,10; 2018,Feb,11; 2018,Jan,8; 2017,Jan,8; 2016,Jan,13

99053   **Service(s) provided between 10:00 PM and 8:00 AM at 24-hour facility, in addition to basic service**

> Code also more than one adjunct code per encounter when appropriate
> Code first basic service provided

📓 0.00   ⚕ 0.00   **FUD** XXX   S B 🖵

AMA: 2018,Dec,10; 2018,Dec,10; 2018,Feb,11; 2018,Jan,8; 2017,Jan,8; 2016,Jan,13

99056   **Service(s) typically provided in the office, provided out of the office at request of patient, in addition to basic service**

> Code also more than one adjunct code per encounter when appropriate
> Code first basic service provided

📓 0.00   ⚕ 0.00   **FUD** XXX   S B 🖵

AMA: 2018,Dec,10; 2018,Dec,10; 2018,Feb,11; 2018,Jan,8; 2017,Jan,8; 2016,Jan,13

99058   **Service(s) provided on an emergency basis in the office, which disrupts other scheduled office services, in addition to basic service**

> Code also more than one adjunct code per encounter when appropriate
> Code first basic service provided

📓 0.00   ⚕ 0.00   **FUD** XXX   S B 🖵

AMA: 2018,Dec,10; 2018,Dec,10; 2018,Feb,11; 2018,Jan,8; 2017,Jan,8; 2016,Jan,13

99060   **Service(s) provided on an emergency basis, out of the office, which disrupts other scheduled office services, in addition to basic service**

> Code also more than one adjunct code per encounter when appropriate
> Code first basic service provided

📓 0.00   ⚕ 0.00   **FUD** XXX   S B 🖵

AMA: 2018,Dec,10; 2018,Dec,10; 2018,Feb,11; 2018,Jan,8; 2017,Jan,8; 2016,Jan,13

99070   **Supplies and materials (except spectacles), provided by the physician or other qualified health care professional over and above those usually included with the office visit or other services rendered (list drugs, trays, supplies, or materials provided)**

> EXCLUDES *Additional supplies, materials, and clinical staff time required for patient symptom review, personal protective equipment (PPE) use, and heightened cleaning processes due to respiratory-transmitted infectious disease during a declared public health emergency (PHE), as defined by law (99072)*
> *Spectacles supply*

📓 0.00   ⚕ 0.00   **FUD** XXX   B 🖵

AMA: 2020,SepSE,1; 2020,SepSE,1; 2019,Apr,10; 2019,Feb,10; 2018,Dec,10; 2018,Dec,10; 2018,Jun,11; 2018,Mar,7; 2018,Jan,3; 2018,Jan,8; 2017,Sep,14; 2017,Jan,8; 2017,Jan,6; 2016,Jan,13

99071   **Educational supplies, such as books, tapes, and pamphlets, for the patient's education at cost to physician or other qualified health care professional**

📓 0.00   ⚕ 0.00   **FUD** XXX   B 🖵

AMA: 2018,Dec,10; 2018,Dec,10; 2018,Jan,8; 2017,Jan,8; 2016,Jan,13

● **99072**   **Additional supplies, materials, and clinical staff time over and above those usually included in an office visit or other nonfacility service(s), when performed during a Public Health Emergency, as defined by law, due to respiratory-transmitted infectious disease**

> INCLUDES *Additional supplies, materials, and clinical staff time required for patient symptom review, personal protective equipment (PPE) use, and heightened cleaning processes due to respiratory-transmitted infectious disease during a declared public health emergency (PHE), as defined by law*
> EXCLUDES *Reporting more than one time per encounter, despite number services provided during encounter*
> *Supplies and materials provided, above those normally included in the encounter, unrelated to a declared PHE (99070)*

AMA: 2020,SepSE,1

99075   **Medical testimony**

📓 0.00   ⚕ 0.00   **FUD** XXX   E 🖵

AMA: 2018,Dec,10; 2018,Dec,10; 2018,Jan,8; 2017,Jan,8; 2016,Jan,13

99078   **Physician or other qualified health care professional qualified by education, training, licensure/regulation (when applicable) educational services rendered to patients in a group setting (eg, prenatal, obesity, or diabetic instructions)**

📓 0.00   ⚕ 0.00   **FUD** XXX   N 🖵

AMA: 2018,Dec,10; 2018,Dec,10; 2018,Jan,8; 2017,Jan,8; 2016,Jan,13

99080   **Special reports such as insurance forms, more than the information conveyed in the usual medical communications or standard reporting form**

> EXCLUDES *Completion workmen's compensation forms (99455-99456)*

📓 0.00   ⚕ 0.00   **FUD** XXX   B 🖵

AMA: 2018,Dec,10; 2018,Dec,10; 2018,Jan,8; 2017,Jan,8; 2016,Jan,13

99082   **Unusual travel (eg, transportation and escort of patient)**

📓 0.00   ⚕ 0.00   **FUD** XXX   B 80 🖵

AMA: 2018,Dec,10; 2018,Dec,10; 2018,Jan,8; 2017,Jan,8; 2016,Jan,13

99091   **Resequenced code. See code following resequenced code 99454.**

26/TC PC/TC Only	A2-Z3 ASC Payment	50 Bilateral	♂ Male Only	♀ Female Only	📓 Facility RVU	⚕ Non-Facility RVU	🖵 CCI	CLIA
FUD Follow-up Days	**CMS:** IOM	**AMA:** CPT Asst	A-Y OPPSI	80/80 Surg Assist Allowed / w/Doc	Lab Crosswalk		Radiology Crosswalk	

530   CPT © 2021 American Medical Association. All Rights Reserved.   © 2021 Optum360, LLC

99100-99140 Modifying Factors for Anesthesia Services

CMS: 100-04,12,140.3 Payment for Qualified Nonphysician Anesthetists; 100-04,12,140.3.3 Billing Modifiers; 100-04,12,140.3.4 General Billing Instructions; 100-04,12,140.4.1 An Anesthesiologist and Qualified Nonphysician Anesthetist Work Together; 100-04,12,140.4.2 Anesthetist and Anesthesiologist in a Single Procedure; 100-04,12,140.4.4 Conversion Factors for Anesthesia Services; 100-04,4,250.3.2 Anesthesia in a Hospital Outpatient Setting

Code first primary anesthesia procedure

+   99100   Anesthesia for patient of extreme age, younger than 1 year and older than 70 (List separately in addition to code for primary anesthesia procedure)   Ⓐ

> EXCLUDES   *Anesthesia services for infants one year old or less (00326, 00561, 00834, 00836)*
>
> 🚑 0.00   ☍ 0.00   **FUD** ZZZ   Ⓑ▱
>
> **AMA:** 2019,Oct,10; 2018,Jan,8; 2017,Dec,8; 2017,Jan,8; 2016,Jan,13

+   99116   Anesthesia complicated by utilization of total body hypothermia (List separately in addition to code for primary anesthesia procedure)

> EXCLUDES   *Anesthesia for procedures on heart/pericardial sac/great vessels chest with pump oxygenator (00561)*
>
> 🚑 0.00   ☍ 0.00   **FUD** ZZZ   Ⓑ▱
>
> **AMA:** 2019,Oct,10; 2018,Jan,8; 2017,Dec,8; 2017,Jan,8; 2016,Jan,13

+   99135   Anesthesia complicated by utilization of controlled hypotension (List separately in addition to code for primary anesthesia procedure)

> EXCLUDES   *Anesthesia for procedures on heart/pericardial sac/great vessels chest with pump oxygenator (00561)*
>
> 🚑 0.00   ☍ 0.00   **FUD** ZZZ   Ⓑ▱
>
> **AMA:** 2019,Oct,10; 2018,Jan,8; 2017,Dec,8; 2017,Jan,8; 2016,Jan,13

+   99140   Anesthesia complicated by emergency conditions (specify) (List separately in addition to code for primary anesthesia procedure)

> INCLUDES   Conditions where treatment delay could be dangerous to life or health
>
> 🚑 0.00   ☍ 0.00   **FUD** ZZZ   Ⓑ▱
>
> **AMA:** 2019,Oct,10; 2018,Jan,8; 2017,Dec,8; 2017,Jan,8; 2016,Jan,13

99151-99157 Moderate Sedation Services

INCLUDES   Intraservice work that begins with sedation administration and ends when procedure complete
Monitoring:
    Patient response to drugs
    Vital signs
Ordering and providing drug to patient (first and subsequent)
Pre- and postservice procedures

99151   Moderate sedation services provided by the same physician or other qualified health care professional performing the diagnostic or therapeutic service that the sedation supports, requiring the presence of an independent trained observer to assist in the monitoring of the patient's level of consciousness and physiological status; initial 15 minutes of intraservice time, patient younger than 5 years of age

> INCLUDES   First 15 minutes intraservice time for patients under age 5
>
> Services provided to patients by same service provider for which moderate sedation necessary with monitoring by trained observer
>
> 🚑 0.72   ☍ 2.12   **FUD** XXX   ⊘Ⓝ▱
>
> **AMA:** 2020,Nov,12; 2019,Feb,10; 2018,Jan,8; 2017,Sep,11; 2017,Jun,3; 2017,Jan,3

99152   initial 15 minutes of intraservice time, patient age 5 years or older

> INCLUDES   First 15 minutes intraservice time for patients age 5 and over
>
> Services provided to patients by same service provider for which moderate sedation necessary with monitoring by trained observer
>
> 🚑 0.35   ☍ 1.44   **FUD** XXX   ⊘Ⓝ▱
>
> **AMA:** 2020,Nov,12; 2019,May,10; 2019,Feb,10; 2018,Jan,8; 2017,Sep,11; 2017,Jun,3; 2017,Jan,3

+   99153   each additional 15 minutes intraservice time (List separately in addition to code for primary service)

> INCLUDES   Services provided to patients by same service provider for which moderate sedation necessary with monitoring by trained observer (99155-99157)
>
> EXCLUDES   *Services provided to patients by physician/other qualified health care professional other than provider rendering service*
>
> Code first (99151-99152)
>
> 🚑 0.30   ☍ 0.30   **FUD** ZZZ   Ⓝ ⓉⒸ ▱
>
> **AMA:** 2020,Nov,12; 2019,May,10; 2019,Feb,10; 2018,Jan,8; 2017,Sep,11; 2017,Jun,3; 2017,Jan,3

99155   Moderate sedation services provided by a physician or other qualified health care professional other than the physician or other qualified health care professional performing the diagnostic or therapeutic service that the sedation supports; initial 15 minutes of intraservice time, patient younger than 5 years of age

> INCLUDES   First 15 minutes intraservice time for patients under age 5
>
> Services provided to patients by physician/other qualified health care professional other than provider rendering service for which moderate sedation necessary
>
> 🚑 2.54   ☍ 2.54   **FUD** XXX   Ⓝ▱
>
> **AMA:** 2020,Nov,12; 2019,Feb,10; 2018,Jan,8; 2017,Sep,11; 2017,Jun,3; 2017,Jan,3

99156   initial 15 minutes of intraservice time, patient age 5 years or older

> INCLUDES   First 15 minutes intraservice time for patients age 5 and over
>
> Services provided to patients by physician/other qualified health care professional other than provider rendering service for which moderate sedation necessary
>
> 🚑 2.24   ☍ 2.24   **FUD** XXX   Ⓝ▱
>
> **AMA:** 2020,Nov,12; 2019,Feb,10; 2018,Jan,8; 2017,Sep,11; 2017,Jun,3; 2017,Jan,3

+   99157   each additional 15 minutes intraservice time (List separately in addition to code for primary service)

> INCLUDES   Each subsequent 15 minutes services
>
> Services provided to patients by physician/other qualified health care professional other than provider rendering service for which moderate sedation necessary (99151-99152)
>
> EXCLUDES   *Services provided to patients by same service provider for which moderate sedation necessary with monitoring by trained observer (99151-99152)*
>
> Code first (99155-99156)
>
> 🚑 1.82   ☍ 1.82   **FUD** ZZZ   Ⓝ▱
>
> **AMA:** 2020,Nov,12; 2019,Feb,10; 2018,Jan,8; 2017,Sep,11; 2017,Jun,3; 2017,Jan,3

99170 Specialized Examination of Child

EXCLUDES   *Moderate sedation (99151-99157)*

99170   Anogenital examination, magnified, in childhood for suspected trauma, including image recording when performed   Ⓐ

> 🚑 2.47   ☍ 4.48   **FUD** 000   Ⓣ▱
>
> **AMA:** 2018,Jan,8; 2017,Jan,8; 2016,Jan,13

● New Code   ▲ Revised Code   ○ Reinstated   ● New Web Release   ▲ Revised Web Release   + Add-on   Unlisted   Not Covered   # Resequenced
㊿ Optum Mod 50 Exempt   ⊘ AMA Mod 51 Exempt   �成 Optum Mod 51 Exempt   ㊢ Mod 63 Exempt   ⚬ Non-FDA Drug   ★ Telemedicine   Ⓜ Maternity   Ⓐ Age Edit

Medicine *(vertical left margin)*

99172 — 99506 *(vertical left margin)*

99172-99173 Visual Acuity Screening Tests

INCLUDES *Graduated visual acuity stimuli that allow quantitative determination/estimation visual acuity*

EXCLUDES *General ophthalmological or E/M services*

99172 **Visual function screening, automated or semi-automated bilateral quantitative determination of visual acuity, ocular alignment, color vision by pseudoisochromatic plates, and field of vision (may include all or some screening of the determination[s] for contrast sensitivity, vision under glare)**

    EXCLUDES *Screening for visual acuity, amblyogenic factors, retinal polarization scan (99173, 99174 [99177], 0469T)*

    🚑 0.00   ⚕ 0.00   **FUD** XXX   E 🖵

    AMA: 2018,Jan,8; 2017,Jan,8; 2016,Jan,13

99173 **Screening test of visual acuity, quantitative, bilateral**

    EXCLUDES *Screening for visual function, amblyogenic factors (99172, 99174, [99177])*

    🚑 0.08   ⚕ 0.08   **FUD** XXX   E 🖵

    AMA: 2018,Jan,8; 2017,Jan,8; 2016,Jan,13

99174-99177 [99177] Screening For Amblyogenic Factors

EXCLUDES *General ophthalmological services (92002-92014)*
Screening for visual acuity (99172-99173, [99177])

99174 **Instrument-based ocular screening (eg, photoscreening, automated-refraction), bilateral; with remote analysis and report**

    EXCLUDES *Ocular screening on-site analysis ([99177])*

    🚑 0.16   ⚕ 0.16   **FUD** XXX   E 🖵

    AMA: 2018,Feb,3; 2018,Jan,8; 2017,Jan,8; 2016,Mar,10; 2016,Jan,13

**99177** **with on-site analysis**

    EXCLUDES *Remote ocular screening (99174)*
                 Retinal polarization scan (0469T)

    🚑 0.13   ⚕ 0.13   **FUD** XXX   E 🖵

    AMA: 2018,Feb,3; 2018,Jan,8; 2017,Jan,8; 2016,Mar,10

99175-99177 [99177] Drug Administration to Induce Vomiting

EXCLUDES *Diagnostic gastric lavage (43754-43755)*
Diagnostic gastric intubation (43754-43755)

99175 **Ipecac or similar administration for individual emesis and continued observation until stomach adequately emptied of poison**

    🚑 0.73   ⚕ 0.73   **FUD** XXX   N 80 🖵

    AMA: 1997,Nov,1

99177 **Resequenced code. See code following 99174.**

99183-99184 Hyperbaric Oxygen Therapy

CMS: 100-03,20.29 Hyperbaric Oxygen Therapy; 100-04,32,30.1 HBO Therapy for Lower Extremity Diabetic Wounds

EXCLUDES *E/M services, when performed*
Other procedures such as wound debridement, when performed

99183 **Physician or other qualified health care professional attendance and supervision of hyperbaric oxygen therapy, per session**

    🚑 3.12   ⚕ 3.12   **FUD** XXX   B 80 26 🖵

    AMA: 2018,Jan,8; 2017,Jan,8; 2016,Jan,13

99184 **Initiation of selective head or total body hypothermia in the critically ill neonate, includes appropriate patient selection by review of clinical, imaging and laboratory data, confirmation of esophageal temperature probe location, evaluation of amplitude EEG, supervision of controlled hypothermia, and assessment of patient tolerance of cooling**   A

    EXCLUDES *Reporting code more than one time per hospitalization*

    🚑 6.33   ⚕ 6.33   **FUD** XXX   C 80 🖵

    AMA: 2018,Jan,8; 2017,Jan,8; 2016,Jan,13

99188 Topical Fluoride Application

99188 **Application of topical fluoride varnish by a physician or other qualified health care professional**

    🚑 0.29   ⚕ 0.35   **FUD** XXX   E 80 🖵

99190-99192 Assemble and Manage Pump with Oxygenator/Heat Exchange

99190 **Assembly and operation of pump with oxygenator or heat exchanger (with or without ECG and/or pressure monitoring); each hour**

    🚑 0.00   ⚕ 0.00   **FUD** XXX   C 🖵

    AMA: 1997,Nov,1

99191 **45 minutes**

    🚑 0.00   ⚕ 0.00   **FUD** XXX   C 🖵

    AMA: 1997,Nov,1

99192 **30 minutes**

    🚑 0.00   ⚕ 0.00   **FUD** XXX   C 🖵

    AMA: 1997,Nov,1

99195-99199 Therapeutic Phlebotomy and Unlisted Procedures

99195 **Phlebotomy, therapeutic (separate procedure)**

    🚑 2.86   ⚕ 2.86   **FUD** XXX   01 80 🖵

    AMA: 2018,Jan,8; 2017,Jan,8; 2016,Jan,13

99199 **Unlisted special service, procedure or report**

    🚑 0.00   ⚕ 0.00   **FUD** XXX   B 80 🖵

    AMA: 2018,Jan,8; 2017,Jan,8; 2016,Jan,13

99500-99602 Home Visit By Non-Physician Professionals

INCLUDES *Services performed by non-physician providers*
Services provided in patient's:
    Assisted living apartment
    Custodial care facility
    Group home
    Nontraditional private home
    Residence
    School

EXCLUDES *Home visits performed by physicians (99341-99350)*
Other services/procedures provided by physicians to patients at home

Code also:
    Home visit E/M codes when health care provider authorized to report (99341-99350)
    Significant separately identifiable E/M service, when performed

99500 **Home visit for prenatal monitoring and assessment to include fetal heart rate, non-stress test, uterine monitoring, and gestational diabetes monitoring**   M ♀

    🚑 0.00   ⚕ 0.00   **FUD** XXX   E 🖵

    AMA: 2018,Jan,8; 2017,Jan,8; 2016,Jan,13

99501 **Home visit for postnatal assessment and follow-up care**   M ♀

    🚑 0.00   ⚕ 0.00   **FUD** XXX   E 🖵

    AMA: 2018,Jan,8; 2017,Jan,8; 2016,Jan,13

99502 **Home visit for newborn care and assessment**   A

    🚑 0.00   ⚕ 0.00   **FUD** XXX   E 🖵

    AMA: 2018,Jan,8; 2017,Jan,8; 2016,Jan,13

99503 **Home visit for respiratory therapy care (eg, bronchodilator, oxygen therapy, respiratory assessment, apnea evaluation)**

    🚑 0.00   ⚕ 0.00   **FUD** XXX   E 🖵

    AMA: 2018,Jan,8; 2017,Jan,8; 2016,Jan,13

99504 **Home visit for mechanical ventilation care**

    🚑 0.00   ⚕ 0.00   **FUD** XXX   E 🖵

    AMA: 2018,Jan,8; 2017,Jan,8; 2016,Jan,13

99505 **Home visit for stoma care and maintenance including colostomy and cystostomy**

    🚑 0.00   ⚕ 0.00   **FUD** XXX   E 🖵

    AMA: 2018,Jan,8; 2017,Jan,8; 2016,Jan,13

99506 **Home visit for intramuscular injections**

    🚑 0.00   ⚕ 0.00   **FUD** XXX   E 🖵

    AMA: 2018,Jan,8; 2017,Jan,8; 2016,Jan,13

26/TC PC/TC Only	A2-Z3 ASC Payment	50 Bilateral	♂ Male Only	♀ Female Only	🚑 Facility RVU	⚕ Non-Facility RVU	🖵 CCI	✕ CLIA
FUD Follow-up Days	**CMS:** IOM	**AMA:** CPT Asst	A-Y OPPSI	80/80 Surg Assist Allowed / w/Doc		🖵 Lab Crosswalk		🖵 Radiology Crosswalk

99507 Home visit for care and maintenance of catheter(s) (eg, urinary, drainage, and enteral)

    0.00   0.00   **FUD** XXX   E ▣

    AMA: 2018,Jan,8; 2017,Jan,8; 2016,Jan,13

99509 Home visit for assistance with activities of daily living and personal care

    EXCLUDES   *Medical nutrition therapy/assessment home services (97802-97804)*

            Self-care/home management training (97535)

            Speech therapy home services (92507-92508)

    0.00   0.00   **FUD** XXX   E ▣

    AMA: 2018,Jan,8; 2017,Jan,8; 2016,Jan,13

99510 Home visit for individual, family, or marriage counseling

    0.00   0.00   **FUD** XXX   E ▣

    AMA: 2018,Jan,8; 2017,Jan,8; 2016,Jan,13

99511 Home visit for fecal impaction management and enema administration

    0.00   0.00   **FUD** XXX   E ▣

    AMA: 2018,Jan,8; 2017,Jan,8; 2016,Jan,13

99512 Home visit for hemodialysis

    EXCLUDES   *Peritoneal dialysis home infusion (99601-99602)*

    0.00   0.00   **FUD** XXX   E ▣

    AMA: 2018,Jan,8; 2017,Jan,8; 2016,Jan,13

99600 Unlisted home visit service or procedure

    0.00   0.00   **FUD** XXX   E ▣

    AMA: 2018,Jan,8; 2017,Jan,8; 2016,Jan,13

99601 Home infusion/specialty drug administration, per visit (up to 2 hours);

    0.00   0.00   **FUD** XXX   E ▣

    AMA: 2005,Nov,1-9; 2003,Oct,7

+ **99602** each additional hour (List separately in addition to code for primary procedure)

    Code first (99601)

    0.00   0.00   **FUD** XXX   E ▣

    AMA: 2005,Nov,1-9; 2003,Oct,7

99605-96607 Medication Management By Pharmacist

INCLUDES   Direct (face-to-face) assessment and intervention by pharmacist:

    Managing medication complications and/or interactions

    Maximizing patient's response to drug therapy

   Documenting required elements:

    Advice given regarding improvement treatment compliance and outcomes

    Medication profile (prescription and nonprescription)

    Review applicable patient history

EXCLUDES   *Routine tasks associated with dispensing and related activities (e.g., providing product information)*

99605 Medication therapy management service(s) provided by a pharmacist, individual, face-to-face with patient, with assessment and intervention if provided; initial 15 minutes, new patient

    0.00   0.00   **FUD** XXX   E ▣

    AMA: 2018,Apr,9; 2018,Jan,8; 2017,Jan,8; 2016,Jan,13

99606 initial 15 minutes, established patient

    0.00   0.00   **FUD** XXX   E ▣

    AMA: 2018,Apr,9; 2018,Jan,8; 2017,Jan,8; 2016,Jan,13

+ **99607** each additional 15 minutes (List separately in addition to code for primary service)

    Code first (99605, 99606)

    0.00   0.00   **FUD** XXX   E ▣

    AMA: 2018,Apr,9; 2018,Jan,8; 2017,Jan,8; 2016,Jan,13

Evaluation and Management Guidelines Common to All E/M Services

Information unique to this section is defined or identified below.

For additional information about evaluation and management services, see Appendix C: Evaluation and Management Extended Guidelines. This appendix includes comprehensive explanations and instructions for the correct selection of an E/M service code based on federal documentation standards.

Classification of Evaluation and Management (E/M) Services

The E/M section is divided into broad categories such as office visits, hospital visits, and consultations. Most of the categories are further divided into two or more subcategories of E/M services. For example, there are two subcategories of office visits (new patient and established patient) and there are two subcategories of hospital visits (initial and subsequent). The subcategories of E/M services are further classified into levels of E/M services that are identified by specific codes.

The basic format of the levels of E/M services is the same for most categories. First, a unique code number is listed. Second, the place and/or type of service is specified, eg, office consultation. Third, the content of the service is defined. Fourth, time is specified. (A detailed discussion of time is provided following the Decision Tree for New vs Established Patients.)

Definitions of Commonly Used Terms

Certain key words and phrases are used throughout the E/M section. The following definitions are intended to reduce the potential for differing interpretations and to increase the consistency of reporting by physicians and other qualified health care professionals. The definitions in the E/M section are provided solely for the basis of code selection.

Some definitions are common to all categories of services, and others are specific to one or more categories only.

New and Established Patient

Solely for the purposes of distinguishing between new and established patients, **professional services** are those face-to-face services rendered by physicians and other qualified health care professionals who may report E/M services with a specific CPT® code or codes. A new patient is one who has not received any professional services from the physician/qualified health care professional or another physician/qualified health care professional of the **exact** same specialty **and subspecialty** who belongs to the same group practice, within the past three years.

An established patient is one who has received professional services from the physician/qualified health care professional or another physician/qualified health care professional of the **exact** same specialty **and subspecialty** who belongs to the same group practice, within the past three years. See the decision tree on the following page.

When a physician/qualified health care professional is on call or covering for another physician/qualified health care professional, the patient's encounter is classified as it would have been by the physician/qualified health care professional who is not available. When advanced practice nurses and physician assistants are working with physicians, they are considered as working in the exact same specialty and exact same subspecialties as the physician.

No distinction is made between new and established patients in the emergency department. E/M services in the emergency department category may be reported for any new or established patient who presents for treatment in the emergency department.

The decision tree on the following page is provided to aid in determining whether to report the E/M service provided as a new or an established patient encounter.

Time

The inclusion of time in the definitions of levels of E/M services has been implicit in prior editions of the CPT codebook. The inclusion of time as an explicit factor beginning in CPT 1992 was done to assist in selecting the most appropriate level of E/M services. Beginning with CPT 2021, except for 99211, time alone may be used to select the appropriate code level for the office or other outpatient E/M services codes (99202, 99203, 99204, 99205, 99212, 99213, 99214, 99215). Different categories of services use time differently. It is important to review the instructions for each category.

Time is **not** a descriptive component for the emergency department levels of E/M services because emergency department services are typically provided on a variable intensity basis, often involving multiple encounters with several patients over an extended period of time. Therefore, it is often difficult to provide accurate estimates of the time spent face-to-face with the patient.

Time may be used to select a code level in office or other outpatient services whether or not counseling and/or coordination of care dominates the service. Time may only be used for selecting the level of the **other** E/M services when counseling and/or coordination of care dominates the service.

When time is used for reporting E/M services codes, the time defined in the service descriptors is used for selecting the appropriate level of services. The E/M services for which these guidelines apply require a face-to-face encounter with the physician or other qualified health care professional. For office or other outpatient services, if the physician's or other qualified health care professional's time is spent in the supervision of clinical staff who perform the face-to-face services of the encounter, use 99211.

A shared or split visit is defined as a visit in which a physician and other qualified health care professional(s) jointly provide the face-to-face and non-face-to-face work related to the visit. When time is being used to select the appropriate level of services for which time-based reporting of shared or split visits is allowed, the time personally spent by the physician and other qualified health care professional(s) assessing and managing the patient on the date of the encounter is summed to define total time. Only distinct time should be summed for shared or split visits (ie, when two or more individuals jointly meet with or discuss the patient, only the time of one individual should be counted).

When prolonged time occurs, the appropriate prolonged services code may be reported. The appropriate time should be documented in the medical record when it is used as the basis for code selection.

Face-to-face time (outpatient consultations [99241, 99242, 99243, 99244, 99245], domiciliary, rest home, or custodial services [99324, 99325, 99326, 99327, 99328, 99334, 99335, 99336, 99337], home services [99341, 99342, 99343, 99344, 99345, 99347, 99348, 99349, 99350], cognitive assessment and care plan services [99483]): For coding purposes, face-to-face time for these services is defined as only that time spent face-to-face with the patient and/or family. This includes the time spent performing such tasks as obtaining a history, examination, and counseling the patient.

Unit/floor time (hospital observation services [99218, 99219, 99220, 99224, 99225, 99226, 99234, 99235, 99236], hospital inpatient services [99221, 99222, 99223, 99231, 99232, 99233], inpatient consultations [99251, 99252, 99253, 99254, 99255], nursing facility services [99304, 99305, 99306, 99307, 99308, 99309, 99310, 99315, 99316, 99318]): For coding purposes, time for these services is defined as unit/floor time, which includes the time present on the patient's hospital unit and at the bedside rendering services for that patient. This includes the time to establish and/or review the patient's chart, examine the patient, write notes, and communicate with other professionals and the patient's family.

Total time on the date of the encounter (office or other outpatient services [99202, 99203, 99204, 99205, 99212, 99213, 99214, 99215]): For coding purposes, time for these services is the total time on the date of the encounter. It includes both the face-to-face and non-face-to-face time personally spent by the physician and/or other qualified health care professional(s) on the day of the encounter (includes time in activities that require the physician or other qualified health care professional and does not include time in activities normally performed by clinical staff).

Physician/other qualified health care professional time includes the following activities, when performed:

- Preparing to see the patient (eg, review of tests)
- Obtaining and/or reviewing separately obtained history
- Performing a medically appropriate examination and/or evaluation
- Counseling and educating the patient/family/caregiver
- Ordering medications, tests, or procedures
- Referring and communicating with other health care professionals (when not separately reported)
- Documenting clinical information in the electronic or other health record
- Independently interpreting results (not separately reported) and communicating results to the patient/family/caregiver
- Care coordination (not separately reported)

Do not count time spent on the following:

- The performance of other services that are reported separately
- Travel
- Teaching that is general and not limited to discussion that is required for the management of a specific patient

Concurrent Care and Transfer of Care

Concurrent care is the provision of similar services (eg, hospital visits) to the same patient by more than one physician or other qualified health care professional on the same day. When concurrent care is provided, no special reporting is required. Transfer of care is the process whereby a physician or other qualified health care professional who is managing some or all of a patient's problems relinquishes this responsibility to another physician or other qualified health care professional who explicitly agrees to accept this responsibility and who, from the initial encounter, is not providing consultative services. The physician or other qualified health care professional transferring care is then no longer providing care for these problems though he or she may continue providing care for other conditions when appropriate. Consultation codes should not be reported by the physician or other qualified health care professional who has agreed to accept transfer of care before an initial evaluation, but they are appropriate to report if the decision to accept transfer of care cannot be made until after the initial consultation evaluation, regardless of site of service.

Decision Tree for New vs Established Patients

Counseling

Counseling is a discussion with a patient and/or family concerning one or more of the following areas:

- Diagnostic results, impressions, and/or recommended diagnostic studies
- Prognosis
- Risks and benefits of management (treatment) options
- Instructions for management (treatment) and/or follow-up
- Importance of compliance with chosen management (treatment) options
- Risk factor reduction
- Patient and family education
  (For psychotherapy, see 90832–90834, 90836–90840)

Services Reported Separately

Any specifically identifiable procedure or service (ie, identified with a specific CPT code) performed on the date of E/M services may be reported separately.

The ordering and actual performance and/or interpretation of diagnostic tests/studies during a patient encounter are not included in determining the levels of E/M services when the professional interpretation of those tests/studies is reported separately by the physician or other qualified health care professional reporting the E/M service. Tests that do not require separate interpretation (eg, tests that are results only) and are analyzed as part of MDM do not count as an independent interpretation, but may be counted as ordered or reviewed for selecting an MDM level. Physician performance of diagnostic tests/studies for which specific CPT codes are available may be reported separately, in addition to the appropriate E/M code. The physician's interpretation of the results of diagnostic tests/studies (ie, professional component) with preparation of a separation distinctly identifiable signed written report may also be reported separately, using the appropriate CPT code and, if required, with modifier 26 appended. If a test/study is independently interpreted in order to manage the patient as part of the E/M service, but is not separately reported, it is part of MDM.

The physician or other qualified health care professional may need to indicate that on the day a procedure or service identified by a CPT code was performed, the patient's condition required a significant separately identifiable E/M service. The E/M service may be caused or prompted by the symptoms or condition for which the procedure and/or service was provided. This circumstance may be reported by adding modifier 25 to the appropriate level of E/M service. As such, different diagnoses are not required for reporting of the procedure and the E/M services on the same date.

Levels of E/M Services

Within each category or subcategory of E/M service, there are three to five levels of E/M services available for reporting purposes. Levels of E/M services are **not** interchangeable among the different categories or subcategories of service. For example, the first level of E/M services in the subcategory of office visit, new patient, does not have the same definition as the first level of E/M services in the subcategory of office visit, established patient. Each level of E/M services may be used by all physicians or other qualified health care professionals.

The levels of E/M services include examinations, evaluations, treatments, conferences with or concerning patients, preventive pediatric and adult health supervision, and similar medical services, such as the determination of the need and/or location for appropriate care. Medical screening includes the history, examination, and medical decision-making required to determine the need and/or location for appropriate care and treatment of the patient (eg, office and other outpatient setting, emergency department, nursing facility). The levels of E/M services encompass the wide variations in skill, effort, time, responsibility, and medical knowledge required for the prevention or diagnosis and treatment of illness or injury and the promotion of optimal health. Each level of E/M services may be used by all physicians or other qualified health care professionals.

The descriptors for the levels of E/M services recognize seven components, six of which are used in defining the levels of E/M services. These components are:

- History
- Examination
- Medical decision making
- Counseling
- Coordination of care
- Nature of presenting problem
- Time

The first three of these components (history, examination, and medical decision making) are considered the **key** components in selecting a level of E/M services. (See "Determine the Extent of History Obtained.")

The next three components (counseling, coordination of care, and the nature of the presenting problem) are considered **contributory** factors in the majority of encounters. Although the first two of these contributory factors are important E/M services, it is not required that these services be provided at every patient encounter.

Coordination of care with other physicians, other qualified health care professionals, or agencies without a patient encounter on that day is reported using the case management codes.

The final component, time, is discussed in detail before the Decision Tree for New vs Established Patients.

Chief Complaint
A chief complaint is a concise statement describing the symptom, problem, condition, diagnosis, or other factor that is the reason for the encounter, usually stated in the patient's words.

History of Present Illness
A chronological description of the development of the patient's present illness from the first sign and/or symptom to the present. This includes a description of location, quality, severity, timing, context, modifying factors, and associated signs and symptoms significantly related to the presenting problem.

Nature of Presenting Problem
A presenting problem is a disease, condition, illness, injury, symptom, sign, finding, complaint, or other reason for encounter, with or without a diagnosis being established at the time of the encounter. The E/M codes recognize five types of presenting problems that are defined as follows:

Minimal: A problem that may not require the presence of the physician or other qualified health care professional, but service is provided under the physician's or other qualified health care professional's supervision.

Self-limited or minor: A problem that runs a definite and prescribed course, is transient in nature, and is not likely to permanently alter health status.

Low severity: A problem where the risk of morbidity without treatment is low; there is little to no risk of mortality without treatment; full recovery without functional impairment is expected.

Moderate severity: A problem where the risk of morbidity without treatment is moderate; there is moderate risk of mortality without treatment; uncertain prognosis OR increased probability of prolonged functional impairment.

High severity: A problem where the risk of morbidity without treatment is high to extreme; there is a moderate to high risk of mortality without treatment OR high probability of severe, prolonged functional impairment.

Past History
A review of the patient's past experiences with illnesses, injuries, and treatments that includes significant information about:

- Prior major illnesses and injuries
- Prior operations
- Prior hospitalizations
- Current medications
- Allergies (eg, drug, food)
- Age appropriate immunization status
- Age appropriate feeding/dietary status

Family History
A review of medical events in the patient's family that includes significant information about:

- The health status of cause of death of parents, siblings, and children
- Specific diseases related to problems identified in the Chief Complaint or History of the Present Illness, and/or System Review
- Diseases of family members that may be hereditary or place the patient at risk

Social History
An age appropriate review of past and current activities that includes significant information about:

- Marital status and/or living arrangements
- Current employment
- Occupational history
- Military history
- Use of drugs, alcohol, and tobacco
- Level of education
- Sexual history
- Other relevant social factors

System Review (Review of Systems)
An inventory of body systems obtained through a series of questions seeking to identify signs and/or symptoms that the patient may be experiencing or has experienced. For the purposes of the CPT codebook the following elements of a system review have been identified:

- Constitutional symptoms (fever, weight loss, etc)
- Eyes
- Ears, nose, mouth, throat
- Cardiovascular
- Respiratory
- Gastrointestinal
- Genitourinary
- Musculoskeletal
- Integumentary (skin and/or breast)
- Neurological
- Psychiatric
- Endocrine
- Hematologic/lymphatic
- Allergic/immunologic

The review of systems helps define the problem, clarify the differential diagnosis, identify needed testing, or serves as baseline data on other systems that might be affected by any possible management options.

Instructions for Selecting a Level of E/M Service

Review the Reporting Instructions for the Selected Category or Subcategory
Most of the categories and many of the subcategories of service have special guidelines or instructions unique to that category or subcategory. Where these are indicated, eg, "Inpatient Hospital Care," special instructions will be presented preceding the levels of E/M services.

Review the Level of E/M Service Descriptors and Examples in the Selected Category or Subcategory

The descriptors for the levels of E/M services recognize seven components, six of which are used in defining the levels of E/M services. These components are:

- History
- Examination
- Medical decision making
- Counseling
- Coordination of care
- Nature of presenting problem
- Time

The first three of these components (ie, history, examination, and medical decision making) should be considered the **key** components in selecting the level of E/M services. An exception to this rule is in the case of visits that consist predominantly of counseling or coordination of care.

The nature of the presenting problem and time are provided in some levels to assist the physician in determining the appropriate level of E/M service.

Determine the Extent of History Obtained

The extent of the history is dependent upon clinical judgment and on the nature of the presenting problem(s). The levels of E/M services recognize four types of history that are defined as follows:

Problem focused: Chief complaint; brief history of present illness or problem.

Expanded problem focused: Chief complaint; brief history of present illness; problem pertinent system review.

Detailed: Chief complaint; extended history of present illness; problem pertinent system review extended to include a review of a limited number of additional systems; pertinent past, family, and/or social history directly related to the patient's problems.

Comprehensive: Chief complaint; extended history of present illness; review of systems that is directly related to the problem(s) identified in the history of the present illness plus a review of all additional body systems; **complete** past, family, and social history.

The comprehensive history obtained as part of the preventive medicine E/M service is not problem-oriented and does not involve a chief complaint or present illness. It does, however, include a comprehensive system review and comprehensive or interval past, family, and social history as well as a comprehensive assessment/history of pertinent risk factors.

Determine the Extent of Examination Performed

The extent of the examination performed is dependent on clinical judgment and on the nature of the presenting problem(s). The levels of E/M services recognize four types of examination that are defined as follows:

Problem focused: A limited examination of the affected body area or organ system.

Expanded problem focused: A limited examination of the affected body area or organ system and other symptomatic or related organ system(s).

Detailed: An extended examination of the affected body area(s) and other symptomatic or related organ system(s).

Comprehensive: A general multisystem examination or a complete examination of a single organ system. **Note:** The comprehensive examination performed as part of the preventive medicine E/M service is multisystem, but its extent is based on age and risk factors identified.

For the purposes of these CPT definitions, the following body areas are recognized:

- Head, including the face
- Neck
- Chest, including breasts and axilla
- Abdomen
- Genitalia, groin, buttocks
- Back
- Each extremity

For the purposes of these CPT definitions, the following organ systems are recognized:

- Eyes
- Ears, nose, mouth, and throat
- Cardiovascular
- Respiratory
- Gastrointestinal
- Genitourinary
- Musculoskeletal
- Skin
- Neurologic
- Psychiatric
- Hematologic/lymphatic/immunologic

Determine the Complexity of Medical Decision Making

Medical decision making refers to the complexity of establishing a diagnosis and/or selecting a management option as measured by:

- The number of possible diagnoses and/or the number of management options that must be considered
- The amount and/or complexity of medical records, diagnostic tests, and/or other information that must be obtained, reviewed, and analyzed
- The risk of significant complications, morbidity, and/or mortality, as well as comorbidities associated with the patient's presenting problem(s), the diagnostic procedure(s), and/or the possible management options

Four types of medical decision making are recognized: straightforward, low complexity, moderate complexity, and high complexity. To qualify for a given type of decision making, two of the three elements in Table 1 must be met or exceeded.

Comorbidities and underlying diseases, in and of themselves, are not considered in selecting a level of E/M services unless their presence significantly increases the complexity of the medical decision making.

Select the Appropriate Level of E/M Services Based on the Following

For the following categories/subcategories, **all of the key components**, ie, history, examination, and medical decision making, must meet or exceed the stated requirements to qualify for a particular level of E/M service: initial observation care; initial hospital care; observation or inpatient hospital care (including admission and discharge services); office or other outpatient consultations; inpatient consultations; emergency department services; initial nursing facility care; other nursing facility services; domiciliary care, new patient; and home services, new patient.

For the following categories/subcategories, **two of the three key components** (ie, history, examination, and medical decision making) must meet or exceed the stated requirements to qualify for a particular level of E/M services: subsequent observation care; subsequent hospital care; subsequent nursing facility care; domiciliary care, established patient; and home services, established patient.

When counseling and/or coordination of care dominates (more than 50 percent) the encounter with the patient and/or family (face-to-face time in the office or other outpatient setting or floor/unit time in the hospital or nursing facility), then **time** shall be considered the key or controlling factor to qualify for a particular level of E/M services. This includes time spent with parties who have assumed responsibility for the care of the patient or decision making whether or not they are family members (eg, foster parents, person acting in loco parentis, legal guardian). The extent of counseling and/or coordination of care must be documented in the medical record.

CONSULTATION CODES AND MEDICARE REIMBURSEMENT

The Centers for Medicare and Medicaid Services (CMS) no longer provides benefits for CPT consultation codes. CMS has, however, redistributed the value of the consultation codes across the other E/M codes for services which are covered by Medicare. CMS has retained codes 99241 - 99251 in the Medicare Physician Fee Schedule for those private payers that use this data for reimbursement. Note that private payers may choose to follow CMS or CPT guidelines, and the use of consultation codes should be verified with individual payers.

Table 1

Complexity of Medical Decision Making

Number of Diagnoses or Management Options	Amount and/or Complexity of Data to Be Reviewed	Risk of Complications and/or Morbidity or Mortality	Type of Decision Making
minimal	minimal or none	minimal	**straightforward**
limited	limited	low	**low complexity**
multiple	moderate	moderate	**moderate complexity**
extensive	extensive	high	**high complexity**

Guidelines for Office or Other Outpatient E/M Services

History and/or Examination

Office or other outpatient services include a medically appropriate history and/or physical examination, when performed. The nature and extent of the history and/or physical examination are determined by the treating physician or other qualified health care professional reporting the service. The care team may collect information and the patient or caregiver may supply information directly (eg, by electronic health record [EHR] portal or questionnaire) that is reviewed by the reporting physician or other qualified health care professional. The extent of history and physical examination is not an element in selection of the level of office or other outpatient code.

Number and Complexity of Problems Addressed at the Encounter

One element used in selecting the level of office or other outpatient services is the number and complexity of the problems that are addressed at an encounter. Multiple new or established conditions may be addressed at the same time and may affect MDM. Symptoms may cluster around a specific diagnosis and each symptom is not necessarily a unique condition. Comorbidities/underlying diseases, in and of themselves, are not considered in selecting a level of E/M services **unless** they are addressed, and their presence increases the amount and/or complexity of data to be reviewed and analyzed or the risk of complications and/or morbidity or mortality of patient management. The final diagnosis for a condition does not, in and of itself, determine the complexity or risk, as extensive evaluation may be required to reach the conclusion that the signs or symptoms do not represent a highly morbid condition. Therefore, presenting symptoms that are likely to represent a highly morbid condition may "drive" MDM even when the ultimate diagnosis is not highly morbid. The evaluation and/or treatment should be consistent with the likely nature of the condition. Multiple problems of a lower severity may, in the aggregate, create higher risk due to interaction. The term "risk" as used in these definitions relates to risk from the condition. While condition risk and management risk may often correlate, the risk from the condition is distinct from the risk of the management.

Definitions for the elements of MDM (see Table 2, Levels of Medical Decision Making) for other office or other outpatient services are:

Problem: A problem is a disease, condition, illness, injury, symptom, sign, finding, complaint, or other matter addressed at the encounter, with or without a diagnosis being established at the time of the encounter.

Problem addressed: A problem is addressed or managed when it is evaluated or treated at the encounter by the physician or other qualified health care professional reporting the service. This includes consideration of further testing or treatment that may not be elected by virtue of risk/benefit analysis or patient/parent/guardian/surrogate choice. Notation in the patient's medical record that another professional is managing the problem without additional assessment or care coordination documented does not qualify as being addressed or managed by the physician or other qualified health care professional reporting the service. Referral without evaluation (by history, examination, or diagnostic study[ies]) or consideration of treatment does not qualify as being addressed or managed by the physician or other qualified health care professional reporting the service.

Minimal problem: A problem that may not require the presence of the physician or other qualified health care professional, but the service is provided under the physician's or other qualified health care professional's supervision (see 99211).

Self-limited or minor problem: A problem that runs a definite and prescribed course, is transient in nature, and is not likely to permanently alter health status.

Stable, chronic illness: A problem with an expected duration of at least one year or until the death of the patient. For the purpose of defining chronicity, conditions are treated as chronic whether or not stage or severity changes (eg, uncontrolled diabetes and controlled diabetes are a single chronic condition). "Stable" for the purposes of categorizing MDM is defined by the specific treatment goals for an individual patient. A patient who is not at his or her treatment goal is not stable, even if the condition has not changed and there is no short\term threat to life or function. For example, in a patient with persistently poorly controlled blood pressure for whom better control is a goal is not stable, even if the pressures are not changing and the patient is asymptomatic, the risk of morbidity **without** treatment is significant. Examples may include well-controlled hypertension, non-insulin dependent diabetes, cataract, or benign prostatic hyperplasia.

Acute, uncomplicated illness or injury: A recent or new short-term problem with low risk of morbidity for which treatment is considered. There is little to no risk of mortality with treatment, and full recovery without functional impairment is expected. A problem that is normally self-limited or minor but is not resolving consistent with a definite and prescribed course is an acute, uncomplicated illness. Examples may include cystitis, allergic rhinitis, or a simple sprain.

Chronic illness with exacerbation, progression, or side effects of treatment: A chronic illness that is acutely worsening, poorly controlled, or progressing with an intent to control progression and requiring additional supportive care or requiring attention to treatment for side effects but that does not require consideration of hospital level of care.

Undiagnosed new problem with uncertain prognosis: A problem in the differential diagnosis that represents a condition likely to result in a high risk of morbidity without treatment. An example may be a lump in the breast.

Acute illness with systemic symptoms: An illness that causes systemic symptoms and has a high risk of morbidity without treatment. For systemic general symptoms, such as fever, body aches, or fatigue in a minor illness that may be treated to alleviate symptoms, shorten the course of illness, or to prevent complications, see the definitions for **self-limited or minor problem** or **acute, uncomplicated illness or injury**. Systemic symptoms may not be general but may be single system. Examples may include pyelonephritis, pneumonitis, or colitis.

Acute, complicated injury: An injury which requires treatment that includes evaluation of body systems that are not directly part of the injured organ, the injury is extensive, or the treatment options are multiple and/or associated with risk of morbidity. An example may be a head injury with brief loss of consciousness.

Chronic illness with severe exacerbation, progression, or side effects of treatment: The severe exacerbation or progression of a chronic illness or severe side effects of treatment that have significant risk of morbidity and may require hospital level of care.

Acute or chronic illness or injury that poses a threat to life or bodily function: An acute illness with systemic symptoms, an acute complicated injury, or a chronic illness or injury with exacerbation and/or progression or side effects of treatment, that poses a threat to life or bodily function in the near term without treatment. Examples may include acute myocardial infarction, pulmonary embolus, severe respiratory distress, progressive severe rheumatoid arthritis, psychiatric illness with potential threat to self or others, peritonitis, acute renal failure, or an abrupt change in neurologic status.

Analyzed: The process of using the data as part of the MDM. The data element itself may not be subject to analysis (eg, glucose), but it is instead included in the thought processes for diagnosis, evaluation, or treatment. Tests ordered are presumed to be analyzed when the results are reported. Therefore, when they are ordered during an encounter, they are counted in that encounter. Tests that are ordered outside of an encounter may be counted in the encounter in which they are analyzed. In the case of a recurring order, each new result may be counted in the encounter in which it is analyzed. For example, an encounter that includes an order for monthly prothrombin times would count for one prothrombin time ordered and reviewed. Additional future results, if analyzed in a subsequent encounter, may be counted as a single test in that subsequent encounter. Any service for which the professional component is separately reported by the physician or other qualified health care professional reporting the E/M services is not counted as a data element ordered, reviewed, analyzed, or independently interpreted for the purposes of determining the level of MDM.

Test: Tests are imaging, laboratory, psychometric, or physiologic data. A clinical laboratory panel (eg, basic metabolic panel [80047]) is a single test. The differentiation between single or multiple tests is defined in accordance with the CPT code set. For the purposes of data reviewed and analyzed, pulse oximetry is not a test.

Unique: A unique test is defined by the CPT code set. When multiple results of the same unique test (eg, serial blood glucose values) are compared during an E/M service, count it as one unique test. Tests that have overlapping elements are not unique, even if they are identified with distinct CPT codes. For example, a CBC with differential would incorporate the set of hemoglobin, CBC without differential, and platelet count. A unique source is defined as a physician or qualified heath care professional in a distinct group or different specialty or subspecialty, or a unique entity. Review of all materials from any unique source counts as one element toward MDM.

Combination of Data Elements: A combination of different data elements, for example, a combination of notes reviewed, tests ordered, tests reviewed, or independent historian, allows these elements to be summed. It does not require each item type or category to be represented. A unique test ordered, plus a note reviewed and an independent historian would be a combination of three elements.

External: External records, communications and/or test results are from an external physician, other qualified health care professional, facility, or health care organization.

External physician or other qualified health care professional: An external physician or other qualified health care professional who is not in the same group practice or is of a different specialty or subspecialty. This includes licensed professionals who are practicing independently. The

individual may also be a facility or organizational provider such as from a hospital, nursing facility, or home health care agency.

Discussion: Discussion requires an interactive exchange. The exchange must be direct and not through intermediaries (eg, clinical staff or trainees). Sending chart notes or written exchanges that are within progress notes does not qualify as an interactive exchange. The discussion does not need to be on the date of the encounter, but it is counted only once and only when it is used in the decision making of the encounter. It may be asynchronous (ie, does not need to be in person), but it must be initiated and completed within a short time period (eg, within a day or two).

Independent historian(s): An individual (eg, parent, guardian, surrogate, spouse, witness) who provides a history in addition to a history provided by the patient who is unable to provide a complete or reliable history (eg, due to developmental stage, dementia, or psychosis) or because a confirmatory history is judged to be necessary. In the case where there may be conflict or poor communication between multiple historians and more than one historian is needed, the independent historian requirement is met. The independent history does not need to be obtained in person but does need to be obtained directly from the historian providing the independent information.

Independent interpretation: The interpretation of a test for which there is a CPT code and an interpretation or report is customary. This does not apply when the physician or other qualified health care professional is reporting the service or has previously report the service for the patient. A form of interpretation should be documented but need not conform to the usual standards of a complete report for the test.

Appropriate source: For the purpose of the discussion of management data element (see Table 2, Levels of Medical Decision Making), an appropriate source includes professionals who are not health care professionals but may be involved in the management of the patient (eg, lawyer, parole officer, case manager, teacher). It does not include discussion with family or informal caregivers.

One element used in selecting the level of service is the risk of complications and/or morbidity or mortality of patient management at an encounter. This is distinct from the risk of the condition itself.

Risk: The probability and/or consequences of an event. The assessment of the level of risk is affected by the nature of the event under consideration. For example, a low probability of death may be high risk, whereas a high chance of a minor, self-limited adverse effect of treatment may be low risk. Definitions of risk are based upon the usual behavior and thought processes of a physician or other qualified health care professional in the same specialty. Trained clinicians apply common language usage meanings to terms such as high, medium, low, or minimal risk and do not require quantification for these definitions (though quantification may be provided when evidence-based medicine has established probabilities). For the purposes of MDM, level of risk is based upon consequences of the problem(s) addressed at the encounter when appropriately treated. Risk also includes MDM related to the need to initiate or forego further testing, treatment, and/or hospitalization. The risk of patient management criteria applies to the patient management decisions made by the reporting physician or other qualified health care professional as part of the reported encounter.

Morbidity: A state of illness or functional impairment that is expected to be of substantial duration during which function is limited, quality of life is impaired, or there is organ damage that may not be transient despite treatment.

Social determinants of health: Economic and social conditions that influence the health of people and communities. Examples may include food and housing insecurity.

Surgery (minor or major, elective, emergency, procedure or patient risk):

- **Surgery—Minor or Major:** The classification of surgery into minor or major is based on the common meaning of such terms when used by trained clinicians, similar to the use of the term "risk." These terms are not defined by a surgical package classification.

- **Surgery—Elective or Emergency:** Elective procedures and emergent or urgent procedures describe the timing of a procedure when the timing is related to the patient's condition. An elective procedure is typically planned in advance (eg, scheduled for weeks later), while an emergent procedure is typically performed immediately or with minimal delay to allow for patient stabilization. Both elective and emergent procedures may be minor or major procedures.

- **Surgery—Risk Factors, Patient or Procedure:** Risk factors are those that are relevant to the patient and procedure. Evidence-based risk calculators may be used, but are not required, in assessing patient and procedure risk.

Drug therapy requiring intensive monitoring for toxicity: A drug that requires intensive monitoring is a therapeutic agent that has the potential to cause serious morbidity or death. The monitoring is performed for assessment of these adverse effects and not primarily for assessment of therapeutic efficacy. The monitoring should be that which is generally accepted practice for the agent but may be patient-specific in some cases. Intensive monitoring may be long-term or short-term. Long-term intensive monitoring is not performed less than quarterly. The monitoring may be performed with a laboratory test, a physiologic test, or imaging. Monitoring by history or examination does not qualify. The monitoring affects the level of MDM in an encounter in which it is considered in the management of the patient. Examples may include monitoring for cytopenia in the use of an antineoplastic agent between dose cycles or the short-term intensive monitoring of electrolytes and renal function in a patient who is undergoing diuresis. Examples of monitoring that do not qualify include monitoring glucose levels during insulin therapy, as the primary reason is the therapeutic effect (unless severe hypoglycemia is a current, significant concern); or annual electrolytes and renal function for a patient on a diuretic, as the frequency does not meet the threshold.

Instructions for Selecting a Level of Office or Other Outpatient E/M Services

Select the appropriate level of E/M services based on the following:

1. The level of the MDM as defined for each service, or

2. The total time for E/M services performed on the date of the encounter.

Medical Decision Making

MDM includes establishing diagnoses, assessing the status of a condition, and/or selecting a management option. MDM in the office or other outpatient services codes is defined by three elements:

- The number and complexity of problem(s) that are addressed during the encounter.

- The amount and/or complexity of data to be reviewed and analyzed. These data include medical records, tests, and/or other information that must be obtained, ordered, reviewed, and analyzed for the encounter. This includes information obtained from multiple sources or interprofessional communications that are not reported separately and interpretation of tests that are not reported separately. Ordering

a test is included in the category of test result(s) and the review of the test result is part of the encounter and not a subsequent encounter. Ordering a test may include those considered, but not selected after shared decision making. For example, a patient may request diagnostic imaging that is not necessary for their condition and discussion of the lack of benefit may be required. Alternatively, a test may normally be performed, but due to the risk for a specific patient it is not ordered. These considerations must be documented.

- Data are divided into three categories:

  — Tests, documents, orders, or independent historian(s). (Each unique test, order, or document is counted to meet a threshold number.)

  — Independent interpretation of tests.

  — Discussion of management or test interpretation with external physician or other qualified health care professional or appropriate source.

- The risk of complications and/or morbidity or mortality of patient management decisions made at the visit, associated with the patient's problem(s), the diagnostic procedure(s), treatment(s). This includes the possible management options selected and those considered but not selected, after shared MDM with the patient and/or family. For example, a decision about hospitalization includes consideration of alternative levels of care. Examples may include a psychiatric patient with a sufficient degree of support in the outpatient setting or the decision to not hospitalize a patient with advanced dementia with an acute condition that would generally warrant inpatient care, but for whom the goal is palliative treatment.

Four types of MDM are recognized: straightforward, low, moderate, and high. The concept of the level of MDM does not apply to 99211. Shared MDM involves eliciting patient and/or family preferences, patient and/or family education, and explaining risks and benefits of management options. MDM may be impacted by role and management responsibility.

When the physician or other qualified health care professional is reporting a separate CPT code that includes interpretation and/or report, the interpretation and/or report should not count toward the MDM when selecting a level of office or other outpatient services. When the physician or other qualified health care professional is reporting a separate service for discussion of management with a physician or another qualified health care professional, the discussion is not counted toward the MDM when selecting a level of office or other outpatient services.

The Levels of Medical Decision Making (MDM) table (Table2) is a guide to assist in selecting the level of MDM for reporting an office or other outpatient E/M services code. The table includes the four levels of MDM (ie, straightforward, low, moderate, high) and the three elements of MDM (ie, number and complexity of problems addressed at the encounter, amount and/or complexity of data reviewed and analyzed, and risk of complications and/or morbidity or mortality of patient management). To qualify for a particular level of MDM, two of the three elements for that level of MDM must be met or exceeded. See Table 2: Levels of Medical Decision Making (MDM) below.

Table 2: Levels of Medical Decision Making (MDM)

Code	Level of MDM (Based on 2 out of 3 Elements of MDM)	Elements of Medical Decision Making		
		Number and Complexity of Problems Addressed	Amount and/or Complexity of Data to be Reviewed and Analyzed	Risk of Complications and/or Morbidity or Mortality of Patient Management
99211	N/A	N/A	N/A	N/A
99202 99212	**Straightforward**	**Minimal** • **1** self-limited or minor problem	**Minimal or none**	**Minimal risk of morbidity from additional diagnostic testing or treatment**
99203 99213	Low	**Low** • **2** or more self-limited or minor problems; **or** • stable chronic illness; **or** • **1** acute, uncomplicated illness or injury	**Limited** *(Must meet the requirements of at least 1 of the 2 categories)* **Category 1: Tests and documents** • Any combination of 2 from the following: 　- Review of prior external note(s) from each unique source*; 　- review of the result(s) of each unique test*; 　- ordering of each unique test* **or** **Category 2: Assessment requiring an independent historian(s)** *(For the categories of independent interpretation of tests and discussion of management or test interpretation, see moderate or high)*	**Low risk of morbidity from additional diagnostic testing or treatment**
99204 99214	**Moderate**	**Moderate** • **1** or more chronic illnesses with exacerbation, progression, or side effects of treatment; **or** • **2** or more stable chronic illnesses; **or** • **1** undiagnosed new problem with uncertain prognosis; **or** • **1** acute illness with systemic symptoms; **or** • **1** acute complicated injury	**Moderate** *(Must meet the requirements of at least 1 out of 3 categories)* **Category 1: Tests, documents, or independent historian(s)** • Any combination of 3 from the following: 　- Review of prior external note(s) from each unique source*; 　- Review of the result(s) of each unique test*; 　- Ordering of each unique test*; 　- Assessment requiring an independent historian(s) **or** **Category 2: Independent interpretation of tests** • Independent interpretation of a test performed by another physician/other qualified health care professional (not separately reported); **or** **Category 3: Discussion of management or test interpretation** Discussion of management or test interpretation with external physician/other qualified health care professional\appropriate source (not separately reported)	**Moderate risk of morbidity from additional diagnostic testing or treatment** *Examples only:* • Prescription drug management • Decision regarding minor surgery with identified patient or procedure risk factors • Decision regarding elective major surgery without identified patient or procedure risk factors Diagnosis or treatment significantly limited by social determinants of health

Each unique test, order, or document contributes to the combination of 2 or combination of 3 in Category 1 below.

Elements of Medical Decision Making

Code	Level of MDM (Based on 2 out of 3 Elements of MDM)	Number and Complexity of Problems Addressed	Amount and/or Complexity of Data to be Reviewed and Analyzed	Risk of Complications and/or Morbidity or Mortality of Patient Management

99205 99215	High	**High**
		
		• **1** or more chronic illnesses with severe exacerbation, progression, or side effects of treatment;
		or
		• **1** acute or chronic illness or injury that poses a threat to life or bodily function
			Extensive
			
			(Must meet the requirements of at least 2 out of 3 categories)
			
			Category 1: Tests, documents, or independent historian(s)
			
			• **Any combination of 3 from the following:**
			  - Review of prior external note(s) from each unique source*;
			  - Review of the result(s) of each unique test*;
			  - Ordering of each unique test*;
			  - Assessment requiring an independent historian(s)
			or
			Category 2: Independent interpretation of tests
			
			• **Independent interpretation of a test performed by another physician/other qualified health care professional (not separately reported);**
			or
			Category 3: Discussion of management or test interpretation
			
			• Discussion of management or test interpretation with external physician/other qualified health care professional/appropriate source (not separately reported)
				High risk of morbidity from additional diagnostic testing or treatment
				
				Examples only:
				• Drug therapy requiring intensive monitoring for toxicity
				• Decision regarding elective major surgery with identified patient or procedure risk factors
				• Decision regarding emergency major surgery
				• Decision regarding hospitalization
				• Decision not to resuscitate or to de-escalate care because of poor prognosis

Each unique test, order, or document contributes to the combination of 2 or combination of 3 in Category 1 below.

Time

For instructions on using time to select the level of office or other outpatient E/M services code, see the *Time* subsection in the *Guidelines Common to All E/M Services.*

Unlisted Service

An E/M service may be provided that is not listed in this section of the CPT codebook. When reporting such a service, the appropriate unlisted code may be used to indicate the service, identifying it by "Special Report," as discussed in the following paragraph. The "Unlisted Services" and accompanying codes for the E/M section are as follows:

99429   **Unlisted preventive** medicine service

99499   **Unlisted evaluation and management** service

Special Report

An unlisted service or one that is unusual, variable, or new may require a special report demonstrating the medical appropriateness of the service. Pertinent information should include an adequate definition or description of the nature, extent, and need for the procedure and the time, effort, and equipment necessary to provide the service. Additional items that may be included are complexity of symptoms, final diagnosis, pertinent physical findings, diagnostic and therapeutic procedures, concurrent problems, and follow-up care.

Clinical Examples

Clinical examples of the codes for E/M services are provided to assist in understanding the meaning of the descriptors and selecting the correct code. The clinical examples are listed in Appendix C. Each example was developed by the specialties shown. The same problem, when seen by different specialties, may involve different amounts of work. Therefore, the appropriate level of encounter should be reported using the descriptors rather than the examples.

99202-99215 Outpatient and Other Visits

INCLUDES Established patients: received prior professional services from physician or qualified health care professional or another physician or qualified health care professional in exact same specialty practice and subspecialty in previous three years (99211-99215)

New patients: have not received professional services from physician or qualified health care professional or any other physician or qualified health care professional in same practice in exact same specialty and subspecialty in previous three years (99202-99205)

Office visits

Outpatient services (including services prior to formal admission to facility)

EXCLUDES Services provided in:
Emergency department (99281-99285)
Hospital observation (99217-99220 [99224, 99225, 99226])
Hospital observation or inpatient with same day admission and discharge (99234-99236)

99202 Office or other outpatient visit for the evaluation and management of a new patient, which requires a medically appropriate history and/or examination and straightforward medical decision making. When using time for code selection, 15-29 minutes of total time is spent on the date of the encounter.

🚑 1.43 ⚕ 2.15 **FUD** XXX ★ Ⓑ 80 ▭

AMA: 2020,Dec,11; 2020,Oct,14; 2020,Nov,3; 2020,Sep,3; 2020,Sep,14; 2020,Jun,3; 2020,May,3; 2020,Feb,3; 2020,Jan,3; 2019,Oct,10; 2019,Feb,3; 2019,Jan,3; 2018,Sep,14; 2018,Apr,10; 2018,Apr,9; 2018,Mar,7; 2018,Jan,8; 2017,Aug,3; 2017,Jun,6; 2017,Jan,8; 2016,Dec,11; 2016,Sep,6; 2016,Mar,10; 2016,Jan,13; 2016,Jan,7

99203 Office or other outpatient visit for the evaluation and management of a new patient, which requires a medically appropriate history and/or examination and low level of medical decision making. When using time for code selection, 30-44 minutes of total time is spent on the date of the encounter.

🚑 2.15 ⚕ 3.05 **FUD** XXX ★ Ⓑ 80 ▭

AMA: 2020,Oct,14; 2020,Nov,3; 2020,Sep,14; 2020,Sep,3; 2020,Jun,3; 2020,May,3; 2020,Feb,3; 2020,Jan,3; 2019,Oct,10; 2019,Feb,3; 2019,Jan,3; 2018,Sep,14; 2018,Apr,9; 2018,Apr,10; 2018,Mar,7; 2018,Jan,8; 2017,Aug,3; 2017,Jun,6; 2017,Jan,8; 2016,Dec,11; 2016,Sep,6; 2016,Mar,10; 2016,Jan,13; 2016,Jan,7

99204 Office or other outpatient visit for the evaluation and management of a new patient, which requires a medically appropriate history and/or examination and moderate level of medical decision making. When using time for code selection, 45-59 minutes of total time is spent on the date of the encounter.

🚑 3.64 ⚕ 4.63 **FUD** XXX ★ Ⓑ 80 ▭

AMA: 2020,Oct,14; 2020,Nov,3; 2020,Nov,12; 2020,Sep,3; 2020,Sep,14; 2020,Jun,3; 2020,May,3; 2020,Feb,3; 2020,Jan,3; 2019,Oct,10; 2019,Feb,3; 2019,Jan,3; 2018,Sep,14; 2018,Apr,10; 2018,Apr,9; 2018,Mar,7; 2018,Jan,8; 2017,Aug,3; 2017,Jun,6; 2017,Jan,8; 2016,Dec,11; 2016,Sep,6; 2016,Mar,10; 2016,Jan,7; 2016,Jan,13

99205 Office or other outpatient visit for the evaluation and management of a new patient, which requires a medically appropriate history and/or examination and high level of medical decision making. When using time for code selection, 60-74 minutes of total time is spent on the date of the encounter.

EXCLUDES Prolonged services (lasting 75 minutes or more) ([99417])

🚑 4.75 ⚕ 5.82 **FUD** XXX ★ Ⓑ 80 ▭

AMA: 2020,Oct,14; 2020,Nov,3; 2020,Nov,12; 2020,Sep,3; 2020,Sep,14; 2020,Jun,3; 2020,May,3; 2020,Feb,3; 2020,Jan,3; 2019,Oct,10; 2019,Feb,3; 2019,Jan,3; 2018,Sep,14; 2018,Apr,10; 2018,Apr,9; 2018,Mar,7; 2018,Jan,8; 2017,Aug,3; 2017,Jun,6; 2017,Jan,8; 2016,Dec,11; 2016,Sep,6; 2016,Mar,10; 2016,Jan,7; 2016,Jan,13

▲ **99211** Office or other outpatient visit for the evaluation and management of an established patient that may not require the presence of a physician or other qualified health care professional

🚑 0.26 ⚕ 0.64 **FUD** XXX ★ Ⓑ 80 ▭

AMA: 2020,Oct,14; 2020,Nov,12; 2020,Nov,3; 2020,Sep,14; 2020,Sep,3; 2020,Jun,3; 2020,May,3; 2020,Feb,3; 2020,Jan,3; 2019,Oct,10; 2019,Feb,3; 2019,Jan,3; 2018,Sep,14; 2018,Apr,9; 2018,Apr,10; 2018,Mar,7; 2018,Jan,8; 2017,Aug,3; 2017,Jun,6; 2017,Mar,10; 2017,Jan,8; 2016,Dec,11; 2016,Sep,6; 2016,Mar,10; 2016,Jan,7; 2016,Jan,13

99212 Office or other outpatient visit for the evaluation and management of an established patient, which requires a medically appropriate history and/or examination and straightforward medical decision making. When using time for code selection, 10-19 minutes of total time is spent on the date of the encounter.

🚑 0.72 ⚕ 1.27 **FUD** XXX ★ Ⓑ 80 ▭

AMA: 2020,Oct,14; 2020,Nov,3; 2020,Sep,14; 2020,Sep,3; 2020,Jun,3; 2020,May,3; 2020,Feb,3; 2020,Jan,3; 2019,Oct,10; 2019,Feb,3; 2019,Jan,3; 2018,Sep,14; 2018,Apr,9; 2018,Apr,10; 2018,Mar,7; 2018,Jan,8; 2017,Oct,5; 2017,Aug,3; 2017,Jun,6; 2017,Jan,8; 2016,Dec,11; 2016,Sep,6; 2016,Mar,10; 2016,Jan,13; 2016,Jan,7

99213 Office or other outpatient visit for the evaluation and management of an established patient, which requires a medically appropriate history and/or examination and low level of medical decision making. When using time for code selection, 20-29 minutes of total time is spent on the date of the encounter.

🚑 1.44 ⚕ 2.09 **FUD** XXX ★ Ⓑ 80 ▭

AMA: 2020,Oct,14; 2020,Nov,3; 2020,Sep,3; 2020,Sep,14; 2020,Jun,3; 2020,May,3; 2020,Feb,3; 2020,Jan,3; 2019,Oct,10; 2019,Feb,3; 2019,Jan,3; 2018,Sep,14; 2018,Apr,10; 2018,Apr,9; 2018,Mar,7; 2018,Jan,8; 2017,Aug,3; 2017,Jun,6; 2017,Jan,8; 2016,Dec,11; 2016,Sep,6; 2016,Mar,10; 2016,Jan,13; 2016,Jan,7

99214 Office or other outpatient visit for the evaluation and management of an established patient, which requires a medically appropriate history and/or examination and moderate level of medical decision making. When using time for code selection, 30-39 minutes of total time is spent on the date of the encounter.

🚑 2.22 ⚕ 3.06 **FUD** XXX ★ Ⓑ 80 ▭

AMA: 2020,Oct,14; 2020,Nov,3; 2020,Nov,12; 2020,Sep,14; 2020,Sep,3; 2020,Jun,3; 2020,May,3; 2020,Feb,3; 2020,Jan,3; 2019,Oct,10; 2019,Feb,3; 2019,Jan,3; 2018,Sep,14; 2018,Apr,9; 2018,Apr,10; 2018,Mar,7; 2018,Jan,8; 2017,Aug,3; 2017,Jun,6; 2017,Jan,8; 2016,Dec,11; 2016,Sep,6; 2016,Mar,10; 2016,Jan,7; 2016,Jan,13

99215 Office or other outpatient visit for the evaluation and management of an established patient, which requires a medically appropriate history and/or examination and high level of medical decision making. When using time for code selection, 40-54 minutes of total time is spent on the date of the encounter.

EXCLUDES Prolonged services (lasting 55 minutes or more) ([99417])

🚑 3.13 ⚕ 4.10 **FUD** XXX ★ Ⓑ 80 ▭

AMA: 2020,Oct,14; 2020,Nov,12; 2020,Nov,3; 2020,Sep,14; 2020,Sep,3; 2020,Jun,3; 2020,May,3; 2020,Feb,3; 2020,Jan,3; 2019,Oct,10; 2019,Feb,3; 2019,Jan,3; 2018,Sep,14; 2018,Apr,9; 2018,Apr,10; 2018,Mar,7; 2018,Jan,8; 2017,Aug,3; 2017,Jun,6; 2017,Jan,8; 2016,Dec,11; 2016,Sep,6; 2016,Mar,10; 2016,Jan,7; 2016,Jan,13

99217-99220 Facility Observation Visits: Initial and Discharge

CMS: 100-04,11,40.1.3 Independent Attending Physician Services; 100-04,12,30.6.4 Services Furnished Incident to Physician's Service; 100-04,12,30.6.8 Payment for Hospital Observation Services; 100-04,12,40.3 Global Surgery Review; 100-04,32,130.1 Billing and Payment of External counterpulsation (ECP)

INCLUDES Services provided on same date in other settings or departments associated with observation status admission (99202-99215, 99281-99285, 99304-99318, 99324-99337, 99341-99350, 99381-99429 [99415, 99416, 99417, 99421, 99422, 99423])

Services provided to new and established patients admitted to hospital specifically for observation (not required to be designated hospital area)

EXCLUDES *Services provided by physicians or another qualified health care professional other than admitting physician ([99224, 99225, 99226], 99241-99245)*

Services provided to patient admitted and discharged from observation status on same date (99234-99236)

Services provided to patient admitted to hospital following observation status (99221-99223)

Services provided to patient discharged from inpatient care (99238-99239)

99217 Observation care discharge day management (This code is to be utilized to report all services provided to a patient on discharge from outpatient hospital "observation status" if the discharge is on other than the initial date of "observation status." To report services to a patient designated as "observation status" or "inpatient status" and discharged on the same date, use the codes for Observation or Inpatient Care Services [including Admission and Discharge Services, 99234-99236 as appropriate.])

INCLUDES Discussing observation admission with patient
Final patient evaluation:
Discharge instructions
Sign off on discharge medical records

🚑 2.06 ⚕ 2.06 **FUD** XXX   B 80 ▦

AMA: 2019,Jul,10; 2018,Jan,8; 2017,Aug,3; 2017,Jun,6; 2017,Jan,8; 2016,Dec,11; 2016,Jan,13; 2016,Jan,7

99218 Initial observation care, per day, for the evaluation and management of a patient which requires these 3 key components: A detailed or comprehensive history; A detailed or comprehensive examination; and Medical decision making that is straightforward or of low complexity. Counseling and/or coordination of care with other physicians, other qualified health care professionals, or agencies are provided consistent with the nature of the problem(s) and the patient's and/or family's needs. Usually, the problem(s) requiring admission to outpatient hospital "observation status" are of low severity. Typically, 30 minutes are spent at the bedside and on the patient's hospital floor or unit.

🚑 2.81 ⚕ 2.81 **FUD** XXX   B 80 ▦

AMA: 2020,Sep,3; 2019,Jul,10; 2018,Dec,8; 2018,Dec,8; 2018,Jan,8; 2017,Aug,3; 2017,Jun,6; 2017,Jan,8; 2016,Dec,11; 2016,Jan,7; 2016,Jan,13

99219 Initial observation care, per day, for the evaluation and management of a patient, which requires these 3 key components: A comprehensive history; A comprehensive examination; and Medical decision making of moderate complexity. Counseling and/or coordination of care with other physicians, other qualified health care professionals, or agencies are provided consistent with the nature of the problem(s) and the patient's and/or family's needs. Usually, the problem(s) requiring admission to outpatient hospital "observation status" are of moderate severity. Typically, 50 minutes are spent at the bedside and on the patient's hospital floor or unit.

🚑 3.83 ⚕ 3.83 **FUD** XXX   B 80 ▦

AMA: 2020,Sep,3; 2019,Jul,10; 2018,Dec,8; 2018,Dec,8; 2018,Jan,8; 2017,Aug,3; 2017,Jun,6; 2017,Jan,8; 2016,Dec,11; 2016,Jan,13; 2016,Jan,7

99220 Initial observation care, per day, for the evaluation and management of a patient, which requires these 3 key components: A comprehensive history; A comprehensive examination; and Medical decision making of high complexity. Counseling and/or coordination of care with other physicians, other qualified health care professionals, or agencies are provided consistent with the nature of the problem(s) and the patient's and/or family's needs. Usually, the problem(s) requiring admission to outpatient hospital "observation status" are of high severity. Typically, 70 minutes are spent at the bedside and on the patient's hospital floor or unit.

🚑 5.23 ⚕ 5.23 **FUD** XXX   B 80 ▦

AMA: 2020,Sep,3; 2019,Jul,10; 2018,Dec,8; 2018,Dec,8; 2018,Jan,8; 2017,Aug,3; 2017,Jun,6; 2017,Jan,8; 2016,Dec,11; 2016,Jan,13; 2016,Jan,7

99224-99226 [99224, 99225, 99226] Facility Observation Visits: Subsequent

CMS: 100-04,11,40.1.3 Independent Attending Physician Services; 100-04,12,30.6.4 Services Furnished Incident to Physician's Service; 100-04,12,30.6.8 Payment for Hospital Observation Services; 100-04,12,30.6.9.1 Initial Hospital Care and Observation or Inpatient Care Services .

INCLUDES Changes in patient's status (e.g., physical condition, history; response to medical management)
Medical record review
Review diagnostic test results
Services provided on same date in other settings or departments associated with observation status admission (99202-99215; 99281-99285, 99304-99318, 99324-99337, 99341-99350, 99381-99429 [99415, 99416, 99417, 99421, 99422, 99423])

EXCLUDES *Observation admission and discharge on same day (99234-99236)*

 # 99224 Subsequent observation care, per day, for the evaluation and management of a patient, which requires at least 2 of these 3 key components: Problem focused interval history; Problem focused examination; Medical decision making that is straightforward or of low complexity. Counseling and/or coordination of care with other physicians, other qualified health care professionals, or agencies are provided consistent with the nature of the problem(s) and the patient's and/or family's needs. Usually, the patient is stable, recovering, or improving. Typically, 15 minutes are spent at the bedside and on the patient's hospital floor or unit.

🚑 1.12 ⚕ 1.12 **FUD** XXX   B 80 ▦

AMA: 2020,Sep,3; 2019,Jul,10; 2018,Jan,8; 2017,Aug,3; 2017,Jun,6; 2017,Jan,8; 2016,Dec,11; 2016,Jan,7; 2016,Jan,13

 # 99225 Subsequent observation care, per day, for the evaluation and management of a patient, which requires at least 2 of these 3 key components: An expanded problem focused interval history; An expanded problem focused examination; Medical decision making of moderate complexity. Counseling and/or coordination of care with other physicians, other qualified health care professionals, or agencies are provided consistent with the nature of the problem(s) and the patient's and/or family's needs. Usually, the patient is responding inadequately to therapy or has developed a minor complication. Typically, 25 minutes are spent at the bedside and on the patient's hospital floor or unit.

🚑 2.06 ⚕ 2.06 **FUD** XXX   B 80 ▦

AMA: 2020,Sep,3; 2019,Jul,10; 2018,Jan,8; 2017,Aug,3; 2017,Jun,6; 2017,Jan,8; 2016,Dec,11; 2016,Jan,7; 2016,Jan,13

Evaluation and Management

99226 — 99233

99226

Subsequent observation care, per day, for the evaluation and management of a patient, which requires at least 2 of these 3 key components: A detailed interval history; A detailed examination; Medical decision making of high complexity. Counseling and/or coordination of care with other physicians, other qualified health care professionals, or agencies are provided consistent with the nature of the problem(s) and the patient's and/or family's needs. Usually, the patient is unstable or has developed a significant complication or a significant new problem. Typically, 35 minutes are spent at the bedside and on the patient's hospital floor or unit.

🔲 2.95   ⅗ 2.95   **FUD** XXX   B 80 ▭

AMA: 2020,Sep,3; 2019,Jul,10; 2018,Jan,8; 2017,Aug,3; 2017,Jun,6; 2017,Jan,8; 2016,Dec,11; 2016,Jan,7; 2016,Jan,13

99221-99233 [99224, 99225, 99226] Inpatient Hospital Visits: Initial and Subsequent

CMS: 100-04,11,40.1.3 Independent Attending Physician Services; 100-04,12,30.6.10 Consultation Services; 100-04,12,30.6.15.1 Prolonged Services With Direct Face-to-Face Patient Contact; 100-04,12,30.6.4 Services Furnished Incident to Physician's Service; 100-04,12,30.6.9 Hospital Visit and Critical Care on Same Day

INCLUDES   Initial physician services provided to patient in hospital or "partial" hospital settings (99221-99223)

Services provided on admission date in other settings or departments associated with observation status admission (99202-99215, 99281-99285, 99304-99318, 99324-99337, 99341-99350, 99381-99397)

Services provided to new or established patient

EXCLUDES   *Inpatient admission and discharge on same date (99234-99236)*
Inpatient E/M services provided by other than admitting physician

99221

Initial hospital care, per day, for the evaluation and management of a patient, which requires these 3 key components: A detailed or comprehensive history; A detailed or comprehensive examination; and Medical decision making that is straightforward or of low complexity. Counseling and/or coordination of care with other physicians, other qualified health care professionals, or agencies are provided consistent with the nature of the problem(s) and the patient's and/or family's needs. Usually, the problem(s) requiring admission are of low severity. Typically, 30 minutes are spent at the bedside and on the patient's hospital floor or unit.

🔲 2.86   ⅗ 2.86   **FUD** XXX   B 80 ▭

AMA: 2020,Oct,14; 2020,Sep,3; 2018,Dec,8; 2018,Dec,8; 2018,Jan,8; 2017,Aug,3; 2017,Jun,6; 2017,Jan,8; 2016,Dec,11; 2016,Mar,10; 2016,Jan,13; 2016,Jan,7

99222

Initial hospital care, per day, for the evaluation and management of a patient, which requires these 3 key components: A comprehensive history; A comprehensive examination; and Medical decision making of moderate complexity. Counseling and/or coordination of care with other physicians, other qualified health care professionals, or agencies are provided consistent with the nature of the problem(s) and the patient's and/or family's needs. Usually, the problem(s) requiring admission are of moderate severity. Typically, 50 minutes are spent at the bedside and on the patient's hospital floor or unit.

🔲 3.86   ⅗ 3.86   **FUD** XXX   B 80 ▭

AMA: 2020,Oct,14; 2020,Sep,3; 2018,Dec,8; 2018,Dec,8; 2018,Jan,8; 2017,Aug,3; 2017,Jun,6; 2017,Jan,8; 2016,Dec,11; 2016,Mar,10; 2016,Jan,13; 2016,Jan,7

99223

Initial hospital care, per day, for the evaluation and management of a patient, which requires these 3 key components: A comprehensive history; A comprehensive examination; and Medical decision making of high complexity. Counseling and/or coordination of care with other physicians, other qualified health care professionals, or agencies are provided consistent with the nature of the problem(s) and the patient's and/or family's needs. Usually, the problem(s) requiring admission are of high severity. Typically, 70 minutes are spent at the bedside and on the patient's hospital floor or unit.

🔲 5.71   ⅗ 5.71   **FUD** XXX   B 80 ▭

AMA: 2020,Oct,14; 2020,Sep,3; 2018,Dec,8; 2018,Dec,8; 2018,Jan,8; 2017,Aug,3; 2017,Jun,6; 2017,Jan,8; 2016,Dec,11; 2016,Mar,10; 2016,Jan,13; 2016,Jan,7

99224   Resequenced code. See code following 99220.

99225   Resequenced code. See code following 99220.

99226   Resequenced code. See code following 99220.

99231

Subsequent hospital care, per day, for the evaluation and management of a patient, which requires at least 2 of these 3 key components: A problem focused interval history; A problem focused examination; Medical decision making that is straightforward or of low complexity. Counseling and/or coordination of care with other physicians, other qualified health care professionals, or agencies are provided consistent with the nature of the problem(s) and the patient's and/or family's needs. Usually, the patient is stable, recovering or improving. Typically, 15 minutes are spent at the bedside and on the patient's hospital floor or unit.

🔲 1.11   ⅗ 1.11   **FUD** XXX   ★ B 80 ▭

AMA: 2020,Sep,3; 2018,Dec,8; 2018,Dec,8; 2018,Jan,8; 2017,Aug,3; 2017,Jun,6; 2017,Jan,8; 2016,Dec,11; 2016,Jan,13; 2016,Jan,7

99232

Subsequent hospital care, per day, for the evaluation and management of a patient, which requires at least 2 of these 3 key components: An expanded problem focused interval history; An expanded problem focused examination; Medical decision making of moderate complexity. Counseling and/or coordination of care with other physicians, other qualified health care professionals, or agencies are provided consistent with the nature of the problem(s) and the patient's and/or family's needs. Usually, the patient is responding inadequately to therapy or has developed a minor complication. Typically, 25 minutes are spent at the bedside and on the patient's hospital floor or unit.

🔲 2.05   ⅗ 2.05   **FUD** XXX   ★ B 80 ▭

AMA: 2020,Sep,3; 2018,Dec,8; 2018,Dec,8; 2018,Jan,8; 2017,Aug,3; 2017,Jun,6; 2017,Jan,8; 2016,Dec,11; 2016,Oct,8; 2016,Jan,13; 2016,Jan,7

99233

Subsequent hospital care, per day, for the evaluation and management of a patient, which requires at least 2 of these 3 key components: A detailed interval history; A detailed examination; Medical decision making of high complexity. Counseling and/or coordination of care with other physicians, other qualified health care professionals, or agencies are provided consistent with the nature of the problem(s) and the patient's and/or family's needs. Usually, the patient is unstable or has developed a significant complication or a significant new problem. Typically, 35 minutes are spent at the bedside and on the patient's hospital floor or unit.

🔲 2.93   ⅗ 2.93   **FUD** XXX   ★ B 80 ▭

AMA: 2020,Sep,3; 2018,Dec,8; 2018,Dec,8; 2018,Jan,8; 2017,Aug,3; 2017,Jun,6; 2017,Jan,8; 2016,Dec,11; 2016,Oct,8; 2016,Jan,13; 2016,Jan,7

28/TC PC/TC Only   42-Z3 ASC Payment   50 Bilateral   ♂ Male Only   ♀ Female Only   🔲 Facility RVU   ⅗ Non-Facility RVU   ▭ CCI   ✖ CLIA
FUD Follow-up Days   CMS: IOM   AMA: CPT Asst   A-Y OPPSI   80/80 Surg Assist Allowed / w/Doc   ▧ Lab Crosswalk   ▨ Radiology Crosswalk

546   CPT © 2021 American Medical Association. All Rights Reserved.   © 2021 Optum360, LLC

99234-99236 Observation/Inpatient Visits: Admitted/Discharged on Same Date

CMS: 100-04,11,40.1.3 Independent Attending Physician Services; 100-04,12,30.6.4 Services Furnished Incident to Physician's Service; 100-04,12,30.6.8 Payment for Hospital Observation Services; 100-04,12,30.6.9 Swing Bed Visits; 100-04,12,30.6.9.1 Initial Hospital Care and Observation or Inpatient Care Services; 100-04,12,30.6.9.2 Hospital Discharge Management; 100-04,12,40.3 Global Surgery Review

INCLUDES Admission and discharge services on same date in observation or inpatient setting

All services provided by admitting physician or other qualified health care professional on same date, even when initiated in another setting (e.g., emergency department, nursing facility, office)

EXCLUDES *Services provided to patients admitted to observation and discharged on different date (99217-99220, [99224, 99225, 99226])*

99234 Observation or inpatient hospital care, for the evaluation and management of a patient including admission and discharge on the same date, which requires these 3 key components: A detailed or comprehensive history; A detailed or comprehensive examination; and Medical decision making that is straightforward or of low complexity. Counseling and/or coordination of care with other physicians, other qualified health care professionals, or agencies are provided consistent with the nature of the problem(s) and the patient's and/or family's needs. Usually the presenting problem(s) requiring admission are of low severity. Typically, 40 minutes are spent at the bedside and on the patient's hospital floor or unit.

🚑 3.75 ⚖ 3.75 **FUD** XXX 🄱 🄼 🖵

AMA: 2020,Sep,3; 2018,Dec,8; 2018,Dec,8; 2018,Apr,10; 2018,Jan,8; 2017,Aug,3; 2017,Jun,6; 2017,Jan,8; 2016,Dec,11; 2016,Jan,13

99235 Observation or inpatient hospital care, for the evaluation and management of a patient including admission and discharge on the same date, which requires these 3 key components: A comprehensive history; A comprehensive examination; and Medical decision making of moderate complexity. Counseling and/or coordination of care with other physicians, other qualified health care professionals, or agencies are provided consistent with the nature of the problem(s) and the patient's and/or family's needs. Usually the presenting problem(s) requiring admission are of moderate severity. Typically, 50 minutes are spent at the bedside and on the patient's hospital floor or unit.

🚑 4.77 ⚖ 4.77 **FUD** XXX 🄱 🄼 🖵

AMA: 2020,Sep,3; 2018,Dec,8; 2018,Dec,8; 2018,Apr,10; 2018,Jan,8; 2017,Aug,3; 2017,Jun,6; 2017,Jan,8; 2016,Dec,11; 2016,Jan,13

99236 Observation or inpatient hospital care, for the evaluation and management of a patient including admission and discharge on the same date, which requires these 3 key components: A comprehensive history; A comprehensive examination; and Medical decision making of high complexity. Counseling and/or coordination of care with other physicians, other qualified health care professionals, or agencies are provided consistent with the nature of the problem(s) and the patient's and/or family's needs. Usually the presenting problem(s) requiring admission are of high severity. Typically, 55 minutes are spent at the bedside and on the patient's hospital floor or unit.

🚑 6.13 ⚖ 6.13 **FUD** XXX 🄱 🄼 🖵

AMA: 2020,Sep,3; 2018,Dec,8; 2018,Dec,8; 2018,Apr,10; 2018,Jan,8; 2017,Aug,3; 2017,Jun,6; 2017,Jan,8; 2016,Dec,11; 2016,Jan,13

99238-99239 Inpatient Hospital Discharge Services

CMS: 100-04,11,40.1.3 Independent Attending Physician Services; 100-04,12,30.6.4 Services Furnished Incident to Physician's Service; 100-04,12,30.6.9 Swing Bed Visits; 100-04,12,30.6.9.1 Initial Hospital Care and Observation or Inpatient Care Services; 100-04,12,30.6.9.2 Hospital Discharge Management; 100-04,12,40.3 Global Surgery Review

INCLUDES All services on discharge day when discharge and admission are not on same day

Discharge instructions

Final patient evaluation

Final preparation patient's medical records

Provision prescriptions/referrals, as needed

Review inpatient admission

EXCLUDES *Admission/discharge on same date (99234-99236)*
Discharge from observation (99217)
Discharge from nursing facility (99315-99316)
Healthy newborn evaluated and discharged on same date (99463)
Services provided by other than attending physician or other qualified health care professional on discharge date (99231-99233)

99238 Hospital discharge day management; 30 minutes or less

🚑 2.06 ⚖ 2.06 **FUD** XXX 🄱 🄼 🖵

AMA: 2018,Dec,8; 2018,Dec,8; 2018,Jan,8; 2017,Aug,3; 2017,Jun,6; 2017,Jan,8; 2016,Dec,11; 2016,Jan,13

99239 more than 30 minutes

🚑 3.02 ⚖ 3.02 **FUD** XXX 🄱 🄼 🖵

AMA: 2018,Dec,8; 2018,Dec,8; 2018,Jan,8; 2017,Aug,3; 2017,Jun,6; 2017,Jan,8; 2016,Dec,11; 2016,Jan,13

99241-99245 Consultations: Office and Outpatient

CMS: 100-04,11,40.1.3 Independent Attending Physician Services; 100-04,12,190.6 Payment Methodology for Physician/Practitioner at the Distant Site ; 100-04,12,190.6.1 Submission of Telehealth Claims for Distant Site Practitioners; 100-04,12,190.7 Contractor Editing of Telehealth Claims; 100-04,12,30.6.10 Consultation Services; 100-04,12,30.6.15.1 Prolonged Services With Direct Face-to-Face Patient Contact; 100-04,12,30.6.4 Services Furnished Incident to Physician's Service; 100-04,12,30.6.9.1 Initial Hospital Care and Observation or Inpatient Care Services; 100-04,12,40.3 Global Surgery Review; 100-04,32,130.1 Billing and Payment of External counterpulsation (ECP); 100-04,4,160 Clinic and Emergency Visits Under OPPS

INCLUDES All outpatient consultations provided in office, outpatient or other ambulatory facility, domiciliary/rest home, emergency department, patient's home, and hospital observation

Documentation consultation request from appropriate source

Documentation need for consultation in patient's medical record

One consultation per consultant

Provision by physician or qualified nonphysician practitioner whose advice, opinion, recommendation, suggestion, direction, or counsel, etc., requested for evaluating/treating patient since that individual's specific medical expertise beyond requesting physician knowledge

Provision written report, findings/recommendations from consultant to referring physician

Third-party mandated consultation; append modifier 32

EXCLUDES *Another appropriately requested and documented consultation pertaining to same/new problem; repeat consultation code reporting*
Any distinctly recognizable procedure/service provided on or following consultation
Care assumption (all or partial); report subsequent codes as appropriate for place of service (99211-99215, 99334-99337, 99347-99350)
Consultation prompted by patient/family; report codes for office, domiciliary/rest home, or home visits instead (99202-99215, 99324-99337, 99341-99350)
Services provided to Medicare patients; E/M code as appropriate for place of service or HCPCS code (99202-99215, 99221-99223, 99231-99233, G0406-G0408, G0425-G0427)

99241 Office consultation for a new or established patient, which requires these 3 key components: A problem focused history; A problem focused examination; and Straightforward medical decision making. Counseling and/or coordination of care with other physicians, other qualified health care professionals, or agencies are provided consistent with the nature of the problem(s) and the patient's and/or family's needs. Usually, the presenting problem(s) are self limited or minor. Typically, 15 minutes are spent face-to-face with the patient and/or family.

🚑 0.92 ⚖ 1.34 **FUD** XXX ★ 🄴 🖵

AMA: 2020,Oct,14; 2020,Nov,3; 2020,Sep,3; 2018,Apr,9; 2018,Apr,10; 2018,Mar,7; 2018,Jan,8; 2017,Aug,3; 2017,Jun,6; 2017,Jan,8; 2016,Dec,11; 2016,Sep,6; 2016,Jan,13; 2016,Jan,7

99242 Office consultation for a new or established patient, which requires these 3 key components: An expanded problem focused history; An expanded problem focused examination; and Straightforward medical decision making. Counseling and/or coordination of care with other physicians, other qualified health care professionals, or agencies are provided consistent with the nature of the problem(s) and the patient's and/or family's needs. Usually, the presenting problem(s) are of low severity. Typically, 30 minutes are spent face-to-face with the patient and/or family.

    1.93   2.52   **FUD** XXX   ★ E ▣

AMA: 2020,Oct,14; 2020,Nov,3; 2020,Sep,3; 2018,Apr,9; 2018,Apr,10; 2018,Mar,7; 2018,Jan,8; 2017,Aug,3; 2017,Jun,8; 2017,Jun,6; 2017,Jan,8; 2016,Dec,11; 2016,Sep,6; 2016,Jan,13; 2016,Jan,7

99243 Office consultation for a new or established patient, which requires these 3 key components: A detailed history; A detailed examination; and Medical decision making of low complexity. Counseling and/or coordination of care with other physicians, other qualified health care professionals, or agencies are provided consistent with the nature of the problem(s) and the patient's and/or family's needs. Usually, the presenting problem(s) are of moderate severity. Typically, 40 minutes are spent face-to-face with the patient and/or family.

    2.70   3.45   **FUD** XXX   ★ E ▣

AMA: 2020,Oct,14; 2020,Nov,3; 2020,Sep,3; 2018,Apr,9; 2018,Apr,10; 2018,Mar,7; 2018,Jan,8; 2017,Aug,3; 2017,Jun,6; 2017,Jan,8; 2016,Dec,11; 2016,Sep,6; 2016,Jan,13; 2016,Jan,7

99244 Office consultation for a new or established patient, which requires these 3 key components: A comprehensive history; A comprehensive examination; and Medical decision making of moderate complexity. Counseling and/or coordination of care with other physicians, other qualified health care professionals, or agencies are provided consistent with the nature of the problem(s) and the patient's and/or family's needs. Usually, the presenting problem(s) are of moderate to high severity. Typically, 60 minutes are spent face-to-face with the patient and/or family.

    4.34   5.16   **FUD** XXX   ★ E ▣

AMA: 2020,Oct,14; 2020,Nov,3; 2020,Sep,3; 2018,Apr,9; 2018,Apr,10; 2018,Mar,7; 2018,Jan,8; 2017,Aug,3; 2017,Jun,6; 2017,Jan,8; 2016,Dec,11; 2016,Sep,6; 2016,Jan,13; 2016,Jan,7

99245 Office consultation for a new or established patient, which requires these 3 key components: A comprehensive history; A comprehensive examination; and Medical decision making of high complexity. Counseling and/or coordination of care with other physicians, other qualified health care professionals, or agencies are provided consistent with the nature of the problem(s) and the patient's and/or family's needs. Usually, the presenting problem(s) are of moderate to high severity. Typically, 80 minutes are spent face-to-face with the patient and/or family.

    5.37   6.29   **FUD** XXX   ★ E ▣

AMA: 2020,Oct,14; 2020,Nov,3; 2020,Sep,3; 2018,Apr,9; 2018,Apr,10; 2018,Mar,7; 2018,Jan,8; 2017,Aug,3; 2017,Jun,6; 2017,Jan,8; 2016,Dec,11; 2016,Sep,6; 2016,Jan,13; 2016,Jan,7

99251-99255 Consultations: Inpatient

CMS: 100-04,11,40.1.3 Independent Attending Physician Services; 100-04,12,190.6 Payment Methodology for Physician/Practitioner at the Distant Site ; 100-04,12,190.6.1 Submission of Telehealth Claims for Distant Site Practitioners; 100-04,12,190.7 Contractor Editing of Telehealth Claims; 100-04,12,30.6.10 Consultation Services; 100-04,12,30.6.15.1 Prolonged Services With Direct Face-to-Face Patient Contact; 100-04,12,30.6.4 Services Furnished Incident to Physician's Service; 100-04,12,30.6.9.1 Initial Hospital Care and Observation or Inpatient Care Services; 100-04,12,40.3 Global Surgery Review

INCLUDES   All outpatient consultations provided in office, outpatient or other ambulatory facility, domiciliary/rest home, emergency department, patient's home, and hospital observation
Documentation consultation request from appropriate source
Documentation need for consultation in patient's medical record
One consultation per consultant
Provision by physician or qualified nonphysician practitioner whose advice, opinion, recommendation, suggestion, direction, or counsel, etc., requested for evaluating/treating patient since that individual's specific medical expertise beyond requesting physician knowledge
Provision written report, findings/recommendations from consultant to referring physician
Third-party mandated consultation; append modifier 32

EXCLUDES   *Another appropriately requested and documented consultation pertaining to same/new problem; repeat consultation code reporting*
Any distinctly recognizable procedure/service provided on or following consultation
Care assumption (all or partial); report subsequent codes as appropriate for place of service (99231-99233, 99307-99310)
Consultation prompted by patient/family; report codes for office, domiciliary/rest home, or home visits instead (99202-99215, 99234-99337, 99341-99350)
Services provided to Medicare patients; E/M code as appropriate for place of service or HCPCS code (99202-99215, 99324-99337, 99341-99350)

99251 Inpatient consultation for a new or established patient, which requires these 3 key components: A problem focused history; A problem focused examination; and Straightforward medical decision making. Counseling and/or coordination of care with other physicians, other qualified health care professionals, or agencies are provided consistent with the nature of the problem(s) and the patient's and/or family's needs. Usually, the presenting problem(s) are self limited or minor. Typically, 20 minutes are spent at the bedside and on the patient's hospital floor or unit.

    1.38   1.38   **FUD** XXX   ★ E ▣

AMA: 2020,Sep,3; 2018,Jan,8; 2017,Aug,3; 2017,Jun,6; 2017,Jan,8; 2016,Dec,11; 2016,Jan,7; 2016,Jan,13

99252 Inpatient consultation for a new or established patient, which requires these 3 key components: An expanded problem focused history; An expanded problem focused examination; and Straightforward medical decision making. Counseling and/or coordination of care with other physicians, other qualified health care professionals, or agencies are provided consistent with the nature of the problem(s) and the patient's and/or family's needs. Usually, the presenting problem(s) are of low severity. Typically, 40 minutes are spent at the bedside and on the patient's hospital floor or unit.

    2.11   2.11   **FUD** XXX   ★ E ▣

AMA: 2020,Sep,3; 2018,Jan,8; 2017,Aug,3; 2017,Jun,6; 2017,Jan,8; 2016,Dec,11; 2016,Jan,13; 2016,Jan,7

99253 Inpatient consultation for a new or established patient, which requires these 3 key components: A detailed history; A detailed examination; and Medical decision making of low complexity. Counseling and/or coordination of care with other physicians, other qualified health care professionals, or agencies are provided consistent with the nature of the problem(s) and the patient's and/or family's needs. Usually, the presenting problem(s) are of moderate severity. Typically, 55 minutes are spent at the bedside and on the patient's hospital floor or unit.

    3.25   3.25   **FUD** XXX   ★ E ▣

AMA: 2020,Sep,3; 2018,Jan,8; 2017,Aug,3; 2017,Jun,6; 2017,Jan,8; 2016,Dec,11; 2016,Jan,13; 2016,Jan,7

| 26/TC PC/TC Only | A2-Z3 ASC Payment | 50 Bilateral | ♂ Male Only | ♀ Female Only | Facility RVU | Non-Facility RVU | ☐ CCI | ☒ CLIA |
| **FUD** Follow-up Days | **CMS:** IOM | **AMA:** CPT Asst | A-Y OPPSI | 80/80 Surg Assist Allowed / w/Doc | Lab Crosswalk | Radiology Crosswalk |

548   CPT © 2021 American Medical Association. All Rights Reserved.   © 2021 Optum360, LLC

99254 Inpatient consultation for a new or established patient, which requires these 3 key components: A comprehensive history; A comprehensive examination; and Medical decision making of moderate complexity. Counseling and/or coordination of care with other physicians, other qualified health care professionals, or agencies are provided consistent with the nature of the problem(s) and the patient's and/or family's needs. Usually, the presenting problem(s) are of moderate to high severity. Typically, 80 minutes are spent at the bedside and on the patient's hospital floor or unit.

4.72 ⚕ 4.72 **FUD** XXX ★Ⓔ▣

AMA: 2020,Sep,3; 2018,Jan,8; 2017,Aug,3; 2017,Jun,6; 2017,Jan,8; 2016,Dec,11; 2016,Jan,7; 2016,Jan,13

99255 Inpatient consultation for a new or established patient, which requires these 3 key components: A comprehensive history; A comprehensive examination; and Medical decision making of high complexity. Counseling and/or coordination of care with other physicians, other qualified health care professionals, or agencies are provided consistent with the nature of the problem(s) and the patient's and/or family's needs. Usually, the presenting problem(s) are of moderate to high severity. Typically, 110 minutes are spent at the bedside and on the patient's hospital floor or unit.

5.76 ⚕ 5.76 **FUD** XXX ★Ⓔ▣

AMA: 2020,Sep,3; 2018,Jan,8; 2017,Aug,3; 2017,Jun,6; 2017,Jan,8; 2016,Dec,11; 2016,Jan,7; 2016,Jan,13

99281-99288 Emergency Department Visits

CMS: 100-04,11,40.1.3 Independent Attending Physician Services; 100-04,12,30.6.11 Emergency Department Visits; 100-04,4,160 Clinic and Emergency Visits Under OPPS

INCLUDES Any time spent with patient, which usually involves multiple encounters while patient in emergency department
Care provided to new and established patients

EXCLUDES Critical care services (99291-99292)
Observation services (99217-99220, 99234-99236)

99281 Emergency department visit for the evaluation and management of a patient, which requires these 3 key components: A problem focused history; A problem focused examination; and Straightforward medical decision making. Counseling and/or coordination of care with other physicians, other qualified health care professionals, or agencies are provided consistent with the nature of the problem(s) and the patient's and/or family's needs. Usually, the presenting problem(s) are self limited or minor.

0.60 ⚕ 0.60 **FUD** XXX Ⓙ⑧⓪▣

AMA: 2020,Oct,13; 2020,Jul,13; 2019,Jul,10; 2018,Jan,8; 2017,Aug,3; 2017,Jun,6; 2017,Jan,8; 2016,Jan,13; 2016,Jan,7

99282 Emergency department visit for the evaluation and management of a patient, which requires these 3 key components: An expanded problem focused history; An expanded problem focused examination; and Medical decision making of low complexity. Counseling and/or coordination of care with other physicians, other qualified health care professionals, or agencies are provided consistent with the nature of the problem(s) and the patient's and/or family's needs. Usually, the presenting problem(s) are of low to moderate severity.

1.17 ⚕ 1.17 **FUD** XXX Ⓙ⑧⓪▣

AMA: 2020,Oct,13; 2020,Jul,13; 2019,Jul,10; 2018,Jan,8; 2017,Aug,3; 2017,Jun,6; 2017,Jan,8; 2016,Jan,13; 2016,Jan,7

99283 Emergency department visit for the evaluation and management of a patient, which requires these 3 key components: An expanded problem focused history; An expanded problem focused examination; and Medical decision making of moderate complexity. Counseling and/or coordination of care with other physicians, other qualified health care professionals, or agencies are provided consistent with the nature of the problem(s) and the patient's and/or family's needs. Usually, the presenting problem(s) are of moderate severity.

1.75 ⚕ 1.75 **FUD** XXX Ⓙ⑧⓪▣

AMA: 2020,Oct,13; 2020,Jul,13; 2019,Jul,10; 2018,Jan,8; 2017,Aug,3; 2017,Jun,6; 2017,Jan,8; 2016,Jan,7; 2016,Jan,13

99284 Emergency department visit for the evaluation and management of a patient, which requires these 3 key components: A detailed history; A detailed examination; and Medical decision making of moderate complexity. Counseling and/or coordination of care with other physicians, other qualified health care professionals, or agencies are provided consistent with the nature of the problem(s) and the patient's and/or family's needs. Usually, the presenting problem(s) are of high severity, and require urgent evaluation by the physician, or other qualified health care professionals but do not pose an immediate significant threat to life or physiologic function.

3.32 ⚕ 3.32 **FUD** XXX Ⓙ⑧⓪▣

AMA: 2020,Oct,13; 2020,Jul,13; 2019,Jul,10; 2018,Jan,8; 2017,Aug,3; 2017,Jun,6; 2017,Jan,8; 2016,Jan,13; 2016,Jan,7

99285 Emergency department visit for the evaluation and management of a patient, which requires these 3 key components within the constraints imposed by the urgency of the patient's clinical condition and/or mental status: A comprehensive history; A comprehensive examination; and Medical decision making of high complexity. Counseling and/or coordination of care with other physicians, other qualified health care professionals, or agencies are provided consistent with the nature of the problem(s) and the patient's and/or family's needs. Usually, the presenting problem(s) are of high severity and pose an immediate significant threat to life or physiologic function.

4.89 ⚕ 4.89 **FUD** XXX Ⓙ⑧⓪▣

AMA: 2020,Oct,13; 2020,Jul,13; 2020,Jan,12; 2019,Jul,10; 2018,Jan,8; 2017,Aug,3; 2017,Jun,6; 2017,Jan,8; 2016,Jan,13; 2016,Jan,7

99288 Physician or other qualified health care professional direction of emergency medical systems (EMS) emergency care, advanced life support

INCLUDES Management provided by emergency/intensive care based physician or other qualified health care professional via voice contact to ambulance/rescue staff for services such as heart monitoring and drug administration

0.00 ⚕ 0.00 **FUD** XXX Ⓑ▣

AMA: 2018,Jan,8; 2017,Aug,3; 2017,Jun,6; 2017,Jan,8; 2016,Jan,13

99291-99292 Critical Care Visits: Patients 72 Months of Age and Older

CMS: 100-04,11,40.1.3 Independent Attending Physician Services; 100-04,12,30.6.4 Services Furnished Incident to Physician's Service; 100-04,12,30.6.9 Payment for Inpatient Hospital Visits - General; 100-04,12,40.3 Global Surgery Review; 100-04,4,160 Clinic and Emergency Visits Under OPPS; 100-04,4,160.1 Critical Care Services

INCLUDES 30 minutes or more direct care provided by physician or other qualified health care professional to critically ill or injured patient, any location
All activities performed outside unit or off floor
All time spent exclusively with patient/family/caregivers on nursing unit or elsewhere
Outpatient critical care provided to neonates and pediatric patients age 71 months or younger
Physician or other qualified health care professional presence during interfacility transfer for critically ill/injured patients age 24 months or older
Professional services for interpretation:
  Blood gases
  Chest films (71045-71046)
  Measurement cardiac output (93598)
  Other computer stored information
  Pulse oximetry (94760-94762)
Professional services:
  Gastric intubation (43752-43753)
  Transcutaneous pacing, temporary (92953)
  Venous access, arterial puncture (36000, 36410, 36415, 36591, 36600)
  Ventilation assistance and management, includes CPAP, CNP (94002-94004, 94660, 94662)

EXCLUDES *All services less than 30 minutes; report appropriate E/M code*
Inpatient critical care services provided to child age 2 through 5 years old (99475-99476)
Inpatient critical care services provided to infants age 29 days through 24 months old (99471-99472)
Inpatient critical care services provided to neonates age 28 days or younger (99468-99469)
Other procedures not listed as included performed by physician or other qualified health care professional rendering critical care
Patients not critically ill but in critical care department (report appropriate E/M code)
Physician or other qualified health care professional presence during interfacility transfer for critically ill/injured patients age 24 months or younger (99466-99467)
Supervisory services control physician during interfacility transfer for critically ill/injured patients age 24 months or younger ([99485, 99486])

99291   **Critical care, evaluation and management of the critically ill or critically injured patient; first 30-74 minutes**
6.28   7.82   **FUD** XXX   J 80
AMA: 2020,Feb,7; 2020,Jan,12; 2019,Dec,14; 2019,Aug,8; 2019,Jul,10; 2018,Dec,8; 2018,Dec,8; 2018,Jun,9; 2018,Jan,8; 2017,Aug,3; 2017,Jun,6; 2017,Jan,8; 2016,Oct,8; 2016,Aug,9; 2016,May,3; 2016,Jan,13

+ 99292   **each additional 30 minutes (List separately in addition to code for primary service)**
Code first (99291)
3.15   3.46   **FUD** ZZZ   N 80
AMA: 2020,Feb,7; 2019,Dec,14; 2019,Aug,8; 2019,Jul,10; 2018,Dec,8; 2018,Dec,8; 2018,Jun,9; 2018,Jan,8; 2017,Aug,3; 2017,Jun,6; 2017,Jan,8; 2016,Aug,9; 2016,May,3; 2016,Jan,13

99304-99310 Nursing Facility Visits

CMS: 100-04,11,40.1.3 Independent Attending Physician Services; 100-04,12,230 Primary Care Incentive Payment Program; 100-04,12,230.1 Definition of Primary Care Practitioners and Services; 100-04,12,230.2 Coordination with Other Payments; 100-04,12,230.3 Claims Processing and Payment; 100-04,12,30.6.10 Consultation Services; 100-04,12,30.6.13 Nursing Facility Visits; 100-04,12,30.6.15.1 Prolonged Services With Direct Face-to-Face Patient Contact; 100-04,12,30.6.4 Services Furnished Incident to Physician's Service; 100-04,12,30.6.9 Payment for Inpatient Hospital Visits - General

INCLUDES All E/M services provided by admitting physician on nursing facility admission date in other locations (e.g., office, emergency department)
Initial care, subsequent care, discharge, and yearly assessments
Initial services include patient assessment and physician participation in developing plan of care (99304-99306)
Services provided in psychiatric residential treatment center
Services provided to new and established patients in nursing facility (skilled, intermediate, and long-term care facilities)
Subsequent services include physician review medical records, reassessment, and review test results (99307-99310)

EXCLUDES *Care plan oversight services (99379-99380)*
Code also hospital discharge services on same admission or readmission date to nursing home (99217, 99234-99236, 99238-99239)

99304   **Initial nursing facility care, per day, for the evaluation and management of a patient, which requires these 3 key components: A detailed or comprehensive history; A detailed or comprehensive examination; and Medical decision making that is straightforward or of low complexity. Counseling and/or coordination of care with other physicians, other qualified health care professionals, or agencies are provided consistent with the nature of the problem(s) and the patient's and/or family's needs. Usually, the problem(s) requiring admission are of low severity. Typically, 25 minutes are spent at the bedside and on the patient's facility floor or unit.**
2.54   2.54   **FUD** XXX   B 80
AMA: 2020,Nov,3; 2020,Sep,3; 2018,Jan,8; 2017,Aug,3; 2017,Jun,6; 2017,Jan,8; 2016,Dec,11; 2016,Jan,7; 2016,Jan,13

99305   **Initial nursing facility care, per day, for the evaluation and management of a patient, which requires these 3 key components: A comprehensive history; A comprehensive examination; and Medical decision making of moderate complexity. Counseling and/or coordination of care with other physicians, other qualified health care professionals, or agencies are provided consistent with the nature of the problem(s) and the patient's and/or family's needs. Usually, the problem(s) requiring admission are of moderate severity. Typically, 35 minutes are spent at the bedside and on the patient's facility floor or unit.**
3.67   3.67   **FUD** XXX   B 80
AMA: 2020,Nov,3; 2020,Sep,3; 2018,Jan,8; 2017,Aug,3; 2017,Jun,6; 2017,Jan,8; 2016,Dec,11; 2016,Jan,7; 2016,Jan,13

99306   **Initial nursing facility care, per day, for the evaluation and management of a patient, which requires these 3 key components: A comprehensive history; A comprehensive examination; and Medical decision making of high complexity. Counseling and/or coordination of care with other physicians, other qualified health care professionals, or agencies are provided consistent with the nature of the problem(s) and the patient's and/or family's needs. Usually, the problem(s) requiring admission are of high severity. Typically, 45 minutes are spent at the bedside and on the patient's facility floor or unit.**
4.71   4.71   **FUD** XXX   B 80
AMA: 2020,Nov,3; 2020,Sep,3; 2018,Jan,8; 2017,Aug,3; 2017,Jun,6; 2017,Jan,8; 2016,Dec,11; 2016,Jan,7; 2016,Jan,13

26/TC PC/TC Only   A2-73 ASC Payment   50 Bilateral   ♂ Male Only   ♀ Female Only   Facility RVU   Non-Facility RVU   CCI   CLIA
FUD Follow-up Days   **CMS:** .IOM   **AMA:** CPT Asst   A-Y OPPSI   80/80 Surg Assist Allowed / w/Doc   Lab Crosswalk   Radiology Crosswalk

99307   Subsequent nursing facility care, per day, for the evaluation and management of a patient, which requires at least 2 of these 3 key components: A problem focused interval history; A problem focused examination; Straightforward medical decision making. Counseling and/or coordination of care with other physicians, other qualified health care professionals, or agencies are provided consistent with the nature of the problem(s) and the patient's and/or family's needs. Usually, the patient is stable, recovering, or improving. Typically, 10 minutes are spent at the bedside and on the patient's facility floor or unit.

📷 1.24   ⚖ 1.24   **FUD** XXX   ★ B 80 ▭

AMA: 2020,Nov,3; 2020,Sep,3; 2018,Jan,8; 2017,Aug,3; 2017,Jun,6; 2017,Jan,8; 2016,Dec,11; 2016,Jan,13; 2016,Jan,7

99308   Subsequent nursing facility care, per day, for the evaluation and management of a patient, which requires at least 2 of these 3 key components: An expanded problem focused interval history; An expanded problem focused examination; Medical decision making of low complexity. Counseling and/or coordination of care with other physicians, other qualified health care professionals, or agencies are provided consistent with the nature of the problem(s) and the patient's and/or family's needs. Usually, the patient is responding inadequately to therapy or has developed a minor complication. Typically, 15 minutes are spent at the bedside and on the patient's facility floor or unit.

📷 1.94   ⚖ 1.94   **FUD** XXX   ★ B 80 ▭

AMA: 2020,Nov,3; 2020,Sep,3; 2018,Jan,8; 2017,Aug,3; 2017,Jun,6; 2017,Jan,8; 2016,Dec,11; 2016,Jan,13; 2016,Jan,7

99309   Subsequent nursing facility care, per day, for the evaluation and management of a patient, which requires at least 2 of these 3 key components: A detailed interval history; A detailed examination; Medical decision making of moderate complexity. Counseling and/or coordination of care with other physicians, other qualified health care professionals, or agencies are provided consistent with the nature of the problem(s) and the patient's and/or family's needs. Usually, the patient has developed a significant complication or a significant new problem. Typically, 25 minutes are spent at the bedside and on the patient's facility floor or unit.

📷 2.58   ⚖ 2.58   **FUD** XXX   ★ B 80 ▭

AMA: 2020,Nov,3; 2020,Sep,3; 2018,Jan,8; 2017,Aug,3; 2017,Jun,6; 2017,Jan,8; 2016,Dec,11; 2016,Jan,13; 2016,Jan,7

99310   Subsequent nursing facility care, per day, for the evaluation and management of a patient, which requires at least 2 of these 3 key components: A comprehensive interval history; A comprehensive examination; Medical decision making of high complexity. Counseling and/or coordination of care with other physicians, other qualified health care professionals, or agencies are provided consistent with the nature of the problem(s) and the patient's and/or family's needs. The patient may be unstable or may have developed a significant new problem requiring immediate physician attention. Typically, 35 minutes are spent at the bedside and on the patient's facility floor or unit.

📷 3.82   ⚖ 3.82   **FUD** XXX   ★ B 80 ▭

AMA: 2020,Nov,3; 2020,Sep,3; 2018,Jan,8; 2017,Aug,3; 2017,Jun,6; 2017,Jan,8; 2016,Dec,11; 2016,Jan,13; 2016,Jan,7

99315-99316 Nursing Home Discharge

CMS: 100-04,11,40.1.3 Independent Attending Physician Services; 100-04,12,230 Primary Care Incentive Payment Program; 100-04,12,230.1 Definition of Primary Care Practitioners and Services; 100-04,12,230.2 Coordination with Other Payments; 100-04,12,230.3 Claims Processing and Payment; 100-04,12,30.6.13 Nursing Facility Visits; 100-04,12,30.6.4 Services Furnished Incident to Physician's Service; 100-04,12,40.3 Global Surgery Review

INCLUDES   Discharge services include all time spent by physician or other qualified health care professional:
Completion discharge records
Discharge instructions for patient and caregivers
Discussion regarding stay in facility
Final patient examination
Provide prescriptions and referrals as appropriate

99315   Nursing facility discharge day management; 30 minutes or less

📷 2.07   ⚖ 2.07   **FUD** XXX   B 80 ▭

AMA: 2020,Nov,3; 2018,Jan,8; 2017,Aug,3; 2017,Jun,6; 2017,Jan,8; 2016,Dec,11; 2016,Jan,7; 2016,Jan,13

99316   more than 30 minutes

📷 2.98   ⚖ 2.98   **FUD** XXX   B 80 ▭

AMA: 2020,Nov,3; 2018,Jan,8; 2017,Aug,3; 2017,Jun,6; 2017,Jan,8; 2016,Dec,11; 2016,Jan,7; 2016,Jan,13

99318 Annual Nursing Home Assessment

CMS: 100-04,11,40.1.3 Independent Attending Physician Services; 100-04,12,230 Primary Care Incentive Payment Program; 100-04,12,230.1 Definition of Primary Care Practitioners and Services; 100-04,12,230.2 Coordination with Other Payments; 100-04,12,230.3 Claims Processing and Payment; 100-04,12,30.6.13 Nursing Facility Visits; 100-04,12,30.6.15.1 Prolonged Services With Direct Face-to-Face Patient Contact; 100-04,12,30.6.4 Services Furnished Incident to Physician's Service; 100-04,12,30.6.9 Payment for Inpatient Hospital Visits - General

INCLUDES   Includes nursing facility visits on same date as (99304-99316)

99318   Evaluation and management of a patient involving an annual nursing facility assessment, which requires these 3 key components: A detailed interval history; A comprehensive examination; and Medical decision making that is of low to moderate complexity. Counseling and/or coordination of care with other physicians, other qualified health care professionals, or agencies are provided consistent with the nature of the problem(s) and the patient's and/or family's needs. Usually, the patient is stable, recovering, or improving. Typically, 30 minutes are spent at the bedside and on the patient's facility floor or unit.

📷 2.70   ⚖ 2.70   **FUD** XXX   B 80 ▭

AMA: 2020,Nov,3; 2018,Jan,8; 2017,Aug,3; 2017,Jun,6; 2017,Jan,8; 2016,Dec,11; 2016,Jan,7; 2016,Jan,13

99324-99337 Domiciliary Care, Rest Home, Assisted Living Visits

CMS: 100-04,12,230 Primary Care Incentive Payment Program; 100-04,12,230.1 Definition of Primary Care Practitioners and Services; 100-04,12,230.2 Coordination with Other Payments; 100-04,12,230.3 Claims Processing and Payment; 100-04,12,30.6.14 Domiciliary Care, Rest Home, Assisted Living Visits; 100-04,12,30.6.15.1 Prolonged Services With Direct Face-to-Face Patient Contact; 100-04,12,30.6.4 Services Furnished Incident to Physician's Service

INCLUDES　E/M services for patients residing in assisted living, domiciliary care, and rest homes where medical care not included
Services provided to new patients or established patients (99324-99328, 99334-99337)

EXCLUDES　*Care plan oversight services provided to patient in rest home under home health agency care (99374-99375)*
Care plan oversight services provided to patient under hospice agency care (99377-99378)

99324　Domiciliary or rest home visit for the evaluation and management of a new patient, which requires these 3 key components: A problem focused history; A problem focused examination; and Straightforward medical decision making. Counseling and/or coordination of care with other physicians, other qualified health care professionals, or agencies are provided consistent with the nature of the problem(s) and the patient's and/or family's needs. Usually, the presenting problem(s) are of low severity. Typically, 20 minutes are spent with the patient and/or family or caregiver.
　1.56　　1.56　　**FUD** XXX　　B 80
　AMA: 2020,Sep,3; 2018,Apr,9; 2018,Jan,8; 2017,Aug,3; 2017,Jun,6; 2017,Jan,8; 2016,Dec,11; 2016,Jan,7; 2016,Jan,13

99325　Domiciliary or rest home visit for the evaluation and management of a new patient, which requires these 3 key components: An expanded problem focused history; An expanded problem focused examination; and Medical decision making of low complexity. Counseling and/or coordination of care with other physicians, other qualified health care professionals, or agencies are provided consistent with the nature of the problem(s) and the patient's and/or family's needs. Usually, the presenting problem(s) are of moderate severity. Typically, 30 minutes are spent with the patient and/or family or caregiver.
　2.26　　2.26　　**FUD** XXX　　B 80
　AMA: 2020,Sep,3; 2018,Apr,9; 2018,Jan,8; 2017,Aug,3; 2017,Jun,6; 2017,Jan,8; 2016,Dec,11; 2016,Jan,7; 2016,Jan,13

99326　Domiciliary or rest home visit for the evaluation and management of a new patient, which requires these 3 key components: A detailed history; A detailed examination; and Medical decision making of moderate complexity. Counseling and/or coordination of care with other physicians, other qualified health care professionals, or agencies are provided consistent with the nature of the problem(s) and the patient's and/or family's needs. Usually, the presenting problem(s) are of moderate to high severity. Typically, 45 minutes are spent with the patient and/or family or caregiver.
　3.92　　3.92　　**FUD** XXX　　B 80
　AMA: 2020,Sep,3; 2018,Apr,9; 2018,Jan,8; 2017,Aug,3; 2017,Jun,6; 2017,Jan,8; 2016,Dec,11; 2016,Jan,7; 2016,Jan,13

99327　Domiciliary or rest home visit for the evaluation and management of a new patient, which requires these 3 key components: A comprehensive history; A comprehensive examination; and Medical decision making of moderate complexity. Counseling and/or coordination of care with other physicians, other qualified health care professionals, or agencies are provided consistent with the nature of the problem(s) and the patient's and/or family's needs. Usually, the presenting problem(s) are of high severity. Typically, 60 minutes are spent with the patient and/or family or caregiver.
　5.26　　5.26　　**FUD** XXX　　B 80
　AMA: 2020,Sep,3; 2018,Apr,9; 2018,Jan,8; 2017,Aug,3; 2017,Jun,6; 2017,Jan,8; 2016,Dec,11; 2016,Jan,7; 2016,Jan,13

99328　Domiciliary or rest home visit for the evaluation and management of a new patient, which requires these 3 key components: A comprehensive history; A comprehensive examination; and Medical decision making of high complexity. Counseling and/or coordination of care with other physicians, other qualified health care professionals, or agencies are provided consistent with the nature of the problem(s) and the patient's and/or family's needs. Usually, the patient is unstable or has developed a significant new problem requiring immediate physician attention. Typically, 75 minutes are spent with the patient and/or family or caregiver.
　6.19　　6.19　　**FUD** XXX　　B 80
　AMA: 2020,Sep,3; 2018,Apr,9; 2018,Jan,8; 2017,Aug,3; 2017,Jun,6; 2017,Jan,8; 2016,Dec,11; 2016,Jan,7; 2016,Jan,13

99334　Domiciliary or rest home visit for the evaluation and management of an established patient, which requires at least 2 of these 3 key components: A problem focused interval history; A problem focused examination; Straightforward medical decision making. Counseling and/or coordination of care with other physicians, other qualified health care professionals, or agencies are provided consistent with the nature of the problem(s) and the patient's and/or family's needs. Usually, the presenting problem(s) are self-limited or minor. Typically, 15 minutes are spent with the patient and/or family or caregiver.
　1.70　　1.70　　**FUD** XXX　　B 80
　AMA: 2020,Sep,3; 2018,Apr,9; 2018,Jan,8; 2017,Aug,3; 2017,Jun,6; 2017,Jan,8; 2016,Dec,11; 2016,Jan,7; 2016,Jan,13

99335　Domiciliary or rest home visit for the evaluation and management of an established patient, which requires at least 2 of these 3 key components: An expanded problem focused interval history; An expanded problem focused examination; Medical decision making of low complexity. Counseling and/or coordination of care with other physicians, other qualified health care professionals, or agencies are provided consistent with the nature of the problem(s) and the patient's and/or family's needs. Usually, the presenting problem(s) are of low to moderate severity. Typically, 25 minutes are spent with the patient and/or family or caregiver.
　2.68　　2.68　　**FUD** XXX　　B 80
　AMA: 2020,Sep,3; 2018,Apr,9; 2018,Jan,8; 2017,Aug,3; 2017,Jun,6; 2017,Jan,8; 2016,Dec,11; 2016,Jan,7; 2016,Jan,13

99336　Domiciliary or rest home visit for the evaluation and management of an established patient, which requires at least 2 of these 3 key components: A detailed interval history; A detailed examination; Medical decision making of moderate complexity. Counseling and/or coordination of care with other physicians, other qualified health care professionals, or agencies are provided consistent with the nature of the problem(s) and the patient's and/or family's needs. Usually, the presenting problem(s) are of moderate to high severity. Typically, 40 minutes are spent with the patient and/or family or caregiver.
　3.82　　3.82　　**FUD** XXX　　B 80
　AMA: 2020,Sep,3; 2018,Apr,9; 2018,Jan,8; 2017,Aug,3; 2017,Jun,6; 2017,Jan,8; 2016,Dec,11; 2016,Jan,7; 2016,Jan,13

99337   Domiciliary or rest home visit for the evaluation and management of an established patient, which requires at least 2 of these 3 key components: A comprehensive interval history; A comprehensive examination; Medical decision making of moderate to high complexity. Counseling and/or coordination of care with other physicians, other qualified health care professionals, or agencies are provided consistent with the nature of the problem(s) and the patient's and/or family's needs. Usually, the presenting problem(s) are of moderate to high severity. The patient may be unstable or may have developed a significant new problem requiring immediate physician attention. Typically, 60 minutes are spent with the patient and/or family or caregiver.

⚕ 5.47   ⚕ 5.47   **FUD** XXX   B 80 ▯

AMA: 2020,Sep,3; 2018,Apr,9; 2018,Jan,8; 2017,Aug,3; 2017,Jun,6; 2017,Jan,8; 2016,Dec,11; 2016,Jan,7; 2016,Jan,13

99339-99340 Care Plan Oversight: Rest Home, Domiciliary Care, Assisted Living, and Home

CMS: 100-04,12,180 Payment of Care Plan Oversight (CPO); 100-04,12,180.1 Billing for Care Plan Oversight (CPO); 100-04,12,230 Primary Care Incentive Payment Program; 100-04,12,230.1 Definition of Primary Care Practitioners and Services; 100-04,12,230.2 Coordination with Other Payments; 100-04,12,230.3 Claims Processing and Payment; 100-04,12,30.6.14 Domiciliary Care, Rest Home, Assisted Living Visits; 100-04,12,30.6.4 Services Furnished Incident to Physician's Service

INCLUDES   Care plan oversight for patients residing in assisted living, domiciliary care, private residences, and rest homes
Online or telephone services during same time frame ([99421, 99422, 99423], 99441-99443, 98966-98968)

EXCLUDES   Care plan oversight services furnished under home health agency, nursing facility, or hospice (99374-99380)
Services during the same time frame:
Chronic/complex chronic care management ([99437], [99439], [99490], [99491], 99487, 99489)
Principal care management ([99424, 99425, 99426, 99427])

99339   Individual physician supervision of a patient (patient not present) in home, domiciliary or rest home (eg, assisted living facility) requiring complex and multidisciplinary care modalities involving regular physician development and/or revision of care plans, review of subsequent reports of patient status, review of related laboratory and other studies, communication (including telephone calls) for purposes of assessment or care decisions with health care professional(s), family member(s), surrogate decision maker(s) (eg, legal guardian) and/or key caregiver(s) involved in patient's care, integration of new information into the medical treatment plan and/or adjustment of medical therapy, within a calendar month; 15-29 minutes

⚕ 2.17   ⚕ 2.17   **FUD** XXX   B ▯

AMA: 2019,Jan,6; 2018,Oct,9; 2018,Jan,8; 2017,Aug,3; 2017,Jun,6; 2017,Jan,8; 2016,Jan,13

99340   **30 minutes or more**

⚕ 3.05   ⚕ 3.05   **FUD** XXX   B ▯

AMA: 2019,Jan,6; 2018,Oct,9; 2018,Jan,8; 2017,Aug,3; 2017,Jun,6; 2017,Jan,8; 2016,Jan,13

99341-99350 Home Visits

CMS: 100-04,11,40.1.3 Independent Attending Physician Services; 100-04,12,230 Primary Care Incentive Payment Program; 100-04,12,230.1 Definition of Primary Care Practitioners and Services; 100-04,12,230.2 Coordination with Other Payments; 100-04,12,230.3 Claims Processing and Payment; 100-04,12,30.6.14 Domiciliary Care, Rest Home, Assisted Living Visits; 100-04,12,30.6.14.1 Home Visits; 100-04,12,30.6.15.1 Prolonged Services With Direct Face-to-Face Patient Contact; 100-04,12,30.6.4 Services Furnished Incident to Physician's Service; 100-04,12,40.3 Global Surgery Review; 100-04,30.6.14.1 Home Services (Codes 99341 - 99350)

INCLUDES   Services for new or established patient (99341-99345, 99347-99350)
Services provided to patient in private home (e.g., private residence, temporary or short-term housing such as campground, cruise ship, hostel, or hotel)

EXCLUDES   Services provided to patients under home health agency or hospice care (99374-99378)

99341   Home visit for the evaluation and management of a new patient, which requires these 3 key components: A problem focused history; A problem focused examination; and Straightforward medical decision making. Counseling and/or coordination of care with other physicians, other qualified health care professionals, or agencies are provided consistent with the nature of the problem(s) and the patient's and/or family's needs. Usually, the presenting problem(s) are of low severity. Typically, 20 minutes are spent face-to-face with the patient and/or family.

⚕ 1.56   ⚕ 1.56   **FUD** XXX   B 80 ▯

AMA: 2020,Nov,3; 2020,Sep,3; 2018,Apr,9; 2018,Jan,8; 2017,Aug,3; 2017,Jun,6; 2017,Jan,8; 2016,Dec,11; 2016,Jan,13; 2016,Jan,7

99342   Home visit for the evaluation and management of a new patient, which requires these 3 key components: An expanded problem focused history; An expanded problem focused examination; and Medical decision making of low complexity. Counseling and/or coordination of care with other physicians, other qualified health care professionals, or agencies are provided consistent with the nature of the problem(s) and the patient's and/or family's needs. Usually, the presenting problem(s) are of moderate severity. Typically, 30 minutes are spent face-to-face with the patient and/or family.

⚕ 2.25   ⚕ 2.25   **FUD** XXX   B 80 ▯

AMA: 2020,Nov,3; 2020,Sep,3; 2018,Apr,9; 2018,Jan,8; 2017,Aug,3; 2017,Jun,6; 2017,Jan,8; 2016,Dec,11; 2016,Jan,7; 2016,Jan,13

99343   Home visit for the evaluation and management of a new patient, which requires these 3 key components: A detailed history; A detailed examination; and Medical decision making of moderate complexity. Counseling and/or coordination of care with other physicians, other qualified health care professionals, or agencies are provided consistent with the nature of the problem(s) and the patient's and/or family's needs. Usually, the presenting problem(s) are of moderate to high severity. Typically, 45 minutes are spent face-to-face with the patient and/or family.

⚕ 3.67   ⚕ 3.67   **FUD** XXX   B 80 ▯

AMA: 2020,Nov,3; 2020,Sep,3; 2018,Apr,9; 2018,Jan,8; 2017,Aug,3; 2017,Jun,6; 2017,Jan,8; 2016,Dec,11; 2016,Jan,13; 2016,Jan,7

99344   Home visit for the evaluation and management of a new patient, which requires these 3 key components: A comprehensive history; A comprehensive examination; and Medical decision making of moderate complexity. Counseling and/or coordination of care with other physicians, other qualified health care professionals, or agencies are provided consistent with the nature of the problem(s) and the patient's and/or family's needs. Usually, the presenting problem(s) are of high severity. Typically, 60 minutes are spent face-to-face with the patient and/or family.

⚕ 5.14   ⚕ 5.14   **FUD** XXX   B 80 ▯

AMA: 2020,Nov,3; 2020,Sep,3; 2018,Apr,9; 2018,Jan,8; 2017,Aug,3; 2017,Jun,6; 2017,Jan,8; 2016,Dec,11; 2016,Jan,13; 2016,Jan,7

99345 Home visit for the evaluation and management of a new patient, which requires these 3 key components: A comprehensive history; A comprehensive examination; and Medical decision making of high complexity. Counseling and/or coordination of care with other physicians, other qualified health care professionals, or agencies are provided consistent with the nature of the problem(s) and the patient's and/or family's needs. Usually, the patient is unstable or has developed a significant new problem requiring immediate physician attention. Typically, 75 minutes are spent face-to-face with the patient and/or family.

🔧 6.25   6.25   **FUD** XXX   B 80 🖵

AMA: 2020,Nov,3; 2020,Sep,3; 2018,Apr,9; 2018,Jan,8; 2017,Aug,3; 2017,Jun,6; 2017,Jan,8; 2016,Dec,11; 2016,Jan,13; 2016,Jan,7

99347 Home visit for the evaluation and management of an established patient, which requires at least 2 of these 3 key components: A problem focused interval history; A problem focused examination; Straightforward medical decision making. Counseling and/or coordination of care with other physicians, other qualified health care professionals, or agencies are provided consistent with the nature of the problem(s) and the patient's and/or family's needs. Usually, the presenting problem(s) are self limited or minor. Typically, 15 minutes are spent face-to-face with the patient and/or family.

🔧 1.56   1.56   **FUD** XXX   B 80 🖵

AMA: 2020,Nov,3; 2020,Sep,3; 2018,Apr,9; 2018,Jan,8; 2017,Aug,3; 2017,Jun,6; 2017,Jan,8; 2016,Dec,11; 2016,Jan,13; 2016,Jan,7

99348 Home visit for the evaluation and management of an established patient, which requires at least 2 of these 3 key components: An expanded problem focused interval history; An expanded problem focused examination; Medical decision making of low complexity. Counseling and/or coordination of care with other physicians, other qualified health care professionals, or agencies are provided consistent with the nature of the problem(s) and the patient's and/or family's needs. Usually, the presenting problem(s) are of low to moderate severity. Typically, 25 minutes are spent face-to-face with the patient and/or family.

🔧 2.37   2.37   **FUD** XXX   B 80 🖵

AMA: 2020,Nov,3; 2020,Sep,3; 2018,Apr,9; 2018,Jan,8; 2017,Aug,3; 2017,Jun,6; 2017,Jan,8; 2016,Dec,11; 2016,Jan,13; 2016,Jan,7

99349 Home visit for the evaluation and management of an established patient, which requires at least 2 of these 3 key components: A detailed interval history; A detailed examination; Medical decision making of moderate complexity. Counseling and/or coordination of care with other physicians, other qualified health care professionals, or agencies are provided consistent with the nature of the problem(s) and the patient's and/or family's needs. Usually, the presenting problem(s) are moderate to high severity. Typically, 40 minutes are spent face-to-face with the patient and/or family.

🔧 3.64   3.64   **FUD** XXX   B 80 🖵

AMA: 2020,Nov,3; 2020,Sep,3; 2018,Apr,9; 2018,Jan,8; 2017,Aug,3; 2017,Jun,6; 2017,Jan,8; 2016,Dec,11; 2016,Jan,13; 2016,Jan,7

99350 Home visit for the evaluation and management of an established patient, which requires at least 2 of these 3 key components: A comprehensive interval history; A comprehensive examination; Medical decision making of moderate to high complexity. Counseling and/or coordination of care with other physicians, other qualified health care professionals, or agencies are provided consistent with the nature of the problem(s) and the patient's and/or family's needs. Usually, the presenting problem(s) are of moderate to high severity. The patient may be unstable or may have developed a significant new problem requiring immediate physician attention. Typically, 60 minutes are spent face-to-face with the patient and/or family.

🔧 5.05   5.05   **FUD** XXX   B 80 🖵

AMA: 2020,Nov,3; 2020,Sep,3; 2018,Apr,9; 2018,Jan,8; 2017,Aug,3; 2017,Jun,6; 2017,Jan,8; 2016,Dec,11; 2016,Jan,13; 2016,Jan,7

99354-99357 Prolonged Services Direct Contact

CMS: 100-04,11,40.1.3 Independent Attending Physician Services; 100-04,12,30.6.15.1 Prolonged Services With Direct Face-to-Face Patient Contact; 100-04,12,30.6.4 Services Furnished Incident to Physician's Service

INCLUDES Personal contact with patient by physician or other qualified health professional

Services extending beyond customary service provided in inpatient, observation, or outpatient setting

Time spent providing additional indirect contact services on floor, hospital unit, or nursing facility during same session as direct contact

Time spent providing prolonged services on service date, even when time not continuous

EXCLUDES *Services less than 30 minutes, less than 15 minutes after first hour, or after final 30 minutes*

Services provided independent from personal contact date with patient (99358-99359)

Code first E/M service code, as appropriate

+ **99354** Prolonged service(s) in the outpatient setting requiring direct patient contact beyond the time of the usual service; first hour (List separately in addition to code for outpatient Evaluation and Management or psychotherapy service, except with office or other outpatient services [99202, 99203, 99204, 99205, 99212, 99213, 99214, 99215])

EXCLUDES *Office or other outpatient visit (99202-99205, 99215-99215)*

Prolonged office/outpatient services ([99417])

Prolonged service provided by clinical staff under supervision ([99415, 99416])

Reporting code more than one time per service date

Code first (99241-99245, 99324-99337, 99341-99350, 90837, 90847)

🔧 3.44   3.67   **FUD** ZZZ   ★ N 80 🖵

AMA: 2020,Dec,11; 2020,Sep,3; 2020,Feb,3; 2019,Oct,10; 2019,Jun,7; 2018,Jan,8; 2017,Jan,8; 2016,Dec,11; 2016,Jan,13

+ **99355** each additional 30 minutes (List separately in addition to code for prolonged service)

EXCLUDES *Office or other outpatient visit (99202-99205, 99212-99215)*

Prolonged office/outpatient services ([99417])

Prolonged service provided by clinical staff under supervision ([99415, 99416])

Code first (99354)

🔧 2.60   2.80   **FUD** ZZZ   ★ N 80 🖵

AMA: 2020,Dec,11; 2020,Sep,3; 2020,Feb,3; 2019,Oct,10; 2019,Jun,7; 2018,Jan,8; 2017,Jan,8; 2016,Dec,11; 2016,Jan,13

+ **99356** Prolonged service in the inpatient or observation setting, requiring unit/floor time beyond the usual service; first hour (List separately in addition to code for inpatient or observation Evaluation and Management service)

EXCLUDES *Reporting code more than one time per service date*

Code first (99218-99223 [99224, 99225, 99226], 99231-99236, 99251-99255, 99304-99310, 90837, 90847)

🔧 2.60   2.60   **FUD** ZZZ   ★ C 80 🖵

AMA: 2020,Dec,11; 2020,Sep,3; 2019,Jun,7; 2018,Jan,8; 2017,Jan,8; 2016,Dec,11; 2016,Jan,13

26/TC PC/TC Only   A2-Z3 ASC Payment   50 Bilateral   ♂ Male Only   ♀ Female Only   🔧 Facility RVU   Non-Facility RVU   CCI   CLIA
FUD Follow-up Days   **CMS:** IOM   **AMA:** CPT Asst   A-Y OPPSI   80/80 Surg Assist Allowed / w/Doc   Lab Crosswalk   Radiology Crosswalk

554   CPT © 2021 American Medical Association. All Rights Reserved.   © 2021 Optum360, LLC

+   99357   each additional 30 minutes (List separately in addition to code for prolonged service)

Code first (99356)

📖 2.61   ⚲ 2.61   **FUD** ZZZ   ★ C 80 🖵

AMA: 2020,Dec,11; 2020,Sep,3; 2019,Jun,7; 2018,Jan,8; 2017,Jan,8; 2016,Dec,11; 2016,Jan,13

99358-99359 Prolonged Services Indirect Contact

CMS: 100-04,11,40.1.3 Independent Attending Physician Services; 100-04,12,30.6.15.2 Prolonged Services Without Face to Face Service; 100-04,12,30.6.4 Services Furnished Incident to Physician's Service

INCLUDES Services extending beyond customary service
Time spent providing indirect contact services by physician or other qualified health care professional in relation to patient management where face-to-face services have or will occur on different date
Time spent providing prolonged services on service date, even when time not continuous

EXCLUDES Any additional unit or floor time in hospital or nursing facility during same evaluation and management session
Behavioral health integration care management services (99484)
Patient management services during same time frame as (99487-99489, 99495-99496)
Psychiatric collaborative care management services during same month (99492-99494)
Reporting code more than one time per service date
Services less than 30 minutes, less than 15 minutes after first hour, or after final 30 minutes
Time without direct patient contact for other services:
   Care plan oversight (99339-99340, 99374-99380)
   Chronic care management services provided during same month ([99491])
   INR monitoring services (93792-93793)
   Medical team conference (99366-99368)
   Online and telephone consultative services (99446-99452 [99451, 99452])
   Online medical services ([99421, 99422, 99423])
   Principal care management services ([99424])
Code also E/M or other services provided, excluding (99202-99205, 99212-99215, 99217)

99358   Prolonged evaluation and management service before and/or after direct patient care; first hour

EXCLUDES Use of code more than one time per date of service

📖 3.15   ⚲ 3.15   **FUD** XXX   N 80 🖵

AMA: 2020,Sep,3; 2020,Feb,3; 2019,Jun,7; 2019,Jan,13; 2018,Oct,9; 2018,Jan,8; 2017,Jan,8; 2016,Jan,13

+   99359   each additional 30 minutes (List separately in addition to code for prolonged service)

Code first (99358)

📖 1.52   ⚲ 1.52   **FUD** ZZZ   N 80 🖵

AMA: 2020,Sep,3; 2020,Feb,3; 2019,Jun,7; 2019,Jan,13; 2018,Oct,9; 2018,Jan,8; 2017,Jan,8; 2016,Jan,13

99415-99417 [99415, 99416, 99417] Prolonged Clinical Staff Services Under Supervision

INCLUDES Time spent by clinical staff providing prolonged face-to-face services extending beyond customary service under physician or other qualified health professional supervision
Time spent by clinical staff providing prolonged services on service date, even when time not continuous

EXCLUDES Prolonged service provided by physician or other qualified health care professional (99354-99355, [99417])

+ #   99415   Prolonged clinical staff service (the service beyond the highest time in the range of total time of the service) during an evaluation and management service in the office or outpatient setting, direct patient contact with physician supervision; first hour (List separately in addition to code for outpatient Evaluation and Management service)

EXCLUDES Reporting code more than one time per service date
Reporting code with ([99417])
Services less than 30 minutes
Services provided to more than two patients at same time

Code first (99202-99205, 99212-99215)

📖 0.28   ⚲ 0.28   **FUD** ZZZ   N 80 TC 🖵

AMA: 2020,Nov,12; 2020,Sep,3; 2020,Feb,3; 2019,Oct,10; 2018,Jan,8; 2017,Jan,8; 2016,Mar,8; 2016,Feb,13; 2016,Jan,13

+ #   99416   each additional 30 minutes (List separately in addition to code for prolonged service)

EXCLUDES Reporting code with ([99417])
Services less than 30 minutes, less than 15 minutes after first hour, or after final 30 minutes
Services provided to more than two patients at same time

Code first ([99415])

📖 0.12   ⚲ 0.12   **FUD** ZZZ   N 80 TC 🖵

AMA: 2020,Nov,12; 2020,Sep,3; 2020,Feb,3; 2019,Oct,10; 2018,Jan,8; 2017,Jan,8; 2016,Mar,8; 2016,Feb,13; 2016,Jan,13

+ #   99417   Prolonged office or other outpatient evaluation and management service(s) beyond the minimum required time of the primary procedure which has been selected using total time, requiring total time with or without direct patient contact beyond the usual service, on the date of the primary service, each 15 minutes of total time (List separately in addition to codes 99205, 99215 for office or other outpatient Evaluation and Management services)

INCLUDES Total time prolonged services provided same date with both direct and indirect patient contact by physician or QHCP

EXCLUDES Services less than 15 minutes

Code first (99205 or 99215)

📖 0.93   ⚲ 0.96   **FUD** XXX   ★

99360 Standby Services

CMS: 100-04,11,40.1.3 Independent Attending Physician Services; 100-04,12,30.6.15.3 Standby Services; 100-04,12,30.6.4 Services Furnished Incident to Physician's Service

INCLUDES Services requested by physician or qualified health care professional that involve no direct patient contact
Total standby time for day

EXCLUDES Delivery attendance (99464)
Less than 30 minutes standby time
On-call services mandated by hospital (99026-99027)
Code also as appropriate (99460, 99465)

99360   Standby service, requiring prolonged attendance, each 30 minutes (eg, operative standby, standby for frozen section, for cesarean/high risk delivery, for monitoring EEG)

📖 1.73   ⚲ 1.73   **FUD** XXX   B 🖵

AMA: 2018,Jan,8; 2017,Jan,8; 2016,Jan,13

99366-99368 Interdisciplinary Conferences

CMS: 100-04,11,40.1.3 Independent Attending Physician Services

INCLUDES Documentation conference participation, contribution, and recommendations
Face-to-face participation by minimum of three qualified people from different specialties or disciplines
Individual patient review from start to conclusion
Only participants who have performed face-to-face evaluations or direct treatment to patient within previous 60 days
Team conferences 30 minutes or more

EXCLUDES Conferences less than 30 minutes (not reportable)
More than one individual from same specialty at same encounter
Patient management services during same month as ([99424, 99425, 99426, 99427], [99437], [99439, 99490, 99491], 99487-99489)
Time spent record keeping or writing report

99366   Medical team conference with interdisciplinary team of health care professionals, face-to-face with patient and/or family, 30 minutes or more, participation by nonphysician qualified health care professional

EXCLUDES Team conferences by physician with patient or family present, see appropriate E/M service code

📖 1.19   ⚲ 1.21   **FUD** XXX   N 🖵

AMA: 2018,Apr,9; 2018,Jan,8; 2017,Jan,8; 2016,Jan,13

99367   Medical team conference with interdisciplinary team of health care professionals, patient and/or family not present, 30 minutes or more; participation by physician

📖 1.60   ⚲ 1.60   **FUD** XXX   N 🖵

AMA: 2019,Dec,14; 2018,Apr,9; 2018,Jan,8; 2017,Jan,8; 2016,Jan,13

Evaluation and Management *(side margin)*

99368 — 99387 *(side margin)*

99368	participation by nonphysician qualified health care professional

    🔲 1.04   ⚖ 1.04   **FUD** XXX   N 🔲

    AMA: 2018,Apr,9; 2018,Jan,8; 2017,Jan,8; 2016,Jan,13

99374-99380 Care Plan Oversight: Patient Under Care of HHA, Hospice, or Nursing Facility

CMS: 100-04,11,40.1.3 Independent Attending Physician Services; 100-04,12,180 Payment of Care Plan Oversight (CPO); 100-04,12,180.1 Billing for Care Plan Oversight (CPO); 100-04,12,30.6.4 Services Furnished Incident to Physician's Service

INCLUDES   Analysis reports, diagnostic tests, treatment plans
    Discussions with other health care providers, outside practice, involved in patient's care
    Establishment and revisions to care plans within 30-day period
    Payment to one physician per month for covered care plan oversight services (must be same one who signed plan of care)

EXCLUDES   *Care plan oversight services provided in hospice agency (99377-99378)*
    Care plan oversight services provided in assisted living, domiciliary care, or private residence, not under home health agency or hospice care (99339-99340)
    Patient management services during same time frame as ([99421, 99422, 99423], 99441-99443, 98966-98968)
    Routine postoperative care provided during global surgery period
    Time discussing treatment with patient and/or caregivers
Code also office/outpatient visits, hospital, home, nursing facility, domiciliary, or non-face-to-face services

99374	Supervision of a patient under care of home health agency (patient not present) in home, domiciliary or equivalent environment (eg, Alzheimer's facility) requiring complex and multidisciplinary care modalities involving regular development and/or revision of care plans by that individual, review of subsequent reports of patient status, review of related laboratory and other studies, communication (including telephone calls) for purposes of assessment or care decisions with health care professional(s), family member(s), surrogate decision maker(s) (eg, legal guardian) and/or key caregiver(s) involved in patient's care, integration of new information into the medical treatment plan and/or adjustment of medical therapy, within a calendar month; 15-29 minutes

    EXCLUDES *Complex chronic care management services during same time frame as (99487, 99489)*

    🔲 1.60   ⚖ 1.96   **FUD** XXX   B 🔲

    AMA: 2019,Jan,6; 2018,Jan,8; 2017,Jan,8; 2016,Jan,13

99375	30 minutes or more

    EXCLUDES *Complex chronic care management services during same time frame as (99487, 99489)*

    🔲 2.50   ⚖ 2.94   **FUD** XXX   E 🔲

    AMA: 2019,Jan,6; 2018,Jan,8; 2017,Jan,8; 2016,Jan,13

99377	Supervision of a hospice patient (patient not present) requiring complex and multidisciplinary care modalities involving regular development and/or revision of care plans by that individual, review of subsequent reports of patient status, review of related laboratory and other studies, communication (including telephone calls) for purposes of assessment or care decisions with health care professional(s), family member(s), surrogate decision maker(s) (eg, legal guardian) and/or key caregiver(s) involved in patient's care, integration of new information into the medical treatment plan and/or adjustment of medical therapy, within a calendar month; 15-29 minutes

    EXCLUDES *Complex chronic care management services during same time frame as (99487, 99489)*

    🔲 1.60   ⚖ 1.96   **FUD** XXX   B 🔲

    AMA: 2019,Jan,6; 2018,Jan,8; 2017,Jan,8; 2016,Jan,13

99378	30 minutes or more

    EXCLUDES *Complex chronic care management services during same time frame as (99487, 99489)*

    🔲 2.50   ⚖ 2.94   **FUD** XXX   E 🔲

    AMA: 2019,Jan,6; 2018,Jan,8; 2017,Jan,8; 2016,Jan,13

99379	Supervision of a nursing facility patient (patient not present) requiring complex and multidisciplinary care modalities involving regular development and/or revision of care plans by that individual, review of subsequent reports of patient status, review of related laboratory and other studies, communication (including telephone calls) for purposes of assessment or care decisions with health care professional(s), family member(s), surrogate decision maker(s) (eg, legal guardian) and/or key caregiver(s) involved in patient's care, integration of new information into the medical treatment plan and/or adjustment of medical therapy, within a calendar month; 15-29 minutes

    🔲 1.60   ⚖ 1.96   **FUD** XXX   B 🔲

    AMA: 2019,Jan,6; 2018,Jan,8; 2017,Jan,8; 2016,Jan,13

99380	30 minutes or more

    🔲 2.50   ⚖ 2.94   **FUD** XXX   B 🔲

    AMA: 2019,Jan,6; 2018,Jan,8; 2017,Jan,8; 2016,Jan,13

99381-99397 Preventive Medicine Visits

CMS: 100-04,11,40.1.3 Independent Attending Physician Services; 100-04,12,30.6.2 Medically Necessary and Preventive Medicine Service on Same Date; 100-04,12,30.6.4 Services Furnished Incident to Physician's Service

INCLUDES   Care for small problem or pre-existing condition that requires no extra work
    New patients or established patients (99381-99387, 99391-99397)
    Regular preventive care (e.g., well-child exams) for all age groups

EXCLUDES   *Behavioral change interventions (99406-99409)*
    Counseling/risk factor reduction interventions not provided with preventive medical examination (99401-99412)
    Diagnostic tests and other procedures

Code also:
    Immunization counseling, administration, and product (90460-90461, 90471-90474, [0001A, 0002A], [0051A, 0052A, 0053A, 0054A], [0071A, 0072A], [0011A, 0012A], [0064A], [0021A, 0022A], [0031A], [0034A], [0041A, 0042A], [91300], [91305], [91307], [91301], [91306], [91302], [91303], [91304], [90619, 90620, 90621, 90625, 90626, 90627, 90630, 90644, 90672, 90673, 90674, 90677, 90694, 90750, 90756, 90758, 90759])
    Significant, separately identifiable E/M service on same date for substantial problems requiring additional work append modifier 25 to (99202-99215)

99381	Initial comprehensive preventive medicine evaluation and management of an individual including an age and gender appropriate history, examination, counseling/anticipatory guidance/risk factor reduction interventions, and the ordering of laboratory/diagnostic procedures, new patient; infant (age younger than 1 year) A

    🔲 2.17   ⚖ 3.13   **FUD** XXX   E 🔲

    AMA: 2018,Jan,8; 2017,Jan,8; 2016,Mar,8; 2016,Jan,13

99382	early childhood (age 1 through 4 years) A

    🔲 2.32   ⚖ 3.28   **FUD** XXX   E 🔲

    AMA: 2018,Jan,8; 2017,Jan,8; 2016,Mar,8; 2016,Jan,13

99383	late childhood (age 5 through 11 years) A

    🔲 2.46   ⚖ 3.41   **FUD** XXX   E 🔲

    AMA: 2018,Jan,8; 2017,Jan,8; 2016,Mar,8; 2016,Jan,13

99384	adolescent (age 12 through 17 years) A

    🔲 2.88   ⚖ 3.85   **FUD** XXX   E 🔲

    AMA: 2018,Jan,8; 2017,Jan,8; 2016,Mar,8; 2016,Jan,13

99385	18-39 years A

    🔲 2.76   ⚖ 3.72   **FUD** XXX   E 🔲

    AMA: 2018,Jan,8; 2017,Jan,8; 2016,Mar,8; 2016,Jan,13

99386	40-64 years A

    🔲 3.36   ⚖ 4.32   **FUD** XXX   E 🔲

    AMA: 2018,Jan,8; 2017,Jan,8; 2016,Mar,8; 2016,Jan,13

99387	65 years and older A

    🔲 3.61   ⚖ 4.68   **FUD** XXX   E 🔲

    AMA: 2018,Jan,8; 2017,Jan,8; 2016,Mar,8; 2016,Jan,13

26/TC PC/TC Only	A2-Z3 ASC Payment	50 Bilateral	♂ Male Only	♀ Female Only	🔲 Facility RVU	⚖ Non-Facility RVU	🔲 CCI	✖ CLIA
FUD Follow-up Days	CMS: IOM	AMA: CPT Asst	A-Y OPPSI	80/80 Surg Assist Allowed / w/Doc	🔲 Lab Crosswalk	🔲 Radiology Crosswalk

556   CPT © 2021 American Medical Association. All Rights Reserved.   © 2021 Optum360, LLC

99391 Periodic comprehensive preventive medicine reevaluation and management of an individual including an age and gender appropriate history, examination, counseling/anticipatory guidance/risk factor reduction interventions, and the ordering of laboratory/diagnostic procedures, established patient; infant (age younger than 1 year)

🔋 1.98 ⚖ 2.82 **FUD** XXX

AMA: 2018,Jan,8; 2017,Jan,8; 2016,Mar,8; 2016,Jan,13

99392 early childhood (age 1 through 4 years)

🔋 2.17 ⚖ 3.01 **FUD** XXX

AMA: 2018,Jan,8; 2017,Jan,8; 2016,Mar,8; 2016,Jan,13

99393 late childhood (age 5 through 11 years)

🔋 2.17 ⚖ 3.00 **FUD** XXX

AMA: 2018,Jan,8; 2017,Jan,8; 2016,Mar,8; 2016,Jan,13

99394 adolescent (age 12 through 17 years)

🔋 2.46 ⚖ 3.29 **FUD** XXX

AMA: 2018,Jan,8; 2017,Jan,8; 2016,Mar,8; 2016,Jan,13

99395 18-39 years

🔋 2.53 ⚖ 3.36 **FUD** XXX

AMA: 2018,Jan,8; 2017,Jan,8; 2016,Mar,8; 2016,Jan,13

99396 40-64 years

🔋 2.74 ⚖ 3.58 **FUD** XXX

AMA: 2018,Jan,8; 2017,Sep,11; 2017,Jan,8; 2016,Mar,8; 2016,Jan,13

99397 65 years and older

🔋 2.88 ⚖ 3.85 **FUD** XXX

AMA: 2018,Jan,8; 2017,Jan,8; 2016,Mar,8; 2016,Jan,13

99401-99423 [99415, 99416, 99417, 99421, 99422, 99423]
Counseling Services: Risk Factor and Behavioral Change Modification

INCLUDES Face-to-face services for new and established patients based on 15- to 60-minute time increments

Health and behavioral services provided on same day (96156-96159 [96164, 96165, 96167, 96168, 96170, 96171])

Issues such as healthy diet, exercise, alcohol, and drug abuse

Services provided by physician or other qualified healthcare professional for promoting health and reducing illness and injury

EXCLUDES *Counseling and risk factor reduction interventions included in preventive medicine services (99381-99397)*

Counseling services provided to patient groups with existing symptoms or illness (99078)

Code also:

Immunization counseling, administration, and product (90460-90461, 90471-90474, [0001A, 0002A], [0051A, 0052A, 0053A, 0054A], [0071A, 0072A], [0011A, 0012A], [0064A], [0021A, 0022A], [0031A], [0034A], [0041A, 0042A], [91300], [91305], [91307], [91301], [91306], [91302], [91303], [91304], [90619, 90620, 90621, 90625, 90626, 90627, 90630, 90644, 90672, 90673, 90674, 90677, 90694, 90750, 90756, 90758, 90759])

Significant, separately identifiable E/M services when performed and append modifier 25 to service

99401 Preventive medicine counseling and/or risk factor reduction intervention(s) provided to an individual (separate procedure); approximately 15 minutes

🔋 0.70 ⚖ 1.10 **FUD** XXX

AMA: 2020,Aug,3; 2018,Jan,8; 2017,Jan,8; 2016,Mar,8; 2016,Jan,13

99402 approximately 30 minutes

🔋 1.42 ⚖ 1.81 **FUD** XXX

AMA: 2020,Aug,3; 2018,Jan,8; 2017,Jan,8; 2016,Mar,8; 2016,Jan,13

99403 approximately 45 minutes

🔋 2.12 ⚖ 2.51 **FUD** XXX

AMA: 2020,Aug,3; 2018,Jan,8; 2017,Jan,8; 2016,Mar,8; 2016,Jan,13

99404 approximately 60 minutes

🔋 2.81 ⚖ 3.21 **FUD** XXX

AMA: 2020,Aug,3; 2018,Jan,8; 2017,Jan,8; 2016,Mar,8; 2016,Jan,13

99406 Smoking and tobacco use cessation counseling visit; intermediate, greater than 3 minutes up to 10 minutes

🔋 0.35 ⚖ 0.42 **FUD** XXX ★ S 80

AMA: 2020,Sep,14; 2020,Aug,3; 2018,Jan,8; 2017,Nov,3; 2017,Jan,8; 2016,Mar,8; 2016,Jan,13

99407 intensive, greater than 10 minutes

INCLUDES Services 11-14 minutes

🔋 0.73 ⚖ 0.80 **FUD** XXX ★ S 80

AMA: 2020,Aug,3; 2018,Jan,8; 2017,Nov,3; 2017,Jan,8; 2016,Mar,8; 2016,Jan,13

99408 Alcohol and/or substance (other than tobacco) abuse structured screening (eg, AUDIT, DAST), and brief intervention (SBI) services; 15 to 30 minutes

INCLUDES Health risk assessment (96160-96161)

Services 15 minutes or more

Only initial screening and brief intervention

🔋 0.94 ⚖ 1.01 **FUD** XXX ★ E

AMA: 2020,Aug,3; 2018,Jan,8; 2017,Nov,3; 2017,Jan,8; 2016,Nov,5; 2016,Mar,8; 2016,Jan,13

99409 greater than 30 minutes

INCLUDES Health risk assessment (96160-96161)

Only initial screening and brief intervention

Services 31 minutes or more

🔋 1.88 ⚖ 1.95 **FUD** XXX ★ E

AMA: 2020,Aug,3; 2018,Jan,8; 2017,Nov,3; 2017,Jan,8; 2016,Nov,5; 2016,Mar,8; 2016,Jan,13

99411 Preventive medicine counseling and/or risk factor reduction intervention(s) provided to individuals in a group setting (separate procedure); approximately 30 minutes

🔋 0.22 ⚖ 0.55 **FUD** XXX

AMA: 2020,Aug,3; 2018,Jan,8; 2017,Jan,8; 2016,Mar,8; 2016,Jan,13

99412 approximately 60 minutes

🔋 0.36 ⚖ 0.69 **FUD** XXX

AMA: 2020,Aug,3; 2018,Jan,8; 2017,Jan,8; 2016,Mar,8; 2016,Jan,13

99415 Resequenced code. See code following 99359.

99416 Resequenced code. See code following 99359.

99417 Resequenced code. See code following 99416.

99421 Resequenced code. See code following 99443.

99422 Resequenced code. See code following 99443.

99423 Resequenced code. See code following 99443.

99424-99439 [99424, 99425, 99426, 99427, 99437, 99439]
Other Preventive Medicine

Code also immunization counseling, administration, and product (90460-90461, 90471-90474, [0001A, 0002A], [0051A, 0052A, 0053A, 0054A], [0071A, 0072A], [0011A, 0012A], [0064A], [0021A, 0022A], [0031A], [0034A], [0041A, 0042A], [91300], [91305], [91307], [91301], [91306], [91302], [91303], [91304], [90619, 90620, 90621, 90625, 90626, 90627, 90630, 90644, 90672, 90673, 90674, 90677, 90694, 90750, 90756, 90758, 90759])

99424 Resequenced code. See code following 99489.

99425 Resequenced code. See code following 99489.

99426 Resequenced code. See code following 99489.

99427 Resequenced code. See code following 99489.

99429 Unlisted preventive medicine service

🔋 0.00 ⚖ 0.00 **FUD** XXX

AMA: 2018,Jan,8; 2017,Jan,8; 2016,Mar,8; 2016,Jan,13

99437 Resequenced code. See code following resequenced code 99491.

99439 Resequenced code. See code following resequenced code 99490.

Evaluation and Management

99441 — 99451

99441-99443 Telephone Calls for Patient Management

CMS: 100-04,11,40.1.3 Independent Attending Physician Services

INCLUDES Care initiated by established patient or patient's guardian
Non-face-to-face E/M services provided by physician or other health care provider qualified to report E/M services
Related E/M services provided within:
Postoperative period
Seven days prior to service

EXCLUDES *Patient management services during same time frame as (99339-99340, 99374-99380, 99487-99489, 99495-99496, 93792-93793)*
Reporting codes more than one time for telephone and online services when reported within 7-day time period by same provider
Services provided by qualified nonphysician health care professional unable to report E/M codes (98966-98968)

99441 **Telephone evaluation and management service by a physician or other qualified health care professional who may report evaluation and management services provided to an established patient, parent, or guardian not originating from a related E/M service provided within the previous 7 days nor leading to an E/M service or procedure within the next 24 hours or soonest available appointment; 5-10 minutes of medical discussion**

0.36   0.39   **FUD** XXX   E 80 ▢

AMA: 2020,JulBULL,1; 2019,Mar,8; 2018,Mar,7; 2018,Jan,8; 2017,Jan,8; 2016,Jan,13

99442 **11-20 minutes of medical discussion**

0.72   0.76   **FUD** XXX   E 80 ▢

AMA: 2020,JulBULL,1; 2019,Mar,8; 2018,Mar,7; 2018,Jan,8; 2017,Jan,8; 2016,Jan,13

99443 **21-30 minutes of medical discussion**

1.08   1.12   **FUD** XXX   E 80 ▢

AMA: 2020,JulBULL,1; 2019,Mar,8; 2018,Mar,7; 2018,Jan,8; 2017,Jan,8; 2016,Jan,13

99421-99423 [99421, 99422, 99423] Digital Evaluation and Management Services

CMS: 100-04,11,40.1.3 Independent Attending Physician Services

INCLUDES Cumulative service time within seven-day time frame needed to evaluate, assess, and manage the patient:
Ordering tests
Prescription generation
Separate digital inquiry for new and unrelated problem
Subsequent communication digitally supported (i.e., email, online, telephone)
Digital service initiated by established patient

EXCLUDES *Clinical staff time*
Digital evaluation by qualified nonphysician health care professional (98970-98972)
Digital evaluation peformed with separately reportable E/M services during same time frame for new or established patient:
Inquiries related to previously completed procedure and within postoperative period
INR monitoring (93792-93793)
Office consultation (99241-99245)
Office or other outpatient visit (99202-99205, 99212-99215)
Patient management services (99339-99340, 99374-99380, [99424, 99425, 99426, 99427], [99437], [99091], [99491], 99487-99489, 99495-99496)
Digital service less than 5 minutes
Reporting code more than one time in 7 days

\# **99421** **Online digital evaluation and management service, for an established patient, for up to 7 days, cumulative time during the 7 days; 5-10 minutes**

0.37   0.43   **FUD** XXX   80 ▢

AMA: 2020,Jan,3

\# **99422** **11-20 minutes**

0.76   0.86   **FUD** XXX   80 ▢

AMA: 2020,Jan,3

\# **99423** **21 or more minutes**

1.21   1.39   **FUD** XXX   80 ▢

AMA: 2020,Jan,3

99446-99452 [99451, 99452] Online and Telephone Consultative Services

INCLUDES Multiple telephone and/or internet contact needed to complete consultation (e.g., test result(s) follow-up)
New or established patient with new problem or exacerbation existing problem and not seen within last 14 days
Review pertinent lab, imaging and/or pathology studies, medical records, medications

EXCLUDES *Any service less than 5 minutes*
Communication with family with or without patient present ([99421, 99422, 99423], 99441-99443, 98966-98967)
Transfer care only

99446 **Interprofessional telephone/Internet/electronic health record assessment and management service provided by a consultative physician, including a verbal and written report to the patient's treating/requesting physician or other qualified health care professional; 5-10 minutes of medical consultative discussion and review**

INCLUDES Verbal and written reports from consultant to requesting provider

EXCLUDES *Prolonged services without direct patient contact (99358-99359)*
Reporting code more than one time in 7 days

0.51   0.51   **FUD** XXX   E 80 ▢

AMA: 2019,Jun,7; 2019,Jan,3; 2018,Jan,8; 2017,Jan,8; 2016,Jan,13

99447 **11-20 minutes of medical consultative discussion and review**

INCLUDES Verbal and written reports from consultant to requesting provider

EXCLUDES *Prolonged services without direct patient contact (99358-99359)*
Reporting code more than one time in 7 days

1.01   1.01   **FUD** XXX   E 80 ▢

AMA: 2019,Jun,7; 2019,Jan,3; 2018,Jan,8; 2017,Jan,8; 2016,Jan,13

99448 **21-30 minutes of medical consultative discussion and review**

INCLUDES Verbal and written reports from consultant to requesting provider

EXCLUDES *Prolonged services without direct patient contact (99358-99359)*
Reporting code more than one time in 7 days

1.52   1.52   **FUD** XXX   E 80 ▢

AMA: 2019,Jun,7; 2019,Jan,3; 2018,Jan,8; 2017,Jan,8; 2016,Jan,13

99449 **31 minutes or more of medical consultative discussion and review**

INCLUDES Verbal and written reports from consultant to requesting provider

EXCLUDES *Prolonged services without direct patient contact (99358-99359)*
Reporting code more than one time in 7 days

2.02   2.02   **FUD** XXX   E 80 ▢

AMA: 2019,Jun,7; 2019,Jan,3; 2018,Jan,8; 2017,Jan,8; 2016,Jan,13

\# **99451** **Interprofessional telephone/Internet/electronic health record assessment and management service provided by a consultative physician, including a written report to the patient's treating/requesting physician or other qualified health care professional, 5 minutes or more of medical consultative time**

INCLUDES Verbal and written reports from consultant to requesting provider

EXCLUDES *Prolonged services without direct patient contact (99358-99359)*
Reporting code more than one time in 7 days

1.04   1.04   **FUD** XXX   80 ▢

AMA: 2019,Jun,7; 2019,Jan,3

| # | 99452 | Interprofessional telephone/Internet/electronic health record referral service(s) provided by a treating/requesting physician or other qualified health care professional, 30 minutes |

INCLUDES Time preparing for referral, 16 to 30 minutes

EXCLUDES *Requesting physician's time 30 minutes over typical E/M service, patient not on site (99358-99359)*
Requesting physician's time 30 minutes over typical E/M service, patient on site (99354-99357)
Reporting code more than one time every 14 days

🚑 1.04 ⚕ 1.04 **FUD** XXX [80] 🖵

AMA: 2020,Jun,3; 2019,Jun,7; 2019,Jan,3

99453-99474 [99091, 99453, 99454, 99473, 99474] Remote Monitoring/Collection Biological Data

| # | 99453 | Remote monitoring of physiologic parameter(s) (eg, weight, blood pressure, pulse oximetry, respiratory flow rate), initial; set-up and patient education on use of equipment |

INCLUDES 30-day period physiologic monitoring parameters such as weight, blood pressure, pulse oximetry
Services ordered by physician or other qualified healthcare professional
Services provided for each care episode (starts when monitoring begins and ends when treatment goals achieved)
Set-up and instructions for use
Treatment with device approved by FDA

EXCLUDES *Monitoring less than 16 days*
Reporting codes when services included in other monitoring services (e.g., 93296, 94760, 95250)

🚑 0.52 ⚕ 0.52 **FUD** XXX [80] 🖵

AMA: 2020,Nov,10; 2020,Apr,5; 2019,Mar,10; 2019,Jan,3; 2019,Jan,6

| # | 99454 | device(s) supply with daily recording(s) or programmed alert(s) transmission, each 30 days |

INCLUDES 30-day period physiologic monitoring parameters such as weight, blood pressure, pulse oximetry
Service ordered by physician or other qualified healthcare professional
Supplying device
Treatment with device approved by FDA

EXCLUDES *Monitoring less than 16 days*
Remote monitoring treatment management ([99457])
Remote therapeutic monitoring (98975-98977)
Reporting codes when services included in other monitoring services (e.g., 93296, 94760, 95250)
Self-measured blood pressure monitoring ([99473, 99474])

🚑 1.73 ⚕ 1.73 **FUD** XXX [80] 🖵

AMA: 2020,Nov,10; 2020,Apr,5; 2019,Oct,3; 2019,Mar,10; 2019,Jan,3; 2019,Jan,6

| # | 99091 | Collection and interpretation of physiologic data (eg, ECG, blood pressure, glucose monitoring) digitally stored and/or transmitted by the patient and/or caregiver to the physician or other qualified health care professional, qualified by education, training, licensure/regulation (when applicable) requiring a minimum of 30 minutes of time, each 30 days |

INCLUDES E/M services provided on same service date

EXCLUDES *Care plan oversight services within same calendar month (99339-99340, 99374-99380)*
Chronic care management services within same calendar month ([99437], [99491], 99487)
Data transfer/interpretation from clinical lab or hospital computers
Principal care management services within same calendar month ([99424, 99425, 99426, 99427])
Remote physiologic monitoring treatment management within same calendar month ([99457, 99458])
Reporting code more than one time in 30 days
Reporting codes when services included in other monitoring services such as (93227, 93272, 95250)
Services for which more specific codes exist, such as:
Ambulatory continuous glucose monitoring (95250)
Electrocardiographic services (93227, 93272)

🚑 1.62 ⚕ 1.62 **FUD** XXX [N] [80] 🖵

AMA: 2020,Nov,10; 2020,Apr,5; 2020,Feb,7; 2019,Oct,3; 2019,Jun,3; 2019,Jan,6; 2018,Dec,10; 2018,Dec,10; 2018,Jun,6; 2018,Mar,5; 2018,Feb,7; 2018,Jan,8; 2017,Jan,8; 2016,Jan,13

| # | 99473 | Self-measured blood pressure using a device validated for clinical accuracy; patient education/training and device calibration |

EXCLUDES *Reporting code more than once per device*
Reporting codes when services included in same calendar month as:
Ambulatory blood pressure monitoring (93784-93790)
Chronic care management services ([99437], [99439, 99490, 99491], 99487-99489)
Principal care management services ([99424, 99425, 99426, 99427])
Remote physiologic monitoring, collection and interpretation ([99453, 99454], [99091], [99457])

🚑 0.31 ⚕ 0.31 **FUD** XXX [80] 🖵

AMA: 2020,Apr,5; 2020,Feb,7; 2020,Jan,3

| # | 99474 | separate self-measurements of two readings one minute apart, twice daily over a 30-day period (minimum of 12 readings), collection of data reported by the patient and/or caregiver to the physician or other qualified health care professional, with report of average systolic and diastolic pressures and subsequent communication of a treatment plan to the patient |

EXCLUDES *Reporting code more than once per device*
Reporting codes when services included in same calendar month as:
Ambulatory blood pressure monitoring (93784-93790)
Chronic care management services ([99437], [99439, 99490, 99491], 99487-99489)
Principal care management services within same calendar month ([99424, 99425, 99426, 99427])
Remote physiologic monitoring, collection and interpretation services ([99453, 99454], [99091], [99457])

🚑 0.25 ⚕ 0.42 **FUD** XXX [80] 🖵

AMA: 2020,Apr,5; 2020,Feb,7; 2020,Jan,3

99457-99458 [99457, 99458] Remote Monitoring Management

CMS: 100-04,11,40.1.3 Independent Attending Physician Services

INCLUDES
Interactive live communication with patient at least 20 minutes per month
Remote monitoring results used for patient management
Reporting code each 30 days no matter number parameters monitored
Service ordered by physician or other qualified healthcare professional
Time managing care when more specific service codes not available
Treatment with device approved by FDA

EXCLUDES
Remote therapeutic monitoring (98980-98981)
Reporting code for services lasting less than 20 minutes
Reporting code on same service date as E/M services (99202-99215, 99221-99223, 99231-99233, 99251-99255, 99324-99328, 99334-99337, 99341-99350)

Code also, when appropriate:
Behavioral health integration services ([99484], 99492-99494)
Chronic care management services ([99437], [99439, 99490, 99491], 99487-99489)
Principal care management services ([99424, 99425, 99426, 99427])
Transitional care management services (99495-99496)

 # 99457 **Remote physiologic monitoring treatment management services, clinical staff/physician/other qualified health care professional time in a calendar month requiring interactive communication with the patient/caregiver during the month; first 20 minutes**

    EXCLUDES *Collection and interpretation physiologic data ([99091])*
    🔧 0.90   ⚕ 1.43   **FUD** XXX   80 🖵
    AMA: 2020,Apr,5; 2020,Feb,7; 2019,Jun,3; 2019,Jan,3; 2019,Jan,6

+ # 99458 **each additional 20 minutes (List separately in addition to code for primary procedure)**

    EXCLUDES *Reporting code when 20 minutes additional treatment time not obtained ([99457])*
    Code first ([99457])
    🔧 0.91   ⚕ 1.17   **FUD** ZZZ   80 🖵
    AMA: 2020,Feb,7

99450-99458 [99451, 99452, 99453, 99454, 99457, 99458] Life/Disability Insurance Eligibility Visits

INCLUDES
Assessment services for insurance eligibility and work-related disability without medical management of the patient's illness/injury
Services provided to new/established patients at any site of service

EXCLUDES
Any additional E&M services or procedures performed on the same date of service: report with appropriate code

99450 **Basic life and/or disability examination that includes: Measurement of height, weight, and blood pressure; Completion of a medical history following a life insurance pro forma; Collection of blood sample and/or urinalysis complying with "chain of custody" protocols; and Completion of necessary documentation/certificates.**

    🔧 0.00   ⚕ 0.00   **FUD** XXX   E 🖵
    AMA: 2019,Jun,7; 2018,Jan,8; 2017,Jan,8; 2016,Jan,13

99451 Resequenced code. See code following 99449.

99452 Resequenced code. See code following 99449.

99453 Resequenced code. See code following 99449.

99454 Resequenced code. See code following 99449.

99455 **Work related or medical disability examination by the treating physician that includes: Completion of a medical history commensurate with the patient's condition; Performance of an examination commensurate with the patient's condition; Formulation of a diagnosis, assessment of capabilities and stability, and calculation of impairment; Development of future medical treatment plan; and Completion of necessary documentation/certificates and report.**

    INCLUDES Special reports (99080)
    🔧 0.00   ⚕ 0.00   **FUD** XXX   B 80 🖵
    AMA: 2018,Jan,8; 2017,Jan,8; 2016,Jan,13

99456 **Work related or medical disability examination by other than the treating physician that includes: Completion of a medical history commensurate with the patient's condition; Performance of an examination commensurate with the patient's condition; Formulation of a diagnosis, assessment of capabilities and stability, and calculation of impairment; Development of future medical treatment plan; and Completion of necessary documentation/certificates and report.**

    INCLUDES Special reports (99080)
    🔧 0.00   ⚕ 0.00   **FUD** XXX   B 80 🖵
    AMA: 2018,Jan,8; 2017,Jan,8; 2016,Jan,13

99457 Resequenced code. See code before 99450.

99458 Resequenced code. See code before 99450.

99460-99463 Evaluation and Management Services for Age 28 Days or Less

CMS: 100-04,12,30.6.4 Services Furnished Incident to Physician's Service

INCLUDES
Family consultation
Healthy newborn history and physical
Medical record documentation
Ordering diagnostic test and treatments
Services provided to healthy newborns age 28 days or younger

EXCLUDES
Neonatal intensive and critical care services (99466-99469 [99485, 99486], 99477-99480)
Newborn follow-up services in office or outpatient setting (99202-99215, 99381, 99391)
Newborn hospital discharge services when provided on date subsequent to admission (99238-99239)
Nonroutine neonatal inpatient evaluation and management services (99221-99233)

Code also:
Attendance at delivery (99464)
Circumcision (54150)
Emergency resuscitation services (99465)

99460 **Initial hospital or birthing center care, per day, for evaluation and management of normal newborn infant**   A

    🔧 2.71   ⚕ 2.71   **FUD** XXX   V 80 🖵
    AMA: 2018,Jan,8; 2017,Jan,8; 2016,Jan,13

99461 **Initial care, per day, for evaluation and management of normal newborn infant seen in other than hospital or birthing center**   A

    🔧 1.78   ⚕ 2.58   **FUD** XXX   M 80 🖵
    AMA: 2018,Jan,8; 2017,Jan,8; 2016,Jan,13

99462 **Subsequent hospital care, per day, for evaluation and management of normal newborn**   A

    🔧 1.19   ⚕ 1.19   **FUD** XXX   C 80 🖵
    AMA: 2018,Jan,8; 2017,Jan,8; 2016,Jan,13

99463 **Initial hospital or birthing center care, per day, for evaluation and management of normal newborn infant admitted and discharged on the same date**   A

    🔧 3.13   ⚕ 3.13   **FUD** XXX   V 80 🖵
    AMA: 2018,Jan,8; 2017,Jan,8; 2016,Jan,13

99464-99465 Newborn Delivery Attendance/Resuscitation

CMS: 100-04,12,30.6.4 Services Furnished Incident to Physician's Service

99464 **Attendance at delivery (when requested by the delivering physician or other qualified health care professional) and initial stabilization of newborn**   A

    EXCLUDES *Resuscitation at delivery (99465)*
    🔧 2.12   ⚕ 2.12   **FUD** XXX   N 80 🖵
    AMA: 2018,Jan,8; 2017,Jan,8; 2016,Jan,13

26/TC PC/TC Only	A2-Z3 ASC Payment	50 Bilateral	♂ Male Only	♀ Female Only	🔧 Facility RVU	⚕ Non-Facility RVU	🖵 CCI	❌ CLIA
FUD Follow-up Days	**CMS:** IOM	**AMA:** CPT Asst	A-Y OPPSI	80/80 Surg Assist Allowed / w/Doc		🔲 Lab Crosswalk		🔲 Radiology Crosswalk

560   CPT © 2021 American Medical Association. All Rights Reserved.   © 2021 Optum360, LLC

99465 Delivery/birthing room resuscitation, provision of positive pressure ventilation and/or chest compressions in the presence of acute inadequate ventilation and/or cardiac output 🄰

> *EXCLUDES* *Attendance at delivery (99464)*
> Code also any necessary procedures performed as resuscitation component
> 🚑 4.13   ⚕ 4.13   **FUD** XXX   🅂 80 🏳

AMA: 2018,Jan,8; 2017,Jan,8; 2016,Jan,13

99466-99467 Critical Care Transport Age 24 Months or Younger

CMS: 100-04,12,30.6.4 Services Furnished Incident to Physician's Service

> *INCLUDES* Face-to-face care starting when physician assumes patient responsibility at referring facility until receiving facility accepts patient
> Physician presence during interfacility transfer critically ill/injured patient age 24 months or younger
> Services provided by physician during transport:
> Blood gases
> Chest x-rays (71045-71046)
> Data stored in computers (e.g., ECGs, blood pressures, hematologic data)
> Gastric intubation (43752-43753)
> Interpretation cardiac output measurements (93598)
> Pulse oximetry (94760-94762)
> Routine monitoring:
> Heart rate
> Respiratory rate
> Temporary transcutaneous pacing (92953)
> Vascular access procedures (36000, 36400, 36405-36406, 36415, 36591, 36600)
> Ventilatory management (94002-94003, 94660, 94662)
> *EXCLUDES* *Neonatal hypothermia (99184)*
> *Patient critical care transport services with personal patient contact less than 30 minutes*
> *Physician directed emergency care via two-way voice communication with transporting staff (99288, [99485, 99486])*
> *Physician services directing transport (control physician) ([99485, 99486])*
> *Services less than 30 minutes in duration (see E/M codes)*
> Code also any services not designated as included in critical care transport service

99466 Critical care face-to-face services, during an interfacility transport of critically ill or critically injured pediatric patient, 24 months of age or younger; first 30-74 minutes of hands-on care during transport 🄰

> 🚑 6.75   ⚕ 6.75   **FUD** XXX   🄽 80 🏳

AMA: 2018,Jun,9; 2018,Jan,8; 2017,Jan,8; 2016,Jan,13

+ 99467 each additional 30 minutes (List separately in addition to code for primary service) 🄰

> Code first (99466)
> 🚑 3.37   ⚕ 3.37   **FUD** ZZZ   🄽 80 🏳

AMA: 2018,Jun,9; 2018,Jan,8; 2017,Jan,8; 2016,Jan,13

99485-99486 [99485, 99486] Critical Care Transport Supervision Age 24 Months or Younger

> *INCLUDES* Advice for treatment to transport team from control physician
> Non face-to-face care starts with first contact by control physician with transport team and ends when patient responsibility assumed by receiving facility
> *EXCLUDES* *Emergency systems physician direction for pediatric patient older than 24 months (99288)*
> *Services less than 15 minutes*
> *Services performed by control physician for same time period*
> *Services performed by same physician providing critical care transport (99466-99467)*
> *Services provided by transport team*

 # 99485 Supervision by a control physician of interfacility transport care of the critically ill or critically injured pediatric patient, 24 months of age or younger, includes two-way communication with transport team before transport, at the referring facility and during the transport, including data interpretation and report; first 30 minutes 🄰

> 🚑 2.17   ⚕ 2.17   **FUD** XXX   🄱 🏳

AMA: 2018,Jun,9; 2018,Jan,8; 2017,Jan,8; 2016,Jan,13

+ # 99486 each additional 30 minutes (List separately in addition to code for primary procedure) 🄰

> Code first ([99485])
> 🚑 1.88   ⚕ 1.88   **FUD** XXX   🄱 🏳

AMA: 2018,Jun,9; 2018,Jan,8; 2017,Jan,8; 2016,Jan,13

99468-99476 [99473, 99474] Critical Care Age 5 Years or Younger

CMS: 100-04,12,30.6.4 Services Furnished Incident to Physician's Service

> *INCLUDES* All services included in codes 99291-99292 as well as (which may be reported by facilities only):
> Administration blood/blood components (36430, 36440)
> Administration intravenous fluids (96360-96361)
> Administration surfactant (94610)
> Bladder aspiration, suprapubic (51100)
> Bladder catheterization (51701, 51702)
> Car seat evaluation (94780-94781)
> Catheterization umbilical artery (36660)
> Catheterization umbilical vein (36510)
> Central venous catheter, centrally inserted (36555)
> Endotracheal intubation (31500)
> Lumbar puncture (62270)
> Oral or nasogastric tube placement (43752)
> Pulmonary function testing, performed at bedside (94375)
> Pulse or ear oximetry (94760-94762)
> Vascular access, arteries (36140, 36620)
> Vascular access, venous (36400-36406, 36420, 36600)
> Ventilatory management (94002-94004, 94660)
> Initial and subsequent care provided to critically ill infant or child
> Other hospital care or intensive care services by same group or individual done on same day patient transferred to initial neonatal/pediatric critical care
> Readmission to critical unit on same day or during same stay (subsequent care)
> *EXCLUDES* *Critical care services for patients age six years or older (99291-99292)*
> *Critical care services provided by second physician or different physician specialty (99291-99292)*
> *Interfacility transport services by same or different individual, same or different specialty or group, on same service date (99466-99467, [99485, 99486])*
> *Neonatal hypothermia (99184)*
> *Services performed by individual in another group receiving patient transferred to lower care level (99231-99233, 99478-99480)*
> *Services performed by individual transferring patient to lower care level (99231-99233, 99291-99292)*
> *Services performed by same or different individual in same group on same day (99291-99292)*
> *Services performed by transferring individual prior to patient transfer to individual in different group (99221-99233, 99291-99292, 99460-99462, 99477-99480)*
> Code also normal newborn care when done on same day by same group or individual providing critical care. Report modifier 25 with initial critical care code (99460-99462)

99468 Initial inpatient neonatal critical care, per day, for the evaluation and management of a critically ill neonate, 28 days of age or younger 🄰

> 🚑 26.0   ⚕ 26.0   **FUD** XXX   🄲 80 🏳

AMA: 2018,Dec,8; 2018,Dec,8; 2018,Jun,9; 2018,Jan,8; 2017,Jan,8; 2016,May,3; 2016,Jan,13

99469 Subsequent inpatient neonatal critical care, per day, for the evaluation and management of a critically ill neonate, 28 days of age or younger 🄰

> 🚑 11.2   ⚕ 11.2   **FUD** XXX   🄲 80 🏳

AMA: 2018,Dec,8; 2018,Dec,8; 2018,Jun,9; 2018,Jan,8; 2017,Jan,8; 2016,May,3; 2016,Jan,13

99471 Initial inpatient pediatric critical care, per day, for the evaluation and management of a critically ill infant or young child, 29 days through 24 months of age 🄰

> 🚑 22.5   ⚕ 22.5   **FUD** XXX   🄲 80 🏳

AMA: 2018,Dec,8; 2018,Dec,8; 2018,Jun,9; 2018,Jan,8; 2017,Jan,8; 2016,May,3; 2016,Jan,13

99472 Subsequent inpatient pediatric critical care, per day, for the evaluation and management of a critically ill infant or young child, 29 days through 24 months of age 🄰

> 🚑 11.5   ⚕ 11.5   **FUD** XXX   🄲 80 🏳

AMA: 2018,Dec,8; 2018,Dec,8; 2018,Jun,9; 2018,Jan,8; 2017,Jan,8; 2016,May,3; 2016,Jan,13

● New Code   ▲ Revised Code   ○ Reinstated   ● New Web Release   ▲ Revised Web Release   + Add-on   Unlisted   Not Covered   # Resequenced
⑤⓪ Optum Mod 50 Exempt   Ⓝ AMA Mod 51 Exempt   ⑤① Optum Mod 51 Exempt   ⑥③ Mod 63 Exempt   ✗ Non-FDA Drug   ★ Telemedicine   Ⓜ Maternity   🄰 Age Edit

99473 Resequenced code. See code before 99450.

99474 Resequenced code. See code before 99450.

99475 Initial inpatient pediatric critical care, per day, for the evaluation and management of a critically ill infant or young child, 2 through 5 years of age Ⓐ

🔧 15.8   ⚕ 15.8   **FUD** XXX   Ⓒ 80 ▫

AMA: 2018,Dec,8; 2018,Dec,8; 2018,Jun,9; 2018,Jan,8; 2017,Jan,8; 2016,May,3; 2016,Jan,13

99476 Subsequent inpatient pediatric critical care, per day, for the evaluation and management of a critically ill infant or young child, 2 through 5 years of age Ⓐ

🔧 9.86   ⚕ 9.86   **FUD** XXX   Ⓒ 80 ▫

AMA: 2018,Dec,8; 2018,Dec,8; 2018,Jun,9; 2018,Jan,8; 2017,Jan,8; 2016,May,3; 2016,Jan,13

99477-99480 Initial Inpatient Neonatal Intensive Care and Other Services

CMS: 100-04,12,30.6.4 Services Furnished Incident to Physician's Service

INCLUDES <insert title here>

INCLUDES All services included in codes 99291-99292 as well as (which may be reported by facilities only):
Adjustments to enteral and/or parenteral nutrition
Airway and ventilator management (31500, 94002-94004, 94375, 94610, 94660)
Bladder catheterization (51701-51702)
Blood transfusion (36430, 36440)
Car seat evaluation (94780-94781)
Constant and/or frequent monitoring vital signs
Continuous observation by the healthcare team
Heat maintenance
Intensive cardiac or respiratory monitoring
Oral or nasogastric tube insertion (43752)
Oxygen saturation (94760-94762)
Spinal puncture (62270)
Suprapubic catheterization (51100)
Vascular access procedures (36000, 36140, 36400, 36405-36406, 36420, 36510, 36555, 36600, 36620, 36660)

EXCLUDES *Critical care services for patient transferred after initial or subsequent intensive care provided (99291-99292)*
Initial day intensive care provided by transferring individual same day neonate/infant transferred to lower care level (99477)
Inpatient neonatal/pediatric critical care services received on same day (99468-99476)
Necessary resuscitation services done as delivery care component prior to admission
Neonatal hypothermia (99184)
Services provided by receiving individual when patient transferred for critical care (99468-99476)
Services for receiving provider when patient improves after initial day and transferred to lower care level (99231-99233, 99478-99480)
Subsequent care sick neonate, under age 28 days, more than 5000 grams, not requiring critical or intensive care services (99231-99233)

Code also:
Care provided by receiving individual when patient transferred to individual in different group (99231-99233, 99462)
Initial neonatal intensive care service when physician or other qualified health care professional present for delivery and/or neonate requires resuscitation (99464-99465); append modifier 25 to (99477)

99477 Initial hospital care, per day, for the evaluation and management of the neonate, 28 days of age or younger, who requires intensive observation, frequent interventions, and other intensive care services Ⓐ

EXCLUDES *Initiation care critically ill neonate (99468)*
Initiation inpatient care normal newborn (99460)

🔧 9.85   ⚕ 9.85   **FUD** XXX   Ⓒ 80 ▫

AMA: 2018,Dec,8; 2018,Dec,8; 2018,Jan,8; 2017,Jan,8; 2016,Jan,13

99478 Subsequent intensive care, per day, for the evaluation and management of the recovering very low birth weight infant (present body weight less than 1500 grams) Ⓐ

🔧 3.87   ⚕ 3.87   **FUD** XXX   Ⓒ 80 ▫

AMA: 2018,Dec,8; 2018,Dec,8; 2018,Jun,11; 2018,Jan,8; 2017,Jan,8; 2016,Jan,13

99479 Subsequent intensive care, per day, for the evaluation and management of the recovering low birth weight infant (present body weight of 1500-2500 grams) Ⓐ

🔧 3.52   ⚕ 3.52   **FUD** XXX   Ⓒ 80 ▫

AMA: 2018,Dec,8; 2018,Dec,8; 2018,Jun,11; 2018,Jan,8; 2017,Jan,8; 2016,Jan,13

99480 Subsequent intensive care, per day, for the evaluation and management of the recovering infant (present body weight of 2501-5000 grams) Ⓐ

🔧 3.37   ⚕ 3.37   **FUD** XXX   Ⓒ 80 ▫

AMA: 2018,Dec,8; 2018,Dec,8; 2018,Jun,11; 2018,Jan,8; 2017,Jan,8; 2016,Jan,13

99483-99486 [99484, 99485, 99486] Cognitive Impairment Services

INCLUDES Assessment and care plan services during same time frame as:
E/M services (99202-99215, 99241-99245, 99324-99337, 99341-99350, 99366-99368, 99497-99498)
Medication management (99605-99607)
Need for services evaluation (e.g., legal, financial, meals, personal care)
Patient and caregiver focused risk assessment (96160-96161)
Psychiatric and psychological services (90785, 90791-90792, [96127])
Psychological or neuropsychological tests (96146)
Consideration other conditions that may cause cognitive impairment (e.g., infection, hydrocephalus, stroke, medications)
Evaluation and care plans for new or existing patients with cognitive impairment symptoms

EXCLUDES *Reporting code more than one time per 180-day period*

▲ **99483** Assessment of and care planning for a patient with cognitive impairment, requiring an independent historian, in the office or other outpatient, home or domiciliary or rest home, with all of the following required elements: Cognition-focused evaluation including a pertinent history and examination, Medical decision making of moderate or high complexity, Functional assessment (eg, basic and instrumental activities of daily living), including decision-making capacity, Use of standardized instruments for staging of dementia (eg, functional assessment staging test [FAST], clinical dementia rating [CDR]), Medication reconciliation and review for high-risk medications, Evaluation for neuropsychiatric and behavioral symptoms, including depression, including use of standardized screening instrument(s), Evaluation of safety (eg, home), including motor vehicle operation, Identification of caregiver(s), caregiver knowledge, caregiver needs, social supports, and the willingness of caregiver to take on caregiving tasks, Development, updating or revision, or review of an Advance Care Plan, Creation of a written care plan, including initial plans to address any neuropsychiatric symptoms, neuro-cognitive symptoms, functional limitations, and referral to community resources as needed (eg, rehabilitation services, adult day programs, support groups) shared with the patient and/or caregiver with initial education and support. Typically, 50 minutes are spent face-to-face with the patient and/or family or caregiver. Ⓢ

🔧 5.12   ⚕ 7.35   **FUD** XXX   Ⓢ 80 ▫

AMA: 2020,Sep,3; 2018,Jul,12; 2018,Apr,9; 2018,Jan,8

99484 Resequenced code. See code following 99498.

99485 Resequenced code. See code following 99467.

99486 Resequenced code. See code following 99467.

26/TC PC/TC Only   A2-Z3 ASC Payment   50 Bilateral   ♂ Male Only   ♀ Female Only   🔧 Facility RVU   ⚕ Non-Facility RVU   ▫ CCI   ✖ CLIA
FUD Follow-up Days   CMS: IOM   AMA: CPT Asst   A-Y OPPSI   80/80 Surg Assist Allowed / w/Doc   Ⓛ Lab Crosswalk   ✚ Radiology Crosswalk

562   CPT © 2021 American Medical Association. All Rights Reserved.   © 2021 Optum360, LLC

99490-99437 [99437, 99439, 99490, 99491] Chronic Care Management Services

INCLUDES Case management services provided to patients that:
Have two or more conditions anticipated to endure more than 12 months or until patient's death
High risk that conditions will result in decompensation, deterioration, or death
Only services given by physician or other qualified health caregiver who has care coordination role for patient for month

EXCLUDES *Patient management services during same time frame as (99339-99340, 99374-99380, [99424, 99425, 99426, 99427], [99437], [99491], 99487-99489, 90951-90970, 99605-99607)*
Service time reported with (99358-99359, 99366-99368, [99421, 99422, 99423], 99441-99443, [99091], [99484], 99492-99494, 93792-93793, 98960-98962, 98966-98968, 99071, 99078, 99080)

▲ # **99490** **Chronic care management services with the following required elements: multiple (two or more) chronic conditions expected to last at least 12 months, or until the death of the patient, chronic conditions that place the patient at significant risk of death, acute exacerbation/decompensation, or functional decline, comprehensive care plan established, implemented, revised, or monitored; first 20 minutes of clinical staff time directed by a physician or other qualified health care professional, per calendar month.**

EXCLUDES *Chronic care management provided personally by physician or other qualified health care professional ([99437], [99491])*
Less than 20 minutes staff time monthly
Qualified nonphysician health care professional online digital assessment and management (98970-98972)
Reporting code more than once per calendar month

🔲 0.90 ⚕ 1.17 **FUD** XXX   [S] [80] 🖿

AMA: 2020,Apr,5; 2020,Feb,7; 2019,Jan,6; 2018,Oct,9; 2018,Jul,12; 2018,Apr,9; 2018,Mar,7; 2018,Mar,5; 2018,Feb,7; 2018,Jan,8; 2017,Jan,8; 2016,Jan,13

▲ + # **99439** **each additional 20 minutes of clinical staff time directed by a physician or other qualified health care professional, per calendar month (List separately in addition to code for primary procedure)**

EXCLUDES *Qualified nonphysician health care professional online digital assessment and management (98970-98972)*
Reporting code more than twice per calendar month
Code first ([99490])

🔲 0.81 ⚕ 1.08 **FUD** ZZZ   [80] 🖿

▲ # **99491** **Chronic care management services with the following required elements: multiple (two or more) chronic conditions expected to last at least 12 months, or until the death of the patient, chronic conditions that place the patient at significant risk of death, acute exacerbation/decompensation, or functional decline, comprehensive care plan established, implemented, revised, or monitored; first 30 minutes provided personally by a physician or other qualified health care professional, per calendar month.**

EXCLUDES *Chronic care management provided by medically directed clinical staff only ([99439], [99490])*
Less than 30 minutes staff time monthly
Reporting code more than once per calendar month
Service time reported for transitional care management services (99495-99496)

🔲 2.33 ⚕ 2.33 **FUD** XXX   [80] 🖿

AMA: 2020,Apr,5

● + # **99437** **each additional 30 minutes by a physician or other qualified health care professional, per calendar month (List separately in addition to code for primary procedure)**
Code first ([99491])
🔲 0.00 ⚕ 0.00 **FUD** 000

99487-99489 Complex Chronic Care Management Services

CMS: 100-04,11,40.1.3 Independent Attending Physician Services

INCLUDES All clinical non-face-to-face time with patient, family, and caregivers
Patient management services during same time frame as (99339-99340, 99374-99380, [99437], [99439, 99490, 99491], 90951-90970, 99605-99607)
Service time reported with (99358-99359, 99366-99368, [99421, 99422, 99423], 99441-99443, [99091], 93792-93793, 98960-98962, 98966-98972, 99071, 99078, 99080, 99605-99607)
Services provided to patients in rest home, domiciliary, assisted living facility, or at home including:
Caregiver education to family or patient, addressing independent living and self-management
Communication with patient and all caregivers and professionals regarding care
Determining which community and health resources benefit patient
Developing and maintaining care plan
Facilitation services and care
Health outcomes data and registry documentation
Providing communication with home health and other patient utilized services
Support for treatment and medication adherence
Services that address activities daily living, psychosocial, and medical needs

EXCLUDES *E/M services by same/different individual during care management services time frame*
Psychiatric collaborative care management (99484, 99492-99494)

▲ **99487** **Complex chronic care management services with the following required elements: multiple (two or more) chronic conditions expected to last at least 12 months, or until the death of the patient, chronic conditions that place the patient at significant risk of death, acute exacerbation/decompensation, or functional decline, comprehensive care plan established, implemented, revised, or monitored, moderate or high complexity medical decision making; first 60 minutes of clinical staff time directed by a physician or other qualified health care professional, per calendar month.**

INCLUDES Clinical services, 60 to 74 minutes, during calendar month
Only services given by physician or other qualified health caregiver who has care coordination role for patient for month

EXCLUDES *Clinical staff time focusing on only one of multiple chronic conditions ([99424, 99425, 99426, 99427])*
Reporting code more than once per calendar month

🔲 1.47 ⚕ 2.58 **FUD** XXX   [S] [80] 🖿

AMA: 2020,Apr,5; 2020,Feb,7; 2019,Jan,6; 2018,Oct,9; 2018,Jul,12; 2018,Apr,9; 2018,Mar,7; 2018,Mar,5; 2018,Feb,7; 2018,Jan,8; 2017,Apr,9; 2017,Jan,8; 2016,Jan,13

▲ + **99489** **each additional 30 minutes of clinical staff time directed by a physician or other qualified health care professional, per calendar month (List separately in addition to code for primary procedure)**

INCLUDES Only services given by physician or other qualified health caregiver who has care coordination role for patient for month

EXCLUDES *Clinical services less than 30 minutes beyond initial 60 minutes, per calendar month*
Code first (99487)
🔲 0.74 ⚕ 1.29 **FUD** ZZZ   [N] [80] 🖿

AMA: 2020,Apr,5; 2020,Feb,7; 2019,Jan,6; 2018,Oct,9; 2018,Jul,12; 2018,Apr,9; 2018,Mar,7; 2018,Mar,5; 2018,Feb,7; 2018,Jan,8; 2017,Apr,9; 2017,Jan,8; 2016,Jan,13

Evaluation and Management

99424 — 99493

99424-99491 [99424, 99425, 99426, 99427, 99490, 99491] Principal Care Management Services

INCLUDES   Establishing, implementing, revising, and monitoring care plan specific to single disease
Medical/psychological need management single, complex chronic condition 3 months duration or longer

● # **99424**   **Principal care management services, for a single high-risk disease, with the following required elements: one complex chronic condition expected to last at least 3 months, and that places the patient at significant risk of hospitalization, acute exacerbation/decompensation, functional decline, or death, the condition requires development, monitoring, or revision of disease-specific care plan, the condition requires frequent adjustments in the medication regimen and/or the management of the condition is unusually complex due to comorbidities, ongoing communication and care coordination between relevant practitioners furnishing care; first 30 minutes provided personally by a physician or other qualified health care professional, per calendar month.**

     EXCLUDES   *Clinical staff time focused on multiple chronic conditions (99487-99489)*
Less than 30 minutes staff time monthly
Principal care management provided by medically directed clinical staff only ([99426, 99427])
Reporting code more than once per calendar month
     🖢 0.00   ⚖ 0.00   **FUD** 000

● + # **99425**   **each additional 30 minutes provided personally by a physician or other qualified health care professional, per calendar month (List separately in addition to code for primary procedure)**
     Code first ([99424])
     🖢 0.00   ⚖ 0.00   **FUD** 000

● # **99426**   **Principal care management services, for a single high-risk disease, with the following required elements: one complex chronic condition expected to last at least 3 months, and that places the patient at significant risk of hospitalization, acute exacerbation/decompensation, functional decline, or death, the condition requires development, monitoring, or revision of disease-specific care plan, the condition requires frequent adjustments in the medication regimen and/or the management of the condition is unusually complex due to comorbidities, ongoing communication and care coordination between relevant practitioners furnishing care; first 30 minutes of clinical staff time directed by physician or other qualified health care professional, per calendar month.**

     EXCLUDES   *Clinical staff time focused on multiple chronic conditions (99487-99489)*
Less than 30 minutes staff time monthly
Principal care management provided personally by physician or other qualified health care professional ([99424, 99425])
Reporting code more than once per calendar month
     🖢 0.00   ⚖ 0.00   **FUD** 000

● + # **99427**   **each additional 30 minutes of clinical staff time directed by a physician or other qualified health care professional, per calendar month (List separately in addition to code for primary procedure)**

     EXCLUDES   *Reporting code more than twice per calendar month*
     Code first ([99426])
     🖢 0.00   ⚖ 0.00   **FUD** 000

99490   Resequenced code. See code before 99487.

99491   Resequenced code. See code before 99487.

99492-99494 Psychiatric Collaborative Care

CMS: 100-02,13,230.2 Chronic Care Management and General Behavioral Health Integration Services

INCLUDES   Services provided during calendar month by physician or other qualified healthcare profession for patients with psychiatric diagnosis
Assessment behavioral health status
Creation and care plan revision
Treatment provided during care episode during which goals may be met, not achieved, or lack of services during six-month period

EXCLUDES   *Additional services provided by behavioral health care manager during same calendar month period (do not count as time for 99492-99494):*
Psychiatric evaluation (90791-90792)
Psychotherapy (99406-99407, 99408-99409, 90832-90834, 90836-90838, 90839-90840, 90846-90847, 90849, 90853)
Services provided by psychiatric consultant (do not count as time for 99492-99494): (E/M services) and psychiatric evaluation (90791-90792)

▲   **99492**   **Initial psychiatric collaborative care management, first 70 minutes in the first calendar month of behavioral health care manager activities, in consultation with a psychiatric consultant, and directed by the treating physician or other qualified health care professional, with the following required elements: outreach to and engagement in treatment of a patient directed by the treating physician or other qualified health care professional, initial assessment of the patient, including administration of validated rating scales, with the development of an individualized treatment plan, review by the psychiatric consultant with modifications of the plan if recommended, entering patient in a registry and tracking patient follow-up and progress using the registry, with appropriate documentation, and participation in weekly caseload consultation with the psychiatric consultant, and provision of brief interventions using evidence-based techniques such as behavioral activation, motivational interviewing, and other focused treatment strategies.**

     EXCLUDES   *Services less than 36 minutes*
Subsequent collaborative care managment in same calendar month (99493)
     🖢 2.50   ⚖ 4.35   **FUD** XXX   [S] [80] 🖃
     AMA: 2020,Feb,7; 2019,Jan,6; 2018,Jul,12; 2018,Mar,5; 2018,Feb,7; 2018,Jan,8; 2017,Nov,3

▲   **99493**   **Subsequent psychiatric collaborative care management, first 60 minutes in a subsequent month of behavioral health care manager activities, in consultation with a psychiatric consultant, and directed by the treating physician or other qualified health care professional, with the following required elements: tracking patient follow-up and progress using the registry, with appropriate documentation, participation in weekly caseload consultation with the psychiatric consultant, ongoing collaboration with and coordination of the patient's mental health care with the treating physician or other qualified health care professional and any other treating mental health providers, additional review of progress and recommendations for changes in treatment, as indicated, including medications, based on recommendations provided by the psychiatric consultant, provision of brief interventions using evidence-based techniques such as behavioral activation, motivational interviewing, and other focused treatment strategies, monitoring of patient outcomes using validated rating scales, and relapse prevention planning with patients as they achieve remission of symptoms and/or other treatment goals and are prepared for discharge from active treatment.**

     EXCLUDES   *Initial collaborative care managment in same calendar month (99492)*
     🖢 2.25   ⚖ 3.50   **FUD** XXX   [S] [80] 🖃
     AMA: 2020,Feb,7; 2019,Jan,6; 2018,Jul,12; 2018,Mar,5; 2018,Feb,7; 2018,Jan,8; 2017,Nov,3

| 26/TC PC/TC Only | A2-Z3 ASC Payment | 50 Bilateral | ♂ Male Only | ♀ Female Only | 🖢 Facility RVU | ⚖ Non-Facility RVU | 🖃 CCI | ☒ CLIA |
| FUD Follow-up Days | CMS: IOM | AMA: CPT Asst | A-Y OPPSI | 80/80 Surg Assist Allowed / w/Doc | 🖃 Lab Crosswalk | | 🖃 Radiology Crosswalk | |

564   CPT © 2021 American Medical Association. All Rights Reserved.   © 2021 Optum360, LLC

+ **99494** Initial or subsequent psychiatric collaborative care management, each additional 30 minutes in a calendar month of behavioral health care manager activities, in consultation with a psychiatric consultant, and directed by the treating physician or other qualified health care professional (List separately in addition to code for primary procedure)

INCLUDES Coordination care with emergency department staff

Code first (99492, 99493)

⚕ 1.20 ⚖ 1.77 **FUD** ZZZ N 80 ▣

AMA: 2020,Feb,7; 2019,Jan,6; 2018,Jul,12; 2018,Mar,5; 2018,Feb,7; 2018,Jan,8; 2017,Nov,3

99495-99496 Management of Transitional Care Services

CMS: 100-02,13,230.1 Transitional Care Management Services; 100-04,11,40.1.3 Independent Attending Physician Services; 100-04,12,190.3 List of Telehealth Services

INCLUDES First interaction (face-to-face, by telephone, or electronic) with patient or his/her caregiver and must be done within two working days from discharge

Initial face-to-face; must be done within code time frame and include medication management

New or established patient with moderate to high complexity medical decision making needs during care transitions

Patient management services during same time frame as (99339-99340, 99358-99359, 99366-99368, 99374-99380, 99441-99443, [99091], 99487-99489, 90951-90970, 93792-93793, 98960-98962, 98966-98968, 99071, 99078, 99080, 99605-99607)

Services from discharge day up to 29 days post discharge

Subsequent discharge within 30 days

Without face-to-face patient care given by physician or other qualified health care professional includes:

Contacting qualified health care professionals for specific patient problems

Discharge information review

Follow-up and referral arrangements with community resources and providers

Need for follow-up care review based on tests and treatments

Patient, family, and caregiver education

Without face-to-face patient care given by staff under physician guidance or other qualified health care professional includes:

Caregiver education to family or patient, addressing independent living and self-management

Communication with patient and all caregivers and professionals regarding care

Determining which community and health resources benefit patient

Facilitation services and care

Providing communication with home health and other patient utilized services

Support for treatment and medication adherence

EXCLUDES E/M services after first face-to-face visit

99495 Transitional Care Management Services with the following required elements: Communication (direct contact, telephone, electronic) with the patient and/or caregiver within 2 business days of discharge Medical decision making of at least moderate complexity during the service period Face-to-face visit, within 14 calendar days of discharge

⚕ 3.11 ⚖ 4.62 **FUD** XXX ★ V 80 ▣

AMA: 2020,Feb,7; 2020,Jan,3; 2019,Jan,6; 2018,Jul,12; 2018,Apr,9; 2018,Mar,5; 2018,Mar,7; 2018,Feb,7; 2018,Jan,8; 2017,Jan,8; 2016,Jan,13

99496 Transitional Care Management Services with the following required elements: Communication (direct contact, telephone, electronic) with the patient and/or caregiver within 2 business days of discharge Medical decision making of high complexity during the service period Face-to-face visit, within 7 calendar days of discharge

⚕ 4.51 ⚖ 6.52 **FUD** XXX ★ V 80 ▣

AMA: 2020,Feb,7; 2020,Jan,3; 2019,Jan,6; 2018,Jul,12; 2018,Apr,9; 2018,Mar,5; 2018,Mar,7; 2018,Feb,7; 2018,Jan,8; 2017,Jan,8; 2016,Jan,13

99497-99498 Advance Directive Guidance

CMS: 100-02,15,280.5.1 Advance Care Planning with an Annual Wellness Visit; 100-04,11,40.1.3 Independent Attending Physician Services; 100-04,18,140.8 Advance Care Planning with an Annual Wellness Visit (AWV); 100-04,4,200.11 Advance Care Planning as an Optional Element of an Annual Wellness Visit

EXCLUDES *Critical care services (99291-99292, 99468-99469, 99471-99472, 99475-99476, 99477-99480)*

Services for cognitive care (99483)

Treatment/management for active problem (see appropriate E/M service)

99497 Advance care planning including the explanation and discussion of advance directives such as standard forms (with completion of such forms, when performed), by the physician or other qualified health care professional; first 30 minutes, face-to-face with the patient, family member(s), and/or surrogate

⚕ 2.23 ⚖ 2.40 **FUD** XXX ★ QI 80 ▣

AMA: 2018,Apr,9; 2018,Jan,8; 2017,Jan,8; 2016,Feb,7; 2016,Jan,13

+ **99498** each additional 30 minutes (List separately in addition to code for primary procedure)

Code first (99497)

⚕ 2.10 ⚖ 2.11 **FUD** ZZZ ★ N 80 ▣

AMA: 2018,Apr,9; 2018,Jan,8; 2017,Jan,8; 2016,Feb,7; 2016,Jan,13

99484 [99484] Behavioral Health Integration Care

CMS: 100-02,13,230.2 Chronic Care Management and General Behavioral Health Integration Services

INCLUDES Care management services requiring 20 minutes or more per calendar month

Coordination of care with emergency department staff

Face to face services when necessary

Provided as outpatient service

Provision services by clinical staff and reported by supervising physician or other qualified healthcare professional

Provision services to patients with ongoing relationship

Treatment plan and specific service components

EXCLUDES *Other services for which time or activities associated with service not used to meet requirements for 99484:*

Behavioral health integration care in same month ([99484])

Chronic care management ([99437], [99439], [99490], 99487-99489)

Principal care management ([99424, 99425, 99426, 99427])

Psychiatric collaborative care in same calendar month (99492-99494)

Psychotherapy services (90785-90899)

Transitional care management (99495-99496)

▲ # **99484** Care management services for behavioral health conditions, at least 20 minutes of clinical staff time, directed by a physician or other qualified health care professional, per calendar month, with the following required elements: initial assessment or follow-up monitoring, including the use of applicable validated rating scales, behavioral health care planning in relation to behavioral/psychiatric health problems, including revision for patients who are not progressing or whose status changes, facilitating and coordinating treatment such as psychotherapy, pharmacotherapy, counseling and/or psychiatric consultation, and continuity of care with a designated member of the care team.

⚕ 0.91 ⚖ 1.33 **FUD** XXX S 80 ▣

AMA: 2020,Feb,7; 2019,Jan,6; 2018,Jul,12; 2018,Mar,5; 2018,Feb,7; 2018,Jan,8

99499 Unlisted Evaluation and Management Services

CMS: 100-04,12,30.6.10 Consultation Services; 100-04,12,30.6.4 Services Furnished Incident to Physician's Service; 100-04,12,30.6.9.1 Initial Hospital Care and Observation or Inpatient Care Services

99499 Unlisted evaluation and management service

⚕ 0.00 ⚖ 0.00 **FUD** XXX B 80 ▣

AMA: 2019,Aug,8; 2018,Jan,8; 2017,Jan,8; 2016,Jan,13

0001F-0015F Quality Measures with Multiple Components

INCLUDES Several measures grouped within single code descriptor to make possible reporting for clinical conditions when all components have been met

0001F Heart failure assessed (includes assessment of all the following components) (CAD): Blood pressure measured (2000F) Level of activity assessed (1003F) Clinical symptoms of volume overload (excess) assessed (1004F) Weight, recorded (2001F) Clinical signs of volume overload (excess) assessed (2002F)

INCLUDES Blood pressure measured (2000F)
Clinical signs volume overload (excess) assessed (2002F)
Clinical symptoms volume overload (excess) assessed (1004F)
Level activity assessed (1003F)
Weight recorded (2001F)

🚑 0.00   ⚕ 0.00   **FUD** XXX   E

AMA: 2018,Jan,8; 2017,Jan,8; 2016,Jan,13

0005F Osteoarthritis assessed (OA) Includes assessment of all the following components: Osteoarthritis symptoms and functional status assessed (1006F) Use of anti-inflammatory or over-the-counter (OTC) analgesic medications assessed (1007F) Initial examination of the involved joint(s) (includes visual inspection, palpation, range of motion) (2004F)

INCLUDES Anti-inflammatory or over-the-counter (OTC) analgesic medication usage assessed (1007F)
Initial examination involved joint(s) (includes visual inspection/palpation/range) (2004F)
Osteoarthritis symptoms and functional status assessed (1006F)

🚑 0.00   ⚕ 0.00   **FUD** XXX   E

AMA: 2005,Oct,1-5

0012F Community-acquired bacterial pneumonia assessment (includes all of the following components) (CAP): Co-morbid conditions assessed (1026F) Vital signs recorded (2010F) Mental status assessed (2014F) Hydration status assessed (2018F)

INCLUDES Co-morbid conditions assessed (1026F)
Hydration status assessed (2018F)
Mental status assessed (2014F)
Vital signs recorded (2010F)

🚑 0.00   ⚕ 0.00   **FUD** XXX   E

0014F Comprehensive preoperative assessment performed for cataract surgery with intraocular lens (IOL) placement (includes assessment of all of the following components) (EC): Dilated fundus evaluation performed within 12 months prior to cataract surgery (2020F) Pre-surgical (cataract) axial length, corneal power measurement and method of intraocular lens power calculation documented (must be performed within 12 months prior to surgery) (3073F) Preoperative assessment of functional or medical indication(s) for surgery prior to the cataract surgery with intraocular lens placement (must be performed within 12 months prior to cataract surgery) (3325F)

INCLUDES Evaluation dilated fundus done within 12 months prior to surgery (2020F)
Preoperative assessment functional or medical indications done within 12 months prior to surgery (3325F)
Presurgical measurement axial length, corneal power, and IOL power calculation performed within 12 months prior to surgery (3073F)

🚑 0.00   ⚕ 0.00   **FUD** XXX   E

AMA: 2008,Mar,8-12

0015F Melanoma follow up completed (includes assessment of all of the following components) (ML): History obtained regarding new or changing moles (1050F) Complete physical skin exam performed (2029F) Patient counseled to perform a monthly self skin examination (5005F)

INCLUDES Complete physical skin exam (2029F)
Counseling to perform monthly skin self-examination (5005F)
History obtained new or changing moles (1050F)

🚑 0.00   ⚕ 0.00   **FUD** XXX   E

AMA: 2008,Mar,8-12

0500F-0584F Care Provided According to Prevailing Guidelines

INCLUDES Utilization measures or patient care provided for certain clinical purposes

0500F Initial prenatal care visit (report at first prenatal encounter with health care professional providing obstetrical care. Report also date of visit and, in a separate field, the date of the last menstrual period [LMP]) (Prenatal)   M ♀

🚑 0.00   ⚕ 0.00   **FUD** XXX   E

AMA: 2018,Jan,8; 2017,Jan,8; 2016,Jan,13

0501F Prenatal flow sheet documented in medical record by first prenatal visit (documentation includes at minimum blood pressure, weight, urine protein, uterine size, fetal heart tones, and estimated date of delivery). Report also: date of visit and, in a separate field, the date of the last menstrual period [LMP] (Note: If reporting 0501F Prenatal flow sheet, it is not necessary to report 0500F Initial prenatal care visit) (Prenatal)   M ♀

🚑 0.00   ⚕ 0.00   **FUD** XXX   E

AMA: 2004,Nov,1

0502F Subsequent prenatal care visit (Prenatal) [Excludes: patients who are seen for a condition unrelated to pregnancy or prenatal care (eg, an upper respiratory infection; patients seen for consultation only, not for continuing care)]   M ♀

EXCLUDES Patients seen for unrelated pregnancy/prenatal care condition (e.g., upper respiratory infection; patients seen for consultation only, not for continuing care)

🚑 0.00   ⚕ 0.00   **FUD** XXX   E

AMA: 2004,Nov,1

0503F Postpartum care visit (Prenatal)   M ♀

🚑 0.00   ⚕ 0.00   **FUD** XXX   E

AMA: 2004,Nov,1

0505F Hemodialysis plan of care documented (ESRD, P-ESRD)

🚑 0.00   ⚕ 0.00   **FUD** XXX   E

AMA: 2008,Mar,8-12

0507F Peritoneal dialysis plan of care documented (ESRD)

🚑 0.00   ⚕ 0.00   **FUD** XXX   E

AMA: 2008,Mar,8-12

0509F Urinary incontinence plan of care documented (GER)

🚑 0.00   ⚕ 0.00   **FUD** XXX   M

0513F Elevated blood pressure plan of care documented (CKD)

🚑 0.00   ⚕ 0.00   **FUD** XXX   M

AMA: 2008,Mar,8-12

0514F Plan of care for elevated hemoglobin level documented for patient receiving Erythropoiesis-Stimulating Agent therapy (ESA) (CKD)

🚑 0.00   ⚕ 0.00   **FUD** XXX   E

AMA: 2008,Mar,8-12

0516F Anemia plan of care documented (ESRD)

🚑 0.00   ⚕ 0.00   **FUD** XXX   E

AMA: 2008,Mar,8-12

0517F Glaucoma plan of care documented (EC)

🚑 0.00   ⚕ 0.00   **FUD** XXX   M

AMA: 2008,Mar,8-12

0518F Falls plan of care documented (GER)
🚑 0.00 ⚖ 0.00 **FUD** XXX M
AMA: 2008,Mar,8-12

0519F Planned chemotherapy regimen, including at a minimum: drug(s) prescribed, dose, and duration, documented prior to initiation of a new treatment regimen (ONC)
🚑 0.00 ⚖ 0.00 **FUD** XXX E
AMA: 2008,Mar,8-12

0520F Radiation dose limits to normal tissues established prior to the initiation of a course of 3D conformal radiation for a minimum of 2 tissue/organ (ONC)
🚑 0.00 ⚖ 0.00 **FUD** XXX M
AMA: 2008,Mar,8-12

0521F Plan of care to address pain documented (COA) (ONC)
🚑 0.00 ⚖ 0.00 **FUD** XXX M
AMA: 2008,Mar,8-12

0525F Initial visit for episode (BkP)
🚑 0.00 ⚖ 0.00 **FUD** XXX E
AMA: 2008,Mar,8-12

0526F Subsequent visit for episode (BkP)
🚑 0.00 ⚖ 0.00 **FUD** XXX M
AMA: 2008,Mar,8-12

0528F Recommended follow-up interval for repeat colonoscopy of at least 10 years documented in colonoscopy report (End/Polyp)
🚑 0.00 ⚖ 0.00 **FUD** XXX M

0529F Interval of 3 or more years since patient's last colonoscopy, documented (End/Polyp)
🚑 0.00 ⚖ 0.00 **FUD** XXX M

0535F Dyspnea management plan of care, documented (Pall Cr)
🚑 0.00 ⚖ 0.00 **FUD** XXX E

0540F Glucorticoid Management Plan Documented (RA)
🚑 0.00 ⚖ 0.00 **FUD** XXX M

0545F Plan for follow-up care for major depressive disorder, documented (MDD ADOL)
🚑 0.00 ⚖ 0.00 **FUD** XXX E

0550F Cytopathology report on routine nongynecologic specimen finalized within two working days of accession date (PATH)
🚑 0.00 ⚖ 0.00 **FUD** XXX E

0551F Cytopathology report on nongynecologic specimen with documentation that the specimen was non-routine (PATH)
🚑 0.00 ⚖ 0.00 **FUD** XXX E

0555F Symptom management plan of care documented (HF)
🚑 0.00 ⚖ 0.00 **FUD** XXX E

0556F Plan of care to achieve lipid control documented (CAD)
🚑 0.00 ⚖ 0.00 **FUD** XXX E

0557F Plan of care to manage anginal symptoms documented (CAD)
🚑 0.00 ⚖ 0.00 **FUD** XXX E

0575F HIV RNA control plan of care, documented (HIV)
🚑 0.00 ⚖ 0.00 **FUD** XXX E

0580F Multidisciplinary care plan developed or updated (ALS)
🚑 0.00 ⚖ 0.00 **FUD** XXX E

0581F Patient transferred directly from anesthetizing location to critical care unit (Peri2)
🚑 0.00 ⚖ 0.00 **FUD** XXX M

0582F Patient not transferred directly from anesthetizing location to critical care unit (Peri2)
🚑 0.00 ⚖ 0.00 **FUD** XXX E

0583F Transfer of care checklist used (Peri2)
🚑 0.00 ⚖ 0.00 **FUD** XXX M

0584F Transfer of care checklist not used (Peri2)
🚑 0.00 ⚖ 0.00 **FUD** XXX E

1000F-1505F Elements of History/Review of Systems

INCLUDES Measures for specific aspects patient history or systems review

1000F Tobacco use assessed (CAD, CAP, COPD, PV) (DM)
🚑 0.00 ⚖ 0.00 **FUD** XXX E
AMA: 2018,Jan,8; 2017,Jan,8; 2016,Jan,13

1002F Anginal symptoms and level of activity assessed (NMA-No Measure Associated)
🚑 0.00 ⚖ 0.00 **FUD** XXX E
AMA: 2004,Nov,1

1003F Level of activity assessed (NMA-No Measure Associated)
🚑 0.00 ⚖ 0.00 **FUD** XXX E
AMA: 2006,Dec,10-12

1004F Clinical symptoms of volume overload (excess) assessed (NMA-No Measure Associated)
🚑 0.00 ⚖ 0.00 **FUD** XXX E
AMA: 2006,Dec,10-12

1005F Asthma symptoms evaluated (includes documentation of numeric frequency of symptoms or patient completion of an asthma assessment tool/survey/questionnaire) (NMA-No Measure Associated)
🚑 0.00 ⚖ 0.00 **FUD** XXX E

1006F Osteoarthritis symptoms and functional status assessed (may include the use of a standardized scale or the completion of an assessment questionnaire, such as the SF-36, AAOS Hip & Knee Questionnaire) (OA) [Instructions: Report when osteoarthritis is addressed during the patient encounter]
INCLUDES Osteoarthritis when addressed during patient encounter
🚑 0.00 ⚖ 0.00 **FUD** XXX M

1007F Use of anti-inflammatory or analgesic over-the-counter (OTC) medications for symptom relief assessed (OA)
🚑 0.00 ⚖ 0.00 **FUD** XXX E

1008F Gastrointestinal and renal risk factors assessed for patients on prescribed or OTC non-steroidal anti-inflammatory drug (NSAID) (OA)
🚑 0.00 ⚖ 0.00 **FUD** XXX E

1010F Severity of angina assessed by level of activity (CAD)
🚑 0.00 ⚖ 0.00 **FUD** XXX E

1011F Angina present (CAD)
🚑 0.00 ⚖ 0.00 **FUD** XXX E

1012F Angina absent (CAD)
🚑 0.00 ⚖ 0.00 **FUD** XXX E

1015F Chronic obstructive pulmonary disease (COPD) symptoms assessed (Includes assessment of at least 1 of the following: dyspnea, cough/sputum, wheezing), or respiratory symptom assessment tool completed (COPD)
🚑 0.00 ⚖ 0.00 **FUD** XXX E

1018F Dyspnea assessed, not present (COPD)
🚑 0.00 ⚖ 0.00 **FUD** XXX E

1019F Dyspnea assessed, present (COPD)
🚑 0.00 ⚖ 0.00 **FUD** XXX E

1022F Pneumococcus immunization status assessed (CAP, COPD)
🚑 0.00 ⚖ 0.00 **FUD** XXX E
AMA: 2010,Jul,3-5; 2008,Mar,8-12

1026F Co-morbid conditions assessed (eg, includes assessment for presence or absence of: malignancy, liver disease, congestive heart failure, cerebrovascular disease, renal disease, chronic obstructive pulmonary disease, asthma, diabetes, other co-morbid conditions) (CAP)
🚑 0.00 ⚖ 0.00 **FUD** XXX E

1030F Influenza immunization status assessed (CAP)
🚑 0.00 ⚖ 0.00 **FUD** XXX E
AMA: 2008,Mar,8-12

1031F Smoking status and exposure to second hand smoke in the home assessed (Asthma)

🖩 0.00   ✀ 0.00   **FUD** XXX   Ⓔ

1032F Current tobacco smoker or currently exposed to secondhand smoke (Asthma)

🖩 0.00   ✀ 0.00   **FUD** XXX   Ⓔ

1033F Current tobacco non-smoker and not currently exposed to secondhand smoke (Asthma)

🖩 0.00   ✀ 0.00   **FUD** XXX   Ⓔ

1034F Current tobacco smoker (CAD, CAP, COPD, PV) (DM)

🖩 0.00   ✀ 0.00   **FUD** XXX   Ⓔ

AMA: 2008,Mar,8-12

1035F Current smokeless tobacco user (eg, chew, snuff) (PV)

🖩 0.00   ✀ 0.00   **FUD** XXX   Ⓔ

AMA: 2008,Mar,8-12

1036F Current tobacco non-user (CAD, CAP, COPD, PV) (DM) (IBD)

🖩 0.00   ✀ 0.00   **FUD** XXX   Ⓜ

AMA: 2008,Mar,8-12

1038F Persistent asthma (mild, moderate or severe) (Asthma)

🖩 0.00   ✀ 0.00   **FUD** XXX   Ⓜ

AMA: 2018,Jan,8; 2017,Jan,8; 2016,Jan,13

1039F Intermittent asthma (Asthma)

🖩 0.00   ✀ 0.00   **FUD** XXX   Ⓜ

AMA: 2018,Jan,8; 2017,Jan,8; 2016,Jan,13

1040F DSM-5 criteria for major depressive disorder documented at the initial evaluation (MDD, MDD ADOL)

🖩 0.00   ✀ 0.00   **FUD** XXX   Ⓔ

AMA: 2008,Mar,8-12

1050F History obtained regarding new or changing moles (ML)

🖩 0.00   ✀ 0.00   **FUD** XXX   Ⓔ

AMA: 2008,Mar,8-12

1052F Type, anatomic location, and activity all assessed (IBD)

🖩 0.00   ✀ 0.00   **FUD** XXX   Ⓔ

1055F Visual functional status assessed (EC)

🖩 0.00   ✀ 0.00   **FUD** XXX   Ⓔ

1060F Documentation of permanent or persistent or paroxysmal atrial fibrillation (STR)

🖩 0.00   ✀ 0.00   **FUD** XXX   Ⓔ

1061F Documentation of absence of permanent and persistent and paroxysmal atrial fibrillation (STR)

🖩 0.00   ✀ 0.00   **FUD** XXX   Ⓔ

1065F Ischemic stroke symptom onset of less than 3 hours prior to arrival (STR)

🖩 0.00   ✀ 0.00   **FUD** XXX   Ⓔ

1066F Ischemic stroke symptom onset greater than or equal to 3 hours prior to arrival (STR)

🖩 0.00   ✀ 0.00   **FUD** XXX   Ⓔ

1070F Alarm symptoms (involuntary weight loss, dysphagia, or gastrointestinal bleeding) assessed; none present (GERD)

🖩 0.00   ✀ 0.00   **FUD** XXX   Ⓔ

1071F 1 or more present (GERD)

🖩 0.00   ✀ 0.00   **FUD** XXX   Ⓔ

1090F Presence or absence of urinary incontinence assessed (GER)

🖩 0.00   ✀ 0.00   **FUD** XXX   Ⓜ

1091F Urinary incontinence characterized (eg, frequency, volume, timing, type of symptoms, how bothersome) (GER)

🖩 0.00   ✀ 0.00   **FUD** XXX   Ⓔ

1100F Patient screened for future fall risk; documentation of 2 or more falls in the past year or any fall with injury in the past year (GER)

🖩 0.00   ✀ 0.00   **FUD** XXX   Ⓜ

AMA: 2008,Mar,8-12

1101F documentation of no falls in the past year or only 1 fall without injury in the past year (GER)

🖩 0.00   ✀ 0.00   **FUD** XXX   Ⓜ

AMA: 2008,Mar,8-12

1110F Patient discharged from an inpatient facility (eg, hospital, skilled nursing facility, or rehabilitation facility) within the last 60 days (GER)

🖩 0.00   ✀ 0.00   **FUD** XXX   Ⓔ

1111F Discharge medications reconciled with the current medication list in outpatient medical record (COA) (GER)

🖩 0.00   ✀ 0.00   **FUD** XXX   Ⓜ

1116F Auricular or periauricular pain assessed (AOE)

🖩 0.00   ✀ 0.00   **FUD** XXX   Ⓔ

AMA: 2008,Mar,8-12

1118F GERD symptoms assessed after 12 months of therapy (GERD)

🖩 0.00   ✀ 0.00   **FUD** XXX   Ⓔ

1119F Initial evaluation for condition (HEP C)(EPI, DSP)

🖩 0.00   ✀ 0.00   **FUD** XXX   Ⓔ

AMA: 2008,Mar,8-12

1121F Subsequent evaluation for condition (HEP C)(EPI)

🖩 0.00   ✀ 0.00   **FUD** XXX   Ⓔ

AMA: 2008,Mar,8-12

1123F Advance Care Planning discussed and documented advance care plan or surrogate decision maker documented in the medical record (DEM) (GER, Pall Cr)

🖩 0.00   ✀ 0.00   **FUD** XXX   Ⓜ

AMA: 2008,Mar,8-12

1124F Advance Care Planning discussed and documented in the medical record, patient did not wish or was not able to name a surrogate decision maker or provide an advance care plan (DEM) (GER, Pall Cr)

🖩 0.00   ✀ 0.00   **FUD** XXX   Ⓜ

AMA: 2008,Mar,8-12

1125F Pain severity quantified; pain present (COA) (ONC)

🖩 0.00   ✀ 0.00   **FUD** XXX   Ⓜ

AMA: 2008,Mar,8-12

1126F no pain present (COA) (ONC)

🖩 0.00   ✀ 0.00   **FUD** XXX   Ⓜ

AMA: 2008,Mar,8-12

1127F New episode for condition (NMA-No Measure Associated)

🖩 0.00   ✀ 0.00   **FUD** XXX   Ⓔ

AMA: 2008,Mar,8-12

1128F Subsequent episode for condition (NMA-No Measure Associated)

🖩 0.00   ✀ 0.00   **FUD** XXX   Ⓔ

AMA: 2008,Mar,8-12

1130F Back pain and function assessed, including all of the following: Pain assessment and functional status and patient history, including notation of presence or absence of "red flags" (warning signs) and assessment of prior treatment and response, and employment status (BkP)

🖩 0.00   ✀ 0.00   **FUD** XXX   Ⓔ

AMA: 2008,Mar,8-12

1134F Episode of back pain lasting 6 weeks or less (BkP)

🖩 0.00   ✀ 0.00   **FUD** XXX   Ⓔ

AMA: 2008,Mar,8-12

1135F Episode of back pain lasting longer than 6 weeks (BkP)

🖩 0.00   ✀ 0.00   **FUD** XXX   Ⓔ

AMA: 2008,Mar,8-12

1136F Episode of back pain lasting 12 weeks or less (BkP)

🖩 0.00   ✀ 0.00   **FUD** XXX   Ⓔ

AMA: 2008,Mar,8-12

● New Code   ▲ Revised Code   ○ Reinstated   ● New Web Release   ▲ Revised Web Release   + Add-on   Unlisted   Not Covered   # Resequenced
㊿ Optum Mod 50 Exempt   Ⓢ AMA Mod 51 Exempt   �51 Optum Mod 51 Exempt   �63 Mod 63 Exempt   ⋏ Non-FDA Drug   ★ Telemedicine   Ⓜ Maternity   Ⓐ Age Edit

CPT © 2021 American Medical Association. All Rights Reserved.

1137F Episode of back pain lasting longer than 12 weeks (BkP)
🚗 0.00 ⚖ 0.00 **FUD** XXX E
AMA: 2008,Mar,8-12

1150F Documentation that a patient has a substantial risk of death within 1 year (Pall Cr)
🚗 0.00 ⚖ 0.00 **FUD** XXX E

1151F Documentation that a patient does not have a substantial risk of death within one year (Pall Cr)
🚗 0.00 ⚖ 0.00 **FUD** XXX E

1152F Documentation of advanced disease diagnosis, goals of care prioritize comfort (Pall Cr)
🚗 0.00 ⚖ 0.00 **FUD** XXX E

1153F Documentation of advanced disease diagnosis, goals of care do not prioritize comfort (Pall Cr)
🚗 0.00 ⚖ 0.00 **FUD** XXX E

1157F Advance care plan or similar legal document present in the medical record (COA)
🚗 0.00 ⚖ 0.00 **FUD** XXX E

1158F Advance care planning discussion documented in the medical record (COA)
🚗 0.00 ⚖ 0.00 **FUD** XXX M

1159F Medication list documented in medical record (COA)
🚗 0.00 ⚖ 0.00 **FUD** XXX E

1160F Review of all medications by a prescribing practitioner or clinical pharmacist (such as, prescriptions, OTCs, herbal therapies and supplements) documented in the medical record (COA)
🚗 0.00 ⚖ 0.00 **FUD** XXX E

1170F Functional status assessed (COA) (RA)
🚗 0.00 ⚖ 0.00 **FUD** XXX M

1175F Functional status for dementia assessed and results reviewed (DEM)
🚗 0.00 ⚖ 0.00 **FUD** XXX E

1180F All specified thromboembolic risk factors assessed (AFIB)
🚗 0.00 ⚖ 0.00 **FUD** XXX E

1181F Neuropsychiatric symptoms assessed and results reviewed (DEM)
🚗 0.00 ⚖ 0.00 **FUD** XXX E

1182F Neuropsychiatric symptoms, one or more present (DEM)
🚗 0.00 ⚖ 0.00 **FUD** XXX E

1183F Neuropsychiatric symptoms, absent (DEM)
🚗 0.00 ⚖ 0.00 **FUD** XXX E

1200F Seizure type(s) and current seizure frequency(ies) documented (EPI)
🚗 0.00 ⚖ 0.00 **FUD** XXX E

1205F Etiology of epilepsy or epilepsy syndrome(s) reviewed and documented (EPI)
🚗 0.00 ⚖ 0.00 **FUD** XXX E

1220F Patient screened for depression (SUD)
🚗 0.00 ⚖ 0.00 **FUD** XXX E

1400F Parkinson's disease diagnosis reviewed (Prkns)
🚗 0.00 ⚖ 0.00 **FUD** XXX E

1450F Symptoms improved or remained consistent with treatment goals since last assessment (HF)
🚗 0.00 ⚖ 0.00 **FUD** XXX E

1451F Symptoms demonstrated clinically important deterioration since last assessment (HF)
🚗 0.00 ⚖ 0.00 **FUD** XXX E

1460F Qualifying cardiac event/diagnosis in previous 12 months (CAD)
🚗 0.00 ⚖ 0.00 **FUD** XXX M

1461F No qualifying cardiac event/diagnosis in previous 12 months (CAD)
🚗 0.00 ⚖ 0.00 **FUD** XXX M

1490F Dementia severity classified, mild (DEM)
🚗 0.00 ⚖ 0.00 **FUD** XXX E

1491F Dementia severity classified, moderate (DEM)
🚗 0.00 ⚖ 0.00 **FUD** XXX E

1493F Dementia severity classified, severe (DEM)
🚗 0.00 ⚖ 0.00 **FUD** XXX E

1494F Cognition assessed and reviewed (DEM)
🚗 0.00 ⚖ 0.00 **FUD** XXX E

1500F Symptoms and signs of distal symmetric polyneuropathy reviewed and documented (DSP)
🚗 0.00 ⚖ 0.00 **FUD** XXX E

1501F Not initial evaluation for condition (DSP)
🚗 0.00 ⚖ 0.00 **FUD** XXX E

1502F Patient queried about pain and pain interference with function using a valid and reliable instrument (DSP)
🚗 0.00 ⚖ 0.00 **FUD** XXX E

1503F Patient queried about symptoms of respiratory insufficiency (ALS)
🚗 0.00 ⚖ 0.00 **FUD** XXX E

1504F Patient has respiratory insufficiency (ALS)
🚗 0.00 ⚖ 0.00 **FUD** XXX E

1505F Patient does not have respiratory insufficiency (ALS)
🚗 0.00 ⚖ 0.00 **FUD** XXX E

2000F-2060F [2033F] Elements of Examination

INCLUDES Components clinical assessment or physical exam

2000F Blood pressure measured (CKD)(DM)
🚗 0.00 ⚖ 0.00 **FUD** XXX M
AMA: 2018,Jan,8; 2017,Jan,8; 2016,Jan,13

2001F Weight recorded (PAG)
🚗 0.00 ⚖ 0.00 **FUD** XXX E
AMA: 2006,Dec,10-12

2002F Clinical signs of volume overload (excess) assessed (NMA-No Measure Associated)
🚗 0.00 ⚖ 0.00 **FUD** XXX E
AMA: 2006,Dec,10-12

2004F Initial examination of the involved joint(s) (includes visual inspection, palpation, range of motion) (OA) [Instructions: Report only for initial osteoarthritis visit or for visits for new joint involvement]
INCLUDES Visits for initial osteoarthritis examination or new joint involvement
🚗 0.00 ⚖ 0.00 **FUD** XXX E
AMA: 2004,Feb,3; 2003,Aug,1

2010F Vital signs (temperature, pulse, respiratory rate, and blood pressure) documented and reviewed (CAP) (EM)
🚗 0.00 ⚖ 0.00 **FUD** XXX E

2014F Mental status assessed (CAP) (EM)
🚗 0.00 ⚖ 0.00 **FUD** XXX E

2015F Asthma impairment assessed (Asthma)
🚗 0.00 ⚖ 0.00 **FUD** XXX E

2016F Asthma risk assessed (Asthma)
🚗 0.00 ⚖ 0.00 **FUD** XXX E

2018F Hydration status assessed (normal/mildly dehydrated/severely dehydrated) (CAP)
🚗 0.00 ⚖ 0.00 **FUD** XXX E

2019F Dilated macular exam performed, including documentation of the presence or absence of macular thickening or hemorrhage and the level of macular degeneration severity (EC)
🚗 0.00 ⚖ 0.00 **FUD** XXX E

2020F Dilated fundus evaluation performed within 12 months prior to cataract surgery (EC)

⚕ 0.00   ⚖ 0.00   **FUD** XXX   E

AMA: 2008,Mar,8-12

2021F Dilated macular or fundus exam performed, including documentation of the presence or absence of macular edema and level of severity of retinopathy (EC)

⚕ 0.00   ⚖ 0.00   **FUD** XXX   E

2022F Dilated retinal eye exam with interpretation by an ophthalmologist or optometrist documented and reviewed; with evidence of retinopathy (DM)

⚕ 0.00   ⚖ 0.00   **FUD** XXX   M

AMA: 2008,Mar,8-12

2023F without evidence of retinopathy (DM)

⚕ 0.00   ⚖ 0.00   **FUD** XXX

2024F 7 standard field stereoscopic retinal photos with interpretation by an ophthalmologist or optometrist documented and reviewed; with evidence of retinopathy (DM)

⚕ 0.00   ⚖ 0.00   **FUD** XXX   M

AMA: 2008,Mar,8-12

2025F without evidence of retinopathy (DM)

⚕ 0.00   ⚖ 0.00   **FUD** XXX

2026F Eye imaging validated to match diagnosis from 7 standard field stereoscopic retinal photos results documented and reviewed; with evidence of retinopathy (DM)

⚕ 0.00   ⚖ 0.00   **FUD** XXX   M

AMA: 2008,Mar,8-12

\# **2033F** without evidence of retinopathy (DM)

⚕ 0.00   ⚖ 0.00   **FUD** XXX

2027F Optic nerve head evaluation performed (EC)

⚕ 0.00   ⚖ 0.00   **FUD** XXX   M

2028F Foot examination performed (includes examination through visual inspection, sensory exam with monofilament, and pulse exam - report when any of the 3 components are completed) (DM)

⚕ 0.00   ⚖ 0.00   **FUD** XXX   E

2029F Complete physical skin exam performed (ML)

⚕ 0.00   ⚖ 0.00   **FUD** XXX   E

AMA: 2008,Mar,8-12

2030F Hydration status documented, normally hydrated (PAG)

⚕ 0.00   ⚖ 0.00   **FUD** XXX   E

2031F Hydration status documented, dehydrated (PAG)

⚕ 0.00   ⚖ 0.00   **FUD** XXX   E

2033F Resequenced code. See code following 2026F.

2035F Tympanic membrane mobility assessed with pneumatic otoscopy or tympanometry (OME)

⚕ 0.00   ⚖ 0.00   **FUD** XXX   E

AMA: 2008,Mar,8-12

2040F Physical examination on the date of the initial visit for low back pain performed, in accordance with specifications (BkP)

⚕ 0.00   ⚖ 0.00   **FUD** XXX   E

2044F Documentation of mental health assessment prior to intervention (back surgery or epidural steroid injection) or for back pain episode lasting longer than 6 weeks (BkP)

⚕ 0.00   ⚖ 0.00   **FUD** XXX   E

AMA: 2008,Mar,8-12

2050F Wound characteristics including size and nature of wound base tissue and amount of drainage prior to debridement documented (CWC)

⚕ 0.00   ⚖ 0.00   **FUD** XXX   E

2060F Patient interviewed directly on or before date of diagnosis of major depressive disorder (MDD ADOL)

⚕ 0.00   ⚖ 0.00   **FUD** XXX   E

3006F-3776F [3051F, 3052F] Findings from Diagnostic or Screening Tests

INCLUDES Results and medical decision making with regards to ordered tests:
Clinical laboratory tests
Other examination procedures
Radiological examinations

3006F Chest X-ray results documented and reviewed (CAP)

⚕ 0.00   ⚖ 0.00   **FUD** XXX   E

AMA: 2018,Jan,8; 2017,Jan,8; 2016,Jan,13

3008F Body Mass Index (BMI), documented (PV)

⚕ 0.00   ⚖ 0.00   **FUD** XXX   E

3011F Lipid panel results documented and reviewed (must include total cholesterol, HDL-C, triglycerides and calculated LDL-C) (CAD)

⚕ 0.00   ⚖ 0.00   **FUD** XXX   E

3014F Screening mammography results documented and reviewed (PV)

⚕ 0.00   ⚖ 0.00   **FUD** XXX   E

AMA: 2008,Mar,8-12

3015F Cervical cancer screening results documented and reviewed (PV)

⚕ 0.00   ⚖ 0.00   **FUD** XXX   ♀

3016F Patient screened for unhealthy alcohol use using a systematic screening method (PV) (DSP)

⚕ 0.00   ⚖ 0.00   **FUD** XXX   E

3017F Colorectal cancer screening results documented and reviewed (PV)

⚕ 0.00   ⚖ 0.00   **FUD** XXX   M

AMA: 2008,Mar,8-12

3018F Pre-procedure risk assessment and depth of insertion and quality of the bowel prep and complete description of polyp(s) found, including location of each polyp, size, number and gross morphology and recommendations for follow-up in final colonoscopy report documented (End/Polyp)

⚕ 0.00   ⚖ 0.00   **FUD** XXX   E

3019F Left ventricular ejection fraction (LVEF) assessment planned post discharge (HF)

⚕ 0.00   ⚖ 0.00   **FUD** XXX   E

3020F Left ventricular function (LVF) assessment (eg, echocardiography, nuclear test, or ventriculography) documented in the medical record (Includes quantitative or qualitative assessment results) (NMA-No Measure Associated)

⚕ 0.00   ⚖ 0.00   **FUD** XXX   E

AMA: 2006,Dec,10-12

3021F Left ventricular ejection fraction (LVEF) less than 40% or documentation of moderately or severely depressed left ventricular systolic function (CAD, HF)

⚕ 0.00   ⚖ 0.00   **FUD** XXX   M

3022F Left ventricular ejection fraction (LVEF) greater than or equal to 40% or documentation as normal or mildly depressed left ventricular systolic function (CAD, HF)

⚕ 0.00   ⚖ 0.00   **FUD** XXX   M

3023F Spirometry results documented and reviewed (COPD)

⚕ 0.00   ⚖ 0.00   **FUD** XXX   M

3025F Spirometry test results demonstrate FEV1/FVC less than 70% with COPD symptoms (eg, dyspnea, cough/sputum, wheezing) (CAP, COPD)

⚕ 0.00   ⚖ 0.00   **FUD** XXX   E

3027F Spirometry test results demonstrate FEV1/FVC greater than or equal to 70% or patient does not have COPD symptoms (COPD)
🚗 0.00   0.00   **FUD** XXX   E

3028F Oxygen saturation results documented and reviewed (includes assessment through pulse oximetry or arterial blood gas measurement) (CAP, COPD) (EM)
🚗 0.00   0.00   **FUD** XXX   E

3035F Oxygen saturation less than or equal to 88% or a PaO2 less than or equal to 55 mm Hg (COPD)
🚗 0.00   0.00   **FUD** XXX   E

3037F Oxygen saturation greater than 88% or PaO2 greater than 55 mm Hg (COPD)
🚗 0.00   0.00   **FUD** XXX   E

3038F Pulmonary function test performed within 12 months prior to surgery (Lung/Esop Cx)
🚗 0.00   0.00   **FUD** XXX   E

3040F Functional expiratory volume (FEV1) less than 40% of predicted value (COPD)
🚗 0.00   0.00   **FUD** XXX   E

3042F Functional expiratory volume (FEV1) greater than or equal to 40% of predicted value (COPD)
🚗 0.00   0.00   **FUD** XXX   E

3044F Most recent hemoglobin A1c (HbA1c) level less than 7.0% (DM)
🚗 0.00   0.00   **FUD** XXX   M

\# **3051F** Most recent hemoglobin A1c (HbA1c) level greater than or equal to 7.0% and less than 8.0% (DM)
🚗 0.00   0.00   **FUD** XXX

\# **3052F** Most recent hemoglobin A1c (HbA1c) level greater than or equal to 8.0% and less than or equal to 9.0% (DM)
🚗 0.00   0.00   **FUD** XXX

3046F Most recent hemoglobin A1c level greater than 9.0% (DM)
EXCLUDES *Hemoglobin A1c less than or equal to 9.0% (3044F, [3051F], [3052F])*
🚗 0.00   0.00   **FUD** XXX   M

3048F Most recent LDL-C less than 100 mg/dL (CAD) (DM)
🚗 0.00   0.00   **FUD** XXX   E

3049F Most recent LDL-C 100-129 mg/dL (CAD) (DM)
🚗 0.00   0.00   **FUD** XXX   E

3050F Most recent LDL-C greater than or equal to 130 mg/dL (CAD) (DM)
🚗 0.00   0.00   **FUD** XXX   E

3051F **Resequenced code. See code following 3044F.**

3052F **Resequenced code. See code before 3046F.**

3055F Left ventricular ejection fraction (LVEF) less than or equal to 35% (HF)
🚗 0.00   0.00   **FUD** XXX   E

3056F Left ventricular ejection fraction (LVEF) greater than 35% or no LVEF result available (HF)
🚗 0.00   0.00   **FUD** XXX   E

3060F Positive microalbuminuria test result documented and reviewed (DM)
🚗 0.00   0.00   **FUD** XXX   M

3061F Negative microalbuminuria test result documented and reviewed (DM)
🚗 0.00   0.00   **FUD** XXX   M

3062F Positive macroalbuminuria test result documented and reviewed (DM)
🚗 0.00   0.00   **FUD** XXX   M

3066F Documentation of treatment for nephropathy (eg, patient receiving dialysis, patient being treated for ESRD, CRF, ARF, or renal insufficiency, any visit to a nephrologist) (DM)
🚗 0.00   0.00   **FUD** XXX   M

3072F Low risk for retinopathy (no evidence of retinopathy in the prior year) (DM)
🚗 0.00   0.00   **FUD** XXX   M
AMA: 2008,Mar,8-12

3073F Pre-surgical (cataract) axial length, corneal power measurement and method of intraocular lens power calculation documented within 12 months prior to surgery (EC)
🚗 0.00   0.00   **FUD** XXX   E
AMA: 2008,Mar,8-12

3074F Most recent systolic blood pressure less than 130 mm Hg (DM), (HTN, CKD, CAD)
🚗 0.00   0.00   **FUD** XXX   E
AMA: 2008,Mar,8-12

3075F Most recent systolic blood pressure 130-139 mm Hg (DM) (HTN, CKD, CAD)
🚗 0.00   0.00   **FUD** XXX   E
AMA: 2008,Mar,8-12

3077F Most recent systolic blood pressure greater than or equal to 140 mm Hg (HTN, CKD, CAD) (DM)
🚗 0.00   0.00   **FUD** XXX   E
AMA: 2008,Mar,8-12

3078F Most recent diastolic blood pressure less than 80 mm Hg (HTN, CKD, CAD) (DM)
🚗 0.00   0.00   **FUD** XXX   E
AMA: 2008,Mar,8-12

3079F Most recent diastolic blood pressure 80-89 mm Hg (HTN, CKD, CAD) (DM)
🚗 0.00   0.00   **FUD** XXX   E
AMA: 2008,Mar,8-12

3080F Most recent diastolic blood pressure greater than or equal to 90 mm Hg (HTN, CKD, CAD) (DM)
🚗 0.00   0.00   **FUD** XXX   E
AMA: 2008,Mar,8-12

3082F Kt/V less than 1.2 (Clearance of urea [Kt]/volume [V]) (ESRD, P-ESRD)
🚗 0.00   0.00   **FUD** XXX   E
AMA: 2008,Mar,8-12

3083F Kt/V equal to or greater than 1.2 and less than 1.7 (Clearance of urea [Kt]/volume [V]) (ESRD, P-ESRD)
🚗 0.00   0.00   **FUD** XXX   E
AMA: 2008,Mar,8-12

3084F Kt/V greater than or equal to 1.7 (Clearance of urea [Kt]/volume [V]) (ESRD, P-ESRD)
🚗 0.00   0.00   **FUD** XXX   E
AMA: 2008,Mar,8-12

3085F Suicide risk assessed (MDD, MDD ADOL)
🚗 0.00   0.00   **FUD** XXX   E

3088F Major depressive disorder, mild (MDD)
🚗 0.00   0.00   **FUD** XXX   E

3089F Major depressive disorder, moderate (MDD)
🚗 0.00   0.00   **FUD** XXX   E

3090F Major depressive disorder, severe without psychotic features (MDD)
🚗 0.00   0.00   **FUD** XXX   E

3091F Major depressive disorder, severe with psychotic features (MDD)
🚗 0.00   0.00   **FUD** XXX   E

3092F Major depressive disorder, in remission (MDD)
🚗 0.00   0.00   **FUD** XXX   E

3093F Documentation of new diagnosis of initial or recurrent episode of major depressive disorder (MDD)
   📷 0.00   ⚖ 0.00   **FUD** XXX   E
   AMA: 2008,Mar,8-12

3095F Central dual-energy X-ray absorptiometry (DXA) results documented (OP)(IBD)
   📷 0.00   ⚖ 0.00   **FUD** XXX   M

3096F Central dual-energy X-ray absorptiometry (DXA) ordered (OP)(IBD)
   📷 0.00   ⚖ 0.00   **FUD** XXX   E

3100F Carotid imaging study report (includes direct or indirect reference to measurements of distal internal carotid diameter as the denominator for stenosis measurement) (STR, RAD)
   📷 0.00   ⚖ 0.00   **FUD** XXX   M
   AMA: 2008,Mar,8-12

3110F Documentation in final CT or MRI report of presence or absence of hemorrhage and mass lesion and acute infarction (STR)
   📷 0.00   ⚖ 0.00   **FUD** XXX   E

3111F CT or MRI of the brain performed in the hospital within 24 hours of arrival or performed in an outpatient imaging center, to confirm initial diagnosis of stroke, TIA or intracranial hemorrhage (STR)
   📷 0.00   ⚖ 0.00   **FUD** XXX   E

3112F CT or MRI of the brain performed greater than 24 hours after arrival to the hospital or performed in an outpatient imaging center for purpose other than confirmation of initial diagnosis of stroke, TIA, or intracranial hemorrhage (STR)
   📷 0.00   ⚖ 0.00   **FUD** XXX   E

3115F Quantitative results of an evaluation of current level of activity and clinical symptoms (HF)
   📷 0.00   ⚖ 0.00   **FUD** XXX   E

3117F Heart failure disease specific structured assessment tool completed (HF)
   📷 0.00   ⚖ 0.00   **FUD** XXX   E

3118F New York Heart Association (NYHA) Class documented (HF)
   📷 0.00   ⚖ 0.00   **FUD** XXX   E

3119F No evaluation of level of activity or clinical symptoms (HF)
   📷 0.00   ⚖ 0.00   **FUD** XXX   E

3120F 12-Lead ECG Performed (EM)
   📷 0.00   ⚖ 0.00   **FUD** XXX   E

3126F Esophageal biopsy report with a statement about dysplasia (present, absent, or indefinite, and if present, contains appropriate grading) (PATH)
   📷 0.00   ⚖ 0.00   **FUD** XXX   M

3130F Upper gastrointestinal endoscopy performed (GERD)
   📷 0.00   ⚖ 0.00   **FUD** XXX   E

3132F Documentation of referral for upper gastrointestinal endoscopy (GERD)
   📷 0.00   ⚖ 0.00   **FUD** XXX   E

3140F Upper gastrointestinal endoscopy report indicates suspicion of Barrett's esophagus (GERD)
   📷 0.00   ⚖ 0.00   **FUD** XXX   E

3141F Upper gastrointestinal endoscopy report indicates no suspicion of Barrett's esophagus (GERD)
   📷 0.00   ⚖ 0.00   **FUD** XXX   E

3142F Barium swallow test ordered (GERD)
   INCLUDES   Documentation barium swallow test
   📷 0.00   ⚖ 0.00   **FUD** XXX   E

3150F Forceps esophageal biopsy performed (GERD)
   📷 0.00   ⚖ 0.00   **FUD** XXX   E

3155F Cytogenetic testing performed on bone marrow at time of diagnosis or prior to initiating treatment (HEM)
   📷 0.00   ⚖ 0.00   **FUD** XXX   M
   AMA: 2008,Mar,8-12

3160F Documentation of iron stores prior to initiating erythropoietin therapy (HEM)
   📷 0.00   ⚖ 0.00   **FUD** XXX   M
   AMA: 2008,Mar,8-12

3170F Baseline flow cytometry studies performed at time of diagnosis or prior to initiating treatment (HEM)
   📷 0.00   ⚖ 0.00   **FUD** XXX   M
   AMA: 2008,Mar,8-12

3200F Barium swallow test not ordered (GERD)
   📷 0.00   ⚖ 0.00   **FUD** XXX   E

3210F Group A Strep Test Performed (PHAR)
   📷 0.00   ⚖ 0.00   **FUD** XXX   M
   AMA: 2008,Mar,8-12

3215F Patient has documented immunity to Hepatitis A (HEP-C)
   📷 0.00   ⚖ 0.00   **FUD** XXX   E
   AMA: 2008,Mar,8-12

3216F Patient has documented immunity to Hepatitis B (HEP-C)(IBD)
   📷 0.00   ⚖ 0.00   **FUD** XXX   E
   AMA: 2008,Mar,8-12

3218F RNA testing for Hepatitis C documented as performed within 6 months prior to initiation of antiviral treatment for Hepatitis C (HEP-C)
   📷 0.00   ⚖ 0.00   **FUD** XXX   E
   AMA: 2008,Mar,8-12

3220F Hepatitis C quantitative RNA testing documented as performed at 12 weeks from initiation of antiviral treatment (HEP-C)
   📷 0.00   ⚖ 0.00   **FUD** XXX   E
   AMA: 2008,Mar,8-12

3230F Documentation that hearing test was performed within 6 months prior to tympanostomy tube insertion (OME)
   📷 0.00   ⚖ 0.00   **FUD** XXX   E
   AMA: 2008,Mar,8-12

3250F Specimen site other than anatomic location of primary tumor (PATH)
   📷 0.00   ⚖ 0.00   **FUD** XXX   M

3260F pT category (primary tumor), pN category (regional lymph nodes), and histologic grade documented in pathology report (PATH)
   📷 0.00   ⚖ 0.00   **FUD** XXX   M

3265F Ribonucleic acid (RNA) testing for Hepatitis C viremia ordered or results documented (HEP C)
   📷 0.00   ⚖ 0.00   **FUD** XXX   E
   AMA: 2008,Mar,8-12

3266F Hepatitis C genotype testing documented as performed prior to initiation of antiviral treatment for Hepatitis C (HEP C)
   📷 0.00   ⚖ 0.00   **FUD** XXX   E
   AMA: 2008,Mar,8-12

3267F Pathology report includes pT category, pN category, Gleason score, and statement about margin status (PATH)
   📷 0.00   ⚖ 0.00   **FUD** XXX   M

3268F Prostate-specific antigen (PSA), and primary tumor (T) stage, and Gleason score documented prior to initiation of treatment (PRCA)
   📷 0.00   ⚖ 0.00   **FUD** XXX   E
   AMA: 2008,Mar,8-12

3269F Bone scan performed prior to initiation of treatment or at any time since diagnosis of prostate cancer (PRCA)
🔧 0.00   ⚕ 0.00   **FUD** XXX   Ⓜ
AMA: 2008,Mar,8-12

3270F Bone scan not performed prior to initiation of treatment nor at any time since diagnosis of prostate cancer (PRCA)
🔧 0.00   ⚕ 0.00   **FUD** XXX   Ⓜ
AMA: 2008,Mar,8-12

3271F Low risk of recurrence, prostate cancer (PRCA)
🔧 0.00   ⚕ 0.00   **FUD** XXX   Ⓔ
AMA: 2008,Mar,8-12

3272F Intermediate risk of recurrence, prostate cancer (PRCA)
🔧 0.00   ⚕ 0.00   **FUD** XXX   Ⓔ
AMA: 2008,Mar,8-12

3273F High risk of recurrence, prostate cancer (PRCA)
🔧 0.00   ⚕ 0.00   **FUD** XXX   Ⓔ
AMA: 2008,Mar,8-12

3274F Prostate cancer risk of recurrence not determined or neither low, intermediate nor high (PRCA)
🔧 0.00   ⚕ 0.00   **FUD** XXX   Ⓔ
AMA: 2008,Mar,8-12

3278F Serum levels of calcium, phosphorus, intact Parathyroid Hormone (PTH) and lipid profile ordered (CKD)
🔧 0.00   ⚕ 0.00   **FUD** XXX   Ⓔ
AMA: 2008,Mar,8-12

3279F Hemoglobin level greater than or equal to 13 g/dL (CKD, ESRD)
🔧 0.00   ⚕ 0.00   **FUD** XXX   Ⓔ
AMA: 2008,Mar,8-12

3280F Hemoglobin level 11 g/dL to 12.9 g/dL (CKD, ESRD)
🔧 0.00   ⚕ 0.00   **FUD** XXX   Ⓔ
AMA: 2008,Mar,8-12

3281F Hemoglobin level less than 11 g/dL (CKD, ESRD)
🔧 0.00   ⚕ 0.00   **FUD** XXX   Ⓔ
AMA: 2008,Mar,8-12

3284F Intraocular pressure (IOP) reduced by a value of greater than or equal to 15% from the pre-intervention level (EC)
🔧 0.00   ⚕ 0.00   **FUD** XXX   Ⓜ
AMA: 2008,Mar,8-12

3285F Intraocular pressure (IOP) reduced by a value less than 15% from the pre-intervention level (EC)
🔧 0.00   ⚕ 0.00   **FUD** XXX   Ⓜ
AMA: 2008,Mar,8-12

3288F Falls risk assessment documented (GER)
🔧 0.00   ⚕ 0.00   **FUD** XXX   Ⓜ
AMA: 2008,Mar,8-12

3290F Patient is D (Rh) negative and unsensitized (Pre-Cr)
🔧 0.00   ⚕ 0.00   **FUD** XXX   Ⓔ
AMA: 2008,Mar,8-12

3291F Patient is D (Rh) positive or sensitized (Pre-Cr)
🔧 0.00   ⚕ 0.00   **FUD** XXX   Ⓔ
AMA: 2008,Mar,8-12

3292F HIV testing ordered or documented and reviewed during the first or second prenatal visit (Pre-Cr)
🔧 0.00   ⚕ 0.00   **FUD** XXX   Ⓔ

3293F ABO and Rh blood typing documented as performed (Pre-Cr)
🔧 0.00   ⚕ 0.00   **FUD** XXX   Ⓔ

3294F Group B Streptococcus (GBS) screening documented as performed during week 35-37 gestation (Pre-Cr)
🔧 0.00   ⚕ 0.00   Ⓔ

3300F American Joint Committee on Cancer (AJCC) stage documented and reviewed (ONC)
🔧 0.00   ⚕ 0.00   **FUD** XXX   Ⓜ
AMA: 2008,Mar,8-12

3301F Cancer stage documented in medical record as metastatic and reviewed (ONC)
EXCLUDES   *Cancer staging measures (3321F-3390F)*
🔧 0.00   ⚕ 0.00   **FUD** XXX   Ⓜ
AMA: 2008,Mar,8-12

3315F Estrogen receptor (ER) or progesterone receptor (PR) positive breast cancer (ONC)
🔧 0.00   ⚕ 0.00   **FUD** XXX   Ⓔ
AMA: 2008,Mar,8-12

3316F Estrogen receptor (ER) and progesterone receptor (PR) negative breast cancer (ONC)
🔧 0.00   ⚕ 0.00   **FUD** XXX   Ⓔ
AMA: 2008,Mar,8-12

3317F Pathology report confirming malignancy documented in the medical record and reviewed prior to the initiation of chemotherapy (ONC)
🔧 0.00   ⚕ 0.00   **FUD** XXX   Ⓔ
AMA: 2008,Mar,8-12

3318F Pathology report confirming malignancy documented in the medical record and reviewed prior to the initiation of radiation therapy (ONC)
🔧 0.00   ⚕ 0.00   **FUD** XXX   Ⓔ
AMA: 2008,Mar,8-12

3319F 1 of the following diagnostic imaging studies ordered: chest x-ray, CT, Ultrasound, MRI, PET, or nuclear medicine scans (ML)
🔧 0.00   ⚕ 0.00   **FUD** XXX   Ⓜ
AMA: 2008,Mar,8-12

3320F None of the following diagnostic imaging studies ordered: chest X-ray, CT, Ultrasound, MRI, PET, or nuclear medicine scans (ML)
🔧 0.00   ⚕ 0.00   **FUD** XXX   Ⓜ
AMA: 2008,Mar,8-12

3321F AJCC Cancer Stage 0 or IA Melanoma, documented (ML)
🔧 0.00   ⚕ 0.00   **FUD** XXX   Ⓜ

3322F Melanoma greater than AJCC Stage 0 or IA (ML)
🔧 0.00   ⚕ 0.00   **FUD** XXX   Ⓜ

3323F Clinical tumor, node and metastases (TNM) staging documented and reviewed prior to surgery (Lung/Esop Cx)
🔧 0.00   ⚕ 0.00   **FUD** XXX   Ⓔ

3324F MRI or CT scan ordered, reviewed or requested (EPI)
🔧 0.00   ⚕ 0.00   **FUD** XXX   Ⓔ

3325F Preoperative assessment of functional or medical indication(s) for surgery prior to the cataract surgery with intraocular lens placement (must be performed within 12 months prior to cataract surgery) (EC)
🔧 0.00   ⚕ 0.00   **FUD** XXX   Ⓔ
AMA: 2008,Mar,8-12

3328F Performance status documented and reviewed within 2 weeks prior to surgery (Lung/Esop Cx)
🔧 0.00   ⚕ 0.00   **FUD** XXX   Ⓔ

3330F Imaging study ordered (BkP)
🔧 0.00   ⚕ 0.00   **FUD** XXX   Ⓔ
AMA: 2008,Mar,8-12

3331F Imaging study not ordered (BkP)
🔧 0.00   ⚕ 0.00   **FUD** XXX   Ⓔ
AMA: 2008,Mar,8-12

3340F Mammogram assessment category of "incomplete: need additional imaging evaluation" documented (RAD)
🔧 0.00   ⚕ 0.00   **FUD** XXX   Ⓜ
AMA: 2008,Mar,8-12

3341F Mammogram assessment category of "negative," documented (RAD)
🔧 0.00   ⚕ 0.00   **FUD** XXX   Ⓜ
AMA: 2008,Mar,8-12

3342F Mammogram assessment category of "benign," documented (RAD)
🔢 0.00 ⚕ 0.00 **FUD** XXX Ⓜ
AMA: 2008,Mar,8-12

3343F Mammogram assessment category of "probably benign," documented (RAD)
🔢 0.00 ⚕ 0.00 **FUD** XXX Ⓜ
AMA: 2008,Mar,8-12

3344F Mammogram assessment category of "suspicious," documented (RAD)
🔢 0.00 ⚕ 0.00 **FUD** XXX Ⓜ
AMA: 2008,Mar,8-12

3345F Mammogram assessment category of "highly suggestive of malignancy," documented (RAD)
🔢 0.00 ⚕ 0.00 **FUD** XXX Ⓜ
AMA: 2008,Mar,8-12

3350F Mammogram assessment category of "known biopsy proven malignancy," documented (RAD)
🔢 0.00 ⚕ 0.00 **FUD** XXX Ⓜ
AMA: 2008,Mar,8-12

3351F Negative screen for depressive symptoms as categorized by using a standardized depression screening/assessment tool (MDD)
🔢 0.00 ⚕ 0.00 **FUD** XXX Ⓔ

3352F No significant depressive symptoms as categorized by using a standardized depression assessment tool (MDD)
🔢 0.00 ⚕ 0.00 **FUD** XXX Ⓔ

3353F Mild to moderate depressive symptoms as categorized by using a standardized depression screening/assessment tool (MDD)
🔢 0.00 ⚕ 0.00 **FUD** XXX Ⓔ

3354F Clinically significant depressive symptoms as categorized by using a standardized depression screening/assessment tool (MDD)
🔢 0.00 ⚕ 0.00 **FUD** XXX Ⓔ

3370F AJCC Breast Cancer Stage 0 documented (ONC)
🔢 0.00 ⚕ 0.00 **FUD** XXX Ⓔ

3372F AJCC Breast Cancer Stage I: T1mic, T1a or T1b (tumor size ≤ 1 cm) documented (ONC)
🔢 0.00 ⚕ 0.00 **FUD** XXX Ⓔ

3374F AJCC Breast Cancer Stage I: T1c (tumor size > 1 cm to 2 cm) documented (ONC)
🔢 0.00 ⚕ 0.00 **FUD** XXX Ⓔ

3376F AJCC Breast Cancer Stage II documented (ONC)
🔢 0.00 ⚕ 0.00 **FUD** XXX Ⓔ

3378F AJCC Breast Cancer Stage III documented (ONC)
🔢 0.00 ⚕ 0.00 **FUD** XXX Ⓔ

3380F AJCC Breast Cancer Stage IV documented (ONC)
🔢 0.00 ⚕ 0.00 **FUD** XXX Ⓔ

3382F AJCC colon cancer, Stage 0 documented (ONC)
🔢 0.00 ⚕ 0.00 **FUD** XXX Ⓔ

3384F AJCC colon cancer, Stage I documented (ONC)
🔢 0.00 ⚕ 0.00 **FUD** XXX Ⓔ

3386F AJCC colon cancer, Stage II documented (ONC)
🔢 0.00 ⚕ 0.00 **FUD** XXX Ⓔ

3388F AJCC colon cancer, Stage III documented (ONC)
🔢 0.00 ⚕ 0.00 **FUD** XXX Ⓔ

3390F AJCC colon cancer, Stage IV documented (ONC)
🔢 0.00 ⚕ 0.00 **FUD** XXX Ⓔ

3394F Quantitative HER2 immunohistochemistry (IHC) evaluation of breast cancer consistent with the scoring system defined in the ASCO/CAP guidelines (PATH)
🔢 0.00 ⚕ 0.00 **FUD** XXX Ⓜ

3395F Quantitative non-HER2 immunohistochemistry (IHC) evaluation of breast cancer (eg, testing for estrogen or progesterone receptors [ER/PR]) performed (PATH)
🔢 0.00 ⚕ 0.00 **FUD** XXX Ⓜ

3450F Dyspnea screened, no dyspnea or mild dyspnea (Pall Cr)
🔢 0.00 ⚕ 0.00 **FUD** XXX Ⓔ

3451F Dyspnea screened, moderate or severe dyspnea (Pall Cr)
🔢 0.00 ⚕ 0.00 **FUD** XXX Ⓔ

3452F Dyspnea not screened (Pall Cr)
🔢 0.00 ⚕ 0.00 **FUD** XXX Ⓔ

3455F TB screening performed and results interpreted within six months prior to initiation of first-time biologic disease modifying anti-rheumatic drug therapy for RA (RA)
🔢 0.00 ⚕ 0.00 **FUD** XXX Ⓜ

3470F Rheumatoid arthritis (RA) disease activity, low (RA)
🔢 0.00 ⚕ 0.00 **FUD** XXX Ⓜ

3471F Rheumatoid arthritis (RA) disease activity, moderate (RA)
🔢 0.00 ⚕ 0.00 **FUD** XXX Ⓜ

3472F Rheumatoid arthritis (RA) disease activity, high (RA)
🔢 0.00 ⚕ 0.00 **FUD** XXX Ⓜ

3475F Disease prognosis for rheumatoid arthritis assessed, poor prognosis documented (RA)
🔢 0.00 ⚕ 0.00 **FUD** XXX Ⓜ

3476F Disease prognosis for rheumatoid arthritis assessed, good prognosis documented (RA)
🔢 0.00 ⚕ 0.00 **FUD** XXX Ⓜ

3490F History of AIDS-defining condition (HIV)
🔢 0.00 ⚕ 0.00 **FUD** XXX Ⓔ

3491F HIV indeterminate (infants of undetermined HIV status born of HIV-infected mothers) (HIV)
🔢 0.00 ⚕ 0.00 **FUD** XXX Ⓔ

3492F History of nadir CD4+ cell count <350 cells/mm3 (HIV)
🔢 0.00 ⚕ 0.00 **FUD** XXX Ⓔ

3493F No history of nadir CD4+ cell count <350 cells/mm3 and no history of AIDS-defining condition (HIV)
🔢 0.00 ⚕ 0.00 **FUD** XXX Ⓔ

3494F CD4+ cell count <200 cells/mm3 (HIV)
🔢 0.00 ⚕ 0.00 **FUD** XXX Ⓔ

3495F CD4+ cell count 200 - 499 cells/mm3 (HIV)
🔢 0.00 ⚕ 0.00 **FUD** XXX Ⓔ

3496F CD4+ cell count ≥ 500 cells/mm3 (HIV)
🔢 0.00 ⚕ 0.00 **FUD** XXX Ⓔ

3497F CD4+ cell percentage <15% (HIV)
🔢 0.00 ⚕ 0.00 **FUD** XXX Ⓔ

3498F CD4+ cell percentage ≥ 15% (HIV)
🔢 0.00 ⚕ 0.00 **FUD** XXX Ⓔ

3500F CD4+ cell count or CD4+ cell percentage documented as performed (HIV)
🔢 0.00 ⚕ 0.00 **FUD** XXX Ⓔ

3502F HIV RNA viral load below limits of quantification (HIV)
🔢 0.00 ⚕ 0.00 **FUD** XXX Ⓔ

3503F HIV RNA viral load not below limits of quantification (HIV)
🔢 0.00 ⚕ 0.00 **FUD** XXX Ⓔ

3510F Documentation that tuberculosis (TB) screening test performed and results interpreted (HIV) (IBD)
🔢 0.00 ⚕ 0.00 **FUD** XXX Ⓔ

3511F Chlamydia and gonorrhea screenings documented as performed (HIV)
🔢 0.00 ⚕ 0.00 **FUD** XXX Ⓔ

3512F Syphilis screening documented as performed (HIV)
🔢 0.00 ⚕ 0.00 **FUD** XXX Ⓔ

● New Code ▲ Revised Code ○ Reinstated ● New Web Release ▲ Revised Web Release + Add-on Unlisted Not Covered # Resequenced
㊿ Optum Mod 50 Exempt ⊘ AMA Mod 51 Exempt �51 Optum Mod 51 Exempt �63 Mod 63 Exempt ✗ Non-FDA Drug ★ Telemedicine Ⓜ Maternity Ⓐ Age Edit

3513F Hepatitis B screening documented as performed (HIV)
🏥 0.00   ⚕ 0.00   **FUD** XXX   E

3514F Hepatitis C screening documented as performed (HIV)
🏥 0.00   ⚕ 0.00   **FUD** XXX   E

3515F Patient has documented immunity to Hepatitis C (HIV)
🏥 0.00   ⚕ 0.00   **FUD** XXX   E

3517F Hepatitis B Virus (HBV) status assessed and results interpreted within one year prior to receiving a first course of anti-TNF (tumor necrosis factor) therapy (IBD)
🏥 0.00   ⚕ 0.00   **FUD** XXX   E

3520F Clostridium difficile testing performed (IBD)
🏥 0.00   ⚕ 0.00   **FUD** XXX   E

3550F Low risk for thromboembolism (AFIB)
🏥 0.00   ⚕ 0.00   **FUD** XXX   E

3551F Intermediate risk for thromboembolism (AFIB)
🏥 0.00   ⚕ 0.00   **FUD** XXX   E

3552F High risk for thromboembolism (AFIB)
🏥 0.00   ⚕ 0.00   **FUD** XXX   E

3555F Patient had International Normalized Ratio (INR) measurement performed (AFIB)
🏥 0.00   ⚕ 0.00   **FUD** XXX   E
AMA: 2010,Jul,3-5

3570F Final report for bone scintigraphy study includes correlation with existing relevant imaging studies (eg, X-ray, MRI, CT) corresponding to the same anatomical region in question (NUC_MED)
🏥 0.00   ⚕ 0.00   **FUD** XXX   M

3572F Patient considered to be potentially at risk for fracture in a weight-bearing site (NUC_MED)
🏥 0.00   ⚕ 0.00   **FUD** XXX   E

3573F Patient not considered to be potentially at risk for fracture in a weight-bearing site (NUC_MED)
🏥 0.00   ⚕ 0.00   **FUD** XXX   E

3650F Electroencephalogram (EEG) ordered, reviewed or requested (EPI)
🏥 0.00   ⚕ 0.00   **FUD** XXX   E

3700F Psychiatric disorders or disturbances assessed (Prkns)
🏥 0.00   ⚕ 0.00   **FUD** XXX   E

3720F Cognitive impairment or dysfunction assessed (Prkns)
🏥 0.00   ⚕ 0.00   **FUD** XXX   M

3725F Screening for depression performed (DEM)
🏥 0.00   ⚕ 0.00   **FUD** XXX   M

3750F Patient not receiving dose of corticosteroids greater than or equal to 10mg/day for 60 or greater consecutive days (IBD)
🏥 0.00   ⚕ 0.00   **FUD** XXX   E

3751F Electrodiagnostic studies for distal symmetric polyneuropathy conducted (or requested), documented, and reviewed within 6 months of initial evaluation for condition (DSP)
🏥 0.00   ⚕ 0.00   **FUD** XXX   E

3752F Electrodiagnostic studies for distal symmetric polyneuropathy not conducted (or requested), documented, or reviewed within 6 months of initial evaluation for condition (DSP)
🏥 0.00   ⚕ 0.00   **FUD** XXX   E

3753F Patient has clear clinical symptoms and signs that are highly suggestive of neuropathy AND cannot be attributed to another condition, AND has an obvious cause for the neuropathy (DSP)
🏥 0.00   ⚕ 0.00   **FUD** XXX   E

3754F Screening tests for diabetes mellitus reviewed, requested, or ordered (DSP)
🏥 0.00   ⚕ 0.00   **FUD** XXX   E

3755F Cognitive and behavioral impairment screening performed (ALS)
🏥 0.00   ⚕ 0.00   **FUD** XXX   E

3756F Patient has pseudobulbar affect, sialorrhea, or ALS-related symptoms (ALS)
🏥 0.00   ⚕ 0.00   **FUD** XXX   E

3757F Patient does not have pseudobulbar affect, sialorrhea, or ALS-related symptoms (ALS)
🏥 0.00   ⚕ 0.00   **FUD** XXX   E

3758F Patient referred for pulmonary function testing or peak cough expiratory flow (ALS)
🏥 0.00   ⚕ 0.00   **FUD** XXX   E

3759F Patient screened for dysphagia, weight loss, and impaired nutrition, and results documented (ALS)
🏥 0.00   ⚕ 0.00   **FUD** XXX   E

3760F Patient exhibits dysphagia, weight loss, or impaired nutrition (ALS)
🏥 0.00   ⚕ 0.00   **FUD** XXX   E

3761F Patient does not exhibit dysphagia, weight loss, or impaired nutrition (ALS)
🏥 0.00   ⚕ 0.00   **FUD** XXX   E

3762F Patient is dysarthric (ALS)
🏥 0.00   ⚕ 0.00   **FUD** XXX   E

3763F Patient is not dysarthric (ALS)
🏥 0.00   ⚕ 0.00   **FUD** XXX   E

3775F Adenoma(s) or other neoplasm detected during screening colonoscopy (SCADR)
🏥 0.00   ⚕ 0.00   **FUD** XXX   E

3776F Adenoma(s) or other neoplasm not detected during screening colonoscopy (SCADR)
🏥 0.00   ⚕ 0.00   **FUD** XXX   E

4000F-4563F Therapies Provided (Includes Preventive Services)

INCLUDES   Behavioral/pharmacologic/procedural therapies
Preventive services including patient education/counseling

4000F Tobacco use cessation intervention, counseling (COPD, CAP, CAD, Asthma) (DM) (PV)
🏥 0.00   ⚕ 0.00   **FUD** XXX   E
AMA: 2018,Jan,8; 2017,Jan,8; 2016,Jan,13

4001F Tobacco use cessation intervention, pharmacologic therapy (COPD, CAD, CAP, PV, Asthma) (DM) (PV)
🏥 0.00   ⚕ 0.00   **FUD** XXX   E
AMA: 2008,Mar,8-12; 2004,Nov,1

4003F Patient education, written/oral, appropriate for patients with heart failure, performed (NMA-No Measure Associated)
🏥 0.00   ⚕ 0.00   **FUD** XXX   E
AMA: 2004,Nov,1

4004F Patient screened for tobacco use and received tobacco cessation intervention (counseling, pharmacotherapy, or both), if identified as a tobacco user (PV, CAD)
🏥 0.00   ⚕ 0.00   **FUD** XXX   M

4005F Pharmacologic therapy (other than minerals/vitamins) for osteoporosis prescribed (OP) (IBD)
🏥 0.00   ⚕ 0.00   **FUD** XXX   E

4008F Beta-blocker therapy prescribed or currently being taken (CAD,HF)
🏥 0.00   ⚕ 0.00   **FUD** XXX   M

4010F Angiotensin Converting Enzyme (ACE) Inhibitor or Angiotensin Receptor Blocker (ARB) therapy prescribed or currently being taken (CAD, CKD, HF) (DM)
🏥 0.00   ⚕ 0.00   **FUD** XXX   M

4011F Oral antiplatelet therapy prescribed (CAD)
 0.00 0.00 **FUD** XXX E
AMA: 2004,Nov,1

4012F Warfarin therapy prescribed (NMA-No Measure Associated)
 0.00 0.00 **FUD** XXX E

4013F Statin therapy prescribed or currently being taken (CAD)
 0.00 0.00 **FUD** XXX E

4014F Written discharge instructions provided to heart failure patients discharged home (Instructions include all of the following components: activity level, diet, discharge medications, follow-up appointment, weight monitoring, what to do if symptoms worsen) (NMA-No Measure Associated)
 0.00 0.00 **FUD** XXX E

4015F Persistent asthma, preferred long term control medication or an acceptable alternative treatment, prescribed (NMA-No Measure Associated)
EXCLUDES *Reporting code with modifier 1P*
Code also modifier 2P for patient reasons for not prescribing
 0.00 0.00 **FUD** XXX E

4016F Anti-inflammatory/analgesic agent prescribed (OA) (Use for prescribed or continued medication[s], including over-the-counter medication[s])
INCLUDES Over-the-counter medication(s)
Prescribed/continued medication(s)
 0.00 0.00 **FUD** XXX E

4017F Gastrointestinal prophylaxis for NSAID use prescribed (OA)
 0.00 0.00 **FUD** XXX E

4018F Therapeutic exercise for the involved joint(s) instructed or physical or occupational therapy prescribed (OA)
 0.00 0.00 **FUD** XXX E

4019F Documentation of receipt of counseling on exercise and either both calcium and vitamin D use or counseling regarding both calcium and vitamin D use (OP)
 0.00 0.00 **FUD** XXX E

4025F Inhaled bronchodilator prescribed (COPD)
 0.00 0.00 **FUD** XXX E

4030F Long-term oxygen therapy prescribed (more than 15 hours per day) (COPD)
 0.00 0.00 **FUD** XXX E

4033F Pulmonary rehabilitation exercise training recommended (COPD)
Code also dyspnea assessed, present (1019F)
 0.00 0.00 **FUD** XXX E

4035F Influenza immunization recommended (COPD) (IBD)
 0.00 0.00 **FUD** XXX E
AMA: 2008,Mar,8-12

4037F Influenza immunization ordered or administered (COPD, PV, CKD, ESRD)(IBD)
 0.00 0.00 **FUD** XXX E
AMA: 2008,Mar,8-12

4040F Pneumococcal vaccine administered or previously received (COPD) (PV), (IBD)
 0.00 0.00 **FUD** XXX M
AMA: 2008,Mar,8-12

4041F Documentation of order for cefazolin OR cefuroxime for antimicrobial prophylaxis (PERI 2)
 0.00 0.00 **FUD** XXX E

4042F Documentation that prophylactic antibiotics were neither given within 4 hours prior to surgical incision nor given intraoperatively (PERI 2)
 0.00 0.00 **FUD** XXX E

4043F Documentation that an order was given to discontinue prophylactic antibiotics within 48 hours of surgical end time, cardiac procedures (PERI 2)
 0.00 0.00 **FUD** XXX E

4044F Documentation that an order was given for venous thromboembolism (VTE) prophylaxis to be given within 24 hours prior to incision time or 24 hours after surgery end time (PERI 2)
 0.00 0.00 **FUD** XXX M

4045F Appropriate empiric antibiotic prescribed (CAP), (EM)
 0.00 0.00 **FUD** XXX E

4046F Documentation that prophylactic antibiotics were given within 4 hours prior to surgical incision or given intraoperatively (PERI 2)
 0.00 0.00 **FUD** XXX E

4047F Documentation of order for prophylactic parenteral antibiotics to be given within 1 hour (if fluoroquinolone or vancomycin, 2 hours) prior to surgical incision (or start of procedure when no incision is required) (PERI 2)
 0.00 0.00 **FUD** XXX E

4048F Documentation that administration of prophylactic parenteral antibiotic was initiated within 1 hour (if fluoroquinolone or vancomycin, 2 hours) prior to surgical incision (or start of procedure when no incision is required) as ordered (PERI 2)
 0.00 0.00 **FUD** XXX E

4049F Documentation that order was given to discontinue prophylactic antibiotics within 24 hours of surgical end time, non-cardiac procedure (PERI 2)
 0.00 0.00 **FUD** XXX E

4050F Hypertension plan of care documented as appropriate (NMA-No Measure Associated)
 0.00 0.00 **FUD** XXX E

4051F Referred for an arteriovenous (AV) fistula (ESRD, CKD)
 0.00 0.00 **FUD** XXX E
AMA: 2008,Mar,8-12

4052F Hemodialysis via functioning arteriovenous (AV) fistula (ESRD)
 0.00 0.00 **FUD** XXX E
AMA: 2008,Mar,8-12

4053F Hemodialysis via functioning arteriovenous (AV) graft (ESRD)
 0.00 0.00 **FUD** XXX E
AMA: 2008,Mar,8-12

4054F Hemodialysis via catheter (ESRD)
 0.00 0.00 **FUD** XXX E
AMA: 2008,Mar,8-12

4055F Patient receiving peritoneal dialysis (ESRD)
 0.00 0.00 **FUD** XXX E
AMA: 2008,Mar,8-12

4056F Appropriate oral rehydration solution recommended (PAG)
 0.00 0.00 **FUD** XXX E

4058F Pediatric gastroenteritis education provided to caregiver (PAG)
 0.00 0.00 **FUD** XXX E

4060F Psychotherapy services provided (MDD, MDD ADOL)
 0.00 0.00 **FUD** XXX E

4062F Patient referral for psychotherapy documented (MDD, MDD ADOL)
 0.00 0.00 **FUD** XXX E

4063F Antidepressant pharmacotherapy considered and not prescribed (MDD ADOL)
 0.00 0.00 **FUD** XXX E

● New Code ▲ Revised Code ○ Reinstated ● New Web Release ▲ Revised Web Release + Add-on Unlisted Not Covered # Resequenced
50 Optum Mod 50 Exempt Ⓢ AMA Mod 51 Exempt 51 Optum Mod 51 Exempt 63 Mod 63 Exempt ∕ Non-FDA Drug ★ Telemedicine M Maternity A Age Edit

4064F Antidepressant pharmacotherapy prescribed (MDD, MDD ADOL)
0.00   0.00   **FUD** XXX   E

4065F Antipsychotic pharmacotherapy prescribed (MDD)
0.00   0.00   **FUD** XXX   E

4066F Electroconvulsive therapy (ECT) provided (MDD)
0.00   0.00   **FUD** XXX   E

4067F Patient referral for electroconvulsive therapy (ECT) documented (MDD)
0.00   0.00   **FUD** XXX   E

4069F Venous thromboembolism (VTE) prophylaxis received (IBD)
0.00   0.00   **FUD** XXX   E

4070F Deep vein thrombosis (DVT) prophylaxis received by end of hospital day 2 (STR)
0.00   0.00   **FUD** XXX   E

4073F Oral antiplatelet therapy prescribed at discharge (STR)
0.00   0.00   **FUD** XXX   E

4075F Anticoagulant therapy prescribed at discharge (STR)
0.00   0.00   **FUD** XXX   E

4077F Documentation that tissue plasminogen activator (t-PA) administration was considered (STR)
0.00   0.00   **FUD** XXX   E

4079F Documentation that rehabilitation services were considered (STR)
0.00   0.00   **FUD** XXX   E

4084F Aspirin received within 24 hours before emergency department arrival or during emergency department stay (EM)
0.00   0.00   **FUD** XXX   E

4086F Aspirin or clopidogrel prescribed or currently being taken (CAD)
0.00   0.00   **FUD** XXX   M

4090F Patient receiving erythropoietin therapy (HEM)
0.00   0.00   **FUD** XXX   M
AMA: 2008,Mar,8-12

4095F Patient not receiving erythropoietin therapy (HEM)
0.00   0.00   **FUD** XXX   E
AMA: 2008,Mar,8-12

4100F Bisphosphonate therapy, intravenous, ordered or received (HEM)
0.00   0.00   **FUD** XXX   M
AMA: 2008,Mar,8-12

4110F Internal mammary artery graft performed for primary, isolated coronary artery bypass graft procedure (CABG)
0.00   0.00   **FUD** XXX   E

4115F Beta blocker administered within 24 hours prior to surgical incision (CABG)
0.00   0.00   **FUD** XXX   M

4120F Antibiotic prescribed or dispensed (URI, PHAR), (A-BRONCH)
0.00   0.00   **FUD** XXX   M
AMA: 2008,Mar,8-12

4124F Antibiotic neither prescribed nor dispensed (URI, PHAR), (A-BRONCH)
0.00   0.00   **FUD** XXX   M
AMA: 2008,Mar,8-12

4130F Topical preparations (including OTC) prescribed for acute otitis externa (AOE)
0.00   0.00   **FUD** XXX   M
AMA: 2010,Jan,6-7; 2008,Mar,8-12

4131F Systemic antimicrobial therapy prescribed (AOE)
0.00   0.00   **FUD** XXX   M
AMA: 2008,Mar,8-12

4132F Systemic antimicrobial therapy not prescribed (AOE)
0.00   0.00   **FUD** XXX   M
AMA: 2008,Mar,8-12

4133F Antihistamines or decongestants prescribed or recommended (OME)
0.00   0.00   **FUD** XXX   E
AMA: 2008,Mar,8-12

4134F Antihistamines or decongestants neither prescribed nor recommended (OME)
0.00   0.00   **FUD** XXX   E
AMA: 2008,Mar,8-12

4135F Systemic corticosteroids prescribed (OME)
0.00   0.00   **FUD** XXX   E
AMA: 2008,Mar,8-12

4136F Systemic corticosteroids not prescribed (OME)
0.00   0.00   **FUD** XXX   E
AMA: 2008,Mar,8-12

4140F Inhaled corticosteroids prescribed (Asthma)
0.00   0.00   **FUD** XXX   E

4142F Corticosteroid sparing therapy prescribed (IBD)
0.00   0.00   **FUD** XXX   E

4144F Alternative long-term control medication prescribed (Asthma)
0.00   0.00   **FUD** XXX   E

4145F Two or more anti-hypertensive agents prescribed or currently being taken (CAD, HTN)
0.00   0.00   **FUD** XXX   E

4148F Hepatitis A vaccine injection administered or previously received (HEP-C)
0.00   0.00   **FUD** XXX   E

4149F Hepatitis B vaccine injection administered or previously received (HEP-C, HIV) (IBD)
0.00   0.00   **FUD** XXX   E

4150F Patient receiving antiviral treatment for Hepatitis C (HEP-C)
0.00   0.00   **FUD** XXX   E
AMA: 2008,Mar,8-12

4151F Patient did not start or is not receiving antiviral treatment for Hepatitis C during the measurement period (HEP-C)
0.00   0.00   **FUD** XXX   E
AMA: 2008,Mar,8-12

4153F Combination peginterferon and ribavirin therapy prescribed (HEP-C)
0.00   0.00   **FUD** XXX   E
AMA: 2008,Mar,8-12

4155F Hepatitis A vaccine series previously received (HEP-C)
0.00   0.00   **FUD** XXX   E
AMA: 2008,Mar,8-12

4157F Hepatitis B vaccine series previously received (HEP-C)
0.00   0.00   **FUD** XXX   E
AMA: 2008,Mar,8-12

4158F Patient counseled about risks of alcohol use (HEP-C)
0.00   0.00   **FUD** XXX   E
AMA: 2008,Mar,8-12

4159F Counseling regarding contraception received prior to initiation of antiviral treatment (HEP-C)
0.00   0.00   **FUD** XXX   E
AMA: 2008,Mar,8-12

4163F Patient counseling at a minimum on all of the following treatment options for clinically localized prostate cancer: active surveillance, and interstitial prostate brachytherapy, and external beam radiotherapy, and radical prostatectomy, provided prior to initiation of treatment (PRCA)
0.00   0.00   **FUD** XXX   E
AMA: 2008,Mar,8-12

4164F Adjuvant (ie, in combination with external beam radiotherapy to the prostate for prostate cancer) hormonal therapy (gonadotropin-releasing hormone [GnRH] agonist or antagonist) prescribed/administered (PRCA)
    📟 0.00   🔱 0.00   **FUD** XXX   E
    AMA: 2008,Mar,8-12

4165F 3-dimensional conformal radiotherapy (3D-CRT) or intensity modulated radiation therapy (IMRT) received (PRCA)
    📟 0.00   🔱 0.00   **FUD** XXX   E
    AMA: 2008,Mar,8-12

4167F Head of bed elevation (30-45 degrees) on first ventilator day ordered (CRIT)
    📟 0.00   🔱 0.00   **FUD** XXX   E
    AMA: 2008,Mar,8-12

4168F Patient receiving care in the intensive care unit (ICU) and receiving mechanical ventilation, 24 hours or less (CRIT)
    📟 0.00   🔱 0.00   **FUD** XXX   E
    AMA: 2008,Mar,8-12

4169F Patient either not receiving care in the intensive care unit (ICU) OR not receiving mechanical ventilation OR receiving mechanical ventilation greater than 24 hours (CRIT)
    📟 0.00   🔱 0.00   **FUD** XXX   E
    AMA: 2008,Mar,8-12

4171F Patient receiving erythropoiesis-stimulating agents (ESA) therapy (CKD)
    📟 0.00   🔱 0.00   **FUD** XXX   E
    AMA: 2008,Mar,8-12

4172F Patient not receiving erythropoiesis-stimulating agents (ESA) therapy (CKD)
    📟 0.00   🔱 0.00   **FUD** XXX   E
    AMA: 2008,Mar,8-12

4174F Counseling about the potential impact of glaucoma on visual functioning and quality of life, and importance of treatment adherence provided to patient and/or caregiver(s) (EC)
    📟 0.00   🔱 0.00   **FUD** XXX   E
    AMA: 2008,Mar,8-12

4175F Best-corrected visual acuity of 20/40 or better (distance or near) achieved within the 90 days following cataract surgery (EC)
    📟 0.00   🔱 0.00   **FUD** XXX   M
    AMA: 2008,Mar,8-12

4176F Counseling about value of protection from UV light and lack of proven efficacy of nutritional supplements in prevention or progression of cataract development provided to patient and/or caregiver(s) (NMA-No Measure Associated)
    📟 0.00   🔱 0.00   **FUD** XXX   E

4177F Counseling about the benefits and/or risks of the Age-Related Eye Disease Study (AREDS) formulation for preventing progression of age-related macular degeneration (AMD) provided to patient and/or caregiver(s) (EC)
    📟 0.00   🔱 0.00   **FUD** XXX   M
    AMA: 2008,Mar,8-12

4178F Anti-D immune globulin received between 26 and 30 weeks gestation (Pre-Cr) M
    📟 0.00   🔱 0.00   **FUD** XXX   E
    AMA: 2008,Mar,8-12

4179F Tamoxifen or aromatase inhibitor (AI) prescribed (ONC)
    📟 0.00   🔱 0.00   **FUD** XXX   E
    AMA: 2008,Mar,8-12

4180F Adjuvant chemotherapy referred, prescribed, or previously received for Stage III colon cancer (ONC)
    📟 0.00   🔱 0.00   **FUD** XXX   E
    AMA: 2008,Mar,8-12

4181F Conformal radiation therapy received (NMA-No Measure Associated)
    📟 0.00   🔱 0.00   **FUD** XXX   E

4182F Conformal radiation therapy not received (NMA-No Measure Associated)
    📟 0.00   🔱 0.00   **FUD** XXX   E

4185F Continuous (12-months) therapy with proton pump inhibitor (PPI) or histamine H2 receptor antagonist (H2RA) received (GERD)
    📟 0.00   🔱 0.00   **FUD** XXX   E
    AMA: 2008,Mar,8-12

4186F No continuous (12-months) therapy with either proton pump inhibitor (PPI) or histamine H2 receptor antagonist (H2RA) received (GERD)
    📟 0.00   🔱 0.00   **FUD** XXX   E
    AMA: 2008,Mar,8-12

4187F Disease modifying anti-rheumatic drug therapy prescribed or dispensed (RA)
    📟 0.00   🔱 0.00   **FUD** XXX   E

4188F Appropriate angiotensin converting enzyme (ACE)/angiotensin receptor blockers (ARB) therapeutic monitoring test ordered or performed (AM)
    📟 0.00   🔱 0.00   **FUD** XXX   E
    AMA: 2008,Mar,8-12

4189F Appropriate digoxin therapeutic monitoring test ordered or performed (AM)
    📟 0.00   🔱 0.00   **FUD** XXX   E
    AMA: 2008,Mar,8-12

4190F Appropriate diuretic therapeutic monitoring test ordered or performed (AM)
    📟 0.00   🔱 0.00   **FUD** XXX   E
    AMA: 2008,Mar,8-12

4191F Appropriate anticonvulsant therapeutic monitoring test ordered or performed (AM)
    📟 0.00   🔱 0.00   **FUD** XXX   E
    AMA: 2008,Mar,8-12

4192F Patient not receiving glucocorticoid therapy (RA)
    📟 0.00   🔱 0.00   **FUD** XXX   M

4193F Patient receiving <10 mg daily prednisone (or equivalent), or RA activity is worsening, or glucocorticoid use is for less than 6 months (RA)
    📟 0.00   🔱 0.00   **FUD** XXX   M

4194F Patient receiving ≥10 mg daily prednisone (or equivalent) for longer than 6 months, and improvement or no change in disease activity (RA)
    📟 0.00   🔱 0.00   **FUD** XXX   M

4195F Patient receiving first-time biologic disease modifying anti-rheumatic drug therapy for rheumatoid arthritis (RA)
    📟 0.00   🔱 0.00   **FUD** XXX   M

4196F Patient not receiving first-time biologic disease modifying anti-rheumatic drug therapy for rheumatoid arthritis (RA)
    📟 0.00   🔱 0.00   **FUD** XXX   M

4200F External beam radiotherapy as primary therapy to prostate with or without nodal irradiation (PRCA)
    📟 0.00   🔱 0.00   **FUD** XXX   E
    AMA: 2008,Mar,8-12

4201F External beam radiotherapy with or without nodal irradiation as adjuvant or salvage therapy for prostate cancer patient (PRCA)
    📟 0.00   🔱 0.00   **FUD** XXX   E
    AMA: 2008,Mar,8-12

4210F Angiotensin converting enzyme (ACE) or angiotensin receptor blockers (ARB) medication therapy for 6 months or more (MM)
    📟 0.00   🔱 0.00   **FUD** XXX   E
    AMA: 2008,Mar,8-12

● New Code   ▲ Revised Code   ○ Reinstated   ● New Web Release   ▲ Revised Web Release   + Add-on   Unlisted   Not Covered   # Resequenced
50 Optum Mod 50 Exempt   ⊘ AMA Mod 51 Exempt   51 Optum Mod 51 Exempt   63 Mod 63 Exempt   ✗ Non-FDA Drug   ★ Telemedicine   M Maternity   A Age Edit

4220F Digoxin medication therapy for 6 months or more (MM)
     0.00   0.00   **FUD** XXX   E
     AMA: 2008,Mar,8-12

4221F Diuretic medication therapy for 6 months or more (MM)
     0.00   0.00   **FUD** XXX   E
     AMA: 2008,Mar,8-12

4230F Anticonvulsant medication therapy for 6 months or more (MM)
     0.00   0.00   **FUD** XXX   E
     AMA: 2008,Mar,8-12

4240F Instruction in therapeutic exercise with follow-up provided to patients during episode of back pain lasting longer than 12 weeks (BkP)
     0.00   0.00   **FUD** XXX   E
     AMA: 2008,Mar,8-12

4242F Counseling for supervised exercise program provided to patients during episode of back pain lasting longer than 12 weeks (BkP)
     0.00   0.00   **FUD** XXX   E
     AMA: 2008,Mar,8-12

4245F Patient counseled during the initial visit to maintain or resume normal activities (BkP)
     0.00   0.00   **FUD** XXX   E
     AMA: 2008,Mar,8-12

4248F Patient counseled during the initial visit for an episode of back pain against bed rest lasting 4 days or longer (BkP)
     0.00   0.00   **FUD** XXX   E
     AMA: 2008,Mar,8-12

4250F Active warming used intraoperatively for the purpose of maintaining normothermia, or at least 1 body temperature equal to or greater than 36 degrees Centigrade (or 96.8 degrees Fahrenheit) recorded within the 30 minutes immediately before or the 15 minutes immediately after anesthesia end time (CRIT)
     0.00   0.00   **FUD** XXX   E
     AMA: 2008,Mar,8-12

4255F Duration of general or neuraxial anesthesia 60 minutes or longer, as documented in the anesthesia record (CRIT) (Peri2)
     0.00   0.00   **FUD** XXX   M

4256F Duration of general or neuraxial anesthesia less than 60 minutes, as documented in the anesthesia record (CRIT) (Peri2)
     0.00   0.00   **FUD** XXX   E

4260F Wound surface culture technique used (CWC)
     0.00   0.00   **FUD** XXX   E

4261F Technique other than surface culture of the wound exudate used (eg, Levine/deep swab technique, semi-quantitative or quantitative swab technique) or wound surface culture technique not used (CWC)
     0.00   0.00   **FUD** XXX   E

4265F Use of wet to dry dressings prescribed or recommended (CWC)
     0.00   0.00   **FUD** XXX   E

4266F Use of wet to dry dressings neither prescribed nor recommended (CWC)
     0.00   0.00   **FUD** XXX   E

4267F Compression therapy prescribed (CWC)
     0.00   0.00   **FUD** XXX   E

4268F Patient education regarding the need for long term compression therapy including interval replacement of compression stockings received (CWC)
     0.00   0.00   **FUD** XXX   E

4269F Appropriate method of offloading (pressure relief) prescribed (CWC)
     0.00   0.00   **FUD** XXX   E

4270F Patient receiving potent antiretroviral therapy for 6 months or longer (HIV)
     0.00   0.00   **FUD** XXX   E

4271F Patient receiving potent antiretroviral therapy for less than 6 months or not receiving potent antiretroviral therapy (HIV)
     0.00   0.00   **FUD** XXX   E

4274F Influenza immunization administered or previously received (HIV) (P-ESRD)
     0.00   0.00   **FUD** XXX   E

4276F Potent antiretroviral therapy prescribed (HIV)
     0.00   0.00   **FUD** XXX   E

4279F Pneumocystis jiroveci pneumonia prophylaxis prescribed (HIV)
     0.00   0.00   **FUD** XXX   E

4280F Pneumocystis jiroveci pneumonia prophylaxis prescribed within 3 months of low CD4+ cell count or percentage (HIV)
     0.00   0.00   **FUD** XXX   E

4290F Patient screened for injection drug use (HIV)
     0.00   0.00   **FUD** XXX   E

4293F Patient screened for high-risk sexual behavior (HIV)
     0.00   0.00   **FUD** XXX   E

4300F Patient receiving warfarin therapy for nonvalvular atrial fibrillation or atrial flutter (AFIB)
     0.00   0.00   **FUD** XXX   E

4301F Patient not receiving warfarin therapy for nonvalvular atrial fibrillation or atrial flutter (AFIB)
     0.00   0.00   **FUD** XXX   E

4305F Patient education regarding appropriate foot care and daily inspection of the feet received (CWC)
     0.00   0.00   **FUD** XXX   E

4306F Patient counseled regarding psychosocial and pharmacologic treatment options for opioid addiction (SUD)
     0.00   0.00   **FUD** XXX   E

4320F Patient counseled regarding psychosocial and pharmacologic treatment options for alcohol dependence (SUD)
     0.00   0.00   **FUD** XXX   E

4322F Caregiver provided with education and referred to additional resources for support (DEM)
     0.00   0.00   **FUD** XXX   M

4324F Patient (or caregiver) queried about Parkinson's disease medication related motor complications (Prkns)
     0.00   0.00   **FUD** XXX   E

4325F Medical and surgical treatment options reviewed with patient (or caregiver) (Prkns)
     0.00   0.00   **FUD** XXX   M

4326F Patient (or caregiver) queried about symptoms of autonomic dysfunction (Prkns)
     0.00   0.00   **FUD** XXX   E

4328F Patient (or caregiver) queried about sleep disturbances (Prkns)
     0.00   0.00   **FUD** XXX   E

4330F Counseling about epilepsy specific safety issues provided to patient (or caregiver(s)) (EPI)
     0.00   0.00   **FUD** XXX   E

4340F Counseling for women of childbearing potential with epilepsy (EPI)
     0.00   0.00   **FUD** XXX   M

26/TC PC/TC Only   A2-Z3 ASC Payment   50 Bilateral   ♂ Male Only   ♀ Female Only   Facility RVU   Non-Facility RVU   CCI   CLIA
FUD Follow-up Days   **CMS:** IOM   **AMA:** CPT Asst   A-Y OPPSI   80/80 Surg Assist Allowed / w/Doc   Lab Crosswalk   Radiology Crosswalk

580   CPT © 2021 American Medical Association. All Rights Reserved.   © 2021 Optum360, LLC

4350F Counseling provided on symptom management, end of life decisions, and palliation (DEM)
🚑 0.00   ⚕ 0.00   **FUD** XXX   E

4400F Rehabilitative therapy options discussed with patient (or caregiver) (Prkns)
🚑 0.00   ⚕ 0.00   **FUD** XXX   M

4450F Self-care education provided to patient (HF)
🚑 0.00   ⚕ 0.00   **FUD** XXX   E

4470F Implantable cardioverter-defibrillator (ICD) counseling provided (HF)
🚑 0.00   ⚕ 0.00   **FUD** XXX   E

4480F Patient receiving ACE inhibitor/ARB therapy and beta-blocker therapy for 3 months or longer (HF)
🚑 0.00   ⚕ 0.00   **FUD** XXX   E

4481F Patient receiving ACE inhibitor/ARB therapy and beta-blocker therapy for less than 3 months or patient not receiving ACE inhibitor/ARB therapy and beta-blocker therapy (HF)
🚑 0.00   ⚕ 0.00   **FUD** XXX   E

4500F Referred to an outpatient cardiac rehabilitation program (CAD)
🚑 0.00   ⚕ 0.00   **FUD** XXX   M

4510F Previous cardiac rehabilitation for qualifying cardiac event completed (CAD)
🚑 0.00   ⚕ 0.00   **FUD** XXX   M

4525F Neuropsychiatric intervention ordered (DEM)
🚑 0.00   ⚕ 0.00   **FUD** XXX   E

4526F Neuropsychiatric intervention received (DEM)
🚑 0.00   ⚕ 0.00   **FUD** XXX   E

4540F Disease modifying pharmacotherapy discussed (ALS)
🚑 0.00   ⚕ 0.00   **FUD** XXX   E

4541F Patient offered treatment for pseudobulbar affect, sialorrhea, or ALS-related symptoms (ALS)
🚑 0.00   ⚕ 0.00   **FUD** XXX   E

4550F Options for noninvasive respiratory support discussed with patient (ALS)
🚑 0.00   ⚕ 0.00   **FUD** XXX   E

4551F Nutritional support offered (ALS)
🚑 0.00   ⚕ 0.00   **FUD** XXX   E

4552F Patient offered referral to a speech language pathologist (ALS)
🚑 0.00   ⚕ 0.00   **FUD** XXX   E

4553F Patient offered assistance in planning for end of life issues (ALS)
🚑 0.00   ⚕ 0.00   **FUD** XXX   E

4554F Patient received inhalational anesthetic agent (Peri2)
🚑 0.00   ⚕ 0.00   **FUD** XXX   M

4555F Patient did not receive inhalational anesthetic agent (Peri2)
🚑 0.00   ⚕ 0.00   **FUD** XXX   E

4556F Patient exhibits 3 or more risk factors for post-operative nausea and vomiting (Peri2)
🚑 0.00   ⚕ 0.00   **FUD** XXX   M

4557F Patient does not exhibit 3 or more risk factors for post-operative nausea and vomiting (Peri2)
🚑 0.00   ⚕ 0.00   **FUD** XXX   E

4558F Patient received at least 2 prophylactic pharmacologic anti-emetic agents of different classes preoperatively and intraoperatively (Peri2)
🚑 0.00   ⚕ 0.00   **FUD** XXX   E

4559F At least 1 body temperature measurement equal to or greater than 35.5 degrees Celsius (or 95.9 degrees Fahrenheit) recorded within the 30 minutes immediately before or the 15 minutes immediately after anesthesia end time (Peri2)
🚑 0.00   ⚕ 0.00   **FUD** XXX   E

4560F Anesthesia technique did not involve general or neuraxial anesthesia (Peri2)
🚑 0.00   ⚕ 0.00   **FUD** XXX   E

4561F Patient has a coronary artery stent (Peri2)
🚑 0.00   ⚕ 0.00   **FUD** XXX   E

4562F Patient does not have a coronary artery stent (Peri2)
🚑 0.00   ⚕ 0.00   **FUD** XXX   E

4563F Patient received aspirin within 24 hours prior to anesthesia start time (Peri2)
🚑 0.00   ⚕ 0.00   **FUD** XXX   E

5005F-5250F Results Conveyed and Documented

INCLUDES   Patient's:
Functional status
Morbidity/mortality
Satisfaction/experience with care
Review/communication test results to patients

5005F Patient counseled on self-examination for new or changing moles (ML)
🚑 0.00   ⚕ 0.00   **FUD** XXX   E
AMA: 2008,Mar,8-12

5010F Findings of dilated macular or fundus exam communicated to the physician or other qualified health care professional managing the diabetes care (EC)
🚑 0.00   ⚕ 0.00   **FUD** XXX   M

5015F Documentation of communication that a fracture occurred and that the patient was or should be tested or treated for osteoporosis (OP)
🚑 0.00   ⚕ 0.00   **FUD** XXX   M

5020F Treatment summary report communicated to physician(s) or other qualified health care professional(s) managing continuing care and to the patient within 1 month of completing treatment (ONC)
🚑 0.00   ⚕ 0.00   **FUD** XXX   E
AMA: 2008,Mar,8-12

5050F Treatment plan communicated to provider(s) managing continuing care within 1 month of diagnosis (ML)
🚑 0.00   ⚕ 0.00   **FUD** XXX   M
AMA: 2008,Mar,8-12

5060F Findings from diagnostic mammogram communicated to practice managing patient's on-going care within 3 business days of exam interpretation (RAD)
🚑 0.00   ⚕ 0.00   **FUD** XXX   E
AMA: 2008,Mar,8-12

5062F Findings from diagnostic mammogram communicated to the patient within 5 days of exam interpretation (RAD)
🚑 0.00   ⚕ 0.00   **FUD** XXX   E
AMA: 2008,Mar,8-12

5100F Potential risk for fracture communicated to the referring physician or other qualified health care professional within 24 hours of completion of the imaging study (NUC_MED)
🚑 0.00   ⚕ 0.00   **FUD** XXX   E

5200F Consideration of referral for a neurological evaluation of appropriateness for surgical therapy for intractable epilepsy within the past 3 years (EPI)
🚑 0.00   ⚕ 0.00   **FUD** XXX   E

5250F Asthma discharge plan provided to patient (Asthma)
🚑 0.00   ⚕ 0.00   **FUD** XXX   E

● New Code   ▲ Revised Code   ○ Reinstated   ● New Web Release   ▲ Revised Web Release   + Add-on   Unlisted   Not Covered   # Resequenced
⑤⓪ Optum Mod 50 Exempt   ⊘ AMA Mod 51 Exempt   ⑤① Optum Mod 51 Exempt   ⑥③ Mod 63 Exempt   ⁄ Non-FDA Drug   ★ Telemedicine   M Maternity   A Age Edit

6005F-6150F Elements Related to Patient Safety Processes

INCLUDES   Patient safety practices

6005F Rationale (eg, severity of illness and safety) for level of care (eg, home, hospital) documented (CAP)

🚑 0.00   ⚖ 0.00   **FUD** XXX   E

AMA: 2018,Jan,8; 2017,Jan,8; 2016,Jan,13

6010F Dysphagia screening conducted prior to order for or receipt of any foods, fluids, or medication by mouth (STR)

🚑 0.00   ⚖ 0.00   **FUD** XXX   E

6015F Patient receiving or eligible to receive foods, fluids, or medication by mouth (STR)

🚑 0.00   ⚖ 0.00   **FUD** XXX   E

6020F NPO (nothing by mouth) ordered (STR)

🚑 0.00   ⚖ 0.00   **FUD** XXX   E

6030F All elements of maximal sterile barrier technique, hand hygiene, skin preparation and, if ultrasound is used, sterile ultrasound techniques followed (CRIT)

🚑 0.00   ⚖ 0.00   **FUD** XXX   M

AMA: 2008,Mar,8-12

6040F Use of appropriate radiation dose reduction devices OR manual techniques for appropriate moderation of exposure, documented (RAD)

🚑 0.00   ⚖ 0.00   **FUD** XXX   E

6045F Radiation exposure or exposure time in final report for procedure using fluoroscopy, documented (RAD)

🚑 0.00   ⚖ 0.00   **FUD** XXX   E

AMA: 2008,Mar,8-12

6070F Patient queried and counseled about anti-epileptic drug (AED) side effects (EPI)

🚑 0.00   ⚖ 0.00   **FUD** XXX   E

6080F Patient (or caregiver) queried about falls (Prkns, DSP)

🚑 0.00   ⚖ 0.00   **FUD** XXX   E

6090F Patient (or caregiver) counseled about safety issues appropriate to patient's stage of disease (Prkns)

🚑 0.00   ⚖ 0.00   **FUD** XXX   E

6100F Timeout to verify correct patient, correct site, and correct procedure, documented (PATH)

🚑 0.00   ⚖ 0.00   **FUD** XXX   E

6101F Safety counseling for dementia provided (DEM)

🚑 0.00   ⚖ 0.00   **FUD** XXX   E

6102F Safety counseling for dementia ordered (DEM)

🚑 0.00   ⚖ 0.00   **FUD** XXX   E

6110F Counseling provided regarding risks of driving and the alternatives to driving (DEM)

🚑 0.00   ⚖ 0.00   **FUD** XXX   E

6150F Patient not receiving a first course of anti-TNF (tumor necrosis factor) therapy (IBD)

🚑 0.00   ⚖ 0.00   **FUD** XXX   E

7010F-7025F Recall/Reminder System in Place

INCLUDES   Measures that address setting or care system provided
           Provider capabilities

7010F Patient information entered into a recall system that includes: target date for the next exam specified and a process to follow up with patients regarding missed or unscheduled appointments (ML)

🚑 0.00   ⚖ 0.00   **FUD** XXX   M

AMA: 2008,Mar,8-12

7020F Mammogram assessment category (eg, Mammography Quality Standards Act [MQSA], Breast Imaging Reporting and Data System [BI-RADS], or FDA approved equivalent categories) entered into an internal database to allow for analysis of abnormal interpretation (recall) rate (RAD)

🚑 0.00   ⚖ 0.00   **FUD** XXX   E

AMA: 2008,Mar,8-12

7025F Patient information entered into a reminder system with a target due date for the next mammogram (RAD)

🚑 0.00   ⚖ 0.00   **FUD** XXX   M

AMA: 2008,Mar,8-12

9001F-9007F No Measure Associated

INCLUDES   Care aspects not associated with measures at current time

9001F Aortic aneurysm less than 5.0 cm maximum diameter on centerline formatted CT or minor diameter on axial formatted CT (NMA-No Measure Associated)

🚑 0.00   ⚖ 0.00   **FUD** XXX   E

9002F Aortic aneurysm 5.0 - 5.4 cm maximum diameter on centerline formatted CT or minor diameter on axial formatted CT (NMA-No Measure Associated)

🚑 0.00   ⚖ 0.00   **FUD** XXX   E

9003F Aortic aneurysm 5.5 - 5.9 cm maximum diameter on centerline formatted CT or minor diameter on axial formatted CT (NMA-No Measure Associated)

🚑 0.00   ⚖ 0.00   **FUD** XXX   M

9004F Aortic aneurysm 6.0 cm or greater maximum diameter on centerline formatted CT or minor diameter on axial formatted CT (NMA-No Measure Associated)

🚑 0.00   ⚖ 0.00   **FUD** XXX   M

9005F Asymptomatic carotid stenosis: No history of any transient ischemic attack or stroke in any carotid or vertebrobasilar territory (NMA-No Measure Associated)

🚑 0.00   ⚖ 0.00   **FUD** XXX   E

9006F Symptomatic carotid stenosis: Ipsilateral carotid territory TIA or stroke less than 120 days prior to procedure (NMA-No Measure Associated)

🚑 0.00   ⚖ 0.00   **FUD** XXX   M

9007F Other carotid stenosis: Ipsilateral TIA or stroke 120 days or greater prior to procedure or any prior contralateral carotid territory or vertebrobasilar TIA or stroke (NMA-No Measure Associated)

🚑 0.00   ⚖ 0.00   **FUD** XXX   M

26/10 PC/TC Only   12-23 ASC Payment   50 Bilateral   ♂ Male Only   ♀ Female Only   🚑 Facility RVU   ⚖ Non-Facility RVU   CCI   CLIA
FUD Follow-up Days   **CMS:** IOM   **AMA:** CPT Asst   A-Y OPPSI   80/80 Surg Assist Allowed / w/Doc   Lab Crosswalk   Radiology Crosswalk

582   CPT © 2021 American Medical Association. All Rights Reserved.   © 2021 Optum360, LLC

0042T

0042T **Cerebral perfusion analysis using computed tomography with contrast administration, including post-processing of parametric maps with determination of cerebral blood flow, cerebral blood volume, and mean transit time**
> 🔧 0.00 ⚖ 0.00 **FUD** XXX N 80 ▱
>
> AMA: 2003,Nov,5

0054T-0055T

+ **0054T** **Computer-assisted musculoskeletal surgical navigational orthopedic procedure, with image-guidance based on fluoroscopic images (List separately in addition to code for primary procedure)**
> Code first primary procedure
> 🔧 0.00 ⚖ 0.00 **FUD** XXX N 80 ▱
>
> AMA: 2018,Jan,8; 2017,Jan,8; 2016,Jan,13

+ **0055T** **Computer-assisted musculoskeletal surgical navigational orthopedic procedure, with image-guidance based on CT/MRI images (List separately in addition to code for primary procedure)**
> INCLUDES Performance both CT and MRI in same session (one unit)
> Code first primary procedure
> 🔧 0.00 ⚖ 0.00 **FUD** XXX N 80 ▱
>
> AMA: 2018,Jan,8; 2017,Jan,8; 2016,Jan,13

0071T-0072T

EXCLUDES *Insertion bladder catheter (51702)*
MRI guidance for parenchymal tissue ablation (77022)

0071T **Focused ultrasound ablation of uterine leiomyomata, including MR guidance; total leiomyomata volume less than 200 cc of tissue** ♀
> 🔧 0.00 ⚖ 0.00 **FUD** XXX J 80 ▱
>
> AMA: 2005,Mar,1-6; 2005,Dec,3-6

0072T **total leiomyomata volume greater or equal to 200 cc of tissue** ♀
> 🔧 0.00 ⚖ 0.00 **FUD** XXX J 80 ▱
>
> AMA: 2005,Mar,1-6; 2005,Dec,3-6

0075T-0076T

INCLUDES All diagnostic services for stenting
Ipsilateral extracranial vertebral selective catheterization when confirming need for stenting
EXCLUDES *Selective catheterization and imaging when stenting not required (report only selective catheterization codes)*

0075T **Transcatheter placement of extracranial vertebral artery stent(s), including radiologic supervision and interpretation, open or percutaneous; initial vessel**
> 🔧 0.00 ⚖ 0.00 **FUD** XXX C 80 ▱
>
> AMA: 2018,Jan,8; 2017,Jan,8; 2016,Jan,13

+ **0076T** **each additional vessel (List separately in addition to code for primary procedure)**
> Code first (0075T)
> 🔧 0.00 ⚖ 0.00 **FUD** XXX C 80 ▱
>
> AMA: 2018,Jan,8; 2017,Jan,8; 2016,Jan,13

0095T-0098T

INCLUDES Fluoroscopy

+ **0095T** **Removal of total disc arthroplasty (artificial disc), anterior approach, each additional interspace, cervical (List separately in addition to code for primary procedure)**
> EXCLUDES *Lumbar disc (0164T)*
> *Revision total disc arthroplasty, cervical (22861)*
> *Revision total disc arthroplasty, lumbar (22862)*
> Code first (22864)
> 🔧 0.00 ⚖ 0.00 **FUD** XXX C 80 ▱
>
> AMA: 2006,Feb,1-6; 2005,Jun,6-8

+ **0098T** **Revision including replacement of total disc arthroplasty (artificial disc), anterior approach, each additional interspace, cervical (List separately in addition to code for primary procedure)**
> EXCLUDES *Application intervertebral biomechanical device(s) at same level (22853-22854, [22859])*
> *Removal total disc arthroplasty (0095T)*
> *Spinal cord decompression (63001-63048)*
> Code first (22861)
> 🔧 0.00 ⚖ 0.00 **FUD** XXX C 80 ▱
>
> AMA: 2006,Feb,1-6; 2005,Jun,6-8

0100T

0100T **Placement of a subconjunctival retinal prosthesis receiver and pulse generator, and implantation of intra-ocular retinal electrode array, with vitrectomy**
> EXCLUDES *Evaluation and initial programming implantable retinal electrode array device (0472T)*
> 🔧 0.00 ⚖ 0.00 **FUD** XXX T J8 80 ▱
>
> AMA: 2018,Feb,3; 2018,Jan,8; 2017,Jan,8; 2016,Jan,13

0101T-0513T [0512T, 0513T]

▲ **0101T** **Extracorporeal shock wave involving musculoskeletal system, not otherwise specified**
> EXCLUDES *Extracorporeal shock wave therapy integumentary system not otherwise specified ([0512T, 0513T])*
> 🔧 0.00 ⚖ 0.00 **FUD** XXX J G2 80 ▱
>
> AMA: 2018,Dec,5; 2018,Dec,5; 2018,Jan,8; 2017,Jan,8; 2016,Jan,13

▲ **0102T** **Extracorporeal shock wave performed by a physician, requiring anesthesia other than local, and involving the lateral humeral epicondyle**
> 🔧 0.00 ⚖ 0.00 **FUD** XXX J G2 80 ▱
>
> AMA: 2019,Jun,11; 2018,Dec,5; 2018,Dec,5; 2018,Jan,8; 2017,Jan,8; 2016,Jan,13

▲ # **0512T** **Extracorporeal shock wave for integumentary wound healing, including topical application and dressing care; initial wound**
> 🔧 0.00 ⚖ 0.00 **FUD** YYY R2 80 ▱
>
> AMA: 2018,Dec,5; 2018,Dec,5

▲ + # **0513T** **each additional wound (List separately in addition to code for primary procedure)**
> Code first ([0512T])
> 🔧 0.00 ⚖ 0.00 **FUD** ZZZ N1 80 ▱
>
> AMA: 2018,Dec,5; 2018,Dec,5

0106T-0110T

0106T **Quantitative sensory testing (QST), testing and interpretation per extremity; using touch pressure stimuli to assess large diameter sensation**
> 🔧 0.00 ⚖ 0.00 **FUD** XXX Q1 80 ▱
>
> AMA: 2018,Jan,8; 2017,Jan,8; 2016,Jan,13

0107T **using vibration stimuli to assess large diameter fiber sensation**
> 🔧 0.00 ⚖ 0.00 **FUD** XXX Q1 80 ▱
>
> AMA: 2018,Jan,8; 2017,Jan,8; 2016,Jan,13

0108T **using cooling stimuli to assess small nerve fiber sensation and hyperalgesia**
> 🔧 0.00 ⚖ 0.00 **FUD** XXX Q1 80 ▱
>
> AMA: 2018,Jan,8; 2017,Jan,8; 2016,Jan,13

0109T **using heat-pain stimuli to assess small nerve fiber sensation and hyperalgesia**
> 🔧 0.00 ⚖ 0.00 **FUD** XXX Q1 80 ▱
>
> AMA: 2018,Jan,8; 2017,Jan,8; 2016,Jan,13

0110T **using other stimuli to assess sensation**
> 🔧 0.00 ⚖ 0.00 **FUD** XXX Q1 80 ▱
>
> AMA: 2018,Jan,8; 2017,Jan,8; 2016,Jan,13

● New Code ▲ Revised Code ○ Reinstated ● New Web Release ▲ Revised Web Release + Add-on Unlisted Not Covered # Resequenced
50 Optum Mod 50 Exempt ⊘ AMA Mod 51 Exempt 51 Optum Mod 51 Exempt 63 Mod 63 Exempt ⁄ Non-FDA Drug ★ Telemedicine M Maternity A Age Edit

Category III Codes

0163T — 0202T

0163T-0165T

CMS: 100-03,150.10 Lumbar Artificial Disc Replacement (LADR)

> **INCLUDES** Fluoroscopy
> **EXCLUDES** *Application intervertebral biomechanical device(s) at same level (22853-22854, [22859])*
> *Cervical disc procedures (22856)*
> *Decompression (63001-63048)*
> *Exploration retroperitoneal area at same level (49010)*

\+ **0163T** **Total disc arthroplasty (artificial disc), anterior approach, including discectomy to prepare interspace (other than for decompression), each additional interspace, lumbar (List separately in addition to code for primary procedure)**
> Code first (22857)
> 🖭 0.00   ⚕ 0.00   **FUD** YYY   C 80 ▭
>
> **AMA:** 2018,Jan,8; 2017,Jan,8; 2016,Jan,13

\+ **0164T** **Removal of total disc arthroplasty, (artificial disc), anterior approach, each additional interspace, lumbar (List separately in addition to code for primary procedure)**
> Code first (22865)
> 🖭 0.00   ⚕ 0.00   **FUD** YYY   C 80 ▭
>
> **AMA:** 2018,Jan,8; 2017,Jan,8; 2016,Jan,13

\+ **0165T** **Revision including replacement of total disc arthroplasty (artificial disc), anterior approach, each additional interspace, lumbar (List separately in addition to code for primary procedure)**
> Code first (22862)
> 🖭 0.00   ⚕ 0.00   **FUD** YYY   C 80 ▭
>
> **AMA:** 2018,Jan,8; 2017,Jan,8; 2016,Jan,13

0174T-0175T

\+ **0174T** **Computer-aided detection (CAD) (computer algorithm analysis of digital image data for lesion detection) with further physician review for interpretation and report, with or without digitization of film radiographic images, chest radiograph(s), performed concurrent with primary interpretation (List separately in addition to code for primary procedure)**
> Code first (71045-71048)
> 🖭 0.00   ⚕ 0.00   **FUD** XXX   N 80 ▭
> **AMA:** 2018,Apr,7

0175T **Computer-aided detection (CAD) (computer algorithm analysis of digital image data for lesion detection) with further physician review for interpretation and report, with or without digitization of film radiographic images, chest radiograph(s), performed remote from primary interpretation**
> **INCLUDES** Chest x-rays (71045-71048)
> 🖭 0.00   ⚕ 0.00   **FUD** XXX   N 80 ▭
> **AMA:** 2018,Apr,7

0184T

0184T **Excision of rectal tumor, transanal endoscopic microsurgical approach (ie, TEMS), including muscularis propria (ie, full thickness)**
> **INCLUDES** Operating microscope (66990)
> Proctosigmoidoscopy (45300, 45308-45309, 45315, 45317, 45320)
> **EXCLUDES** *Nonendoscopic excision rectal tumor (45160, 45171-45172)*
> 🖭 0.00   ⚕ 0.00   **FUD** XXX   J 62 80 ▭
>
> **AMA:** 2018,Feb,11; 2018,Jan,8; 2017,Jan,8; 2016,Feb,12; 2016,Jan,13

0671T-0253T [0253T, 0376T, 0671T]

● # **0671T** **Insertion of anterior segment aqueous drainage device into the trabecular meshwork, without external reservoir, and without concomitant cataract removal, one or more**
> **EXCLUDES** *Aqueous drainage device insertion, external approach (66183)*
> *Aqueous drainage device insertion, internal approach:*
> *Subconjunctival space (0449T-0450T)*
> *Suprachoroidal space ([0253T])*
> *Supraciliary space (0474T)*
> *With extracapsular cataract removal and insertion of intraocular prosthesis during same session ([66989], [66987], [66991], [66988])*
> *Extracapsular cataract removal with IOL implant without aqueous drainage device during same session (66982, 66984)*
> 🖭 0.00   ⚕ 0.00   **FUD** 000

~~**0191T** **Insertion of anterior segment aqueous drainage device, without extraocular reservoir, internal approach, into the trabecular meshwork; initial insertion**~~
> To report, see ([66989], [66991], [0671T])

~~**0376T** **each additional device insertion (List separately in addition to code for primary procedure)**~~
> To report, see ([66989], [66991], [0671T])

\# **0253T** **Insertion of anterior segment aqueous drainage device, without extraocular reservoir, internal approach, into the suprachoroidal space**
> **EXCLUDES** *Aqueous drainage device insertion, external approach (66183)*
> *Aqueous drainage device insertion, internal approach:*
> *Subconjunctival space (0449T-0450T)*
> *Supraciliary space (0474T)*
> *Trabecular meshwork ([0671T])*
> 🖭 0.00   ⚕ 0.00   **FUD** YYY   J J8 80 ▭
> **AMA:** 2018,Jul,3

0198T

0198T **Measurement of ocular blood flow by repetitive intraocular pressure sampling, with interpretation and report**
> 🖭 0.00   ⚕ 0.00   **FUD** XXX   01 80 ▭
> **AMA:** 2018,Jan,8; 2017,Jan,8; 2016,Jan,13

0200T-0201T

> **INCLUDES** Deep bone biopsy (20225)

0200T **Percutaneous sacral augmentation (sacroplasty), unilateral injection(s), including the use of a balloon or mechanical device, when used, 1 or more needles, includes imaging guidance and bone biopsy, when performed**
> 🖭 0.00   ⚕ 0.00   **FUD** XXX   J 62 80 50 ▭
> **AMA:** 2018,Jan,8; 2017,Jan,8; 2016,Jan,13

0201T **Percutaneous sacral augmentation (sacroplasty), bilateral injections, including the use of a balloon or mechanical device, when used, 2 or more needles, includes imaging guidance and bone biopsy, when performed**
> 🖭 0.00   ⚕ 0.00   **FUD** XXX   J 62 80 ▭
> **AMA:** 2018,Jan,8; 2017,Jan,8; 2016,Jan,13

0202T-0563T [0563T]

0202T **Posterior vertebral joint(s) arthroplasty (eg, facet joint[s] replacement), including facetectomy, laminectomy, foraminotomy, and vertebral column fixation, injection of bone cement, when performed, including fluoroscopy, single level, lumbar spine**
> **INCLUDES** Instrumentation (22840, 22853-22854, [22859])
> Laminectomy (63005, 63012, 63017, 63047)
> Laminotomy (63030, 63042)
> Lumbar arthroplasty (22857)
> Percutaneous lumbar vertebral augmentation (22514)
> Percutaneous vertebroplasty (22511)
> Spinal cord decompression (63056)
> 🖭 0.00   ⚕ 0.00   **FUD** XXX   C 80 ▭

26/TC PC/TC Only   A2-Z3 ASC Payment   50 Bilateral   ♂ Male Only   ♀ Female Only   🖭 Facility RVU   ⚕ Non-Facility RVU   ▭ CCI   ✖ CLIA
FUD Follow-up Days   CMS: IOM   AMA: CPT Asst   A-Y OPPSI   80/80 Surg Assist Allowed / w/Doc   ▭ Lab Crosswalk   ▭ Radiology Crosswalk

584   CPT © 2021 American Medical Association. All Rights Reserved.   © 2021 Optum360, LLC

0207T Evacuation of meibomian glands, automated, using heat and intermittent pressure, unilateral

> EXCLUDES Evacuation using:
> Heat through wearable device ([0563T])
> Manual expression only, report appropriate E/M code

🔲 0.00 🔲 0.00 **FUD** XXX 〔Q1〕〔80〕〔TC〕🔲

AMA: 2018,Jan,8; 2017,Jan,8; 2016,Jan,13

**0563T** Evacuation of meibomian glands, using heat delivered through wearable, open-eye eyelid treatment devices and manual gland expression, bilateral

> EXCLUDES Evacuation using:
> Heat and intermittent pressure (0207T)
> Manual expression only, report appropriate E/M code

🔲 0.00 🔲 0.00 **FUD** YYY 〔80〕🔲

0208T-0212T

> EXCLUDES Manual audiometric testing by qualified health care professional, using audiometers (92551-92557)

0208T Pure tone audiometry (threshold), automated; air only

🔲 0.00 🔲 0.00 **FUD** XXX 〔Q1〕〔80〕〔TC〕🔲

AMA: 2018,Jan,8; 2017,Jan,8; 2016,Jan,13

0209T air and bone

🔲 0.00 🔲 0.00 **FUD** ·XXX 〔Q1〕〔80〕〔TC〕🔲

AMA: 2018,Jan,8; 2017,Jan,8; 2016,Jan,13

0210T Speech audiometry threshold, automated;

🔲 0.00 🔲 0.00 **FUD** XXX 〔Q1〕〔80〕〔TC〕🔲

AMA: 2014,Aug,3

0211T with speech recognition

🔲 0.00 🔲 0.00 **FUD** XXX 〔Q1〕〔80〕〔TC〕🔲

AMA: 2018,Jan,8; 2017,Jan,8; 2016,Jan,13

0212T Comprehensive audiometry threshold evaluation and speech recognition (0209T, 0211T combined), automated

🔲 0.00 🔲 0.00 **FUD** XXX 〔Q1〕〔80〕〔TC〕🔲

AMA: 2018,Jan,8; 2017,Jan,8; 2016,Jan,13

0213T-0215T

> INCLUDES Ultrasound guidance (76942)

0213T Injection(s), diagnostic or therapeutic agent, paravertebral facet (zygapophyseal) joint (or nerves innervating that joint) with ultrasound guidance, cervical or thoracic; single level

🔲 0.00 🔲 0.00 **FUD** XXX 〔T〕〔R2〕〔80〕〔50〕🔲

AMA: 2018,Jan,8; 2017,Jan,8; 2016,Jan,13

+ **0214T** second level (List separately in addition to code for primary procedure)

> EXCLUDES Reporting with modifier 50. Report once for each side when performed bilaterally
> Code first (0213T)

🔲 0.00 🔲 0.00 **FUD** ZZZ 〔N〕〔N1〕〔80〕🔲

AMA: 2018,Jan,8; 2017,Jan,8; 2016,Jan,13

+ **0215T** third and any additional level(s) (List separately in addition to code for primary procedure)

> EXCLUDES Reporting code more than one time per service date
> Reporting with modifier 50. Report once for each side when performed bilaterally
> Code first (0213T-0214T)

🔲 0.00 🔲 0.00 **FUD** ZZZ 〔N〕〔N1〕〔80〕🔲

AMA: 2018,Jan,8; 2017,Jan,8; 2016,Jan,13

0216T-0218T

> INCLUDES Ultrasound guidance (76942)
> EXCLUDES Injection with CT or fluoroscopic guidance (64490-64495)

0216T Injection(s), diagnostic or therapeutic agent, paravertebral facet (zygapophyseal) joint (or nerves innervating that joint) with ultrasound guidance, lumbar or sacral; single level

🔲 0.00 🔲 0.00 **FUD** XXX 〔T〕〔R2〕〔80〕〔50〕🔲

AMA: 2018,Jan,8; 2017,Jan,8; 2016,Jan,13

+ **0217T** second level (List separately in addition to code for primary procedure)

> EXCLUDES Reporting with modifier 50. Report once for each side when performed bilaterally
> Code first (0216T)

🔲 0.00 🔲 0.00 **FUD** ZZZ 〔N〕〔N1〕〔80〕🔲

AMA: 2018,Jan,8; 2017,Jan,8; 2016,Jan,13

+ **0218T** third and any additional level(s) (List separately in addition to code for primary procedure)

> EXCLUDES Reporting code more than one time per service date
> Reporting with modifier 50. Report once for each side when performed bilaterally
> Code first (0216T-0217T)

🔲 0.00 🔲 0.00 **FUD** ZZZ 〔N〕〔N1〕〔80〕🔲

AMA: 2018,Jan,8; 2017,Jan,8; 2016,Jan,13

0219T-0222T

> INCLUDES Allografts at same level (20930-20931)
> Application intervertebral biomechanical device(s) at same level (22853-22854, [22859])
> Arthrodesis at same level (22600-22614)
> Instrumentation at same level (22840)
> Radiologic services

0219T Placement of a posterior intrafacet implant(s), unilateral or bilateral, including imaging and placement of bone graft(s) or synthetic device(s), single level; cervical

🔲 0.00 🔲 0.00 **FUD** XXX 〔C〕〔80〕🔲

AMA: 2018,Jan,8; 2017,Jan,8; 2016,Jan,13

0220T thoracic

🔲 0.00 🔲 0.00 **FUD** XXX 〔C〕〔80〕🔲

AMA: 2018,Jan,8; 2017,Jan,8; 2016,Jan,13

0221T lumbar

🔲 0.00 🔲 0.00 **FUD** XXX 〔J〕〔G2〕〔80〕🔲

AMA: 2018,Jan,8; 2017,Jan,8; 2016,Jan,13

+ **0222T** each additional vertebral segment (List separately in addition to code for primary procedure)

> Code first (0219T-0221T)

🔲 0.00 🔲 0.00 **FUD** ZZZ 〔N〕〔80〕🔲

AMA: 2018,Jan,8; 2017,Jan,8; 2016,Jan,13

0232T

> INCLUDES Arthrocentesis (20600-20611)
> Blood collection (36415, 36592)
> Fat and other soft tissue grafts ([15769], 15771-15774)
> Imaging guidance (76942, 77002, 77012, 77021)
> Injections (20550-20551)
> Platelet/blood product pooling (86965)
> EXCLUDES Aspiration bone marrow for grafting, biopsy, harvesting for transplant (38220-38221, 38230)
> Injections white cell concentrate (0481T)

0232T Injection(s), platelet rich plasma, any site, including image guidance, harvesting and preparation when performed

🔲 0.00 🔲 0.00 **FUD** XXX 〔Q1〕〔N1〕🔲

AMA: 2019,Oct,5; 2019,Apr,10; 2018,May,3; 2018,Jan,8; 2017,Jan,8; 2016,Jan,13

0234T-0253T [0253T]

> INCLUDES Atherectomy by any technique in arteries above inguinal ligaments
> Radiology supervision and interpretation
> EXCLUDES Accessing and catheterization vessel
> Atherectomy performed below inguinal ligaments (37225, 37227, 37229, 37231, 37233, 37235)
> Closure arteriotomy by any technique
> Negotiating lesion
> Other interventions to same or different vessels
> Protection from embolism

0234T Transluminal peripheral atherectomy, open or percutaneous, including radiological supervision and interpretation; renal artery

🔲 0.00 🔲 0.00 **FUD** YYY 〔J〕〔80〕🔲

AMA: 2018,Jan,8; 2017,Jan,8; 2016,Jan,13

0235T visceral artery (except renal), each vessel

🔲 0.00 🔲 0.00 **FUD** YYY 〔C〕〔80〕🔲

AMA: 2018,Jan,8; 2017,Jan,8; 2016,Jan,13

	abdominal aorta				
0236T		🖢 0.00	⚕ 0.00	**FUD** YYY	J 80 ▭

AMA: 2018,Jan,8; 2017,Jan,8; 2016,Jan,13

0237T	brachiocephalic trunk and branches, each vessel
	🖢 0.00 ⚕ 0.00 **FUD** YYY J 80 ▭

AMA: 2018,Jan,8; 2017,Jan,8; 2016,Jan,13

0238T	iliac artery, each vessel
	🖢 0.00 ⚕ 0.00 **FUD** YYY J J8 80 ▭

AMA: 2018,Jan,8; 2017,Jan,8; 2016,Jan,13

0253T   **Resequenced code. See code before 0198T.**

0263T-0265T

EXCLUDES   *Bone marrow and stem cell services (38204-38242 [38243])*

0263T   **Intramuscular autologous bone marrow cell therapy, with preparation of harvested cells, multiple injections, one leg, including ultrasound guidance, if performed; complete procedure including unilateral or bilateral bone marrow harvest**

     INCLUDES   Duplex scan (93925-93926)
               Ultrasound guidance (76942)
     🖢 0.00   ⚕ 0.00   **FUD** XXX   S 62 80 ▭

0264T   **complete procedure excluding bone marrow harvest**

     INCLUDES   Bone marrow harvest only (0265T)
               Duplex scan (93925-93926)
               Ultrasound guidance (76942)
     🖢 0.00   ⚕ 0.00   **FUD** XXX   S 62 80 ▭

0265T   **unilateral or bilateral bone marrow harvest only for intramuscular autologous bone marrow cell therapy**

     EXCLUDES   *Complete procedure (0263T-0264T)*
     🖢 0.00   ⚕ 0.00   **FUD** XXX   S 62 80 ▭

0266T-0273T

0266T   **Implantation or replacement of carotid sinus baroreflex activation device; total system (includes generator placement, unilateral or bilateral lead placement, intra-operative interrogation, programming, and repositioning, when performed)**

     INCLUDES   Components complete procedure (0267T-0268T)
     🖢 0.00   ⚕ 0.00   **FUD** YYY   C J8 80 ▭

0267T   **lead only, unilateral (includes intra-operative interrogation, programming, and repositioning, when performed)**

     EXCLUDES   *Complete procedure (0266T)*
               Device interrogation (0272T-0273T)
               Removal/revision device or components (0269T-0271T)
     🖢 0.00   ⚕ 0.00   **FUD** YYY   T 62 80 ▭

0268T   **pulse generator only (includes intra-operative interrogation, programming, and repositioning, when performed)**

     EXCLUDES   *Complete procedure (0266T)*
               Device interrogation (0272T-0273T)
               Removal/revision device or components (0269T-0271T)
     🖢 0.00   ⚕ 0.00   **FUD** YYY   J J8 80 ▭

0269T   **Revision or removal of carotid sinus baroreflex activation device; total system (includes generator placement, unilateral or bilateral lead placement, intra-operative interrogation, programming, and repositioning, when performed)**

     EXCLUDES   *Device interrogation (0272T-0273T)*
               Implantation/replacement device and/or components (0266T-0268T)
               Removal/revision device or components (0270T-0271T)
     🖢 0.00   ⚕ 0.00   **FUD** YYY   Q2 62 80 ▭

0270T   **lead only, unilateral (includes intra-operative interrogation, programming, and repositioning, when performed)**

     EXCLUDES   *Device interrogation (0272T-0273T)*
               Implantation/replacement device and/or components (0266T-0269T)
               Removal/revision device or components (0271T)
     🖢 0.00   ⚕ 0.00   **FUD** XXX   Q2 62 80 ▭

0271T   **pulse generator only (includes intra-operative interrogation, programming, and repositioning, when performed)**

     EXCLUDES   *Device interrogation (0272T-0273T)*
               Implantation/replacement device and/or components (0266T-0268T)
               Removal/revision device or components (0271T-0273T)
     🖢 0.00   ⚕ 0.00   **FUD** XXX   Q2 62 80 ▭

0272T   **Interrogation device evaluation (in person), carotid sinus baroreflex activation system, including telemetric iterative communication with the implantable device to monitor device diagnostics and programmed therapy values, with interpretation and report (eg, battery status, lead impedance, pulse amplitude, pulse width, therapy frequency, pathway mode, burst mode, therapy start/stop times each day);**

     EXCLUDES   *Device interrogation (0273T)*
               Implantation/replacement device and/or components (0266T-0268T)
               Removal/revision device or components (0269T-0271T)
     🖢 0.00   ⚕ 0.00   **FUD** XXX   S 80 ▭

0273T   **with programming**

     EXCLUDES   *Device interrogation (0272T)*
               Implantation/replacement device and/or components (0266T-0268T)
               Removal/revision device or components (0269T-0271T)
     🖢 0.00   ⚕ 0.00   **FUD** XXX   S 80 ▭

0274T-0275T

EXCLUDES   *Laminotomy/hemilaminectomy by open and endoscopically assisted approach (63020-63035)*
               Percutaneous decompression nucleus pulposus intervertebral disc by needle-based technique (62287)

0274T   **Percutaneous laminotomy/laminectomy (interlaminar approach) for decompression of neural elements, (with or without ligamentous resection, discectomy, facetectomy and/or foraminotomy), any method, under indirect image guidance (eg, fluoroscopic, CT), single or multiple levels, unilateral or bilateral; cervical or thoracic**

     🖢 0.00   ⚕ 0.00   **FUD** YYY   J 62 80 ▭

AMA: 2018,Jan,8; 2017,Feb,12; 2017,Jan,8; 2016,Jan,13

0275T   **lumbar**

     🖢 0.00   ⚕ 0.00   **FUD** YYY   J J8 80 ▭

AMA: 2018,Jan,8; 2017,Feb,12; 2017,Jan,8; 2016,Jan,13

0278T

0278T   **Transcutaneous electrical modulation pain reprocessing (eg, scrambler therapy), each treatment session (includes placement of electrodes)**

     🖢 0.00   ⚕ 0.00   **FUD** XXX   Q1 N1 80 ▭

0290T

0290T   ~~Corneal incisions in the recipient cornea created using a laser, in preparation for penetrating or lamellar keratoplasty (List separately in addition to code for primary procedure)~~

     To report, see (66999)

26/TC PC/TC Only	A2-Z3 ASC Payment	50 Bilateral	♂ Male Only	♀ Female Only	🖢 Facility RVU	⚕ Non-Facility RVU	▭ CCI	✖ CLIA
FUD Follow-up Days	**CMS:** IOM	**AMA:** CPT Asst	A-Y OPPSI	80/80 Surg Assist Allowed / w/Doc		Lab Crosswalk		Radiology Crosswalk

586   CPT © 2021 American Medical Association. All Rights Reserved.   © 2021 Optum360, LLC

0308T

0308T Insertion of ocular telescope prosthesis including removal of crystalline lens or intraocular lens prosthesis

> INCLUDES Injection procedures (66020, 66030)
> Iridectomy when performed (66600-66635, 66761)
> Operating microscope (69990)
> Repositioning intraocular lens (66825)
>
> EXCLUDES Cataract extraction (66982-66986 [66987, 66988, 66989, 66991])
>
> ⚙ 0.00   ⚕ 0.00   **FUD** YYY   J J8 50
>
> **AMA:** 2019,Dec,6; 2018,Jan,8; 2017,Jan,8; 2016,Jan,13

0312T-0317T

> EXCLUDES Analysis and/or programming (or reprogramming) vagus nerve stimulator (95970, 95976-95977)
> Implantation, replacement, removal, and/or revision vagus nerve neurostimulator (electrode array and/or pulse generator) for stimulation vagus nerve other than at esophagogastric junction (64568-64570)

0312T Vagus nerve blocking therapy (morbid obesity); laparoscopic implantation of neurostimulator electrode array, anterior and posterior vagal trunks adjacent to esophagogastric junction (EGJ), with implantation of pulse generator, includes programming

> ⚙ 0.00   ⚕ 0.00   **FUD** XXX   J G2 80
>
> **AMA:** 2018,Jan,8; 2017,Jan,8; 2016,Jan,13

0313T laparoscopic revision or replacement of vagal trunk neurostimulator electrode array, including connection to existing pulse generator

> ⚙ 0.00   ⚕ 0.00   **FUD** XXX   T J8 80
>
> **AMA:** 2018,Jan,8; 2017,Jan,8; 2016,Jan,13

0314T laparoscopic removal of vagal trunk neurostimulator electrode array and pulse generator

> ⚙ 0.00   ⚕ 0.00   **FUD** XXX   Q2 G2 80
>
> **AMA:** 2018,Jan,8; 2017,Jan,8; 2016,Jan,13

0315T removal of pulse generator

> EXCLUDES Removal with replacement pulse generator (0316T)
>
> ⚙ 0.00   ⚕ 0.00   **FUD** XXX   Q2 G2 80
>
> **AMA:** 2018,Jan,8; 2017,Jan,8; 2016,Jan,13

0316T replacement of pulse generator

> EXCLUDES Removal without replacement pulse generator (0315T)
>
> ⚙ 0.00   ⚕ 0.00   **FUD** XXX   J J8 80
>
> **AMA:** 2018,Jan,8; 2017,Jan,8; 2016,Jan,13

0317T neurostimulator pulse generator electronic analysis, includes reprogramming when performed

> EXCLUDES Analysis and/or programming (or reprogramming) vagus nerve stimulator (95970, 95976-95977)
>
> ⚙ 0.00   ⚕ 0.00   **FUD** XXX   01 80
>
> **AMA:** 2018,Jan,8; 2017,Jan,8; 2016,Jan,13

0329T-0330T

0329T Monitoring of intraocular pressure for 24 hours or longer, unilateral or bilateral, with interpretation and report

> ⚙ 0.00   ⚕ 0.00   **FUD** YYY   E
>
> **AMA:** 2018,Jan,8; 2017,Jan,8; 2016,Jan,13

0330T Tear film imaging, unilateral or bilateral, with interpretation and report

> ⚙ 0.00   ⚕ 0.00   **FUD** YYY   01 N1
>
> **AMA:** 2018,Jan,8; 2017,Jan,8; 2016,Jan,13

0331T-0332T

> EXCLUDES Myocardial infarction avid imaging (78466, 78468, 78469)

0331T Myocardial sympathetic innervation imaging, planar qualitative and quantitative assessment;

> ⚙ 0.00   ⚕ 0.00   **FUD** YYY   S Z2
>
> **AMA:** 2018,Jan,8; 2017,Jan,8; 2016,Jan,13

0332T with tomographic SPECT

> ⚙ 0.00   ⚕ 0.00   **FUD** YYY   S Z2
>
> **AMA:** 2018,Jan,8; 2017,Jan,8; 2016,Jan,13

0333T-0464T [0464T]

0333T Visual evoked potential, screening of visual acuity, automated, with report

> EXCLUDES Visual evoked potential testing for glaucoma ([0464T])
>
> ⚙ 0.00   ⚕ 0.00   **FUD** YYY   E
>
> **AMA:** 2018,Feb,3; 2018,Jan,8; 2017,Jan,8; 2016,Jan,13

\# **0464T** Visual evoked potential, testing for glaucoma, with interpretation and report

> EXCLUDES Visual evoked potential for visual acuity (0333T)
>
> ⚙ 0.00   ⚕ 0.00   **FUD** YYY   S
>
> **AMA:** 2018,Feb,3

0335T-0511T [0510T, 0511T]

0335T Insertion of sinus tarsi implant

> EXCLUDES Arthroscopic subtalar arthrodesis (29907)
> Open talotarsal joint dislocation repair (28585)
> Subtalar arthrodesis (28725)
>
> ⚙ 0.00   ⚕ 0.00   **FUD** YYY   J J8

\# **0510T** Removal of sinus tarsi implant

> ⚙ 0.00   ⚕ 0.00   **FUD** YYY   G2 50

\# **0511T** Removal and reinsertion of sinus tarsi implant

> ⚙ 0.00   ⚕ 0.00   **FUD** YYY   J8 50

0338T-0339T

> INCLUDES Selective catheter placement renal arteries (36251-36254)

0338T Transcatheter renal sympathetic denervation, percutaneous approach including arterial puncture, selective catheter placement(s) renal artery(ies), fluoroscopy, contrast injection(s), intraprocedural roadmapping and radiological supervision and interpretation, including pressure gradient measurements, flush aortogram and diagnostic renal angiography when performed; unilateral

> ⚙ 0.00   ⚕ 0.00   **FUD** YYY   J G2

0339T bilateral

> ⚙ 0.00   ⚕ 0.00   **FUD** YYY   J G2

0342T

0342T Therapeutic apheresis with selective HDL delipidation and plasma reinfusion

> ⚙ 0.00   ⚕ 0.00   **FUD** YYY   S G2

0345T

0345T Transcatheter mitral valve repair percutaneous approach via the coronary sinus

> INCLUDES Coronary angiography (93563-93564)
> Fluoroscopy (76000)
>
> EXCLUDES Diagnostic cardiac catheterization procedures integral to valve procedure (93451-93461, 93593-93598)
> Repair mitral valve including transseptal puncture (33418-33419)
> Transcatheter implantation/replacement mitral valve (TMVI) (0483T-0484T)
> Transcatheter mitral valve annulus reconstruction (0544T)
>
> Code also diagnostic cardiac catheterization/angiography procedures, and append modifier 59, if patient's condition (clinical indication) changed since intervention or prior study, no available prior catheter-based diagnostic study in treatment zone, or prior study not adequate (93451-93461, 93593-93598)
> Code also transvascular ventricular support, when performed:
> Balloon pump insertion (33967, 33970, 33973)
> Ventricular assist device ([33995], 33990-33993, [33997])
>
> ⚙ 0.00   ⚕ 0.00   **FUD** YYY   C
>
> **AMA:** 2018,Jan,8; 2017,Jan,8; 2016,Jan,13

0347T

0347T Placement of interstitial device(s) in bone for radiostereometric analysis (RSA)

> ⚙ 0.00   ⚕ 0.00   **FUD** YYY   01 N1
>
> **AMA:** 2018,Jan,8; 2017,Jan,8; 2016,Jan,13

0348T-0350T

0348T Radiologic examination, radiostereometric analysis (RSA); spine, (includes cervical, thoracic and lumbosacral, when performed)

🔧 0.00   ⚕ 0.00   **FUD** YYY   Q1 N1 ▣

AMA: 2018,Jan,8; 2017,Jan,8; 2016,Jan,13

0349T upper extremity(ies), (includes shoulder, elbow, and wrist, when performed)

🔧 0.00   ⚕ 0.00   **FUD** YYY   Q1 N1 ▣

AMA: 2018,Jan,8; 2017,Jan,8; 2016,Jan,13

0350T lower extremity(ies), (includes hip, proximal femur, knee, and ankle, when performed)

🔧 0.00   ⚕ 0.00   **FUD** YYY   Q1 N1 ▣

AMA: 2018,Jan,8; 2017,Jan,8; 2016,Jan,13

0351T-0354T

0351T Optical coherence tomography of breast or axillary lymph node, excised tissue, each specimen; real-time intraoperative

INCLUDES Interpretation and report (0352T)

🔧 0.00   ⚕ 0.00   **FUD** YYY   N N1 ▣

AMA: 2018,Jan,8; 2017,Jan,8; 2016,Jan,13

0352T interpretation and report, real-time or referred

INCLUDES Interpretation and report (0351T)

🔧 0.00   ⚕ 0.00   **FUD** YYY   B ▣

AMA: 2018,Jan,8; 2017,Jan,8; 2016,Jan,13

0353T Optical coherence tomography of breast, surgical cavity; real-time intraoperative

INCLUDES Interpretation and report (0354T)

EXCLUDES Reporting code more than one time per session

🔧 0.00   ⚕ 0.00   **FUD** YYY   N N1 ▣

AMA: 2018,Jan,8; 2017,Jan,8; 2016,Jan,13

0354T interpretation and report, real time or referred

🔧 0.00   ⚕ 0.00   **FUD** YYY   B ▣

AMA: 2018,Jan,8; 2017,Jan,8; 2016,Jan,13

0355T-0358T

0355T ~~Gastrointestinal tract imaging, intraluminal (eg, capsule endoscopy), colon, with interpretation and report~~

To report, see ([91113])

0356T ~~Insertion of drug-eluting implant (including punctal dilation and implant removal when performed) into lacrimal canaliculus, each~~

To report, see (68841, 0444T-0445T)

0358T Bioelectrical impedance analysis whole body composition assessment, with interpretation and report

🔧 0.00   ⚕ 0.00   **FUD** YYY   Q1 ▣

0362T-0376T [0376T]

INCLUDES Only one technician time when more than one technician in attendance

Provided by physician/other qualified healthcare professional while on-site (immediately available during procedure), but does not need to be face-to-face

Provided in environment appropriate for patient

Provided to patients with destructive behaviors

EXCLUDES Adaptive behavior services ([97153, 97154, 97155, 97156, 97157, 97158])

Aphasia assessment (96105)

Behavioral/developmental screening/testing (96110-96113, [96127])

Behavior/health assessment (96156-96159 [96164, 96165, 96167, 96168, 96170, 96171])

Cognitive testing ([96125])

Neurobehavioral testing (96116-96121)

Psychiatric evaluations/psychotherapy/interactive complexity (90785-90899)

Psychological/neuropsychological evaluation/testing (96130-96146)

0362T Behavior identification supporting assessment, each 15 minutes of technicians' time face-to-face with a patient, requiring the following components: administration by the physician or other qualified health care professional who is on site; with the assistance of two or more technicians; for a patient who exhibits destructive behavior; completion in an environment that is customized to the patient's behavior.

INCLUDES Comprises:

Functional analysis and behavioral assessment

Procedures and instruments to assess functional impairment and behavior levels

Structured observation with data collection not including direct patient involvement

EXCLUDES Conferences by medical team (99366-99368)

Occupational therapy evaluation ([97165, 97166, 97167, 97168])

Speech evaluation (92521-92524)

Code also when performed on different days until behavioral and supporting assessments complete

🔧 0.00   ⚕ 0.00   **FUD** YYY   S ▣

AMA: 2018,Nov,3; 2018,Jan,8; 2017,Jan,8; 2016,Jan,13

0373T Adaptive behavior treatment with protocol modification, each 15 minutes of technicians' time face-to-face with a patient, requiring the following components: administration by the physician or other qualified health care professional who is on site; with the assistance of two or more technicians; for a patient who exhibits destructive behavior; completion in an environment that is customized to the patient's behavior.

🔧 0.00   ⚕ 0.00   **FUD** YYY   S ▣

AMA: 2018,Nov,3; 2018,Jan,8; 2017,Jan,8; 2016,Jan,13

0378T-0379T

0378T Visual field assessment, with concurrent real time data analysis and accessible data storage with patient initiated data transmitted to a remote surveillance center for up to 30 days; review and interpretation with report by a physician or other qualified health care professional

🔧 0.00   ⚕ 0.00   **FUD** XXX   B 80 ▣

AMA: 2018,Jan,8; 2017,Jan,8; 2016,Jan,13

0379T technical support and patient instructions, surveillance, analysis and transmission of daily and emergent data reports as prescribed by a physician or other qualified health care professional

🔧 0.00   ⚕ 0.00   **FUD** XXX   Q1 N1 80 ▣

AMA: 2018,Jan,8; 2017,Jan,8; 2016,Jan,13

0394T-0395T

EXCLUDES Radiation oncology procedures (77261-77263, 77300, 77306-77307, 77316-77318, 77332-77334, 77336, 77427-77499, 77761-77772, 77778, 77789)

0394T High dose rate electronic brachytherapy, skin surface application, per fraction, includes basic dosimetry, when performed

EXCLUDES Superficial non-brachytherapy radiation (77401)

🔧 0.00   ⚕ 0.00   **FUD** XXX   S 72 80 ▣

0395T High dose rate electronic brachytherapy, interstitial or intracavitary treatment, per fraction, includes basic dosimetry, when performed

> *EXCLUDES* High dose rate skin surface application (0394T)
> 🔧 0.00   ✂ 0.00   **FUD** XXX   [S] [Z2] [80] [▣]

0397T-0398T

+ 0397T Endoscopic retrograde cholangiopancreatography (ERCP), with optical endomicroscopy (List separately in addition to code for primary procedure)

> *INCLUDES* Optical endomicroscopic image(s) (88375)
> *EXCLUDES* Reporting code more than one time per operative session
> Code first (43260-43265, [43274], [43275], [43276], [43277], [43278])
> 🔧 0.00   ✂ 0.00   **FUD** XXX   [N] [M1] [80] [▣]

0398T Magnetic resonance image guided high intensity focused ultrasound (MRgFUS), stereotactic ablation lesion, intracranial for movement disorder including stereotactic navigation and frame placement when performed

> *INCLUDES* Application stereotactic headframe (61800)
> Stereotactic computer-assisted navigation (61781)
> 🔧 0.00   ✂ 0.00   **FUD** XXX   [S] [80] [▣]

0402T

0402T Collagen cross-linking of cornea, including removal of the corneal epithelium and intraoperative pachymetry, when performed (Report medication separately)

> *INCLUDES* Corneal epithelium removal (65435)
> Corneal pachymetry (76514)
> Operating microscope (69990)
> 🔧 0.00   ✂ 0.00   **FUD** XXX   [J] [R2] [80] [▣]
> **AMA:** 2018,Jun,11; 2018,Jan,8; 2017,Jan,8; 2016,Feb,12

0403T-0488T [0488T]

> *INCLUDES* Intensive behavioral counseling by trained lifestyle coach
> Standardized course with emphasis on weight, exercise, stress management, and nutrition

0403T Preventive behavior change, intensive program of prevention of diabetes using a standardized diabetes prevention program curriculum, provided to individuals in a group setting, minimum 60 minutes, per day

> *EXCLUDES* Online/electronic diabetes prevention program ([0488T])
> Self-management training and education by nonphysician health care professional (98960-98962)
> 🔧 0.00   ✂ 0.00   **FUD** XXX   [E] [80] [▣]
> **AMA:** 2020,Jul,7; 2018,Aug,6

 # 0488T Preventive behavior change, online/electronic structured intensive program for prevention of diabetes using a standardized diabetes prevention program curriculum, provided to an individual, per 30 days

> *INCLUDES* In person elements when appropriate
> *EXCLUDES* Group diabetes prevention program (0403T)
> Self-management training and education by nonphysician health care professional (98960-98962)
> 🔧 0.00   ✂ 0.00   **FUD** XXX   [E] [▣]
> **AMA:** 2020,Jul,7; 2018,Aug,6

0404T

0404T Transcervical uterine fibroid(s) ablation with ultrasound guidance, radiofrequency   ♀

> 🔧 0.00   ✂ 0.00   **FUD** XXX   [J] [J8] [80] [▣]

0408T-0418T

0408T Insertion or replacement of permanent cardiac contractility modulation system, including contractility evaluation when performed, and programming of sensing and therapeutic parameters; pulse generator with transvenous electrodes

> *INCLUDES* Device evaluation (93286-93287, 0415T, 0417T-0418T)
> Insertion or replacement entire system
> *EXCLUDES* Cardiac catheterization (93452-93453, 93456-93461)
> Code also removal each electrode when pulse generator and electrodes removed and replaced (0410T-0411T)
> 🔧 0.00   ✂ 0.00   **FUD** XXX   [J] [J8] [80] [▣]

0409T pulse generator only

> *INCLUDES* Device evaluation (93286-93287, 0415T, 0417T-0418T)
> *EXCLUDES* Cardiac catheterization (93452-93453, 93456-93461)
> 🔧 0.00   ✂ 0.00   **FUD** XXX   [J] [J8] [80] [▣]

0410T atrial electrode only

> *INCLUDES* Device evaluation (93286-93287, 0415T, 0417T-0418T)
> Each atrial electrode inserted or replaced
> *EXCLUDES* Cardiac catheterization (93452-93453, 93456-93461)
> 🔧 0.00   ✂ 0.00   **FUD** XXX   [J] [J8] [80] [▣]

0411T ventricular electrode only

> *INCLUDES* Device evaluation (93286-93287, 0415T, 0417T-0418T)
> Each ventricular electrode inserted or replaced
> *EXCLUDES* Cardiac catheterization (93452-93453, 93456-93461)
> Insertion or replacement complete CCM system (0408T)
> 🔧 0.00   ✂ 0.00   **FUD** XXX   [J] [J8] [80] [▣]

0412T Removal of permanent cardiac contractility modulation system; pulse generator only

> *EXCLUDES* Device evaluation (0417T-0418T)
> Insertion or replacement complete CCM system (0408T)
> 🔧 0.00   ✂ 0.00   **FUD** XXX   [Q2] [G2] [80] [▣]

0413T transvenous electrode (atrial or ventricular)

> *INCLUDES* Each electrode removed
> *EXCLUDES* Device evaluation (0417T-0418T)
> Insertion or replacement complete CCM system (0408T)
> Code also:
> Removal and replacement electrode(s), as appropriate (0410T-0411T)
> Removal pulse generator when leads also removed (0412T)
> 🔧 0.00   ✂ 0.00   **FUD** XXX   [Q2] [G2] [80] [▣]

0414T Removal and replacement of permanent cardiac contractility modulation system pulse generator only

> *INCLUDES* Device evaluation (93286-93287, 0417T-0418T)
> *EXCLUDES* Cardiac catheterization (93452-93453, 93456-93461)
> Code also replacement pulse generator when leads also removed and replaced (0408T, 0412T-0413T)
> 🔧 0.00   ✂ 0.00   **FUD** XXX   [J] [J8] [80] [▣]

0415T Repositioning of previously implanted cardiac contractility modulation transvenous electrode, (atrial or ventricular lead)

> *INCLUDES* Device evaluation (93286-93287, 0417T-0418T)
> *EXCLUDES* Cardiac catheterization (93452-93453, 93456-93461)
> Insertion or replacement entire system or components (0408T-0411T)
> 🔧 0.00   ✂ 0.00   **FUD** XXX   [T] [G2] [80] [▣]

0416T Relocation of skin pocket for implanted cardiac contractility modulation pulse generator

> 🔧 0.00   ✂ 0.00   **FUD** XXX   [T] [G2] [80] [▣]

0417T Programming device evaluation (in person) with iterative adjustment of the implantable device to test the function of the device and select optimal permanent programmed values with analysis, including review and report, implantable cardiac contractility modulation system

> *EXCLUDES* Insertion/replacement/removal/repositioning device or components (0408T-0415T, 0418T)
> 🔧 0.00   ✂ 0.00   **FUD** XXX   [Q1] [80] [▣]

0418T Interrogation device evaluation (in person) with analysis, review and report, includes connection, recording and disconnection per patient encounter, implantable cardiac contractility modulation system

> EXCLUDES Insertion/replacement/removal/repositioning device or components (0408T-0415T, 0417T)

🛏 0.00 ⚕ 0.00 **FUD** XXX 〔Q1〕〔80〕🖵

0419T-0420T

> EXCLUDES Neurofibroma excision (64792)
> Reporting code more than one time per session

0419T Destruction of neurofibroma, extensive (cutaneous, dermal extending into subcutaneous); face, head and neck, greater than 50 neurofibromas

🛏 0.00 ⚕ 0.00 **FUD** XXX 〔T〕〔R2〕〔80〕🖵

AMA: 2018,Jan,8; 2017,Jan,8; 2016,Apr,3

0420T trunk and extremities, extensive, greater than 100 neurofibromas

🛏 0.00 ⚕ 0.00 **FUD** XXX 〔T〕〔R2〕〔80〕🖵

AMA: 2018,Jan,8; 2017,Jan,8; 2016,Apr,3

0421T-0423T

0421T Transurethral waterjet ablation of prostate, including control of post-operative bleeding, including ultrasound guidance, complete (vasectomy, meatotomy, cystourethroscopy, urethral calibration and/or dilation, and internal urethrotomy are included when performed) ♂

> EXCLUDES Transrectal ultrasound (76872)
> Transurethral prostate resection (52500, 52630)

🛏 0.00 ⚕ 0.00 **FUD** XXX 〔J〕〔G2〕〔80〕🖵

AMA: 2020,Aug,6

0422T Tactile breast imaging by computer-aided tactile sensors, unilateral or bilateral

🛏 0.00 ⚕ 0.00 **FUD** XXX 〔Q1〕〔Z2〕〔80〕🖵

~~**0423T** Secretory type II phospholipase A2 (sPLA2-IIA)~~
To report, see (84999)

0424T-0436T

> INCLUDES Phrenic nerve stimulation system includes:
> Pulse generator
> Sensing lead (placed in azygos vein)
> Stimulation lead (placed into right brachiocephalic vein or left pericardiophrenic vein)

0424T Insertion or replacement of neurostimulator system for treatment of central sleep apnea; complete system (transvenous placement of right or left stimulation lead, sensing lead, implantable pulse generator)

> INCLUDES Device evaluation (0434T-0436T)
> Insertion or replacement system components (0425T-0427T)
> Repositioning leads (0432T-0433T)
> Code also when pulse generator and all leads removed and replaced (0428T-0430T)

🛏 0.00 ⚕ 0.00 **FUD** XXX 〔J〕〔G2〕〔80〕🖵

0425T sensing lead only

> EXCLUDES Device evaluation (0434T-0436T)
> Insertion/replacement complete system (0424T)
> Repositioning leads (0432T-0433T)

🛏 0.00 ⚕ 0.00 **FUD** XXX 〔J〕〔G2〕〔80〕🖵

0426T stimulation lead only

> EXCLUDES Device evaluation (0434T-0436T)
> Insertion/replacement complete system (0424T)
> Repositioning leads (0432T-0433T)

🛏 0.00 ⚕ 0.00 **FUD** XXX 〔J〕〔G2〕〔80〕🖵

0427T pulse generator only

> EXCLUDES Device evaluation (0434T-0436T)
> Insertion/replacement complete system (0424T)
> Repositioning leads (0432T-0433T)

🛏 0.00 ⚕ 0.00 **FUD** XXX 〔J〕〔J8〕〔80〕🖵

0428T Removal of neurostimulator system for treatment of central sleep apnea; pulse generator only

> EXCLUDES Device evaluation (0434T-0436T)
> Removal with replacement of pulse generator and all leads (0424T, 0429T-0430T)
> Repositioning leads (0432T-0433T)
> Code also when lead removed (0429T-0430T)

🛏 0.00 ⚕ 0.00 **FUD** XXX 〔Q2〕〔G2〕〔80〕🖵

0429T sensing lead only

> INCLUDES Removal one sensing lead
> EXCLUDES Device evaluation (0434T-0436T)

🛏 0.00 ⚕ 0.00 **FUD** XXX 〔Q2〕〔G2〕〔80〕🖵

0430T stimulation lead only

> INCLUDES Removal one stimulation lead
> EXCLUDES Device evaluation (0434T-0436T)

🛏 0.00 ⚕ 0.00 **FUD** XXX 〔Q2〕〔G2〕〔80〕🖵

AMA: 2015,Aug,4

0431T Removal and replacement of neurostimulator system for treatment of central sleep apnea, pulse generator only

> EXCLUDES Device evaluation (0434T-0436T)
> Removal with replacement generator and all three leads (0424T, 0428T-0430T)

🛏 0.00 ⚕ 0.00 **FUD** XXX 〔J〕〔J8〕〔80〕🖵

0432T Repositioning of neurostimulator system for treatment of central sleep apnea; stimulation lead only

> EXCLUDES Device evaluation (0434T-0436T)
> Insertion/replacement complete system or components (0424T-0427T)

🛏 0.00 ⚕ 0.00 **FUD** XXX 〔T〕〔G2〕〔80〕🖵

0433T sensing lead only

> EXCLUDES Device evaluation (0434T-0436T)
> Insertion/replacement complete system or components (0424T-0427T)

🛏 0.00 ⚕ 0.00 **FUD** XXX 〔T〕〔G2〕〔80〕🖵

0434T Interrogation device evaluation implanted neurostimulator pulse generator system for central sleep apnea

> EXCLUDES Insertion/replacement complete system or components (0424T-0427T)
> Removal system or components (0428T-0431T)
> Repositioning leads (0432T-0433T)

🛏 0.00 ⚕ 0.00 **FUD** XXX 〔S〕〔G2〕〔80〕🖵

0435T Programming device evaluation of implanted neurostimulator pulse generator system for central sleep apnea; single session

> EXCLUDES Device evaluation (0436T)
> Insertion/replacement complete system or components (0424T-0427T)
> Removal system or components (0428T-0431T)
> Repositioning leads (0432T-0433T)

🛏 0.00 ⚕ 0.00 **FUD** XXX 〔S〕〔80〕🖵

0436T during sleep study

> EXCLUDES Device evaluation (0435T)
> Insertion/replacement complete system or components (0424T-0427T)
> Removal system or components (0428T-0431T)
> Reporting code more than one time for each sleep study
> Repositioning leads (0432T-0433T)

🛏 0.00 ⚕ 0.00 **FUD** XXX 〔S〕〔80〕🖵

26/TC PC/TC Only   A2-Z3 ASC Payment   50 Bilateral   ♂ Male Only   ♀ Female Only   🛏 Facility RVU   ⚕ Non-Facility RVU   🖵 CCI   ❌ CLIA
FUD Follow-up Days   CMS: IOM   AMA: CPT Asst   A-Y OPPSI   80/80 Surg Assist Allowed / w/Doc   Lab Crosswalk   Radiology Crosswalk

590   CPT © 2021 American Medical Association. All Rights Reserved.   © 2021 Optum360, LLC

0437T-0439T

+ **0437T** Implantation of non-biologic or synthetic implant (eg, polypropylene) for fascial reinforcement of the abdominal wall (List separately in addition to code for primary procedure)

> EXCLUDES *Implantation mesh, other material for repair incisional or ventral hernia (49560-49561, 49565-49566, 49568)*
> *Insertion mesh, other material for closure wound caused by necrotizing soft tissue infection (11004-11006, 49568)*

Code first primary procedure

🚘 0.00   ⚕ 0.00   **FUD** ZZZ   N N1 80 ▣

+ **0439T** Myocardial contrast perfusion echocardiography, at rest or with stress, for assessment of myocardial ischemia or viability (List separately in addition to code for primary procedure)

Code first (93306-93308, 93350-93351)

🚘 0.00   ⚕ 0.00   **FUD** ZZZ   N N1 80 ▣

AMA: 2018,Jan,8; 2017,Jan,8; 2016,Apr,8

0440T-0442T

0440T Ablation, percutaneous, cryoablation, includes imaging guidance; upper extremity distal/peripheral nerve

🚘 0.00   ⚕ 0.00   **FUD** YYY   J G2 80 ▣

AMA: 2019,Apr,9; 2018,Jan,8

0441T lower extremity distal/peripheral nerve

🚘 0.00   ⚕ 0.00   **FUD** YYY   J G2 80 ▣

AMA: 2019,Apr,9; 2018,Jan,8

0442T nerve plexus or other truncal nerve (eg, brachial plexus, pudendal nerve)

🚘 0.00   ⚕ 0.00   **FUD** YYY   J J8 80 ▣

AMA: 2019,Apr,9; 2018,Jan,8

0443T

+ **0443T** Real-time spectral analysis of prostate tissue by fluorescence spectroscopy, including imaging guidance (List separately in addition to code for primary procedure)   ♂

> EXCLUDES *Reporting code more than one time for each session*

Code first (55700)

🚘 0.00   ⚕ 0.00   **FUD** ZZZ   N N1 80 ▣

0444T-0445T

> EXCLUDES *Insertion/removal drug-eluting stent into canaliculus (68841)*

0444T Initial placement of a drug-eluting ocular insert under one or more eyelids, including fitting, training, and insertion, unilateral or bilateral

🚘 0.00   ⚕ 0.00   **FUD** YYY   N N1 80 ▣

AMA: 2018,Jan,8; 2017,Aug,7

0445T Subsequent placement of a drug-eluting ocular insert under one or more eyelids, including re-training, and removal of existing insert, unilateral or bilateral

🚘 0.00   ⚕ 0.00   **FUD** YYY   N N1 80 ▣

AMA: 2018,Jan,8; 2017,Aug,7

0446T-0448T

> EXCLUDES *Placement non-implantable interstitial glucose sensor without pocket (95250)*

0446T Creation of subcutaneous pocket with insertion of implantable interstitial glucose sensor, including system activation and patient training

> EXCLUDES *Interpretation/report ambulatory glucose monitoring interstitial tissue (95251)*
> *Removal interstitial glucose sensor (0447T-0448T)*

🚘 0.00   ⚕ 0.00   **FUD** YYY   T G2 ▣

AMA: 2018,Jun,6

0447T Removal of implantable interstitial glucose sensor from subcutaneous pocket via incision

🚘 0.00   ⚕ 0.00   **FUD** YYY   02 G2 ▣

0448T Removal of implantable interstitial glucose sensor with creation of subcutaneous pocket at different anatomic site and insertion of new implantable sensor, including system activation

> EXCLUDES *Initial insertion sensor (0446T)*
> *Removal sensor (0447T)*

🚘 0.00   ⚕ 0.00   **FUD** YYY   T G2 ▣

0449T-0450T

> EXCLUDES *Insertion anterior segment aqueous drainage device ([0671T])*
> *Removal by internal approach aqueous drainage device without extraocular reservoir in subconjunctival space (92499)*

0449T Insertion of aqueous drainage device, without extraocular reservoir, internal approach, into the subconjunctival space; initial device

🚘 0.00   ⚕ 0.00   **FUD** YYY   J J8 ▣

AMA: 2018,Sep,3; 2018,Jul,3

+ **0450T** each additional device (List separately in addition to code for primary procedure)

Code first (0449T)

🚘 0.00   ⚕ 0.00   **FUD** YYY   N N1 ▣

AMA: 2018,Jul,3

0451T-0463T

0451T ~~Insertion or replacement of a permanently implantable aortic counterpulsation ventricular assist system, endovascular approach, and programming of sensing and therapeutic parameters; complete system (counterpulsation device, vascular graft, implantable vascular hemostatic seal, mechano-electrical skin interface and subcutaneous electrodes)~~

To report, see (33999)

0452T ~~aortic counterpulsation device and vascular hemostatic seal~~

To report, see (33999)

0453T ~~mechano-electrical skin interface~~

To report, see (33999)

0454T ~~subcutaneous electrode~~

To report, see (33999)

0455T ~~Removal of permanently implantable aortic counterpulsation ventricular assist system; complete system (aortic counterpulsation device, vascular hemostatic seal, mechano-electrical skin interface and electrodes)~~

To report, see (33999)

0456T ~~aortic counterpulsation device and vascular hemostatic seal~~

To report, see (33999)

0457T ~~mechano-electrical skin interface~~

To report, see (33999)

0458T ~~subcutaneous electrode~~

To report, see (33999)

0459T ~~Relocation of skin pocket with replacement of implanted aortic counterpulsation ventricular assist device, mechano-electrical skin interface and electrodes~~

To report, see (33999)

0460T ~~Repositioning of previously implanted aortic counterpulsation ventricular assist device; subcutaneous electrode~~

To report, see (33999)

0461T ~~aortic counterpulsation device~~

To report, see (33999)

0462T ~~Programming device evaluation (in person) with iterative adjustment of the implantable mechano-electrical skin interface and/or external driver to test the function of the device and select optimal permanent programmed values with analysis, including review and report, implantable aortic counterpulsation ventricular assist system, per day~~

To report, see (33999)

● New Code   ▲ Revised Code   ○ Reinstated   ● New Web Release   ▲ Revised Web Release   + Add-on   Unlisted   Not Covered   # Resequenced

50 Optum Mod 50 Exempt   ⚕ AMA Mod 51 Exempt   51 Optum Mod 51 Exempt   63 Mod 63 Exempt   ∕ Non-FDA Drug   ★ Telemedicine   M Maternity   A Age Edit

© 2021 Optum360, LLC   CPT © 2021 American Medical Association. All Rights Reserved.   591

0463T ~~Interrogation device evaluation (in person) with analysis, review and report, includes connection, recording and disconnection per patient encounter, implantable aortic counterpulsation ventricular assist system, per day~~

　　　To report, see (33999)

0464T [0464T]

0464T **Resequenced code. See code following 0333T.**

0465T-0469T

EXCLUDES *Replacement/revision cranial nerve neurostimulator electrode array (64569)*

0465T **Suprachoroidal injection of a pharmacologic agent (does not include supply of medication)**

　　　EXCLUDES *Intravitreal implantation or injection (67025-67028)*

　　　🚗 0.00　🔧 0.00　**FUD** YYY　　　T R2 🖵

　　　AMA: 2018,Feb,3

0466T ~~Insertion of chest wall respiratory sensor electrode or electrode array, including connection to pulse generator (List separately in addition to code for primary procedure)~~

　　　To report, see (64582-64584)

0467T ~~Revision or replacement of chest wall respiratory sensor electrode or electrode array, including connection to existing pulse generator~~

　　　To report, see (64582-64584)

0468T ~~Removal of chest wall respiratory sensor electrode or electrode array~~

　　　To report, see (64582-64584)

0469T **Retinal polarization scan, ocular screening with on-site automated results, bilateral**

　　　INCLUDES Ophthalmic medical services (92002-92014)

　　　EXCLUDES *Ocular screening (99174, [99177])*

　　　🚗 0.00　🔧 0.00　**FUD** XXX　　　E 🖵

　　　AMA: 2018,Feb,3

0470T-0471T

EXCLUDES *Optical coherence tomography coronary vessel or graft (92978-92979)*
Reflectance confocal microscopy (RCM) for cellular and subcellular skin imaging (96931-96936)

0470T **Optical coherence tomography (OCT) for microstructural and morphological imaging of skin, image acquisition, interpretation, and report; first lesion**

　　　🚗 0.00　🔧 0.00　**FUD** XXX　　　M 🖵

+ 0471T **each additional lesion (List separately in addition to code for primary procedure)**

　　　Code first (0470T)

　　　🚗 0.00　🔧 0.00　**FUD** XXX　　　N N1 🖵

0472T-0474T

0472T **Device evaluation, interrogation, and initial programming of intraocular retinal electrode array (eg, retinal prosthesis), in person, with iterative adjustment of the implantable device to test functionality, select optimal permanent programmed values with analysis, including visual training, with review and report by a qualified health care professional**

　　　🚗 0.00　🔧 0.00　**FUD** XXX　　　Q1 🖵

　　　AMA: 2018,Feb,3

0473T **Device evaluation and interrogation of intraocular retinal electrode array (eg, retinal prosthesis), in person, including reprogramming and visual training, when performed, with review and report by a qualified health care professional**

　　　INCLUDES Reprogramming device (0473T)

　　　EXCLUDES *Placement intraocular retinal electrode display (0100T)*

　　　🚗 0.00　🔧 0.00　**FUD** XXX　　　Q1 🖵

　　　AMA: 2018,Feb,3

0474T **Insertion of anterior segment aqueous drainage device, with creation of intraocular reservoir, internal approach, into the supraciliary space**

　　　🚗 0.00　🔧 0.00　**FUD** XXX　　　J 🖵

　　　AMA: 2018,Dec,8; 2018,Dec,8; 2018,Jul,3; 2018,Feb,3

0475T-0478T

0475T **Recording of fetal magnetic cardiac signal using at least 3 channels; patient recording and storage, data scanning with signal extraction, technical analysis and result, as well as supervision, review, and interpretation of report by a physician or other qualified health care professional**

　　　🚗 0.00　🔧 0.00　**FUD** XXX　　　M 🖵

0476T **patient recording, data scanning, with raw electronic signal transfer of data and storage**

　　　🚗 0.00　🔧 0.00　**FUD** XXX　　　Q1 🖵

0477T **signal extraction, technical analysis, and result**

　　　🚗 0.00　🔧 0.00　**FUD** XXX　　　Q1 🖵

0478T **review, interpretation, report by physician or other qualified health care professional**

　　　🚗 0.00　🔧 0.00　**FUD** XXX　　　M 🖵

0479T-0480T

EXCLUDES *Ablative laser treatment for additional square cm open wound (0492T)*
Cicatricial lesion excision (11400-11446)
Reporting code more than one time per day

0479T **Fractional ablative laser fenestration of burn and traumatic scars for functional improvement; first 100 cm2 or part thereof, or 1% of body surface area of infants and children**

　　　🚗 0.00　🔧 0.00　**FUD** 000　　　T 62 🖵

　　　AMA: 2018,Jan,8; 2017,Dec,13

+ 0480T **each additional 100 cm2, or each additional 1% of body surface area of infants and children, or part thereof (List separately in addition to code for primary procedure)**

　　　Code first (0479T)

　　　🚗 0.00　🔧 0.00　**FUD** ZZZ　　　N N1 🖵

　　　AMA: 2018,Jan,8; 2017,Dec,13

0481T

0481T **Injection(s), autologous white blood cell concentrate (autologous protein solution), any site, including image guidance, harvesting and preparation, when performed**

　　　INCLUDES Radiologic guidance (76942, 77002, 77012, 77021)

　　　EXCLUDES *Blood collection (36415, 36592)*
Bone marrow procedures (38220-38222, 38230)
Injection platelet rich plasma (0232T)
Injections to tendon, ligament, or fascia (20550-20551)
Joint aspiration or injection (20600-20611)
Other tissue grafts ([15769], 15771-15774)
Pooling platelets (86965)

　　　🚗 0.00　🔧 0.00　**FUD** 000　　　Q1 🖵

　　　AMA: 2019,Oct,5

0483T-0484T

INCLUDES Access and closure
Angiography
Balloon valvuloplasty
Contrast injections
Fluoroscopy
Radiological supervision and interpretation
Valve deployment and repositioning
Ventriculography

EXCLUDES *Diagnostic heart catheterization (93451-93453, 93456-93461, 93593-93598)*
Transcatheter mitral valve annulus reconstruction (0544T)
Transcatheter mitral valve repair through coronary sinus (0345T)
Transcatheter mitral valve repair with transseptal puncture, when performed (33418-33419)
Transcatheter tricuspid valve annulus reconstruction (0545T)

Code also:
　　Cardiopulmonary bypass, when provided (33367-33369)
　　Diagnostic cardiac catheterization/angiography procedures, and append modifier 59, if patient's condition (clinical indication) changed since intervention or prior study, no available prior catheter-based diagnostic study in treatment zone, or prior study not adequate (93451-93461, 93563-93564, 93593-93598)

0483T **Transcatheter mitral valve implantation/replacement (TMVI) with prosthetic valve; percutaneous approach, including transseptal puncture, when performed**

　　　🚗 0.00　🔧 0.00　**FUD** 000　　　C 80 🖵

26/TC PC/TC Only　　A2-Z3 ASC Payment　　50 Bilateral　　♂ Male Only　　♀ Female Only　　🚗 Facility RVU　　🔧 Non-Facility RVU　　🖵 CCI　　❌ CLIA
FUD Follow-up Days　　**CMS:** IOM　　**AMA:** CPT Asst　　A-Y OPPSI　　80/80 Surg Assist Allowed / w/Doc　　🖵 Lab Crosswalk　　Radiology Crosswalk

592　　　　　　　　　　　CPT © 2021 American Medical Association. All Rights Reserved.　　　　　　　　　　　© 2021 Optum360, LLC

0484T　　transthoracic exposure (eg, thoracotomy, transapical)
🚑 0.00　🔪 0.00　**FUD** 000
[C] [80] 🖥

0485T-0486T

0485T　**Optical coherence tomography (OCT) of middle ear, with interpretation and report; unilateral**
🚑 0.00　🔪 0.00　**FUD** XXX
[01] [50] 🖥

0486T　**bilateral**
🚑 0.00　🔪 0.00　**FUD** XXX
[01] 🖥

0487T-0488T [0488T]

0487T　**Biomechanical mapping, transvaginal, with report**
🚑 0.00　🔪 0.00　**FUD** XXX
[01] [N1] 🖥

0488T　Resequenced code. See code following 0403T.

0489T-0490T

EXCLUDES　Joint injection/aspiration (20600, 20604)
　　　　　Liposuction procedures (15876-15879)
　　　　　Tissue grafts ([15769], 15771-15774)
Code also for complete procedure report both codes (0489T-0490T)

0489T　**Autologous adipose-derived regenerative cell therapy for scleroderma in the hands; adipose tissue harvesting, isolation and preparation of harvested cells including incubation with cell dissociation enzymes, removal of non-viable cells and debris, determination of concentration and dilution of regenerative cells**
🚑 0.00　🔪 0.00　**FUD** 000
[E] 🖥
AMA: 2019,Oct,5; 2018,Sep,12

0490T　**multiple injections in one or both hands**
EXCLUDES　Single injections
🚑 0.00　🔪 0.00　**FUD** 000
[E] 🖥
AMA: 2019,Oct,5; 2018,Sep,12

0491T-0642T [0640T, 0641T, 0642T]

0491T　**Ablative laser treatment, non-contact, full field and fractional ablation, open wound, per day, total treatment surface area; first 20 sq cm or less**
🚑 0.00　🔪 0.00　**FUD** 000
[T] [G2] 🖥

+　**0492T**　**each additional 20 sq cm, or part thereof (List separately in addition to code for primary procedure)**
EXCLUDES　Laser fenestration scars (0479T-0480T)
Code first (0491T)
🚑 0.00　🔪 0.00　**FUD** ZZZ
[N] [N1] 🖥

▲　**0493T**　**Contact near-infrared spectroscopy studies of lower extremity wounds (eg, for oxyhemoglobin measurement)**
EXCLUDES　Noncontact near-infrared spectroscopy studies ([0640T, 0641T, 0642T])
🚑 0.00　🔪 0.00　**FUD** XXX
[N] [N1] 🖥

● **#**　**0640T**　**Noncontact near-infrared spectroscopy studies of flap or wound (eg, for measurement of deoxyhemoglobin, oxyhemoglobin, and ratio of tissue oxygenation [StO$_2$]); image acquisition, interpretation and report, each flap or wound**
INCLUDES　All complete test components ([0640T], [0641T], [0642T])
EXCLUDES　Contact near-infrared spectroscopy studies (0493T)
　　　　　Image acquisition or interpretation and report only ([0641T], [0642T])
🚑 0.00　🔪 0.00　**FUD** XXX
[80]

● **#**　**0641T**　**image acquisition only, each flap or wound**
EXCLUDES　Complete noncontact-infrared spectroscopy study ([0640T])
　　　　　Contact near-infrared spectroscopy studies (0493T)
　　　　　Interpretation and report only ([0642T])
🚑 0.00　🔪 0.00　**FUD** XXX
[80] [TC]

● **#**　**0642T**　**interpretation and report only, each flap or wound**
EXCLUDES　Complete noncontact-infrared spectroscopy study ([0640T])
　　　　　Contact near-infrared spectroscopy studies (0493T)
　　　　　Image acquisition only ([0641T])
🚑 0.00　🔪 0.00　**FUD** XXX
[80] [26]

0494T-0496T

0494T　**Surgical preparation and cannulation of marginal (extended) cadaver donor lung(s) to ex vivo organ perfusion system, including decannulation, separation from the perfusion system, and cold preservation of the allograft prior to implantation, when performed**
🚑 0.00　🔪 0.00　**FUD** XXX
[C] [80] 🖥

0495T　**Initiation and monitoring marginal (extended) cadaver donor lung(s) organ perfusion system by physician or qualified health care professional, including physiological and laboratory assessment (eg, pulmonary artery flow, pulmonary artery pressure, left atrial pressure, pulmonary vascular resistance, mean/peak and plateau airway pressure, dynamic compliance and perfusate gas analysis), including bronchoscopy and X ray when performed; first two hours in sterile field**
🚑 0.00　🔪 0.00　**FUD** XXX
[C] 🖥

+　**0496T**　**each additional hour (List separately in addition to code for primary procedure)**
Code first (0495T)
🚑 0.00　🔪 0.00　**FUD** ZZZ
[C] 🖥

0497T-0498T

EXCLUDES　ECG event monitoring (93268, 93271-93272)
　　　　　ECG rhythm strips (93040-93042)
　　　　　Remote telemetry (93228-93229)

0497T　**External patient-activated, physician- or other qualified health care professional-prescribed, electrocardiographic rhythm derived event recorder without 24 hour attended monitoring; in-office connection**
🚑 0.00　🔪 0.00　**FUD** XXX
[01] [TC] 🖥
AMA: 2020,Nov,10

0498T　**review and interpretation by a physician or other qualified health care professional per 30 days with at least one patient-generated triggered event**
🚑 0.00　🔪 0.00　**FUD** XXX
[M] [26] 🖥
AMA: 2020,Nov,10

0499T-0500T

0499T　**Cystourethroscopy, with mechanical dilation and urethral therapeutic drug delivery for urethral stricture or stenosis, including fluoroscopy, when performed**
EXCLUDES　Cystourethroscopy for stricture (52281, 52283)
🚑 0.00　🔪 0.00　**FUD** 000
[E] [G2] 🖥

0500T　**Infectious agent detection by nucleic acid (DNA or RNA), human papillomavirus (HPV) for five or more separately reported high-risk HPV types (eg, 16, 18, 31, 33, 35, 39, 45, 51, 52, 56, 58, 59, 68) (ie, genotyping)**
EXCLUDES　Less than five high-risk HPV types ([87624, 87625])
🚑 0.00　🔪 0.00　**FUD** XXX
[A] 🖥

0501T-0523T [0523T, 0623T, 0624T, 0625T, 0626T]

EXCLUDES *Reporting code more than one time for each CT angiogram*

0501T Noninvasive estimated coronary fractional flow reserve (FFR) derived from coronary computed tomography angiography data using computation fluid dynamics physiologic simulation software analysis of functional data to assess the severity of coronary artery disease; data preparation and transmission, analysis of fluid dynamics and simulated maximal coronary hyperemia, generation of estimated FFR model, with anatomical data review in comparison with estimated FFR model to reconcile discordant data, interpretation and report

  INCLUDES All complete test components (0501T-0504T)

  EXCLUDES *Automated coronary plaque characterization/quantification using coronary CT angiography data ([0623T, 0624T, 0625T, 0626T])*

  🚗 0.00   ⚕ 0.00   **FUD** XXX   M ▢

  AMA: 2018,Sep,10

0502T data preparation and transmission

  EXCLUDES *Automated coronary plaque characterization/quantification using coronary CT angiography data ([0623T, 0624T, 0625T, 0626T])*

  🚗 0.00   ⚕ 0.00   **FUD** XXX   N N1 TC ▢

  AMA: 2018,Sep,10

0503T analysis of fluid dynamics and simulated maximal coronary hyperemia, and generation of estimated FFR model

  EXCLUDES *Automated coronary plaque characterization/quantification using coronary CT angiography data ([0623T, 0624T, 0625T, 0626T])*

  🚗 0.00   ⚕ 0.00   **FUD** XXX   S N1 TC ▢

  AMA: 2018,Sep,10

0504T anatomical data review in comparison with estimated FFR model to reconcile discordant data, interpretation and report

  EXCLUDES *Automated coronary plaque characterization/quantification using coronary CT angiography data ([0623T, 0624T, 0625T, 0626T])*

  🚗 0.00   ⚕ 0.00   **FUD** XXX   M 26 ▢

  AMA: 2018,Sep,10

 # 0623T Automated quantification and characterization of coronary atherosclerotic plaque to assess severity of coronary disease, using data from coronary computed tomographic angiography; data preparation and transmission, computerized analysis of data, with review of computerized analysis output to reconcile discordant data, interpretation and report

  INCLUDES All complete test components ([0623T, 0624T, 0625T, 0626T])

  EXCLUDES *3D rendering (76376-76377)*

  Noninvasive estimated coronary fractional flow reserve (FFR) (0501T-0504T)

  Report coronary computed tomographic angiography (CTA) separately from automated analysis (75574)

  🚗 0.00   ⚕ 0.00   **FUD** XXX   80 ▢

 # 0624T data preparation and transmission

  EXCLUDES *3D rendering (76376-76377)*

  Noninvasive estimated coronary fractional flow reserve (FFR) (0501T-0504T)

  🚗 0.00   ⚕ 0.00   **FUD** XXX   80 TC ▢

 # 0625T computerized analysis of data from coronary computed tomographic angiography

  EXCLUDES *3D rendering (76376-76377)*

  Noninvasive estimated coronary fractional flow reserve (FFR) (0501T-0504T)

  🚗 0.00   ⚕ 0.00   **FUD** XXX   80 TC ▢

 # 0626T review of computerized analysis output to reconcile discordant data, interpretation and report

  EXCLUDES *3D rendering (76376-76377)*

  Noninvasive estimated coronary fractional flow reserve (FFR) (0501T-0504T)

  🚗 0.00   ⚕ 0.00   **FUD** XXX   80 26 ▢

+ # 0523T Intraprocedural coronary fractional flow reserve (FFR) with 3D functional mapping of color-coded FFR values for the coronary tree, derived from coronary angiogram data, for real-time review and interpretation of possible atherosclerotic stenosis(es) intervention (List separately in addition to code for primary procedure)

  EXCLUDES *3D rendering (76376-76377)*

  Coronary artery doppler studies (93571-93572)

  Noninvasive estimated coronary fractional flow reserve (FFR) (0501T-0504T)

  Procedure reported more than one time each session

  Code first (93454-93461)

  🚗 0.00   ⚕ 0.00   **FUD** ZZZ   N1 80 ▢

0505T-0514T [0510T, 0511T, 0512T, 0513T, 0620T]

0505T Endovenous femoral-popliteal arterial revascularization, with transcatheter placement of intravascular stent graft(s) and closure by any method, including percutaneous or open vascular access, ultrasound guidance for vascular access when performed, all catheterization(s) and intraprocedural roadmapping and imaging guidance necessary to complete the intervention, all associated radiological supervision and interpretation, when performed, with crossing of the occlusive lesion in an extraluminal fashion

  INCLUDES All procedures performed on same side:
    Catheterization (arterial and venous)
    Diagnostic imaging for arteriography
    Radiologic supervision and interpretation
  Ultrasound guidance (76937)

  EXCLUDES *Balloon angioplasty arteries other than dialysis circuit ([37248, 37249])*

  Revascularization femoral or popliteal artery (37224-37227)

  Venous stenting (37238-37239)

  🚗 0.00   ⚕ 0.00   **FUD** YYY   J8 80 ▢

 # 0620T Endovascular venous arterialization, tibial or peroneal vein, with transcatheter placement of intravascular stent graft(s) and closure by any method, including percutaneous or open vascular access, ultrasound guidance for vascular access when performed, all catheterization(s) and intraprocedural roadmapping and imaging guidance necessary to complete the intervention, all associated radiological supervision and interpretation, when performed

  INCLUDES All procedures performed on same side:
    Catheterization (arterial and venous)
    Diagnostic imaging for arteriography
    Radiologic supervision and interpretation

  EXCLUDES *When performed within tibial-peroneal segment:*
    Endovascular revascularization procedures (37228-37231)
    Transcatheter intravascular stent placement (37238-37239)
    Transluminal balloon angioplasty ([37248, 37249])

  🚗 0.00   ⚕ 0.00   **FUD** YYY   J8 80 50 ▢

0506T Macular pigment optical density measurement by heterochromatic flicker photometry, unilateral or bilateral, with interpretation and report

  🚗 0.00   ⚕ 0.00   **FUD** XXX   80 ▢

  AMA: 2018,Dec,6; 2018,Dec,6

0507T Near-infrared dual imaging (ie, simultaneous reflective and trans-illuminated light) of meibomian glands, unilateral or bilateral, with interpretation and report

  EXCLUDES *External ocular photography (92285)*

  Tear film imaging (0330T)

  🚗 0.00   ⚕ 0.00   **FUD** XXX   80 ▢

26/TC PC/TC Only   A2-Z3 ASC Payment   50 Bilateral   ♂ Male Only   ♀ Female Only   🚗 Facility RVU   ⚕ Non-Facility RVU   ▢ CCI   ✖ CLIA
FUD Follow-up Days   CMS: IOM   AMA: CPT Asst   A-Y OPPSI   80/80 Surg Assist Allowed / w/Doc   ▨ Lab Crosswalk   ▨ Radiology Crosswalk

594   CPT © 2021 American Medical Association. All Rights Reserved.   © 2021 Optum360, LLC

0508T Pulse-echo ultrasound bone density measurement resulting in indicator of axial bone mineral density, tibia
    🚐 0.00   ✂ 0.00   **FUD** XXX   [Z2] [80] 🖼

0509T Electroretinography (ERG) with interpretation and report, pattern (PERG)
    EXCLUDES   *Full field ERG (92273)*
               Multifocal ERG (92274)
    🚐 2.24   ✂ 2.24   **FUD** XXX   [80] 🖼
    AMA: 2019,Jan,12

0510T **Resequenced code. See code following 0335T.**

0511T **Resequenced code. See code following 0335T.**

0512T **Resequenced code. See code following 0102T.**

0513T **Resequenced code. See code following 0102T.**

+ 0514T Intraoperative visual axis identification using patient fixation (List separately in addition to code for primary procedure)
    Code first (66982, 66984)
    🚐 0.00   ✂ 0.00   **FUD** ZZZ   [N1] 🖼
    AMA: 2018,Dec,6; 2018,Dec,6

0515T-0523T [0523T]

INCLUDES   Complete system with two components
        Pulse generator including battery and transmitter
        Wireless endocardial left ventricular electrode

0515T Insertion of wireless cardiac stimulator for left ventricular pacing, including device interrogation and programming, and imaging supervision and interpretation, when performed; complete system (includes electrode and generator [transmitter and battery])
    INCLUDES   Catheterization (93452-93453, 93458-93461, 93595-93597)
            Creation pockets
            Electrode insertion
            Imaging guidance (76000, 76998, 93303-93355 [93319, 93356])
            Insertion complete wireless cardiac stimulator system
            Interrogation device (0521T)
            Programming device (0522T)
            Pulse generator (battery and transmitter) (0517T)
            Revision and repositioning
    EXCLUDES   *Insertion electrode as separate procedure (0516T)*
            Removal/replacement device or components (0518T-0520T)
    🚐 0.00   ✂ 0.00   **FUD** YYY   [J8] 🖼

0516T electrode only
    INCLUDES   Catheterization (93452-93453, 93458-93461, 93595-93597)
            Imaging guidance (76000, 76998, 93303-93355 [93319, 93356])
            Interrogation device (0521T)
            Programming device (0522T)
    EXCLUDES   *Removal/replacement device or components (0518T-0520T)*
    🚐 0.00   ✂ 0.00   **FUD** YYY   [G2] 🖼

0517T pulse generator component(s) (battery and/or transmitter) only
    INCLUDES   Catheterization (93452-93453, 93458-93461, 93595-93597)
            Imaging guidance (76000, 76998, 93303-93355 [93319, 93356])
            Interrogation device (0521T)
            Programming device (0522T)
    EXCLUDES   *Removal/replacement device or components (0518T-0520T)*
    🚐 0.00   ✂ 0.00   **FUD** YYY   [J8] 🖼

0518T Removal of only pulse generator component(s) (battery and/or transmitter) of wireless cardiac stimulator for left ventricular pacing
    INCLUDES   Catheterization (93452-93453, 93458-93461, 93595-93597)
            Imaging guidance (76000, 76998, 93303-93355 [93319, 93356])
            Interrogation device (0521T)
            Programming device (0522T)
            Pulse generator (battery and transmitter) (0517T)
    EXCLUDES   *Complete procedure (0515T)*
            Insertion electrode only (0516T)
            Removal/replacement device or components (0519T-0520T)
    🚐 0.00   ✂ 0.00   **FUD** YYY   [G2] 🖼

0519T Removal and replacement of wireless cardiac stimulator for left ventricular pacing; pulse generator component(s) (battery and/or transmitter)
    INCLUDES   Catheterization (93452-93453, 93458-93461, 93595-93597)
            Imaging guidance (76000, 76998, 93303-93355 [93319, 93356])
            Interrogation device (0521T)
            Programming device (0522T)
            Pulse generator (battery and transmitter) (0517T)
    EXCLUDES   *Complete procedure (0515T)*
            Insertion electrode only (0516T)
            Removal/replacement device or components (0518T)
    🚐 0.00   ✂ 0.00   **FUD** YYY   [J8] 🖼

0520T pulse generator component(s) (battery and/or transmitter), including placement of a new electrode
    INCLUDES   Catheterization (93452-93453, 93458-93461, 93595-93597)
            Imaging guidance (76000, 76998, 93303-93355 [93319, 93356])
            Interrogation device (0521T)
            Programming device (0522T)
            Pulse generator (battery and transmitter) (0517T)
    EXCLUDES   *Complete procedure (0515T)*
            Insertion electrode only (0516T)
            Removal only device or components (0518T)
    🚐 0.00   ✂ 0.00   **FUD** YYY   [J8] 🖼

0521T Interrogation device evaluation (in person) with analysis, review and report, includes connection, recording, and disconnection per patient encounter, wireless cardiac stimulator for left ventricular pacing
    INCLUDES   Programming device (0522T)
            Pulse generator (battery and transmitter) (0517T)
    EXCLUDES   *Complete procedure (0515T)*
            Insertion electrode only (0516T)
            Removal/replacement device or components (0518T-0520T)
    🚐 0.00   ✂ 0.00   **FUD** XXX   🖼

0522T Programming device evaluation (in person) with iterative adjustment of the implantable device to test the function of the device and select optimal permanent programmed values with analysis, including review and report, wireless cardiac stimulator for left ventricular pacing
    INCLUDES   Interrogation device (0521T)
            Pulse generator (battery and transmitter) (0517T)
    EXCLUDES   *Complete procedure (0515T)*
            Insertion electrode only (0516T)
            Removal/replacement device or components (0518T-0520T)
    🚐 0.00   ✂ 0.00   **FUD** XXX   🖼

0523T **Resequenced code. See code before 0505T.**

● New Code   ▲ Revised Code   ○ Reinstated   ● New Web Release   ▲ Revised Web Release   + Add-on   Unlisted   Not Covered   # Resequenced
 Optum Mod 50 Exempt   AMA Mod 51 Exempt   ⑤① Optum Mod 51 Exempt   ㊚ Mod 63 Exempt   ✗ Non-FDA Drug   ★ Telemedicine   Ⓜ Maternity   Ⓐ Age Edit

0524T

0524T Endovenous catheter directed chemical ablation with balloon isolation of incompetent extremity vein, open or percutaneous, including all vascular access, catheter manipulation, diagnostic imaging, imaging guidance and monitoring

🚑 0.00   🔪 0.00   **FUD** YYY   G2 50 ▣

0525T-0532T

0525T Insertion or replacement of intracardiac ischemia monitoring system, including testing of the lead and monitor, initial system programming, and imaging supervision and interpretation; complete system (electrode and implantable monitor)

INCLUDES   Electrocardiography (93000, 93005, 93010)
Interrogation device (0529T)
Programming device (0528T)

EXCLUDES   Removal intracardiac ischemia monitor or components (0530T-0532T)

🚑 0.00   🔪 0.00   **FUD** YYY   J8 ▣

0526T electrode only

INCLUDES   Electrocardiography (93000, 93005, 93010)
Interrogation device (0529T)
Programming device (0528T)

EXCLUDES   Removal intracardiac ischemia monitor or components (0530T-0532T)

🚑 0.00   🔪 0.00   **FUD** YYY   J8 ▣

0527T implantable monitor only

INCLUDES   Electrocardiography (93000, 93005, 93010)
Interrogation device (0529T)
Programming device (0528T)

EXCLUDES   Removal intracardiac ischemia monitor or components (0530T-0532T)

🚑 0.00   🔪 0.00   **FUD** YYY   G2 ▣

0528T Programming device evaluation (in person) of intracardiac ischemia monitoring system with iterative adjustment of programmed values, with analysis, review, and report

INCLUDES   Electrocardiography (93000, 93005, 93010)

EXCLUDES   Insertion/replacement intracardiac ischemia monitor or components (0525T-0527T)
Interrogation device (0529T)
Removal intracardiac ischemia monitor or components (0530T-0532T)

🚑 0.00   🔪 0.00   **FUD** XXX   ▣

0529T Interrogation device evaluation (in person) of intracardiac ischemia monitoring system with analysis, review, and report

INCLUDES   Electrocardiography (93000, 93005, 93010)

EXCLUDES   Insertion/replacement electrode only (0526T)
Insertion/replacement intracardiac ischemia monitor or components (0525T-0527T)
Programming device (0528T)
Removal intracardiac ischemia monitor or components (0530T-0532T)

🚑 0.00   🔪 0.00   **FUD** XXX   ▣

0530T Removal of intracardiac ischemia monitoring system, including all imaging supervision and interpretation; complete system (electrode and implantable monitor)

EXCLUDES   Interrogation device (0529T)
Programming device (0528T)

🚑 0.00   🔪 0.00   **FUD** YYY   G2 ▣

0531T electrode only

EXCLUDES   Interrogation device (0529T)
Programming device (0528T)

🚑 0.00   🔪 0.00   **FUD** YYY   G2 ▣

0532T implantable monitor only

EXCLUDES   Interrogation device (0529T)
Programming device (0528T)

🚑 0.00   🔪 0.00   **FUD** YYY   G2 ▣

0533T-0536T

0533T Continuous recording of movement disorder symptoms, including bradykinesia, dyskinesia, and tremor for 6 days up to 10 days; includes set-up, patient training, configuration of monitor, data upload, analysis and initial report configuration, download review, interpretation and report

🚑 0.00   🔪 0.00   **FUD** XXX   ▣

0534T set-up, patient training, configuration of monitor

🚑 0.00   🔪 0.00   **FUD** XXX   ▣

0535T data upload, analysis and initial report configuration

🚑 0.00   🔪 0.00   **FUD** XXX   ▣

0536T download review, interpretation and report

🚑 0.00   🔪 0.00   **FUD** XXX   ▣

0537T-0540T

CMS: 100-04,32,400 Chimeric Antigen Receptor (CAR) T-cell therapy; 100-04,32,400.1 Coverage Requirements; 100-04,32,400.2 Billing Requirements; 100-04,32,400.2.1 A/B Medicare Administrative Contractor (MAC) (A) Bill Types; 100-04,32,400.2.2 A/B MAC (A) Revenue Code; 100-04,32,400.2.3 A/B MAC Billing HCPCS Codes; 100-04,32,400.2.4 A/B MAC Diagnosis Requirements; 100-04,32,400.3 Payment Requirements; 100-04,32,400.4 Claim Adjustment Reason Codes (CARCs), Remittance Advice Remark Codes (RARCs), Group Codes, and Medicare Summary Notice (MSN) Messages; 100-04,32,400.5 Claims Editing

INCLUDES   Administration genetically modified cells for treatment serious diseases (e.g., cancer)
Evaluation prior to, during, and after CAR-T cell administration
Infusion fluids and supportive medications provided with administration
Management clinical staff
Management untoward events (e.g., nausea)
Physician certification, processing cells
Physician presence during cell administration
Code also care provided not directly related to CAR-T cell administration (e.g., other medical problems) may be reported separately using appropriate E/M code and appending modifier 25

0537T Chimeric antigen receptor T-cell (CAR-T) therapy; harvesting of blood-derived T lymphocytes for development of genetically modified autologous CAR-T cells, per day

EXCLUDES   Reporting more than one time per day despite times cells are collected

🚑 0.00   🔪 0.00   **FUD** XXX   ▣

AMA: 2019,Jun,5

0538T preparation of blood-derived T lymphocytes for transportation (eg, cryopreservation, storage)

🚑 0.00   🔪 0.00   **FUD** XXX   ▣

AMA: 2019,Jun,5

0539T receipt and preparation of CAR-T cells for administration

🚑 0.00   🔪 0.00   **FUD** XXX   ▣

AMA: 2019,Jun,5

0540T CAR-T cell administration, autologous

EXCLUDES   Reporting more than one time per day despite units administered

🚑 0.00   🔪 0.00   **FUD** YYY   ▣

AMA: 2019,Jun,5

0541T-0542T

0541T Myocardial imaging by magnetocardiography (MCG) for detection of cardiac ischemia, by signal acquisition using minimum 36 channel grid, generation of magnetic-field time-series images, quantitative analysis of magnetic dipoles, machine learning-derived clinical scoring, and automated report generation, single study;

🚑 0.00   🔪 0.00   **FUD** XXX   TC ▣

0542T interpretation and report

🚑 0.00   🔪 0.00   **FUD** XXX   26 ▣

0543T

EXCLUDES *Transesophageal echocardiography (93355)*

0543T **Transapical mitral valve repair, including transthoracic echocardiography, when performed, with placement of artificial chordae tendineae**
🚗 0.00   ⚕ 0.00   **FUD** YYY   [80] [▢]

0544T-0643T [0643T]

INCLUDES   Adjustment/deployment reconstruction device
Catheterization
Fluoroscopic guidance (76000)
Insertion temporary pacemaker
Vascular access and closure

EXCLUDES *Diagnostic cardiac catheterization procedures integral to valve procedure (93451-93461, 93565-93566, 93593-93598)*
Percutaneous mitral valve repair (0345T)

Code also diagnostic cardiac catheterization/angiography procedures, and append modifier 59, if patient's condition (clinical indication) changed since intervention or prior study, no available prior catheter-based diagnostic study in treatment zone, or prior study not adequate (93451-93461, 93563-93564, 93593-93598)
Code also transcatheter implantation/replacement mitral valve (0483T)
Code also when performed:
Balloon pump insertion (33967, 33970, 33973)
Central bypass (33369)
Peripheral bypass (33367-33368)
Ventricular assist device (33990-33993)

0544T **Transcatheter mitral valve annulus reconstruction, with implantation of adjustable annulus reconstruction device, percutaneous approach including transseptal puncture**

EXCLUDES *Transcatheter mitral valve repair (33418-33419)*
Transcatheter mitral valve repair via coronary sinus (0345T)
🚗 0.00   ⚕ 0.00   **FUD** YYY   [80] [▢]

0545T **Transcatheter tricuspid valve annulus reconstruction with implantation of adjustable annulus reconstruction device, percutaneous approach**

EXCLUDES *Left ventricular restoration device not necessitating transseptal puncture ([0643T])*
Repositioning/plication tricuspid valve (33468)
🚗 0.00   ⚕ 0.00   **FUD** YYY   [80] [▢]

● # **0643T** **Transcatheter left ventricular restoration device implantation including right and left heart catheterization and left ventriculography when performed, arterial approach**

INCLUDES   Guide catheter(s) and snare wire(s), when performed
Left ventriculography (93565)
Primary and contralateral arterial access

EXCLUDES *Transcatheter mitral valve annulus reconstruction (0544T)*
🚗 0.00   ⚕ 0.00   **FUD** YYY   [80]

0546T

EXCLUDES *Reporting code for re-excision of site*
Reporting code more than one time per partial mastectomy site

0546T **Radiofrequency spectroscopy, real time, intraoperative margin assessment, at the time of partial mastectomy, with report**
🚗 0.00   ⚕ 0.00   **FUD** YYY   [80] [▢]
AMA: 2020,May,9

0547T

0547T **Bone-material quality testing by microindentation(s) of the tibia(s), with results reported as a score**
🚗 0.00   ⚕ 0.00   **FUD** XXX   [80]

0548T-0551T

~~0548T~~   ~~Transperineal periurethral balloon continence device; bilateral placement, including cystoscopy and fluoroscopy~~
To report, see (53451-53454)

~~0549T~~   ~~unilateral placement, including cystoscopy and fluoroscopy~~
To report, see (53451-53454)

~~0550T~~   ~~removal, each balloon~~
To report, see (53451-53454)

~~0551T~~   ~~adjustment of balloon(s) fluid volume~~
To report, see (53451-53454)

0552T

0552T **Low-level laser therapy, dynamic photonic and dynamic thermokinetic energies, provided by a physician or other qualified health care professional**
🚗 0.00   ⚕ 0.00   **FUD** YYY   [80] [▢]

0553T

EXCLUDES *Angiography extremity (75710)*
Endovascular revascularization (37220-37221, 37224, 37226, 37238)
Injection for venography (36005)
Insertion catheter/needle, upper or lower extremity artery (36140)
Selective catheter placement (36011-36012, 36245-36246)
Transluminal balloon angioplasty ([37248])
Venography (75820)

0553T **Percutaneous transcatheter placement of iliac arteriovenous anastomosis implant, inclusive of all radiological supervision and interpretation, intraprocedural roadmapping, and imaging guidance necessary to complete the intervention**
🚗 0.00   ⚕ 0.00   **FUD** YYY   [80] [▢]

0554T-0557T

EXCLUDES *Automated analysis existing CT study for vertebral fracture(s) (0691T)*

0554T **Bone strength and fracture risk using finite element analysis of functional data, and bone-mineral density, utilizing data from a computed tomography scan; retrieval and transmission of the scan data, assessment of bone strength and fracture risk and bone mineral density, interpretation and report**

INCLUDES   Assessment, interpretation and report, and retrieval and transmission of data (0555T-0557T)
🚗 0.00   ⚕ 0.00   **FUD** XXX   [80] [▢]
AMA: 2020,Sep,11

0555T **retrieval and transmission of the scan data**
🚗 0.00   ⚕ 0.00   **FUD** XXX   [80]
AMA: 2020,Sep,11

0556T **assessment of bone strength and fracture risk and bone mineral density**
🚗 0.00   ⚕ 0.00   **FUD** XXX   [80]
AMA: 2020,Sep,11

0557T **interpretation and report**
🚗 0.00   ⚕ 0.00   **FUD** XXX   [80]
AMA: 2020,Sep,11

0558T

EXCLUDES *Automated analysis existing CT study for vertebral fracture(s) (0691T)*
Computed tomography:
Abdominal aorta (75635)
Abdomen/pelvis (72191-72194, 74150-74178)
Chest/thorax (71250-71270, 71275)
Colonography (74261-74263)
Heart (75571-75574)
Spine (72125-72133)
Whole body (78816)

0558T **Computed tomography scan taken for the purpose of biomechanical computed tomography analysis**
🚗 0.00   ⚕ 0.00   **FUD** XXX   [Z2] [80] [▢]
AMA: 2020,Sep,11

0559T-0562T

EXCLUDES *3D rendering (76376-76377)*

0559T **Anatomic model 3D-printed from image data set(s); first individually prepared and processed component of an anatomic structure**

INCLUDES   3D printed anatomical model production
🚗 0.00   ⚕ 0.00   **FUD** XXX   [80] [▢]

+ **0560T** **each additional individually prepared and processed component of an anatomic structure (List separately in addition to code for primary procedure)**

INCLUDES   3D printed anatomical model production
Code first (0559T)
🚗 0.00   ⚕ 0.00   **FUD** ZZZ   [80] [▢]

0561T   Anatomic guide 3D-printed and designed from image data set(s); first anatomic guide

> INCLUDES   3D printed cutting or drilling guides for use during surgery
>
> 🖭 0.00   ✂ 0.00   **FUD** XXX   80 ▭

+ **0562T**   each additional anatomic guide (List separately in addition to code for primary procedure)

> INCLUDES   3D printed cutting or drilling guides for use during surgery
>
> Code first (0561T)
>
> 🖭 0.00   ✂ 0.00   **FUD** ZZZ   80 ▭

0563T-0564T [0563T]

0563T   Resequenced code. See code before code 0207T.

0564T   Oncology, chemotherapeutic drug cytotoxicity assay of cancer stem cells (CSCs), from cultured CSCs and primary tumor cells, categorical drug response reported based on percent of cytotoxicity observed, a minimum of 14 drugs or drug combinations

> 🖭 0.00   ✂ 0.00   **FUD** YYY   80

0565T-0566T

0565T   Autologous cellular implant derived from adipose tissue for the treatment of osteoarthritis of the knees; tissue harvesting and cellular implant creation

> EXCLUDES   Other tissue grafts ([15769], 15771-15774)
>
> 🖭 0.00   ✂ 0.00   **FUD** YYY   80 ▭

0566T   injection of cellular implant into knee joint including ultrasound guidance, unilateral

> INCLUDES   Guidance for needle placement:
>   Fluoroscopy (77002)
>   Ultrasound (76942)
>
> EXCLUDES   Arthrocentesis, with or without imaging guidance (20610-20611)
>
> 🖭 0.00   ✂ 0.00   **FUD** YYY   R2 80 ▭

0567T-0568T

0567T   Permanent fallopian tube occlusion with degradable biopolymer implant, transcervical approach, including transvaginal ultrasound   ♀

> INCLUDES   Transvaginal ultrasound (76830)
>
> EXCLUDES   Catheter insertion and introduction saline/contrast for sonohysterography or hysterosalpingography (58340)
>   Hysterosalpingography (74740)
>   Nonobstetric pelvic ultrasound (76856-76857)
>   Surgical hysteroscopy with bilateral occlusion fallopian tube (58565)
>   Transcervical catheterization fallopian tube (74742)
>
> 🖭 0.00   ✂ 0.00   **FUD** YYY   80 ▭

0568T   Introduction of mixture of saline and air for sonosalpingography to confirm occlusion of fallopian tubes, transcervical approach, including transvaginal ultrasound and pelvic ultrasound   ♀

> INCLUDES   Transvaginal ultrasound (76830)
>
> EXCLUDES   Catheter insertion and introduction saline/contrast for sonohysterography or hysterosalpingography (58340)
>   Hysterosalpingography (74740)
>   Nonobstetric pelvic ultrasound (76856-76857)
>   Sonohysterography (SIS) (76831)
>   Surgical hysteroscopy with bilateral occlusion fallopian tube (58565)
>   Transcervical catheterization fallopian tube (74742)
>
> 🖭 0.00   ✂ 0.00   **FUD** YYY   80 ▭

0569T-0646T [0646T]

> INCLUDES   Adjustment/deployment prosthetic device
>   Catheterization
>   Fluoroscopic guidance (76000)
>   Intracardiac echocardiography (93662)
>   Vascular access and closure
>
> EXCLUDES   Open tricuspid valve procedures (33460, 33463-33465, 33468)

Code also diagnostic cardiac catheterization/angiography procedures, and append modifer 59, if patient's condition (clinical indication) changed since intervention or prior study, no available prior catheter-based diagnostic study in treatment zone, or prior study not adequate (93451-93461, 93563-93564, 93593-93598)

Code also when performed:
     Balloon pump insertion (33967, 33970, 33973)
     Central bypass (33369)
     Peripheral bypass (33367-33368)
     Ventricular assist device (33990-33993)
     TEE, when done by different operator (93355)

0569T   Transcatheter tricuspid valve repair, percutaneous approach; initial prosthesis

> EXCLUDES   Reporting code more than once per session
>
> 🖭 0.00   ✂ 0.00   **FUD** YYY   80 ▭

+ **0570T**   each additional prosthesis during same session (List separately in addition to code for primary procedure)

> Code first (0569T)
>
> 🖭 0.00   ✂ 0.00   **FUD** ZZZ   80 ▭

● # **0646T**   Transcatheter tricuspid valve implantation (TTVI)/replacement with prosthetic valve, percutaneous approach, including right heart catheterization, temporary pacemaker insertion, and selective right ventricular or right atrial angiography, when performed

> INCLUDES   Temporary pacemaker insertion (33210-33211)
>
> EXCLUDES   Tricuspid valve:
>   Transcatheter,
>   Reconstruction (0545T)
>   Repair (0569T-0570T)
>
> 🖭 0.00   ✂ 0.00   **FUD** YYY   80

0571T-0614T [0614T]

> EXCLUDES   Defibrillator or pacemaker device evaluations (93279-93284, 93285-93289, 93290-93298)
>   Implantable defibrillator procedures (33215-33220, 33223-33226, 33240-33249 [33230, 33231, 33262, 33263, 33264])
>   Pacemaker procedures (33202-33220 [33221], 33222-33226, 33233-33238 [33227, 33228, 33229])
>   Subcutaneous implantable defibrillator system procedures:
>   Electrophysiological evaluation (93644)
>   Insertion electrode ([33271])
>   Insertion/replacement entire system ([33270])
>   Interrogation ([93261])
>   Programming ([93260])
>   Removal electrode ([33272])
>   Repositioning electrode ([33273])
>   Transcatheter permanent leadless pacemaker procedures:
>   Insertion or replacement ([33274])

0571T   Insertion or replacement of implantable cardioverter-defibrillator system with substernal electrode(s), including all imaging guidance and electrophysiological evaluation (includes defibrillation threshold evaluation, induction of arrhythmia, evaluation of sensing for arrhythmia termination, and programming or reprogramming of sensing or therapeutic parameters), when performed

> INCLUDES   Imaging guidance
>   Programming, interrogation, and electrophysiological evaluations (0575T-0577T)
>
> EXCLUDES   Substernal electrode insertion only (0572T)

Code also removal implantable cardioverter-defibrillator generator and substernal electrode(s), when total system replaced:
     Electrode(s) (0573T)
     Generator (0580T)

> 🖭 0.00   ✂ 0.00   **FUD** YYY   80 ▭

26/TC PC/TC Only   A2-Z3 ASC Payment   50 Bilateral   ♂ Male Only   ♀ Female Only   🖭 Facility RVU   ✂ Non-Facility RVU   ▭ CCI   ✖ CLIA

FUD Follow-up Days   **CMS:** IOM   **AMA:** CPT Asst   A-Y OPPSI   80/80 Surg Assist Allowed / w/Doc   ▭ Lab Crosswalk   ▭ Radiology Crosswalk

598   CPT © 2021 American Medical Association. All Rights Reserved.   © 2021 Optum360, LLC

0572T   Insertion of substernal implantable defibrillator electrode

> INCLUDES   Imaging guidance
>
> EXCLUDES   *Insertion generator and electrode (0571T)*
>
> *Programming, interrogation, and electrophysiological evaluations (0575T-0577T)*
>
> *Removal generator only (0580T)*
>
> 🚑 0.00   ⚕ 0.00   **FUD** YYY   80 ▢

0573T   Removal of substernal implantable defibrillator electrode

> INCLUDES   Imaging guidance
>
> EXCLUDES   *Programming, interrogation, and electrophysiological evaluations (0575T-0577T)*
>
> Code also removal implantable cardioverter-defibrillator generator and insertion new generator/electrode, when total system replaced:
>
> Insertion new system (0571T)
>
> Removal generator (0580T)
>
> Code also removal generator when system not replaced (0580T)
>
> 🚑 0.00   ⚕ 0.00   **FUD** YYY   80 ▢

0574T   Repositioning of previously implanted substernal implantable defibrillator-pacing electrode

> INCLUDES   Imaging guidance
>
> EXCLUDES   *Programming, interrogation, and electrophysiological evaluations (0575T-0577T)*
>
> *Substernal electrode insertion only (0572T)*
>
> 🚑 0.00   ⚕ 0.00   **FUD** YYY   80 ▢

0575T   Programming device evaluation (in person) of implantable cardioverter-defibrillator system with substernal electrode, with iterative adjustment of the implantable device to test the function of the device and select optimal permanent programmed values with analysis, review and report by a physician or other qualified health care professional

> EXCLUDES   *Interrogation and programming device (93260 [93260], 93282, 93287, 0576T)*
>
> *Programming during:*
>
> *Electrode insertion (0572T)*
>
> *Electrode removal (0573T)*
>
> *Electrode repositioning (0574T)*
>
> *Generator removal (0580T)*
>
> *Insertion/replacement entire system (0571T)*
>
> *Removal and replacement generator ([0614T])*
>
> 🚑 0.00   ⚕ 0.00   **FUD** YYY   80 ▢

0576T   Interrogation device evaluation (in person) of implantable cardioverter-defibrillator system with substernal electrode, with analysis, review and report by a physician or other qualified health care professional, includes connection, recording and disconnection per patient encounter

> EXCLUDES   *Interrogation and programming device (93261 [93261], 93289, 0575T)*
>
> *Interrogation during:*
>
> *Electrode insertion (0572T)*
>
> *Electrode removal (0573T)*
>
> *Electrode repositioning (0574T)*
>
> *Generator removal (0580T)*
>
> *Insertion/replacement entire system (0571T)*
>
> *Removal and replacement generator ([0614T])*
>
> 🚑 0.00   ⚕ 0.00   **FUD** YYY   80 ▢

0577T   Electrophysiologic evaluation of implantable cardioverter-defibrillator system with substernal electrode (includes defibrillation threshold evaluation, induction of arrhythmia, evaluation of sensing for arrhythmia termination, and programming or reprogramming of sensing or therapeutic parameters)

> EXCLUDES   *Electrophysiologic evaluation during:*
>
> *Electrode insertion (0572T)*
>
> *Electrode removal (0573T)*
>
> *Electrode repositioning (0574T)*
>
> *Generator removal (0580T)*
>
> *Insertion/replacement entire system (0571T)*
>
> *Removal and replacement generator ([0614T])*
>
> *Electrophysiologic evaluation of subcutaneous implantable defibrillator (93644)*
>
> 🚑 0.00   ⚕ 0.00   **FUD** YYY   80 ▢

0578T   Interrogation device evaluation(s) (remote), up to 90 days, substernal lead implantable cardioverter-defibrillator system with interim analysis, review(s) and report(s) by a physician or other qualified health care professional

> EXCLUDES   *In person device interrogation (0576T)*
>
> *Reporting code more than once per 90 days*
>
> 🚑 0.00   ⚕ 0.00   **FUD** YYY   80 ▢

0579T   Interrogation device evaluation(s) (remote), up to 90 days, substernal lead implantable cardioverter-defibrillator system, remote data acquisition(s), receipt of transmissions and technician review, technical support and distribution of results

> EXCLUDES   *In person device interrogation (0576T)*
>
> *Reporting code more than once per 90 days*
>
> 🚑 0.00   ⚕ 0.00   **FUD** YYY   80 ▢

0580T   Removal of substernal implantable defibrillator pulse generator only

> INCLUDES   Removal generator when system not replaced
>
> EXCLUDES   *Programming, interrogation, and electrophysiological evaluations (0575T-0577T)*
>
> *Removal and replacement generator ([33262])*
>
> Code also removal substernal electrode and insertion new generator/electrode, when total system replaced:
>
> Insertion new system (0571T)
>
> 🚑 0.00   ⚕ 0.00   **FUD** YYY   80 ▢

0614T   Removal and replacement of substernal implantable defibrillator pulse generator

> EXCLUDES   *Electrode insertion (0572T)*
>
> *Insertion/replacement entire system (0571T)*
>
> *Programming, interrogation, and electrophysiological evaluations (0575T-0577T)*
>
> *Removal generator only (0580T)*
>
> *Removal/replacement single lead system ([33262])*
>
> 🚑 0.00   ⚕ 0.00   **FUD** YYY   J8 80 ▢

0581T-0582T

0581T   Ablation, malignant breast tumor(s), percutaneous, cryotherapy, including imaging guidance when performed, unilateral

> INCLUDES   Ultrasound for:
>
> Breast imaging (76641-76642)
>
> Monitoring tissue ablation (76940)
>
> Needle placement (76942)
>
> EXCLUDES   *Cryoablation for breast fibroadenoma(s) (19105)*
>
> *Reporting code more than once per treated breast*
>
> 🚑 0.00   ⚕ 0.00   **FUD** YYY   80 ▢

0572T — 0581T

Category III Codes

0582T — 0592T

0582T   Transurethral ablation of malignant prostate tissue by high-energy water vapor thermotherapy, including intraoperative imaging and needle guidance ♂

INCLUDES   3D rendering (76376-76377)
Cystourethroscopy (52000)
MRI pelvis (72195-72197)
Radiologic guidance for:
  Needle placement (76942, 77021)
  Tissue ablation monitoring (76940, 77022)
Transrectal ultrasound (76872)

EXCLUDES   *Destruction by radiofrequency-generated water vapor thermotherapy for benign prostatic hypertrophy (BPH) (53854)*

🚗 0.00   ⚕ 0.00   **FUD** YYY   80 ▭

0583T

0583T   Tympanostomy (requiring insertion of ventilating tube), using an automated tube delivery system, iontophoresis local anesthesia

INCLUDES   Binocular microscopy (92504)
Iontophoresis (97033)
Operating microscope (69990)

EXCLUDES   *Myringotomy (69420-69421)*
Removal impacted cerumen (69209-69210)
Tympanostomy without automated delivery system (69433, 69436)

🚗 0.00   ⚕ 0.00   **FUD** YYY   J8 80 ▭

0584T-0586T

0584T   Islet cell transplant, includes portal vein catheterization and infusion, including all imaging, including guidance, and radiological supervision and interpretation, when performed; percutaneous

🚗 0.00   ⚕ 0.00   **FUD** YYY   80 ▭

0585T   laparoscopic

🚗 0.00   ⚕ 0.00   **FUD** YYY   80 ▭

0586T   open

🚗 0.00   ⚕ 0.00   **FUD** YYY   80 ▭

0587T-0590T

0587T   Percutaneous implantation or replacement of integrated single device neurostimulation system including electrode array and receiver or pulse generator, including analysis, programming, and imaging guidance when performed, posterior tibial nerve

INCLUDES   Electronic analysis (95970-95972, 0589T-0590T)

EXCLUDES   *Insertion other neurostimulator devices (64555, 64566, 64575, 64590)*
Revision or removal integrated neurostimulation system (0588T)

🚗 0.00   ⚕ 0.00   **FUD** YYY   J8 80 ▭

0588T   Revision or removal of integrated single device neurostimulation system including electrode array and receiver or pulse generator, including analysis, programming, and imaging guidance when performed, posterior tibial nerve

INCLUDES   Electronic analysis (95970-95972, 0589T-0590T)

EXCLUDES   *Initial insertion or replacement integrated neurostimulation system (0587T)*
Insertion other neurostimulator devices (64555, 64566, 64575, 64590)

🚗 0.00   ⚕ 0.00   **FUD** YYY   R2 80 ▭

0589T   Electronic analysis with simple programming of implanted integrated neurostimulation system (eg, electrode array and receiver), including contact group(s), amplitude, pulse width, frequency (Hz), on/off cycling, burst, dose lockout, patient-selectable parameters, responsive neurostimulation, detection algorithms, closed-loop parameters, and passive parameters, when performed by physician or other qualified health care professional, posterior tibial nerve, 1-3 parameters

EXCLUDES   *Electronic analysis other implanted neurostimulators (95970-95977, [95983, 95984])*
Electronic analysis with complex programming (0590T)
Reporting code during insertion, replacement, revision, or removal integrated neurostimulation system (0587T-0588T)
Reporting code during insertion, replacement, revision, or removal other neurostimulator device (generator and/or electrode) (43647-43648, 43881-43882, 61850-61888, 63650, 63655, 63661-63688, 64553-64595)

🚗 0.00   ⚕ 0.00   **FUD** YYY   80 ▭

0590T   Electronic analysis with complex programming of implanted integrated neurostimulation system (eg, electrode array and receiver), including contact group(s), amplitude, pulse width, frequency (Hz), on/off cycling, burst, dose lockout, patient-selectable parameters, responsive neurostimulation, detection algorithms, closed-loop parameters, and passive parameters, when performed by physician or other qualified health care professional, posterior tibial nerve, 4 or more parameters

EXCLUDES   *Electronic analysis other implanted neurostimulators (95970-95977, [95983, 95984])*
Electronic analysis with simple programming (0589T)
Reporting code during insertion, replacement, revision, or removal integrated neurostimulation system (0587T-0588T)
Reporting code during insertion, replacement, revision, or removal other neurostimulator device (generator and/or electrode) (43647-43648, 43881-43882, 61850-61888, 63650, 63655, 63661-63688, 64553-64595)

🚗 0.00   ⚕ 0.00   **FUD** YYY   80 ▭

0591T-0593T

INCLUDES   Nonphysician health care professional coach trained to assist patients in obtaining improved health and well-being goals through:
Accountability
Active learning processes
Self-discovery

0591T   Health and well-being coaching face-to-face; individual, initial assessment

EXCLUDES   *Health and well-being coaching, follow-up session (0592T)*
Health and well-being coaching, group session (0593T)

🚗 0.00   ⚕ 0.00   **FUD** YYY   80 ▭

AMA: 2020,Jul,7

0592T   individual, follow-up session, at least 30 minutes

EXCLUDES   *Diabetic preventative behavior change program ([0488T])*
Education/training for self-management (98960)
Health and well-being coaching, group session (0593T)
Health and well-being coaching, initial session (0591T)
Health behavior assessment/intervention (96156-96159)
Medical nutrition therapy (97802-97804)

🚗 0.00   ⚕ 0.00   **FUD** YYY   80 ▭

AMA: 2020,Jul,7

26/TC PC/TC Only   A2-Z3 ASC Payment   50 Bilateral   ♂ Male Only   ♀ Female Only   🚗 Facility RVU   ⚕ Non-Facility RVU   ▭ CCI   ❌ CLIA
FUD Follow-up Days   **CMS:** IOM   **AMA:** CPT Asst   A-Y OPPSI   80/80 Surg Assist Allowed / w/Doc   ◼ Lab Crosswalk   ▦ Radiology Crosswalk

600   CPT © 2021 American Medical Association. All Rights Reserved.   © 2021 Optum360, LLC

0593T   **group (2 or more individuals), at least 30 minutes**

    EXCLUDES   *Diabetic preventative behavior change program (0403T)*
Education/training for self-management (98961-98962)
Group therapy procedure (97150)
Health and well-being coaching, individual (0591T-0592T)
Health behavior assessment/intervention ([96164, 96165])

    🚲 0.00   ✂ 0.00   **FUD** YYY   80 🔲

    AMA: 2020,Jul,7

0594T

0594T   **Osteotomy, humerus, with insertion of an externally controlled intramedullary lengthening device, including intraoperative imaging, initial and subsequent alignment assessments, computations of adjustment schedules, and management of the intramedullary lengthening device**

    EXCLUDES   *Application multiplane external fixation device (20696)*
Osteoplasty, humerus (24420)
Osteotomy, humerus (24400-24410)
Revision externally controlled intramedullary lengthening device (24999)
Treatment humeral shaft fracture (24516)

    🚲 0.00   ✂ 0.00   **FUD** YYY   J8 80 🔲

0596T-0597T

    EXCLUDES   *Bladder irrigation (51700)*
Change cystostomy tube (51705)
Injection retrograde urethrocystography (51610)
Insertion bladder catheter (51701-51703)

0596T   **Temporary female intraurethral valve-pump (ie, voiding prosthesis); initial insertion, including urethral measurement**

    🚲 0.00   ✂ 0.00   **FUD** YYY   ♀ R2 80 🔲

0597T   **replacement**

    🚲 0.00   ✂ 0.00   **FUD** YYY   ♀ R2 80 🔲

0598T-0599T

0598T   **Noncontact real-time fluorescence wound imaging, for bacterial presence, location, and load, per session; first anatomic site (eg, lower extremity)**

    🚲 0.00   ✂ 0.00   **FUD** YYY   Z2 80 🔲

+   0599T   **each additional anatomic site (eg, upper extremity) (List separately in addition to code for primary procedure)**

    Code first (0598T)

    🚲 0.00   ✂ 0.00   **FUD** YYY   N1 80 🔲

0600T-0601T

0600T   **Ablation, irreversible electroporation; 1 or more tumors per organ, including imaging guidance, when performed, percutaneous**

    INCLUDES   Radiological guidance (76940, 77002, 77013, 77022)

    🚲 0.00   ✂ 0.00   **FUD** YYY   J8 80 🔲

0601T   **1 or more tumors, including fluoroscopic and ultrasound guidance, when performed, open**

    INCLUDES   Fluoroscopic guidance (76940)
Ultrasound guidance (77002)

    🚲 0.00   ✂ 0.00   **FUD** YYY   J8 80 🔲

0602T-0603T

0602T   **Glomerular filtration rate (GFR) measurement(s), transdermal, including sensor placement and administration of a single dose of fluorescent pyrazine agent**

    EXCLUDES   *Glomerular filtration rate (GFR) monitoring (0603T)*

    🚲 0.00   ✂ 0.00   **FUD** YYY   80 🔲

0603T   **Glomerular filtration rate (GFR) monitoring, transdermal, including sensor placement and administration of more than one dose of fluorescent pyrazine agent, each 24 hours**

    EXCLUDES   *Glomerular filtration rate (GFR) measurement(s) (0602T)*

    🚲 0.00   ✂ 0.00   **FUD** YYY   80 🔲

0604T-0606T

    EXCLUDES   *Remote physiologic monitoring treatment management services ([99457], [99458])*

0604T   **Optical coherence tomography (OCT) of retina, remote, patient-initiated image capture and transmission to a remote surveillance center unilateral or bilateral; initial device provision, set-up and patient education on use of equipment**

    🚲 0.00   ✂ 0.00   **FUD** YYY   80 🔲

0605T   **remote surveillance center technical support, data analyses and reports, with a minimum of 8 daily recordings, each 30 days**

    🚲 0.00   ✂ 0.00   **FUD** YYY   80 🔲

0606T   **review, interpretation and report by the prescribing physician or other qualified health care professional of remote surveillance center data analyses, each 30 days**

    🚲 0.00   ✂ 0.00   **FUD** YYY   80 🔲

0607T-0608T

    EXCLUDES   *During same monitoring period:*
Cardiac event monitor (93268-93272)
External mobile cardiovascular telemetry (93228-93229)
Holter monitor procedures (93224-93227)
Interrogation cardiovasular physiologic monitoring system (93297)
Remote monitoring pulmonary artery pressure sensor ([93264])

0607T   **Remote monitoring of an external continuous pulmonary fluid monitoring system, including measurement of radiofrequency-derived pulmonary fluid levels, heart rate, respiration rate, activity, posture, and cardiovascular rhythm (eg, ECG data), transmitted to a remote 24-hour attended surveillance center; set-up and patient education on use of equipment**

    EXCLUDES   *Remote monitoring physiologic parameters, initial during same monitoring period ([99453])*

    🚲 0.00   ✂ 0.00   **FUD** YYY   80

0608T   **analysis of data received and transmission of reports to the physician or other qualified health care professional**

    EXCLUDES   *Remote monitoring physiologic parameters, each 30 days, during same monitoring period ([99454])*
Reporting more than once per 30 days

    🚲 0.00   ✂ 0.00   **FUD** YYY   80

0609T-0612T

    EXCLUDES   *Magnetic resonance angiography, spine (72159)*
Magnetic resonance imaging, spine (72141-72158)
Other magnetic spectroscopy (76390)

0609T   **Magnetic resonance spectroscopy, determination and localization of discogenic pain (cervical, thoracic, or lumbar); acquisition of single voxel data, per disc, on biomarkers (ie, lactic acid, carbohydrate, alanine, laal, propionic acid, proteoglycan, and collagen) in at least 3 discs**

    🚲 0.00   ✂ 0.00   **FUD** YYY   Z2 80 🔲

0610T   **transmission of biomarker data for software analysis**

    🚲 0.00   ✂ 0.00   **FUD** YYY   80 🔲

0611T   **postprocessing for algorithmic analysis of biomarker data for determination of relative chemical differences between discs**

    🚲 0.00   ✂ 0.00   **FUD** YYY   Z2 80 🔲

0612T   **interpretation and report**

    🚲 0.00   ✂ 0.00   **FUD** YYY   80 🔲

0613T

EXCLUDES *Heart catheterization (93451-93453, 93456-93462)*
Heart catheterization for congenital defect(s) (93593-93598)
Intracardiac echocardiography (93662)
Transcatheter/transvenous procedures atrial septectomy/septostomy (33741-33746)
Transesophageal echocardiography procedures (93313-93314, 93318, 93355)
Ultrasound guidance (76937)

0613T Percutaneous transcatheter implantation of interatrial septal shunt device, including right and left heart catheterization, intracardiac echocardiography, and imaging guidance by the proceduralist, when performed
0.00   0.00   **FUD** YYY   80

0614T-0615T [0614T]

0614T **Resequenced code. See code following code 0580T.**

0615T **Eye-movement analysis without spatial calibration, with interpretation and report**
EXCLUDES *Vestibular function tests (92540-92542, 92544-92547)*
0.00   0.00   **FUD** YYY   80

0616T-0618T

EXCLUDES *Iridectomy (66600)*
Repair/suture iris (66680, 66682)

0616T Insertion of iris prosthesis, including suture fixation and repair or removal of iris, when performed; without removal of crystalline lens or intraocular lens, without insertion of intraocular lens
0.00   0.00   **FUD** YYY   J8 80

0617T with removal of crystalline lens and insertion of intraocular lens
EXCLUDES *Cataract extraction/removal:*
Extracapsular (66982, 66984)
Intracapsular (66983)
0.00   0.00   **FUD** YYY   J8 80

0618T with secondary intraocular lens placement or intraocular lens exchange
EXCLUDES *Intraocular lens:*
Exchange (66986)
Insertion, secondary implant (66985)
0.00   0.00   **FUD** YYY   J8 80

0619T

INCLUDES Cystourethroscopy (separate procedure) (52000)
EXCLUDES *Cystourethroscopy:*
with insertion transprostatic implant (52441-52442)
with mechanical dilation/drug delivery (0499T)
Laser:
Coagulation (52647)
Enucleation (52649)
Vaporization (52648)
Prostate, transurethral:
Destruction (53850-53854)
Incision (52450)
Resection (52500, 52601, 52630, 52640)
Transrectal ultrasound (76872)

0619T Cystourethroscopy with transurethral anterior prostate commissurotomy and drug delivery, including transrectal ultrasound and fluoroscopy, when performed ♂
0.00   0.00   **FUD** YYY   J8 80

0620T-0622T [0620T]

0620T **Resequenced code. See code following 0505T.**

0621T **Trabeculostomy ab interno by laser**
EXCLUDES *Gonioscopy (92020)*
0.00   0.00   **FUD** YYY   80 50

0622T with use of ophthalmic endoscope
EXCLUDES *Gonioscopy (92020)*
0.00   0.00   **FUD** YYY   80 50

0623T-0626T [0623T, 0624T, 0625T, 0626T]

0623T **Resequenced code. See code following 0504T.**

0624T **Resequenced code. See code following 0504T.**

0625T **Resequenced code. See code following 0504T.**

0626T **Resequenced code. See code following 0504T.**

0627T-0630T

0627T Percutaneous injection of allogeneic cellular and/or tissue-based product, intervertebral disc, unilateral or bilateral injection, with fluoroscopic guidance, lumbar; first level
INCLUDES Fluoroscopic guidance (77003)
0.00   0.00   **FUD** YYY   G2 80

+ 0628T each additional level (List separately in addition to code for primary procedure)
EXCLUDES *Fluoroscopic guidance (77003)*
Code first (0627T)
0.00   0.00   **FUD** ZZZ   N1 80

0629T Percutaneous injection of allogeneic cellular and/or tissue-based product, intervertebral disc, unilateral or bilateral injection, with CT guidance, lumbar; first level
INCLUDES CT guidance (77012)
0.00   0.00   **FUD** YYY   G2 80

+ 0630T each additional level (List separately in addition to code for primary procedure)
INCLUDES CT guidance (77012)
Code first (0629T)
0.00   0.00   **FUD** ZZZ   N1 80

0631T

EXCLUDES *Pulse oximetry (94760-94762)*
Transcutaneous biomarker measurement (0061U)

0631T Transcutaneous visible light hyperspectral imaging measurement of oxyhemoglobin, deoxyhemoglobin, and tissue oxygenation, with interpretation and report, per extremity
0.00   0.00   **FUD** XXX   80

0632T

0632T Percutaneous transcatheter ultrasound ablation of nerves innervating the pulmonary arteries, including right heart catheterization, pulmonary artery angiography, and all imaging guidance
INCLUDES Heart catheterization (93451, 93453, 93456, 93460, 93593-93594, 93596-93597)
Pulmonary artery angiography/injection (75741, 75743, 75746, 93568)
Pulmonary artery catheterization (36013-36015)
Swan-Ganz catheter insertion (93503)
EXCLUDES *Endomyocardial biopsy (93505)*
0.00   0.00   **FUD** YYY   J8 80

0633T-0638T

INCLUDES 3D rendering (76376-76377)
EXCLUDES *Diagnostic/interventional CT (76497)*
Limited/localized follow-up CT (76380)

0633T Computed tomography, breast, including 3D rendering, when performed, unilateral; without contrast material
0.00   0.00   **FUD** XXX   Z2 80

0634T with contrast material(s)
0.00   0.00   **FUD** XXX   Z2 80

0635T without contrast, followed by contrast material(s)
0.00   0.00   **FUD** XXX   Z2 80

0636T Computed tomography, breast, including 3D rendering, when performed, bilateral; without contrast material(s)
0.00   0.00   **FUD** XXX   Z2 80

0637T with contrast material(s)
0.00   0.00   **FUD** XXX   Z2 80

0638T without contrast, followed by contrast material(s)
0.00   0.00   **FUD** XXX   Z2 80

 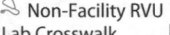

0639T

EXCLUDES *Ultrasound guidance (76998-76999)*

● 0639T **Wireless skin sensor thermal anisotropy measurement(s) and assessment of flow in cerebrospinal fluid shunt, including ultrasound guidance, when performed**
🔧 0.00   ✂ 0.00   **FUD** XXX   80 💻

0640T-0643T [0640T, 0641T, 0642T, 0643T]

0640T **Resequenced code. See code following 0493T.**

0641T **Resequenced code. See code following 0493T.**

0642T **Resequenced code. See code following 0493T.**

0643T **Resequenced code. See code following 0545T.**

0644T

● 0644T **Transcatheter removal or debulking of intracardiac mass (eg, vegetations, thrombus) via suction (eg, vacuum, aspiration) device, percutaneous approach, with intraoperative reinfusion of aspirated blood, including imaging guidance, when performed**

INCLUDES Access with insertion and positioning of device
Arterial closure device, when used
Blood vessel dilation
Embolic protection, when used
Fluoroscopy (76000)
Imaging guidance
Initial extracorporeal circuit for intraoperative reinfusion aspirated blood
Percutaneous venous thrombectomy (37187-37188)
Selective and nonselective catheterizations
Code also, when performed:
Axillary, femoral, or iliac conduit required for catheter access facilitation (34714, [34833], 34716)
Balloon pump insertion (33967, 33970, 33973)
Central or peripheral bypass (33367-33369)
Extensive repair/replacement blood vessel
Other interventional procedures performed during same operative session (i.e., placement dialysis catheters, removal infected pacemaker wires, removal tunneled catheters, repair/replacement valve)
Prolonged extracorporeal membrane oxygenation (ECMO) or extracorporeal life support (ECLS) required when procedure complete may be separately reported (33946-33947, 33951-33956, [33965], [33966], [33969], [33984], [33985], [33986])
Ventricular assist device (33975-33976, [33995], 33990-33993 [33997], 33999)
🔧 0.00   ✂ 0.00   **FUD** YYY   J8 80

0645T-0646T [0646T]

● 0645T **Transcatheter implantation of coronary sinus reduction device including vascular access and closure, right heart catheterization, venous angiography, coronary sinus angiography, imaging guidance, and supervision and interpretation, when performed**

INCLUDES Access with insertion and positioning of device
Angiography
Arterial closure device, when used
Balloon angioplasty ([37246, 37247])
Coronary sinus catheterization and interventions
Diagnostic right heart catheterization (93451, 93453, 93456-93457, 93460-93461, 93566, 93593-93594, 93596-93597, 93662)
Imaging guidance (76000, 76499, 76937, 77001)
Intracardiac echocardiography (93662)
Intravascular ultrasound during evaluation/intervention (37252-37253)
Introduction/selective catheter placement (36010-36013)
Venography (75827, 75860)

EXCLUDES *Indicator dilution studies (93598)*
Code also, when performed:
Diagnostic right and left heart catheterization and angiography performed:
AND previous study available but documentation states patient's condition changed since previous study; visualization insufficient; or change necessitates re-evaluation; append modifier 59
OR when no previous study available and complete diagnostic study performed; append modifier 59
Code also transesophageal echocardiography by separate operator for guidance, when performed (93355)
🔧 0.00   ✂ 0.00   **FUD** YYY   80

0646T **Resequenced code. See code following 0570T.**

0647T

● 0647T **Insertion of gastrostomy tube, percutaneous, with magnetic gastropexy, under ultrasound guidance, image documentation and report**

INCLUDES Ultrasound guidance (76942)
🔧 0.00   ✂ 0.00   **FUD** YYY   J8 80

0648T-0698T [0697T, 0698T]

▲ 0648T **Quantitative magnetic resonance for analysis of tissue composition (eg, fat, iron, water content), including multiparametric data acquisition, data preparation and transmission, interpretation and report, obtained without diagnostic MRI examination of the same anatomy (eg, organ, gland, tissue, target structure) during the same session; single organ**

EXCLUDES *Diagnostic MRI on same gland, organ, tissue or target area during same session (70540-70543, 70551-70553, 71550-71552, 72141-72142, 72146-72149, 72156-72158, 72195-72197, 73218-73223, 73718-73723, 74181-74183, 75557-75563, 76498, 77046-77049, 0398T)*
Quantitative magnetic resonance for analysis of tissue composition with MRI (0649T)
🔧 0.00   ✂ 0.00   **FUD** XXX   Z2 80

● # 0697T   **multiple organs**
🔧 0.00   ✂ 0.00   **FUD** 000

Category III Codes

0649T — 0666T

▲ + **0649T** Quantitative magnetic resonance for analysis of tissue composition (eg, fat, iron, water content), including multiparametric data acquisition, data preparation and transmission, interpretation and report, obtained with diagnostic MRI examination of the same anatomy (eg, organ, gland, tissue, target structure); single organ (List separately in addition to code for primary procedure)

> EXCLUDES *Quantitative magnetic resonance for analysis of tissue composition without MRI (0648T)*
> Code also diagnostic MRI on same gland, organ, tissue or target area during same session (70540-70543, 70551-70553, 71550-71552, 72141-72142, 72146-72149, 72156-72158, 72195-72197, 73218-73223, 73718-73723, 74181-74183, 75557-75563, 76498, 77046-77049, 0398T)
> 🚑 0.00   ⚕ 0.00   **FUD** ZZZ   80

● + # **0698T** multiple organs (List separately in addition to code for primary procedure)
> 🚑 0.00   ⚕ 0.00   **FUD** 000

0650T

● **0650T** Programming device evaluation (remote) of subcutaneous cardiac rhythm monitor system, with iterative adjustment of the implantable device to test the function of the device and select optimal permanently programmed values with analysis, review and report by a physician or other qualified health care professional

> INCLUDES In-person evaluation, interrogation, programming ([93260], 93279-93282, 93284, 93285, 93291)
> EXCLUDES *Insertion subcutaneous cardiac rhythm monitor (33285)*
> Code also remote interrogation during the 30-day remote interrogation device evaluation period, when performed (93298)
> 🚑 0.00   ⚕ 0.00   **FUD** XXX   80

0651T

● **0651T** Magnetically controlled capsule endoscopy, esophagus through stomach, including intraprocedural positioning of capsule, with interpretation and report

> EXCLUDES *Intraluminal gastrointestinal tract imaging (91110, 91111)*
> 🚑 0.00   ⚕ 0.00   **FUD** YYY   J8 80

0652T-0654T

> EXCLUDES Transnasal:
> Diagnostic esophagoscopy, flexible (43197)
> Esophagoscopy with biopsy(ies), flexible (43198)
> Other esophagogastroduodenoscopy (43499, 43999, 44799)
> Transoral:
> Esophagoscopy, flexible (43200-43232 [43210, 43211, 43212, 43213, 43214])
> Esophagogastroduodenoscopy, rigid (43235-43259 [43233, 43266, 43270])
> Esophagoscopy, rigid (43191-43195)

● **0652T** Esophagogastroduodenoscopy, flexible, transnasal; diagnostic, including collection of specimen(s) by brushing or washing, when performed (separate procedure)
> 🚑 0.00   ⚕ 0.00   **FUD** YYY   J8

● **0653T** with biopsy, single or multiple
> 🚑 0.00   ⚕ 0.00   **FUD** YYY   J8

● **0654T** with insertion of intraluminal tube or catheter
> 🚑 0.00   ⚕ 0.00   **FUD** YYY   J8

0655T

● **0655T** Transperineal focal laser ablation of malignant prostate tissue, including transrectal imaging guidance, with MR-fused images or other enhanced ultrasound imaging   ♂

> INCLUDES 3D rendering (76376-76377)
> Cystourethroscopy (52000)
> Imaging guidance (76872, 76940, 76942, 76998)
> 🚑 0.00   ⚕ 0.00   **FUD** YYY   G2

0656T-0657T

> EXCLUDES Arthrodesis (22800-22812)
> Instrumentation, anterior (22845-22847)
> Kyphectomy (22818-22819)

● **0656T** Vertebral body tethering, anterior; up to 7 vertebral segments
> 🚑 0.00   ⚕ 0.00   **FUD** YYY   80

● **0657T** 8 or more vertebral segments
> 🚑 0.00   ⚕ 0.00   **FUD** YYY   80

0658T

● **0658T** Electrical impedance spectroscopy of 1 or more skin lesions for automated melanoma risk score
> 🚑 0.00   ⚕ 0.00   **FUD** XXX   80 TC

0659T

● **0659T** Transcatheter intracoronary infusion of supersaturated oxygen in conjunction with percutaneous coronary revascularization during acute myocardial infarction, including catheter placement, imaging guidance (eg, fluoroscopy), angiography, and radiologic supervision and interpretation

> EXCLUDES *Percutaneous angioplasty or atherectomy ([92920], [92924], [92928], [92933])*
> *Percutaneous revascularization excluding with acute myocardial infarction ([92937], [92943])*
> Code also percutaneous coronary revascularization during acute myocardial infarction ([92941])
> 🚑 0.00   ⚕ 0.00   **FUD** YYY   80

0660T-0661T

Code also drug(s) administered

● **0660T** Implantation of anterior segment intraocular nonbiodegradable drug-eluting system, internal approach
> 🚑 0.00   ⚕ 0.00   **FUD** YYY   50

● **0661T** Removal and reimplantation of anterior segment intraocular nonbiodegradable drug-eluting implant
> 🚑 0.00   ⚕ 0.00   **FUD** YYY   50

0662T-0663T

> EXCLUDES *Selective head/total body hypothermia for critically ill neonate (99184)*

● **0662T** Scalp cooling, mechanical; initial measurement and calibration of cap
> EXCLUDES *Reporting more than one time per chemotherapy treatment period*
> 🚑 0.00   ⚕ 0.00   **FUD** XXX   80

● + **0663T** placement of device, monitoring, and removal of device
> EXCLUDES *Reporting more than one time per chemotherapy session*
> Code also chemotherapy administration (96409, 96411, 96413, 96415, 96416, 96417)
> 🚑 0.00   ⚕ 0.00   **FUD** ZZZ   80

0664T-0670T

● **0664T** Donor hysterectomy (including cold preservation); open, from cadaver donor   ♀
> INCLUDES Harvesting uterus allograft from cadaver donor and cold-preservation solution/maintenance
> 🚑 0.00   ⚕ 0.00   **FUD** XXX

● **0665T** open, from living donor   ♀
> INCLUDES Care for donor
> Harvesting uterus allograft from living donor and cold-preservation solution/maintenance
> 🚑 0.00   ⚕ 0.00   **FUD** XXX

● **0666T** laparoscopic or robotic, from living donor   ♀
> INCLUDES Care for donor
> Harvesting uterus allograft from living donor and cold-preservation solution/maintenance
> 🚑 0.00   ⚕ 0.00   **FUD** XXX

● **0667T**   recipient uterus allograft transplantation from cadaver or living donor ♀
> INCLUDES   Care for recipient
> Transplantation uterine allograft
> 🔲 0.00   ⬠ 0.00   **FUD** XXX

● **0668T**   Backbench standard preparation of cadaver or living donor uterine allograft prior to transplantation, including dissection and removal of surrounding soft tissues and preparation of uterine vein(s) and uterine artery(ies), as necessary ♀
> INCLUDES   Standard preparation cadaver/living uterus allograft (i.e., preparation uterine vein(s) and artery(ies), removal of surrounding soft tissue, as needed)
> EXCLUDES   Reconstruction uterine allograft (i.e., venous or arterial anastomosis(es) (0669T-0670T)
> 🔲 0.00   ⬠ 0.00   **FUD** YYY   80

● **0669T**   Backbench reconstruction of cadaver or living donor uterus allograft prior to transplantation; venous anastomosis, each ♀
> EXCLUDES   Standard preparation cadaver/living uterus allograft (i.e., preparation uterine vein(s) and artery(ies), removal of surrounding soft tissue, as needed) (0668T)
> 🔲 0.00   ⬠ 0.00   **FUD** YYY   80

● **0670T**   arterial anastomosis, each ♀
> EXCLUDES   Standard preparation cadaver/living uterus allograft (i.e., preparation uterine vein(s) and artery(ies), removal of surrounding soft tissue, as needed) (0668T)
> 🔲 0.00   ⬠ 0.00   **FUD** YYY   80

0671T-0672T [0671T]

0671T   Resequenced code. See code following 0184T.

● **0672T**   Endovaginal cryogen-cooled, monopolar radiofrequency remodeling of the tissues surrounding the female bladder neck and proximal urethra for urinary incontinence

0673T

● **0673T**   Ablation, benign thyroid nodule(s), percutaneous, laser, including imaging guidance
> INCLUDES   Radiological guidance for:
> Needle placement (76942)
> Tissue ablation monitoring (76940, 77013, 77022)

0674T-0685T

● **0674T**   Laparoscopic insertion of new or replacement of permanent implantable synchronized diaphragmatic stimulation system for augmentation of cardiac function, including an implantable pulse generator and diaphragmatic lead(s)
> INCLUDES   Complete SDS system insertion/replacement
> Device evaluation, interrogation, and programming (0683T-0685T)
> EXCLUDES   Diaphragmatic lead(s) only:
> Insertion/replacement (0675T-0676T)
> Removal (0679T)
> Repositioning/relocation (0677T-0678T)
> Pulse generator only:
> Insertion/replacement (0680T)
> Removal (0682T)
> Repositioning/relocation (0681T)

● **0675T**   Laparoscopic insertion of new or replacement of diaphragmatic lead(s), permanent implantable synchronized diaphragmatic stimulation system for augmentation of cardiac function, including connection to an existing pulse generator; first lead
> INCLUDES   Device evaluation, interrogation, and programming (0683T-0685T)
> EXCLUDES   Diaphragmatic lead:
> Removal (0679T)
> Repositioning/relocation (0677T)
> Insertion/replacement of complete SDS system (0674T)
> Procedures performed on pulse generator only (0680T-0682T)

● + **0676T**   each additional lead (List separately in addition to
> INCLUDES   Device evaluation, interrogation, and programming (0683T-0685T)
> EXCLUDES   Additional diaphragmatic lead:
> Removal (0679T)
> Repositioning/relocation (0678T)
> Code first (0675T)
> 🔲 0.00   ⬠ 0.00   **FUD** 000

● **0677T**   Laparoscopic repositioning of diaphragmatic lead(s), permanent implantable synchronized diaphragmatic stimulation system for augmentation of cardiac function, including connection to an existing pulse generator; first repositioned lead
> INCLUDES   Device evaluation, interrogation, and programming (0683T-0685T)
> EXCLUDES   Diaphragmatic lead:
> Insertion/replacement (0675T)
> Removal (0679T)
> Insertion/replacement of complete SDS system (0674T)
> Procedures performed on pulse generator only (0680T-0682T)

● + **0678T**   each additional repositioned lead (List separately in
> INCLUDES   Device evaluation, interrogation, and programming (0683T-0685T)
> EXCLUDES   Additional diaphragmatic lead:
> Insertion/replacement (0676T)
> Removal (0679T)
> Code first (0677T)
> 🔲 0.00   ⬠ 0.00   **FUD** 000

● **0679T**   Laparoscopic removal of diaphragmatic lead(s), permanent implantable synchronized diaphragmatic stimulation system for augmentation of cardiac function
> EXCLUDES   Device evaluation, interrogation, and programming (0683T-0685T)
> Insertion/replacement of complete SDS system (0674T)
> Procedures performed on pulse generator only (0680T-0682T)
> Reporting more than once when more than one lead removed
> Repositioning/relocation of lead (0677T)

● **0680T**   Insertion or replacement of pulse generator only, permanent implantable synchronized diaphragmatic stimulation system for augmentation of cardiac function, with connection to existing lead(s)
> INCLUDES   Device evaluation, interrogation, and programming (0683T-0685T)
> EXCLUDES   Insertion/replacement of complete SDS system (0674T)
> Procedures performed on diaphragmatic lead(s) only (0675T-0679T)
> Pulse generator:
> Removal (0682T)
> Repositioning/relocation (0681T)

Category III Codes

0681T — 0695T

● **0681T** Relocation of pulse generator only, permanent implantable synchronized diaphragmatic stimulation system for augmentation of cardiac function, with connection to existing dual leads

INCLUDES Device evaluation, interrogation, and programming (0683T-0685T)

EXCLUDES *Insertion/replacement of complete SDS system (0674T)*
Procedures performed on diaghragmatic lead(s) only (0675T-0679T)
Pulse generator:
Insertion/replacement (0680T)
Removal (0682T)

● **0682T** Removal of pulse generator only, permanent implantable synchronized diaphragmatic stimulation system for augmentation of cardiac function

EXCLUDES *Device evaluation, interrogation, and programming (0683T-0685T)*
Insertion/replacement of complete SDS system (0674T)
Procedures performed on diaghragmatic lead(s) only (0675T-0679T)
Pulse generator:
Insertion/replacement (0680T)
Repositioning/relocation (0681T)

● **0683T** Programming device evaluation (in-person) with iterative adjustment of the implantable device to test the function of the device and select optimal permanent programmed values with analysis, review and report by a physician or other qualified health care professional, permanent implantable synchronized diaphragmatic stimulation system for augmentation of cardiac function

EXCLUDES *Reporting when performed by the same provider as:*
Complete SDS system or individual component procedures (0674T-0682T)
Device evaluation and programming before and after surgery (0684T)
Device interrogation with analysis (0685T)

● **0684T** Peri-procedural device evaluation (in-person) and programming of device system parameters before or after a surgery, procedure, or test with analysis, review, and report by a physician or other qualified health care professional, permanent implantable synchronized diaphragmatic stimulation system for augmentation of cardiac function

EXCLUDES *Reporting when performed by the same provider as:*
Complete SDS system or individual component procedures (0674T-0675T, 0677T, 0679T-0682T)
Device interrogation with analysis (0685T)
Device programming (0683T)

● **0685T** Interrogation device evaluation (in-person) with analysis, review and report by a physician or other qualified health care professional, including connection, recording and disconnection per patient encounter, permanent implantable synchronized diaphragmatic stimulation system for augmentation of cardiac function

EXCLUDES *Reporting when performed by the same provider as:*
Complete SDS system or individual component procedures (0674T-0675T, 0677T, 0679T-0682T)
Device evaluation and programming before and after surgery (0684T)
Device programming (0683T)

0686T

● **0686T** Histotripsy (ie, non-thermal ablation via acoustic energy delivery) of malignant hepatocellular tissue, including image guidance

0687T-0688T

EXCLUDES *Orthoptic training services on same day (92065)*

● **0687T** Treatment of amblyopia using an online digital program; device supply, educational set-up, and initial session

● **0688T** assessment of patient performance and program data by physician or other qualified health care professional, with report, per calendar month

0689T-0690T

● **0689T** Quantitative ultrasound tissue characterization (non-elastographic), including interpretation and report, obtained without diagnostic ultrasound examination of the same anatomy (eg, organ, gland, tissue, target structure)

EXCLUDES *Quantitative ultrasound with diagnostic ultrasound examination, same anatomy (0690T)*
Ultrasound (76536, 76604, 76641-76642, 76700-76705, 76770-76775, 76830, 76856-76857, 76870, 76872, 76881, 76882, 76981-76983, 76999)
Vascular studies (93880, 93882, 93998)

● + **0690T** Quantitative ultrasound tissue characterization (non-elastographic), including interpretation and report, obtained with diagnostic ultrasound examination of the same anatomy (eg, organ, gland, tissue, target structure) (List separately in addition to code for primary procedure)

EXCLUDES *Quantitative ultrasound without diagnostic ultrasound examination, same anatomy (0689T)*
Vascular studies (93880, 93882, 93998)

Code first (76536, 76604, 76641-76642, 76700-76705, 76770-76775, 76830, 76856-76857, 76870, 76872, 76881, 76882, 76981-76982, 76999, 93880, 93882, 93998)

📋 0.00   ⚖ 0.00   **FUD** 000

0691T

● **0691T** Automated analysis of an existing computed tomography study for vertebral fracture(s), including assessment of bone density when performed, data preparation, interpretation, and report

EXCLUDES *Computed tomography:*
Abdominal aorta (75635)
Abdomen/pelvis (72191-72194, 74150-74178)
Biomechanical analysis (0558T)
Bone strength and fracture risk analysis (0554T-0557T)
Chest/thorax (71250-71271, 71275)
Colonography (74261-74263)
Heart (75571-75574)
Spine (72125-72133)
Positron emission tomography (PET) with computed tomography (78814-78816)

0692T

● **0692T** Therapeutic ultrafiltration

EXCLUDES *Apheresis, therapeutic (36511-36516)*
Dialysis/hemodialysis (90935, 90937, 90945, 90947)
Photophoresis, extracorporeal (36522)
Reporting more than once per day

0693T

● **0693T** Comprehensive full body computer-based markerless 3D kinematic and kinetic motion analysis and report

0694T

● **0694T** 3-dimensional volumetric imaging and reconstruction of breast or axillary lymph node tissue, each excised specimen, 3-dimensional automatic specimen reorientation, interpretation and report, real-time intraoperative

INCLUDES Reporting once per specimen

EXCLUDES *Radiological examination (76098)*

0695T-0696T

● **0695T** Body surface-activation mapping of pacemaker or pacing cardioverter-defibrillator lead(s) to optimize electrical synchrony, cardiac resynchronization therapy device, including connection, recording, disconnection, review, and report; at time of implant or replacement

Code also insertion or repositioning pacing electrode for cardiac venous system (33224-33226)

● 0696T **at time of follow-up interrogation or programming device evaluation**

> Code also pacemaker/defibrillator device evaluation, programming, interrogation (93281, 93284, 93286-93289)

0697T-0699T [0697T, 0698T]

0697T **Resequenced code. See code following 0648T.**

0698T **Resequenced code. See code following 0649T.**

● 0699T **Injection, posterior chamber of eye, medication**

0700T-0701T

● 0700T **Molecular fluorescent imaging of suspicious nevus; first lesion**

● + 0701T **each additional lesion (List separately in addition to code for primary procedure)**

> Code first (0700T)
>
> 🚑 0.00   ⚖ 0.00   **FUD** 000

0702T-0703T

EXCLUDES *Behavioral health services:*
Intervention, individual (96158-96159)
Integration ([99484], 99492-99494)
Chronic care management services ([99437])
Collection and interpretation physiologic data ([99091])
Principal care management services ([99424, 99425, 99426, 99427])
Remote physiologic monitoring services ([99453, 99454])
Remote physiologic monitoring treatment management services ([99457, 99458])
Remote therapeutic monitoring (98975-98977)

● 0702T **Remote therapeutic monitoring of a standardized online digital cognitive behavioral therapy program ordered by a physician or other qualified health care professional; supply and technical support, per 30 days**

● 0703T **management services by physician or other qualified health care professional, per calendar month**

0704T-0706T

EXCLUDES *Amblyopia treatment using online digital program during same time period (0687T-0688T)*
Orthoptic training services on same day (92065)

● 0704T **Remote treatment of amblyopia using an eye tracking device; device supply with initial set-up and patient education on use of equipment**

● 0705T **surveillance center technical support including data transmission with analysis, with a minimum of 18 training hours, each 30 days**

● 0706T **interpretation and report by physician or other qualified health care professional, per calendar month**

0707T

● 0707T **Injection(s), bone-substitute material (eg, calcium phosphate) into subchondral bone defect (ie, bone marrow lesion, bone bruise, stress injury, microtrabecular fracture), including imaging guidance and arthroscopic assistance for joint visualization**

> INCLUDES Diagnostic arthroscopy of:
> Hip (29860)
> Knee (29870)
> Shoulder (29805)
> Fluoroscopy (77002)

0708T-0709T

EXCLUDES *Injection procedure (96372)*

● 0708T **Intradermal cancer immunotherapy; preparation and initial injection**

● + 0709T **each additional injection (List separately in addition to code for primary procedure)**

> Code first (0708T)
>
> 🚑 0.00   ⚖ 0.00   **FUD** 000

0710T-0713T

EXCLUDES *Automated coronary plaque characterization/quantification using coronary CT angiography data ([0623T, 0624T, 0625T, 0626T])*
Noninvasive estimated coronary fractional flow reserve (FFR) (0501T-0504T)

● 0710T **Noninvasive arterial plaque analysis using software processing of data from non-coronary computerized tomography angiography; including data preparation and transmission, quantification of the structure and composition of the vessel wall and assessment for lipid-rich necrotic core plaque to assess atherosclerotic plaque stability, data review, interpretation and report**

> INCLUDES Data preparation/transmission (0711T)
> Interpretation and report (0713T)
> Vessel wall structure and composition quantification (0712T)

● 0711T **data preparation and transmission**

● 0712T **quantification of the structure and composition of the vessel wall and assessment for lipid-rich necrotic core plaque to assess atherosclerotic plaque stability**

● 0713T **data review, interpretation and report**

● New Code   ▲ Revised Code   ○ Reinstated   ● New Web Release   ▲ Revised Web Release   + Add-on   Unlisted   Not Covered   # Resequenced
㊿ Optum Mod 50 Exempt   ⊘ AMA Mod 51 Exempt   �51 Optum Mod 51 Exempt   �63 Mod 63 Exempt   ⚢ Non-FDA Drug   ★ Telemedicine   Ⓜ Maternity   Ⓐ Age Edit

Appendix A — Modifiers

CPT Modifiers

A modifier is a two-position alpha or numeric code appended to a CPT® code to clarify the services being billed. Modifiers provide a means by which a service can be altered without changing the procedure code. They add more information, such as the anatomical site, to the code. In addition, they help to eliminate the appearance of duplicate billing and unbundling. Modifiers are used to increase accuracy in reimbursement, coding consistency, editing, and to capture payment data.

22 **Increased Procedural Services:** When the work required to provide a service is substantially greater than typically required, it may be identified by adding modifier 22 to the usual procedure code. Documentation must support the substantial additional work and the reason for the additional work (ie, increased intensity, time, technical difficulty of procedure, severity of patient's condition, physical and mental effort required).
Note: This modifier should not be appended to an E/M service.

23 **Unusual Anesthesia:** Occasionally, a procedure, which usually requires either no anesthesia or local anesthesia, because of unusual circumstances must be done under general anesthesia. This circumstance may be reported by adding modifier 23 to the procedure code of the basic service.

24 **Unrelated Evaluation and Management Service by the Same Physician or Other Qualified Health Care Professional During a Postoperative Period:** The physician or other qualified health care professional may need to indicate that an evaluation and management service was performed during a postoperative period for a reason(s) unrelated to the original procedure. This circumstance may be reported by adding modifier 24 to the appropriate level of E/M service.

25 **Significant, Separately Identifiable Evaluation and Management Service by the Same Physician or Other Qualified Health Care Professional on the Same Day of the Procedure or Other Service:** It may be necessary to indicate that on the day a procedure or service identified by a CPT code was performed, the patient's condition required a significant, separately identifiable E/M service above and beyond the other service provided or beyond the usual preoperative and postoperative care associated with the procedure that was performed. A significant, separately identifiable E/M service is defined or substantiated by documentation that satisfies the relevant criteria for the respective E/M service to be reported (see Evaluation and Management Services Guidelines for instructions on determining level of E/M service). The E/M service may be prompted by the symptom or condition for which the procedure and/or service was provided. As such, different diagnoses are not required for reporting of the E/M services on the same date. This circumstance may be reported by adding modifier 25 to the appropriate level of E/M service.
Note: This modifier is not used to report an E/M service that resulted in a decision to perform surgery. See modifier 57. For significant, separately identifiable non-E/M services, see modifier 59.

26 **Professional Component:** Certain procedures are a combination of a physician or other qualified health care professional component and a technical component. When the physician or other qualified health care professional component is reported separately, the service may be identified by adding modifier 26 to the usual procedure number.

32 **Mandated Services:** Services related to *mandated* consultation and/or related services (eg, third party payer, governmental, legislative or regulatory requirement) may be identified by adding modifier 32 to the basic procedure.

33 **Preventive Services:** When the primary purpose of the service is the delivery of an evidence based service in accordance with a US Preventive Services Task Force A or B rating in effect and other preventive services identified in preventive services mandates (legislative or regulatory), the service may be identified by adding 33 to the procedure. For separately reported services specifically identified as preventive, the modifier should not be used.

47 **Anesthesia by Surgeon:** Regional or general anesthesia provided by the surgeon may be reported by adding modifier 47 to the basic service. (This does not include local anesthesia.)
Note: Modifier 47 would not be used as a modifier for the anesthesia procedures.

50 **Bilateral Procedure:** Unless otherwise identified in the listings, bilateral procedures that are performed at the same session should be identified by adding modifier 50 to the appropriate 5 digit code.
Note: This modifier should not be appended to designated "add-on" codes (see Appendix F).

51 **Multiple Procedures:** When multiple procedures, other than E/M services, Physical Medicine and Rehabilitation services or provision of supplies (eg, vaccines), are performed at the same session by the same individual, the primary procedure or service may be reported as listed. The additional procedure(s) or service(s) may be identified by appending modifier 51 to the additional procedure or service code(s).
Note: This modifier should not be appended to designated "add-on" codes (see Appendix F).

52 **Reduced Services:** Under certain circumstances a service or procedure is partially reduced or eliminated at the discretion of the physician or other qualified health care professional. Under these circumstances the service provided can be identified by its usual procedure number and the addition of modifier 52, signifying that the service is reduced. This provides a means of reporting reduced services without disturbing the identification of the basic service.
Note: For hospital outpatient reporting of a previously scheduled procedure/service that is partially reduced or cancelled as a result of extenuating circumstances or those that threaten the well-being of the patient prior to or after administration of anesthesia, see modifiers 73 and 74 (see modifiers approved for ASC hospital outpatient use).

53 **Discontinued Procedure:** Under certain circumstances, the physician or other qualified health care professional may elect to terminate a surgical or diagnostic procedure. Due to extenuating circumstances or those that threaten the well being of the patient, it may be necessary to indicate that a surgical or diagnostic procedure was started but discontinued. This circumstance may be reported by adding modifier 53 to the code reported by the physician for the discontinued procedure.
Note: This modifier is not used to report the elective cancellation of a procedure prior to the patient's anesthesia induction and/or surgical preparation in the operating suite. For outpatient hospital/ambulatory surgery center (ASC) reporting of a previously scheduled procedure/service that is partially reduced or cancelled as a result of extenuating circumstances or those that threaten the well being of the patient prior to or after administration of anesthesia, see modifiers 73 and 74 (see modifiers approved for ASC hospital outpatient use).

54 **Surgical Care Only:** When 1 physician or other qualified health care professional performs a surgical procedure and another provides preoperative and/or postoperative management, surgical services may be identified by adding modifier 54 to the usual procedure number.

55 **Postoperative Management Only:** When 1 physician or other qualified health care professional performed the postoperative management and another performed the surgical procedure, the postoperative component may be identified by adding modifier 55 to the usual procedure number.

56 **Preoperative Management Only:** When 1 physician or other qualified health care professional performed the preoperative care and evaluation and another performed the surgical procedure, the preoperative component may be identified by adding modifier 56 to the usual procedure number.

57 **Decision for Surgery:** An evaluation and management service that resulted in the initial decision to perform the surgery may be identified by adding modifier 57 to the appropriate level of E/M service.

58   **Staged or Related Procedure or Service by the Same Physician or Other Qualified Health Care Professional During the Postoperative Period:** It may be necessary to indicate that the performance of a procedure or service during the postoperative period was (a) planned or anticipated (staged); (b) more extensive than the original procedure; or (c) for therapy following a surgical procedure. This circumstance may be reported by adding modifier 58 to the staged or related procedure. **Note:** For treatment of a problem that requires a return to the operating/procedure room (eg, unanticipated clinical condition), see modifier 78.

59   **Distinct Procedural Service:** Under certain circumstances, it may be necessary to indicate that a procedure or service was distinct or independent from other non-E/M services performed on the same day. Modifier 59 is used to identify procedures/services, other than E/M services, that are not normally reported together but are appropriate under the circumstances. Documentation must support a different session, different procedure or surgery, different site or organ system, separate incision/excision, separate lesion, or separate injury (or area of injury in extensive injuries) not ordinarily encountered or performed on the same day by the same individual. However, when another already established modifier is appropriate it should be used rather than modifier 59. Only if no more descriptive modifier is available, and the use of modifier 59 best explains the circumstances, should modifier 59 be used. **Note:** Modifier 59 should not be appended to an E/M service. To report a separate and distinct E/M service with a non-E/M service performed on the same date, see modifier 25.

62   **Two Surgeons:** When 2 surgeons work together as primary surgeons performing distinct part(s) of a procedure, each surgeon should report his/her distinct operative work by adding modifier 62 to the procedure code and any associated add-on code(s) for that procedure as long as both surgeons continue to work together as primary surgeons. Each surgeon should report the co-surgery once using the same procedure code. If additional procedure(s) (including add-on procedure[s]) are performed during the same surgical session, separate code(s) may also be reported with modifier 62 added. **Note:** If a co-surgeon acts as an assistant in the performance of additional procedure(s), other than those reported with the modifier 62, during the same surgical session, those services may be reported using separate procedure code(s) with modifier 80 or modifier 82 added, as appropriate.

63   **Procedure Performed on Infants less than 4 kg:** Procedures performed on neonates and infants up to a present body weight of 4 kg may involve significantly increased complexity and physician or other qualified health care professional work commonly associated with these patients. This circumstance may be reported by adding modifier 63 to the procedure number. **Note:** Unless otherwise designated, this modifier may only be appended to procedures/services listed in the 20100-69990 code series and 92920, 92928, 92953, 92960, 92986, 92987, 92990, 92997, 92998, 93312, 93313, 93314, 93315, 93316, 93317, 93318, 93452, 93505, 93563, 93564, 93568, 93580, 93582, 93590, 93591, 93592, 93593, 93594, 93595, 93596, 93597, 93598, 93615, 93616 from the Medicine/Cardiovascular section.

Modifier 63 should not be appended to any CPT codes listed in the Evaluation and Management Services, Anesthesia, Radiology, Pathology/Laboratory, or Medicine sections (other than those identified above from the Medicine/Cardiovascular section).

66   **Surgical Team:** Under some circumstances, highly complex procedures (requiring the concomitant services of several physicians or other qualified health care professionals, often of different specialties, plus other highly skilled, specially trained personnel, various types of complex equipment) are carried out under the "surgical team" concept. Such circumstances may be identified by each participating individual with the addition of modifier 66 to the basic procedure number used for reporting services.

76   **Repeat Procedure or Service by Same Physician or Other Qualified Health Care Professional:** It may be necessary to indicate that a procedure or service was repeated by the same physician or other qualified health care professional subsequent to the original procedure or service. This circumstance may be reported by adding modifier 76 to the repeated procedure or service. **Note:** This modifier should not be appended to an E/M service.

77   **Repeat Procedure by Another Physician or Other Qualified Health Care Professional:** It may be necessary to indicate that a basic procedure or service was repeated by another physician or other qualified health care professional subsequent to the original procedure or service. This circumstance may be reported by adding modifier 77 to the repeated procedure or service. **Note:** This modifier should not be appended to an E/M service.

78   **Unplanned Return to the Operating/Procedure Room by the Same Physician or Other Qualified Health Care Professional Following Initial Procedure for a Related Procedure During the Postoperative Period:** It may be necessary to indicate that another procedure was performed during the postoperative period of the initial procedure (unplanned procedure following initial procedure). When this procedure is related to the first, and requires the use of an operating/procedure room, it may be reported by adding modifier 78 to the related procedure. (For repeat procedures, see modifier 76.)

79   **Unrelated Procedure or Service by the Same Physician or Other Qualified Health Care Professional During the Postoperative Period:** The individual may need to indicate that the performance of a procedure or service during the postoperative period was unrelated to the original procedure. This circumstance may be reported by using modifier 79. (For repeat procedures on the same day, see modifier 76.)

80   **Assistant Surgeon:** Surgical assistant services may be identified by adding modifier 80 to the usual procedure number(s).

81   **Minimum Assistant Surgeon:** Minimum surgical assistant services are identified by adding modifier 81 to the usual procedure number.

82   **Assistant Surgeon (when qualified resident surgeon not available):** The unavailability of a qualified resident surgeon is a prerequisite for use of modifier 82 appended to the usual procedure code number(s).

90   **Reference (Outside) Laboratory:** When laboratory procedures are performed by a party other than the treating or reporting physician or other qualified health care professional, the procedure may be identified by adding modifier 90 to the usual procedure number.

91   **Repeat Clinical Diagnostic Laboratory Test:** In the course of treatment of the patient, it may be necessary to repeat the same laboratory test on the same day to obtain subsequent (multiple) test results. Under these circumstances, the laboratory test performed can be identified by its usual procedure number and the addition of modifier 91. **Note:** This modifier may not be used when tests are rerun to confirm initial results; due to testing problems with specimens or equipment; or for any other reason when a normal, one-time, reportable result is all that is required. This modifier may not be used when other code(s) describe a series of test results (eg, glucose tolerance tests, evocative/suppression testing). This modifier may only be used for laboratory test(s) performed more than once on the same day on the same patient.

92   **Alternative Laboratory Platform Testing:** When laboratory testing is being performed using a kit or transportable instrument that wholly or in part consists of a single use, disposable analytical chamber, the service may be identified by adding modifier 92 to the usual laboratory procedure code (HIV testing 86701-86703, and 87389). The test does not require permanent dedicated space, hence by its design may be hand carried or transported to the vicinity of the patient for immediate testing at that site, although location of the testing is not in itself determinative of the use of this modifier.

95 **Synchronous Telemedicine Service Rendered Via a Real-Time Interactive Audio and Video Telecommunications System:** Synchronous telemedicine service is defined as a **real-time** interaction between a physician or other qualified health care professional and a patient who is located at a distant site from the physician or other qualified health care professional. The totality of the communication of information exchanged between the physician or other qualified health care professional and patient during the course of the synchronous telemedicine service must be of an amount and nature that would be sufficient to meet the key components and/or requirements of the same service when rendered via a face-to-face interaction. Modifier 95 may only be appended to the services listed in Appendix F. Appendix F is the list of CPT codes for services that are typically performed face-to-face, but may be rendered via real-time (synchronous) interactive audio and video telecommunications system.

96 **Habilitative Services:** When a service or procedure that may be either habilitative or rehabilitative in nature is provided for habilitative purposes, the physician or other qualified health care professional may add modifier 96 to the service or procedure code to indicate that the service or procedure provided was a habilitative service. Habilitative services help an individual learn skills and functioning for daily living that the individual has not yet developed, and then keep and/or improve those learned skills. Habilitative services also help an individual keep, learn, or improve skills and functioning for daily living.

97 **Rehabilitative Services:** When a service or procedure that may be either habilitative or rehabilitative in nature is provided for rehabilitative purposes, the physician or other qualified health care professional may add modifier 97 to the service or procedure code to indicate that the service or procedure provided was a rehabilitative service. Rehabilitative services help an individual keep, get back, or improve skills and functioning for daily living that have been lost or impaired because the individual was sick, hurt, or disabled.

99 **Multiple Modifiers:** Under certain circumstances 2 or more modifiers may be necessary to completely delineate a service. In such situations modifier 99 should be added to the basic procedure, and other applicable modifiers may be listed as part of the description of the service.

Anesthesia Physical Status Modifiers

All anesthesia services are reported by use of the five-digit anesthesia procedure code with the appropriate physical status modifier appended.

Under certain circumstances, when other modifier(s) are appropriate, they should be reported in addition to the physical status modifier.

P1 A normal healthy patient

P2 A patient with mild systemic disease

P3 A patient with severe systemic disease

P4 A patient with severe systemic disease that is a constant threat to life

P5 A moribund patient who is not expected to survive without the operation

P6 A declared brain-dead patient whose organs are being removed for donor purposes

Modifiers Approved for Ambulatory Surgery Center (ASC) Hospital Outpatient Use

CPT Level I Modifiers

25 **Significant, Separately Identifiable Evaluation and Management Service by the Same Physician or Other Qualified Health Care Professional on the Same Day of the Procedure or Other Service:** It may be necessary to indicate that on the day a procedure or service identified by a CPT code was performed, the patient's condition required a significant, separately identifiable E/M service above and beyond the other service provided or beyond the usual preoperative and postoperative care associated with the procedure that was performed. A significant, separately identifiable E/M service is defined or substantiated by documentation that satisfies the relevant criteria for the respective E/M service to be reported (see Evaluation and Management Services Guidelines for instructions on determining level of E/M service). The E/M service may be prompted by the symptom or condition for which the procedure and/or service was provided. As such, different diagnoses are not required for reporting of the E/M services on the same date. This circumstance may be reported by adding modifier 25 to the appropriate level of E/M service. **Note:** This modifier is not used to report an E/M service that resulted in a decision to perform surgery. See modifier 57. For significant, separately identifiable non-E/M services, see modifier 59.

27 **Multiple Outpatient Hospital E/M Encounters on the Same Date:** For hospital outpatient reporting purposes, utilization of hospital resources related to separate and distinct E/M encounters performed in multiple outpatient hospital settings on the same date may be reported by adding modifier 27 to each appropriate level outpatient and/or emergency department E/M code(s). This modifier provides a means of reporting circumstances involving evaluation and management services provided by a physician(s) in more than one (multiple) outpatient hospital setting(s) (eg, hospital emergency department, clinic). **Note:** This modifier is not to be used for physician reporting of multiple E/M services performed by the same physician on the same date. For physician reporting of all outpatient evaluation and management services provided by the same physician on the same date and performed in multiple outpatient settings (eg, hospital emergency department, clinic), see Evaluation and Management, Emergency Department, or Preventive Medicine Services codes.

33 **Preventive Services:** When the primary purpose of the service is the delivery of an evidence based service in accordance with a US Preventive Services Task Force A or B rating in effect and other preventive services identified in preventive services mandates (legislative or regulatory), the service may be identified by adding 33 to the procedure. For separately reported services specifically identified as preventive, the modifier should not be used.

50 **Bilateral Procedure:** Unless otherwise identified in the listings, bilateral procedures that are performed at the same session should be identified by adding modifier 50 to the appropriate 5 digit code. **Note:** This modifier should not be appended to designated "add-on" codes (see appendix F).

52 **Reduced Services:** Under certain circumstances a service or procedure is partially reduced or eliminated at the discretion of the physician or other qualified health care professional. Under these circumstances the service provided can be identified by its usual procedure number and the addition of modifier 52, signifying that the service is reduced. This provides a means of reporting reduced services without disturbing the identification of the basic service. **Note:** For hospital outpatient reporting of a previously scheduled procedure/service that is partially reduced or cancelled as a result of extenuating circumstances or those that threaten the well-being of the patient prior to or after administration of anesthesia, see modifiers 73 and 74 (see modifiers approved for ASC hospital outpatient use).

58 **Staged or Related Procedure or Service by the Same Physician or Other Qualified Health Care Professional During the Postoperative Period:** It may be necessary to indicate that the performance of a procedure or service during the postoperative period was (a) planned or anticipated (staged); (b) more extensive than the original procedure; or (c) for therapy following a surgical procedure. This circumstance may be reported by adding modifier 58 to the staged or related procedure. **Note:** For treatment of a problem that requires a return to the operating or procedure room (eg, unanticipated clinical condition), see modifier 78.

59 **Distinct Procedural Service:** Under certain circumstances, it may be necessary to indicate that a procedure or service was distinct or independent from other non-E/M services performed on the same day. Modifier 59 is used to identify procedures/services, other than E/M services, that are not normally reported together but are appropriate under the circumstances. Documentation must support a different session, different procedure or surgery, different site or organ system, separate incision/excision, separate lesion, or

separate injury (or area of injury in extensive injuries) not ordinarily encountered or performed on the same day by the same individual. However, when another already established modifier is appropriate it should be used rather than modifier 59. Only if no more descriptive modifier is available, and the use of modifier 59 best explains the circumstances, should modifier 59 be used.
Note: Modifier 59 should not be appended to an E/M service. To report a separate and distinct E/M service with a non-E/M service performed on the same date, see modifier 25.

73   Discontinued Out-Patient Hospital/Ambulatory Surgery Center (ASC) Procedure Prior to the Administration of Anesthesia: Due to extenuating circumstances or those that threaten the well being of the patient, the physician may cancel a surgical or diagnostic procedure subsequent to the patient's surgical preparation (including sedation when provided, and being taken to the room where the procedure is to be performed), but prior to the administration of anesthesia (local, regional block(s) or general). Under these circumstances, the intended service that is prepared for but cancelled can be reported by its usual procedure number and the addition of modifier 73.
Note: The elective cancellation of a service prior to the administration of anesthesia and/or surgical preparation of the patient should not be reported. For physician reporting of a discontinued procedure, see modifier 53.

74   Discontinued Out-Patient Hospital/Ambulatory Surgery Center (ASC) Procedure After Administration of Anesthesia: Due to extenuating circumstances or those that threaten the well being of the patient, the physician may terminate a surgical or diagnostic procedure after the administration of anesthesia (local, regional block(s), general) or after the procedure was started (incision made, intubation started, scope inserted, etc.). Under these circumstances, the procedure started but terminated can be reported by its usual procedure number and the addition of modifier 74.
Note: The elective cancellation of a service prior to the administration of anesthesia and/or surgical preparation of the patient should not be reported. For physician reporting of a discontinued procedure, see modifier 53.

76   Repeat Procedure or Service by Same Physician or Other Qualified Health Care Professional: It may be necessary to indicate that a procedure or service was repeated by the same physician or other qualified health care professional subsequent to the original procedure or service. This circumstance may be reported by adding modifier 76 to the repeated procedure or service.
Note: This modifier should not be appended to an E/M service.

77   Repeat Procedure by Another Physician or Other Qualified Health Care Professional: It may be necessary to indicate that a basic procedure or service was repeated by another physician or other qualified health care professional subsequent to the original procedure or service. This circumstance may be reported by adding modifier 77 to the repeated procedure or service.
Note: This modifier should not be appended to an E/M service.

78   Unplanned Return to the Operating/Procedure Room by the Same Physician or Other Qualified Health Care Professional Following Initial Procedure for a Related Procedure During the Postoperative Period: It may be necessary to indicate that another procedure was performed during the postoperative period of the initial procedure (unplanned procedure following initial procedure). When this procedure is related to the first, and requires the use of an operating/procedure room, it may be reported by adding modifier 78 to the related procedure. (For repeat procedures, see modifier 76.)

79   Unrelated Procedure or Service by the Same Physician During the Postoperative Period: The individual may need to indicate that the performance of a procedure or service during the postoperative period was unrelated to the original procedure. This circumstance may be reported by using modifier 79. (For repeat procedures on the same day, see modifier 76.)

91   Repeat Clinical Diagnostic Laboratory Test: In the course of treatment of the patient, it may be necessary to repeat the same laboratory test on the same day to obtain subsequent (multiple) test results. Under these circumstances, the laboratory test performed can be identified by its usual procedure number and the addition of modifier 91.
Note: This modifier may not be used when tests are rerun to confirm initial results; due to testing problems with specimens or equipment; or for any other reason when a normal, one-time, reportable result is all that is required. This modifier may not be used when other code(s) describe a series of test results (eg, glucose tolerance tests, evocative/suppression testing). This modifier may only be used for laboratory test(s) performed more than once on the same day on the same patient.

Level II (HCPCS/National) Modifiers

The HCPCS Level II modifiers included here are those most commonly used when coding procedures. See your 2022 HCPCS Level II book for a complete listing.

Anatomical Modifiers

E1	Upper left, eyelid
E2	Lower left, eyelid
E3	Upper right, eyelid
E4	Lower right, eyelid
FA	Left hand, thumb
F1	Left hand, second digit
F2	Left hand, third digit
F3	Left hand, fourth digit
F4	Left hand, fifth digit
F5	Right hand, thumb
F6	Right hand, second digit
F7	Right hand, third digit
F8	Right hand, fourth digit
F9	Right hand, fifth digit
LT	Left side (used to identify procedures performed on the left side of the body)
RT	Right side (used to identify procedures performed on the right side of the body)
TA	Left foot, great toe
T1	Left foot, second digit
T2	Left foot, third digit
T3	Left foot, fourth digit
T4	Left foot, fifth digit
T5	Right foot, great toe
T6	Right foot, second digit
T7	Right foot, third digit
T8	Right foot, fourth digit
T9	Right foot, fifth digit

Anesthesia Modifiers

AA	Anesthesia services performed personally by anesthesiologist
AD	Medical supervision by a physician: more than four concurrent anesthesia procedures
G8	Monitored anesthesia care (MAC) for deep complex, complicated, or markedly invasive surgical procedure
G9	Monitored anesthesia care for patient who has history of severe cardiopulmonary condition
QK	Medical direction of two, three, or four concurrent anesthesia procedures involving qualified individuals
QS	Monitored anesthesiology care service
QX	CRNA service: with medical direction by a physician
QY	Medical direction of one certified registered nurse anesthetist (CRNA) by an anesthesiologist
QZ	CRNA service: without medical direction by a physician

Coronary Artery Modifiers

LC Left circumflex coronary artery

LD Left anterior descending coronary artery

LM Left main coronary artery

RC Right coronary artery

RI Ramus intermedius coronary artery

Other Modifiers

CS Cost-sharing waived for specified COVID-19 testing-related services that result in an order for, or administration of, a COVID-19 test and/or used for cost-sharing waived preventive services furnished via telehealth in Rural Health Clinics and Federally Qualified Health Centers during the COVID-19 public health emergency

CT Computed tomography services furnished using equipment that does not meet each of the attributes of the national electrical manufacturers association (NEMA) XR-29-2013 standard

EA Erythropoetic stimulating agent (ESA) administered to treat anemia due to anticancer chemotherapy

EB Erythropoetic stimulating agent (ESA) administered to treat anemia due to anticancer radiotherapy

EC Erythropoetic stimulating agent (ESA) administered to treat anemia not due to anticancer radiotherapy or anticancer chemotherapy

FP Service provided as part of family planning program

FX X-ray taken using film

G7 Pregnancy resulted from rape or incest or pregnancy certified by physician as life threatening

GA Waiver of liability statement issued as required by payer policy, individual case

GG Performance and payment of a screening mammogram and diagnostic mammogram on the same patient, same day

GH Diagnostic mammogram converted from screening mammogram on same day

GQ Via asynchronous telecommunications system

GT Via interactive audio and video telecommunication systems

GU Waiver of liability statement issued as required by payer policy, routine notice

GX Notice of liability issued, voluntary under payer policy

GY Item or service statutorily excluded, does not meet the definition of any Medicare benefit or, for non-Medicare insurers, is not a contract benefit

GZ Item or service expected to be denied as not reasonable and necessary

PI Positron emission tomography (PET) or PET/computed tomography (CT) to inform the initial treatment strategy of tumors that are biopsy proven or strongly suspected of being cancerous based on other diagnostic testing

PS Positron emission tomography (PET) or PET/computed tomography (CT) to inform the subsequent treatment strategy of cancerous tumors when the beneficiary's treating physician determines that the PET study is needed to inform subsequent antitumor strategy

PT Colorectal cancer screening test; converted to diagnostic test or other procedure

Q7 One Class A finding

Q8 Two Class B findings

Q9 One Class B and two Class C findings

QC Single channel monitoring

QM Ambulance service provided under arrangement by a provider of services

QN Ambulance service furnished directly by a provider of services

QW CLIA waived test

TC Technical component; under certain circumstances, a charge may be made for the technical component alone; under those circumstances the technical component charge is identified by adding modifier TC to the usual procedure number; technical component charges are institutional charges and not billed separately by physicians; however, portable x-ray suppliers only bill for technical component and should utilize modifier TC; the charge data from portable x-ray suppliers will then be used to build customary and prevailing profiles

* **XE** Separate encounter, a service that is distinct because it occurred during a separate encounter

* **XP** Separate practitioner, a service that is distinct because it was performed by a different practitioner

* **XS** Separate structure, a service that is distinct because it was performed on a separate organ/structure

* **XU** Unusual nonoverlapping service, the use of a service that is distinct because it does not overlap usual components of the main service

* CMS instituted additional HCPCS modifiers to define explicit subsets of modifier 59 Distinct Procedural Service.

Category II Modifiers

1P Performance Measure Exclusion Modifier due to Medical Reasons

Reasons include:

- Not indicated (absence of organ/limb, already received/performed, other)
- Contraindicated (patient allergic history, potential adverse drug interaction, other)
- Other medical reasons

2P Performance Measure Exclusion Modifier due to Patient Reasons

Reasons include:

- Patient declined
- Economic, social, or religious reasons
- Other patient reasons

3P Performance Measure Exclusion Modifier due to System Reasons

Reasons include:

- Resources to perform the services not available
- Insurance coverage/payor-related limitations
- Other reasons attributable to health care delivery system

~~Modifier 8P is intended to be used as a "reporting modifier" to allow the reporting of circumstances when an action described in a measure's numerator is not performed and the reason is not otherwise specified.~~

~~8P~~ ~~Performance measure reporting modifier-action not performed, reason not otherwise specified~~

Appendix B — New, Revised, and Deleted Codes

New Codes

01937 Anesthesia for percutaneous image-guided injection, drainage or aspiration procedures on the spine or spinal cord; cervical or thoracic

01938   lumbar or sacral

01939 Anesthesia for percutaneous image-guided destruction procedures by neurolytic agent on the spine or spinal cord; cervical or thoracic

01940   lumbar or sacral

01941 Anesthesia for percutaneous image-guided neuromodulation or intravertebral procedures (eg, kyphoplasty, vertebroplasty) on the spine or spinal cord; cervical or thoracic

01942   lumbar or sacral

33267 Exclusion of left atrial appendage, open, any method (eg, excision, isolation via stapling, oversewing, ligation, plication, clip)

33268 Exclusion of left atrial appendage, open, performed at the time of other sternotomy or thoracotomy procedure(s), any method (eg, excision, isolation via stapling, oversewing, ligation, plication, clip) (List separately in addition to code for primary procedure)

33269 Exclusion of left atrial appendage, thoracoscopic, any method (eg, excision, isolation via stapling, oversewing, ligation, plication, clip)

33370 Transcatheter placement and subsequent removal of cerebral embolic protection device(s), including arterial access, catheterization, imaging, and radiological supervision and interpretation, percutaneous (List separately in addition to code for primary procedure)

33509 Harvest of upper extremity artery, 1 segment, for coronary artery bypass procedure, endoscopic

33894 Endovascular stent repair of coarctation of the ascending, transverse, or descending thoracic or abdominal aorta, involving stent placement; across major side branches

33895   not crossing major side branches

33897 Percutaneous transluminal angioplasty of native or recurrent coarctation of the aorta

42975 Drug-induced sleep endoscopy, with dynamic evaluation of velum, pharynx, tongue base, and larynx for evaluation of sleep-disordered breathing, flexible, diagnostic

43497 Lower esophageal myotomy, transoral (ie, peroral endoscopic myotomy [POEM])

53451 Periurethral transperineal adjustable balloon continence device; bilateral insertion, including cystourethroscopy and imaging guidance

53452   unilateral insertion, including cystourethroscopy and imaging guidance

53453   removal, each balloon

53454   percutaneous adjustment of balloon(s) fluid volume

61736 Laser interstitial thermal therapy (LITT) of lesion, intracranial, including burr hole(s), with magnetic resonance imaging guidance, when performed; single trajectory for 1 simple lesion

61737   multiple trajectories for multiple or complex lesion(s)

63052 Laminectomy, facetectomy, or foraminotomy (unilateral or bilateral with decompression of spinal cord, cauda equina and/or nerve root[s] [eg, spinal or lateral recess stenosis]), during posterior interbody arthrodesis, lumbar; single vertebral segment (List separately in addition to code for primary procedure)

63053   each additional segment (List separately in addition to code for primary procedure)

64582 Open implantation of hypoglossal nerve neurostimulator array, pulse generator, and distal respiratory sensor electrode or electrode array

64583 Revision or replacement of hypoglossal nerve neurostimulator array and distal respiratory sensor electrode or electrode array, including connection to existing pulse generator

64584 Removal of hypoglossal nerve neurostimulator array, pulse generator, and distal respiratory sensor electrode or electrode array

64628 Thermal destruction of intraosseous basivertebral nerve, including all imaging guidance; first 2 vertebral bodies, lumbar or sacral

64629   each additional vertebral body, lumbar or sacral (List separately in addition to code for primary procedure)

66989   with insertion of intraocular (eg, trabecular meshwork, supraciliary, suprachoroidal) anterior segment aqueous drainage device, without extraocular reservoir, internal approach, one or more

66991   with insertion of intraocular (eg, trabecular meshwork, supraciliary, suprachoroidal) anterior segment aqueous drainage device, without extraocular reservoir, internal approach, one or more

68841 Insertion of drug-eluting implant, including punctal dilation when performed, into lacrimal canaliculus, each

69716   with magnetic transcutaneous attachment to external speech processor

69719   with magnetic transcutaneous attachment to external speech processor

69726 Removal, osseointegrated implant, skull; with percutaneous attachment to external speech processor

69727   with magnetic transcutaneous attachment to external speech processor

77089 Trabecular bone score (TBS), structural condition of the bone microarchitecture; using dual X-ray absorptiometry (DXA) or other imaging data on gray-scale variogram, calculation, with interpretation and report on fracture-risk

77090   technical preparation and transmission of data for analysis to be performed elsewhere

77091   technical calculation only

77092   interpretation and report on fracture-risk only by other qualified health care professional

80220 Hydroxychloroquine

80503 Pathology clinical consultation; for a clinical problem, with limited review of patient's history and medical records and straightforward medical decision making

80504   for a moderately complex clinical problem, with review of patient's history and medical records and moderate level of medical decision making

80505   for a highly complex clinical problem, with comprehensive review of patient's history and medical records and high level of medical decision making

80506   prolonged service, each additional 30 minutes (List separately in addition to code for primary procedure)

81349   interrogation of genomic regions for copy number and loss-of-heterozygosity variants, low-pass sequencing analysis

81523 Oncology (breast), mRNA, next-generation sequencing gene profiling of 70 content genes and 31 housekeeping genes, utilizing formalin-fixed paraffin-embedded tissue, algorithm reported as index related to risk to distant metastasis

81560 Transplantation medicine (allograft rejection, pediatric liver and small bowel), measurement of donor and third-party-induced CD154+T-cytotoxic memory cells, utilizing whole peripheral blood, algorithm reported as a rejection risk score

82653   quantitative

83521 Immunoglobulin light chains (ie, kappa, lambda), free, each

83529 Interleukin-6 (IL-6)

86015 Actin (smooth muscle) antibody (ASMA), each

86036 Antineutrophil cytoplasmic antibody (ANCA); screen, each antibody

86037   titer, each antibody

86051 Aquaporin-4 (neuromyelitis optica [NMO]) antibody; enzyme-linked immunosorbent immunoassay (ELISA)

86052   cell-based immunofluorescence assay (CBA), each

86053   flow cytometry (ie, fluorescence-activated cell sorting [FACS]), each

86231 Endomysial antibody (EMA), each immunoglobulin (Ig) class

86258 Gliadin (deamidated) (DGP) antibody, each immunoglobulin (Ig) class

86362 Myelin oligodendrocyte glycoprotein (MOG-IgG1) antibody; cell-based immunofluorescence assay (CBA), each

86363 Myelin oligodendrocyte glycoprotein (MOG-IgG1) antibody; cell-based immunofluorescence assay (CBA), each

86364 Tissue transglutaminase, each immunoglobulin (Ig) class

86381 Mitochondrial antibody (eg, M2), each

86408 Neutralizing antibody, severe acute respiratory syndrome coronavirus 2 (SARS-CoV-2) (coronavirus disease [COVID-19]); screen

86409   titer

86413 Severe acute respiratory syndrome coronavirus 2 (SARS-CoV-2) (coronavirus disease [COVID-19]) antibody, quantitative

86596 Voltage-gated calcium channel antibody, each

87154   identification of blood pathogen and resistance typing, when performed, by nucleic acid (DNA or RNA) probe, multiplexed amplified probe technique including multiplex reverse transcription, when performed, per culture or isolate, 6 or more targets

87428 Infectious agent antigen detection by immunoassay technique, (eg, enzyme immunoassay [EIA], enzyme-linked immunosorbent assay [ELISA], fluorescence immunoassay [FIA], immunochemiluminometric assay [IMCA]) qualitative or semiquantitative; severe acute respiratory syndrome coronavirus (eg, SARS-CoV, SARS-CoV-2 [COVID-19]) and influenza virus types A and B

87636   severe acute respiratory syndrome coronavirus 2 (SARS-CoV-2) (coronavirus disease [COVID-19]) and influenza virus types A and B, multiplex amplified probe technique

87637   severe acute respiratory syndrome coronavirus 2 (SARS-CoV-2) (coronavirus disease [COVID-19]), influenza virus types A and B, and respiratory syncytial virus, multiplex amplified probe technique

87811   severe acute respiratory syndrome coronavirus 2 (SARS-CoV-2) (coronavirus disease [COVID-19])

90626 Tick-borne encephalitis virus vaccine, inactivated; 0.25 mL dosage, for intramuscular use

90627 Tick-borne encephalitis virus vaccine, inactivated; 0.5 mL dosage, for intramuscular use

90671 Pneumococcal conjugate vaccine, 15 valent (PCV15), for intramuscular use

90677 Pneumococcal conjugate vaccine, 20 valent (PCV20), for intramuscular use

90758 Zaire ebolavirus vaccine, live, for intramuscular use

90759 Hepatitis B vaccine (HepB), 3-antigen (S, Pre-S1, Pre-S2), 10 mcg dosage, 3 dose schedule, for intramuscular use

91113 Gastrointestinal tract imaging, intraluminal (eg, capsule endoscopy), colon, with interpretation and report

91300 Severe acute respiratory syndrome coronavirus 2 (SARS-CoV-2) (coronavirus disease [COVID-19]) vaccine, mRNA-LNP, spike protein, preservative free, 30 mcg/0.3.mL dosage, diluent reconstituted, for intramuscular use

91301 Severe acute respiratory syndrome coronavirus 2 (SARS-CoV-2) (coronavirus disease [COVID-19]) vaccine, mRNA-LNP, spike protein, preservative free, 100 mcg/0.5mL dosage, for intramuscular use

91302 Severe acute respiratory syndrome coronavirus 2 (SARS-CoV-2) (coronavirus disease [COVID-19]) vaccine, DNA, spike protein, chimpanzee adenovirus Oxford 1 (ChAdOx1) vector, preservative free, $5x10^{10}$ viral particles/0.5mL dosage, for intramuscular use

91303 Severe acute respiratory syndrome coronavirus 2 (SARS-CoV-2) (coronavirus disease [COVID-19]) vaccine, DNA, spike protein, adenovirus type 26 (Ad26) vector, preservative free, $5x10^{10}$ viral particles/0.5mL dosage, for intramuscular use

91304 Severe acute respiratory syndrome coronavirus 2 (SARS-CoV-2) (coronavirus disease [COVID-19]) vaccine, recombinant spike protein nanoparticle, saponin-based adjuvant, preservative free, 5 mcg/0.5mL dosage, for intramuscular use

93319 3D echocardiographic imaging and postprocessing during transesophageal echocardiography, or during transthoracic echocardiography for congenital cardiac anomalies, for the assessment of cardiac structure(s) (eg, cardiac chambers and valves, left atrial appendage, interatrial septum, interventricular septum) and function, when performed (List separately in addition to code for echocardiographic imaging)

93593 Right heart catheterization for congenital heart defect(s) including imaging guidance by the proceduralist to advance the catheter to the target zone; normal native connections

93594   abnormal native connections

93595 Left heart catheterization for congenital heart defect(s) including imaging guidance by the proceduralist to advance the catheter to the target zone, normal or abnormal native connections

93596 Right and left heart catheterization for congenital heart defect(s) including imaging guidance by the proceduralist to advance the catheter to the target zone(s); normal native connections

93597   abnormal native connections

93598 Cardiac output measurement(s), thermodilution or other indicator dilution method, performed during cardiac catheterization for the evaluation of congenital heart defects (List separately in addition to code for primary procedure)

94625 Physician or other qualified health care professional services for outpatient pulmonary rehabilitation; without continuous oximetry monitoring (per session)

94626   with continuous oximetry monitoring (per session)

98975 Remote therapeutic monitoring (eg, respiratory system status, musculoskeletal system status, therapy adherence, therapy response); initial set-up and patient education on use of equipment

98976   device(s) supply with scheduled (eg, daily) recording(s) and/or programmed alert(s) transmission to monitor respiratory system, each 30 days

98977   device(s) supply with scheduled (eg, daily) recording(s) and/or programmed alert(s) transmission to monitor musculoskeletal system, each 30 days

98980 Remote therapeutic monitoring treatment management services, physician or other qualified health care professional time in a calendar month requiring at least one interactive communication with the patient or caregiver during the calendar month; first 20 minutes

98981   each additional 20 minutes (List separately in addition to code for primary procedure)

99072 Additional supplies, materials, and clinical staff time over and above those usually included in an office visit or other nonfacility service(s), when performed during a Public Health Emergency, as defined by law, due to respiratory-transmitted infectious disease

99424 Principal care management services, for a single high-risk disease, with the following required elements: one complex chronic condition expected to last at least 3 months, and that places the patient at significant risk of hospitalization, acute exacerbation/decompensation, functional decline, or death, the condition requires development, monitoring, or revision of disease-specific care plan, the condition requires frequent adjustments in the medication regimen and/or the management of the condition is unusually complex due to comorbidities, ongoing communication and care coordination between relevant practitioners furnishing care; first 30 minutes provided personally by a physician or other qualified health care professional, per calendar month.

99425   each additional 30 minutes provided personally by a physician or other qualified health care professional, per calendar month (List separately in addition to code for primary procedure)

99426 Principal care management services, for a single high-risk disease, with the following required elements: one complex chronic condition expected to last at least 3 months, and that places the patient at significant risk of hospitalization, acute exacerbation/decompensation, functional decline, or death, the condition requires development, monitoring, or revision of disease-specific care plan, the condition requires frequent adjustments in the medication regimen and/or the management of the condition is unusually complex due to comorbidities, ongoing communication and care coordination between relevant practitioners furnishing care; first 30 minutes of clinical staff time directed by physician or other qualified health care professional, per calendar month.

99427   each additional 30 minutes of clinical staff time directed by a physician or other qualified health care professional, per calendar month (List separately in addition to code for primary procedure)

99437 Chronic care management services with the following required elements: multiple (two or more) chronic conditions expected to last at least 12 months, or until the death of the patient, chronic conditions that place the patient at significant risk of death, acute exacerbation/decompensation, or functional decline, comprehensive care plan established, implemented, revised, or monitored; each additional 30 minutes by a physician or other qualified health care professional, per calendar month (List separately in addition to code for primary procedure)

0001A Immunization administration by intramuscular injection of severe acute respiratory syndrome coronavirus 2 (SARS-CoV-2) (coronavirus disease [COVID-19]) vaccine, mRNA-LNP, spike protein, preservative free, 30 mcg/0.3mL dosage, diluent reconstituted; first dose

0002A Immunization administration by intramuscular injection of severe acute respiratory syndrome coronavirus 2 (SARS-CoV-2) (coronavirus disease [COVID-19]) vaccine, mRNA-LNP, spike protein, preservative free, 30 mcg/0.3mL dosage, diluent reconstituted; second dose

0011A Immunization administration by intramuscular injection of severe acute respiratory syndrome coronavirus 2 (SARS-CoV-2) (coronavirus disease [COVID-19]) vaccine, mRNA-LNP, spike protein, preservative free, 100 mcg/0.5mL dosage; first dose

0012A Immunization administration by intramuscular injection of severe acute respiratory syndrome coronavirus 2 (SARS-CoV-2) (coronavirus disease [COVID-19] vaccine, mRNA-LNP, spike protein, preservative free, 100 mcg/0.5mL dosage; second dose

0021A Immunization administration by intramuscular injection of severe acute respiratory syndrome coronavirus 2 (SARS-CoV-2) (coronavirus disease [COVID-19]) vaccine, DNA, spike protein, chimpanzee adenovirus Oxford 1 (ChAdOx1) vector, preservative free, 5×10^{10} viral particles/0.5mL dosage; first dose

0022A Immunization administration by intramuscular injection of severe acute respiratory syndrome coronavirus 2 (SARS-CoV-2) (coronavirus disease [COVID-19]) vaccine, DNA, spike protein, chimpanzee adenovirus Oxford 1 (ChAdOx1) vector, preservative free, 5×10^{10} viral particles/0.5mL dosage; second dose

0031A Immunization administration by intramuscular injection of severe acute respiratory syndrome coronavirus 2 (SARS-CoV-2) (coronavirus disease [COVID-19]) vaccine, DNA, spike protein, adenovirus type 26 (Ad26) vector, preservative free, 5×10^{10} viral particles/0.5mL dosage, single dose

0041A Immunization administration by intramuscular injection of severe acute respiratory syndrome coronavirus 2 (SARS-CoV-2) (coronavirus disease [COVID-19]) vaccine, recombinant spike protein nanoparticle, saponin-based adjuvant, preservative free, 5 mcg/0.5mL dosage; first dose

0042A Immunization administration by intramuscular injection of severe acute respiratory syndrome coronavirus 2 (SARS-CoV-2) (coronavirus disease [COVID-19]) vaccine, recombinant spike protein nanoparticle, saponin-based adjuvant, preservative free, 5 mcg/0.5mL dosage; second dose

0223U Infectious disease (bacterial or viral respiratory tract infection), pathogen-specific nucleic acid (DNA or RNA), 22 targets including severe acute respiratory syndrome coronavirus 2 (SARS-CoV-2), qualitative RT-PCR, nasopharyngeal swab, each pathogen reported as detected or not detected

0224U Antibody, severe acute respiratory syndrome coronavirus 2 (SARS-CoV-2) (coronavirus disease [COVID-19]), includes titer(s), when performed

0225U Infectious disease (bacterial or viral respiratory tract infection) pathogen-specific DNA and RNA, 21 targets, including severe acute respiratory syndrome coronavirus 2 (SARS-CoV-2), amplified probe technique, including multiplex reverse transcription for RNA targets, each analyte reported as detected or not detected

0226U Surrogate viral neutralization test (sVNT), severe acute respiratory syndrome coronavirus 2 (SARS-CoV-2) (coronavirus disease [COVID-19]), ELISA, plasma, serum

0227U Drug assay, presumptive, 30 or more drugs or metabolites, urine, liquid chromatography with tandem mass spectrometry (LC-MS/MS) using multiple reaction monitoring (MRM), with drug or metabolite description, includes sample validation

0228U Oncology (prostate), multianalyte molecular profile by photometric detection of macromolecules adsorbed on nanosponge array slides with machine learning, utilizing first morning voided urine, algorithm reported as likelihood of prostate cancer

0229U BCAT1 (Branched chain amino acid transaminase 1) or IKZF1 (IKAROS family zinc finger 1) (eg, colorectal cancer) promoter methylation analysis

0230U AR (androgen receptor) (eg, spinal and bulbar muscular atrophy, Kennedy disease, X chromosome inactivation), full sequence analysis, including small sequence changes in exonic and intronic regions, deletions, duplications, short tandem repeat (STR) expansions, mobile element insertions, and variants in non-uniquely mappable regions

0231U CACNA1A (calcium voltage-gated channel subunit alpha 1A) (eg, spinocerebellar ataxia), full gene analysis, including small sequence changes in exonic and intronic regions, deletions, duplications, short tandem repeat (STR) gene expansions, mobile element insertions, and variants in non-uniquely mappable regions

0232U CSTB (cystatin B) (eg, progressive myoclonic epilepsy type 1A, Unverricht-Lundborg disease), full gene analysis, including small sequence changes in exonic and intronic regions, deletions, duplications, short tandem repeat (STR) expansions, mobile element insertions, and variants in non-uniquely mappable regions

0233U FXN (frataxin) (eg, Friedreich ataxia), gene analysis, including small sequence changes in exonic and intronic regions, deletions, duplications, short tandem repeat (STR) expansions, mobile element insertions, and variants in non-uniquely mappable regions

0234U MECP2 (methyl CpG binding protein 2) (eg, Rett syndrome), full gene analysis, including small sequence changes in exonic and intronic regions, deletions, duplications, mobile element insertions, and variants in non-uniquely mappable regions

0235U PTEN (phosphatase and tensin homolog) (eg, Cowden syndrome, PTEN hamartoma tumor syndrome), full gene analysis, including small sequence changes in exonic and intronic regions, deletions, duplications, mobile element insertions, and variants in non-uniquely mappable regions

0236U SMN1 (survival of motor neuron 1, telomeric) and SMN2 (survival of motor neuron 2, centromeric) (eg, spinal muscular atrophy) full gene analysis, including small sequence changes in exonic and intronic regions, duplications, deletions, and mobile element insertions

0237U Cardiac ion channelopathies (eg, Brugada syndrome, long QT syndrome, short QT syndrome, catecholaminergic polymorphic ventricular tachycardia), genomic sequence analysis panel including ANK2, CASQ2, CAV3, KCNE1, KCNE2, KCNH2, KCNJ2, KCNQ1, RYR2, and SCN5A, including small sequence changes in exonic and intronic regions, deletions, duplications, mobile element insertions, and variants in non-uniquely mappable regions

0238U Oncology (Lynch syndrome), genomic DNA sequence analysis of MLH1, MSH2, MSH6, PMS2, and EPCAM, including small sequence changes in exonic and intronic regions, deletions, duplications, mobile element insertions, and variants in non-uniquely mappable regions

0239U Targeted genomic sequence analysis panel, solid organ neoplasm, cell-free DNA, analysis of 311 or more genes, interrogation for sequence variants, including substitutions, insertions, deletions, select rearrangements, and copy number variations

0240U Infectious disease (viral respiratory tract infection), pathogen-specific RNA, 3 targets (severe acute respiratory syndrome coronavirus 2 [SARS-CoV-2], influenza A, influenza B), upper respiratory specimen, each pathogen reported as detected or not detected

0241U Infectious disease (viral respiratory tract infection), pathogen-specific RNA, 4 targets (severe acute respiratory syndrome coronavirus 2 [SARS-CoV-2], influenza A, influenza B, respiratory syncytial virus [RSV]), upper respiratory specimen, each pathogen reported as detected or not detected

0242U Targeted genomic sequence analysis panel, solid organ neoplasm, cell-free circulating DNA analysis of 55-74 genes, interrogation for sequence variants, gene copy number amplifications, and gene rearrangements

0243U Obstetrics (preeclampsia), biochemical assay of placental-growth factor, time-resolved fluorescence immunoassay, maternal serum, predictive algorithm reported as a risk score for preeclampsia

0244U Oncology (solid organ), DNA, comprehensive genomic profiling, 257 genes, interrogation for single-nucleotide variants, insertions/deletions, copy number alterations, gene rearrangements, tumor-mutational burden and microsatellite instability, utilizing formalin-fixed paraffin-embedded tumor tissue

0245U Oncology (thyroid), mutation analysis of 10 genes and 37 RNA fusions and expression of 4 mRNA markers using next-generation sequencing, fine needle aspirate, report includes associated risk of malignancy expressed as a percentage

0246U Red blood cell antigen typing, DNA, genotyping of at least 16 blood groups with phenotype prediction of at least 51 red blood cell antigens

0247U Obstetrics (preterm birth), insulin-like growth factor–binding protein 4 (IBP4), sex hormone–binding globulin (SHBG), quantitative measurement by LC-MS/MS, utilizing maternal serum, combined with clinical data, reported as predictive-risk stratification for spontaneous preterm birth

0248U Oncology (brain), spheroid cell culture in a 3D microenvironment, 12 drug panel, tumor-response prediction for each drug

0249U Oncology (breast), semiquantitative analysis of 32 phosphoproteins and protein analytes, includes laser capture microdissection, with algorithmic analysis and interpretative report

0250U Oncology (solid organ neoplasm), targeted genomic sequence DNA analysis of 505 genes, interrogation for somatic alterations (SNVs [single nucleotide variant], small insertions and deletions, one amplification, and four translocations), microsatellite instability and tumor-mutation burden

0251U Hepcidin-25, enzyme-linked immunosorbent assay (ELISA), serum or plasma

0252U Fetal aneuploidy short tandem–repeat comparative analysis, fetal DNA from products of conception, reported as normal (euploidy), monosomy, trisomy, or partial deletion/duplications, mosaicism, and segmental aneuploidy

0253U Reproductive medicine (endometrial receptivity analysis), RNA gene expression profile, 238 genes by next-generation sequencing, endometrial tissue, predictive algorithm reported as endometrial window of implantation (eg, pre-receptive, receptive, post-receptive)

0254U Reproductive medicine (preimplantation genetic assessment), analysis of 24 chromosomes using embryonic DNA genomic sequence analysis for aneuploidy, and a mitochondrial DNA score in euploid embryos, results reported as normal (euploidy), monosomy, trisomy, or partial deletion/duplications, mosaicism, and segmental aneuploidy, per embryo tested

0255U Andrology (infertility), sperm-capacitation assessment of ganglioside GM1 distribution patterns, fluorescence microscopy, fresh or frozen specimen, reported as percentage of capacitated sperm and probability of generating a pregnancy score

0256U Trimethylamine/trimethylamine N-oxide (TMA/TMAO) profile, tandem mass spectrometry (MS/MS), urine, with algorithmic analysis and interpretive report

0257U Very long chain acyl-coenzyme A (CoA) dehydrogenase (VLCAD), leukocyte enzyme activity, whole blood

0258U Autoimmune (psoriasis), mRNA, next-generation sequencing, gene expression profiling of 50-100 genes, skin-surface collection using adhesive patch, algorithm reported as likelihood of response to psoriasis biologics

0259U Nephrology (chronic kidney disease), nuclear magnetic resonance spectroscopy measurement of myo-inositol, valine, and creatinine, algorithmically combined with cystatin C (by immunoassay) and demographic data to determine estimated glomerular filtration rate (GFR), serum, quantitative

0260U Rare diseases (constitutional/heritable disorders), identification of copy number variations, inversions, insertions, translocations, and other structural variants by optical genome mapping

0261U Oncology (colorectal cancer), image analysis with artificial intelligence assessment of 4 histologic and immunohistochemical features (CD3 and CD8 within tumor-stroma border and tumor core), tissue, reported as immune response and recurrence-risk score

0262U Oncology (solid tumor), gene expression profiling by real-time RT-PCR of 7 gene pathways (ER, AR, PI3K, MAPK, HH, TGFB, Notch), formalin-fixed paraffin-embedded (FFPE), algorithm reported as gene pathway activity score

0263U Neurology (autism spectrum disorder [ASD]), quantitative measurements of 16 central carbon metabolites (ie, α-ketoglutarate, alanine, lactate, phenylalanine, pyruvate, succinate, carnitine, citrate, fumarate, hypoxanthine, inosine, malate, S-sulfocysteine, taurine, urate, and xanthine), liquid chromatography tandem mass spectrometry (LC-MS/MS), plasma, algorithmic analysis with result reported as negative or positive (with metabolic subtypes of ASD)

0264U Rare diseases (constitutional/heritable disorders), identification of copy number variations, inversions, insertions, translocations, and other structural variants by optical genome mapping

0265U Rare constitutional and other heritable disorders, whole genome and mitochondrial DNA sequence analysis, blood, frozen and formalin-fixed paraffin-embedded (FFPE) tissue, saliva, buccal swabs or cell lines, identification of single nucleotide and copy number variants

0266U Unexplained constitutional or other heritable disorders or syndromes, tissue-specific gene expression by whole-transcriptome and next-generation sequencing, blood, formalin-fixed paraffin-embedded (FFPE) tissue or fresh frozen tissue, reported as presence or absence of splicing or expression changes

0267U Rare constitutional and other heritable disorders, identification of copy number variations, inversions, insertions, translocations, and other structural variants by optical genome mapping and whole genome sequencing

0268U Hematology (atypical hemolytic uremic syndrome [aHUS]), genomic sequence analysis of 15 genes, blood, buccal swab, or amniotic fluid

0269U Hematology (autosomal dominant congenital thrombocytopenia), genomic sequence analysis of 14 genes, blood, buccal swab, or amniotic fluid

0270U Hematology (congenital coagulation disorders), genomic sequence analysis of 20 genes, blood, buccal swab, or amniotic fluid

0271U Hematology (congenital neutropenia), genomic sequence analysis of 23 genes, blood, buccal swab, or amniotic fluid

0272U Hematology (genetic bleeding disorders), genomic sequence analysis of 51 genes, blood, buccal swab, or amniotic fluid, comprehensive

0273U Hematology (genetic hyperfibrinolysis, delayed bleeding), genomic sequence analysis of 8 genes (F13A1, F13B, FGA, FGB, FGG, SERPINA1, SERPINE1, SERPINF2, PLAU), blood, buccal swab, or amniotic fluid

0274U Hematology (genetic platelet disorders), genomic sequence analysis of 43 genes, blood, buccal swab, or amniotic fluid

0275U Hematology (heparin-induced thrombocytopenia), platelet antibody reactivity by flow cytometry, serum

0276U Hematology (inherited thrombocytopenia), genomic sequence analysis of 23 genes, blood, buccal swab, or amniotic fluid

0277U Hematology (genetic platelet function disorder), genomic sequence analysis of 31 genes, blood, buccal swab, or amniotic fluid

0278U Hematology (genetic thrombosis), genomic sequence analysis of 12 genes, blood, buccal swab, or amniotic fluid

0279U Hematology (von Willebrand disease [VWD]), von Willebrand factor (VWF) and collagen III binding by enzyme-linked immunosorbent assays (ELISA), plasma, report of collagen III binding

0280U Hematology (von Willebrand disease [VWD]), von Willebrand factor (VWF) and collagen IV binding by enzyme-linked immunosorbent assays (ELISA), plasma, report of collagen IV binding

0281U Hematology (von Willebrand disease [VWD]), von Willebrand propeptide, enzyme-linked immunosorbent assays (ELISA), plasma, diagnostic report of von Willebrand factor (VWF) propeptide antigen level

0282U Red blood cell antigen typing, DNA, genotyping of 12 blood group system genes to predict 44 red blood cell antigen phenotypes

0283U von Willebrand factor (VWF), type 2B, platelet-binding evaluation, radioimmunoassay, plasma

0284U von Willebrand factor (VWF), type 2N, factor VIII and VWF binding evaluation, enzyme-linked immunosorbent assays (ELISA), plasma

0640T Noncontact near-infrared spectroscopy studies of flap or wound (eg, for measurement of deoxyhemoglobin, oxyhemoglobin, and ratio of tissue oxygenation [StO2]); image acquisition, interpretation and report, each flap or wound

0641T Noncontact near-infrared spectroscopy studies of flap or wound (eg, for measurement of deoxyhemoglobin, oxyhemoglobin, and ratio of tissue oxygenation [StO2]); image acquisition only, each flap or wound

0642T Noncontact near-infrared spectroscopy studies of flap or wound (eg, for measurement of deoxyhemoglobin, oxyhemoglobin, and ratio of tissue oxygenation [StO2]); interpretation and report only, each flap or wound

0643T Transcatheter left ventricular restoration device implantation including right and left heart catheterization and left ventriculography when performed, arterial approach

0644T Transcatheter removal or debulking of intracardiac mass (eg, vegetations, thrombus) via suction (eg, vacuum, aspiration) device, percutaneous approach, with intraoperative reinfusion of aspirated blood, including imaging guidance, when performed

0645T Transcatheter implantation of coronary sinus reduction device including vascular access and closure, right heart catheterization, venous angiography, coronary sinus angiography, imaging guidance, and supervision and interpretation, when performed

0646T Transcatheter tricuspid valve implantation/replacement (TTVI) with prosthetic valve, percutaneous approach, including right heart catheterization, temporary pacemaker insertion, and selective right ventricular or right atrial angiography, when performed

0647T Insertion of gastrostomy tube, percutaneous, with magnetic gastropexy, under ultrasound guidance, image documentation and report

0648T Quantitative magnetic resonance for analysis of tissue composition (eg, fat, iron, water content), including multiparametric data acquisition, data preparation and transmission, interpretation and report, obtained without diagnostic MRI examination of the same anatomy (eg, organ, gland, tissue, target structure) during the same session

0649T Quantitative magnetic resonance for analysis of tissue composition (eg, fat, iron, water content), including multiparametric data acquisition, data preparation and transmission, interpretation and report, obtained with diagnostic MRI examination of the same anatomy (eg, organ, gland, tissue, target structure) (List separately in addition to code for primary procedure)

0650T Programming device evaluation (remote) of subcutaneous cardiac rhythm monitor system, with iterative adjustment of the implantable device to test the function of the device and select optimal permanently programmed values with analysis, review and report by a physician or other qualified health care professional

0651T Magnetically controlled capsule endoscopy, esophagus through stomach, including intraprocedural positioning of capsule, with interpretation and report

0652T Esophagogastroduodenoscopy, flexible, transnasal; diagnostic, including collection of specimen(s) by brushing or washing, when performed (separate procedure)

0653T Esophagogastroduodenoscopy, flexible, transnasal; with biopsy, single or multiple

0654T Esophagogastroduodenoscopy, flexible, transnasal; with insertion of intraluminal tube or catheter

0655T Transperineal focal laser ablation of malignant prostate tissue, including transrectal imaging guidance, with MR-fused images or other enhanced ultrasound imaging

0656T Vertebral body tethering, anterior; up to 7 vertebral segments

0657T Vertebral body tethering, anterior; 8 or more vertebral segments

0658T Electrical impedance spectroscopy of 1 or more skin lesions for automated melanoma risk score

0659T Transcatheter intracoronary infusion of supersaturated oxygen in conjunction with percutaneous coronary revascularization during acute myocardial infarction, including catheter placement, imaging guidance (eg, fluoroscopy), angiography, and radiologic supervision and interpretation

0660T Implantation of anterior segment intraocular nonbiodegradable drug-eluting system, internal approach

0661T Removal and reimplantation of anterior segment intraocular nonbiodegradable drug-eluting implant

0662T Scalp cooling, mechanical; initial measurement and calibration of cap

0663T Scalp cooling, mechanical; placement of device, monitoring, and removal of device (List separately in addition to code for primary procedure)

0664T Donor hysterectomy (including cold preservation); open, from cadaver donor

0665T Donor hysterectomy (including cold preservation); open, from living donor

0666T Donor hysterectomy (including cold preservation); laparoscopic or robotic, from living donor

0667T Donor hysterectomy (including cold preservation); recipient uterus allograft transplantation from cadaver or living donor

0668T Backbench standard preparation of cadaver or living donor uterine allograft prior to transplantation, including dissection and removal of surrounding soft tissues and preparation of uterine vein(s) and uterine artery(ies), as necessary

0669T Backbench reconstruction of cadaver or living donor uterus allograft prior to transplantation; venous anastomosis, each

0670T Backbench reconstruction of cadaver or living donor uterus allograft prior to transplantation; arterial anastomosis, each

0671T Insertion of anterior segment aqueous drainage device into the trabecular meshwork, without external reservoir, and without concomitant cataract removal, one or more

0672T Endovaginal cryogen-cooled, monopolar radiofrequency remodeling of the tissues surrounding the female bladder neck and proximal urethra for urinary incontinence

0673T Ablation, benign thyroid nodule(s), percutaneous, laser, including imaging guidance

0674T Laparoscopic insertion of new or replacement of permanent implantable synchronized diaphragmatic stimulation system for augmentation of cardiac function, including an implantable pulse generator and diaphragmatic lead(s)

0675T Laparoscopic insertion of new or replacement of diaphragmatic lead(s), permanent implantable synchronized diaphragmatic stimulation system for augmentation of cardiac function, including connection to an existing pulse generator; first lead

0676T Laparoscopic insertion of new or replacement of diaphragmatic lead(s), permanent implantable synchronized diaphragmatic stimulation system for augmentation of cardiac function, including connection to an existing pulse generator; each additional lead (List separately in addition to code for primary procedure)

0677T Laparoscopic repositioning of diaphragmatic lead(s), permanent implantable synchronized diaphragmatic stimulation system for augmentation of cardiac function, including connection to an existing pulse generator; first repositioned lead

0678T Laparoscopic repositioning of diaphragmatic lead(s), permanent implantable synchronized diaphragmatic stimulation system for augmentation of cardiac function, including connection to an existing pulse generator; each additional repositioned lead (List separately in addition to code for primary procedure)

0679T Laparoscopic removal of diaphragmatic lead(s), permanent implantable synchronized diaphragmatic stimulation system for augmentation of cardiac function

0680T Insertion or replacement of pulse generator only, permanent implantable synchronized diaphragmatic stimulation system for augmentation of cardiac function, with connection to existing lead(s)

0681T Relocation of pulse generator only, permanent implantable synchronized diaphragmatic stimulation system for augmentation of cardiac function, with connection to existing dual leads

0682T Removal of pulse generator only, permanent implantable synchronized diaphragmatic stimulation system for augmentation of cardiac function

0683T Programming device evaluation (in-person) with iterative adjustment of the implantable device to test the function of the device and select optimal permanent programmed values with analysis, review and report by a physician or other qualified health care professional, permanent implantable synchronized diaphragmatic stimulation system for augmentation of cardiac function

0684T Peri-procedural device evaluation (in-person) and programming of device system parameters before or after a surgery, procedure, or test with analysis, review, and report by a physician or other qualified health care professional, permanent implantable synchronized diaphragmatic stimulation system for augmentation of cardiac function

0685T Interrogation device evaluation (in-person) with analysis, review and report by a physician or other qualified health care professional, including connection, recording and disconnection per patient encounter, permanent implantable synchronized diaphragmatic stimulation system for augmentation of cardiac function

0686T Histotripsy (ie, non-thermal ablation via acoustic energy delivery) of malignant hepatocellular tissue, including image guidance

0687T Treatment of amblyopia using an online digital program; device supply, educational set-up, and initial session

0688T Treatment of amblyopia using an online digital program; assessment of patient performance and program data by physician or other qualified health care professional, with report, per calendar month

0689T Quantitative ultrasound tissue characterization (non-elastographic), including interpretation and report, obtained without diagnostic ultrasound examination of the same anatomy (eg, organ, gland, tissue, target structure)

0690T Quantitative ultrasound tissue characterization (non-elastographic), including interpretation and report, obtained with diagnostic ultrasound examination of the same anatomy (eg, organ, gland, tissue, target structure) (List separately in addition to code for primary procedure)

0691T Automated analysis of an existing computed tomography study for vertebral fracture(s), including assessment of bone density when performed, data preparation, interpretation, and report

0692T Therapeutic ultrafiltration

0693T Comprehensive full body computer-based markerless 3D kinematic and kinetic motion analysis and report

0694T 3-dimensional volumetric imaging and reconstruction of breast or axillary lymph node tissue, each excised specimen, 3-dimensional automatic specimen reorientation, interpretation and report, real-time intraoperative

0695T Body surface–activation mapping of pacemaker or pacing cardioverter-defibrillator lead(s) to optimize electrical synchrony, cardiac resynchronization therapy device, including connection, recording, disconnection, review, and report; at time of implant or replacement

0696T Body surface–activation mapping of pacemaker or pacing cardioverter-defibrillator lead(s) to optimize electrical synchrony, cardiac resynchronization therapy device, including connection, recording, disconnection, review, and report; at time of follow-up interrogation or programming device evaluation

0697T multiple organs

0698T multiple organs (List separately in addition to code for primary procedure)

0699T Injection, posterior chamber of eye, medication

0700T Molecular fluorescent imaging of suspicious nevus; first lesion

0701T Molecular fluorescent imaging of suspicious nevus; each additional lesion (List separately in addition to code for primary procedure)

0702T Remote therapeutic monitoring of a standardized online digital cognitive behavioral therapy program ordered by a physician or other qualified health care professional; supply and technical support, per 30 days

0703T Remote therapeutic monitoring of a standardized online digital cognitive behavioral therapy program ordered by a physician or other qualified health care professional; management services by physician or other qualified health care professional, per calendar month

0704T Remote treatment of amblyopia using an eye tracking device; device supply with initial set-up and patient education on use of equipment

0705T Remote treatment of amblyopia using an eye tracking device; surveillance center technical support including data transmission with analysis, with a minimum of 18 training hours, each 30 days

0706T Remote treatment of amblyopia using an eye tracking device; interpretation and report by physician or other qualified health care professional, per calendar month

0707T Injection(s), bone substitute material (eg, calcium phosphate) into subchondral bone defect (ie, bone marrow lesion, bone bruise, stress injury, microtrabecular fracture), including imaging guidance and arthroscopic assistance for joint visualization

0708T Intradermal cancer immunotherapy; preparation and initial injection

0709T Intradermal cancer immunotherapy; each additional injection (List separately in addition to code for primary procedure)

0710T Noninvasive arterial plaque analysis using software processing of data from non-coronary computerized tomography angiography; including data preparation and transmission, quantification of the structure and composition of the vessel wall and assessment for lipid-rich necrotic core plaque to assess atherosclerotic plaque stability, data review, interpretation and report

0711T Noninvasive arterial plaque analysis using software processing of data from non-coronary computerized tomography angiography; data preparation and transmission

0712T Noninvasive arterial plaque analysis using software processing of data from non-coronary computerized tomography angiography; quantification of the structure and composition of the vessel wall and assessment for lipid-rich necrotic core plaque to assess atherosclerotic plaque stability

0713T Noninvasive arterial plaque analysis using software processing of data from non-coronary computerized tomography angiography; data review, interpretation and report

0017M Oncology (diffuse large B-cell lymphoma [DLBCL]), mRNA, gene expression profiling by fluorescent probe hybridization of 20 genes, formalin-fixed paraffin-embedded tissue, algorithm reported as cell of origin

0018M Transplantation medicine (allograft rejection, renal), measurement of donor and third-party-induced CD154+T-cytotoxic memory cells, utilizing whole peripheral blood, algorithm reported as a rejection risk score

Revised Codes

11981 Insertion, ~~non-biodegradable~~ drug-delivery implant (ie, bioresorbable, biodegradable, non-biodegradable)

21315 Closed treatment of nasal bone fracture with manipulation; without stabilization

21320 Closed treatment of nasal bone fracture with manipulation; with~~out~~ stabilization

22600 Arthrodesis, posterior or posterolateral technique, single ~~level~~ interspace; cervical below C2 segment

22610 Arthrodesis, posterior or posterolateral technique, single ~~level~~ interspace; thoracic (with lateral transverse technique, when performed)

22612 Arthrodesis, posterior or posterolateral technique, single ~~level~~ interspace; lumbar (with lateral transverse technique, when performed)

22614 Arthrodesis, posterior or posterolateral technique, single level interspace; each additional ~~vertebral segment~~ interspace (List separately in addition to code for primary procedure)

22633 Arthrodesis, combined posterior or posterolateral technique with posterior interbody technique including laminectomy and/or discectomy sufficient to prepare interspace (other than for decompression), single interspace ~~and segment~~; lumbar

22634 Arthrodesis, combined posterior or posterolateral technique with posterior interbody technique including laminectomy and/or discectomy sufficient to prepare interspace (other than for decompression), single interspace and segment; each additional interspace ~~and segment~~ (List separately in addition to code for primary procedure)

33471 Valvotomy, pulmonary valve, closed heart~~;~~, via pulmonary artery

35600 Harvest of upper extremity artery, 1 segment, for coronary artery bypass procedure, open ~~(List separately in addition to code for primary procedure)~~

54340 Repair of hypospadias complication(s) (ie, fistula, stricture, diverticula); by closure, incision, or excision, simple

54344 Repair of hypospadias complication(s) (ie, fistula, stricture, diverticula); requiring mobilization of skin flaps and urethroplasty with flap or patch graft

54348 Repair of hypospadias complication(s) (ie, fistula, stricture, diverticula); requiring extensive dissection, and urethroplasty with flap, patch or tubed graft (include inges urinary diversion, when performed)

54352 Revision of prior hypospadias repair~~Repair of hypospadias cripple~~ requiring extensive dissection and excision of previously constructed structures including re-release of chordee and reconstruction of urethra and penis by use of local skin as grafts and island flaps and skin brought in as flaps or grafts

63048 Laminectomy, facetectomy and foraminotomy (unilateral or bilateral with decompression of spinal cord, cauda equina and/or nerve root[s], [eg, spinal or lateral recess stenosis]), single vertebral segment; each additional vertebral segment, cervical, thoracic, or lumbar (List separately in addition to code for primary procedure)

63197 Laminectomy with cordotomy, with section of both spinothalamic tracts, 1 stage~~;~~, thoracic

64568 ~~Incision for~~ Open implantation of cranial nerve (eg, vagus nerve) neurostimulator electrode array and pulse generator

64575 ~~Incision for~~ Open implantation of neurostimulator electrode array; peripheral nerve (excludes sacral nerve)

64580 ~~Incision for~~ Open implantation of neurostimulator electrode array; neuromuscular

64581 ~~Incision for~~ Open implantation of neurostimulator electrode array; sacral nerve (transforaminal placement)

67141 Prophylaxis of retinal detachment (eg, retinal break, lattice degeneration) without drainage, ~~1 or more sessions~~; cryotherapy, diathermy

67145 Prophylaxis of retinal detachment (eg, retinal break, lattice degeneration) without drainage, ~~1 or more sessions~~; photocoagulation ~~(laser or xenon arc)~~

69714 Implantation, osseointegrated implant, ~~temporal bone~~ skull, ~~with percutaneous attachment to external speech processor/cochlear stimulator;without mastoidectomy~~ with percutaneous attachment to external speech processor

69717 Revision or r~~R~~eplacement (including removal of existing device), osseointegrated implant, ~~temporal bone~~ skull, ~~with percutaneous attachment to external speech processor/cochlear stimulator;~~ with percutaneous attachment to external speech processor~~without mastoidectomy~~

75573 Computed tomography, heart, with contrast material, for evaluation of cardiac structure and morphology in the setting of congenital heart disease (including 3D image postprocessing, assessment of left ventricular [LV] cardiac function, right ventricular [RV] structure and function and evaluation of ~~venous~~ vascular structures, if performed)

81228 Cytogenomic ~~constitutional~~ (genome-wide) ~~microarray~~ analysis for constitutional chromosomal abnormalities; interrogation of genomic regions for copy number variants, ~~(eg, bacterial artificial chromosome [BAC] or oligo-based comparative~~ genomic hybridization ([CGH]) microarray analysis)

81229 Cytogenomic ~~constitutional~~ (genome-wide) ~~microarray~~ analysis for constitutional chromosomal abnormalities; interrogation of genomic regions for copy number and single nucleotide polymorphism (SNP) variants, ~~for chromosomal abnormalities~~ comparative genomic hybridization (CGH) microarray analysis

81405 Molecular pathology procedure, Level 6 (eg, analysis of 6-10 exons by DNA sequence analysis, mutation scanning or duplication/deletion variants of 11-25 exons, regionally targeted cytogenomic array analysis)

82656 Elastase, pancreatic (EL-1), fecal,~~ qualitative or semi-quantitative~~ ; qualitative or semi-quantitative

87301 Infectious agent antigen detection by immunoassay technique, (eg, enzyme immunoassay [EIA], enzyme-linked immunosorbent assay [ELISA], fluorescence immunoassay [FIA], immunochemiluminometric assay [IMCA]), qualitative or semiquantitative, ~~multiple-step method~~; adenovirus enteric types 40/41

87305 Infectious agent antigen detection by immunoassay technique, (eg, enzyme immunoassay [EIA], enzyme-linked immunosorbent assay [ELISA], fluorescence immunoassay [FIA], immunochemiluminometric assay [IMCA]), qualitative or semiquantitative~~, multiple-step method~~; Aspergillus

87320 Infectious agent antigen detection by immunoassay technique, (eg, enzyme immunoassay [EIA], enzyme-linked immunosorbent assay [ELISA], fluorescence immunoassay [FIA], immunochemiluminometric assay [IMCA]), qualitative or semiquantitative~~, multiple-step method~~; Chlamydia trachomatis

87324 Infectious agent antigen detection by immunoassay technique, (eg, enzyme immunoassay [EIA], enzyme-linked immunosorbent assay [ELISA], fluorescence immunoassay [FIA], immunochemiluminometric assay [IMCA]), qualitative or semiquantitative~~, multiple-step method~~; Clostridium difficile toxin(s)

87327	Infectious agent antigen detection by immunoassay technique, (eg, enzyme immunoassay [EIA], enzyme-linked immunosorbent assay [ELISA], fluorescence immunoassay [FIA], immunochemiluminometric assay [IMCA]), qualitative or semiquantitative, multiple-step method; Cryptococcus neoformans

87328	Infectious agent antigen detection by immunoassay technique, (eg, enzyme immunoassay [EIA], enzyme-linked immunosorbent assay [ELISA], fluorescence immunoassay [FIA], immunochemiluminometric assay [IMCA]), qualitative or semiquantitative, multiple-step method; cryptosporidium

87329	Infectious agent antigen detection by immunoassay technique, (eg, enzyme immunoassay [EIA], enzyme-linked immunosorbent assay [ELISA], fluorescence immunoassay [FIA], immunochemiluminometric assay [IMCA]), qualitative or semiquantitative, multiple-step method; giardia

87332	Infectious agent antigen detection by immunoassay technique, (eg, enzyme immunoassay [EIA], enzyme-linked immunosorbent assay [ELISA], fluorescence immunoassay [FIA], immunochemiluminometric assay [IMCA]), qualitative or semiquantitative, multiple-step method; cytomegalovirus

87335	Infectious agent antigen detection by immunoassay technique, (eg, enzyme immunoassay [EIA], enzyme-linked immunosorbent assay [ELISA], fluorescence immunoassay [FIA], immunochemiluminometric assay [IMCA]), qualitative or semiquantitative, multiple-step method; Escherichia coli 0157

87336	Infectious agent antigen detection by immunoassay technique, (eg, enzyme immunoassay [EIA], enzyme-linked immunosorbent assay [ELISA], fluorescence immunoassay [FIA], immunochemiluminometric assay [IMCA]), qualitative or semiquantitative, multiple-step method; Entamoeba histolytica dispar group

87337	Infectious agent antigen detection by immunoassay technique, (eg, enzyme immunoassay [EIA], enzyme-linked immunosorbent assay [ELISA], fluorescence immunoassay [FIA], immunochemiluminometric assay [IMCA]), qualitative or semiquantitative, multiple-step method; Entamoeba histolytica group

87338	Infectious agent antigen detection by immunoassay technique, (eg, enzyme immunoassay [EIA], enzyme-linked immunosorbent assay [ELISA], fluorescence immunoassay [FIA], immunochemiluminometric assay [IMCA]), qualitative or semiquantitative, multiple-step method; Helicobacter pylori, stool

87339	Infectious agent antigen detection by immunoassay technique, (eg, enzyme immunoassay [EIA], enzyme-linked immunosorbent assay [ELISA], fluorescence immunoassay [FIA], immunochemiluminometric assay [IMCA]), qualitative or semiquantitative, multiple-step method; Helicobacter pylori

87340	Infectious agent antigen detection by immunoassay technique, (eg, enzyme immunoassay [EIA], enzyme-linked immunosorbent assay [ELISA], fluorescence immunoassay [FIA], immunochemiluminometric assay [IMCA]), qualitative or semiquantitative, multiple-step method; hepatitis B surface antigen (HBsAg)

87341	Infectious agent antigen detection by immunoassay technique, (eg, enzyme immunoassay [EIA], enzyme-linked immunosorbent assay [ELISA], fluorescence immunoassay [FIA], immunochemiluminometric assay [IMCA]), qualitative or semiquantitative, multiple-step method; hepatitis B surface antigen (HBsAg) neutralization

87350	Infectious agent antigen detection by immunoassay technique, (eg, enzyme immunoassay [EIA], enzyme-linked immunosorbent assay [ELISA], fluorescence immunoassay [FIA], immunochemiluminometric assay [IMCA]), qualitative or semiquantitative, multiple-step method; hepatitis Be antigen (HBeAg)

87380	Infectious agent antigen detection by immunoassay technique, (eg, enzyme immunoassay [EIA], enzyme-linked immunosorbent assay [ELISA], fluorescence immunoassay [FIA], immunochemiluminometric assay [IMCA]), qualitative or semiquantitative, multiple-step method; hepatitis, delta agent

87385	Infectious agent antigen detection by immunoassay technique, (eg, enzyme immunoassay [EIA], enzyme-linked immunosorbent assay [ELISA], fluorescence immunoassay [FIA], immunochemiluminometric assay [IMCA]), qualitative or semiquantitative, multiple-step method; Histoplasma capsulatum

87389	Infectious agent antigen detection by immunoassay technique, (eg, enzyme immunoassay [EIA], enzyme-linked immunosorbent assay [ELISA], fluorescence immunoassay [FIA], immunochemiluminometric assay [IMCA]), qualitative or semiquantitative, multiple-step method; HIV-1 antigen(s), with HIV-1 and HIV-2 antibodies, single result

87390	Infectious agent antigen detection by immunoassay technique, (eg, enzyme immunoassay [EIA], enzyme-linked immunosorbent assay [ELISA], fluorescence immunoassay [FIA], immunochemiluminometric assay [IMCA]), qualitative or semiquantitative, multiple-step method; HIV-1

87391	Infectious agent antigen detection by immunoassay technique, (eg, enzyme immunoassay [EIA], enzyme-linked immunosorbent assay [ELISA], fluorescence immunoassay [FIA], immunochemiluminometric assay [IMCA]), qualitative or semiquantitative, multiple-step method; HIV-2

87400	Infectious agent antigen detection by immunoassay technique, (eg, enzyme immunoassay [EIA], enzyme-linked immunosorbent assay [ELISA], fluorescence immunoassay [FIA], immunochemiluminometric assay [IMCA]), qualitative or semiquantitative, multiple-step method; Influenza, A or B, each

87420	Infectious agent antigen detection by immunoassay technique, (eg, enzyme immunoassay [EIA], enzyme-linked immunosorbent assay [ELISA], fluorescence immunoassay [FIA], immunochemiluminometric assay [IMCA]), qualitative or semiquantitative, multiple-step method; respiratory syncytial virus

87425	Infectious agent antigen detection by immunoassay technique, (eg, enzyme immunoassay [EIA], enzyme-linked immunosorbent assay [ELISA], fluorescence immunoassay [FIA], immunochemiluminometric assay [IMCA]), qualitative or semiquantitative, multiple-step method; rotavirus

87426	Infectious agent antigen detection by immunoassay technique, (eg, enzyme immunoassay [EIA], enzyme-linked immunosorbent assay [ELISA], fluorescence immunoassay [FIA], immunochemiluminometric assay [IMCA]), qualitative or semiquantitative, multiple-step method; severe acute respiratory syndrome coronavirus (eg, SARS-CoV, SARS-CoV-2 [COVID-19])

87427	Infectious agent antigen detection by immunoassay technique, (eg, enzyme immunoassay [EIA], enzyme-linked immunosorbent assay [ELISA], fluorescence immunoassay [FIA], immunochemiluminometric assay [IMCA]), qualitative or semiquantitative, multiple-step method; Shiga-like toxin

87430	Infectious agent antigen detection by immunoassay technique, (eg, enzyme immunoassay [EIA], enzyme-linked immunosorbent assay [ELISA], fluorescence immunoassay [FIA], immunochemiluminometric assay [IMCA]), qualitative or semiquantitative, multiple-step method; Streptococcus, group A

87449	Infectious agent antigen detection by immunoassay technique, (eg, enzyme immunoassay [EIA], enzymelinked immunosorbent assay [ELISA], immunochemiluminometric assay [IMCA]), qualitative or semiquantitative; multiple-step method,; not otherwise specified, each organism

87451	Infectious agent antigen detection by immunoassay technique, (eg, enzyme immunoassay [EIA], enzymelinked immunosorbent assay [ELISA], immunochemiluminometric assay [IMCA]), qualitative or semiquantitative; multiple-step method,; polyvalent for multiple organisms, each polyvalent antiserum

87802	Infectious agent antigen detection by immunoassay with direct optical (ie, visual) observation; Streptococcus, group B

87803	Infectious agent antigen detection by immunoassay with direct optical (ie, visual) observation; Clostridium difficile toxin A

87804	Infectious agent antigen detection by immunoassay with direct optical (ie, visual) observation; Influenza

87806	Infectious agent antigen detection by immunoassay with direct optical (ie, visual) observation; HIV-1 antigen(s), with HIV-1 and HIV-2 antibodies

87807   Infectious agent antigen detection by immunoassay with direct optical (ie, visual) observation; respiratory syncytial virus

87808   Infectious agent antigen detection by immunoassay with direct optical (ie, visual) observation; Trichomonas vaginalis

87809   Infectious agent antigen detection by immunoassay with direct optical (ie, visual) observation; adenovirus

87810   Infectious agent antigen detection by immunoassay with direct optical (ie, visual) observation; Chlamydia trachomatis

87850   Infectious agent antigen detection by immunoassay with direct optical (ie, visual) observation; Neisseria gonorrhoeae

87880   Infectious agent antigen detection by immunoassay with direct optical (ie, visual) observation; Streptococcus, group A

87899   Infectious agent antigen detection by immunoassay with direct optical (ie, visual) observation; not otherwise specified

92065   Orthoptic and/or pleoptic training, with continuing medical direction and evaluation

93653   Comprehensive electrophysiologic evaluation including with insertion and repositioning of multiple electrode catheters, with induction or attempted induction of an arrhythmia with right atrial pacing and recording and catheter ablation of arrhythmogenic focus, including intracardiac electrophysiologic 3-dimensional mapping, right ventricular pacing and recording (when necessary), left atrial pacing and recording from coronary sinus or left atrium, and His bundle recording , when performed (when necessary) with intracardiac catheter ablation of arrhythmogenic focus; with treatment of supraventricular tachycardia by ablation of fast or slow atrioventricular pathway, accessory atrioventricular connection, cavo-tricuspid isthmus or other single atrial focus or source of atrial re-entry

93654   Comprehensive electrophysiologic evaluation including with insertion and repositioning of multiple electrode catheters, with induction or attempted induction of an arrhythmia with right atrial pacing and recording and catheter ablation of arrhythmogenic focus, including intracardiac electrophysiologic 3-dimensional mapping, right ventricular pacing and recording (when necessary), left atrial pacing and recording from coronary sinus or left atrium, and His bundle recording , when performed (when necessary) with intracardiac catheter ablation of arrhythmogenic focus; with treatment of ventricular tachycardia or focus of ventricular ectopy including intracardiac electrophysiologic 3D mapping, when performed, and left ventricular pacing and recording, when performed

93656   Comprehensive electrophysiologic evaluation including transseptal catheterizations, insertion and repositioning of multiple electrode catheters with intracardiac catheter ablation of atrial fibrillation by pulmonary vein isolation, including intracardiac electrophysiologic 3-dimensional mapping, intracardiac echocardiography including imaging supervision and interpretation, induction or attempted induction of an arrhythmia including left or right atrial pacing/recording when necessary, right ventricular pacing/recording when necessary, and His bundle recording, when necessary performed with intracardiac catheter ablation of atrial fibrillation by pulmonary vein isolation

99072   Additional supplies, materials, and clinical staff time over and above those usually included in an office visit or other nonfacility service(s), when performed during a Public Health Emergency, as defined by law, due to respiratory-transmitted infectious disease

99211   Office or other outpatient visit for the evaluation and management of an established patient, that may not require the presence of a physician or other qualified health care professional. Usually, the presenting problem(s) are minimal.

99439   Chronic care management services with the following required elements: multiple (two or more) chronic conditions expected to last at least 12 months, or until the death of the patient, chronic conditions that place the patient at significant risk of death, acute exacerbation/decompensation, or functional decline, comprehensive care plan established, implemented, revised, or monitored; each additional 20 minutes of clinical staff time directed by a physician or other qualified health care professional, per calendar month (List separately in addition to code for primary procedure)

99483   Assessment of and care planning for a patient with cognitive impairment, requiring an independent historian, in the office or other outpatient, home or domiciliary or rest home, with all of the following required elements: Cognition-focused evaluation including a pertinent history and examination, ; Medical decision making of moderate or high complexity, ; Functional assessment (eg, basic and instrumental activities of daily living), including decision-making capacity, ; Use of standardized instruments for staging of dementia (eg, functional assessment staging test [FAST], clinical dementia rating [CDR]), ; Medication reconciliation and review for high-risk medications, ; Evaluation for neuropsychiatric and behavioral symptoms, including depression, including use of standardized screening instrument(s) , ; Evaluation of safety (eg, home), including motor vehicle operation, ; Identification of caregiver(s), caregiver knowledge, caregiver needs, social supports, and the willingness of caregiver to take on caregiving tasks, ; Development, updating or revision, or review of an Advance Care Plan, ; Creation of a written care plan, including initial plans to address any neuropsychiatric symptoms, neuro-cognitive symptoms, functional limitations, and referral to community resources as needed (eg, rehabilitation services, adult day programs, support groups) shared with the patient and/or caregiver with initial education and support. Typically, 50 minutes are spent face-to-face with the patient and/or family or caregiver.

99484   Care management services for behavioral health conditions, at least 20 minutes of clinical staff time, directed by a physician or other qualified health care professional, per calendar month, with the following required elements: initial assessment or follow-up monitoring, including the use of applicable validated rating scales, ; behavioral health care planning in relation to behavioral/psychiatric health problems, including revision for patients who are not progressing or whose status changes, ; facilitating and coordinating treatment such as psychotherapy, pharmacotherapy, counseling and/or psychiatric consultation, ; and continuity of care with a designated member of the care team.

99487   Complex chronic care management services with the following required elements: multiple (two or more) chronic conditions expected to last at least 12 months, or until the death of the patient, chronic conditions that place the patient at significant risk of death, acute exacerbation/decompensation, or functional decline, comprehensive care plan established, implemented, revised, or monitored, moderate or high complexity medical decision making; first 60 minutes of clinical staff time directed by a physician or other qualified health care professional, per calendar month.

99489   Complex chronic care management services with the following required elements: multiple (two or more) chronic conditions expected to last at least 12 months, or until the death of the patient, chronic conditions that place the patient at significant risk of death, acute exacerbation/decompensation, or functional decline, comprehensive care plan established, implemented, revised, or monitored, moderate or high complexity medical decision making; each additional 30 minutes of clinical staff time directed by a physician or other qualified health care professional, per calendar month (List separately in addition to code for primary procedure)

99490   Chronic care management services with the following required elements: multiple (two or more) chronic conditions expected to last at least 12 months, or until the death of the patient, chronic conditions that place the patient at significant risk of death, acute exacerbation/decompensation, or functional decline, comprehensive care plan established, implemented, revised, or monitored; first 20 minutes of clinical staff time directed by a physician or other qualified health care professional, per calendar month.

99491   Chronic care management services, provided personally by a physician or other qualified health care professional, at least 30 minutes of physician or other qualified health care professional time, per calendar month, with the following required elements: multiple (two or more) chronic conditions expected to last at least 12 months, or until the death of the patient]), ; chronic conditions that place the patient at significant risk of death, acute exacerbation/decompensation, or functional decline, ; comprehensive care plan established, implemented, revised, or monitored]), ; first 30 minutes provided personally by a physician or other qualified health care professional, per calendar month.

99492 Initial psychiatric collaborative care management, first 70 minutes in the first calendar month of behavioral health care manager activities, in consultation with a psychiatric consultant, and directed by the treating physician or other qualified health care professional, with the following required elements: outreach to and engagement in treatment of a patient directed by the treating physician or other qualified health care professional]), ; initial assessment of the patient, including administration of validated rating scales, with the development of an individualized treatment plan, ; review by the psychiatric consultant with modifications of the plan if recommended]), ; entering patient in a registry and tracking patient follow-up and progress using the registry, with appropriate documentation, and participation in weekly caseload consultation with the psychiatric consultant]), ; and provision of brief interventions using evidence-based techniques such as behavioral activation, motivational interviewing, and other focused treatment strategies.

99493 Subsequent psychiatric collaborative care management, first 60 minutes in a subsequent month of behavioral health care manager activities, in consultation with a psychiatric consultant, and directed by the treating physician or other qualified health care professional, with the following required elements: tracking patient follow-up and progress using the registry, with appropriate documentation]), ; participation in weekly caseload consultation with the psychiatric consultant, ; ongoing collaboration with and coordination of the patient's mental health care with the treating physician or other qualified health care professional and any other treating mental health providers, ; additional review of progress and recommendations for changes in treatment, as indicated, including medications, based on recommendations provided by the psychiatric consultant, ; provision of brief interventions using evidence-based techniques such as behavioral activation, motivational interviewing, and other focused treatment strategies, ; monitoring of patient outcomes using validated rating scales, ; and relapse prevention planning with patients as they achieve remission of symptoms and/or other treatment goals and are prepared for discharge from active treatment.

0101T Extracorporeal shock wave involving musculoskeletal system, not otherwise specified, high energy

0102T Extracorporeal shock wave, high energy, performed by a physician, requiring anesthesia other than local, and involving the lateral humeral epicondyle

0493T Contact N near-infrared spectroscopy studies of lower extremity wounds (eg, for oxyhemoglobin measurement)

0512T Extracorporeal shock wave for integumentary wound healing , high energy, including topical application and dressing care; initial wound

0513T Extracorporeal shock wave for integumentary wound healing, high energy, including topical application and dressing care; each additional wound (List separately in addition to code for primary procedure)

0646T Transcatheter tricuspid valve implantation (TTVI)/replacement (TTVI) with prosthetic valve, percutaneous approach, including right heart catheterization, temporary pacemaker insertion, and selective right ventricular or right atrial angiography, when performed

0648T Quantitative magnetic resonance for analysis of tissue composition (eg, fat, iron, water content), including multiparametric data acquisition, data preparation and transmission, interpretation and report, obtained without diagnostic MRI examination of the same anatomy (eg, organ, gland, tissue, target structure) during the same session; single organ

0649T Quantitative magnetic resonance for analysis of tissue composition (eg, fat, iron, water content), including multiparametric data acquisition, data preparation and transmission, interpretation and report, obtained with diagnostic MRI examination of the same anatomy (eg, organ, gland, tissue, target structure); single organ (List separately in addition to code for primary procedure)

0051U Prescription drug monitoring, evaluation of drugs present by liquid chromatography tandem mass spectrometry (LC-MS/MS),urine or blood, 31 drug panel, reported as quantitative results, detected or not detected, per date of service

0152U Infectious disease (bacteria, fungi, parasites, and DNA viruses), microbial cell-free DNA, PCR and plasma, untargeted next-generation sequencing, plasma, detection of >1,000 potential microbial organisms report for significant positive pathogens

Deleted Codes

01935	01936	21310	33470	33722	43850	43855
59135	63194	63195	63196	63198	63199	69715
69718	72275	76101	76102	80500	80502	87450
92559	92560	92561	92564	93530	93531	93532
92533	93561	93562	95943	0191T	0290T	0355T
0356T	0376T	0423T	0451T	0452T	0453T	0454T
0455T	0456T	0457T	0458T	0459T	0460T	0461T
0462T	0463T	0466T	0467T	0468T	0548T	0549T
0550T	0551T	0098U	0099U	0100U	0139U	0168U

Resequenced Icon Added

33267	33268	33269	63052	63053	64628	64629
66989	66991	69714	69716	69717	69719	69726
69727	80220	81349	82653	83529	86015	86051
86052	86053	86362	86363	86364	86408	86409
86413	87154	87428	87806	87811	90626	90627
90677	90758	90759	91113	91300	91301	91302
91303	91304	91305	91306	91307	93319	99424
99425	99426	99427	99437	0640T	0641T	0642T
0643T	0646T	0671T	0697T	0698T		

Web Release New, Revised, and Deleted Codes

Codes indicated as "Web Release" codes indicate CPT codes that are in *Current Procedural Coding Expert* for the current year, but will not be in the AMA CPT book until the following year. This can also include those codes designated by the AMA as new or revised for 2022 but that actually appeared in the 2021 Optum360 book. These codes will have the appropriate new or revised icon appended to match the CPT code book, however. See the complete list that follows:

New codes, deleted codes, and revisions to codes in the 2022 *Current Procedural Coding Expert* that will not appear in the CPT code book until 2023

These codes are indicated with the following icons: ● ▲ These icons will be green in the body of the book.

New Codes

0285U Oncology, response to radiation, cell-free DNA, quantitative branched chain DNA amplification, plasma, reported as a radiation toxicity score

0286U *CEP72 (centrosomal protein, 72-KDa), NUDT15 (nudix hydrolase 15)* and*TPMT (thiopurine S-methyltransferase)* (eg, drug metabolism) gene analysis, common variants

0287U Oncology (thyroid), DNA and mRNA, next-generation sequencing analysis of 112 genes, fine needle aspirate or formalin-fixed paraffin-embedded (FFPE) tissue, algorithmic prediction of cancer recurrence, reported as a categorical risk result (low, intermediate, high)

0288U Oncology (lung), mRNA, quantitative PCR analysis of 11 genes *(BAG1, BRCA1, CDC6, CDK2AP1, ERBB3, FUT3, IL11, LCK, RND3, SH3BGR, WNT3A)* and 3 reference genes *(ESD, TBP, YAP1),* formalin-fixed paraffin-embedded (FFPE) tumor tissue, algorithmic interpretation reported as a recurrence risk score

0289U Neurology (Alzheimer disease), mRNA, gene expression profiling by RNA sequencing of 24 genes, whole blood, algorithm reported as predictive risk score

0290U Pain management, mRNA, gene expression profiling by RNA sequencing of 36 genes, whole blood, algorithm reported as predictive risk score

0291U Psychiatry (mood disorders), mRNA, gene expression profiling by RNA sequencing of 144 genes, whole blood, algorithm reported as predictive risk score

0292U Psychiatry (stress disorders), mRNA, gene expression profiling by RNA sequencing of 72 genes, whole blood, algorithm reported as predictive risk score

0293U Psychiatry (suicidal ideation), mRNA, gene expression profiling by RNA sequencing of 54 genes, whole blood, algorithm reported as predictive risk score

0294U Longevity and mortality risk, mRNA, gene expression profiling by RNA sequencing of 18 genes, whole blood, algorithm reported as predictive risk score

0295U Oncology (breast ductal carcinoma in situ), protein expression profiling by immunohistochemistry of 7 proteins (COX2, FOXA1, HER2, Ki-67, p16, PR, SIAH2), with 4 clinicopathologic factors (size, age, margin status, palpability), utilizing formalin-fixed paraffin-embedded (FFPE) tissue, algorithm reported as a recurrence risk score

0296U Oncology (oral and/or oropharyngeal cancer), gene expression profiling by RNA sequencing at least 20 molecular features (eg, human and/or microbial mRNA), saliva, algorithm reported as positive or negative for signature associated with malignancy

0297U Oncology (pan tumor), whole genome sequencing of paired malignant and normal DNA specimens, fresh or formalin-fixed paraffin-embedded (FFPE) tissue, blood or bone marrow, comparative sequence analyses and variant identification

0298U Oncology (pan tumor), whole transcriptome sequencing of paired malignant and normal RNA specimens, fresh or formalin-fixed paraffin-embedded (FFPE) tissue, blood or bone marrow, comparative sequence analyses and expression level and chimeric transcript identification

0299U Oncology (pan tumor), whole genome optical genome mapping of paired malignant and normal DNA specimens, fresh frozen tissue, blood, or bone marrow, comparative structural variant identification

0300U Oncology (pan tumor), whole genome sequencing and optical genome mapping of paired malignant and normal DNA specimens, fresh tissue, blood, or bone marrow, comparative sequence analyses and variant identification

0301U Infectious agent detection by nucleic acid (DNA or RNA), Bartonella henselae and Bartonella quintana, droplet digital PCR (ddPCR);

0302U   following liquid enhancement

0303U Hematology, red blood cell (RBC) adhesion to endothelial/subendothelial adhesion molecules, functional assessment, whole blood, with algorithmic analysis and result reported as an RBC adhesion index; hypoxic

0304U   normoxic

0305U Hematology, red blood cell (RBC) functionality and deformity as a function of shear stress, whole blood, reported as a maximum elongation index

91305 Severe acute respiratory syndrome coronavirus 2 (SARS-CoV-2) (coronavirus disease [COVID-19]) vaccine, mRNA-LNP, spike protein, preservative free, 30 mcg/0.3 mL dosage, tris-sucrose formulation, for intramuscular use

91306 Severe acute respiratory syndrome coronavirus 2 (SARS-CoV-2) (coronavirus disease [COVID-19]) vaccine, mRNA-LNP, spike protein, preservative free, 50 mcg/0.25 mL dosage, for intramuscular use

91307 Severe acute respiratory syndrome coronavirus 2 (SARS-CoV-2) (coronavirus disease [COVID-19]) vaccine, mRNA-LNP, spike protein, preservative free, 10 mcg/0.2 mL dosage, diluent reconstituted, tris-sucrose formulation, for intramuscular use

0003A   third dose

0004A   booster dose

0013A   third dose

0034A   booster dose

0051A Immunization administration by intramuscular injection of severe acute respiratory syndrome coronavirus 2 (SARS-CoV-2) (coronavirus disease [COVID-19]) vaccine, mRNA-LNP, spike protein, preservative free, 30 mcg/0.3 mL dosage, tris-sucrose formulation; first dose

0052A   second dose

0053A   third dose

0054A   booster dose

0064A   Immunization administration by intramuscular injection of severe acute respiratory syndrome coronavirus 2 (SARS-CoV-2) (coronavirus disease [COVID-19]) vaccine, mRNA-LNP, spike protein, preservative free, 50 mcg/0.25 mL dosage, booster dose

0071A Immunization administration by intramuscular injection of severe acute respiratory syndrome coronavirus 2 (SARS-CoV-2) (coronavirus disease [COVID-19]) vaccine, mRNA-LNP, spike protein, preservative free, 10 mcg/0.2 mL dosage, diluent reconstituted, tris-sucrose formulation; first dose

0072A   second dose

Revised Codes

0090U Oncology (cutaneous melanoma), mRNA gene expression profiling by RT-PCR of 23 genes (14 content and 9 housekeeping), utilizing formalin-fixed paraffin-embedded (FFPE) tissue, algorithm reported as a categorical result (ie, benign, ~~indeterminate~~ intermediate, malignant)

Deleted Codes

0208U Oncology (medullary thyroid carcinoma), mRNA, gene expression analysis of 108 genes, utilizing fine needle aspirate, algorithm reported as positive or negative for medullary thyroid carcinoma

Appendix C — Evaluation and Management Extended Guidelines

This appendix provides an overview of evaluation and management (E/M) services, tables that identify the documentation elements associated with each code, the 2021 changes to some E/M services, and the federal documentation guidelines with emphasis on the 1997 exam guidelines. The 1997 version identifies both general multi-system physical examinations and single-system examinations, but providers may also use the original 1995 version of the E/M guidelines; both are currently supported by the Centers for Medicare and Medicaid Services (CMS) for audit purposes when reporting 99217–99499.

The levels of E/M services define the wide variations in skill, effort, and time and are required for preventing and/or diagnosing and treating illness or injury, and promoting optimal health. These codes are intended to represent physician work, and because much of this work involves the amount of training, experience, expertise, and knowledge that a provider may employ when treating a given patient, the true indications of the level of this work may be difficult to recognize without some explanation.

Providers

The AMA advises coders that while a particular service or procedure may be assigned to a specific section, the service or procedure itself is not limited to use only by that specialty group (see paragraphs 2 and 3 under "Instructions for Use of the CPT® Codebook" on page xiv of the AMA CPT book). Additionally, the procedures and services listed throughout the book are for use by any qualified physician or other qualified health care professional or entity (e.g., hospitals, laboratories, or home health agencies).

The use of the phrase "physician or other qualified health care professional" (OQHCP) was adopted to identify a health care provider other than a physician. This type of provider is further described in CPT as an individual "qualified by education, training, licensure/regulation (when applicable), and facility privileging (when applicable)." State licensure guidelines determine the scope of practice and an OQHCP must practice within these guidelines, even if more restrictive than the CPT guidelines. The OQHCP may report services independently or under incident-to guidelines. The professionals within this definition are separate from "clinical staff" and are able to practice independently. CPT defines clinical staff as "a person who works under the supervision of a physician or OQHCP and who is allowed, by law, regulation, and facility policy to perform or assist in the performance of a specified professional service, but who does not individually report that professional service." Keep in mind that there may be other policies or guidance that can affect who may report a specific service.

Types of E/M Services

When approaching E/M, the first choice that a provider must make is what type of code to use. The following tables outline the E/M codes for different levels of care for:

- Office or other outpatient services—new patient
- Office or other outpatient services—established patient
- Hospital observation services—initial care, subsequent, and discharge
- Hospital inpatient services—initial care, subsequent, and discharge
- Observation or inpatient care (including admission and discharge services)
- Consultations—office or other outpatient
- Consultations—inpatient
- Emergency department services
- Critical care
- Nursing facility—initial services
- Nursing facility—subsequent services
- Nursing facility—discharge and annual assessment
- Domiciliary, rest home, or custodial care—new patient
- Domiciliary, rest home, or custodial care—established patient
- Home services—new patient
- Home services—established patient
- Newborn care services
- Neonatal and pediatric interfacility transport
- Neonatal and pediatric critical care—inpatient
- Neonate and infant intensive care services—initial and continuing
- Care management

The specifics of the code components that determine code selection are listed in the table and discussed in the next section. Before a level of service is decided upon, the correct type of service is identified.

A new patient is a patient who has not received any face-to-face professional services from the physician or OQHCP within the past three years. An established patient is a patient who has received face-to-face professional services from the physician or OQHCP within the past three years. In the case of group practices, if a physician or OQHCP of the exact same specialty or subspecialty has seen the patient within three years, the patient is considered established.

If a physician or OQHCP is on call or covering for another physician or OQHCP, the patient's encounter is classified as it would have been by the physician or OQHCP who is not available. Thus, a locum tenens physician or OQHCP who sees a patient on behalf of the patient's attending physician or OQHCP may not bill a new patient code unless the attending physician or OQHCP has not seen the patient for any problem within three years.

Office or other outpatient services are E/M services provided in the physician or OQHCP office, the outpatient area, or other ambulatory facility. Until the patient is admitted to a health care facility, he/she is considered to be an outpatient. Hospital observation services are E/M services provided to patients who are designated or admitted as "observation status" in a hospital.

Codes 99218-99220 are used to indicate initial observation care. These codes include the initiation of the observation status, supervision of patient care including writing orders, and the performance of periodic reassessments. These codes are used only by the provider "admitting" the patient for observation.

Codes 99234-99236 are used to indicate evaluation and management services to a patient who is admitted to and discharged from observation status or hospital inpatient on the same day. If the patient is admitted as an inpatient from observation on the same day, use the appropriate level of Initial Hospital Care (99221-99223).

Code 99217 indicates discharge from observation status. It includes the final physical examination of the patient, instructions, and preparation of the discharge records. It should not be used when admission and discharge are on the same date of service. As mentioned above, report codes 99234-99236 to appropriately describe same day observation services.

If a patient is in observation longer than one day, subsequent observation care codes 99224-99226 should be reported. If the patient is discharged on the second day, observation discharge code 99217 should be reported. If the patient status is changed to inpatient on a subsequent date, the appropriate inpatient code, 99221-99233, should be reported.

Initial hospital care is defined as E/M services provided during the first hospital inpatient encounter with the patient by the admitting provider. (If a physician other than the admitting physician performs the initial inpatient encounter, refer to consultations or subsequent hospital care in the CPT book.) Subsequent hospital care includes all follow-up encounters with the patient by all physicians or OQHCP. As there may only be one admitting physician, HCPCS Level II modifier AI Principal physician of record, should be appended to the initial hospital care code by the attending physician or OQHCP.

A consultation is the provision of a physician or OQHCP's opinion or advice about a patient for a specific problem at the request of another physician or other appropriate source. CPT also states that a consultation may be performed when a physician or OQHCP is determining whether to accept the transfer of patient care at the request of another physician or appropriate source. An office or other outpatient consultation is a consultation provided in the consultant's office, in the emergency department, or in an outpatient or other ambulatory facility including hospital observation services, home services, domiciliary, rest home, or custodial care. An inpatient consultation is a consultation provided in the hospital or partial hospital nursing facility setting. Report only one inpatient consultation by a consultant for each admission to the hospital or nursing facility.

If a consultant participates in the patient's management after the opinion or advice is provided, use codes for subsequent hospital or observation care or for office or other outpatient services (established patient), as appropriate.

Under CMS guidelines, the inpatient and office/outpatient consultation codes contained in the CPT manual are not covered services.

All outpatient consultation services should be reported for Medicare using the appropriate new or established evaluation and management (E/M) codes. Inpatient consultation services for the initial encounter should be reported by the physician providing the service using initial hospital care codes 99221–99223, and subsequent inpatient care codes 99231–99233.

Codes 99439, 99487, 99489, 99490, 99491, and 99347 are used to report evaluation and management services for chronic care management. These codes represent management and support services provided by clinical staff, under the direction of a physician or OQHCP, to patients residing at home or in a domiciliary, rest home, or assisted living facility. The qualified provider oversees the management and/or coordination of services for all

medical conditions, psychosocial needs, and activities of daily living. These codes are reported only once per calendar month and have specific time-based thresholds.

Codes 99424–99427 are used to report principal care management services for complex chronic conditions for medical and/or psychological needs. These codes represent management and support services provided by clinical staff, a physician, or OQHCP for patients with a single, complex chronic condition that is expected to last at least three months. The qualified provider oversees the establishment, implementation, revision, or monitoring of a specific plan of care for that single condition. These codes are reported only once per month and have specific time-based thresholds.

Codes 99497-99498 are used to report the discussion and explanation of advanced directives by a physician or OQHCP. These codes represent a face-to-face service between the provider and a patient, family member, or surrogate. These codes are time-based codes and, since no active management of the problem(s) is undertaken during this time, may be reported on the same day as another E/M service.

Certain codes that CPT considers appropriate telehealth services are identified with the ★ icon and reported with modifier 95 Synchronous telemedicine service rendered via a real-time interactive audio and video telecommunications system. Medicare recognizes certain CPT and HCPCS Level II G codes as telehealth services reported with modifier GT. Check with individual payers for telehealth modifier guidance.

E/M Code	History	Exam	Medical Decision Making	Time Spent Face-to-Face (avg.)
99202	Medically appropriate	Medically appropriate	Straightforward	15–29 min.
99203	Medically appropriate	Medically appropriate	Low	30–44 min.
99204	Medically appropriate	Medically appropriate	Moderate	45–59 min.
99205	Medically appropriate	Medically appropriate	High	60–74 min.

Office or Other Outpatient Services—Established Patient[1]

E/M Code	History	Exam	Medical Decision Making	Time Spent Face-to-Face (avg.)
99211	—	—	Physician supervision, but presence not required	—
99212	Medically appropriate	Medically appropriate	Straightforward	10–19 min.
99213	Medically appropriate	Medically appropriate	Low	20–29 min.
99214	Medically appropriate	Medically appropriate	Moderate	30–39 min.
99215	Medically appropriate	Medically appropriate	High	40–54 min.

1 Includes follow-up, periodic reevaluation, and evaluation and management of new problems.

Hospital Observation Services

E/M Code	History[1]	Exam[1]	Medical Decision Making[1]	Problem Severity	Coordination of Care; Counseling	Time Spent Bedside and on Unit/Floor (avg.)
99217	Observation care discharge day management					
99218	Detailed or comprehensive	Detailed or comprehensive	Straightforward or low complexity	Low	Consistent with problem(s) and patient's needs	30 min.
99219	Comprehensive	Comprehensive	Moderate complexity	Moderate	Consistent with problem(s) and patient's needs	50 min.
99220	Comprehensive	Comprehensive	High complexity	High	Consistent with problem(s) and patient's needs	70 min.

1 Key component. All three components (history, exam, and medical decision making) are crucial for selecting the correct code.

Subsequent Hospital Observation Services[1]

E/M Code[2]	History[3]	Exam[3]	Medical Decision Making[3]	Problem Severity	Coordination of Care; Counseling	Time Spent Bedside and on Unit/Floor (avg.)
99224	Problem-focused interval	Problem-focused	Straightforward or low complexity	Stable, recovering, or improving	Consistent with problem(s) and patient's needs	15 min.
99225	Expanded problem-focused interval	Expanded problem-focused	Moderate complexity	Inadequate response to treatment; minor complications	Consistent with problem(s) and patient's needs	25 min.
99226	Detailed interval	Detailed	High complexity	Unstable; significant new problem or significant complication	Consistent with problem(s) and patient's needs	35 min.

1 All subsequent levels of service include reviewing the medical record, diagnostic studies, and changes in the patient's status, such as history, physical condition, and response to treatment since the last assessment.

2 These codes are resequenced in CPT and are printed following codes 99217-99220.

3 Key component. For subsequent care, at least two of the three components (history, exam, and medical decision making) are needed to select the correct code.

Hospital Inpatient Services—Initial Care[1]

E/M Code	History[2]	Exam[2]	Medical Decision Making[2]	Problem Severity	Coordination of Care; Counseling	Time Spent Bedside and on Unit/Floor (avg.)
99221	Detailed or comprehensive	Detailed or comprehensive	Straightforward or low complexity	Low	Consistent with problem(s) and patient's needs	30 min.
99222	Comprehensive	Comprehensive	Moderate complexity	Moderate	Consistent with problem(s) and patient's needs	50 min.
99223	Comprehensive	Comprehensive	High complexity	High	Consistent with problem(s) and patient's needs	70 min.

1 The admitting physician should append modifier AI, Principal physician of record, for Medicare patients

2 Key component. For initial care, all three components (history, exam, and medical decision making) are crucial for selecting the correct code.

Hospital Inpatient Services—Subsequent Care[1]

E/M Code	History[2]	Exam[2]	Medical Decision Making[2]	Problem Severity	Coordination of Care; Counseling	Time Spent Bedside and on Unit/Floor (avg.)
99231	Problem-focused interval	Problem-focused	Straightforward or low complexity	Stable, recovering or Improving	Consistent with problem(s) and patient's needs	15 min.
99232	Expanded problem-focused interval	Expanded problem-focused	Moderate complexity	Inadequate response to treatment; minor complications	Consistent with problem(s) and patient's needs	25 min.
99233	Detailed interval	Detailed	High complexity	Unstable; significant new problem or significant complication	Consistent with problem(s) and patient's needs	35 min.
99238	Hospital discharge day management					30 min. or less
99239	Hospital discharge day management					> 30 min.

1 All subsequent levels of service include reviewing the medical record, diagnostic studies, and changes in the patient's status, such as history, physical condition, and response to treatment since the last assessment.

2 Key component. For subsequent care, at least two of the three components (history, exam, and medical decision making) are needed to select the correct code.

Observation or Inpatient Care Services (Including Admission and Discharge Services)

E/M Code	History[1]	Exam[1]	Medical Decision Making[1]	Problem Severity	Coordination of Care; Counseling	Time
99234	Detailed or comprehensive	Detailed or comprehensive	Straightforward or low complexity	Low	Consistent with problem(s) and patient's needs	40 min.
99235	Comprehensive	Comprehensive	Moderate	Moderate	Consistent with problem(s) and patient's needs	50 min.
99236	Comprehensive	Comprehensive	High	High	Consistent with problem(s) and patient's needs	55 min.

1 Key component. All three components (history, exam, and medical decision making) are crucial for selecting the correct code.

Consultations—Office or Other Outpatient

E/M Code	History[1]	Exam[1]	Medical Decision Making[1]	Problem Severity	Coordination of Care; Counseling	Time Spent Face-to-Face (avg.)
99241	Problem-focused	Problem-focused	Straightforward	Minor or self-limited	Consistent with problem(s) and patient's needs	15 min.
99242	Expanded problem-focused	Expanded problem-focused	Straightforward	Low	Consistent with problem(s) and patient's needs	30 min.
99243	Detailed	Detailed	Low complexity	Moderate	Consistent with problem(s) and patient's needs	40 min.
99244	Comprehensive	Comprehensive	Moderate complexity	Moderate to high	Consistent with problem(s) and patient's needs	60 min.
99245	Comprehensive	Comprehensive	High complexity	Moderate to high	Consistent with problem(s) and patient's needs	80 min.

1 Key component. For office or other outpatient consultations, all three components (history, exam, and medical decision making) are crucial for selecting the correct code.

Consultations—Inpatient[1]

E/M Code	History[2]	Exam[2]	Medical Decision Making[2]	Problem Severity	Coordination of Care; Counseling	Time Spent Bedside and on Unit/Floor (avg.)
99251	Problem-focused	Problem-focused	Straightforward	Minor or self-limited	Consistent with problem(s) and patient's needs	20 min.
99252	Expanded problem-focused	Expanded problem-focused	Straightforward	Low	Consistent with problem(s) and patient's needs	40 min.
99253	Detailed	Detailed	Low complexity	Moderate	Consistent with problem(s) and patient's needs	55 min.
99254	Comprehensive	Comprehensive	Moderate complexity	Moderate to high	Consistent with problem(s) and patient's needs	80 min.
99255	Comprehensive	Comprehensive	High complexity	Moderate to high	Consistent with problem(s) and patient's needs	110 min.

1 These codes are used for hospital inpatients, residents of nursing facilities or patients in a partial hospital setting.
2 Key component. For initial inpatient consultations, all three components (history, exam, and medical decision making) are crucial for selecting the correct code.

Emergency Department Services, New or Established Patient

E/M Code	History[1]	Exam[1]	Medical Decision Making[1]	Problem Severity[3]	Coordination of Care; Counseling	Time Spent[2] Face-to-Face (avg.)
99281	Problem-focused	Problem-focused	Straightforward	Minor or self-limited	Consistent with problem(s) and patient's needs	N/A
99282	Expanded problem-focused	Expanded problem-focused	Low complexity	Low to moderate	Consistent with problem(s) and patient's needs	N/A
99283	Expanded problem-focused	Expanded problem-focused	Moderate complexity	Moderate	Consistent with problem(s) and patient's needs	N/A
99284	Detailed	Detailed	Moderate complexity	High; requires urgent evaluation	Consistent with problem(s) and patient's needs	N/A
99285	Comprehensive	Comprehensive	High complexity	High; poses immediate/significant threat to life or physiologic function	Consistent with problem(s) and patient's needs	N/A
99288[4]			High complexity			N/A

1 Key component. For emergency department services, all three components (history, exam, and medical decision making) are crucial for selecting the correct code and must be adequately documented in the medical record to substantiate the level of service reported.

2 Typical times have not been established for this category of services.

3 NOTE: The severity of the patient's problem, while taken into consideration when evaluating and treating the patient, does not automatically determine the level of E/M service unless the medical record documentation reflects the severity of the patient's illness, injury, or condition in the details of the history, physical examination, and medical decision making process. Federal auditors will "downcode" the level of E/M service despite the nature of the patient's problem when the documentation does not support the E/M code reported.

4 Code 99288 is used to report two-way communication with emergency medical services personnel in the field.

Critical Care

E/M Code	Patient Status	Physician Attendance	Time[1]
99291	Critically ill or critically injured	Constant	First 30–74 minutes
99292	Critically ill or critically injured	Constant	Each additional 30 minutes beyond the first 74 minutes

1 Per the guidelines for time in *CPT 2016 page xv*, "A unit of time is attained when the mid-point is passed. For example, an hour is attained when 31 minutes have elapsed (more than midway between zero and 60 minutes)."

Nursing Facility Services—Initial Nursing Facility Care[1]

E/M Code	History[1]	Exam[1]	Medical Decision Making[1]	Problem Severity	Coordination of Care; Counseling
99304	Detailed or comprehensive	Detailed or comprehensive	Straightforward or low complexity	Low	25 min.
99305	Comprehensive	Comprehensive	Moderate complexity	Moderate	35 min.
99306	Comprehensive	Comprehensive	High complexity	High	45 min.

1 These services must be performed by the physician. See CPT Corrections Document – CPT 2013 page 3 or guidelines CPT 2016 page 26.

2 Key component. For new patients, all three components (history, exam, and medical decision making) are crucial for selecting the correct code.

Nursing Facility Services—Subsequent Nursing Facility Care

E/M Code	History[1]	Exam[1]	Medical Decision Making[2]	Problem Severity	Coordination of Care; Counseling
99307	Problem-focused interval	Problem-focused	Straightforward	Stable, recovering or improving	10 min.
99308	Expanded problem-focused interval	Expanded problem-focused	Low complexity	Responding inadequately or has developed a minor complication	15 min.
99309	Detailed interval	Detailed	Moderate complexity	Significant complication or a significant new problem	25 min.
99310	Comprehensive interval	Comprehensive	High complexity	Developed a significant new problem requiring immediate attention	35 min.

1 Key component. For established patients, at least two of the three components (history, exam, and medical decision making) are needed for selecting the correct code.

Nursing Facility Discharge and Annual Assessment

E/M Code	History[1]	Exam[1]	Medical Decision Making[1]	Problem Severity	Time Spent Bedside and on Unit/Floor (avg.)
99315	Nursing facility discharge day management				30 min. or less
99316	Nursing facility discharge day management				more than 30 min.
99318	Detailed interval	Comprehensive	Low to moderate complexity	Stable, recovering or improving	30 min.

1 Key component. For annual nursing facility assessment, all three components (history, exam, and medical decision making) are crucial for selecting the correct code.

Domiciliary, Rest Home (e.g., Boarding Home) or Custodial Care Services—New Patient

E/M Code	History[1]	Exam[1]	Medical Decision Making[1]	Problem Severity	Coordination of Care; Counseling	Time Spent Face-to-Face (avg.)
99324	Problem-focused	Problem-focused	Straightforward	Low	Consistent with problem(s) and patient's needs	20 min.
99325	Expanded problem-focused	Expanded problem-focused	Low complexity	Moderate	Consistent with problem(s) and patient's needs	30 min.
99326	Detailed	Detailed	Moderate complexity	Moderate to high	Consistent with problem(s) and patient's needs	45 min.
99327	Comprehensive	Comprehensive	Moderate complexity	High	Consistent with problem(s) and patient's needs	60 min.
99328	Comprehensive	Comprehensive	High complexity	Unstable or developed a new problem requiring immediate physician attention	Consistent with problem(s) and patient's needs	75 min.

1 Key component. For new patients, all three components (history, exam, and medical decision making) are crucial for selecting the correct code and must be adequately documented in the medical record to substantiate the level of service reported.

Domiciliary, Rest Home (e.g., Boarding Home) or Custodial Care Services— Established Patient

E/M Code	History[1]	Exam[1]	Medical Decision Making[1]	Problem Severity	Coordination of Care; Counseling	Time Spent Face-to-Face (avg.)
99334	Problem-focused interval	Problem-focused	Straightforward	Minor or self-limited	Consistent with problem(s) and patient's needs	15 min.
99335	Expanded problem-focused interval	Expanded problem-focused	Low complexity	Low to moderate	Consistent with problem(s) and patient's needs	25 min.
99336	Detailed interval	Detailed	Moderate complexity	Moderate to high	Consistent with problem(s) and patient's needs	40 min.
99337	Comprehensive interval	Comprehensive	Moderate to high complexity	Moderate to high	Consistent with problem(s) and patient's needs	60 min.

1 Key component. For established patients, at least two of the three components (history, exam, and medical decision making) are needed for selecting the correct code.

Domiciliary, Rest Home (e.g., Assisted Living Facility), or Home Care Plan Oversight Services

E/M Code	Intent of Service	Presence of Patient	Time
99339	Individual physician supervision of a patient (patient not present) in home, domiciliary or rest home (e.g., assisted living facility) requiring complex and multidisciplinary care modalities involving regular physician development and/or revision of care plans, review of subsequent reports of patient status, review of related laboratory and other studies, communication (including telephone calls) for purposes of assessment or care decisions with health care professional(s), family member(s), surrogate decision maker(s) (e.g., legal guardian) and/or key caregiver(s) involved in patient's care, integration of new information into the medical treatment plan and/or adjustment of medical therapy, within a calendar month	Patient not present	15–29 min.
99340	Same as 99339	Patient not present	30 min. or more

Home Services—New Patient

E/M Code	History[1]	Exam[1]	Medical Decision Making[1]	Problem Severity	Coordination of Care; Counseling	Time Spent Face-to-Face (avg.)
99341	Problem-focused	Problem-focused	Straightforward complexity	Low	Consistent with problem(s) and patient's needs	20 min.
99342	Expanded problem-focused	Expanded problem-focused	Low complexity	Moderate	Consistent with problem(s) and patient's needs	30 min.
99343	Detailed	Detailed	Moderate complexity	Moderate to high	Consistent with problem(s) and patient's needs	45 min.
99344	Comprehensive	Comprehensive	Moderate complexity	High	Consistent with problem(s) and patient's needs	60 min.
99345	Comprehensive	Comprehensive	High complexity	Usually the patient has developed a significant new problem requiring immediate physician attention	Consistent with problem(s) and patient's needs	75 min.

1 Key component. For new patients, all three components (history, exam, and medical decision making) are crucial for selecting the correct code and must be adequately documented in the medical record to substantiate the level of service reported.

Home Services—Established Patient

E/M Code	History[1]	Exam[1]	Medical Decision Making[1]	Problem Severity	Coordination of Care; Counseling	Time Spent Face-to-Face (avg.)
99347	Problem-focused interval	Problem-focused	Straightforward	Minor or self-limited	Consistent with problem(s) and patient's needs	15 min.
99348	Expanded problem-focused interval	Expanded problem-focused	Low complexity	Low to moderate	Consistent with problem(s) and patient's needs	25 min.
99349	Detailed interval	Detailed	Moderate complexity	Moderate to high	Consistent with problem(s) and patient's needs	40 min.
99350	Comprehensive interval	Comprehensive	Moderate to high complexity	Moderate to high Usually the patient has developed a significant new problem requiring immediate physician attention	Consistent with problem(s) and patient's needs	60 min.

1 Key component. For established patients, at least two of the three components (history, exam, and medical decision making) are needed for selecting the correct code.

Newborn Care Services

E/M Code	Patient Status	Type of Visit
99460	Normal newborn	Inpatient initial inpatient hospital or birthing center per day
99461	Normal newborn	Inpatient initial treatment not in hospital or birthing center per day
99462	Normal newborn	Inpatient subsequent per day
99463	Normal newborn	Inpatient initial inpatient and discharge in hospital or birthing center per day
99464	Unstable newborn	Attendance at delivery
99465	High-risk newborn at delivery	Resuscitation, ventilation, and cardiac treatment

Neonatal and Pediatric Interfacility Transportation

E/M Code	Patient Status	Type of Visit
99466	Critically ill or injured infant or young child, to 24 months	Face-to-face transportation from one facility to another, initial 30-74 minutes
99467	Critically ill or injured infant or young child, to 24 months	Face-to-face transportation from one facility to another, each additional 30 minutes
99485[1]	Critically ill or injured infant or young child, to 24 months	Supervision of patient transport from one facility to another, initial 30 minutes
99486[1]	Critically ill or injured infant or young child, to 24 months	Supervision of patient transport from one facility to another, each additional 30 minutes

1 These codes are resequenced in CPT and are printed following codes 99466-99467.

Inpatient Neonatal and Pediatric Critical Care

E/M Code	Patient Status	Type of Visit
99468[1]	Critically ill neonate, aged 28 days or less	Inpatient initial per day
99469[2]	Critically ill neonate, aged 28 days or less	Inpatient subsequent per day
99471	Critically ill infant or young child, aged 29 days to 24 months	Inpatient initial per day
99472	Critically ill infant or young child, aged 29 days to 24 months	Inpatient subsequent per day
99475	Critically ill infant or young child, 2 to 5 years[3]	Inpatient initial per day
99476	Critically ill infant or young child, 2 to 5 years	Inpatient subsequent per day

1 Codes 99468, 99471, and 99475 may be reported only once per admission.
2 Codes 99469, 99472, and 99476 may be reported only once per day and by only one provider.
3 See 99291-99292 for patients 6 years of age and older.

Neonate and Infant Initial and Continuing Intensive Care Services

E/M Code	Patient Status	Type of Visit
99477	Neonate, aged 28 days or less	Inpatient initial per day
99478	Infant with present body weight of less than 1500 grams, no longer critically ill	Inpatient subsequent per day
99479	Infant with present body weight of 1500-2500 grams, no longer critically ill	Inpatient subsequent per day
99480	Infant with present body weight of 2501-5000 grams, no longer critically ill	Inpatient subsequent per day

Reporting Levels of E/M Services Codes 99202–99215

A medically appropriate history and physical examination, as determined by the treating provider, should be documented. The level of history and physical examination are no longer used when determining the level of service. Codes should be selected based upon the CPT 2022 Medical Decision Making (MDM) table or time as documented in the patient record.

The 2022 Medical Decision Making (MDM) table requires two of three levels of the three elements be met or exceeded to determine the level of code reported. The three elements are:

- Number and complexity of problems addressed at the encounter
- Amount and/or complexity of data to be reviewed and analyzed
- Risk of complications and/or morbidity or mortality of patient management

Instructions and examples of each element are given in the table to enable accurate selection of the level of MDM and E/M service to be reported for codes 99202–99215.

Alternately time alone may be used to select the appropriate level of service. Total time for reporting these services included face-to-face and non-face-to-face time personally spent by the physician or other qualified health care professional on the date of the encounter. The E/M codes 99202–99205 and 99212–99215 include specific time ranges used to select the appropriate code. Report 99417 for prolonged services when the time for code 99205 or 99215 is exceeded. Report 99417 for each minimum of 15 minutes additional prolonged services.

Code 99211 is used to report the E/M service that does not require the presence of the physician or other qualified health care professional.

Levels of E/M Services Codes 99217–99499

Confusion may be experienced when first approaching E/M codes 99217–99499 due to the way that each description of a code component or element seems to have another layer of description beneath. The three key components—history, exam, and decision making—are each comprised of elements that combine to create varying levels of that component.

For example, an expanded problem-focused history includes the chief complaint, a brief history of the present illness, and a system review focusing on the patient's problems. The level of exam is not made up of different elements but rather distinguished by the extent of exam across body areas or organ systems.

The single largest source of confusion are the "labels" or names applied to the varying degrees of history, exam, and decision-making. Terms such as expanded problem-focused, detailed, and comprehensive are somewhat meaningless unless they are defined. The lack of definition in CPT guidelines relative to these terms is precisely what caused the first set of federal guidelines to be developed in 1995 and again in 1997.

Documentation Guidelines for Evaluation and Management Services

Both versions of the federal guidelines go well beyond CPT guidelines in defining specific code requirements. The current version of the CPT guidelines does not explain the number of history of present illness (HPI) elements or the specific number of organ systems or body areas to be examined as they are in the federal guidelines. Adherence to some version of the guidelines is required when billing E/M to federal payers, but at this time, the CPT guidelines do not incorporate this level of detail into the code definitions. Although that could be interpreted to mean that non-governmental payers have a lesser documentation standard, it is best to adopt one set of the federal versions for all payer types for both consistency and ease of use.

The 1997 guidelines supply a great amount of detail relative to history and exam and will give the provider clear direction to follow when documenting elements. With that stated, the 1995 guidelines are equally valid and place a lesser documentation burden on the provider in regard to the physical exam.

The 1995 guidelines ask only for a notation of "normal" on systems with normal findings. The only narrative required is for abnormal findings. The 1997 version calls for much greater detail, or an "elemental" or "bullet-point" approach to organ systems, although a notation of normal is sufficient when addressing the elements within a system. The 1997 version works well in a template or electronic health record (EHR) format for recording E/M services.

The 1997 version did produce the single system specialty exam guidelines. When reviewing the complete guidelines listed below, note the differences between exam requirements in the 1995 and 1997 versions.

A Comparison of 1995 and 1997 Exam Guidelines

There are four types of exams indicated in the levels of E/M codes. Although the descriptors or labels are the same under 1995 and 1997 guidelines, the degree of detail required is different. The remaining content on this topic references the 1997 general multi-system specialty examination, at the end of this chapter.

The levels under each set of guidelines are:

1995 Exam Guidelines:

Problem focused:	One body area or system
Expanded problem focused:	Two to seven body areas or organ systems
Detailed:	Two to seven body areas or organ systems
Comprehensive:	Eight or more organ systems or a complete single-system examination

1997 Exam Guidelines:

Problem-focused:	Perform and document examination of one to five bullet point elements in one or more organ systems/body areas from the general multi-system examination
OR	
	Perform or document examination of one to five bullet point elements from one of the 10 single-organ-system examinations, shaded or unshaded boxes
Expanded problem-focused:	Perform and document examination of at least six bullet point elements in one or more organ systems from the general multi-system examination
OR	
	Perform and document examination of at least six bullet point elements from one of the 10 single-organ-system examinations, shaded or unshaded boxes
Detailed:	Perform and document examination of at least six organ systems or body areas, including at least two bullet point elements for each organ system or body area from the general multi-system examination
OR	
	Perform and document examination of at least 12 bullet point elements in two or more organ systems or body areas from the general multisystem examination

OR	
	Perform and document examination of at least 12 bullet elements from one of the single-organ-system examinations, shaded or unshaded boxes
Comprehensive:	Perform and document examination of at least nine organ systems or body areas, with all bullet elements for each organ system or body area (unless specific instructions are expected to limit examination content with at least two bullet elements for each organ system or body area) from the general multi-system examination
OR	
	Perform and document examination of all bullet point elements from one of the 10 single-organ system examinations with documentation of every element in shaded boxes and at least one element in each unshaded box from the single-organ-system examination.

The Documentation Guidelines

The following guidelines were developed jointly by the American Medical Association (AMA) and the Centers for Medicare and Medicaid Services (CMS). Their mutual goal was to provide physicians and claims reviewers with advice about preparing or reviewing documentation for Evaluation and Management (E/M) services.

I. Introduction

What is Documentation and Why Is It Important?

Medical record documentation is required to record pertinent facts, findings, and observations about an individual's health history, including past and present illnesses, examinations, tests, treatments, and outcomes. The medical record chronologically documents the care of the patient and is an important element contributing to high quality care. The medical record facilitates:

- The ability of the physician and other health care professionals to evaluate and plan the patient's immediate treatment and to monitor his/her health care over time
- Communication and continuity of care among physicians and other health care professionals involved in the patient's care
- Accurate and timely claims review and payment
- Appropriate utilization review and quality of care evaluations
- Collection of data that may be useful for research and education

An appropriately documented medical record can reduce many of the problems associated with claims processing and may serve as a legal document to verify the care provided, if necessary.

What Do Payers Want and Why?

Because payers have a contractual obligation to enrollees, they may require reasonable documentation that services are consistent with the insurance coverage provided. They may request information to validate:

- The site of service
- The medical necessity and appropriateness of the diagnostic and/or therapeutic services provided
- Services provided have been accurately reported

II. General Principles of Medical Record Documentation

The principles of documentation listed below are applicable to all types of medical and surgical services in all settings. For Evaluation and Management (E/M) services, the nature and amount of physician work and documentation varies by type of service, place of service, and the patient's status. The general principles listed below may be modified to account for these variable circumstances in providing E/M services.

- The medical record should be complete and legible
- The documentation of each patient encounter should include:

- A reason for the encounter and relevant history, physical examination findings, and prior diagnostic test results
- Assessment, clinical impression, or diagnosis
- Plan for care
- Date and legible identity of the practitioner
- If not documented, the rationale for ordering diagnostic and other ancillary services should be easily inferred
- Past and present diagnoses should be accessible to the treating and/or consulting physician
- Appropriate health risk factors should be identified
- The patient's progress, response to, and changes in treatment and revision of diagnosis should be documented
- The CPT and ICD-9-CM codes reported on the health insurance claim form or billing statement should be supported by the documentation in the medical record

III. Documentation of E/M Services 1995 and 1997

The following information provides definitions and documentation guidelines for the three key components of E/M services and for visits that consist predominately of counseling or coordination of care. The three key components—history, examination, and medical decision making—appear in the descriptors for office and other outpatient services, hospital observation services, hospital inpatient services, consultations, emergency department services, nursing facility services, domiciliary care services, and home services. While some of the text of the CPT guidelines has been repeated in this document, the reader should refer to CMS or CPT for the complete descriptors for E/M services and instructions for selecting a level of service. Documentation guidelines are identified by the symbol DG.

The descriptors for the levels of E/M services recognize seven components that are used in defining the levels of E/M services. These components are:

- History
- Examination
- Medical decision making
- Counseling
- Coordination of care
- Nature of presenting problem
- Time

The first three of these components (i.e., history, examination, and medical decision making) are the key components in selecting the level of E/M services. In the case of visits that consist predominately of counseling or coordination of care, time is the key or controlling factor to qualify for a particular level of E/M service.

Because the level of E/M service is dependent on two or three key components, performance and documentation of one component (e.g., examination) at the highest level does not necessarily mean that the encounter in its entirety qualifies for the highest level of E/M service.

These Documentation Guidelines for E/M services reflect the needs of the typical adult population. For certain groups of patients, the recorded information may vary slightly from that described here. Specifically, the medical records of infants, children, adolescents, and pregnant women may have additional or modified information, as appropriate, recorded in each history and examination area.

As an example, newborn records may include under history of the present illness (HPI) the details of the mother's pregnancy and the infant's status at birth; social history will focus on family structure; and family history will focus on congenital anomalies and hereditary disorders in the family. In addition, the content of a pediatric examination will vary with the age and development of the child. Although not specifically defined in these documentation guidelines, these patient group variations on history and examination are appropriate.

A. Documentation of History

The levels of E/M services are based on four types of history (Problem Focused, Expanded Problem Focused, Detailed, and Comprehensive). Each type of history includes some or all of the following elements:

- Chief complaint (CC)
- History of present illness (HPI)
- Review of systems (ROS)

- Past, family, and/or social history (PFSH)

The extent of history of present illness, review of systems, and past, family, and/or social history that is obtained and documented is dependent upon clinical judgment and the nature of the presenting problem.

The chart below shows the progression of the elements required for each type of history. To qualify for a given type of history all three elements in the table must be met. (A chief complaint is indicated at all levels.)

- DG: The CC, ROS, and PFSH may be listed as separate elements of history or they may be included in the description of the history of present illness

- DG: A ROS and/or a PFSH obtained during an earlier encounter does not need to be re-recorded if there is evidence that the physician reviewed and updated the previous information. This may occur when a physician updates his/her own record or in an institutional setting or group practice where many physicians use a common record. The review and update may be documented by:

  - Describing any new ROS and/or PFSH information or noting there has been no change in the information

  - Noting the date and location of the earlier ROS and/or PFSH

- DG: The ROS and/or PFSH may be recorded by ancillary staff or on a form completed by the patient. To document that the physician reviewed the information, there must be a notation supplementing or confirming the information recorded by others

- DG: If the physician is unable to obtain a history from the patient or other source, the record should describe the patient's condition or other circumstance that precludes obtaining a history

Definitions and specific documentation guidelines for each of the elements of history are listed below.

Chief Complaint (CC)

The CC is a concise statement describing the symptom, problem, condition, diagnosis, physician recommended return, or other factor that is the reason for the encounter, usually stated in the patient's words.

- DG: The medical record should clearly reflect the chief complaint

History of Present Illness (HPI)

The HPI is a chronological description of the development of the patient's present illness from the first sign and/or symptom or from the previous encounter to the present. It includes the following elements:

- Location
- Quality
- Severity
- Duration
- Timing
- Context
- Modifying factors
- Associated signs and symptoms

Brief and extended HPIs are distinguished by the amount of detail needed to accurately characterize the clinical problem.

A brief HPI consists of one to three elements of the HPI.

- DG: The medical record should describe one to three elements of the present illness (HPI)

An extended HPI consists of at least four elements of the HPI or the status of at least three chronic or inactive conditions.

- DG: The medical record should describe at least four elements of the present illness (HPI) or the status of at least three chronic or inactive conditions

Beginning with services performed on or after September 10, 2013, CMS has stated that physicians and OQHCP will be able to use the 1997 guidelines for an extended history of present illness (HPI) in combination with other elements from the 1995 documentation guidelines to document a particular level of evaluation and management service.

History of Present Illness	Review of systems (ROS)	PFSH	Type of History
Brief	N/A	N/A	Problem-focused
Brief	Problem Pertinent	N/A	Expanded Problem-Focused
Extended	Extended	Pertinent	Detailed
Extended	Complete	Complete	Comprehensive

Review of Systems (ROS)

A ROS is an inventory of body systems obtained through a series of questions seeking to identify signs and/or symptoms that the patient may be experiencing or has experienced. For purposes of ROS, the following systems are recognized:

- Constitutional symptoms (e.g., fever, weight loss)
- Eyes
- Ears, nose, mouth, throat
- Cardiovascular
- Respiratory
- Gastrointestinal
- Genitourinary
- Musculoskeletal
- Integumentary (skin and/or breast)
- Neurological
- Psychiatric
- Endocrine
- Hematologic/lymphatic
- Allergic/immunologic

A problem pertinent ROS inquires about the system directly related to the problem identified in the HPI.

- DG: The patient's positive responses and pertinent negatives for the system related to the problem should be documented

An extended ROS inquires about the system directly related to the problem identified in the HPI and a limited number of additional systems.

- DG: The patient's positive responses and pertinent negatives for two to nine systems should be documented

A complete ROS inquires about the system directly related to the problem identified in the HPI plus all additional body systems.

- DG: At least 10 organ systems must be reviewed. Those systems with positive or pertinent negative responses must be individually documented. For the remaining systems, a notation indicating all other systems are negative is permissible. In the absence of such a notation, at least 10 systems must be individually documented

Past, Family, and/or Social History (PFSH)

The PFSH consists of a review of three areas:

- Past history (the patient's past experiences with illnesses, operations, injuries, and treatment)
- Family history (a review of medical events in the patient's family, including diseases that may be hereditary or place the patient at risk)
- Social history (an age appropriate review of past and current activities)

For certain categories of E/M services that include only an interval history, it is not necessary to record information about the PFSH. Those categories are subsequent hospital care, follow-up inpatient consultations, and subsequent nursing facility care.

A pertinent PFSH is a review of the history area directly related to the problem identified in the HPI.

- DG: At least one specific item from any of the three history areas must be documented for a pertinent PFSH

A complete PFSH is a review of two or all three of the PFSH history areas, depending on the category of the E/M service. A review of all three history areas is required for services that by their nature include a comprehensive

assessment or reassessment of the patient. A review of two of the three history areas is sufficient for other services.

- DG: A least one specific item from two of the three history areas must be documented for a complete PFSH for the following categories of E/M services: office or other outpatient services, established patient; emergency department; domiciliary care, established patient; and home care, established patient

- DG: At least one specific item from each of the three history areas must be documented for a complete PFSH for the following categories of E/M services: office or other outpatient services, new patient; hospital observation services; hospital inpatient services, initial care; consultations; comprehensive nursing facility assessments; domiciliary care, new patient; and home care, new patient

B.   Documentation of Examination 1997 Guidelines

The levels of E/M services are based on four types of examination:

- Problem Focused: A limited examination of the affected body area or organ system
- Expanded Problem Focused: A limited examination of the affected body area or organ system and any other symptomatic or related body area or organ system
- Detailed: An extended examination of the affected body area or organ system and any other symptomatic or related body area or organ system
- Comprehensive: A general multi-system examination or complete examination of a single organ system and other symptomatic or related body area or organ system

These types of examinations have been defined for general multi-system and the following single organ systems:

- Cardiovascular
- Ears, nose, mouth, and throat
- Eyes
- Genitourinary (Female)
- Genitourinary (Male)
- Hematologic/lymphatic/immunologic
- Musculoskeletal
- Neurological
- Psychiatric
- Respiratory
- Skin

Any physician regardless of specialty may perform a general multi-system examination or any of the single organ system examinations. The type (general multi-system or single organ system) and content of examination are selected by the examining physician and are based upon clinical judgment, the patient's history, and the nature of the presenting problem.

The content and documentation requirements for each type and level of examination are summarized below and described in detail in a table found later on in this document. In the table, organ systems and body areas recognized by CPT for purposes of describing examinations are shown in the left column. The content, or individual elements, of the examination pertaining to that body area or organ system are identified by bullets (•) in the right column.

Parenthetical examples "(e.g., ...)," have been used for clarification and to provide guidance regarding documentation. Documentation for each element must satisfy any numeric requirements (such as "Measurement of any three of the following seven...") included in the description of the element. Elements with multiple components but with no specific numeric requirement (such as "Examination of liver and spleen") require documentation of at least one component. It is possible for a given examination to be expanded beyond what is defined here. When that occurs, findings related to the additional systems and/or areas should be documented.

- DG: Specific abnormal and relevant negative findings from the examination of the affected or symptomatic body area or organ system should be documented. A notation of "abnormal" without elaboration is insufficient

- DG: Abnormal or unexpected findings from the examination of any asymptomatic body area or organ system should be described

- DG: A brief statement or notation indicating "negative" or "normal" is sufficient to document normal findings related to an unaffected areas or asymptomatic organ system

General Multi-System Examinations

General multi-system examinations are described in detail later in this document. To qualify for a given level of multi-system examination, the following content and documentation requirements should be met:

- Problem Focused Examination: It should include performance and documentation of one to five elements identified by a bullet (·) in one or more organ systems or body areas .
- Expanded Problem Focused Examination: It should include performance and documentation of at least six elements identified by a bullet (·) in one or more organ systems or body areas
- Detailed Examination: It should include at least six organ systems or body areas. For each system/area selected, performance and

documentation of at least two elements identified by a bullet (·) is expected. Alternatively, a detailed examination may include performance and documentation of at least 12 elements identified by a bullet (·) in two or more organ systems or body areas
- Comprehensive Examination: It should include at least nine organ systems or body areas. For each system/area selected, all elements of the examination identified by a bullet (·) should be performed, unless specific directions limit the content of the examination. For each area/system, documentation of at least two elements identified by a bullet (·) is expected

Single Organ System Examinations

The single organ system examinations recognized by CMS include eyes; ears, nose, mouth, and throat; cardiovascular; respiratory; genitourinary (male and female); musculoskeletal; neurologic; hematologic, lymphatic, and immunologic; skin; and psychiatric. Note that for each specific single organ examination type, the performance and documentation of the stated number of elements, identified by a bullet (·) should be included, whether in a box with a shaded or unshaded border. The following content and documentation requirements must be met to qualify for a given level:

- Problem Focused Examination: one to five elements
- Expanded Problem Focused Examination: at least six elements
- Detailed Examination: at least 12 elements (other than eye and psychiatric examinations)
- Comprehensive Examination: all elements (Documentation of every element in a box with a shaded border and at least one element in a box with an unshaded border is expected)

Content and Documentation Requirements

General Multisystem Examination 1997

System/Body Area	Elements of Examination
Constitutional	• Measurement of any three of the following seven vital signs: 1) sitting or standing blood pressure, 2) supine blood pressure, 3) pulse rate and regularity, 4) respiration, 5) temperature, 6) height, 7) weight (May be measured and recorded by ancillary staff). • General appearance of patient (e.g., development, nutrition, body habitus, deformities attention to grooming)
Eyes	• Inspection of conjunctivae and lids • Examination of pupils and irises (e.g., reaction to light and accommodation, size and symmetry) • Ophthalmoscopic examination of optic discs (e.g., size, C/D ratio, appearance) and posterior segments (e.g., vessel changes, exudates, hemorrhages)
Ears, nose, mouth, and throat	• External inspection of ears and nose (e.g., overall appearance, scars, lesions, masses) • Otoscopic examination of external auditory canals and tympanic membranes • Assessment of hearing (e.g., whispered voice, finger rub, tuning fork) • Inspection of nasal mucosa, septum and turbinates • Inspection of lips, teeth and gums • Examination of oropharynx: oral mucosa, salivary glands, hard and soft palates, tongue, tonsils and posterior pharynx
Neck	• Examination of neck (e.g., masses, overall appearance, symmetry, tracheal position, crepitus) • Examination of thyroid (e.g., enlargement, tenderness, mass)
Respiratory	• Assessment of respiratory effort (e.g., intercostal retractions, use of accessory muscles, diaphragmatic movement) • Percussion of chest (e.g., dullness, flatness, hyperresonance) • Palpation of chest (e.g., tactile fremitus) • Auscultation of lungs (e.g., breath sounds, adventitious sounds, rubs)
Cardiovascular	• Palpation of heart (e.g., location, size, thrills) • Auscultation of heart with notation of abnormal sounds and murmurs • Examination of: — carotid arteries (e.g., pulse amplitude, bruits) — abdominal aorta (e.g., size, bruits) — femoral arteries (e.g., pulse amplitude, bruits) — pedal pulses (e.g., pulse amplitude) — extremities for edema and/or varicosities
Chest (Breasts)	• Inspection of breasts (e.g., symmetry, nipple discharge) • Palpation of breasts and axillae (e.g., masses or lumps, tenderness)

System/Body Area	Elements of Examination
Gastrointestinal (Abdomen)	• Examination of abdomen with notation of presence of masses or tenderness • Examination of liver and spleen • Examination for presence or absence of hernia • Examination (when indicated) of anus, perineum and rectum, including sphincter tone, presence of hemorrhoids, rectal masses • Obtain stool sample for occult blood test when indicated

Genitourinary	**Male:**
	• Examination of the scrotal contents (e.g., hydrocele, spermatocele, tenderness of cord, testicular mass)
	• Examination of the penis
	• Digital rectal examination of prostate gland (e.g., size, symmetry, nodularity tenderness)
	Female:
	• Pelvic examination (with or without specimen collection for smears and cultures), including:
	  — examination of external genitalia (e.g., general appearance, hair distribution, lesions) and vagina (e.g., general appearance, estrogen effect, discharge, lesions, pelvic support, cystocele, rectocele)
	  — examination of urethra (e.g., masses, tenderness, scarring)
	  — examination of bladder (e.g., fullness, masses, tenderness)
	• Cervix (e.g., general appearance, lesions, discharge)
	• Uterus (e.g., size, contour, position, mobility, tenderness, consistency, descent or support)
	• Adnexa/parametria (e.g., masses, tenderness)

Lymphatic	Palpation of lymph nodes in **two or more** areas: • Neck • Groin • Axillae • Other
Musculoskeletal	• Examination of gait and station *(if circled, add to total at bottom of column to the left) • Inspection and/or palpation of digits and nails (e.g., clubbing, cyanosis, inflammatory conditions, petechiae, ischemia, infections, nodes) *(if circled, add to total at bottom of column to the left) Examination of joints, bones and muscles of **one or more of the following six** areas: 1) head and neck; 2) spine, ribs, and pelvis; 3) right upper extremity; 4) left upper extremity; 5) right lower extremity; and 6) left lower extremity. The examination of a given area includes: • Inspection and/or palpation with notation of presence of any misalignment, asymmetry, crepitation, defects, tenderness, masses, effusions • Assessment of range of motion with notation of any pain, crepitation or contracture • Assessment of stability with notation of any dislocation (luxation), subluxation, or laxity • Assessment of muscle strength and tone (e.g., flaccid, cog wheel, spastic) with notation of any atrophy or abnormal movements
Skin	• Inspection of skin and subcutaneous tissue (e.g., rashes, lesions, ulcers) • Palpation of skin and subcutaneous tissue (e.g., induration, subcutaneous nodules, tightening)
Neurologic	• Test cranial nerves with notation of any deficits • Examination of deep tendon reflexes with notation of pathological reflexes (e.g., Babinski) • Examination of sensation (e.g., by touch, pin, vibration, proprioception)

Psychiatric	• Description of patient's judgment and insight
	• Brief assessment of mental status including:
	  — Orientation to time, place and person
	  — Recent and remote memory
	  — Mood and affect (e.g., depression, anxiety, agitation)

Content and Documentation Requirements

Level of exam	Perform and document
Problem focused	**One to five** elements identified by a bullet
Expanded problem focused	**At least six** elements identified by a bullet
Detailed	**At least 12** elements identified by a bullet, whether in a box with a shaded or unshaded border
Comprehensive	Performance of **all** elements identified by a bullet; whether in a box or with a shaded or unshaded box. Documentation of every element in each with a shaded border and at least one element in a box with an unshaded border is expected

Number of Diagnoses or Management Options	Amount and/or Complexity of Data to be Reviewed	Risk of Complications and/or Morbidity or Mortality	Type of Decision Making
Minimal	Minimal or None	Minimal	Straightforward
Limited	Limited	Low	Low Complexity
Multiple	Moderate	Moderate	Moderate Complexity
Extensive	Extensive	High	High Complexity

C. Documentation of the Complexity of Medical Decision Making 1995 and 1997

The levels of E/M services recognize four types of medical decision-making (straightforward, low complexity, moderate complexity, and high complexity). Medical decision-making refers to the complexity of establishing a diagnosis and/or selecting a management option as measured by:

- The number of possible diagnoses and/or the number of management options that must be considered
- The amount and/or complexity of medical records, diagnostic tests, and/or other information that must be obtained, reviewed, and analyzed
- The risk of significant complications, morbidity, and/or mortality, as well as comorbidities, associated with the patient's presenting problem, the diagnostic procedure, and/or the possible management options

The following chart shows the progression of the elements required for each level of medical decision-making. To qualify for a given type of decision-making, two of the three elements in the table must be either met or exceeded.

Each of the elements of medical decision-making is described below.

Number of Diagnoses or Management Options

The number of possible diagnoses and/or the number of management options that must be considered is based on the number and types of problems addressed during the encounter, the complexity of establishing a diagnosis, and the management decisions that are made by the physician.

Generally, decision making with respect to a diagnosed problem is easier than that for an identified but undiagnosed problem. The number and type of diagnostic tests employed may be an indicator of the number of possible diagnoses. Problems that are improving or resolving are less complex than those that are worsening or failing to change as expected. The need to seek advice from others is another indicator of complexity of diagnostic or management problems.

- DG: For each encounter, an assessment, clinical impression, or diagnosis should be documented. It may be explicitly stated or implied in documented decisions regarding management plans and/or further evaluation

  - For a presenting problem with an established diagnosis, the record should reflect whether the problem is: a) improved, well controlled, resolving, or resolved; or b) inadequately controlled, worsening, or failing to change as expected

  - For a presenting problem without an established diagnosis, the assessment or clinical impression may be stated in the form of a differential diagnosis or as a "possible," "probable," or "rule-out" (R/O) diagnosis

- DG: The initiation of, or changes in, treatment should be documented. Treatment includes a wide range of management options including patient instructions, nursing instructions, therapies, and medications

- DG: If referrals are made, consultations requested, or advice sought, the record should indicate to whom or where the referral or consultation is made or from whom the advice is requested

Amount and/or Complexity of Data to be Reviewed

The amount and complexity of data to be reviewed is based on the types of diagnostic testing ordered or reviewed. A decision to obtain and review old medical records and/or obtain history from sources other than the patient increases the amount and complexity of data to be reviewed.

Discussion of contradictory or unexpected test results with the physician who performed or interpreted the test is an indication of the complexity of data being reviewed. On occasion, the physician who ordered a test may personally review the image, tracing, or specimen to supplement information from the physician who prepared the test report or interpretation; this is another indication of the complexity of data being reviewed.

- DG: If a diagnostic service (test or procedure) is ordered, planned, scheduled, or performed at the time of the E/M encounter, the type of service (e.g., lab or x-ray) should be documented

- DG: The review of lab, radiology, and/or other diagnostic tests should be documented. A simple notation such as WBC elevated" or "chest x-ray unremarkable" is acceptable. Alternatively, the review may be documented by initialing and dating the report containing the test results

- DG: A decision to obtain old records or a decision to obtain additional history from the family, caretaker, or other source to supplement that obtained from the patient should be documented

- DG: Relevant findings from the review of old records and/or the receipt of additional history from the family, caretaker, or other source to supplement that obtained from the patient should be documented. If there is no relevant information beyond that already obtained, that fact should be documented. A notation of "old records reviewed" or "additional history obtained from family" without elaboration is insufficient

- DG: The results of discussion of laboratory, radiology, or other diagnostic tests with the physician who performed or interpreted the study should be documented

- DG: The direct visualization and independent interpretation of an image, tracing, or specimen previously or subsequently interpreted by another physician should be documented

Risk of Significant Complications, Morbidity, and/or Mortality

The risk of significant complications, morbidity, and/or mortality is based on the risks associated with the presenting problem, the diagnostic procedure, and the possible management options.

- DG: Comorbidities/underlying disease or other factors that increase the complexity of medical decision making by increasing the risk of complications, morbidity, and/or mortality should be documented

- DG: If a surgical or invasive diagnostic procedure is ordered, planned, or scheduled at the time of the E/M encounter, the type of procedure (e.g., laparoscopy) should be documented

- DG: If a surgical or invasive diagnostic procedure is performed at the time of the E/M encounter, the specific procedure should be documented

- DG: The referral for or decision to perform a surgical or invasive diagnostic procedure on an urgent basis should be documented or implied

The following Table of Risk may be used to help determine whether the risk of significant complications, morbidity, and/or mortality is minimal, low, moderate, or high. Because the determination of risk is complex and not readily quantifiable, the table includes common clinical examples rather than absolute measures of risk. The assessment of risk of the presenting problem is based on the risk related to the disease process anticipated between the present encounter and the next one. The assessment of risk of selecting diagnostic procedures and management options is based on the risk during and immediately following any procedures or treatment. The highest level of risk in any one category (presenting problem, diagnostic procedure, or management options) determines the overall risk.

Table of Risk

Level of Risk	Presenting Problem(s)	Diagnostic Procedure(s) Ordered	Management Options Selected
Minimal	One self-limited or minor problem (e.g., cold, insect bite, tinea corporis)	Laboratory test requiring venipuncture Chest x-rays EKG/EEG Urinalysis Ultrasound (e.g., echocardiography) KOH prep	Rest Gargles Elastic bandages Superficial dressings
Low	Two or more self-limited or minor problems One stable chronic illness (e.g., well controlled hypertension, non-insulin dependent diabetes, cataract, BPH) Acute, uncomplicated illness or injury (e.g., cystitis, allergic rhinitis, simple sprain)	Physiologic tests not under stress (e.g., pulmonary function tests) Non-cardiovascular imaging studies with contrast (e.g., barium enema) Superficial needle biopsies Clinical laboratory tests requiring arterial puncture Skin biopsies	Over-the-counter drugs Minor surgery with no identified risk factors Physical therapy Occupational therapy IV fluids without additives
Moderate	One or more chronic illnesses with mild exacerbation, progression or side effects of treatment Two or more stable chronic illnesses Undiagnosed new problem with uncertain prognosis (e.g., lump in breast) Acute illness with systemic symptoms (e.g., pyelonephritis, pneumonitis, colitis) Acute complicated injury (e.g., head injury with brief loss of consciousness)	Physiologic tests not under stress (e.g., cardiac stress test, fetal contraction stress test) Diagnostic endoscopies with no identified risk factors Deep needle or incisional biopsy Cardiovascular imaging studies with contrast and no identified risk factors (e.g., arteriogram, cardiac catheterization) Obtain fluid from body cavity (e.g., lumbar puncture, thoracentesis, culdocentesis)	Minor surgery with identified risk factors Effective major surgery (open, percutaneous or endoscopic) with no identified risk factors Prescription drug management Therapeutic nuclear medicine IV fluids with additives Closed treatment of fracture or dislocation without manipulation
High	One or more chronic illnesses with severe exacerbation, progression or side effects of treatment Acute/chronic illnesses that may pose a threat to life or bodily function (e.g., multiple trauma, acute MI, pulmonary embolus, severe respiratory distress, progressive severe rheumatoid arthritis, psychiatric illness with potential threat to self or others, peritonitis, acute renal failure An abrupt change in neurologic status (e.g., seizure, TIA, weakness or sensory loss)	Cardiovascular imaging studies with contrast with identified risk factors Cardiac electrophysiological tests Diagnostic endoscopies with identified risk factors Discography	Elective major surgery (open, percutaneous or endoscopic) with identified risk factors Emergency major surgery (open, percutaneous or endoscopic) Parenteral controlled substances Drug therapy requiring intensive monitoring for toxicity Decision not to resuscitate or to de-escalate care because of poor prognosis

D.   Documentation of an Encounter Dominated by Counseling or Coordination of Care

In the case where counseling and/or coordination of care dominates (more than 50 percent) the physician/patient and/or family encounter (face-to-face time in the office or other outpatient setting or floor-unit time in the hospital or nursing facility), time is considered the key or controlling factor to qualify for a particular level of E/M service.

- DG: If the physician elects to report the level of service based on counseling and/or coordination of care, the total length of time of the encounter (face-to-face or floor time, as appropriate) should be documented and the record should describe the counseling and/or activities to coordinate care

Appendix D — Crosswalk of Deleted Codes

The deleted code crosswalk is meant to be used as a reference tool to find active codes that could be used in place of the deleted code. This will not always be an exact match. Please review the code descriptions and guidelines before selecting a code.

Code	Cross reference
01935	To report, see 01937, 01938, 01939, 01940, 01941, 01942
01936	To report, see 01937, 01938, 01939, 01940, 01941, 01942
69715	To report, see 69501-69530, 69535-69554, 69601-69604, 69610-69646, 69650-69662, 69666-69676
69718	To report, see 69501-69530, 69535-69554, 69601-69604, 69610-69646, 69650-69662, 69666-69676
72275	To report, see 62281, 62282, 62321, 62323, 62325, 62327, 64479, 64480, 64483, 64484
80500	To report, see 80503, 80504, 80505, 80506
80502	To report, see 80503, 80504, 80505, 80506
87450	To report, see 87301-87451, 87802-87899
92559	To report, see 92700
92560	To report, see 92700

Code	Cross reference
92561	To report, see 92700
92564	To report, see 92700
93530	To report, see 93593, 93594
93531	To report, see 93462, 93596, 93597
93532	To report, see 93462, 93596, 93597
93533	To report, see 93462, 93596, 93597
93561	To report, see 93598
93562	To report, see 93598
95943	To report, see 95999
0191T	To report, see [66989], [66991], [0671T]
0290T	To report, see 66999
0355T	To report, see [91113]
0356T	To report, see 68841
0376T	To report, see [66989], [66991], [0671T]
0423T	To report, see 84999
0451T	To report, see 33999
0452T	To report, see 33999
0453T	To report, see 33999

Code	Cross reference
0454T	To report, see 33999
0454T	To report, see 33999
0455T	To report, see 33999
0456T	To report, see 33999
0457T	To report, see 33999
0458T	To report, see 33999
0459T	To report, see 33999
0460T	To report, see 33999
0461T	To report, see 33999
0462T	To report, see 33999
0463T	To report, see 33999
0466T	To report, see 64582-64584
0467T	To report, see 64582-64584
0468T	To report, see 64582-64584
0548T	To report, see 53451-53454
0549T	To report, see 53451-53454
0550T	To report, see 53451-53454
0551T	To report, see 53451-53454

Appendix E — Resequenced Codes

This appendix contains a list of codes that are not in numeric order in the book. AMA resequenced some code numbers to relocate codes in the same category but not in numeric sequence. In addition to the list of resequenced codes, the page number where the code may be found is provided for ease of use.

Code	Page	Reference
10004	13	See code following 10021.
10005	13	See code following 10021.
10006	13	See code following 10021.
10007	13	See code following 10021.
10008	13	See code following 10021.
10009	13	See code following 10021.
10010	13	See code following 10021.
10011	13	See code following 10021.
10012	13	See code following 10021.
11045	15	See code following 11042.
11046	15	See code following 11043.
15769	27	See code following 15770.
20560	38	See code following 20553.
20561	38	See code before 20555.
21552	49	See code following 21555.
21554	49	See code following 21556.
22858	58	See code following 22856.
22859	58	See code following 22854.
23071	60	See code following 23075.
23073	60	See code following 23076.
24071	63	See code following 24075.
24073	64	See code following 24076.
25071	68	See code following 25075.
25073	68	See code following 25076.
26111	73	See code following 26115.
26113	73	See code following 26116.
27043	79	See code following 27047.
27045	79	See code following 27048.
27059	79	See code following 27049.
27329	85	See code following 27360.
27337	84	See code following 27327.
27339	84	See code before 27330.
27632	90	See code following 27618.
27634	90	See code following 27619.
28039	94	See code following 28043.
28041	94	See code following 28045.
28295	97	See code following 28296.
29914	103	See code following 29863.
29915	103	See code following 29863.
29916	103	See code before 29866.
31253	110	See code following 31255.
31257	110	See code following 31255.
31259	110	See code following 31255.
31551	114	See code following 31580.
31552	114	See code following 31580.
31553	114	See code following 31580.
31554	114	See code following 31580.
31572	114	See code following 31578.

Code	Page	Reference
31573	114	See code following 31578.
31574	114	See code following 31578.
31651	116	See code following 31647.
32994	122	See code following 32998.
33221	125	See code following 33213.
33227	126	See code following 33233.
33228	126	See code following 33233.
33229	126	See code before 33234.
33230	127	See code following 33240.
33231	127	See code before 33241.
33262	128	See code following 33241.
33263	128	See code following 33241.
33264	128	See code before 33243.
33267	130	See code following 33261.
33268	130	See code following 33261.
33269	131	See code following 33261.
33270	129	See code following 33249.
33271	129	See code following 33249.
33272	129	See code following 33249.
33273	129	See code following 33249.
33274	129	See code following 33249.
33275	129	See code following 33249.
33440	133	See code following 33410.
33962	144	See code following 33959.
33963	145	See code following 33959.
33964	145	See code following 33959.
33965	145	See code following 33959.
33966	145	See code following 33959.
33969	145	See code following 33959.
33984	145	See code following 33959.
33985	145	See code following 33959.
33986	145	See code following 33959.
33987	145	See code following 33959.
33988	145	See code following 33959.
33989	145	See code following 33959.
33995	147	See code following 33983.
33997	147	See code following 33992.
34717	149	See code following 34708.
34718	149	See code following 34709.
34812	150	See code following 34713.
34820	150	See code following 34714.
34833	150	See code following 34714.
34834	150	See code following 34714.
36465	162	See code following 36471.
36466	162	See code following 36471.
36482	163	See code following 36479.
36483	163	See code following 36479.
36572	165	See code following 36569.

Code	Page	Reference
36573	165	See code following 36569.
37246	172	See code following 37235.
37247	173	See code following 37235.
37248	173	See code following 37235.
37249	173	See code following 37235.
38243	177	See code following 38241.
43210	194	See code following 43259.
43211	190	See code following 43217.
43212	190	See code following 43217.
43213	190	See code following 43220.
43214	190	See code following 43220.
43233	193	See code following 43249.
43266	194	See code following 43255.
43270	194	See code following 43257.
43274	195	See code following numeric code 43270.
43275	195	See code following numeric code 43270.
43276	195	See code following numeric code 43270.
43277	195	See code following numeric code 43270.
43278	195	See code following numeric code 43270.
44381	206	See code following 44382.
44401	206	See code following 44392.
45346	210	See code following 45338.
45388	211	See code following 45382.
45390	212	See code following 45392.
45398	212	See code following 45393.
45399	213	See code before 45990.
46220	214	See code before 46230.
46320	214	See code following 46230.
46945	214	See code following 46221.
46946	214	See code following resequenced code 46945.
46947	216	See code following 46761.
46948	214	See code before resequenced code 46220.
50430	231	See code following 50396.
50431	231	See code following 50396.
50432	232	See code following 50396.
50433	232	See code following 50396.
50434	232	See code following 50396.
50435	232	See code following 50396.
50436	231	See code following 50391.
50437	231	See code following 50391.
51797	238	See code following 51729.
52356	242	See code following 52353.
58674	260	See code before 58541.

Code	Page	Reference
62328	283	See code following 62270.
62329	283	See code following 62272.
63052	286	See code following 63048.
63053	286	See code following 63048.
64461	292	See code following 64484.
64462	292	See code following 64484.
64463	292	See code following 64484.
64624	294	See code following 64610.
64625	294	See code before 64611.
64628	294	See code before 64611.
64629	294	See code before 64611.
64633	295	See code following 64620.
64634	295	See code following 64620.
64635	295	See code following 64620.
64636	295	See code before 64630.
66987	306	See code following 66982. Resequenced code. See code following resequenced code 66989.
66988	307	See code following 66984. Resequenced code. See code following resequenced code 66991.
66989	306	See code following 66982.
66991	307	See code following 66984.
67810	311	See code following 67715.
69714	317	See code following 69676.
69716	317	See code following 69676.
69717	317	See code following 69676.
69719	317	See code following 69676.
69726	317	See code following 69676.
69727	317	See code following 69676.
77085	344	See code following 77081.
77086	344	See code before 77084.
77295	344	See code before 77300.
77385	346	See code following 77417.
77386	346	See code following 77417.
77387	346	See code following 77417.
77424	346	See code following 77417.
77425	346	See code following 77417.
78429	350	See code following 78459.
78430	350	See code following 78491.
78431	351	See code following 78492.
78432	351	See code following 78492.
78433	351	See code following 78492.
78434	351	See code following 78492.
78804	352	See code following 78802.
78830	352	See code following numeric code 78804.
78831	353	See code following numeric code 78804.
78832	353	See code following numeric code 78804.
78835	353	See code following numeric code 78804.
80081	357	See code following 80055.
80161	360	See code following 80157.

Code	Page	Reference
80164	361	See code following 80201.
80165	361	See code following 80201.
80167	360	See code following 80169.
80171	360	See code before 80170.
80176	361	See code following 80177.
80179	361	See code before 80195.
80181	360	See code following resequenced code 80167.
80189	360	See code following resequenced code 80230.
80193	360	See code before 80177.
80204	361	See code following 80178.
80210	361	See code following 80194.
80220	360	See code following 80173.
80230	360	See code following 80173.
80235	360	See code before 80175.
80280	361	See code following 80202.
80285	361	See code before 80203.
80305	358	See code before 80143.
80306	358	See code before 80143.
80307	358	See code before 80143.
80320	358	See code before 80143.
80321	358	See code before 80143.
80322	358	See code before 80143.
80323	358	See code before 80143.
80324	358	See code before 80143.
80325	358	See code before 80143.
80326	358	See code before 80143.
80327	358	See code before 80143.
80328	358	See code before 80143.
80329	358	See code before 80143.
80330	358	See code before 80143.
80331	358	See code before 80143.
80332	358	See code before 80143.
80333	359	See code before 80143.
80334	359	See code before 80143.
80335	359	See code before 80143.
80336	359	See code before 80143.
80337	359	See code before 80143.
80338	359	See code before 80143.
80339	359	See code before 80143.
80340	359	See code following resequenced code 80339.
80341	359	See code before 80143.
80342	359	See code before 80143.
80343	359	See code before 80143.
80344	359	See code before 80143.
80345	359	See code before 80143.
80346	359	See code before 80143.
80347	359	See code before 80143.
80348	359	See code before 80143.
80349	359	See code before 80143.
80350	359	See code before 80143.
80351	359	See code before 80143.
80352	359	See code before 80143.

Code	Page	Reference
80353	359	See code before 80143.
80354	359	See code before 80143.
80355	359	See code before 80143.
80356	359	See code before 80143.
80357	359	See code before 80143.
80358	359	See code before 80143.
80359	359	See code before 80143.
80360	359	See code before 80143.
80361	359	See code before 80143.
80362	359	See code before 80143.
80363	359	See code before 80143.
80364	359	See code before 80143.
80365	359	See code before 80143.
80366	359	See code before 80143.
80367	359	See code before 80143.
80368	359	See code before 80143.
80369	359	See code before 80143.
80370	359	See code before 80143.
80371	360	See code before 80143.
80372	360	See code before 80143.
80373	360	See code before 80143.
80374	360	See code before 80143.
80375	360	See code before 80143.
80376	360	See code before 80143.
80377	360	See code before 80143.
81105	369	See code before 81260.
81106	370	See code before 81260.
81107	370	See code before 81260.
81108	370	See code before 81260.
81109	370	See code before 81260.
81110	370	See code before 81260.
81111	370	See code before 81260.
81112	370	See code before 81260.
81120	370	See code before 81260.
81121	370	See code before 81260.
81161	368	See code following numeric code 81231.
81162	366	See code following resequenced code 81210.
81163	366	See code following resequenced code 81210.
81164	366	See code before 81212.
81165	366	See code following 81212.
81166	366	See code following 81212.
81167	366	See code following 81216.
81168	367	See code before 81218.
81173	365	See code following resequenced code 81204.
81174	365	See code following resequenced code 81204.
81184	367	See code following resequenced code 81233.
81185	367	See code following resequenced code 81233.
81186	367	See code following resequenced code 81233.

Code	Page	Reference
81187	367	See code following resequenced code 81268.
81188	367	See code following resequenced code 81266.
81189	367	See code following resequenced code 81266.
81190	367	See code following resequenced code 81266.
81191	372	See code following numeric code 81312.
81192	372	See code following numeric code 81312.
81193	372	See code following numeric code 81312.
81194	372	See code following numeric code 81312.
81200	365	See code before 81175.
81201	365	See code following numeric code 81174.
81202	365	See code following numeric code 81174.
81203	365	See code following numeric code 81174.
81204	365	See code following numeric code 81174.
81205	366	See code following numeric code 81210.
81206	366	See code following numeric code 81210.
81207	366	See code following numeric code 81210.
81208	366	See code following numeric code 81210.
81209	366	See code following numeric code 81210.
81210	366	See code following numeric code 81210.
81219	367	See code before 81218.
81227	367	See code before 81225.
81230	367	See code following numeric code 81227.
81231	367	See code following numeric code 81227.
81233	366	See code following 81217.
81234	368	See code following numeric code 81231.
81238	368	See code following 81241.
81239	368	See code before 81232.
81245	368	See code following 81242.
81246	368	See code following 81242.
81250	369	See code before 81247.
81257	369	See code following 81254.
81258	369	See code following 81254.
81259	369	See code following 81254.
81261	370	See code before 81260.
81262	370	See code before 81260.
81263	370	See code before 81260.
81264	370	See code before 81260.
81265	367	See code following resequenced code 81187.
81266	367	See code following resequenced code 81265.
81267	367	See code following 81224.
81268	367	See code following 81224.
81269	369	See code following resequenced code 81259.
81271	369	See code following numeric code 81259.
81274	369	See code following resequenced code 81271.
81277	368	See code following 81229.
81278	370	See code following resequenced code 81263.
81279	370	See code following 81270.
81283	370	See code following resequenced code 81121.
81284	369	See code following numeric code 81246.
81285	369	See code following numeric code 81246.
81286	369	See code following numeric code 81246.
81287	371	See code following resequenced code 81304.
81288	371	See code following resequenced code 81292.
81289	369	See code following numeric code 81246.
81291	371	See code before 81305.
81292	371	See code before numeric code 81291.
81293	371	See code before numeric code 81291.
81294	371	See code before numeric code 81291.
81295	371	See code before numeric code 81291.
81301	371	See code following resequenced code 81287.
81302	371	See code following 81290.
81303	371	See code following 81290.
81304	371	See code following 81290.
81306	372	See code following resequenced code 81194.
81307	372	See code before 81313.
81308	372	See code before 81313.
81309	372	See code following 81314.
81312	372	See code before resequenced code 81307.
81320	372	See code before 81315.
81324	372	See code following 81316.
81325	372	See code following 81316.
81326	372	See code following 81316.
81332	373	See code following 81327.
81334	373	See code following numeric code 81326.
81336	373	See code following 81329.
81337	373	See code following 81329.
81338	371	See code following resequenced code 81294.
81339	371	See code before resequenced code 81295.
81343	372	See code following numeric code 81320.
81344	373	See code following numeric code 81332.
81345	373	See code following numeric code 81332.
81347	373	See code before 81328.
81348	373	See code following numeric code 81332.
81349	368	See code following 81229.
81351	373	See code before 81335.
81352	373	See code before 81335.
81353	373	See code before 81335.
81357	374	See code before 81350.
81361	369	See code following 81254.
81362	369	See code following 81254.
81363	369	See code following 81254.
81364	369	See code following 81254.
81419	386	See code following 81414.
81443	386	See code following 81422.
81448	387	See code following 81438.
81479	386	See code following 81408.
81500	389	See code following 81538.
81503	389	See code before 81539.
81504	390	See code following resequenced code 81546.
81522	389	See code following 81518.
81540	390	See code before 81552.
81546	390	See code following 81551.
81595	388	See code following 81490.
81596	389	See code following 81514.
82042	391	See code following 82045.
82652	393	See code following 82306.
82653	395	See code following 82656.
82681	396	See code following 82670.
83529	399	See code following 83527.
83992	359	See code following resequenced code 80365.
86015	409	See code before 86000.
86051	409	See code following 86063.
86052	409	See code following 86063.
86053	409	See code following 86063.
86152	410	See code following 86147.
86153	410	See code before 86148.
86328	411	See code following 86318.
86362	411	See code following 86356.
86363	411	See code following 86356.
86364	411	See code following 86357.
86408	412	See code following 86382.
86409	412	See code following 86382.
86413	412	See code following resequenced code 86409.

Code	Page	Reference
87154	419	See code following 87150.
87428	422	See code following 87426.
87623	424	See code following 87539.
87624	424	See code following 87539.
87625	424	See code before 87540.
87806	426	See code following 87803.
87811	426	See code following 87807.
87906	426	See code following 87901.
87910	426	See code following 87900.
87912	426	See code before 87902.
88177	428	See code following 88173.
88341	432	See code following 88342.
88350	432	See code following 88346.
88364	433	See code following 88365.
88373	433	See code following 88367.
88374	433	See code following 88367.
88377	433	See code following 88369.
0051A	454	See code following 0004A.
0052A	454	See code following 0004A.
0053A	454	See code following 0004A.
0054A	454	See code following 0004A.
0064A	454	See code following 0013A.
0071A	454	See code following 0004A.
0072A	454	See code following 0004A.
90619	459	See code following 90734.
90620	459	See code following 90734.
90621	460	See code following 90734.
90625	459	See code following 90723.
90626	459	See code following 90715.
90627	459	See code following 90715.
90630	457	See code following 90654.
90644	459	See code following 90732.
90672	457	See code following 90660.
90673	457	See code before 90662.
90674	457	See code following 90661.
90677	458	See code following 90671.
90694	458	See code following 90689.
90750	460	See code following 90736.
90756	457	See code following 90661.
90758	460	See code following 90748.
90759	460	See code following 90746.
91113	466	See code following 91111.
91300	455	See code before 90476.
91301	456	See code before 90476.
91302	456	See code before 90476.
91303	456	See code before 90476.
91304	456	See code before 90476.
91305	456	See code following resequenced code 91300.
91306	456	See code following resequenced code 91301.
91307	456	See code following resequenced code 91305.
92517	472	See code following 92549.
92518	472	See code following 92549.

Code	Page	Reference
92519	472	See code following 92549.
92558	473	See code before 92587.
92597	473	See code following 92604.
92618	473	See code following 92605.
92650	473	See code following 92584.
92651	473	See code following 92584.
92652	473	See code following 92584.
92653	473	See code following 92584.
92920	476	See code following 92998.
92921	476	See code following 92998.
92924	476	See code following 92998.
92925	476	See code following 92998.
92928	476	See code following 92998.
92929	476	See code following 92998.
92933	476	See code following 92998.
92934	477	See code following 92998.
92937	477	See code following 92998.
92938	477	See code following 92998.
92941	477	See code following 92998.
92943	477	See code following 92998.
92944	477	See code following 92998.
92973	477	See code following 92998.
92974	477	See code following 92998.
92975	477	See code following 92998.
92977	477	See code following 92998.
92978	477	See code following 92998.
92979	477	See code following 92998.
93241	479	See code following 93227.
93242	479	See code following 93227.
93243	479	See code following 93227.
93244	479	See code following 93227.
93245	479	See code following 93227.
93246	479	See code following 93227.
93247	479	See code following 93227.
93248	479	See code following 93227.
93260	481	See code following 93284.
93261	482	See code following 93289.
93264	480	See code before 93279.
93319	484	See code following 93317.
93356	484	See code following 93351.
94619	497	See code following 94617.
95249	501	See code following 95250.
95700	508	See code following 95967.
95705	508	See code following 95967.
95706	508	See code following 95967.
95707	508	See code following 95967.
95708	508	See code following 95967.
95709	508	See code following 95967.
95710	508	See code following 95967.
95711	508	See code following 95967.
95712	509	See code following 95967.
95713	509	See code following 95967.
95714	509	See code following 95967.
95715	509	See code following 95967.

Code	Page	Reference
95716	509	See code following 95967.
95717	509	See code following 95967.
95718	509	See code following 95967.
95719	509	See code following 95967.
95720	509	See code following 95967.
95721	509	See code following 95967.
95722	509	See code following 95967.
95723	509	See code following 95967.
95724	509	See code following 95967.
95725	509	See code following 95967.
95726	509	See code following 95967.
95782	502	See code following 95811.
95783	502	See code following 95811.
95800	502	See code following 95806.
95801	502	See code following 95806.
95829	503	See code following 95830.
95836	504	See code following 95830.
95885	504	See code following 95872.
95886	505	See code following 95872.
95887	505	See code before 95873.
95938	507	See code following 95926.
95939	507	See code following 95929.
95940	506	See code following 95913.
95941	506	See code following 95913.
95983	510	See code following 95977.
95984	510	See code following 95977.
96125	513	See code following 96105.
96127	513	See code following 96113.
96164	514	See code following 96159.
96165	514	See code following 96159.
96167	514	See code following 96159.
96168	514	See code following 96159.
96170	514	See code following 96159.
96171	514	See code following 96159.
97151	511	See code following 96040.
97152	512	See code following 96040.
97153	512	See code following 96040.
97154	512	See code following 96040.
97155	512	See code following 96040.
97156	512	See code following 96040.
97157	512	See code following 96040.
97158	513	See code following 96040.
97161	521	See code before 97010.
97162	522	See code before 97010.
97163	522	See code before 97010.
97164	522	See code before 97010.
97165	522	See code before 97010.
97166	522	See code before 97010.
97167	523	See code before 97010.
97168	523	See code before 97010.
97169	523	See code before 97010.
97170	523	See code before 97010.
97171	523	See code before 97010.
97172	523	See code before 97010.

Code	Page	Reference
99091	559	See code following resequenced code 99454.
99177	532	See code following 99174.
99224	545	See code following 99220.
99225	545	See code following 99220.
99226	546	See code following 99220.
99415	555	See code following 99359.
99416	555	See code following 99359.
99417	555	See code following resequenced code 99416.
99421	558	See code following 99443.
99422	558	See code following 99443.
99423	558	See code following 99443.
99424	564	See code following 99489.
99425	564	See code following 99489.
99426	564	See code following 99489.
99427	564	See code following 99489.
99437	563	See code following resequenced code 99491.
99439	563	See code following resequenced code 99490.
99451	558	See code following 99449.

Code	Page	Reference
99452	559	See code following 99449.
99453	559	See code following 99449.
99454	559	See code following 99449.
99457	560	See code before 99450.
99458	560	See code before 99450.
99473	559	See code before 99450.
99474	559	See code before 99450.
99484	565	See code following 99498.
99485	561	See code following 99467.
99486	561	See code following 99467.
99490	563	See code before 99487.
99491	563	See code before 99487.
2033F	571	See code following 2026F.
3051F	572	See code following 3044F.
3052F	572	See code before 3046F.
0253T	584	See code before 0198T.
0464T	587	See code following 0333T.
0488T	589	See code following 0403T.
0510T	587	See code following 0335T.
0511T	587	See code following 0335T.
0512T	583	See code following 0102T.

Code	Page	Reference
0513T	583	See code following 0102T.
0523T	594	See code before 0505T.
0563T	585	See code following 0207T.
0614T	599	See code following 0580T.
0620T	594	See code following 0505T.
0623T	594	See code following 0504T.
0624T	594	See code following 0504T.
0625T	594	See code following 0504T.
0626T	594	See code following 0504T.
0640T	593	See code following 0493T
0641T	593	See code following 0493T
0642T	593	See code following 0493T
0643T	597	See code following 0545T
0646T	598	See code following 0570T
0671T	584	See code following 0184T.
0697T	603	See code following 0648T.
0698T	604	See code following 0649T.

Appendix F — Add-on Codes, Optum Modifier 50 Exempt, Modifier 51 Exempt, Optum Modifier 51 Exempt, Modifier 63 Exempt, and Modifier 95 Telemedicine Services

Codes specified as add-on, exempt from modifiers 50, 51 and 63, and modifier 95 (telemedicine services) are listed. The lists are designed to be read left to right rather than vertically.

Add-on Codes

0054T	0055T	0076T	0095T	0098T	0163T	0164T
0165T	0174T	0214T	0215T	0217T	0218T	0222T
0397T	0437T	0439T	0443T	0450T	0471T	0480T
0492T	0496T	0513T	0514T	0523T	0560T	0562T
0570T	0599T	0628T	0630T	0649T	0663T	0676T
0678T	0690T	0698T	0701T	0709T	0071U	0072U
0073U	0074U	0075U	0076U	0130U	0131U	0132U
0133U	0134U	0135U	0136U	0137U	0138U	0157U
0158U	0159U	0160U	0161U	0162U	0207U	01953
01968	01969	10004	10006	10008	10010	10012
10036	11001	11008	11045	11046	11047	11103
11105	11107	11201	11732	11922	13102	13122
13133	13153	14302	15003	15005	15101	15111
15116	15121	15131	15136	15151	15152	15156
15157	15201	15221	15241	15261	15272	15274
15276	15278	15772	15774	15777	15787	15847
16036	17003	17312	17314	17315	19001	19082
19084	19086	19126	19282	19284	19286	19288
19294	19297	20700	20701	20702	20703	20704
20705	20930	20931	20932	20933	20934	20936
20937	20938	20939	20985	22103	22116	22208
22216	22226	22328	22512	22515	22527	22534
22552	22585	22614	22632	22634	22840	22841
22842	22843	22844	22845	22846	22847	22848
22853	22854	22858	22859	22868	22870	26125
26861	26863	27358	27692	29826	31627	31632
31633	31637	31649	31651	31654	32501	32506
32507	32667	32668	32674	33141	33225	33257
33258	33259	33268	33367	33368	33369	33370
33419	33508	33517	33518	33519	33521	33522
33523	33530	33572	33746	33768	33866	33884
33924	33929	33987	34709	34711	34713	34714
34715	34716	34717	34808	34812	34813	34820
34833	34834	35306	35390	35400	35500	35572
35681	35682	35683	35685	35686	35697	35700
36218	36227	36228	36248	36474	36476	36479
36483	36907	36908	36909	37185	37186	37222
37223	37232	37233	37234	37235	37237	37239
37247	37249	37252	37253	38102	38746	38747
38900	43273	43283	43338	43635	44015	44121
44128	44139	44203	44213	44701	44955	47001
47542	47543	47544	47550	48400	49326	49327
49412	49435	49568	49905	50606	50705	50706
51797	52442	56606	57267	57465	58110	58611
59525	60512	61316	61517	61611	61641	61642
61651	61781	61782	61783	61797	61799	61800
61864	61868	62148	62160	63035	63043	63044
63048	63052	63053	63057	63066	63076	63078
63082	63086	63088	63091	63103	63295	63308
63621	64421	64462	64480	64484	64491	64492
64494	64495	64629	64634	64636	64643	64645
64727	64778	64783	64787	64832	64837	64859
64872	64874	64876	64901	64902	64913	65757
66990	67225	67320	67331	67332	67334	67335
67340	69990	74248	74301	74713	75565	75774
76125	76802	76810	76812	76814	76937	76979
76983	77001	77002	77003	77063	77293	78020
78434	78496	78730	78835	80506	81266	81416
81426	81536	82952	86826	87187	87503	87904
88155	88177	88185	88311	88314	88332	88334
88341	88350	88364	88369	88373	88388	90461
90472	90474	90785	90833	90836	90838	90840
90863	90913	91013	92547	92608	92618	92621
92627	92921	92925	92929	92934	92938	92944
92973	92974	92978	92979	92998	93319	93320
93321	93325	93352	93356	93462	93463	93464
93563	93564	93565	93566	93567	93568	93571
93572	93592	93598	93609	93613	93621	93622
93623	93655	93657	93662	94645	94729	94781
95079	95873	95874	95885	95886	95887	95940
95941	95962	95967	95984	96113	96121	96131
96133	96137	96139	96159	96165	96168	96171
96361	96366	96367	96368	96370	96371	96375
96376	96411	96415	96417	96423	96570	96571
96934	96935	96936	97130	97546	97598	97811
97814	98981	99100	99116	99135	99140	99153
99157	99292	99354	99355	99356	99357	99359
99415	99416	99417	99425	99427	99437	99439
99458	99467	99486	99489	99494	99498	99602
99607						

Optum Modifier 50 Exempt Codes

0214T	0215T	0217T	0218T	15777	20939	34713
34714	34715	34716	34717	34812	34820	34833
34834	35572	49568	63035	63043	63044	64421
64480	64484	64491	64492	64494	64495	64634
64636						

AMA Modifier 51 Exempt Codes

20697	20974	20975	33509	35600	44500	61107
93600	93602	93603	93610	93612	93615	93616
93618	94610	95905	99151	99152		

Optum Modifier 51 Exempt Codes

22585	22614	22632	69990	90281	90283	90284
90287	90288	90291	90296	90371	90375	90376
90377	90378	90384	90385	90386	90389	90393
90396	90399	90476	90477	90581	90585	90586
90587	90619	90620	90621	90625	90630	90632
90633	90634	90636	90644	90647	90648	90649
90650	90651	90653	90654	90655	90656	90657
90658	90660	90661	90662	90664	90666	90667
90668	90670	90672	90673	90674	90675	90676
90680	90681	90682	90685	90686	90687	90688
90689	90690	90691	90694	90696	90697	90698
90700	90702	90707	90710	90713	90714	90715
90716	90717	90723	90732	90733	90734	90736
90738	90739	90740	90743	90744	90746	90747
90748	90749	90750	90756	97010	97012	97014
97016	97018	97022	97024	97026	97028	97032
97033	97034	97035	97036	97110	97112	97113
97116	97124	97129	97130	97140	97150	97161
97162	97163	97164	97165	97166	97167	97168
97169	97170	97171	97172	97530	97533	97535
97537	97542	97545	97546	97597	97598	97602
97605	97606	97607	97608	97610	97750	97755
97760	97761	97763	99050	99051	99053	99056
99058	99060					

Modifier 63 Exempt Codes

30540	30545	31520	33502	33503	33505	33506
33610	33611	33619	33647	33670	33690	33694
33730	33732	33735	33736	33741	33750	33755
33762	33778	33786	33922	33946	33947	33948

33949	36415	36420	36450	36456	36460	36510
36660	39503	43313	43314	43520	43831	44055
44126	44127	44128	46070	46705	46715	46716
46730	46735	46740	46742	46744	47700	47701
49215	49491	49492	49495	49496	49600	49605
49606	49610	49611	53025	54000	54150	54160
63700	63702	63704	63706	65820		

Telemedicine Services Codes

The codes on the following list may be used to report telemedicine services when modifier 95 Synchronous Telemedicine Service Rendered via a Real-Time Interactive Audio and Visual Telecommunications System, is appended.

90785	90791	90792	90832	90833	90834	90836
90837	90838	90839	90840	90845	90846	90847
90863	90951	90952	90954	90955	90957	90958
90960	90961	90963	90964	90965	90966	90967
90968	90969	90970	92227	92228	93228	93229

93268	93270	93271	93272	96040	96116	96160
96161	97110	97112	97116	97161	97162	97165
97166	97530	97535	97750	97755	97760	97761
97802	97803	97804	98960	98961	98962	99202
99203	99204	99205	99211	99212	99213	99214
99215	99231	99232	99233	*99241	*99242	*99243
*99244	*99245	*99251	*99252	*99253	*99254	*99255
99307	99308	99309	99310	99354	99355	99356
99357	99406	99407	99408	99409	99417	99495
99496	99497	99498				

* Consultations are noncovered by Medicare

Appendix G — Medicare Internet-only Manuals (IOMs)

The Centers for Medicare and Medicaid Services restructured its paper-based manual system as a web-based system on October 1, 2003. Called the online CMS manual system, it combines all of the various program instructions into internet-only manuals (IOMs), which are used by all CMS programs and contractors. In many instances, the references from the online manuals in appendix G contain a mention of the old paper manuals from which the current information was obtained when the manuals were converted. This information is shown in the header of the text, in the following format, when applicable, as A3-3101, HO-210, and B3-2049.

Effective with implementation of the IOMs, the former method of publishing program memoranda (PMs) to communicate program instructions was replaced by the following four templates:

- One-time notification
- Manual revisions
- Business requirements
- Confidential requirements

The web-based system has been organized by functional area (e.g., eligibility, entitlement, claims processing, benefit policy, program integrity) in an effort to eliminate redundancy within the manuals, simplify updating, and make CMS program instructions available more quickly. The web-based system contains the functional areas included below:

Pub. 100	Introduction
Pub. 100-01	Medicare General Information, Eligibility and Entitlement Manual
Pub. 100-02	Medicare Benefit Policy Manual
Pub. 100-03	Medicare National Coverage Determinations (NCD) Manual
Pub. 100-04	Medicare Claims Processing Manual
Pub. 100-05	Medicare Secondary Payer Manual
Pub. 100-06	Medicare Financial Management Manual
Pub. 100-07	State Operations Manual
Pub. 100-08	Medicare Program Integrity Manual
Pub. 100-09	Medicare Contractor Beneficiary and Provider Communications Manual
Pub. 100-10	Quality Improvement Organization Manual
Pub. 100-11	Programs of All-Inclusive Care for the Elderly (PACE) Manual
Pub. 100-12	State Medicaid Manual (under development)
Pub. 100-13	Medicaid State Children's Health Insurance Program (under development)
Pub. 100-14	Medicare ESRD Network Organizations Manual
Pub. 100-15	Medicaid Integrity Program (MIP)
Pub. 100-16	Medicare Managed Care Manual
Pub. 100-17	CMS/Business Partners Systems Security Manual
Pub. 100-18	Medicare Prescription Drug Benefit Manual
Pub. 100-19	Demonstrations
Pub. 100-20	One-Time Notification
Pub. 100-21	Reserved
Pub. 100-22	Medicare Quality Reporting Incentive Programs Manual
Pub. 100-24	State Buy-In Manual
Pub. 100-25	Information Security Acceptable Risk Safeguards Manual

A brief description of the Medicare manuals primarily used for *CPC Expert* follows:

The *National Coverage Determinations Manual* (NCD), is organized according to categories such as diagnostic services, supplies, and medical procedures. The table of contents lists each category and subject within that category. Revision transmittals identify any new or background material, recap the changes, and provide an effective date for the change. The manual contains four sections and is organized in accordance with CPT category sequence and contains a list of HCPCS codes related to coverage determinations, where appropriate.

The *Medicare Benefit Policy Manual* contains Medicare general coverage instructions that are not national coverage determinations. As a general rule, in the past these instructions have been found in chapter II of the *Medicare Carriers Manual,* the *Medicare Intermediary Manual*, other provider manuals, and program memoranda.

The *Medicare Claims Processing Manual* contains instructions for processing claims for contractors and providers.

The *Medicare Program Integrity Manual* communicates the priorities and standards for the Medicare integrity programs.

Medicare IOM References

A printed version of the Medicare IOM references will no longer be published in Optum360's *Current Procedural Coding* product. Complete versions of all the manuals can be found online at https://www.cms.gov/Regulations-and-Guidance/Guidance/Manuals/Internet-Only-Manuals-IOMs.

Appendix H — Quality Payment Program

In 2015, Congress passed the Medicare Access and CHIP Reauthorization Act (MACRA), which included sweeping changes for practitioners who provide services reimbursed under the Medicare physician fee schedule (MPFS). The act focused on repealing the faulty Medicare sustainable growth rate, focusing on quality of patient outcomes, and controlling Medicare spending.

A MACRA final rule in October 2016 established the Quality Payment Program (QPP), which was effective January 1, 2017. This value-based payment model rewards eligible clinicians (ECs) who provide high-quality care and reduce the payments for those who fail to meet specific performance standards.

ECs can receive incentives under the QPP. Once the performance threshold is established, all ECs who score above that threshold are eligible to receive a positive payment adjustment. Keep in mind that the key requirement is that an EC **submit data** to avoid the negative payment adjustment and receive the incentives. The Centers for Medicare and Medicaid Services (CMS) has redesigned the scoring so that clinicians are able to know how well they are doing in the program, as benchmarks are known in advance of participating.

The QPP consists of two tracks that clinicians may choose from based on their practice size, location, specialty, or patient population:

*   The merit-based incentive payment system (MIPS)

*   Alternative payment models (APMs)

The 2017 QPP final rule established regulations for MIPS and APMs as well as related policies applicable to eligible clinicians who participate in the Shared Savings Program. These policies included requirements for Shared Savings Program accountable care organizations (ACOs) regarding reporting for the MIPS Quality performance category and a policy that gave ACOs full credit for the MIPS Improvement Activities performance category based on their participation in the Shared Savings Program. Since that time, revisions and modifications have been made to allow more focus on measurement efforts and to reduce barriers to entry into advanced APMs. Refinements will continue in order to reduce reporting burden and focus on patient outcomes.

MIPS provides specified performance categories under which payment adjustments may be earned for Part B covered professional services. Eligible clinicians can obtain a composite performance score (CPS) of up to 100 points from these weighted performance categories, which focus on patient care quality and cost, improvements in patient engagement and clinical care processes, and use of certified electronic health record technology (CEHRT). This performance score then defines the payment adjustments in the second calendar year after the year the score is obtained. For instance, the score obtained for the 2020 performance year is linked to payment for Medicare Part B services in 2022.

ECs currently have three available reporting frameworks, depending on individual needs and eligibility—traditional MIPS, MIPS Value Pathways (MVPs), and the alternative payment model (APM) performance pathway (APP). The majority of the proposed updates for CY 2022 focus on MIPS.

Traditional MIPS currently consists of the following performance categories:

*   Quality

*   Improvement Activities

*   Promoting Interoperability (PI)

*   Cost

MVPs, which were added as a result of complaints by some physicians of confusing quality measures, allow clinicians to report only on those measures that apply to their specialty. The CY 2022 proposed rule includes seven MVPs for the 2023 performance year related to the following clinical areas: anesthesia, chronic disease management, emergency medicine, heart disease, lower extremity joint repair, rheumatology, and stroke care and prevention. Additional MVPs will gradually be implemented for more specialties and subspecialties that participate in the program.

The APP is intended for MIPS-eligible ECs who also participate in MIPS APMs. Performance is measured across three areas (Quality, Improvement Activities, and Promoting Interoperability) in this reporting and scoring pathway, which aims to decrease reporting burden, encourage APM participation, and create new opportunities for scoring for existing MIPS APM participants. For performance year 2021, the APP Quality performance category accounted for 50 percent of the MIPS final score; the PI performance category weight was 30 percent; and the Improvement Activities performance category weight was 20 percent.

Proposed 2022/2023 Changes

As noted earlier, the majority of the proposed updates for CY 2022 focus on MIPS. In addition to the seven MVPs proposed for the 2023 performance year, other proposals in the CY 2022 proposed rule include:

*   Additions to the MVP development criteria beginning with the 2022 performance year/2024 payment year related to relevant outcome measures, high-priority measures, outcomes-based administrative claims measures, and a qualified clinical data registry (QCDR) measure

*   Timelines for transitioning to MVPs and for participant registration

*   Establishment of subgroup reporting to provide more granular and comprehensive information that will be more clinically meaningful. Subgroup reporting is proposed to be limited to only those clinicians reporting through MVPs or APP

*   MVP scoring policies by performance category and updating of the scoring hierarchy to include subgroups

*   Revision of the definition of an MIPS-eligible clinician to include certified nurse midwives and clinical social workers

*   Revision of the performance threshold

*   Revisions and updates to the existing performance categories included in the traditional MIPS framework

*   Proposals specific to the transition timeframe of accountable care organizations (ACOs) for reporting specific quality measures

Additionally, a request for public comments was made regarding an incremental timeline to transition to mandatory MVP reporting that will coincide with the sunset of traditional MIPS. The timeline currently being considered is the end of the CY 2027 performance period/2029 MIPS payment year, although this is not an official proposal at this time.

Detailed information regarding the Quality Payment Program may be found at https://qpp.cms.gov/. This website will also announce the final CMS determinations of advanced APMs and MIPS APMs for the 2022 performance period.

Appendix I — Medically Unlikely Edits (MUEs)

The Centers for Medicare & Medicaid Services (CMS) began to publish many of the edits used in the medically unlikely edits (MUE) program for the first time effective October 2008. What follows below is a list of the published CPT codes that have MUEs assigned to them and the number of units allowed with each code. CMS publishes the updates on a quarterly basis. Not all MUEs will be published, however. MUEs intended to detect and discourage any questionable payments will not be published as the agency feels the efficacy of these edits would be compromised. CMS added another component to the MUEs—the MUE Adjudication Indicator (MAI). The appropriate MAI can be found in parentheses following the MUE in this table and specify the maximum units of service (UOS) for a CPT/HCPCS code for the service. The MAI designates whether the UOS edit is applied to the line or claim.

The three MAIs are defined as follows:

MAI 1 (Line Edit) This MAI will continue to be adjudicated as the line edit on the claim and is auto-adjudicated by the contractor.

MAI 2 (Date of Service Edit, Policy) This MAI is considered to be the "absolute date of service edit" and is based on policy. The total unit of services (UOS) for that CPT code and that date of service (DOS) are combined for this edit. Medicare contractors are required to review all claims for the same patient, same date of service, and same provider.

MAI 3 (Date of Service Edit: Clinical) This MAI is also a date-of-service edit but is based upon clinical standards. The review takes current and previously submitted claims for the same patient, same date of service, and same provider into account. When medical necessity is clearly documented, the edit may be bypassed or the claim resubmitted.

The quarterly updates are published on the CMS website at https://www.cms.gov/Medicare/Coding/NationalCorrectCodInitEd/MUE. The following was updated on 10/01/2021.

Practitioner

CPT	MUE	CPT	MUE	CPT	MUE	CPT	MUE	CPT	MUE	CPT	MUE	CPT	MUE	CPT	MUE
0001A	1(2)	0032U	1(2)	0071U	1(2)	0109U	1(3)	0157U	1(2)	0209T	1(3)	0237T	2(3)	0345T	1(2)
0001U	1(2)	0033U	1(2)	0072T	1(2)	0110T	4(2)	0158U	1(2)	0209U	1(2)	0237U	1(2)	0347T	1(3)
0002A	1(2)	0034U	1(2)	0072U	1(2)	0110U	1(2)	0159U	1(2)	0210T	1(3)	0238T	2(3)	0348T	1(3)
0002M	1(3)	0035U	1(2)	0073U	1(2)	0111U	1(2)	0160U	1(2)	0210U	2(3)	0238U	1(2)	0349T	1(3)
0002U	1(2)	0036U	1(3)	0074U	1(2)	0112U	1(3)	0161U	1(2)	0211T	1(3)	0239U	1(2)	0350T	1(3)
0003M	1(3)	0037U	1(3)	0075T	1(2)	0113U	1(2)	0162U	1(2)	0211U	2(3)	0240U	1(3)	0351T	5(3)
0003U	1(2)	0038U	1(2)	0075U	1(2)	0114U	1(2)	0163T	1(3)	0212T	1(3)	0241U	1(3)	0352T	5(3)
0004M	1(2)	0039U	1(2)	0076T	1(2)	0115U	1(3)	0163U	0(3)	0212U	1(2)	0242U	1(2)	0353T	2(3)
0005U	1(2)	0040U	1(2)	0076U	1(2)	0116U	1(2)	0164T	4(2)	0213T	1(2)	0243U	1(2)	0354T	2(3)
0006M	1(2)	0041A	1(2)	0077U	2(2)	0117U	1(2)	0164U	1(2)	0213U	1(3)	0244U	1(3)	0355T	1(2)
0007M	1(2)	0041U	1(2)	0078U	1(2)	0118U	1(2)	0165T	4(2)	0214T	1(2)	0245U	2(3)	0356T	4(2)
0007U	1(2)	0042A	1(2)	0079U	0(3)	0119U	1(2)	0165U	1(2)	0214U	1(2)	0247U	1(2)	0358T	1(2)
0008U	1(3)	0042T	1(3)	0080U	1(2)	0120U	1(2)	0166U	1(2)	0215T	1(2)	0253T	1(3)	0362T	16(3)
0009U	2(3)	0042U	1(2)	0082U	1(2)	0121U	1(2)	0167U	1(2)	0215U	1(3)	0263T	1(3)	0373T	24(3)
0010U	2(3)	0043U	1(2)	0083U	1(3)	0122U	1(2)	0168U	1(2)	0216T	1(2)	0264T	1(3)	0376T	2(3)
0011A	1(2)	0044U	1(2)	0084U	1(2)	0123U	1(2)	0169U	1(2)	0216U	1(2)	0265T	1(3)	0378T	1(2)
0011M	1(2)	0045U	1(3)	0086U	1(3)	0129U	1(2)	0170U	1(2)	0217T	1(2)	0266T	1(2)	0379T	1(2)
0011U	1(2)	0046U	1(3)	0087U	1(2)	0130U	1(2)	0171U	1(2)	0217U	1(2)	0267T	1(3)	0394T	2(3)
0012A	1(2)	0047U	1(3)	0088U	1(2)	0131U	1(2)	0172U	1(2)	0218T	1(2)	0268T	1(3)	0395T	2(3)
0012M	1(2)	0048U	1(3)	0089U	1(3)	0132U	1(2)	0173U	1(2)	0218U	1(2)	0269T	1(2)	0397T	1(3)
0012U	1(2)	0049U	1(3)	0090U	1(2)	0133U	1(2)	0174T	1(3)	0219T	1(2)	0270T	1(3)	0398T	1(3)
0013M	1(2)	0050U	1(3)	0091U	1(2)	0134U	1(2)	0174U	1(2)	0219U	1(2)	0271T	1(3)	0402T	2(2)
0013U	1(3)	0051U	1(2)	0092U	1(2)	0135U	1(2)	0175T	1(3)	0220T	1(2)	0272T	1(3)	0403T	1(2)
0014M	1(2)	0052U	1(2)	0093U	1(2)	0136U	1(2)	0175U	1(2)	0220U	1(2)	0273T	1(3)	0404T	1(2)
0014U	1(3)	0053U	1(3)	0094U	1(2)	0137U	1(2)	0176U	1(3)	0221T	1(2)	0274T	1(2)	0408T	1(3)
0015M	1(2)	0054T	1(3)	0095T	1(3)	0138U	1(2)	0177U	1(3)	0222T	1(3)	0275T	1(2)	0409T	1(3)
0016M	2(3)	0054U	1(2)	0095U	1(2)	0139U	1(2)	0178U	1(2)	0223U	1(3)	0278T	1(3)	0410T	1(3)
0016U	1(3)	0055T	1(3)	0096U	1(2)	0140U	1(2)	0179U	1(3)	0224U	3(3)	0290T	1(3)	0411T	1(3)
0017U	1(3)	0055U	1(2)	0097U	1(2)	0141U	1(2)	0184T	1(3)	0225U	1(3)	0308T	1(3)	0412T	1(2)
0018U	2(3)	0056U	1(3)	0098T	2(3)	0142U	1(2)	0191T	2(2)	0226U	1(2)	0312T	1(3)	0413T	1(2)
0019U	1(3)	0058U	1(2)	0100T	1(2)	0143U	1(2)	0198T	2(2)	0227U	1(2)	0313T	1(3)	0414T	1(2)
0021A	1(2)	0059U	1(2)	0101T	1(3)	0144U	1(2)	01996	1(2)	0228U	1(2)	0314T	1(3)	0415T	1(3)
0021U	1(2)	0060U	1(2)	0101U	1(2)	0145U	1(2)	0200T	1(2)	0229U	1(2)	0315T	1(3)	0416T	1(3)
0022A	1(2)	0061U	2(3)	0102T	2(2)	0146U	1(2)	0201T	1(2)	0230U	1(2)	0316T	1(3)	0417T	1(3)
0022U	2(3)	0062U	1(2)	0102U	1(2)	0147U	1(2)	0202T	1(3)	0231U	1(2)	0317T	1(3)	0418T	1(3)
0023U	1(2)	0063U	1(2)	0103U	1(2)	0148U	1(2)	0202U	1(3)	0232T	1(3)	0329T	1(2)	0419T	1(2)
0024U	1(2)	0064U	2(3)	0105U	1(2)	0149U	1(2)	0203U	1(2)	0232U	1(2)	0330T	1(2)	0420T	1(2)
0025U	1(2)	0065U	2(3)	0106T	4(2)	0150U	1(2)	0204U	1(3)	0233U	1(2)	0331T	1(3)	0421T	1(2)
0026U	2(3)	0066U	1(3)	0106U	1(2)	0151U	1(2)	0205U	1(2)	0234T	2(2)	0332T	1(3)	0422T	1(3)
0027U	1(2)	0067U	2(3)	0107T	4(2)	0152U	1(2)	0206U	1(3)	0234U	1(2)	0333T	1(2)	0423T	1(3)
0029U	1(2)	0068U	1(3)	0107U	1(3)	0153U	1(2)	0207T	2(2)	0235T	2(3)	0335T	2(2)	0424T	1(3)
0030U	1(2)	0069U	1(3)	0108T	4(2)	0154U	1(2)	0207U	1(2)	0235U	1(2)	0338T	1(2)	0425T	1(3)
0031A	1(2)	0070U	1(3)	0108U	1(2)	0155U	1(2)	0208T	1(3)	0236T	1(2)	0339T	1(3)	0426T	1(3)
0031U	1(2)	0071T	1(2)	0109T	4(2)	0156U	1(2)	0208U	1(3)	0236U	1(2)	0342T	1(3)	0427T	1(3)

CPT	MUE	CPT	MUE	CPT	MUE	CPT	MUE	CPT	MUE	CPT	MUE	CPT	MUE	CPT	MUE
0428T	1(2)	0496T	4(3)	0562T	1(3)	0629T	1(2)	11307	3(3)	11922	1(3)	14060	2(3)	15769	1(3)
0429T	1(2)	0497T	1(3)	0563T	1(2)	0630T	4(2)	11308	2(3)	11950	1(2)	14061	2(3)	15770	2(3)
0430T	1(2)	0498T	1(2)	0564T	1(2)	0631T	4(2)	11310	4(3)	11951	1(2)	14301	2(3)	15771	1(2)
0431T	1(2)	0499T	1(2)	0565T	1(2)	0632T	1(2)	11311	4(3)	11952	1(2)	14302	8(3)	15772	9(3)
0432T	1(3)	0500T	1(3)	0566T	1(2)	0633T	1(2)	11312	3(3)	11954	1(3)	14350	2(3)	15773	1(3)
0433T	1(3)	0501T	1(2)	0567T	1(2)	0634T	1(2)	11313	3(3)	11960	2(3)	15002	1(2)	15774	3(3)
0434T	1(3)	0502T	1(2)	0568T	1(2)	0635T	1(2)	11400	3(3)	11970	2(3)	15003	60(3)	15775	1(2)
0435T	1(3)	0503T	1(2)	0569T	1(2)	0636T	1(2)	11401	3(3)	11971	2(3)	15004	1(2)	15776	1(2)
0436T	1(3)	0504T	1(2)	0570T	1(3)	0637T	1(2)	11402	3(3)	11976	1(2)	15005	19(3)	15777	1(3)
0437T	1(3)	0505T	1(3)	0571T	1(2)	0638T	1(2)	11403	2(3)	11980	1(2)	15040	1(2)	15780	1(2)
0439T	1(3)	0506T	1(2)	0572T	1(2)	0639T	1(3)	11404	2(3)	11981	1(3)	15050	1(3)	15781	1(3)
0440T	3(3)	0507T	1(2)	0573T	1(2)	10004	3(3)	11406	2(3)	11982	1(3)	15100	1(2)	15782	1(3)
0441T	3(3)	0508T	1(3)	0574T	1(2)	10005	1(2)	11420	3(3)	11983	1(3)	15101	40(3)	15783	1(3)
0442T	3(3)	0509T	1(2)	0575T	1(2)	10006	3(3)	11421	3(3)	12001	1(2)	15110	1(2)	15786	1(2)
0443T	1(2)	0510T	1(2)	0576T	1(2)	10007	1(2)	11422	3(3)	12002	1(2)	15111	5(3)	15787	2(3)
0444T	1(2)	0511T	1(2)	0577T	1(2)	10008	2(3)	11423	2(3)	12004	1(2)	15115	1(2)	15788	1(2)
0445T	1(2)	0512T	1(2)	0578T	1(2)	10009	1(2)	11424	2(3)	12005	1(2)	15116	2(3)	15789	1(2)
0446T	1(3)	0513T	2(3)	0579T	1(2)	10010	3(3)	11426	2(3)	12006	1(2)	15120	1(2)	15792	1(3)
0447T	1(3)	0514T	2(2)	0580T	1(2)	10011	1(2)	11440	4(3)	12007	1(2)	15121	8(3)	15793	1(3)
0448T	1(3)	0515T	1(3)	0581T	0(3)	10012	3(3)	11441	3(3)	12011	1(2)	15130	1(2)	15819	1(2)
0449T	1(2)	0516T	1(3)	0582T	0(3)	10021	1(2)	11442	3(3)	12013	1(2)	15131	2(3)	15820	1(2)
0450T	1(3)	0517T	1(3)	0583T	2(2)	10030	2(3)	11443	2(3)	12014	1(2)	15135	1(2)	15821	1(2)
0451T	1(3)	0518T	1(3)	0584T	1(2)	10035	1(2)	11444	2(3)	12015	1(2)	15136	1(2)	15822	1(2)
0452T	1(3)	0519T	1(3)	0585T	1(2)	10036	2(3)	11446	2(3)	12016	1(2)	15150	1(2)	15823	1(2)
0453T	1(3)	0520T	1(3)	0586T	1(2)	10040	1(2)	11450	1(2)	12017	1(2)	15151	1(2)	15824	1(2)
0454T	3(3)	0521T	1(3)	0587T	1(2)	10060	1(2)	11451	1(2)	12018	1(2)	15152	5(3)	15825	1(2)
0455T	1(3)	0522T	1(3)	0588T	1(2)	10061	1(2)	11462	1(2)	12020	2(3)	15155	1(2)	15826	1(2)
0456T	1(3)	0523T	1(3)	0589T	1(2)	10080	1(3)	11463	1(2)	12021	3(3)	15156	1(2)	15828	1(2)
0457T	1(3)	0524T	3(3)	0590T	1(2)	10081	1(3)	11470	3(2)	12031	1(2)	15157	1(3)	15829	1(2)
0458T	3(3)	0525T	1(3)	0591T	1(2)	10120	3(3)	11471	2(3)	12032	1(2)	15200	1(2)	15830	1(2)
0459T	1(3)	0526T	1(3)	0592T	1(2)	10121	2(3)	11600	2(3)	12034	1(2)	15201	7(3)	15832	1(2)
0460T	3(3)	0527T	1(3)	0593T	1(2)	10140	2(3)	11601	2(3)	12035	1(2)	15220	1(2)	15833	1(2)
0461T	1(3)	0528T	1(3)	0594T	2(2)	10160	3(3)	11602	3(3)	12036	1(2)	15221	9(3)	15834	1(2)
0462T	1(2)	0529T	1(3)	0596T	1(2)	10180	2(3)	11603	2(3)	12037	1(2)	15240	1(2)	15835	1(3)
0463T	1(2)	0530T	1(3)	0597T	1(2)	11000	1(2)	11604	2(3)	12041	1(2)	15241	9(3)	15836	1(2)
0464T	1(2)	0531T	1(3)	0598T	1(2)	11001	1(3)	11606	2(3)	12042	1(2)	15260	1(2)	15837	2(3)
0465T	1(3)	0532T	1(3)	0599T	1(3)	11004	1(2)	11620	2(3)	12044	1(2)	15261	6(3)	15838	1(2)
0466T	1(3)	0533T	1(2)	0600T	3(3)	11005	1(2)	11621	2(3)	12045	1(2)	15271	1(2)	15839	2(3)
0467T	1(3)	0534T	1(2)	0601T	3(3)	11006	1(2)	11622	2(3)	12046	1(2)	15272	3(3)	15840	1(3)
0468T	1(3)	0535T	1(2)	0602T	1(2)	11008	1(2)	11623	2(3)	12047	1(2)	15273	1(2)	15841	1(3)
0469T	1(2)	0536T	1(2)	0603T	1(2)	11010	2(3)	11624	2(3)	12051	1(2)	15274	60(3)	15842	2(3)
0470T	1(2)	0537T	1(3)	0604T	1(2)	11011	2(3)	11626	2(3)	12052	1(2)	15275	1(2)	15845	2(3)
0471T	2(1)	0538T	1(3)	0605T	1(2)	11012	2(3)	11640	2(3)	12053	1(2)	15276	3(2)	15847	1(2)
0472T	1(2)	0539T	1(3)	0606T	1(2)	11042	1(2)	11641	2(3)	12054	1(2)	15277	1(2)	15850	0(3)
0473T	1(2)	0540T	1(3)	0607T	1(2)	11043	1(2)	11642	3(3)	12055	1(2)	15278	15(3)	15851	1(2)
0474T	2(2)	0541T	1(3)	0608T	1(2)	11044	1(2)	11643	2(3)	12056	1(2)	15570	2(3)	15852	1(3)
0475T	1(3)	0542T	1(3)	0609T	1(3)	11045	12(3)	11644	2(3)	12057	1(2)	15572	2(3)	15860	1(3)
0476T	1(3)	0543T	1(2)	0610T	1(3)	11046	10(3)	11646	2(3)	13100	1(2)	15574	2(3)	15876	1(2)
0477T	1(3)	0544T	1(2)	0611T	1(3)	11047	10(3)	11719	1(2)	13101	1(2)	15576	2(3)	15877	1(2)
0478T	1(3)	0545T	1(2)	0612T	1(2)	11055	1(2)	11720	1(2)	13102	9(3)	15600	2(3)	15878	1(2)
0479T	1(2)	0546T	2(2)	0613T	1(2)	11056	1(2)	11721	1(2)	13120	1(2)	15610	2(3)	15879	1(2)
0480T	4(1)	0547T	1(2)	0614T	1(3)	11057	1(2)	11730	1(2)	13121	1(2)	15620	2(3)	15920	1(3)
0481T	1(3)	0548T	1(2)	0615T	1(3)	11102	1(2)	11732	4(3)	13122	9(3)	15630	2(3)	15922	1(3)
0483T	1(2)	0549T	1(2)	0616T	2(2)	11103	6(3)	11740	2(3)	13131	1(2)	15650	1(3)	15931	1(3)
0484T	1(2)	0550T	2(3)	0617T	2(2)	11104	1(2)	11750	6(3)	13132	1(2)	15730	1(3)	15933	1(3)
0485T	1(2)	0551T	1(2)	0618T	2(2)	11105	3(3)	11755	2(3)	13133	7(3)	15731	1(3)	15934	1(3)
0486T	1(2)	0552T	1(3)	0619T	1(2)	11106	1(2)	11760	4(3)	13151	1(2)	15733	2(3)	15935	1(3)
0487T	1(3)	0553T	2(2)	0620T	2(2)	11107	2(3)	11762	2(3)	13152	1(2)	15734	4(3)	15936	1(3)
0488T	1(2)	0554T	1(2)	0621T	2(2)	11200	1(2)	11765	4(3)	13153	2(3)	15736	2(3)	15937	1(3)
0489T	1(2)	0555T	1(2)	0622T	2(2)	11201	1(3)	11770	1(3)	13160	2(3)	15738	3(3)	15940	2(3)
0490T	1(2)	0556T	1(2)	0623T	1(2)	11300	5(3)	11771	1(3)	14000	2(3)	15740	2(3)	15941	2(3)
0491T	1(2)	0557T	1(2)	0624T	1(2)	11301	6(3)	11772	1(3)	14001	2(3)	15750	2(3)	15944	2(3)
0492T	4(3)	0558T	1(2)	0625T	1(2)	11302	4(3)	11900	1(2)	14020	2(3)	15756	2(3)	15945	2(3)
0493T	1(3)	0559T	1(2)	0626T	1(2)	11303	3(3)	11901	1(2)	14021	2(3)	15757	2(3)	15946	2(3)
0494T	1(2)	0560T	1(3)	0627T	1(2)	11305	4(3)	11920	1(2)	14040	2(3)	15758	2(3)	15950	2(3)
0495T	1(2)	0561T	1(2)	0628T	4(2)	11306	4(3)	11921	1(2)	14041	3(3)	15760	2(3)	15951	2(3)

CPT	MUE	CPT	MUE	CPT	MUE	CPT	MUE	CPT	MUE	CPT	MUE	CPT	MUE	CPT	MUE
15952	2(3)	19282	2(3)	20604	4(3)	20985	2(3)	21179	1(2)	21386	1(2)	21820	1(2)	22630	1(2)
15953	2(3)	19283	1(2)	20605	2(3)	20999	1(3)	21180	1(2)	21387	1(2)	21825	1(2)	22632	4(2)
15956	2(3)	19284	2(3)	20606	2(3)	21010	1(2)	21181	1(3)	21390	1(2)	21899	1(3)	22633	1(2)
15958	2(3)	19285	1(2)	20610	2(3)	21011	4(3)	21182	1(2)	21395	1(2)	21920	2(3)	22634	4(2)
15999	1(3)	19286	2(3)	20611	2(3)	21012	3(3)	21183	1(2)	21400	1(2)	21925	2(3)	22800	1(2)
16000	1(2)	19287	1(2)	20612	2(3)	21013	2(3)	21184	1(2)	21401	1(2)	21930	5(3)	22802	1(2)
16020	1(2)	19288	2(3)	20615	1(3)	21014	2(3)	21188	1(2)	21406	1(2)	21931	3(3)	22804	1(2)
16025	1(3)	19294	2(3)	20650	4(3)	21015	1(3)	21193	1(2)	21407	1(2)	21932	2(3)	22808	1(2)
16030	1(3)	19296	1(3)	20660	1(2)	21016	2(3)	21194	1(2)	21408	1(2)	21933	2(3)	22810	1(2)
16035	1(2)	19297	2(3)	20661	1(2)	21025	2(3)	21195	1(2)	21421	1(2)	21935	1(3)	22812	1(2)
16036	8(3)	19298	1(2)	20662	1(2)	21026	2(3)	21196	1(2)	21422	1(2)	21936	1(3)	22818	1(2)
17000	1(2)	19300	1(2)	20663	1(2)	21029	1(3)	21198	1(3)	21423	1(2)	22010	2(3)	22819	1(2)
17003	13(2)	19301	1(3)	20664	1(2)	21030	1(3)	21199	1(2)	21431	1(2)	22015	2(3)	22830	1(2)
17004	1(2)	19302	1(2)	20665	1(2)	21031	2(3)	21206	1(3)	21432	1(2)	22100	1(2)	22840	1(3)
17106	1(2)	19303	1(2)	20670	3(3)	21032	1(3)	21208	1(3)	21433	1(2)	22101	1(2)	22841	1(2)
17107	1(2)	19305	1(2)	20680	3(3)	21034	1(3)	21209	1(3)	21435	1(2)	22102	1(2)	22842	1(3)
17108	1(2)	19306	1(2)	20690	2(3)	21040	2(3)	21210	2(3)	21436	1(2)	22103	3(3)	22843	1(3)
17110	1(2)	19307	1(2)	20692	2(3)	21044	1(3)	21215	2(3)	21440	2(3)	22110	1(2)	22844	1(3)
17111	1(2)	19316	1(2)	20693	2(3)	21045	1(3)	21230	2(3)	21445	2(3)	22112	1(2)	22845	1(3)
17250	4(3)	19318	1(2)	20694	2(3)	21046	2(3)	21235	2(3)	21450	1(2)	22114	1(2)	22846	1(3)
17260	7(3)	19325	1(2)	20696	2(3)	21047	2(3)	21240	1(2)	21451	1(2)	22116	3(3)	22847	1(3)
17261	7(3)	19328	1(2)	20697	4(3)	21048	2(3)	21242	1(2)	21452	1(2)	22206	1(2)	22848	1(2)
17262	6(3)	19330	1(2)	20700	1(3)	21049	1(3)	21243	1(2)	21453	1(2)	22207	1(2)	22849	1(2)
17263	3(3)	19340	1(2)	20701	1(3)	21050	1(2)	21244	1(2)	21454	1(2)	22208	5(3)	22850	1(2)
17264	3(3)	19342	1(2)	20702	1(3)	21060	1(2)	21245	2(3)	21461	1(2)	22210	1(2)	22852	1(2)
17266	2(3)	19350	1(2)	20703	1(3)	21070	1(2)	21246	1(3)	21462	1(2)	22212	1(2)	22853	4(3)
17270	6(3)	19355	1(2)	20704	1(3)	21073	1(2)	21247	1(2)	21465	1(2)	22214	1(2)	22854	4(3)
17271	4(3)	19357	1(2)	20705	1(3)	21076	1(2)	21248	2(3)	21470	1(2)	22216	6(3)	22855	1(2)
17272	5(3)	19361	1(2)	20802	1(2)	21077	1(2)	21249	2(3)	21480	1(2)	22220	1(2)	22856	1(2)
17273	4(3)	19364	1(3)	20805	1(2)	21079	1(2)	21255	1(2)	21485	1(2)	22222	1(2)	22857	1(2)
17274	2(3)	19367	1(2)	20808	1(2)	21080	1(2)	21256	1(2)	21490	1(2)	22224	1(2)	22858	1(2)
17276	2(3)	19368	1(2)	20816	3(3)	21081	1(2)	21260	1(2)	21497	1(2)	22226	4(3)	22859	4(3)
17280	6(3)	19369	1(2)	20822	3(3)	21082	1(2)	21261	1(2)	21499	1(3)	22310	1(2)	22861	1(2)
17281	5(3)	19370	1(2)	20824	1(2)	21083	1(2)	21263	1(2)	21501	3(3)	22315	1(2)	22862	1(2)
17282	4(3)	19371	1(2)	20827	1(2)	21084	1(2)	21267	1(2)	21502	1(3)	22318	1(2)	22864	1(2)
17283	4(3)	19380	1(2)	20838	1(2)	21085	1(3)	21268	1(2)	21510	1(3)	22319	1(2)	22865	1(2)
17284	2(3)	19396	1(2)	20900	2(3)	21086	1(2)	21270	1(2)	21550	2(3)	22325	1(2)	22867	1(2)
17286	2(3)	19499	1(3)	20902	2(3)	21087	1(2)	21275	1(2)	21552	2(3)	22326	1(2)	22868	1(2)
17311	4(3)	20100	2(3)	20910	1(3)	21088	1(2)	21280	1(2)	21554	2(3)	22327	1(2)	22869	1(2)
17312	6(3)	20101	2(3)	20912	1(3)	21089	1(3)	21282	1(2)	21555	2(3)	22328	6(3)	22870	1(2)
17313	3(3)	20102	3(3)	20920	1(3)	21100	1(2)	21295	1(2)	21556	2(3)	22505	1(2)	22899	1(3)
17314	4(3)	20103	3(3)	20922	1(3)	21110	2(3)	21296	1(2)	21557	1(3)	22510	1(2)	22900	3(3)
17315	15(3)	20150	2(3)	20924	2(3)	21116	1(2)	21299	1(3)	21558	1(3)	22511	1(2)	22901	2(3)
17340	1(2)	20200	2(3)	20930	0(3)	21120	1(2)	21310	1(2)	21600	5(3)	22512	3(3)	22902	4(3)
17360	1(2)	20205	3(3)	20931	1(2)	21121	1(2)	21315	1(2)	21601	2(3)	22513	1(2)	22903	3(3)
17380	1(3)	20206	3(3)	20932	1(3)	21122	1(2)	21320	1(2)	21602	1(3)	22514	1(2)	22904	1(3)
17999	1(3)	20220	3(3)	20933	1(3)	21123	1(2)	21325	1(2)	21603	1(3)	22515	4(3)	22905	1(3)
19000	2(3)	20225	2(3)	20934	1(3)	21125	2(2)	21330	1(2)	21610	1(3)	22526	0(3)	22999	1(3)
19001	5(3)	20240	4(3)	20936	0(3)	21127	2(3)	21335	1(2)	21615	1(2)	22527	0(3)	23000	1(2)
19020	2(3)	20245	3(3)	20937	1(2)	21137	1(2)	21336	1(2)	21616	1(2)	22532	1(2)	23020	1(2)
19030	1(2)	20250	1(3)	20938	1(2)	21138	1(2)	21337	1(2)	21620	1(2)	22533	1(2)	23030	2(3)
19081	1(2)	20251	2(3)	20939	1(3)	21139	1(2)	21338	1(2)	21627	1(2)	22534	3(3)	23031	1(3)
19082	2(3)	20500	2(3)	20950	2(3)	21141	1(2)	21339	1(2)	21630	1(2)	22548	1(2)	23035	1(3)
19083	1(2)	20501	2(3)	20955	1(3)	21142	1(2)	21340	1(2)	21632	1(2)	22551	1(2)	23040	1(2)
19084	2(3)	20520	2(3)	20956	1(3)	21143	1(2)	21343	1(2)	21685	1(2)	22552	5(3)	23044	1(3)
19085	2(3)	20525	4(3)	20957	1(3)	21145	1(2)	21344	1(2)	21700	1(2)	22554	1(2)	23065	2(3)
19086	2(3)	20526	1(2)	20962	1(3)	21146	1(2)	21345	1(2)	21705	1(2)	22556	1(2)	23066	2(3)
19100	4(3)	20527	2(3)	20969	2(3)	21147	1(2)	21346	1(2)	21720	1(3)	22558	1(2)	23071	2(3)
19101	3(3)	20550	5(3)	20970	1(3)	21150	1(2)	21347	1(2)	21725	1(3)	22585	5(3)	23073	2(3)
19105	2(3)	20551	5(3)	20972	2(3)	21151	1(2)	21348	1(2)	21740	1(2)	22586	1(2)	23075	2(3)
19110	1(3)	20552	1(2)	20973	1(2)	21154	1(2)	21355	1(2)	21742	1(2)	22590	1(2)	23076	2(3)
19112	2(3)	20553	1(2)	20974	1(3)	21155	1(2)	21356	1(2)	21743	1(2)	22595	1(2)	23077	1(3)
19120	1(2)	20555	1(3)	20975	1(3)	21159	1(2)	21360	1(2)	21750	1(2)	22600	1(2)	23078	1(3)
19125	1(2)	20560	1(2)	20979	1(3)	21160	1(2)	21365	1(2)	21811	1(2)	22610	1(2)	23100	1(2)
19126	3(3)	20561	1(2)	20982	1(2)	21172	1(3)	21366	1(2)	21812	1(2)	22612	1(2)	23101	1(3)
19281	1(2)	20600	6(3)	20983	1(2)	21175	1(2)	21385	1(2)	21813	1(2)	22614	13(3)	23105	1(2)

CPT	MUE	CPT	MUE	CPT	MUE	CPT	MUE	CPT	MUE	CPT	MUE	CPT	MUE	CPT	MUE
23106	1(2)	23600	1(2)	24331	1(3)	24931	1(2)	25310	5(3)	25650	1(2)	26205	1(3)	26525	4(3)
23107	1(2)	23605	1(2)	24332	1(2)	24935	1(2)	25312	4(3)	25651	1(2)	26210	2(3)	26530	4(3)
23120	1(2)	23615	1(2)	24340	1(2)	24940	1(2)	25315	1(3)	25652	1(2)	26215	2(3)	26531	4(3)
23125	1(2)	23616	1(2)	24341	2(3)	24999	1(3)	25316	1(3)	25660	1(2)	26230	2(3)	26535	3(3)
23130	1(2)	23620	1(2)	24342	2(3)	25000	2(3)	25320	1(2)	25670	1(2)	26235	2(3)	26536	4(3)
23140	1(3)	23625	1(2)	24343	1(2)	25001	1(3)	25332	1(2)	25671	1(2)	26236	2(3)	26540	4(3)
23145	1(3)	23630	1(2)	24344	1(2)	25020	1(2)	25335	1(2)	25675	1(2)	26250	2(3)	26541	4(3)
23146	1(3)	23650	1(2)	24345	1(2)	25023	1(2)	25337	1(2)	25676	1(2)	26260	1(3)	26542	4(3)
23150	1(3)	23655	1(2)	24346	1(2)	25024	1(2)	25350	1(3)	25680	1(2)	26262	1(3)	26545	4(3)
23155	1(3)	23660	1(2)	24357	1(3)	25025	1(2)	25355	1(3)	25685	1(2)	26320	4(3)	26546	2(3)
23156	1(3)	23665	1(2)	24358	1(3)	25028	4(3)	25360	1(3)	25690	1(2)	26340	4(3)	26548	3(3)
23170	1(3)	23670	1(2)	24359	2(3)	25031	2(3)	25365	1(3)	25695	1(2)	26341	2(3)	26550	1(2)
23172	1(3)	23675	1(2)	24360	1(2)	25035	2(3)	25370	1(2)	25800	1(2)	26350	6(3)	26551	1(2)
23174	1(3)	23680	1(2)	24361	1(2)	25040	1(3)	25375	1(2)	25805	1(2)	26352	2(3)	26553	1(3)
23180	1(3)	23700	1(2)	24362	1(2)	25065	2(3)	25390	1(2)	25810	1(2)	26356	4(3)	26554	1(3)
23182	1(3)	23800	1(2)	24363	1(2)	25066	2(3)	25391	1(2)	25820	1(2)	26357	2(3)	26555	2(3)
23184	1(3)	23802	1(2)	24365	1(2)	25071	3(3)	25392	1(2)	25825	1(2)	26358	2(3)	26556	2(3)
23190	1(3)	23900	1(2)	24366	1(2)	25073	2(3)	25393	1(2)	25830	1(2)	26370	3(3)	26560	2(3)
23195	1(2)	23920	1(2)	24370	1(2)	25075	6(3)	25394	1(3)	25900	1(2)	26372	1(3)	26561	2(3)
23200	1(3)	23921	1(2)	24371	1(2)	25076	3(3)	25400	1(2)	25905	1(2)	26373	2(3)	26562	2(3)
23210	1(3)	23929	1(3)	24400	1(3)	25077	1(3)	25405	1(2)	25907	1(2)	26390	2(3)	26565	2(3)
23220	1(3)	23930	2(3)	24410	1(2)	25078	1(3)	25415	1(2)	25909	1(2)	26392	2(3)	26567	3(3)
23330	2(3)	23931	2(3)	24420	1(2)	25085	1(2)	25420	1(2)	25915	1(2)	26410	4(3)	26568	2(3)
23333	1(3)	23935	2(3)	24430	1(3)	25100	1(2)	25425	1(2)	25920	1(2)	26412	3(3)	26580	1(2)
23334	1(2)	24000	1(2)	24435	1(3)	25101	1(2)	25426	1(2)	25922	1(2)	26415	2(3)	26587	2(3)
23335	1(2)	24006	1(2)	24470	1(2)	25105	1(2)	25430	1(3)	25924	1(2)	26416	2(3)	26590	2(3)
23350	1(2)	24065	2(3)	24495	1(2)	25107	1(2)	25431	1(3)	25927	1(2)	26418	4(3)	26591	4(3)
23395	1(2)	24066	2(3)	24498	1(2)	25109	4(3)	25440	1(2)	25929	1(2)	26420	3(3)	26593	8(3)
23397	1(3)	24071	2(3)	24500	1(2)	25110	2(3)	25441	1(2)	25931	1(2)	26426	4(3)	26596	1(3)
23400	1(2)	24073	2(3)	24505	1(2)	25111	1(3)	25442	1(2)	25999	1(3)	26428	2(3)	26600	2(3)
23405	2(3)	24075	5(3)	24515	1(2)	25112	1(3)	25443	1(2)	26010	2(3)	26432	2(3)	26605	3(3)
23406	1(3)	24076	4(3)	24516	1(2)	25115	1(3)	25444	1(2)	26011	3(3)	26433	2(3)	26607	2(3)
23410	1(2)	24077	1(3)	24530	1(2)	25116	1(3)	25445	1(2)	26020	4(3)	26434	2(3)	26608	4(3)
23412	1(2)	24079	1(3)	24535	1(2)	25118	5(3)	25446	1(2)	26025	1(2)	26437	4(3)	26615	3(3)
23415	1(2)	24100	1(2)	24538	1(2)	25119	1(2)	25447	4(3)	26030	1(2)	26440	6(3)	26641	1(2)
23420	1(2)	24101	1(2)	24545	1(2)	25120	1(3)	25449	1(2)	26034	2(3)	26442	5(3)	26645	1(2)
23430	1(2)	24102	1(2)	24546	1(2)	25125	1(3)	25450	1(2)	26035	1(3)	26445	5(3)	26650	1(2)
23440	1(2)	24105	1(2)	24560	1(3)	25126	1(3)	25455	1(2)	26037	1(3)	26449	5(3)	26665	1(2)
23450	1(2)	24110	1(3)	24565	1(3)	25130	1(3)	25490	1(2)	26040	1(2)	26450	6(3)	26670	2(3)
23455	1(2)	24115	1(3)	24566	1(3)	25135	1(3)	25491	1(2)	26045	1(2)	26455	6(3)	26675	1(3)
23460	1(2)	24116	1(3)	24575	1(3)	25136	1(3)	25492	1(2)	26055	5(3)	26460	4(3)	26676	2(3)
23462	1(2)	24120	1(3)	24576	1(3)	25145	1(3)	25500	1(2)	26060	5(3)	26471	4(3)	26685	3(3)
23465	1(2)	24125	1(3)	24577	1(3)	25150	1(3)	25505	1(2)	26070	2(3)	26474	4(3)	26686	3(3)
23466	1(2)	24126	1(3)	24579	1(3)	25151	1(3)	25515	1(2)	26075	3(3)	26476	4(3)	26700	1(2)
23470	1(2)	24130	1(2)	24582	1(3)	25170	1(3)	25520	1(2)	26080	3(3)	26477	2(3)	26705	3(3)
23472	1(2)	24134	1(3)	24586	1(3)	25210	2(3)	25525	1(2)	26100	1(3)	26478	6(3)	26706	2(3)
23473	1(2)	24136	1(3)	24587	1(2)	25215	1(2)	25526	1(2)	26105	2(3)	26479	4(3)	26715	3(3)
23474	1(2)	24138	1(3)	24600	1(2)	25230	1(2)	25530	1(2)	26110	2(3)	26480	4(3)	26720	4(3)
23480	1(2)	24140	1(3)	24605	1(2)	25240	1(2)	25535	1(2)	26111	4(3)	26483	4(3)	26725	3(3)
23485	1(2)	24145	1(3)	24615	1(2)	25246	1(2)	25545	1(2)	26113	3(3)	26485	4(3)	26727	3(3)
23490	1(2)	24147	1(2)	24620	1(2)	25248	3(3)	25560	1(2)	26115	4(3)	26489	2(3)	26735	4(3)
23491	1(2)	24149	1(2)	24635	1(2)	25250	1(2)	25565	1(2)	26116	2(3)	26490	3(3)	26740	3(3)
23500	1(2)	24150	1(3)	24640	1(2)	25251	1(2)	25574	1(2)	26117	2(3)	26492	2(3)	26742	3(3)
23505	1(2)	24152	1(3)	24650	1(2)	25259	1(2)	25575	1(2)	26118	1(3)	26494	1(3)	26746	3(3)
23515	1(2)	24155	1(2)	24655	1(2)	25260	9(3)	25600	1(2)	26121	1(2)	26496	1(3)	26750	3(3)
23520	1(2)	24160	1(2)	24665	1(2)	25263	4(3)	25605	1(2)	26123	1(2)	26497	2(3)	26755	2(3)
23525	1(2)	24164	1(2)	24666	1(2)	25265	4(3)	25606	1(2)	26125	4(3)	26498	1(3)	26756	2(3)
23530	1(2)	24200	3(3)	24670	1(2)	25270	8(3)	25607	1(2)	26130	1(3)	26499	2(3)	26765	3(3)
23532	1(2)	24201	3(3)	24675	1(2)	25272	4(3)	25608	1(2)	26135	4(3)	26500	3(3)	26770	3(3)
23540	1(2)	24220	1(2)	24685	1(2)	25274	4(3)	25609	1(2)	26140	2(3)	26502	2(3)	26775	2(3)
23545	1(2)	24300	1(2)	24800	1(2)	25275	2(3)	25622	1(2)	26145	6(3)	26508	1(2)	26776	4(3)
23550	1(2)	24301	2(3)	24802	1(2)	25280	9(3)	25624	1(2)	26160	4(3)	26510	4(3)	26785	3(3)
23552	1(2)	24305	4(3)	24900	1(2)	25290	10(3)	25628	1(2)	26170	4(3)	26516	1(2)	26820	1(2)
23570	1(2)	24310	2(3)	24920	1(2)	25295	9(3)	25630	1(3)	26180	4(3)	26517	1(2)	26841	1(2)
23575	1(2)	24320	2(3)	24925	1(2)	25300	1(2)	25635	1(3)	26185	1(3)	26518	1(2)	26842	1(2)
23585	1(2)	24330	1(3)	24930	1(2)	25301	1(2)	25645	1(3)	26200	2(3)	26520	4(3)	26843	2(3)

CPT	MUE	CPT	MUE	CPT	MUE	CPT	MUE	CPT	MUE	CPT	MUE	CPT	MUE	CPT	MUE
26844	2(3)	27132	1(2)	27301	3(3)	27440	1(2)	27596	1(2)	27724	1(2)	28010	4(3)	28238	1(2)
26850	5(3)	27134	1(2)	27303	2(3)	27441	1(2)	27598	1(2)	27725	1(2)	28011	4(3)	28240	1(2)
26852	2(3)	27137	1(2)	27305	1(2)	27442	1(2)	27599	1(3)	27726	1(2)	28020	2(3)	28250	1(2)
26860	1(2)	27138	1(2)	27306	1(2)	27443	1(2)	27600	1(2)	27727	1(2)	28022	3(3)	28260	1(2)
26861	4(3)	27140	1(2)	27307	1(2)	27445	1(2)	27601	1(2)	27730	1(2)	28024	4(3)	28261	1(3)
26862	1(2)	27146	1(3)	27310	1(2)	27446	1(2)	27602	1(2)	27732	1(2)	28035	1(2)	28262	1(2)
26863	2(3)	27147	1(3)	27323	2(3)	27447	1(2)	27603	2(3)	27734	1(2)	28039	2(3)	28264	1(2)
26910	4(3)	27151	1(3)	27324	3(3)	27448	1(3)	27604	2(3)	27740	1(2)	28041	2(3)	28270	6(3)
26951	8(3)	27156	1(2)	27325	1(2)	27450	1(3)	27605	1(2)	27742	1(2)	28043	4(3)	28272	6(3)
26952	4(3)	27158	1(2)	27326	1(2)	27454	1(2)	27606	1(2)	27745	1(2)	28045	4(3)	28280	1(2)
26989	1(3)	27161	1(2)	27327	5(3)	27455	1(3)	27607	2(3)	27750	1(2)	28046	1(3)	28285	4(3)
26990	2(3)	27165	1(2)	27328	3(3)	27457	1(3)	27610	1(2)	27752	1(2)	28047	1(3)	28286	1(2)
26991	1(3)	27170	1(2)	27329	1(3)	27465	1(2)	27612	1(2)	27756	1(2)	28050	2(3)	28288	4(3)
26992	2(3)	27175	1(2)	27330	1(2)	27466	1(2)	27613	3(3)	27758	1(2)	28052	2(3)	28289	1(2)
27000	1(3)	27176	1(2)	27331	1(2)	27468	1(2)	27614	3(3)	27759	1(2)	28054	2(3)	28291	1(2)
27001	1(3)	27177	1(2)	27332	1(2)	27470	1(2)	27615	1(3)	27760	1(2)	28055	1(3)	28292	1(2)
27003	1(3)	27178	1(2)	27333	1(2)	27472	1(2)	27616	1(3)	27762	1(2)	28060	1(2)	28295	1(2)
27005	1(2)	27179	1(2)	27334	1(2)	27475	1(2)	27618	3(3)	27766	1(2)	28062	1(2)	28296	1(2)
27006	1(2)	27181	1(2)	27335	1(2)	27477	1(2)	27619	2(3)	27767	1(2)	28070	2(3)	28297	1(2)
27025	1(3)	27185	1(2)	27337	3(3)	27479	1(2)	27620	1(2)	27768	1(2)	28072	4(3)	28298	1(2)
27027	1(2)	27187	1(2)	27339	4(3)	27485	1(2)	27625	1(2)	27769	1(2)	28080	3(3)	28299	1(2)
27030	1(2)	27197	1(2)	27340	1(2)	27486	1(2)	27626	1(2)	27780	1(2)	28086	2(3)	28300	1(3)
27033	1(2)	27198	1(2)	27345	1(2)	27487	1(2)	27630	2(3)	27781	1(2)	28088	2(3)	28302	1(2)
27035	1(2)	27200	1(2)	27347	1(2)	27488	1(2)	27632	3(3)	27784	1(2)	28090	2(3)	28304	1(3)
27036	1(2)	27202	1(2)	27350	1(2)	27495	1(2)	27634	2(3)	27786	1(2)	28092	2(3)	28305	1(3)
27040	2(3)	27215	0(3)	27355	1(3)	27496	1(2)	27635	1(3)	27788	1(2)	28100	1(3)	28306	1(2)
27041	3(3)	27216	0(3)	27356	1(3)	27497	1(2)	27637	1(3)	27792	1(2)	28102	1(3)	28307	1(2)
27043	2(3)	27217	0(3)	27357	1(3)	27498	1(2)	27638	1(3)	27808	1(2)	28103	1(3)	28308	4(3)
27045	3(3)	27218	0(3)	27358	1(3)	27499	1(2)	27640	1(3)	27810	1(2)	28104	2(3)	28309	1(2)
27047	2(3)	27220	1(2)	27360	2(3)	27500	1(2)	27641	1(3)	27814	1(2)	28106	1(3)	28310	1(2)
27048	2(3)	27222	1(2)	27364	1(3)	27501	1(2)	27645	1(3)	27816	1(2)	28107	1(3)	28312	4(3)
27049	1(3)	27226	1(2)	27365	1(3)	27502	1(2)	27646	1(3)	27818	1(2)	28108	2(3)	28313	4(3)
27050	1(2)	27227	1(2)	27369	1(2)	27503	1(2)	27647	1(3)	27822	1(2)	28110	1(2)	28315	1(2)
27052	1(2)	27228	1(2)	27372	2(3)	27506	1(2)	27648	1(2)	27823	1(2)	28111	1(2)	28320	1(2)
27054	1(2)	27230	1(2)	27380	1(2)	27507	1(2)	27650	1(2)	27824	1(2)	28112	4(3)	28322	2(3)
27057	1(2)	27232	1(2)	27381	1(2)	27508	1(2)	27652	1(2)	27825	1(2)	28113	1(2)	28340	2(3)
27059	1(2)	27235	1(2)	27385	2(3)	27509	1(2)	27654	1(2)	27826	1(2)	28114	1(2)	28341	2(3)
27060	1(2)	27236	1(2)	27386	2(3)	27510	1(2)	27656	1(3)	27827	1(2)	28116	1(2)	28344	1(2)
27062	1(2)	27238	1(2)	27390	1(2)	27511	1(2)	27658	2(3)	27828	1(2)	28118	1(2)	28345	2(3)
27065	1(3)	27240	1(2)	27391	1(2)	27513	1(2)	27659	2(3)	27829	1(2)	28119	1(2)	28360	1(2)
27066	1(3)	27244	1(2)	27392	1(2)	27514	1(2)	27664	2(3)	27830	1(2)	28120	2(3)	28400	1(2)
27067	1(3)	27245	1(2)	27393	1(2)	27516	1(2)	27665	2(3)	27831	1(2)	28122	4(3)	28405	1(2)
27070	1(3)	27246	1(2)	27394	1(2)	27517	1(2)	27675	1(2)	27832	1(2)	28124	4(3)	28406	1(2)
27071	1(3)	27248	1(2)	27395	1(3)	27519	1(2)	27676	1(2)	27840	1(2)	28126	4(3)	28415	1(2)
27075	1(3)	27250	1(2)	27396	1(2)	27520	1(2)	27680	2(3)	27842	1(2)	28130	1(2)	28420	1(2)
27076	1(2)	27252	1(2)	27397	1(2)	27524	1(2)	27681	1(2)	27846	1(2)	28140	3(3)	28430	1(2)
27077	1(2)	27253	1(2)	27400	1(2)	27530	1(2)	27685	2(3)	27848	1(2)	28150	4(3)	28435	1(2)
27078	1(2)	27254	1(2)	27403	1(3)	27532	1(2)	27686	3(3)	27860	1(2)	28153	4(3)	28436	1(2)
27080	1(2)	27256	1(2)	27405	1(3)	27535	1(2)	27687	1(2)	27870	1(2)	28160	5(3)	28445	1(2)
27086	1(3)	27257	1(2)	27407	1(3)	27536	1(2)	27690	2(3)	27871	1(3)	28171	1(3)	28446	1(2)
27087	1(3)	27258	1(2)	27409	1(2)	27538	1(2)	27691	2(3)	27880	1(2)	28173	2(3)	28450	2(3)
27090	1(2)	27259	1(2)	27412	1(2)	27540	1(2)	27692	4(3)	27881	1(2)	28175	2(3)	28455	3(3)
27091	1(2)	27265	1(2)	27415	1(2)	27550	1(2)	27695	1(2)	27882	1(2)	28190	3(3)	28456	2(3)
27093	1(2)	27266	1(2)	27416	1(2)	27552	1(2)	27696	1(2)	27884	1(2)	28192	2(3)	28465	3(3)
27095	1(2)	27267	1(2)	27418	1(2)	27556	1(2)	27698	2(3)	27886	1(2)	28193	2(3)	28470	2(3)
27096	1(2)	27268	1(2)	27420	1(2)	27557	1(2)	27700	1(2)	27888	1(2)	28200	4(3)	28475	5(3)
27097	1(3)	27269	1(2)	27422	1(2)	27558	1(2)	27702	1(2)	27889	1(2)	28202	2(3)	28476	4(3)
27098	1(2)	27275	2(2)	27424	1(2)	27560	1(2)	27703	1(2)	27892	1(2)	28208	4(3)	28485	5(3)
27100	1(2)	27279	1(2)	27425	1(2)	27562	1(2)	27704	1(2)	27893	1(2)	28210	2(3)	28490	1(2)
27105	1(3)	27280	1(2)	27427	1(2)	27566	1(2)	27705	1(3)	27894	1(2)	28220	1(2)	28495	1(2)
27110	1(2)	27282	1(2)	27428	1(2)	27570	1(2)	27707	1(3)	27899	1(3)	28222	1(2)	28496	1(2)
27111	1(2)	27284	1(2)	27429	1(2)	27580	1(2)	27709	1(3)	28001	2(3)	28225	1(2)	28505	1(2)
27120	1(2)	27286	1(2)	27430	1(2)	27590	1(2)	27712	1(2)	28002	3(3)	28226	1(2)	28510	4(3)
27122	1(2)	27290	1(2)	27435	1(2)	27591	1(2)	27715	1(2)	28003	2(3)	28230	1(2)	28515	4(3)
27125	1(2)	27295	1(2)	27437	1(2)	27592	1(2)	27720	1(2)	28005	3(3)	28232	6(3)	28525	4(3)
27130	1(2)	27299	1(3)	27438	1(2)	27594	1(2)	27722	1(2)	28008	2(3)	28234	6(3)	28530	1(2)

CPT	MUE	CPT	MUE	CPT	MUE	CPT	MUE	CPT	MUE	CPT	MUE	CPT	MUE	CPT	MUE
28531	1(2)	29365	1(3)	29874	1(2)	30545	1(2)	31300	1(2)	31614	1(2)	32160	1(3)	32800	1(3)
28540	1(3)	29405	1(3)	29875	1(2)	30560	1(2)	31360	1(2)	31615	1(3)	32200	2(3)	32810	1(3)
28545	1(3)	29425	1(3)	29876	1(2)	30580	2(3)	31365	1(2)	31622	1(3)	32215	1(2)	32815	1(3)
28546	1(3)	29435	1(3)	29877	1(2)	30600	1(3)	31367	1(2)	31623	1(3)	32220	1(2)	32820	1(3)
28555	1(3)	29440	1(2)	29879	1(2)	30620	1(2)	31368	1(2)	31624	1(3)	32225	1(2)	32850	1(2)
28570	1(2)	29445	1(3)	29880	1(2)	30630	1(2)	31370	1(2)	31625	1(2)	32310	1(3)	32851	1(2)
28575	1(2)	29450	1(3)	29881	1(2)	30801	1(2)	31375	1(2)	31626	1(2)	32320	1(3)	32852	1(2)
28576	1(2)	29505	1(2)	29882	1(2)	30802	1(2)	31380	1(2)	31627	1(3)	32400	2(3)	32853	1(2)
28585	1(3)	29515	1(2)	29883	1(2)	30901	1(3)	31382	1(2)	31628	1(2)	32408	2(3)	32854	1(2)
28600	2(3)	29520	1(2)	29884	1(2)	30903	1(3)	31390	1(2)	31629	1(2)	32440	1(2)	32855	1(2)
28605	2(3)	29530	1(2)	29885	1(2)	30905	1(3)	31395	1(2)	31630	1(3)	32442	1(2)	32856	1(2)
28606	3(3)	29540	1(2)	29886	1(2)	30906	1(3)	31400	1(3)	31631	1(2)	32445	1(2)	32900	1(2)
28615	5(3)	29550	1(2)	29887	1(2)	30915	1(3)	31420	1(2)	31632	2(3)	32480	1(2)	32905	1(2)
28630	2(3)	29580	1(2)	29888	1(2)	30920	1(3)	31500	2(3)	31633	2(3)	32482	1(2)	32906	1(2)
28635	2(3)	29581	1(2)	29889	1(2)	30930	1(2)	31502	1(3)	31634	1(3)	32484	2(3)	32940	1(3)
28636	4(3)	29584	1(2)	29891	1(2)	30999	1(3)	31505	1(3)	31635	1(3)	32486	1(3)	32960	1(2)
28645	4(3)	29700	2(3)	29892	1(2)	31000	1(2)	31510	1(2)	31636	1(2)	32488	1(2)	32994	1(2)
28660	4(3)	29705	1(3)	29893	1(2)	31002	1(2)	31511	1(3)	31637	2(3)	32491	1(2)	32997	1(2)
28665	3(3)	29710	1(2)	29894	1(2)	31020	1(2)	31512	1(3)	31638	1(3)	32501	1(3)	32998	1(2)
28666	4(3)	29720	1(2)	29895	1(2)	31030	1(2)	31513	1(3)	31640	1(3)	32503	1(2)	32999	1(3)
28675	3(3)	29730	1(3)	29897	1(2)	31032	1(2)	31515	1(3)	31641	1(3)	32504	1(2)	33016	1(3)
28705	1(2)	29740	1(3)	29898	1(2)	31040	1(2)	31520	1(3)	31643	1(2)	32505	1(2)	33017	1(3)
28715	1(2)	29750	1(3)	29899	1(2)	31050	1(2)	31525	1(3)	31645	1(2)	32506	3(3)	33018	1(3)
28725	1(2)	29799	1(3)	29900	2(3)	31051	1(2)	31526	1(3)	31646	2(3)	32507	2(3)	33019	1(3)
28730	1(2)	29800	1(2)	29901	2(3)	31070	1(2)	31527	1(2)	31647	1(2)	32540	1(3)	33020	1(3)
28735	1(2)	29804	1(2)	29902	2(3)	31075	1(2)	31528	1(2)	31648	1(2)	32550	2(3)	33025	1(2)
28737	1(2)	29805	1(2)	29904	1(2)	31080	1(2)	31529	1(3)	31649	2(3)	32551	2(3)	33030	1(2)
28740	1(2)	29806	1(2)	29905	1(2)	31081	1(2)	31530	1(3)	31651	3(3)	32552	2(2)	33031	1(2)
28750	1(2)	29807	1(2)	29906	1(2)	31084	1(2)	31531	1(3)	31652	1(2)	32553	1(2)	33050	1(2)
28755	1(2)	29819	1(2)	29907	1(2)	31085	1(2)	31535	1(3)	31653	1(2)	32554	2(3)	33120	1(3)
28760	1(2)	29820	1(2)	29914	1(2)	31086	1(2)	31536	1(3)	31654	1(3)	32555	2(3)	33130	1(3)
28800	1(2)	29821	1(2)	29915	1(2)	31087	1(2)	31540	1(3)	31660	1(2)	32556	2(3)	33140	1(2)
28805	1(2)	29822	1(2)	29916	1(2)	31090	1(2)	31541	1(3)	31661	1(2)	32557	2(3)	33141	1(2)
28810	5(3)	29823	1(2)	29999	1(3)	31200	1(2)	31545	1(2)	31717	1(3)	32560	1(3)	33202	1(2)
28820	6(3)	29824	1(2)	30000	1(3)	31201	1(2)	31546	1(2)	31720	1(3)	32561	1(2)	33203	1(2)
28825	8(3)	29825	1(2)	30020	1(3)	31205	1(2)	31551	1(2)	31725	1(3)	32562	1(2)	33206	1(3)
28890	1(2)	29826	1(2)	30100	2(3)	31225	1(2)	31552	1(2)	31730	1(3)	32601	1(3)	33207	1(3)
28899	1(3)	29827	1(3)	30110	1(2)	31230	1(2)	31553	1(2)	31750	1(2)	32604	1(3)	33208	1(3)
29000	1(3)	29828	1(2)	30115	1(2)	31231	1(2)	31554	1(2)	31755	1(2)	32606	1(3)	33210	1(3)
29010	1(3)	29830	1(2)	30117	2(3)	31233	1(2)	31560	1(2)	31760	1(2)	32607	1(3)	33211	1(3)
29015	1(3)	29834	1(2)	30118	1(3)	31235	1(2)	31561	1(2)	31766	1(2)	32608	1(3)	33212	1(3)
29035	1(3)	29835	1(2)	30120	1(2)	31237	1(2)	31570	1(2)	31770	2(3)	32609	1(3)	33213	1(3)
29040	1(3)	29836	1(2)	30124	2(3)	31238	1(3)	31571	1(2)	31775	1(3)	32650	1(2)	33214	1(3)
29044	1(3)	29837	1(2)	30125	1(3)	31239	1(2)	31572	1(2)	31780	1(2)	32651	1(2)	33215	2(3)
29046	1(3)	29838	1(2)	30130	1(2)	31240	1(2)	31573	1(2)	31781	1(2)	32652	1(2)	33216	1(3)
29049	1(3)	29840	1(2)	30140	1(2)	31241	1(2)	31574	1(2)	31785	1(3)	32653	1(3)	33217	1(3)
29055	1(3)	29843	1(2)	30150	1(2)	31253	1(2)	31575	1(3)	31786	1(3)	32654	1(3)	33218	1(3)
29058	1(3)	29844	1(2)	30160	1(2)	31254	1(2)	31576	1(3)	31800	1(3)	32655	1(3)	33220	1(3)
29065	1(3)	29845	1(2)	30200	1(2)	31255	1(2)	31577	1(3)	31805	1(3)	32656	1(2)	33221	1(3)
29075	1(3)	29846	1(2)	30210	1(3)	31256	1(2)	31578	1(3)	31820	1(2)	32658	1(3)	33222	1(3)
29085	1(3)	29847	1(2)	30220	1(2)	31257	1(2)	31579	1(2)	31825	1(2)	32659	1(2)	33223	1(3)
29086	2(3)	29848	1(2)	30300	1(3)	31259	1(2)	31580	1(2)	31830	1(2)	32661	1(3)	33224	1(3)
29105	1(2)	29850	1(2)	30310	1(3)	31267	1(2)	31584	1(2)	31899	1(3)	32662	1(3)	33225	1(3)
29125	1(2)	29851	1(2)	30320	1(3)	31276	1(2)	31587	1(2)	32035	1(2)	32663	1(3)	33226	1(3)
29126	1(2)	29855	1(2)	30400	1(2)	31287	1(2)	31590	1(2)	32036	1(3)	32664	1(2)	33227	1(3)
29130	3(3)	29856	1(2)	30410	1(2)	31288	1(2)	31591	1(2)	32096	1(3)	32665	1(3)	33228	1(3)
29131	2(3)	29860	1(2)	30420	1(2)	31290	1(2)	31592	1(2)	32097	1(3)	32666	1(3)	33229	1(3)
29200	1(2)	29861	1(2)	30430	1(2)	31291	1(2)	31599	1(3)	32098	1(2)	32667	3(3)	33230	1(3)
29240	1(2)	29862	1(2)	30435	1(2)	31292	1(2)	31600	1(2)	32100	1(3)	32668	2(3)	33231	1(3)
29260	1(3)	29863	1(2)	30450	1(2)	31293	1(2)	31601	1(2)	32110	1(3)	32669	2(3)	33233	1(2)
29280	2(3)	29866	1(2)	30460	1(2)	31294	1(2)	31603	1(2)	32120	1(3)	32670	1(2)	33234	1(2)
29305	1(3)	29867	1(2)	30462	1(2)	31295	1(2)	31605	1(2)	32124	1(3)	32671	1(2)	33235	1(2)
29325	1(3)	29868	1(3)	30465	1(2)	31296	1(2)	31610	1(2)	32140	1(3)	32672	1(3)	33236	1(2)
29345	1(3)	29870	1(2)	30468	1(2)	31297	1(2)	31611	1(2)	32141	1(3)	32673	1(2)	33237	1(2)
29355	1(3)	29871	1(2)	30520	1(2)	31298	1(2)	31612	1(3)	32150	1(3)	32674	1(2)	33238	1(2)
29358	1(3)	29873	1(2)	30540	1(2)	31299	1(3)	31613	1(2)	32151	1(3)	32701	1(2)	33240	1(3)

CPT	MUE	CPT	MUE	CPT	MUE	CPT	MUE	CPT	MUE	CPT	MUE	CPT	MUE	CPT	MUE
33241	1(2)	33430	1(2)	33677	1(2)	33883	1(2)	33993	1(3)	35082	1(2)	35515	1(3)	35701	1(2)
33243	1(2)	33440	1(2)	33681	1(2)	33884	2(3)	33995	1(3)	35091	1(2)	35516	1(3)	35702	2(2)
33244	1(2)	33460	1(2)	33684	1(2)	33886	1(2)	33997	1(3)	35092	1(2)	35518	1(3)	35703	2(2)
33249	1(3)	33463	1(2)	33688	1(2)	33889	1(2)	33999	1(3)	35102	1(2)	35521	1(3)	35800	2(3)
33250	1(2)	33464	1(2)	33690	1(2)	33891	1(2)	34001	1(3)	35103	1(2)	35522	1(3)	35820	2(3)
33251	1(2)	33465	1(2)	33692	1(2)	33910	1(3)	34051	1(3)	35111	1(2)	35523	1(3)	35840	2(3)
33254	1(2)	33468	1(2)	33694	1(2)	33915	1(3)	34101	1(3)	35112	1(2)	35525	1(3)	35860	2(3)
33255	1(2)	33470	1(2)	33697	1(2)	33916	1(3)	34111	2(3)	35121	1(3)	35526	1(3)	35870	1(3)
33256	1(2)	33471	1(2)	33702	1(2)	33917	1(2)	34151	1(3)	35122	1(3)	35531	1(3)	35875	2(3)
33257	1(2)	33474	1(2)	33710	1(2)	33920	1(2)	34201	1(3)	35131	1(2)	35533	1(3)	35876	2(3)
33258	1(2)	33475	1(2)	33720	1(2)	33922	1(2)	34203	1(2)	35132	1(3)	35535	1(3)	35879	2(3)
33259	1(2)	33476	1(2)	33722	1(3)	33924	1(2)	34401	1(3)	35141	1(2)	35536	1(3)	35881	1(3)
33261	1(2)	33477	1(2)	33724	1(2)	33925	1(2)	34421	1(3)	35142	1(2)	35537	1(3)	35883	1(3)
33262	1(3)	33478	1(2)	33726	1(2)	33926	1(2)	34451	1(3)	35151	1(2)	35538	1(3)	35884	1(3)
33263	1(3)	33496	1(3)	33730	1(2)	33927	1(3)	34471	1(2)	35152	1(2)	35539	1(3)	35901	1(3)
33264	1(3)	33500	1(3)	33732	1(2)	33928	1(3)	34490	1(2)	35180	2(3)	35540	1(3)	35903	2(3)
33265	1(2)	33501	1(3)	33735	1(2)	33929	1(3)	34501	1(2)	35182	2(3)	35556	1(3)	35905	1(3)
33266	1(2)	33502	1(3)	33736	1(2)	33930	1(2)	34502	1(2)	35184	2(3)	35558	1(3)	35907	1(3)
33270	1(3)	33503	1(3)	33737	1(2)	33933	1(2)	34510	2(3)	35188	2(3)	35560	1(3)	36000	4(3)
33271	1(3)	33504	1(3)	33741	1(3)	33935	1(2)	34520	1(3)	35189	1(3)	35563	1(3)	36002	2(3)
33272	1(3)	33505	1(3)	33745	2(2)	33940	1(2)	34530	1(2)	35190	2(3)	35565	1(3)	36005	2(3)
33273	1(3)	33506	1(3)	33746	1(3)	33944	1(2)	34701	1(2)	35201	2(3)	35566	1(3)	36010	2(3)
33274	1(3)	33507	1(3)	33750	1(3)	33945	1(2)	34702	1(2)	35206	2(3)	35570	1(3)	36011	4(3)
33275	1(3)	33508	1(2)	33755	1(2)	33946	1(2)	34703	1(2)	35207	3(3)	35571	1(3)	36012	4(3)
33285	1(3)	33510	1(2)	33762	1(2)	33947	1(2)	34704	1(2)	35211	3(3)	35572	2(3)	36013	2(3)
33286	1(2)	33511	1(2)	33764	1(3)	33948	1(2)	34705	1(2)	35216	2(3)	35583	1(2)	36014	2(3)
33289	1(3)	33512	1(2)	33766	1(2)	33949	1(2)	34706	1(2)	35221	3(3)	35585	2(3)	36015	4(3)
33300	1(3)	33513	1(2)	33767	1(2)	33951	1(3)	34707	1(2)	35226	3(3)	35587	1(3)	36100	2(3)
33305	1(3)	33514	1(2)	33768	1(2)	33952	1(3)	34708	1(2)	35231	2(3)	35600	2(3)	36140	3(3)
33310	1(2)	33516	1(2)	33770	1(2)	33953	1(3)	34709	3(3)	35236	2(3)	35601	1(3)	36160	2(3)
33315	1(2)	33517	1(2)	33771	1(2)	33954	1(3)	34710	1(2)	35241	2(3)	35606	1(3)	36200	2(3)
33320	1(3)	33518	1(2)	33774	1(2)	33955	1(3)	34711	2(3)	35246	2(3)	35612	1(3)	36215	6(3)
33321	1(3)	33519	1(2)	33775	1(2)	33956	1(3)	34712	1(2)	35251	2(3)	35616	1(3)	36216	4(3)
33322	1(3)	33521	1(2)	33776	1(2)	33957	1(3)	34713	1(2)	35256	2(3)	35621	1(3)	36217	2(3)
33330	1(3)	33522	1(2)	33777	1(2)	33958	1(3)	34714	1(2)	35261	1(3)	35623	1(3)	36218	6(3)
33335	1(3)	33523	1(2)	33778	1(2)	33959	1(3)	34715	1(2)	35266	2(3)	35626	3(3)	36221	1(3)
33340	1(2)	33530	1(2)	33779	1(2)	33962	1(3)	34716	1(2)	35271	2(3)	35631	4(3)	36222	1(3)
33361	1(2)	33533	1(2)	33780	1(2)	33963	1(3)	34717	2(2)	35276	2(3)	35632	1(3)	36223	1(3)
33362	1(2)	33534	1(2)	33781	1(2)	33964	1(3)	34718	2(2)	35281	2(3)	35633	1(3)	36224	1(3)
33363	1(2)	33535	1(2)	33782	1(2)	33965	1(3)	34808	1(3)	35286	2(3)	35634	1(3)	36225	1(3)
33364	1(2)	33536	1(2)	33783	1(2)	33966	1(3)	34812	1(2)	35301	2(3)	35636	1(3)	36226	1(3)
33365	1(2)	33542	1(2)	33786	1(2)	33967	1(3)	34813	1(2)	35302	1(2)	35637	1(3)	36227	2(2)
33366	1(3)	33545	1(2)	33788	1(2)	33968	1(3)	34820	1(2)	35303	1(2)	35638	1(3)	36228	4(3)
33367	1(2)	33548	1(2)	33800	1(2)	33969	1(3)	34830	1(2)	35304	1(2)	35642	1(3)	36245	6(3)
33368	1(2)	33572	3(2)	33802	1(3)	33970	1(3)	34831	1(2)	35305	1(2)	35645	1(3)	36246	4(3)
33369	1(2)	33600	1(3)	33803	1(3)	33971	1(3)	34832	1(2)	35306	2(3)	35646	1(3)	36247	3(3)
33390	1(3)	33602	1(3)	33813	1(2)	33973	1(3)	34833	1(2)	35311	1(2)	35647	1(3)	36248	6(3)
33391	1(2)	33606	1(2)	33814	1(2)	33974	1(3)	34834	1(2)	35321	1(2)	35650	1(3)	36251	1(3)
33404	1(2)	33608	1(2)	33820	1(2)	33975	1(3)	34839	1(2)	35331	1(2)	35654	1(3)	36252	1(3)
33405	1(2)	33610	1(2)	33822	1(2)	33976	1(3)	34841	1(2)	35341	3(3)	35656	1(3)	36253	1(3)
33406	1(2)	33611	1(2)	33824	1(2)	33977	1(3)	34842	1(2)	35351	1(3)	35661	1(3)	36254	1(3)
33410	1(2)	33612	1(2)	33840	1(2)	33978	1(3)	34843	1(2)	35355	1(2)	35663	1(3)	36260	1(2)
33411	1(2)	33615	1(2)	33845	1(2)	33979	1(3)	34844	1(2)	35361	1(2)	35665	1(3)	36261	1(2)
33412	1(2)	33617	1(2)	33851	1(2)	33980	1(3)	34845	1(2)	35363	1(2)	35666	2(3)	36262	1(2)
33413	1(2)	33619	1(2)	33852	1(2)	33981	1(3)	34846	1(2)	35371	1(2)	35671	2(3)	36299	1(3)
33414	1(2)	33620	1(2)	33853	1(2)	33982	1(3)	34847	1(2)	35372	1(2)	35681	1(3)	36400	1(3)
33415	1(2)	33621	1(3)	33858	1(2)	33983	1(3)	34848	1(2)	35390	1(2)	35682	1(2)	36405	1(3)
33416	1(2)	33622	1(2)	33859	1(2)	33984	1(3)	35001	1(2)	35400	1(3)	35683	1(3)	36406	1(3)
33417	1(2)	33641	1(2)	33863	1(2)	33985	1(3)	35002	1(2)	35500	2(3)	35685	2(3)	36410	3(3)
33418	1(2)	33645	1(2)	33864	1(2)	33986	1(3)	35005	1(2)	35501	1(3)	35686	1(3)	36415	2(3)
33419	1(2)	33647	1(2)	33866	1(2)	33987	1(3)	35011	1(2)	35506	1(3)	35691	1(3)	36416	0(3)
33420	1(2)	33660	1(2)	33871	1(2)	33988	1(3)	35013	1(2)	35508	1(3)	35693	1(3)	36420	2(3)
33422	1(2)	33665	1(2)	33875	1(2)	33989	1(3)	35021	1(2)	35509	1(3)	35694	1(3)	36425	2(3)
33425	1(2)	33670	1(2)	33877	1(2)	33990	1(3)	35022	1(2)	35510	1(3)	35695	1(3)	36430	1(3)
33426	1(2)	33675	1(2)	33880	1(2)	33991	1(3)	35045	1(3)	35511	1(3)	35697	2(3)	36440	1(3)
33427	1(2)	33676	1(2)	33881	1(2)	33992	1(2)	35081	1(2)	35512	1(3)	35700	2(3)	36450	1(3)

Appendix I — Medically Unlikely Edits (MUEs)—Practitioner

CPT	MUE	CPT	MUE	CPT	MUE	CPT	MUE	CPT	MUE	CPT	MUE	CPT	MUE	CPT	MUE
36455	1(3)	36815	1(3)	37236	1(2)	38240	1(3)	40652	2(3)	41800	2(3)	42650	2(3)	43197	1(3)
36456	1(3)	36818	1(3)	37237	2(3)	38241	1(2)	40654	2(3)	41805	1(3)	42660	2(3)	43198	1(3)
36460	2(3)	36819	1(3)	37238	1(2)	38242	1(2)	40700	1(2)	41806	1(3)	42665	2(3)	43200	1(3)
36465	1(2)	36820	1(3)	37239	2(3)	38243	1(3)	40701	1(2)	41820	4(2)	42699	1(3)	43201	1(2)
36466	1(2)	36821	2(3)	37241	2(3)	38300	1(3)	40702	1(2)	41821	2(3)	42700	2(3)	43202	1(2)
36468	2(3)	36823	1(3)	37242	2(3)	38305	1(3)	40720	1(2)	41822	1(2)	42720	1(3)	43204	1(2)
36470	1(2)	36825	1(3)	37243	1(3)	38308	1(3)	40761	1(2)	41823	1(2)	42725	1(3)	43205	1(2)
36471	1(2)	36830	2(3)	37244	2(3)	38380	1(2)	40799	1(3)	41825	2(3)	42800	3(3)	43206	1(2)
36473	1(3)	36831	1(3)	37246	1(2)	38381	1(2)	40800	2(3)	41826	2(3)	42804	1(3)	43210	1(2)
36474	1(3)	36832	2(3)	37247	2(3)	38382	1(2)	40801	2(3)	41827	2(3)	42806	1(3)	43211	1(3)
36475	1(3)	36833	1(3)	37248	1(2)	38500	2(3)	40804	1(3)	41828	4(2)	42808	2(3)	43212	1(3)
36476	2(3)	36835	1(3)	37249	3(3)	38505	2(3)	40805	2(3)	41830	2(3)	42809	1(3)	43213	1(2)
36478	1(3)	36838	1(3)	37252	1(2)	38510	1(2)	40806	2(2)	41850	2(3)	42810	1(3)	43214	1(3)
36479	2(3)	36860	2(3)	37253	5(3)	38520	1(2)	40808	2(3)	41870	2(3)	42815	1(3)	43215	1(3)
36481	1(3)	36861	2(3)	37500	1(3)	38525	1(2)	40810	2(3)	41872	4(2)	42820	1(2)	43216	1(2)
36482	1(3)	36901	1(3)	37501	1(3)	38530	1(2)	40812	2(3)	41874	4(2)	42821	1(2)	43217	1(2)
36483	2(3)	36902	1(3)	37565	1(2)	38531	1(2)	40814	4(3)	41899	1(3)	42825	1(2)	43220	1(3)
36500	4(3)	36903	1(3)	37600	1(3)	38542	1(2)	40816	2(3)	42000	1(3)	42826	1(2)	43226	1(3)
36510	1(3)	36904	1(3)	37605	1(3)	38550	1(3)	40818	2(3)	42100	2(3)	42830	1(2)	43227	1(3)
36511	1(3)	36905	1(3)	37606	1(3)	38555	1(3)	40819	2(2)	42104	2(3)	42831	1(2)	43229	1(3)
36512	1(3)	36906	1(3)	37607	1(3)	38562	1(2)	40820	2(3)	42106	2(3)	42835	1(2)	43231	1(2)
36513	1(3)	36907	1(3)	37609	1(2)	38564	1(2)	40830	2(3)	42107	2(3)	42836	1(2)	43232	1(2)
36514	1(3)	36908	1(3)	37615	2(3)	38570	1(2)	40831	2(3)	42120	1(2)	42842	1(3)	43233	1(2)
36516	1(3)	36909	1(3)	37616	1(3)	38571	1(2)	40840	1(2)	42140	1(2)	42844	1(3)	43235	1(2)
36522	1(3)	37140	1(2)	37617	3(3)	38572	1(2)	40842	1(2)	42145	1(2)	42845	1(3)	43236	1(2)
36555	2(3)	37145	1(3)	37618	2(3)	38573	1(2)	40843	1(2)	42160	1(3)	42860	1(3)	43237	1(2)
36556	2(3)	37160	1(3)	37619	1(2)	38589	1(3)	40844	1(2)	42180	1(3)	42870	1(3)	43238	1(2)
36557	2(3)	37180	1(2)	37650	1(2)	38700	1(2)	40845	1(3)	42182	1(3)	42890	1(2)	43239	1(2)
36558	2(3)	37181	1(2)	37660	1(2)	38720	1(2)	40899	1(3)	42200	1(2)	42892	1(3)	43240	1(2)
36560	2(3)	37182	1(2)	37700	1(2)	38724	1(2)	41000	1(3)	42205	1(2)	42894	1(3)	43241	1(3)
36561	2(3)	37183	1(2)	37718	1(2)	38740	1(2)	41005	1(3)	42210	1(2)	42900	1(3)	43242	1(2)
36563	1(3)	37184	1(2)	37722	1(2)	38745	1(2)	41006	2(3)	42215	1(2)	42950	1(2)	43243	1(2)
36565	1(3)	37185	2(3)	37735	1(2)	38746	1(2)	41007	2(3)	42220	1(2)	42953	1(3)	43244	1(2)
36566	1(3)	37186	2(3)	37760	1(2)	38747	1(2)	41008	2(3)	42225	1(2)	42955	1(3)	43245	1(2)
36568	2(3)	37187	1(3)	37761	1(2)	38760	1(2)	41009	2(3)	42226	1(2)	42960	1(3)	43246	1(2)
36569	2(3)	37188	1(3)	37765	1(2)	38765	1(2)	41010	1(2)	42227	1(2)	42961	1(3)	43247	1(2)
36570	2(3)	37191	1(3)	37766	1(2)	38770	1(2)	41015	2(3)	42235	1(2)	42962	1(3)	43248	1(3)
36571	2(3)	37192	1(3)	37780	1(2)	38780	1(2)	41016	1(3)	42260	1(3)	42970	1(3)	43249	1(3)
36572	1(3)	37193	1(3)	37785	1(2)	38790	1(2)	41017	2(3)	42280	1(2)	42971	1(3)	43250	1(2)
36573	1(3)	37195	1(3)	37788	1(2)	38792	1(3)	41018	1(2)	42281	1(2)	42972	1(3)	43251	1(2)
36575	2(3)	37197	2(3)	37790	1(2)	38794	1(2)	41019	1(2)	42299	1(3)	42999	1(3)	43252	1(2)
36576	2(3)	37200	2(3)	37799	1(3)	38900	1(3)	41100	2(3)	42300	2(3)	43020	1(2)	43253	1(3)
36578	2(3)	37211	1(2)	38100	1(2)	38999	1(3)	41105	2(3)	42305	2(3)	43030	1(2)	43254	1(3)
36580	2(3)	37212	1(2)	38101	1(3)	39000	1(2)	41108	2(3)	42310	2(3)	43045	1(2)	43255	2(3)
36581	2(3)	37213	1(2)	38102	1(3)	39010	1(2)	41110	2(3)	42320	2(3)	43100	1(3)	43257	1(2)
36582	2(3)	37214	1(2)	38115	1(3)	39200	1(2)	41112	2(3)	42330	1(3)	43101	1(3)	43259	1(2)
36583	2(3)	37215	1(2)	38120	1(2)	39220	1(2)	41113	2(3)	42335	2(2)	43107	1(2)	43260	1(3)
36584	2(3)	37216	0(3)	38129	1(3)	39401	1(3)	41114	2(3)	42340	1(2)	43108	1(2)	43261	1(2)
36585	2(3)	37217	1(2)	38200	1(3)	39402	1(3)	41115	1(2)	42400	2(3)	43112	1(2)	43262	2(2)
36589	2(3)	37218	1(2)	38204	0(3)	39499	1(3)	41116	2(3)	42405	2(3)	43113	1(2)	43263	1(2)
36590	2(3)	37220	1(2)	38205	1(3)	39501	1(3)	41120	1(2)	42408	1(3)	43116	1(2)	43264	1(2)
36591	2(3)	37221	1(2)	38206	1(3)	39503	1(2)	41130	1(2)	42409	1(3)	43117	1(2)	43265	1(2)
36592	1(3)	37222	2(2)	38207	0(3)	39540	1(2)	41135	1(2)	42410	1(2)	43118	1(2)	43266	1(3)
36593	2(3)	37223	2(2)	38208	0(3)	39541	1(2)	41140	1(2)	42415	1(2)	43121	1(2)	43270	1(3)
36595	2(3)	37224	1(2)	38209	0(3)	39545	1(2)	41145	1(2)	42420	1(2)	43122	1(2)	43273	1(2)
36596	2(3)	37225	1(2)	38210	0(3)	39560	1(3)	41150	1(2)	42425	1(2)	43123	1(2)	43274	2(3)
36597	2(3)	37226	1(2)	38211	0(3)	39561	1(3)	41153	1(2)	42426	1(2)	43124	1(2)	43275	1(3)
36598	2(3)	37227	1(2)	38212	0(3)	39599	1(3)	41155	1(2)	42440	1(2)	43130	1(3)	43276	2(3)
36600	4(3)	37228	1(2)	38213	0(3)	40490	2(3)	41250	2(3)	42450	1(3)	43135	1(3)	43277	3(3)
36620	3(3)	37229	1(2)	38214	0(3)	40500	2(3)	41251	2(3)	42500	2(3)	43180	1(2)	43278	1(3)
36625	2(3)	37230	1(2)	38215	0(3)	40510	2(3)	41252	2(3)	42505	2(3)	43191	1(3)	43279	1(2)
36640	1(3)	37231	1(2)	38220	1(3)	40520	2(3)	41510	1(2)	42507	1(2)	43192	1(3)	43280	1(2)
36660	1(3)	37232	2(3)	38221	1(3)	40525	2(3)	41512	1(2)	42509	1(2)	43193	1(3)	43281	1(2)
36680	1(3)	37233	2(3)	38222	1(3)	40527	2(3)	41520	1(3)	42510	1(2)	43194	1(3)	43282	1(2)
36800	1(3)	37234	2(3)	38230	1(2)	40530	2(3)	41530	1(3)	42550	2(3)	43195	1(3)	43283	1(2)
36810	1(3)	37235	2(3)	38232	1(2)	40650	2(3)	41599	1(3)	42600	1(3)	43196	1(3)	43284	1(2)

CPT	MUE	CPT	MUE	CPT	MUE	CPT	MUE	CPT	MUE	CPT	MUE	CPT	MUE	CPT	MUE
43285	1(2)	43659	1(3)	44140	2(3)	44394	1(2)	45305	1(2)	46040	2(3)	46942	1(3)	47564	1(2)
43286	1(2)	43752	2(3)	44141	1(3)	44401	1(2)	45307	1(3)	46045	2(3)	46945	1(2)	47570	1(2)
43287	1(2)	43753	1(3)	44143	1(2)	44402	1(3)	45308	1(2)	46050	2(3)	46946	1(2)	47579	1(3)
43288	1(2)	43754	1(3)	44144	1(3)	44403	1(3)	45309	1(2)	46060	2(3)	46947	1(2)	47600	1(2)
43289	1(3)	43755	1(3)	44145	1(2)	44404	1(3)	45315	1(2)	46070	1(2)	46948	1(2)	47605	1(2)
43300	1(2)	43756	1(2)	44146	1(2)	44405	1(3)	45317	1(3)	46080	1(2)	46999	1(3)	47610	1(2)
43305	1(2)	43757	1(2)	44147	1(3)	44406	1(3)	45320	1(2)	46083	2(3)	47000	3(3)	47612	1(2)
43310	1(2)	43761	2(3)	44150	1(2)	44407	1(2)	45321	1(2)	46200	1(3)	47001	3(3)	47620	1(2)
43312	1(2)	43762	2(3)	44151	1(2)	44408	1(2)	45327	1(2)	46220	1(2)	47010	1(3)	47700	1(2)
43313	1(2)	43763	2(3)	44155	1(2)	44500	1(3)	45330	1(3)	46221	1(2)	47015	1(2)	47701	1(2)
43314	1(2)	43770	1(2)	44156	1(2)	44602	1(2)	45331	1(2)	46230	1(2)	47100	3(3)	47711	1(2)
43320	1(2)	43771	1(2)	44157	1(2)	44603	1(2)	45332	1(3)	46250	1(2)	47120	2(3)	47712	1(2)
43325	1(2)	43772	1(2)	44158	1(2)	44604	1(2)	45333	1(2)	46255	1(2)	47122	1(2)	47715	1(2)
43327	1(2)	43773	1(2)	44160	1(2)	44605	1(2)	45334	1(3)	46257	1(2)	47125	1(2)	47720	1(2)
43328	1(2)	43774	1(2)	44180	1(2)	44615	3(3)	45335	1(2)	46258	1(2)	47130	1(2)	47721	1(2)
43330	1(2)	43775	1(2)	44186	1(2)	44620	2(3)	45337	1(2)	46260	1(2)	47133	1(2)	47740	1(2)
43331	1(2)	43800	1(2)	44187	1(3)	44625	1(3)	45338	1(2)	46261	1(2)	47135	1(2)	47741	1(2)
43332	1(2)	43810	1(2)	44188	1(3)	44626	1(3)	45340	1(2)	46262	1(2)	47140	1(2)	47760	1(2)
43333	1(2)	43820	1(2)	44202	1(2)	44640	2(3)	45341	1(2)	46270	1(3)	47141	1(2)	47765	1(2)
43334	1(2)	43825	1(2)	44203	2(3)	44650	2(3)	45342	1(2)	46275	1(3)	47142	1(2)	47780	1(2)
43335	1(2)	43830	1(2)	44204	2(3)	44660	1(3)	45346	1(2)	46280	1(2)	47143	1(2)	47785	1(2)
43336	1(2)	43831	1(2)	44205	1(2)	44661	1(3)	45347	1(3)	46285	1(3)	47144	1(2)	47800	1(2)
43337	1(2)	43832	1(2)	44206	1(2)	44680	1(3)	45349	1(3)	46288	1(3)	47145	1(2)	47801	1(3)
43338	1(2)	43840	2(3)	44207	1(2)	44700	1(2)	45350	1(2)	46320	2(3)	47146	2(3)	47802	1(2)
43340	1(2)	43842	0(3)	44208	1(2)	44701	1(2)	45378	1(3)	46500	1(2)	47147	1(3)	47900	1(2)
43341	1(2)	43843	1(2)	44210	1(2)	44705	1(3)	45379	1(3)	46505	1(2)	47300	2(3)	47999	1(3)
43351	1(2)	43845	1(2)	44211	1(2)	44715	1(2)	45380	1(2)	46600	1(3)	47350	1(3)	48000	1(2)
43352	1(2)	43846	1(2)	44212	1(2)	44720	2(3)	45381	1(2)	46601	1(3)	47360	1(3)	48001	1(2)
43360	1(2)	43847	1(2)	44213	1(2)	44721	2(3)	45382	1(2)	46604	1(2)	47361	1(2)	48020	1(3)
43361	1(2)	43848	1(2)	44227	1(3)	44799	1(3)	45384	1(2)	46606	1(2)	47362	1(3)	48100	1(3)
43400	1(2)	43850	1(2)	44238	1(3)	44800	1(3)	45385	1(2)	46607	1(2)	47370	1(2)	48102	1(3)
43405	1(2)	43855	1(2)	44300	1(3)	44820	1(3)	45386	1(2)	46608	1(3)	47371	1(2)	48105	1(2)
43410	1(3)	43860	1(2)	44310	2(3)	44850	1(3)	45388	1(2)	46610	1(2)	47379	1(3)	48120	1(3)
43415	1(3)	43865	1(2)	44312	1(2)	44899	1(3)	45389	1(3)	46611	1(2)	47380	1(2)	48140	1(2)
43420	1(3)	43870	1(2)	44314	1(2)	44900	1(2)	45390	1(3)	46612	1(2)	47381	1(2)	48145	1(2)
43425	1(3)	43880	1(3)	44316	1(2)	44950	1(2)	45391	1(2)	46614	1(3)	47382	1(2)	48146	1(2)
43450	1(3)	43881	1(3)	44320	1(2)	44955	1(2)	45392	1(2)	46615	1(2)	47383	1(2)	48148	1(2)
43453	1(3)	43882	1(3)	44322	1(2)	44960	1(2)	45393	1(3)	46700	1(2)	47399	1(3)	48150	1(2)
43460	1(3)	43886	1(2)	44340	1(2)	44970	1(2)	45395	1(2)	46705	1(2)	47400	1(3)	48152	1(2)
43496	1(3)	43887	1(2)	44345	1(2)	44979	1(3)	45397	1(2)	46706	1(3)	47420	1(2)	48153	1(2)
43499	1(3)	43888	1(2)	44346	1(2)	45000	1(3)	45398	1(2)	46707	1(3)	47425	1(2)	48154	1(2)
43500	1(2)	43999	1(3)	44360	1(3)	45005	1(3)	45399	1(3)	46710	1(3)	47460	1(2)	48155	1(2)
43501	1(3)	44005	1(2)	44361	1(2)	45020	1(3)	45400	1(2)	46712	1(3)	47480	1(2)	48160	0(3)
43502	1(2)	44010	1(2)	44363	1(3)	45100	2(3)	45402	1(2)	46715	1(2)	47490	1(2)	48400	1(3)
43510	1(2)	44015	1(2)	44364	1(2)	45108	1(2)	45499	1(3)	46716	1(2)	47531	2(3)	48500	1(3)
43520	1(2)	44020	2(3)	44365	1(2)	45110	1(2)	45500	1(2)	46730	1(2)	47532	1(3)	48510	1(3)
43605	1(2)	44021	1(3)	44366	1(3)	45111	1(2)	45505	1(2)	46735	1(2)	47533	1(3)	48520	1(3)
43610	2(3)	44025	1(3)	44369	1(2)	45112	1(2)	45520	1(2)	46740	1(2)	47534	2(3)	48540	1(3)
43611	2(3)	44050	1(2)	44370	1(2)	45113	1(2)	45540	1(2)	46742	1(2)	47535	1(3)	48545	1(3)
43620	1(2)	44055	1(2)	44372	1(2)	45114	1(2)	45541	1(2)	46744	1(2)	47536	2(3)	48547	1(2)
43621	1(2)	44100	1(2)	44373	1(2)	45116	1(2)	45550	1(2)	46746	1(2)	47537	1(3)	48548	1(2)
43622	1(2)	44110	1(2)	44376	1(3)	45119	1(2)	45560	1(2)	46748	1(2)	47538	2(3)	48550	1(2)
43631	1(2)	44111	1(2)	44377	1(2)	45120	1(2)	45562	1(2)	46750	1(2)	47539	2(3)	48551	1(2)
43632	1(2)	44120	1(2)	44378	1(3)	45121	1(2)	45563	1(2)	46751	1(2)	47540	2(3)	48552	2(3)
43633	1(2)	44121	2(3)	44379	1(2)	45123	1(2)	45800	1(3)	46753	1(2)	47541	1(3)	48554	1(2)
43634	1(2)	44125	1(2)	44380	1(3)	45126	1(2)	45805	1(3)	46754	1(3)	47542	2(3)	48556	1(2)
43635	1(2)	44126	1(2)	44381	1(3)	45130	1(2)	45820	1(3)	46760	1(2)	47543	1(3)	48999	1(3)
43640	1(2)	44127	1(2)	44382	1(2)	45135	1(2)	45825	1(3)	46761	1(2)	47544	1(3)	49000	1(2)
43641	1(2)	44128	2(3)	44384	1(3)	45136	1(2)	45900	1(2)	46900	1(2)	47550	1(3)	49002	1(3)
43644	1(2)	44130	2(3)	44385	1(3)	45150	1(2)	45905	1(2)	46910	1(2)	47552	1(3)	49010	1(3)
43645	1(2)	44132	1(2)	44386	1(3)	45160	1(2)	45910	1(2)	46916	1(2)	47553	1(2)	49013	1(2)
43647	1(2)	44133	1(2)	44388	1(3)	45171	2(3)	45915	1(2)	46917	1(2)	47554	1(2)	49014	1(3)
43648	1(2)	44135	1(2)	44389	1(2)	45172	2(3)	45990	1(2)	46922	1(2)	47555	1(2)	49020	2(3)
43651	1(2)	44136	1(2)	44390	1(3)	45190	1(3)	45999	1(3)	46924	1(2)	47556	1(2)	49040	2(3)
43652	1(2)	44137	1(2)	44391	1(3)	45300	1(3)	46020	2(3)	46930	1(2)	47562	1(2)	49060	2(3)
43653	1(2)	44139	1(2)	44392	1(2)	45303	1(3)	46030	1(3)	46940	1(2)	47563	1(2)	49062	1(3)

CPT	MUE	CPT	MUE	CPT	MUE	CPT	MUE	CPT	MUE	CPT	MUE	CPT	MUE	CPT	MUE
49082	1(3)	49561	1(3)	50370	1(2)	50705	2(3)	51595	1(2)	52290	1(2)	53431	1(2)	54308	1(2)
49083	2(3)	49565	2(3)	50380	1(2)	50706	2(3)	51596	1(2)	52300	1(2)	53440	1(2)	54312	1(2)
49084	1(3)	49566	2(3)	50382	1(3)	50715	1(2)	51597	1(2)	52301	1(2)	53442	1(2)	54316	1(2)
49180	2(3)	49568	2(3)	50384	1(3)	50722	1(2)	51600	1(3)	52305	1(2)	53444	1(3)	54318	1(2)
49185	2(3)	49570	1(3)	50385	1(3)	50725	1(3)	51605	1(3)	52310	1(3)	53445	1(2)	54322	1(2)
49203	1(2)	49572	1(3)	50386	1(3)	50727	1(3)	51610	1(3)	52315	2(3)	53446	1(2)	54324	1(2)
49204	1(2)	49580	1(2)	50387	1(3)	50728	1(3)	51700	1(3)	52317	1(3)	53447	1(2)	54326	1(2)
49205	1(2)	49582	1(2)	50389	1(3)	50740	1(2)	51701	2(3)	52318	1(3)	53448	1(2)	54328	1(2)
49215	1(2)	49585	1(2)	50390	2(3)	50750	1(2)	51702	2(3)	52320	1(2)	53449	1(2)	54332	1(2)
49250	1(2)	49587	1(2)	50391	1(3)	50760	1(2)	51703	2(3)	52325	1(3)	53450	1(2)	54336	1(2)
49255	1(2)	49590	1(2)	50396	1(3)	50770	1(2)	51705	1(3)	52327	1(2)	53460	1(2)	54340	1(2)
49320	1(3)	49600	1(2)	50400	1(2)	50780	1(2)	51710	1(3)	52330	1(2)	53500	1(2)	54344	1(2)
49321	1(2)	49605	1(2)	50405	1(2)	50782	1(2)	51715	1(2)	52332	1(2)	53502	1(3)	54348	1(2)
49322	1(2)	49606	1(2)	50430	2(3)	50783	1(2)	51720	1(3)	52334	1(2)	53505	1(3)	54352	1(2)
49323	1(2)	49610	1(2)	50431	2(3)	50785	1(2)	51725	1(3)	52341	1(2)	53510	1(3)	54360	1(2)
49324	1(2)	49611	1(2)	50432	2(3)	50800	1(2)	51726	1(3)	52342	1(2)	53515	1(3)	54380	1(2)
49325	1(2)	49650	1(2)	50433	2(3)	50810	1(3)	51727	1(3)	52343	1(2)	53520	1(3)	54385	1(2)
49326	1(2)	49651	1(2)	50434	2(3)	50815	1(2)	51728	1(3)	52344	1(2)	53600	1(3)	54390	1(2)
49327	1(2)	49652	2(3)	50435	2(3)	50820	1(2)	51729	1(3)	52345	1(2)	53601	1(3)	54400	1(2)
49329	1(3)	49653	2(3)	50436	1(3)	50825	1(3)	51736	1(3)	52346	1(2)	53605	1(3)	54401	1(2)
49400	1(3)	49654	1(3)	50437	1(3)	50830	1(3)	51741	1(3)	52351	1(3)	53620	1(2)	54405	1(2)
49402	1(3)	49655	1(3)	50500	1(3)	50840	1(2)	51784	1(3)	52352	1(2)	53621	1(3)	54406	1(2)
49405	2(3)	49656	1(3)	50520	1(3)	50845	1(2)	51785	1(3)	52353	1(2)	53660	1(2)	54408	1(2)
49406	2(3)	49657	1(3)	50525	1(3)	50860	1(2)	51792	1(3)	52354	1(3)	53661	1(3)	54410	1(2)
49407	1(3)	49659	1(3)	50526	1(3)	50900	1(3)	51797	1(3)	52355	1(3)	53665	1(3)	54411	1(2)
49411	1(2)	49900	1(3)	50540	1(2)	50920	2(3)	51798	1(3)	52356	1(2)	53850	1(2)	54415	1(2)
49412	1(2)	49904	1(3)	50541	1(2)	50930	2(3)	51800	1(2)	52400	1(2)	53852	1(2)	54416	1(2)
49418	1(3)	49905	1(3)	50542	1(2)	50940	1(2)	51820	1(2)	52402	1(2)	53854	1(2)	54417	1(2)
49419	1(2)	49906	1(3)	50543	1(2)	50945	1(2)	51840	1(2)	52441	1(2)	53855	1(2)	54420	1(2)
49421	1(2)	49999	1(3)	50544	1(2)	50947	1(2)	51841	1(2)	52442	6(3)	53860	1(2)	54430	1(2)
49422	1(2)	50010	1(2)	50545	1(2)	50948	1(2)	51845	1(2)	52450	1(2)	53899	1(3)	54435	1(2)
49423	2(3)	50020	1(3)	50546	1(2)	50949	1(3)	51860	1(3)	52500	1(2)	54000	1(2)	54437	1(2)
49424	3(3)	50040	1(2)	50547	1(2)	50951	1(3)	51865	1(3)	52601	1(2)	54001	1(2)	54438	1(2)
49425	1(2)	50045	1(2)	50548	1(2)	50953	1(3)	51880	1(2)	52630	1(2)	54015	1(3)	54440	1(2)
49426	1(3)	50060	1(2)	50549	1(3)	50955	1(2)	51900	1(3)	52640	1(2)	54050	1(2)	54450	1(2)
49427	1(3)	50065	1(2)	50551	1(3)	50957	1(2)	51920	1(3)	52647	1(2)	54055	1(2)	54500	1(3)
49428	1(2)	50070	1(2)	50553	1(3)	50961	1(3)	51925	1(2)	52648	1(2)	54056	1(2)	54505	1(3)
49429	1(2)	50075	1(2)	50555	1(3)	50970	1(3)	51940	1(2)	52649	1(2)	54057	1(2)	54512	1(3)
49435	1(2)	50080	1(2)	50557	1(3)	50972	1(3)	51960	1(2)	52700	1(3)	54060	1(2)	54520	1(2)
49436	1(2)	50081	1(2)	50561	1(3)	50974	1(2)	51980	1(2)	53000	1(2)	54065	1(2)	54522	1(2)
49440	1(3)	50100	1(2)	50562	1(3)	50976	1(2)	51990	1(2)	53010	1(2)	54100	2(3)	54530	1(2)
49441	1(3)	50120	1(2)	50570	1(3)	50980	1(2)	51992	1(2)	53020	1(2)	54105	2(3)	54535	1(2)
49442	1(3)	50125	1(2)	50572	1(3)	51020	1(2)	51999	1(3)	53025	1(2)	54110	1(2)	54550	1(2)
49446	1(2)	50130	1(2)	50574	1(2)	51030	1(2)	52000	1(3)	53040	1(3)	54111	1(2)	54560	1(2)
49450	1(3)	50135	1(2)	50575	1(2)	51040	1(3)	52001	1(3)	53060	1(3)	54112	1(3)	54600	1(2)
49451	1(3)	50200	1(3)	50576	1(2)	51045	2(3)	52005	2(3)	53080	1(3)	54115	1(3)	54620	1(2)
49452	1(3)	50205	1(3)	50580	1(2)	51050	1(3)	52007	1(2)	53085	1(3)	54120	1(2)	54640	1(2)
49460	1(3)	50220	1(2)	50590	1(2)	51060	1(3)	52010	1(2)	53200	1(3)	54125	1(2)	54650	1(2)
49465	1(3)	50225	1(2)	50592	1(2)	51065	1(3)	52204	1(2)	53210	1(2)	54130	1(2)	54660	1(2)
49491	1(2)	50230	1(2)	50593	1(2)	51080	1(3)	52214	1(2)	53215	1(2)	54135	1(2)	54670	1(3)
49492	1(2)	50234	1(2)	50600	1(3)	51100	1(3)	52224	1(2)	53220	1(3)	54150	1(2)	54680	1(2)
49495	1(2)	50236	1(2)	50605	1(3)	51101	1(3)	52234	1(2)	53230	1(3)	54160	1(2)	54690	1(2)
49496	1(2)	50240	1(2)	50606	1(3)	51102	1(3)	52235	1(2)	53235	1(3)	54161	1(2)	54692	1(2)
49500	1(2)	50250	1(3)	50610	1(2)	51500	1(2)	52240	1(2)	53240	1(3)	54162	1(2)	54699	1(3)
49501	1(2)	50280	1(2)	50620	1(2)	51520	1(2)	52250	1(2)	53250	1(3)	54163	1(2)	54700	1(3)
49505	1(2)	50290	1(3)	50630	1(2)	51525	1(2)	52260	1(2)	53260	1(2)	54164	1(2)	54800	1(2)
49507	1(2)	50300	1(2)	50650	1(2)	51530	1(2)	52265	1(2)	53265	1(3)	54200	1(2)	54830	1(2)
49520	1(2)	50320	1(2)	50660	1(3)	51535	1(2)	52270	1(2)	53270	1(2)	54205	1(2)	54840	1(2)
49521	1(2)	50323	1(2)	50684	1(3)	51550	1(2)	52275	1(2)	53275	1(2)	54220	1(3)	54860	1(2)
49525	1(2)	50325	1(2)	50686	1(3)	51555	1(2)	52276	1(2)	53400	1(2)	54230	1(3)	54861	1(2)
49540	1(2)	50327	2(3)	50688	2(3)	51565	1(2)	52277	1(2)	53405	1(2)	54231	1(3)	54865	1(3)
49550	1(2)	50328	1(3)	50690	2(3)	51570	1(2)	52281	1(2)	53410	1(2)	54235	1(3)	54900	1(2)
49553	1(2)	50329	1(3)	50693	2(3)	51575	1(2)	52282	1(2)	53415	1(2)	54240	1(2)	54901	1(2)
49555	1(2)	50340	1(2)	50694	2(3)	51580	1(2)	52283	1(2)	53420	1(2)	54250	1(2)	55000	1(3)
49557	1(2)	50360	1(2)	50695	2(3)	51585	1(2)	52285	1(2)	53425	1(2)	54300	1(2)	55040	1(2)
49560	2(3)	50365	1(2)	50700	1(2)	51590	1(2)	52287	1(2)	53430	1(2)	54304	1(2)	55041	1(2)

CPT	MUE	CPT	MUE	CPT	MUE	CPT	MUE	CPT	MUE	CPT	MUE	CPT	MUE	CPT	MUE
55060	1(2)	56637	1(2)	57415	1(3)	58400	1(3)	58957	1(2)	59870	1(2)	61330	1(2)	61600	1(3)
55100	2(3)	56640	1(2)	57420	1(3)	58410	1(2)	58958	1(2)	59871	1(2)	61333	1(2)	61601	1(3)
55110	1(2)	56700	1(2)	57421	1(3)	58520	1(2)	58960	1(2)	59897	1(3)	61340	1(2)	61605	1(3)
55120	1(3)	56740	1(3)	57423	1(2)	58540	1(3)	58970	1(3)	59898	1(3)	61343	1(2)	61606	1(3)
55150	1(2)	56800	1(2)	57425	1(2)	58541	1(3)	58974	1(3)	59899	1(3)	61345	1(3)	61607	1(3)
55175	1(2)	56805	1(2)	57426	1(2)	58542	1(2)	58976	2(3)	60000	1(3)	61450	1(3)	61608	1(3)
55180	1(2)	56810	1(2)	57452	1(3)	58543	1(3)	58999	1(3)	60100	3(3)	61458	1(2)	61611	1(3)
55200	1(2)	56820	1(2)	57454	1(3)	58544	1(2)	59000	2(3)	60200	2(3)	61460	1(2)	61613	1(3)
55250	1(2)	56821	1(2)	57455	1(3)	58545	1(2)	59001	2(3)	60210	1(2)	61500	1(3)	61615	1(3)
55300	1(2)	57000	1(3)	57456	1(3)	58546	1(2)	59012	2(3)	60212	1(2)	61501	1(3)	61616	1(3)
55400	1(2)	57010	1(3)	57460	1(3)	58548	1(2)	59015	2(3)	60220	1(3)	61510	1(3)	61618	2(3)
55500	1(2)	57020	1(3)	57461	1(3)	58550	1(3)	59020	2(3)	60225	1(2)	61512	1(3)	61619	2(3)
55520	1(2)	57022	1(3)	57465	1(3)	58552	1(3)	59025	2(3)	60240	1(2)	61514	2(3)	61623	2(3)
55530	1(2)	57023	1(3)	57500	1(3)	58553	1(3)	59030	2(3)	60252	1(2)	61516	1(3)	61624	2(3)
55535	1(2)	57061	1(2)	57505	1(3)	58554	1(2)	59050	2(3)	60254	1(2)	61517	1(3)	61626	2(3)
55540	1(2)	57065	1(2)	57510	1(3)	58555	1(3)	59051	2(3)	60260	1(2)	61518	1(3)	61630	1(3)
55550	1(2)	57100	2(3)	57511	1(3)	58558	1(3)	59070	2(3)	60270	1(2)	61519	1(3)	61635	2(3)
55559	1(3)	57105	2(3)	57513	1(3)	58559	1(3)	59072	2(3)	60271	1(2)	61520	1(3)	61640	0(3)
55600	1(2)	57106	1(2)	57520	1(3)	58560	1(3)	59074	2(3)	60280	1(2)	61521	1(3)	61641	0(3)
55605	1(2)	57107	1(2)	57522	1(3)	58561	1(3)	59076	2(3)	60281	1(2)	61522	1(3)	61642	0(3)
55650	1(2)	57109	1(2)	57530	1(3)	58562	1(3)	59100	1(2)	60300	2(3)	61524	2(3)	61645	1(3)
55680	1(3)	57110	1(2)	57531	1(2)	58563	1(3)	59120	1(3)	60500	1(2)	61526	1(3)	61650	1(2)
55700	1(2)	57111	1(2)	57540	1(2)	58565	1(2)	59121	1(3)	60502	1(3)	61530	1(3)	61651	2(2)
55705	1(2)	57120	1(2)	57545	1(3)	58570	1(3)	59130	1(3)	60505	1(3)	61531	1(2)	61680	1(3)
55706	1(2)	57130	1(2)	57550	1(3)	58571	1(2)	59135	1(3)	60512	1(3)	61533	2(3)	61682	1(3)
55720	1(3)	57135	2(3)	57555	1(2)	58572	1(3)	59136	1(3)	60520	1(2)	61534	1(3)	61684	1(3)
55725	1(3)	57150	1(3)	57556	1(2)	58573	1(3)	59140	1(3)	60521	1(2)	61535	2(3)	61686	1(3)
55801	1(2)	57155	1(3)	57558	1(2)	58575	1(2)	59150	1(3)	60522	1(2)	61536	1(3)	61690	1(3)
55810	1(2)	57156	1(3)	57700	1(3)	58578	1(3)	59151	1(3)	60540	1(2)	61537	1(3)	61692	1(3)
55812	1(2)	57160	1(2)	57720	1(3)	58579	1(3)	59160	1(2)	60545	1(2)	61538	1(2)	61697	2(3)
55815	1(2)	57170	1(2)	57800	1(3)	58600	1(2)	59200	1(3)	60600	1(3)	61539	1(3)	61698	1(3)
55821	1(2)	57180	1(3)	58100	1(3)	58605	1(2)	59300	1(2)	60605	1(3)	61540	1(3)	61700	2(3)
55831	1(2)	57200	1(3)	58110	1(3)	58611	1(2)	59320	1(2)	60650	1(2)	61541	1(2)	61702	1(3)
55840	1(2)	57210	1(3)	58120	1(3)	58615	1(2)	59325	1(2)	60659	1(3)	61543	1(2)	61703	1(3)
55842	1(2)	57220	1(2)	58140	1(3)	58660	1(2)	59350	1(2)	60699	1(3)	61544	1(3)	61705	1(3)
55845	1(2)	57230	1(2)	58145	1(3)	58661	1(2)	59400	1(2)	61000	1(2)	61545	1(2)	61708	1(3)
55860	1(2)	57240	1(2)	58146	1(3)	58662	1(2)	59409	2(3)	61001	1(2)	61546	1(2)	61710	1(3)
55862	1(2)	57250	1(2)	58150	1(3)	58670	1(2)	59410	1(2)	61020	2(3)	61548	1(2)	61711	1(3)
55865	1(2)	57260	1(2)	58152	1(2)	58671	1(2)	59412	1(3)	61026	2(3)	61550	1(2)	61720	1(3)
55866	1(2)	57265	1(2)	58180	1(3)	58672	1(2)	59414	1(3)	61050	1(3)	61552	1(2)	61735	1(3)
55870	1(2)	57267	2(3)	58200	1(2)	58673	1(2)	59425	1(2)	61055	1(3)	61556	1(3)	61750	2(3)
55873	1(2)	57268	1(2)	58210	1(2)	58674	1(2)	59426	1(2)	61070	2(3)	61557	1(2)	61751	2(3)
55874	1(2)	57270	1(2)	58240	1(2)	58679	1(3)	59430	1(2)	61105	1(3)	61558	1(3)	61760	1(2)
55875	1(2)	57280	1(2)	58260	1(3)	58700	1(2)	59510	1(2)	61107	1(3)	61559	1(3)	61770	1(2)
55876	1(2)	57282	1(2)	58262	1(3)	58720	1(2)	59514	1(2)	61108	1(3)	61563	2(3)	61781	1(3)
55880	1(2)	57283	1(2)	58263	1(2)	58740	1(2)	59515	1(2)	61120	1(3)	61564	1(2)	61782	1(3)
55899	1(3)	57284	1(2)	58267	1(2)	58750	1(2)	59525	1(2)	61140	1(3)	61566	1(3)	61783	1(3)
55920	1(2)	57285	1(2)	58270	1(2)	58752	1(2)	59610	1(2)	61150	1(3)	61567	1(2)	61790	1(2)
55970	1(2)	57287	1(2)	58275	1(2)	58760	1(2)	59612	2(3)	61151	1(3)	61570	1(3)	61791	1(2)
55980	1(2)	57288	1(2)	58280	1(2)	58770	1(2)	59614	1(2)	61154	1(3)	61571	1(3)	61796	1(2)
56405	2(3)	57289	1(2)	58285	1(3)	58800	1(2)	59618	1(2)	61156	1(3)	61575	1(2)	61797	4(3)
56420	1(3)	57291	1(2)	58290	1(3)	58805	1(2)	59620	1(2)	61210	1(3)	61576	1(2)	61798	1(2)
56440	1(3)	57292	1(2)	58291	1(2)	58820	1(3)	59622	1(2)	61215	1(3)	61580	1(2)	61799	4(3)
56441	1(2)	57295	1(2)	58292	1(2)	58822	1(2)	59812	1(2)	61250	1(3)	61581	1(2)	61800	1(2)
56442	1(2)	57296	1(2)	58294	1(2)	58825	1(2)	59820	1(2)	61253	1(3)	61582	1(2)	61850	1(3)
56501	1(2)	57300	1(3)	58300	0(3)	58900	1(2)	59821	1(2)	61304	1(3)	61583	1(2)	61860	1(3)
56515	1(2)	57305	1(3)	58301	1(3)	58920	1(2)	59830	1(2)	61305	1(3)	61584	1(2)	61863	1(2)
56605	1(2)	57307	1(3)	58321	1(2)	58925	1(3)	59840	1(2)	61312	2(3)	61585	1(2)	61864	1(3)
56606	6(3)	57308	1(3)	58322	1(2)	58940	1(2)	59841	1(2)	61313	2(3)	61586	1(2)	61867	1(2)
56620	1(2)	57310	1(3)	58323	1(2)	58943	1(2)	59850	1(2)	61314	2(3)	61590	1(2)	61868	2(3)
56625	1(2)	57311	1(3)	58340	1(3)	58950	1(2)	59851	1(2)	61315	1(3)	61591	1(2)	61880	1(2)
56630	1(2)	57320	1(3)	58345	1(3)	58951	1(2)	59852	1(2)	61316	1(3)	61592	1(2)	61885	1(3)
56631	1(2)	57330	1(3)	58346	1(2)	58952	1(2)	59855	1(2)	61320	2(3)	61595	1(2)	61886	1(3)
56632	1(2)	57335	1(2)	58350	1(2)	58953	1(2)	59856	1(2)	61321	1(3)	61596	1(2)	61888	1(3)
56633	1(2)	57400	1(2)	58353	1(3)	58954	1(2)	59857	1(2)	61322	1(3)	61597	1(2)	62000	1(3)
56634	1(2)	57410	1(2)	58356	1(3)	58956	1(2)	59866	1(2)	61323	1(3)	61598	1(3)	62005	1(3)

Appendix I — Medically Unlikely Edits (MUEs)—Practitioner

CPT	MUE	CPT	MUE	CPT	MUE	CPT	MUE	CPT	MUE	CPT	MUE	CPT	MUE	CPT	MUE
62010	1(3)	62360	1(2)	63265	1(3)	64446	1(2)	64647	1(2)	64865	1(3)	65750	1(2)	66821	1(2)
62100	1(3)	62361	1(2)	63266	1(3)	64447	1(3)	64650	1(2)	64866	1(3)	65755	1(2)	66825	1(2)
62115	1(2)	62362	1(2)	63267	1(3)	64448	1(2)	64653	1(2)	64868	1(3)	65756	1(2)	66830	1(2)
62117	1(2)	62365	1(2)	63268	1(3)	64449	1(2)	64680	1(2)	64872	1(3)	65757	1(3)	66840	1(2)
62120	1(2)	62367	1(3)	63270	1(3)	64450	10(3)	64681	1(2)	64874	1(3)	65760	0(3)	66850	1(2)
62121	1(2)	62368	1(3)	63271	1(3)	64451	2(2)	64702	2(3)	64876	1(3)	65765	0(3)	66852	1(2)
62140	1(3)	62369	1(3)	63272	1(3)	64454	2(2)	64704	4(3)	64885	1(3)	65767	0(3)	66920	1(2)
62141	1(3)	62370	1(3)	63273	1(3)	64455	1(2)	64708	3(3)	64886	1(3)	65770	1(2)	66930	1(2)
62142	2(3)	62380	2(3)	63275	1(3)	64461	1(2)	64712	1(2)	64890	2(3)	65771	0(3)	66940	1(2)
62143	2(3)	63001	1(2)	63276	1(3)	64462	1(2)	64713	1(2)	64891	2(3)	65772	1(2)	66982	1(2)
62145	2(3)	63003	1(2)	63277	1(3)	64463	1(3)	64714	1(2)	64892	2(3)	65775	1(2)	66983	1(2)
62146	2(3)	63005	1(2)	63278	1(3)	64479	1(2)	64716	2(3)	64893	2(3)	65778	1(2)	66984	1(2)
62147	1(3)	63011	1(2)	63280	1(3)	64480	4(3)	64718	1(2)	64895	2(3)	65779	1(2)	66985	1(2)
62148	1(3)	63012	1(2)	63281	1(3)	64483	1(2)	64719	1(2)	64896	2(3)	65780	1(2)	66986	1(2)
62160	1(3)	63015	1(2)	63282	1(3)	64484	4(3)	64721	1(2)	64897	2(3)	65781	1(2)	66987	2(2)
62161	1(3)	63016	1(2)	63283	1(3)	64486	1(3)	64722	4(3)	64898	2(3)	65782	1(2)	66988	2(2)
62162	1(3)	63017	1(2)	63285	1(3)	64487	1(2)	64726	2(3)	64901	2(3)	65785	1(2)	66990	1(3)
62164	1(3)	63020	1(2)	63286	1(3)	64488	1(3)	64727	2(3)	64902	1(3)	65800	1(2)	66999	1(3)
62165	1(2)	63030	1(2)	63287	1(3)	64489	1(2)	64732	1(2)	64905	1(3)	65810	1(2)	67005	1(2)
62180	1(3)	63035	4(3)	63290	1(3)	64490	1(2)	64734	1(2)	64907	1(3)	65815	1(3)	67010	1(2)
62190	1(3)	63040	1(2)	63295	1(2)	64491	1(2)	64736	1(2)	64910	3(3)	65820	1(2)	67015	1(2)
62192	1(3)	63042	1(2)	63300	1(2)	64492	1(2)	64738	1(2)	64911	1(3)	65850	1(2)	67025	1(2)
62194	1(3)	63043	4(3)	63301	1(2)	64493	1(2)	64740	1(2)	64912	3(3)	65855	1(2)	67027	1(2)
62200	1(2)	63044	4(2)	63302	1(2)	64494	1(2)	64742	1(2)	64913	3(3)	65860	1(2)	67028	1(3)
62201	1(2)	63045	1(2)	63303	1(2)	64495	1(2)	64744	1(2)	64999	1(3)	65865	1(2)	67030	1(2)
62220	1(3)	63046	1(2)	63304	1(2)	64505	1(3)	64746	1(2)	65091	1(2)	65870	1(2)	67031	1(2)
62223	1(3)	63047	1(2)	63305	1(2)	64510	1(3)	64755	1(2)	65093	1(2)	65875	1(2)	67036	1(2)
62225	2(3)	63048	5(3)	63306	1(2)	64517	1(3)	64760	1(2)	65101	1(2)	65880	1(2)	67039	1(2)
62230	2(3)	63050	1(2)	63307	1(2)	64520	1(3)	64763	1(2)	65103	1(2)	65900	1(3)	67040	1(2)
62252	2(3)	63051	1(2)	63308	3(3)	64530	1(3)	64766	1(2)	65105	1(2)	65920	1(2)	67041	1(2)
62256	1(3)	63055	1(2)	63600	2(3)	64553	1(3)	64771	2(3)	65110	1(2)	65930	1(3)	67042	1(2)
62258	1(3)	63056	1(2)	63610	1(3)	64555	2(3)	64772	2(3)	65112	1(2)	66020	1(3)	67043	1(2)
62263	1(2)	63057	3(3)	63620	1(2)	64561	1(3)	64774	2(3)	65114	1(2)	66030	1(3)	67101	1(2)
62264	1(2)	63064	1(2)	63621	2(2)	64566	1(3)	64776	1(2)	65125	1(2)	66130	1(3)	67105	1(2)
62267	2(3)	63066	1(3)	63650	2(3)	64568	1(3)	64778	1(3)	65130	1(2)	66150	1(2)	67107	1(2)
62268	1(3)	63075	1(2)	63655	1(3)	64569	1(3)	64782	2(2)	65135	1(2)	66155	1(2)	67108	1(2)
62269	2(3)	63076	3(3)	63661	1(2)	64570	1(3)	64783	2(3)	65140	1(2)	66160	1(2)	67110	1(2)
62270	2(3)	63077	1(2)	63662	1(2)	64575	2(3)	64784	3(3)	65150	1(2)	66170	1(2)	67113	1(2)
62272	1(3)	63078	3(3)	63663	1(3)	64580	2(3)	64786	1(3)	65155	1(2)	66172	1(2)	67115	1(2)
62273	2(3)	63081	1(2)	63664	1(3)	64581	2(3)	64787	4(3)	65175	1(2)	66174	1(2)	67120	1(2)
62280	1(3)	63082	6(2)	63685	1(3)	64585	2(3)	64788	5(3)	65205	1(3)	66175	1(2)	67121	1(2)
62281	1(3)	63085	1(2)	63688	1(3)	64590	1(3)	64790	1(3)	65210	1(3)	66179	1(2)	67141	1(2)
62282	1(3)	63086	2(3)	63700	1(3)	64595	1(3)	64792	2(3)	65220	1(3)	66180	1(2)	67145	1(2)
62284	1(3)	63087	1(2)	63702	1(3)	64600	2(3)	64795	2(3)	65222	1(3)	66183	1(3)	67208	1(2)
62287	1(2)	63088	3(3)	63704	1(3)	64605	1(2)	64802	1(2)	65235	1(3)	66184	1(2)	67210	1(2)
62290	5(2)	63090	1(2)	63706	1(3)	64610	1(2)	64804	1(2)	65260	1(3)	66185	1(2)	67218	1(2)
62291	4(3)	63091	3(3)	63707	1(3)	64611	1(2)	64809	1(2)	65265	1(3)	66225	1(2)	67220	1(2)
62292	1(2)	63101	1(2)	63709	1(3)	64612	1(2)	64818	1(2)	65270	1(3)	66250	1(2)	67221	1(2)
62294	1(3)	63102	1(2)	63710	1(3)	64615	1(2)	64820	4(3)	65272	1(3)	66500	1(2)	67225	1(2)
62302	1(3)	63103	3(3)	63740	1(3)	64616	1(2)	64821	1(2)	65273	1(3)	66505	1(2)	67227	1(2)
62303	1(3)	63170	1(3)	63741	1(3)	64617	1(2)	64822	1(2)	65275	1(3)	66600	1(2)	67228	1(2)
62304	1(3)	63172	1(3)	63744	1(3)	64620	5(3)	64823	1(2)	65280	1(3)	66605	1(2)	67229	1(2)
62305	1(3)	63173	1(3)	63746	1(2)	64624	2(2)	64831	1(2)	65285	1(3)	66625	1(2)	67250	1(2)
62320	1(3)	63185	1(2)	64400	4(3)	64625	2(2)	64832	3(3)	65286	1(3)	66630	1(2)	67255	1(2)
62321	1(3)	63190	1(2)	64405	1(3)	64630	1(3)	64834	1(2)	65290	1(3)	66635	1(2)	67299	1(3)
62322	1(3)	63191	1(2)	64408	1(3)	64632	1(2)	64835	1(2)	65400	1(3)	66680	1(2)	67311	1(2)
62323	1(3)	63194	1(2)	64415	1(3)	64633	1(2)	64836	1(2)	65410	1(3)	66682	1(2)	67312	1(2)
62324	1(3)	63195	1(2)	64416	1(2)	64634	4(3)	64837	2(3)	65420	1(2)	66700	1(2)	67314	1(2)
62325	1(3)	63196	1(2)	64417	1(3)	64635	1(2)	64840	1(2)	65426	1(2)	66710	1(2)	67316	1(2)
62326	1(3)	63197	1(2)	64418	1(3)	64636	4(3)	64856	2(3)	65430	1(2)	66711	1(2)	67318	1(2)
62327	1(3)	63198	1(2)	64420	2(2)	64640	5(3)	64857	2(3)	65435	1(2)	66720	1(2)	67320	2(3)
62328	2(3)	63199	1(2)	64421	3(3)	64642	1(2)	64858	1(2)	65436	1(2)	66740	1(2)	67331	1(2)
62329	1(3)	63200	1(2)	64425	1(3)	64643	3(2)	64859	2(3)	65450	1(3)	66761	1(2)	67332	1(2)
62350	1(3)	63250	1(3)	64430	1(3)	64644	1(2)	64861	1(2)	65600	1(3)	66762	1(2)	67334	1(2)
62351	1(3)	63251	1(3)	64435	1(3)	64645	3(2)	64862	1(2)	65710	1(2)	66770	1(3)	67335	1(2)
62355	1(3)	63252	1(3)	64445	1(3)	64646	1(2)	64864	2(3)	65730	1(2)	66820	1(2)	67340	2(2)

CPT	MUE	CPT	MUE	CPT	MUE	CPT	MUE	CPT	MUE	CPT	MUE	CPT	MUE	CPT	MUE
67343	1(2)	67975	1(2)	69300	1(2)	69915	1(3)	70552	2(3)	72194	1(3)	73660	2(3)	74485	2(3)
67345	1(3)	67999	1(3)	69310	1(2)	69930	1(2)	70553	2(3)	72195	1(3)	73700	2(3)	74710	1(3)
67346	1(3)	68020	1(3)	69320	1(2)	69949	1(3)	70554	1(3)	72196	1(3)	73701	2(3)	74712	1(3)
67399	1(3)	68040	1(2)	69399	1(3)	69950	1(2)	70555	1(3)	72197	1(3)	73702	2(3)	74713	2(3)
67400	1(2)	68100	1(3)	69420	1(2)	69955	1(2)	70557	1(3)	72198	1(3)	73706	2(3)	74740	1(3)
67405	1(2)	68110	1(3)	69421	1(2)	69960	1(2)	70558	1(3)	72200	2(3)	73718	2(3)	74742	2(2)
67412	1(2)	68115	1(3)	69424	1(2)	69970	1(3)	70559	1(3)	72202	1(3)	73719	2(3)	74775	1(2)
67413	1(2)	68130	1(3)	69433	1(2)	69979	1(3)	71045	4(3)	72220	1(3)	73720	2(3)	75557	1(3)
67414	1(2)	68135	1(3)	69436	1(2)	69990	1(3)	71046	2(3)	72240	1(2)	73721	3(3)	75559	1(3)
67415	1(3)	68200	1(3)	69440	1(2)	70010	1(3)	71047	1(3)	72255	1(2)	73722	2(3)	75561	1(3)
67420	1(2)	68320	1(2)	69450	1(2)	70015	1(3)	71048	1(3)	72265	1(2)	73723	2(3)	75563	1(3)
67430	1(2)	68325	1(2)	69501	1(3)	70030	2(2)	71100	2(3)	72270	1(2)	73725	2(3)	75565	1(3)
67440	1(2)	68326	1(2)	69502	1(2)	70100	2(3)	71101	2(3)	72275	1(3)	74018	3(3)	75571	1(3)
67445	1(2)	68328	1(2)	69505	1(2)	70110	2(3)	71110	1(3)	72285	4(3)	74019	2(3)	75572	1(3)
67450	1(2)	68330	1(3)	69511	1(2)	70120	1(3)	71111	1(3)	72295	5(3)	74021	2(3)	75573	1(3)
67500	1(3)	68335	1(3)	69530	1(2)	70130	1(3)	71120	1(3)	73000	2(3)	74022	2(3)	75574	1(3)
67505	1(3)	68340	1(3)	69535	1(2)	70134	1(3)	71130	1(3)	73010	2(3)	74150	1(3)	75600	1(3)
67515	1(3)	68360	1(3)	69540	1(3)	70140	2(3)	71250	2(3)	73020	2(3)	74160	1(3)	75605	1(3)
67550	1(2)	68362	1(3)	69550	1(3)	70150	1(3)	71260	2(3)	73030	4(3)	74170	1(3)	75625	1(3)
67560	1(2)	68371	1(3)	69552	1(2)	70160	1(3)	71270	1(3)	73040	2(2)	74174	1(3)	75630	1(3)
67570	1(2)	68399	1(3)	69554	1(2)	70170	2(2)	71271	1(2)	73050	1(3)	74175	1(3)	75635	1(3)
67599	1(3)	68400	1(2)	69601	1(2)	70190	1(2)	71275	1(3)	73060	2(3)	74176	2(3)	75705	20(3)
67700	2(3)	68420	1(2)	69602	1(2)	70200	2(3)	71550	1(3)	73070	2(3)	74177	2(3)	75710	2(3)
67710	1(2)	68440	2(3)	69603	1(2)	70210	1(3)	71551	1(3)	73080	2(3)	74178	1(3)	75716	1(3)
67715	1(3)	68500	1(2)	69604	1(2)	70220	1(3)	71552	1(3)	73085	2(2)	74181	1(3)	75726	3(3)
67800	1(2)	68505	1(2)	69610	1(2)	70240	1(2)	71555	1(3)	73090	2(3)	74182	1(3)	75731	1(3)
67801	1(2)	68510	1(2)	69620	1(2)	70250	2(3)	72020	4(3)	73092	2(3)	74183	1(3)	75733	1(3)
67805	1(2)	68520	1(2)	69631	1(2)	70260	1(3)	72040	3(3)	73100	2(3)	74185	1(3)	75736	2(3)
67808	1(2)	68525	1(2)	69632	1(3)	70300	1(3)	72050	1(3)	73110	3(3)	74190	1(3)	75741	1(3)
67810	2(3)	68530	1(2)	69633	1(2)	70310	1(3)	72052	1(3)	73115	2(2)	74210	1(3)	75743	1(3)
67820	1(2)	68540	1(2)	69635	1(3)	70320	1(3)	72070	1(3)	73120	2(3)	74220	1(3)	75746	1(3)
67825	1(2)	68550	1(2)	69636	1(3)	70328	1(3)	72072	1(3)	73130	3(3)	74221	1(3)	75756	2(3)
67830	1(2)	68700	1(2)	69637	1(3)	70330	1(3)	72074	1(3)	73140	3(3)	74230	1(3)	75774	7(3)
67835	1(2)	68705	2(3)	69641	1(2)	70332	2(3)	72080	1(3)	73200	2(3)	74235	1(3)	75801	1(3)
67840	3(3)	68720	1(2)	69642	1(2)	70336	1(3)	72081	1(3)	73201	2(3)	74240	2(3)	75803	1(3)
67850	3(3)	68745	1(2)	69643	1(2)	70350	1(3)	72082	1(3)	73202	2(3)	74246	1(3)	75805	1(2)
67875	1(2)	68750	1(2)	69644	1(2)	70355	1(3)	72083	1(3)	73206	2(3)	74248	1(2)	75807	1(2)
67880	1(2)	68760	4(2)	69645	1(2)	70360	2(3)	72084	1(3)	73218	2(3)	74250	1(3)	75809	1(3)
67882	1(2)	68761	4(2)	69646	1(2)	70370	1(3)	72100	2(3)	73219	2(3)	74251	1(3)	75810	1(3)
67900	1(2)	68770	1(3)	69650	1(2)	70371	1(2)	72110	1(3)	73220	2(3)	74261	1(2)	75820	2(3)
67901	1(2)	68801	4(2)	69660	1(2)	70380	2(3)	72114	1(3)	73221	2(3)	74262	1(2)	75822	1(3)
67902	1(2)	68810	1(2)	69661	1(2)	70390	2(3)	72120	1(3)	73222	2(3)	74263	0(3)	75825	1(3)
67903	1(2)	68811	1(2)	69662	1(2)	70450	3(3)	72125	1(3)	73223	2(3)	74270	1(3)	75827	1(3)
67904	1(2)	68815	1(2)	69666	1(2)	70460	1(3)	72126	1(3)	73225	2(3)	74280	1(3)	75831	1(3)
67906	1(2)	68816	1(2)	69667	1(2)	70470	2(3)	72127	1(3)	73501	2(3)	74283	1(3)	75833	1(3)
67908	1(2)	68840	1(2)	69670	1(2)	70480	1(3)	72128	1(3)	73502	2(3)	74290	1(3)	75840	1(3)
67909	1(2)	68850	1(3)	69676	1(2)	70481	1(3)	72129	1(3)	73503	2(3)	74300	1(3)	75842	1(3)
67911	2(3)	68899	1(3)	69700	1(3)	70482	1(3)	72130	1(3)	73521	2(3)	74301	1(3)	75860	2(3)
67912	1(2)	69000	1(3)	69705	1(2)	70486	1(3)	72131	1(3)	73522	2(3)	74328	1(3)	75870	1(3)
67914	2(3)	69005	1(3)	69706	1(2)	70487	1(3)	72132	1(3)	73523	2(3)	74329	1(3)	75872	1(3)
67915	2(3)	69020	1(3)	69710	0(3)	70488	1(3)	72133	1(3)	73525	2(2)	74330	1(3)	75880	1(3)
67916	2(3)	69090	0(3)	69711	1(2)	70490	1(3)	72141	1(3)	73551	2(3)	74340	1(3)	75885	1(3)
67917	2(3)	69100	3(3)	69714	1(2)	70491	1(3)	72142	1(3)	73552	2(3)	74355	1(3)	75887	1(3)
67921	2(3)	69105	1(3)	69715	1(3)	70492	1(3)	72146	1(3)	73560	4(3)	74360	1(3)	75889	1(3)
67922	2(3)	69110	1(2)	69717	1(2)	70496	2(3)	72147	1(3)	73562	3(3)	74363	2(3)	75891	1(3)
67923	2(3)	69120	1(3)	69718	1(2)	70498	2(3)	72148	1(3)	73564	4(3)	74400	1(3)	75893	2(3)
67924	2(3)	69140	1(2)	69720	1(2)	70540	1(3)	72149	1(3)	73565	1(3)	74410	1(3)	75894	2(3)
67930	2(3)	69145	1(3)	69725	1(2)	70542	1(3)	72156	1(3)	73580	2(2)	74415	1(3)	75898	2(3)
67935	2(3)	69150	1(3)	69740	1(2)	70543	1(3)	72157	1(3)	73590	3(3)	74420	2(3)	75901	1(3)
67938	2(3)	69155	1(3)	69745	1(2)	70544	2(3)	72158	1(3)	73592	2(3)	74425	2(3)	75902	2(3)
67950	2(2)	69200	1(2)	69799	1(3)	70545	1(3)	72159	1(3)	73600	2(3)	74430	1(3)	75956	1(2)
67961	2(3)	69205	1(3)	69801	1(3)	70546	1(3)	72170	2(3)	73610	3(3)	74440	1(2)	75957	1(2)
67966	2(3)	69209	1(2)	69805	1(3)	70547	1(3)	72190	1(3)	73615	2(3)	74445	1(2)	75958	2(3)
67971	1(2)	69210	1(2)	69806	1(3)	70548	1(3)	72191	1(3)	73620	2(3)	74450	1(3)	75959	1(2)
67973	1(2)	69220	1(2)	69905	1(2)	70549	1(3)	72192	1(3)	73630	3(3)	74455	1(3)	75970	1(3)
67974	1(2)	69222	1(2)	69910	1(2)	70551	2(3)	72193	1(3)	73650	2(3)	74470	2(2)	75984	2(3)

Appendix I — Medically Unlikely Edits (MUEs)—Practitioner

CPT	MUE	CPT	MUE	CPT	MUE	CPT	MUE	CPT	MUE	CPT	MUE	CPT	MUE	CPT	MUE
75989	2(3)	76873	1(2)	77299	1(3)	78020	1(3)	78466	1(3)	80047	2(3)	80307	1(2)	80415	1(3)
76000	3(3)	76881	2(3)	77300	10(3)	78070	1(2)	78468	1(3)	80048	2(3)	80320	1(3)	80416	1(3)
76010	2(3)	76882	2(3)	77301	1(3)	78071	1(3)	78469	1(3)	80050	0(3)	80321	1(3)	80417	1(3)
76080	3(3)	76885	1(2)	77306	1(3)	78072	1(3)	78472	1(2)	80051	2(3)	80322	1(3)	80418	1(3)
76098	3(3)	76886	1(2)	77307	1(3)	78075	1(3)	78473	1(2)	80053	1(3)	80323	1(3)	80420	1(3)
76100	2(3)	76932	1(2)	77316	1(3)	78099	1(3)	78481	1(3)	80055	1(3)	80324	1(3)	80422	1(3)
76101	1(3)	76936	1(3)	77317	1(3)	78102	1(2)	78483	1(2)	80061	1(3)	80325	1(3)	80424	1(3)
76102	1(3)	76937	2(3)	77318	1(3)	78103	1(2)	78491	1(3)	80069	1(3)	80326	1(3)	80426	1(3)
76120	1(3)	76940	1(3)	77321	1(2)	78104	1(2)	78492	1(2)	80074	1(2)	80327	1(3)	80428	1(3)
76125	1(3)	76941	3(3)	77331	3(3)	78110	1(2)	78494	1(3)	80076	1(3)	80328	1(3)	80430	1(3)
76140	0(3)	76942	1(3)	77332	4(3)	78111	1(2)	78496	1(3)	80081	1(2)	80329	1(3)	80432	1(3)
76145	1(2)	76945	1(3)	77333	2(3)	78120	1(2)	78499	1(3)	80143	2(3)	80330	1(3)	80434	1(3)
76376	2(3)	76946	1(3)	77334	10(3)	78121	1(2)	78579	1(3)	80145	1(3)	80331	1(3)	80435	1(3)
76377	2(3)	76948	1(2)	77336	1(2)	78122	1(2)	78580	1(3)	80150	2(3)	80332	1(3)	80436	1(3)
76380	2(3)	76965	2(3)	77338	1(3)	78130	1(2)	78582	1(3)	80151	1(3)	80333	1(3)	80438	1(3)
76390	1(3)	76975	1(3)	77370	1(3)	78140	1(3)	78597	1(3)	80155	1(3)	80334	1(3)	80439	1(3)
76391	1(3)	76977	1(2)	77371	1(2)	78185	1(2)	78598	1(3)	80156	2(3)	80335	1(3)	80500	1(3)
76496	1(3)	76978	1(2)	77372	1(2)	78191	1(2)	78599	1(3)	80157	2(3)	80336	1(3)	80502	1(3)
76497	1(3)	76979	3(3)	77373	1(3)	78195	1(2)	78600	1(3)	80158	1(3)	80337	1(3)	81000	2(3)
76498	1(3)	76981	1(3)	77385	1(3)	78199	1(3)	78601	1(3)	80159	2(3)	80338	1(3)	81001	2(3)
76499	1(3)	76982	1(2)	77386	1(3)	78201	1(3)	78605	1(3)	80161	1(3)	80339	1(3)	81002	2(3)
76506	1(2)	76983	2(3)	77387	1(3)	78202	1(3)	78606	1(3)	80162	2(3)	80340	1(3)	81003	2(3)
76510	2(2)	76998	1(3)	77399	1(3)	78215	1(3)	78608	1(3)	80163	1(3)	80341	1(3)	81005	2(3)
76511	2(2)	76999	1(3)	77401	1(2)	78216	1(3)	78609	0(3)	80164	2(3)	80342	1(3)	81007	1(3)
76512	2(2)	77001	2(3)	77402	2(3)	78226	1(3)	78610	1(3)	80165	1(3)	80343	1(3)	81015	2(3)
76513	1(2)	77002	1(3)	77407	2(3)	78227	1(3)	78630	1(3)	80167	1(3)	80344	1(3)	81020	1(3)
76514	1(2)	77003	1(3)	77412	1(3)	78230	1(3)	78635	1(3)	80168	2(3)	80345	1(3)	81025	1(3)
76516	1(2)	77011	1(3)	77417	1(2)	78231	1(3)	78645	1(3)	80169	1(3)	80346	1(3)	81050	2(3)
76519	2(2)	77012	1(3)	77423	1(3)	78232	1(3)	78650	1(3)	80170	2(3)	80347	1(3)	81099	1(3)
76529	2(2)	77013	1(3)	77424	1(2)	78258	1(2)	78660	1(2)	80171	1(3)	80348	1(3)	81105	1(2)
76536	1(3)	77014	2(3)	77425	1(3)	78261	1(2)	78699	1(3)	80173	2(3)	80349	1(3)	81106	1(2)
76604	1(3)	77021	1(3)	77427	1(2)	78262	1(2)	78700	1(3)	80175	1(3)	80350	1(3)	81107	1(2)
76641	2(2)	77022	1(3)	77431	1(2)	78264	1(2)	78701	1(3)	80176	1(3)	80351	1(3)	81108	1(2)
76642	2(2)	77046	1(2)	77432	1(2)	78265	1(2)	78707	1(2)	80177	1(3)	80352	1(3)	81109	1(2)
76700	1(3)	77047	1(2)	77435	1(2)	78266	1(2)	78708	1(2)	80178	2(3)	80353	1(3)	81110	1(2)
76705	2(3)	77048	1(2)	77469	1(2)	78267	1(2)	78709	1(2)	80179	2(3)	80354	1(3)	81111	1(2)
76706	1(2)	77049	1(2)	77470	1(2)	78268	1(2)	78725	1(3)	80180	1(3)	80355	1(3)	81112	1(2)
76770	1(3)	77053	2(2)	77499	1(3)	78278	2(3)	78730	1(2)	80181	1(3)	80356	1(3)	81120	1(3)
76775	2(3)	77054	2(2)	77520	1(3)	78282	1(2)	78740	1(2)	80183	1(3)	80357	1(3)	81121	1(3)
76776	2(3)	77061	1(2)	77522	1(3)	78290	1(3)	78761	1(2)	80184	2(3)	80358	1(3)	81161	1(3)
76800	1(3)	77062	1(2)	77523	1(3)	78291	1(3)	78799	1(3)	80185	2(3)	80359	1(3)	81162	1(2)
76801	1(2)	77063	1(2)	77525	1(3)	78299	1(3)	78800	1(2)	80186	2(3)	80360	1(3)	81163	1(2)
76802	1(2)	77065	1(2)	77600	1(3)	78300	1(2)	78801	1(2)	80187	1(3)	80361	1(3)	81164	1(2)
76805	1(2)	77066	1(2)	77605	1(3)	78305	1(2)	78802	1(2)	80188	2(3)	80362	1(3)	81165	1(2)
76810	2(3)	77067	1(2)	77610	1(3)	78306	1(2)	78803	1(2)	80189	1(3)	80363	1(3)	81166	1(2)
76811	1(2)	77071	1(3)	77615	1(3)	78315	1(2)	78804	1(2)	80190	2(3)	80364	1(3)	81167	1(2)
76812	2(3)	77072	1(2)	77620	1(3)	78350	0(3)	78808	1(2)	80192	2(3)	80365	1(3)	81168	1(3)
76813	1(2)	77073	1(2)	77750	1(3)	78351	0(3)	78811	1(2)	80193	1(3)	80366	1(3)	81170	1(2)
76814	2(3)	77074	1(2)	77761	1(3)	78399	1(3)	78812	1(2)	80194	2(3)	80367	1(3)	81171	1(2)
76815	1(2)	77075	1(2)	77762	1(3)	78414	1(2)	78813	1(2)	80195	2(3)	80368	1(3)	81172	1(2)
76816	2(3)	77076	1(2)	77763	1(3)	78428	1(3)	78814	1(2)	80197	2(3)	80369	1(3)	81173	1(2)
76817	1(3)	77077	1(2)	77767	2(3)	78429	1(2)	78815	1(2)	80198	2(3)	80370	1(3)	81174	1(2)
76818	2(3)	77078	1(2)	77768	2(3)	78430	1(2)	78816	1(2)	80199	1(3)	80371	1(3)	81175	1(3)
76819	2(3)	77080	1(2)	77770	2(3)	78431	1(2)	78830	1(2)	80200	2(3)	80372	1(3)	81176	1(3)
76820	3(3)	77081	1(2)	77771	2(3)	78432	1(2)	78831	1(2)	80201	2(3)	80373	1(3)	81177	1(2)
76821	2(3)	77084	1(2)	77772	2(3)	78433	1(2)	78832	1(2)	80202	2(3)	80374	1(3)	81178	1(2)
76825	2(3)	77085	1(2)	77778	1(3)	78434	1(2)	78835	4(3)	80203	1(3)	80375	1(3)	81179	1(2)
76826	2(3)	77086	1(2)	77789	2(3)	78445	1(2)	78999	1(3)	80204	1(3)	80376	1(3)	81180	1(2)
76827	2(3)	77261	1(3)	77790	1(3)	78451	1(2)	79005	1(3)	80210	1(3)	80377	1(3)	81181	1(2)
76828	2(3)	77262	1(3)	77799	1(3)	78452	1(2)	79101	1(3)	80230	1(3)	80400	1(3)	81182	1(2)
76830	1(3)	77263	1(3)	78012	1(3)	78453	1(2)	79200	1(3)	80235	1(3)	80402	1(3)	81183	1(2)
76831	1(3)	77280	2(3)	78013	1(3)	78454	1(2)	79300	1(3)	80280	1(3)	80406	1(3)	81184	1(2)
76856	1(3)	77285	1(3)	78014	1(2)	78456	1(3)	79403	1(3)	80285	1(3)	80408	1(3)	81185	1(2)
76857	1(3)	77290	1(3)	78015	1(3)	78457	1(2)	79440	1(3)	80299	3(3)	80410	1(3)	81186	1(2)
76870	1(2)	77293	1(3)	78016	1(3)	78458	1(2)	79445	1(3)	80305	1(2)	80412	1(3)	81187	1(2)
76872	1(3)	77295	1(3)	78018	1(2)	78459	1(3)	79999	1(3)	80306	1(2)	80414	1(3)	81188	1(2)

CPT	MUE	CPT	MUE	CPT	MUE	CPT	MUE	CPT	MUE	CPT	MUE	CPT	MUE	CPT	MUE
81189	1(2)	81263	1(3)	81332	1(3)	81431	1(2)	82043	1(3)	82390	1(2)	82760	1(3)	83505	1(3)
81190	1(2)	81264	1(3)	81333	1(2)	81432	1(2)	82044	1(3)	82397	3(3)	82775	1(3)	83516	4(3)
81191	1(3)	81265	1(3)	81334	1(3)	81433	1(2)	82045	1(3)	82415	1(3)	82776	1(2)	83518	1(3)
81192	1(3)	81266	2(3)	81335	1(2)	81434	1(2)	82075	2(3)	82435	1(3)	82777	1(3)	83519	5(3)
81193	1(3)	81267	1(3)	81336	1(2)	81435	1(2)	82077	1(3)	82436	1(3)	82784	6(3)	83520	9(3)
81194	1(3)	81268	4(3)	81337	1(3)	81436	1(2)	82085	1(3)	82438	1(3)	82785	1(3)	83525	4(3)
81200	1(2)	81269	1(2)	81338	1(3)	81437	1(2)	82088	2(3)	82441	1(2)	82787	4(3)	83527	1(3)
81201	1(2)	81270	1(2)	81339	1(2)	81438	1(2)	82103	1(3)	82465	1(3)	82800	1(3)	83528	1(3)
81202	1(3)	81271	1(2)	81340	1(3)	81439	1(2)	82104	1(2)	82480	2(3)	82803	2(3)	83540	2(3)
81203	1(3)	81272	1(3)	81341	1(3)	81440	1(2)	82105	1(3)	82482	1(3)	82805	2(3)	83550	1(3)
81204	1(2)	81273	1(3)	81342	1(3)	81442	1(2)	82106	2(3)	82485	1(3)	82810	2(3)	83570	1(3)
81205	1(3)	81274	1(2)	81343	1(2)	81443	1(2)	82107	1(3)	82495	1(2)	82820	1(3)	83582	1(3)
81206	1(3)	81275	1(3)	81344	1(2)	81445	1(2)	82108	1(3)	82507	1(3)	82930	1(3)	83586	1(3)
81207	1(3)	81276	1(3)	81345	1(3)	81448	1(2)	82120	1(3)	82523	1(3)	82938	1(3)	83593	1(3)
81208	1(3)	81277	1(2)	81346	1(2)	81450	1(2)	82127	1(3)	82525	2(3)	82941	1(3)	83605	1(3)
81209	1(3)	81278	1(3)	81347	1(2)	81455	1(2)	82128	2(3)	82528	1(3)	82943	1(3)	83615	2(3)
81210	1(3)	81279	1(2)	81348	1(2)	81460	1(2)	82131	2(3)	82530	4(3)	82945	4(3)	83625	1(3)
81212	1(2)	81283	1(2)	81350	1(3)	81465	1(2)	82135	1(3)	82533	5(3)	82946	1(2)	83630	1(3)
81215	1(2)	81284	1(2)	81351	1(2)	81470	1(2)	82136	2(3)	82540	1(3)	82947	5(3)	83631	1(3)
81216	1(2)	81285	1(2)	81352	1(2)	81471	1(2)	82139	2(3)	82542	6(3)	82948	2(3)	83632	1(3)
81217	1(2)	81286	1(2)	81353	1(2)	81479	3(3)	82140	2(3)	82550	3(3)	82950	3(3)	83633	1(3)
81218	1(3)	81287	1(3)	81355	1(3)	81490	1(2)	82143	2(3)	82552	3(3)	82951	1(2)	83655	2(3)
81219	1(3)	81288	1(3)	81357	1(2)	81493	1(2)	82150	2(3)	82553	3(3)	82952	3(3)	83661	3(3)
81220	1(3)	81289	1(2)	81360	1(2)	81500	1(2)	82154	1(3)	82554	1(3)	82955	1(2)	83662	4(3)
81221	1(3)	81290	1(3)	81361	1(2)	81503	1(2)	82157	1(3)	82565	2(3)	82960	1(2)	83663	3(3)
81222	1(3)	81291	1(3)	81362	1(2)	81504	1(2)	82160	1(3)	82570	3(3)	82962	2(3)	83664	3(3)
81223	1(2)	81292	1(2)	81363	1(2)	81506	1(2)	82163	1(3)	82575	1(3)	82963	1(3)	83670	1(3)
81224	1(3)	81293	1(3)	81364	1(2)	81507	1(2)	82164	1(3)	82585	1(2)	82965	1(3)	83690	2(3)
81225	1(3)	81294	1(3)	81370	1(2)	81508	1(2)	82172	2(3)	82595	1(3)	82977	1(3)	83695	1(3)
81226	1(3)	81295	1(2)	81371	1(2)	81509	1(2)	82175	2(3)	82600	1(3)	82978	1(3)	83698	1(3)
81227	1(3)	81296	1(3)	81372	1(2)	81510	1(2)	82180	1(2)	82607	1(2)	82979	1(3)	83700	1(2)
81228	1(3)	81297	1(3)	81373	2(2)	81511	1(2)	82190	2(3)	82608	1(2)	82985	1(3)	83701	1(3)
81229	1(3)	81298	1(2)	81374	1(3)	81512	1(2)	82232	2(3)	82610	1(3)	83001	1(3)	83704	1(3)
81230	1(2)	81299	1(3)	81375	1(2)	81513	1(2)	82239	1(3)	82615	1(3)	83002	1(3)	83718	1(3)
81231	1(2)	81300	1(3)	81376	5(3)	81514	1(2)	82240	1(3)	82626	1(3)	83003	5(3)	83719	1(3)
81232	1(2)	81301	1(3)	81377	2(3)	81518	1(2)	82247	2(3)	82627	1(3)	83006	1(2)	83721	1(3)
81233	1(3)	81302	1(3)	81378	1(2)	81519	1(2)	82248	2(3)	82633	1(3)	83009	1(3)	83722	1(2)
81234	1(2)	81303	1(3)	81379	1(2)	81520	1(2)	82252	1(3)	82634	1(3)	83010	1(3)	83727	1(3)
81235	1(3)	81304	1(3)	81380	2(2)	81521	1(2)	82261	1(3)	82638	1(3)	83012	1(2)	83735	4(3)
81236	1(3)	81305	1(3)	81381	3(3)	81522	1(2)	82270	1(3)	82642	1(2)	83013	1(3)	83775	1(3)
81237	1(3)	81306	1(2)	81382	6(3)	81525	1(2)	82271	1(3)	82652	1(2)	83014	1(2)	83785	1(3)
81238	1(2)	81307	1(2)	81383	1(3)	81528	1(2)	82272	1(3)	82656	1(3)	83015	1(3)	83789	4(3)
81239	1(3)	81308	1(2)	81400	2(3)	81529	1(3)	82274	1(2)	82657	2(3)	83018	4(3)	83825	2(3)
81240	1(2)	81309	1(2)	81401	2(3)	81535	1(2)	82286	1(3)	82658	2(3)	83020	1(3)	83835	2(3)
81241	1(2)	81310	1(3)	81402	1(3)	81536	11(3)	82300	1(3)	82664	2(3)	83021	2(3)	83857	1(3)
81242	1(3)	81311	1(3)	81403	4(3)	81538	1(2)	82306	1(2)	82668	1(3)	83026	1(3)	83861	2(2)
81243	1(3)	81312	1(2)	81404	5(3)	81539	1(2)	82308	1(3)	82670	1(3)	83030	1(3)	83864	1(2)
81244	1(3)	81313	1(3)	81405	2(3)	81540	1(2)	82310	2(3)	82671	1(3)	83033	1(3)	83872	2(3)
81245	1(3)	81314	1(3)	81406	2(3)	81541	1(2)	82330	2(3)	82672	1(3)	83036	1(2)	83873	1(3)
81246	1(3)	81315	1(3)	81407	1(3)	81542	1(2)	82331	1(3)	82677	1(3)	83037	1(2)	83874	2(3)
81247	1(2)	81316	1(2)	81408	2(3)	81546	2(3)	82340	1(3)	82679	1(3)	83045	1(3)	83876	1(3)
81248	1(3)	81317	1(2)	81410	1(2)	81551	1(2)	82355	2(3)	82681	1(3)	83050	1(3)	83880	1(3)
81249	1(2)	81318	1(3)	81411	1(2)	81552	1(2)	82360	2(3)	82693	2(3)	83051	1(3)	83883	4(3)
81250	1(3)	81319	1(2)	81412	1(2)	81554	1(2)	82365	2(3)	82696	1(3)	83060	1(3)	83885	2(3)
81251	1(3)	81320	1(3)	81413	1(2)	81595	1(2)	82370	2(3)	82705	1(3)	83065	1(2)	83915	1(3)
81252	1(3)	81321	1(3)	81414	1(2)	81596	1(2)	82373	1(3)	82710	1(3)	83068	1(2)	83916	2(3)
81253	1(3)	81322	1(3)	81415	1(2)	81599	1(3)	82374	1(3)	82715	3(3)	83069	1(3)	83918	2(3)
81254	1(3)	81323	1(3)	81416	2(3)	82009	1(3)	82375	1(3)	82725	1(3)	83070	1(2)	83919	1(3)
81255	1(3)	81324	1(3)	81417	1(3)	82010	1(3)	82376	1(3)	82726	1(3)	83080	2(3)	83921	2(3)
81256	1(2)	81325	1(3)	81419	1(3)	82013	1(3)	82378	1(3)	82728	1(3)	83088	1(3)	83930	2(3)
81257	1(2)	81326	1(3)	81420	1(2)	82016	1(3)	82379	1(3)	82731	1(3)	83090	2(3)	83935	1(3)
81258	1(2)	81327	1(2)	81422	1(2)	82017	1(3)	82380	1(3)	82735	1(3)	83150	1(3)	83937	1(3)
81259	1(2)	81328	1(2)	81425	1(2)	82024	4(3)	82382	1(2)	82746	1(2)	83491	1(3)	83945	2(3)
81260	1(3)	81329	1(2)	81426	2(3)	82030	1(3)	82383	1(3)	82747	1(2)	83497	1(3)	83950	1(3)
81261	1(3)	81330	1(3)	81427	1(3)	82040	1(3)	82384	2(3)	82757	1(2)	83498	2(3)	83951	1(2)
81262	1(3)	81331	1(3)	81430	1(2)	82042	2(3)	82387	1(3)	82759	1(3)	83500	1(3)	83970	2(3)

CPT	MUE	CPT	MUE	CPT	MUE	CPT	MUE	CPT	MUE	CPT	MUE	CPT	MUE	CPT	MUE
83986	2(3)	84305	1(3)	85007	1(3)	85441	1(2)	86256	9(3)	86618	2(3)	86769	3(3)	86970	1(3)
83987	1(3)	84307	1(3)	85008	1(3)	85445	1(2)	86277	1(3)	86619	2(3)	86771	2(3)	86971	1(3)
83992	2(3)	84311	2(3)	85009	1(3)	85460	1(3)	86280	1(3)	86622	2(3)	86774	2(3)	86972	1(3)
83993	1(3)	84315	1(3)	85013	1(3)	85461	1(2)	86294	1(3)	86625	1(3)	86777	2(3)	86975	1(3)
84030	1(2)	84375	1(3)	85014	2(3)	85475	1(3)	86300	2(3)	86628	3(3)	86778	2(3)	86976	1(3)
84035	1(2)	84376	1(3)	85018	2(3)	85520	1(3)	86301	1(2)	86631	6(3)	86780	2(3)	86977	1(3)
84060	1(3)	84377	1(3)	85025	2(3)	85525	2(3)	86304	1(2)	86632	3(3)	86784	1(3)	86978	1(3)
84066	1(3)	84378	2(3)	85027	2(3)	85530	1(3)	86305	1(2)	86635	4(3)	86787	2(3)	86985	1(3)
84075	2(3)	84379	1(3)	85032	1(3)	85536	1(2)	86308	1(2)	86638	6(3)	86788	2(3)	86999	1(3)
84078	1(2)	84392	1(3)	85041	1(3)	85540	1(2)	86309	1(2)	86641	2(3)	86789	2(3)	87003	1(3)
84080	1(3)	84402	1(3)	85044	1(2)	85547	1(2)	86310	1(2)	86644	2(3)	86790	4(3)	87015	3(3)
84081	1(3)	84403	2(3)	85045	1(2)	85549	1(3)	86316	2(3)	86645	1(3)	86793	2(3)	87040	2(3)
84085	1(2)	84410	1(2)	85046	1(2)	85555	1(2)	86317	6(3)	86648	2(3)	86794	1(3)	87045	3(3)
84087	1(3)	84425	1(2)	85048	2(3)	85557	1(2)	86318	2(3)	86651	2(3)	86800	1(3)	87046	6(3)
84100	2(3)	84430	1(3)	85049	2(3)	85576	7(3)	86320	1(2)	86652	2(3)	86803	1(3)	87070	3(3)
84105	1(3)	84431	1(3)	85055	1(3)	85597	1(3)	86325	2(3)	86653	2(3)	86804	1(2)	87071	2(3)
84106	1(2)	84432	1(2)	85060	1(3)	85598	1(3)	86327	1(3)	86654	2(3)	86805	2(3)	87073	2(3)
84110	1(3)	84436	1(2)	85097	2(3)	85610	4(3)	86328	3(3)	86658	12(3)	86806	2(3)	87075	6(3)
84112	1(3)	84437	1(2)	85130	1(3)	85611	2(3)	86329	3(3)	86663	2(3)	86807	2(3)	87076	2(3)
84119	1(2)	84439	1(2)	85170	1(3)	85612	1(3)	86331	12(3)	86664	2(3)	86808	1(3)	87077	4(3)
84120	1(3)	84442	1(2)	85175	1(3)	85613	3(3)	86332	1(3)	86665	2(3)	86812	1(2)	87081	2(3)
84126	1(3)	84443	4(2)	85210	2(3)	85635	1(3)	86334	2(2)	86666	4(3)	86813	1(2)	87084	1(3)
84132	2(3)	84445	1(2)	85220	2(3)	85651	1(2)	86335	2(3)	86668	2(3)	86816	1(2)	87086	3(3)
84133	2(3)	84446	1(3)	85230	2(3)	85652	1(2)	86336	1(3)	86671	3(3)	86817	1(2)	87088	3(3)
84134	1(3)	84449	1(3)	85240	2(3)	85660	2(3)	86337	1(2)	86674	3(3)	86821	1(3)	87101	2(3)
84135	1(3)	84450	1(3)	85244	1(3)	85670	2(3)	86340	1(2)	86677	3(3)	86825	1(3)	87102	4(3)
84138	1(3)	84460	1(3)	85245	2(3)	85675	1(3)	86341	4(3)	86682	2(3)	86826	2(3)	87103	2(3)
84140	1(3)	84466	1(3)	85246	2(3)	85705	1(3)	86343	1(3)	86684	2(3)	86828	1(3)	87106	3(3)
84143	2(3)	84478	1(3)	85247	2(3)	85730	4(3)	86344	1(2)	86687	1(3)	86829	1(3)	87107	4(3)
84144	1(3)	84479	1(2)	85250	2(3)	85732	4(3)	86352	1(3)	86688	1(3)	86830	2(3)	87109	2(3)
84145	1(3)	84480	1(2)	85260	2(3)	85810	2(3)	86353	7(3)	86689	2(3)	86831	2(3)	87110	2(3)
84146	3(3)	84481	1(2)	85270	2(3)	85999	1(3)	86355	1(2)	86692	2(3)	86832	2(3)	87116	2(3)
84150	2(3)	84482	1(2)	85280	2(3)	86000	6(3)	86356	7(3)	86694	2(3)	86833	1(3)	87118	3(3)
84152	1(2)	84484	2(3)	85290	2(3)	86001	20(3)	86357	1(2)	86695	2(3)	86834	1(3)	87140	3(3)
84153	1(2)	84485	1(3)	85291	1(3)	86005	2(3)	86359	1(2)	86696	2(3)	86835	1(3)	87143	2(3)
84154	1(2)	84488	1(3)	85292	1(3)	86008	20(3)	86360	1(2)	86698	3(3)	86849	1(3)	87149	4(3)
84155	1(3)	84490	1(2)	85293	1(3)	86021	1(2)	86361	1(2)	86701	1(3)	86850	3(3)	87150	12(3)
84156	1(3)	84510	1(3)	85300	2(3)	86022	1(2)	86367	1(3)	86702	2(3)	86860	2(3)	87152	1(3)
84157	2(3)	84512	1(3)	85301	1(3)	86023	3(3)	86376	2(3)	86703	1(2)	86870	2(3)	87153	3(3)
84160	2(3)	84520	1(3)	85302	1(3)	86038	1(3)	86382	3(3)	86704	1(2)	86880	4(3)	87158	1(3)
84163	1(3)	84525	1(3)	85303	1(3)	86039	1(3)	86384	1(3)	86705	1(2)	86885	2(3)	87164	2(3)
84165	1(2)	84540	2(3)	85305	2(3)	86060	1(3)	86386	1(2)	86706	2(3)	86886	3(3)	87166	2(3)
84166	2(3)	84545	1(3)	85306	2(3)	86063	1(3)	86403	2(3)	86707	1(3)	86890	1(3)	87168	2(3)
84181	3(3)	84550	1(3)	85307	2(3)	86077	1(2)	86406	2(3)	86708	1(2)	86891	1(3)	87169	2(3)
84182	6(3)	84560	2(3)	85335	2(3)	86078	1(3)	86408	1(3)	86709	1(2)	86900	1(3)	87172	1(3)
84202	1(2)	84577	1(3)	85337	1(3)	86079	1(3)	86409	1(3)	86710	4(3)	86901	1(3)	87176	2(3)
84203	1(2)	84578	1(3)	85345	1(3)	86140	1(2)	86413	3(3)	86711	2(3)	86902	6(3)	87177	3(3)
84206	1(2)	84580	1(3)	85347	3(3)	86141	1(2)	86430	2(3)	86713	3(3)	86904	2(3)	87181	12(3)
84207	1(2)	84583	1(3)	85348	1(3)	86146	3(3)	86431	2(3)	86717	8(3)	86905	8(3)	87184	8(3)
84210	1(3)	84585	1(2)	85360	1(3)	86147	4(3)	86480	1(3)	86720	2(3)	86906	1(2)	87185	4(3)
84220	1(3)	84586	1(2)	85362	2(3)	86148	3(3)	86481	1(3)	86723	2(3)	86910	0(3)	87186	12(3)
84228	1(3)	84588	1(3)	85366	1(3)	86152	1(3)	86485	1(2)	86727	2(3)	86911	0(3)	87187	3(3)
84233	1(3)	84590	1(2)	85370	1(3)	86153	1(3)	86486	2(3)	86732	2(3)	86920	9(3)	87188	6(3)
84234	1(3)	84591	1(3)	85378	1(3)	86155	1(3)	86490	1(2)	86735	2(3)	86921	2(3)	87190	9(3)
84235	1(3)	84597	1(3)	85379	2(3)	86156	1(2)	86510	1(2)	86738	2(3)	86922	5(3)	87197	1(3)
84238	3(3)	84600	2(3)	85380	1(3)	86157	1(2)	86580	1(2)	86741	2(3)	86923	10(3)	87205	3(3)
84244	2(3)	84620	1(2)	85384	2(3)	86160	4(3)	86590	1(3)	86744	2(3)	86927	2(3)	87206	6(3)
84252	1(2)	84630	2(3)	85385	1(3)	86161	2(3)	86592	2(3)	86747	2(3)	86930	0(3)	87207	3(3)
84255	2(3)	84681	1(3)	85390	3(3)	86162	1(2)	86593	2(3)	86750	4(3)	86931	1(3)	87209	4(3)
84260	1(3)	84702	2(3)	85396	1(2)	86171	2(3)	86602	3(3)	86753	3(3)	86932	1(3)	87210	4(3)
84270	1(3)	84703	1(3)	85397	2(3)	86200	1(3)	86603	2(3)	86756	2(3)	86940	1(3)	87220	3(3)
84275	1(3)	84704	1(3)	85400	1(3)	86215	1(3)	86609	14(3)	86757	6(3)	86941	1(3)	87230	2(3)
84285	1(3)	84830	1(2)	85410	1(3)	86225	1(3)	86611	4(3)	86759	2(3)	86945	2(3)	87250	1(3)
84295	1(3)	84999	1(3)	85415	2(3)	86226	1(3)	86612	2(3)	86762	2(3)	86950	1(3)	87252	2(3)
84300	2(3)	85002	1(3)	85420	2(3)	86235	10(3)	86615	6(3)	86765	2(3)	86960	1(3)	87253	2(3)
84302	1(3)	85004	1(3)	85421	1(3)	86255	5(3)	86617	2(3)	86768	5(3)	86965	1(3)	87254	7(3)

CPT	MUE	CPT	MUE	CPT	MUE	CPT	MUE	CPT	MUE	CPT	MUE	CPT	MUE	CPT	MUE
87255	2(3)	87493	2(3)	87650	1(3)	88153	1(3)	88334	5(3)	89320	1(2)	90655	1(2)	90840	3(3)
87260	1(3)	87495	1(3)	87651	1(3)	88155	1(3)	88341	13(3)	89321	1(2)	90656	1(2)	90845	1(2)
87265	1(3)	87496	1(3)	87652	1(3)	88160	4(3)	88342	4(3)	89322	1(2)	90657	1(2)	90846	1(3)
87267	1(3)	87497	2(3)	87653	1(3)	88161	4(3)	88344	6(3)	89325	1(2)	90658	1(2)	90847	1(3)
87269	1(3)	87498	1(3)	87660	1(3)	88162	3(3)	88346	2(3)	89329	1(2)	90660	1(2)	90849	1(3)
87270	1(3)	87500	1(3)	87661	1(3)	88164	1(3)	88348	1(3)	89330	1(2)	90661	1(2)	90853	1(3)
87271	1(3)	87501	1(3)	87662	2(3)	88165	1(3)	88350	9(3)	89331	1(2)	90662	1(2)	90863	1(3)
87272	1(3)	87502	1(3)	87797	3(3)	88166	1(3)	88355	1(3)	89335	1(3)	90664	1(2)	90865	1(3)
87273	1(3)	87503	1(3)	87798	13(3)	88167	1(3)	88356	3(3)	89337	1(2)	90666	1(2)	90867	1(2)
87274	1(3)	87505	1(2)	87799	3(3)	88172	5(3)	88358	2(3)	89342	1(2)	90667	1(2)	90868	1(3)
87275	1(3)	87506	1(2)	87800	2(3)	88173	5(3)	88360	6(3)	89343	1(2)	90668	1(2)	90869	1(3)
87276	1(3)	87507	1(2)	87801	3(3)	88174	1(3)	88361	6(3)	89344	1(2)	90670	1(2)	90870	2(3)
87278	1(3)	87510	1(3)	87802	2(3)	88175	1(3)	88362	1(3)	89346	1(2)	90672	1(2)	90875	1(3)
87279	1(3)	87511	1(3)	87803	3(3)	88177	6(3)	88363	2(3)	89352	1(2)	90673	1(2)	90876	0(3)
87280	1(3)	87512	1(3)	87804	3(3)	88182	2(3)	88364	3(3)	89353	1(3)	90674	1(2)	90880	1(3)
87281	1(3)	87516	1(3)	87806	1(2)	88184	2(3)	88365	4(3)	89354	1(3)	90675	1(2)	90882	0(3)
87283	1(3)	87517	1(3)	87807	2(3)	88185	35(3)	88366	2(3)	89356	2(3)	90676	1(2)	90885	0(3)
87285	1(3)	87520	1(3)	87808	1(3)	88187	2(3)	88367	3(3)	89398	1(3)	90680	1(2)	90887	0(3)
87290	1(3)	87521	1(3)	87809	2(3)	88188	2(3)	88368	3(3)	90281	0(3)	90681	1(2)	90889	0(3)
87299	1(3)	87522	1(3)	87810	2(3)	88189	2(3)	88369	3(3)	90283	0(3)	90682	1(2)	90899	1(3)
87300	2(3)	87525	1(3)	87811	3(3)	88199	1(3)	88371	1(3)	90284	0(3)	90685	1(2)	90901	1(3)
87301	1(3)	87526	1(3)	87850	1(3)	88230	2(3)	88372	1(3)	90287	0(3)	90686	1(2)	90912	1(3)
87305	1(3)	87527	1(3)	87880	2(3)	88233	2(3)	88373	3(3)	90288	0(3)	90687	1(2)	90913	3(3)
87320	1(3)	87528	1(3)	87899	4(3)	88235	2(3)	88374	5(3)	90291	0(3)	90688	1(2)	90935	1(3)
87324	2(3)	87529	2(3)	87900	1(2)	88237	4(3)	88375	1(3)	90296	1(2)	90689	1(2)	90937	1(3)
87327	1(3)	87530	2(3)	87901	1(2)	88239	3(3)	88377	5(3)	90371	10(3)	90690	1(2)	90940	1(3)
87328	2(3)	87531	1(3)	87902	1(2)	88240	1(3)	88380	1(3)	90375	20(3)	90691	1(2)	90945	1(3)
87329	2(3)	87532	1(3)	87903	1(2)	88241	3(3)	88381	1(3)	90376	20(3)	90694	1(2)	90947	1(3)
87332	1(3)	87533	1(3)	87904	14(3)	88245	1(2)	88387	2(3)	90377	20(3)	90696	1(2)	90951	1(2)
87335	1(3)	87534	1(3)	87905	2(3)	88248	1(2)	88388	1(3)	90378	4(3)	90697	1(2)	90952	1(2)
87336	1(3)	87535	1(3)	87906	2(3)	88249	1(2)	88399	1(3)	90384	0(3)	90698	1(2)	90953	1(2)
87337	1(3)	87536	1(3)	87910	1(3)	88261	2(3)	88720	1(3)	90385	1(2)	90700	1(2)	90954	1(2)
87338	1(3)	87537	1(3)	87912	1(3)	88262	2(3)	88738	1(3)	90386	0(3)	90702	1(2)	90955	1(2)
87339	1(3)	87538	1(3)	87999	1(3)	88263	1(3)	88740	1(2)	90389	0(3)	90707	1(2)	90956	1(2)
87340	1(2)	87539	1(3)	88000	0(3)	88264	1(3)	88741	1(2)	90393	1(2)	90710	1(2)	90957	1(2)
87341	1(2)	87540	1(3)	88005	0(3)	88267	2(3)	88749	1(3)	90396	1(2)	90713	1(2)	90958	1(2)
87350	1(2)	87541	1(3)	88007	0(3)	88269	2(3)	89049	1(3)	90399	0(3)	90714	1(2)	90959	1(2)
87380	1(2)	87542	1(3)	88012	0(3)	88271	16(3)	89050	2(3)	90460	9(3)	90715	1(2)	90960	1(2)
87385	2(3)	87550	1(3)	88014	0(3)	88272	12(3)	89051	2(3)	90461	8(3)	90716	1(2)	90961	1(2)
87389	1(3)	87551	2(3)	88016	0(3)	88273	3(3)	89055	2(3)	90471	1(2)	90717	1(2)	90962	1(2)
87390	1(3)	87552	1(3)	88020	0(3)	88274	5(3)	89060	2(3)	90472	8(3)	90723	0(3)	90963	1(2)
87391	1(3)	87555	1(3)	88025	0(3)	88275	12(3)	89125	2(3)	90473	1(2)	90732	1(2)	90964	1(2)
87400	2(3)	87556	1(3)	88027	0(3)	88280	1(3)	89160	1(3)	90474	1(3)	90733	1(2)	90965	1(2)
87420	1(3)	87557	1(3)	88028	0(3)	88283	5(3)	89190	1(3)	90476	1(2)	90734	1(2)	90966	1(2)
87425	1(3)	87560	1(3)	88029	0(3)	88285	10(3)	89220	2(3)	90477	1(2)	90736	1(2)	90967	1(2)
87426	3(3)	87561	1(3)	88036	0(3)	88289	1(3)	89230	1(2)	90581	1(2)	90738	1(2)	90968	1(2)
87427	2(3)	87562	1(3)	88037	0(3)	88291	1(3)	89240	1(3)	90585	1(2)	90739	1(2)	90969	1(2)
87428	3(3)	87563	3(3)	88040	0(3)	88299	1(3)	89250	1(2)	90586	1(2)	90740	1(2)	90970	1(2)
87430	1(3)	87580	1(3)	88045	0(3)	88300	4(3)	89251	1(2)	90587	1(2)	90743	1(2)	90989	1(2)
87449	3(3)	87581	1(3)	88099	0(3)	88302	4(3)	89253	1(3)	90619	1(2)	90744	1(2)	90993	1(3)
87450	2(3)	87582	1(3)	88104	5(3)	88304	5(3)	89254	1(3)	90620	1(2)	90746	1(2)	90997	1(3)
87451	2(3)	87590	1(3)	88106	5(3)	88305	16(3)	89255	1(3)	90621	1(2)	90747	1(2)	90999	1(3)
87471	1(3)	87591	3(3)	88108	6(3)	88307	8(3)	89257	1(3)	90625	1(2)	90748	0(3)	91010	1(2)
87472	1(3)	87592	1(3)	88112	6(3)	88309	3(3)	89258	1(2)	90630	1(2)	90749	1(3)	91013	1(3)
87475	1(3)	87623	1(2)	88120	2(3)	88311	4(3)	89259	1(2)	90632	1(2)	90750	1(2)	91020	1(2)
87476	1(3)	87624	1(3)	88121	2(3)	88312	9(3)	89260	1(2)	90633	1(2)	90756	1(2)	91022	1(2)
87480	1(3)	87625	1(3)	88125	1(3)	88313	8(3)	89261	1(2)	90634	1(2)	90785	3(3)	91030	1(2)
87481	5(3)	87631	1(3)	88130	1(2)	88314	6(3)	89264	1(3)	90636	1(2)	90791	1(3)	91034	1(2)
87482	1(3)	87632	1(3)	88140	1(2)	88319	11(3)	89268	1(2)	90644	1(2)	90792	1(3)	91035	1(2)
87483	1(2)	87633	1(3)	88141	1(3)	88321	1(2)	89272	1(2)	90647	1(2)	90832	2(3)	91037	1(2)
87485	1(3)	87634	1(3)	88142	1(3)	88323	1(2)	89280	1(2)	90648	1(2)	90833	2(3)	91038	1(2)
87486	1(3)	87635	2(3)	88143	1(3)	88325	1(2)	89281	1(2)	90649	1(2)	90834	2(3)	91040	1(2)
87487	1(3)	87636	3(3)	88147	1(3)	88329	2(3)	89290	1(2)	90650	1(2)	90836	2(3)	91065	2(2)
87490	1(3)	87637	3(3)	88148	1(3)	88331	11(3)	89291	1(2)	90651	1(2)	90837	2(3)	91110	1(2)
87491	3(3)	87640	1(3)	88150	1(3)	88332	13(3)	89300	1(2)	90653	1(2)	90838	2(3)	91111	1(2)
87492	1(3)	87641	1(3)	88152	1(3)	88333	4(3)	89310	1(2)	90654	1(2)	90839	1(2)	91112	1(3)

Appendix I — Medically Unlikely Edits (MUEs)—Practitioner

CPT	MUE	CPT	MUE	CPT	MUE	CPT	MUE	CPT	MUE	CPT	MUE	CPT	MUE	CPT	MUE
91117	1(2)	92342	0(3)	92584	1(2)	92979	2(3)	93312	1(3)	93623	1(3)	94013	1(3)	95132	0(3)
91120	1(2)	92352	0(3)	92587	1(2)	92986	1(2)	93313	1(3)	93624	1(3)	94014	1(2)	95133	0(3)
91122	1(2)	92353	0(3)	92588	1(2)	92987	1(2)	93314	1(3)	93631	1(3)	94015	1(2)	95134	0(3)
91132	1(3)	92354	0(3)	92590	0(3)	92990	1(2)	93315	1(3)	93640	1(3)	94016	1(2)	95144	30(3)
91133	1(3)	92355	0(3)	92591	0(3)	92997	1(2)	93316	1(3)	93641	1(2)	94060	1(3)	95145	10(3)
91200	1(2)	92358	0(3)	92592	0(3)	92998	2(3)	93317	1(3)	93642	1(3)	94070	1(2)	95146	10(3)
91299	1(3)	92370	0(3)	92593	0(3)	93000	3(3)	93318	1(3)	93644	1(3)	94150	0(3)	95147	10(3)
91300	1(2)	92371	0(3)	92594	0(3)	93005	3(3)	93320	2(3)	93650	1(2)	94200	1(3)	95148	10(3)
91301	1(2)	92499	1(3)	92595	0(3)	93010	5(3)	93321	1(3)	93653	1(3)	94375	1(3)	95149	10(3)
91302	1(2)	92502	1(3)	92596	1(2)	93015	1(3)	93325	2(3)	93654	1(3)	94450	1(3)	95165	30(3)
91303	1(2)	92504	1(3)	92597	1(3)	93016	1(3)	93350	1(2)	93655	2(3)	94452	1(2)	95170	10(3)
91304	1(2)	92507	1(3)	92601	1(3)	93017	1(3)	93351	1(2)	93656	1(3)	94453	1(2)	95180	6(3)
92002	1(2)	92508	1(3)	92602	1(3)	93018	1(3)	93352	1(3)	93657	2(3)	94610	2(3)	95199	1(3)
92004	1(2)	92511	1(3)	92603	1(3)	93024	1(3)	93355	1(3)	93660	1(3)	94617	1(3)	95249	1(2)
92012	1(3)	92512	1(2)	92604	1(3)	93025	1(2)	93356	1(3)	93662	1(3)	94618	1(3)	95250	1(2)
92014	1(3)	92516	1(3)	92605	0(3)	93040	3(3)	93451	1(3)	93668	1(3)	94619	1(3)	95251	1(2)
92015	0(3)	92517	1(2)	92606	0(3)	93041	2(3)	93452	1(3)	93701	1(2)	94621	1(3)	95700	1(2)
92018	1(2)	92518	1(2)	92607	1(3)	93042	3(3)	93453	1(3)	93702	1(2)	94640	4(3)	95705	1(2)
92019	1(2)	92519	1(2)	92608	4(3)	93050	1(3)	93454	1(3)	93724	1(3)	94642	1(3)	95706	1(2)
92020	1(2)	92520	1(2)	92609	1(3)	93224	1(2)	93455	1(3)	93740	0(3)	94644	1(2)	95707	1(2)
92025	1(2)	92521	1(2)	92610	1(2)	93225	1(2)	93456	1(3)	93745	1(2)	94645	2(3)	95708	4(3)
92060	1(2)	92522	1(2)	92611	1(3)	93226	1(2)	93457	1(3)	93750	4(3)	94660	1(3)	95709	4(3)
92065	1(2)	92523	1(2)	92612	1(3)	93227	1(2)	93458	1(3)	93770	0(3)	94662	1(2)	95710	4(3)
92071	2(2)	92524	1(2)	92613	1(2)	93228	1(2)	93459	1(3)	93784	1(2)	94664	1(3)	95711	1(2)
92072	1(2)	92526	1(2)	92614	1(3)	93229	1(2)	93460	1(3)	93786	1(2)	94667	1(2)	95712	1(2)
92081	1(2)	92531	0(3)	92615	1(2)	93241	1(2)	93461	1(3)	93788	1(2)	94668	2(3)	95713	1(2)
92082	1(2)	92532	0(3)	92616	1(3)	93242	1(2)	93462	1(3)	93790	1(2)	94669	2(3)	95714	4(3)
92083	1(2)	92533	0(3)	92617	1(2)	93243	1(2)	93463	1(3)	93792	1(2)	94680	1(3)	95715	4(3)
92100	1(2)	92534	0(3)	92618	1(3)	93244	1(2)	93464	1(3)	93793	1(2)	94681	1(3)	95716	4(3)
92132	1(2)	92537	1(2)	92620	1(2)	93245	1(2)	93503	2(3)	93797	2(2)	94690	1(3)	95717	1(2)
92133	1(2)	92538	1(2)	92621	2(3)	93246	1(2)	93505	1(2)	93798	2(2)	94726	1(3)	95718	1(2)
92134	1(2)	92540	1(3)	92625	1(2)	93247	1(2)	93530	1(3)	93799	1(3)	94727	1(3)	95719	1(2)
92136	2(2)	92541	1(3)	92626	1(2)	93248	1(2)	93531	1(3)	93880	1(3)	94728	1(3)	95720	1(2)
92145	1(2)	92542	1(3)	92627	6(3)	93260	1(2)	93532	1(3)	93882	1(3)	94729	1(3)	95721	1(2)
92201	1(2)	92544	1(3)	92630	0(3)	93261	1(3)	93533	1(3)	93886	1(3)	94760	1(3)	95722	1(2)
92202	1(2)	92545	1(3)	92633	0(3)	93264	1(2)	93561	1(3)	93888	1(3)	94761	1(2)	95723	1(2)
92227	1(2)	92546	1(3)	92640	1(3)	93268	1(2)	93562	1(3)	93890	1(3)	94762	1(2)	95724	1(2)
92228	1(2)	92547	1(3)	92650	1(2)	93270	1(2)	93563	1(3)	93892	1(3)	94772	1(2)	95725	1(2)
92229	1(2)	92548	1(3)	92651	1(2)	93271	1(2)	93564	1(3)	93893	1(3)	94774	1(2)	95726	1(2)
92230	2(2)	92549	1(3)	92652	1(2)	93272	1(2)	93565	1(3)	93895	1(3)	94775	1(2)	95782	1(2)
92235	1(2)	92550	1(3)	92653	1(2)	93278	1(3)	93566	1(3)	93922	2(2)	94776	1(2)	95783	1(2)
92240	1(2)	92551	0(3)	92700	1(3)	93279	1(3)	93567	1(3)	93923	2(2)	94777	1(2)	95800	1(2)
92242	1(2)	92552	1(2)	92920	3(3)	93280	1(3)	93568	1(3)	93924	1(2)	94780	1(2)	95801	1(2)
92250	1(2)	92553	1(2)	92921	6(2)	93281	1(3)	93571	1(3)	93925	1(3)	94781	2(3)	95803	1(2)
92260	1(2)	92555	1(2)	92924	2(3)	93282	1(3)	93572	2(3)	93926	1(3)	94799	1(3)	95805	1(2)
92265	1(2)	92556	1(2)	92925	6(2)	93283	1(3)	93580	1(3)	93930	1(3)	95004	80(3)	95806	1(2)
92270	1(2)	92557	1(2)	92928	3(3)	93284	1(3)	93581	1(3)	93931	1(3)	95012	2(3)	95807	1(2)
92273	1(2)	92558	0(3)	92929	2(3)	93285	1(3)	93582	1(2)	93970	1(3)	95017	27(3)	95808	1(2)
92274	1(2)	92559	0(3)	92933	2(3)	93286	2(3)	93583	1(2)	93971	1(3)	95018	19(3)	95810	1(2)
92283	1(2)	92560	0(3)	92934	2(3)	93287	2(3)	93590	1(2)	93975	1(3)	95024	40(3)	95811	1(2)
92284	1(2)	92561	1(2)	92937	2(3)	93288	1(3)	93591	1(2)	93976	1(3)	95027	90(3)	95812	1(3)
92285	1(2)	92562	1(2)	92938	2(3)	93289	1(3)	93592	2(3)	93978	1(3)	95028	30(3)	95813	1(3)
92286	1(2)	92563	1(2)	92941	1(3)	93290	1(3)	93600	1(3)	93979	1(3)	95044	80(3)	95816	1(3)
92287	1(2)	92564	1(2)	92943	2(3)	93291	1(3)	93602	1(3)	93980	1(3)	95052	20(3)	95819	1(3)
92310	0(3)	92565	1(2)	92944	2(3)	93292	1(3)	93603	1(3)	93981	1(3)	95056	1(2)	95822	1(3)
92311	1(2)	92567	1(2)	92950	2(3)	93293	1(2)	93609	1(3)	93985	1(3)	95060	1(2)	95824	1(3)
92312	1(2)	92568	1(2)	92953	2(3)	93294	1(2)	93610	1(3)	93986	1(3)	95065	1(3)	95829	1(3)
92313	1(3)	92570	1(2)	92960	2(3)	93295	1(2)	93612	1(3)	93990	2(3)	95070	1(3)	95830	1(3)
92314	0(3)	92571	1(2)	92961	1(3)	93296	1(2)	93613	1(3)	93998	1(3)	95076	1(2)	95836	1(2)
92315	1(2)	92572	1(2)	92970	1(3)	93297	1(2)	93615	1(3)	94002	1(2)	95079	2(3)	95851	3(3)
92316	1(2)	92575	1(2)	92971	1(3)	93298	1(2)	93616	1(3)	94003	1(2)	95115	1(2)	95852	1(3)
92317	1(3)	92576	1(2)	92973	2(3)	93303	1(3)	93618	1(3)	94004	1(2)	95117	1(2)	95857	1(2)
92325	1(3)	92577	1(2)	92974	1(3)	93304	1(3)	93619	1(3)	94005	1(3)	95120	0(3)	95860	1(3)
92326	2(2)	92579	1(2)	92975	1(3)	93306	1(3)	93620	1(3)	94010	1(3)	95125	0(3)	95861	1(3)
92340	0(3)	92582	1(2)	92977	1(3)	93307	1(3)	93621	1(3)	94011	1(3)	95130	0(3)	95863	1(3)
92341	0(3)	92583	1(2)	92978	1(3)	93308	1(3)	93622	1(3)	94012	1(3)	95131	0(3)	95864	1(3)

CPT	MUE	CPT	MUE	CPT	MUE	CPT	MUE	CPT	MUE	CPT	MUE	CPT	MUE	CPT	MUE
95865	1(3)	96020	1(2)	96542	1(3)	97171	0(3)	99091	1(2)	99285	1(3)	99403	0(3)	99498	3(3)
95866	1(3)	96040	4(3)	96549	1(3)	97172	0(3)	99100	1(3)	99288	0(3)	99404	0(3)	99499	1(3)
95867	1(3)	96105	3(3)	96567	1(3)	97530	6(3)	99116	0(3)	99291	1(2)	99406	1(2)	99500	0(3)
95868	1(3)	96110	3(3)	96570	1(2)	97533	4(3)	99135	0(3)	99292	8(3)	99407	1(2)	99501	0(3)
95869	1(3)	96112	1(2)	96571	2(3)	97535	8(3)	99140	0(3)	99304	1(2)	99408	0(3)	99502	0(3)
95870	4(3)	96113	6(3)	96573	1(2)	97537	6(3)	99151	1(3)	99305	1(2)	99409	0(3)	99503	0(3)
95872	4(3)	96116	1(2)	96574	1(2)	97542	8(3)	99152	2(3)	99306	1(2)	99411	0(3)	99504	0(3)
95873	1(2)	96121	3(3)	96900	1(3)	97545	1(2)	99153	9(3)	99307	1(2)	99412	0(3)	99505	0(3)
95874	1(2)	96125	2(3)	96902	0(3)	97546	2(3)	99155	1(3)	99308	1(2)	99415	1(2)	99506	0(3)
95875	2(3)	96127	2(3)	96904	1(2)	97597	1(3)	99156	1(3)	99309	1(2)	99416	3(3)	99507	0(3)
95885	4(2)	96130	1(2)	96910	1(3)	97598	8(3)	99157	6(3)	99310	1(2)	99417	4(3)	99509	0(3)
95886	4(2)	96131	7(3)	96912	1(3)	97602	0(3)	99170	1(3)	99315	1(2)	99421	1(2)	99510	0(3)
95887	1(2)	96132	1(2)	96913	1(3)	97605	1(3)	99172	0(3)	99316	1(2)	99422	1(2)	99511	0(3)
95905	2(3)	96133	7(3)	96920	1(2)	97606	1(3)	99173	0(3)	99318	1(2)	99423	1(2)	99512	0(3)
95907	1(2)	96136	1(2)	96921	1(2)	97607	1(3)	99174	0(3)	99324	1(2)	99429	0(3)	99600	0(3)
95908	1(2)	96137	11(3)	96922	1(2)	97608	1(3)	99175	1(3)	99325	1(2)	99439	2(2)	99601	0(3)
95909	1(2)	96138	1(2)	96931	1(2)	97610	1(2)	99177	1(2)	99326	1(2)	99441	1(2)	99602	0(3)
95910	1(2)	96139	11(3)	96932	1(2)	97750	8(3)	99183	1(3)	99327	1(2)	99442	1(2)	99605	0(2)
95911	1(2)	96146	1(2)	96933	1(2)	97755	1(3)	99184	1(2)	99328	1(2)	99443	1(2)	99606	0(3)
95912	1(2)	96156	1(3)	96934	2(3)	97760	6(3)	99188	1(3)	99334	1(3)	99446	1(2)	99607	0(3)
95913	1(2)	96158	1(2)	96935	2(3)	97761	6(3)	99190	1(3)	99335	1(3)	99447	1(2)	A0021	0(3)
95921	1(3)	96159	4(3)	96936	2(3)	97763	6(3)	99191	1(3)	99336	1(3)	99448	1(2)	A0080	0(3)
95922	1(3)	96160	3(3)	96999	1(3)	97799	1(3)	99192	1(3)	99337	1(3)	99449	1(2)	A0090	0(3)
95923	1(3)	96161	1(3)	97010	0(3)	97802	8(3)	99195	2(3)	99339	0(3)	99450	0(3)	A0100	0(3)
95924	1(3)	96164	1(2)	97012	1(3)	97803	8(3)	99199	1(3)	99340	0(3)	99451	1(2)	A0110	0(3)
95925	1(3)	96165	6(3)	97014	0(3)	97804	6(3)	99202	1(2)	99341	1(2)	99452	1(2)	A0120	0(3)
95926	1(3)	96167	1(2)	97016	1(3)	97810	1(2)	99203	1(2)	99342	1(2)	99453	1(2)	A0130	0(3)
95927	1(3)	96168	6(3)	97018	1(3)	97811	2(3)	99204	1(2)	99343	1(2)	99454	1(2)	A0140	0(3)
95928	1(3)	96170	1(3)	97022	1(3)	97813	1(2)	99205	1(2)	99344	1(2)	99455	1(3)	A0160	0(3)
95929	1(3)	96171	2(3)	97024	1(3)	97814	2(3)	99211	1(3)	99345	1(2)	99456	1(3)	A0170	0(3)
95930	1(3)	96360	1(3)	97026	1(3)	98925	1(2)	99212	2(3)	99347	1(3)	99457	1(2)	A0180	0(3)
95933	1(3)	96361	8(3)	97028	1(3)	98926	1(2)	99213	2(3)	99348	1(3)	99458	3(3)	A0190	0(3)
95937	4(3)	96365	1(3)	97032	4(3)	98927	1(2)	99214	2(3)	99349	1(3)	99460	1(2)	A0200	0(3)
95938	1(3)	96366	8(3)	97033	4(3)	98928	1(2)	99215	1(3)	99350	1(3)	99461	1(2)	A0210	0(3)
95939	1(3)	96367	4(3)	97034	2(3)	98929	1(2)	99217	1(2)	99354	1(2)	99462	1(2)	A0225	0(3)
95940	32(3)	96368	1(2)	97035	2(3)	98940	1(2)	99218	1(2)	99355	4(3)	99463	1(2)	A0380	0(3)
95941	0(3)	96369	1(2)	97036	3(3)	98941	1(2)	99219	1(2)	99356	1(2)	99464	1(2)	A0382	0(3)
95943	1(3)	96370	3(3)	97039	1(3)	98942	1(2)	99220	1(2)	99357	4(3)	99465	1(2)	A0384	0(3)
95954	1(3)	96371	1(3)	97110	6(3)	98943	0(3)	99221	1(3)	99358	1(2)	99466	1(2)	A0390	0(3)
95955	1(3)	96372	4(3)	97112	4(3)	98960	0(3)	99222	1(3)	99359	2(3)	99467	4(3)	A0392	0(3)
95957	1(3)	96373	2(3)	97113	6(3)	98961	0(3)	99223	1(3)	99360	1(3)	99468	1(2)	A0394	0(3)
95958	1(3)	96374	1(3)	97116	4(3)	98962	0(3)	99224	1(2)	99366	0(3)	99469	1(2)	A0396	0(3)
95961	1(2)	96375	6(3)	97124	4(3)	98966	1(2)	99225	1(2)	99367	0(3)	99471	1(2)	A0398	0(3)
95962	5(3)	96376	0(3)	97129	1(2)	98967	1(2)	99226	1(2)	99368	0(3)	99472	1(2)	A0420	0(3)
95965	1(3)	96377	1(3)	97130	7(3)	98968	1(2)	99231	1(3)	99374	0(3)	99473	1(2)	A0422	0(3)
95966	1(3)	96379	1(3)	97139	1(3)	98970	1(2)	99232	1(3)	99375	0(3)	99474	1(2)	A0424	0(3)
95967	3(3)	96401	3(3)	97140	6(3)	98971	1(2)	99233	1(3)	99377	0(3)	99475	1(2)	A0425	250(1)
95970	1(3)	96402	2(3)	97150	1(3)	98972	1(2)	99234	1(3)	99378	0(3)	99476	1(2)	A0426	2(3)
95971	1(3)	96405	1(2)	97151	8(3)	99000	0(3)	99235	1(3)	99379	0(3)	99477	1(2)	A0427	2(3)
95972	1(3)	96406	1(2)	97152	16(3)	99001	0(3)	99236	1(3)	99380	0(3)	99478	1(2)	A0428	2(3)
95976	1(3)	96409	1(3)	97153	32(3)	99002	0(3)	99238	1(3)	99381	0(3)	99479	1(2)	A0429	2(3)
95977	1(3)	96411	3(3)	97154	18(3)	99024	1(3)	99239	1(3)	99382	0(3)	99480	1(2)	A0430	1(3)
95980	1(3)	96413	1(3)	97155	24(3)	99026	0(3)	99241	0(3)	99383	0(3)	99483	1(2)	A0431	1(3)
95981	1(3)	96415	8(3)	97156	16(3)	99027	0(3)	99242	0(3)	99384	0(3)	99484	1(2)	A0432	1(3)
95982	1(3)	96416	1(3)	97157	16(3)	99050	0(3)	99243	0(3)	99385	0(3)	99485	1(2)	A0433	1(3)
95983	1(2)	96417	3(3)	97158	16(3)	99051	0(3)	99244	0(3)	99386	0(3)	99486	4(1)	A0434	2(3)
95984	11(3)	96420	1(3)	97161	1(2)	99053	0(3)	99245	0(3)	99387	0(3)	99487	1(2)	A0435	999(3)
95990	1(3)	96422	2(3)	97162	1(2)	99056	0(3)	99251	0(3)	99391	0(3)	99489	10(3)	A0436	300(3)
95991	1(3)	96423	1(3)	97163	1(2)	99058	0(3)	99252	0(3)	99392	0(3)	99490	1(2)	A0888	0(3)
95992	1(2)	96425	1(3)	97164	1(2)	99060	0(3)	99253	0(3)	99393	0(3)	99491	1(2)	A0998	0(3)
95999	1(3)	96440	1(3)	97165	1(2)	99070	0(3)	99254	0(3)	99394	0(3)	99492	1(2)	A0999	1(3)
96000	1(2)	96446	1(3)	97166	1(2)	99071	0(3)	99255	0(3)	99395	0(3)	99493	1(2)	A4206	0(3)
96001	1(2)	96450	1(3)	97167	1(2)	99075	0(3)	99281	1(3)	99396	0(3)	99494	2(3)	A4207	0(3)
96002	1(3)	96521	2(3)	97168	1(2)	99078	0(3)	99282	1(3)	99397	0(3)	99495	1(2)	A4208	0(3)
96003	1(3)	96522	1(3)	97169	0(3)	99080	0(3)	99283	1(3)	99401	0(3)	99496	1(2)	A4209	0(3)
96004	1(2)	96523	1(3)	97170	0(3)	99082	1(3)	99284	1(3)	99402	0(3)	99497	1(2)	A4210	0(3)

CPT	MUE	CPT	MUE	CPT	MUE	CPT	MUE	CPT	MUE	CPT	MUE	CPT	MUE	CPT	MUE
A4211	0(3)	A4326	0(3)	A4408	1(3)	A4604	0(3)	A4755	0(3)	A6022	0(3)	A6402	0(3)	A7012	0(3)
A4212	0(3)	A4327	0(3)	A4409	1(3)	A4605	0(3)	A4760	0(3)	A6023	0(3)	A6403	0(3)	A7013	0(3)
A4213	0(3)	A4328	0(3)	A4410	2(3)	A4606	0(3)	A4765	0(3)	A6024	0(3)	A6404	0(3)	A7014	0(3)
A4215	0(3)	A4330	0(3)	A4411	1(3)	A4608	0(3)	A4766	0(3)	A6025	0(3)	A6407	0(3)	A7015	0(3)
A4216	0(3)	A4331	1(3)	A4412	1(3)	A4611	0(3)	A4770	0(3)	A6154	0(3)	A6410	2(3)	A7016	0(3)
A4217	0(3)	A4332	2(3)	A4413	2(3)	A4612	0(3)	A4771	0(3)	A6196	0(3)	A6411	0(3)	A7017	0(3)
A4218	0(3)	A4333	1(3)	A4414	1(3)	A4613	0(3)	A4772	0(3)	A6197	0(3)	A6412	0(3)	A7018	0(3)
A4220	1(3)	A4334	2(3)	A4415	1(3)	A4614	0(3)	A4773	0(3)	A6198	0(3)	A6413	0(3)	A7020	0(3)
A4221	0(3)	A4335	0(3)	A4416	2(3)	A4615	0(3)	A4774	0(3)	A6199	0(3)	A6441	0(3)	A7025	0(3)
A4222	0(3)	A4336	1(3)	A4417	2(3)	A4616	0(3)	A4802	0(3)	A6203	0(3)	A6442	0(3)	A7026	0(3)
A4223	0(3)	A4337	0(3)	A4418	2(3)	A4617	0(3)	A4860	0(3)	A6204	0(3)	A6443	0(3)	A7027	0(3)
A4224	0(3)	A4338	0(3)	A4419	2(3)	A4618	1(3)	A4870	0(3)	A6205	0(3)	A6444	0(3)	A7028	0(3)
A4225	0(3)	A4340	0(3)	A4420	1(3)	A4619	0(3)	A4890	0(3)	A6206	0(3)	A6445	0(3)	A7029	0(3)
A4226	0(3)	A4344	0(3)	A4422	7(3)	A4620	0(3)	A4911	0(3)	A6207	0(3)	A6446	0(3)	A7030	0(3)
A4230	0(3)	A4346	0(3)	A4423	2(3)	A4623	0(3)	A4913	0(3)	A6208	0(3)	A6447	0(3)	A7031	0(3)
A4231	0(3)	A4349	1(3)	A4424	1(3)	A4624	0(3)	A4918	0(3)	A6209	0(3)	A6448	0(3)	A7032	0(3)
A4232	0(3)	A4351	0(3)	A4425	1(3)	A4625	30(3)	A4927	0(3)	A6210	0(3)	A6449	0(3)	A7033	0(3)
A4233	0(3)	A4352	0(3)	A4426	2(3)	A4626	0(3)	A4928	0(3)	A6211	0(3)	A6450	0(3)	A7034	0(3)
A4234	0(3)	A4353	1(3)	A4427	1(3)	A4627	0(3)	A4929	0(3)	A6212	0(3)	A6451	0(3)	A7035	0(3)
A4235	0(3)	A4354	0(3)	A4428	1(3)	A4628	0(3)	A4930	0(3)	A6213	0(3)	A6452	0(3)	A7036	0(3)
A4236	0(3)	A4355	0(3)	A4429	2(3)	A4629	0(3)	A4931	0(3)	A6214	0(3)	A6453	0(3)	A7037	0(3)
A4244	0(3)	A4356	0(3)	A4430	1(3)	A4630	0(3)	A4932	0(3)	A6215	0(3)	A6454	0(3)	A7038	0(3)
A4245	0(3)	A4357	0(3)	A4431	1(3)	A4633	0(3)	A5051	0(3)	A6216	0(3)	A6455	0(3)	A7039	0(3)
A4246	0(3)	A4358	0(3)	A4432	2(3)	A4634	0(3)	A5052	0(3)	A6217	0(3)	A6456	0(3)	A7040	2(3)
A4247	0(3)	A4360	1(3)	A4433	1(3)	A4635	0(3)	A5053	0(3)	A6218	0(3)	A6457	0(3)	A7041	2(3)
A4248	0(3)	A4361	0(3)	A4434	1(3)	A4636	0(3)	A5054	0(3)	A6219	0(3)	A6460	1(1)	A7044	0(3)
A4250	0(3)	A4362	0(3)	A4435	2(3)	A4637	0(3)	A5055	0(3)	A6220	0(3)	A6461	1(1)	A7045	0(3)
A4252	0(3)	A4363	1(3)	A4450	0(3)	A4638	0(3)	A5056	90(3)	A6221	0(3)	A6501	0(3)	A7046	0(3)
A4253	0(3)	A4364	0(3)	A4452	0(3)	A4639	0(3)	A5057	90(3)	A6222	0(3)	A6502	0(3)	A7047	0(3)
A4255	0(3)	A4366	1(3)	A4455	0(3)	A4640	0(3)	A5061	0(3)	A6223	0(3)	A6503	0(3)	A7048	2(3)
A4256	0(3)	A4367	0(3)	A4458	0(3)	A4642	1(3)	A5062	0(3)	A6224	0(3)	A6504	0(3)	A7501	0(3)
A4257	0(3)	A4368	1(3)	A4459	0(3)	A4648	5(3)	A5063	0(3)	A6228	0(3)	A6505	0(3)	A7502	0(3)
A4258	0(3)	A4369	1(3)	A4461	2(3)	A4649	1(3)	A5071	0(3)	A6229	0(3)	A6506	0(3)	A7503	0(3)
A4259	0(3)	A4371	1(3)	A4463	0(3)	A4650	3(3)	A5072	0(3)	A6230	0(3)	A6507	0(3)	A7504	0(3)
A4261	0(3)	A4372	1(3)	A4465	0(3)	A4651	0(3)	A5073	0(3)	A6231	0(3)	A6508	0(3)	A7505	0(3)
A4262	0(3)	A4373	1(3)	A4467	0(3)	A4652	0(3)	A5081	0(3)	A6232	0(3)	A6509	0(3)	A7506	0(3)
A4263	0(3)	A4375	2(3)	A4470	0(3)	A4653	0(3)	A5082	0(3)	A6233	0(3)	A6510	0(3)	A7507	0(3)
A4264	0(3)	A4376	2(3)	A4480	0(3)	A4657	0(3)	A5083	5(3)	A6234	0(3)	A6511	0(3)	A7508	0(3)
A4265	0(3)	A4377	2(3)	A4481	0(3)	A4660	0(3)	A5093	0(3)	A6235	0(3)	A6513	0(3)	A7509	0(3)
A4266	0(3)	A4378	2(3)	A4483	0(3)	A4663	0(3)	A5102	0(3)	A6236	0(3)	A6530	0(3)	A7520	0(3)
A4267	0(3)	A4379	2(3)	A4490	0(3)	A4670	0(3)	A5105	0(3)	A6237	0(3)	A6531	0(3)	A7521	0(3)
A4268	0(3)	A4380	2(3)	A4495	0(3)	A4671	0(3)	A5112	0(3)	A6238	0(3)	A6532	0(3)	A7522	0(3)
A4269	0(3)	A4381	2(3)	A4500	0(3)	A4672	0(3)	A5113	0(3)	A6239	0(3)	A6533	0(3)	A7523	0(3)
A4270	0(3)	A4382	2(3)	A4510	0(3)	A4673	0(3)	A5114	0(3)	A6240	0(3)	A6534	0(3)	A7524	0(3)
A4280	0(3)	A4383	2(3)	A4520	0(3)	A4674	0(3)	A5120	150(3)	A6241	0(3)	A6535	0(3)	A7525	8(3)
A4281	0(3)	A4384	2(3)	A4550	0(3)	A4680	0(3)	A5121	0(3)	A6242	0(3)	A6536	0(3)	A7526	0(3)
A4282	0(3)	A4385	2(3)	A4553	0(3)	A4690	0(3)	A5122	0(3)	A6243	0(3)	A6537	0(3)	A7527	0(3)
A4283	0(3)	A4387	1(3)	A4554	0(3)	A4706	0(3)	A5126	0(3)	A6244	0(3)	A6538	0(3)	A8000	0(3)
A4284	0(3)	A4388	1(3)	A4555	0(3)	A4707	0(3)	A5131	0(3)	A6245	0(3)	A6539	0(3)	A8001	0(3)
A4285	0(3)	A4389	2(3)	A4556	0(3)	A4708	0(3)	A5200	2(3)	A6246	0(3)	A6540	0(3)	A8002	0(3)
A4286	0(3)	A4390	1(3)	A4557	0(3)	A4709	0(3)	A5500	0(3)	A6247	0(3)	A6541	0(3)	A8003	0(3)
A4290	2(3)	A4391	1(3)	A4558	0(3)	A4714	0(3)	A5501	0(3)	A6248	0(3)	A6544	0(3)	A8004	0(3)
A4300	0(3)	A4392	2(3)	A4559	0(3)	A4719	0(3)	A5503	0(3)	A6250	0(3)	A6545	0(3)	A9152	0(3)
A4301	1(2)	A4393	1(3)	A4561	1(3)	A4720	0(3)	A5504	0(3)	A6251	0(3)	A6549	0(3)	A9153	0(3)
A4305	0(3)	A4394	1(3)	A4562	1(3)	A4721	0(3)	A5505	0(3)	A6252	0(3)	A6550	0(3)	A9155	1(3)
A4306	0(3)	A4395	3(3)	A4563	1(2)	A4722	0(3)	A5506	0(3)	A6253	0(3)	A7000	0(3)	A9180	0(3)
A4310	0(3)	A4396	2(3)	A4565	2(3)	A4723	0(3)	A5507	0(3)	A6254	0(3)	A7001	0(3)	A9270	0(3)
A4311	0(3)	A4397	0(3)	A4566	0(3)	A4724	0(3)	A5508	0(3)	A6255	0(3)	A7002	0(3)	A9272	0(3)
A4312	0(3)	A4398	0(3)	A4570	0(3)	A4725	0(3)	A5510	0(3)	A6256	0(3)	A7003	0(3)	A9273	0(3)
A4313	0(3)	A4399	0(3)	A4575	0(3)	A4726	0(3)	A5512	0(3)	A6257	0(3)	A7004	0(3)	A9274	0(3)
A4314	0(3)	A4400	0(3)	A4580	0(3)	A4728	0(3)	A5513	0(3)	A6258	0(3)	A7005	0(3)	A9275	0(3)
A4315	0(3)	A4402	0(3)	A4590	0(3)	A4730	0(3)	A5514	0(3)	A6259	0(3)	A7006	0(3)	A9276	0(3)
A4316	0(3)	A4404	0(3)	A4595	0(3)	A4736	0(3)	A6000	0(3)	A6260	0(3)	A7007	0(3)	A9277	0(3)
A4320	0(3)	A4405	1(3)	A4600	0(3)	A4737	0(3)	A6010	0(3)	A6261	0(3)	A7008	0(3)	A9278	0(3)
A4321	1(3)	A4406	1(3)	A4601	0(3)	A4740	0(3)	A6011	0(3)	A6262	0(3)	A7009	0(3)	A9279	0(3)
A4322	0(3)	A4407	2(3)	A4602	0(3)	A4750	0(3)	A6021	0(3)	A6266	0(3)	A7010	0(3)	A9280	0(3)

CPT	MUE	CPT	MUE	CPT	MUE	CPT	MUE	CPT	MUE	CPT	MUE	CPT	MUE	CPT	MUE
A9281	0(3)	A9576	40(3)	B5200	0(3)	C1813	1(3)	C2635	124(3)	C9352	3(3)	D0150	1(3)	E0112	0(3)
A9282	0(3)	A9577	50(3)	B9002	0(3)	C1814	2(3)	C2636	690(3)	C9353	4(3)	D0240	1(3)	E0113	0(3)
A9283	0(3)	A9578	50(3)	B9004	0(3)	C1815	1(3)	C2637	0(3)	C9354	300(3)	D0250	2(3)	E0114	0(3)
A9284	0(3)	A9579	100(3)	B9006	0(3)	C1816	2(3)	C2638	150(3)	C9355	3(3)	D0270	1(3)	E0116	0(3)
A9285	0(3)	A9580	1(3)	B9998	0(3)	C1817	1(3)	C2639	150(3)	C9356	125(3)	D0272	1(3)	E0117	0(3)
A9286	0(3)	A9581	20(3)	B9999	0(3)	C1818	2(3)	C2640	150(3)	C9358	800(3)	D0274	1(3)	E0118	0(3)
A9300	0(3)	A9582	1(3)	C1052	1(3)	C1819	4(3)	C2641	150(3)	C9359	30(3)	D0277	1(3)	E0130	0(3)
A9500	3(3)	A9583	18(3)	C1062	2(3)	C1820	2(3)	C2642	120(3)	C9360	300(3)	D0412	0(3)	E0135	0(3)
A9501	1(3)	A9584	1(3)	C1713	20(3)	C1821	4(3)	C2643	120(3)	C9361	10(3)	D0416	1(3)	E0140	0(3)
A9502	3(3)	A9585	300(3)	C1714	4(3)	C1822	1(3)	C2644	500(1)	C9362	60(3)	D0431	1(3)	E0141	0(3)
A9503	1(3)	A9586	1(3)	C1715	45(3)	C1823	1(3)	C2645	4608(3)	C9363	500(3)	D0460	1(2)	E0143	0(3)
A9504	1(3)	A9587	54(3)	C1716	4(3)	C1824	1(2)	C5271	1(2)	C9364	600(3)	D0484	1(2)	E0144	0(3)
A9505	4(3)	A9588	10(3)	C1717	10(3)	C1825	1(2)	C5272	3(2)	C9460	1(3)	D0485	1(2)	E0147	0(3)
A9507	1(3)	A9589	1(3)	C1719	99(3)	C1830	2(3)	C5273	1(2)	C9462	600(3)	D0601	1(3)	E0148	0(3)
A9508	2(3)	A9590	675(3)	C1721	1(3)	C1839	2(2)	C5274	35(3)	C9482	150(3)	D0602	1(2)	E0149	0(3)
A9509	5(3)	A9591	6(3)	C1722	1(3)	C1840	1(3)	C5275	1(2)	C9488	20(3)	D0603	1(2)	E0153	0(3)
A9510	1(3)	A9600	7(3)	C1724	5(3)	C1841	1(2)	C5276	3(2)	C9600	3(3)	D1510	2(2)	E0154	0(3)
A9512	30(3)	A9604	1(3)	C1725	9(3)	C1842	1(2)	C5277	1(2)	C9601	2(3)	D1516	1(2)	E0155	0(3)
A9513	200(3)	A9606	224(3)	C1726	5(3)	C1874	5(3)	C5278	15(3)	C9602	2(3)	D1517	1(2)	E0156	0(3)
A9515	1(3)	A9698	2(3)	C1727	4(3)	C1875	4(3)	C8900	1(3)	C9603	2(3)	D1520	2(2)	E0157	0(3)
A9516	4(3)	A9700	2(3)	C1728	5(3)	C1876	5(3)	C8901	1(3)	C9604	2(3)	D1526	1(2)	E0158	0(3)
A9517	200(3)	A9900	1(3)	C1729	6(3)	C1877	5(3)	C8902	1(3)	C9605	2(3)	D1527	1(2)	E0159	2(2)
A9520	1(3)	A9901	0(3)	C1730	4(3)	C1878	2(3)	C8903	1(3)	C9606	1(3)	D1551	1(2)	E0160	0(3)
A9521	2(3)	A9999	1(3)	C1731	1(3)	C1880	2(3)	C8905	1(3)	C9607	2(3)	D1552	1(2)	E0161	0(3)
A9524	10(3)	B4034	0(3)	C1732	3(3)	C1881	2(3)	C8906	1(3)	C9608	2(3)	D1553	2(2)	E0162	0(3)
A9526	2(3)	B4035	0(3)	C1733	3(3)	C1882	1(3)	C8908	1(3)	C9725	1(3)	D1575	4(2)	E0163	0(3)
A9527	195(3)	B4036	0(3)	C1734	2(3)	C1883	4(3)	C8909	1(3)	C9726	2(3)	D4260	4(2)	E0165	0(3)
A9528	10(3)	B4081	0(3)	C1748	1(3)	C1884	4(3)	C8910	1(3)	C9727	1(2)	D4263	4(2)	E0167	0(3)
A9529	10(3)	B4082	0(3)	C1749	1(3)	C1885	2(3)	C8911	1(3)	C9728	1(2)	D4264	3(3)	E0168	0(3)
A9530	200(3)	B4083	0(3)	C1750	2(3)	C1886	1(3)	C8912	1(3)	C9733	1(3)	D4270	4(3)	E0170	0(3)
A9531	100(3)	B4087	0(3)	C1751	3(3)	C1887	7(3)	C8913	1(3)	C9734	1(3)	D4273	1(2)	E0171	0(3)
A9532	10(3)	B4088	0(3)	C1752	2(3)	C1888	2(3)	C8914	1(3)	C9738	1(3)	D4277	1(2)	E0172	0(3)
A9536	1(3)	B4100	0(3)	C1753	2(3)	C1889	1(3)	C8918	1(3)	C9739	1(2)	D4278	3(3)	E0175	0(3)
A9537	1(3)	B4102	0(3)	C1754	2(3)	C1890	1(3)	C8919	1(3)	C9740	1(2)	D4355	1(2)	E0181	0(3)
A9538	1(3)	B4103	0(3)	C1755	2(3)	C1891	1(3)	C8920	1(3)	C9751	1(3)	D4381	12(3)	E0182	0(3)
A9539	2(3)	B4104	0(3)	C1756	2(3)	C1892	6(3)	C8921	1(3)	C9752	1(2)	D5282	0(3)	E0184	0(3)
A9540	2(3)	B4149	0(3)	C1757	6(3)	C1893	6(3)	C8922	1(3)	C9753	3(3)	D5283	0(3)	E0185	0(3)
A9541	1(3)	B4150	0(3)	C1758	2(3)	C1894	6(3)	C8923	1(3)	C9756	1(3)	D5876	0(3)	E0186	0(3)
A9542	1(3)	B4152	0(3)	C1759	2(3)	C1895	2(3)	C8924	1(3)	C9757	2(2)	D5911	1(3)	E0187	0(3)
A9543	1(3)	B4153	0(3)	C1760	4(3)	C1896	2(3)	C8925	1(3)	C9758	1(2)	D5912	1(2)	E0188	0(3)
A9546	1(3)	B4154	0(3)	C1762	4(3)	C1897	2(3)	C8926	1(3)	C9759	1(3)	D5983	1(3)	E0189	0(3)
A9547	2(3)	B4155	0(3)	C1763	4(3)	C1898	2(3)	C8927	1(3)	C9760	1(2)	D5984	1(3)	E0190	0(3)
A9548	2(3)	B4157	0(3)	C1764	1(3)	C1899	2(3)	C8928	1(2)	C9761	2(2)	D5985	1(3)	E0191	0(3)
A9550	1(3)	B4158	0(3)	C1765	4(3)	C1900	1(3)	C8929	1(3)	C9762	1(3)	D7111	20(3)	E0193	0(3)
A9551	1(3)	B4159	0(3)	C1766	4(3)	C1982	1(3)	C8930	1(2)	C9763	1(3)	D7140	32(2)	E0194	0(3)
A9552	1(3)	B4160	0(3)	C1767	2(3)	C2596	1(3)	C8931	1(3)	C9764	2(3)	D7210	32(2)	E0196	0(3)
A9553	1(3)	B4161	0(3)	C1768	3(3)	C2613	2(3)	C8932	1(3)	C9765	2(3)	D7220	6(3)	E0197	0(3)
A9554	1(3)	B4162	0(3)	C1769	9(3)	C2614	3(3)	C8933	1(3)	C9766	2(3)	D7230	6(3)	E0198	0(3)
A9555	2(3)	B4164	0(3)	C1770	3(3)	C2615	2(3)	C8934	2(3)	C9767	2(3)	D7240	6(3)	E0199	0(3)
A9556	10(3)	B4168	0(3)	C1771	1(3)	C2616	1(3)	C8935	2(3)	C9768	1(3)	D7241	6(3)	E0200	0(3)
A9557	2(3)	B4172	0(3)	C1772	1(3)	C2617	4(3)	C8936	2(3)	C9769	1(2)	D7250	32(2)	E0202	0(3)
A9558	7(3)	B4176	0(3)	C1773	3(3)	C2618	4(3)	C8937	2(2)	C9770	2(2)	D7260	1(3)	E0203	0(3)
A9559	1(3)	B4178	0(3)	C1776	10(3)	C2619	1(3)	C8957	2(3)	C9771	1(2)	D7261	1(3)	E0205	0(3)
A9560	2(3)	B4180	0(3)	C1777	2(3)	C2620	1(3)	C9046	160(3)	C9772	2(2)	D7283	4(3)	E0210	0(3)
A9561	1(3)	B4185	0(3)	C1778	4(3)	C2621	1(3)	C9047	22(3)	C9773	2(2)	D7288	2(3)	E0215	0(3)
A9562	2(3)	B4187	0(3)	C1779	2(3)	C2622	1(3)	C9065	40(3)	C9774	2(2)	D7321	4(2)	E0217	0(3)
A9563	10(3)	B4189	0(3)	C1780	2(3)	C2623	2(3)	C9067	500(3)	C9775	2(2)	D9110	1(3)	E0218	0(3)
A9564	20(3)	B4193	0(3)	C1781	4(3)	C2624	1(3)	C9113	10(3)	C9803	2(3)	D9130	0(3)	E0221	0(3)
A9566	1(3)	B4197	0(3)	C1782	1(3)	C2625	4(3)	C9132	5500(3)			D9230	1(3)	E0225	0(3)
A9567	2(3)	B4199	0(3)	C1783	2(3)	C2626	1(3)	C9248	25(3)			D9248	1(3)	E0231	0(3)
A9568	0(3)	B4216	0(3)	C1784	2(3)	C2627	2(3)	C9250	1(3)			D9613	0(3)	E0232	0(3)
A9569	1(3)	B4220	0(3)	C1785	1(3)	C2628	4(3)	C9254	400(3)			D9930	1(2)	E0235	0(3)
A9570	1(3)	B4222	0(3)	C1786	1(3)	C2629	4(3)	C9257	10(2)			D9944	0(3)	E0236	0(3)
A9571	1(3)	B4224	0(3)	C1787	2(3)	C2630	3(3)	C9285	2(3)			D9945	0(3)	E0239	0(3)
A9572	1(3)	B5000	0(3)	C1788	2(3)	C2631	1(3)	C9290	266(3)			D9946	0(3)	E0240	0(3)
A9575	300(3)	B5100	0(3)	C1789	2(3)	C2634	24(3)	C9293	700(3)			D9950	1(3)	E0241	0(3)
												D9951	1(3)		
												D9952	1(3)		
												D9961	0(3)		
												D9990	0(3)		
												E0100	0(3)		
												E0105	0(3)		
												E0110	0(3)		
												E0111	0(3)		

CPT	MUE	CPT	MUE	CPT	MUE	CPT	MUE	CPT	MUE	CPT	MUE	CPT	MUE	CPT	MUE
E0242	0(3)	E0446	0(3)	E0657	0(3)	E0935	0(3)	E1037	0(3)	E1355	0(3)	E2204	0(3)	E2371	0(3)
E0243	0(3)	E0447	0(3)	E0660	0(3)	E0936	0(3)	E1038	0(3)	E1356	0(3)	E2205	0(3)	E2372	0(3)
E0244	0(3)	E0455	0(3)	E0665	0(3)	E0940	0(3)	E1039	0(3)	E1357	0(3)	E2206	0(3)	E2373	0(3)
E0245	0(3)	E0457	0(3)	E0666	0(3)	E0941	0(3)	E1050	0(3)	E1358	0(3)	E2207	0(3)	E2374	0(3)
E0246	0(3)	E0459	0(3)	E0667	0(3)	E0942	0(3)	E1060	0(3)	E1372	0(3)	E2208	0(3)	E2375	0(3)
E0247	0(3)	E0462	0(3)	E0668	0(3)	E0944	0(3)	E1070	0(3)	E1390	0(3)	E2209	0(3)	E2376	0(3)
E0248	0(3)	E0465	0(3)	E0669	0(3)	E0945	0(3)	E1083	0(3)	E1391	0(3)	E2210	0(3)	E2377	0(3)
E0249	0(3)	E0466	0(3)	E0670	0(3)	E0946	0(3)	E1084	0(3)	E1392	0(3)	E2211	0(3)	E2378	0(3)
E0250	0(3)	E0467	0(3)	E0671	0(3)	E0947	0(3)	E1085	0(3)	E1399	1(3)	E2212	0(3)	E2381	0(3)
E0251	0(3)	E0470	0(3)	E0672	0(3)	E0948	0(3)	E1086	0(3)	E1405	0(3)	E2213	0(3)	E2382	0(3)
E0255	0(3)	E0471	0(3)	E0673	0(3)	E0950	0(3)	E1087	0(3)	E1406	0(3)	E2214	0(3)	E2383	0(3)
E0256	0(3)	E0472	0(3)	E0675	0(3)	E0951	0(3)	E1088	0(3)	E1500	0(3)	E2215	0(3)	E2384	0(3)
E0260	0(3)	E0480	0(3)	E0676	1(3)	E0952	0(3)	E1089	0(3)	E1510	0(3)	E2216	0(3)	E2385	0(3)
E0261	0(3)	E0481	0(3)	E0691	0(3)	E0953	0(3)	E1090	0(3)	E1520	0(3)	E2217	0(3)	E2386	0(3)
E0265	0(3)	E0482	0(3)	E0692	0(3)	E0954	0(3)	E1092	0(3)	E1530	0(3)	E2218	0(3)	E2387	0(3)
E0266	0(3)	E0483	0(3)	E0693	0(3)	E0955	0(3)	E1093	0(3)	E1540	0(3)	E2219	0(3)	E2388	0(3)
E0270	0(3)	E0484	0(3)	E0694	0(3)	E0956	0(3)	E1100	0(3)	E1550	0(3)	E2220	0(3)	E2389	0(3)
E0271	0(3)	E0485	0(3)	E0700	0(3)	E0957	0(3)	E1110	0(3)	E1560	0(3)	E2221	0(3)	E2390	0(3)
E0272	0(3)	E0486	0(3)	E0705	0(3)	E0958	0(3)	E1130	0(3)	E1570	0(3)	E2222	0(3)	E2391	0(3)
E0273	0(3)	E0487	0(3)	E0710	0(3)	E0959	0(3)	E1140	0(3)	E1575	0(3)	E2224	0(3)	E2392	0(3)
E0274	0(3)	E0500	0(3)	E0720	0(3)	E0960	0(3)	E1150	0(3)	E1580	0(3)	E2225	0(3)	E2394	0(3)
E0275	0(3)	E0550	0(3)	E0730	0(3)	E0961	0(3)	E1160	0(3)	E1590	0(3)	E2226	0(3)	E2395	0(3)
E0276	0(3)	E0555	0(3)	E0731	0(3)	E0966	0(3)	E1161	0(3)	E1592	0(3)	E2227	0(3)	E2396	0(3)
E0277	0(3)	E0560	0(3)	E0740	0(3)	E0967	0(3)	E1170	0(3)	E1594	0(3)	E2228	0(3)	E2397	0(3)
E0280	0(3)	E0561	0(3)	E0744	0(3)	E0968	0(3)	E1171	0(3)	E1600	0(3)	E2230	0(3)	E2398	0(3)
E0290	0(3)	E0562	0(3)	E0745	0(3)	E0969	0(3)	E1172	0(3)	E1610	0(3)	E2231	0(3)	E2402	0(3)
E0291	0(3)	E0565	0(3)	E0746	1(3)	E0970	0(3)	E1180	0(3)	E1615	0(3)	E2291	1(2)	E2500	0(3)
E0292	0(3)	E0570	0(3)	E0747	0(3)	E0971	0(3)	E1190	0(3)	E1620	0(3)	E2292	1(2)	E2502	0(3)
E0293	0(3)	E0572	0(3)	E0748	0(3)	E0973	0(3)	E1195	0(3)	E1625	0(3)	E2293	1(2)	E2504	0(3)
E0294	0(3)	E0574	0(3)	E0749	1(3)	E0974	0(3)	E1200	0(3)	E1630	0(3)	E2294	1(2)	E2506	0(3)
E0295	0(3)	E0575	0(3)	E0755	0(3)	E0978	0(3)	E1220	0(3)	E1632	0(3)	E2295	0(3)	E2508	0(3)
E0296	0(3)	E0580	0(3)	E0760	0(3)	E0980	0(3)	E1221	0(3)	E1634	0(3)	E2300	0(3)	E2510	0(3)
E0297	0(3)	E0585	0(3)	E0761	0(3)	E0981	0(3)	E1222	0(3)	E1635	0(3)	E2301	0(3)	E2511	0(3)
E0300	0(3)	E0600	0(3)	E0762	0(3)	E0982	0(3)	E1223	0(3)	E1636	0(3)	E2310	0(3)	E2512	0(3)
E0301	0(3)	E0601	0(3)	E0764	0(3)	E0983	0(3)	E1224	0(3)	E1637	0(3)	E2311	0(3)	E2599	0(3)
E0302	0(3)	E0602	0(3)	E0765	0(3)	E0984	0(3)	E1225	0(3)	E1639	0(3)	E2312	0(3)	E2601	0(3)
E0303	0(3)	E0603	0(3)	E0766	0(3)	E0985	0(3)	E1226	0(3)	E1699	0(3)	E2313	0(3)	E2602	0(3)
E0304	0(3)	E0604	0(3)	E0769	0(3)	E0986	0(3)	E1227	0(3)	E1700	0(3)	E2321	0(3)	E2603	0(3)
E0305	0(3)	E0605	0(3)	E0770	1(3)	E0988	0(3)	E1228	0(3)	E1701	0(3)	E2322	0(3)	E2604	0(3)
E0310	0(3)	E0606	0(3)	E0776	0(3)	E0990	0(3)	E1229	0(3)	E1702	0(3)	E2323	0(3)	E2605	0(3)
E0315	0(3)	E0607	0(3)	E0779	0(3)	E0992	0(3)	E1230	0(3)	E1800	0(3)	E2324	0(3)	E2606	0(3)
E0316	0(3)	E0610	0(3)	E0780	0(3)	E0994	0(3)	E1231	0(3)	E1801	0(3)	E2325	0(3)	E2607	0(3)
E0325	0(3)	E0615	0(3)	E0781	1(2)	E0995	0(3)	E1232	0(3)	E1802	0(3)	E2326	0(3)	E2608	0(3)
E0326	0(3)	E0616	1(2)	E0782	1(2)	E1002	0(3)	E1233	0(3)	E1805	0(3)	E2327	0(3)	E2609	0(3)
E0328	0(3)	E0617	0(3)	E0783	1(2)	E1003	0(3)	E1234	0(3)	E1806	0(3)	E2328	0(3)	E2610	0(3)
E0329	0(3)	E0618	0(3)	E0784	0(3)	E1004	0(3)	E1235	0(3)	E1810	0(3)	E2329	0(3)	E2611	0(3)
E0350	0(3)	E0619	0(3)	E0785	1(2)	E1005	0(3)	E1236	0(3)	E1811	0(3)	E2330	0(3)	E2612	0(3)
E0352	0(3)	E0620	0(3)	E0786	1(2)	E1006	0(3)	E1237	0(3)	E1812	0(3)	E2331	0(3)	E2613	0(3)
E0370	0(3)	E0621	0(3)	E0787	0(3)	E1007	0(3)	E1238	0(3)	E1815	0(3)	E2340	0(3)	E2614	0(3)
E0371	0(3)	E0625	0(3)	E0791	0(3)	E1008	0(3)	E1239	0(3)	E1816	0(3)	E2341	0(3)	E2615	0(3)
E0372	0(3)	E0627	0(3)	E0830	0(3)	E1009	0(3)	E1240	0(3)	E1818	0(3)	E2342	0(3)	E2616	0(3)
E0373	0(3)	E0629	0(3)	E0840	0(3)	E1010	0(3)	E1250	0(3)	E1820	0(3)	E2343	0(3)	E2617	0(3)
E0424	0(3)	E0630	0(3)	E0849	0(3)	E1011	0(3)	E1260	0(3)	E1821	0(3)	E2351	0(3)	E2619	0(3)
E0425	0(3)	E0635	0(3)	E0850	0(3)	E1012	0(3)	E1270	0(3)	E1825	0(3)	E2358	0(3)	E2620	0(3)
E0430	0(3)	E0636	0(3)	E0855	0(3)	E1014	0(3)	E1280	0(3)	E1830	0(3)	E2359	0(3)	E2621	0(3)
E0431	0(3)	E0637	0(3)	E0856	0(3)	E1015	0(3)	E1285	0(3)	E1831	0(3)	E2360	0(3)	E2622	0(3)
E0433	0(3)	E0638	0(3)	E0860	0(3)	E1016	0(3)	E1290	0(3)	E1840	0(3)	E2361	0(3)	E2623	0(3)
E0434	0(3)	E0639	0(3)	E0870	0(3)	E1017	0(3)	E1295	0(3)	E1841	0(3)	E2362	0(3)	E2624	0(3)
E0435	0(3)	E0640	0(3)	E0880	0(3)	E1018	0(3)	E1296	0(3)	E1902	0(3)	E2363	0(3)	E2625	0(3)
E0439	0(3)	E0641	0(3)	E0890	0(3)	E1020	0(3)	E1297	0(3)	E2000	0(3)	E2364	0(3)	E2626	0(3)
E0440	0(3)	E0642	0(3)	E0900	0(3)	E1028	0(3)	E1298	0(3)	E2100	0(3)	E2365	0(3)	E2627	0(3)
E0441	0(3)	E0650	0(3)	E0910	0(3)	E1029	0(3)	E1300	0(3)	E2101	0(3)	E2366	0(3)	E2628	0(3)
E0442	0(3)	E0651	0(3)	E0911	0(3)	E1030	0(3)	E1310	0(3)	E2120	0(3)	E2367	0(3)	E2629	0(3)
E0443	0(3)	E0652	0(3)	E0912	0(3)	E1031	0(3)	E1352	0(3)	E2201	0(3)	E2368	0(3)	E2630	0(3)
E0444	0(3)	E0655	0(3)	E0920	0(3)	E1035	0(3)	E1353	0(3)	E2202	0(3)	E2369	0(3)	E2631	0(3)
E0445	0(3)	E0656	0(3)	E0930	0(3)	E1036	0(3)	E1354	0(3)	E2203	0(3)	E2370	0(3)	E2632	0(3)

CPT	MUE	CPT	MUE	CPT	MUE	CPT	MUE	CPT	MUE	CPT	MUE	CPT	MUE	CPT	MUE
E2633	0(3)	G0255	0(3)	G0422	6(2)	G2001	1(3)	G9149	1(3)	J0288	0(3)	J0690	12(3)	J1162	1(3)
E8000	0(3)	G0257	0(3)	G0423	6(2)	G2002	1(3)	G9150	1(3)	J0289	50(3)	J0691	300(3)	J1165	50(3)
E8001	0(3)	G0259	2(3)	G0424	2(2)	G2003	1(3)	G9151	1(3)	J0290	24(3)	J0692	12(3)	J1170	350(3)
E8002	0(3)	G0260	2(3)	G0425	1(3)	G2004	1(3)	G9152	1(3)	J0291	500(3)	J0693	1600(3)	J1180	0(3)
G0008	1(2)	G0268	1(2)	G0426	1(3)	G2005	1(3)	G9153	1(3)	J0295	12(3)	J0694	8(3)	J1190	8(3)
G0009	1(2)	G0269	0(3)	G0427	1(3)	G2006	1(3)	G9156	1(2)	J0300	8(3)	J0695	60(3)	J1200	8(3)
G0010	1(3)	G0270	8(3)	G0428	0(3)	G2007	1(3)	G9157	1(2)	J0330	10(3)	J0696	16(3)	J1201	20(3)
G0027	1(2)	G0271	4(3)	G0429	1(2)	G2008	1(3)	G9187	1(3)	J0348	200(3)	J0697	4(3)	J1205	4(3)
G0071	1(3)	G0276	1(3)	G0432	1(2)	G2009	1(3)	G9480	1(3)	J0350	0(3)	J0698	10(3)	J1212	1(3)
G0076	1(3)	G0277	5(3)	G0433	1(2)	G2010	1(3)	G9481	1(3)	J0360	2(3)	J0702	18(3)	J1230	3(3)
G0077	1(3)	G0278	1(2)	G0435	1(2)	G2011	1(2)	G9482	1(3)	J0364	6(3)	J0706	1(3)	J1240	6(3)
G0078	1(3)	G0279	1(2)	G0438	1(2)	G2012	1(3)	G9483	1(3)	J0365	0(3)	J0710	0(3)	J1245	10(3)
G0079	1(3)	G0281	1(3)	G0439	1(2)	G2013	1(3)	G9484	1(3)	J0380	1(3)	J0712	120(3)	J1250	2(3)
G0080	1(3)	G0282	0(3)	G0442	1(2)	G2014	1(3)	G9485	1(3)	J0390	0(3)	J0713	12(3)	J1260	2(3)
G0081	1(3)	G0283	1(3)	G0443	1(2)	G2015	1(3)	G9486	1(3)	J0395	0(3)	J0714	12(3)	J1265	20(3)
G0082	1(3)	G0288	1(2)	G0444	1(2)	G2023	2(3)	G9487	1(3)	J0400	39(3)	J0715	0(3)	J1267	150(3)
G0083	1(3)	G0289	1(2)	G0445	1(2)	G2024	2(3)	G9488	1(3)	J0401	400(3)	J0716	4(3)	J1270	8(3)
G0084	1(3)	G0293	1(2)	G0446	1(3)	G2025	1(3)	G9489	1(3)	J0456	4(3)	J0717	400(3)	J1290	30(3)
G0085	1(3)	G0294	1(2)	G0447	2(3)	G2064	1(2)	G9490	1(3)	J0461	200(3)	J0720	15(3)	J1300	120(3)
G0086	1(3)	G0295	0(3)	G0448	1(3)	G2065	1(2)	G9678	1(2)	J0470	2(3)	J0725	10(3)	J1301	60(3)
G0087	1(3)	G0296	1(2)	G0451	1(2)	G2066	1(2)	G9685	1(3)	J0475	8(3)	J0735	50(3)	J1303	360(3)
G0101	1(2)	G0302	1(2)	G0452	6(3)	G2067	1(2)	G9978	1(3)	J0476	2(3)	J0740	2(3)	J1320	0(3)
G0102	1(2)	G0303	1(2)	G0453	40(3)	G2068	1(2)	G9979	1(3)	J0480	1(3)	J0742	500(3)	J1322	150(3)
G0103	1(2)	G0304	1(2)	G0454	1(2)	G2069	1(2)	G9980	1(3)	J0485	1500(3)	J0743	16(3)	J1324	108(3)
G0104	1(2)	G0305	1(2)	G0455	1(2)	G2070	1(2)	G9981	1(3)	J0490	160(3)	J0744	6(3)	J1325	1(3)
G0105	1(2)	G0306	1(3)	G0458	1(3)	G2071	1(2)	G9982	1(3)	J0500	4(3)	J0745	2(3)	J1327	1(3)
G0106	1(2)	G0307	1(3)	G0459	1(3)	G2072	1(2)	G9983	1(3)	J0515	3(3)	J0770	5(3)	J1330	1(3)
G0108	6(3)	G0328	1(2)	G0460	1(3)	G2073	1(2)	G9984	1(3)	J0517	30(3)	J0775	180(3)	J1335	2(3)
G0109	12(3)	G0329	1(3)	G0463	0(3)	G2074	1(2)	G9985	1(3)	J0520	0(3)	J0780	4(3)	J1364	2(3)
G0117	1(2)	G0333	0(3)	G0466	1(2)	G2075	1(2)	G9986	1(3)	J0558	24(3)	J0791	160(3)	J1380	4(3)
G0118	1(2)	G0337	1(2)	G0467	1(3)	G2076	1(2)	G9987	1(3)	J0561	24(3)	J0795	100(3)	J1410	4(3)
G0120	1(2)	G0339	1(2)	G0468	1(2)	G2078	3(3)	J0120	1(3)	J0565	200(3)	J0800	3(3)	J1428	450(3)
G0121	1(2)	G0340	1(3)	G0469	1(2)	G2079	3(3)	J0121	200(3)	J0567	300(3)	J0834	3(3)	J1429	450(3)
G0122	0(3)	G0341	1(2)	G0470	1(3)	G2081	1(2)	J0122	300(3)	J0570	4(3)	J0840	6(3)	J1430	10(3)
G0123	1(3)	G0342	1(2)	G0471	2(3)	G2082	1(2)	J0129	100(3)	J0571	0(3)	J0841	20(3)	J1435	1(3)
G0124	1(3)	G0343	1(2)	G0472	1(2)	G2083	1(2)	J0130	4(3)	J0572	0(3)	J0850	9(3)	J1436	0(3)
G0127	1(2)	G0372	1(2)	G0473	1(2)	G2086	1(3)	J0131	400(3)	J0573	0(3)	J0875	300(3)	J1437	100(3)
G0128	1(2)	G0378	0(3)	G0475	1(2)	G2087	2(3)	J0132	12(3)	J0574	0(3)	J0878	1500(3)	J1438	2(3)
G0130	1(2)	G0379	0(3)	G0476	1(2)	G2170	1(3)	J0133	1200(3)	J0575	0(3)	J0881	500(3)	J1439	750(3)
G0141	1(3)	G0380	0(3)	G0480	1(2)	G2171	1(3)	J0135	8(3)	J0583	250(3)	J0882	300(3)	J1442	1500(3)
G0143	1(3)	G0381	0(3)	G0481	1(2)	G2212	4(3)	J0153	180(3)	J0584	90(3)	J0883	1125(3)	J1443	272(3)
G0144	1(3)	G0382	0(3)	G0482	1(2)	G2213	1(2)	J0171	20(3)	J0585	600(3)	J0884	1125(3)	J1444	272(3)
G0145	1(3)	G0383	0(3)	G0483	1(2)	G2214	1(2)	J0178	4(2)	J0586	300(3)	J0885	60(3)	J1447	960(3)
G0147	1(3)	G0384	0(3)	G0490	1(3)	G2250	1(2)	J0179	12(2)	J0587	300(3)	J0887	360(3)	J1450	4(3)
G0148	1(3)	G0390	0(3)	G0491	1(3)	G2251	1(2)	J0180	140(3)	J0588	600(3)	J0888	360(3)	J1451	1(3)
G0166	2(3)	G0396	1(2)	G0492	1(3)	G2252	1(2)	J0185	130(3)	J0591	100(3)	J0890	0(3)	J1452	0(3)
G0168	2(3)	G0397	1(2)	G0493	1(3)	G6001	2(3)	J0190	0(3)	J0592	6(3)	J0894	100(3)	J1453	150(3)
G0175	1(3)	G0398	1(2)	G0494	1(3)	G6002	2(3)	J0200	0(3)	J0593	300(3)	J0895	12(3)	J1454	1(3)
G0177	0(3)	G0399	1(2)	G0495	1(3)	G6003	2(3)	J0202	12(3)	J0594	320(3)	J0896	1100(3)	J1455	18(3)
G0179	1(2)	G0400	1(2)	G0496	1(3)	G6004	2(3)	J0205	0(3)	J0595	8(3)	J0897	120(3)	J1457	0(3)
G0180	1(2)	G0402	1(2)	G0498	1(2)	G6005	2(3)	J0207	4(3)	J0596	840(3)	J0945	4(3)	J1458	100(3)
G0181	1(2)	G0403	1(2)	G0499	1(2)	G6006	2(3)	J0210	4(3)	J0597	250(3)	J1000	1(3)	J1459	300(3)
G0182	1(2)	G0404	1(2)	G0500	1(3)	G6007	2(3)	J0215	30(3)	J0598	100(3)	J1020	8(3)	J1460	10(2)
G0186	1(2)	G0405	1(2)	G0501	0(3)	G6008	2(3)	J0220	1(3)	J0599	900(3)	J1030	8(3)	J1554	240(3)
G0219	0(3)	G0406	1(3)	G0506	1(2)	G6009	2(3)	J0221	250(3)	J0600	3(3)	J1040	4(3)	J1555	480(3)
G0235	1(3)	G0407	1(3)	G0508	1(2)	G6010	2(3)	J0222	300(3)	J0606	150(3)	J1050	1000(3)	J1556	300(3)
G0237	8(3)	G0408	1(3)	G0509	1(2)	G6011	2(3)	J0223	756(3)	J0610	15(3)	J1071	400(3)	J1557	300(3)
G0238	8(3)	G0410	4(3)	G0511	1(2)	G6012	2(3)	J0256	1600(3)	J0620	1(3)	J1094	0(3)	J1558	480(3)
G0239	1(3)	G0411	4(3)	G0512	1(2)	G6013	2(3)	J0257	1400(3)	J0630	1(3)	J1095	1034(2)	J1559	300(3)
G0245	1(2)	G0412	1(2)	G0513	1(2)	G6014	2(3)	J0270	32(3)	J0636	100(3)	J1096	8(2)	J1560	1(2)
G0246	1(2)	G0413	1(2)	G0514	1(1)	G6015	2(3)	J0275	1(3)	J0637	20(3)	J1097	4(3)	J1561	300(3)
G0247	1(2)	G0414	1(2)	G0516	1(2)	G6016	2(3)	J0278	15(3)	J0638	300(3)	J1100	120(3)	J1562	0(3)
G0248	1(2)	G0415	1(2)	G0517	1(2)	G6017	2(3)	J0280	7(3)	J0640	24(3)	J1110	3(3)	J1566	300(3)
G0249	3(3)	G0416	1(2)	G0518	1(2)	G9143	1(2)	J0282	5(3)	J0641	1200(3)	J1120	2(3)	J1568	300(3)
G0250	1(2)	G0420	2(3)	G0659	1(2)	G9147	0(3)	J0285	5(3)	J0642	1200(3)	J1130	300(3)	J1569	300(3)
G0252	0(3)	G0421	2(3)	G2000	1(3)	G9148	1(3)	J0287	50(3)	J0670	10(3)	J1160	2(3)	J1570	4(3)

Appendix I — Medically Unlikely Edits (MUEs)—Practitioner

CPT	MUE	CPT	MUE	CPT	MUE	CPT	MUE	CPT	MUE	CPT	MUE	CPT	MUE	CPT	MUE
J1571	20(3)	J1956	4(3)	J2562	48(3)	J3230	2(3)	J7131	500(3)	J7330	1(3)	J7649	0(3)	J9045	22(3)
J1572	300(3)	J1960	0(3)	J2590	3(3)	J3240	1(3)	J7169	180(3)	J7331	40(3)	J7650	0(3)	J9047	160(3)
J1573	130(3)	J1980	2(3)	J2597	45(3)	J3241	300(3)	J7170	1800(3)	J7332	40(3)	J7657	0(3)	J9050	6(3)
J1575	650(3)	J1990	0(3)	J2650	0(3)	J3243	150(3)	J7175	9000(1)	J7336	1120(3)	J7658	0(3)	J9055	150(3)
J1580	9(3)	J2001	60(3)	J2670	0(3)	J3245	100(3)	J7177	10500(1)	J7340	1(3)	J7659	0(3)	J9057	60(3)
J1595	1(3)	J2010	10(3)	J2675	1(3)	J3246	1(3)	J7178	7700(1)	J7342	10(3)	J7660	0(3)	J9060	24(3)
J1599	300(3)	J2020	6(3)	J2680	4(3)	J3250	2(3)	J7179	7500(1)	J7345	200(3)	J7665	0(3)	J9065	100(3)
J1600	2(3)	J2060	4(3)	J2690	4(3)	J3260	8(3)	J7180	6000(1)	J7351	20(2)	J7667	0(3)	J9070	55(3)
J1602	300(3)	J2062	10(3)	J2700	48(3)	J3262	800(3)	J7181	3850(1)	J7352	16(3)	J7668	0(3)	J9098	5(3)
J1610	2(3)	J2150	8(3)	J2704	80(3)	J3265	0(3)	J7182	22000(1)	J7500	0(3)	J7669	0(3)	J9100	120(3)
J1620	0(3)	J2170	8(3)	J2710	2(3)	J3280	0(3)	J7183	7500(1)	J7501	1(3)	J7670	0(3)	J9118	750(3)
J1626	30(3)	J2175	4(3)	J2720	5(3)	J3285	1(3)	J7185	22000(1)	J7502	0(3)	J7674	100(3)	J9119	350(3)
J1627	100(3)	J2180	0(3)	J2724	3500(3)	J3300	160(3)	J7186	7500(1)	J7503	0(3)	J7676	0(3)	J9120	5(3)
J1628	100(3)	J2182	300(3)	J2725	0(3)	J3301	16(3)	J7187	7500(1)	J7504	15(3)	J7677	175(3)	J9130	24(3)
J1630	5(3)	J2185	60(3)	J2730	2(3)	J3302	0(3)	J7188	22000(1)	J7505	1(3)	J7680	0(3)	J9144	180(3)
J1631	9(3)	J2186	600(3)	J2760	2(3)	J3303	24(3)	J7189	13000(1)	J7507	0(3)	J7681	0(3)	J9145	240(3)
J1632	700(3)	J2210	1(3)	J2765	10(3)	J3304	64(2)	J7190	22000(1)	J7508	0(3)	J7682	2(3)	J9150	12(3)
J1640	672(3)	J2212	240(3)	J2770	6(3)	J3305	0(3)	J7191	0(3)	J7509	0(3)	J7683	0(3)	J9151	12(3)
J1642	100(3)	J2248	150(3)	J2778	10(2)	J3310	0(3)	J7192	22000(1)	J7510	0(3)	J7684	0(3)	J9153	132(3)
J1644	40(3)	J2250	22(3)	J2780	16(3)	J3315	6(3)	J7193	4000(1)	J7511	9(3)	J7685	0(3)	J9155	240(3)
J1645	10(3)	J2260	4(3)	J2783	60(3)	J3316	6(3)	J7194	9000(1)	J7512	0(3)	J7686	1(3)	J9160	7(3)
J1650	30(3)	J2265	400(3)	J2785	4(3)	J3320	0(3)	J7195	6000(1)	J7513	0(3)	J7699	1(3)	J9165	0(3)
J1652	20(3)	J2270	9(3)	J2786	500(3)	J3350	0(3)	J7196	175(3)	J7515	0(3)	J7799	2(3)	J9171	240(3)
J1655	0(3)	J2274	250(3)	J2787	2(3)	J3355	1(3)	J7197	6300(1)	J7516	1(3)	J7999	2(3)	J9173	150(3)
J1670	1(3)	J2278	1000(3)	J2788	1(3)	J3357	90(3)	J7198	6000(1)	J7517	0(3)	J8498	0(3)	J9175	10(3)
J1675	0(3)	J2280	4(3)	J2790	1(3)	J3358	520(3)	J7200	20000(1)	J7518	0(3)	J8499	0(3)	J9176	3000(3)
J1700	0(3)	J2300	4(3)	J2791	15(3)	J3360	6(3)	J7201	9000(1)	J7520	0(3)	J8501	0(3)	J9177	520(3)
J1710	0(3)	J2310	4(3)	J2792	450(3)	J3364	0(3)	J7202	11550(1)	J7525	2(3)	J8510	0(3)	J9178	150(3)
J1720	10(3)	J2315	380(3)	J2793	320(3)	J3365	0(3)	J7203	12000(1)	J7527	0(3)	J8515	0(3)	J9179	50(3)
J1726	28(3)	J2320	4(3)	J2794	100(3)	J3370	12(3)	J7204	19500(1)	J7599	1(3)	J8520	0(3)	J9181	100(3)
J1729	25(3)	J2323	300(3)	J2795	200(3)	J3380	300(3)	J7205	9750(1)	J7604	0(3)	J8521	0(3)	J9185	2(3)
J1730	0(3)	J2325	0(3)	J2796	150(3)	J3385	80(3)	J7207	22500(1)	J7605	2(3)	J8530	0(3)	J9190	20(3)
J1738	30(3)	J2326	120(3)	J2797	333(3)	J3396	150(3)	J7208	12000(1)	J7606	2(3)	J8540	0(3)	J9198	38(3)
J1740	3(3)	J2350	600(3)	J2798	240(3)	J3397	600(3)	J7209	7500(1)	J7607	0(3)	J8560	0(3)	J9200	5(3)
J1741	8(3)	J2353	60(3)	J2800	3(3)	J3398	150(2)	J7210	22000(1)	J7608	3(3)	J8562	0(3)	J9201	20(3)
J1742	2(3)	J2354	60(3)	J2805	3(3)	J3399	1(3)	J7211	22000(1)	J7609	0(3)	J8565	0(3)	J9202	3(3)
J1743	66(3)	J2355	2(3)	J2810	5(3)	J3400	0(3)	J7212	90000(1)	J7610	0(3)	J8597	0(3)	J9203	180(3)
J1744	30(3)	J2357	120(3)	J2820	15(3)	J3410	8(3)	J7296	0(3)	J7611	10(3)	J8600	0(3)	J9204	160(3)
J1745	150(3)	J2358	405(3)	J2840	160(3)	J3411	4(3)	J7297	0(3)	J7612	10(3)	J8610	0(3)	J9205	215(3)
J1746	200(3)	J2360	2(3)	J2850	16(3)	J3415	6(3)	J7298	0(3)	J7613	10(3)	J8650	0(3)	J9206	42(3)
J1750	45(3)	J2370	2(3)	J2860	170(3)	J3420	1(3)	J7300	0(3)	J7614	10(3)	J8655	1(3)	J9207	90(3)
J1756	500(3)	J2400	4(3)	J2910	0(3)	J3430	25(3)	J7301	0(3)	J7615	0(3)	J8670	0(3)	J9208	15(3)
J1786	680(3)	J2405	64(3)	J2916	20(3)	J3465	40(3)	J7303	0(3)	J7620	6(3)	J8700	0(3)	J9209	55(3)
J1790	2(3)	J2407	120(3)	J2920	25(3)	J3470	3(3)	J7304	0(3)	J7622	0(3)	J8705	0(3)	J9210	1500(3)
J1800	6(3)	J2410	2(3)	J2930	25(3)	J3471	999(1)	J7306	0(3)	J7624	0(3)	J8999	0(3)	J9211	6(3)
J1810	0(3)	J2425	125(3)	J2940	0(3)	J3472	2(3)	J7307	0(3)	J7626	2(3)	J9000	20(3)	J9212	0(3)
J1815	8(3)	J2426	819(3)	J2941	8(3)	J3473	450(3)	J7308	3(3)	J7627	0(3)	J9015	1(3)	J9213	12(3)
J1817	0(3)	J2430	3(3)	J2950	0(3)	J3475	20(3)	J7309	1(3)	J7628	0(3)	J9017	30(3)	J9214	100(3)
J1823	300(3)	J2440	4(3)	J2993	2(3)	J3480	40(3)	J7310	0(3)	J7629	0(3)	J9019	60(3)	J9215	0(3)
J1826	1(3)	J2460	0(3)	J2995	0(3)	J3485	160(3)	J7311	118(2)	J7631	4(3)	J9020	0(3)	J9216	2(3)
J1830	1(3)	J2469	10(3)	J2997	8(3)	J3486	4(3)	J7312	14(2)	J7632	0(3)	J9022	168(3)	J9217	6(3)
J1833	372(3)	J2501	2(3)	J3000	2(3)	J3489	5(3)	J7313	38(2)	J7633	0(3)	J9023	140(3)	J9218	1(3)
J1835	0(3)	J2502	60(3)	J3010	100(3)	J3520	0(3)	J7314	36(2)	J7634	0(3)	J9025	300(3)	J9219	1(3)
J1840	3(3)	J2503	2(3)	J3030	1(3)	J3530	0(3)	J7315	2(3)	J7635	0(3)	J9027	100(3)	J9223	120(3)
J1850	4(3)	J2504	15(3)	J3031	675(3)	J3535	0(3)	J7316	3(3)	J7636	0(3)	J9030	50(3)	J9225	1(3)
J1885	8(3)	J2505	1(3)	J3032	300(3)	J3570	0(3)	J7318	120(3)	J7637	0(3)	J9032	300(3)	J9226	1(3)
J1890	0(3)	J2507	8(3)	J3060	760(3)	J7030	5(3)	J7320	50(3)	J7638	0(3)	J9033	300(3)	J9227	150(3)
J1930	120(3)	J2510	4(3)	J3070	3(3)	J7040	6(3)	J7321	2(2)	J7639	3(3)	J9034	360(3)	J9228	1100(3)
J1931	377(3)	J2513	1(3)	J3090	200(3)	J7042	6(3)	J7322	48(3)	J7640	0(3)	J9035	180(3)	J9229	27(3)
J1940	6(3)	J2515	1(3)	J3095	150(3)	J7050	10(3)	J7323	2(2)	J7641	0(3)	J9036	360(3)	J9230	5(3)
J1943	675(3)	J2540	75(3)	J3101	50(3)	J7060	10(3)	J7324	2(2)	J7642	0(3)	J9039	210(3)	J9245	9(3)
J1944	1064(3)	J2543	16(3)	J3105	2(3)	J7070	4(3)	J7325	96(3)	J7643	0(3)	J9040	4(3)	J9250	25(3)
J1945	0(3)	J2545	1(3)	J3110	2(3)	J7100	2(3)	J7326	2(2)	J7644	3(3)	J9041	35(3)	J9260	20(3)
J1950	12(3)	J2547	600(3)	J3111	210(3)	J7110	2(3)	J7327	2(2)	J7645	0(3)	J9042	200(3)	J9261	80(3)
J1953	300(3)	J2550	3(3)	J3121	400(3)	J7120	4(3)	J7328	336(3)	J7647	0(3)	J9043	60(3)	J9262	700(3)
J1955	11(3)	J2560	1(3)	J3145	750(3)	J7121	4(3)	J7329	50(2)	J7648	0(3)	J9044	35(3)		

CPT	MUE	CPT	MUE	CPT	MUE	CPT	MUE	CPT	MUE	CPT	MUE	CPT	MUE	CPT	MUE
J9263	700(3)	K0020	0(3)	K0826	0(3)	L0120	0(3)	L0820	0(3)	L1833	0(3)	L2200	0(3)	L2830	0(3)
J9264	600(3)	K0037	0(3)	K0827	0(3)	L0130	0(3)	L0830	0(3)	L1834	0(3)	L2210	0(3)	L2840	0(3)
J9266	2(3)	K0038	0(3)	K0828	0(3)	L0140	0(3)	L0859	0(3)	L1836	0(3)	L2220	0(3)	L2850	0(3)
J9267	750(3)	K0039	0(3)	K0829	0(3)	L0150	0(3)	L0861	0(3)	L1840	0(3)	L2230	0(3)	L2861	0(3)
J9268	1(3)	K0040	0(3)	K0830	0(3)	L0160	0(3)	L0970	0(3)	L1843	0(3)	L2232	0(3)	L2999	0(3)
J9269	200(3)	K0041	0(3)	K0831	0(3)	L0170	0(3)	L0972	0(3)	L1844	0(3)	L2240	0(3)	L3000	0(3)
J9270	0(3)	K0042	0(3)	K0835	0(3)	L0172	0(3)	L0974	0(3)	L1845	0(3)	L2250	0(3)	L3001	0(3)
J9271	400(3)	K0043	0(3)	K0836	0(3)	L0174	0(3)	L0976	0(3)	L1846	0(3)	L2260	0(3)	L3002	0(3)
J9280	12(3)	K0044	0(3)	K0837	0(3)	L0180	0(3)	L0978	0(3)	L1847	0(3)	L2265	0(3)	L3003	0(3)
J9281	80(3)	K0045	0(3)	K0838	0(3)	L0190	0(3)	L0980	0(3)	L1848	0(3)	L2270	0(3)	L3010	0(3)
J9285	200(3)	K0046	0(3)	K0839	0(3)	L0200	0(3)	L0982	0(3)	L1850	0(3)	L2275	0(3)	L3020	0(3)
J9293	8(3)	K0047	0(3)	K0840	0(3)	L0220	0(3)	L0984	0(3)	L1851	0(3)	L2280	0(3)	L3030	0(3)
J9295	800(3)	K0050	0(3)	K0841	0(3)	L0450	0(3)	L0999	0(3)	L1852	0(3)	L2300	0(3)	L3031	0(3)
J9299	480(3)	K0051	0(3)	K0842	0(3)	L0452	0(3)	L1000	0(3)	L1860	0(3)	L2310	0(3)	L3040	0(3)
J9301	100(3)	K0052	0(3)	K0843	0(3)	L0454	0(3)	L1001	0(3)	L1900	0(3)	L2320	0(3)	L3050	0(3)
J9302	200(3)	K0053	0(3)	K0848	0(3)	L0455	0(3)	L1005	0(3)	L1902	0(3)	L2330	0(3)	L3060	0(3)
J9303	90(3)	K0056	0(3)	K0849	0(3)	L0456	0(3)	L1010	0(3)	L1904	0(3)	L2335	0(3)	L3070	0(3)
J9304	150(3)	K0065	0(3)	K0850	0(3)	L0457	0(3)	L1020	0(3)	L1906	0(3)	L2340	0(3)	L3080	0(3)
J9305	150(3)	K0069	0(3)	K0851	0(3)	L0458	0(3)	L1025	0(3)	L1907	0(3)	L2350	0(3)	L3090	0(3)
J9306	840(3)	K0070	0(3)	K0852	0(3)	L0460	0(3)	L1030	0(3)	L1910	0(3)	L2360	0(3)	L3100	0(3)
J9307	60(3)	K0071	0(3)	K0853	0(3)	L0462	0(3)	L1040	0(3)	L1920	0(3)	L2370	0(3)	L3140	0(3)
J9308	280(3)	K0072	0(3)	K0854	0(3)	L0464	0(3)	L1050	0(3)	L1930	0(3)	L2375	0(3)	L3150	0(3)
J9309	280(3)	K0073	0(3)	K0855	0(3)	L0466	0(3)	L1060	0(3)	L1932	0(3)	L2380	0(3)	L3160	0(3)
J9311	160(3)	K0077	0(3)	K0856	0(3)	L0467	0(3)	L1070	0(3)	L1940	0(3)	L2385	0(3)	L3170	0(3)
J9312	150(3)	K0098	0(3)	K0857	0(3)	L0468	0(3)	L1080	0(3)	L1945	0(3)	L2387	0(3)	L3201	0(3)
J9313	600(3)	K0105	0(3)	K0858	0(3)	L0469	0(3)	L1085	0(3)	L1950	0(3)	L2390	0(3)	L3202	0(3)
J9315	40(3)	K0108	0(3)	K0859	0(3)	L0470	0(3)	L1090	0(3)	L1951	0(3)	L2395	0(3)	L3203	0(3)
J9316	120(3)	K0195	0(3)	K0860	0(3)	L0472	0(3)	L1100	0(3)	L1960	0(3)	L2397	0(3)	L3204	0(3)
J9317	648(3)	K0455	0(3)	K0861	0(3)	L0480	0(3)	L1110	0(3)	L1970	0(3)	L2405	0(3)	L3206	0(3)
J9320	4(3)	K0462	0(3)	K0862	0(3)	L0482	0(3)	L1120	0(3)	L1971	0(3)	L2415	0(3)	L3207	0(3)
J9325	400(3)	K0553	0(3)	K0863	0(3)	L0484	0(3)	L1200	0(3)	L1980	0(3)	L2425	0(3)	L3208	0(3)
J9328	400(3)	K0554	0(3)	K0864	0(3)	L0486	0(3)	L1210	0(3)	L1990	0(3)	L2430	0(3)	L3209	0(3)
J9330	50(3)	K0602	0(3)	K0868	0(3)	L0488	0(3)	L1220	0(3)	L2000	0(3)	L2492	0(3)	L3211	0(3)
J9340	4(3)	K0604	0(3)	K0869	0(3)	L0490	0(3)	L1230	0(3)	L2005	0(3)	L2500	0(3)	L3212	0(3)
J9351	120(3)	K0605	0(3)	K0870	0(3)	L0491	0(3)	L1240	0(3)	L2006	0(3)	L2510	0(3)	L3213	0(3)
J9352	40(3)	K0606	0(3)	K0871	0(3)	L0492	0(3)	L1250	0(3)	L2010	0(3)	L2520	0(3)	L3214	0(3)
J9354	600(3)	K0607	0(3)	K0877	0(3)	L0621	0(3)	L1260	0(3)	L2020	0(3)	L2525	0(3)	L3215	0(3)
J9355	105(3)	K0608	0(3)	K0878	0(3)	L0622	0(3)	L1270	0(3)	L2030	0(3)	L2526	0(3)	L3216	0(3)
J9356	60(3)	K0609	0(3)	K0879	0(3)	L0623	0(3)	L1280	0(3)	L2034	0(3)	L2530	0(3)	L3217	0(3)
J9357	4(3)	K0669	0(3)	K0880	0(3)	L0624	0(3)	L1290	0(3)	L2035	0(3)	L2540	0(3)	L3219	0(3)
J9358	900(3)	K0672	0(3)	K0884	0(3)	L0625	0(3)	L1300	0(3)	L2036	0(3)	L2550	0(3)	L3221	0(3)
J9360	40(3)	K0730	0(3)	K0885	0(3)	L0626	0(3)	L1310	0(3)	L2037	0(3)	L2570	0(3)	L3222	0(3)
J9370	4(3)	K0733	0(3)	K0886	0(3)	L0627	0(3)	L1499	1(3)	L2038	0(3)	L2580	0(3)	L3224	0(3)
J9371	5(3)	K0738	0(3)	K0890	0(3)	L0628	0(3)	L1600	0(3)	L2040	0(3)	L2600	0(3)	L3225	0(3)
J9390	36(3)	K0740	0(3)	K0891	0(3)	L0629	0(3)	L1610	0(3)	L2050	0(3)	L2610	0(3)	L3230	0(3)
J9395	20(3)	K0743	0(3)	K0898	1(2)	L0630	0(3)	L1620	0(3)	L2060	0(3)	L2620	0(3)	L3250	0(3)
J9400	500(3)	K0744	0(3)	K0899	0(3)	L0631	0(3)	L1630	0(3)	L2070	0(3)	L2622	0(3)	L3251	0(3)
J9600	4(3)	K0745	0(3)	K0900	0(3)	L0632	0(3)	L1640	0(3)	L2080	0(3)	L2624	0(3)	L3252	0(3)
K0001	0(3)	K0746	0(3)	K1001	1(3)	L0633	0(3)	L1650	0(3)	L2090	0(3)	L2627	0(3)	L3253	0(3)
K0002	0(3)	K0800	0(3)	K1002	1(3)	L0634	0(3)	L1652	0(3)	L2106	0(3)	L2628	0(3)	L3254	0(3)
K0003	0(3)	K0801	0(3)	K1003	1(3)	L0635	0(3)	L1660	0(3)	L2108	0(3)	L2630	0(3)	L3255	0(3)
K0004	0(3)	K0802	0(3)	K1004	1(3)	L0636	0(3)	L1680	0(3)	L2112	0(3)	L2640	0(3)	L3257	0(3)
K0005	0(3)	K0806	0(3)	K1005	1(3)	L0637	0(3)	L1685	0(3)	L2114	0(3)	L2650	0(3)	L3260	0(3)
K0006	0(3)	K0807	0(3)	K1006	1(2)	L0638	0(3)	L1686	0(3)	L2116	0(3)	L2660	0(3)	L3265	0(3)
K0007	0(3)	K0808	0(3)	K1007	1(2)	L0639	0(3)	L1690	0(3)	L2126	0(3)	L2670	0(3)	L3300	0(3)
K0008	0(3)	K0812	0(3)	K1009	1(2)	L0640	0(3)	L1700	0(3)	L2128	0(3)	L2680	0(3)	L3310	0(3)
K0009	0(3)	K0813	0(3)	K1013	1(3)	L0641	0(3)	L1710	0(3)	L2132	0(3)	L2750	0(3)	L3320	0(3)
K0010	0(3)	K0814	0(3)	K1014	1(3)	L0642	0(3)	L1720	0(3)	L2134	0(3)	L2755	0(3)	L3330	0(3)
K0011	0(3)	K0815	0(3)	K1015	2(2)	L0643	0(3)	L1730	0(3)	L2136	0(3)	L2760	0(3)	L3332	0(3)
K0012	0(3)	K0816	0(3)	K1016	1(2)	L0648	0(3)	L1755	0(3)	L2180	0(3)	L2768	0(3)	L3334	0(3)
K0013	0(3)	K0820	0(3)	K1017	3(2)	L0649	0(3)	L1810	0(3)	L2182	0(3)	L2780	0(3)	L3340	0(3)
K0014	0(3)	K0821	0(3)	K1018	1(2)	L0650	0(3)	L1812	0(3)	L2184	0(3)	L2785	0(3)	L3350	0(3)
K0015	0(3)	K0822	0(3)	K1019	3(2)	L0651	0(3)	L1820	0(3)	L2186	0(3)	L2795	0(3)	L3360	0(3)
K0017	0(3)	K0823	0(3)	K1020	1(2)	L0700	0(3)	L1830	0(3)	L2188	0(3)	L2800	0(3)	L3370	0(3)
K0018	0(3)	K0824	0(3)	L0112	0(3)	L0710	0(3)	L1831	0(3)	L2190	0(3)	L2810	0(3)	L3380	0(3)
K0019	0(3)	K0825	0(3)	L0113	0(3)	L0810	0(3)	L1832	0(3)	L2192	0(3)	L2820	0(3)	L3390	0(3)

CPT	MUE	CPT	MUE	CPT	MUE	CPT	MUE	CPT	MUE	CPT	MUE	CPT	MUE	CPT	MUE
L3400	0(3)	L3919	0(3)	L5160	0(3)	L5653	0(3)	L5828	0(3)	L6388	0(3)	L6708	0(3)	L8000	0(3)
L3410	0(3)	L3921	0(3)	L5200	0(3)	L5654	0(3)	L5830	0(3)	L6400	0(3)	L6709	0(3)	L8001	0(3)
L3420	0(3)	L3923	0(3)	L5210	0(3)	L5655	0(3)	L5840	0(3)	L6450	0(3)	L6711	0(3)	L8002	0(3)
L3430	0(3)	L3924	0(3)	L5220	0(3)	L5656	0(3)	L5845	0(3)	L6500	0(3)	L6712	0(3)	L8010	0(3)
L3440	0(3)	L3925	0(3)	L5230	0(3)	L5658	0(3)	L5848	0(3)	L6550	0(3)	L6713	0(3)	L8015	0(3)
L3450	0(3)	L3927	0(3)	L5250	0(3)	L5661	0(3)	L5850	0(3)	L6570	0(3)	L6714	0(3)	L8020	0(3)
L3455	0(3)	L3929	0(3)	L5270	0(3)	L5665	0(3)	L5855	0(3)	L6580	0(3)	L6715	0(3)	L8030	0(3)
L3460	0(3)	L3930	0(3)	L5280	0(3)	L5666	0(3)	L5856	0(3)	L6582	0(3)	L6721	0(3)	L8031	0(3)
L3465	0(3)	L3931	0(3)	L5301	0(3)	L5668	0(3)	L5857	0(3)	L6584	0(3)	L6722	0(3)	L8032	0(3)
L3470	0(3)	L3933	0(3)	L5312	0(3)	L5670	0(3)	L5858	0(3)	L6586	0(3)	L6805	0(3)	L8033	0(3)
L3480	0(3)	L3935	0(3)	L5321	0(3)	L5671	0(3)	L5859	0(3)	L6588	0(3)	L6810	0(3)	L8035	0(3)
L3485	0(3)	L3956	0(3)	L5331	0(3)	L5672	0(3)	L5910	0(3)	L6590	0(3)	L6880	0(3)	L8039	0(3)
L3500	0(3)	L3960	0(3)	L5341	0(3)	L5673	0(3)	L5920	0(3)	L6600	0(3)	L6881	0(3)	L8040	0(3)
L3510	0(3)	L3961	0(3)	L5400	0(3)	L5676	0(3)	L5925	0(3)	L6605	0(3)	L6882	0(3)	L8041	0(3)
L3520	0(3)	L3962	0(3)	L5410	0(3)	L5677	0(3)	L5930	0(3)	L6610	0(3)	L6883	0(3)	L8042	0(3)
L3530	0(3)	L3967	0(3)	L5420	0(3)	L5678	0(3)	L5940	0(3)	L6611	0(3)	L6884	0(3)	L8043	0(3)
L3540	0(3)	L3971	0(3)	L5430	0(3)	L5679	0(3)	L5950	0(3)	L6615	0(3)	L6885	0(3)	L8044	0(3)
L3550	0(3)	L3973	0(3)	L5450	0(3)	L5680	0(3)	L5960	0(3)	L6616	0(3)	L6890	0(3)	L8045	0(3)
L3560	0(3)	L3975	0(3)	L5460	0(3)	L5681	0(3)	L5961	0(3)	L6620	0(3)	L6895	0(3)	L8046	0(3)
L3570	0(3)	L3976	0(3)	L5500	0(3)	L5682	0(3)	L5962	0(3)	L6621	0(3)	L6900	0(3)	L8047	0(3)
L3580	0(3)	L3977	0(3)	L5505	0(3)	L5683	0(3)	L5964	0(3)	L6623	0(3)	L6905	0(3)	L8048	1(3)
L3590	0(3)	L3978	0(3)	L5510	0(3)	L5684	0(3)	L5966	0(3)	L6624	0(3)	L6910	0(3)	L8049	0(3)
L3595	0(3)	L3980	0(3)	L5520	0(3)	L5685	0(3)	L5968	0(3)	L6625	0(3)	L6915	0(3)	L8300	0(3)
L3600	0(3)	L3981	0(3)	L5530	0(3)	L5686	0(3)	L5969	0(3)	L6628	0(3)	L6920	0(3)	L8310	0(3)
L3610	0(3)	L3982	0(3)	L5535	0(3)	L5688	0(3)	L5970	0(3)	L6629	0(3)	L6925	0(3)	L8320	0(3)
L3620	0(3)	L3984	0(3)	L5540	0(3)	L5690	0(3)	L5971	0(3)	L6630	0(3)	L6930	0(3)	L8330	0(3)
L3630	0(3)	L3995	0(3)	L5560	0(3)	L5692	0(3)	L5972	0(3)	L6632	0(3)	L6935	0(3)	L8400	0(3)
L3640	0(3)	L3999	0(3)	L5570	0(3)	L5694	0(3)	L5973	0(3)	L6635	0(3)	L6940	0(3)	L8410	0(3)
L3649	0(3)	L4000	0(3)	L5580	0(3)	L5695	0(3)	L5974	0(3)	L6637	0(3)	L6945	0(3)	L8415	0(3)
L3650	0(3)	L4002	0(3)	L5585	0(3)	L5696	0(3)	L5975	0(3)	L6638	0(3)	L6950	0(3)	L8417	0(3)
L3660	0(3)	L4010	0(3)	L5590	0(3)	L5697	0(3)	L5976	0(3)	L6640	0(3)	L6955	0(3)	L8420	0(3)
L3670	0(3)	L4020	0(3)	L5595	0(3)	L5698	0(3)	L5978	0(3)	L6641	0(3)	L6960	0(3)	L8430	0(3)
L3671	0(3)	L4030	0(3)	L5600	0(3)	L5699	0(3)	L5979	0(3)	L6642	0(3)	L6965	0(3)	L8435	0(3)
L3674	0(3)	L4040	0(3)	L5610	0(3)	L5700	0(3)	L5980	0(3)	L6645	0(3)	L6970	0(3)	L8440	0(3)
L3675	0(3)	L4045	0(3)	L5611	0(3)	L5701	0(3)	L5981	0(3)	L6646	0(3)	L6975	0(3)	L8460	0(3)
L3677	0(3)	L4050	0(3)	L5613	0(3)	L5702	0(3)	L5982	0(3)	L6647	0(3)	L7007	0(3)	L8465	0(3)
L3678	0(3)	L4055	0(3)	L5614	0(3)	L5703	0(3)	L5984	0(3)	L6648	0(3)	L7008	0(3)	L8470	0(3)
L3702	0(3)	L4060	0(3)	L5616	0(3)	L5704	0(3)	L5985	0(3)	L6650	0(3)	L7009	0(3)	L8480	0(3)
L3710	0(3)	L4070	0(3)	L5617	0(3)	L5705	0(3)	L5986	0(3)	L6655	0(3)	L7040	0(3)	L8485	0(3)
L3720	0(3)	L4080	0(3)	L5618	0(3)	L5706	0(3)	L5987	0(3)	L6660	0(3)	L7045	0(3)	L8499	1(3)
L3730	0(3)	L4090	0(3)	L5620	0(3)	L5707	0(3)	L5988	0(3)	L6665	0(3)	L7170	0(3)	L8500	0(3)
L3740	0(3)	L4100	0(3)	L5622	0(3)	L5710	0(3)	L5990	0(3)	L6670	0(3)	L7180	0(3)	L8501	0(3)
L3760	0(3)	L4110	0(3)	L5624	0(3)	L5711	0(3)	L5999	0(3)	L6672	0(3)	L7181	0(3)	L8505	0(3)
L3761	0(3)	L4130	0(3)	L5626	0(3)	L5712	0(3)	L6000	0(3)	L6675	0(3)	L7185	0(3)	L8507	0(3)
L3762	0(3)	L4205	0(3)	L5628	0(3)	L5714	0(3)	L6010	0(3)	L6676	0(3)	L7186	0(3)	L8509	1(3)
L3763	0(3)	L4210	0(3)	L5629	0(3)	L5716	0(3)	L6020	0(3)	L6677	0(3)	L7190	0(3)	L8510	0(3)
L3764	0(3)	L4350	0(3)	L5630	0(3)	L5718	0(3)	L6026	0(3)	L6680	0(3)	L7191	0(3)	L8511	1(3)
L3765	0(3)	L4360	0(3)	L5631	0(3)	L5722	0(3)	L6050	0(3)	L6682	0(3)	L7259	0(3)	L8512	1(3)
L3766	0(3)	L4361	0(3)	L5632	0(3)	L5724	0(3)	L6055	0(3)	L6684	0(3)	L7360	0(3)	L8513	1(3)
L3806	0(3)	L4370	0(3)	L5634	0(3)	L5726	0(3)	L6100	0(3)	L6686	0(3)	L7362	0(3)	L8514	1(3)
L3807	0(3)	L4386	0(3)	L5636	0(3)	L5728	0(3)	L6110	0(3)	L6687	0(3)	L7364	0(3)	L8515	1(3)
L3808	0(3)	L4387	0(3)	L5637	0(3)	L5780	0(3)	L6120	0(3)	L6688	0(3)	L7366	0(3)	L8600	2(3)
L3809	0(3)	L4392	0(3)	L5638	0(3)	L5781	0(3)	L6130	0(3)	L6689	0(3)	L7367	0(3)	L8603	4(3)
L3891	0(3)	L4394	0(3)	L5639	0(3)	L5782	0(3)	L6200	0(3)	L6690	0(3)	L7368	0(3)	L8604	3(3)
L3900	0(3)	L4396	0(3)	L5640	0(3)	L5785	0(3)	L6205	0(3)	L6691	0(3)	L7400	0(3)	L8605	4(3)
L3901	0(3)	L4397	0(3)	L5642	0(3)	L5790	0(3)	L6250	0(3)	L6692	0(3)	L7401	0(3)	L8606	5(3)
L3904	0(3)	L4398	0(3)	L5643	0(3)	L5795	0(3)	L6300	0(3)	L6693	0(3)	L7402	0(3)	L8607	20(3)
L3905	0(3)	L4631	0(3)	L5644	0(3)	L5810	0(3)	L6310	0(3)	L6694	0(3)	L7403	0(3)	L8609	1(3)
L3906	0(3)	L5000	0(3)	L5645	0(3)	L5811	0(3)	L6320	0(3)	L6695	0(3)	L7404	0(3)	L8610	1(3)
L3908	0(3)	L5010	0(3)	L5646	0(3)	L5812	0(3)	L6350	0(3)	L6696	0(3)	L7405	0(3)	L8612	1(3)
L3912	0(3)	L5020	0(3)	L5647	0(3)	L5814	0(3)	L6360	0(3)	L6697	0(3)	L7499	0(3)	L8613	1(3)
L3913	0(3)	L5050	0(3)	L5648	0(3)	L5816	0(3)	L6370	0(3)	L6698	0(3)	L7510	4(3)	L8614	1(3)
L3915	0(3)	L5060	0(3)	L5649	0(3)	L5818	0(3)	L6380	0(3)	L6703	0(3)	L7600	0(3)	L8615	2(3)
L3916	0(3)	L5100	0(3)	L5650	0(3)	L5822	0(3)	L6382	0(3)	L6704	0(3)	L7700	0(3)	L8616	2(3)
L3917	0(3)	L5105	0(3)	L5651	0(3)	L5824	0(3)	L6384	0(3)	L6706	0(3)	L7900	0(3)	L8617	2(3)
L3918	0(3)	L5150	0(3)	L5652	0(3)	L5826	0(3)	L6386	0(3)	L6707	0(3)	L7902	0(3)	L8618	2(3)

　　CPT © 2021 American Medical Association. All Rights Reserved.　　© 2021 Optum360, LLC

CPT	MUE	CPT	MUE	CPT	MUE	CPT	MUE	CPT	MUE	CPT	MUE	CPT	MUE	CPT	MUE
L8619	2(3)	P9021	3(3)	Q0167	0(3)	Q2037	1(2)	Q9954	18(3)	V2212	0(3)	V2630	2(2)	V5221	0(3)
L8621	360(3)	P9022	2(3)	Q0169	0(3)	Q2038	1(2)	Q9955	0(3)	V2213	0(3)	V2631	2(2)	V5230	0(3)
L8622	2(3)	P9023	2(3)	Q0173	0(3)	Q2039	1(2)	Q9956	9(3)	V2214	0(3)	V2632	2(2)	V5240	0(3)
L8625	1(3)	P9031	12(3)	Q0174	0(3)	Q2043	1(2)	Q9957	3(3)	V2215	0(3)	V2700	0(3)	V5241	0(3)
L8627	2(2)	P9032	12(3)	Q0175	0(3)	Q2049	10(3)	Q9958	300(3)	V2218	0(3)	V2702	0(3)	V5242	0(3)
L8628	2(2)	P9033	12(3)	Q0177	0(3)	Q2050	14(3)	Q9959	0(3)	V2219	0(3)	V2710	0(3)	V5243	0(3)
L8629	2(2)	P9034	2(3)	Q0180	0(3)	Q2052	1(3)	Q9960	250(3)	V2220	0(3)	V2715	0(3)	V5244	0(3)
L8631	1(3)	P9035	2(3)	Q0181	0(3)	Q3014	1(3)	Q9961	200(3)	V2221	0(3)	V2718	0(3)	V5245	0(3)
L8641	4(3)	P9036	2(3)	Q0243	1(3)	Q3027	30(3)	Q9962	150(3)	V2299	0(3)	V2730	0(3)	V5246	0(3)
L8642	2(3)	P9037	2(3)	Q0244	1(3)	Q3028	0(3)	Q9963	240(3)	V2300	0(3)	V2744	0(3)	V5247	0(3)
L8658	2(3)	P9038	2(3)	Q0245	1(3)	Q3031	1(3)	Q9964	0(3)	V2301	0(3)	V2745	0(3)	V5248	0(3)
L8659	2(3)	P9039	2(3)	Q0247	1(2)	Q4001	1(3)	Q9966	250(3)	V2302	0(3)	V2750	0(3)	V5249	0(3)
L8670	2(3)	P9040	3(3)	Q0477	1(1)	Q4002	1(3)	Q9967	300(3)	V2303	0(3)	V2755	0(3)	V5250	0(3)
L8679	1(3)	P9041	5(3)	Q0478	1(3)	Q4003	2(3)	Q9969	3(3)	V2304	0(3)	V2756	0(3)	V5251	0(3)
L8681	1(3)	P9043	5(3)	Q0479	1(3)	Q4004	2(3)	Q9982	1(3)	V2305	0(3)	V2760	0(3)	V5252	0(3)
L8682	2(3)	P9044	10(3)	Q0480	1(3)	Q4012	2(3)	Q9983	1(3)	V2306	0(3)	V2761	0(2)	V5253	0(3)
L8683	1(3)	P9045	20(3)	Q0481	1(2)	Q4013	2(3)	Q9991	1(2)	V2307	0(3)	V2762	0(3)	V5254	0(3)
L8684	1(3)	P9046	25(3)	Q0482	1(3)	Q4014	2(3)	Q9992	1(2)	V2308	0(3)	V2770	0(3)	V5255	0(3)
L8685	1(3)	P9047	20(3)	Q0483	1(3)	Q4018	2(3)	R0070	2(3)	V2309	0(3)	V2780	0(3)	V5256	0(3)
L8686	2(3)	P9048	1(3)	Q0484	1(3)	Q4021	2(3)	R0075	2(3)	V2310	0(3)	V2781	0(2)	V5257	0(3)
L8687	1(3)	P9050	1(3)	Q0485	1(3)	Q4025	1(3)	R0076	1(3)	V2311	0(3)	V2782	0(3)	V5258	0(3)
L8688	1(3)	P9051	2(3)	Q0486	1(3)	Q4026	1(3)	U0001	2(3)	V2312	0(3)	V2783	0(3)	V5259	0(3)
L8689	1(3)	P9052	2(3)	Q0487	1(3)	Q4027	1(3)	U0002	2(3)	V2313	0(3)	V2784	0(3)	V5260	0(3)
L8690	2(2)	P9053	2(3)	Q0488	1(3)	Q4028	1(3)	U0003	2(3)	V2314	0(3)	V2785	2(2)	V5261	0(3)
L8691	1(3)	P9054	2(3)	Q0489	1(3)	Q4030	2(3)	U0004	2(3)	V2315	0(3)	V2786	0(3)	V5262	0(3)
L8692	0(3)	P9055	2(3)	Q0490	1(3)	Q4037	2(3)	U0005	1(3)	V2318	0(3)	V2787	0(3)	V5263	0(3)
L8693	1(3)	P9056	2(3)	Q0491	1(3)	Q4042	2(3)	V2020	0(3)	V2319	0(3)	V2788	0(3)	V5264	0(3)
L8694	1(3)	P9057	2(3)	Q0492	1(3)	Q4046	2(3)	V2025	0(3)	V2320	0(3)	V2790	1(3)	V5265	0(3)
L8695	1(3)	P9058	2(3)	Q0493	1(3)	Q4050	2(3)	V2100	0(3)	V2321	0(3)	V2797	0(3)	V5266	0(3)
L8696	1(3)	P9059	2(3)	Q0494	1(3)	Q4051	2(3)	V2101	0(3)	V2399	0(3)	V5008	0(3)	V5267	0(3)
L8701	0(3)	P9060	2(3)	Q0495	1(3)	Q4074	3(3)	V2102	0(3)	V2410	0(3)	V5010	0(3)	V5268	0(3)
L8702	0(3)	P9070	2(3)	Q0496	1(3)	Q4081	100(3)	V2103	0(3)	V2430	0(3)	V5011	0(3)	V5269	0(3)
M0075	0(3)	P9071	2(3)	Q0497	2(3)	Q5101	1500(3)	V2104	0(3)	V2499	2(3)	V5014	0(3)	V5270	0(3)
M0076	0(3)	P9073	2(3)	Q0498	1(3)	Q5103	150(3)	V2105	0(3)	V2500	0(3)	V5020	0(3)	V5271	0(3)
M0100	0(3)	P9099	1(3)	Q0499	1(3)	Q5104	150(3)	V2106	0(3)	V2501	0(3)	V5030	0(3)	V5272	0(3)
M0201	1(2)	P9100	2(3)	Q0501	1(3)	Q5105	100(3)	V2107	0(3)	V2502	0(3)	V5040	0(3)	V5273	0(3)
M0243	1(2)	P9603	300(3)	Q0502	1(3)	Q5106	60(3)	V2108	0(3)	V2503	0(3)	V5050	0(3)	V5274	0(3)
M0244	1(2)	P9604	2(3)	Q0503	3(3)	Q5107	170(3)	V2109	0(3)	V2510	0(3)	V5060	0(3)	V5275	0(3)
M0245	1(2)	P9612	1(3)	Q0504	1(3)	Q5108	12(3)	V2110	0(3)	V2511	0(3)	V5070	0(3)	V5281	0(3)
M0246	1(2)	P9615	1(3)	Q0506	8(3)	Q5109	150(3)	V2111	0(3)	V2512	0(3)	V5080	0(3)	V5282	0(3)
M0247	1(2)	Q0035	1(3)	Q0507	1(3)	Q5110	1500(3)	V2112	0(3)	V2513	0(3)	V5090	0(3)	V5283	0(3)
M0248	1(2)	Q0081	1(3)	Q0508	4(3)	Q5111	12(3)	V2113	0(3)	V2520	2(3)	V5095	0(3)	V5284	0(3)
M0300	0(3)	Q0083	1(3)	Q0509	2(3)	Q5112	120(3)	V2114	0(3)	V2521	2(3)	V5100	0(3)	V5285	0(3)
M0301	0(3)	Q0084	1(3)	Q0510	0(3)	Q5113	120(3)	V2115	0(3)	V2522	2(3)	V5110	0(3)	V5286	0(3)
P2028	1(2)	Q0085	1(3)	Q0511	0(3)	Q5114	120(3)	V2118	0(3)	V2523	2(3)	V5120	0(3)	V5287	0(3)
P2029	1(2)	Q0091	1(3)	Q0512	0(3)	Q5115	150(3)	V2121	0(3)	V2524	2(3)	V5130	0(3)	V5288	0(3)
P2031	0(3)	Q0111	2(3)	Q0513	0(3)	Q5116	120(3)	V2199	2(3)	V2530	0(3)	V5140	0(3)	V5289	0(3)
P2033	1(2)	Q0112	3(3)	Q0514	0(3)	Q5117	120(3)	V2200	0(3)	V2531	0(3)	V5150	0(3)	V5290	0(3)
P2038	1(2)	Q0113	1(3)	Q0515	0(3)	Q5118	230(3)	V2201	0(3)	V2599	2(3)	V5160	0(3)	V5298	0(3)
P3000	1(3)	Q0114	1(3)	Q1004	2(2)	Q5119	150(3)	V2202	0(3)	V2600	0(2)	V5171	0(3)	V5299	1(3)
P3001	1(3)	Q0115	1(3)	Q1005	2(2)	Q5120	12(3)	V2203	0(3)	V2610	0(2)	V5172	0(3)	V5336	0(3)
P7001	0(3)	Q0138	510(3)	Q2004	1(3)	Q5121	150(3)	V2204	0(3)	V2615	0(2)	V5181	0(3)	V5362	0(3)
P9010	2(3)	Q0139	510(3)	Q2009	100(3)	Q5122	12(3)	V2205	0(3)	V2623	0(3)	V5190	0(3)	V5363	0(3)
P9011	2(3)	Q0144	0(3)	Q2017	12(3)	Q9001	1(3)	V2206	0(3)	V2624	0(3)	V5200	0(3)	V5364	0(3)
P9012	8(3)	Q0161	0(3)	Q2026	30(3)	Q9002	1(3)	V2207	0(3)	V2625	0(3)	V5211	0(3)		
P9016	3(3)	Q0162	0(3)	Q2028	1470(3)	Q9003	1(3)	V2208	0(3)	V2626	0(3)	V5212	0(3)		
P9017	2(3)	Q0163	0(3)	Q2034	1(3)	Q9950	5(3)	V2209	0(3)	V2627	0(3)	V5213	0(3)		
P9019	2(3)	Q0164	0(3)	Q2035	1(2)	Q9951	0(3)	V2210	0(3)	V2628	0(3)	V5214	0(3)		
P9020	2(3)	Q0166	0(3)	Q2036	1(2)	Q9953	10(3)	V2211	0(3)	V2629	0(3)	V5215	0(3)		

OPPS

CPT	MUE	CPT	MUE	CPT	MUE	CPT	MUE	CPT	MUE	CPT	MUE	CPT	MUE	CPT	MUE
0001A	1(2)	0050U	1(3)	0108U	1(2)	0173U	1(2)	0235T	2(3)	0394T	2(3)	0467T	1(3)	0533T	1(2)
0001U	1(2)	0051U	1(2)	0109T	4(2)	0174T	1(3)	0235U	1(2)	0395T	2(3)	0468T	1(3)	0534T	1(2)
0002A	1(2)	0052U	1(2)	0109U	1(3)	0174U	1(2)	0236T	1(2)	0397T	1(3)	0469T	1(2)	0535T	1(2)
0002M	1(3)	0053U	1(3)	0110T	4(2)	0175T	1(3)	0236U	1(2)	0398T	1(3)	0470T	1(2)	0536T	1(2)
0002U	1(2)	0054T	1(3)	0110U	1(2)	0175U	1(2)	0237T	2(3)	0402T	2(2)	0471T	2(1)	0537T	1(3)
0003M	1(3)	0054U	1(2)	0111U	1(2)	0176U	1(3)	0237U	1(2)	0403T	0(3)	0472T	1(2)	0538T	1(3)
0003U	1(2)	0055T	1(3)	0112U	1(3)	0177U	1(3)	0238T	2(3)	0404T	1(2)	0473T	1(2)	0539T	1(3)
0004M	1(2)	0055U	1(2)	0113U	1(2)	0178U	1(2)	0238U	1(2)	0408T	1(3)	0474T	0(3)	0540T	1(3)
0005U	1(2)	0056U	1(3)	0114U	1(2)	0179U	1(2)	0239U	1(2)	0409T	1(3)	0475T	1(3)	0541T	1(3)
0006M	1(2)	0058U	1(2)	0115U	1(2)	0184T	1(3)	0240U	1(3)	0410T	1(3)	0476T	1(3)	0542T	1(3)
0007M	1(2)	0059U	1(3)	0116U	1(2)	0191T	2(2)	0241U	1(3)	0411T	1(3)	0477T	1(3)	0543T	1(2)
0007U	1(2)	0060U	1(2)	0117U	1(2)	0198T	2(2)	0242U	1(2)	0412T	1(2)	0478T	1(3)	0544T	1(2)
0008U	1(3)	0061U	2(3)	0118U	1(2)	01996	1(2)	0243U	1(2)	0413T	1(3)	0479T	1(2)	0545T	1(2)
0009U	2(3)	0062U	1(2)	0119U	1(2)	0200T	1(2)	0244U	1(3)	0414T	1(2)	0480T	4(1)	0546T	2(2)
0010U	2(3)	0063U	1(2)	0120U	1(2)	0201T	1(2)	0245U	2(3)	0415T	1(3)	0481T	1(3)	0547T	1(2)
0011A	1(2)	0064U	2(3)	0121U	1(2)	0202T	1(3)	0247U	1(2)	0416T	1(3)	0483T	1(2)	0548T	1(2)
0011M	1(2)	0065U	2(3)	0122U	1(2)	0202U	1(3)	0253T	1(3)	0417T	1(3)	0484T	1(2)	0549T	1(2)
0011U	1(2)	0066U	1(3)	0123U	1(2)	0203U	1(2)	0263T	1(3)	0418T	1(3)	0485T	1(2)	0550T	2(3)
0012A	1(2)	0067U	2(3)	0129U	1(2)	0204U	1(3)	0264T	1(3)	0419T	1(2)	0486T	1(2)	0551T	1(2)
0012M	1(2)	0068U	1(3)	0130U	1(2)	0205U	1(2)	0265T	1(3)	0420T	1(2)	0487T	1(3)	0552T	0(3)
0012U	1(2)	0069U	1(3)	0131U	1(2)	0206U	1(3)	0266T	1(2)	0421T	1(2)	0488T	1(2)	0553T	0(3)
0013M	1(2)	0070U	1(2)	0132U	1(2)	0207T	2(2)	0267T	1(3)	0422T	1(3)	0489T	1(2)	0554T	0(3)
0013U	1(3)	0071T	1(2)	0133U	1(2)	0207U	1(2)	0268T	1(3)	0423T	1(3)	0490T	1(2)	0555T	1(2)
0014M	1(2)	0071U	1(2)	0134U	1(2)	0208T	1(3)	0269T	1(2)	0424T	1(3)	0491T	1(2)	0556T	1(2)
0014U	1(3)	0072T	1(2)	0135U	1(2)	0208U	1(3)	0270T	1(3)	0425T	1(3)	0492T	4(3)	0557T	0(3)
0015M	1(2)	0072U	1(2)	0136U	1(2)	0209T	1(3)	0271T	1(3)	0426T	1(3)	0493T	1(3)	0558T	1(2)
0016M	2(3)	0073U	1(2)	0137U	1(2)	0209U	1(2)	0272T	1(3)	0427T	1(3)	0494T	1(3)	0559T	1(2)
0016U	1(3)	0074U	1(2)	0138U	1(2)	0210T	1(3)	0273T	1(3)	0428T	1(2)	0495T	1(2)	0560T	1(3)
0017U	1(3)	0075T	1(2)	0139U	1(2)	0210U	2(3)	0274T	1(2)	0429T	1(2)	0496T	4(3)	0561T	1(2)
0018U	2(3)	0075U	1(2)	0140U	1(2)	0211T	1(3)	0275T	1(2)	0430T	1(2)	0497T	1(3)	0562T	1(3)
0019U	1(3)	0076T	1(2)	0141U	1(2)	0211U	2(3)	0278T	1(3)	0431T	1(2)	0498T	1(2)	0563T	1(2)
0021A	1(2)	0076U	1(2)	0142U	1(2)	0212T	1(3)	0290T	1(3)	0432T	1(3)	0499T	1(2)	0564T	1(2)
0021U	1(2)	0077U	2(2)	0143U	1(2)	0212U	1(2)	0308T	1(3)	0433T	1(3)	0500T	1(3)	0565T	1(2)
0022A	1(2)	0078U	1(2)	0144U	1(2)	0213T	1(3)	0312T	1(3)	0434T	1(3)	0501T	1(2)	0566T	1(2)
0022U	2(3)	0079U	0(3)	0145U	1(2)	0213U	1(3)	0313T	1(3)	0435T	1(3)	0502T	1(2)	0567T	1(2)
0023U	1(2)	0080U	1(2)	0146U	1(2)	0214T	1(2)	0314T	1(3)	0436T	1(3)	0503T	1(2)	0568T	1(2)
0024U	1(2)	0082U	1(2)	0147U	1(2)	0214U	1(2)	0315T	1(3)	0437T	1(3)	0504T	1(2)	0569T	1(2)
0025U	1(2)	0083U	1(3)	0148U	1(2)	0215T	1(2)	0316T	1(3)	0439T	1(3)	0505T	1(3)	0570T	1(3)
0026U	2(3)	0084U	1(2)	0149U	1(2)	0215U	1(3)	0317T	1(3)	0440T	3(3)	0506T	1(2)	0571T	1(2)
0027U	1(2)	0086U	1(3)	0150U	1(2)	0216T	1(2)	0329T	0(3)	0441T	3(3)	0507T	1(2)	0572T	1(2)
0029U	1(2)	0087U	1(2)	0151U	1(2)	0216U	1(2)	0330T	1(2)	0442T	3(3)	0508T	1(3)	0573T	1(2)
0030U	1(2)	0088U	1(2)	0152U	1(2)	0217T	1(2)	0331T	1(3)	0443T	1(2)	0509T	1(2)	0574T	1(2)
0031A	1(2)	0089U	1(3)	0153U	1(2)	0217U	1(2)	0332T	1(3)	0444T	1(2)	0510T	1(2)	0575T	1(2)
0031U	1(2)	0090U	1(2)	0154U	1(2)	0218T	1(2)	0333T	0(3)	0445T	1(3)	0511T	1(2)	0576T	1(2)
0032U	1(2)	0091U	1(2)	0155U	1(2)	0218U	1(2)	0335T	2(2)	0446T	1(3)	0512T	1(2)	0577T	1(2)
0033U	1(2)	0092U	1(2)	0156U	1(2)	0219T	1(2)	0338T	1(3)	0447T	1(3)	0513T	2(3)	0578T	1(2)
0034U	1(2)	0093U	1(2)	0157U	1(2)	0219U	1(2)	0339T	1(2)	0448T	1(3)	0514T	2(2)	0579T	1(2)
0035U	1(2)	0094U	1(2)	0158U	1(2)	0220T	1(2)	0342T	1(3)	0449T	1(2)	0515T	1(3)	0580T	1(2)
0036U	1(3)	0095T	1(3)	0159U	1(2)	0220U	1(2)	0345T	1(2)	0450T	1(3)	0516T	1(3)	0581T	0(3)
0037U	1(3)	0095U	1(2)	0160U	1(2)	0221T	1(2)	0347T	1(3)	0451T	1(3)	0517T	1(3)	0582T	0(3)
0038U	1(3)	0096U	1(2)	0161U	1(2)	0222T	1(3)	0348T	1(3)	0452T	1(3)	0518T	1(3)	0583T	2(2)
0039U	1(2)	0097U	1(2)	0162U	1(2)	0223U	1(3)	0349T	1(3)	0453T	1(3)	0519T	1(3)	0584T	1(2)
0040U	1(2)	0098T	2(3)	0163T	1(3)	0224U	3(3)	0350T	1(3)	0454T	3(3)	0520T	1(3)	0585T	1(2)
0041A	1(2)	0100T	1(2)	0163U	0(3)	0225U	1(3)	0351T	5(3)	0455T	1(3)	0521T	1(3)	0586T	1(2)
0041U	1(2)	0101T	1(3)	0164T	4(2)	0226U	1(3)	0352T	5(3)	0456T	1(3)	0522T	1(3)	0587T	1(2)
0042A	1(2)	0101U	1(2)	0164U	1(2)	0227U	1(2)	0353T	2(3)	0457T	1(3)	0523T	1(3)	0588T	1(2)
0042T	1(3)	0102T	2(2)	0165T	4(2)	0228U	1(2)	0354T	2(3)	0458T	3(3)	0524T	3(3)	0589T	1(2)
0042U	1(2)	0102U	1(2)	0165U	1(2)	0229U	1(2)	0355T	1(2)	0459T	1(3)	0525T	1(3)	0590T	1(2)
0043U	1(2)	0103U	1(2)	0166U	1(2)	0230U	1(2)	0356T	4(2)	0460T	3(3)	0526T	1(3)	0591T	1(2)
0044U	1(2)	0105U	1(2)	0167U	1(2)	0231U	1(2)	0358T	1(2)	0461T	1(3)	0527T	1(3)	0592T	1(2)
0045U	1(3)	0106T	4(2)	0168U	1(2)	0232T	1(3)	0362T	16(3)	0462T	1(2)	0528T	1(3)	0593T	1(2)
0046U	1(3)	0106U	1(2)	0169U	1(2)	0232U	1(2)	0373T	24(3)	0463T	1(3)	0529T	1(3)	0594T	2(2)
0047U	1(3)	0107T	4(2)	0170U	1(2)	0233U	1(3)	0376T	2(3)	0464T	1(2)	0530T	1(3)	0596T	1(2)
0048U	1(3)	0107U	1(3)	0171U	1(3)	0234T	2(2)	0378T	1(2)	0465T	1(3)	0531T	1(3)	0597T	1(2)
0049U	1(3)	0108T	4(2)	0172U	1(2)	0234U	1(2)	0379T	1(2)	0466T	1(3)	0532T	1(3)	0598T	1(2)

CPT	MUE	CPT	MUE	CPT	MUE	CPT	MUE	CPT	MUE	CPT	MUE	CPT	MUE	CPT	MUE
0599T	1(3)	11004	1(2)	11620	2(3)	12044	1(2)	15261	6(3)	15838	1(2)	17284	2(3)	19396	1(2)
0600T	3(3)	11005	1(2)	11621	2(3)	12045	1(2)	15271	1(2)	15839	2(3)	17286	2(3)	19499	1(3)
0601T	3(3)	11006	1(2)	11622	2(3)	12046	1(2)	15272	3(3)	15840	1(3)	17311	4(3)	20100	2(3)
0602T	1(2)	11008	1(2)	11623	2(3)	12047	1(2)	15273	1(2)	15841	2(3)	17312	6(3)	20101	2(3)
0603T	1(2)	11010	2(3)	11624	2(3)	12051	1(2)	15274	6(3)	15842	2(3)	17313	3(3)	20102	3(3)
0604T	1(2)	11011	2(3)	11626	2(3)	12052	1(2)	15275	1(2)	15845	2(3)	17314	4(3)	20103	3(3)
0605T	1(2)	11012	2(3)	11640	2(3)	12053	1(2)	15276	3(2)	15847	1(2)	17315	15(3)	20150	2(3)
0606T	0(3)	11042	1(2)	11641	2(3)	12054	1(2)	15277	1(2)	15850	1(2)	17340	1(2)	20200	2(3)
0607T	1(2)	11043	1(2)	11642	3(3)	12055	1(2)	15278	3(3)	15851	1(2)	17360	1(2)	20205	3(3)
0608T	1(2)	11044	1(2)	11643	2(3)	12056	1(2)	15570	2(3)	15852	1(3)	17380	1(3)	20206	2(3)
0609T	1(3)	11045	12(3)	11644	2(3)	12057	1(2)	15572	2(3)	15860	1(3)	17999	1(3)	20220	3(3)
0610T	1(3)	11046	4(3)	11646	2(3)	13100	1(2)	15574	2(3)	15876	1(2)	19000	2(3)	20225	2(3)
0611T	1(3)	11047	4(3)	11719	1(2)	13101	1(2)	15576	2(3)	15877	1(2)	19001	5(3)	20240	4(3)
0612T	0(3)	11055	1(2)	11720	1(2)	13102	9(3)	15600	2(3)	15878	1(2)	19020	2(3)	20245	3(3)
0613T	0(3)	11056	1(2)	11721	1(2)	13120	1(2)	15610	2(3)	15879	1(2)	19030	1(2)	20250	1(3)
0614T	1(3)	11057	1(2)	11730	1(2)	13121	1(2)	15620	2(3)	15920	1(3)	19081	1(2)	20251	2(3)
0615T	1(3)	11102	1(2)	11732	4(3)	13122	9(3)	15630	2(3)	15922	1(3)	19082	2(3)	20500	2(3)
0616T	2(2)	11103	6(3)	11740	2(3)	13131	1(2)	15650	1(3)	15931	1(3)	19083	1(2)	20501	2(3)
0617T	2(2)	11104	1(2)	11750	6(3)	13132	1(2)	15730	1(3)	15933	1(3)	19084	2(3)	20520	2(3)
0618T	2(2)	11105	3(3)	11755	2(3)	13133	7(3)	15731	1(3)	15934	1(3)	19085	1(2)	20525	4(3)
0619T	1(2)	11106	1(2)	11760	4(3)	13151	1(2)	15733	2(3)	15935	1(3)	19086	2(3)	20526	1(2)
0620T	2(2)	11107	2(3)	11762	2(3)	13152	1(2)	15734	4(3)	15936	1(3)	19100	4(3)	20527	2(3)
0621T	2(2)	11200	1(2)	11765	4(3)	13153	2(3)	15736	2(3)	15937	1(3)	19101	3(3)	20550	5(3)
0622T	2(2)	11201	1(3)	11770	1(3)	13160	2(3)	15738	3(3)	15940	2(3)	19105	2(3)	20551	5(3)
0623T	1(2)	11300	5(3)	11771	1(3)	14000	2(3)	15740	2(3)	15941	2(3)	19110	1(3)	20552	1(2)
0624T	1(2)	11301	6(3)	11772	1(3)	14001	2(3)	15750	2(3)	15944	2(3)	19112	2(3)	20553	1(2)
0625T	1(2)	11302	4(3)	11900	1(2)	14020	2(3)	15756	2(3)	15945	2(3)	19120	1(2)	20555	1(3)
0626T	1(2)	11303	3(3)	11901	1(2)	14021	2(3)	15757	2(3)	15946	2(3)	19125	1(2)	20560	1(2)
0627T	1(2)	11305	4(3)	11920	1(2)	14040	2(3)	15758	2(3)	15950	2(3)	19126	3(3)	20561	1(2)
0628T	4(2)	11306	4(3)	11921	1(2)	14041	3(3)	15760	2(3)	15951	2(3)	19281	1(2)	20600	6(3)
0629T	1(2)	11307	3(3)	11922	1(3)	14060	2(3)	15769	1(3)	15952	2(3)	19282	2(3)	20604	4(3)
0630T	4(2)	11308	2(3)	11950	1(2)	14061	2(3)	15770	2(3)	15953	2(3)	19283	1(2)	20605	2(3)
0631T	4(2)	11310	4(3)	11951	1(2)	14301	2(3)	15771	1(2)	15956	2(3)	19284	2(3)	20606	2(3)
0632T	1(2)	11311	4(3)	11952	1(2)	14302	8(3)	15772	9(3)	15958	2(3)	19285	1(2)	20610	2(3)
0633T	1(2)	11312	3(3)	11954	1(3)	14350	2(3)	15773	1(2)	15999	1(3)	19286	2(3)	20611	2(3)
0634T	1(2)	11313	3(3)	11960	2(3)	15002	1(2)	15774	3(3)	16000	1(2)	19287	1(2)	20612	2(3)
0635T	1(2)	11400	3(3)	11970	2(3)	15003	9(3)	15775	1(2)	16020	1(3)	19288	2(3)	20615	1(3)
0636T	1(2)	11401	3(3)	11971	2(3)	15004	1(2)	15776	1(2)	16025	1(3)	19294	2(3)	20650	4(3)
0637T	1(2)	11402	3(3)	11976	1(2)	15005	2(3)	15777	1(3)	16030	1(3)	19296	1(3)	20660	1(2)
0638T	1(2)	11403	2(3)	11980	1(2)	15040	1(2)	15780	1(2)	16035	1(2)	19297	2(3)	20661	1(2)
0639T	1(3)	11404	2(3)	11981	1(3)	15050	1(3)	15781	1(3)	16036	2(3)	19298	1(2)	20662	1(2)
10004	3(3)	11406	2(3)	11982	1(3)	15100	1(2)	15782	1(3)	17000	1(2)	19300	1(2)	20663	1(2)
10005	1(2)	11420	3(3)	11983	1(3)	15101	9(3)	15783	1(3)	17003	13(2)	19301	1(3)	20664	1(2)
10006	3(3)	11421	3(3)	12001	1(2)	15110	1(2)	15786	1(2)	17004	1(2)	19302	1(2)	20665	1(2)
10007	1(2)	11422	3(3)	12002	1(2)	15111	2(3)	15787	2(3)	17106	1(2)	19303	1(2)	20670	3(3)
10008	2(3)	11423	2(3)	12004	1(2)	15115	1(2)	15788	1(2)	17107	1(2)	19305	1(2)	20680	3(3)
10009	1(2)	11424	2(3)	12005	1(2)	15116	2(3)	15789	1(3)	17108	1(2)	19306	1(2)	20690	1(2)
10010	3(3)	11426	2(3)	12006	1(2)	15120	1(2)	15792	1(3)	17110	1(2)	19307	1(2)	20692	2(3)
10011	1(2)	11440	4(3)	12007	1(2)	15121	5(3)	15793	1(3)	17111	1(2)	19316	1(2)	20693	2(3)
10012	3(3)	11441	3(3)	12011	1(2)	15130	1(2)	15819	1(2)	17250	4(3)	19318	1(2)	20694	2(3)
10021	1(2)	11442	3(3)	12013	1(2)	15131	2(3)	15820	1(2)	17260	7(3)	19325	1(2)	20696	2(3)
10030	2(3)	11443	2(3)	12014	1(2)	15135	1(2)	15821	1(2)	17261	7(3)	19328	1(2)	20697	4(3)
10035	1(2)	11444	2(3)	12015	1(2)	15136	1(3)	15822	1(2)	17262	6(3)	19330	1(2)	20700	1(3)
10036	3(3)	11446	2(3)	12016	1(2)	15150	1(2)	15823	1(2)	17263	3(3)	19340	1(2)	20701	1(3)
10040	1(2)	11450	1(2)	12017	1(2)	15151	1(2)	15824	1(2)	17264	3(3)	19342	1(2)	20702	1(3)
10060	1(2)	11451	1(2)	12018	1(2)	15152	2(3)	15825	1(2)	17266	2(3)	19350	1(2)	20703	1(3)
10061	1(2)	11462	1(2)	12020	2(3)	15155	1(2)	15826	1(2)	17270	6(3)	19355	1(2)	20704	1(3)
10080	1(3)	11463	1(2)	12021	3(3)	15156	1(2)	15828	1(2)	17271	4(3)	19357	1(2)	20705	1(3)
10081	1(3)	11470	3(2)	12031	1(2)	15157	1(3)	15829	1(2)	17272	5(3)	19361	1(2)	20802	1(2)
10120	3(3)	11471	2(3)	12032	1(2)	15200	1(2)	15830	1(2)	17273	4(3)	19364	1(3)	20805	1(2)
10121	2(3)	11600	2(3)	12034	1(2)	15201	7(3)	15832	1(2)	17274	2(3)	19367	1(2)	20808	1(2)
10140	2(3)	11601	2(3)	12035	1(2)	15220	1(2)	15833	1(2)	17276	2(3)	19368	1(2)	20816	3(3)
10160	3(3)	11602	3(3)	12036	1(2)	15221	9(3)	15834	1(2)	17280	6(3)	19369	1(2)	20822	3(3)
10180	2(3)	11603	2(3)	12037	1(2)	15240	1(2)	15835	1(3)	17281	5(3)	19370	1(2)	20824	1(2)
11000	1(2)	11604	2(3)	12041	1(2)	15241	9(3)	15836	1(2)	17282	4(3)	19371	1(2)	20827	1(2)
11001	1(3)	11606	2(3)	12042	1(2)	15260	1(2)	15837	2(3)	17283	4(3)	19380	1(2)	20838	1(2)

CPT	MUE	CPT	MUE	CPT	MUE	CPT	MUE	CPT	MUE	CPT	MUE	CPT	MUE	CPT	MUE
20900	2(3)	21086	1(2)	21270	1(2)	21550	2(3)	22325	1(2)	22867	1(2)	23430	1(2)	24102	1(2)
20902	2(3)	21087	1(2)	21275	1(2)	21552	2(3)	22326	1(2)	22868	1(2)	23440	1(2)	24105	1(2)
20910	1(3)	21088	1(2)	21280	1(2)	21554	2(3)	22327	1(2)	22869	1(2)	23450	1(2)	24110	1(3)
20912	1(3)	21089	1(3)	21282	1(2)	21555	2(3)	22328	6(3)	22870	1(2)	23455	1(2)	24115	1(3)
20920	1(3)	21100	1(2)	21295	1(2)	21556	2(3)	22505	1(2)	22899	1(3)	23460	1(2)	24116	1(3)
20922	1(3)	21110	2(3)	21296	1(2)	21557	1(3)	22510	1(2)	22900	3(3)	23462	1(2)	24120	1(3)
20924	2(3)	21116	1(2)	21299	1(3)	21558	1(3)	22511	1(2)	22901	2(3)	23465	1(2)	24125	1(3)
20930	1(3)	21120	1(2)	21310	1(2)	21600	5(3)	22512	3(3)	22902	4(3)	23466	1(2)	24126	1(3)
20931	1(2)	21121	1(2)	21315	1(2)	21601	2(3)	22513	1(2)	22903	3(3)	23470	1(2)	24130	1(2)
20932	1(3)	21122	1(2)	21320	1(2)	21602	1(3)	22514	1(2)	22904	1(3)	23472	1(2)	24134	1(3)
20933	1(3)	21123	1(2)	21325	1(2)	21603	1(3)	22515	4(3)	22905	1(3)	23473	1(2)	24136	1(3)
20934	1(3)	21125	2(2)	21330	1(2)	21610	1(3)	22526	0(3)	22999	1(3)	23474	1(2)	24138	1(3)
20936	1(3)	21127	2(3)	21335	1(2)	21615	1(2)	22527	0(3)	23000	1(2)	23480	1(2)	24140	1(3)
20937	1(2)	21137	1(2)	21336	1(2)	21616	1(2)	22532	1(2)	23020	1(2)	23485	1(2)	24145	1(3)
20938	1(2)	21138	1(2)	21337	1(2)	21620	1(2)	22533	1(2)	23030	2(3)	23490	1(2)	24147	1(2)
20939	1(3)	21139	1(2)	21338	1(2)	21627	1(2)	22534	3(3)	23031	1(3)	23491	1(2)	24149	1(2)
20950	2(3)	21141	1(2)	21339	1(2)	21630	1(2)	22548	1(2)	23035	1(3)	23500	1(2)	24150	1(3)
20955	1(3)	21142	1(2)	21340	1(2)	21632	1(2)	22551	1(2)	23040	1(2)	23505	1(2)	24152	1(3)
20956	1(3)	21143	1(2)	21343	1(2)	21685	1(2)	22552	5(3)	23044	1(3)	23515	1(2)	24155	1(2)
20957	1(3)	21145	1(2)	21344	1(2)	21700	1(2)	22554	1(2)	23065	2(3)	23520	1(2)	24160	1(2)
20962	1(3)	21146	1(2)	21345	1(2)	21705	1(2)	22556	1(2)	23066	2(3)	23525	1(2)	24164	1(2)
20969	2(3)	21147	1(2)	21346	1(2)	21720	1(3)	22558	1(2)	23071	2(3)	23530	1(2)	24200	3(3)
20970	1(3)	21150	1(2)	21347	1(2)	21725	1(3)	22585	5(3)	23073	2(3)	23532	1(2)	24201	3(3)
20972	2(3)	21151	1(2)	21348	1(2)	21740	1(2)	22586	1(2)	23075	2(3)	23540	1(2)	24220	1(2)
20973	1(2)	21154	1(2)	21355	1(2)	21742	1(2)	22590	1(2)	23076	2(3)	23545	1(2)	24300	1(2)
20974	1(2)	21155	1(2)	21356	1(2)	21743	1(2)	22595	1(2)	23077	1(3)	23550	1(2)	24301	2(3)
20975	1(3)	21159	1(2)	21360	1(2)	21750	1(2)	22600	1(2)	23078	1(3)	23552	1(2)	24305	4(3)
20979	1(3)	21160	1(2)	21365	1(2)	21811	1(2)	22610	1(2)	23100	1(2)	23570	1(2)	24310	2(3)
20982	1(2)	21172	1(3)	21366	1(2)	21812	1(2)	22612	1(2)	23101	1(3)	23575	1(2)	24320	2(3)
20983	1(2)	21175	1(2)	21385	1(2)	21813	1(2)	22614	13(3)	23105	1(2)	23585	1(2)	24330	1(3)
20985	2(3)	21179	1(2)	21386	1(2)	21820	1(2)	22630	1(2)	23106	1(2)	23600	1(2)	24331	1(3)
20999	1(3)	21180	1(2)	21387	1(2)	21825	1(2)	22632	4(2)	23107	1(2)	23605	1(2)	24332	1(2)
21010	1(2)	21181	1(3)	21390	1(2)	21899	1(3)	22633	1(2)	23120	1(2)	23615	1(2)	24340	1(2)
21011	4(3)	21182	1(2)	21395	1(2)	21920	2(3)	22634	4(2)	23125	1(2)	23616	1(2)	24341	2(3)
21012	3(3)	21183	1(2)	21400	1(2)	21925	2(3)	22800	1(2)	23130	1(2)	23620	1(2)	24342	2(3)
21013	2(3)	21184	1(2)	21401	1(2)	21930	5(3)	22802	1(2)	23140	1(3)	23625	1(2)	24343	1(2)
21014	2(3)	21188	1(2)	21406	1(2)	21931	3(3)	22804	1(2)	23145	1(3)	23630	1(2)	24344	1(2)
21015	1(3)	21193	1(2)	21407	1(2)	21932	2(3)	22808	1(2)	23146	1(3)	23650	1(2)	24345	1(2)
21016	2(3)	21194	1(2)	21408	1(2)	21933	2(3)	22810	1(2)	23150	1(3)	23655	1(2)	24346	1(2)
21025	2(3)	21195	1(2)	21421	1(2)	21935	1(3)	22812	1(2)	23155	1(3)	23660	1(2)	24357	1(3)
21026	2(3)	21196	1(2)	21422	1(2)	21936	1(3)	22818	1(2)	23156	1(3)	23665	1(2)	24358	1(3)
21029	1(3)	21198	1(3)	21423	1(2)	22010	2(3)	22819	1(2)	23170	1(3)	23670	1(2)	24359	2(3)
21030	1(3)	21199	1(2)	21431	1(2)	22015	2(3)	22830	1(2)	23172	1(3)	23675	1(2)	24360	1(2)
21031	2(3)	21206	1(3)	21432	1(2)	22100	1(2)	22840	1(3)	23174	1(3)	23680	1(2)	24361	1(2)
21032	1(3)	21208	1(3)	21433	1(2)	22101	1(2)	22841	1(2)	23180	1(3)	23700	1(2)	24362	1(2)
21034	1(3)	21209	1(3)	21435	1(2)	22102	1(2)	22842	1(3)	23182	1(3)	23800	1(2)	24363	1(2)
21040	2(3)	21210	2(3)	21436	1(2)	22103	3(3)	22843	1(3)	23184	1(3)	23802	1(2)	24365	1(2)
21044	1(3)	21215	2(3)	21440	2(3)	22110	1(2)	22844	1(3)	23190	1(3)	23900	1(2)	24366	1(2)
21045	1(3)	21230	2(3)	21445	2(3)	22112	1(2)	22845	1(3)	23195	1(2)	23920	1(2)	24370	1(2)
21046	2(3)	21235	2(3)	21450	1(2)	22114	1(2)	22846	1(3)	23200	1(3)	23921	1(2)	24371	1(2)
21047	2(3)	21240	1(2)	21451	1(2)	22116	3(3)	22847	1(3)	23210	1(3)	23929	1(3)	24400	1(3)
21048	2(3)	21242	1(2)	21452	1(2)	22206	1(2)	22848	1(2)	23220	1(3)	23930	2(3)	24410	1(2)
21049	1(3)	21243	1(2)	21453	1(2)	22207	1(2)	22849	1(2)	23330	2(3)	23931	2(3)	24420	1(2)
21050	1(2)	21244	1(2)	21454	1(2)	22208	5(3)	22850	1(2)	23333	1(3)	23935	2(3)	24430	1(3)
21060	1(2)	21245	2(3)	21461	1(2)	22210	1(2)	22852	1(2)	23334	1(2)	24000	1(2)	24435	1(3)
21070	1(2)	21246	1(3)	21462	1(2)	22212	1(2)	22853	4(3)	23335	1(2)	24006	1(2)	24470	1(2)
21073	1(2)	21247	1(2)	21465	1(2)	22214	1(2)	22854	4(3)	23350	1(2)	24065	2(3)	24495	1(2)
21076	1(2)	21248	2(3)	21470	1(2)	22216	6(3)	22855	1(2)	23395	1(2)	24066	2(3)	24498	1(2)
21077	1(2)	21249	2(3)	21480	1(2)	22220	1(2)	22856	1(2)	23397	1(3)	24071	2(3)	24500	1(2)
21079	1(2)	21255	1(2)	21485	1(2)	22222	1(2)	22857	1(2)	23400	1(2)	24073	2(3)	24505	1(2)
21080	1(2)	21256	1(2)	21490	1(2)	22224	1(2)	22858	1(2)	23405	2(3)	24075	5(3)	24515	1(2)
21081	1(2)	21260	1(2)	21497	1(2)	22226	4(3)	22859	4(3)	23406	1(2)	24076	4(3)	24516	1(2)
21082	1(2)	21261	1(2)	21499	1(3)	22310	1(2)	22861	1(2)	23410	1(2)	24077	1(3)	24530	1(2)
21083	1(2)	21263	1(2)	21501	3(3)	22315	1(2)	22862	1(2)	23412	1(2)	24079	1(3)	24535	1(2)
21084	1(2)	21267	1(2)	21502	1(3)	22318	1(2)	22864	1(2)	23415	1(2)	24100	1(2)	24538	1(2)
21085	1(3)	21268	1(2)	21510	1(3)	22319	1(2)	22865	1(2)	23420	1(2)	24101	1(2)	24545	1(2)

CPT	MUE	CPT	MUE	CPT	MUE	CPT	MUE	CPT	MUE	CPT	MUE	CPT	MUE	CPT	MUE
24546	1(2)	25125	1(3)	25450	1(2)	26035	1(3)	26445	5(3)	26650	1(2)	27059	1(3)	27235	1(2)
24560	1(3)	25126	1(3)	25455	1(2)	26037	1(3)	26449	5(3)	26665	1(2)	27060	1(2)	27236	1(2)
24565	1(3)	25130	1(3)	25490	1(2)	26040	1(2)	26450	6(3)	26670	2(3)	27062	1(2)	27238	1(2)
24566	1(3)	25135	1(3)	25491	1(2)	26045	1(2)	26455	6(3)	26675	1(3)	27065	1(3)	27240	1(2)
24575	1(3)	25136	1(3)	25492	1(2)	26055	5(3)	26460	4(3)	26676	2(3)	27066	1(3)	27244	1(2)
24576	1(3)	25145	1(3)	25500	1(2)	26060	5(3)	26471	4(3)	26685	3(3)	27067	1(3)	27245	1(2)
24577	1(3)	25150	1(3)	25505	1(2)	26070	2(3)	26474	4(3)	26686	3(3)	27070	1(3)	27246	1(2)
24579	1(3)	25151	1(3)	25515	1(2)	26075	3(3)	26476	4(3)	26700	2(3)	27071	1(3)	27248	1(2)
24582	1(3)	25170	1(3)	25520	1(2)	26080	3(3)	26477	2(3)	26705	3(3)	27075	1(3)	27250	1(2)
24586	1(3)	25210	2(3)	25525	1(2)	26100	1(3)	26478	6(3)	26706	2(3)	27076	1(2)	27252	1(2)
24587	1(2)	25215	1(2)	25526	1(2)	26105	2(3)	26479	4(3)	26715	3(3)	27077	1(2)	27253	1(2)
24600	1(2)	25230	1(2)	25530	1(2)	26110	2(3)	26480	4(3)	26720	4(3)	27078	1(2)	27254	1(2)
24605	1(2)	25240	1(2)	25535	1(2)	26111	4(3)	26483	4(3)	26725	3(3)	27080	1(2)	27256	1(2)
24615	1(2)	25246	1(2)	25545	1(2)	26113	3(3)	26485	4(3)	26727	3(3)	27086	1(3)	27257	1(2)
24620	1(2)	25248	3(3)	25560	1(2)	26115	4(3)	26489	2(3)	26735	4(3)	27087	1(3)	27258	1(2)
24635	1(2)	25250	1(2)	25565	1(2)	26116	2(3)	26490	3(3)	26740	3(3)	27090	1(2)	27259	1(2)
24640	1(2)	25251	1(2)	25574	1(2)	26117	2(3)	26492	2(3)	26742	3(3)	27091	1(2)	27265	1(2)
24650	1(2)	25259	1(2)	25575	1(2)	26118	1(3)	26494	1(3)	26746	3(3)	27093	1(2)	27266	1(2)
24655	1(2)	25260	7(3)	25600	1(2)	26121	1(2)	26496	1(3)	26750	3(3)	27095	1(2)	27267	1(2)
24665	1(2)	25263	4(3)	25605	1(2)	26123	1(2)	26497	2(3)	26755	2(3)	27096	1(2)	27268	1(2)
24666	1(2)	25265	4(3)	25606	1(2)	26125	4(3)	26498	1(3)	26756	2(3)	27097	1(3)	27269	1(2)
24670	1(2)	25270	8(3)	25607	1(2)	26130	1(3)	26499	2(3)	26765	3(3)	27098	1(2)	27275	2(2)
24675	1(2)	25272	4(3)	25608	1(2)	26135	4(3)	26500	3(3)	26770	3(3)	27100	1(2)	27279	1(2)
24685	1(2)	25274	4(3)	25609	1(2)	26140	2(3)	26502	2(3)	26775	2(3)	27105	1(3)	27280	1(2)
24800	1(2)	25275	2(3)	25622	1(2)	26145	6(3)	26508	1(2)	26776	4(3)	27110	1(2)	27282	1(2)
24802	1(2)	25280	9(3)	25624	1(2)	26160	4(3)	26510	4(3)	26785	3(3)	27111	1(2)	27284	1(2)
24900	1(2)	25290	10(3)	25628	1(2)	26170	4(3)	26516	1(2)	26820	1(2)	27120	1(2)	27286	1(2)
24920	1(2)	25295	9(3)	25630	1(3)	26180	4(3)	26517	1(2)	26841	1(2)	27122	1(2)	27290	1(2)
24925	1(2)	25300	1(2)	25635	1(3)	26185	1(3)	26518	1(2)	26842	1(2)	27125	1(2)	27295	1(2)
24930	1(2)	25301	1(2)	25645	1(3)	26200	2(3)	26520	4(3)	26843	2(3)	27130	1(2)	27299	1(3)
24931	1(2)	25310	5(3)	25650	1(2)	26205	1(3)	26525	4(3)	26844	2(3)	27132	1(2)	27301	3(3)
24935	1(2)	25312	4(3)	25651	1(2)	26210	2(3)	26530	4(3)	26850	5(3)	27134	1(2)	27303	2(3)
24940	1(2)	25315	1(3)	25652	1(2)	26215	2(3)	26531	4(3)	26852	2(3)	27137	1(2)	27305	1(2)
24999	1(3)	25316	1(3)	25660	1(2)	26230	2(3)	26535	3(3)	26860	1(2)	27138	1(2)	27306	1(2)
25000	2(3)	25320	1(2)	25670	1(2)	26235	2(3)	26536	4(3)	26861	4(3)	27140	1(2)	27307	1(2)
25001	1(3)	25332	1(2)	25671	1(2)	26236	2(3)	26540	4(3)	26862	1(2)	27146	1(3)	27310	1(2)
25020	1(2)	25335	1(2)	25675	1(2)	26250	2(3)	26541	4(3)	26863	2(3)	27147	1(3)	27323	2(3)
25023	1(2)	25337	1(2)	25676	1(2)	26260	1(3)	26542	4(3)	26910	4(3)	27151	1(3)	27324	3(3)
25024	1(2)	25350	1(3)	25680	1(2)	26262	1(3)	26545	4(3)	26951	8(3)	27156	1(2)	27325	1(2)
25025	1(2)	25355	1(3)	25685	1(2)	26320	4(3)	26546	2(3)	26952	4(3)	27158	1(2)	27326	1(2)
25028	4(3)	25360	1(3)	25690	1(2)	26340	4(3)	26548	3(3)	26989	1(3)	27161	1(2)	27327	5(3)
25031	2(3)	25365	1(3)	25695	1(2)	26341	2(3)	26550	1(2)	26990	2(3)	27165	1(2)	27328	3(3)
25035	2(3)	25370	1(2)	25800	1(2)	26350	6(3)	26551	1(2)	26991	1(3)	27170	1(2)	27329	1(3)
25040	1(3)	25375	1(2)	25805	1(2)	26352	2(3)	26553	1(3)	26992	2(3)	27175	1(2)	27330	1(2)
25065	2(3)	25390	1(2)	25810	1(2)	26356	4(3)	26554	1(3)	27000	1(3)	27176	1(2)	27331	1(2)
25066	2(3)	25391	1(2)	25820	1(2)	26357	2(3)	26555	2(3)	27001	1(3)	27177	1(2)	27332	1(2)
25071	3(3)	25392	1(2)	25825	1(2)	26358	2(3)	26556	2(3)	27003	1(2)	27178	1(2)	27333	1(2)
25073	2(3)	25393	1(2)	25830	1(2)	26370	3(3)	26560	2(3)	27005	1(2)	27179	1(2)	27334	1(2)
25075	6(3)	25394	1(3)	25900	1(2)	26372	1(3)	26561	2(3)	27006	1(2)	27181	1(2)	27335	1(2)
25076	3(3)	25400	1(2)	25905	1(2)	26373	2(3)	26562	2(3)	27025	1(3)	27185	1(2)	27337	3(3)
25077	1(3)	25405	1(2)	25907	1(2)	26390	2(3)	26565	2(3)	27027	1(2)	27187	1(2)	27339	4(3)
25078	1(3)	25415	1(2)	25909	1(2)	26392	2(3)	26567	3(3)	27030	1(2)	27197	1(2)	27340	1(2)
25085	1(2)	25420	1(2)	25915	1(2)	26410	4(3)	26568	2(3)	27033	1(2)	27198	1(2)	27345	1(2)
25100	1(2)	25425	1(2)	25920	1(2)	26412	3(3)	26580	1(2)	27035	1(2)	27200	1(2)	27347	1(2)
25101	1(2)	25426	1(2)	25922	1(2)	26415	2(3)	26587	2(3)	27036	1(2)	27202	1(2)	27350	1(2)
25105	1(2)	25430	1(3)	25924	1(2)	26416	2(3)	26590	2(3)	27040	2(3)	27215	0(3)	27355	1(3)
25107	1(2)	25431	1(3)	25927	1(2)	26418	4(3)	26591	4(3)	27041	3(3)	27216	0(3)	27356	1(3)
25109	4(3)	25440	1(2)	25929	1(2)	26420	3(3)	26593	8(3)	27043	2(3)	27217	0(3)	27357	1(3)
25110	2(3)	25441	1(2)	25931	1(2)	26426	4(3)	26596	1(3)	27045	3(3)	27218	0(3)	27358	1(3)
25111	1(3)	25442	1(2)	25999	1(3)	26428	2(3)	26600	2(3)	27047	2(3)	27220	1(2)	27360	2(3)
25112	1(3)	25443	1(2)	26010	2(3)	26432	2(3)	26605	3(3)	27048	2(3)	27222	1(2)	27364	1(3)
25115	1(3)	25444	1(2)	26011	3(3)	26433	2(3)	26607	2(3)	27049	1(3)	27226	1(2)	27365	1(3)
25116	1(3)	25445	1(2)	26020	4(3)	26434	2(3)	26608	4(3)	27050	1(2)	27227	1(2)	27369	1(2)
25118	5(3)	25446	1(2)	26025	1(2)	26437	4(3)	26615	3(3)	27052	1(2)	27228	1(2)	27372	2(3)
25119	1(2)	25447	4(3)	26030	1(2)	26440	6(3)	26641	1(2)	27054	1(2)	27230	1(2)	27380	1(2)
25120	1(3)	25449	1(2)	26034	2(3)	26442	5(3)	26645	1(2)	27057	1(2)	27232	1(2)	27381	1(2)

CPT	MUE	CPT	MUE	CPT	MUE	CPT	MUE	CPT	MUE	CPT	MUE	CPT	MUE	CPT	MUE
27385	2(3)	27509	1(2)	27654	1(2)	27826	1(2)	28114	1(2)	28341	2(3)	28890	1(2)	29826	1(2)
27386	2(3)	27510	1(2)	27656	1(3)	27827	1(2)	28116	1(2)	28344	1(2)	28899	1(3)	29827	1(2)
27390	1(2)	27511	1(2)	27658	2(3)	27828	1(2)	28118	1(2)	28345	2(3)	29000	1(3)	29828	1(2)
27391	1(2)	27513	1(2)	27659	2(3)	27829	1(2)	28119	1(2)	28360	1(2)	29010	1(3)	29830	1(2)
27392	1(2)	27514	1(2)	27664	2(3)	27830	1(2)	28120	2(3)	28400	1(2)	29015	1(3)	29834	1(2)
27393	1(2)	27516	1(2)	27665	2(3)	27831	1(2)	28122	4(3)	28405	1(2)	29035	1(3)	29835	1(2)
27394	1(2)	27517	1(2)	27675	1(2)	27832	1(2)	28124	4(3)	28406	1(2)	29040	1(3)	29836	1(2)
27395	1(2)	27519	1(2)	27676	1(2)	27840	1(2)	28126	4(3)	28415	1(2)	29044	1(3)	29837	1(2)
27396	1(2)	27520	1(2)	27680	2(3)	27842	1(2)	28130	1(2)	28420	1(2)	29046	1(3)	29838	1(2)
27397	1(2)	27524	1(2)	27681	1(2)	27846	1(2)	28140	3(3)	28430	1(2)	29049	1(3)	29840	1(2)
27400	1(2)	27530	1(2)	27685	2(3)	27848	1(2)	28150	4(3)	28435	1(2)	29055	1(3)	29843	1(2)
27403	1(3)	27532	1(2)	27686	3(3)	27860	1(2)	28153	4(3)	28436	1(2)	29058	1(3)	29844	1(2)
27405	1(3)	27535	1(2)	27687	1(2)	27870	1(2)	28160	5(3)	28445	1(2)	29065	1(3)	29845	1(2)
27407	1(3)	27536	1(2)	27690	2(3)	27871	1(3)	28171	1(3)	28446	1(2)	29075	1(3)	29846	1(2)
27409	1(2)	27538	1(2)	27691	2(3)	27880	1(2)	28173	2(3)	28450	2(3)	29085	1(3)	29847	1(2)
27412	1(2)	27540	1(2)	27692	4(3)	27881	1(2)	28175	2(3)	28455	3(3)	29086	2(3)	29848	1(2)
27415	1(2)	27550	1(2)	27695	1(2)	27882	1(2)	28190	3(3)	28456	2(3)	29105	1(2)	29850	1(2)
27416	1(2)	27552	1(2)	27696	1(2)	27884	1(2)	28192	2(3)	28465	3(3)	29125	1(2)	29851	1(2)
27418	1(2)	27556	1(2)	27698	2(2)	27886	1(2)	28193	2(3)	28470	2(3)	29126	1(2)	29855	1(2)
27420	1(2)	27557	1(2)	27700	1(2)	27888	1(2)	28200	4(3)	28475	5(3)	29130	3(3)	29856	1(2)
27422	1(2)	27558	1(2)	27702	1(2)	27889	1(2)	28202	2(3)	28476	4(3)	29131	2(3)	29860	1(2)
27424	1(2)	27560	1(2)	27703	1(2)	27892	1(2)	28208	4(3)	28485	5(3)	29200	1(2)	29861	1(2)
27425	1(2)	27562	1(2)	27704	1(2)	27893	1(2)	28210	2(3)	28490	1(2)	29240	1(2)	29862	1(2)
27427	1(2)	27566	1(2)	27705	1(3)	27894	1(2)	28220	1(2)	28495	1(2)	29260	1(3)	29863	1(2)
27428	1(2)	27570	1(2)	27707	1(3)	27899	1(3)	28222	1(2)	28496	1(2)	29280	2(3)	29866	1(2)
27429	1(2)	27580	1(2)	27709	1(3)	28001	2(3)	28225	1(2)	28505	1(2)	29305	1(3)	29867	1(2)
27430	1(2)	27590	1(2)	27712	1(2)	28002	3(3)	28226	1(2)	28510	4(3)	29325	1(3)	29868	1(3)
27435	1(2)	27591	1(2)	27715	1(2)	28003	2(3)	28230	1(2)	28515	4(3)	29345	1(3)	29870	1(2)
27437	1(2)	27592	1(2)	27720	1(2)	28005	3(3)	28232	6(3)	28525	4(3)	29355	1(3)	29871	1(2)
27438	1(2)	27594	1(2)	27722	1(2)	28008	2(3)	28234	6(3)	28530	1(2)	29358	1(3)	29873	1(2)
27440	1(2)	27596	1(2)	27724	1(2)	28010	4(3)	28238	1(2)	28531	1(2)	29365	1(3)	29874	1(2)
27441	1(2)	27598	1(2)	27725	1(2)	28011	4(3)	28240	1(2)	28540	1(3)	29405	1(3)	29875	1(2)
27442	1(2)	27599	1(3)	27726	1(2)	28020	2(3)	28250	1(2)	28545	1(3)	29425	1(3)	29876	1(2)
27443	1(2)	27600	1(2)	27727	1(2)	28022	3(3)	28260	1(2)	28546	1(3)	29435	1(3)	29877	1(2)
27445	1(2)	27601	1(2)	27730	1(2)	28024	4(3)	28261	1(3)	28555	1(3)	29440	1(2)	29879	1(2)
27446	1(2)	27602	1(2)	27732	1(2)	28035	1(2)	28262	1(2)	28570	1(2)	29445	1(3)	29880	1(2)
27447	1(2)	27603	2(3)	27734	1(2)	28039	2(3)	28264	1(2)	28575	1(2)	29450	1(3)	29881	1(2)
27448	1(3)	27604	2(3)	27740	1(2)	28041	2(3)	28270	6(3)	28576	1(2)	29505	1(2)	29882	1(2)
27450	1(3)	27605	1(2)	27742	1(2)	28043	4(3)	28272	6(3)	28585	1(3)	29515	1(2)	29883	1(2)
27454	1(2)	27606	1(2)	27745	1(2)	28045	4(3)	28280	1(2)	28600	2(3)	29520	1(2)	29884	1(2)
27455	1(3)	27607	2(3)	27750	1(2)	28046	1(3)	28285	4(3)	28605	2(3)	29530	1(2)	29885	1(2)
27457	1(3)	27610	1(2)	27752	1(2)	28047	1(3)	28286	1(2)	28606	3(3)	29540	1(2)	29886	1(2)
27465	1(2)	27612	1(2)	27756	1(2)	28050	2(3)	28288	4(3)	28615	5(3)	29550	1(2)	29887	1(2)
27466	1(2)	27613	3(3)	27758	1(2)	28052	2(3)	28289	1(2)	28630	2(3)	29580	1(2)	29888	1(2)
27468	1(2)	27614	3(3)	27759	1(2)	28054	2(3)	28291	1(2)	28635	2(3)	29581	1(2)	29889	1(2)
27470	1(2)	27615	1(3)	27760	1(2)	28055	1(3)	28292	1(2)	28636	4(3)	29584	1(2)	29891	1(2)
27472	1(2)	27616	1(3)	27762	1(2)	28060	1(2)	28295	1(2)	28645	4(3)	29700	2(3)	29892	1(2)
27475	1(2)	27618	3(3)	27766	1(2)	28062	1(2)	28296	1(2)	28660	4(3)	29705	1(3)	29893	1(2)
27477	1(2)	27619	2(3)	27767	1(2)	28070	2(3)	28297	1(2)	28665	3(3)	29710	1(2)	29894	1(2)
27479	1(2)	27620	1(2)	27768	1(2)	28072	4(3)	28298	1(2)	28666	4(3)	29720	1(2)	29895	1(2)
27485	1(2)	27625	1(2)	27769	1(2)	28080	3(3)	28299	1(2)	28675	3(3)	29730	1(3)	29897	1(2)
27486	1(2)	27626	1(2)	27780	1(2)	28086	2(3)	28300	1(3)	28705	1(2)	29740	1(3)	29898	1(2)
27487	1(2)	27630	2(3)	27781	1(2)	28088	2(3)	28302	1(2)	28715	1(2)	29750	1(3)	29899	1(2)
27488	1(2)	27632	3(3)	27784	1(2)	28090	2(3)	28304	1(3)	28725	1(2)	29799	1(3)	29900	2(3)
27495	1(2)	27634	2(3)	27786	1(2)	28092	2(3)	28305	1(3)	28730	1(2)	29800	1(2)	29901	2(3)
27496	1(2)	27635	1(3)	27788	1(2)	28100	1(3)	28306	1(2)	28735	1(2)	29804	1(2)	29902	2(3)
27497	1(2)	27637	1(3)	27792	1(2)	28102	1(3)	28307	1(2)	28737	1(2)	29805	1(2)	29904	1(2)
27498	1(2)	27638	1(3)	27808	1(2)	28103	1(3)	28308	4(3)	28740	1(2)	29806	1(2)	29905	1(2)
27499	1(2)	27640	1(3)	27810	1(2)	28104	2(3)	28309	1(2)	28750	1(2)	29807	1(2)	29906	1(2)
27500	1(2)	27641	1(3)	27814	1(2)	28106	1(3)	28310	1(2)	28755	1(2)	29819	1(2)	29907	1(2)
27501	1(2)	27645	1(3)	27816	1(2)	28107	1(3)	28312	4(3)	28760	1(2)	29820	1(2)	29914	1(2)
27502	1(2)	27646	1(3)	27818	1(2)	28108	2(3)	28313	4(3)	28800	1(2)	29821	1(2)	29915	1(2)
27503	1(2)	27647	1(3)	27822	1(2)	28110	1(2)	28315	1(2)	28805	1(2)	29822	1(2)	29916	1(2)
27506	1(2)	27648	1(2)	27823	1(2)	28111	1(2)	28320	1(2)	28810	5(3)	29823	1(2)	29999	1(3)
27507	1(2)	27650	1(2)	27824	1(2)	28112	4(3)	28322	2(3)	28820	6(3)	29824	1(2)	30000	1(3)
27508	1(2)	27652	1(2)	27825	1(2)	28113	1(2)	28340	2(3)	28825	8(3)	29825	1(2)	30020	1(3)

Appendix I — Medically Unlikely Edits (MUEs)—OPPS

CPT	MUE	CPT	MUE	CPT	MUE	CPT	MUE	CPT	MUE	CPT	MUE	CPT	MUE	CPT	MUE
30100	2(3)	31225	1(2)	31552	1(2)	31730	1(3)	32601	1(3)	33207	1(3)	33340	1(2)	33530	1(2)
30110	1(2)	31230	1(2)	31553	1(2)	31750	1(2)	32604	1(3)	33208	1(3)	33361	1(2)	33533	1(2)
30115	1(2)	31231	1(2)	31554	1(2)	31755	1(2)	32606	1(3)	33210	1(3)	33362	1(2)	33534	1(2)
30117	2(3)	31233	1(2)	31560	1(2)	31760	1(2)	32607	1(3)	33211	1(3)	33363	1(2)	33535	1(2)
30118	1(3)	31235	1(2)	31561	1(2)	31766	1(2)	32608	1(3)	33212	1(3)	33364	1(2)	33536	1(2)
30120	1(2)	31237	1(2)	31570	1(2)	31770	2(3)	32609	1(3)	33213	1(3)	33365	1(2)	33542	1(2)
30124	2(3)	31238	1(3)	31571	1(2)	31775	1(3)	32650	1(2)	33214	1(3)	33366	1(2)	33545	1(2)
30125	1(3)	31239	1(2)	31572	1(2)	31780	1(2)	32651	1(2)	33215	2(3)	33367	1(2)	33548	1(2)
30130	1(2)	31240	1(2)	31573	1(2)	31781	1(2)	32652	1(2)	33216	1(3)	33368	1(2)	33572	3(2)
30140	1(2)	31241	1(2)	31574	1(2)	31785	1(3)	32653	1(3)	33217	1(3)	33369	1(2)	33600	1(3)
30150	1(2)	31253	1(2)	31575	1(3)	31786	1(3)	32654	1(3)	33218	1(3)	33390	1(2)	33602	1(3)
30160	1(2)	31254	1(2)	31576	1(3)	31800	1(3)	32655	1(3)	33220	1(3)	33391	1(2)	33606	1(2)
30200	1(2)	31255	1(2)	31577	1(3)	31805	1(3)	32656	1(2)	33221	1(3)	33404	1(2)	33608	1(2)
30210	1(3)	31256	1(2)	31578	1(3)	31820	1(2)	32658	1(3)	33222	1(3)	33405	1(2)	33610	1(2)
30220	1(2)	31257	1(2)	31579	1(2)	31825	1(2)	32659	1(2)	33223	1(3)	33406	1(2)	33611	1(2)
30300	1(3)	31259	1(2)	31580	1(2)	31830	1(2)	32661	1(3)	33224	1(3)	33410	1(2)	33612	1(2)
30310	1(3)	31267	1(2)	31584	1(2)	31899	1(3)	32662	1(3)	33225	1(3)	33411	1(2)	33615	1(2)
30320	1(3)	31276	1(2)	31587	1(2)	32035	1(2)	32663	1(3)	33226	1(3)	33412	1(2)	33617	1(2)
30400	1(2)	31287	1(2)	31590	1(2)	32036	1(3)	32664	1(2)	33227	1(3)	33413	1(2)	33619	1(2)
30410	1(2)	31288	1(2)	31591	1(2)	32096	1(3)	32665	1(2)	33228	1(3)	33414	1(2)	33620	1(2)
30420	1(2)	31290	1(2)	31592	1(2)	32097	1(3)	32666	1(3)	33229	1(3)	33415	1(2)	33621	1(3)
30430	1(2)	31291	1(2)	31599	1(3)	32098	1(2)	32667	3(3)	33230	1(3)	33416	1(2)	33622	1(2)
30435	1(2)	31292	1(2)	31600	1(2)	32100	1(3)	32668	2(3)	33231	1(3)	33417	1(2)	33641	1(2)
30450	1(2)	31293	1(2)	31601	1(2)	32110	1(3)	32669	2(3)	33233	1(2)	33418	1(3)	33645	1(2)
30460	1(2)	31294	1(2)	31603	1(2)	32120	1(2)	32670	1(2)	33234	1(2)	33419	1(2)	33647	1(2)
30462	1(2)	31295	1(2)	31605	1(2)	32124	1(3)	32671	1(3)	33235	1(3)	33420	1(2)	33660	1(2)
30465	1(2)	31296	1(2)	31610	1(2)	32140	1(3)	32672	1(3)	33236	1(2)	33422	1(2)	33665	1(2)
30468	1(2)	31297	1(2)	31611	1(2)	32141	1(3)	32673	1(2)	33237	1(2)	33425	1(2)	33670	1(2)
30520	1(2)	31298	1(2)	31612	1(3)	32150	1(3)	32674	1(2)	33238	1(2)	33426	1(2)	33675	1(2)
30540	1(2)	31299	1(3)	31613	1(2)	32151	1(3)	32701	1(2)	33240	1(3)	33427	1(2)	33676	1(2)
30545	1(2)	31300	1(2)	31614	1(2)	32160	1(3)	32800	1(3)	33241	1(2)	33430	1(2)	33677	1(2)
30560	1(2)	31360	1(2)	31615	1(3)	32200	2(3)	32810	1(3)	33243	1(2)	33440	1(2)	33681	1(2)
30580	2(3)	31365	1(2)	31622	1(3)	32215	1(2)	32815	1(3)	33244	1(2)	33460	1(2)	33684	1(2)
30600	1(3)	31367	1(2)	31623	1(3)	32220	1(2)	32820	1(2)	33249	1(3)	33463	1(2)	33688	1(2)
30620	1(2)	31368	1(2)	31624	1(3)	32225	1(2)	32850	1(2)	33250	1(2)	33464	1(2)	33690	1(2)
30630	1(2)	31370	1(2)	31625	1(2)	32310	1(3)	32851	1(2)	33251	1(2)	33465	1(2)	33692	1(2)
30801	1(2)	31375	1(2)	31626	1(2)	32320	1(3)	32852	1(2)	33254	1(2)	33468	1(2)	33694	1(2)
30802	1(2)	31380	1(2)	31627	1(3)	32400	2(3)	32853	1(2)	33255	1(2)	33470	1(2)	33697	1(2)
30901	1(3)	31382	1(2)	31628	1(2)	32408	2(3)	32854	1(2)	33256	1(2)	33471	1(2)	33702	1(2)
30903	1(3)	31390	1(2)	31629	1(2)	32440	1(2)	32855	1(2)	33257	1(2)	33474	1(2)	33710	1(2)
30905	1(2)	31395	1(2)	31630	1(2)	32442	1(2)	32856	1(2)	33258	1(2)	33475	1(2)	33720	1(2)
30906	1(3)	31400	1(3)	31631	1(2)	32445	1(2)	32900	1(2)	33259	1(2)	33476	1(2)	33722	1(3)
30915	1(3)	31420	1(2)	31632	2(3)	32480	1(2)	32905	1(2)	33261	1(2)	33477	1(2)	33724	1(2)
30920	1(3)	31500	2(3)	31633	2(3)	32482	1(2)	32906	1(2)	33262	1(3)	33478	1(2)	33726	1(2)
30930	1(2)	31502	1(3)	31634	1(3)	32484	2(3)	32940	1(3)	33263	1(3)	33496	1(3)	33730	1(2)
30999	1(3)	31505	1(3)	31635	1(3)	32486	1(3)	32960	1(2)	33264	1(3)	33500	1(3)	33732	1(2)
31000	1(2)	31510	1(2)	31636	1(2)	32488	1(2)	32994	1(2)	33265	1(2)	33501	1(3)	33735	1(2)
31002	1(2)	31511	1(3)	31637	2(3)	32491	1(2)	32997	1(2)	33266	1(2)	33502	1(3)	33736	1(2)
31020	1(2)	31512	1(3)	31638	1(3)	32501	1(3)	32998	1(2)	33270	1(3)	33503	1(3)	33737	1(2)
31030	1(2)	31513	1(3)	31640	1(3)	32503	1(2)	32999	1(3)	33271	1(3)	33504	1(3)	33741	1(3)
31032	1(2)	31515	1(3)	31641	1(3)	32504	1(2)	33016	1(3)	33272	1(3)	33505	1(3)	33745	2(2)
31040	1(2)	31520	1(3)	31643	1(2)	32505	1(2)	33017	1(3)	33273	1(3)	33506	1(3)	33746	1(3)
31050	1(2)	31525	1(3)	31645	1(2)	32506	3(3)	33018	1(3)	33274	1(3)	33507	1(3)	33750	1(3)
31051	1(2)	31526	1(3)	31646	2(3)	32507	2(3)	33019	1(3)	33275	1(3)	33508	1(2)	33755	1(2)
31070	1(2)	31527	1(2)	31647	1(2)	32540	1(3)	33020	1(3)	33285	1(3)	33510	1(2)	33762	1(2)
31075	1(2)	31528	1(2)	31648	1(2)	32550	2(3)	33025	1(2)	33286	1(3)	33511	1(2)	33764	1(3)
31080	1(2)	31529	1(3)	31649	2(3)	32551	2(3)	33030	1(2)	33289	1(3)	33512	1(2)	33766	1(2)
31081	1(2)	31530	1(3)	31651	3(3)	32552	2(2)	33031	1(2)	33300	1(3)	33513	1(2)	33767	1(2)
31084	1(2)	31531	1(3)	31652	1(2)	32553	1(2)	33050	1(2)	33305	1(2)	33514	1(2)	33768	1(2)
31085	1(2)	31535	1(3)	31653	1(2)	32554	2(3)	33120	1(3)	33310	1(2)	33516	1(2)	33770	1(2)
31086	1(2)	31536	1(3)	31654	1(3)	32555	2(3)	33130	1(3)	33315	1(3)	33517	1(2)	33771	1(2)
31087	1(2)	31540	1(3)	31660	1(2)	32556	2(3)	33140	1(2)	33320	1(3)	33518	1(2)	33774	1(2)
31090	1(2)	31541	1(3)	31661	1(2)	32557	2(3)	33141	1(2)	33321	1(3)	33519	1(2)	33775	1(2)
31200	1(2)	31545	1(2)	31717	1(3)	32560	1(3)	33202	1(2)	33322	1(3)	33521	1(2)	33776	1(2)
31201	1(2)	31546	1(2)	31720	3(3)	32561	1(2)	33203	1(2)	33330	1(3)	33522	1(2)	33777	1(2)
31205	1(2)	31551	1(2)	31725	1(3)	32562	1(2)	33206	1(3)	33335	1(3)	33523	1(2)	33778	1(2)

CPT	MUE	CPT	MUE	CPT	MUE	CPT	MUE	CPT	MUE	CPT	MUE	CPT	MUE	CPT	MUE
33779	1(2)	33962	1(3)	34716	1(2)	35271	2(3)	35631	4(3)	36222	1(3)	36570	2(3)	37191	1(3)
33780	1(2)	33963	1(3)	34717	2(2)	35276	2(3)	35632	1(3)	36223	1(3)	36571	2(3)	37192	1(3)
33781	1(2)	33964	1(3)	34718	2(2)	35281	2(3)	35633	1(3)	36224	1(3)	36572	1(3)	37193	1(3)
33782	1(2)	33965	1(3)	34808	1(3)	35286	2(3)	35634	1(3)	36225	1(3)	36573	1(3)	37195	1(3)
33783	1(2)	33966	1(3)	34812	1(2)	35301	2(3)	35636	1(3)	36226	1(3)	36575	2(3)	37197	2(3)
33786	1(2)	33967	1(3)	34813	1(2)	35302	1(2)	35637	1(3)	36227	2(2)	36576	2(3)	37200	2(3)
33788	1(2)	33968	1(3)	34820	1(2)	35303	1(2)	35638	1(3)	36228	2(3)	36578	2(3)	37211	1(2)
33800	1(2)	33969	1(3)	34830	1(2)	35304	1(2)	35642	1(3)	36245	3(3)	36580	2(3)	37212	1(2)
33802	1(3)	33970	1(3)	34831	1(2)	35305	1(2)	35645	1(3)	36246	4(3)	36581	2(3)	37213	1(2)
33803	1(3)	33971	1(3)	34832	1(2)	35306	2(3)	35646	1(3)	36247	2(3)	36582	2(3)	37214	1(2)
33813	1(2)	33973	1(3)	34833	1(2)	35311	1(2)	35647	1(3)	36248	2(3)	36583	2(3)	37215	1(2)
33814	1(2)	33974	1(3)	34834	1(2)	35321	1(2)	35650	1(3)	36251	1(3)	36584	2(3)	37216	0(3)
33820	1(2)	33975	1(3)	34839	1(2)	35331	1(2)	35654	1(3)	36252	1(3)	36585	2(3)	37217	1(2)
33822	1(2)	33976	1(3)	34841	1(2)	35341	3(3)	35656	1(3)	36253	1(3)	36589	2(3)	37218	1(2)
33824	1(2)	33977	1(3)	34842	1(2)	35351	1(3)	35661	1(3)	36254	1(3)	36590	2(3)	37220	1(2)
33840	1(2)	33978	1(3)	34843	1(2)	35355	1(2)	35663	1(3)	36260	1(2)	36591	2(3)	37221	1(2)
33845	1(2)	33979	1(3)	34844	1(2)	35361	1(2)	35665	1(3)	36261	1(2)	36592	1(3)	37222	2(2)
33851	1(2)	33980	1(3)	34845	1(2)	35363	1(2)	35666	2(3)	36262	1(2)	36593	2(3)	37223	2(2)
33852	1(2)	33981	1(3)	34846	1(2)	35371	1(2)	35671	2(3)	36299	1(3)	36595	2(3)	37224	1(2)
33853	1(2)	33982	1(3)	34847	1(2)	35372	1(2)	35681	1(3)	36400	1(3)	36596	2(3)	37225	1(2)
33858	1(2)	33983	1(3)	34848	1(2)	35390	1(3)	35682	1(2)	36405	1(3)	36597	2(3)	37226	1(2)
33859	1(2)	33984	1(3)	35001	1(2)	35400	1(3)	35683	1(2)	36406	1(3)	36598	2(3)	37227	1(2)
33863	1(2)	33985	1(3)	35002	1(2)	35500	2(3)	35685	2(3)	36410	3(3)	36600	4(3)	37228	1(2)
33864	1(2)	33986	1(3)	35005	1(2)	35501	1(3)	35686	1(3)	36415	2(3)	36620	3(3)	37229	1(2)
33866	1(2)	33987	1(3)	35011	1(2)	35506	1(3)	35691	1(3)	36416	6(3)	36625	2(3)	37230	1(2)
33871	1(2)	33988	1(3)	35013	1(2)	35508	1(3)	35693	1(3)	36420	2(3)	36640	1(3)	37231	1(2)
33875	1(2)	33989	1(3)	35021	1(2)	35509	1(3)	35694	1(3)	36425	2(3)	36660	1(3)	37232	2(3)
33877	1(2)	33990	1(3)	35022	1(2)	35510	1(3)	35695	1(3)	36430	1(3)	36680	1(3)	37233	2(3)
33880	1(2)	33991	1(3)	35045	1(3)	35511	1(3)	35697	2(3)	36440	1(3)	36800	1(3)	37234	2(3)
33881	1(2)	33992	1(2)	35081	1(2)	35512	1(3)	35700	2(3)	36450	1(3)	36810	1(3)	37235	2(3)
33883	1(2)	33993	1(3)	35082	1(2)	35515	1(3)	35701	1(2)	36455	1(3)	36815	1(3)	37236	1(2)
33884	2(3)	33995	1(3)	35091	1(2)	35516	1(3)	35702	2(2)	36456	1(3)	36818	1(3)	37237	2(3)
33886	1(2)	33997	1(3)	35092	1(2)	35518	1(3)	35703	2(2)	36460	2(3)	36819	1(3)	37238	1(2)
33889	1(2)	33999	1(3)	35102	1(2)	35521	1(3)	35800	2(3)	36465	1(2)	36820	1(3)	37239	2(3)
33891	1(2)	34001	1(3)	35103	1(2)	35522	1(3)	35820	2(3)	36466	1(2)	36821	2(3)	37241	2(3)
33910	1(3)	34051	1(3)	35111	1(2)	35523	1(3)	35840	2(3)	36468	2(3)	36823	1(3)	37242	2(3)
33915	1(3)	34101	1(3)	35112	1(2)	35525	1(3)	35860	2(3)	36470	1(2)	36825	1(3)	37243	1(3)
33916	1(3)	34111	2(3)	35121	1(3)	35526	1(3)	35870	1(3)	36471	1(2)	36830	2(3)	37244	2(3)
33917	1(2)	34151	1(3)	35122	1(3)	35531	1(3)	35875	2(3)	36473	1(3)	36831	1(3)	37246	1(2)
33920	1(2)	34201	1(3)	35131	1(2)	35533	1(3)	35876	2(3)	36474	1(3)	36832	2(3)	37247	2(3)
33922	1(2)	34203	1(2)	35132	1(2)	35535	1(3)	35879	2(3)	36475	1(3)	36833	1(3)	37248	1(2)
33924	1(2)	34401	1(3)	35141	1(2)	35536	1(3)	35881	1(3)	36476	2(3)	36835	1(3)	37249	3(3)
33925	1(2)	34421	1(3)	35142	1(2)	35537	1(3)	35883	1(3)	36478	1(3)	36838	1(3)	37252	1(2)
33926	1(2)	34451	1(3)	35151	1(2)	35538	1(3)	35884	1(3)	36479	2(3)	36860	2(3)	37253	5(3)
33927	1(3)	34471	1(2)	35152	1(2)	35539	1(3)	35901	1(3)	36481	1(3)	36861	2(3)	37500	1(3)
33928	1(3)	34490	1(2)	35180	2(3)	35540	1(3)	35903	2(3)	36482	1(3)	36901	1(3)	37501	1(3)
33929	1(3)	34501	1(2)	35182	2(3)	35556	1(3)	35905	1(3)	36483	2(3)	36902	1(3)	37565	1(2)
33930	1(2)	34502	1(2)	35184	2(3)	35558	1(3)	35907	1(3)	36500	4(3)	36903	1(3)	37600	1(3)
33933	1(2)	34510	2(3)	35188	2(3)	35560	1(3)	36000	4(3)	36510	1(3)	36904	1(3)	37605	1(3)
33935	1(2)	34520	1(3)	35189	1(3)	35563	1(3)	36002	2(3)	36511	1(3)	36905	1(3)	37606	1(3)
33940	1(2)	34530	1(2)	35190	2(3)	35565	1(3)	36005	2(3)	36512	1(3)	36906	1(3)	37607	1(3)
33944	1(2)	34701	1(2)	35201	2(3)	35566	1(3)	36010	2(3)	36513	1(3)	36907	1(3)	37609	1(2)
33945	1(2)	34702	1(2)	35206	2(3)	35570	1(3)	36011	4(3)	36514	1(3)	36908	1(3)	37615	2(3)
33946	1(2)	34703	1(2)	35207	3(3)	35571	1(3)	36012	4(3)	36516	1(3)	36909	1(3)	37616	1(3)
33947	1(2)	34704	1(2)	35211	3(3)	35572	2(3)	36013	2(3)	36522	1(3)	37140	1(2)	37617	3(3)
33948	1(2)	34705	1(2)	35216	2(3)	35583	1(2)	36014	2(3)	36555	2(3)	37145	1(3)	37618	2(3)
33949	1(2)	34706	1(2)	35221	3(3)	35585	2(3)	36015	4(3)	36556	2(3)	37160	1(3)	37619	1(2)
33951	1(3)	34707	1(2)	35226	3(3)	35587	1(3)	36100	2(3)	36557	2(3)	37180	1(2)	37650	1(2)
33952	1(3)	34708	1(2)	35231	2(3)	35600	2(3)	36140	3(3)	36558	2(3)	37181	1(2)	37660	1(2)
33953	1(3)	34709	3(3)	35236	2(3)	35601	1(3)	36160	2(3)	36560	2(3)	37182	1(2)	37700	1(2)
33954	1(3)	34710	1(2)	35241	2(3)	35606	1(3)	36200	2(3)	36561	2(3)	37183	1(2)	37718	1(2)
33955	1(3)	34711	2(3)	35246	2(3)	35612	1(3)	36215	2(3)	36563	1(3)	37184	1(2)	37722	1(2)
33956	1(3)	34712	1(2)	35251	2(3)	35616	1(3)	36216	2(3)	36565	1(3)	37185	2(3)	37735	1(2)
33957	1(3)	34713	1(2)	35256	2(3)	35621	1(3)	36217	2(3)	36566	1(3)	37186	2(3)	37760	1(2)
33958	1(3)	34714	1(2)	35261	1(3)	35623	1(3)	36218	2(3)	36568	2(3)	37187	1(3)	37761	1(2)
33959	1(3)	34715	1(2)	35266	2(3)	35626	3(3)	36221	1(3)	36569	2(3)	37188	1(3)	37765	1(2)

CPT	MUE	CPT	MUE	CPT	MUE	CPT	MUE	CPT	MUE	CPT	MUE	CPT	MUE	CPT	MUE
37766	1(2)	38770	1(2)	41015	2(3)	42235	1(2)	42962	1(3)	43248	1(3)	43450	1(3)	43881	1(3)
37780	1(2)	38780	1(2)	41016	1(3)	42260	1(3)	42970	1(3)	43249	1(3)	43453	1(3)	43882	1(3)
37785	1(2)	38790	1(2)	41017	2(3)	42280	1(2)	42971	1(3)	43250	1(2)	43460	1(3)	43886	1(2)
37788	1(2)	38792	1(3)	41018	2(3)	42281	1(2)	42972	1(3)	43251	1(2)	43496	1(3)	43887	1(2)
37790	1(2)	38794	1(2)	41019	1(3)	42299	1(3)	42999	1(3)	43252	1(2)	43499	1(3)	43888	1(2)
37799	1(3)	38900	1(3)	41100	2(3)	42300	2(3)	43020	1(2)	43253	1(3)	43500	1(2)	43999	1(3)
38100	1(2)	38999	1(3)	41105	2(3)	42305	2(3)	43030	1(2)	43254	1(3)	43501	1(3)	44005	1(2)
38101	1(3)	39000	1(2)	41108	2(3)	42310	2(3)	43045	1(2)	43255	2(3)	43502	1(2)	44010	1(2)
38102	1(2)	39010	1(2)	41110	2(3)	42320	2(3)	43100	1(3)	43257	1(2)	43510	1(2)	44015	1(2)
38115	1(3)	39200	1(2)	41112	2(3)	42330	1(3)	43101	1(3)	43259	1(2)	43520	1(2)	44020	2(3)
38120	1(2)	39220	1(2)	41113	2(3)	42335	2(2)	43107	1(2)	43260	1(3)	43605	1(2)	44021	1(3)
38129	1(3)	39401	1(3)	41114	2(3)	42340	1(2)	43108	1(2)	43261	1(2)	43610	2(3)	44025	1(3)
38200	1(3)	39402	1(3)	41115	1(2)	42400	2(3)	43112	1(2)	43262	2(2)	43611	2(3)	44050	1(2)
38204	1(2)	39499	1(3)	41116	2(3)	42405	2(3)	43113	1(2)	43263	1(2)	43620	1(2)	44055	1(2)
38205	1(3)	39501	1(3)	41120	1(2)	42408	1(3)	43116	1(2)	43264	1(2)	43621	1(2)	44100	1(2)
38206	1(3)	39503	1(2)	41130	1(2)	42409	1(3)	43117	1(2)	43265	1(2)	43622	1(2)	44110	1(2)
38207	1(3)	39540	1(2)	41135	1(2)	42410	1(2)	43118	1(2)	43266	1(3)	43631	1(2)	44111	1(2)
38208	1(3)	39541	1(2)	41140	1(2)	42415	1(2)	43121	1(2)	43270	1(3)	43632	1(2)	44120	1(2)
38209	1(3)	39545	1(2)	41145	1(2)	42420	1(2)	43122	1(2)	43273	1(3)	43633	1(2)	44121	2(3)
38210	1(3)	39560	1(3)	41150	1(2)	42425	1(2)	43123	1(2)	43274	2(3)	43634	1(2)	44125	1(2)
38211	1(3)	39561	1(3)	41153	1(2)	42426	1(2)	43124	1(2)	43275	1(3)	43635	1(2)	44126	1(2)
38212	1(3)	39599	1(3)	41155	1(2)	42440	1(2)	43130	1(3)	43276	2(3)	43640	1(2)	44127	1(2)
38213	1(3)	40490	2(3)	41250	2(3)	42450	1(3)	43135	1(3)	43277	3(3)	43641	1(2)	44128	2(3)
38214	1(3)	40500	2(3)	41251	2(3)	42500	2(3)	43180	1(3)	43278	1(3)	43644	1(2)	44130	2(3)
38215	1(3)	40510	2(3)	41252	2(3)	42505	2(3)	43191	1(3)	43279	1(2)	43645	1(2)	44132	1(2)
38220	1(3)	40520	2(3)	41510	1(2)	42507	1(2)	43192	1(3)	43280	1(2)	43647	1(2)	44133	1(2)
38221	1(3)	40525	2(3)	41512	1(2)	42509	1(2)	43193	1(3)	43281	1(2)	43648	1(2)	44135	1(2)
38222	1(2)	40527	2(3)	41520	1(3)	42510	1(2)	43194	1(3)	43282	1(2)	43651	1(2)	44136	1(2)
38230	1(2)	40530	2(3)	41530	1(3)	42550	2(3)	43195	1(3)	43283	1(2)	43652	1(2)	44137	1(2)
38232	1(2)	40650	2(3)	41599	1(3)	42600	1(3)	43196	1(3)	43284	1(2)	43653	1(2)	44139	1(2)
38240	1(3)	40652	2(3)	41800	2(3)	42650	2(3)	43197	1(3)	43285	1(2)	43659	1(3)	44140	2(3)
38241	1(2)	40654	2(3)	41805	1(3)	42660	2(3)	43198	1(3)	43286	1(2)	43752	2(3)	44141	1(3)
38242	1(2)	40700	1(2)	41806	1(3)	42665	2(3)	43200	1(3)	43287	1(2)	43753	1(3)	44143	1(2)
38243	1(3)	40701	1(2)	41820	4(2)	42699	1(3)	43201	1(2)	43288	1(2)	43754	1(3)	44144	1(3)
38300	1(3)	40702	1(2)	41821	2(3)	42700	2(3)	43202	1(2)	43289	1(2)	43755	1(3)	44145	1(2)
38305	1(3)	40720	1(2)	41822	1(2)	42720	1(3)	43204	1(2)	43300	1(2)	43756	1(2)	44146	1(2)
38308	1(3)	40761	1(2)	41823	1(2)	42725	1(3)	43205	1(2)	43305	1(2)	43757	1(2)	44147	1(3)
38380	1(2)	40799	1(3)	41825	2(3)	42800	3(3)	43206	1(2)	43310	1(2)	43761	2(3)	44150	1(2)
38381	1(2)	40800	2(3)	41826	2(3)	42804	1(3)	43210	1(2)	43312	1(2)	43762	2(3)	44151	1(2)
38382	1(2)	40801	2(3)	41827	2(3)	42806	1(3)	43211	1(3)	43313	1(2)	43763	2(3)	44155	1(2)
38500	2(3)	40804	1(3)	41828	4(2)	42808	2(3)	43212	1(3)	43314	1(2)	43770	1(2)	44156	1(2)
38505	2(3)	40805	2(3)	41850	2(3)	42809	1(3)	43213	1(2)	43320	1(2)	43771	1(2)	44157	1(2)
38510	1(2)	40806	2(2)	41870	2(3)	42810	1(3)	43214	1(2)	43325	1(2)	43772	1(2)	44158	1(2)
38520	1(2)	40808	2(3)	41872	4(2)	42815	1(3)	43215	1(3)	43327	1(2)	43773	1(2)	44160	1(2)
38525	1(2)	40810	2(3)	41874	4(2)	42820	1(2)	43216	1(2)	43328	1(2)	43774	1(2)	44180	1(2)
38530	1(2)	40812	2(3)	41899	1(3)	42821	1(2)	43217	1(2)	43330	1(2)	43775	1(2)	44186	1(2)
38531	1(2)	40814	4(3)	42000	1(3)	42825	1(2)	43220	1(3)	43331	1(2)	43800	1(2)	44187	1(3)
38542	1(2)	40816	2(3)	42100	2(3)	42826	1(2)	43226	1(3)	43332	1(2)	43810	1(2)	44188	1(3)
38550	1(3)	40818	2(3)	42104	2(3)	42830	1(2)	43227	1(3)	43333	1(2)	43820	1(2)	44202	1(2)
38555	1(3)	40819	2(2)	42106	2(3)	42831	1(2)	43229	1(3)	43334	1(2)	43825	1(2)	44203	2(3)
38562	1(2)	40820	2(3)	42107	2(3)	42835	1(2)	43231	1(2)	43335	1(2)	43830	1(2)	44204	2(3)
38564	1(2)	40830	2(3)	42120	1(2)	42836	1(2)	43232	1(2)	43336	1(2)	43831	1(2)	44205	1(2)
38570	1(2)	40831	2(3)	42140	1(2)	42842	1(3)	43233	1(3)	43337	1(2)	43832	1(2)	44206	1(2)
38571	1(2)	40840	1(2)	42145	1(2)	42844	1(3)	43235	1(3)	43338	1(2)	43840	2(3)	44207	1(2)
38572	1(2)	40842	1(2)	42160	1(3)	42845	1(3)	43236	1(2)	43340	1(2)	43842	0(3)	44208	1(2)
38573	1(2)	40843	1(2)	42180	1(3)	42860	1(3)	43237	1(2)	43341	1(2)	43843	1(2)	44210	1(2)
38589	1(3)	40844	1(2)	42182	1(3)	42870	1(3)	43238	1(2)	43351	1(2)	43845	1(2)	44211	1(2)
38700	1(2)	40845	1(3)	42200	1(2)	42890	1(2)	43239	1(2)	43352	1(2)	43846	1(2)	44212	1(2)
38720	1(2)	40899	1(3)	42205	1(2)	42892	1(3)	43240	1(2)	43360	1(2)	43847	1(2)	44213	1(2)
38724	1(2)	41000	1(3)	42210	1(2)	42894	1(3)	43241	1(3)	43361	1(2)	43848	1(2)	44227	1(2)
38740	1(2)	41005	1(3)	42215	1(2)	42900	1(3)	43242	1(2)	43400	1(2)	43850	1(2)	44238	1(3)
38745	1(2)	41006	2(3)	42220	1(2)	42950	1(2)	43243	1(2)	43405	1(2)	43855	1(2)	44300	1(3)
38746	1(2)	41007	2(3)	42225	1(2)	42953	1(3)	43244	1(2)	43410	1(3)	43860	1(2)	44310	2(3)
38747	1(2)	41008	2(3)	42226	1(2)	42955	1(2)	43245	1(2)	43415	1(3)	43865	1(2)	44312	1(2)
38760	1(2)	41009	2(3)	42227	1(2)	42960	1(3)	43246	1(2)	43420	1(3)	43870	1(2)	44314	1(2)
38765	1(2)	41010	1(2)					42961	1(3)	43247	1(2)	43425	1(3)	43880	1(3)	44316	1(2)

CPT	MUE	CPT	MUE	CPT	MUE	CPT	MUE	CPT	MUE	CPT	MUE	CPT	MUE	CPT	MUE
44320	1(2)	44955	1(2)	45392	1(2)	46615	1(2)	47383	1(2)	48148	1(2)	49428	1(2)	50070	1(2)
44322	1(2)	44960	1(2)	45393	1(3)	46700	1(2)	47399	1(3)	48150	1(2)	49429	1(2)	50075	1(2)
44340	1(2)	44970	1(2)	45395	1(2)	46705	1(2)	47400	1(3)	48152	1(2)	49435	1(2)	50080	1(2)
44345	1(2)	44979	1(3)	45397	1(2)	46706	1(3)	47420	1(2)	48153	1(2)	49436	1(2)	50081	1(2)
44346	1(2)	45000	1(3)	45398	1(2)	46707	1(3)	47425	1(2)	48154	1(2)	49440	1(3)	50100	1(2)
44360	1(3)	45005	1(3)	45399	1(3)	46710	1(3)	47460	1(2)	48155	1(2)	49441	1(3)	50120	1(2)
44361	1(2)	45020	1(3)	45400	1(2)	46712	1(3)	47480	1(2)	48160	0(3)	49442	1(3)	50125	1(2)
44363	1(3)	45100	2(3)	45402	1(2)	46715	1(3)	47490	1(2)	48400	1(3)	49446	1(2)	50130	1(2)
44364	1(2)	45108	1(2)	45499	1(3)	46716	1(2)	47531	2(3)	48500	1(3)	49450	1(3)	50135	1(2)
44365	1(2)	45110	1(2)	45500	1(2)	46730	1(2)	47532	1(3)	48510	1(3)	49451	1(3)	50200	1(3)
44366	1(3)	45111	1(2)	45505	1(2)	46735	1(2)	47533	1(3)	48520	1(3)	49452	1(3)	50205	1(3)
44369	1(2)	45112	1(2)	45520	1(2)	46740	1(2)	47534	2(3)	48540	1(3)	49460	1(3)	50220	1(2)
44370	1(2)	45113	1(2)	45540	1(2)	46742	1(2)	47535	1(3)	48545	1(3)	49465	1(3)	50225	1(2)
44372	1(2)	45114	1(2)	45541	1(2)	46744	1(2)	47536	2(3)	48547	1(2)	49491	1(2)	50230	1(2)
44373	1(2)	45116	1(2)	45550	1(2)	46746	1(2)	47537	1(3)	48548	1(2)	49492	1(2)	50234	1(2)
44376	1(3)	45119	1(2)	45560	1(2)	46748	1(2)	47538	2(3)	48550	1(2)	49495	1(2)	50236	1(2)
44377	1(2)	45120	1(2)	45562	1(2)	46750	1(2)	47539	2(3)	48551	1(2)	49496	1(2)	50240	1(2)
44378	1(3)	45121	1(2)	45563	1(2)	46751	1(2)	47540	2(3)	48552	2(3)	49500	1(2)	50250	1(3)
44379	1(2)	45123	1(2)	45800	1(3)	46753	1(2)	47541	1(3)	48554	1(2)	49501	1(2)	50280	1(2)
44380	1(3)	45126	1(2)	45805	1(3)	46754	1(3)	47542	2(3)	48556	1(2)	49505	1(2)	50290	1(3)
44381	1(3)	45130	1(2)	45820	1(3)	46760	1(2)	47543	1(3)	48999	1(3)	49507	1(2)	50300	1(2)
44382	1(2)	45135	1(2)	45825	1(3)	46761	1(2)	47544	1(3)	49000	1(2)	49520	1(2)	50320	1(2)
44384	1(3)	45136	1(2)	45900	1(2)	46900	1(2)	47550	1(3)	49002	1(3)	49521	1(2)	50323	1(2)
44385	1(3)	45150	1(2)	45905	1(2)	46910	1(2)	47552	1(3)	49010	1(3)	49525	1(2)	50325	1(2)
44386	1(2)	45160	1(3)	45910	1(2)	46916	1(2)	47553	1(2)	49013	1(2)	49540	1(2)	50327	2(3)
44388	1(3)	45171	2(3)	45915	1(2)	46917	1(2)	47554	1(2)	49014	1(3)	49550	1(2)	50328	1(3)
44389	1(3)	45172	2(3)	45990	1(2)	46922	1(2)	47555	1(2)	49020	2(3)	49553	1(2)	50329	1(3)
44390	1(3)	45190	1(3)	45999	1(3)	46924	1(2)	47556	1(2)	49040	2(3)	49555	1(2)	50340	1(2)
44391	1(3)	45300	1(3)	46020	2(3)	46930	1(2)	47562	1(2)	49060	2(3)	49557	1(2)	50360	1(2)
44392	1(2)	45303	1(3)	46030	1(3)	46940	1(2)	47563	1(2)	49062	1(3)	49560	2(3)	50365	1(2)
44394	1(2)	45305	1(2)	46040	2(3)	46942	1(3)	47564	1(2)	49082	1(3)	49561	1(3)	50370	1(2)
44401	1(2)	45307	1(3)	46045	2(3)	46945	1(2)	47570	1(2)	49083	2(3)	49565	2(3)	50380	1(2)
44402	1(3)	45308	1(2)	46050	2(3)	46946	1(2)	47579	1(3)	49084	1(3)	49566	2(3)	50382	1(3)
44403	1(3)	45309	1(2)	46060	2(3)	46947	1(2)	47600	1(2)	49180	2(3)	49568	2(3)	50384	1(3)
44404	1(3)	45315	1(2)	46070	1(2)	46948	1(2)	47605	1(2)	49185	2(3)	49570	1(3)	50385	1(3)
44405	1(3)	45317	1(3)	46080	1(2)	46999	1(3)	47610	1(2)	49203	1(2)	49572	1(3)	50386	1(3)
44406	1(3)	45320	1(2)	46083	2(3)	47000	3(3)	47612	1(2)	49204	1(2)	49580	1(2)	50387	1(3)
44407	1(2)	45321	1(2)	46200	1(3)	47001	3(3)	47620	1(2)	49205	1(2)	49582	1(2)	50389	1(3)
44408	1(3)	45327	1(2)	46220	1(2)	47010	1(3)	47700	1(2)	49215	1(2)	49585	1(2)	50390	2(3)
44500	1(3)	45330	1(3)	46221	1(2)	47015	1(2)	47701	1(2)	49250	1(2)	49587	1(2)	50391	1(3)
44602	1(2)	45331	1(2)	46230	1(2)	47100	3(3)	47711	1(2)	49255	1(2)	49590	1(2)	50396	1(3)
44603	1(2)	45332	1(3)	46250	1(2)	47120	2(3)	47712	1(2)	49320	1(3)	49600	1(2)	50400	1(2)
44604	1(2)	45333	1(2)	46255	1(2)	47122	1(2)	47715	1(2)	49321	1(2)	49605	1(2)	50405	1(2)
44605	1(2)	45334	1(3)	46257	1(2)	47125	1(2)	47720	1(2)	49322	1(2)	49606	1(2)	50430	2(3)
44615	3(3)	45335	1(2)	46258	1(2)	47130	1(2)	47721	1(2)	49323	1(2)	49610	1(2)	50431	2(3)
44620	2(3)	45337	1(2)	46260	1(2)	47133	1(2)	47740	1(2)	49324	1(2)	49611	1(2)	50432	2(3)
44625	1(3)	45338	1(2)	46261	1(2)	47135	1(2)	47741	1(2)	49325	1(2)	49650	1(2)	50433	2(3)
44626	1(3)	45340	1(2)	46262	1(2)	47140	1(2)	47760	1(2)	49326	1(2)	49651	1(2)	50434	2(3)
44640	2(3)	45341	1(2)	46270	1(3)	47141	1(2)	47765	1(2)	49327	1(2)	49652	2(3)	50435	2(3)
44650	2(3)	45342	1(2)	46275	1(3)	47142	1(2)	47780	1(2)	49329	1(3)	49653	2(3)	50436	1(3)
44660	1(3)	45346	1(2)	46280	1(2)	47143	1(2)	47785	1(2)	49400	1(3)	49654	1(3)	50437	1(3)
44661	1(3)	45347	1(3)	46285	1(3)	47144	1(2)	47800	1(2)	49402	1(3)	49655	1(3)	50500	1(3)
44680	1(3)	45349	1(3)	46288	1(3)	47145	1(2)	47801	1(3)	49405	2(3)	49656	1(3)	50520	1(3)
44700	1(2)	45350	1(2)	46320	2(3)	47146	2(3)	47802	1(2)	49406	2(3)	49657	1(3)	50525	1(3)
44701	1(2)	45378	1(3)	46500	1(2)	47147	1(3)	47900	1(2)	49407	1(3)	49659	1(3)	50526	1(3)
44705	1(3)	45379	1(3)	46505	1(2)	47300	2(3)	47999	1(3)	49411	1(2)	49900	1(3)	50540	1(2)
44715	1(2)	45380	1(2)	46600	1(3)	47350	1(3)	48000	1(2)	49412	1(2)	49904	1(3)	50541	1(2)
44720	2(3)	45381	1(2)	46601	1(3)	47360	1(3)	48001	1(2)	49418	1(3)	49905	1(3)	50542	1(2)
44721	2(3)	45382	1(3)	46604	1(2)	47361	1(3)	48020	1(3)	49419	1(2)	49906	1(3)	50543	1(2)
44799	1(3)	45384	1(2)	46606	1(2)	47362	1(3)	48100	1(3)	49421	1(2)	49999	1(3)	50544	1(2)
44800	1(2)	45385	1(2)	46607	1(2)	47370	1(2)	48102	1(3)	49422	1(2)	50010	1(2)	50545	1(2)
44820	1(3)	45386	1(2)	46608	1(3)	47371	1(2)	48105	1(3)	49423	2(3)	50020	1(3)	50546	1(2)
44850	1(3)	45388	1(2)	46610	1(2)	47379	1(3)	48120	1(3)	49424	3(3)	50040	1(2)	50547	1(2)
44899	1(3)	45389	1(3)	46611	1(2)	47380	1(2)	48140	1(2)	49425	1(2)	50045	1(2)	50548	1(2)
44900	1(2)	45390	1(3)	46612	1(2)	47381	1(2)	48145	1(2)	49426	1(3)	50060	1(2)	50549	1(3)
44950	1(2)	45391	1(2)	46614	1(3)	47382	1(2)	48146	1(2)	49427	1(3)	50065	1(2)	50551	1(3)

CPT	MUE	CPT	MUE	CPT	MUE	CPT	MUE	CPT	MUE	CPT	MUE	CPT	MUE	CPT	MUE
50553	1(3)	50961	1(2)	51925	1(2)	52648	1(2)	54056	1(2)	54505	1(3)	55860	1(2)	57240	1(2)
50555	1(2)	50970	1(3)	51940	1(2)	52649	1(2)	54057	1(2)	54512	1(3)	55862	1(2)	57250	1(2)
50557	1(2)	50972	1(3)	51960	1(2)	52700	1(3)	54060	1(2)	54520	1(2)	55865	1(2)	57260	1(2)
50561	1(2)	50974	1(2)	51980	1(2)	53000	1(2)	54065	1(2)	54522	1(2)	55866	1(2)	57265	1(2)
50562	1(3)	50976	1(2)	51990	1(2)	53010	1(2)	54100	2(3)	54530	1(2)	55870	1(2)	57267	2(3)
50570	1(3)	50980	1(2)	51992	1(2)	53020	1(2)	54105	2(3)	54535	1(2)	55873	1(2)	57268	1(2)
50572	1(3)	51020	1(2)	51999	1(3)	53025	1(2)	54110	1(2)	54550	1(2)	55874	1(2)	57270	1(2)
50574	1(2)	51030	1(2)	52000	1(3)	53040	1(3)	54111	1(2)	54560	1(2)	55875	1(2)	57280	1(2)
50575	1(2)	51040	1(3)	52001	1(3)	53060	1(3)	54112	1(3)	54600	1(2)	55876	1(2)	57282	1(2)
50576	1(2)	51045	2(3)	52005	2(3)	53080	1(3)	54115	1(3)	54620	1(2)	55880	1(2)	57283	1(2)
50580	1(2)	51050	1(3)	52007	1(2)	53085	1(3)	54120	1(2)	54640	1(2)	55899	1(3)	57284	1(2)
50590	1(2)	51060	1(3)	52010	1(2)	53200	1(3)	54125	1(2)	54650	1(2)	55920	1(2)	57285	1(2)
50592	1(2)	51065	1(3)	52204	1(2)	53210	1(2)	54130	1(2)	54660	1(2)	55970	1(2)	57287	1(2)
50593	1(2)	51080	1(3)	52214	1(2)	53215	1(2)	54135	1(2)	54670	1(3)	55980	1(2)	57288	1(2)
50600	1(3)	51100	1(3)	52224	1(2)	53220	1(3)	54150	1(2)	54680	1(2)	56405	2(3)	57289	1(2)
50605	1(3)	51101	1(3)	52234	1(2)	53230	1(3)	54160	1(2)	54690	1(2)	56420	1(3)	57291	1(2)
50606	1(3)	51102	1(3)	52235	1(2)	53235	1(3)	54161	1(2)	54692	1(2)	56440	1(3)	57292	1(2)
50610	1(2)	51500	1(2)	52240	1(2)	53240	1(3)	54162	1(2)	54699	1(3)	56441	1(2)	57295	1(2)
50620	1(2)	51520	1(2)	52250	1(2)	53250	1(3)	54163	1(2)	54700	1(3)	56442	1(2)	57296	1(2)
50630	1(2)	51525	1(2)	52260	1(2)	53260	1(2)	54164	1(2)	54800	1(2)	56501	1(2)	57300	1(3)
50650	1(2)	51530	1(2)	52265	1(2)	53265	1(3)	54200	1(2)	54830	1(2)	56515	1(2)	57305	1(3)
50660	1(3)	51535	1(2)	52270	1(2)	53270	1(2)	54205	1(2)	54840	1(2)	56605	1(2)	57307	1(3)
50684	1(3)	51550	1(2)	52275	1(2)	53275	1(2)	54220	1(3)	54860	1(2)	56606	6(3)	57308	1(3)
50686	2(3)	51555	1(2)	52276	1(2)	53400	1(2)	54230	1(2)	54861	1(2)	56620	1(2)	57310	1(3)
50688	2(3)	51565	1(2)	52277	1(2)	53405	1(2)	54231	1(3)	54865	1(3)	56625	1(2)	57311	1(3)
50690	2(3)	51570	1(2)	52281	1(2)	53410	1(2)	54235	1(3)	54900	1(2)	56630	1(2)	57320	1(3)
50693	2(3)	51575	1(2)	52282	1(2)	53415	1(2)	54240	1(2)	54901	1(2)	56631	1(2)	57330	1(3)
50694	2(3)	51580	1(2)	52283	1(2)	53420	1(2)	54250	1(2)	55000	1(3)	56632	1(2)	57335	1(2)
50695	2(3)	51585	1(2)	52285	1(2)	53425	1(2)	54300	1(2)	55040	1(2)	56633	1(2)	57400	1(2)
50700	1(2)	51590	1(2)	52287	1(2)	53430	1(2)	54304	1(2)	55041	1(2)	56634	1(2)	57410	1(2)
50705	2(3)	51595	1(2)	52290	1(2)	53431	1(2)	54308	1(2)	55060	1(2)	56637	1(2)	57415	1(3)
50706	2(3)	51596	1(2)	52300	1(2)	53440	1(2)	54312	1(2)	55100	2(3)	56640	1(2)	57420	1(3)
50715	1(2)	51597	1(2)	52301	1(2)	53442	1(2)	54316	1(2)	55110	1(2)	56700	1(2)	57421	1(3)
50722	1(2)	51600	1(3)	52305	1(2)	53444	1(3)	54318	1(2)	55120	1(3)	56740	1(3)	57423	1(2)
50725	1(3)	51605	1(3)	52310	1(3)	53445	1(2)	54322	1(2)	55150	1(2)	56800	1(2)	57425	1(2)
50727	1(3)	51610	1(3)	52315	2(3)	53446	1(2)	54324	1(2)	55175	1(2)	56805	1(2)	57426	1(2)
50728	1(3)	51700	1(3)	52317	1(3)	53447	1(2)	54326	1(2)	55180	1(2)	56810	1(2)	57452	1(3)
50740	1(2)	51701	2(3)	52318	1(3)	53448	1(2)	54328	1(2)	55200	1(2)	56820	1(2)	57454	1(3)
50750	1(2)	51702	2(3)	52320	1(2)	53449	1(2)	54332	1(2)	55250	1(2)	56821	1(2)	57455	1(3)
50760	1(2)	51703	2(3)	52325	1(3)	53450	1(2)	54336	1(2)	55300	1(2)	57000	1(3)	57456	1(3)
50770	1(2)	51705	2(3)	52327	1(2)	53460	1(2)	54340	1(2)	55400	1(2)	57010	1(3)	57460	1(3)
50780	1(2)	51710	1(3)	52330	1(2)	53500	1(2)	54344	1(2)	55500	1(2)	57020	1(3)	57461	1(3)
50782	1(2)	51715	1(2)	52332	1(2)	53502	1(3)	54348	1(2)	55520	1(2)	57022	1(3)	57465	1(3)
50783	1(2)	51720	1(3)	52334	1(2)	53505	1(3)	54352	1(2)	55530	1(2)	57023	1(3)	57500	1(3)
50785	1(2)	51725	1(3)	52341	1(2)	53510	1(3)	54360	1(2)	55535	1(2)	57061	1(2)	57505	1(3)
50800	1(2)	51726	1(3)	52342	1(2)	53515	1(3)	54380	1(2)	55540	1(2)	57065	1(2)	57510	1(3)
50810	1(3)	51727	1(3)	52343	1(2)	53520	1(3)	54385	1(2)	55550	1(2)	57100	2(3)	57511	1(3)
50815	1(2)	51728	1(3)	52344	1(2)	53600	1(3)	54390	1(2)	55559	1(3)	57105	2(3)	57513	1(3)
50820	1(2)	51729	1(3)	52345	1(2)	53601	1(3)	54400	1(2)	55600	1(2)	57106	1(2)	57520	1(3)
50825	1(3)	51736	1(3)	52346	1(2)	53605	1(3)	54401	1(2)	55605	1(2)	57107	1(2)	57522	1(3)
50830	1(3)	51741	1(3)	52351	1(3)	53620	1(2)	54405	1(2)	55650	1(2)	57109	1(2)	57530	1(3)
50840	1(2)	51784	1(3)	52352	1(2)	53621	1(3)	54406	1(2)	55680	1(3)	57110	1(2)	57531	1(2)
50845	1(2)	51785	1(3)	52353	1(2)	53660	1(2)	54408	1(2)	55700	1(2)	57111	1(2)	57540	1(2)
50860	1(2)	51792	1(3)	52354	1(3)	53661	1(3)	54410	1(2)	55705	1(2)	57120	1(2)	57545	1(3)
50900	1(3)	51797	1(3)	52355	1(3)	53665	1(3)	54411	1(2)	55706	1(2)	57130	1(2)	57550	1(3)
50920	2(3)	51798	1(3)	52356	1(2)	53850	1(2)	54415	1(2)	55720	1(3)	57135	2(3)	57555	1(3)
50930	2(3)	51800	1(2)	52400	1(2)	53852	1(2)	54416	1(2)	55725	1(3)	57150	1(3)	57556	1(2)
50940	1(2)	51820	1(2)	52402	1(2)	53854	1(2)	54417	1(2)	55801	1(2)	57155	1(3)	57558	1(3)
50945	1(2)	51840	1(2)	52441	1(2)	53855	1(2)	54420	1(2)	55810	1(2)	57156	1(3)	57700	1(3)
50947	1(2)	51841	1(2)	52442	6(3)	53860	1(2)	54430	1(2)	55812	1(2)	57160	1(2)	57720	1(3)
50948	1(2)	51845	1(2)	52450	1(2)	53899	1(3)	54435	1(2)	55815	1(2)	57170	1(2)	57800	1(3)
50949	1(3)	51860	1(3)	52500	1(2)	54000	1(2)	54437	1(2)	55821	1(2)	57180	1(3)	58100	1(3)
50951	1(3)	51865	1(3)	52601	1(2)	54001	1(2)	54438	1(2)	55831	1(2)	57200	1(3)	58110	1(3)
50953	1(3)	51880	1(2)	52630	1(2)	54015	1(3)	54440	1(2)	55840	1(2)	57210	1(3)	58120	1(3)
50955	1(2)	51900	1(3)	52640	1(2)	54050	1(2)	54450	1(2)	55842	1(2)	57220	1(2)	58140	1(3)
50957	1(2)	51920	1(3)	52647	1(2)	54055	1(2)	54500	1(3)	55845	1(2)	57230	1(2)	58145	1(3)

CPT	MUE	CPT	MUE	CPT	MUE	CPT	MUE	CPT	MUE	CPT	MUE	CPT	MUE	CPT	MUE
58146	1(3)	58662	1(2)	59409	2(3)	61001	1(2)	61546	1(2)	61710	1(3)	62269	2(3)	63076	3(3)
58150	1(3)	58670	1(2)	59410	1(2)	61020	2(3)	61548	1(2)	61711	1(3)	62270	2(3)	63077	1(2)
58152	1(2)	58671	1(2)	59412	1(3)	61026	2(3)	61550	1(2)	61720	1(3)	62272	2(3)	63078	3(3)
58180	1(3)	58672	1(2)	59414	1(3)	61050	1(3)	61552	1(2)	61735	1(3)	62273	2(3)	63081	1(2)
58200	1(2)	58673	1(2)	59425	1(2)	61055	1(3)	61556	1(3)	61750	2(3)	62280	1(3)	63082	6(2)
58210	1(3)	58674	1(2)	59426	1(2)	61070	2(3)	61557	1(2)	61751	2(3)	62281	1(3)	63085	1(2)
58240	1(2)	58679	1(3)	59430	1(2)	61105	1(3)	61558	1(3)	61760	1(2)	62282	1(3)	63086	2(3)
58260	1(3)	58700	1(2)	59510	1(2)	61107	1(3)	61559	1(3)	61770	1(2)	62284	1(3)	63087	1(2)
58262	1(3)	58720	1(2)	59514	1(3)	61108	1(3)	61563	2(3)	61781	1(3)	62287	1(2)	63088	3(3)
58263	1(2)	58740	1(2)	59515	1(2)	61120	1(3)	61564	1(2)	61782	1(3)	62290	5(2)	63090	1(2)
58267	1(2)	58750	1(2)	59525	1(2)	61140	1(3)	61566	1(3)	61783	1(3)	62291	4(3)	63091	3(3)
58270	1(2)	58752	1(2)	59610	1(2)	61150	1(3)	61567	1(2)	61790	1(2)	62292	1(2)	63101	1(2)
58275	1(2)	58760	1(2)	59612	2(3)	61151	1(3)	61570	1(3)	61791	1(2)	62294	1(3)	63102	1(2)
58280	1(2)	58770	1(2)	59614	1(2)	61154	1(3)	61571	1(3)	61796	1(2)	62302	1(3)	63103	3(3)
58285	1(3)	58800	1(2)	59618	1(2)	61156	1(3)	61575	1(2)	61797	4(3)	62303	1(3)	63170	1(3)
58290	1(3)	58805	1(2)	59620	1(2)	61210	1(3)	61576	1(2)	61798	1(2)	62304	1(3)	63172	1(3)
58291	1(2)	58820	1(3)	59622	1(2)	61215	1(3)	61580	1(2)	61799	4(3)	62305	1(3)	63173	1(3)
58292	1(2)	58822	1(3)	59812	1(2)	61250	1(3)	61581	1(2)	61800	1(2)	62320	1(3)	63185	1(2)
58294	1(2)	58825	1(2)	59820	1(2)	61253	1(3)	61582	1(2)	61850	1(3)	62321	1(3)	63190	1(2)
58300	0(3)	58900	1(2)	59821	1(2)	61304	1(3)	61583	1(2)	61860	1(3)	62322	1(3)	63191	1(2)
58301	1(3)	58920	1(2)	59830	1(2)	61305	1(3)	61584	1(2)	61863	1(2)	62323	1(3)	63194	1(2)
58321	1(2)	58925	1(3)	59840	1(2)	61312	2(3)	61585	1(2)	61864	1(3)	62324	1(3)	63195	1(2)
58322	1(2)	58940	1(2)	59841	1(2)	61313	2(3)	61586	1(3)	61867	1(2)	62325	1(3)	63196	1(2)
58323	1(3)	58943	1(2)	59850	1(2)	61314	2(3)	61590	1(2)	61868	2(3)	62326	1(3)	63197	1(2)
58340	1(3)	58950	1(2)	59851	1(2)	61315	1(3)	61591	1(2)	61880	1(2)	62327	1(3)	63198	1(2)
58345	1(3)	58951	1(2)	59852	1(2)	61316	1(3)	61592	1(2)	61885	1(3)	62328	2(3)	63199	1(2)
58346	1(2)	58952	1(2)	59855	1(2)	61320	2(3)	61595	1(2)	61886	1(3)	62329	1(3)	63200	1(2)
58350	1(2)	58953	1(2)	59856	1(2)	61321	1(3)	61596	1(2)	61888	1(3)	62350	1(3)	63250	1(3)
58353	1(3)	58954	1(2)	59857	1(2)	61322	1(3)	61597	1(2)	62000	1(3)	62351	1(3)	63251	1(3)
58356	1(3)	58956	1(2)	59866	1(2)	61323	1(3)	61598	1(3)	62005	1(3)	62355	1(3)	63252	1(3)
58400	1(3)	58957	1(2)	59870	1(2)	61330	1(2)	61600	1(3)	62010	1(3)	62360	1(2)	63265	1(3)
58410	1(2)	58958	1(2)	59871	1(2)	61333	1(2)	61601	1(3)	62100	1(3)	62361	1(2)	63266	1(3)
58520	1(2)	58960	1(2)	59897	1(3)	61340	1(2)	61605	1(3)	62115	1(2)	62362	1(2)	63267	1(3)
58540	1(3)	58970	1(3)	59898	1(3)	61343	1(2)	61606	1(3)	62117	1(2)	62365	1(2)	63268	1(3)
58541	1(3)	58974	1(3)	59899	1(3)	61345	1(3)	61607	1(3)	62120	1(2)	62367	1(3)	63270	1(3)
58542	1(2)	58976	2(3)	60000	1(3)	61450	1(3)	61608	1(3)	62121	1(3)	62368	1(3)	63271	1(3)
58543	1(3)	58999	1(3)	60100	3(3)	61458	1(2)	61611	1(3)	62140	1(3)	62369	1(3)	63272	1(3)
58544	1(2)	59000	2(3)	60200	2(3)	61460	1(2)	61613	1(3)	62141	1(3)	62370	1(3)	63273	1(3)
58545	1(2)	59001	2(3)	60210	1(2)	61500	1(3)	61615	1(3)	62142	2(3)	62380	2(3)	63275	1(3)
58546	1(2)	59012	2(3)	60212	1(2)	61501	1(3)	61616	1(3)	62143	2(3)	63001	1(2)	63276	1(3)
58548	1(2)	59015	2(3)	60220	1(2)	61510	1(3)	61618	2(3)	62145	2(3)	63003	1(2)	63277	1(3)
58550	1(3)	59020	2(3)	60225	1(2)	61512	1(3)	61619	2(3)	62146	2(3)	63005	1(2)	63278	1(3)
58552	1(3)	59025	2(3)	60240	1(2)	61514	2(3)	61623	2(3)	62147	1(3)	63011	1(2)	63280	1(3)
58553	1(3)	59030	2(3)	60252	1(2)	61516	1(3)	61624	2(3)	62148	1(3)	63012	1(2)	63281	1(3)
58554	1(2)	59050	2(3)	60254	1(2)	61517	1(3)	61626	2(3)	62160	1(3)	63015	1(2)	63282	1(3)
58555	1(3)	59051	2(3)	60260	1(2)	61518	1(3)	61630	1(3)	62161	1(3)	63016	1(2)	63283	1(3)
58558	1(3)	59070	2(3)	60270	1(2)	61519	1(3)	61635	2(3)	62162	1(3)	63017	1(2)	63285	1(3)
58559	1(3)	59072	2(3)	60271	1(2)	61520	1(3)	61640	0(3)	62164	1(3)	63020	1(2)	63286	1(3)
58560	1(3)	59074	2(3)	60280	1(3)	61521	1(3)	61641	0(3)	62165	1(2)	63030	1(2)	63287	1(3)
58561	1(3)	59076	2(3)	60281	1(3)	61522	1(3)	61642	0(3)	62180	1(3)	63035	4(3)	63290	1(3)
58562	1(3)	59100	1(2)	60300	2(3)	61524	2(3)	61645	1(3)	62190	1(3)	63040	1(2)	63295	1(2)
58563	1(3)	59120	1(3)	60500	1(2)	61526	1(3)	61650	1(2)	62192	1(3)	63042	1(2)	63300	1(2)
58565	1(2)	59121	1(3)	60502	1(3)	61530	1(3)	61651	2(2)	62194	1(3)	63043	4(3)	63301	1(2)
58570	1(3)	59130	1(3)	60505	1(3)	61531	1(3)	61680	1(3)	62200	1(2)	63044	4(2)	63302	1(2)
58571	1(2)	59135	1(3)	60512	1(3)	61533	2(3)	61682	1(3)	62201	1(2)	63045	1(2)	63303	1(2)
58572	1(3)	59136	1(3)	60520	1(3)	61534	1(3)	61684	1(3)	62220	1(3)	63046	1(2)	63304	1(2)
58573	1(2)	59140	1(2)	60521	1(2)	61535	2(3)	61686	1(3)	62223	1(3)	63047	1(2)	63305	1(2)
58575	1(2)	59150	1(3)	60522	1(2)	61536	1(3)	61690	1(3)	62225	2(3)	63048	5(3)	63306	1(2)
58578	1(3)	59151	1(3)	60540	1(2)	61537	1(3)	61692	1(3)	62230	2(3)	63050	1(2)	63307	1(2)
58579	1(3)	59160	1(2)	60545	1(2)	61538	1(2)	61697	2(3)	62252	2(3)	63051	1(2)	63308	3(3)
58600	1(2)	59200	1(3)	60600	1(3)	61539	1(3)	61698	1(3)	62256	1(3)	63055	1(2)	63600	2(3)
58605	1(2)	59300	1(2)	60605	1(3)	61540	1(3)	61700	2(3)	62258	1(3)	63056	1(2)	63610	1(3)
58611	1(2)	59320	1(2)	60650	1(2)	61541	1(2)	61702	1(3)	62263	1(2)	63057	3(3)	63620	1(2)
58615	1(2)	59325	1(2)	60659	1(3)	61543	1(2)	61703	1(3)	62264	1(2)	63064	1(2)	63621	2(2)
58660	1(2)	59350	1(2)	60699	1(3)	61544	1(3)	61705	1(3)	62267	2(3)	63066	1(3)	63650	2(3)
58661	1(2)	59400	1(2)	61000	1(2)	61545	1(2)	61708	1(3)	62268	1(3)	63075	1(2)	63655	1(3)

CPT	MUE	CPT	MUE	CPT	MUE	CPT	MUE	CPT	MUE	CPT	MUE	CPT	MUE	CPT	MUE
63661	1(2)	64570	1(3)	64783	2(3)	65140	1(2)	66160	1(2)	67110	1(2)	67875	1(2)	68750	1(2)
63662	1(2)	64575	2(3)	64784	3(3)	65150	1(2)	66170	1(2)	67113	1(2)	67880	1(2)	68760	4(2)
63663	1(3)	64580	2(3)	64786	1(3)	65155	1(2)	66172	1(2)	67115	1(2)	67882	1(2)	68761	4(2)
63664	1(3)	64581	2(3)	64787	4(3)	65175	1(2)	66174	1(2)	67120	1(2)	67900	1(2)	68770	1(3)
63685	1(3)	64585	2(3)	64788	5(3)	65205	1(3)	66175	1(2)	67121	1(2)	67901	1(2)	68801	4(2)
63688	1(3)	64590	1(3)	64790	1(2)	65210	1(3)	66179	1(2)	67141	1(2)	67902	1(2)	68810	1(2)
63700	1(3)	64595	1(3)	64792	2(3)	65220	1(3)	66180	1(2)	67145	1(2)	67903	1(2)	68811	1(2)
63702	1(3)	64600	2(3)	64795	2(3)	65222	1(3)	66183	1(3)	67208	1(2)	67904	1(2)	68815	1(2)
63704	1(3)	64605	1(2)	64802	1(2)	65235	1(3)	66184	1(2)	67210	1(2)	67906	1(2)	68816	1(2)
63706	1(3)	64610	1(2)	64804	1(2)	65260	1(3)	66185	1(2)	67218	1(2)	67908	1(2)	68840	1(2)
63707	1(3)	64611	1(2)	64809	1(2)	65265	1(3)	66225	1(2)	67220	1(2)	67909	1(2)	68850	1(3)
63709	1(3)	64612	1(2)	64818	1(2)	65270	1(3)	66250	1(2)	67221	1(2)	67911	2(3)	68899	1(3)
63710	1(3)	64615	1(2)	64820	4(3)	65272	1(3)	66500	1(2)	67225	1(2)	67912	1(2)	69000	1(3)
63740	1(3)	64616	1(2)	64821	1(2)	65273	1(3)	66505	1(2)	67227	1(2)	67914	2(3)	69005	1(3)
63741	1(3)	64617	1(2)	64822	1(2)	65275	1(3)	66600	1(2)	67228	1(2)	67915	2(3)	69020	1(3)
63744	1(3)	64620	5(3)	64823	1(2)	65280	1(3)	66605	1(2)	67229	1(2)	67916	2(3)	69090	0(3)
63746	1(2)	64624	2(2)	64831	1(2)	65285	1(3)	66625	1(2)	67250	1(2)	67917	2(3)	69100	3(3)
64400	4(3)	64625	2(2)	64832	3(3)	65286	1(3)	66630	1(2)	67255	1(2)	67921	2(3)	69105	1(3)
64405	1(3)	64630	1(3)	64834	1(2)	65290	1(3)	66635	1(2)	67299	1(3)	67922	2(3)	69110	1(2)
64408	1(3)	64632	1(2)	64835	1(2)	65400	1(3)	66680	1(2)	67311	1(2)	67923	2(3)	69120	1(3)
64415	1(3)	64633	1(2)	64836	1(2)	65410	1(3)	66682	1(2)	67312	1(2)	67924	2(3)	69140	1(2)
64416	1(2)	64634	4(3)	64837	2(3)	65420	1(2)	66700	1(2)	67314	1(2)	67930	2(3)	69145	1(3)
64417	1(3)	64635	1(2)	64840	1(2)	65426	1(2)	66710	1(2)	67316	1(2)	67935	2(3)	69150	1(3)
64418	1(3)	64636	4(3)	64856	2(3)	65430	1(2)	66711	1(2)	67318	1(2)	67938	2(3)	69155	1(3)
64420	2(2)	64640	5(3)	64857	2(3)	65435	1(2)	66720	1(2)	67320	2(3)	67950	2(2)	69200	1(2)
64421	3(3)	64642	1(2)	64858	1(2)	65436	1(2)	66740	1(2)	67331	1(2)	67961	2(3)	69205	1(3)
64425	1(3)	64643	3(2)	64859	2(3)	65450	1(3)	66761	1(2)	67332	1(2)	67966	2(3)	69209	1(2)
64430	1(3)	64644	1(2)	64861	1(2)	65600	1(2)	66762	1(2)	67334	1(2)	67971	1(2)	69210	1(2)
64435	1(3)	64645	3(2)	64862	1(2)	65710	1(3)	66770	1(3)	67335	1(2)	67973	1(2)	69220	1(2)
64445	1(3)	64646	1(2)	64864	2(3)	65730	1(2)	66820	1(2)	67340	2(2)	67974	1(2)	69222	1(2)
64446	1(2)	64647	1(2)	64865	1(3)	65750	1(2)	66821	1(2)	67343	1(2)	67975	1(2)	69300	1(2)
64447	1(3)	64650	1(2)	64866	1(3)	65755	1(2)	66825	1(2)	67345	1(3)	67999	1(3)	69310	1(2)
64448	1(2)	64653	1(2)	64868	1(3)	65756	1(2)	66830	1(2)	67346	1(3)	68020	1(3)	69320	1(2)
64449	1(2)	64680	1(2)	64872	1(3)	65757	1(3)	66840	1(2)	67399	1(3)	68040	1(2)	69399	1(3)
64450	10(3)	64681	1(2)	64874	1(3)	65760	0(3)	66850	1(2)	67400	1(2)	68100	1(3)	69420	1(2)
64451	2(2)	64702	2(3)	64876	1(3)	65765	0(3)	66852	1(2)	67405	1(2)	68110	1(3)	69421	1(2)
64454	2(2)	64704	4(3)	64885	1(3)	65767	0(3)	66920	1(2)	67412	1(2)	68115	1(3)	69424	1(2)
64455	1(3)	64708	3(3)	64886	1(3)	65770	1(2)	66930	1(2)	67413	1(2)	68130	1(3)	69433	1(2)
64461	1(2)	64712	1(2)	64890	2(3)	65771	0(3)	66940	1(2)	67414	1(2)	68135	1(3)	69436	1(2)
64462	1(2)	64713	1(2)	64891	2(3)	65772	1(2)	66982	1(2)	67415	1(3)	68200	1(3)	69440	1(2)
64463	1(3)	64714	1(2)	64892	2(3)	65775	1(2)	66983	1(2)	67420	1(2)	68320	1(2)	69450	1(2)
64479	1(2)	64716	2(3)	64893	2(3)	65778	1(2)	66984	1(2)	67430	1(2)	68325	1(2)	69501	1(3)
64480	4(3)	64718	1(2)	64895	2(3)	65779	1(2)	66985	1(2)	67440	1(2)	68326	1(2)	69502	1(2)
64483	1(2)	64719	1(2)	64896	2(3)	65780	1(2)	66986	1(2)	67445	1(2)	68328	1(2)	69505	1(2)
64484	4(3)	64721	1(2)	64897	2(3)	65781	1(2)	66987	2(2)	67450	1(2)	68330	1(3)	69511	1(2)
64486	1(3)	64722	4(3)	64898	2(3)	65782	1(2)	66988	2(2)	67500	1(3)	68335	1(3)	69530	1(2)
64487	1(2)	64726	2(3)	64901	2(3)	65785	1(2)	66990	1(3)	67505	1(3)	68340	1(3)	69535	1(2)
64488	1(3)	64727	2(3)	64902	1(3)	65800	1(2)	66999	1(3)	67515	1(3)	68360	1(3)	69540	1(3)
64489	1(2)	64732	1(2)	64905	1(3)	65810	1(2)	67005	1(2)	67550	1(2)	68362	1(3)	69550	1(3)
64490	1(2)	64734	1(2)	64907	1(3)	65815	1(3)	67010	1(2)	67560	1(2)	68371	1(3)	69552	1(2)
64491	1(2)	64736	1(2)	64910	3(3)	65820	1(2)	67015	1(2)	67570	1(2)	68399	1(3)	69554	1(2)
64492	1(2)	64738	1(2)	64911	2(3)	65850	1(2)	67025	1(2)	67599	1(3)	68400	1(2)	69601	1(2)
64493	1(2)	64740	1(2)	64912	3(3)	65855	1(2)	67027	1(2)	67700	2(3)	68420	1(2)	69602	1(2)
64494	1(2)	64742	1(2)	64913	3(3)	65860	1(2)	67028	1(3)	67710	1(2)	68440	2(3)	69603	1(2)
64495	1(2)	64744	1(2)	64999	1(3)	65865	1(2)	67030	1(2)	67715	1(3)	68500	1(2)	69604	1(2)
64505	1(3)	64746	1(2)	65091	1(2)	65870	1(2)	67031	1(2)	67800	1(2)	68505	1(2)	69610	1(2)
64510	1(3)	64755	1(2)	65093	1(2)	65875	1(2)	67036	1(2)	67801	1(2)	68510	1(2)	69620	1(2)
64517	1(3)	64760	1(2)	65101	1(2)	65880	1(2)	67039	1(2)	67805	1(2)	68520	1(2)	69631	1(2)
64520	1(3)	64763	1(2)	65103	1(2)	65900	1(3)	67040	1(2)	67808	1(2)	68525	1(2)	69632	1(2)
64530	1(3)	64766	1(2)	65105	1(2)	65920	1(2)	67041	1(2)	67810	2(3)	68530	1(2)	69633	1(2)
64553	1(3)	64771	2(3)	65110	1(2)	65930	1(3)	67042	1(2)	67820	1(2)	68540	1(2)	69635	1(3)
64555	2(3)	64772	2(3)	65112	1(2)	66020	1(3)	67043	1(2)	67825	1(2)	68550	1(2)	69636	1(3)
64561	1(3)	64774	2(3)	65114	1(2)	66030	1(3)	67101	1(2)	67830	1(2)	68700	1(2)	69637	1(3)
64566	1(3)	64776	1(2)	65125	1(2)	66130	1(3)	67105	1(2)	67835	1(2)	68705	2(3)	69641	1(2)
64568	1(3)	64778	1(3)	65130	1(2)	66150	1(2)	67107	1(2)	67840	3(3)	68720	1(2)	69642	1(2)
64569	1(3)	64782	2(2)	65135	1(2)	66155	1(2)	67108	1(2)	67850	3(3)	68745	1(2)	69643	1(2)

CPT	MUE	CPT	MUE	CPT	MUE	CPT	MUE	CPT	MUE	CPT	MUE	CPT	MUE	CPT	MUE
69644	1(2)	70355	1(3)	72083	1(3)	73206	2(3)	74248	1(2)	75807	1(2)	76706	1(2)	77049	1(2)
69645	1(2)	70360	2(3)	72084	1(3)	73218	2(3)	74250	1(3)	75809	1(3)	76770	1(3)	77053	2(2)
69646	1(2)	70370	1(3)	72100	2(3)	73219	2(3)	74251	1(3)	75810	1(3)	76775	2(3)	77054	2(2)
69650	1(2)	70371	1(2)	72110	1(3)	73220	2(3)	74261	1(2)	75820	2(3)	76776	2(3)	77061	1(2)
69660	1(2)	70380	2(3)	72114	1(3)	73221	2(3)	74262	1(2)	75822	1(3)	76800	1(3)	77062	1(2)
69661	1(2)	70390	2(3)	72120	1(3)	73222	2(3)	74263	0(3)	75825	1(3)	76801	1(2)	77063	1(2)
69662	1(2)	70450	3(3)	72125	1(3)	73223	2(3)	74270	1(3)	75827	1(3)	76802	2(3)	77065	1(2)
69666	1(2)	70460	1(3)	72126	1(3)	73225	2(3)	74280	1(3)	75831	1(3)	76805	1(2)	77066	1(2)
69667	1(2)	70470	2(3)	72127	1(3)	73501	2(3)	74283	1(3)	75833	1(3)	76810	2(3)	77067	1(2)
69670	1(2)	70480	1(3)	72128	1(3)	73502	2(3)	74290	1(3)	75840	1(3)	76811	1(2)	77071	1(3)
69676	1(2)	70481	1(3)	72129	1(3)	73503	2(3)	74300	1(3)	75842	1(3)	76812	2(3)	77072	1(2)
69700	1(3)	70482	1(3)	72130	1(3)	73521	2(3)	74301	1(3)	75860	2(3)	76813	1(2)	77073	1(2)
69705	1(2)	70486	1(3)	72131	1(3)	73522	2(3)	74328	1(3)	75870	1(3)	76814	2(3)	77074	1(2)
69706	1(2)	70487	1(3)	72132	1(3)	73523	2(3)	74329	1(3)	75872	1(3)	76815	1(2)	77075	1(2)
69710	0(3)	70488	1(3)	72133	1(3)	73525	2(2)	74330	1(3)	75880	1(3)	76816	2(3)	77076	1(2)
69711	1(2)	70490	1(3)	72141	1(3)	73551	2(3)	74340	1(3)	75885	1(3)	76817	1(3)	77077	1(2)
69714	1(2)	70491	1(3)	72142	1(3)	73552	2(3)	74355	1(3)	75887	1(3)	76818	2(3)	77078	1(2)
69715	1(3)	70492	1(3)	72146	1(3)	73560	4(3)	74360	1(3)	75889	1(3)	76819	2(3)	77080	1(2)
69717	1(2)	70496	2(3)	72147	1(3)	73562	3(3)	74363	2(3)	75891	1(3)	76820	3(3)	77081	1(2)
69718	1(2)	70498	2(3)	72148	1(3)	73564	4(3)	74400	1(3)	75893	2(3)	76821	2(3)	77084	1(2)
69720	1(2)	70540	1(3)	72149	1(3)	73565	1(3)	74410	1(3)	75894	2(3)	76825	2(3)	77085	1(2)
69725	1(2)	70542	1(3)	72156	1(3)	73580	2(2)	74415	1(3)	75898	2(3)	76826	2(3)	77086	1(2)
69740	1(2)	70543	1(3)	72157	1(3)	73590	3(3)	74420	2(3)	75901	1(3)	76827	2(3)	77261	1(3)
69745	1(2)	70544	2(3)	72158	1(3)	73592	2(3)	74425	2(3)	75902	2(3)	76828	2(3)	77262	1(3)
69799	1(3)	70545	1(3)	72159	1(3)	73600	2(3)	74430	1(3)	75956	1(2)	76830	1(3)	77263	1(3)
69801	1(3)	70546	1(3)	72170	2(3)	73610	3(3)	74440	1(2)	75957	1(2)	76831	1(3)	77280	2(3)
69805	1(3)	70547	1(3)	72190	1(3)	73615	2(2)	74445	1(2)	75958	2(3)	76856	1(3)	77285	1(3)
69806	1(3)	70548	1(3)	72191	1(3)	73620	2(3)	74450	1(3)	75959	1(2)	76857	1(3)	77290	1(3)
69905	1(2)	70549	1(3)	72192	1(3)	73630	3(3)	74455	1(3)	75970	1(3)	76870	1(2)	77293	1(3)
69910	1(2)	70551	2(3)	72193	1(3)	73650	2(3)	74470	2(2)	75984	2(3)	76872	1(3)	77295	1(3)
69915	1(3)	70552	2(3)	72194	1(3)	73660	2(3)	74485	2(3)	75989	2(3)	76873	1(2)	77299	1(3)
69930	1(2)	70553	2(3)	72195	1(3)	73700	2(3)	74710	1(3)	76000	3(3)	76881	2(3)	77300	10(3)
69949	1(3)	70554	1(3)	72196	1(3)	73701	2(3)	74712	1(3)	76010	2(3)	76882	2(3)	77301	1(3)
69950	1(2)	70555	1(3)	72197	1(3)	73702	2(3)	74713	2(3)	76080	3(3)	76885	1(2)	77306	1(3)
69955	1(2)	70557	1(3)	72198	1(3)	73706	2(3)	74740	1(3)	76098	3(3)	76886	1(2)	77307	1(3)
69960	1(2)	70558	1(3)	72200	2(3)	73718	2(3)	74742	2(2)	76100	2(3)	76932	1(2)	77316	1(3)
69970	1(3)	70559	1(3)	72202	1(3)	73719	2(3)	74775	1(2)	76101	1(3)	76936	1(3)	77317	1(3)
69979	1(3)	71045	4(3)	72220	1(3)	73720	2(3)	75557	1(3)	76102	1(3)	76937	2(3)	77318	1(3)
69990	1(3)	71046	3(3)	72240	1(2)	73721	3(3)	75559	1(3)	76120	1(3)	76940	1(3)	77321	1(2)
70010	1(3)	71047	2(3)	72255	1(2)	73722	2(3)	75561	1(3)	76125	1(3)	76941	3(3)	77331	3(3)
70015	1(3)	71048	1(3)	72265	1(2)	73723	2(3)	75563	1(3)	76140	0(3)	76942	1(3)	77332	4(3)
70030	2(2)	71100	2(3)	72270	1(2)	73725	2(3)	75565	1(3)	76145	1(2)	76945	1(3)	77333	2(3)
70100	2(3)	71101	2(3)	72275	1(3)	74018	3(3)	75571	1(3)	76376	2(3)	76946	1(3)	77334	10(3)
70110	2(3)	71110	1(3)	72285	4(3)	74019	2(3)	75572	1(3)	76377	2(3)	76948	1(2)	77336	1(2)
70120	1(3)	71111	1(3)	72295	5(3)	74021	2(3)	75573	1(3)	76380	2(3)	76965	2(3)	77338	1(3)
70130	1(3)	71120	1(3)	73000	2(3)	74022	2(3)	75574	1(3)	76390	1(3)	76975	1(3)	77370	1(3)
70134	1(3)	71130	1(3)	73010	2(3)	74150	1(3)	75600	1(3)	76391	1(3)	76977	1(2)	77371	1(2)
70140	2(3)	71250	2(3)	73020	2(3)	74160	1(3)	75605	1(3)	76496	1(3)	76978	1(2)	77372	1(2)
70150	1(3)	71260	2(3)	73030	4(3)	74170	1(3)	75625	1(3)	76497	1(3)	76979	3(3)	77373	1(3)
70160	1(3)	71270	1(3)	73040	2(2)	74174	1(3)	75630	1(3)	76498	1(3)	76981	1(3)	77385	2(3)
70170	2(2)	71271	1(2)	73050	1(3)	74175	1(3)	75635	1(3)	76499	1(3)	76982	1(2)	77386	2(3)
70190	1(2)	71275	1(3)	73060	2(3)	74176	2(3)	75705	20(3)	76506	1(2)	76983	2(3)	77387	2(3)
70200	2(3)	71550	1(3)	73070	2(3)	74177	2(3)	75710	2(3)	76510	2(2)	76998	1(3)	77399	1(3)
70210	1(3)	71551	1(3)	73080	2(3)	74178	1(3)	75716	1(3)	76511	2(2)	76999	1(3)	77401	1(2)
70220	1(3)	71552	1(3)	73085	2(2)	74181	1(3)	75726	3(3)	76512	2(2)	77001	2(3)	77402	2(3)
70240	1(2)	71555	1(3)	73090	2(3)	74182	1(3)	75731	1(3)	76513	1(2)	77002	1(3)	77407	2(3)
70250	2(3)	72020	4(3)	73092	2(3)	74183	1(3)	75733	1(3)	76514	1(2)	77003	1(3)	77412	2(3)
70260	1(3)	72040	3(3)	73100	2(3)	74185	1(3)	75736	2(3)	76516	1(2)	77011	1(3)	77417	1(3)
70300	1(3)	72050	1(3)	73110	3(3)	74190	1(3)	75741	1(3)	76519	1(3)	77012	1(3)	77423	1(3)
70310	1(3)	72052	1(3)	73115	2(2)	74210	1(3)	75743	1(3)	76529	2(2)	77013	1(3)	77424	1(2)
70320	1(3)	72070	1(3)	73120	2(3)	74220	1(3)	75746	1(3)	76536	1(3)	77014	2(3)	77425	1(3)
70328	1(3)	72072	1(3)	73130	3(3)	74221	1(3)	75756	1(3)	76604	1(3)	77021	1(3)	77427	1(2)
70330	1(3)	72074	1(3)	73140	3(3)	74230	1(3)	75774	7(3)	76641	2(2)	77022	1(3)	77431	1(2)
70332	2(3)	72080	1(3)	73200	2(3)	74235	1(3)	75801	1(3)	76642	2(2)	77046	1(2)	77432	1(2)
70336	1(3)	72081	1(3)	73201	2(3)	74240	2(3)	75803	1(3)	76700	1(3)	77047	1(2)	77435	1(2)
70350	1(3)	72082	1(3)	73202	2(3)	74246	1(3)	75805	1(2)	76705	2(3)	77048	1(2)	77469	1(2)

CPT	MUE	CPT	MUE	CPT	MUE	CPT	MUE	CPT	MUE	CPT	MUE	CPT	MUE	CPT	MUE
77470	1(2)	78268	1(2)	78725	1(3)	80180	1(3)	80355	1(3)	81112	1(2)	81233	1(3)	81302	1(3)
77499	1(3)	78278	2(3)	78730	1(2)	80181	1(3)	80356	1(3)	81120	1(3)	81234	1(2)	81303	1(3)
77520	2(3)	78282	1(2)	78740	1(2)	80183	1(3)	80357	1(3)	81121	1(3)	81235	1(3)	81304	1(3)
77522	2(3)	78290	1(3)	78761	1(2)	80184	2(3)	80358	1(3)	81161	1(3)	81236	1(3)	81305	1(3)
77523	2(3)	78291	1(3)	78799	1(3)	80185	2(3)	80359	1(3)	81162	1(2)	81237	1(3)	81306	1(2)
77525	2(3)	78299	1(3)	78800	1(2)	80186	2(3)	80360	1(3)	81163	1(2)	81238	1(2)	81307	1(2)
77600	1(3)	78300	1(2)	78801	1(2)	80187	1(3)	80361	2(3)	81164	1(2)	81239	1(2)	81308	1(2)
77605	1(3)	78305	1(2)	78802	1(2)	80188	2(3)	80362	1(3)	81165	1(2)	81240	1(2)	81309	1(2)
77610	1(3)	78306	1(2)	78803	1(2)	80189	1(3)	80363	1(3)	81166	1(2)	81241	1(2)	81310	1(3)
77615	1(3)	78315	1(2)	78804	1(2)	80190	2(3)	80364	1(3)	81167	1(2)	81242	1(3)	81311	1(3)
77620	1(3)	78350	0(3)	78808	1(2)	80192	2(3)	80365	2(3)	81168	1(3)	81243	1(3)	81312	1(2)
77750	1(3)	78351	0(3)	78811	1(2)	80193	1(3)	80366	1(3)	81170	1(2)	81244	1(3)	81313	1(3)
77761	1(3)	78399	1(3)	78812	1(2)	80194	2(3)	80367	1(3)	81171	1(2)	81245	1(3)	81314	1(3)
77762	1(3)	78414	1(2)	78813	1(2)	80195	2(3)	80368	1(3)	81172	1(2)	81246	1(3)	81315	1(3)
77763	1(3)	78428	1(3)	78814	1(2)	80197	2(3)	80369	1(3)	81173	1(2)	81247	1(2)	81316	1(2)
77767	2(3)	78429	1(2)	78815	1(2)	80198	2(3)	80370	1(3)	81174	1(2)	81248	1(2)	81317	1(2)
77768	2(3)	78430	1(2)	78816	1(2)	80199	1(3)	80371	1(3)	81175	1(3)	81249	1(2)	81318	1(3)
77770	2(3)	78431	1(2)	78830	1(2)	80200	2(3)	80372	1(3)	81176	1(3)	81250	1(3)	81319	1(2)
77771	2(3)	78432	1(2)	78831	1(2)	80201	2(3)	80373	1(3)	81177	1(2)	81251	1(3)	81320	1(3)
77772	2(3)	78433	1(2)	78832	1(2)	80202	2(3)	80374	1(3)	81178	1(2)	81252	1(3)	81321	1(3)
77778	1(3)	78434	1(2)	78835	4(3)	80203	1(3)	80375	1(3)	81179	1(2)	81253	1(3)	81322	1(3)
77789	2(3)	78445	1(3)	78999	1(3)	80204	1(3)	80376	1(3)	81180	1(2)	81254	1(3)	81323	1(3)
77790	1(3)	78451	1(2)	79005	1(3)	80210	1(3)	80377	1(3)	81181	1(2)	81255	1(3)	81324	1(3)
77799	1(3)	78452	1(2)	79101	1(3)	80230	1(3)	80400	1(3)	81182	1(2)	81256	1(2)	81325	1(3)
78012	1(3)	78453	1(2)	79200	1(3)	80235	1(3)	80402	1(3)	81183	1(2)	81257	1(2)	81326	1(3)
78013	1(3)	78454	1(2)	79300	1(3)	80280	1(3)	80406	1(3)	81184	1(2)	81258	1(2)	81327	1(2)
78014	1(2)	78456	1(3)	79403	1(3)	80285	1(3)	80408	1(3)	81185	1(2)	81259	1(2)	81328	1(2)
78015	1(3)	78457	1(2)	79440	1(3)	80299	3(3)	80410	1(3)	81186	1(2)	81260	1(3)	81329	1(2)
78016	1(3)	78458	1(2)	79445	1(3)	80305	1(2)	80412	1(3)	81187	1(2)	81261	1(3)	81330	1(3)
78018	1(2)	78459	1(3)	79999	1(3)	80306	1(2)	80414	1(3)	81188	1(2)	81262	1(3)	81331	1(3)
78020	1(3)	78466	1(3)	80047	2(3)	80307	1(2)	80415	1(3)	81189	1(2)	81263	1(3)	81332	1(3)
78070	1(2)	78468	1(3)	80048	2(3)	80320	2(3)	80416	1(3)	81190	1(2)	81264	1(3)	81333	1(2)
78071	1(3)	78469	1(3)	80050	0(3)	80321	1(3)	80417	1(3)	81191	1(3)	81265	1(3)	81334	1(3)
78072	1(3)	78472	1(2)	80051	4(3)	80322	1(3)	80418	1(3)	81192	1(3)	81266	2(3)	81335	1(2)
78075	1(2)	78473	1(2)	80053	1(3)	80323	1(3)	80420	1(2)	81193	1(3)	81267	1(3)	81336	1(2)
78099	1(3)	78481	1(2)	80055	1(3)	80324	1(3)	80422	1(3)	81194	1(3)	81268	4(3)	81337	1(2)
78102	1(2)	78483	1(2)	80061	1(3)	80325	1(3)	80424	1(3)	81200	1(2)	81269	1(2)	81338	1(3)
78103	1(2)	78491	1(3)	80069	1(3)	80326	1(3)	80426	1(3)	81201	1(2)	81270	1(2)	81339	1(2)
78104	1(2)	78492	1(2)	80074	1(2)	80327	1(3)	80428	1(3)	81202	1(3)	81271	1(2)	81340	1(3)
78110	1(2)	78494	1(3)	80076	1(3)	80328	1(3)	80430	1(3)	81203	1(3)	81272	1(3)	81341	1(3)
78111	1(2)	78496	1(3)	80081	1(2)	80329	2(3)	80432	1(3)	81204	1(2)	81273	1(3)	81342	1(3)
78120	1(2)	78499	1(3)	80143	2(3)	80330	1(3)	80434	1(3)	81205	1(3)	81274	1(2)	81343	1(2)
78121	1(2)	78579	1(3)	80145	1(3)	80331	1(3)	80435	1(3)	81206	1(3)	81275	1(3)	81344	1(2)
78122	1(2)	78580	1(3)	80150	2(3)	80332	1(3)	80436	1(3)	81207	1(3)	81276	1(3)	81345	1(3)
78130	1(3)	78582	1(3)	80151	1(3)	80333	1(3)	80438	1(3)	81208	1(3)	81277	1(2)	81346	1(2)
78140	1(3)	78597	1(3)	80155	1(3)	80334	1(3)	80439	1(3)	81209	1(3)	81278	1(2)	81347	1(2)
78185	1(2)	78598	1(3)	80156	2(3)	80335	1(3)	80500	1(3)	81210	1(3)	81279	1(2)	81348	1(2)
78191	1(2)	78599	1(3)	80157	2(3)	80336	1(3)	80502	1(3)	81212	1(2)	81283	1(2)	81350	1(3)
78195	1(2)	78600	1(3)	80158	2(3)	80337	1(3)	81000	2(3)	81215	1(2)	81284	1(2)	81351	1(2)
78199	1(3)	78601	1(3)	80159	2(3)	80338	1(3)	81001	2(3)	81216	1(2)	81285	1(2)	81352	1(2)
78201	1(3)	78605	1(3)	80161	1(3)	80339	2(3)	81002	2(3)	81217	1(2)	81286	1(2)	81353	1(2)
78202	1(3)	78606	1(3)	80162	2(3)	80340	1(3)	81003	2(3)	81218	1(3)	81287	1(3)	81355	1(3)
78215	1(3)	78608	1(3)	80163	1(3)	80341	1(3)	81005	2(3)	81219	1(3)	81288	1(3)	81357	1(2)
78216	1(3)	78609	0(3)	80164	2(3)	80342	1(3)	81007	1(3)	81220	1(3)	81289	1(2)	81360	1(2)
78226	1(3)	78610	1(3)	80165	1(3)	80343	1(3)	81015	2(3)	81221	1(3)	81290	1(3)	81361	1(2)
78227	1(3)	78630	1(3)	80167	1(3)	80344	1(3)	81020	1(3)	81222	1(3)	81291	1(3)	81362	1(2)
78230	1(3)	78635	1(3)	80168	2(3)	80345	2(3)	81025	1(3)	81223	1(2)	81292	1(2)	81363	1(2)
78231	1(3)	78645	1(3)	80169	2(3)	80346	1(3)	81050	2(3)	81224	1(3)	81293	1(3)	81364	1(2)
78232	1(3)	78650	1(3)	80170	2(3)	80347	1(3)	81099	1(3)	81225	1(3)	81294	1(3)	81370	1(2)
78258	1(2)	78660	1(2)	80171	1(3)	80348	1(3)	81105	1(2)	81226	1(3)	81295	1(2)	81371	1(2)
78261	1(2)	78699	1(3)	80173	2(3)	80349	1(3)	81106	1(2)	81227	1(3)	81296	1(3)	81372	1(2)
78262	1(2)	78700	1(3)	80175	1(3)	80350	1(3)	81107	1(2)	81228	1(3)	81297	1(3)	81373	2(2)
78264	1(2)	78701	1(3)	80176	1(3)	80351	1(3)	81108	1(2)	81229	1(3)	81298	1(2)	81374	1(3)
78265	1(2)	78707	1(2)	80177	1(3)	80352	1(3)	81109	1(2)	81230	1(2)	81299	1(3)	81375	1(2)
78266	1(2)	78708	1(3)	80178	2(3)	80353	1(3)	81110	1(2)	81231	1(2)	81300	1(3)	81376	5(3)
78267	1(2)	78709	1(2)	80179	2(3)	80354	1(3)	81111	1(2)	81232	1(2)	81301	1(3)	81377	2(3)

CPT	MUE	CPT	MUE	CPT	MUE	CPT	MUE	CPT	MUE	CPT	MUE	CPT	MUE	CPT	MUE
81378	1(2)	81519	1(2)	82248	2(3)	82633	1(3)	83013	1(3)	83775	1(3)	84160	2(3)	84520	2(3)
81379	1(2)	81520	1(2)	82252	1(3)	82634	1(3)	83014	1(2)	83785	1(3)	84163	1(3)	84525	1(3)
81380	2(2)	81521	1(2)	82261	1(3)	82638	1(3)	83015	1(2)	83789	4(3)	84165	1(2)	84540	2(3)
81381	3(3)	81522	1(2)	82270	1(3)	82642	1(2)	83018	4(3)	83825	2(3)	84166	2(3)	84545	1(3)
81382	6(3)	81525	1(2)	82271	3(3)	82652	1(2)	83020	2(3)	83835	2(3)	84181	3(3)	84550	1(3)
81383	1(3)	81528	1(2)	82272	1(3)	82656	1(3)	83021	2(3)	83857	1(3)	84182	6(3)	84560	2(3)
81400	2(3)	81529	1(2)	82274	1(3)	82657	2(3)	83026	1(3)	83861	2(2)	84202	1(2)	84577	1(3)
81401	3(3)	81535	1(2)	82286	1(3)	82658	2(3)	83030	1(3)	83864	1(2)	84203	1(2)	84578	1(3)
81402	1(3)	81536	11(3)	82300	1(3)	82664	2(3)	83033	1(3)	83872	2(3)	84206	1(2)	84580	1(3)
81403	3(3)	81538	1(2)	82306	1(2)	82668	1(3)	83036	1(2)	83873	1(3)	84207	1(2)	84583	1(3)
81404	3(3)	81539	1(2)	82308	1(3)	82670	1(3)	83037	1(2)	83874	4(3)	84210	1(3)	84585	1(2)
81405	2(3)	81540	1(2)	82310	4(3)	82671	1(3)	83045	1(3)	83876	1(3)	84220	1(3)	84586	1(2)
81406	3(3)	81541	1(2)	82330	4(3)	82672	1(3)	83050	2(3)	83880	1(3)	84228	1(3)	84588	1(3)
81407	1(3)	81542	1(2)	82331	1(3)	82677	1(3)	83051	1(3)	83883	4(3)	84233	1(3)	84590	1(2)
81408	1(3)	81546	2(3)	82340	1(3)	82679	1(3)	83060	1(3)	83885	2(3)	84234	1(3)	84591	1(3)
81410	1(2)	81551	1(2)	82355	2(3)	82681	1(3)	83065	1(2)	83915	1(3)	84235	1(3)	84597	1(3)
81411	1(2)	81552	1(2)	82360	2(3)	82693	2(3)	83068	1(2)	83916	2(3)	84238	3(3)	84600	2(3)
81412	1(2)	81554	1(2)	82365	2(3)	82696	1(3)	83069	1(3)	83918	2(3)	84244	2(3)	84620	1(2)
81413	1(2)	81595	1(2)	82370	2(3)	82705	1(3)	83070	1(2)	83919	1(3)	84252	1(2)	84630	2(3)
81414	1(2)	81596	1(2)	82373	1(3)	82710	1(3)	83080	2(3)	83921	2(3)	84255	2(3)	84681	1(3)
81415	1(2)	81599	1(3)	82374	2(3)	82715	3(3)	83088	1(3)	83930	2(3)	84260	1(3)	84702	2(3)
81416	2(3)	82009	3(3)	82375	4(3)	82725	1(3)	83090	2(3)	83935	2(3)	84270	1(3)	84703	1(3)
81417	1(3)	82010	3(3)	82376	2(3)	82726	1(3)	83150	1(3)	83937	1(3)	84275	1(3)	84704	1(3)
81419	1(2)	82013	1(3)	82378	1(3)	82728	1(3)	83491	1(3)	83945	2(3)	84285	1(3)	84830	1(3)
81420	1(2)	82016	1(3)	82379	1(3)	82731	1(3)	83497	1(3)	83950	1(2)	84295	2(3)	84999	1(3)
81422	1(2)	82017	1(3)	82380	1(3)	82735	1(3)	83498	2(3)	83951	1(2)	84300	2(3)	85002	1(3)
81425	1(2)	82024	4(3)	82382	1(2)	82746	1(2)	83500	1(3)	83970	4(3)	84302	1(3)	85004	2(3)
81426	2(3)	82030	1(3)	82383	1(3)	82747	1(2)	83505	1(3)	83986	2(3)	84305	1(3)	85007	1(3)
81427	1(3)	82040	1(3)	82384	2(3)	82757	1(2)	83516	5(3)	83987	1(3)	84307	1(3)	85008	1(3)
81430	1(2)	82042	2(3)	82387	1(3)	82759	1(3)	83518	1(3)	83992	2(3)	84311	2(3)	85009	1(3)
81431	1(2)	82043	1(3)	82390	1(2)	82760	1(3)	83519	5(3)	83993	1(3)	84315	1(3)	85013	1(3)
81432	1(2)	82044	1(3)	82397	4(3)	82775	1(3)	83520	9(3)	84030	1(2)	84375	1(3)	85014	4(3)
81433	1(2)	82045	1(3)	82415	1(3)	82776	1(2)	83525	4(3)	84035	1(2)	84376	1(3)	85018	4(3)
81434	1(2)	82075	2(3)	82435	2(3)	82777	1(3)	83527	1(3)	84060	1(3)	84377	1(3)	85025	4(3)
81435	1(2)	82077	1(3)	82436	1(3)	82784	6(3)	83528	1(3)	84066	1(3)	84378	2(3)	85027	4(3)
81436	1(2)	82085	1(3)	82438	1(3)	82785	1(3)	83540	2(3)	84075	2(3)	84379	1(3)	85032	2(3)
81437	1(2)	82088	2(3)	82441	1(2)	82787	4(3)	83550	1(3)	84078	1(2)	84392	1(3)	85041	1(3)
81438	1(2)	82103	1(3)	82465	1(3)	82800	2(3)	83570	1(3)	84080	1(3)	84402	1(3)	85044	1(2)
81439	1(2)	82104	1(2)	82480	2(3)	82805	3(3)	83582	1(3)	84081	1(3)	84403	2(3)	85045	1(2)
81440	1(2)	82105	1(3)	82482	1(3)	82810	4(3)	83586	1(3)	84085	1(2)	84410	1(2)	85046	1(2)
81442	1(2)	82106	2(3)	82485	1(3)	82820	1(3)	83593	1(3)	84087	1(3)	84425	1(2)	85048	2(3)
81443	1(2)	82107	1(3)	82495	1(3)	82930	1(3)	83605	2(3)	84100	2(3)	84430	1(3)	85049	2(3)
81445	1(2)	82108	1(3)	82507	1(3)	82938	1(3)	83615	3(3)	84105	1(3)	84431	1(3)	85055	1(3)
81448	1(2)	82120	1(3)	82523	1(3)	82941	1(3)	83625	1(3)	84106	1(2)	84432	1(2)	85060	1(3)
81450	1(2)	82127	1(3)	82525	2(3)	82943	1(3)	83630	1(3)	84110	1(3)	84436	1(2)	85097	2(3)
81455	1(2)	82128	2(3)	82528	1(3)	82945	4(3)	83631	1(3)	84112	1(3)	84437	1(2)	85130	1(3)
81460	1(2)	82131	2(3)	82530	4(3)	82946	1(2)	83632	1(3)	84119	1(2)	84439	1(2)	85170	1(3)
81465	1(2)	82135	1(3)	82533	5(3)	82947	5(3)	83633	1(3)	84120	1(3)	84442	1(2)	85175	1(3)
81470	1(2)	82136	2(3)	82540	1(3)	82950	3(3)	83655	2(3)	84126	1(3)	84443	4(2)	85210	2(3)
81471	1(2)	82139	2(3)	82542	6(3)	82951	1(2)	83661	3(3)	84132	3(3)	84445	1(2)	85220	2(3)
81479	3(3)	82140	2(3)	82550	3(3)	82952	3(3)	83662	4(3)	84133	2(3)	84446	1(2)	85230	2(3)
81490	1(2)	82143	2(3)	82552	3(3)	82955	1(2)	83663	3(3)	84134	1(3)	84449	1(3)	85240	2(3)
81493	1(2)	82150	4(3)	82553	3(3)	82960	1(2)	83664	3(3)	84135	1(3)	84450	1(3)	85244	1(3)
81500	1(2)	82154	1(3)	82554	2(3)	82963	1(3)	83670	1(3)	84138	1(3)	84460	1(3)	85245	2(3)
81503	1(2)	82157	1(3)	82565	2(3)	82965	1(3)	83690	2(3)	84140	1(3)	84466	1(3)	85246	2(3)
81504	1(2)	82160	1(3)	82570	3(3)	82977	1(3)	83695	1(3)	84143	2(3)	84478	1(3)	85247	2(3)
81506	1(2)	82163	1(3)	82575	1(3)	82978	1(3)	83698	1(3)	84144	1(3)	84479	1(2)	85250	2(3)
81507	1(2)	82164	1(3)	82585	1(2)	82979	1(3)	83700	1(2)	84145	1(3)	84480	1(2)	85260	2(3)
81508	1(2)	82172	2(3)	82595	1(3)	82985	1(3)	83701	1(3)	84146	3(3)	84481	1(2)	85270	2(3)
81509	1(2)	82175	2(3)	82600	1(3)	83001	1(3)	83704	1(3)	84150	2(3)	84482	1(2)	85280	2(3)
81510	1(2)	82180	1(2)	82607	1(2)	83002	1(3)	83718	1(3)	84152	1(2)	84484	4(3)	85290	2(3)
81511	1(2)	82190	2(3)	82608	1(2)	83003	5(3)	83719	1(3)	84153	1(2)	84485	1(3)	85291	1(3)
81512	1(2)	82232	2(3)	82610	1(3)	83006	1(2)	83721	1(3)	84154	1(2)	84488	1(3)	85292	1(3)
81513	1(2)	82239	1(3)	82615	1(3)	83009	1(3)	83722	1(2)	84155	1(3)	84490	1(2)	85293	1(3)
81514	1(2)	82240	1(3)	82626	1(3)	83010	1(3)	83727	1(3)	84156	1(3)	84510	1(3)	85300	2(3)
81518	1(2)	82247	2(3)	82627	1(3)	83012	1(2)	83735	4(3)	84157	2(3)	84512	3(3)	85301	1(3)

CPT	MUE	CPT	MUE	CPT	MUE	CPT	MUE	CPT	MUE	CPT	MUE	CPT	MUE	CPT	MUE
85302	1(3)	86038	1(3)	86382	3(3)	86704	1(2)	86880	4(3)	87185	4(3)	87450	2(3)	87582	1(3)
85303	2(3)	86039	1(3)	86384	1(3)	86705	1(2)	86885	3(3)	87186	12(3)	87451	2(3)	87590	1(3)
85305	2(3)	86060	1(3)	86386	1(2)	86706	2(3)	86886	3(3)	87187	3(3)	87471	1(3)	87591	3(3)
85306	2(3)	86063	1(3)	86403	3(3)	86707	1(3)	86890	2(3)	87188	14(3)	87472	1(3)	87592	1(3)
85307	2(3)	86077	1(2)	86406	2(3)	86708	1(2)	86891	2(3)	87190	10(3)	87475	1(3)	87623	1(2)
85335	2(3)	86078	1(3)	86408	1(3)	86709	1(2)	86900	3(3)	87197	1(3)	87476	1(3)	87624	1(3)
85337	1(3)	86079	1(3)	86409	1(3)	86710	4(3)	86901	3(3)	87206	6(3)	87480	1(3)	87625	1(3)
85345	1(3)	86140	1(2)	86413	3(3)	86711	2(3)	86902	40(3)	87207	3(3)	87481	6(3)	87631	1(3)
85347	9(3)	86141	1(2)	86430	2(3)	86713	3(3)	86905	28(3)	87209	4(3)	87482	1(3)	87632	1(3)
85348	4(3)	86146	3(3)	86431	2(3)	86717	8(3)	86906	1(2)	87210	4(3)	87483	1(2)	87633	1(3)
85360	1(3)	86147	4(3)	86480	1(3)	86720	2(3)	86910	0(3)	87220	3(3)	87485	1(3)	87634	1(3)
85362	2(3)	86148	3(3)	86481	1(3)	86723	2(3)	86911	0(3)	87230	2(3)	87486	1(3)	87635	2(3)
85366	1(3)	86152	1(3)	86485	1(2)	86727	2(3)	86920	19(3)	87250	1(3)	87487	1(3)	87636	3(3)
85370	1(3)	86153	1(3)	86486	2(3)	86732	2(3)	86922	10(3)	87252	4(3)	87490	1(3)	87637	3(3)
85378	2(3)	86155	1(3)	86490	1(2)	86735	2(3)	86923	10(3)	87253	3(3)	87491	3(3)	87640	1(3)
85379	2(3)	86156	1(2)	86510	1(2)	86738	2(3)	86930	3(3)	87254	10(3)	87492	1(3)	87641	1(3)
85380	2(3)	86157	1(2)	86580	1(2)	86741	2(3)	86931	4(3)	87255	2(3)	87493	2(3)	87650	1(3)
85384	2(3)	86160	4(3)	86590	1(3)	86744	2(3)	86940	3(3)	87260	1(3)	87495	1(3)	87651	1(3)
85385	1(3)	86161	2(3)	86592	2(3)	86747	2(3)	86941	3(3)	87265	1(3)	87496	1(3)	87652	1(3)
85390	3(3)	86162	1(2)	86593	2(3)	86750	4(3)	86945	5(3)	87267	1(3)	87497	2(3)	87653	1(3)
85396	1(2)	86171	2(3)	86602	3(3)	86753	3(3)	86950	1(3)	87269	1(3)	87498	1(3)	87660	1(3)
85397	2(3)	86200	1(3)	86603	2(3)	86756	2(3)	86960	3(3)	87270	1(3)	87500	1(3)	87661	1(3)
85400	1(3)	86215	1(3)	86609	14(3)	86757	6(3)	86965	4(3)	87271	1(3)	87501	1(3)	87662	2(3)
85410	1(3)	86225	1(3)	86611	4(3)	86759	2(3)	86971	6(3)	87272	1(3)	87502	1(3)	87797	3(3)
85415	2(3)	86226	1(3)	86612	2(3)	86762	2(3)	86972	2(3)	87273	1(3)	87503	1(3)	87798	21(3)
85420	2(3)	86235	10(3)	86615	6(3)	86765	2(3)	86975	2(3)	87274	1(3)	87505	1(2)	87799	3(3)
85421	1(3)	86255	5(3)	86617	2(3)	86768	5(3)	86976	2(3)	87275	1(3)	87506	1(2)	87800	2(3)
85441	1(2)	86256	9(3)	86618	2(3)	86769	3(3)	86977	2(3)	87276	1(3)	87507	1(2)	87801	3(3)
85445	1(2)	86277	1(3)	86619	2(3)	86771	2(3)	86999	1(3)	87278	1(3)	87510	1(3)	87802	2(3)
85460	1(3)	86280	1(3)	86622	2(3)	86774	2(3)	87003	1(3)	87279	1(3)	87511	1(3)	87803	3(3)
85461	1(2)	86294	1(3)	86625	1(3)	86777	2(3)	87015	3(3)	87280	1(3)	87512	1(3)	87804	3(3)
85475	1(3)	86300	2(3)	86628	3(3)	86778	2(3)	87040	4(3)	87281	1(3)	87516	1(3)	87806	1(2)
85520	3(3)	86301	1(2)	86631	6(3)	86780	2(3)	87045	3(3)	87283	1(3)	87517	1(3)	87807	2(3)
85525	2(3)	86304	1(2)	86632	3(3)	86784	1(3)	87046	6(3)	87285	1(3)	87520	1(3)	87808	1(3)
85530	1(3)	86305	1(2)	86635	4(3)	86787	2(3)	87071	2(3)	87290	1(3)	87521	1(3)	87809	2(3)
85536	1(2)	86308	1(2)	86638	6(3)	86788	2(3)	87073	2(3)	87299	1(3)	87522	1(3)	87810	2(3)
85540	1(2)	86309	1(2)	86641	2(3)	86789	2(3)	87075	6(3)	87300	2(3)	87525	1(3)	87811	3(3)
85547	1(2)	86310	1(2)	86644	2(3)	86790	4(3)	87076	4(3)	87301	1(3)	87526	1(3)	87850	1(3)
85549	1(3)	86316	2(3)	86645	1(3)	86793	2(3)	87077	6(3)	87305	1(3)	87527	1(3)	87880	2(3)
85555	1(2)	86317	6(3)	86648	2(3)	86794	1(3)	87081	4(3)	87320	1(3)	87528	1(3)	87899	6(3)
85557	1(2)	86318	2(3)	86651	2(3)	86800	1(3)	87084	1(3)	87324	2(3)	87529	2(3)	87900	1(2)
85576	7(3)	86320	1(2)	86652	2(3)	86803	1(3)	87086	3(3)	87327	1(3)	87530	2(3)	87901	1(2)
85597	1(3)	86325	2(3)	86653	2(3)	86804	1(2)	87088	3(3)	87328	2(3)	87531	1(3)	87902	1(2)
85598	1(3)	86327	1(3)	86654	2(3)	86805	12(3)	87101	3(3)	87329	2(3)	87532	1(3)	87903	1(2)
85610	4(3)	86328	3(3)	86658	12(3)	86806	2(3)	87102	4(3)	87332	1(3)	87533	1(3)	87904	14(3)
85611	2(3)	86329	3(3)	86663	2(3)	86807	2(3)	87103	2(3)	87335	1(3)	87534	1(3)	87905	2(3)
85612	1(3)	86331	12(3)	86664	2(3)	86808	1(3)	87106	4(3)	87336	1(3)	87535	1(3)	87906	2(3)
85613	3(3)	86332	1(3)	86665	2(3)	86812	1(2)	87107	4(3)	87337	1(3)	87536	1(3)	87910	1(3)
85635	1(3)	86334	2(2)	86666	4(3)	86813	1(2)	87109	2(3)	87338	1(3)	87537	1(3)	87912	1(3)
85651	1(2)	86335	2(3)	86668	2(3)	86816	1(2)	87110	2(3)	87339	1(3)	87538	1(3)	87999	1(3)
85652	1(2)	86336	1(3)	86671	3(3)	86817	1(2)	87118	3(3)	87340	1(2)	87539	1(3)	88000	0(3)
85660	2(3)	86337	1(2)	86674	3(3)	86821	1(3)	87140	3(3)	87341	1(2)	87540	1(3)	88005	0(3)
85670	2(3)	86340	1(2)	86677	3(3)	86825	1(3)	87143	2(3)	87350	1(2)	87541	1(3)	88007	0(3)
85675	1(3)	86341	4(3)	86682	2(3)	86826	8(3)	87149	11(3)	87380	1(2)	87542	1(3)	88012	0(3)
85705	1(3)	86343	1(3)	86684	2(3)	86828	2(3)	87150	12(3)	87385	2(3)	87550	1(3)	88014	0(3)
85730	4(3)	86344	1(2)	86687	1(3)	86829	2(3)	87152	1(3)	87389	1(3)	87551	2(3)	88016	0(3)
85732	4(3)	86352	1(3)	86688	1(3)	86830	2(3)	87153	3(3)	87390	1(3)	87552	1(3)	88020	0(3)
85810	2(3)	86353	7(3)	86689	2(3)	86831	2(3)	87164	2(3)	87391	1(3)	87555	1(3)	88025	0(3)
85999	1(3)	86355	1(2)	86692	2(3)	86832	2(3)	87166	2(3)	87400	2(3)	87556	1(3)	88027	0(3)
86000	6(3)	86356	7(3)	86694	2(3)	86833	1(3)	87168	2(3)	87420	1(3)	87557	1(3)	88028	0(3)
86001	20(3)	86357	1(2)	86695	2(3)	86834	1(3)	87169	2(3)	87425	1(3)	87560	1(3)	88029	0(3)
86005	6(3)	86359	1(2)	86696	2(3)	86835	1(3)	87172	1(3)	87426	3(3)	87561	1(3)	88036	0(3)
86008	20(3)	86360	1(2)	86698	3(3)	86849	1(3)	87176	3(3)	87427	2(3)	87562	1(3)	88037	0(3)
86021	1(2)	86361	1(2)	86701	1(3)	86850	3(3)	87177	3(3)	87428	3(3)	87563	3(3)	88040	0(3)
86022	1(2)	86367	2(3)	86702	2(3)	86860	2(3)	87181	12(3)	87430	1(3)	87580	1(3)	88045	0(3)
86023	3(3)	86376	2(3)	86703	1(2)	86870	6(3)	87184	8(3)	87449	3(3)	87581	1(3)	88099	0(3)

CPT	MUE	CPT	MUE	CPT	MUE	CPT	MUE	CPT	MUE	CPT	MUE	CPT	MUE	CPT	MUE
88104	5(3)	88304	5(3)	89254	1(3)	90620	1(2)	90746	1(2)	90997	1(3)	92284	1(2)	92561	1(2)
88106	5(3)	88305	16(3)	89255	1(3)	90621	1(2)	90747	1(2)	90999	1(3)	92285	1(2)	92562	1(2)
88108	6(3)	88307	8(3)	89257	1(3)	90625	1(2)	90748	0(3)	91010	1(2)	92286	1(2)	92563	1(2)
88112	6(3)	88309	3(3)	89258	1(2)	90630	1(2)	90749	1(3)	91013	1(3)	92287	1(2)	92564	1(2)
88120	2(3)	88311	4(3)	89259	1(2)	90632	1(2)	90750	1(2)	91020	1(2)	92310	0(3)	92565	1(2)
88121	2(3)	88312	9(3)	89260	1(2)	90633	1(2)	90756	1(2)	91022	1(2)	92311	1(2)	92567	1(2)
88125	1(3)	88313	8(3)	89261	1(2)	90634	1(2)	90785	3(3)	91030	1(2)	92312	1(2)	92568	1(2)
88130	1(2)	88314	6(3)	89264	1(3)	90636	1(2)	90791	1(3)	91034	1(2)	92313	1(3)	92570	1(2)
88140	1(2)	88319	11(3)	89268	1(2)	90644	1(2)	90792	2(3)	91035	1(2)	92314	0(3)	92571	1(2)
88141	1(3)	88321	1(2)	89272	1(2)	90647	1(2)	90832	3(3)	91037	1(2)	92315	1(2)	92572	1(2)
88142	1(3)	88323	1(2)	89280	1(2)	90648	1(2)	90833	3(3)	91038	1(2)	92316	1(2)	92575	1(2)
88143	1(3)	88325	1(2)	89281	1(2)	90649	1(2)	90834	3(3)	91040	1(2)	92317	1(3)	92576	1(2)
88147	1(3)	88329	2(3)	89290	1(2)	90650	1(2)	90836	3(3)	91065	2(2)	92325	1(3)	92577	1(2)
88148	1(3)	88331	11(3)	89291	1(2)	90651	1(2)	90837	3(3)	91110	1(2)	92326	2(2)	92579	1(2)
88150	1(3)	88332	13(3)	89300	1(2)	90653	1(2)	90838	3(3)	91111	1(2)	92340	0(3)	92582	1(2)
88152	1(3)	88333	4(3)	89310	1(2)	90654	1(2)	90839	1(2)	91112	1(3)	92341	0(3)	92583	1(2)
88153	1(3)	88334	5(3)	89320	1(2)	90655	1(2)	90840	4(3)	91117	1(2)	92342	0(3)	92584	1(2)
88155	1(3)	88341	13(3)	89321	1(2)	90656	1(2)	90845	1(2)	91120	1(2)	92352	1(3)	92587	1(2)
88160	4(3)	88342	4(3)	89322	1(2)	90657	1(2)	90846	2(3)	91122	1(2)	92353	1(3)	92588	1(2)
88161	4(3)	88344	6(3)	89325	1(2)	90658	1(2)	90847	2(3)	91132	1(2)	92354	1(3)	92590	0(3)
88162	3(3)	88346	2(3)	89329	1(2)	90660	1(2)	90849	2(3)	91133	1(3)	92355	1(3)	92591	0(3)
88164	1(3)	88348	1(3)	89330	1(2)	90661	1(2)	90853	4(3)	91200	1(2)	92358	1(3)	92592	0(3)
88165	1(3)	88350	9(3)	89331	1(2)	90662	1(2)	90863	1(3)	91299	1(3)	92370	0(3)	92593	0(3)
88166	1(3)	88355	1(3)	89335	1(3)	90664	1(2)	90865	1(3)	91300	1(2)	92371	1(3)	92594	0(3)
88167	1(3)	88356	3(3)	89337	1(2)	90666	1(2)	90867	1(2)	91301	1(2)	92499	1(3)	92595	0(3)
88172	7(3)	88358	2(3)	89342	1(2)	90667	1(2)	90868	1(3)	91302	1(2)	92502	1(3)	92596	1(2)
88173	7(3)	88360	6(3)	89343	1(2)	90668	1(2)	90869	1(3)	91303	1(2)	92504	1(3)	92597	1(3)
88174	1(3)	88361	6(3)	89344	1(2)	90670	1(2)	90870	2(3)	91304	1(2)	92507	1(3)	92601	1(3)
88175	1(3)	88362	1(3)	89346	1(2)	90672	1(2)	90875	1(3)	92002	1(2)	92508	1(3)	92602	1(3)
88177	6(3)	88363	2(3)	89352	1(2)	90673	1(2)	90876	0(3)	92004	1(2)	92511	1(3)	92603	1(3)
88182	2(3)	88364	3(3)	89353	1(3)	90674	1(2)	90880	1(3)	92012	1(3)	92512	1(2)	92604	1(3)
88184	2(3)	88365	4(3)	89354	1(3)	90675	1(2)	90882	0(3)	92014	1(3)	92516	1(3)	92605	1(2)
88185	35(3)	88366	2(3)	89356	2(3)	90676	1(2)	90885	1(3)	92015	0(3)	92517	1(2)	92606	1(2)
88187	2(3)	88367	3(3)	89398	1(3)	90680	1(2)	90887	1(3)	92018	1(2)	92518	1(2)	92607	1(3)
88188	2(3)	88368	3(3)	90281	0(3)	90681	1(2)	90889	1(3)	92019	1(2)	92519	1(2)	92608	4(3)
88189	2(3)	88369	3(3)	90283	0(3)	90682	1(2)	90899	1(3)	92020	1(2)	92520	1(2)	92609	1(3)
88199	1(3)	88371	1(3)	90284	0(3)	90685	1(2)	90901	1(3)	92025	1(2)	92521	1(2)	92610	1(2)
88230	2(3)	88372	1(3)	90287	0(3)	90686	1(2)	90912	1(2)	92060	1(2)	92522	1(2)	92611	1(3)
88233	2(3)	88373	3(3)	90288	0(3)	90687	1(2)	90913	3(3)	92065	1(2)	92523	1(2)	92612	1(3)
88235	2(3)	88374	5(3)	90291	0(3)	90688	1(2)	90935	1(3)	92071	2(2)	92524	1(2)	92613	1(2)
88237	4(3)	88375	1(3)	90296	1(2)	90689	1(2)	90937	1(3)	92072	1(2)	92526	1(2)	92614	1(3)
88239	3(3)	88377	5(3)	90371	10(3)	90690	1(2)	90940	1(3)	92081	1(2)	92531	1(3)	92615	1(2)
88240	3(3)	88380	1(3)	90375	20(3)	90691	1(2)	90945	1(3)	92082	1(2)	92532	1(3)	92616	1(3)
88241	3(3)	88381	1(3)	90376	20(3)	90694	1(2)	90947	1(3)	92083	1(2)	92533	4(2)	92617	1(2)
88245	1(2)	88387	2(3)	90377	20(3)	90696	1(2)	90951	1(2)	92100	1(2)	92534	1(3)	92618	1(3)
88248	1(2)	88388	1(3)	90378	4(3)	90697	1(2)	90952	1(2)	92132	1(2)	92537	1(2)	92620	1(2)
88249	1(2)	88399	1(3)	90384	0(3)	90698	1(2)	90953	1(2)	92133	1(2)	92538	1(2)	92621	4(3)
88261	2(3)	88720	1(3)	90385	1(2)	90700	1(2)	90954	1(2)	92134	1(2)	92540	1(3)	92625	1(2)
88262	2(3)	88738	1(3)	90386	0(3)	90702	1(2)	90955	1(2)	92136	1(3)	92541	1(3)	92626	1(2)
88263	1(3)	88740	1(2)	90389	0(3)	90707	1(2)	90956	1(2)	92145	1(2)	92542	1(3)	92627	6(3)
88264	1(3)	88741	1(2)	90393	1(2)	90710	1(2)	90957	1(2)	92201	1(2)	92544	1(3)	92630	0(3)
88267	2(3)	88749	1(3)	90396	1(2)	90713	1(2)	90958	1(2)	92202	1(2)	92545	1(3)	92633	0(3)
88269	2(3)	89049	1(3)	90399	0(3)	90714	1(2)	90959	1(2)	92227	1(2)	92546	1(3)	92640	1(3)
88271	16(3)	89050	2(3)	90460	9(3)	90715	1(2)	90960	1(2)	92228	1(2)	92547	1(3)	92650	1(2)
88272	12(3)	89051	2(3)	90461	8(3)	90716	1(2)	90961	1(2)	92229	1(2)	92548	1(3)	92651	1(2)
88273	3(3)	89055	2(3)	90471	1(2)	90717	1(2)	90962	1(2)	92230	2(2)	92549	1(3)	92652	1(2)
88274	5(3)	89060	2(3)	90472	8(3)	90723	0(3)	90963	1(2)	92235	1(2)	92550	1(2)	92653	1(2)
88275	12(3)	89125	2(3)	90473	1(2)	90732	1(2)	90964	1(2)	92240	1(2)	92551	0(3)	92700	1(3)
88280	1(3)	89160	1(3)	90474	1(3)	90733	1(2)	90965	1(2)	92242	1(2)	92552	1(2)	92920	3(3)
88283	5(3)	89190	1(3)	90476	1(2)	90734	1(2)	90966	1(2)	92250	1(2)	92553	1(2)	92921	6(2)
88285	10(3)	89220	2(3)	90477	1(2)	90736	1(2)	90967	1(2)	92260	1(2)	92555	1(2)	92924	2(3)
88289	1(3)	89230	1(2)	90581	1(2)	90738	1(2)	90968	1(2)	92265	1(2)	92556	1(2)	92925	6(2)
88291	0(3)	89240	1(3)	90585	1(2)	90739	1(2)	90969	1(2)	92270	1(2)	92557	1(2)	92928	3(3)
88299	1(3)	89250	1(2)	90586	1(2)	90740	1(2)	90970	1(2)	92273	1(2)	92558	0(3)	92929	2(3)
88300	4(3)	89251	1(2)	90587	1(2)	90743	1(2)	90989	1(2)	92274	1(2)	92559	0(3)	92933	2(3)
88302	4(3)	89253	1(3)	90619	1(2)	90744	1(2)	90993	1(3)	92283	1(2)	92560	0(3)	92934	2(3)

CPT	MUE	CPT	MUE	CPT	MUE	CPT	MUE	CPT	MUE	CPT	MUE	CPT	MUE	CPT	MUE
92937	2(3)	93288	1(3)	93591	1(2)	93976	1(3)	95027	90(3)	95812	1(3)	95976	1(3)	96409	1(3)
92938	2(3)	93289	1(3)	93592	2(3)	93978	1(3)	95028	30(3)	95813	1(3)	95977	1(3)	96411	3(3)
92941	1(3)	93290	1(3)	93600	1(3)	93979	1(3)	95044	80(3)	95816	1(3)	95980	1(3)	96413	1(3)
92943	2(3)	93291	1(3)	93602	1(3)	93980	1(3)	95052	20(3)	95819	1(3)	95981	1(3)	96415	8(3)
92944	2(3)	93292	1(3)	93603	1(3)	93981	1(3)	95056	1(2)	95822	1(3)	95982	1(3)	96416	1(3)
92950	2(3)	93293	1(2)	93609	1(3)	93985	1(3)	95060	1(2)	95824	1(3)	95983	1(2)	96417	3(3)
92953	2(3)	93294	1(2)	93610	1(3)	93986	1(3)	95065	1(3)	95829	1(3)	95984	11(3)	96420	2(3)
92960	2(3)	93295	1(2)	93612	1(3)	93990	2(3)	95070	1(3)	95830	1(3)	95990	1(3)	96422	2(3)
92961	1(3)	93296	1(2)	93613	1(3)	93998	1(3)	95076	1(2)	95836	1(2)	95991	1(3)	96423	2(3)
92970	1(3)	93297	1(2)	93615	1(3)	94002	1(2)	95079	2(3)	95851	3(3)	95992	1(2)	96425	1(3)
92971	1(3)	93298	1(2)	93616	1(3)	94003	1(2)	95115	1(2)	95852	1(3)	95999	1(3)	96440	1(3)
92973	2(3)	93303	1(3)	93618	1(3)	94004	1(2)	95117	1(2)	95857	1(2)	96000	1(2)	96446	1(3)
92974	1(3)	93304	1(3)	93619	1(3)	94005	1(3)	95120	0(3)	95860	1(3)	96001	1(2)	96450	1(3)
92975	1(3)	93306	1(3)	93620	1(3)	94010	1(3)	95125	0(3)	95861	1(3)	96002	1(3)	96521	2(3)
92977	1(3)	93307	1(3)	93621	1(3)	94011	1(3)	95130	0(3)	95863	1(3)	96003	1(3)	96522	1(3)
92978	1(3)	93308	1(3)	93622	1(3)	94012	1(3)	95131	0(3)	95864	1(3)	96004	1(2)	96523	2(3)
92979	2(3)	93312	1(3)	93623	1(3)	94013	1(3)	95132	0(3)	95865	1(3)	96020	1(2)	96542	1(3)
92986	1(2)	93313	1(3)	93624	1(3)	94014	1(2)	95133	0(3)	95866	1(3)	96040	4(3)	96549	1(3)
92987	1(2)	93314	1(3)	93631	1(3)	94015	1(2)	95134	0(3)	95867	1(3)	96105	3(3)	96567	1(3)
92990	1(2)	93315	1(3)	93640	1(3)	94016	1(2)	95144	30(3)	95868	1(3)	96110	3(3)	96570	1(2)
92997	1(2)	93316	1(3)	93641	1(2)	94060	1(3)	95145	10(3)	95869	1(3)	96112	1(2)	96571	2(3)
92998	2(3)	93317	1(3)	93642	1(3)	94070	1(2)	95146	10(3)	95870	4(3)	96113	6(3)	96573	1(2)
93000	3(3)	93318	1(3)	93644	1(3)	94150	2(3)	95147	10(3)	95872	4(3)	96116	1(2)	96574	1(2)
93005	5(3)	93320	2(3)	93650	1(3)	94200	1(3)	95148	10(3)	95873	1(2)	96121	3(3)	96900	1(3)
93010	5(3)	93321	1(3)	93653	1(3)	94375	1(3)	95149	10(3)	95874	1(2)	96125	1(2)	96902	1(3)
93015	1(3)	93325	2(3)	93654	1(3)	94450	1(3)	95165	30(3)	95875	2(3)	96127	2(3)	96904	1(2)
93016	1(3)	93350	1(2)	93655	2(3)	94452	1(2)	95170	10(3)	95885	4(2)	96130	1(2)	96910	1(3)
93017	1(3)	93351	1(2)	93656	1(3)	94453	1(2)	95180	8(3)	95886	4(2)	96131	7(3)	96912	1(3)
93018	1(3)	93352	1(3)	93657	2(3)	94610	2(3)	95199	1(3)	95887	1(2)	96132	1(2)	96913	1(3)
93024	1(3)	93355	1(3)	93660	1(3)	94617	1(3)	95249	1(2)	95905	2(3)	96133	7(3)	96920	1(2)
93025	1(2)	93356	1(3)	93662	1(3)	94618	1(3)	95250	1(2)	95907	1(2)	96136	1(2)	96921	1(2)
93040	3(3)	93451	1(3)	93668	1(3)	94619	1(3)	95251	1(2)	95908	1(2)	96137	11(3)	96922	1(2)
93041	3(3)	93452	1(3)	93701	1(2)	94621	1(3)	95700	1(2)	95909	1(2)	96138	1(2)	96931	1(2)
93042	3(3)	93453	1(3)	93702	1(2)	94640	1(3)	95705	1(2)	95910	1(2)	96139	11(3)	96932	1(2)
93050	1(3)	93454	1(3)	93724	1(3)	94642	1(3)	95706	1(2)	95911	1(2)	96146	1(2)	96933	1(2)
93224	1(2)	93455	1(3)	93740	1(3)	94644	1(2)	95707	1(2)	95912	1(2)	96156	1(3)	96934	2(3)
93225	1(2)	93456	1(3)	93745	1(2)	94645	4(3)	95708	4(3)	95913	1(2)	96158	1(2)	96935	2(3)
93226	1(2)	93457	1(3)	93750	1(3)	94660	1(2)	95709	4(3)	95921	1(3)	96159	4(3)	96936	2(3)
93227	1(2)	93458	1(3)	93770	1(3)	94662	1(2)	95710	4(3)	95922	1(3)	96160	3(3)	96999	1(3)
93228	1(2)	93459	1(3)	93784	1(3)	94664	1(2)	95711	1(2)	95923	1(3)	96161	1(2)	97010	1(3)
93229	1(2)	93460	1(3)	93786	1(2)	94667	1(2)	95712	1(2)	95924	1(3)	96165	6(3)	97012	1(3)
93241	1(2)	93461	1(3)	93788	1(2)	94668	5(3)	95713	1(2)	95925	1(3)	96167	1(2)	97014	0(3)
93242	1(2)	93462	1(3)	93790	1(2)	94669	4(3)	95714	4(3)	95926	1(3)	96168	6(3)	97016	1(3)
93243	1(2)	93463	1(3)	93792	1(2)	94680	1(3)	95715	4(3)	95927	1(3)	96170	1(3)	97018	1(3)
93244	1(2)	93464	1(3)	93793	1(2)	94681	1(3)	95716	4(3)	95928	1(3)	96171	2(3)	97022	1(3)
93245	1(2)	93503	2(3)	93797	2(2)	94690	1(3)	95717	1(2)	95929	1(3)	96360	2(3)	97024	1(3)
93246	1(2)	93505	1(2)	93798	2(2)	94726	1(3)	95718	1(2)	95930	1(3)	96361	24(3)	97026	1(3)
93247	1(2)	93530	1(3)	93799	1(3)	94727	1(3)	95719	1(2)	95933	1(3)	96365	2(3)	97028	1(3)
93248	1(2)	93531	1(3)	93880	1(3)	94728	1(3)	95720	1(2)	95937	4(3)	96366	24(3)	97032	4(3)
93260	1(2)	93532	1(3)	93882	1(3)	94729	1(3)	95721	1(2)	95938	1(3)	96367	4(3)	97033	4(3)
93261	1(3)	93533	1(3)	93886	1(3)	94760	1(3)	95722	1(2)	95939	1(3)	96368	1(2)	97034	2(3)
93264	1(2)	93561	1(3)	93888	1(3)	94761	1(2)	95723	1(2)	95940	20(3)	96369	1(2)	97035	2(3)
93268	1(2)	93562	1(3)	93890	1(3)	94762	1(2)	95724	1(2)	95941	8(3)	96370	3(3)	97036	3(3)
93270	1(2)	93563	1(3)	93892	1(3)	94772	1(2)	95725	1(2)	95943	1(3)	96371	1(3)	97039	1(3)
93271	1(2)	93564	1(3)	93893	1(3)	94774	1(2)	95726	1(2)	95954	1(3)	96372	5(3)	97110	8(3)
93272	1(2)	93565	1(3)	93895	1(3)	94775	1(2)	95782	1(2)	95955	1(3)	96373	3(3)	97112	6(3)
93278	1(3)	93566	1(3)	93922	2(2)	94776	1(2)	95783	1(2)	95957	1(3)	96374	1(3)	97113	6(3)
93279	1(3)	93567	1(3)	93923	2(2)	94777	1(2)	95800	1(2)	95958	1(3)	96375	6(3)	97116	4(3)
93280	1(3)	93568	1(3)	93924	1(2)	94780	1(2)	95801	1(2)	95961	1(2)	96376	10(3)	97124	4(3)
93281	1(3)	93571	1(3)	93925	1(3)	94781	2(3)	95803	1(2)	95962	3(3)	96377	1(3)	97129	1(2)
93282	1(3)	93572	2(3)	93926	1(3)	94799	1(3)	95805	1(2)	95965	1(3)	96379	2(3)	97130	7(3)
93283	1(3)	93580	1(3)	93930	1(3)	95004	80(3)	95806	1(2)	95966	1(3)	96401	4(3)	97139	1(3)
93284	1(3)	93581	1(3)	93931	1(3)	95012	2(3)	95807	1(2)	95967	3(3)	96402	2(3)	97140	6(3)
93285	1(3)	93582	1(2)	93970	1(3)	95017	27(3)	95808	1(2)	95970	1(3)	96405	1(2)	97150	2(3)
93286	2(3)	93583	1(2)	93971	1(3)	95018	19(3)	95810	1(2)	95971	1(3)	96406	1(2)	97151	8(3)
93287	2(3)	93590	1(2)	93975	1(3)	95024	40(3)	95811	1(2)	95972	1(3)			97152	16(3)

CPT	MUE	CPT	MUE	CPT	MUE	CPT	MUE	CPT	MUE	CPT	MUE	CPT	MUE	CPT	MUE
97153	32(3)	99002	1(3)	99238	0(3)	99381	0(3)	99479	1(2)	A0429	2(3)	A4286	0(3)	A4392	2(3)
97154	18(3)	99024	1(3)	99239	0(3)	99382	0(3)	99480	1(2)	A0430	1(3)	A4290	2(3)	A4393	1(3)
97155	24(3)	99026	0(3)	99241	0(3)	99383	0(3)	99483	1(2)	A0431	1(3)	A4300	4(3)	A4394	1(3)
97156	16(3)	99027	0(3)	99242	0(3)	99384	0(3)	99484	1(2)	A0432	1(3)	A4301	1(2)	A4395	3(3)
97157	16(3)	99050	1(3)	99243	0(3)	99385	0(3)	99485	1(3)	A0433	1(3)	A4305	2(3)	A4396	2(3)
97158	16(3)	99051	1(3)	99244	0(3)	99386	0(3)	99486	4(1)	A0434	2(3)	A4306	2(3)	A4397	1(3)
97161	1(2)	99053	1(3)	99245	0(3)	99387	0(3)	99487	1(2)	A0435	999(3)	A4310	2(3)	A4398	2(3)
97162	1(2)	99056	1(3)	99251	0(3)	99391	0(3)	99489	4(3)	A0436	300(3)	A4311	2(3)	A4399	1(3)
97163	1(2)	99058	1(3)	99252	0(3)	99392	0(3)	99490	1(2)	A0888	0(3)	A4312	1(3)	A4400	1(3)
97164	1(2)	99060	1(3)	99253	0(3)	99393	0(3)	99491	1(2)	A0998	0(3)	A4313	1(3)	A4402	1(3)
97165	1(2)	99070	1(3)	99254	0(3)	99394	0(3)	99492	1(2)	A0999	1(3)	A4314	2(3)	A4404	1(3)
97166	1(2)	99071	1(3)	99255	0(3)	99395	0(3)	99493	1(2)	A4206	1(3)	A4315	2(3)	A4405	1(3)
97167	1(2)	99075	0(3)	99281	2(3)	99396	0(3)	99494	2(3)	A4207	1(3)	A4316	1(3)	A4406	1(3)
97168	1(2)	99078	3(3)	99282	2(3)	99397	0(3)	99495	1(2)	A4208	4(3)	A4320	2(3)	A4407	2(3)
97169	0(3)	99080	1(3)	99283	2(3)	99401	0(3)	99496	1(2)	A4209	6(3)	A4321	1(3)	A4408	1(3)
97170	0(3)	99082	1(3)	99284	2(3)	99402	0(3)	99497	1(2)	A4210	0(3)	A4322	2(3)	A4409	1(3)
97171	0(3)	99091	1(2)	99285	2(3)	99403	0(3)	99498	3(3)	A4211	1(3)	A4326	1(3)	A4410	2(3)
97172	0(3)	99100	1(3)	99288	1(3)	99404	0(3)	99499	1(3)	A4212	2(3)	A4327	2(3)	A4411	1(3)
97530	6(3)	99116	1(3)	99291	1(2)	99406	1(2)	99500	0(3)	A4213	5(3)	A4328	1(3)	A4412	1(3)
97533	4(3)	99135	1(3)	99292	8(3)	99407	1(2)	99501	0(3)	A4215	9(3)	A4330	1(3)	A4413	2(3)
97535	8(3)	99140	2(3)	99304	1(2)	99408	0(3)	99502	0(3)	A4216	25(3)	A4331	3(3)	A4414	1(3)
97537	8(3)	99151	1(3)	99305	1(2)	99409	0(3)	99503	0(3)	A4217	4(3)	A4332	2(3)	A4415	1(3)
97542	8(3)	99152	2(3)	99306	1(2)	99411	0(3)	99504	0(3)	A4218	20(3)	A4334	3(3)	A4416	2(3)
97545	1(2)	99153	12(3)	99307	1(2)	99412	0(3)	99505	0(3)	A4220	1(3)	A4335	1(3)	A4417	2(3)
97546	2(3)	99155	1(3)	99308	1(2)	99415	1(2)	99506	0(3)	A4221	1(3)	A4336	1(3)	A4418	2(3)
97597	1(3)	99156	1(3)	99309	1(2)	99416	3(3)	99507	0(3)	A4222	2(3)	A4337	2(3)	A4419	2(3)
97598	8(3)	99157	6(3)	99310	1(2)	99417	4(3)	99509	0(3)	A4223	1(3)	A4338	3(3)	A4420	1(3)
97602	1(3)	99170	1(3)	99315	1(2)	99421	1(2)	99510	0(3)	A4224	1(2)	A4340	2(3)	A4423	2(3)
97605	1(3)	99172	0(3)	99316	1(2)	99422	1(2)	99511	0(3)	A4225	1(3)	A4344	2(3)	A4424	1(3)
97606	1(3)	99173	0(3)	99318	1(2)	99423	1(2)	99512	0(3)	A4226	0(3)	A4346	2(3)	A4425	1(3)
97607	1(3)	99174	0(3)	99324	1(2)	99429	0(3)	99600	0(3)	A4230	1(3)	A4351	2(3)	A4426	2(3)
97608	1(3)	99175	1(3)	99325	1(2)	99439	2(2)	99601	0(3)	A4231	1(3)	A4352	2(3)	A4427	1(3)
97610	1(2)	99177	1(2)	99326	1(2)	99441	1(2)	99602	0(3)	A4232	0(3)	A4353	3(3)	A4428	1(3)
97750	8(3)	99183	1(3)	99327	1(2)	99442	1(2)	99605	0(2)	A4233	0(3)	A4354	2(3)	A4429	2(3)
97755	8(3)	99184	1(2)	99328	1(2)	99443	1(2)	99606	0(3)	A4234	0(3)	A4355	2(3)	A4430	1(3)
97760	6(3)	99188	1(2)	99334	1(3)	99446	1(2)	99607	0(3)	A4235	1(3)	A4356	2(3)	A4431	1(3)
97761	6(3)	99190	1(3)	99335	1(3)	99447	1(2)	A0021	0(3)	A4236	0(3)	A4357	2(3)	A4432	2(3)
97763	6(3)	99191	1(3)	99336	1(3)	99448	1(2)	A0080	0(3)	A4244	1(3)	A4358	6(3)	A4433	1(3)
97799	1(3)	99192	1(3)	99337	1(3)	99449	1(2)	A0090	0(3)	A4245	1(3)	A4360	1(3)	A4434	1(3)
97802	8(3)	99195	2(3)	99339	1(2)	99450	0(3)	A0100	0(3)	A4246	1(3)	A4361	1(3)	A4435	2(3)
97803	8(3)	99199	1(3)	99340	1(2)	99451	1(2)	A0110	0(3)	A4247	1(3)	A4362	2(3)	A4450	20(3)
97804	6(3)	99202	1(2)	99341	1(2)	99452	1(2)	A0120	0(3)	A4248	10(3)	A4363	0(3)	A4452	4(3)
97810	1(2)	99203	1(2)	99342	1(2)	99453	1(2)	A0130	0(3)	A4250	0(3)	A4364	2(3)	A4455	1(3)
97811	2(3)	99204	1(2)	99343	1(2)	99454	1(2)	A0140	0(3)	A4252	0(3)	A4366	1(3)	A4458	1(3)
97813	1(2)	99205	1(2)	99344	1(2)	99455	1(3)	A0160	0(3)	A4253	0(3)	A4367	1(3)	A4459	1(3)
97814	2(3)	99211	2(3)	99345	1(2)	99456	1(3)	A0170	0(3)	A4255	0(3)	A4368	1(3)	A4461	2(3)
98925	1(2)	99212	2(3)	99347	1(3)	99457	1(2)	A0180	0(3)	A4256	1(3)	A4369	1(3)	A4463	2(3)
98926	1(2)	99213	2(3)	99348	1(3)	99458	3(3)	A0190	0(3)	A4257	0(3)	A4371	1(3)	A4465	1(3)
98927	1(2)	99214	2(3)	99349	1(3)	99460	1(2)	A0200	0(3)	A4258	0(3)	A4372	1(3)	A4467	0(3)
98928	1(2)	99215	2(3)	99350	1(3)	99461	1(2)	A0210	0(3)	A4259	0(3)	A4373	1(3)	A4470	1(3)
98929	1(2)	99217	1(2)	99354	1(2)	99462	1(2)	A0225	0(3)	A4261	0(3)	A4375	2(3)	A4480	1(3)
98940	1(2)	99218	1(2)	99355	4(3)	99463	1(2)	A0380	0(3)	A4262	4(2)	A4376	2(3)	A4481	2(3)
98941	1(2)	99219	1(2)	99356	1(2)	99464	1(2)	A0382	0(3)	A4263	4(2)	A4377	2(3)	A4483	1(3)
98942	1(2)	99220	1(2)	99357	1(3)	99465	1(2)	A0384	0(3)	A4264	0(3)	A4378	2(3)	A4490	0(3)
98943	0(3)	99221	0(3)	99358	1(2)	99466	1(2)	A0390	0(3)	A4265	1(3)	A4379	2(3)	A4495	0(3)
98960	0(3)	99222	0(3)	99359	1(3)	99467	4(3)	A0392	0(3)	A4266	0(3)	A4380	2(3)	A4500	0(3)
98961	0(3)	99223	0(3)	99360	1(3)	99468	1(2)	A0394	0(3)	A4267	0(3)	A4381	2(3)	A4510	0(3)
98962	0(3)	99224	1(2)	99366	2(3)	99469	1(2)	A0396	0(3)	A4268	0(3)	A4382	2(3)	A4520	0(3)
98966	1(2)	99225	1(2)	99367	1(3)	99471	1(2)	A0398	0(3)	A4269	0(3)	A4383	2(3)	A4550	3(3)
98967	1(2)	99226	1(2)	99368	2(3)	99472	1(2)	A0420	0(3)	A4270	3(3)	A4384	2(3)	A4553	0(3)
98968	1(2)	99231	0(3)	99374	1(2)	99473	1(2)	A0422	0(3)	A4280	1(3)	A4385	2(3)	A4554	0(3)
98970	1(2)	99232	0(3)	99375	0(3)	99474	1(2)	A0424	0(3)	A4281	0(3)	A4387	1(3)	A4555	0(3)
98971	1(2)	99233	0(3)	99377	1(3)	99475	1(2)	A0425	250(1)	A4282	0(3)	A4388	1(3)	A4556	2(3)
98972	1(2)	99234	1(3)	99378	0(3)	99476	1(2)	A0426	2(3)	A4283	0(3)	A4389	2(3)	A4557	2(3)
99000	0(3)	99235	1(3)	99379	1(2)	99477	1(2)	A0427	2(3)	A4284	0(3)	A4390	1(3)	A4558	1(3)
99001	0(3)	99236	1(3)	99380	1(2)	99478	1(2)	A0428	2(3)	A4285	0(3)	A4391	1(3)	A4559	1(3)

CPT	MUE	CPT	MUE	CPT	MUE	CPT	MUE	CPT	MUE	CPT	MUE	CPT	MUE	CPT	MUE
A4561	1(3)	A4721	0(3)	A5505	0(3)	A6511	1(3)	A7508	0(3)	A9541	1(3)	B4150	0(3)	C1758	2(3)
A4562	1(3)	A4722	0(3)	A5506	0(3)	A6513	1(3)	A7509	0(3)	A9542	1(3)	B4152	0(3)	C1759	2(3)
A4563	1(2)	A4723	0(3)	A5507	0(3)	A6530	0(3)	A7520	1(3)	A9543	1(3)	B4153	0(3)	C1760	4(3)
A4565	2(3)	A4724	0(3)	A5508	0(3)	A6531	2(3)	A7521	1(3)	A9546	1(3)	B4154	0(3)	C1762	4(3)
A4566	0(3)	A4725	0(3)	A5510	0(3)	A6532	2(3)	A7522	0(3)	A9547	2(3)	B4155	0(3)	C1763	4(3)
A4570	0(3)	A4726	0(3)	A5512	0(3)	A6533	0(3)	A7523	0(3)	A9548	2(3)	B4157	0(3)	C1764	1(3)
A4575	0(3)	A4728	0(3)	A5513	0(3)	A6534	0(3)	A7524	1(3)	A9550	1(3)	B4158	0(3)	C1765	4(3)
A4580	0(3)	A4730	0(3)	A5514	0(3)	A6535	0(3)	A7525	8(3)	A9551	1(3)	B4159	0(3)	C1766	4(3)
A4590	0(3)	A4736	0(3)	A6000	0(3)	A6536	0(3)	A7526	0(3)	A9552	1(3)	B4160	0(3)	C1767	2(3)
A4595	2(3)	A4737	0(3)	A6010	3(3)	A6537	0(3)	A7527	1(3)	A9553	1(3)	B4161	0(3)	C1768	3(3)
A4600	0(3)	A4740	0(3)	A6011	20(3)	A6538	0(3)	A8000	0(3)	A9554	1(3)	B4162	0(3)	C1769	9(3)
A4601	0(3)	A4750	0(3)	A6024	1(3)	A6539	0(3)	A8001	0(3)	A9555	2(3)	B4164	0(3)	C1770	3(3)
A4602	1(3)	A4755	0(3)	A6025	4(3)	A6540	0(3)	A8002	0(3)	A9556	10(3)	B4168	0(3)	C1771	1(3)
A4604	1(3)	A4760	0(3)	A6154	1(3)	A6541	0(3)	A8003	0(3)	A9557	2(3)	B4172	0(3)	C1772	1(3)
A4605	1(3)	A4765	0(3)	A6205	1(3)	A6544	0(3)	A8004	0(3)	A9558	7(3)	B4176	0(3)	C1773	3(3)
A4606	1(3)	A4766	0(3)	A6221	9(3)	A6545	2(3)	A9152	0(3)	A9559	1(3)	B4178	0(3)	C1776	10(3)
A4608	1(3)	A4770	0(3)	A6228	2(3)	A6549	0(3)	A9153	0(3)	A9560	2(3)	B4180	0(3)	C1777	2(3)
A4611	0(3)	A4771	0(3)	A6230	1(3)	A6550	1(3)	A9155	1(3)	A9561	1(3)	B4185	0(3)	C1778	4(3)
A4612	0(3)	A4772	0(3)	A6236	1(3)	A7000	0(3)	A9180	0(3)	A9562	2(3)	B4187	0(3)	C1779	2(3)
A4613	0(3)	A4773	0(3)	A6238	3(3)	A7001	0(3)	A9270	0(3)	A9563	10(3)	B4189	0(3)	C1780	2(3)
A4614	1(2)	A4774	0(3)	A6239	1(3)	A7002	0(3)	A9272	0(3)	A9564	0(3)	B4193	0(3)	C1781	4(3)
A4615	2(3)	A4802	0(3)	A6240	2(3)	A7003	0(3)	A9273	0(3)	A9566	1(3)	B4197	0(3)	C1782	1(3)
A4616	1(3)	A4860	0(3)	A6241	1(3)	A7004	0(3)	A9274	0(3)	A9567	2(3)	B4199	0(3)	C1783	2(3)
A4617	1(3)	A4870	0(3)	A6244	1(3)	A7005	0(3)	A9275	0(3)	A9568	0(3)	B4216	0(3)	C1784	2(3)
A4618	1(3)	A4890	0(3)	A6246	3(3)	A7006	0(3)	A9276	0(3)	A9569	1(3)	B4220	0(3)	C1785	1(3)
A4619	1(3)	A4911	0(3)	A6247	2(3)	A7007	0(3)	A9277	0(3)	A9570	1(3)	B4222	0(3)	C1786	1(3)
A4620	1(3)	A4913	0(3)	A6250	1(3)	A7008	0(3)	A9278	0(3)	A9571	1(3)	B4224	0(3)	C1787	2(3)
A4623	10(3)	A4918	0(3)	A6256	3(3)	A7009	0(3)	A9279	0(3)	A9572	1(3)	B5000	0(3)	C1788	2(3)
A4624	2(3)	A4927	0(3)	A6259	3(3)	A7010	0(3)	A9280	0(3)	A9575	300(3)	B5100	0(3)	C1789	2(3)
A4625	30(3)	A4928	0(3)	A6261	3(3)	A7012	0(3)	A9281	0(3)	A9576	100(3)	B5200	0(3)	C1813	1(3)
A4626	1(3)	A4929	0(3)	A6262	3(3)	A7013	0(3)	A9282	0(3)	A9577	50(3)	B9002	0(3)	C1814	2(3)
A4627	0(3)	A4930	0(3)	A6404	2(3)	A7014	0(3)	A9283	0(3)	A9578	50(3)	B9004	0(3)	C1815	1(3)
A4628	1(3)	A4931	0(3)	A6407	4(3)	A7015	0(3)	A9284	0(3)	A9579	100(3)	B9006	0(3)	C1816	2(3)
A4629	1(3)	A4932	0(3)	A6410	2(3)	A7016	0(3)	A9285	0(3)	A9580	1(3)	B9998	0(3)	C1817	1(3)
A4630	0(3)	A5051	1(3)	A6411	2(3)	A7017	0(3)	A9286	0(3)	A9581	20(3)	B9999	0(3)	C1818	2(3)
A4633	0(3)	A5052	1(3)	A6412	2(3)	A7018	0(3)	A9300	0(3)	A9582	1(3)	C1052	1(3)	C1819	4(3)
A4634	1(3)	A5053	2(3)	A6413	0(3)	A7020	0(3)	A9500	3(3)	A9583	18(3)	C1062	2(3)	C1820	2(3)
A4635	0(3)	A5054	1(3)	A6441	8(3)	A7025	0(3)	A9501	1(3)	A9584	1(3)	C1713	20(3)	C1821	4(3)
A4636	0(3)	A5055	1(3)	A6442	8(3)	A7026	0(3)	A9502	3(3)	A9585	300(3)	C1714	4(3)	C1822	1(3)
A4637	0(3)	A5056	90(3)	A6443	8(3)	A7027	0(3)	A9503	1(3)	A9586	1(3)	C1715	45(3)	C1823	1(3)
A4638	0(3)	A5057	90(3)	A6444	4(3)	A7028	0(3)	A9504	1(3)	A9587	54(3)	C1716	4(3)	C1824	1(2)
A4639	0(3)	A5061	2(3)	A6445	8(3)	A7029	0(3)	A9505	4(3)	A9588	10(3)	C1717	10(3)	C1825	1(2)
A4640	0(3)	A5062	1(3)	A6446	14(3)	A7030	0(3)	A9507	1(3)	A9589	1(3)	C1719	99(3)	C1830	2(3)
A4642	1(3)	A5063	1(3)	A6447	6(3)	A7031	0(3)	A9508	2(3)	A9590	675(3)	C1721	1(3)	C1839	2(2)
A4648	3(3)	A5071	2(3)	A6448	24(3)	A7032	0(3)	A9509	5(3)	A9591	6(3)	C1722	1(3)	C1840	1(3)
A4650	3(3)	A5072	1(3)	A6449	12(3)	A7033	0(3)	A9510	1(3)	A9600	7(3)	C1724	5(3)	C1841	1(2)
A4651	2(3)	A5073	1(3)	A6450	8(3)	A7034	0(3)	A9512	30(3)	A9604	1(3)	C1725	9(3)	C1842	1(2)
A4652	2(3)	A5081	2(3)	A6451	8(3)	A7035	0(3)	A9513	200(3)	A9606	224(3)	C1726	5(3)	C1874	5(3)
A4653	0(3)	A5082	1(3)	A6452	22(3)	A7036	0(3)	A9515	1(3)	A9698	3(3)	C1727	4(3)	C1875	4(3)
A4657	0(3)	A5083	5(3)	A6453	6(3)	A7037	0(3)	A9516	4(3)	A9700	2(3)	C1728	5(3)	C1876	5(3)
A4660	0(3)	A5093	2(3)	A6454	25(3)	A7038	0(3)	A9517	200(3)	A9900	0(3)	C1729	6(3)	C1877	5(3)
A4663	0(3)	A5102	1(3)	A6455	4(3)	A7039	0(3)	A9520	1(3)	A9901	0(3)	C1730	4(3)	C1878	2(3)
A4670	0(3)	A5105	1(3)	A6456	20(3)	A7040	2(3)	A9521	2(3)	A9999	0(3)	C1731	2(3)	C1880	2(3)
A4671	0(3)	A5112	2(3)	A6457	12(3)	A7041	2(3)	A9524	10(3)	B4034	0(3)	C1732	3(3)	C1881	2(3)
A4672	0(3)	A5113	0(3)	A6460	1(1)	A7044	0(3)	A9526	2(3)	B4035	0(3)	C1733	3(3)	C1882	1(3)
A4673	0(3)	A5114	0(3)	A6461	1(1)	A7045	0(3)	A9527	195(3)	B4036	0(3)	C1734	2(3)	C1883	4(3)
A4674	0(3)	A5120	150(3)	A6501	1(3)	A7046	0(3)	A9528	10(3)	B4081	0(3)	C1748	1(3)	C1884	4(3)
A4680	0(3)	A5121	1(3)	A6502	1(3)	A7047	1(3)	A9529	10(3)	B4082	0(3)	C1749	1(3)	C1885	2(3)
A4690	0(3)	A5122	1(3)	A6503	1(3)	A7048	2(3)	A9530	200(3)	B4083	0(3)	C1750	2(3)	C1886	1(3)
A4706	0(3)	A5126	2(3)	A6504	2(3)	A7501	1(3)	A9531	100(3)	B4087	0(3)	C1751	3(3)	C1887	7(3)
A4707	0(3)	A5131	1(3)	A6505	2(3)	A7502	1(3)	A9532	10(3)	B4088	0(3)	C1752	2(3)	C1888	2(3)
A4708	0(3)	A5200	2(3)	A6506	2(3)	A7503	1(3)	A9536	1(3)	B4100	0(3)	C1753	2(3)	C1889	2(3)
A4709	0(3)	A5500	0(3)	A6507	2(3)	A7504	180(3)	A9537	1(3)	B4102	0(3)	C1754	2(3)	C1890	1(3)
A4714	0(3)	A5501	0(3)	A6508	2(3)	A7505	1(3)	A9538	1(3)	B4103	0(3)	C1755	2(3)	C1891	1(3)
A4719	0(3)	A5503	0(3)	A6509	1(3)	A7506	0(3)	A9539	2(3)	B4104	0(3)	C1756	2(3)	C1892	6(3)
A4720	0(3)	A5504	0(3)	A6510	1(3)	A7507	200(3)	A9540	2(3)	B4149	0(3)	C1757	6(3)	C1893	6(3)

CPT	MUE	CPT	MUE	CPT	MUE	CPT	MUE	CPT	MUE	CPT	MUE	CPT	MUE	CPT	MUE
C1894	6(3)	C8923	1(3)	C9756	1(3)	D5985	1(3)	E0181	0(3)	E0300	0(3)	E0600	0(3)	E0762	1(3)
C1895	2(3)	C8924	1(3)	C9757	2(2)	D6052	0(3)	E0182	0(3)	E0301	0(3)	E0601	0(3)	E0764	0(3)
C1896	2(3)	C8925	1(3)	C9758	1(2)	D7111	20(3)	E0184	0(3)	E0302	0(3)	E0602	0(3)	E0765	0(3)
C1897	2(3)	C8926	1(3)	C9759	1(3)	D7140	32(2)	E0185	0(3)	E0303	0(3)	E0603	0(3)	E0766	0(3)
C1898	2(3)	C8927	1(3)	C9760	1(2)	D7210	32(2)	E0186	0(3)	E0304	0(3)	E0604	0(3)	E0769	0(3)
C1899	2(3)	C8928	1(2)	C9761	2(2)	D7220	6(3)	E0187	0(3)	E0305	0(3)	E0605	0(3)	E0770	1(3)
C1900	1(3)	C8929	1(3)	C9762	1(3)	D7230	6(3)	E0188	0(3)	E0310	0(3)	E0606	0(3)	E0776	0(3)
C1982	1(3)	C8930	1(2)	C9763	1(3)	D7240	6(3)	E0189	0(3)	E0315	0(3)	E0607	0(3)	E0779	0(3)
C2596	1(3)	C8931	1(3)	C9764	2(3)	D7241	6(3)	E0190	0(3)	E0316	0(3)	E0610	0(3)	E0780	0(3)
C2613	2(3)	C8932	1(3)	C9765	2(3)	D7250	32(2)	E0191	0(3)	E0325	0(3)	E0615	0(3)	E0781	1(3)
C2614	3(3)	C8933	1(3)	C9766	2(3)	D7260	1(3)	E0193	0(3)	E0326	0(3)	E0616	1(2)	E0782	1(2)
C2615	2(3)	C8934	2(3)	C9767	2(3)	D7261	1(3)	E0194	0(3)	E0328	0(3)	E0617	0(3)	E0783	1(2)
C2616	1(3)	C8935	2(3)	C9768	1(3)	D7283	4(3)	E0196	0(3)	E0329	0(3)	E0618	0(3)	E0784	0(3)
C2617	4(3)	C8936	2(3)	C9769	1(2)	D7288	2(3)	E0197	0(3)	E0350	0(3)	E0619	0(3)	E0785	1(2)
C2618	4(3)	C8937	2(2)	C9770	2(2)	D7321	4(2)	E0198	0(3)	E0352	0(3)	E0620	0(3)	E0786	1(2)
C2619	1(3)	C8957	2(3)	C9771	1(2)	D9110	1(3)	E0199	0(3)	E0370	0(3)	E0621	0(3)	E0787	0(3)
C2620	1(3)	C9046	160(3)	C9772	2(2)	D9130	0(3)	E0200	0(3)	E0371	0(3)	E0625	0(3)	E0791	0(3)
C2621	1(3)	C9047	22(3)	C9773	2(2)	D9230	1(3)	E0202	0(3)	E0372	0(3)	E0627	0(3)	E0830	0(3)
C2622	1(3)	C9065	40(3)	C9774	2(2)	D9248	1(3)	E0203	0(3)	E0373	0(3)	E0629	0(3)	E0840	0(3)
C2623	4(3)	C9067	500(3)	C9775	2(2)	D9613	0(3)	E0205	0(3)	E0424	0(3)	E0630	0(3)	E0849	0(3)
C2624	1(3)	C9113	10(3)	C9803	2(3)	D9930	1(2)	E0210	0(3)	E0425	0(3)	E0635	0(3)	E0850	0(3)
C2625	4(3)	C9132	5500(3)	C9898	1(3)	D9944	2(2)	E0215	0(3)	E0430	0(3)	E0636	0(3)	E0855	0(3)
C2626	1(3)	C9248	25(3)	D0150	1(3)	D9945	2(2)	E0217	0(3)	E0431	0(3)	E0637	0(3)	E0856	0(3)
C2627	2(3)	C9250	5(3)	D0240	1(3)	D9946	2(2)	E0218	0(3)	E0433	0(3)	E0638	0(3)	E0860	0(3)
C2628	4(3)	C9254	400(3)	D0250	2(3)	D9950	1(3)	E0221	0(3)	E0434	0(3)	E0639	0(3)	E0870	0(3)
C2629	4(3)	C9257	10(2)	D0270	1(3)	D9951	1(3)	E0225	0(3)	E0435	0(3)	E0640	0(3)	E0880	0(3)
C2630	3(3)	C9285	2(3)	D0272	1(3)	D9952	1(3)	E0231	0(3)	E0439	0(3)	E0641	0(3)	E0890	0(3)
C2631	1(3)	C9290	266(3)	D0274	1(3)	D9961	0(3)	E0232	0(3)	E0440	0(3)	E0642	0(3)	E0900	0(3)
C2634	24(3)	C9293	700(3)	D0277	1(3)	D9990	0(3)	E0235	0(3)	E0441	0(3)	E0650	0(3)	E0910	0(3)
C2635	124(3)	C9352	3(3)	D0412	0(3)	E0100	0(3)	E0236	0(3)	E0442	0(3)	E0651	0(3)	E0911	0(3)
C2636	690(3)	C9353	4(3)	D0416	1(3)	E0105	0(3)	E0239	0(3)	E0443	0(3)	E0652	0(3)	E0912	0(3)
C2637	0(3)	C9354	300(3)	D0431	1(3)	E0110	0(3)	E0240	0(3)	E0444	0(3)	E0655	0(3)	E0920	0(3)
C2638	150(3)	C9355	3(3)	D0460	1(2)	E0111	0(3)	E0241	0(3)	E0445	0(3)	E0656	0(3)	E0930	0(3)
C2639	150(3)	C9356	125(3)	D0484	1(2)	E0112	0(3)	E0242	0(3)	E0446	0(3)	E0657	0(3)	E0935	0(3)
C2640	150(3)	C9358	800(3)	D0485	1(2)	E0113	0(3)	E0243	0(3)	E0447	0(3)	E0660	0(3)	E0936	0(3)
C2641	150(3)	C9359	30(3)	D0601	0(3)	E0114	0(3)	E0244	0(3)	E0455	0(3)	E0665	0(3)	E0940	0(3)
C2642	120(3)	C9360	300(3)	D0602	0(3)	E0116	0(3)	E0245	0(3)	E0457	0(3)	E0666	0(3)	E0941	0(3)
C2643	120(3)	C9361	10(3)	D0603	0(3)	E0117	0(3)	E0246	0(3)	E0459	0(3)	E0667	0(3)	E0942	0(3)
C2644	0(3)	C9362	60(3)	D1510	2(2)	E0118	0(3)	E0247	0(3)	E0462	0(3)	E0668	0(3)	E0944	0(3)
C2645	4608(3)	C9363	500(3)	D1516	1(2)	E0130	0(3)	E0248	0(3)	E0465	0(3)	E0669	0(3)	E0945	0(3)
C5271	1(2)	C9364	600(3)	D1517	1(2)	E0135	0(3)	E0249	0(3)	E0466	0(3)	E0670	0(3)	E0946	0(3)
C5272	3(2)	C9460	100(3)	D1520	2(2)	E0140	0(3)	E0250	0(3)	E0467	0(3)	E0671	0(3)	E0947	0(3)
C5273	1(2)	C9462	600(3)	D1526	1(2)	E0141	0(3)	E0251	0(3)	E0470	0(3)	E0672	0(3)	E0948	0(3)
C5274	35(3)	C9482	300(3)	D1527	1(2)	E0143	0(3)	E0255	0(3)	E0471	0(3)	E0673	0(3)	E0950	0(3)
C5275	1(2)	C9488	40(3)	D1551	1(2)	E0144	0(3)	E0256	0(3)	E0472	0(3)	E0675	0(3)	E0951	0(3)
C5276	3(2)	C9600	3(3)	D1552	1(2)	E0147	0(3)	E0260	0(3)	E0480	0(3)	E0676	1(3)	E0952	0(3)
C5277	1(2)	C9601	2(3)	D1553	2(2)	E0148	0(3)	E0261	0(3)	E0481	0(3)	E0691	0(3)	E0953	0(3)
C5278	15(3)	C9602	2(3)	D1575	4(2)	E0149	0(3)	E0265	0(3)	E0482	0(3)	E0692	0(3)	E0954	0(3)
C8900	1(3)	C9603	2(3)	D1999	0(3)	E0153	0(3)	E0266	0(3)	E0483	0(3)	E0693	0(3)	E0955	0(3)
C8901	1(3)	C9604	2(3)	D4260	4(2)	E0154	0(3)	E0270	0(3)	E0484	0(3)	E0694	0(3)	E0956	0(3)
C8902	1(3)	C9605	2(3)	D4263	4(2)	E0155	0(3)	E0271	0(3)	E0485	0(3)	E0700	0(3)	E0957	0(3)
C8903	1(3)	C9606	1(3)	D4264	3(3)	E0156	0(3)	E0272	0(3)	E0486	0(3)	E0705	1(2)	E0958	0(3)
C8905	1(3)	C9607	2(3)	D4270	4(3)	E0157	0(3)	E0273	0(3)	E0487	0(3)	E0710	0(3)	E0959	2(2)
C8906	1(3)	C9608	2(3)	D4273	1(2)	E0158	0(3)	E0274	0(3)	E0500	0(3)	E0720	0(3)	E0960	0(3)
C8908	1(3)	C9725	1(3)	D4277	0(3)	E0159	1(3)	E0275	0(3)	E0550	0(3)	E0730	0(3)	E0961	2(2)
C8909	1(3)	C9726	2(3)	D4278	0(3)	E0160	0(3)	E0276	0(3)	E0555	0(3)	E0731	0(3)	E0966	1(2)
C8910	1(3)	C9727	1(2)	D4355	1(2)	E0161	0(3)	E0277	0(3)	E0560	0(3)	E0740	0(3)	E0967	0(3)
C8911	1(3)	C9728	1(2)	D4381	12(3)	E0162	0(3)	E0280	0(3)	E0561	0(3)	E0744	0(3)	E0968	0(3)
C8912	1(3)	C9733	1(3)	D5282	0(3)	E0163	0(3)	E0290	0(3)	E0562	0(3)	E0745	0(3)	E0969	0(3)
C8913	1(3)	C9734	1(3)	D5283	0(3)	E0165	0(3)	E0291	0(3)	E0565	0(3)	E0746	1(3)	E0970	0(3)
C8914	1(3)	C9738	1(3)	D5876	0(3)	E0167	0(3)	E0292	0(3)	E0570	0(3)	E0747	0(3)	E0971	2(3)
C8918	1(3)	C9739	1(2)	D5911	1(3)	E0168	0(3)	E0293	0(3)	E0572	0(3)	E0748	0(3)	E0973	2(2)
C8919	1(3)	C9740	1(2)	D5912	1(2)	E0170	0(3)	E0294	0(3)	E0574	0(3)	E0749	1(3)	E0974	2(2)
C8920	1(3)	C9751	1(3)	D5951	0(3)	E0171	0(3)	E0295	0(3)	E0575	0(3)	E0755	0(3)	E0978	1(3)
C8921	1(3)	C9752	1(2)	D5983	1(3)	E0172	0(3)	E0296	0(3)	E0580	0(3)	E0760	0(3)	E0980	0(3)
C8922	1(3)	C9753	3(3)	D5984	1(3)	E0175	0(3)	E0297	0(3)	E0585	0(3)	E0761	0(3)	E0981	0(3)

CPT	MUE	CPT	MUE	CPT	MUE	CPT	MUE	CPT	MUE	CPT	MUE	CPT	MUE	CPT	MUE
E0982	0(3)	E1223	0(3)	E1636	0(3)	E2310	0(3)	E2512	0(3)	G0122	0(3)	G0339	1(2)	G0469	1(2)
E0983	0(3)	E1224	0(3)	E1637	0(3)	E2311	0(3)	E2599	0(3)	G0123	1(3)	G0340	1(3)	G0470	1(3)
E0984	0(3)	E1225	0(3)	E1639	0(3)	E2312	0(3)	E2601	0(3)	G0124	1(3)	G0341	1(2)	G0471	2(3)
E0985	0(3)	E1226	1(2)	E1699	1(3)	E2313	0(3)	E2602	0(3)	G0127	1(2)	G0342	1(2)	G0472	1(2)
E0986	0(3)	E1227	0(3)	E1700	0(3)	E2321	0(3)	E2603	0(3)	G0128	1(3)	G0343	1(2)	G0473	1(3)
E0988	0(3)	E1228	0(3)	E1701	0(3)	E2322	0(3)	E2604	0(3)	G0129	6(3)	G0372	1(2)	G0475	1(2)
E0990	2(2)	E1229	0(3)	E1702	0(3)	E2323	0(3)	E2605	0(3)	G0130	1(2)	G0379	1(2)	G0476	1(2)
E0992	1(2)	E1230	0(3)	E1800	0(3)	E2324	0(3)	E2606	0(3)	G0141	1(3)	G0380	2(3)	G0480	1(2)
E0994	0(3)	E1231	0(3)	E1801	0(3)	E2325	0(3)	E2607	0(3)	G0143	1(3)	G0381	2(3)	G0481	1(2)
E0995	2(2)	E1232	0(3)	E1802	0(3)	E2326	0(3)	E2608	0(3)	G0144	1(3)	G0382	2(3)	G0482	1(2)
E1002	0(3)	E1233	0(3)	E1805	0(3)	E2327	0(3)	E2609	0(3)	G0145	1(3)	G0383	2(3)	G0483	1(2)
E1003	0(3)	E1234	0(3)	E1806	0(3)	E2328	0(3)	E2610	1(3)	G0147	1(3)	G0384	2(3)	G0490	1(3)
E1004	0(3)	E1235	0(3)	E1810	0(3)	E2329	0(3)	E2611	0(3)	G0148	1(3)	G0390	1(2)	G0491	1(3)
E1005	0(3)	E1236	0(3)	E1811	0(3)	E2330	0(3)	E2612	0(3)	G0166	2(3)	G0396	1(2)	G0492	1(3)
E1006	0(3)	E1237	0(3)	E1812	0(3)	E2331	0(3)	E2613	0(3)	G0168	2(3)	G0397	1(2)	G0493	1(3)
E1007	0(3)	E1238	0(3)	E1815	0(3)	E2340	0(3)	E2614	0(3)	G0175	1(3)	G0398	1(2)	G0494	1(3)
E1008	0(3)	E1239	0(3)	E1816	0(3)	E2341	0(3)	E2615	0(3)	G0176	5(3)	G0399	1(2)	G0495	1(3)
E1009	0(3)	E1240	0(3)	E1818	0(3)	E2342	0(3)	E2616	0(3)	G0177	5(3)	G0400	1(2)	G0496	1(2)
E1010	0(3)	E1250	0(3)	E1820	0(3)	E2343	0(3)	E2617	0(3)	G0179	1(2)	G0402	1(2)	G0498	1(2)
E1011	0(3)	E1260	0(3)	E1821	0(3)	E2351	0(3)	E2619	0(3)	G0180	1(2)	G0403	1(2)	G0499	1(2)
E1012	0(3)	E1270	0(3)	E1825	0(3)	E2358	0(3)	E2620	0(3)	G0181	1(2)	G0404	1(2)	G0500	1(3)
E1014	0(3)	E1280	0(3)	E1830	0(3)	E2359	0(3)	E2621	0(3)	G0182	1(2)	G0405	1(2)	G0501	1(3)
E1015	0(3)	E1285	0(3)	E1831	0(3)	E2360	0(3)	E2622	0(3)	G0186	1(2)	G0406	1(3)	G0506	1(2)
E1016	0(3)	E1290	0(3)	E1840	0(3)	E2361	0(3)	E2623	0(3)	G0219	0(3)	G0407	1(3)	G0508	1(2)
E1017	0(3)	E1295	0(3)	E1841	0(3)	E2362	0(3)	E2624	0(3)	G0235	1(3)	G0408	1(3)	G0509	1(2)
E1018	0(3)	E1296	0(3)	E1902	0(3)	E2363	0(3)	E2625	0(3)	G0237	8(3)	G0410	6(3)	G0511	1(2)
E1020	0(3)	E1297	0(3)	E2000	0(3)	E2364	0(3)	E2626	0(3)	G0238	8(3)	G0411	6(3)	G0512	1(2)
E1028	0(3)	E1298	0(3)	E2100	0(3)	E2365	0(3)	E2627	0(3)	G0239	2(3)	G0412	1(2)	G0513	1(2)
E1029	0(3)	E1300	0(3)	E2101	0(3)	E2366	0(3)	E2628	0(3)	G0245	1(2)	G0413	1(2)	G0514	1(1)
E1030	0(3)	E1310	0(3)	E2120	0(3)	E2367	0(3)	E2629	0(3)	G0246	1(2)	G0414	1(2)	G0516	1(2)
E1031	0(3)	E1352	0(3)	E2201	0(3)	E2368	0(3)	E2630	0(3)	G0247	1(2)	G0415	1(2)	G0517	1(2)
E1035	0(3)	E1353	0(3)	E2202	0(3)	E2369	0(3)	E2631	0(3)	G0248	1(2)	G0416	1(2)	G0518	1(2)
E1036	0(3)	E1354	0(3)	E2203	0(3)	E2370	0(3)	E2632	0(3)	G0249	3(3)	G0420	2(3)	G0659	1(2)
E1037	0(3)	E1355	0(3)	E2204	0(3)	E2371	0(3)	E2633	0(3)	G0250	1(2)	G0421	2(3)	G2000	1(3)
E1038	0(3)	E1356	0(3)	E2205	0(3)	E2372	0(3)	E8000	0(3)	G0252	0(3)	G0422	6(2)	G2001	1(3)
E1039	0(3)	E1357	0(3)	E2206	0(3)	E2373	0(3)	E8001	0(3)	G0255	0(3)	G0423	6(3)	G2002	1(3)
E1050	0(3)	E1358	0(3)	E2207	0(3)	E2374	0(3)	E8002	0(3)	G0257	1(3)	G0424	2(2)	G2003	1(3)
E1060	0(3)	E1372	0(3)	E2208	0(3)	E2375	0(3)	G0008	1(2)	G0259	2(3)	G0425	1(3)	G2004	1(3)
E1070	0(3)	E1390	0(3)	E2209	0(3)	E2376	0(3)	G0009	1(2)	G0260	2(3)	G0426	1(3)	G2005	1(3)
E1083	0(3)	E1391	0(3)	E2210	0(3)	E2377	0(3)	G0010	1(3)	G0268	1(2)	G0427	1(3)	G2006	1(3)
E1084	0(3)	E1392	0(3)	E2211	0(3)	E2378	0(3)	G0027	1(2)	G0269	2(3)	G0428	0(3)	G2007	1(3)
E1085	0(3)	E1399	0(3)	E2212	0(3)	E2381	0(3)	G0071	1(3)	G0270	8(3)	G0429	1(2)	G2008	1(3)
E1086	0(3)	E1405	0(3)	E2213	0(3)	E2382	0(3)	G0076	1(3)	G0271	4(3)	G0432	1(2)	G2009	1(3)
E1087	0(3)	E1406	0(3)	E2214	0(3)	E2383	0(3)	G0077	1(3)	G0276	1(3)	G0433	1(2)	G2010	1(3)
E1088	0(3)	E1500	0(3)	E2215	0(3)	E2384	0(3)	G0078	1(3)	G0277	5(3)	G0435	1(2)	G2011	1(2)
E1089	0(3)	E1510	0(3)	E2216	0(3)	E2385	0(3)	G0079	1(3)	G0278	1(2)	G0438	1(2)	G2012	1(3)
E1090	0(3)	E1520	0(3)	E2217	0(3)	E2386	0(3)	G0080	1(3)	G0279	1(2)	G0439	1(2)	G2013	1(3)
E1092	0(3)	E1530	0(3)	E2218	0(3)	E2387	0(3)	G0081	1(3)	G0281	1(3)	G0442	1(2)	G2014	1(3)
E1093	0(3)	E1540	0(3)	E2219	0(3)	E2388	0(3)	G0082	1(3)	G0282	0(3)	G0443	1(2)	G2015	1(3)
E1100	0(3)	E1550	0(3)	E2220	0(3)	E2389	0(3)	G0083	1(3)	G0283	1(3)	G0444	1(2)	G2023	2(3)
E1110	0(3)	E1560	0(3)	E2221	0(3)	E2390	0(3)	G0084	1(3)	G0288	1(2)	G0445	1(2)	G2024	2(3)
E1130	0(3)	E1570	0(3)	E2222	0(3)	E2391	0(3)	G0085	1(3)	G0289	1(2)	G0446	1(3)	G2025	1(3)
E1140	0(3)	E1575	0(3)	E2224	0(3)	E2392	0(3)	G0086	1(3)	G0293	1(2)	G0447	2(3)	G2064	1(2)
E1150	0(3)	E1580	0(3)	E2225	0(3)	E2394	0(3)	G0087	1(3)	G0294	1(2)	G0448	1(3)	G2065	1(2)
E1160	0(3)	E1590	0(3)	E2226	0(3)	E2395	0(3)	G0101	1(2)	G0295	0(3)	G0451	1(3)	G2066	1(2)
E1161	0(3)	E1592	0(3)	E2227	0(3)	E2396	0(3)	G0102	1(2)	G0296	1(2)	G0452	1(3)	G2067	1(2)
E1170	0(3)	E1594	0(3)	E2228	0(3)	E2397	0(3)	G0103	1(2)	G0302	1(2)	G0453	10(3)	G2068	1(2)
E1171	0(3)	E1600	0(3)	E2230	0(3)	E2398	0(3)	G0104	1(2)	G0303	1(2)	G0454	1(2)	G2069	1(2)
E1172	0(3)	E1610	0(3)	E2231	0(3)	E2402	0(3)	G0105	1(2)	G0304	1(2)	G0455	1(2)	G2070	1(2)
E1180	0(3)	E1615	0(3)	E2291	1(2)	E2500	0(3)	G0106	1(2)	G0305	1(2)	G0458	1(3)	G2071	1(2)
E1190	0(3)	E1620	0(3)	E2292	1(2)	E2502	0(3)	G0108	8(3)	G0306	4(3)	G0459	1(3)	G2072	1(2)
E1195	0(3)	E1625	0(3)	E2293	1(2)	E2504	0(3)	G0109	12(3)	G0307	4(3)	G0460	1(3)	G2073	1(2)
E1200	0(3)	E1630	0(3)	E2294	1(2)	E2506	0(3)	G0117	1(2)	G0328	1(2)	G0463	4(3)	G2074	1(2)
E1220	0(3)	E1632	0(3)	E2295	0(3)	E2508	0(3)	G0118	1(2)	G0329	1(3)	G0466	1(2)	G2075	1(2)
E1221	0(3)	E1634	0(3)	E2300	0(3)	E2510	0(3)	G0120	1(2)	G0333	0(3)	G0467	1(3)	G2076	1(2)
E1222	0(3)	E1635	0(3)	E2301	0(3)	E2511	0(3)	G0121	1(2)	G0337	1(2)	G0468	1(2)	G2078	3(3)

Appendix I — Medically Unlikely Edits (MUEs)—OPPS

CPT	MUE	CPT	MUE	CPT	MUE	CPT	MUE	CPT	MUE	CPT	MUE	CPT	MUE	CPT	MUE
G2079	3(3)	J0121	200(3)	J0567	300(3)	J0834	3(3)	J1429	450(3)	J1738	30(3)	J2326	120(3)	J2797	333(3)
G2081	1(2)	J0122	300(3)	J0570	4(3)	J0840	18(3)	J1430	10(3)	J1740	3(3)	J2350	600(3)	J2798	240(3)
G2082	1(2)	J0129	100(3)	J0571	0(3)	J0841	24(3)	J1435	0(3)	J1741	32(3)	J2353	60(3)	J2800	3(3)
G2083	1(2)	J0130	6(3)	J0572	0(3)	J0850	9(3)	J1436	0(3)	J1742	4(3)	J2354	60(3)	J2805	3(3)
G2086	1(3)	J0131	400(3)	J0573	0(3)	J0875	300(3)	J1437	100(3)	J1743	66(3)	J2355	2(3)	J2810	20(3)
G2087	2(3)	J0132	300(3)	J0574	0(3)	J0878	1500(3)	J1438	2(3)	J1744	90(3)	J2357	120(3)	J2820	10(3)
G2170	1(3)	J0133	1200(3)	J0575	0(3)	J0881	500(3)	J1439	750(3)	J1745	150(3)	J2358	405(3)	J2840	160(3)
G2171	1(3)	J0135	8(3)	J0583	1250(3)	J0882	300(3)	J1442	1500(3)	J1746	200(3)	J2360	3(3)	J2850	48(3)
G2212	4(3)	J0153	180(3)	J0584	90(3)	J0883	1250(3)	J1443	0(3)	J1750	45(3)	J2370	30(3)	J2860	170(3)
G2213	1(2)	J0171	120(3)	J0585	600(3)	J0884	1250(3)	J1444	272(3)	J1756	500(3)	J2400	4(3)	J2910	0(3)
G2214	1(2)	J0178	4(2)	J0586	300(3)	J0885	60(3)	J1447	960(3)	J1786	680(3)	J2405	64(3)	J2916	20(3)
G2250	1(2)	J0179	12(2)	J0587	300(3)	J0887	360(3)	J1450	4(3)	J1790	2(3)	J2407	120(3)	J2920	25(3)
G2251	1(2)	J0180	140(3)	J0588	600(3)	J0888	360(3)	J1451	200(3)	J1800	12(3)	J2410	2(3)	J2930	25(3)
G2252	1(2)	J0185	130(3)	J0591	100(3)	J0890	0(3)	J1452	0(3)	J1810	0(3)	J2425	125(3)	J2940	0(3)
G6001	2(3)	J0190	0(3)	J0592	12(3)	J0894	100(3)	J1453	150(3)	J1815	200(3)	J2426	819(3)	J2941	8(3)
G6002	2(3)	J0200	0(3)	J0593	300(3)	J0895	12(3)	J1454	1(3)	J1817	0(3)	J2430	3(3)	J2950	0(3)
G6003	2(3)	J0202	12(3)	J0594	320(3)	J0896	1100(3)	J1455	18(3)	J1823	300(3)	J2440	4(3)	J2993	2(3)
G6004	2(3)	J0205	0(3)	J0595	12(3)	J0897	120(3)	J1457	0(3)	J1826	1(3)	J2460	0(3)	J2995	0(3)
G6005	2(3)	J0207	4(3)	J0596	840(3)	J0945	4(3)	J1458	100(3)	J1830	1(3)	J2469	10(3)	J2997	100(3)
G6006	2(3)	J0210	16(3)	J0597	250(3)	J1000	1(3)	J1459	300(3)	J1833	1116(3)	J2501	25(3)	J3000	2(3)
G6007	2(3)	J0215	0(3)	J0598	100(3)	J1020	8(3)	J1460	10(2)	J1835	0(3)	J2502	60(3)	J3010	100(3)
G6008	2(3)	J0220	20(3)	J0599	900(3)	J1030	8(3)	J1554	240(3)	J1840	3(3)	J2503	2(3)	J3030	2(3)
G6009	2(3)	J0221	300(3)	J0600	3(3)	J1040	4(3)	J1555	480(3)	J1850	14(3)	J2504	15(3)	J3031	675(3)
G6010	2(3)	J0222	300(3)	J0606	150(3)	J1050	1000(3)	J1556	300(3)	J1885	8(3)	J2505	1(3)	J3032	300(3)
G6011	2(3)	J0223	756(3)	J0610	15(3)	J1071	400(3)	J1557	300(3)	J1890	0(3)	J2507	8(3)	J3060	760(3)
G6012	2(3)	J0256	1600(3)	J0620	1(3)	J1094	0(3)	J1558	480(3)	J1930	120(3)	J2510	4(3)	J3070	3(3)
G6013	2(3)	J0257	1400(3)	J0630	8(3)	J1095	1034(2)	J1559	300(3)	J1931	609(3)	J2513	1(3)	J3090	200(3)
G6014	2(3)	J0270	32(3)	J0636	100(3)	J1096	8(2)	J1560	1(2)	J1940	10(3)	J2515	8(3)	J3095	150(3)
G6015	2(3)	J0275	1(3)	J0637	20(3)	J1097	4(3)	J1561	300(3)	J1943	675(3)	J2540	75(3)	J3101	50(3)
G6016	2(3)	J0278	15(3)	J0638	300(3)	J1100	120(3)	J1562	0(3)	J1944	1064(3)	J2543	20(3)	J3105	4(3)
G6017	2(3)	J0280	10(3)	J0640	24(3)	J1110	3(3)	J1566	300(3)	J1945	0(3)	J2545	1(3)	J3110	2(3)
G9143	1(2)	J0282	70(3)	J0641	1200(3)	J1120	2(3)	J1568	300(3)	J1950	12(3)	J2547	600(3)	J3111	210(3)
G9147	0(3)	J0285	5(3)	J0642	1200(3)	J1130	300(3)	J1569	300(3)	J1953	300(3)	J2550	3(3)	J3121	400(3)
G9148	0(3)	J0287	60(3)	J0670	10(3)	J1160	3(3)	J1570	4(3)	J1955	11(3)	J2560	16(3)	J3145	750(3)
G9149	0(3)	J0288	0(3)	J0690	16(3)	J1162	10(3)	J1571	20(3)	J1956	4(3)	J2562	48(3)	J3230	6(3)
G9150	0(3)	J0289	115(3)	J0691	300(3)	J1165	50(3)	J1572	300(3)	J1960	0(3)	J2590	15(3)	J3240	1(3)
G9151	0(3)	J0290	24(3)	J0692	12(3)	J1170	50(3)	J1573	130(3)	J1980	8(3)	J2597	45(3)	J3241	300(3)
G9152	0(3)	J0291	500(3)	J0693	1600(3)	J1180	0(3)	J1575	650(3)	J1990	0(3)	J2650	0(3)	J3243	200(3)
G9153	0(3)	J0295	12(3)	J0694	12(3)	J1190	8(3)	J1580	9(3)	J2001	400(3)	J2670	0(3)	J3245	100(3)
G9156	1(2)	J0300	8(3)	J0695	60(3)	J1200	8(3)	J1595	2(3)	J2010	10(3)	J2675	1(3)	J3246	100(3)
G9157	1(2)	J0330	50(3)	J0696	16(3)	J1201	20(3)	J1599	300(3)	J2020	6(3)	J2680	4(3)	J3250	4(3)
G9187	0(3)	J0348	200(3)	J0697	12(3)	J1205	4(3)	J1600	0(3)	J2060	10(3)	J2690	4(3)	J3260	12(3)
G9480	1(3)	J0350	0(3)	J0698	12(3)	J1212	1(3)	J1602	300(3)	J2062	10(3)	J2700	48(3)	J3262	800(3)
G9481	2(3)	J0360	6(3)	J0702	20(3)	J1230	5(3)	J1610	3(3)	J2150	8(3)	J2704	400(3)	J3265	0(3)
G9482	2(3)	J0364	6(3)	J0706	16(3)	J1240	6(3)	J1620	0(3)	J2170	8(3)	J2710	10(3)	J3280	0(3)
G9483	2(3)	J0365	0(3)	J0710	0(3)	J1245	10(3)	J1626	30(3)	J2175	6(3)	J2720	10(3)	J3285	9(3)
G9484	2(3)	J0380	1(3)	J0712	180(3)	J1250	4(3)	J1627	100(3)	J2180	0(3)	J2724	3500(3)	J3300	160(3)
G9485	2(3)	J0390	0(3)	J0713	12(3)	J1260	2(3)	J1628	100(3)	J2182	300(3)	J2725	0(3)	J3301	16(3)
G9486	2(3)	J0395	0(3)	J0714	12(3)	J1265	100(3)	J1630	7(3)	J2185	60(3)	J2730	2(3)	J3302	0(3)
G9487	2(3)	J0400	120(3)	J0715	0(3)	J1267	150(3)	J1631	9(3)	J2186	600(3)	J2760	2(3)	J3303	24(3)
G9488	2(3)	J0401	400(3)	J0716	4(1)	J1270	16(3)	J1632	700(3)	J2210	5(3)	J2765	18(3)	J3304	64(2)
G9489	2(3)	J0456	4(3)	J0717	400(3)	J1290	60(3)	J1640	672(3)	J2212	240(3)	J2770	7(3)	J3305	0(3)
G9490	2(3)	J0461	800(3)	J0720	15(3)	J1300	120(3)	J1644	50(3)	J2248	300(3)	J2778	10(2)	J3310	0(3)
G9678	1(2)	J0470	2(3)	J0725	10(3)	J1301	60(3)	J1645	10(3)	J2250	30(3)	J2780	16(3)	J3315	6(3)
G9685	1(3)	J0475	8(3)	J0735	50(3)	J1303	360(3)	J1650	30(3)	J2260	16(3)	J2783	60(3)	J3316	6(3)
G9978	2(3)	J0476	2(3)	J0740	2(3)	J1320	0(3)	J1652	20(3)	J2265	400(3)	J2785	4(3)	J3320	0(3)
G9979	2(3)	J0480	1(3)	J0742	500(3)	J1322	150(3)	J1655	0(3)	J2270	15(3)	J2786	500(3)	J3350	0(3)
G9980	2(3)	J0485	1500(3)	J0743	16(3)	J1324	0(3)	J1670	2(3)	J2274	100(3)	J2787	2(3)	J3355	0(3)
G9981	2(3)	J0490	160(3)	J0744	8(3)	J1325	18(3)	J1675	0(3)	J2278	1000(3)	J2788	1(3)	J3357	90(3)
G9982	2(3)	J0500	4(3)	J0745	8(3)	J1327	99(3)	J1700	0(3)	J2280	8(3)	J2790	3(3)	J3358	520(3)
G9983	2(3)	J0515	6(3)	J0770	5(3)	J1330	0(3)	J1710	0(3)	J2300	10(3)	J2791	15(3)	J3360	6(3)
G9984	2(3)	J0517	30(3)	J0775	180(3)	J1335	2(3)	J1720	10(3)	J2310	10(3)	J2792	450(3)	J3364	0(3)
G9985	2(3)	J0520	0(3)	J0780	10(3)	J1364	8(3)	J1726	28(3)	J2315	380(3)	J2793	320(3)	J3365	0(3)
G9986	2(3)	J0558	24(3)	J0791	160(3)	J1380	4(3)	J1729	25(3)	J2320	4(3)	J2794	100(3)	J3370	12(3)
G9987	2(3)	J0561	24(3)	J0795	100(3)	J1410	4(3)	J1730	0(3)	J2323	300(3)	J2795	2400(3)	J3380	300(3)
J0120	1(3)	J0565	200(3)	J0800	3(3)	J1428	450(3)			J2325	34(3)	J2796	150(3)	J3385	80(3)

CPT	MUE	CPT	MUE	CPT	MUE	CPT	MUE	CPT	MUE	CPT	MUE	CPT	MUE	CPT	MUE
J3396	150(3)	J7208	18000(1)	J7606	0(3)	J8540	48(3)	J9198	38(3)	J9330	50(3)	K0554	0(3)	K0868	0(3)
J3397	600(3)	J7209	7500(1)	J7607	0(3)	J8560	6(3)	J9200	20(3)	J9340	4(3)	K0601	0(3)	K0869	0(3)
J3398	150(2)	J7210	22000(1)	J7608	0(3)	J8562	12(3)	J9201	20(3)	J9351	120(3)	K0602	0(3)	K0870	0(3)
J3399	1(3)	J7211	22000(1)	J7609	0(3)	J8565	0(3)	J9202	3(3)	J9352	40(3)	K0603	0(3)	K0871	0(3)
J3400	0(3)	J7212	90000(1)	J7610	0(3)	J8597	4(3)	J9203	180(3)	J9354	600(3)	K0604	0(3)	K0877	0(3)
J3410	16(3)	J7296	0(3)	J7611	0(3)	J8600	40(3)	J9204	160(3)	J9355	105(3)	K0605	0(3)	K0878	0(3)
J3411	8(3)	J7297	0(3)	J7612	0(3)	J8610	20(3)	J9205	215(3)	J9356	60(3)	K0606	0(3)	K0879	0(3)
J3415	6(3)	J7298	0(3)	J7613	0(3)	J8650	0(3)	J9206	42(3)	J9357	4(3)	K0607	0(3)	K0880	0(3)
J3420	1(3)	J7300	0(3)	J7614	0(3)	J8655	1(3)	J9207	90(3)	J9358	900(3)	K0608	0(3)	K0884	0(3)
J3430	50(3)	J7301	0(3)	J7615	0(3)	J8670	180(3)	J9208	15(3)	J9360	40(3)	K0609	0(3)	K0885	0(3)
J3465	120(3)	J7303	0(3)	J7620	0(3)	J8700	120(3)	J9209	55(3)	J9370	4(3)	K0669	0(3)	K0886	0(3)
J3470	3(3)	J7304	0(3)	J7622	0(3)	J8705	22(3)	J9210	1500(3)	J9371	5(3)	K0672	4(3)	K0890	0(3)
J3471	999(1)	J7306	0(3)	J7624	0(3)	J8999	2(3)	J9211	6(3)	J9390	36(3)	K0730	0(3)	K0891	0(3)
J3472	2(3)	J7307	0(3)	J7626	0(3)	J9000	20(3)	J9212	0(3)	J9395	20(3)	K0733	0(3)	K0898	1(2)
J3473	450(3)	J7308	3(3)	J7627	0(3)	J9015	1(3)	J9213	12(3)	J9400	500(3)	K0738	0(3)	K0899	0(3)
J3475	80(3)	J7309	0(3)	J7628	0(3)	J9017	30(3)	J9214	100(3)	J9600	4(3)	K0740	0(3)	K0900	0(3)
J3480	200(3)	J7310	0(3)	J7629	0(3)	J9019	60(3)	J9215	0(3)	K0001	0(3)	K0743	0(3)	K1001	1(3)
J3485	160(3)	J7311	118(2)	J7631	0(3)	J9020	0(3)	J9216	0(3)	K0002	0(3)	K0800	0(3)	K1002	1(3)
J3486	4(3)	J7312	14(2)	J7632	0(3)	J9022	168(3)	J9217	6(3)	K0003	0(3)	K0801	0(3)	K1003	1(3)
J3489	5(3)	J7313	38(2)	J7633	0(3)	J9023	140(3)	J9218	1(3)	K0004	0(3)	K0802	0(3)	K1004	1(3)
J3520	0(3)	J7314	36(2)	J7634	0(3)	J9025	300(3)	J9219	0(3)	K0005	0(3)	K0806	0(3)	K1005	1(3)
J3530	0(3)	J7315	2(3)	J7635	0(3)	J9027	100(3)	J9223	120(3)	K0006	0(3)	K0807	0(3)	K1006	1(2)
J3535	0(3)	J7316	3(3)	J7636	0(3)	J9030	50(3)	J9225	1(3)	K0007	0(3)	K0808	0(3)	K1007	1(2)
J3570	0(3)	J7318	120(3)	J7637	0(3)	J9032	300(3)	J9226	1(3)	K0008	0(3)	K0812	0(3)	K1009	1(2)
J7030	20(3)	J7320	50(3)	J7638	0(3)	J9033	300(3)	J9227	150(3)	K0009	0(3)	K0813	0(3)	K1013	1(3)
J7040	12(3)	J7321	2(2)	J7639	0(3)	J9034	360(3)	J9228	1100(3)	K0010	0(3)	K0814	0(3)	K1014	1(3)
J7042	12(3)	J7322	48(3)	J7640	0(3)	J9035	180(3)	J9229	27(3)	K0011	0(3)	K0815	0(3)	K1015	2(2)
J7050	20(3)	J7323	2(2)	J7641	0(3)	J9036	360(3)	J9230	5(3)	K0012	0(3)	K0816	0(3)	K1016	1(2)
J7060	10(3)	J7324	2(2)	J7642	0(3)	J9039	210(3)	J9245	11(3)	K0013	0(3)	K0820	0(3)	K1017	3(2)
J7070	7(3)	J7325	96(3)	J7643	0(3)	J9040	4(3)	J9246	300(3)	K0014	0(3)	K0821	0(3)	K1018	1(2)
J7100	2(3)	J7326	2(2)	J7644	0(3)	J9041	35(3)	J9250	50(3)	K0015	0(3)	K0822	0(3)	K1019	3(2)
J7110	3(3)	J7327	2(2)	J7645	0(3)	J9042	200(3)	J9260	20(3)	K0017	0(3)	K0823	0(3)	K1020	1(2)
J7120	20(3)	J7328	336(3)	J7647	0(3)	J9043	60(3)	J9261	80(3)	K0018	0(3)	K0824	0(3)	L0112	1(2)
J7121	5(3)	J7329	50(2)	J7648	0(3)	J9044	35(3)	J9262	700(3)	K0019	0(3)	K0825	0(3)	L0113	1(2)
J7131	500(3)	J7330	1(3)	J7649	0(3)	J9045	22(3)	J9263	700(3)	K0020	0(3)	K0826	0(3)	L0120	1(2)
J7169	180(3)	J7331	40(3)	J7650	0(3)	J9047	160(3)	J9264	600(3)	K0037	0(3)	K0827	0(3)	L0130	1(2)
J7170	1800(3)	J7332	40(3)	J7657	0(3)	J9050	6(3)	J9266	2(3)	K0038	0(3)	K0828	0(3)	L0140	1(2)
J7175	9000(1)	J7336	1120(3)	J7658	0(3)	J9055	150(3)	J9267	750(3)	K0039	0(3)	K0829	0(3)	L0150	1(2)
J7177	10500(3)	J7340	1(3)	J7659	0(3)	J9057	60(3)	J9268	1(3)	K0040	0(3)	K0830	0(3)	L0160	1(2)
J7178	7700(1)	J7342	10(3)	J7660	0(3)	J9060	24(3)	J9269	200(3)	K0041	0(3)	K0831	0(3)	L0170	1(2)
J7179	9600(1)	J7345	200(3)	J7665	0(3)	J9065	100(3)	J9270	0(3)	K0042	0(3)	K0835	0(3)	L0172	1(2)
J7180	6000(1)	J7351	20(2)	J7667	0(3)	J9070	55(3)	J9271	400(3)	K0043	0(3)	K0836	0(3)	L0174	1(2)
J7181	3850(1)	J7352	16(3)	J7668	0(3)	J9098	5(3)	J9280	12(3)	K0044	0(3)	K0837	0(3)	L0180	1(2)
J7182	22000(1)	J7500	15(3)	J7669	0(3)	J9100	120(3)	J9281	80(3)	K0045	0(3)	K0838	0(3)	L0190	1(2)
J7183	9600(1)	J7501	8(3)	J7670	0(3)	J9118	750(3)	J9285	200(3)	K0046	0(3)	K0839	0(3)	L0200	1(2)
J7185	22000(1)	J7502	60(3)	J7674	100(3)	J9119	350(3)	J9293	8(3)	K0047	0(3)	K0840	0(3)	L0220	1(3)
J7186	9600(1)	J7503	120(3)	J7676	0(3)	J9120	5(3)	J9295	800(3)	K0050	0(3)	K0841	0(3)	L0450	1(2)
J7187	9600(1)	J7504	15(3)	J7677	175(3)	J9130	24(3)	J9299	480(3)	K0051	0(3)	K0842	0(3)	L0452	1(2)
J7188	22000(1)	J7505	1(3)	J7680	0(3)	J9144	180(3)	J9301	100(3)	K0052	0(3)	K0843	0(3)	L0454	1(2)
J7189	26000(1)	J7507	40(3)	J7681	0(3)	J9145	240(3)	J9302	200(3)	K0053	0(3)	K0848	0(3)	L0455	1(2)
J7190	22000(1)	J7508	300(3)	J7682	0(3)	J9150	12(3)	J9303	90(3)	K0056	0(3)	K0849	0(3)	L0456	1(2)
J7191	0(3)	J7509	60(3)	J7683	0(3)	J9151	12(3)	J9304	150(3)	K0065	0(3)	K0850	0(3)	L0457	1(2)
J7192	22000(1)	J7510	60(3)	J7684	0(3)	J9153	132(3)	J9305	150(3)	K0069	0(3)	K0851	0(3)	L0458	1(2)
J7193	20000(1)	J7511	9(3)	J7685	0(3)	J9155	240(3)	J9306	840(3)	K0070	0(3)	K0852	0(3)	L0460	1(2)
J7194	9000(1)	J7512	300(3)	J7686	0(3)	J9160	0(3)	J9307	80(3)	K0071	0(3)	K0853	0(3)	L0462	1(2)
J7195	20000(1)	J7513	0(3)	J7699	0(3)	J9165	0(3)	J9308	280(3)	K0072	0(3)	K0854	0(3)	L0464	1(2)
J7196	175(3)	J7515	90(3)	J7799	2(3)	J9171	240(3)	J9309	280(3)	K0073	0(3)	K0855	0(3)	L0466	1(2)
J7197	6300(1)	J7516	4(3)	J7999	6(3)	J9173	150(3)	J9311	160(3)	K0077	0(3)	K0856	0(3)	L0467	1(2)
J7198	30000(1)	J7517	16(3)	J8498	1(3)	J9175	10(3)	J9312	150(3)	K0098	0(3)	K0857	0(3)	L0468	1(2)
J7200	20000(1)	J7518	12(3)	J8499	0(3)	J9176	3000(3)	J9313	600(3)	K0105	0(3)	K0858	0(3)	L0469	1(2)
J7201	9000(1)	J7520	40(3)	J8501	57(3)	J9177	520(3)	J9315	40(3)	K0108	0(3)	K0859	0(3)	L0470	1(2)
J7202	11550(1)	J7525	2(3)	J8510	5(3)	J9178	150(3)	J9316	120(3)	K0195	0(3)	K0860	0(3)	L0472	1(2)
J7203	12000(1)	J7527	20(3)	J8515	0(3)	J9179	50(3)	J9317	648(3)	K0455	0(3)	K0861	0(3)	L0480	1(2)
J7204	19500(1)	J7599	1(3)	J8520	50(3)	J9181	100(3)	J9320	4(3)	K0462	0(3)	K0862	0(3)	L0482	1(2)
J7205	9750(1)	J7604	0(3)	J8521	15(3)	J9185	2(3)	J9325	400(3)	K0552	0(3)	K0863	0(3)	L0484	1(2)
J7207	22500(1)	J7605	0(3)	J8530	60(3)	J9190	20(3)	J9328	400(3)	K0553	0(3)	K0864	0(3)	L0486	1(2)

CPT	MUE	CPT	MUE	CPT	MUE	CPT	MUE	CPT	MUE	CPT	MUE	CPT	MUE	CPT	MUE
L0488	1(2)	L1220	1(3)	L2000	2(2)	L2492	4(2)	L3213	1(3)	L3677	1(2)	L4055	2(2)	L5614	2(2)
L0490	1(2)	L1230	1(2)	L2005	2(2)	L2500	2(2)	L3214	1(3)	L3678	1(2)	L4060	2(2)	L5616	2(2)
L0491	1(2)	L1240	1(3)	L2006	0(3)	L2510	2(2)	L3215	0(3)	L3702	2(2)	L4070	2(3)	L5617	2(3)
L0492	1(2)	L1250	2(3)	L2010	2(2)	L2520	2(2)	L3216	0(3)	L3710	2(2)	L4080	2(2)	L5618	4(3)
L0621	1(2)	L1260	1(3)	L2020	2(2)	L2525	2(2)	L3217	0(3)	L3720	2(2)	L4090	4(2)	L5620	4(3)
L0622	1(2)	L1270	3(3)	L2030	2(2)	L2526	2(2)	L3219	0(3)	L3730	2(2)	L4100	2(2)	L5622	4(3)
L0623	1(2)	L1280	2(3)	L2034	2(2)	L2530	2(2)	L3221	0(3)	L3740	2(2)	L4110	4(2)	L5624	4(3)
L0624	1(2)	L1290	2(3)	L2035	2(2)	L2540	2(2)	L3222	0(3)	L3760	2(2)	L4130	2(2)	L5626	4(3)
L0625	1(2)	L1300	1(2)	L2036	2(2)	L2550	2(2)	L3224	2(2)	L3761	2(2)	L4205	8(3)	L5628	2(3)
L0626	1(2)	L1310	1(2)	L2037	2(2)	L2570	2(2)	L3225	2(2)	L3762	2(2)	L4210	4(3)	L5629	2(2)
L0627	1(2)	L1499	1(3)	L2038	2(2)	L2580	2(2)	L3230	2(2)	L3763	2(2)	L4350	2(2)	L5630	2(2)
L0628	1(2)	L1600	1(2)	L2040	1(2)	L2600	2(2)	L3250	2(2)	L3764	2(2)	L4360	2(2)	L5631	2(2)
L0629	1(2)	L1610	1(2)	L2050	1(2)	L2610	2(2)	L3251	2(2)	L3765	2(2)	L4361	2(2)	L5632	2(2)
L0630	1(2)	L1620	1(2)	L2060	1(2)	L2620	2(2)	L3252	2(2)	L3766	2(2)	L4370	2(2)	L5634	2(2)
L0631	1(2)	L1630	1(2)	L2070	1(2)	L2622	2(2)	L3253	2(2)	L3806	2(2)	L4386	2(2)	L5636	2(2)
L0632	1(2)	L1640	1(2)	L2080	1(2)	L2624	2(2)	L3254	1(3)	L3807	2(2)	L4387	2(2)	L5637	2(2)
L0633	1(2)	L1650	1(2)	L2090	1(2)	L2627	1(3)	L3255	1(3)	L3808	2(2)	L4392	2(3)	L5638	2(2)
L0634	1(2)	L1652	1(2)	L2106	2(2)	L2628	1(3)	L3257	1(3)	L3809	2(2)	L4394	2(3)	L5639	2(2)
L0635	1(2)	L1660	1(2)	L2108	2(2)	L2630	1(2)	L3260	0(3)	L3891	0(3)	L4396	2(2)	L5640	2(2)
L0636	1(2)	L1680	1(2)	L2112	2(2)	L2640	1(2)	L3265	1(3)	L3900	2(2)	L4397	2(2)	L5642	2(2)
L0637	1(2)	L1685	1(2)	L2114	2(2)	L2650	2(3)	L3300	4(3)	L3901	2(2)	L4398	2(2)	L5643	2(2)
L0638	1(2)	L1686	1(3)	L2116	2(2)	L2660	1(3)	L3310	4(3)	L3904	2(2)	L4631	2(2)	L5644	2(2)
L0639	1(2)	L1690	1(2)	L2126	2(2)	L2670	2(3)	L3330	2(2)	L3905	2(2)	L5000	2(3)	L5645	2(2)
L0640	1(2)	L1700	1(2)	L2128	2(2)	L2680	2(3)	L3332	2(2)	L3906	2(2)	L5010	2(2)	L5646	2(2)
L0641	1(2)	L1710	1(2)	L2132	2(2)	L2750	8(3)	L3334	4(3)	L3908	2(2)	L5020	2(2)	L5647	2(2)
L0642	1(2)	L1720	2(2)	L2134	2(2)	L2755	8(3)	L3340	2(2)	L3912	2(3)	L5050	2(2)	L5648	2(2)
L0643	1(2)	L1730	1(2)	L2136	2(2)	L2760	8(2)	L3350	2(2)	L3913	2(2)	L5060	2(2)	L5649	2(2)
L0648	1(2)	L1755	2(2)	L2180	2(2)	L2768	4(2)	L3360	2(2)	L3915	2(2)	L5100	2(2)	L5650	2(2)
L0649	1(2)	L1810	2(2)	L2182	4(2)	L2780	8(3)	L3370	2(2)	L3916	2(3)	L5105	2(2)	L5651	2(2)
L0650	1(2)	L1812	2(2)	L2184	4(2)	L2785	4(2)	L3380	2(2)	L3917	2(2)	L5150	2(2)	L5652	2(2)
L0651	1(2)	L1820	2(2)	L2186	4(2)	L2795	2(2)	L3390	2(2)	L3918	2(2)	L5160	2(2)	L5653	2(2)
L0700	1(2)	L1830	2(2)	L2188	2(2)	L2800	2(2)	L3400	2(2)	L3919	2(2)	L5200	2(2)	L5654	2(2)
L0710	1(2)	L1831	2(2)	L2190	2(2)	L2810	4(2)	L3410	2(2)	L3921	2(2)	L5210	2(2)	L5655	2(2)
L0810	1(2)	L1832	2(2)	L2192	2(2)	L2820	2(3)	L3420	2(2)	L3923	2(2)	L5220	2(2)	L5656	2(2)
L0820	1(2)	L1833	2(2)	L2200	4(2)	L2830	2(2)	L3430	2(2)	L3924	2(2)	L5230	2(2)	L5658	2(2)
L0830	1(2)	L1834	2(2)	L2210	4(2)	L2861	0(3)	L3440	2(2)	L3925	4(3)	L5250	2(2)	L5661	2(2)
L0859	1(2)	L1836	2(2)	L2220	4(2)	L2999	2(3)	L3450	2(2)	L3927	4(3)	L5270	2(2)	L5665	2(2)
L0861	1(2)	L1840	2(2)	L2230	2(2)	L3000	2(3)	L3455	2(2)	L3929	2(2)	L5280	2(2)	L5666	2(2)
L0970	1(2)	L1843	2(2)	L2232	2(2)	L3001	2(3)	L3460	2(2)	L3930	2(2)	L5301	2(2)	L5668	2(2)
L0972	1(2)	L1844	2(2)	L2240	2(2)	L3002	2(3)	L3465	2(2)	L3931	2(2)	L5312	2(2)	L5670	2(2)
L0974	1(2)	L1845	2(2)	L2250	2(2)	L3003	2(3)	L3470	2(2)	L3933	3(3)	L5321	2(2)	L5671	2(2)
L0976	1(2)	L1846	2(2)	L2260	2(2)	L3010	2(3)	L3480	2(2)	L3935	3(3)	L5331	2(2)	L5672	2(2)
L0978	2(3)	L1847	2(2)	L2265	2(2)	L3020	2(3)	L3485	2(2)	L3956	4(3)	L5341	2(2)	L5673	4(3)
L0980	1(2)	L1848	2(2)	L2270	2(3)	L3030	2(3)	L3500	2(2)	L3960	1(3)	L5400	2(2)	L5676	2(2)
L0982	1(3)	L1850	2(2)	L2275	2(3)	L3031	2(3)	L3510	2(2)	L3961	1(3)	L5410	2(2)	L5677	2(2)
L0984	3(3)	L1851	2(2)	L2280	2(2)	L3040	2(3)	L3520	2(2)	L3962	1(3)	L5420	2(2)	L5678	2(2)
L0999	1(3)	L1852	2(2)	L2300	1(2)	L3050	2(3)	L3530	2(2)	L3967	1(3)	L5430	2(2)	L5679	4(3)
L1000	1(2)	L1860	2(2)	L2310	1(2)	L3060	2(3)	L3540	2(2)	L3971	1(3)	L5450	2(2)	L5680	2(2)
L1001	1(2)	L1900	2(2)	L2320	2(3)	L3070	2(3)	L3550	2(2)	L3973	1(3)	L5460	2(2)	L5681	2(2)
L1005	1(2)	L1902	2(2)	L2330	2(3)	L3080	2(3)	L3560	2(2)	L3975	1(3)	L5500	2(2)	L5682	2(2)
L1010	2(2)	L1904	2(2)	L2335	2(2)	L3090	2(3)	L3570	2(2)	L3976	1(3)	L5505	2(2)	L5683	2(2)
L1020	2(3)	L1906	2(2)	L2340	2(2)	L3100	2(2)	L3580	2(2)	L3977	1(3)	L5510	2(2)	L5684	2(3)
L1025	1(3)	L1907	2(2)	L2350	2(2)	L3140	1(2)	L3590	2(2)	L3978	1(3)	L5520	2(2)	L5685	4(3)
L1030	1(3)	L1910	2(2)	L2360	2(2)	L3150	1(2)	L3595	2(2)	L3980	2(2)	L5530	2(2)	L5686	2(2)
L1040	1(3)	L1920	2(2)	L2370	2(2)	L3160	2(2)	L3600	2(2)	L3981	2(2)	L5535	2(2)	L5688	2(3)
L1050	1(3)	L1930	2(2)	L2375	2(2)	L3170	2(2)	L3610	2(2)	L3982	2(2)	L5540	2(2)	L5690	2(3)
L1060	1(3)	L1932	2(2)	L2380	2(3)	L3201	1(3)	L3620	2(2)	L3984	2(2)	L5560	2(2)	L5692	2(2)
L1070	2(2)	L1940	2(2)	L2385	4(2)	L3202	1(3)	L3630	2(2)	L3999	2(3)	L5570	2(2)	L5694	2(2)
L1080	2(2)	L1945	2(2)	L2387	4(2)	L3203	1(3)	L3640	1(2)	L4000	1(2)	L5580	2(2)	L5695	2(3)
L1085	1(2)	L1950	2(2)	L2390	4(2)	L3204	1(3)	L3649	2(3)	L4002	4(3)	L5585	2(2)	L5696	2(2)
L1090	1(3)	L1951	2(2)	L2395	4(2)	L3206	1(3)	L3650	2(2)	L4010	2(2)	L5590	2(2)	L5697	2(2)
L1100	2(2)	L1960	2(2)	L2397	4(3)	L3207	1(3)	L3660	2(2)	L4020	2(2)	L5595	2(2)	L5698	2(2)
L1110	2(2)	L1970	2(2)	L2405	4(2)	L3208	1(3)	L3670	1(3)	L4030	2(2)	L5600	2(2)	L5699	2(3)
L1120	3(3)	L1971	2(2)	L2415	4(2)	L3209	1(3)	L3671	1(3)	L4040	2(2)	L5610	2(2)	L5700	2(2)
L1200	1(2)	L1980	2(2)	L2425	4(2)	L3211	1(3)	L3674	1(3)	L4045	2(2)	L5611	2(2)	L5701	2(2)
L1210	2(3)	L1990	2(2)	L2430	4(2)	L3212	1(3)	L3675	1(2)	L4050	2(2)	L5613	2(2)	L5702	2(2)

CPT	MUE	CPT	MUE	CPT	MUE	CPT	MUE	CPT	MUE	CPT	MUE	CPT	MUE	CPT	MUE
L5703	2(2)	L5984	2(2)	L6648	2(2)	L7008	2(2)	L8470	14(3)	M0243	1(2)	Q0084	2(3)	Q1005	0(3)
L5704	2(2)	L5985	2(2)	L6650	2(2)	L7009	2(2)	L8480	12(3)	M0244	1(2)	Q0085	2(3)	Q2004	1(3)
L5705	2(2)	L5986	2(2)	L6655	4(3)	L7040	2(2)	L8485	12(3)	M0245	1(2)	Q0091	1(3)	Q2009	100(3)
L5706	2(2)	L5987	2(2)	L6660	4(3)	L7045	2(2)	L8499	1(3)	M0246	1(2)	Q0092	2(3)	Q2017	12(3)
L5707	2(2)	L5988	2(2)	L6665	4(3)	L7170	2(2)	L8500	1(2)	M0247	1(2)	Q0111	2(3)	Q2026	30(3)
L5710	2(2)	L5990	2(2)	L6670	2(2)	L7180	2(2)	L8501	2(3)	M0248	1(2)	Q0112	3(3)	Q2028	1470(3)
L5711	2(2)	L5999	2(3)	L6672	2(2)	L7181	2(2)	L8507	3(3)	M0300	0(3)	Q0113	1(3)	Q2034	1(2)
L5712	2(2)	L6000	2(2)	L6675	2(2)	L7185	2(2)	L8509	1(3)	M0301	0(3)	Q0114	1(3)	Q2035	1(2)
L5714	2(2)	L6010	2(2)	L6676	2(2)	L7186	2(2)	L8510	1(2)	P2028	1(2)	Q0115	1(3)	Q2036	1(2)
L5716	2(2)	L6020	2(2)	L6677	2(2)	L7190	2(2)	L8511	1(3)	P2029	1(2)	Q0138	510(3)	Q2037	1(2)
L5718	2(2)	L6026	2(2)	L6680	4(3)	L7191	2(2)	L8512	1(3)	P2031	0(3)	Q0139	510(3)	Q2038	1(2)
L5722	2(2)	L6050	2(2)	L6682	4(3)	L7259	2(2)	L8513	1(3)	P2033	1(2)	Q0144	0(3)	Q2039	1(2)
L5724	2(2)	L6055	2(2)	L6684	4(3)	L7360	1(3)	L8514	1(3)	P2038	1(2)	Q0161	66(3)	Q2043	1(2)
L5726	2(2)	L6100	2(2)	L6686	2(2)	L7362	1(2)	L8515	1(3)	P3000	1(3)	Q0162	24(3)	Q2049	10(3)
L5728	2(2)	L6110	2(2)	L6687	2(2)	L7364	1(3)	L8600	2(3)	P3001	1(3)	Q0163	6(3)	Q2050	20(3)
L5780	2(2)	L6120	2(2)	L6688	2(2)	L7366	1(2)	L8603	4(3)	P7001	0(3)	Q0164	8(3)	Q2052	0(3)
L5781	2(2)	L6130	2(2)	L6689	2(2)	L7367	2(3)	L8604	3(3)	P9010	4(3)	Q0166	2(3)	Q3014	2(3)
L5782	2(2)	L6200	2(2)	L6690	2(2)	L7368	2(2)	L8605	4(3)	P9011	4(3)	Q0167	108(3)	Q3027	30(3)
L5785	2(2)	L6205	2(2)	L6691	2(3)	L7400	2(2)	L8606	5(3)	P9012	12(3)	Q0169	12(3)	Q3028	0(3)
L5790	2(2)	L6250	2(2)	L6692	2(3)	L7401	2(2)	L8607	20(3)	P9016	12(3)	Q0173	5(3)	Q3031	1(3)
L5795	2(2)	L6300	2(2)	L6693	2(2)	L7402	2(2)	L8609	1(3)	P9017	24(3)	Q0174	0(3)	Q4001	1(3)
L5810	2(2)	L6310	2(2)	L6694	2(3)	L7403	2(2)	L8610	2(3)	P9019	12(3)	Q0175	6(3)	Q4002	1(3)
L5811	2(2)	L6320	2(2)	L6695	2(3)	L7404	2(2)	L8612	1(3)	P9020	5(3)	Q0177	16(3)	Q4003	2(3)
L5812	2(2)	L6350	2(2)	L6696	2(2)	L7405	2(2)	L8613	2(3)	P9021	8(3)	Q0180	1(3)	Q4004	2(3)
L5814	2(2)	L6360	2(2)	L6697	2(2)	L7499	2(3)	L8614	2(3)	P9022	12(3)	Q0181	2(3)	Q4012	2(3)
L5816	2(2)	L6370	2(2)	L6698	2(2)	L7510	4(3)	L8615	2(3)	P9023	15(3)	Q0243	1(3)	Q4013	2(3)
L5818	2(2)	L6380	2(2)	L6703	2(2)	L7600	0(3)	L8616	2(3)	P9031	12(3)	Q0244	1(3)	Q4014	2(3)
L5822	2(2)	L6382	2(2)	L6704	2(2)	L7700	2(1)	L8617	2(3)	P9032	12(3)	Q0245	1(3)	Q4018	2(3)
L5824	2(2)	L6384	2(2)	L6706	2(2)	L7900	0(3)	L8618	2(3)	P9033	12(3)	Q0247	1(2)	Q4021	2(3)
L5826	2(2)	L6386	2(2)	L6707	2(2)	L7902	0(3)	L8619	2(3)	P9034	4(3)	Q0477	1(1)	Q4025	1(3)
L5828	2(2)	L6388	2(2)	L6708	2(2)	L8000	6(3)	L8621	360(3)	P9035	4(3)	Q0478	1(3)	Q4026	1(3)
L5830	2(2)	L6400	2(2)	L6709	2(2)	L8001	4(3)	L8622	2(3)	P9036	4(3)	Q0479	1(3)	Q4027	1(3)
L5840	2(2)	L6450	2(2)	L6711	2(2)	L8002	4(3)	L8625	1(3)	P9037	4(3)	Q0480	1(3)	Q4028	1(3)
L5845	2(2)	L6500	2(2)	L6712	2(2)	L8010	4(3)	L8627	2(2)	P9038	4(3)	Q0481	1(2)	Q4030	2(3)
L5848	2(2)	L6550	2(2)	L6713	2(2)	L8015	4(3)	L8628	2(2)	P9039	2(3)	Q0482	1(3)	Q4037	2(3)
L5850	2(2)	L6570	2(2)	L6714	2(2)	L8020	4(3)	L8629	2(2)	P9040	8(3)	Q0483	1(3)	Q4042	2(3)
L5855	2(2)	L6580	2(2)	L6715	5(3)	L8030	2(3)	L8631	2(3)	P9041	100(3)	Q0484	1(3)	Q4046	2(3)
L5856	2(2)	L6582	2(2)	L6721	2(2)	L8031	2(3)	L8641	4(3)	P9043	10(3)	Q0485	1(3)	Q4050	2(3)
L5857	2(2)	L6584	2(2)	L6722	2(2)	L8032	2(2)	L8642	2(3)	P9044	20(3)	Q0486	1(3)	Q4051	2(3)
L5858	2(2)	L6586	2(2)	L6805	2(2)	L8033	0(3)	L8658	3(3)	P9045	20(3)	Q0487	1(3)	Q4074	0(3)
L5859	2(2)	L6588	2(2)	L6810	2(3)	L8035	2(3)	L8659	4(3)	P9046	40(3)	Q0488	1(3)	Q4081	400(3)
L5910	2(2)	L6590	2(2)	L6880	2(2)	L8039	2(3)	L8670	3(3)	P9047	20(3)	Q0489	1(3)	Q5101	1500(3)
L5920	2(2)	L6600	2(2)	L6881	2(2)	L8040	1(2)	L8679	3(3)	P9048	2(3)	Q0490	1(3)	Q5103	150(3)
L5925	2(3)	L6605	2(2)	L6882	2(2)	L8041	1(2)	L8680	0(3)	P9050	1(3)	Q0491	1(3)	Q5104	150(3)
L5930	2(2)	L6610	2(2)	L6883	2(2)	L8042	2(2)	L8681	1(3)	P9051	4(3)	Q0492	1(3)	Q5105	400(3)
L5940	2(2)	L6611	2(3)	L6884	2(2)	L8043	1(2)	L8682	2(3)	P9052	3(3)	Q0493	1(3)	Q5106	60(3)
L5950	2(2)	L6615	2(2)	L6885	2(2)	L8044	1(2)	L8683	1(3)	P9053	3(3)	Q0494	1(3)	Q5107	170(3)
L5960	2(2)	L6616	2(2)	L6890	2(3)	L8045	2(2)	L8684	1(3)	P9054	2(3)	Q0495	1(3)	Q5108	12(3)
L5961	1(3)	L6620	2(2)	L6895	2(3)	L8046	1(3)	L8685	0(3)	P9055	2(3)	Q0497	2(3)	Q5109	150(3)
L5962	2(2)	L6621	2(2)	L6900	2(2)	L8047	1(2)	L8686	0(3)	P9056	3(3)	Q0498	1(3)	Q5110	1500(3)
L5964	2(2)	L6623	2(2)	L6905	2(2)	L8048	1(3)	L8687	0(3)	P9057	4(3)	Q0499	1(3)	Q5111	12(3)
L5966	2(2)	L6624	2(2)	L6910	2(2)	L8049	6(3)	L8688	0(3)	P9058	4(3)	Q0501	1(3)	Q5112	120(3)
L5968	2(2)	L6625	2(2)	L6915	2(3)	L8300	1(3)	L8689	1(3)	P9059	15(3)	Q0502	1(3)	Q5113	120(3)
L5969	0(3)	L6628	2(2)	L6920	2(2)	L8310	1(3)	L8690	2(2)	P9060	4(3)	Q0503	3(3)	Q5114	120(3)
L5970	2(2)	L6629	2(2)	L6925	2(2)	L8320	2(3)	L8691	1(3)	P9070	15(3)	Q0504	1(3)	Q5115	150(3)
L5971	2(2)	L6630	2(2)	L6930	2(2)	L8330	2(3)	L8692	0(3)	P9071	15(3)	Q0506	8(3)	Q5116	120(3)
L5972	2(2)	L6632	4(3)	L6935	2(2)	L8400	12(3)	L8693	1(3)	P9073	4(3)	Q0507	1(3)	Q5117	120(3)
L5973	2(3)	L6635	2(2)	L6940	2(2)	L8410	12(3)	L8694	1(3)	P9099	1(3)	Q0508	24(3)	Q5118	230(3)
L5974	2(2)	L6637	2(2)	L6945	2(2)	L8415	6(3)	L8695	1(3)	P9100	12(3)	Q0509	2(3)	Q5119	150(3)
L5975	2(2)	L6638	2(2)	L6950	2(2)	L8417	12(3)	L8696	1(3)	P9603	100(3)	Q0510	1(2)	Q5120	12(3)
L5976	2(2)	L6640	2(2)	L6955	2(2)	L8420	14(3)	L8701	1(3)	P9604	2(3)	Q0511	1(2)	Q5121	150(3)
L5978	2(2)	L6641	2(3)	L6960	2(2)	L8430	12(3)	L8702	1(3)	P9612	1(3)	Q0512	4(3)	Q5122	12(3)
L5979	2(2)	L6642	2(3)	L6965	2(2)	L8435	12(3)	M0075	0(3)	P9615	1(3)	Q0513	1(2)	Q9001	1(3)
L5980	2(2)	L6645	2(2)	L6970	2(2)	L8440	4(3)	M0076	0(3)	Q0035	1(3)	Q0514	1(2)	Q9002	1(3)
L5981	2(2)	L6646	2(2)	L6975	2(2)	L8460	4(3)	M0100	0(3)	Q0081	2(3)	Q0515	0(3)	Q9003	1(3)
L5982	2(2)	L6647	2(2)	L7007	2(2)	L8465	4(3)	M0201	1(2)	Q0083	2(3)	Q1004	0(3)	Q9950	5(3)

CPT	MUE	CPT	MUE	CPT	MUE	CPT	MUE	CPT	MUE	CPT	MUE	CPT	MUE	CPT	MUE
Q9951	0(3)	V2100	2(3)	V2211	2(3)	V2399	2(3)	V2630	2(2)	V5010	0(3)	V5230	0(3)	V5269	0(3)
Q9953	10(3)	V2101	2(3)	V2212	2(3)	V2410	2(3)	V2631	2(2)	V5011	0(3)	V5240	0(3)	V5270	0(3)
Q9954	18(3)	V2102	2(3)	V2213	2(3)	V2430	2(3)	V2632	2(2)	V5014	0(3)	V5241	0(3)	V5271	0(3)
Q9955	0(3)	V2103	2(3)	V2214	2(3)	V2499	2(3)	V2700	2(3)	V5020	0(3)	V5242	0(3)	V5272	0(3)
Q9956	9(3)	V2104	2(3)	V2215	2(3)	V2500	2(3)	V2702	0(3)	V5030	0(3)	V5243	0(3)	V5273	0(3)
Q9957	3(3)	V2105	2(3)	V2218	2(3)	V2501	2(3)	V2710	2(3)	V5040	0(3)	V5244	0(3)	V5274	0(3)
Q9958	600(3)	V2106	2(3)	V2219	2(3)	V2502	2(3)	V2715	4(3)	V5050	0(3)	V5245	0(3)	V5275	0(3)
Q9959	0(3)	V2107	2(3)	V2220	2(3)	V2503	2(3)	V2718	2(3)	V5060	0(3)	V5246	0(3)	V5281	0(3)
Q9960	250(3)	V2108	2(3)	V2221	2(3)	V2510	2(3)	V2730	2(3)	V5070	0(3)	V5247	0(3)	V5282	0(3)
Q9961	200(3)	V2109	2(3)	V2299	2(3)	V2511	2(3)	V2744	2(3)	V5080	0(3)	V5248	0(3)	V5283	0(3)
Q9962	200(3)	V2110	2(3)	V2300	2(3)	V2512	2(3)	V2745	2(3)	V5090	0(3)	V5249	0(3)	V5284	0(3)
Q9963	240(3)	V2111	2(3)	V2301	2(3)	V2513	2(3)	V2750	2(3)	V5095	0(3)	V5250	0(3)	V5285	0(3)
Q9964	0(3)	V2112	2(3)	V2302	2(3)	V2520	2(3)	V2755	2(3)	V5100	0(3)	V5251	0(3)	V5286	0(3)
Q9966	250(3)	V2113	2(3)	V2303	2(3)	V2521	2(3)	V2756	0(3)	V5110	0(3)	V5252	0(3)	V5287	0(3)
Q9967	300(3)	V2114	2(3)	V2304	2(3)	V2522	2(3)	V2760	0(3)	V5120	0(3)	V5253	0(3)	V5288	0(3)
Q9969	3(3)	V2115	2(3)	V2305	2(3)	V2523	2(3)	V2761	0(2)	V5130	0(3)	V5254	0(3)	V5289	0(3)
Q9982	1(3)	V2118	2(3)	V2306	2(3)	V2524	2(3)	V2762	2(3)	V5140	0(3)	V5255	0(3)	V5290	0(3)
Q9983	1(3)	V2121	2(3)	V2307	2(3)	V2530	2(3)	V2770	2(3)	V5150	0(3)	V5256	0(3)	V5298	0(3)
Q9991	1(2)	V2199	2(3)	V2308	2(3)	V2531	2(3)	V2780	2(3)	V5160	0(3)	V5257	0(3)	V5299	1(3)
Q9992	1(2)	V2200	2(3)	V2309	2(3)	V2599	2(3)	V2781	0(2)	V5171	0(3)	V5258	0(3)	V5336	0(3)
R0070	2(3)	V2201	2(3)	V2310	2(3)	V2600	0(2)	V2782	2(3)	V5172	0(3)	V5259	0(3)	V5362	0(3)
R0075	2(3)	V2202	2(3)	V2311	2(3)	V2610	0(2)	V2783	2(3)	V5181	0(3)	V5260	0(3)	V5363	0(3)
R0076	1(3)	V2203	2(3)	V2312	2(3)	V2615	0(2)	V2784	2(3)	V5190	0(3)	V5261	0(3)	V5364	0(3)
U0001	2(3)	V2204	2(3)	V2313	2(3)	V2623	2(2)	V2785	2(2)	V5200	0(3)	V5262	0(3)		
U0002	2(3)	V2205	2(3)	V2314	2(3)	V2624	2(2)	V2786	0(3)	V5211	0(3)	V5263	0(3)		
U0003	2(3)	V2206	2(3)	V2315	2(3)	V2625	2(2)	V2787	0(3)	V5212	0(3)	V5264	0(3)		
U0004	2(3)	V2207	2(3)	V2318	2(3)	V2626	2(2)	V2788	0(3)	V5213	0(3)	V5265	0(3)		
U0005	1(3)	V2208	2(3)	V2319	2(3)	V2627	2(2)	V2790	1(3)	V5214	0(3)	V5266	0(3)		
V2020	1(3)	V2209	2(3)	V2320	2(3)	V2628	2(3)	V2797	0(3)	V5215	0(3)	V5267	0(3)		
V2025	0(3)	V2210	2(3)	V2321	2(3)	V2629	2(2)	V5008	0(3)	V5221	0(3)	V5268	0(3)		

CPT © 2021 American Medical Association. All Rights Reserved.

Inpatient Only Procedures—This appendix identifies services with the status indicator C. Medicare will not pay an OPPS hospital or ASC when they are performed on a Medicare patient as an outpatient. Physicians should refer to this list when scheduling Medicare patients for surgical procedures. CMS updates this list quarterly. The following was updated 10/01/2021.

00176 Anesth pharyngeal surgery	0569T Ttvr perq appr 1st prosth	32150 Removal of lung lesion(s)
00211 Anesth cran surg hematoma	0570T Ttvr perq ea addl prosth	32151 Remove lung foreign body
00214 Anesth skull drainage	0584T Perq islet cell transplant	32160 Open chest heart massage
00215 Anesth skull repair/fract	0585T Laps islet cell transplant	32200 Drain open lung lesion
00474 Anesth surgery of rib	0586T Open islet cell transplant	32215 Treat chest lining
00524 Anesth chest drainage	11004 Debride genitalia & perineum	32220 Release of lung
00540 Anesth chest surgery	11005 Debride abdom wall	32225 Partial release of lung
00542 Anesthesia removal pleura	11006 Debride genit/per/abdom wall	32310 Removal of chest lining
00546 Anesth lung chest wall surg	11008 Remove mesh from abd wall	32320 Free/remove chest lining
00560 Anesth heart surg w/o pump	15756 Free myo/skin flap microvasc	32440 Remove lung pneumonectomy
00561 Anesth heart surg <1 yr	15757 Free skin flap microvasc	32442 Sleeve pneumonectomy
00562 Anesth hrt surg w/pmp age 1+	15758 Free fascial flap microvasc	32445 Removal of lung extrapleural
00567 Anesth CABG w/pump	16036 Escharotomy addl incision	32480 Partial removal of lung
00580 Anesth heart/lung transplnt	19305 Mast radical	32482 Bilobectomy
00632 Anesth removal of nerves	19306 Mast rad urban type	32484 Segmentectomy
0075T Perq stent/chest vert art	19361 Breast reconstr w/lat flap	32486 Sleeve lobectomy
0076T S&i stent/chest vert art	19364 Breast reconstruction	32488 Completion pneumonectomy
00792 Anesth hemorr/excise liver	19367 Breast reconstruction	32491 Lung volume reduction
00794 Anesth pancreas removal	19368 Breast reconstruction	32501 Repair bronchus add-on
00796 Anesth for liver transplant	19369 Breast reconstruction	32503 Resect apical lung tumor
00844 Anesth pelvis surgery	31225 Removal of upper jaw	32504 Resect apical lung tum/chest
00846 Anesth hysterectomy	31230 Removal of upper jaw	32505 Wedge resect of lung initial
00848 Anesth pelvic organ surg	31290 Nasal/sinus endoscopy surg	32506 Wedge resect of lung add-on
00864 Anesth removal of bladder	31291 Nasal/sinus endoscopy surg	32507 Wedge resect of lung diag
00866 Anesth removal of adrenal	31360 Removal of larynx	32540 Removal of lung lesion
00868 Anesth kidney transplant	31365 Removal of larynx	32650 Thoracoscopy w/pleurodesis
00882 Anesth major vein ligation	31367 Partial removal of larynx	32651 Thoracoscopy remove cortex
00908 Anesth removal of prostate	31368 Partial removal of larynx	32652 Thoracoscopy rem totl cortex
00932 Anesth amputation of penis	31370 Partial removal of larynx	32653 Thoracoscopy remov fb/fibrin
00934 Anesth penis nodes removal	31375 Partial removal of larynx	32654 Thoracoscopy contrl bleeding
00936 Anesth penis nodes removal	31380 Partial removal of larynx	32655 Thoracoscopy resect bullae
01272 Anesth femoral artery surg	31382 Partial removal of larynx	32656 Thoracoscopy w/pleurectomy
01442 Anesth knee artery surg	31390 Removal of larynx & pharynx	32658 Thoracoscopy w/sac fb remove
01444 Anesth knee artery repair	31395 Reconstruct larynx & pharynx	32659 Thoracoscopy w/sac drainage
01502 Anesth lwr leg embolectomy	31725 Clearance of airways	32661 Thoracoscopy w/pericard exc
01652 Anesth shoulder vessel surg	31760 Repair of windpipe	32662 Thoracoscopy w/mediast exc
01654 Anesth shoulder vessel surg	31766 Reconstruction of windpipe	32663 Thoracoscopy w/lobectomy
01656 Anesth arm-leg vessel surg	31770 Repair/graft of bronchus	32664 Thoracoscopy w/ th nrv exc
01990 Support for organ donor	31775 Reconstruct bronchus	32665 Thoracoscop w/esoph musc exc
0235T Trluml perip athrc visceral	31780 Reconstruct windpipe	32666 Thoracoscopy w/wedge resect
0345T Transcath mtral vlve repair	31781 Reconstruct windpipe	32667 Thoracoscopy w/w resect addl
0451T Insj/rplcmt aortic ventr sys	31786 Remove windpipe lesion	32668 Thoracoscopy w/w resect diag
0452T Insj/rplcmt dev vasc seal	31800 Repair of windpipe injury	32669 Thoracoscopy remove segment
0455T Remvl aortic ventr cmpl sys	31805 Repair of windpipe injury	32670 Thoracoscopy bilobectomy
0456T Remvl aortic dev vasc seal	32035 Thoracostomy w/rib resection	32671 Thoracoscopy pneumonectomy
0459T Relocaj rplcmt aortic ventr	32036 Thoracostomy w/flap drainage	32672 Thoracoscopy for lvrs
0461T Repos aortic contrpulsj dev	32096 Open wedge/bx lung infiltr	32673 Thoracoscopy w/thymus resect
0483T Tmvi percutaneous approach	32097 Open wedge/bx lung nodule	32674 Thoracoscopy lymph node exc
0484T Tmvi transthoracic exposure	32098 Open biopsy of lung pleura	32800 Repair lung hernia
0494T Prep & cannulj cdvr don lung	32100 Exploration of chest	32810 Close chest after drainage
0495T Mntr cdvr don lng 1st 2 hrs	32110 Explore/repair chest	32815 Close bronchial fistula
0496T Mntr cdvr don lng ea addl hr	32120 Re-exploration of chest	32820 Reconstruct injured chest
0543T Ta mv rpr w/artif chord tend	32124 Explore chest free adhesions	32850 Donor pneumonectomy
0544T Tcat mv annulus rcnstj	32140 Removal of lung lesion(s)	32851 Lung transplant single
0545T Tcat tv annulus rcnstj	32141 Remove/treat lung lesions	32852 Lung transplant with bypass

32853 Lung transplant double	33406 Replacement of aortic valve	33606 Anastomosis/artery-aorta
32854 Lung transplant with bypass	33410 Replacement of aortic valve	33608 Repair anomaly w/conduit
32855 Prepare donor lung single	33411 Replacement of aortic valve	33610 Repair by enlargement
32856 Prepare donor lung double	33412 Replacement of aortic valve	33611 Repair double ventricle
32900 Removal of rib(s)	33413 Replacement of aortic valve	33612 Repair double ventricle
32905 Revise & repair chest wall	33414 Repair of aortic valve	33615 Repair modified fontan
32906 Revise & repair chest wall	33415 Revision subvalvular tissue	33617 Repair single ventricle
32940 Revision of lung	33416 Revise ventricle muscle	33619 Repair single ventricle
32997 Total lung lavage	33417 Repair of aortic valve	33620 Apply r&l pulm art bands
33017 Prcrd drg 6yr+ w/o cgen car	33418 Repair tcat mitral valve	33621 Transthor cath for stent
33018 Prcrd drg 0-5yr or w/anomly	33420 Revision of mitral valve	33622 Redo compl cardiac anomaly
33019 Perq prcrd drg insj cath ct	33422 Revision of mitral valve	33641 Repair heart septum defect
33020 Incision of heart sac	33425 Repair of mitral valve	33645 Revision of heart veins
33025 Incision of heart sac	33426 Repair of mitral valve	33647 Repair heart septum defects
33030 Partial removal of heart sac	33427 Repair of mitral valve	33660 Repair of heart defects
33031 Partial removal of heart sac	33430 Replacement of mitral valve	33665 Repair of heart defects
33050 Resect heart sac lesion	33440 Rplcmt a-valve tlcj autol pv	33670 Repair of heart chambers
33120 Removal of heart lesion	33460 Revision of tricuspid valve	33675 Close mult vsd
33130 Removal of heart lesion	33463 Valvuloplasty tricuspid	33676 Close mult vsd w/resection
33140 Heart revascularize (tmr)	33464 Valvuloplasty tricuspid	33677 Cl mult vsd w/rem pul band
33141 Heart tmr w/other procedure	33465 Replace tricuspid valve	33681 Repair heart septum defect
33202 Insert epicard eltrd open	33468 Revision of tricuspid valve	33684 Repair heart septum defect
33203 Insert epicard eltrd endo	33470 Revision of pulmonary valve	33688 Repair heart septum defect
33236 Remove electrode/thoracotomy	33471 Valvotomy pulmonary valve	33690 Reinforce pulmonary artery
33237 Remove electrode/thoracotomy	33474 Revision of pulmonary valve	33692 Repair of heart defects
33238 Remove electrode/thoracotomy	33475 Replacement pulmonary valve	33694 Repair of heart defects
33243 Remove eltrd/thoracotomy	33476 Revision of heart chamber	33697 Repair of heart defects
33250 Ablate heart dysrhythm focus	33477 Implant tcat pulm vlv perq	33702 Repair of heart defects
33251 Ablate heart dysrhythm focus	33478 Revision of heart chamber	33710 Repair of heart defects
33254 Ablate atria lmtd	33496 Repair prosth valve clot	33720 Repair of heart defect
33255 Ablate atria w/o bypass ext	33500 Repair heart vessel fistula	33722 Repair of heart defect
33256 Ablate atria w/bypass exten	33501 Repair heart vessel fistula	33724 Repair venous anomaly
33257 Ablate atria lmtd add-on	33502 Coronary artery correction	33726 Repair pul venous stenosis
33258 Ablate atria x10sv add-on	33503 Coronary artery graft	33730 Repair heart-vein defect(s)
33259 Ablate atria w/bypass add-on	33504 Coronary artery graft	33732 Repair heart-vein defect
33261 Ablate heart dysrhythm focus	33505 Repair artery w/tunnel	33735 Revision of heart chamber
33265 Ablate atria lmtd endo	33506 Repair artery translocation	33736 Revision of heart chamber
33266 Ablate atria x10sv endo	33507 Repair art intramural	33737 Revision of heart chamber
33300 Repair of heart wound	33510 Cabg vein single	33741 Tas congenital car anomal
33305 Repair of heart wound	33511 Cabg vein two	33745 Tis cgen car anomal 1st shnt
33310 Exploratory heart surgery	33512 Cabg vein three	33746 Tis cgen car anomal ea addl
33315 Exploratory heart surgery	33513 Cabg vein four	33750 Major vessel shunt
33320 Repair major blood vessel(s)	33514 Cabg vein five	33755 Major vessel shunt
33321 Repair major vessel	33516 Cabg vein six or more	33762 Major vessel shunt
33322 Repair major blood vessel(s)	33517 Cabg artery-vein single	33764 Major vessel shunt & graft
33330 Insert major vessel graft	33518 Cabg artery-vein two	33766 Major vessel shunt
33335 Insert major vessel graft	33519 Cabg artery-vein three	33767 Major vessel shunt
33340 Perq clsr tcat l atr apndge	33521 Cabg artery-vein four	33768 Cavopulmonary shunting
33361 Replace aortic valve perq	33522 Cabg artery-vein five	33770 Repair great vessels defect
33362 Replace aortic valve open	33523 Cabg art-vein six or more	33771 Repair great vessels defect
33363 Replace aortic valve open	33530 Coronary artery bypass/reop	33774 Repair great vessels defect
33364 Replace aortic valve open	33533 Cabg arterial single	33775 Repair great vessels defect
33365 Replace aortic valve open	33534 Cabg arterial two	33776 Repair great vessels defect
33366 Trcath replace aortic valve	33535 Cabg arterial three	33777 Repair great vessels defect
33367 Replace aortic valve w/byp	33536 Cabg arterial four or more	33778 Repair great vessels defect
33368 Replace aortic valve w/byp	33542 Removal of heart lesion	33779 Repair great vessels defect
33369 Replace aortic valve w/byp	33545 Repair of heart damage	33780 Repair great vessels defect
33390 Valvuloplasty aortic valve	33548 Restore/remodel ventricle	33781 Repair great vessels defect
33391 Valvuloplasty aortic valve	33572 Open coronary endarterectomy	33782 Nikaidoh proc
33404 Prepare heart-aorta conduit	33600 Closure of valve	33783 Nikaidoh proc w/ostia implt
33405 Replacement of aortic valve	33602 Closure of valve	33786 Repair arterial trunk

CPT © 2021 American Medical Association. All Rights Reserved.   © 2021 Optum360, LLC

33788 Revision of pulmonary artery	33964 Ecmo/ecls repos perph cnula	34842 Endovasc visc aorta 2 graft
33800 Aortic suspension	33965 Ecmo/ecls rmvl perph cannula	34843 Endovasc visc aorta 3 graft
33802 Repair vessel defect	33966 Ecmo/ecls rmvl prph cannula	34844 Endovasc visc aorta 4 graft
33803 Repair vessel defect	33967 Insert i-aort percut device	34845 Visc & infraren abd 1 prosth
33813 Repair septal defect	33968 Remove aortic assist device	34846 Visc & infraren abd 2 prosth
33814 Repair septal defect	33969 Ecmo/ecls rmvl perph cannula	34847 Visc & infraren abd 3 prosth
33820 Revise major vessel	33970 Aortic circulation assist	34848 Visc & infraren abd 4+ prost
33822 Revise major vessel	33971 Aortic circulation assist	35001 Repair defect of artery
33824 Revise major vessel	33973 Insert balloon device	35002 Repair artery rupture neck
33840 Remove aorta constriction	33974 Remove intra-aortic balloon	35005 Repair defect of artery
33845 Remove aorta constriction	33975 Implant ventricular device	35013 Repair artery rupture arm
33851 Remove aorta constriction	33976 Implant ventricular device	35021 Repair defect of artery
33852 Repair septal defect	33977 Remove ventricular device	35022 Repair artery rupture chest
33853 Repair septal defect	33978 Remove ventricular device	35081 Repair defect of artery
33858 As-aort grf f/aortic dsj	33979 Insert intracorporeal device	35082 Repair artery rupture aorta
33859 As-aort grf f/ds oth/thn dsj	33980 Remove intracorporeal device	35091 Repair defect of artery
33863 Ascending aortic graft	33981 Replace vad pump ext	35092 Repair artery rupture aorta
33864 Ascending aortic graft	33982 Replace vad intra w/o bp	35102 Repair defect of artery
33871 Transvrs a-arch grf hypthrm	33983 Replace vad intra w/bp	35103 Repair artery rupture aorta
33875 Thoracic aortic graft	33984 Ecmo/ecls rmvl prph cannula	35111 Repair defect of artery
33877 Thoracoabdominal graft	33985 Ecmo/ecls rmvl ctr cannula	35112 Repair artery rupture spleen
33880 Endovasc taa repr incl subcl	33986 Ecmo/ecls rmvl ctr cannula	35121 Repair defect of artery
33881 Endovasc taa repr w/o subcl	33987 Artery expos/graft artery	35122 Repair artery rupture belly
33883 Insert endovasc prosth taa	33988 Insertion of left heart vent	35131 Repair defect of artery
33884 Endovasc prosth taa add-on	33989 Removal of left heart vent	35132 Repair artery rupture groin
33886 Endovasc prosth delayed	33990 Insert vad artery access	35141 Repair defect of artery
33889 Artery transpose/endovas taa	33991 Insert vad art&vein access	35142 Repair artery rupture thigh
33891 Car-car bp grft/endovas taa	33992 Remove vad different session	35151 Repair defect of artery
33910 Remove lung artery emboli	33993 Reposition vad diff session	35152 Repair ruptd popliteal art
33915 Remove lung artery emboli	33995 Insj perq vad r hrt venous	35182 Repair blood vessel lesion
33916 Surgery of great vessel	33997 Rmvl perq right heart vad	35189 Repair blood vessel lesion
33917 Repair pulmonary artery	34001 Removal of artery clot	35211 Repair blood vessel lesion
33920 Repair pulmonary atresia	34051 Removal of artery clot	35216 Repair blood vessel lesion
33922 Transect pulmonary artery	34151 Removal of artery clot	35221 Repair blood vessel lesion
33924 Remove pulmonary shunt	34401 Removal of vein clot	35241 Repair blood vessel lesion
33925 Rpr pul art unifocal w/o cpb	34451 Removal of vein clot	35246 Repair blood vessel lesion
33926 Repr pul art unifocal w/cpb	34502 Reconstruct vena cava	35251 Repair blood vessel lesion
33927 Impltj tot rplcmt hrt sys	34701 Evasc rpr a-ao ndgft	35271 Repair blood vessel lesion
33928 Rmvl & rplcmt tot hrt sys	34702 Evasc rpr a-ao ndgft rpt	35276 Repair blood vessel lesion
33929 Rmvl rplcmt hrt sys f/trnspl	34703 Evasc rpr a-unilac ndgft	35281 Repair blood vessel lesion
33930 Removal of donor heart/lung	34704 Evasc rpr a-unilac ndgft rpt	35301 Rechanneling of artery
33933 Prepare donor heart/lung	34705 Evac rpr a-biiliac ndgft	35302 Rechanneling of artery
33935 Transplantation heart/lung	34706 Evasc rpr a-biiliac rpt	35303 Rechanneling of artery
33940 Removal of donor heart	34707 Evasc rpr ilio-iliac ndgft	35304 Rechanneling of artery
33944 Prepare donor heart	34708 Evasc rpr ilio-iliac rpt	35305 Rechanneling of artery
33945 Transplantation of heart	34709 Plmt xtn prosth evasc rpr	35306 Rechanneling of artery
33946 Ecmo/ecls initiation venous	34710 Dlyd plmt xtn prosth 1st vsl	35311 Rechanneling of artery
33947 Ecmo/ecls initiation artery	34711 Dlyd plmt xtn prosth ea addl	35331 Rechanneling of artery
33948 Ecmo/ecls daily mgmt-venous	34712 Tcat dlvr enhncd fixj dev	35341 Rechanneling of artery
33949 Ecmo/ecls daily mgmt artery	34717 Evasc rpr a-iliac ndgft	35351 Rechanneling of artery
33951 Ecmo/ecls insj prph cannula	34718 Evasc rpr n/a a-iliac ndgft	35355 Rechanneling of artery
33952 Ecmo/ecls insj prph cannula	34808 Endovas iliac a device addon	35361 Rechanneling of artery
33953 Ecmo/ecls insj prph cannula	34812 Xpose for endoprosth femorl	35363 Rechanneling of artery
33954 Ecmo/ecls insj prph cannula	34813 Femoral endovas graft add-on	35371 Rechanneling of artery
33955 Ecmo/ecls insj ctr cannula	34820 Xpose for endoprosth iliac	35390 Reoperation carotid add-on
33956 Ecmo/ecls insj ctr cannula	34830 Open aortic tube prosth repr	35400 Angioscopy
33957 Ecmo/ecls repos perph cnula	34831 Open aortoiliac prosth repr	35501 Art byp grft ipsilat carotid
33958 Ecmo/ecls repos perph cnula	34832 Open aortofemor prosth repr	35506 Art byp grft subclav-carotid
33959 Ecmo/ecls repos perph cnula	34833 Xpose for endoprosth iliac	35508 Art byp grft carotid-vertbrl
33962 Ecmo/ecls repos perph cnula	34834 Xpose endoprosth brachial	35509 Art byp grft contral carotid
33963 Ecmo/ecls repos perph cnula	34841 Endovasc visc aorta 1 graft	35510 Art byp grft carotid-brchial

35511 Art byp grft subclav-subclav	35694 Art trnsposj subclav carotid	42426 Excise parotid gland/lesion
35512 Art byp grft subclav-brchial	35695 Art trnsposj carotid subclav	42845 Extensive surgery of throat
35515 Art byp grft subclav-vertbrl	35697 Reimplant artery each	42894 Revision of pharyngeal walls
35516 Art byp grft subclav-axilary	35700 Reoperation bypass graft	42953 Repair throat esophagus
35518 Art byp grft axillary-axilry	35701 Exploration carotid artery	42961 Control throat bleeding
35521 Art byp grft axill-femoral	35702 Expl n/flwd surg uxtr art	42971 Control nose/throat bleeding
35522 Art byp grft axill-brachial	35703 Expl n/flwd surg lxtr art	43045 Incision of esophagus
35523 Art byp grft brchl-ulnr-rdl	35820 Explore chest vessels	43100 Excision of esophagus lesion
35525 Art byp grft brachial-brchl	35840 Explore abdominal vessels	43101 Excision of esophagus lesion
35526 Art byp grft aor/carot/innom	35870 Repair vessel graft defect	43107 Removal of esophagus
35531 Art byp grft aorcel/aormesen	35901 Excision graft neck	43108 Removal of esophagus
35533 Art byp grft axill/fem/fem	35905 Excision graft thorax	43112 Removal of esophagus
35535 Art byp grft hepatorenal	35907 Excision graft abdomen	43113 Removal of esophagus
35536 Art byp grft splenorenal	36660 Insertion catheter artery	43116 Partial removal of esophagus
35537 Art byp grft aortoiliac	36823 Insertion of cannula(s)	43117 Partial removal of esophagus
35538 Art byp grft aortobi-iliac	37140 Revision of circulation	43118 Partial removal of esophagus
35539 Art byp grft aortofemoral	37145 Revision of circulation	43121 Partial removal of esophagus
35540 Art byp grft aortbifemoral	37160 Revision of circulation	43122 Partial removal of esophagus
35556 Art byp grft fem-popliteal	37180 Revision of circulation	43123 Partial removal of esophagus
35558 Art byp grft fem-femoral	37181 Splice spleen/kidney veins	43124 Removal of esophagus
35560 Art byp grft aortorenal	37215 Transcath stent cca w/eps	43135 Removal of esophagus pouch
35563 Art byp grft ilioiliac	37217 Stent placemt retro carotid	43279 Lap myotomy heller
35565 Art byp grft iliofemoral	37218 Stent placemt ante carotid	43283 Lap esoph lengthening
35566 Art byp fem-ant-post tib/prl	37616 Ligation of chest artery	43286 Esphg tot w/laps moblj
35570 Art byp tibial-tib/peroneal	37618 Ligation of extremity artery	43287 Esphg dstl 2/3 w/laps moblj
35571 Art byp pop-tibl-prl-other	37660 Revision of major vein	43288 Esphg thrsc moblj
35583 Vein byp grft fem-popliteal	37788 Revascularization penis	43300 Repair of esophagus
35585 Vein byp fem-tibial peroneal	38100 Removal of spleen total	43305 Repair esophagus and fistula
35587 Vein byp pop-tibl peroneal	38101 Removal of spleen partial	43310 Repair of esophagus
35600 Harvest art for cabg add-on	38102 Removal of spleen total	43312 Repair esophagus and fistula
35601 Art byp common ipsi carotid	38115 Repair of ruptured spleen	43313 Esophagoplasty congenital
35606 Art byp carotid-subclavian	38380 Thoracic duct procedure	43314 Tracheo-esophagoplasty cong
35612 Art byp subclav-subclavian	38381 Thoracic duct procedure	43320 Fuse esophagus & stomach
35616 Art byp subclav-axillary	38382 Thoracic duct procedure	43325 Revise esophagus & stomach
35621 Art byp axillary-femoral	38564 Removal abdomen lymph nodes	43327 Esoph fundoplasty lap
35623 Art byp axillary-pop-tibial	38724 Removal of lymph nodes neck	43328 Esoph fundoplasty thor
35626 Art byp aorsubcl/carot/innom	38746 Remove thoracic lymph nodes	43330 Esophagomyotomy abdominal
35631 Art byp aor-celiac-msn-renal	38747 Remove abdominal lymph nodes	43331 Esophagomyotomy thoracic
35632 Art byp ilio-celiac	38765 Remove groin lymph nodes	43332 Transab esoph hiat hern rpr
35633 Art byp ilio-mesenteric	38770 Remove pelvis lymph nodes	43333 Transab esoph hiat hern rpr
35634 Art byp iliorenal	38780 Remove abdomen lymph nodes	43334 Transthor diaphrag hern rpr
35636 Art byp spenorenal	39000 Exploration of chest	43335 Transthor diaphrag hern rpr
35637 Art byp aortoiliac	39010 Exploration of chest	43336 Thorabd diaphr hern repair
35638 Art byp aortobi-iliac	39200 Resect mediastinal cyst	43337 Thorabd diaphr hern repair
35642 Art byp carotid-vertebral	39220 Resect mediastinal tumor	43338 Esoph lengthening
35645 Art byp subclav-vertebrl	39499 Chest procedure	43340 Fuse esophagus & intestine
35646 Art byp aortobifemoral	39501 Repair diaphragm laceration	43341 Fuse esophagus & intestine
35647 Art byp aortofemoral	39503 Repair of diaphragm hernia	43351 Surgical opening esophagus
35650 Art byp axillary-axillary	39540 Repair of diaphragm hernia	43352 Surgical opening esophagus
35654 Art byp axill-fem-femoral	39541 Repair of diaphragm hernia	43360 Gastrointestinal repair
35656 Art byp femoral-popliteal	39545 Revision of diaphragm	43361 Gastrointestinal repair
35661 Art byp femoral-femoral	39560 Resect diaphragm simple	43400 Ligate esophagus veins
35663 Art byp ilioiliac	39561 Resect diaphragm complex	43405 Ligate/staple esophagus
35665 Art byp iliofemoral	39599 Diaphragm surgery procedure	43410 Repair esophagus wound
35666 Art byp fem-ant-post tib/prl	41130 Partial removal of tongue	43415 Repair esophagus wound
35671 Art byp pop-tibl-prl-other	41135 Tongue and neck surgery	43425 Repair esophagus opening
35681 Composite byp grft pros&vein	41140 Removal of tongue	43460 Pressure treatment esophagus
35682 Composite byp grft 2 veins	41145 Tongue removal neck surgery	43496 Free jejunum flap microvasc
35683 Composite byp grft 3/> segmt	41150 Tongue mouth jaw surgery	43500 Surgical opening of stomach
35691 Art trnsposj vertbrl carotid	41153 Tongue mouth neck surgery	43501 Surgical repair of stomach
35693 Art trnsposj subclavian	41155 Tongue jaw & neck surgery	43502 Surgical repair of stomach

43520 Incision of pyloric muscle	44144 Partial removal of colon	45126 Pelvic exenteration
43605 Biopsy of stomach	44145 Partial removal of colon	45130 Excision of rectal prolapse
43610 Excision of stomach lesion	44146 Partial removal of colon	45135 Excision of rectal prolapse
43611 Excision of stomach lesion	44147 Partial removal of colon	45136 Excise ileoanal reservior
43620 Removal of stomach	44150 Removal of colon	45395 Lap removal of rectum
43621 Removal of stomach	44151 Removal of colon/ileostomy	45397 Lap remove rectum w/pouch
43622 Removal of stomach	44155 Removal of colon/ileostomy	45400 Laparoscopic proc
43631 Removal of stomach partial	44156 Removal of colon/ileostomy	45402 Lap proctopexy w/sig resect
43632 Removal of stomach partial	44157 Colectomy w/ileoanal anast	45540 Correct rectal prolapse
43633 Removal of stomach partial	44158 Colectomy w/neo-rectum pouch	45550 Repair rectum/remove sigmoid
43634 Removal of stomach partial	44160 Removal of colon	45562 Exploration/repair of rectum
43635 Removal of stomach partial	44187 Lap ileo/jejuno-stomy	45563 Exploration/repair of rectum
43640 Vagotomy & pylorus repair	44188 Lap colostomy	45800 Repair rect/bladder fistula
43641 Vagotomy & pylorus repair	44202 Lap enterectomy	45805 Repair fistula w/colostomy
43644 Lap gastric bypass/roux-en-y	44203 Lap resect s/intestine addl	45820 Repair rectourethral fistula
43645 Lap gastr bypass incl smll i	44204 Laparo partial colectomy	45825 Repair fistula w/colostomy
43771 Lap revise gastr adj device	44205 Lap colectomy part w/ileum	46705 Repair of anal stricture
43775 Lap sleeve gastrectomy	44206 Lap part colectomy w/stoma	46710 Repr per/vag pouch sngl proc
43800 Reconstruction of pylorus	44207 L colectomy/coloproctostomy	46712 Repr per/vag pouch dbl proc
43810 Fusion of stomach and bowel	44208 L colectomy/coloproctostomy	46715 Rep perf anoper fistu
43820 Fusion of stomach and bowel	44210 Laparo total proctocolectomy	46716 Rep perf anoper/vestib fistu
43825 Fusion of stomach and bowel	44211 Lap colectomy w/proctectomy	46730 Construction of absent anus
43832 Place gastrostomy tube	44212 Laparo total proctocolectomy	46735 Construction of absent anus
43843 Gastroplasty w/o v-band	44213 Lap mobil splenic fl add-on	46740 Construction of absent anus
43845 Gastroplasty duodenal switch	44227 Lap close enterostomy	46742 Repair of imperforated anus
43846 Gastric bypass for obesity	44310 Ileostomy/jejunostomy	46744 Repair of cloacal anomaly
43847 Gastric bypass incl small i	44316 Devise bowel pouch	46746 Repair of cloacal anomaly
43848 Revision gastroplasty	44320 Colostomy	46748 Repair of cloacal anomaly
43850 Revise stomach-bowel fusion	44322 Colostomy with biopsies	46751 Repair of anal sphincter
43855 Revise stomach-bowel fusion	44603 Suture small intestine	47010 Open drainage liver lesion
43860 Revise stomach-bowel fusion	44604 Suture large intestine	47015 Inject/aspirate liver cyst
43865 Revise stomach-bowel fusion	44605 Repair of bowel lesion	47100 Wedge biopsy of liver
43880 Repair stomach-bowel fistula	44615 Intestinal stricturoplasty	47120 Partial removal of liver
43881 Impl/redo electrd antrum	44620 Repair bowel opening	47122 Extensive removal of liver
43882 Revise/remove electrd antrum	44625 Repair bowel opening	47125 Partial removal of liver
44005 Freeing of bowel adhesion	44626 Repair bowel opening	47130 Partial removal of liver
44010 Incision of small bowel	44640 Repair bowel-skin fistula	47133 Removal of donor liver
44015 Insert needle cath bowel	44650 Repair bowel fistula	47135 Transplantation of liver
44020 Explore small intestine	44660 Repair bowel-bladder fistula	47140 Partial removal donor liver
44021 Decompress small bowel	44661 Repair bowel-bladder fistula	47141 Partial removal donor liver
44025 Incision of large bowel	44680 Surgical revision intestine	47142 Partial removal donor liver
44050 Reduce bowel obstruction	44700 Suspend bowel w/prosthesis	47143 Prep donor liver whole
44055 Correct malrotation of bowel	44715 Prepare donor intestine	47144 Prep donor liver 3-segment
44110 Excise intestine lesion(s)	44720 Prep donor intestine/venous	47145 Prep donor liver lobe split
44111 Excision of bowel lesion(s)	44721 Prep donor intestine/artery	47146 Prep donor liver/venous
44120 Removal of small intestine	44800 Excision of bowel pouch	47147 Prep donor liver/arterial
44121 Removal of small intestine	44820 Excision of mesentery lesion	47300 Surgery for liver lesion
44125 Removal of small intestine	44850 Repair of mesentery	47350 Repair liver wound
44126 Enterectomy w/o taper cong	44899 Bowel surgery procedure	47360 Repair liver wound
44127 Enterectomy w/taper cong	44900 Drain appendix abscess open	47361 Repair liver wound
44128 Enterectomy cong add-on	44960 Appendectomy	47362 Repair liver wound
44130 Bowel to bowel fusion	45110 Removal of rectum	47380 Open ablate liver tumor rf
44132 Enterectomy cadaver donor	45111 Partial removal of rectum	47381 Open ablate liver tumor cryo
44133 Enterectomy live donor	45112 Removal of rectum	47400 Incision of liver duct
44135 Intestine transplnt cadaver	45113 Partial proctectomy	47420 Incision of bile duct
44136 Intestine transplant live	45114 Partial removal of rectum	47425 Incision of bile duct
44137 Remove intestinal allograft	45116 Partial removal of rectum	47460 Incise bile duct sphincter
44139 Mobilization of colon	45119 Remove rectum w/reservoir	47480 Incision of gallbladder
44140 Partial removal of colon	45120 Removal of rectum	47550 Bile duct endoscopy add-on
44141 Partial removal of colon	45121 Removal of rectum and colon	47570 Laparo cholecystoenterostomy
44143 Partial removal of colon	45123 Partial proctectomy	47600 Removal of gallbladder

47605	Removal of gallbladder	49425	Insert abdomen-venous drain	50660	Removal of ureter
47610	Removal of gallbladder	49428	Ligation of shunt	50700	Revision of ureter
47612	Removal of gallbladder	49605	Repair umbilical lesion	50715	Release of ureter
47620	Removal of gallbladder	49606	Repair umbilical lesion	50722	Release of ureter
47700	Exploration of bile ducts	49610	Repair umbilical lesion	50725	Release/revise ureter
47701	Bile duct revision	49611	Repair umbilical lesion	50728	Revise ureter
47711	Excision of bile duct tumor	49900	Repair of abdominal wall	50740	Fusion of ureter & kidney
47712	Excision of bile duct tumor	49904	Omental flap extra-abdom	50750	Fusion of ureter & kidney
47715	Excision of bile duct cyst	49905	Omental flap intra-abdom	50760	Fusion of ureters
47720	Fuse gallbladder & bowel	49906	Free omental flap microvasc	50770	Splicing of ureters
47721	Fuse upper gi structures	50010	Exploration of kidney	50780	Reimplant ureter in bladder
47740	Fuse gallbladder & bowel	50040	Drainage of kidney	50782	Reimplant ureter in bladder
47741	Fuse gallbladder & bowel	50045	Exploration of kidney	50783	Reimplant ureter in bladder
47760	Fuse bile ducts and bowel	50060	Removal of kidney stone	50785	Reimplant ureter in bladder
47765	Fuse liver ducts & bowel	50065	Incision of kidney	50800	Implant ureter in bowel
47780	Fuse bile ducts and bowel	50070	Incision of kidney	50810	Fusion of ureter & bowel
47785	Fuse bile ducts and bowel	50075	Removal of kidney stone	50815	Urine shunt to intestine
47800	Reconstruction of bile ducts	50100	Revise kidney blood vessels	50820	Construct bowel bladder
47801	Placement bile duct support	50120	Exploration of kidney	50825	Construct bowel bladder
47802	Fuse liver duct & intestine	50125	Explore and drain kidney	50830	Revise urine flow
47900	Suture bile duct injury	50130	Removal of kidney stone	50840	Replace ureter by bowel
48000	Drainage of abdomen	50135	Exploration of kidney	50845	Appendico-vesicostomy
48001	Placement of drain pancreas	50205	Renal biopsy open	50860	Transplant ureter to skin
48020	Removal of pancreatic stone	50220	Remove kidney open	50900	Repair of ureter
48100	Biopsy of pancreas open	50225	Removal kidney open complex	50920	Closure ureter/skin fistula
48105	Resect/debride pancreas	50230	Removal kidney open radical	50930	Closure ureter/bowel fistula
48120	Removal of pancreas lesion	50234	Removal of kidney & ureter	50940	Release of ureter
48140	Partial removal of pancreas	50236	Removal of kidney & ureter	51525	Removal of bladder lesion
48145	Partial removal of pancreas	50240	Partial removal of kidney	51530	Removal of bladder lesion
48146	Pancreatectomy	50250	Cryoablate renal mass open	51550	Partial removal of bladder
48148	Removal of pancreatic duct	50280	Removal of kidney lesion	51555	Partial removal of bladder
48150	Partial removal of pancreas	50290	Removal of kidney lesion	51565	Revise bladder & ureter(s)
48152	Pancreatectomy	50300	Remove cadaver donor kidney	51570	Removal of bladder
48153	Pancreatectomy	50320	Remove kidney living donor	51575	Removal of bladder & nodes
48154	Pancreatectomy	50323	Prep cadaver renal allograft	51580	Remove bladder/revise tract
48155	Removal of pancreas	50325	Prep donor renal graft	51585	Removal of bladder & nodes
48400	Injection intraop add-on	50327	Prep renal graft/venous	51590	Remove bladder/revise tract
48500	Surgery of pancreatic cyst	50328	Prep renal graft/arterial	51595	Remove bladder/revise tract
48510	Drain pancreatic pseudocyst	50329	Prep renal graft/ureteral	51596	Remove bladder/create pouch
48520	Fuse pancreas cyst and bowel	50340	Removal of kidney	51597	Removal of pelvic structures
48540	Fuse pancreas cyst and bowel	50360	Transplantation of kidney	51800	Revision of bladder/urethra
48545	Pancreatorrhaphy	50365	Transplantation of kidney	51820	Revision of urinary tract
48547	Duodenal exclusion	50370	Remove transplanted kidney	51841	Attach bladder/urethra
48548	Fuse pancreas and bowel	50380	Reimplantation of kidney	51865	Repair of bladder wound
48551	Prep donor pancreas	50400	Revision of kidney/ureter	51900	Repair bladder/vagina lesion
48552	Prep donor pancreas/venous	50405	Revision of kidney/ureter	51920	Close bladder-uterus fistula
48554	Transpl allograft pancreas	50500	Repair of kidney wound	51925	Hysterectomy/bladder repair
48556	Removal allograft pancreas	50520	Close kidney-skin fistula	51940	Correction of bladder defect
49000	Exploration of abdomen	50525	Close nephrovisceral fistula	51960	Revision of bladder & bowel
49002	Reopening of abdomen	50526	Close nephrovisceral fistula	51980	Construct bladder opening
49013	Prpertl pel pack hemrrg trma	50540	Revision of horseshoe kidney	53415	Reconstruction of urethra
49014	Reexploration pelvic wound	50545	Laparo radical nephrectomy	53448	Remov/replc ur sphinctr comp
49020	Drainage abdom abscess open	50546	Laparoscopic nephrectomy	54125	Removal of penis
49040	Drain open abdom abscess	50547	Laparo removal donor kidney	54130	Remove penis & nodes
49060	Drain open retroperi abscess	50548	Laparo remove w/ureter	54135	Remove penis & nodes
49062	Drain to peritoneal cavity	50600	Exploration of ureter	54390	Repair penis and bladder
49203	Exc abd tum 5 cm or less	50605	Insert ureteral support	54430	Revision of penis
49204	Exc abd tum over 5 cm	50610	Removal of ureter stone	54438	Replantation of penis
49205	Exc abd tum over 10 cm	50620	Removal of ureter stone	55605	Incise sperm duct pouch
49215	Excise sacral spine tumor	50630	Removal of ureter stone	55650	Remove sperm duct pouch
49412	Ins device for rt guide open	50650	Removal of ureter	55801	Removal of prostate

55810 Extensive prostate surgery	58953 Tah rad dissect for debulk	61450 Incise skull for surgery
55812 Extensive prostate surgery	58954 Tah rad debulk/lymph remove	61458 Incise skull for brain wound
55815 Extensive prostate surgery	58956 Bso omentectomy w/tah	61460 Incise skull for surgery
55821 Removal of prostate	58957 Resect recurrent gyn mal	61500 Removal of skull lesion
55831 Removal of prostate	58958 Resect recur gyn mal w/lym	61501 Remove infected skull bone
55840 Extensive prostate surgery	58960 Exploration of abdomen	61510 Removal of brain lesion
55842 Extensive prostate surgery	59120 Treat ectopic pregnancy	61512 Remove brain lining lesion
55845 Extensive prostate surgery	59121 Treat ectopic pregnancy	61514 Removal of brain abscess
55862 Extensive prostate surgery	59130 Treat ectopic pregnancy	61516 Removal of brain lesion
55865 Extensive prostate surgery	59135 Treat ectopic pregnancy	61517 Implt brain chemotx add-on
56631 Extensive vulva surgery	59136 Treat ectopic pregnancy	61518 Removal of brain lesion
56632 Extensive vulva surgery	59140 Treat ectopic pregnancy	61519 Remove brain lining lesion
56633 Extensive vulva surgery	59325 Revision of cervix	61520 Removal of brain lesion
56634 Extensive vulva surgery	59350 Repair of uterus	61521 Removal of brain lesion
56637 Extensive vulva surgery	59514 Cesarean delivery only	61522 Removal of brain abscess
56640 Extensive vulva surgery	59525 Remove uterus after cesarean	61524 Removal of brain lesion
57110 Remove vagina wall complete	59620 Attempted vbac delivery only	61526 Removal of brain lesion
57111 Remove vagina tissue compl	59830 Treat uterus infection	61530 Removal of brain lesion
57270 Repair of bowel pouch	59850 Abortion	61531 Implant brain electrodes
57280 Suspension of vagina	59851 Abortion	61533 Implant brain electrodes
57296 Revise vag graft open abd	59852 Abortion	61534 Removal of brain lesion
57305 Repair rectum-vagina fistula	59855 Abortion	61535 Remove brain electrodes
57307 Fistula repair & colostomy	59856 Abortion	61536 Removal of brain lesion
57308 Fistula repair transperine	59857 Abortion	61537 Removal of brain tissue
57311 Repair urethrovaginal lesion	60254 Extensive thyroid surgery	61538 Removal of brain tissue
57531 Removal of cervix radical	60270 Removal of thyroid	61539 Removal of brain tissue
57540 Removal of residual cervix	60505 Explore parathyroid glands	61540 Removal of brain tissue
57545 Remove cervix/repair pelvis	60521 Removal of thymus gland	61541 Incision of brain tissue
58140 Myomectomy abdom method	60522 Removal of thymus gland	61543 Removal of brain tissue
58146 Myomectomy abdom complex	60540 Explore adrenal gland	61544 Remove & treat brain lesion
58150 Total hysterectomy	60545 Explore adrenal gland	61545 Excision of brain tumor
58152 Total hysterectomy	60600 Remove carotid body lesion	61546 Removal of pituitary gland
58180 Partial hysterectomy	60605 Remove carotid body lesion	61548 Removal of pituitary gland
58200 Extensive hysterectomy	60650 Laparoscopy adrenalectomy	61550 Release of skull seams
58210 Extensive hysterectomy	61105 Twist drill hole	61552 Release of skull seams
58240 Removal of pelvis contents	61107 Drill skull for implantation	61556 Incise skull/sutures
58267 Vag hyst w/urinary repair	61108 Drill skull for drainage	61557 Incise skull/sutures
58275 Hysterectomy/revise vagina	61120 Burr hole for puncture	61558 Excision of skull/sutures
58280 Hysterectomy/revise vagina	61140 Pierce skull for biopsy	61559 Excision of skull/sutures
58285 Extensive hysterectomy	61150 Pierce skull for drainage	61563 Excision of skull tumor
58400 Suspension of uterus	61151 Pierce skull for drainage	61564 Excision of skull tumor
58410 Suspension of uterus	61154 Pierce skull & remove clot	61566 Removal of brain tissue
58520 Repair of ruptured uterus	61156 Pierce skull for drainage	61567 Incision of brain tissue
58540 Revision of uterus	61210 Pierce skull implant device	61570 Remove foreign body brain
58548 Lap radical hyst	61250 Pierce skull & explore	61571 Incise skull for brain wound
58575 Laps tot hyst resj mal	61253 Pierce skull & explore	61575 Skull base/brainstem surgery
58605 Division of fallopian tube	61304 Open skull for exploration	61576 Skull base/brainstem surgery
58611 Ligate oviduct(s) add-on	61305 Open skull for exploration	61580 Craniofacial approach skull
58700 Removal of fallopian tube	61312 Open skull for drainage	61581 Craniofacial approach skull
58720 Removal of ovary/tube(s)	61313 Open skull for drainage	61582 Craniofacial approach skull
58740 Adhesiolysis tube ovary	61314 Open skull for drainage	61583 Craniofacial approach skull
58750 Repair oviduct	61315 Open skull for drainage	61584 Orbitocranial approach/skull
58752 Revise ovarian tube(s)	61316 Implt cran bone flap to abdo	61585 Orbitocranial approach/skull
58760 Fimbrioplasty	61320 Open skull for drainage	61586 Resect nasopharynx skull
58822 Drain ovary abscess percut	61321 Open skull for drainage	61590 Infratemporal approach/skull
58825 Transposition ovary(s)	61322 Decompressive craniotomy	61591 Infratemporal approach/skull
58940 Removal of ovary(s)	61323 Decompressive lobectomy	61592 Orbitocranial approach/skull
58943 Removal of ovary(s)	61333 Explore orbit/remove lesion	61595 Transtemporal approach/skull
58950 Resect ovarian malignancy	61340 Subtemporal decompression	61596 Transcochlear approach/skull
58951 Resect ovarian malignancy	61343 Incise skull (press relief)	61597 Transcondylar approach/skull
58952 Resect ovarian malignancy	61345 Relieve cranial pressure	61598 Transpetrosal approach/skull

Appendix J — Inpatient-Only Procedures

Code	Description
61600	Resect/excise cranial lesion
61601	Resect/excise cranial lesion
61605	Resect/excise cranial lesion
61606	Resect/excise cranial lesion
61607	Resect/excise cranial lesion
61608	Resect/excise cranial lesion
61611	Transect artery sinus
61613	Remove aneurysm sinus
61615	Resect/excise lesion skull
61616	Resect/excise lesion skull
61618	Repair dura
61619	Repair dura
61630	Intracranial angioplasty
61635	Intracran angioplsty w/stent
61645	Perq art m-thrombect &/nfs
61650	Evasc prlng admn rx agnt 1st
61651	Evasc prlng admn rx agnt add
61680	Intracranial vessel surgery
61682	Intracranial vessel surgery
61684	Intracranial vessel surgery
61686	Intracranial vessel surgery
61690	Intracranial vessel surgery
61692	Intracranial vessel surgery
61697	Brain aneurysm repr complx
61698	Brain aneurysm repr complx
61700	Brain aneurysm repr simple
61702	Inner skull vessel surgery
61703	Clamp neck artery
61705	Revise circulation to head
61708	Revise circulation to head
61710	Revise circulation to head
61711	Fusion of skull arteries
61735	Incise skull/brain surgery
61750	Incise skull/brain biopsy
61751	Brain biopsy w/ct/mr guide
61760	Implant brain electrodes
61850	Implant neuroelectrodes
61860	Implant neuroelectrodes
61863	Implant neuroelectrode
61864	Implant neuroelectrde addl
61867	Implant neuroelectrode
61868	Implant neuroelectrde addl
62005	Treat skull fracture
62010	Treatment of head injury
62100	Repair brain fluid leakage
62115	Reduction of skull defect
62117	Reduction of skull defect
62120	Repair skull cavity lesion
62121	Incise skull repair
62140	Repair of skull defect
62141	Repair of skull defect
62142	Remove skull plate/flap
62143	Replace skull plate/flap
62145	Repair of skull & brain
62146	Repair of skull with graft
62147	Repair of skull with graft
62148	Retr bone flap to fix skull
62161	Dissect brain w/scope
62162	Remove colloid cyst w/scope
62164	Remove brain tumor w/scope
62165	Remove pituit tumor w/scope
62180	Establish brain cavity shunt
62190	Establish brain cavity shunt
62192	Establish brain cavity shunt
62200	Establish brain cavity shunt
62201	Brain cavity shunt w/scope
62220	Establish brain cavity shunt
62223	Establish brain cavity shunt
62256	Remove brain cavity shunt
62258	Replace brain cavity shunt
63050	Cervical laminoplsty 2/> seg
63051	C-laminoplasty w/graft/plate
63077	Spine disk surgery thorax
63078	Spine disk surgery thorax
63081	Remove vert body dcmprn crvl
63082	Remove vertebral body add-on
63085	Remove vert body dcmprn thrc
63086	Remove vertebral body add-on
63087	Remov vertbr dcmprn thrclmbr
63088	Remove vertebral body add-on
63090	Remove vert body dcmprn lmbr
63091	Remove vertebral body add-on
63101	Remove vert body dcmprn thrc
63102	Remove vert body dcmprn lmbr
63103	Remove vertebral body add-on
63170	Incise spinal cord tract(s)
63172	Drainage of spinal cyst
63173	Drainage of spinal cyst
63185	Incise spine nrv half segmnt
63190	Incise spine nrv >2 segmnts
63191	Incise spine accessory nerve
63194	Incise spine & cord cervical
63195	Incise spine & cord thoracic
63196	Incise spine&cord 2 trx crvl
63197	Incise spine&cord 2 trx thrc
63198	Incise spin&cord 2 stgs crvl
63199	Incise spin&cord 2 stgs thrc
63200	Release spinal cord lumbar
63250	Revise spinal cord vsls crvl
63251	Revise spinal cord vsls thrc
63252	Revise spine cord vsl thrlmb
63270	Excise intrspinl lesion crvl
63271	Excise intrspinl lesion thrc
63272	Excise intrspinl lesion lmbr
63273	Excise intrspinl lesion scrl
63275	Bx/exc xdrl spine lesn crvl
63276	Bx/exc xdrl spine lesn thrc
63277	Bx/exc xdrl spine lesn lmbr
63278	Bx/exc xdrl spine lesn scrl
63280	Bx/exc idrl spine lesn crvl
63281	Bx/exc idrl spine lesn thrc
63282	Bx/exc idrl spine lesn lmbr
63283	Bx/exc idrl spine lesn scrl
63285	Bx/exc idrl imed lesn cervl
63286	Bx/exc idrl imed lesn thrc
63287	Bx/exc idrl imed lesn thrlmb
63290	Bx/exc xdrl/idrl lsn any lvl
63295	Repair laminectomy defect
63300	Remove vert xdrl body crvcl
63301	Remove vert xdrl body thrc
63302	Remove vert xdrl body thrlmb
63303	Remov vert xdrl bdy lmbr/sac
63304	Remove vert idrl body crvcl
63305	Remove vert idrl body thrc
63306	Remov vert idrl bdy thrclmbr
63307	Remov vert idrl bdy lmbr/sac
63308	Remove vertebral body add-on
63700	Repair of spinal herniation
63702	Repair of spinal herniation
63704	Repair of spinal herniation
63706	Repair of spinal herniation
63707	Repair spinal fluid leakage
63709	Repair spinal fluid leakage
63710	Graft repair of spine defect
63740	Install spinal shunt
64755	Incision of stomach nerves
64760	Incision of vagus nerve
64809	Remove sympathetic nerves
64818	Remove sympathetic nerves
64866	Fusion of facial/other nerve
64868	Fusion of facial/other nerve
65273	Repair of eye wound
69155	Extensive ear/neck surgery
69535	Remove part of temporal bone
69554	Remove ear lesion
69950	Incise inner ear nerve
75956	Xray endovasc thor ao repr
75957	Xray endovasc thor ao repr
75958	Xray place prox ext thor ao
75959	Xray place dist ext thor ao
92941	Prq card revasc mi 1 vsl
92970	Cardioassist internal
92971	Cardioassist external
92975	Dissolve clot heart vessel
93583	Perq transcath septal reduxn
99184	Hypothermia ill neonate
99190	Special pump services
99191	Special pump services
99192	Special pump services
99356	Prolonged service inpatient
99357	Prolonged service inpatient
99462	Sbsq nb em per day hosp
99468	Neonate crit care initial
99469	Neonate crit care subsq
99471	Ped critical care initial
99472	Ped critical care subsq
99475	Ped crit care age 2-5 init
99476	Ped crit care age 2-5 subsq
99477	Init day hosp neonate care
99478	Ic lbw inf < 1500 gm subsq
99479	Ic lbw inf 1500-2500 g subsq
99480	Ic inf pbw 2501-5000 g subsq
C9606	PC H rev ac tot/subtot occl 1 ves
G0341	Percutaneous islet celltrans
G0342	Laparoscopy islet cell trans
G0343	Laparotomy islet cell transp
0656T	Vrt bdy tethering ant
0657T	Vrt bdy tethering ant 8+ seg
0659T	Tcat intra-c nfs supersat o2

Appendix K — Place of Service and Type of Service

Place-of-Service Codes for Professional Claims

Listed below are place of service codes and descriptions. These codes should be used on professional claims to specify the entity where service(s) were rendered. Check with individual payers (e.g., Medicare, Medicaid, other private insurance) for reimbursement policies regarding these codes. Comments or questions regarding place-of-service codes or descriptions should be directed to your Medicare administrative contractor (MAC).

01 Pharmacy — A facility or location where drugs and other medically related items and services are sold, dispensed, or otherwise provided directly to patients.

02 Telehealth Provided Other than in Patient's Home — The location where health services and health related services are provided or received, through telecommunication technology. Patient is not located in their home when receiving health services or health related services through telecommunication technology.

03 School — A facility whose primary purpose is education.

04 Homeless Shelter — A facility or location whose primary purpose is to provide temporary housing to homeless individuals (e.g., emergency shelters, individual or family shelters).

05 Indian Health Service Free-Standing Facility — A facility or location, owned and operated by the Indian Health Service, which provides diagnostic, therapeutic (surgical and non-surgical), and rehabilitation services to American Indians and Alaska Natives who do not require hospitalization.

06 Indian Health Service Provider-based Facility — A facility or location, owned and operated by the Indian Health Service, which provides diagnostic, therapeutic (surgical and nonsurgical), and rehabilitation services rendered by, or under the supervision of, physicians to American Indians and Alaska Natives admitted as inpatients or outpatients.

07 Tribal 638 Free-Standing Facility — A facility or location owned and operated by a federally recognized American Indian or Alaska Native tribe or tribal organization under a 638 agreement, which provides diagnostic, therapeutic (surgical and nonsurgical), and rehabilitation services to tribal members who do not require hospitalization.

08 Tribal 638 Provider-based Facility — A facility or location owned and operated by a federally recognized American Indian or Alaska Native tribe or tribal organization under a 638 agreement, which provides diagnostic, therapeutic (surgical and nonsurgical), and rehabilitation services to tribal members admitted as inpatients or outpatients.

09 Prison/Correctional Facility — A prison, jail, reformatory, work farm, detention center, or any other similar facility maintained by either Federal, State or local authorities for the purpose of confinement or rehabilitation of adult or juvenile criminal offenders.

10 Telehealth Provided in Patient's Home — The location where health services and health related services are provided or received, through telecommunication technology. Patient is located in their home (which is a location other than a hospital or other facility where the patient receives care in a private residence) when receiving health services or health related services through telecommunication technology.

11 Office — Location, other than a hospital, skilled nursing facility (SNF), military treatment facility, community health center, State or local public health clinic, or intermediate care facility (ICF), where the health professional routinely provides health examinations, diagnosis, and treatment of illness or injury on an ambulatory basis.

12 Home — Location, other than a hospital or other facility, where the patient receives care in a private residence.

13 Assisted Living Facility — Congregate residential facility with self-contained living units providing assessment of each resident's needs and on-site support 24 hours a day, 7 days a week, with the capacity to deliver or arrange for services including some health care and other services.

14 Group Home — A residence, with shared living areas, where clients receive supervision and other services such as social and/or behavioral services, custodial service, and minimal services (e.g., medication administration).

15 Mobile Unit — A facility/unit that moves from place-to-place equipped to provide preventive, screening, diagnostic, and/or treatment services.

16 Temporary Lodging — A short-term accommodation such as a hotel, campground, hostel, cruise ship or resort where the patient receives care, and which is not identified by any other POS code.

17 Walk-in Retail Health Clinic — A walk-in health clinic, other than an office, urgent care facility, pharmacy, or independent clinic and not described by any other place of service code, that is located within a retail operation and provides, on an ambulatory basis, preventive and primary care services.

18 Place of Employment-Worksite — A location, not described by any other POS code, owned or operated by a public or private entity where the patient is employed, and where a health professional provides on-going or episodic occupational medical, therapeutic or rehabilitative services to the individual.

Code	Name	Description
19	Off Campus-Outpatient Hospital	A portion of an off-campus hospital provider based department which provides diagnostic, therapeutic (both surgical and nonsurgical), and rehabilitation services to sick or injured persons who do not require hospitalization or institutionalization.
20	Urgent Care Facility	Location, distinct from a hospital emergency room, an office, or a clinic, whose purpose is to diagnose and treat illness or injury for unscheduled, ambulatory patients seeking immediate medical attention.
21	Inpatient Hospital	A facility, other than psychiatric, which primarily provides diagnostic, therapeutic (both surgical and nonsurgical), and rehabilitation services by, or under, the supervision of physicians to patients admitted for a variety of medical conditions.
22	On Campus-Outpatient Hospital	A portion of a hospital's main campus which provides diagnostic, therapeutic (both surgical and nonsurgical), and rehabilitation services to sick or injured persons who do not require hospitalization or institutionalization.
23	Emergency Room—Hospital	A portion of a hospital where emergency diagnosis and treatment of illness or injury is provided.
24	Ambulatory Surgical Center	A freestanding facility, other than a physician's office, where surgical and diagnostic services are provided on an ambulatory basis.
25	Birthing Center	A facility, other than a hospital's maternity facilities or a physician's office, which provides a setting for labor, delivery, and immediate post-partum care as well as immediate care of new born infants.
26	Military Treatment Facility	A medical facility operated by one or more of the Uniformed Services. Military Treatment Facility (MTF) also refers to certain former U.S. Public Health Service (USPHS) facilities now designated as Uniformed Service Treatment Facilities (USTF).
27-30	Unassigned	N/A
31	Skilled Nursing Facility	A facility which primarily provides inpatient skilled nursing care and related services to patients who require medical, nursing, or rehabilitative services but does not provide the level of care or treatment available in a hospital.
32	Nursing Facility	A facility which primarily provides to residents skilled nursing care and related services for the rehabilitation of injured, disabled, or sick persons, or, on a regular basis, health-related care services above the level of custodial care to individuals other than those with intellectual disabilities.
33	Custodial Care Facility	A facility which provides room, board, and other personal assistance services, generally on a long-term basis, and which does not include a medical component.
34	Hospice	A facility, other than a patient's home, in which palliative and supportive care for terminally ill patients and their families is provided.
35-40	Unassigned	N/A
41	Ambulance—Land	A land vehicle specifically designed, equipped and staffed for lifesaving and transporting the sick or injured.
42	Ambulance—Air or Water	An air or water vehicle specifically designed, equipped and staffed for lifesaving and transporting the sick or injured.
43-48	Unassigned	N/A
49	Independent Clinic	A location, not part of a hospital and not described by any other Place of Service code, that is organized and operated to provide preventive, diagnostic, therapeutic, rehabilitative, or palliative services to outpatients only.
50	Federally Qualified Health Center	A facility located in a medically underserved area that provides Medicare beneficiaries with preventive primary medical care under the general direction of a physician.
51	Inpatient Psychiatric Facility	A facility that provides inpatient psychiatric services for the diagnosis and treatment of mental illness on a 24-hour basis, by or under the supervision of a physician.
52	Psychiatric Facility-Partial Hospitalization	A facility for the diagnosis and treatment of mental illness that provides a planned therapeutic program for patients who do not require full time hospitalization, but who need broader programs than are possible from outpatient visits to a hospital-based or hospital-affiliated facility.
53	Community Mental Health Center	A facility that provides the following services: outpatient services, including specialized outpatient services for children, the elderly, individuals who are chronically ill, and residents of the CMHC's mental health services area who have been discharged from inpatient treatment at a mental health facility; 24 hour a day emergency care services; day treatment, other partial hospitalization services, or psychosocial rehabilitation services; screening for patients being considered for admission to State mental health facilities to determine the appropriateness of such admission; and consultation and education services.
54	Intermediate Care Facility/Individuals with Intellectual Disabilities	A facility which primarily provides health-related care and services above the level of custodial care to individuals but does not provide the level of care or treatment available in a hospital or SNF.
55	Residential Substance Abuse Treatment Facility	A facility which provides treatment for substance (alcohol and drug) abuse to live-in residents who do not require acute medical care. Services include individual and group therapy and counseling, family counseling, laboratory tests, drugs and supplies, psychological testing, and room and board.
56	Psychiatric Residential Treatment Center	A facility or distinct part of a facility for psychiatric care which provides a total 24-hour therapeutically planned and professionally staffed group living and learning environment.

57	Non-residential Substance Abuse Treatment Facility	A location which provides treatment for substance (alcohol and drug) abuse on an ambulatory basis. Services include individual and group therapy and counseling, family counseling, laboratory tests, drugs and supplies, and psychological testing.
58	Non-residential Opioid Treatment Facility	A location that provides treatment for opioid use disorder on an ambulatory basis. Services include methadone and other forms of Medication Assisted Treatment (MAT).
59	Unassigned	N/A
60	Mass Immunization Center	A location where providers administer pneumococcal pneumonia and influenza virus vaccinations and submit these services as electronic media claims, paper claims, or using the roster billing method. This generally takes place in a mass immunization setting, such as, a public health center, pharmacy, or mall but may include a physician office setting.
61	Comprehensive Inpatient Rehabilitation Facility	A facility that provides comprehensive rehabilitation services under the supervision of a physician to inpatients with physical disabilities. Services include physical therapy, occupational therapy, speech pathology, social or psychological services, and orthotics and prosthetics services.
62	Comprehensive Outpatient Rehabilitation Facility	A facility that provides comprehensive rehabilitation services under the supervision of a physician to outpatients with physical disabilities. Services include physical therapy, occupational therapy, and speech pathology services.
63-64	Unassigned	N/A
65	End-Stage Renal Disease Treatment Facility	A facility other than a hospital, which provides dialysis treatment, maintenance, and/or training to patients or caregivers on an ambulatory or home-care basis.
66-70	Unassigned	N/A
71	Public Health Clinic	A facility maintained by either State or local health departments that provides ambulatory primary medical care under the general direction of a physician.
72	Rural Health Clinic	A certified facility which is located in a rural medically underserved area that provides ambulatory primary medical care under the general direction of a physician.
73-80	Unassigned	N/A
81	Independent Laboratory	A laboratory certified to perform diagnostic and/or clinical tests independent of an institution or a physician's office.
82-98	Unassigned	N/A
99	Other Place of Service	Other place of service not identified above.

Type of Service

Common Working File Type of Service (TOS) Indicators

For submitting a claim to the Common Working File (CWF), use the following table to assign the proper TOS. Some procedures may have more than one applicable TOS. CWF will reject codes with incorrect TOS designations. CWF will produce alerts on codes with incorrect TOS designations.

The only exceptions to this annual update are:

- Surgical services billed for dates of service through December 31, 2007, containing the ASC facility service modifier SG must be reported as TOS F. Effective for services on or after January 1, 2008, the SG modifier is no longer applicable for Medicare services. ASC providers should discontinue applying the SG modifier on ASC facility claims. The indicator F does not appear in the TOS table because its use depends upon claims submitted with POS 24 (ASC facility) from an ASC (specialty 49). This became effective for dates of service January 1, 2008, or after.

- Surgical services billed with an assistant-at-surgery modifier (80-82, AS) must be reported with TOS 8. The 8 indicator does not appear on the TOS table because its use is dependent upon the use of the appropriate modifier. (See Pub. 100-4 *Medicare Claims Processing Manual,* chapter 12, "Physician/Practitioner Billing," for instructions on when assistant-at-surgery is allowable.)

- TOS H appears in the list of descriptors. However, it does not appear in the table. In CWF, "H" is used only as an indicator for hospice. The contractor should not submit TOS H to CWF at this time.

- For outpatient services, when a transfusion medicine code appears on a claim that also contains a blood product, the service is paid under reasonable charge at 80 percent; coinsurance and deductible apply. When transfusion medicine codes are paid under the clinical laboratory fee schedule they are paid at 100 percent; coinsurance and deductible do not apply.

Note: For injection codes with more than one possible TOS designation, use the following guidelines when assigning the TOS:

When the choice is L or 1:

- Use TOS L when the drug is used related to ESRD; or
- Use TOS 1 when the drug is not related to ESRD and is administered in the office.

When the choice is G or 1:

- Use TOS G when the drug is an immunosuppressive drug; or
- Use TOS 1 when the drug is used for other than immunosuppression.

When the choice is P or 1:

- Use TOS P if the drug is administered through durable medical equipment (DME); or
- Use TOS 1 if the drug is administered in the office.

The place of service or diagnosis may be considered when determining the appropriate TOS. The descriptors for each of the TOS codes listed in the annual HCPCS update are:

0	Whole blood
1	Medical care
2	Surgery
3	Consultation
4	Diagnostic radiology
5	Diagnostic laboratory
6	Therapeutic radiology
7	Anesthesia
8	Assistant at surgery
9	Other medical items or services
A	Used durable medical equipment (DME)
D	Ambulance
E	Enteral/parenteral nutrients/supplies
F	Ambulatory surgical center (facility usage for surgical services)
G	Immunosuppressive drugs
J	Diabetic shoes
K	Hearing items and services
L	ESRD supplies
M	Monthly capitation payment for dialysis
N	Kidney donor

P   Lump sum purchase of DME, prosthetics, orthotics
Q   Vision items or services
R   Rental of DME
S   Surgical dressings or other medical supplies

T   Outpatient mental health limitation
U   Occupational therapy
V   Pneumococcal/flu vaccine
W   Physical therapy

Appendix L — Multianalyte Assays with Algorithmic Analyses

The following tables contain the Administrative Codes for Multianalyte Assays with Algorithmic Analyses (MAAA), Category I codes for MAAA and the most current list of Proprietary Laboratory Analysis (PLA) codes.

The following is a list of MAAA procedures that are usually exclusive to one single clinical laboratory or manufacturer. These tests use the results from several different assays, including molecular pathology assays, fluorescent in situ hybridization assays, and nonnucleic acid-based assays (e.g., proteins, polypeptides, lipids, and carbohydrates) to perform an algorithmic analysis that is reported as a numeric score or probability. Although the laboratory report may list results of individual component tests of the MAAAs, these assays are not separately reportable.

The following list includes the proprietary name and clinical laboratory/manufacturer, an alphanumeric code, and the code descriptor.

The format for the code descriptor usually includes:

- Type of disease (e.g., oncology, autoimmune, tissue rejection)
- Chemical(s) analyzed (e.g., DNA, RNA, protein, antibody)
- Number of markers (e.g., number of genes, number of proteins)

- Methodology(s) (e.g., microarray, real-time [RT]-PCR, in situ hybridization [ISH], enzyme linked immunosorbent assays [ELISA])
- Number of functional domains (when indicated)
- Type of specimen (e.g., blood, fresh tissue, formalin-fixed paraffin embedded)
- Type of algorithm result (e.g., prognostic, diagnostic)
- Report (e.g., probability index, risk score)

MAAA procedures with a Category I code are noted on the following list and can also be found in code range 81500–81599 in the pathology and laboratory chapter. If a specific MAAA test does not have a Category I code, it is denoted with a four-digit number and the letter M. Use code 81599 if an MAAA test is not included on the following list or in the Category I codes. The codes on the list are exclusive to the assays identified by proprietary name. Report code 81599 also when an analysis is performed that may possibly fall within a specific descriptor but the proprietary name is not included in the list. The list does not contain all MAAA procedures.

Proprietary Name/Clinical Laboratory/Manufacturer	Code	Descriptor
Administrative Codes for Multianalyte Assays with Algorithmic Analyses (MAAA)		
ASH FibroSURE™, BioPredictive S.A.S	0002M	Liver disease, ten biochemical assays (ALT, A2-macroglobulin, apolipoprotein A-1, total bilirubin, GGT, haptoglobin, AST, glucose, total cholesterol and triglycerides) utilizing serum, prognostic algorithm reported as quantitative scores for fibrosis, steatosis and alcoholic steatohepatitis (ASH)
NASH FibroSURE™, BioPredictive S.A.S	0003M	Liver disease, ten biochemical assays (ALT, A2-macroglobulin, apolipoprotein A-1, total bilirubin, GGT, haptoglobin, AST, glucose, total cholesterol and triglycerides) utilizing serum, prognostic algorithm reported as quantitative scores for fibrosis, steatosis and nonalcoholic steatohepatitis (NASH)
ScoliScore™ Transgenomic	0004M	Scoliosis, DNA analysis of 53 single nucleotide polymorphisms (SNPs), using saliva, prognostic algorithm reported as a risk score
HeproDX™, GoPath Laboratories, LLC	0006M	Oncology (hepatic), mRNA expression levels of 161 genes, utilizing fresh hepatocellular carcinoma tumor tissue, with alpha-fetoprotein level, algorithm reported as a risk classifier
NETest, Wren Laboratories, LLC	0007M	Oncology (gastrointestinal neuroendocrine tumors), real-time PCR expression analysis of 51 genes, utilizing whole peripheral blood, algorithm reported as a nomogram of tumor disease index
	(0009M has been deleted)	
NeoLAB™ Prostate Liquid Biopsy, NeoGenomics Laboratories	0011M	Oncology, prostate cancer, mRNA expression assay of 12 genes (10 content and 2 housekeeping), RT-PCR test utilizing blood plasma and urine, algorithms to predict high-grade prostate cancer risk
Cxbladder™ Detect, Pacific Edge Diagnostics USA, Ltd	0012M	Oncology (urothelial), mRNA, gene expression profiling by real-time quantitative PCR of five genes (*MDK, HOXA13, CDC2 [CDK1], IGFBP5,* and *CXCR2*), utilizing urine, algorithm reported as a risk score for having urothelial carcinoma
Cxbladder™ Monitor, Pacific Edge Diagnostics USA, Ltd	0013M	Oncology (urothelial), mRNA, gene expression profiling by real-time quantitative PCR of five genes (*MDK, HOXA13, CDC2 [CDK1], IGFBP5,* and *CXCR2*), utilizing urine, algorithm reported as a risk score for having recurrent urothelial carcinoma
Enhanced Liver Fibrosis™ (ELF™) Test, Siemens Healthcare Diagnostics Inc/Siemens Healthcare Laboratory LLC	0014M	Liver disease, analysis of 3 biomarkers (hyaluronic acid [HA], procollagen III amino terminal peptide [PIIINP], tissue inhibitor of metalloproteinase 1 [TIMP-1]), using immunoassays, utilizing serum, prognostic algorithm reported as a risk score and risk of liver fibrosis and liver-related clinical events within 5 years
Adrenal Mass Panel, 24 Hour, Urine, Mayo Clinic Laboratories (MCL), Mayo Clinic	0015M	Adrenal cortical tumor, biochemical assay of 25 steroid markers, utilizing 24-hour urine specimen and clinical parameters, prognostic algorithm reported as a clinical risk and integrated clinical steroid risk for adrenal cortical carcinoma, adenoma, or other adrenal malignancy
Decipher Bladder TURBT®, Decipher Biosciences, Inc	0016M	Oncology (bladder), mRNA, microarray gene expression profiling of 209 genes, utilizing formalin fixed paraffin-embedded tissue, algorithm reported as molecular subtype (luminal, luminal infiltrated, basal, basal claudin-low, neuroendocrine-like)
Lymph2Cx, Mayo Clinic Arizona Molecular Diagnostics Laboratory CPT Excludes: Lymph3Cx Lymphoma Molecular Subtyping Assay, Mayo Clinic, Laboratory Developed Test (0120U)	● 0017M	Oncology (diffuse large B-cell lymphoma [DLBCL]), mRNA, gene expression profiling by fluorescent probe hybridization of 20 genes, formalin-fixed paraffin-embedded tissue, algorithm reported as cell of origin

Proprietary Name/Clinical Laboratory/Manufacturer		Code	Descriptor
Pleximark™ Plexision, Inc CPT Excludes: Blood count (85032); Cryopreservation (88240); Flow cytometry (88184-88185, 88187); HLA typing (86821); Lymphocyte transformation, mitogen, antigen induced blastogenesis (86353); Thawing, expansion frozen cells (88241); Tissue cultures, nonneoplastic disorders (88230); Transplantation rejection risk score (81560)	●	0018M	Transplantation medicine (allograft rejection, renal), measurement of donor and third-party-induced CD154+T-cytotoxic memory cells, utilizing whole peripheral blood, algorithm reported as a rejection risk score

Category I Codes for Multianalyte Assays with Algorithmic Analyses (MAAA)

Proprietary Name/Clinical Laboratory/Manufacturer		Code	Descriptor
Vectra® DA, Crescendo Bioscience, Inc		81490	Autoimmune (rheumatoid arthritis), analysis of 12 biomarkers using immunoassays, utilizing serum, prognostic algorithm reported as a disease activity score
AlloMap®, CareDx, Inc	#	81595	Cardiology (heart transplant), mRNA, gene expression profiling by real-time quantitative PCR of 20 genes (11 content and 9 housekeeping), utilizing subfraction of peripheral blood, algorithm reported as a rejection risk score
Corus® CAD, CardioDx, Inc		81493	Coronary artery disease, mRNA, gene expression profiling by real-time RT-PCR of 23 genes, utilizing whole peripheral blood, algorithm reported as a risk score
PreDx Diabetes Risk Score™, Tethys Clinical Laboratory		81506	Endocrinology (type 2 diabetes), biochemical assays of seven analytes (glucose, HbA1c, insulin, hs-CRP, adiponectin, ferritin, interleukin 2-receptor alpha), utilizing serum or plasma, algorithm reporting a risk score
Harmony™ Prenatal Test, Ariosa Diagnostics		81507	Fetal aneuploidy (trisomy 21, 18, and 13) DNA sequence analysis of selected regions using maternal plasma, algorithm reported as a risk score for each trisomy
No proprietary name and clinical laboratory or manufacturer. Maternal serum screening procedures are performed by many labs and are not exclusive to a single facility.		81508	Fetal congenital abnormalities, biochemical assays of two proteins (PAPP-A, hCG [any form]), utilizing maternal serum, algorithm reported as a risk score
		81509	Fetal congenital abnormalities, biochemical assays of three proteins (PAPP-A, hCG [any form], DIA), utilizing maternal serum, algorithm reported as a risk score
		81510	Fetal congenital abnormalities, biochemical assays of three analytes (AFP, uE3, hCG [any form]), utilizing maternal serum, algorithm reported as a risk score
		81511	Fetal congenital abnormalities, biochemical assays of four analytes (AFP, uE3, hCG [any form], DIA) utilizing maternal serum, algorithm reported as a risk score (may include additional results from previous biochemical testing)
		81512	Fetal congenital abnormalities, biochemical assays of five analytes (AFP, uE3, total hCG, hyperglycosylated hCG, DIA) utilizing maternal serum, algorithm reported as a risk score
Aptima® BV Assay, Hologic, Inc		81513	Infectious disease, bacterial vaginosis, quantitative real-time amplification of RNA markers for Atopobium vaginae, Gardnerella vaginalis, and Lactobacillus species, utilizing vaginal-fluid specimens, algorithm reported as a positive or negative result for bacterial vaginosis
BD MAX™ Vaginal Panel, Becton Dickson and Company		81514	Infectious disease, bacterial vaginosis and vaginitis, quantitative real-time amplification of DNA markers for Gardnerella vaginalis, Atopobium vaginae, Megasphaera type 1, Bacterial Vaginosis Associated Bacteria-2 (BVAB-2), and Lactobacillus species (L. crispatus and L. jensenii), utilizing vaginal-fluid specimens, algorithm reported as a positive or negative for high likelihood of bacterial vaginosis, includes separate detection of Trichomonas vaginalis and/or Candida species (C. albicans, C. tropicalis, C. parapsilosis, C. dubliniensis), Candida glabrata, Candida krusei, when reported
HCV FibroSURE™, FibroTest™, BioPredictive S.A.S.	#	81596	Infectious disease, chronic hepatitis C virus (HCV) infection, six biochemical assays (ALT, A2-macroglobulin, apolipoprotein A-1, total bilirubin, GGT, and haptoglobin) utilizing serum, prognostic algorithm reported as scores for fibrosis and necroinflammatory activity in liver
Breast Cancer Index, Biotheranostics, Inc		81518	Oncology (breast), mRNA, gene expression profiling by real-time RT-PCR of 11 genes (7 content and 4 housekeeping), utilizing formalin-fixed paraffin-embedded tissue, algorithms reported as percentage risk for metastatic recurrence and likelihood of benefit from extended endocrine therapy
EndoPredict®, Myriad Genetic Laboratories, Inc	#	81522	Oncology (breast), mRNA, gene expression profiling by RT-PCR of 12 genes (8 content and 4 housekeeping), utilizing formalin-fixed paraffin-embedded tissue, algorithm reported as recurrence risk score
Oncotype DX® Genomic Health		81519	Oncology (breast), mRNA, gene expression profiling by real-time RT-PCR of 21 genes, utilizing formalin-fixed paraffin embedded tissue, algorithm reported as recurrence score
Prosigna® Breast Cancer Assay, NanoString Technologies, Inc		81520	Oncology (breast), mRNA gene expression profiling by hybrid capture of 58 genes (50 content and 8 housekeeping), utilizing formalin-fixed paraffin-embedded tissue, algorithm reported as a recurrence risk score
MammaPrint®, Agendia, Inc		81521	Oncology (breast), mRNA, microarray gene expression profiling of 70 content genes and 465 housekeeping genes, utilizing fresh frozen or formalin-fixed paraffin-embedded tissue, algorithm reported as index related to risk of distant metastasis
MammaPrint®, Agendia, Inc	●	81523	Oncology (breast), mRNA, next-generation sequencing gene expression profiling of 70 content genes and 31 housekeeping genes, utilizing formalin-fixed paraffin-embedded tissue, algorithm reported as index related to risk to distant metastasis

Proprietary Name/Clinical Laboratory/Manufacturer	Code	Descriptor
Oncotype DX® Colon Cancer Assay, Genomic Health CPT Excludes: Oncology (breast), mRNA, next-generation sequencing gene expression profiling, when performed on same specimen (81523).	81525	Oncology (colon), mRNA, gene expression profiling by real-time RT-PCR of 12 genes (7 content and 5 housekeeping), utilizing formalin-fixed paraffin-embedded tissue, algorithm reported as a recurrence score
Cologuard™, Exact Sciences, Inc	81528	Oncology (colorectal) screening, quantitative real-time target and signal amplification of 10 DNA markers (*KRAS* mutations, promoter methylation of *NDRG4* and *BMP3*) and fecal hemoglobin, utilizing stool, algorithm reported as a positive or negative result
DecisionDx® Melanoma, Castle Biosciences, Inc	81529	Oncology (cutaneous melanoma), mRNA, gene expression profiling by real-time RT-PCR of 31 genes (28 content and 3 housekeeping), utilizing formalin-fixed paraffin-embedded tissue, algorithm reported as recurrence risk, including likelihood of sentinel lymph node metastasis
ChemoFX®, Helomics, Corp	81535	Oncology (gynecologic), live tumor cell culture and chemotherapeutic response by DAPI stain and morphology, predictive algorithm reported as a drug response score; first single drug or drug combination
ChemoFX®, Helomics, Corp	+ 81536	each additional single drug or drug combination (List separately in addition to code for primary procedure)
VeriStrat, Biodesix, Inc	81538	Oncology (lung), mass spectrometric 8-protein signature, including amyloid A, utilizing serum, prognostic and predictive algorithm reported as good versus poor overall survival
Risk of Ovarian Malignancy Algorithm (ROMA)™, Fujirebio Diagnostics	# 81500	Oncology (ovarian), biochemical assays of two proteins (CA-125 and HE4), utilizing serum, with menopausal status, algorithm reported as a risk score
OVA1™, Vermillion, Inc	# 81503	Oncology (ovarian), biochemical assays of five proteins (CA-125, apolipoprotein A1, beta-2 microglobulin, transferrin, and pre-albumin), utilizing serum, algorithm reported as a risk score
4Kscore test, OPKO Health, Inc	81539	Oncology (high-grade prostate cancer), biochemical assay of four proteins (Total PSA, Free PSA, Intact PSA, and human kallikrein-2 [hK2]), utilizing plasma or serum, prognostic algorithm reported as a probability score
Prolaris®, Myriad Genetic Laboratories, Inc	81541	Oncology (prostate), mRNA gene expression profiling by real-time RT-PCR of 46 genes (31 content and 15 housekeeping), utilizing formalin-fixed paraffin-embedded tissue, algorithm reported as a disease-specific mortality risk score
Decipher® Prostate, Decipher® Biosciences	81542	Oncology (prostate), mRNA, microarray gene expression profiling of 22 content genes, utilizing formalin-fixed paraffin-embedded tissue, algorithm reported as metastasis risk score
	(81545 has been deleted)	
ConfirmMDx® for Prostate Cancer, MDxHealth, Inc	81551	Oncology (prostate), promoter methylation profiling by real-time PCR of 3 genes (*GSTP1, APC, RASSF1*), utilizing formalin-fixed paraffin-embedded tissue, algorithm reported as a likelihood of prostate cancer detection on repeat biopsy
Afirma® Genomic Sequencing Classifier, Veracyte, Inc	# 81546	Oncology (thyroid), mRNA, gene expression analysis of 10,196 genes, utilizing fine needle aspirate, algorithm reported as a categorical result (eg, benign or suspicious)
Tissue of Origin Test, Kit-FFPE, Cancer Genetics, Inc	# 81504	Oncology (tissue of origin), microarray gene expression profiling of >2000 genes, utilizing formalin-fixed paraffin-embedded tissue, algorithm reported as tissue similarity scores
CancerTYPE ID, bioTheranostics, Inc	# 81540	Oncology (tumor of unknown origin), mRNA, gene expression profiling by real-time RT-PCR of 92 genes (87 content and 5 housekeeping) to classify tumor into main cancer type and subtype, utilizing formalin-fixed paraffin-embedded tissue, algorithm reported as a probability of a predicted main cancer type and subtype
DecisionDx®-UM test, Castle Biosciences, Inc	81552	Oncology (uveal melanoma), mRNA, gene expression profiling by real-time RT-PCR of 15 genes (12 content and 3 housekeeping), utilizing fine needle aspirate or formalin-fixed paraffin-embedded tissue, algorithm reported as risk of metastasis
Envisia® Genomic Classifier, Veracyte, Inc	81554	Pulmonary disease (idiopathic pulmonary fibrosis [IPF]), mRNA, gene expression analysis of 190 genes, utilizing transbronchial biopsies, diagnostic algorithm reported as categorical result (eg, positive or negative for high probability of usual interstitial pneumonia [UIP])
Pleximmune™; Plexision, Inc	● 81560	Transplantation medicine (allograft rejection, pediatric liver and small bowel), measurement of donor and third-party-induced CD154+T-cytotoxic memory cells, utilizing whole peripheral blood, algorithm reported as a rejection risk score
	81599	Unlisted multianalyte assay with algorithmic analysis

Proprietary Laboratory Analyses (PLA)

Proprietary Name/Clinical Laboratory/Manufacturer	Code	Descriptor
PreciseType® HEA Test, Immucor, Inc	0001U	Red blood cell antigen typing, DNA, human erythrocyte antigen gene analysis of 35 antigens from 11 blood groups, utilizing whole blood, common RBC alleles reported
PolypDX™, Atlantic Diagnostic Laboratories, LLC, Metabolomic Technologies, Inc	0002U	Oncology (colorectal), quantitative assessment of three urine metabolites (ascorbic acid, succinic acid and carnitine) by liquid chromatography with tandem mass spectrometry (LC-MS/MS) using multiple reaction monitoring acquisition, algorithm reported as likelihood of adenomatous polyps

Proprietary Name/Clinical Laboratory/Manufacturer	Code	Descriptor
Overa (OVA1 Next Generation), Aspira Labs, Inc, Vermillion, Inc	0003U	Oncology (ovarian) biochemical assays of five proteins (apolipoprotein A-1, CA 125 II, follicle stimulating hormone, human epididymis protein 4, transferrin), utilizing serum, algorithm reported as a likelihood score
ExosomeDx®, Prostate (IntelliScore), Exosome Diagnostics, Inc, Exosome Diagnostics, Inc	0005U	Oncology (prostate) gene expression profile by real-time RT-PCR of 3 genes *ERG, PCA3,* and *SPDEF*), urine, algorithm reported as risk score
	(0006U has been deleted)	
ToxProtect, Genotox Laboratories LTD	0007U	Drug test(s), presumptive, with definitive confirmation of positive results, any number of drug classes, urine, includes specimen verification including DNA authentication in comparison to buccal DNA, per date of service.
AmHPR® H. pylori Antibiotic Resistance Panel, American Molecular Laboratories, Inc	0008U	Helicobacter pylori detection and antibiotic resistance, DNA, 16S and 23S rRNA, gyrA, pbp1,rdxA and rpoB, next generation sequencing, formalin-fixed paraffin-embedded or fresh tissue or fecal sample, predictive, reported as positive or negative for resistance to clarithromycin, fluoroquinolones, metronidazole, amoxicillin, tetracycline, and rifabutin
DEPArray™ HER2, PacificDx	0009U	Oncology (breast cancer), *ERBB2* (HER2) copy number by FISH, tumor cells from formalin-fixed paraffin-embedded tissue isolated using image-based dielectrophoresis (DEP) sorting, reported as *ERBB2* gene amplified or non-amplified
Bacterial Typing by Whole Genome Sequencing, Mayo Clinic	0010U	Infectious disease (bacterial), strain typing by whole genome sequencing, phylogenetic-based report of strain relatedness, per submitted isolate
Cordant CORE™, Cordant Health Solutions	0011U	Prescription drug monitoring, evaluation of drugs present by LC-MS/MS, using oral fluid, reported as a comparison to an estimated steady-state range, per date of service including all drug compounds and metabolites
MatePair Targeted Rearrangements, Congenital, Mayo Clinic	0012U	Germline disorders, gene rearrangement detection by whole genome next-generation sequencing, DNA, whole blood, report of specific gene rearrangement(s)
MatePair Targeted Rearrangements, Oncology, Mayo Clinic	0013U	Oncology (solid organ neoplasia), gene rearrangement detection by whole genome next-generation sequencing, DNA, fresh or frozen tissue or cells, report of specific gene rearrangement(s)
MatePair Targeted Rearrangements, Hematologic, Mayo Clinic	0014U	Hematology (hematolymphoid neoplasia), gene rearrangement detection by whole genome next-generation sequencing, DNA, whole blood or bone marrow, report of specific gene rearrangement(s)
BCR-ABL1 major and minor breakpoint fusion transcripts, University of Iowa, Department of Pathology, Asuragen	0016U	Oncology (hematolymphoid neoplasia), RNA, *BCR/ABL1* major and minor breakpoint fusion transcripts, quantitative PCR amplification, blood or bone marrow, report of fusion not detected or detected with quantitation
JAK2 Mutation, University of Iowa, Department of Pathology	0017U	Oncology (hematolymphoid neoplasia), *JAK2* mutation, DNA, PCR amplification of exons 12-14 and sequence analysis, blood or bone marrow, report of *JAK2* mutation not detected or detected
ThyraMIR™, Interpace Diagnostics	0018U	Oncology (thyroid), microRNA profiling by RT-PCR of 10 microRNA sequences, utilizing fine needle aspirate, algorithm reported as a positive or negative result for moderate to high risk of malignancy
OncoTarget/OncoTreat, Columbia University Department of Pathology and Cell Biology, Darwin Health	0019U	Oncology, RNA, gene expression by whole transcriptome sequencing, formalin-fixed paraffin embedded tissue or fresh frozen tissue, predictive algorithm reported as potential targets for therapeutic agents
	(0020U has been deleted)	
Apifiny®, Armune BioScience, Inc	0021U	Oncology (prostate), detection of 8 autoantibodies (ARF 6, NKX3-1, 5'-UTR-BMI1, CEP 164, 3'-UTR-Ropporin, Desmocollin, AURKAIP-1, CSNK2A2), multiplexed immunoassay and flow cytometry serum, algorithm reported as risk score
Oncomine™ Dx Target Test, Thermo Fisher Scientific	0022U	Targeted genomic sequence analysis panel, non-small cell lung neoplasia, DNA and RNA analysis, 23 genes, interrogation for sequence variants and rearrangements, reported as presence/absence of variants and associated therapy(ies) to consider
LeukoStrat® CDx *FLT3* Mutation Assay, LabPMM LLC, an Invivoscribe Technologies, Inc Company, Invivoscribe Technologies, Inc	0023U	Oncology (acute myelogenous leukemia), DNA, genotyping of internal tandem duplication, p.D835, p.I836, using mononuclear cells, reported as detection or non-detection of *FLT3* mutation and indication for or against the use of midostaurin
GlycA, Laboratory Corporation of America, Laboratory Corporation of America	0024U	Glycosylated acute phase proteins (GlycA), nuclear magnetic resonance spectroscopy, quantitative
UrSure Tenofovir Quantification Test, Synergy Medical Laboratories, UrSure Inc	0025U	Tenofovir, by liquid chromatography with tandem mass spectrometry (LC-MS/MS), urine, quantitative
Thyroseq Genomic Classifier, CBLPath, Inc, University of Pittsburgh Medical Center	0026U	Oncology (thyroid), DNA and mRNA of 112 genes, next-generation sequencing, fine needle aspirate of thyroid nodule, algorithmic analysis reported as a categorical result ("Positive, high probability of malignancy" or "Negative, low probability of malignancy")
JAK2 Exons 12 to 15 Sequencing, Mayo Clinic, Mayo Clinic	0027U	*JAK2 (Janus kinase 2)* (eg, myeloproliferative disorder) gene analysis, targeted sequence analysis exons 12-15
	(0028U has been deleted)	
Focused Pharmacogenomics Panel, Mayo Clinic, Mayo Clinic	0029U	Drug metabolism (adverse drug reactions and drug response), targeted sequence analysis (ie, *CYP1A2, CYP2C19, CYP2C9, CYP2D6, CYP3A4, CYP3A5, CYP4F2, SLCO1B1, VKORC1* and rs12777823)

Proprietary Name/Clinical Laboratory/Manufacturer	Code	Descriptor
Warfarin Response Genotype, Mayo Clinic, Mayo Clinic	0030U	Drug metabolism (warfarin drug response), targeted sequence analysis (i.e., *CYP2C9, CYP4F2, VKORC1,* rs12777823)
Cytochrome P450 1A2 Genotype, Mayo Clinic, Mayo Clinic	0031U	*CYP1A2 (cytochrome P450 family 1, subfamily A, member 2)* (eg, drug metabolism) gene analysis, common variants (ie, *1F, *1K, *6, *7)
Catechol-O-Methyltransferase *(COMT)* Genotype, Mayo Clinic, Mayo Clinic	0032U	*COMT (catechol-O-methyltransferase)* (eg, drug metabolism) gene analysis, c.472G>A (rs4680) variant
Serotonin Receptor Genotype *(HTR2A* and *HTR2C)*, Mayo Clinic, Mayo Clinic	0033U	*HTR2A (5-hydroxytryptamine receptor 2A), HTR2C (5-hydroxytryptamine receptor 2C)* (eg, citalopram metabolism) gene analysis, common variants (i.e., *HTR2A* rs7997012 [c.614-2211T>C], *HTR2C* rs3813929 [c.- 759C>T] and rs1414334 [c.551-3008C>G])
Thiopurine Methyltransferase *(TPMT)* and Nudix Hydrolase *(NUDT15)* Genotyping, Mayo Clinic, Mayo Clinic	0034U	*TPMT (thiopurine S-methyltransferase), NUDT15 (nudix hydroxylase 15)* (eg, thiopurine metabolism) gene analysis, common variants (i.e., *TPMT *2, *3A, *3B, *3C, *4, *5, *6, *8, *12; NUDT15 *3, *4, *5)*
Real-time quaking-induced conversion for prion detection (RT QuIC), National Prion Disease Pathology Surveillance Center	0035U	Neurology (prion disease), cerebrospinal fluid, detection of prion protein by quaking induced conformational conversion, qualitative
EXaCT-1 Whole Exome Testing, Lab of Oncology-Molecular Detection, Weill Cornell Medicine- Clinical Genomics Laboratory	0036U	Exome (ie, somatic mutations), paired formalin-fixed paraffin-embedded tumor tissue and normal specimen, sequence analyses
FoundationOne CDx™ (F1CDx), Foundation Medicine, Inc, Foundation Medicine, Inc	0037U	Targeted genomic sequence analysis, solid organ neoplasm, DNA analysis of 324 genes, interrogation for sequence variants, gene copy number amplifications, gene rearrangements, microsatellite instability and tumor mutational burden
Sensieva ™ Droplet 25OH Vitamin D2/D3 Microvolume LC/MS Assay, InSource Diagnostics, InSource Diagnostics	0038U	Vitamin D, 25 hydroxy D2 and D3, by LC- MS/MS, serum microsample, quantitative
Anti-dsDNA, High Salt/Avidity, University of Washington, Department of Laboratory Medicine, Bio-Rad	0039U	Deoxyribonucleic acid (DNA) antibody, double stranded, high avidity
MRDx BCR-ABL Test, MolecularMD, MolecularMD	0040U	*BCR/ABL1 (t(9;22))* (eg, chronic myelogenous leukemia) translocation analysis, major breakpoint, quantitative
Lyme ImmunoBlot IgM, IGeneX Inc, ID-FISH Technology Inc (ASR) (Lyme ImmunoBlot IgM Strips Only)	0041U	Borrelia burgdorferi, antibody detection of 5 recombinant protein groups, by immunoblot, IgM
Lyme ImmunoBlot IgG, IGeneX Inc, ID-FISH Technology Inc (ASR) (Lyme ImmunoBlot IgG Strips Only)	0042U	Borrelia burgdorferi, antibody detection of 12 recombinant protein groups, by immunoblot, IgG
Tick-Borne Relapsing Fever (TBRF) Borrelia ImmunoBlots IgM Test, IGeneX Inc, ID-FISH Technology Inc (Provides TBRF ImmunoBlot IgM Strips)	0043U	Tick-borne relapsing fever Borrelia group, antibody detection to 4 recombinant protein groups, by immunoblot, IgM
Tick-Borne Relapsing Fever (TBRF) Borrelia ImmunoBlots IgG Test, IGeneX Inc, ID-FISH Technology Inc (Provides TBRF ImmunoBlot IgG Strips)	0044U	Tick-borne relapsing fever Borrelia group, antibody detection to 4 recombinant protein groups, by immunoblot, IgG
The Oncotype DX® Breast DCIS Score™ Test, Genomic Health, Inc, Genomic Health, Inc	0045U	Oncology (breast ductal carcinoma in situ), mRNA, gene expression profiling by real- time RT-PCR of 12 genes (7 content and 5 housekeeping), utilizing formalin-fixed paraffin-embedded tissue, algorithm reported as recurrence score
FLT3 ITD MRD by NGS, LabPMM LLC, an Invivoscribe Technologies, Inc Company	0046U	*FLT3 (fms-related tyrosine kinase 3)* (eg, acute myeloid leukemia) internal tandem duplication (ITD) variants, quantitative
Oncotype DX Genomic Prostate Score, Genomic Health, Inc, Genomic Health, Inc	0047U	Oncology (prostate), mRNA, gene expression profiling by real-time RT-PCR of 17 genes (12 content and 5 housekeeping), utilizing formalin-fixed paraffin-embedded tissue, algorithm reported as a risk score
MSK-IMPACT (Integrated Mutation Profiling of Actionable Cancer Targets), Memorial Sloan Kettering Cancer Center	0048U	Oncology (solid organ neoplasia), DNA, targeted sequencing of protein-coding exons of 468 cancer-associated genes, including interrogation for somatic mutations and microsatellite instability, matched with normal specimens, utilizing formalin-fixed paraffin-embedded tumor tissue, report of clinically significant mutation(s)
NPM1 MRD by NGS, LabPMM LLC, an Invivoscribe Technologies, Inc Company	0049U	*NPM1 (nucleophosmin)* (eg, acute myeloid leukemia) gene analysis, quantitative
MyAML NGS Panel, LabPMM LLC, an Invivoscribe Technologies, Inc Company	0050U	Targeted genomic sequence analysis panel, acute myelogenous leukemia, DNA analysis, 194 genes, interrogation for sequence variants, copy number variants or rearrangements
UCompliDx, Elite Medical Laboratory Solutions, LLC, Elite Medical Laboratory Solutions, LLC (LDT)	▲ 0051U	Prescription drug monitoring, evaluation of drugs present by liquid chromatography tandem mass spectrometry (LC-MS/MS), urine or blood, 31 drug panel, reported as quantitative results, detected or not detected, per date of service
VAP Cholesterol Test, VAP Diagnostics Laboratory, Inc, VAP Diagnostics Laboratory, Inc	0052U	Lipoprotein, blood, high resolution fractionation and quantitation of lipoproteins, including all five major lipoprotein classes and subclasses of HDL, LDL, and VLDL by vertical auto profile ultracentrifugation
Prostate Cancer Risk Panel, Mayo Clinic, Laboratory Developed Test	0053U	Oncology (prostate cancer), FISH analysis of 4 genes (*ASAP1, HDAC9, CHD1* and *PTEN*), needle biopsy specimen, algorithm reported as probability of higher tumor grade
AssuranceRx Micro Serum, Firstox Laboratories, LLC, Firstox Laboratories, LLC	0054U	Prescription drug monitoring, 14 or more classes of drugs and substances, definitive tandem mass spectrometry with chromatography, capillary blood, quantitative report with therapeutic and toxic ranges, including steady-state range for the prescribed dose when detected, per date of service

Proprietary Name/Clinical Laboratory/Manufacturer	Code	Descriptor
myTAIHEART, TAI Diagnostics, Inc, TAI Diagnostics, Inc	0055U	Cardiology (heart transplant), cell-free DNA, PCR assay of 96 DNA target sequences (94 single nucleotide polymorphism targets and two control targets), plasma
MatePair Acute Myeloid Leukemia Panel, Mayo Clinic, Laboratory Developed Test	0056U	Hematology (acute myelogenous leukemia), DNA, whole genome next- generation sequencing to detect gene rearrangement(s), blood or bone marrow, report of specific gene rearrangement(s)
	(0057U has been deleted)	
Merkel SmT Oncoprotein Antibody Titer, University of Washington, Department of Laboratory Medicine	0058U	Oncology (Merkel cell carcinoma), detection of antibodies to the Merkel cell polyoma virus oncoprotein (small T antigen), serum, quantitative
Merkel Virus VP1 Capsid Antibody, University of Washington, Department of Laboratory Medicine	0059U	Oncology (Merkel cell carcinoma), detection of antibodies to the Merkel cell polyoma virus capsid protein (VP1), serum, reported as positive or negative
Twins Zygosity PLA, Natera, Inc, Natera, Inc	0060U	Twin zygosity, genomic-targeted sequence analysis of chromosome 2, using circulating cell-free fetal DNA in maternal blood
Transcutaneous multispectral measurement of tissue oxygenation and hemoglobin using spatial frequency domain imaging (SFDI), Modulated Imaging, Inc, Modulated Imaging, Inc	0061U	Transcutaneous measurement of five biomarkers (tissue oxygenation [StO2], oxyhemoglobin [ctHbO2], deoxyhemoglobin [ctHbR], papillary and reticular dermal hemoglobin concentrations [ctHb1 and ctHb2]), using spatial frequency domain imaging (SFDI) and multi-spectral analysis
SLE-key® Rule Out, Veracis Inc, Veracis Inc	0062U	Autoimmune (systemic lupus erythematosus), IgG and IgM analysis of 80 biomarkers, utilizing serum, algorithm reported with a risk score
NPDX ASD ADM Panel I, Stemina Biomarker Discovery, Inc, Stemina Biomarker Discovery, Inc d/b/a NeuroPointDX	0063U	Neurology (autism), 32 amines by LC-MS/MS, using plasma, algorithm reported as metabolic signature associated with autism spectrum disorder
BioPlex 2200 Syphilis Total & RPR Assay, Bio-Rad Laboratories, Bio-Rad Laboratories	0064U	Antibody, Treponema pallidum, total and rapid plasma reagin (RPR), immunoassay, qualitative
BioPlex 2200 RPR Assay, Bio-Rad Laboratories, Bio-Rad Laboratories	0065U	Syphilis test, non-treponemal antibody, immunoassay, qualitative (RPR)
PartoSure™ Test, Parsagen Diagnostics, Inc, Parsagen Diagnostics, Inc, a QIAGEN Company	0066U	Placental alpha-micro globulin-1 (PAMG-1), immunoassay with direct optical observation, cervico-vaginal fluid, each specimen
BBDRisk Dx™, Silbiotech, Inc, Silbiotech, Inc	0067U	Oncology (breast), immunohistochemistry, protein expression profiling of 4 biomarkers (matrix metalloproteinase-1 [MMP-1], carcinoembryonic antigen-related cell adhesion molecule 6 [CEACAM6], hyaluronoglucosaminidase [HYAL1], highly expressed in cancer protein [HEC1]), formalin-fixed paraffin-embedded precancerous breast tissue, algorithm reported as carcinoma risk score
MYCODART-PCR™ Dual Amplification Real Time PCR Panel for 6 Candida species, RealTime Laboratories, Inc/MycoDART, Inc, RealTime Laboratories, Inc	0068U	Candida species panel (*C. albicans, C. glabrata, C. parapsilosis, C. kruseii, C tropicalis, and C. auris*), amplified probe technique with qualitative report of the presence or absence of each species
miR-31now™, GoPath Laboratories, GoPath Laboratories	0069U	Oncology (colorectal), microRNA, RT-PCR expression profiling of miR-31-3p, formalin-fixed paraffin-embedded tissue, algorithm reported as an expression score
CYP2D6 Common Variants and Copy Number, Mayo Clinic, Laboratory Developed Test	0070U	*CYP2D6 (cytochrome P450, family 2, subfamily D, polypeptide 6)* (eg, drug metabolism) gene analysis, common and select rare variants (ie, *2, *3, *4, *4N, *5, *6, *7, *8, *9, *10, *11, *12, *13, *14A, *14B, *15, *17, *29, *35, *36, *41, *57, *61, *63, *68, *83, *xN)
CYP2D6 Full Gene Sequencing, Mayo Clinic, Laboratory Developed Test	+ 0071U	*CYP2D6 (cytochrome P450, family 2, subfamily D, polypeptide 6)* (eg, drug metabolism) gene analysis, full gene sequence (List separately in addition to code for primary procedure)
CYP2D6-2D7 Hybrid Gene Targeted Sequence Analysis, Mayo Clinic, Laboratory Developed Test	+ 0072U	*CYP2D6 (cytochrome P450, family 2, subfamily D, polypeptide 6)* (eg, drug metabolism) gene analysis, targeted sequence analysis (ie, CYP2D6-2D7 hybrid gene) (List separately in addition to code for primary procedure)
CYP2D7-2D6 Hybrid Gene Targeted Sequence Analysis, Mayo Clinic, Laboratory Developed Test	+ 0073U	*CYP2D6 (cytochrome P450, family 2, subfamily D, polypeptide 6)* (eg, drug metabolism) gene analysis, targeted sequence analysis (ie, CYP2D7-2D6 hybrid gene) (List separately in addition to code for primary procedure)
CYP2D6 trans-duplication/multiplication non-duplicated gene targeted sequence analysis, Mayo Clinic, Laboratory Developed Test	+ 0074U	*CYP2D6 (cytochrome P450, family 2, subfamily D, polypeptide 6)* (eg, drug metabolism) gene analysis, targeted sequence analysis (ie, non-duplicated gene when duplication/multiplication is trans) (List separately in addition to code for primary procedure)
CYP2D6 5' gene duplication/multiplication targeted sequence analysis, Mayo Clinic, Laboratory Developed Test	+ 0075U	*CYP2D6 (cytochrome P450, family 2, subfamily D, polypeptide 6)* (eg, drug metabolism) gene analysis, targeted sequence analysis (ie, 5' gene duplication/multiplication) (List separately in addition to code for primary procedure)
CYP2D6 3' gene duplication/multiplication targeted sequence analysis, Mayo Clinic, Laboratory Developed Test	+ 0076U	*CYP2D6 (cytochrome P450, family 2, subfamily D, polypeptide 6)* (eg, drug metabolism) gene analysis, targeted sequence analysis (ie, 3' gene duplication/multiplication) (List separately in addition to code for primary procedure)
M-Protein Detection and Isotyping by MALDI-TOF Mass Spectrometry, Mayo Clinic, Laboratory Developed Test	0077U	Immunoglobulin paraprotein (M-protein), qualitative, immunoprecipitation and mass spectrometry, blood or urine, including isotype
INFINITI® Neural Response Panel, PersonalizeDx Labs, AutoGenomics Inc	0078U	Pain management (opioid-use disorder) genotyping panel, 16 common variants (ie, *ABCB1, COMT, DAT1, DBH, DOR, DRD1, DRD2, DRD4, GABA, GAL, HTR2A, HTTLPR, MTHFR, MUOR, OPRK1, OPRM1*), buccal swab or other germline tissue sample, algorithm reported as positive or negative risk of opioid-use disorder
ToxLok™, InSource Diagnostics, InSource Diagnostics	0079U	Comparative DNA analysis using multiple selected single-nucleotide polymorphisms (SNPs), urine and buccal DNA, for specimen identity verification

Proprietary Name/Clinical Laboratory/Manufacturer	Code	Descriptor
BDX-XL2, Biodesix®, Inc, Biodesix®, Inc	0080U	Oncology (lung), mass spectrometric analysis of galectin-3-binding protein and scavenger receptor cysteine-rich type 1 protein M130, with five clinical risk factors (age, smoking status, nodule diameter, nodule-spiculation status and nodule location), utilizing plasma, algorithm reported as a categorical probability of malignancy
	(0081U has been deleted. To report, use 81552)	
NextGen Precision™ Testing, Precision Diagnostics, Precision Diagnostics LBN Precision Toxicology, LLC	0082U	Drug test(s), definitive, 90 or more drugs or substances, definitive chromatography with mass spectrometry, and presumptive, any number of drug classes, by instrument chemistry analyzer (utilizing immunoassay), urine, report of presence or absence of each drug, drug metabolite or substance with description and severity of significant interactions per date of service
Onco4D™, Animated Dynamics, Inc, Animated Dynamics, Inc	0083U	Oncology, response to chemotherapy drugs using motility contrast tomography, fresh or frozen tissue, reported as likelihood of sensitivity or resistance to drugs or drug combinations
BLOODchip®, ID CORE XT™, Grifols Diagnostic Solutions Inc	0084U	Red blood cell antigen typing, DNA, genotyping of 10 blood groups with phenotype prediction of 37 red blood cell antigens
	(0085U has been deleted)	
Accelerate PhenoTest™ BC kit, Accelerate Diagnostics, Inc	0086U	Infectious disease (bacterial and fungal), organism identification, blood culture, using rRNA FISH, 6 or more organism targets, reported as positive or negative with phenotypic minimum inhibitory concentration (MIC)-based antimicrobial susceptibility
Molecular Microscope® MMDx—Heart, Kashi Clinical Laboratories	0087U	Cardiology (heart transplant), mRNA gene expression profiling by microarray of 1283 genes, transplant biopsy tissue, allograft rejection and injury algorithm reported as a probability score
Molecular Microscope® MMDx—Kidney, Kashi Clinical Laboratories	0088U	Transplantation medicine (kidney allograft rejection), microarray gene expression profiling of 1494 genes, utilizing transplant biopsy tissue, algorithm reported as a probability score for rejection
Pigmented Lesion Assay (PLA), DermTech	0089U	Oncology (melanoma), gene expression profiling by RTqPCR, *PRAME* and *LINC00518*, superficial collection using adhesive patch(es)
myPath® Melanoma, Myriad Genetic Laboratories	0090U	Oncology (cutaneous melanoma), mRNA gene expression profiling by RT-PCR of 23 genes (14 content and 9 housekeeping), utilizing formalin-fixed paraffin-embedded tissue, algorithm reported as a categorical result (ie, benign, indeterminate, malignant)
FirstSight^CRC, CellMax Life	0091U	Oncology (colorectal) screening, cell enumeration of circulating tumor cells, utilizing whole blood, algorithm, for the presence of adenoma or cancer, reported as a positive or negative result
REVEAL Lung Nodule Characterization, MagArray, Inc	0092U	Oncology (lung), three protein biomarkers, immunoassay using magnetic nanosensor technology, plasma, algorithm reported as risk score for likelihood of malignancy
ComplyRX, Claro Labs	0093U	Prescription drug monitoring, evaluation of 65 common drugs by LC-MS/MS, urine, each drug reported detected or not detected
RCIGM Rapid Whole Genome Sequencing, Rady Children's Institute for Genomic Medicine (RCIGM)	0094U	Genome (eg, unexplained constitutional or heritable disorder or syndrome), rapid sequence analysis
Esophageal String Test™ (EST), Cambridge Biomedical, Inc	0095U	Inflammation (eosinophilic esophagitis), ELISA analysis of eotaxin-3 *(CCL26 [C-C motif chemokine ligand 26])* and major basic protein *(PRG2 [proteoglycan 2, pro eosinophil major basic protein])*, specimen obtained by swallowed nylon string, algorithm reported as predictive probability index for active eosinophilic esophagitis
HPV, High-Risk, Male Urine, Molecular Testing Labs	0096U	Human papillomavirus (HPV), high-risk types (ie, 16, 18, 31, 33, 35, 39, 45, 51, 52, 56, 58, 59, 66, 68), male urine
BioFire® FilmArray® Gastrointestinal (GI) Panel, BioFire® Diagnostics	0097U	Gastrointestinal pathogen, multiplex reverse transcription and multiplex amplified probe technique, multiple types or subtypes, 22 targets (Campylobacter [C. jejuni/C. coli/C. upsaliensis], Clostridium difficile [C. difficile] toxin A/B, Plesiomonas shigelloides, Salmonella, Vibrio [V. parahaemolyticus/V. vulnificus/V. cholerae], including specific identification of Vibrio cholerae, Yersinia enterocolitica, Enteroaggregative Escherichia coli [EAEC], Enteropathogenic Escherichia coli [EPEC], Enterotoxigenic Escherichia coli [ETEC] lt/st, Shiga-like toxin-producing Escherichia coli [STEC] stx1/stx2 [including specific identification of the E. coli O157 serogroup within STEC], Shigella/Enteroinvasive Escherichia coli [EIEC], Cryptosporidium, Cyclospora cayetanensis, Entamoeba histolytica, Giardia lamblia [also known as G. intestinalis and G. duodenalis], adenovirus F 40/41, astrovirus, norovirus GI/GII, rotavirus A, sapovirus [Genogroups I, II, IV, and V])
	(0098U has been deleted)	
	(0099U has been deleted)	
	(0100U has been deleted)	
ColoNext®, Ambry Genetics®, Ambry Genetics®	0101U	Hereditary colon cancer disorders (eg, Lynch syndrome, *PTEN* hamartoma syndrome, Cowden syndrome, familial adenomatosis polyposis), genomic sequence analysis panel utilizing a combination of NGS, Sanger, MLPA, and array CGH, with MRNA analytics to resolve variants of unknown significance when indicated (15 genes [sequencing and deletion/duplication], *EPCAM* and *GREM1* [deletion/duplication only])

Proprietary Name/Clinical Laboratory/Manufacturer	Code	Descriptor
BreastNext®, Ambry Genetics®, Ambry Genetics®	0102U	Hereditary breast cancer-related disorders (eg, hereditary breast cancer, hereditary ovarian cancer, hereditary endometrial cancer), genomic sequence analysis panel utilizing a combination of NGS, Sanger, MLPA, and array CGH, with MRNA analytics to resolve variants of unknown significance when indicated (17 genes [sequencing and deletion/duplication])
OvaNext®, Ambry Genetics®, Ambry Genetics®	0103U	Hereditary ovarian cancer (eg, hereditary ovarian cancer, hereditary endometrial cancer), genomic sequence analysis panel utilizing a combination of NGS, Sanger, MLPA, and array CGH, with MRNA analytics to resolve variants of unknown significance when indicated (24 genes [sequencing and deletion/duplication], *EPCAM* [deletion/duplication only])
	(0104U has been deleted)	
KidneyIntelX™, RenalytixAI, RenalytixAI	0105U	Nephrology (chronic kidney disease), multiplex electrochemiluminescent immunoassay (ECLIA) of tumor necrosis factor receptor 1A, receptor superfamily 2 (*TNFR1, TNFR2*), and kidney injury molecule-1 (KIM-1) combined with longitudinal clinical data, including *APOL1* genotype if available, and plasma (isolated fresh or frozen), algorithm reported as probability score for rapid kidney function decline (RKFD)
13C-Spirulina Gastric Emptying Breath Test (GEBT), Cairn Diagnostics d/b/a Advanced Breath Diagnostics, LLC, Cairn Diagnostics d/b/a Advanced Breath Diagnostics, LLC	0106U	Gastric emptying, serial collection of 7 timed breath specimens, non-radioisotope carbon-13 (^{13}C) spirulina substrate, analysis of each specimen by gas isotope ratio mass spectrometry, reported as rate of $^{13}CO_2$ excretion
Singulex Clarity C.diff toxins A/B Assay, Singulex	0107U	Clostridium difficile toxin(s) antigen detection by immunoassay technique, stool, qualitative, multiple-step method
TissueCypher® Barrett's Esophagus Assay, Cernostics, Cernostics	0108U	Gastroenterology (Barrett's esophagus), whole slide-digital imaging, including morphometric analysis, computer-assisted quantitative immunolabeling of 9 protein biomarkers (p16, AMACR, p53, CD68, COX-2, CD45RO, HIF1a, HER-2, K20) and morphology, formalin-fixed paraffin-embedded tissue, algorithm reported as risk of progression to high-grade dysplasia or cancer
MYCODART Dual Amplification Real Time PCR Panel for 4 Aspergillus species, RealTime Laboratories, Inc/MycoDART, Inc	0109U	Infectious disease (Aspergillus species), real-time PCR for detection of DNA from 4 species (*A. fumigatus, A. terreus, A. niger,* and *A. flavus*), blood, lavage fluid, or tissue, qualitative reporting of presence or absence of each species
Oral OncolyticAssuranceRX, Firstox Laboratories, LLC, Firstox Laboratories, LLC	0110U	Prescription drug monitoring, one or more oral oncology drug(s) and substances, definitive tandem mass spectrometry with chromatography, serum or plasma from capillary blood or venous blood, quantitative report with steady-state range for the prescribed drug(s) when detected
Praxis™ Extended RAS Panel, Illumina, Illumina	0111U	Oncology (colon cancer), targeted *KRAS* (codons 12, 13, and 61) and *NRAS* (codons 12, 13, and 61) gene analysis utilizing formalin-fixed paraffin-embedded tissue
MicroGenDX qPCR & NGS For Infection, MicroGenDX, MicroGenDX	0112U	Infectious agent detection and identification, targeted sequence analysis (16S and 18S rRNA genes) with drug-resistance gene
MiPS (Mi-Prostate Score), MLabs, MLabs	0113U	Oncology (prostate), measurement of *PCA3* and *TMPRSS2-ERG* in urine and PSA in serum following prostatic massage, by RNA amplification and fluorescence-based detection, algorithm reported as risk score
EsoGuard™, Lucid Diagnostics, Lucid Diagnostics	0114U	Gastroenterology (Barrett's esophagus), *VIM* and *CCNA1* methylation analysis, esophageal cells, algorithm reported as likelihood for Barrett's esophagus
ePlex Respiratory Pathogen (RP) Panel, GenMark Diagnostics, Inc, GenMark Diagnostics, Inc	0115U	Respiratory infectious agent detection by nucleic acid (DNA and RNA), 18 viral types and subtypes and 2 bacterial targets, amplified probe technique, including multiplex reverse transcription for RNA targets, each analyte reported as detected or not detected
Snapshot Oral Fluid Compliance, Ethos Laboratories	0116U	Prescription drug monitoring, enzyme immunoassay of 35 or more drugs confirmed with LC-MS/MS, oral fluid, algorithm results reported as a patient-compliance measurement with risk of drug to drug interactions for prescribed medications
Foundation PI℠, Ethos Laboratories	0117U	Pain management, analysis of 11 endogenous analytes (methylmalonic acid, xanthurenic acid, homocysteine, pyroglutamic acid, vanilmandelate, 5-hydroxyindoleacetic acid, hydroxymethylglutarate, ethylmalonate, 3-hydroxypropyl mercapturic acid (3-HPMA), quinolinic acid, kynurenic acid), LC-MS/MS, urine, algorithm reported as a pain-index score with likelihood of atypical biochemical function associated with pain
Viracor TRAC™ dd-cfDNA, Viracor Eurofins, Viracor Eurofins	0118U	Transplantation medicine, quantification of donor-derived cell-free DNA using whole genome next-generation sequencing, plasma, reported as percentage of donor-derived cell-free DNA in the total cell-free DNA
MI-HEART Ceramides, Plasma, Mayo Clinic, Laboratory Developed Test	0119U	Cardiology, ceramides by liquid chromatography-tandem mass spectrometry, plasma, quantitative report with risk score for major cardiovascular events
Lymph3Cx Lymphoma Molecular Subtyping Assay, Mayo Clinic, Laboratory Developed Test CPT Excludes: Oncology (diffuse large B-cell lymphoma [DLBCL]), mRNA, gene expression profiling by fluorescent probe hybridization of 20 genes (0017M)	0120U	Oncology (B-cell lymphoma classification), mRNA, gene expression profiling by fluorescent probe hybridization of 58 genes (45 content and 13 housekeeping genes), formalin-fixed paraffin-embedded tissue, algorithm reported as likelihood for primary mediastinal B-cell lymphoma (PMBCL) and diffuse large B-cell lymphoma (DLBCL) with cell of origin subtyping in the latter
Flow Adhesion of Whole Blood on VCAM-1 (FAB-V), Functional Fluidics, Functional Fluidics	0121U	Sickle cell disease, microfluidic flow adhesion (VCAM-1), whole blood
Flow Adhesion of Whole Blood to P-SELECTIN (WB-PSEL), Functional Fluidics, Functional Fluidics	0122U	Sickle cell disease, microfluidic flow adhesion (P-Selectin), whole blood

Proprietary Name/Clinical Laboratory/Manufacturer	Code	Descriptor
Mechanical Fragility, RBC by shear stress profiling and spectral analysis, Functional Fluidics, Functional Fluidics	0123U	Mechanical fragility, RBC, shear stress and spectral analysis profiling
	(0124U has been deleted)	
	(0125U has been deleted)	
	(0126U has been deleted)	
	(0127U has been deleted)	
	(0128U has been deleted)	
BRCAplus, Ambry Genetics	0129U	Hereditary breast cancer-related disorders (eg, hereditary breast cancer, hereditary ovarian cancer, hereditary endometrial cancer), genomic sequence analysis and deletion/duplication analysis panel *(ATM, BRCA1, BRCA2, CDH1, CHEK2, PALB2, PTEN, and TP53)*
+RNAinsight™ for ColoNext®, Ambry Genetics	+ 0130U	Hereditary colon cancer disorders (eg, Lynch syndrome, PTEN hamartoma syndrome, Cowden syndrome, familial adenomatosis polyposis), targeted mRNA sequence analysis panel *(APC, CDH1, CHEK2, MLH1, MSH2, MSH6, MUTYH, PMS2, PTEN,* and *TP53)* (List separately in addition to code for primary procedure)
+RNAinsight™ for BreastNext®, Ambry Genetics	+ 0131U	Hereditary breast cancer-related disorders (eg, hereditary breast cancer, hereditary ovarian cancer, hereditary endometrial cancer), targeted mRNA sequence analysis panel (13 genes) (List separately in addition to code for primary procedure)
+RNAinsight™ for OvaNext®, Ambry Genetics	+ 0132U	Hereditary ovarian cancer-related disorders (eg, hereditary breast cancer, hereditary ovarian cancer, hereditary endometrial cancer), targeted mRNA sequence analysis panel (17 genes) (List separately in addition to code for primary procedure)
+RNAinsight™ for ProstateNext®, Ambry Genetics	+ 0133U	Hereditary prostate cancer-related disorders, targeted mRNA sequence analysis panel (11 genes) (List separately in addition to code for primary procedure)
+RNAinsight™ for CancerNext®, Ambry Genetics	+ 0134U	Hereditary pan cancer (eg, hereditary breast and ovarian cancer, hereditary endometrial cancer, hereditary colorectal cancer), targeted mRNA sequence analysis panel (18 genes) (List separately in addition to code for primary procedure)
+RNAinsight™ for GYNPlus®, Ambry Genetics	+ 0135U	Hereditary gynecological cancer (eg, hereditary breast and ovarian cancer, hereditary endometrial cancer, hereditary colorectal cancer), targeted mRNA sequence analysis panel (12 genes) (List separately in addition to code for primary procedure)
+RNAinsight™ for *ATM*, Ambry Genetics	+ 0136U	*ATM (ataxia telangiectasia mutated)* (eg, ataxia telangiectasia) mRNA sequence analysis (List separately in addition to code for primary procedure)
+RNAinsight™ for *PALB2*, Ambry Genetics	+ 0137U	*PALB2 (partner and localizer of BRCA2)* (eg, breast and pancreatic cancer) mRNA sequence analysis (List separately in addition to code for primary procedure)
+RNAinsight™ for *BRCA1/2*, Ambry Genetics	+ 0138U	*BRCA1 (BRCA1, DNA repair associated), BRCA2 (BRCA2, DNA repair associated)* (eg, hereditary breast and ovarian cancer) mRNA sequence analysis (List separately in addition to code for primary procedure)
	(0139U has been deleted)	
ePlex® BCID Fungal Pathogens Panel, GenMark Diagnostics, Inc, GenMark Diagnostics, Inc	0140U	Infectious disease (fungi), fungal pathogen identification, DNA (15 fungal targets), blood culture, amplified probe technique, each target reported as detected or not detected
ePlex® BCID Gram-Positive Panel, GenMark Diagnostics, Inc, GenMark Diagnostics, Inc	0141U	Infectious disease (bacteria and fungi), gram-positive organism identification and drug resistance element detection, DNA (20 gram-positive bacterial targets, 4 resistance genes, 1 pan gram-negative bacterial target, 1 pan Candida target), blood culture, amplified probe technique, each target reported as detected or not detected
ePlex® BCID Gram-Negative Panel, GenMark Diagnostics, Inc, GenMark Diagnostics, Inc	0142U	Infectious disease (bacteria and fungi), gram-negative bacterial identification and drug resistance element detection, DNA (21 gram-negative bacterial targets, 6 resistance genes, 1 pan gram-positive bacterial target, 1 pan Candida target), amplified probe technique, each target reported as detected or not detected
CareViewRx, Newstar Medical Laboratories, LLC, Newstar Medical Laboratories, LLC CPT Excludes: PsychViewRx Plus analysis by Newstar Medical Laboratories, LLC. (0150U)	0143U	Drug assay, definitive, 120 or more drugs or metabolites, urine, quantitative liquid chromatography with tandem mass spectrometry (LC-MS/MS) using multiple reaction monitoring (MRM), with drug or metabolite description, comments including sample validation, per date of service
CareViewRx Plus, Newstar Medical Laboratories, LLC, Newstar Medical Laboratories, LLC	0144U	Drug assay, definitive, 160 or more drugs or metabolites, urine, quantitative liquid chromatography with tandem mass spectrometry (LC-MS/MS) using multiple reaction monitoring (MRM), with drug or metabolite description, comments including sample validation, per date of service
PainViewRx, Newstar Medical Laboratories, LLC, Newstar Medical Laboratories, LLC	0145U	Drug assay, definitive, 65 or more drugs or metabolites, urine, quantitative liquid chromatography with tandem mass spectrometry (LC-MS/MS) using multiple reaction monitoring (MRM), with drug or metabolite description, comments including sample validation, per date of service
PainViewRx Plus, Newstar Medical Laboratories, LLC, Newstar Medical Laboratories, LLC	0146U	Drug assay, definitive, 80 or more drugs or metabolites, urine, by quantitative liquid chromatography with tandem mass spectrometry (LC-MS/MS) using multiple reaction monitoring (MRM), with drug or metabolite description, comments including sample validation, per date of service

Appendix L — Multianalyte Assays with Algorithmic Analyses

Proprietary Name/Clinical Laboratory/Manufacturer	Code	Descriptor
RiskViewRx, Newstar Medical Laboratories, LLC, Newstar Medical Laboratories, LLC	0147U	Drug assay, definitive, 85 or more drugs or metabolites, urine, quantitative liquid chromatography with tandem mass spectrometry (LC-MS/MS) using multiple reaction monitoring (MRM), with drug or metabolite description, comments including sample validation, per date of service
RiskViewRx Plus, Newstar Medical Laboratories, LLC, Newstar Medical Laboratories, LLC	0148U	Drug assay, definitive, 100 or more drugs or metabolites, urine, quantitative liquid chromatography with tandem mass spectrometry (LC-MS/MS) using multiple reaction monitoring (MRM), with drug or metabolite description, comments including sample validation, per date of service
PsychViewRx, Newstar Medical Laboratories, LLC, Newstar Medical Laboratories, LLC	0149U	Drug assay, definitive, 60 or more drugs or metabolites, urine, quantitative liquid chromatography with tandem mass spectrometry (LC-MS/MS) using multiple reaction monitoring (MRM), with drug or metabolite description, comments including sample validation, per date of service
PsychViewRx Plus, Newstar Medical Laboratories, LLC, Newstar Medical Laboratories, LLC CPT Excludes: CareViewRx analysis by Newstar Medical Laboratories, LLC. (0143U)	0150U	Drug assay, definitive, 120 or more drugs or metabolites, urine, quantitative liquid chromatography with tandem mass spectrometry (LC-MS/MS) using multiple reaction monitoring (MRM), with drug or metabolite description, comments including sample validation, per date of service
BioFire® FilmArray® Pneumonia Panel, BioFire® Diagnostics, BioFire® Diagnostics	0151U	Infectious disease (bacterial or viral respiratory tract infection), pathogen specific nucleic acid (DNA or RNA), 33 targets, real-time semi-quantitative PCR, bronchoalveolar lavage, sputum, or endotracheal aspirate, detection of 33 organismal and antibiotic resistance genes with limited semi-quantitative results
Karius® Test, Karius Inc, Karius Inc	▲ 0152U	Infectious disease (bacteria, fungi, parasites, and DNA viruses), microbial cell-free DNA, plasma, untargeted next-generation sequencing, report for significant positive pathogens
Insight TNBCtype™, Insight Molecular Labs	0153U	Oncology (breast), mRNA, gene expression profiling by next-generation sequencing of 101 genes, utilizing formalin-fixed paraffin-embedded tissue, algorithm reported as a triple negative breast cancer clinical subtype(s) with information on immune cell involvement
therascreen® FGFR RGQ RT-PCR Kit, QIAGEN, QIAGEN GmbH	0154U	Oncology (urothelial cancer), RNA, analysis by real-time RT-PCR of the *FGFR3 (fibroblast growth factor receptor3)* gene analysis (ie, p.R248C [c.742C>T], p.S249C [c.746C>G], p.G370C [c.1108G>T], p.Y373C [c.1118A>G], FGFR3-TACC3v1, and FGFR3-TACC3v3) utilizing formalin-fixed paraffin-embedded urothelial cancer tumor tissue, reported as *FGFR* gene alteration status
therascreen PIK3CA RGQ PCR Kit, QIAGEN, QIAGEN GmbH	0155U	Oncology (breast cancer), DNA, *PIK3CA (phosphatidylinositol-4,5-bisphosphate 3-kinase, catalytic subunit alpha)* (eg, breast cancer) gene analysis (ie, p.C420R, p.E542K, p.E545A, p.E545D [g.1635G>T only], p.E545G, p.E545K, p.Q546E, p.Q546R, p.H1047L, p.H1047R, p.H1047Y), utilizing formalin-fixed paraffin-embedded breast tumor tissue, reported as *PIK3CA* gene mutation status
SMASH™, New York Genome Center, Marvel Genomics™	0156U	Copy number (eg, intellectual disability, dysmorphology), sequence analysis
CustomNext + RNA: APC, Ambry Genetics®, Ambry Genetics®	✚ 0157U	*APC (APC regulator of WNT signaling pathway)* (eg, familial adenomatosis polyposis [FAP]) mRNA sequence analysis (List separately in addition to code for primary procedure)
CustomNext + RNA: *MLH1*, Ambry Genetics®, Ambry Genetics®	✚ 0158U	*MLH1 (mutL homolog 1)* (eg, hereditary non-polyposis colorectal cancer, Lynch syndrome) mRNA sequence analysis (List separately in addition to code for primary procedure)
CustomNext + RNA: *MSH2*, Ambry Genetics®, Ambry Genetics®	✚ 0159U	*MSH2 (mutS homolog 2)* (eg, hereditary colon cancer, Lynch syndrome) mRNA sequence analysis (List separately in addition to code for primary procedure)
CustomNext + RNA: *MSH6*, Ambry Genetics®, Ambry Genetics®	✚ 0160U	*MSH6 (mutS homolog 6)* (eg, hereditary colon cancer, Lynch syndrome) mRNA sequence analysis (List separately in addition to code for primary procedure)
CustomNext + RNA: *PMS2*, Ambry Genetics®, Ambry Genetics®	✚ 0161U	*PMS2 (PMS1 homolog 2, mismatch repair system component)* (eg, hereditary non-polyposis colorectal cancer, Lynch syndrome) mRNA sequence analysis (List separately in addition to code for primary procedure)
CustomNext + RNA: Lynch *(MLH1, MSH2, MSH6, PMS2)*, Ambry Genetics®, Ambry Genetics®	✚ 0162U	Hereditary colon cancer (Lynch syndrome), targeted mRNA sequence analysis panel *(MLH1, MSH2, MSH6, PMS2)* (List separately in addition to code for primary procedure)
BeScreened™-CRC, Beacon Biomedical Inc, Beacon Biomedical Inc	0163U	Oncology (colorectal) screening, biochemical enzyme-linked immunosorbent assay (ELISA) of 3 plasma or serum proteins (teratocarcinoma derived growth factor-1 [TDGF-1, Cripto-1], carcinoembryonic antigen [CEA], extracellular matrix protein [ECM]), with demographic data (age, gender, CRC-screening compliance) using a proprietary algorithm and reported as likelihood of CRC or advanced adenomas
ibs-smart™, Gemelli Biotech, Gemelli Biotech	0164U	Gastroenterology (irritable bowel syndrome [IBS]), immunoassay for anti-CdtB and anti-vinculin antibodies, utilizing plasma, algorithm for elevated or not elevated qualitative results
VeriMAP™ Peanut Dx—Bead-based Epitope Assay, AllerGenis™ Clinical Laboratory, AllerGenis™ LLC	0165U	Peanut allergen-specific quantitative assessment of multiple epitopes using enzyme-linked immunosorbent assay (ELISA), blood, individual epitope results and interpretation probability of peanut allergy
LiverFASt™, Fibronostics, Fibronostics	0166U	Liver disease, 10 biochemical assays (a2-macroglobulin, haptoglobin, apolipoprotein A1, bilirubin, GGT, ALT, AST, triglycerides, cholesterol, fasting glucose) and biometric and demographic data, utilizing serum, algorithm reported as scores for fibrosis, necroinflammatory activity, and steatosis with a summary interpretation
ADEXUSDx hCG Test, NOWDiagnostics, NOWDiagnostics	0167U	Gonadotropin, chorionic (hCG), immunoassay with direct optical observation, blood

     CPT © 2021 American Medical Association. All Rights Reserved.   © 2021 Optum360, LLC

Proprietary Name/Clinical Laboratory/Manufacturer	Code	Descriptor
	(0168U has been deleted)	
NT (*NUDT15* and *TPMT*) genotyping panel, RPRD Diagnostics	0169U	*NUDT15 (nudix hydrolase 15)* and *TPMT (thiopurine S-methyltransferase)* (eg, drug metabolism) gene analysis, common variants
Clarifi™, Quadrant Biosciences, Inc, Quadrant Biosciences, Inc	0170U	Neurology (autism spectrum disorder [ASD]), RNA, next-generation sequencing, saliva, algorithmic analysis, and results reported as predictive probability of ASD diagnosis
MyMRD® NGS Panel, Laboratory for Personalized Molecular Medicine, Laboratory for Personalized Molecular Medicine	0171U	Targeted genomic sequence analysis panel, acute myeloid leukemia, myelodysplastic syndrome, and myeloproliferative neoplasms, DNA analysis, 23 genes, interrogation for sequence variants, rearrangements and minimal residual disease, reported as presence/absence
myChoice® CDx, Myriad Genetics Laboratories, Inc, Myriad Genetics Laboratories, Inc	0172U	Oncology (solid tumor as indicated by the label), somatic mutation analysis of *BRCA1 (BRCA1, DNA repair associated), BRCA2 (BRCA2, DNA repair associated)* and analysis of homologous recombination deficiency pathways, DNA, formalin-fixed paraffin-embedded tissue, algorithm quantifying tumor genomic instability score
Psych HealthPGx Panel, RPRD Diagnostics, RPRD Diagnostics	0173U	Psychiatry (ie, depression, anxiety), genomic analysis panel, includes variant analysis of 14 genes
LC-MS/MS Targeted Proteomic Assay, OncoOmicDx Laboratory, LDT	0174U	Oncology (solid tumor), mass spectrometric 30 protein targets, formalin-fixed paraffin-embedded tissue, prognostic and predictive algorithm reported as likely, unlikely, or uncertain benefit of 39 chemotherapy and targeted therapeutic oncology agents
Genomind® Professional PGx Express™ CORE, Genomind, Inc, Genomind, Inc	0175U	Psychiatry (eg, depression, anxiety), genomic analysis panel, variant analysis of 15 genes
IBSchek®, Commonwealth Diagnostics International, Inc, Commonwealth Diagnostics International, Inc	0176U	Cytolethal distending toxin B (CdtB) and vinculin IgG antibodies by immunoassay (ie, ELISA)
therascreen® *PIK3CA* RGQ PCR Kit, QIAGEN, QIAGEN GmbH	0177U	Oncology (breast cancer), DNA, *PIK3CA (phosphatidylinositol-4,5-bisphosphate 3-kinase catalytic subunit alpha)* gene analysis of 11 gene variants utilizing plasma, reported as PIK3CA gene mutation status
VeriMAP™ Peanut Reactivity Threshold Bead Based Epitope Assay, AllerGenis™ Clinical Laboratory, AllerGenis™ LLC	0178U	Peanut allergen-specific quantitative assessment of multiple epitopes using enzyme-linked immunosorbent assay (ELISA), blood, report of minimum eliciting exposure for a clinical reaction
Resolution ctDx Lung™, Resolution Bioscience, Resolution Bioscience, Inc	0179U	Oncology (non-small cell lung cancer), cell-free DNA, targeted sequence analysis of 23 genes (single nucleotide variations, insertions and deletions, fusions without prior knowledge of partner/breakpoint, copy number variations), with report of significant mutation(s)
Navigator ABO Sequencing, Grifols Immunohematology Center, Grifols Immunohematology Center	0180U	Red cell antigen (ABO blood group) genotyping *(ABO), gene analysis Sanger/chain termination/conventional sequencing, ABO (ABO, alpha 1-3-N-acetylgalactosaminyltransferase and alpha 1-3-galactosyltransferase)* gene, including subtyping, 7 exons
Navigator CO Sequencing, Grifols Immunohematology Center, Grifols Immunohematology Center	0181U	Red cell antigen (Colton blood group) genotyping (CO), gene analysis, *AQP1 (aquaporin 1 [Colton blood group])* exon 1
Navigator CROM Sequencing, Grifols Immunohematology Center, Grifols Immunohematology Center	0182U	Red cell antigen (Cromer blood group) genotyping (CROM), gene analysis, *CD55 (CD55 molecule [Cromer blood group])* exons 1-10
Navigator DI Sequencing, Grifols Immunohematology Center, Grifols Immunohematology Center	0183U	Red cell antigen (Diego blood group) genotyping (DI), gene analysis, *SLC4A1 (solute carrier family 4 member 1 [Diego blood group])* exon 19
Navigator DO Sequencing, Grifols Immunohematology Center, Grifols Immunohematology Center	0184U	Red cell antigen (Dombrock blood group) genotyping (DO), gene analysis, *ART4 (ADP-ribosyltransferase 4 [Dombrock blood group])* exon 2
Navigator FUT1 Sequencing, Grifols Immunohematology Center, Grifols Immunohematology Center	0185U	Red cell antigen (H blood group) genotyping (FUT1), gene analysis, *FUT1 (fucosyltransferase 1 [H blood group])* exon 4
Navigator FUT2 Sequencing, Grifols Immunohematology Center, Grifols Immunohematology Center	0186U	Red cell antigen (H blood group) genotyping (FUT2), gene analysis, *FUT2 (fucosyltransferase 2)* exon 2
Navigator FY Sequencing, Grifols Immunohematology Center, Grifols Immunohematology Center	0187U	Red cell antigen (Duffy blood group) genotyping (FY), gene analysis, *ACKR1 (atypical chemokine receptor 1 [Duffy blood group])* exons 1-2
Navigator GE Sequencing, Grifols Immunohematology Center, Grifols Immunohematology Center	0188U	Red cell antigen (Gerbich blood group) genotyping (GE), gene analysis, *GYPC (glycophorin C [Gerbich blood group])* exons 1-4
Navigator GYPA Sequencing, Grifols Immunohematology Center, Grifols Immunohematology Center	0189U	Red cell antigen (MNS blood group) genotyping (GYPA), gene analysis, *GYPA (glycophorin A [MNS blood group])* introns 1, 5, exon 2
Navigator GYPB Sequencing, Grifols Immunohematology Center, Grifols Immunohematology Center	0190U	Red cell antigen (MNS blood group) genotyping (GYPB), gene analysis, *GYPB (glycophorin B [MNS blood group])* introns 1, 5, pseudoexon 3
Navigator IN Sequencing, Grifols Immunohematology Center, Grifols Immunohematology Center	0191U	Red cell antigen (Indian blood group) genotyping (IN), gene analysis, *CD44 (CD44 molecule [Indian blood group])* exons 2, 3, 6
Navigator JK Sequencing, Grifols Immunohematology Center, Grifols Immunohematology Center	0192U	Red cell antigen (Kidd blood group) genotyping (JK), gene analysis, *SLC14A1 (solute carrier family 14 member 1 [Kidd blood group])* gene promoter, exon 9
Navigator JR Sequencing, Grifols Immunohematology Center, Grifols Immunohematology Center	0193U	Red cell antigen (JR blood group) genotyping (JR), gene analysis, *ABCG2 (ATP binding cassette subfamily G member 2 [Junior blood group])* exons 2-26
Navigator KEL Sequencing, Grifols Immunohematology Center, Grifols Immunohematology Center	0194U	Red cell antigen (Kell blood group) genotyping (KEL), gene analysis, *KEL (Kell metallo-endopeptidase [Kell blood group])* exon 8
Navigator *KLF1* Sequencing, Grifols Immunohematology Center, Grifols Immunohematology Center	0195U	*KLF1 (Kruppel-like factor 1)*, targeted sequencing (ie, exon 13)

Proprietary Name/Clinical Laboratory/Manufacturer	Code	Descriptor
Navigator LU Sequencing, Grifols Immunohematology Center, Grifols Immunohematology Center	0196U	Red cell antigen (Lutheran blood group) genotyping (LU), gene analysis, *BCAM (basal cell adhesion molecule [Lutheran blood group])* exon 3
Navigator LW Sequencing, Grifols Immunohematology Center, Grifols Immunohematology Center	0197U	Red cell antigen (Landsteiner-Wiener blood group) genotyping (LW), gene analysis, *ICAM4 (intercellular adhesion molecule 4 [Landsteiner-Wiener blood group])* exon 1
Navigator RHD/CE Sequencing, Grifols Immunohematology Center, Grifols Immunohematology Center	0198U	Red cell antigen (RH blood group) genotyping (RHD and RHCE), gene analysis Sanger/chain termination/conventional sequencing, *RHD (Rh blood group D antigen)* exons 1-10 and *RHCE (Rh blood group CcEe antigens)* exon 5
Navigator SC Sequencing, Grifols Immunohematology Center, Grifols Immunohematology Center	0199U	Red cell antigen (Scianna blood group) genotyping (SC), gene analysis, *ERMAP (erythroblast membrane associated protein [Scianna blood group])* exons 4, 12
Navigator XK Sequencing, Grifols Immunohematology Center, Grifols Immunohematology Center	0200U	Red cell antigen (Kx blood group) genotyping (XK), gene analysis, *XK (X-linked Kx blood group)* exons 1-3
Navigator YT Sequencing, Grifols Immunohematology Center, Grifols Immunohematology Center	0201U	Red cell antigen (Yt blood group) genotyping (YT), gene analysis, *ACHE (acetylcholinesterase [Cartwright blood group])* exon 2
BioFire® Respiratory Panel 2.1 (RP2.1), BioFire® Diagnostics, BioFire® Diagnostics, LLC CPT Excludes: QIAstat-Dx Respiratory SARS CoV-2 Panel, QIAGEN Sciences, QIAGEN GmbH. (0223U)	0202U	Infectious disease (bacterial or viral respiratory tract infection), pathogen-specific nucleic acid (DNA or RNA), 22 targets including severe acute respiratory syndrome coronavirus 2 (SARS-CoV-2), qualitative RT-PCR, nasopharyngeal swab, each pathogen reported as detected or not detected
PredictSURE IBD™ Test, KSL Diagnostics, PredictImmune Ltd	0203U	Autoimmune (inflammatory bowel disease), mRNA, gene expression profiling by quantitative RT-PCR, 17 genes (15 target and 2 reference genes), whole blood, reported as a continuous risk score and classification of inflammatory bowel disease aggressiveness
Afirma Xpression Atlas, Veracyte, Inc, Veracyte, Inc	0204U	Oncology (thyroid), mRNA, gene expression analysis of 593 genes (including *BRAF, RAS, RET, PAX8,* and *NTRK*) for sequence variants and rearrangements, utilizing fine needle aspirate, reported as detected or not detected
Vita Risk®, Arctic Medical Laboratories, Arctic Medical Laboratories	0205U	Ophthalmology (age-related macular degeneration), analysis of 3 gene variants (2 *CFH* gene, 1 *ARMS2* gene), using PCR and MALDI-TOF, buccal swab, reported as positive or negative for neovascular age-related macular-degeneration risk associated with zinc supplements
DISCERN™, NeuroDiagnostics, NeuroDiagnostics	0206U	Neurology (Alzheimer disease); cell aggregation using morphometric imaging and protein kinase C-epsilon (PKCe) concentration in response to amylospheroid treatment by ELISA, cultured skin fibroblasts, each reported as positive or negative for Alzheimer disease
DISCERN™, NeuroDiagnostics, NeuroDiagnostics	+ 0207U	quantitative imaging of phosphorylated *ERK1* and *ERK2* in response to bradykinin treatment by in situ immunofluorescence, using cultured skin fibroblasts, reported as a probability index for Alzheimer disease (List separately in addition to code for primary procedure)
Afirma Medullary Thyroid Carcinoma (MTC) Classifier, Veracyte, Inc, Veracyte, Inc	0208U	Oncology (medullary thyroid carcinoma), mRNA, gene expression analysis of 108 genes, utilizing fine needle aspirate, algorithm reported as positive or negative for medullary thyroid carcinoma
CNGnome™, PerkinElmer Genomics, PerkinElmer Genomics	0209U	Cytogenomic constitutional (genome-wide) analysis, interrogation of genomic regions for copy number, structural changes and areas of homozygosity for chromosomal abnormalities
BioPlex 2200 RPR Assay - Quantitative, Bio-Rad Laboratories, Bio-Rad Laboratories	0210U	Syphilis test, non-treponemal antibody, immunoassay, quantitative (RPR)
MI Cancer Seek™ - NGS Analysis, Caris MPI d/b/a Caris Life Sciences, Caris MPI d/b/a Caris Life Sciences	0211U	Oncology (pan-tumor), DNA and RNA by next-generation sequencing, utilizing formalin-fixed paraffin-embedded tissue, interpretative report for single nucleotide variants, copy number alterations, tumor mutational burden, and microsatellite instability, with therapy association
Genomic Unity® Whole Genome Analysis—Proband, Variantyx Inc, Variantyx Inc	0212U	Rare diseases (constitutional/heritable disorders), whole genome and mitochondrial DNA sequence analysis, including small sequence changes, deletions, duplications, short tandem repeat gene expansions, and variants in non-uniquely mappable regions, blood or saliva, identification and categorization of genetic variants, proband
Genomic Unity® Whole Genome Analysis - Comparator, Variantyx Inc, Variantyx Inc	0213U	Rare diseases (constitutional/heritable disorders), whole genome and mitochondrial DNA sequence analysis, including small sequence changes, deletions, duplications, short tandem repeat gene expansions, and variants in non-uniquely mappable regions, blood or saliva, identification and categorization of genetic variants, each comparator genome (eg, parent, sibling)
Genomic Unity® Exome Plus Analysis - Proband, Variantyx Inc, Variantyx Inc	0214U	Rare diseases (constitutional/heritable disorders), whole exome and mitochondrial DNA sequence analysis, including small sequence changes, deletions, duplications, short tandem repeat gene expansions, and variants in non-uniquely mappable regions, blood or saliva, identification and categorization of genetic variants, proband
Genomic Unity® Exome Plus Analysis - Comparator, Variantyx Inc, Variantyx Inc	0215U	Rare diseases (constitutional/heritable disorders), whole exome and mitochondrial DNA sequence analysis, including small sequence changes, deletions, duplications, short tandem repeat gene expansions, and variants in non-uniquely mappable regions, blood or saliva, identification and categorization of genetic variants, each comparator exome (eg, parent, sibling)
Genomic Unity® Ataxia Repeat Expansion and Sequence Analysis, Variantyx Inc, Variantyx Inc	0216U	Neurology (inherited ataxias), genomic DNA sequence analysis of 12 common genes including small sequence changes, deletions, duplications, short tandem repeat gene expansions, and variants in non-uniquely mappable regions, blood or saliva, identification and categorization of genetic variants

Proprietary Name/Clinical Laboratory/Manufacturer	Code	Descriptor
Genomic Unity® Comprehensive Ataxia Repeat Expansion and Sequence Analysis, Variantyx Inc, Variantyx Inc	0217U	Neurology (inherited ataxias), genomic DNA sequence analysis of 51 genes including small sequence changes, deletions, duplications, short tandem repeat gene expansions, and variants in non-uniquely mappable regions, blood or saliva, identification and categorization of genetic variants
Genomic Unity® DMD Analysis, Variantyx Inc, Variantyx Inc	0218U	Neurology (muscular dystrophy), *DMD* gene sequence analysis, including small sequence changes, deletions, duplications, and variants in non-uniquely mappable regions, blood or saliva, identification and characterization of genetic variants
Sentosa® SQ HIV-1 Genotyping Assay, Vela Diagnostics USA, Inc, Vela Operations Singapore Pte Ltd	0219U	Infectious agent (human immunodeficiency virus), targeted viral next-generation sequence analysis (ie, protease [PR], reverse transcriptase [RT], integrase [INT]), algorithm reported as prediction of antiviral drug susceptibility
PreciseDx™ Breast Cancer Test, PreciseDx, PreciseDx	0220U	Oncology (breast cancer), image analysis with artificial intelligence assessment of 12 histologic and immunohistochemical features, reported as a recurrence score
Navigator ABO Blood Group NGS, Grifols Immunohematology Center, Grifols Immunohematology Center	0221U	Red cell antigen (ABO blood group) genotyping (ABO), gene analysis, next-generation sequencing, *ABO (ABO, alpha 1-3-N-acetylgalactosaminyltransferase and alpha 1-3-galactosyltransferase)* gene
Navigator Rh Blood Group NGS, Grifols Immunohematology Center, Grifols Immunohematology Center	0222U	Red cell antigen (RH blood group) genotyping (RHD and RHCE), gene analysis, next-generation sequencing, RH proximal promoter, exons 1-10, portions of introns 2-3
QIAstat-Dx Respiratory SARS CoV-2 Panel, QIAGEN Sciences, QIAGEN GmbH CPT Excludes: BioFire® Respiratory Panel 2.1 (RP2.1), BioFire® Diagnostics, BioFire® Diagnostics, LLC. (0202U)	● 0223U	Infectious disease (bacterial or viral respiratory tract infection), pathogen-specific nucleic acid (DNA or RNA), 22 targets including severe acute respiratory syndrome coronavirus 2 (SARS-CoV-2), qualitative RT-PCR, nasopharyngeal swab, each pathogen reported as detected or not detected
COVID-19 Antibody Test, Mt Sinai, Mount Sinai Laboratory	● 0224U	Antibody, severe acute respiratory syndrome coronavirus 2 (SARS-CoV-2) (Coronavirus disease [COVID-19]), includes titer(s), when performed
ePlex® Respiratory Pathogen Panel 2, GenMark Dx, GenMark Diagnostics, Inc	● 0225U	Infectious disease (bacterial or viral respiratory tract infection) pathogen-specific DNA and RNA, 21 targets, including severe acute respiratory syndrome coronavirus 2 (SARS-CoV-2), amplified probe technique, including multiplex reverse transcription for RNA targets, each analyte reported as detected or not detected
Tru-Immune™, Ethos Laboratories, GenScript® USA Inc	● 0226U	Surrogate viral neutralization test (sVNT), severe acute respiratory syndrome coronavirus 2 (SARS-CoV-2) (Coronavirus disease [COVID-19]), ELISA, plasma, serum
Comprehensive Screen, Aspenti Health	● 0227U	Drug assay, presumptive, 30 or more drugs or metabolites, urine, liquid chromatography with tandem mass spectrometry (LC-MS/MS) using multiple reaction monitoring (MRM), with drug or metabolite description, includes sample validation
PanGIA Prostate, Genetics Institute of America, Entopsis, LLC	● 0228U	Oncology (prostate), multianalyte molecular profile by photometric detection of macromolecules adsorbed on nanosponge array slides with machine learning, utilizing first morning voided urine, algorithm reported as likelihood of prostate cancer
Colvera®, Clinical Genomic Pathology Inc	● 0229U	*BCAT1 (Branched chain amino acid transaminase 1)* or *IKZF1 (IKAROS family zinc finger 1)* (eg, colorectal cancer) promoter methylation analysis
Genomic Unity® AR Analysis, Variantyx Inc, Variantyx Inc	● 0230U	*AR (androgen receptor)* (eg, spinal and bulbar muscular atrophy, Kennedy disease, X chromosome inactivation), full sequence analysis, including small sequence changes in exonic and intronic regions, deletions, duplications, short tandem repeat (STR) expansions, mobile element insertions, and variants in non-uniquely mappable regions
Genomic Unity® CACNA1A Analysis, Variantyx Inc, Variantyx Inc	● 0231U	*CACNA1A (calcium voltage-gated channel subunit alpha 1A)* (eg, spinocerebellar ataxia), full gene analysis, including small sequence changes in exonic and intronic regions, deletions, duplications, short tandem repeat (STR) gene expansions, mobile element insertions, and variants in non-uniquely mappable regions
Genomic Unity® CSTB Analysis, Variantyx Inc, Variantyx Inc	● 0232U	*CSTB (cystatin B)* (eg, progressive myoclonic epilepsy type 1A, Unverricht-Lundborg disease), full gene analysis, including small sequence changes in exonic and intronic regions, deletions, duplications, short tandem repeat (STR) expansions, mobile element insertions, and variants in non-uniquely mappable regions
Genomic Unity® FXN Analysis, Variantyx Inc, Variantyx Inc	● 0233U	*FXN (frataxin)* (eg, Friedreich ataxia), gene analysis, including small sequence changes in exonic and intronic regions, deletions, duplications, short tandem repeat (STR) expansions, mobile element insertions, and variants in non-uniquely mappable regions
Genomic Unity® MECP2 Analysis, Variantyx Inc, Variantyx Inc	● 0234U	*MECP2 (methyl CpG binding protein 2)* (eg, Rett syndrome), full gene analysis, including small sequence changes in exonic and intronic regions, deletions, duplications, mobile element insertions, and variants in non-uniquely mappable regions
Genomic Unity® PTEN Analysis, Variantyx Inc, Variantyx Inc	● 0235U	*PTEN (phosphatase and tensin homolog)* (eg, Cowden syndrome, PTEN hamartoma tumor syndrome), full gene analysis, including small sequence changes in exonic and intronic regions, deletions, duplications, mobile element insertions, and variants in non-uniquely mappable regions
Genomic Unity® SMN1/2 Analysis, Variantyx Inc, Variantyx Inc	● 0236U	*SMN1 (survival of motor neuron 1, telomeric)* and *SMN2 (survival of motor neuron 2, centromeric)* (eg, spinal muscular atrophy) full gene analysis, including small sequence changes in exonic and intronic regions, duplications, deletions, and mobile element insertions

Proprietary Name/Clinical Laboratory/Manufacturer		Code	Descriptor
Genomic Unity® Cardiac Ion Channelopathies Analysis, Variantyx Inc, Variantyx Inc	●	0237U	Cardiac ion channelopathies (eg, Brugada syndrome, long QT syndrome, short QT syndrome, catecholaminergic polymorphic ventricular tachycardia), genomic sequence analysis panel including ANK2, CASQ2, CAV3, KCNE1, KCNE2, KCNH2, KCNJ2, KCNQ1, RYR2, and SCN5A, including small sequence changes in exonic and intronic regions, deletions, duplications, mobile element insertions, and variants in non-uniquely mappable regions
Genomic Unity® Lynch Syndrome Analysis, Variantyx Inc, Variantyx Inc	●	0238U	Oncology (Lynch syndrome), genomic DNA sequence analysis of MLH1, MSH2, MSH6, PMS2, and EPCAM, including small sequence changes in exonic and intronic regions, deletions, duplications, mobile element insertions, and variants in non-uniquely mappable regions
FoundationOne® Liquid CDx, Foundation Medicine Inc, Foundation Medicine Inc	●	0239U	Targeted genomic sequence analysis panel, solid organ neoplasm, cell-free DNA, analysis of 311 or more genes, interrogation for sequence variants, including substitutions, insertions, deletions, select rearrangements, and copy number variations
Xpert® Xpress SARS-CoV-2/Flu/RSV (SARS-CoV-2 & Flu targets only), Cepheid	●	0240U	Infectious disease (viral respiratory tract infection), pathogen-specific RNA, 3 targets (severe acute respiratory syndrome coronavirus 2 [SARS-CoV-2], influenza A, influenza B), upper respiratory specimen, each pathogen reported as detected or not detected
Xpert® Xpress SARS-CoV-2/Flu/RSV (all targets), Cepheid	●	0241U	Infectious disease (viral respiratory tract infection), pathogen-specific RNA, 4 targets (severe acute respiratory syndrome coronavirus 2 [SARS-CoV-2], influenza A, influenza B, respiratory syncytial virus [RSV]), upper respiratory specimen, each pathogen reported as detected or not detected
Guardant360® CDx, Guardant Health Inc, Guardant Health Inc	●	0242U	Targeted genomic sequence analysis panel, solid organ neoplasm, cell-free circulating DNA analysis of 55-74 genes, interrogation for sequence variants, gene copy number amplifications, and gene rearrangements
PIGF Preeclampsia Screen, PerkinElmer Genetics, PerkinElmer Genetics, Inc	●	0243U	Obstetrics (preeclampsia), biochemical assay of placental-growth factor, time-resolved fluorescence immunoassay, maternal serum, predictive algorithm reported as a risk score for preeclampsia
Oncotype MAP® Pan-Cancer Tissue Test, Paradigm Diagnostics, Inc, Paradigm Diagnostics, Inc	●	0244U	Oncology (solid organ), DNA, comprehensive genomic profiling, 257 genes, interrogation for single-nucleotide variants, insertions/deletions, copy number alterations, gene rearrangements, tumor-mutational burden and microsatellite instability, utilizing formalin-fixed paraffin-embedded tumor tissue
ThyGeNEXT® Thyroid Oncogene Panel, Interpace Diagnostics, Interpace Diagnostics	●	0245U	Oncology (thyroid), mutation analysis of 10 genes and 37 RNA fusions and expression of 4 mRNA markers using next-generation sequencing, fine needle aspirate, report includes associated risk of malignancy expressed as a percentage
PrecisionBlood™, San Diego Blood Bank, San Diego Blood Bank	●	0246U	Red blood cell antigen typing, DNA, genotyping of at least 16 blood groups with phenotype prediction of at least 51 red blood cell antigens
PreTRM®, Sera Prognostics, Sera Prognostics, Inc®	●	0247U	Obstetrics (preterm birth), insulin-like growth factor-binding protein 4 (IBP4), sex hormone-binding globulin (SHBG), quantitative measurement by LC-MS/MS, utilizing maternal serum, combined with clinical data, reported as predictive-risk stratification for spontaneous preterm birth
3D Predict Glioma, KIYATEC®, Inc	●	0248U	Oncology (brain), spheroid cell culture in a 3D microenvironment, 12 drug panel, tumor-response prediction for each drug
Theralink® Reverse Phase Protein Array (RPPA), Theralink® Technologies, Inc, Theralink® Technologies, Inc	●	0249U	Oncology (breast), semiquantitative analysis of 32 phosphoproteins and protein analytes, includes laser capture microdissection, with algorithmic analysis and interpretative report
PGDx elio™ tissue complete, Personal Genome Diagnostics, Inc, Personal Genome Diagnostics, Inc	●	0250U	Oncology (solid organ neoplasm), targeted genomic sequence DNA analysis of 505 genes, interrogation for somatic alterations (SNVs [single nucleotide variant], small insertions and deletions, one amplification, and four translocations), microsatellite instability and tumor-mutation burden
Intrinsic Hepcidin IDx™ Test, IntrinsicDx, Intrinsic LifeSciences™ LLC	●	0251U	Hepcidin-25, enzyme-linked immunosorbent assay (ELISA), serum or plasma
POC (Products of Conception), Igenomix®, Igenomix® USA	●	0252U	Fetal aneuploidy short tandem-repeat comparative analysis, fetal DNA from products of conception, reported as normal (euploidy), monosomy, trisomy, or partial deletion/duplications, mosaicism, and segmental aneuploidy
ERA® (Endometrial Receptivity Analysis), Igenomix®, Igenomix® USA	●	0253U	Reproductive medicine (endometrial receptivity analysis), RNA gene expression profile, 238 genes by next-generation sequencing, endometrial tissue, predictive algorithm reported as endometrial window of implantation (eg, pre-receptive, receptive, post-receptive)
SMART PGT-A (Pre-implantation Genetic Testing — Aneuploidy), Igenomix®, Igenomix® USA	●	0254U	Reproductive medicine (preimplantation genetic assessment), analysis of 24 chromosomes using embryonic DNA genomic sequence analysis for aneuploidy, and a mitochondrial DNA score in euploid embryos, results reported as normal (euploidy), monosomy, trisomy, or partial deletion/duplications, mosaicism, and segmental aneuploidy, per embryo tested
Cap-Score™ Test, Androvia LifeSciences, Avantor Clinical Services (previously known as Therapak)	●	0255U	Andrology (infertility), sperm-capacitation assessment of ganglioside GM1 distribution patterns, fluorescence microscopy, fresh or frozen specimen, reported as percentage of capacitated sperm and probability of generating a pregnancy score
Trimethylamine (TMA) and TMA N-Oxide, Children's Hospital Colorado Laboratory	●	0256U	Trimethylamine/trimethylamine N-oxide (TMA/TMAO) profile, tandem mass spectrometry (MS/MS), urine, with algorithmic analysis and interpretive report
Very-Long Chain Acyl-CoA Dehydrogenase (VLCAD) Enzyme Activity, Children's Hospital Colorado Laboratory	●	0257U	Very long chain acyl-coenzyme A (CoA) dehydrogenase (VLCAD), leukocyte enzyme activity, whole blood

Proprietary Name/Clinical Laboratory/Manufacturer		Code	Descriptor
Mind.Px, Mindera, Mindera Corporation	●	0258U	Autoimmune (psoriasis), mRNA, nextgeneration sequencing, gene expression profiling of 50-100 genes, skin-surface collection using adhesive patch, algorithm reported as likelihood of response to psoriasis biologics
GFR by NMR, Labtech™ Diagnostics	●	0259U	Nephrology (chronic kidney disease), nuclear magnetic resonance spectroscopy measurement of myo-inositol, valine, and creatinine, algorithmically combined with cystatin C (by immunoassay) and demographic data to determine estimated glomerular filtration rate (GFR), serum, quantitative
Augusta Optical Genome Mapping, Georgia Esoteric and Molecular (GEM) CPT Excludes: Praxis Optical Genome Mapping, Praxis Genomics LLC (0264U)	●	0260U	Rare diseases (constitutional/heritable disorders), identification of copy number variations, inversions, insertions, translocations, and other structural variants by optical genome mapping
Immunoscore®, HalioDx, HalioDx	●	0261U	Oncology (colorectal cancer), image analysis with artificial intelligence assessment of 4 histologic and immunohistochemical features (CD3 and CD8 within tumor-stroma border and tumor core), tissue, reported as immune response and recurrence-risk score
OncoSignal 7 Pathway Signal, Protean BioDiagnostics, Philips Electronics Nederland BV	●	0262U	Oncology (solid tumor), gene expression profiling by real-time RT-PCR of 7 gene pathways *(ER, AR, PI3K, MAPK, HH, TGFB,* Notch), formalin-fixed paraffin-embedded (FFPE), algorithm reported as gene pathway activity score
NPDX ASD and Central Carbon Energy Metabolism, Stemina Biomarker Discovery, Inc, Stemina Biomarker Discovery, Inc	●	0263U	Neurology (autism spectrum disorder [ASD]), quantitative measurements of 16 central carbon metabolites (ie, a-ketoglutarate, alanine, lactate, phenylalanine, pyruvate, succinate, carnitine, citrate, fumarate, hypoxanthine, inosine, malate, S-sulfocysteine, taurine, urate, and xanthine), liquid chromatography tandem mass spectrometry (LC-MS/MS), plasma, algorithmic analysis with result reported as negative or positive (with metabolic subtypes of ASD)
Praxis Optical Genome Mapping, Praxis Genomics LLC CPT Excludes: Augusta Optical Genome Mapping, Georgia Esoteric and Molecular (GEM) Laboratory, LLC, Bionano Genomics Inc (0260U)	●	0264U	Rare diseases (constitutional/heritable disorders), identification of copy number variations, inversions, insertions, translocations, and other structural variants by optical genome mapping
Praxis Whole Genome Sequencing, Praxis Genomics LLC	●	0265U	Rare constitutional and other heritable disorders, whole genome and mitochondrial DNA sequence analysis, blood, frozen and formalin-fixed paraffin-embedded (FFPE) tissue, saliva, buccal swabs or cell lines, identification of single nucleotide and copy number variants
Praxis Transcriptome, Praxis Genomics LLC	●	0266U	Unexplained constitutional or other heritable disorders or syndromes, tissue-specific gene expression by whole-transcriptome and next-generation sequencing, blood, formalin-fixed paraffin-embedded (FFPE) tissue or fresh frozen tissue, reported as presence or absence of splicing or expression changes
Praxis Combined Whole Genome Sequencing and Optical Genome Mapping, Praxis Genomics LLC	●	0267U	Rare constitutional and other heritable disorders, identification of copy number variations, inversions, insertions, translocations, and other structural variants by optical genome mapping and whole genome sequencing
Versiti™ aHUS Genetic Evaluation, Versiti™ Diagnostic Laboratories, Versiti™	●	0268U	Hematology (atypical hemolytic uremic syndrome [aHUS]), genomic sequence analysis of 15 genes, blood, buccal swab, or amniotic fluid
Versiti™ Autosomal Dominant Thrombocytopenia Panel, Versiti™ Diagnostic Laboratories, Versiti™	●	0269U	Hematology (autosomal dominant congenital thrombocytopenia), genomic sequence analysis of 14 genes, blood, buccal swab, or amniotic fluid
Versiti™ Coagulation Disorder Panel, Versiti™ Diagnostic Laboratories, Versiti™	●	0270U	Hematology (congenital coagulation disorders), genomic sequence analysis of 20 genes, blood, buccal swab, or amniotic fluid
Versiti™ Congenital Neutropenia Panel, Versiti™ Diagnostic Laboratories, Versiti™	●	0271U	Hematology (congenital neutropenia), genomic sequence analysis of 23 genes, blood, buccal swab, or amniotic fluid
Versiti™ Comprehensive Bleeding Disorder Panel, Versiti™ Diagnostic Laboratories, Versiti™	●	0272U	Hematology (genetic bleeding disorders), genomic sequence analysis of 51 genes, blood, buccal swab, or amniotic fluid, comprehensive
Versiti™ Fibrinolytic Disorder Panel, Versiti™ Diagnostic Laboratories, Versiti™	●	0273U	Hematology (genetic hyperfibrinolysis, delayed bleeding), genomic sequence analysis of 8 genes *(F13A1, F13B, FGA, FGB, FGG, SERPINA1, SERPINE1, SERPINF2, PLAU),* blood, buccal swab, or amniotic fluid
Versiti™ Comprehensive Platelet Disorder Panel, Versiti™ Diagnostic Laboratories, Versiti™	●	0274U	Hematology (genetic platelet disorders), genomic sequence analysis of 43 genes, blood, buccal swab, or amniotic fluid
Versiti™ Heparin-Induced Thrombocytopenia Evaluation — PEA, Versiti™ Diagnostic Laboratories, Versiti™	●	0275U	Hematology (heparin-induced thrombocytopenia), platelet antibody reactivity by flow cytometry, serum
Versiti™ Inherited Thrombocytopenia Panel, Versiti™ Diagnostic Laboratories, Versiti™	●	0276U	Hematology (inherited thrombocytopenia), genomic sequence analysis of 23 genes, blood, buccal swab, or amniotic fluid
Versiti™ Platelet Function Disorder Panel, Versiti™ Diagnostic Laboratories, Versiti™	●	0277U	Hematology (genetic platelet function disorder), genomic sequence analysis of 31 genes, blood, buccal swab, or amniotic fluid
Versiti™ Thrombosis Panel, Versiti™ Diagnostic Laboratories, Versiti™	●	0278U	Hematology (genetic thrombosis), genomic sequence analysis of 12 genes, blood, buccal swab, or amniotic fluid
Versiti™ VWF Collagen III Binding, Versiti™ Diagnostic Laboratories, Versiti™	●	0279U	Hematology (von Willebrand disease [VWD]), von Willebrand factor (VWF) and collagen III binding by enzyme-linked immunosorbent assays (ELISA), plasma, report of collagen III binding
Versiti™ VWF Collagen IV Binding, Versiti™ Diagnostic Laboratories, Versiti™	●	0280U	Hematology (von Willebrand disease [VWD]), von Willebrand factor (VWF) and collagen IV binding by enzyme-linked immunosorbent assays (ELISA), plasma, report of collagen IV binding

Proprietary Name/Clinical Laboratory/Manufacturer		Code	Descriptor
Versiti™ VWF Propeptide Antigen, Versiti™ Diagnostic Laboratories, Versiti™	●	0281U	Hematology (von Willebrand disease [VWD]), von Willebrand propeptide, enzyme-linked immunosorbent assays (ELISA), plasma, diagnostic report of von Willebrand factor (VWF) propeptide antigen level
Versiti™ Red Cell Genotyping Panel, Versiti™ Diagnostic Laboratories, Versiti™	●	0282U	Red blood cell antigen typing, DNA, genotyping of 12 blood group system genes to predict 44 red blood cell antigen phenotypes
Versiti™ VWD Type 2B Evaluation, Versiti™ Diagnostic Laboratories, Versiti™	●	0283U	von Willebrand factor (VWF), type 2B, platelet-binding evaluation, radioimmunoassay, plasma
Versiti™ VWD Type 2N Binding, Versiti™ Diagnostic Laboratories, Versiti™	●	0284U	von Willebrand factor (VWF), type 2N, factor VIII and VWF binding evaluation, enzyme-linked immunosorbent assays (ELISA), plasma
RadTox™ cfDNA test, DiaCarta Clinical Lab, DiaCarta Inc	●	0285U	Oncology, response to radiation, cell-free DNA, quantitative branched chain DNA amplification, plasma, reported as a radiation toxicity score
CNT CEP72, TPMT and NUDT15) genotyping panel, RPRD Diagnostics	●	0286U	CEP72 (centrosomal protein, 72-KDa), NUDT15 (nudix hydrolase 15) and TPMT (thiopurine S-methyltransferase) (eg, drug metabolism) gene analysis, common variants
ThyroSeq® CRC, CBLPath, Inc, University of Pittsburgh Medical Center	●	0287U	Oncology (thyroid), DNA and mRNA, next-generation sequencing analysis of 112 genes, fine needle aspirate or formalin-fixed paraffin-embedded (FFPE) tissue, algorithmic prediction of cancer recurrence, reported as a categorical risk result (low, intermediate, high)
DetermaRx™, Oncocyte Corporation	●	0288U	Oncology (lung), mRNA, quantitative PCR analysis of 11 genes (BAG1, BRCA1, CDC6, CDK2AP1, ERBB3, FUT3, IL11, LCK, RND3, SH3BGR, WNT3A) and 3 reference genes (ESD, TBP, YAP1), formalin-fixed paraffin-embedded (FFPE) tumor tissue, algorithmic interpretation reported as a recurrence risk score
MindX Blood Test™ — Memory/Alzheimer's, MindX Sciences™ Laboratory, MindX Sciences™ Inc	●	0289U	Neurology (Alzheimer disease), mRNA, gene expression profiling by RNA sequencing of 24 genes, whole blood, algorithm reported as predictive risk score
MindX Blood Test™ — Pain, MindX Sciences™ Laboratory, MindX Sciences™ Inc	●	0290U	Pain management, mRNA, gene expression profiling by RNA sequencing of 36 genes, whole blood, algorithm reported as predictive risk score
MindX Blood Test™ — Mood, MindX Sciences™ Laboratory, MindX Sciences™ Inc	●	0291U	Psychiatry (mood disorders), mRNA, gene expression profiling by RNA sequencing of 144 genes, whole blood, algorithm reported as predictive risk score
MindX Blood Test™ — Stress, MindX Sciences™ Laboratory, MindX Sciences™ Inc	●	0292U	Psychiatry (stress disorders), mRNA, gene expression profiling by RNA sequencing of 72 genes, whole blood, algorithm reported as predictive risk score
MindX Blood Test™ — Suicidality, MindX Sciences™ Laboratory, MindX Sciences™ Inc	●	0293U	Psychiatry (suicidal ideation), mRNA, gene expression profiling by RNA sequencing of 54 genes, whole blood, algorithm reported as predictive risk score
MindX Blood Test™ — Longevity, MindX Sciences™ Laboratory, MindX Sciences™ Inc	●	0294U	Longevity and mortality risk, mRNA, gene expression profiling by RNA sequencing of 18 genes, whole blood, algorithm reported as predictive risk score
DCISionRT®, PreludeDx™, Prelude Corporation	●	0295U	Oncology (breast ductal carcinoma in situ), protein expression profiling by immunohistochemistry of 7 proteins (COX2, FOXA1, HER2, Ki-67, p16, PR, SIAH2), with 4 clinicopathologic factors (size, age, margin status, palpability), utilizing formalin-fixed paraffin-embedded (FFPE) tissue, algorithm reported as a recurrence risk score
mRNA CancerDetect™, Viome Life Sciences, Inc, Viome Life Sciences, Inc	●	0296U	Oncology (oral and/or oropharyngeal cancer), gene expression profiling by RNA sequencing at least 20 molecular features (eg, human and/or microbial mRNA), saliva, algorithm reported as positive or negative for signature associated with malignancy
Praxis Somatic Whole Genome Sequencing, Praxis Genomics LLC	●	0297U	Oncology (pan tumor), whole genome sequencing of paired malignant and normal DNA specimens, fresh or formalin-fixed paraffin-embedded (FFPE) tissue, blood or bone marrow, comparative sequence analyses and variant identification
Praxis Somatic Transcriptome, Praxis Genomics LLC	●	0298U	Oncology (pan tumor), whole transcriptome sequencing of paired malignant and normal RNA specimens, fresh or formalin-fixed paraffin-embedded (FFPE) tissue, blood or bone marrow, comparative sequence analyses and expression level and chimeric transcript identification
Praxis Somatic Optical Genome Mapping, Praxis Genomics LLC	●	0299U	Oncology (pan tumor), whole genome optical genome mapping of paired malignant and normal DNA specimens, fresh frozen tissue, blood, or bone marrow, comparative structural variant identification
Praxis Somatic Combined Whole Genome Sequencing and Optical Genome Mapping, Praxis Genomics LLC	●	0300U	Oncology (pan tumor), whole genome sequencing and optical genome mapping of paired malignant and normal DNA specimens, fresh tissue, blood, or bone marrow, comparative sequence analyses and variant identification
Bartonella ddPCR, Galaxy Diagnostics Inc	●	0301U	Infectious agent detection by nucleic acid (DNA or RNA), Bartonella henselae and Bartonella quintana, droplet digital PCR (ddPCR);
Bartonella Digital ePCR™, Galaxy Diagnostics Inc	●	0302U	following liquid enhancement
Hypoxic BioChip Adhesion, BioChip Labs™, BioChip Labs™	●	0303U	Hematology, red blood cell (RBC) adhesion to endothelial/subendothelial adhesion molecules, functional assessment, whole blood, with algorithmic analysis and result reported as an RBC adhesion index; hypoxic
Normoxic BioChip Adhesion, BioChip Labs™, BioChip Labs™	●	0304U	normoxic
Ektacytometry, BioChip Labs™, BioChip Labs™	●	0305U	Hematology, red blood cell (RBC) functionality and deformity as a function of shear stress, whole blood, reported as a maximum elongation index

Appendix M — Glossary

-centesis. Puncture, as with a needle, trocar, or aspirator; often done for withdrawing fluid from a cavity.

-ectomy. Excision, removal.

-orrhaphy. Suturing.

-ostomy. Indicates a surgically created artificial opening.

-otomy. Making an incision or opening.

-plasty. Indicates surgically formed or molded.

abdominal lymphadenectomy. Surgical removal of the abdominal lymph nodes grouping, with or without para-aortic and vena cava nodes.

ablation. Removal or destruction of a body part or tissue or its function. Ablation may be performed by surgical means, hormones, drugs, radiofrequency, heat, chemical application, or other methods.

abnormal alleles. Form of gene that includes disease-related variations.

absorbable sutures. Strands prepared from collagen or a synthetic polymer and capable of being absorbed by tissue over time. Examples include surgical gut and collagen sutures; or synthetics like polydioxanone (PDS), polyglactin 910 (Vicryl), poliglecaprone 25 (Monocryl), polyglyconate (Maxon), and polyglycolic acid (Dexon).

acetabuloplasty. Surgical repair or reconstruction of the large cup-shaped socket in the hipbone (acetabulum) with which the head of the femur articulates.

Achilles tendon. Tendon attached to the back of the heel bone (calcaneus) that flexes the foot downward.

acromioclavicular joint. Junction between the clavicle and the scapula. The acromion is the projection from the back of the scapula that forms the highest point of the shoulder and connects with the clavicle. Trauma or injury to the acromioclavicular joint is often referred to as a dislocation of the shoulder. This is not correct, however, as a dislocation of the shoulder is a disruption of the glenohumeral joint.

acromionectomy. Surgical treatment for acromioclavicular arthritis in which the distal portion of the acromion process is removed.

acromioplasty. Repair of the part of the shoulder blade that connects to the deltoid muscles and clavicle.

actigraphy. Science of monitoring activity levels, particularly during sleep. In most cases, the patient wears a wristband that records motion while sleeping. The data are recorded, analyzed, and interpreted to study sleep/wake patterns and circadian rhythms.

air conduction. Transportation of sound from the air, through the external auditory canal, to the tympanic membrane and ossicular chain. Air conduction hearing is tested by presenting an acoustic stimulus through earphones or a loudspeaker to the ear.

air puff device. Instrument that measures intraocular pressure by evaluating the force of a reflected amount of air blown against the cornea.

alleles. Form of gene usually arising from a mutation responsible for a hereditary variation.

allogeneic collection. Collection of blood or blood components from one person for the use of another. Allogeneic collection was formerly termed homologous collection.

allograft. Graft from one individual to another of the same species.

amniocentesis. Surgical puncture through the abdominal wall, with a specialized needle and under ultrasonic guidance, into the interior of the pregnant uterus and directly into the amniotic sac to collect fluid for diagnostic analysis or therapeutic reduction of fluid levels.

anastomosis. Surgically created connection between ducts, blood vessels, or bowel segments to allow flow from one to the other.

anesthesia time. Time period factored into anesthesia procedures beginning with the anesthesiologist preparing the patient for surgery and ending when the patient is turned over to the recovery department.

Angelman syndrome. Early childhood emergence of a pattern of interrupted development, stiff, jerky gait, absence or impairment of speech, excessive laughter, and seizures.

angioplasty. Reconstruction or repair of a diseased or damaged blood vessel.

annuloplasty. Surgical plication of weakened tissue of the heart, to improve its muscular function. Annuli are thick, fibrous rings and one is found surrounding each of the cardiac chambers. The atrial and ventricular muscle fibers attach to the annuli. In annuloplasty, weakened annuli may be surgically plicated, or tucked, to improve muscular functions.

anorectal anometry. Measurement of pressure generated by anal sphincter to diagnose incontinence.

anterior chamber lenses. Lenses inserted into the anterior chamber following intracapsular cataract extraction.

applanation tonometer. Instrument that measures intraocular pressure by recording the force required to flatten an area of the cornea.

appropriateness of care. Proper setting of medical care that best meets the patient's care or diagnosis, as defined by a health care plan or other legal entity.

aqueous humor. Fluid within the anterior and posterior chambers of the eye that is continually replenished as it diffuses out into the blood. When the flow of aqueous is blocked, a build-up of fluid in the eye causes increased intraocular pressure and leads to glaucoma and blindness.

arteriogram. Radiograph of arteries.

arteriovenous fistula. Connecting passage between an artery and a vein.

arteriovenous malformation. Connecting passage between an artery and a vein.

arthrotomy. Surgical incision into a joint that may include exploration, drainage, or removal of a foreign body.

ASA. 1) Acetylsalicylic acid. Synonym(s): aspirin. 2) American Society of Anesthesiologists. National organization for anesthesiology that maintains and publishes the guidelines and relative values for anesthesia coding.

aspirate. To withdraw fluid or air from a body cavity by suction.

assay. Chemical analysis of a substance to establish the presence and strength of its components. A therapeutic drug assay is used to determine if a drug is within the expected therapeutic range for a patient.

asynchronous services. Those that allow a physician or other qualified health care professional (QHP) to share a patient's clinical data, medical history, radiographic images, laboratory results, and/or pathology reports with a specialist physician in order to obtain their expertise in diagnosis and treatment. They also allow the patient to share health information with their physician or other QHP. These services utilize an electronic health record (EHR), encrypted email, a secure Web server, or specially designed software (store-and-forward).

atrial septal defect. Cardiac anomaly consisting of a patent opening in the atrial septum due to a fusion failure, classified as ostium secundum type, ostium primum defect, or endocardial cushion defect.

attended surveillance. Ability of a technician at a remote surveillance center or location to respond immediately to patient transmissions regarding rhythm or device alerts as they are produced and received at the remote location. These transmissions may originate from wearable or implanted therapy or monitoring devices.

auricle. External ear, which is a single elastic cartilage covered in skin and normal adnexal features (hair follicles, sweat glands, and sebaceous glands), shaped to channel sound waves into the acoustic meatus.

autogenous transplant. Tissue, such as bone, that is harvested from the patient and used for transplantation back into the same patient.

autograft. Any tissue harvested from one anatomical site of a person and grafted to another anatomical site of the same person. Most commonly, blood vessels, skin, tendons, fascia, and bone are used as autografts.

autologous. Tissue, cells, or structure obtained from the same individual.

AVF. Arteriovenous fistula.

AVM. Arteriovenous malformation. Clusters of abnormal blood vessels that grow in the brain comprised of a blood vessel "nidus" or nest through which arteries and veins connect directly without going through the capillaries. As time passes, the nidus may enlarge resulting in the formation of a mass that may bleed. AVMs are more prone to bleeding in patients ages 10 to 55. Once older than age 55, the possibility of bleeding is reduced dramatically.

backbench preparation. Procedures performed on a donor organ following procurement to prepare the organ for transplant into the recipient. Excess fat and other tissue may be removed, the organ may be perfused, and vital arteries may be sized, repaired, or modified to fit the patient. These procedures are done on a back table in the operating room before transplantation can begin.

Bartholin's gland. Mucous-producing gland found in the vestibular bulbs on either side of the vaginal orifice and connected to the mucosal membrane at the opening by a duct.

Bartholin's gland abscess. Pocket of pus and surrounding cellulitis caused by infection of the Bartholin's gland and causing localized swelling and pain in the posterior labia majora that may extend into the lower vagina.

basic value. Relative weighted value based upon the usual anesthesia services and the relative work or cost of the specific anesthesia service assigned to each anesthesia-specific procedure code.

Berman locator. Small, sensitive tool used to detect the location of a metallic foreign body in the eye.

bifurcated. Having two branches or divisions, such as the left pulmonary veins that split off from the left atrium to carry oxygenated blood away from the heart.

Billroth's operation. Anastomosis of the stomach to the duodenum or jejunum.

bioprosthetic heart valve. Replacement cardiac valve made of biological tissue. Allograft, xenograft or engineered tissue.

biopsy. Tissue or fluid removed for diagnostic purposes through analysis of the cells in the biopsy material.

Blalock-Hanlon procedure. Atrial septectomy procedure to allow free mixing of the blood from the right and left atria.

Blalock-Taussig procedure. Anastomosis of the left subclavian artery to the left pulmonary artery or the right subclavian artery to the right pulmonary artery in order to shunt some of the blood flow from the systemic to the pulmonary circulation.

blepharochalasis. Loss of elasticity and relaxation of skin of the eyelid, thickened or indurated skin on the eyelid associated with recurrent episodes of edema, and intracellular atrophy.

blepharoplasty. Plastic surgery of the eyelids to remove excess fat and redundant skin weighting down the lid. The eyelid is pulled tight and sutured to support sagging muscles.

blepharoptosis. Droop or displacement of the upper eyelid, caused by paralysis, muscle problems, or outside mechanical forces.

blepharorrhaphy. Suture of a portion or all of the opposing eyelids to shorten the palpebral fissure or close it entirely.

bone conduction. Transportation of sound through the bones of the skull to the inner ear.

bone mass measurement. Radiologic or radioisotopic procedure or other procedure approved by the FDA for identifying bone mass, detecting bone loss, or determining bone quality. The procedure includes a physician's interpretation of the results. Qualifying individuals must be an estrogen-deficient woman at clinical risk for osteoporosis with vertebral abnormalities.

brachytherapy. Form of radiation therapy in which radioactive pellets or seeds are implanted directly into the tissue being treated to deliver their dose of radiation in a more directed fashion. Brachytherapy provides radiation to the prescribed body area while minimizing exposure to normal tissue.

breakpoint. Point at which a chromosome breaks.

Bristow procedure. Anterior capsulorrhaphy prevents chronic separation of the shoulder. In this procedure, the bone block is affixed to the anterior glenoid rim with a screw.

buccal mucosa. Tissue from the mucous membrane on the inside of the cheek.

bundle of His. Bundle of modified cardiac fibers that begins at the atrioventricular node and passes through the right atrioventricular fibrous ring to the interventricular septum, where it divides into two branches. Bundle of His recordings are taken for intracardiac electrograms.

Caldwell-Luc operation. Intraoral antrostomy approach into the maxillary sinus for the removal of tooth roots or tissue, or for packing the sinus to reduce zygomatic fractures by creating a window above the teeth in the canine fossa area.

canthorrhaphy. Suturing of the palpebral fissure, the juncture between the eyelids, at either end of the eye.

canthotomy. Horizontal incision at the canthus (junction of upper and lower eyelids) to divide the outer canthus and enlarge lid margin separation.

cardio-. Relating to the heart.

cardiopulmonary bypass. Venous blood is diverted to a heart-lung machine, which mechanically pumps and oxygenates the blood temporarily so the heart can be bypassed while an open procedure on the heart or coronary arteries is performed. During bypass, the lungs are deflated and immobile.

cardioverter-defibrillator. Device that uses both low energy cardioversion or defibrillating shocks and antitachycardia pacing to treat ventricular tachycardia or ventricular fibrillation.

care plan oversight services. Physician's ongoing review and revision of a patient's care plan involving complex or multidisciplinary care modalities.

case management services. Physician case management is a process of involving direct patient care as well as coordinating and controlling access to the patient or initiating and/or supervising other necessary health care services.

cataract extraction. Surgical removal of the cataract or cloudy lens. Anterior chamber lenses are inserted in conjunction with intracapsular cataract extraction and posterior chamber lenses are inserted in conjunction with extracapsular cataract extraction.

catheter. Flexible tube inserted into an area of the body for introducing or withdrawing fluid.

Centers for Medicare and Medicaid Services. Federal agency that oversees the administration of the public health programs such as Medicare, Medicaid, and State Children's Insurance Program.

certified nurse midwife. Registered nurse who has successfully completed a program of study and clinical experience or has been certified by a recognized organization for the care of pregnant or delivering patients.

CFR. Code of Federal Regulations.

CGMS. Continuous glucose monitoring system.

CHAMPUS. Civilian Health and Medical Program of the Uniformed Services. See Tricare.

CHAMPVA. Civilian Health and Medical Program of the Department of Veterans Affairs.

chemodenervation. Chemical destruction of nerves. A substance, for example, Botox, is used to temporarily inhibit the transfer of chemicals at the presynaptic membrane, blocking the neuromuscular junctions.

chemoembolization. Administration of chemotherapeutic agents directly to a tumor in combination with the percutaneous administration of an occlusive substance into a vessel to deprive the tumor of its blood supply. This ensures a prolonged level of therapy directed at the tumor. Chemoembolization is primarily being used for cancers of the liver and endocrine system.

chemosurgery. Application of chemical agents to destroy tissue, originally referring to the in situ chemical fixation of premalignant or malignant lesions to facilitate surgical excision.

Chiari osteotomy. Top of the femur is altered to correct a dislocated hip caused by congenital conditions or cerebral palsy. Plate and screws are often used.

chimera. Organ or anatomic structure consisting of tissues of diverse genetic constitution.

choanal atresia. Congenital, membranous, or bony closure of one or both posterior nostrils due to failure of the embryonic bucconasal membrane to rupture and open up the nasal passageway.

chondromalacia. Condition in which the articular cartilage softens, seen in various body sites but most often in the patella, and may be congenital or acquired.

chorionic villus sampling. Aspiration of a placental sample through a catheter, under ultrasonic guidance. The specialized needle is placed transvaginally through the cervix or transabdominally into the uterine cavity.

chronic pain management services. Distinct services frequently performed by anesthesiologists who have additional training in pain management procedures. Pain management services include initial and subsequent evaluation and management (E/M) services, trigger point injections, spine and spinal cord injections, and nerve blocks.

cineplastic amputation. Amputation in which muscles and tendons of the remaining portion of the extremity are arranged so that they may be utilized for motor functions. Following this type of amputation, a specially constructed prosthetic device allows the individual to execute more complex movements because the muscles and tendons are able to communicate independent movements to the device.

circadian. Relating to a cyclic, 24-hour period.

CLIA. Clinical Laboratory Improvement Amendments. Requirements set in 1988, CLIA imposes varying levels of federal regulations on clinical procedures. Few laboratories, including those in physician offices, are exempt. Adopted by Medicare and Medicaid, CLIA regulations redefine laboratory testing in regard to laboratory certification and accreditation, proficiency testing, quality assurance, personnel standards, and program administration.

clinical social worker. Individual who possesses a master's or doctor's degree in social work and, after obtaining the degree, has performed at least two years of supervised clinical social work. A clinical social worker must be licensed by the state or, in the case of states without licensure, must completed at least two years or 3,000 hours of post-master's degree supervised clinical social work practice under the supervision of a master's level social worker.

clinical staff. Someone who works for, or under, the direction of a physician or qualified health care professional and does not bill services separately. The person may be licensed or regulated to help the physician perform specific duties.

clonal. Originating from one cell.

CMS. Centers for Medicare and Medicaid Services. Federal agency that administers the public health programs.

CO₂ laser. Carbon dioxide laser that emits an invisible beam and vaporizes water-rich tissue. The vapor is suctioned from the site.

codons. Series of three adjoining bases in one polynucleotide chain of a DNA or RNA molecule that provides the codes for a specific amino acid.

cognitive. Being aware by drawing from knowledge, such as judgment, reason, perception, and memory.

colostomy. Artificial surgical opening anywhere along the length of the colon to the skin surface for the diversion of feces.

commissurotomy. Surgical division or disruption of any two parts that are joined to form a commissure in order to increase the opening. The procedure most often refers to opening the adherent leaflet bands of fibrous tissue in a stenosed mitral valve.

common variants. Nucleotide sequence differences associated with abnormal gene function. Tests are usually performed in a single series of laboratory testing (in a single, typically multiplex, assay arrangement or using more than one assay to include all variants to be examined). Variants are representative of a mutation that mainly causes a single disease, such as cystic fibrosis. Other uncommon variants could provide additional information. Tests may be performed based on society recommendations and guidelines.

community mental health center. Facility providing outpatient mental health day treatment, assessments, and education as appropriate to community members.

component code. In the National Correct Coding Initiative (NCCI), the column II code that cannot be charged to Medicare when the column I code is reported.

comprehensive code. In the National Correct Coding Initiative (NCCI), the column I code that is reported to Medicare and precludes reporting column II codes.

computerized corneal topography. Digital imaging and analysis by computer of the shape of the corneal.

conjunctiva. Mucous membrane lining of the eyelids and covering of the exposed, anterior sclera.

conjunctivodacryocystostomy. Surgical connection of the lacrimal sac directly to the conjunctival sac.

conjunctivorhinostomy. Correction of an obstruction of the lacrimal canal achieved by suturing the posterior flaps and removing any lacrimal obstruction, preserving the conjunctiva.

constitutional. Cells containing genetic code that may be passed down to future generations. May also be referred to as germline.

consultation. Advice or opinion regarding diagnosis and treatment or determination to accept transfer of care of a patient rendered by a medical professional at the request of the primary care provider.

continuous positive airway pressure device. Pressurized device used to maintain the patient's airway for spontaneous or mechanically aided breathing. Often used for patients with mild to moderate sleep apnea.

core needle biopsy. Large-bore biopsy needle inserted into a mass and a core of tissue is removed for diagnostic study.

corpectomy. Removal of the body of a bone, such as a vertebra.

costochondral. Pertaining to the ribs and the scapula.

COTD. Cardiac output thermodilution. Cardiac output measured by thermodilution method that requires heart catheterization and then injection of a thermal indicator, usually iced saline. A computer calculates the cardiac output using an equation that incorporates body temperature, injectate volume and temperature, time, and other calculated ratios over a denominator of the integral of the change in blood temperature during the cold injection, reflected by the area of the inscribed curve.

CPT. 1) Chest physical therapy. 2) Cold pressor test. 3) Current Procedural Terminology.

craniosynostosis. Congenital condition in which one or more of the cranial sutures fuse prematurely, creating a deformed or aberrant head shape.

craterization. Excision of a portion of bone creating a crater-like depression to facilitate drainage from infected areas of bone.

cricoid. Circular cartilage around the trachea.

CRNA. Certified registered nurse anesthetist. Nurse trained and specializing in the administration of anesthesia.

cryolathe. Tool used for reshaping a button of corneal tissue.

cryosurgery. Application of intense cold, usually produced using liquid nitrogen, to locally freeze diseased or unwanted tissue and induce tissue necrosis without causing harm to adjacent tissue.

CT. Computed tomography.

cutdown. Small, incised opening in the skin to expose a blood vessel, especially over a vein (venous cutdown) to allow venipuncture and permit a needle or cannula to be inserted for the withdrawal of blood or administration of fluids.

cyclophotocoagulation. Procedure done to prevent vision loss from glaucoma in which a neodymium: YAG laser is used to burn and destroy a portion of the ciliary body in order to decrease the amount of aqueous humor being produced in the eye. This procedure is only done when creating a drain for aqueous humor to reduce intraocular pressure would not be successful. Destroying portions of the ciliary body reduces the amount of fluid present in the eye.

cytogenetic studies. Procedures in CPT that are related to the branch of genetics that studies cellular (cyto) structure and function as it relates to heredity (genetics). White blood cells, specifically T-lymphocytes, are the most commonly used specimen for chromosome analysis.

cytogenomic. Chromosomic evaluation using molecular methods.

dacryocystotome. Instrument used for incising the lacrimal duct strictures.

DBS. Deep brain stimulation. Treatment for disabling neurological symptoms associated with diseases including Parkinson's. DBS requires three components: the implanted electrode, extension, and neurostimulator. Electrical impulses are sent from the neurostimulator to the implant to block tremors.

debride. To remove all foreign objects and devitalized or infected tissue from a burn or wound to prevent infection and promote healing.

definitive drug testing. Drug tests used to further analyze or confirm the presence or absence of specific drugs or classes of drugs used by the patient. These tests are able to provide more conclusive information regarding the concentration of the drug and their metabolites. May be used for medical, workplace, or legal purposes.

definitive identification. Identification of microorganisms using additional tests to specify the genus or species (e.g., slide cultures or biochemical panels).

dentoalveolar structure. Area of alveolar bone surrounding the teeth and adjacent tissue.

Department of Health and Human Services. Cabinet department that oversees the operating divisions of the federal government responsible for health and welfare. HHS oversees the Centers for Medicare and Medicaid Services, Food and Drug Administration, Public Health Service, and other such entities.

Department of Justice. Attorneys from the DOJ and the United States Attorney's Office have, under the memorandum of understanding, the same direct access to contractor data and records as the OIG and the Federal Bureau of Investigation (FBI). DOJ is responsible for prosecution of fraud and civil or criminal cases presented.

dermis. Skin layer found under the epidermis that contains a papillary upper layer and the deep reticular layer of collagen, vascular bed, and nerves.

dermis graft. Skin graft that has been separated from the epidermal tissue and the underlying subcutaneous fat, used primarily as a substitute for fascia grafts in plastic surgery.

desensitization. 1) Administration of extracts of allergens periodically to build immunity in the patient. 2) Application of medication to decrease the symptoms, usually pain, associated with a dental condition or disease.

destruction. Ablation or eradication of a structure or tissue.

diabetes outpatient self-management training services. Educational and training services furnished by a certified provider in an outpatient setting. The physician managing the individual's diabetic condition must certify that the services are needed under a comprehensive plan of care and provide the patient with the skills and knowledge necessary for therapeutic program compliance (including skills related to the self-administration of injectable drugs). The provider must meet applicable standards established by the National Diabetes Advisory or be recognized by an organization that represents individuals with diabetes as meeting standards for furnishing the services.

diagnostic procedures. Procedure performed on a patient to obtain information to assess the medical condition of the patient or to identify a disease and to determine the nature and severity of an illness or injury.

dialysis. Artificial filtering of the blood to remove contaminating waste elements and restore normal balance.

diaphragm. 1) Muscular wall separating the thorax and its structures from the abdomen. 2) Flexible disk inserted into the vagina and against the cervix as a method of birth control.

diaphysectomy. Surgical removal of a portion of the shaft of a long bone, often done to facilitate drainage from infected bone.

diathermy. Applying heat to body tissues by various methods for therapeutic treatment or surgical purposes to coagulate and seal tissue.

digital medicine services. Those that utilize technology in various forms to provide patient health services.

dilation. Artificial increase in the diameter of an opening or lumen made by medication or by instrumentation.

dissect. Cut apart or separate tissue for surgical purposes or for visual or microscopic study.

DNA. Deoxyribonucleic acid. Chemical containing the genetic information necessary to produce and propagate living organisms. Molecules are comprised of two twisting paired strands, called a double helix.

DNA marker. Specific gene sequence within a chromosome indicating the inheritance of a certain trait.

dorsal. Pertaining to the back or posterior aspect.

drugs and biologicals. Drugs and biologicals included - or approved for inclusion - in the United States Pharmacopoeia, the National Formulary, the United States Homeopathic Pharmacopoeia, in New Drugs or Accepted Dental Remedies, or approved by the pharmacy and drug therapeutics committee of the medical staff of the hospital. Also included are medically accepted and FDA approved drugs used in an anticancer chemotherapeutic regimen. The carrier determines medical acceptance based on supportive clinical evidence.

dual-lead device. Implantable cardiac device (pacemaker or implantable cardioverter-defibrillator [ICD]) in which pacing and sensing components are placed in only two chambers of the heart.

duplex scan. Noninvasive vascular diagnostic technique that uses ultrasonic scanning to identify the pattern and direction of blood flow within arteries or veins displayed in real time images. Duplex scanning combines B-mode two-dimensional pictures of the vessel structure with spectra and/or color flow Doppler mapping or imaging of the blood as it moves through the vessels.

duplication/deletion (DUP/DEL). Term used in molecular testing which examines genomic regions to determine if there are extra chromosomes (duplication) or missing chromosomes (deletions). Normal gene dosage is two copies per cell except for the sex chromosomes which have one per cell.

DuToit staple capsulorrhaphy. Reattachment of the capsule of the shoulder and glenoid labrum to the glenoid lip using staples to anchor the avulsed capsule and glenoid labrum.

Dx. Diagnosis.

DXA. Dual energy x-ray absorptiometry. Radiological technique for bone density measurement using a two-dimensional projection system in which two x-ray beams with different levels of energy are pulsed alternately and the results are given in two scores, reported as standard deviations from peak bone mass density.

dynamic mutation. Unstable or changing polynucleotides resulting in repeats related to genes that can undergo disease-producing increases or decreases in the repeats that differ within tissues or over generations.

ECMO. Extracorporeal membrane oxygenation.

ectropion. Drooping of the lower eyelid away from the eye or outward turning or eversion of the edge of the eyelid, exposing the palpebral conjunctiva and causing irritation.

Eden-Hybinette procedure. Anterior shoulder repair using an anterior bone block to augment the bony anterior glenoid lip.

EDTA. Drug used to inhibit damage to the cornea by collagenase. EDTA is especially effective in alkali burns as it neutralizes soluble alkali, including lye.

effusion. Escape of fluid from within a body cavity.

electrocardiographic rhythm derived. Analysis of data obtained from readings of the heart's electrical activation, including heart rate and rhythm, variability of heart rate, ST analysis, and T-wave alternans. Other data may also be assessed when warranted.

electrocautery. Division or cutting of tissue using high-frequency electrical current to produce heat, which destroys cells.

electrode array. Electronic device containing more than one contact whose function can be adjusted during programming services. Electrodes are specialized for a particular electrochemical reaction that acts as a medium between a body surface and another instrument.

Appendix M — Glossary

electromyography. Test that measures muscle response to nerve stimulation determining if muscle weakness is present and if it is related to the muscles themselves or a problem with the nerves that supply the muscles.

electrooculogram (EOG). Record of electrical activity associated with eye movements.

electrophysiologic studies. Electrical stimulation and monitoring to diagnose heart conduction abnormalities that predispose patients to bradyarrhythmias and to determine a patient's chance for developing ventricular and supraventricular tachyarrhythmias.

embolization. Placement of a clotting agent, such as a coil, plastic particles, gel, foam, etc., into an area of hemorrhage to stop the bleeding or to block blood flow to a problem area, such as an aneurysm or a tumor.

emergency. Serious medical condition or symptom (including severe pain) resulting from injury, sickness, or mental illness that arises suddenly and requires immediate care and treatment, generally received within 24 hours of onset, to avoid jeopardy to the life, limb, or health of a covered person.

empyema. Accumulation of pus within the respiratory, or pleural, cavity.

EMTALA. Emergency Medical Treatment and Active Labor Act.

end-stage renal disease. Chronic, advanced kidney disease requiring renal dialysis or a kidney transplant to prevent imminent death.

endarterectomy. Removal of the thickened, endothelial lining of a diseased or damaged artery.

endomicroscopy. Diagnostic technology that allows for the examination of tissue at the cellular level during endoscopy. The technology decreases the need for biopsy with histological examination for some types of lesions.

endovascular embolization. Procedure whereby vessels are occluded by a variety of therapeutic substances for the treatment of abnormal blood vessels by inhibiting the flow of blood to a tumor, arteriovenous malformations, lymphatic malformation, and to prevent or stop hemorrhage.

entropion. Inversion of the eyelid, turning the edge in toward the eyeball and causing irritation from contact of the lashes with the surface of the eye.

enucleation. Removal of a growth or organ cleanly so as to extract it in one piece.

enzyme immunoassay. Any of several diagnostic immunoassay methods in which an enzyme is bound to an antigen or antibody and acts as a label.

enzyme-linked immunosorbent assay. A laboratory immunoassay technique used in the diagnosis of certain diseases in which antibodies bound to enzymes reveal and quantify the amount of a substance in a solution, such as serum. It is performed using a solid surface to which the antibodies and other molecules adhere. In the last step, an enzymatic reaction occurs that results in a color change that can be read using a specialized instrument.

epidermis. Outermost, nonvascular layer of skin that contains four to five differentiated layers depending on its body location: stratum corneum, lucidum, granulosum, spinosum, and basale.

epiphysiodesis. Surgical fusion of an epiphysis performed to prematurely stop further bone growth.

escharotomy. Surgical incision into the scab or crust resulting from a severe burn in order to relieve constriction and allow blood flow to the distal unburned tissue.

established patient. 1) Patient who has received professional services in a face-to-face setting within the last three years from the same physician/qualified health care professional or another physician/qualified health care professional of the exact same specialty and subspecialty who belongs to the same group practice. 2) For OPPS hospitals, patient who has been registered as an inpatient or outpatient in a hospital's provider-based clinic or emergency department within the past three years.

evacuation. Removal or purging of waste material.

evaluation and management codes. Assessment and management of a patient's health care.

evaluation and management service components. Key components of history, examination, and medical decision making that are key to selecting the correct E/M codes. Other non-key components include counseling, coordination of care, nature of presenting problem, and time.

event recorder. Portable, ambulatory heart monitor worn by the patient that makes electrocardiographic recordings of the length and frequency of aberrant cardiac rhythm to help diagnose heart conditions and to assess pacemaker functioning or programming.

exenteration. Surgical removal of the entire contents of a body cavity, such as the pelvis or orbit.

exon. One of multiple nucleic acid sequences used to encode information for a gene polypeptide or protein. Exons are separated from other exons by non-protein-coding sequences known as introns.

extended care services. Items and services provided to an inpatient of a skilled nursing facility, including nursing care, physical or occupational therapy, speech pathology, drugs and supplies, and medical social services.

external electrical capacitor device. External electrical stimulation device designed to promote bone healing. This device may also promote neural regeneration, revascularization, epiphyseal growth, and ligament maturation.

external pulsating electromagnetic field. External stimulation device designed to promote bone healing. This device may also promote neural regeneration, revascularization, epiphyseal growth, and ligament maturation.

extracorporeal. Located or taking place outside the body.

Eyre-Brook capsulorrhaphy. Reattachment of the capsule of the shoulder and glenoid labrum to the glenoid lip.

False Claims Act. Governs civil actions for filing false claims. Liability under this act pertains to any person who knowingly presents or causes to be presented a false or fraudulent claim to the government for payment or approval.

fascia. Fibrous sheet or band of tissue that envelops organs, muscles, and groupings of muscles.

fasciectomy. Excision of fascia or strips of fascial tissue.

fasciotomy. Incision or transection of fascial tissue.

fat graft. Graft composed of fatty tissue completely freed from surrounding tissue that is used primarily to fill in depressions.

FDA. Food and Drug Administration. Federal agency responsible for protecting public health by substantiating the safety, efficacy, and security of human and veterinary drugs, biological products, medical devices, national food supply, cosmetics, and items that give off radiation.

filtered speech test. Test most commonly used to identify central auditory dysfunction in which the patient is presented monosyllabic words that are low pass filtered, allowing only the parts of each word below a certain pitch to be presented. A score is given on the number of correct responses. This may be a subset of a standard battery of tests provided during a single encounter.

fissure. Deep furrow, groove, or cleft in tissue structures.

fistulization. Creation of a communication between two structures that were not previously connected.

flexor digitorum profundus tendon. Tendon originating in the proximal forearm and extending to the index finger and wrist. A thickened FDP sheath, usually caused by age, illness, or injury, can fill the carpal canal and lead to impingement of the median nerve.

fluorescence immunoassay. A form of immunoassay that uses a fluorescent compound as the detection reagent. This compound absorbs light or energy at a particular wavelength and then emits light or energy at a different wavelength.

fluoroscopy. Radiology technique that allows visual examination of part of the body or a function of an organ using a device that projects an x-ray image on a fluorescent screen.

focal length. Distance between the object in focus and the lens.

focused medical review. Process of targeting and directing medical review efforts on Medicare claims where the greatest risk of inappropriate program payment exists. The goal is to reduce the number of noncovered claims or unnecessary services. CMS analyzes national data such as internal billing, utilization, and payment data and provides its findings to the FI. Local medical review policies are developed identifying aberrances, abuse, and overutilized services. Providers are responsible for knowing national Medicare coverage and billing guidelines and local medical review policies, and for determining whether the services provided to Medicare beneficiaries are covered by Medicare.

fragile X syndrome. Intellectual disabilities, enlarged testes, big jaw, high forehead, and long ears in males. In females, fragile X presents with mild intellectual disabilities and heterozygous sexual structures. In some families, males have shown no symptoms but carry the gene.

free flap. Tissue that is completely detached from the donor site and transplanted to the recipient site, receiving its blood supply from capillary ingrowth at the recipient site.

free microvascular flap. Tissue that is completely detached from the donor site following careful dissection and preservation of the blood vessels, then attached to the recipient site with the transferred blood vessels anastomosed to the vessels in the recipient bed.

fulguration. Destruction of living tissue by using sparks from a high-frequency electric current.

gas tamponade. Absorbable gas may be injected to force the retina against the choroid. Common gases include room air, short-acting sulfahexafluoride, intermediate-acting perfluoroethane, or long-acting perfluorooctane.

Gaucher disease. Genetic metabolic disorder in which fat deposits may accumulate in the spleen, liver, lungs, bone marrow, and brain.

gene. Basic unit of heredity that contains nucleic acid. Genes are arranged in different and unique sequences or strings that determine the gene's function. Human genes usually include multiple protein coding regions such as exons separated by introns which are nonprotein coding sections.

genome. Complete set of DNA of an organism. Each cell in the human body is comprised of a complete copy of the approximately three billion DNA base pairs that constitute the human genome.

habilitative services. Procedures or services provided to assist a patient in learning, keeping, and improving new skills needed to perform daily living activities. Habilitative services assist patients in acquiring a skill for the first time.

HCPCS. Healthcare Common Procedure Coding System.

HCPCS Level I. Healthcare Common Procedure Coding System Level I. Numeric coding system used by physicians, facility outpatient departments, and ambulatory surgery centers (ASC) to code ambulatory, laboratory, radiology, and other diagnostic services for Medicare billing. This coding system contains only the American Medical Association's Physicians' Current Procedural Terminology (CPT) codes. The AMA updates codes annually.

HCPCS Level II. Healthcare Common Procedure Coding System Level II. National coding system, developed by CMS, that contains alphanumeric codes for physician and nonphysician services not included in the CPT coding system. HCPCS Level II covers such things as ambulance services, durable medical equipment, and orthotic and prosthetic devices.

HCPCS modifiers. Two-character code (AA-ZZ) that identifies circumstances that alter or enhance the description of a service or supply. They are recognized by carriers nationally and are updated annually by CMS.

Hct. Hematocrit.

health care provider. Entity that administers diagnostic and therapeutic services.

hemilaminectomy. Excision of a portion of the vertebral lamina.

hemodialysis. Cleansing of wastes and contaminating elements from the blood by virtue of different diffusion rates through a semipermeable membrane, which separates blood from a filtration solution that diffuses other elements out of the blood. The blood is slowly filtered extracorporeally through special dialysis equipment and returned to the body. Synonym(s): renal dialysis.

hemodialysis. Cleansing of wastes and contaminating elements from the blood by virtue of different diffusion rates through a semipermeable membrane, which separates blood from a filtration solution that diffuses other elements out of the blood.

hemoperitoneum. Effusion of blood into the peritoneal cavity, the space between the continuous membrane lining the abdominopelvic walls and encasing the visceral organs.

heterograft. Surgical graft of tissue from one animal species to a different animal species. A common type of heterograft is porcine (pig) tissue, used for temporary wound closure.

heterotopic transplant. Tissue transplanted from a different anatomical site for usage as is natural for that tissue, for example, buccal mucosa to a conjunctival site.

HGNC. HUGO gene nomenclature committee.

HGVS. Human genome variation society.

Hickman catheter. Central venous catheter used for long-term delivery of medications, such as antibiotics, nutritional substances, or chemotherapeutic agents.

HLA. Human leukocyte antigen.

home health services. Services furnished to patients in their homes under the care of physicians. These services include part-time or intermittent skilled nursing care, physical therapy, medical social services, medical supplies, and some rehabilitation equipment. Home health supplies and services must be prescribed by a physician, and the beneficiary must be confined at home in order for Medicare to pay the benefits in full.

homograft. Graft from one individual to another of the same species.

hospice care. Items and services provided to a terminally ill individual by a hospice program under a written plan established and periodically reviewed by the individual's attending physician and by the medical director: Nursing care provided by or under the supervision of a registered professional nurse; Physical or occupational therapy or speech-language pathology services; Medical social services under the direction of a physician; Services of a home health aide who has successfully completed a training program; Medical supplies (including drugs and biologicals) and the use of medical appliances; Physicians' services; Short-term inpatient care (including both respite care and procedures necessary for pain control and acute and chronic symptom management) in an inpatient facility on an intermittent basis and not consecutively over longer than five days; Counseling (including dietary counseling) with respect to care of the terminally ill individual and adjustment to his death; Any item or service which is specified in the plan and for which payment may be made.

hospital. Institution that provides, under the supervision of physicians, diagnostic, therapeutic, and rehabilitation services for medical diagnosis, treatment, and care of patients. Hospitals receiving federal funds must maintain clinical records on all patients, provide 24-hour nursing services, and have a discharge planning process in place. The term "hospital" also includes religious nonmedical health care institutions and facilities of 50 beds or less located in rural areas.

HUGO. Human genome organization

IA. Intra-arterial.

ICD. Implantable cardioverter defibrillator.

ICD-10-CM. International Classification of Diseases, 10th Revision, Clinical Modification. Clinical modification of the alphanumeric classification of diseases used by the World Health Organization, already in use in much of the world, and used for mortality reporting in the United States. The implementation date for ICD-10-CM diagnostic coding system to replace ICD-9-CM in the United States was October 1, 2015.

ICD-10-PCS. International Classification of Diseases, 10th Revision, Procedure Coding System. Beginning October 1, 2015, inpatient hospital services and surgical procedures must be coded using ICD-10-PCS codes, replacing ICD-9-CM, Volume 3 for procedures.

ICM. Implantable cardiovascular monitor.

ileostomy. Artificial surgical opening that brings the end of the ileum out through the abdominal wall to the skin surface for the diversion of feces through a stoma.

iliopsoas tendon. Fibrous tissue that connects muscle to bone in the pelvic region, common to the iliacus and psoas major.

ILR. Implantable loop recorder.

IM. 1) Infectious mononucleosis. 2) Internal medicine. 3) Intramuscular.

immunochemiluminometric assay. A form of immunoassay in which the antigen-antibody complex is measured using light emission produced from a chemical reaction.

immunotherapy. Therapeutic use of serum or gamma globulin.

implant. Material or device inserted or placed within the body for therapeutic, reconstructive, or diagnostic purposes.

implantable cardiovascular monitor. Implantable electronic device that stores cardiovascular physiologic data such as intracardiac pressure waveforms collected from internal sensors or data such as weight and blood pressure collected from external sensors. The information stored in these devices is used as an aid in managing patients with heart failure and other cardiac conditions that are non-rhythm related. The data may be transmitted via local telemetry or remotely to a surveillance technician or an internet-based file server.

implantable cardioverter-defibrillator. Implantable electronic cardiac device used to control rhythm abnormalities such as tachycardia, fibrillation, or bradycardia by producing high- or low-energy stimulation and pacemaker functions. It may also have the capability to provide the functions of an implantable loop recorder or implantable cardiovascular monitor.

implantable loop recorder. Implantable electronic cardiac device that constantly monitors and records electrocardiographic rhythm. It may be triggered by the patient when a symptomatic episode occurs or activated automatically by rapid or slow heart rates. This may be the sole purpose of the device or it may be a component of another cardiac device, such as a pacemaker or implantable cardioverter-defibrillator. The data can be transmitted via local telemetry or remotely to a surveillance technician or an internet-based file server.

implantable venous access device. Catheter implanted for continuous access to the venous system for long-term parenteral feeding or for the administration of fluids or medications.

IMRT. Intensity modulated radiation therapy. External beam radiation therapy delivery using computer planning to specify the target dose and to modulate the radiation intensity, usually as a treatment for a malignancy. The delivery system approaches the patient from multiple angles, minimizing damage to normal tissue.

in situ. Located in the natural position or contained within the origin site, not spread into neighboring tissue.

incontinence. Inability to control urination or defecation.

infundibulectomy. Excision of the anterosuperior portion of the right ventricle of the heart.

internal direct current stimulator. Electrostimulation device placed directly into the surgical site designed to promote bone regeneration by encouraging cellular healing response in bone and ligaments.

interrogation device evaluation. Assessment of an implantable cardiac device (pacemaker, cardioverter-defibrillator, cardiovascular monitor, or loop recorder) in which collected data about the patient's heart rate and rhythm, battery and pulse generator function, and any leads or sensors present, are retrieved and evaluated. Determinations regarding device programming and appropriate treatment settings are made based on the findings. CPT provides required components for evaluation of the various types of devices.

intramedullary implants. Nail, rod, or pin placed into the intramedullary canal at the fracture site. Intramedullary implants not only provide a method of aligning the fracture, they also act as a splint and may reduce fracture pain. Implants may be rigid or flexible. Rigid implants are preferred for prophylactic treatment of diseased bone, while flexible implants are preferred for traumatic injuries.

intraocular lens. Artificial lens implanted into the eye to replace a damaged natural lens or cataract.

intravenous. Within a vein or veins.

introducer. Instrument, such as a catheter, needle, or tube, through which another instrument or device is introduced into the body.

intron. Nonprotein section of a gene that separates exons in human genes. Contains vital sequences that allow splicing of exons to produce a functional protein from a gene. Sometimes referred to as intervening sequences (IVS).

IP. 1) Interphalangeal. 2) Intraperitoneal.

irrigation. To wash out or cleanse a body cavity, wound, or tissue with water or other fluid.

Kayser-Fleischer ring. Condition found in Wilson's disease in which deposits of copper cause a pigmented ring around the cornea's outer border in the deep epithelial layers.

keratoprosthesis. Surgical procedure in which the physician creates a new anterior chamber with a plastic optical implant to replace a severely damaged cornea that cannot be repaired.

keratotomy. Surgical incision of the cornea.

krypton laser. Laser light energy that uses ionized krypton by electric current as the active source, has a radiation beam between the visible yellow-red spectrum, and is effective in photocoagulation of retinal bleeding, macular lesions, and vessel aberrations of the choroid.

lacrimal. Tear-producing gland or ducts that provides lubrication and flushing of the eyes and nasal cavities.

lacrimal punctum. Opening of the lacrimal papilla of the eyelid through which tears flow to the canaliculi to the lacrimal sac.

lacrimotome. Knife for cutting the lacrimal sac or duct.

lacrimotomy. Incision of the lacrimal sac or duct.

laparotomy. Incision through the flank or abdomen for therapeutic or diagnostic purposes.

laryngoscopy. Examination of the hypopharynx, larynx, and tongue base with an endoscope.

larynx. Musculocartilaginous structure between the trachea and the pharynx that functions as the valve preventing food and other particles from entering the respiratory tract, as well as the voice mechanism. Also called the voicebox, the larynx is composed of three single cartilages: cricoid, epiglottis, and thyroid; and three paired cartilages: arytenoid, corniculate, and cuneiform.

laser surgery. Use of concentrated, sharply defined light beams to cut, cauterize, coagulate, seal, or vaporize tissue.

LEEP. Loop electrode excision procedure. Biopsy specimen or cone shaped wedge of cervical tissue is removed using a hot cautery wire loop with an electrical current running through it.

levonorgestrel. Drug inhibiting ovulation and preventing sperm from penetrating cervical mucus. It is delivered subcutaneously in polysiloxone capsules. The capsules can be effective for up to five years, and provide a cumulative pregnancy rate of less than 2 percent. The capsules are not biodegradable, and therefore must be removed. Removal is more difficult than insertion of levonorgestrel capsules because fibrosis develops around the capsules. Normal hormonal activity and a return to fertility begins immediately upon removal.

ligament. Band or sheet of fibrous tissue that connects the articular surfaces of bones or supports visceral organs.

ligation. Tying off a blood vessel or duct with a suture or a soft, thin wire.

light chains. Proteins produced by plasma (immune) cells; also called kappa and lambda light chains.

lymphadenectomy. Dissection of lymph nodes free from the vessels and removal for examination by frozen section in a separate procedure to detect early-stage metastases.

lysis. Destruction, breakdown, dissolution, or decomposition of cells or substances by a specific catalyzing agent.

Magnuson-Stack procedure. Treatment for recurrent anterior dislocation of the shoulder that involves tightening and realigning the subscapularis tendon.

maintenance of wakefulness test. Attended study determining the patient's ability to stay awake.

Manchester operation. Preservation of the uterus following prolapse by amputating the vaginal portion of the cervix, shortening the cardinal ligaments, and performing a colpoperineorrhaphy posteriorly.

mapping. Multidimensional depiction of a tachycardia that identifies its site of origin and its electrical conduction pathway after tachycardia has been induced. The recording is made from multiple catheter sites within the heart, obtaining electrograms simultaneously or sequentially.

marsupialization. Creation of a pouch in surgical treatment of a cyst in which one wall is resected and the remaining cut edges are sutured to adjacent tissue creating an open pouch of the previously enclosed cyst.

mastectomy. Surgical removal of one or both breasts.

McDonald procedure. Polyester tape is placed around the cervix with a running stitch to assist in the prevention of pre-term delivery. Tape is removed at term for vaginal delivery.

MCP. Metacarpophalangeal.

medial. Middle or midline.

mediastinotomy. Incision into the mediastinum for purposes of exploration, foreign body removal, drainage, or biopsy.

medical review. Review by a Medicare administrative contractor, carrier, and/or quality improvement organization (QIO) of services and items provided by physicians, other health care practitioners, and providers of health care services under Medicare. The review determines if the items and services are reasonable and necessary and meet Medicare coverage requirements, whether the quality meets professionally recognized standards of health care, and whether the services are medically appropriate in an inpatient, outpatient, or other setting as supported by documentation.

Medicare contractor. Medicare Part A fiscal intermediary, Medicare Part B carrier, Medicare administrative contractor (MAC), or a durable medical equipment Medicare administrative contractor (DME MAC).

Medicare physician fee schedule. List of payments Medicare allows by procedure or service. Payments may vary through geographic adjustments. The MPFS is based on the resource-based relative value scale (RBRVS). A national total relative value unit (RVU) is given to each procedure (HCPCS Level I CPT, Level II national codes). Each total RVU has three components: physician work, practice expense, and malpractice insurance.

meibomian gland. Sebaceous gland located in the tarsal plates along the eyelid margins that produces the lipid components found in tears.

metabolite. Chemical compound resulting from the natural process of metabolism. In drug testing, the metabolite of the drug may endure in a higher concentration or for a longer duration than the initial "parent" drug.

methylation. Mechanism used to regulate genes and protect DNA from some types of cleavage.

microarray. Small surface onto which multiple specific nucleic acid sequences can be attached to be used for analysis. Microarray may also be known as a gene chip or DNA chip. Tests can be run on the sequences for any variants that may be present.

mitral valve. Valve with two cusps that is between the left atrium and left ventricle of the heart.

moderate sedation. Medically controlled state of depressed consciousness, with or without analgesia, while maintaining the patient's airway, protective reflexes, and ability to respond to stimulation or verbal commands.

Mohs micrographic surgery. Special technique used to treat complex or ill-defined skin cancer and requires a single physician to provide two distinct services. The first service is surgical and involves the destruction of the lesion by a combination of chemosurgery and excision. The second service is that of a pathologist and includes mapping, color coding of specimens, microscopic examination of specimens, and complete histopathologic preparation.

monitored anesthesia care. Sedation, with or without analgesia, used to achieve a medically controlled state of depressed consciousness while maintaining the patient's airway, protective reflexes, and ability to respond to stimulation or verbal commands. In dental conscious sedation, the patient is rendered free of fear, apprehension, and anxiety through the use of pharmacological agents.

monoclonal. Relating to a single clone of cells.

mosaicplasty. Multiple, small grafts composed of bone and cartilage placed to treat osteochondral defects of the knee. The grafts are cylindrical in shape and are placed in corresponding size holes made to the desired depth to fill the defect and allow for a more naturally shaped reconstruction.

multiple sleep latency test (MSLT). Attended study to determine the tendency of the patient to fall asleep.

multiple-lead device. Implantable cardiac device (pacemaker or implantable cardioverter-defibrillator [ICD]) in which pacing and sensing components are placed in at least three chambers of the heart.

Mustard procedure. Corrective measure for transposition of great vessels involves an intra-atrial baffle made of pericardial tissue or synthetic material. The baffle is secured between pulmonary veins and mitral valve and between mitral and tricuspid valves. The baffle directs systemic venous flow into the left ventricle and lungs and pulmonary venous flow into the right ventricle and aorta.

mutation. Alteration in gene function that results in changes to a gene or chromosome. Can cause deficits or disease that can be inherited, can have beneficial effects, or result in no noticeable change.

mutation scanning. Process normally used on multiple polymerase chain reaction (PCR) amplicons to determine DNA sequence variants by differences in characteristics compared to normal. Specific DNA variants can then be studied further.

myotomy. Surgical cutting of a muscle to gain access to underlying tissues or for therapeutic reasons.

myringotomy. Incision in the eardrum done to prevent spontaneous rupture precipitated by fluid pressure build-up behind the tympanic membrane and to prevent stagnant infection and erosion of the ossicles.

nasal polyp. Fleshy outgrowth projecting from the mucous membrane of the nose or nasal sinus cavity that may obstruct ventilation or affect the sense of smell.

nasal sinus. Air-filled cavities in the cranial bones lined with mucous membrane and continuous with the nasal cavity, draining fluids through the nose.

nasogastric tube. Long, hollow, cylindrical catheter made of soft rubber or plastic that is inserted through the nose down into the stomach, and is used for feeding, instilling medication, or withdrawing gastric contents.

nasolacrimal punctum. Opening of the lacrimal duct near the nose.

nasopharynx. Membranous passage above the level of the soft palate.

Nd:YAG laser. Laser light energy that uses an yttrium, aluminum, and garnet crystal doped with neodymium ions as the active source, has a radiation beam nearing the infrared spectrum, and is effective in photocoagulation, photoablation, cataract extraction, and lysis of vitreous strands.

nebulizer. Latin for mist, a device that converts liquid into a fine spray and is commonly used to deliver medicine to the upper respiratory, bronchial, and lung areas.

nerve conduction study. Diagnostic test performed to assess muscle or nerve damage. Nerves are stimulated with electric shocks along the course of the muscle. Sensors are utilized to measure and record nerve functions, including conduction and velocity.

neurectomy. Excision of all or a portion of a nerve.

neuromuscular junction. Nerve synapse at the meeting point between the terminal end of a nerve (motor neuron) and a muscle fiber.

neuropsychological testing. Evaluation of a patient's behavioral abilities wherein a physician or other health care professional administers a series of tests in thinking, reasoning, and judgment.

new patient. Patient who is receiving face-to-face care from a provider/qualified health care professional or another physician/qualified health care professional of the exact same specialty and subspecialty who belongs to the same group practice for the first time in three years. For OPPS hospitals, a patient who has not been registered as an inpatient or outpatient, including off-campus provider based clinic or emergency department, within the past three years.

Niemann-Pick syndrome. Accumulation of phospholipid in histiocytes in the bone marrow, liver, lymph nodes, and spleen, cerebral involvement, and red macular spots similar to Tay-Sachs disease. Most commonly found in Jewish infants.

Nissen fundoplasty. Surgical repair technique that involves the fundus of the stomach being wrapped around the lower end of the esophagus to treat reflux esophagitis.

nonabsorbable sutures. Strands of natural or synthetic material that resist absorption into living tissue and are removed once healing is under way. Nonabsorbable sutures are commonly used to close skin wounds and repair tendons or collagenous tissue.

obturator. Prosthesis used to close an acquired or congenital opening in the palate that aids in speech and chewing.

obturator nerve. Lumbar plexus nerve with anterior and posterior divisions that innervate the adductor muscles (e.g., adductor longus, adductor brevis) of the leg and the skin over the medial area of the thigh or a sacral plexus nerve with anterior and posterior divisions that innervate the superior gemellus muscles.

occult blood test. Chemical or microscopic test to determine the presence of blood in a specimen.

ocular implant. Implant inside muscular cone.

oophorectomy. Surgical removal of all or part of one or both ovaries, either as open procedure or laparoscopically. Menstruation and childbearing ability continues when one ovary is removed.

orthosis. Derived from a Greek word meaning "to make straight," it is an artificial appliance that supports, aligns, or corrects an anatomical deformity or improves the use of a moveable body part. Unlike a prosthesis, an orthotic device is always functional in nature.

osteo-. Having to do with bone.

osteogenesis stimulator. Device used to stimulate the growth of bone by electrical impulses or ultrasound.

osteotomy. Surgical cutting of a bone.

ostomy. Artificial (surgical) opening in the body used for drainage or for delivery of medications or nutrients.

pacemaker. Implantable cardiac device that controls the heart's rhythm and maintains regular beats by artificial electric discharges. This device consists of the pulse generator with a battery and the electrodes, or leads, which are placed in single or dual chambers of the heart, usually transvenously.

palmaris longus tendon. Tendon located in the hand that flexes the wrist joint.

paracentesis. Surgical puncture of a body cavity with a specialized needle or hollow tubing to aspirate fluid for diagnostic or therapeutic reasons.

paratenon graft. Graft composed of the fatty tissue found between a tendon and its sheath.

passive mobilization. Pressure, movement, or pulling of a limb or body part utilizing an apparatus or device.

pedicle flap. Full-thickness skin and subcutaneous tissue for grafting that remains partially attached to the donor site by a pedicle or stem in which the blood vessels supplying the flap remain intact.

Pemberton osteotomy. Osteotomy is performed to position triradiate cartilage as a hinge for rotating the acetabular roof in cases of dysplasia of the hip in children.

penetrance. Being formed by, or pertaining to, a single clone.

percutaneous intradiscal electrothermal annuloplasty. Procedure corrects tears in the vertebral annulus by applying heat to the collagen disc walls percutaneously through a catheter. The heat contracts and thickens the wall, which may contract and close any annular tears.

percutaneous skeletal fixation. Treatment that is neither open nor closed and the injury site is not directly visualized. Fixation devices (pins, screws) are placed through the skin to stabilize the dislocation using x-ray guidance.

pericardium. Thin and slippery case in which the heart lies that is lined with fluid so that the heart is free to pulse and move as it beats.

peripheral arterial tonometry (PAT). Pulsatile volume changes in a digit are measured to determine activity in the sympathetic nervous system for respiratory analysis.

peritoneal. Space between the lining of the abdominal wall, or parietal peritoneum, and the surface layer of the abdominal organs, or visceral peritoneum. It contains a thin, watery fluid that keeps the peritoneal surfaces moist.

peritoneal dialysis. Dialysis that filters waste from blood inside the body using the peritoneum, the natural lining of the abdomen, as the semipermeable membrane across which ultrafiltration is accomplished. A special catheter is inserted into the abdomen and a dialysis solution is drained into the abdomen. This solution extracts fluids and wastes, which are then discarded when the fluid is drained. Various forms of peritoneal dialysis include CAPD, CCPD, and NIDP.

peritoneal effusion. Persistent escape of fluid within the peritoneal cavity.

pessary. Device placed in the vagina to support and reposition a prolapsing or retropositioned uterus, rectum, or vagina.

phacoemulsification. Cataract extraction in which the lens is fragmented by ultrasonic vibrations and simultaneously irrigated and aspirated.

phenotype. Physical expression of a trait or characteristic as determined by an individual's genetic makeup or genotype.

photocoagulation. Application of an intense laser beam of light to disrupt tissue and condense protein material to a residual mass, used especially for treating ocular conditions.

physical status modifiers. Alphanumeric modifier used to identify the patient's health status as it affects the work related to providing the anesthesia service.

physical therapy modality. Therapeutic agent or regimen applied or used to provide appropriate treatment of the musculoskeletal system.

physician. Legally authorized practitioners including a doctor of medicine or osteopathy, a doctor of dental surgery or of dental medicine, a doctor of podiatric medicine, a doctor of optometry, and a chiropractor only with respect to treatment by means of manual manipulation of the spine (to correct a subluxation).

PICC. Peripherally inserted central catheter. PICC is inserted into one of the large veins of the arm and threaded through the vein until the tip sits in a large vein just above the heart.

PKR. Photorefractive therapy. Procedure involving the removal of the surface layer of the cornea (epithelium) by gentle scraping and use of a computer-controlled excimer laser to reshape the stroma.

plasma. The liquid portion of normal unclotted blood that contains red cells, white cells, and platelets.

pleurodesis. Injection of a sclerosing agent into the pleural space for creating adhesions between the parietal and the visceral pleura to treat a collapsed lung caused by air trapped in the pleural cavity, or severe cases of pleural effusion.

plication. Surgical technique involving folding, tucking, or pleating to reduce the size of a hollow structure or organ.

polyclonal. Containing one or more cells.

polymorphism. Genetic variation in the same species that does not harm the gene function or create disease.

polypeptide. Chain of amino acids held together by covalent bonds. Proteins are made up of amino acids.

polysomnography. Test involving monitoring of respiratory, cardiac, muscle, brain, and ocular function during sleep.

Potts-Smith-Gibson procedure. Side-to-side anastomosis of the aorta and left pulmonary artery creating a shunt that enlarges as the child grows.

Prader-Willi syndrome. Rounded face, almond-shaped eyes, strabismus, low forehead, hypogonadism, hypotonia, intellectual disabilities, and an insatiable appetite.

presumptive drug testing. Drug screening tests to identify the presence or absence of drugs in a patient's system. Tests are usually able to identify low concentrations of the drug. These tests may be used for medical, workplace, or legal purposes.

presumptive identification. Identification of microorganisms using media growth, colony morphology, gram stains, or up to three specific tests (e.g., catalase, indole, oxidase, urease).

professional component. Portion of a charge for health care services that represents the physician's (or other practitioner's) work in providing the service, including interpretation and report of the procedure. This component of the service usually is charged for and billed separately from the inpatient hospital charges.

profunda. Denotes a part of a structure that is deeper from the surface of the body than the rest of the structure.

prolonged physician services. Extended pre- or post-service care provided to a patient whose condition requires services beyond the usual.

prostate. Male gland surrounding the bladder neck and urethra that secretes a substance into the seminal fluid.

prosthetic. Device that replaces all or part of an internal body organ or body part, or that replaces part of the function of a permanently inoperable or malfunctioning internal body organ or body part.

provider of services. Institution, individual, or organization that provides health care.

proximal. Located closest to a specified reference point, usually the midline or trunk.

psychiatric hospital. Specialized institution that provides, under the supervision of physicians, services for the diagnosis and treatment of mentally ill persons.

pterygium. Benign, wedge-shaped, conjunctival thickening that advances from the inner corner of the eye toward the cornea.

pterygomaxillary fossa. Wide depression on the external surface of the maxilla above and to the side of the canine tooth socket.

pulmonary artery banding. Surgical constriction of the pulmonary artery to prevent irreversible pulmonary vascular obstructive changes and overflow into the left ventricle.

Putti-Platt procedure. Realignment of the subscapularis tendon to treat recurrent anterior dislocation, thereby partially eliminating external rotation. The anterior capsule is also tightened and reinforced.

pyloroplasty. Enlargement and reconstruction of the lower portion of the stomach opening into the duodenum performed after vagotomy to speed gastric emptying and treat duodenal ulcers.

qualified health care professional. Educated, licensed or certified, and regulated professional operating under a specified scope of practice to provide patient services that are separate and distinct from other clinical staff. Services may be billed independently or under the facility's services.

RAC. Recovery audit contractor. National program using CMS-affiliated contractors to review claims prior to payment as well as for payments on claims already processed, including overpayments and underpayments.

radiation therapy simulation. Radiation therapy simulation. Procedure by which the specific body area to be treated with radiation is defined and marked. A CT scan is performed to define the body contours and these images are used to create a plan customized treatment for the patient, targeting the area to be treated while sparing adjacent tissue. The center of the area to be treated is marked and an immobilization device (e.g., cradle, mold) is created to make sure the patient is in the same position each time for treatment. Complexity of treatment depends on the number of treatment areas and the use of tools to isolate the area of treatment.

radioactive substances. Materials used in the diagnosis and treatment of disease that emit high-speed particles and energy-containing rays.

radiology services. Services that include diagnostic and therapeutic radiology, nuclear medicine, CT scan procedures, magnetic resonance imaging services, ultrasound, and other imaging procedures.

radiotherapy afterloading. Part of the radiation therapy process in which the chemotherapy agent is actually instilled into the tumor area subsequent to surgery and placement of an expandable catheter into the void remaining after tumor excision. The specialized catheter remains in place and the patient may come in for multiple treatments with radioisotope placed to treat the margin of tissue surrounding the excision. After the radiotherapy is completed, the patient returns to have the catheter emptied and removed. This is a new therapy in breast cancer treatment.

Rashkind procedure. Transvenous balloon atrial septectomy or septostomy performed by cardiac catheterization. A balloon catheter is inserted into the heart either to create or enlarge an opening in the interatrial septal wall.

rehabilitation services. Therapy services provided primarily for assisting in a rehabilitation program of evaluation and service including cardiac rehabilitation, medical social services, occupational therapy, physical therapy, respiratory therapy, skilled nursing, speech therapy, psychiatric rehabilitation, and alcohol and substance abuse rehabilitation.

respiratory airflow (ventilation). Assessment of air movement during inhalation and exhalation as measured by nasal pressure sensors and thermistor.

respiratory analysis. Assessment of components of respiration obtained by other methods such as airflow or peripheral arterial tone.

respiratory effort. Measurement of diaphragm and/or intercostal muscle for airflow using transducers to estimate thoracic and abdominal motion.

respiratory movement. Measurement of chest and abdomen movement during respiration.

ribbons. In oncology, small plastic tubes containing radioactive sources for interstitial placement that may be cut into specific lengths tailored to the size of the area receiving ionizing radiation treatment.

Ridell sinusotomy. Frontal sinus tissue is destroyed to eliminate tumors.

RNA. Ribonucleic acid.

rural health clinic. Clinic in an area where there is a shortage of health services staffed by a nurse practitioner, physician assistant, or certified nurse midwife under physician direction that provides routine diagnostic services, including clinical laboratory services, drugs, and biologicals and that has prompt access to additional diagnostic services from facilities meeting federal requirements.

Salter osteotomy. Innominate bone of the hip is cut, removed, and repositioned to repair a congenital dislocation, subluxation, or deformity.

saucerization. Creation of a shallow, saucer-like depression in the bone to facilitate drainage of infected areas.

Schiotz tonometer. Instrument that measures intraocular pressure by recording the depth of an indentation on the cornea by a plunger of known weight.

screening mammography. Radiologic images taken of the female breast for the early detection of breast cancer.

screening pap smear. Diagnostic laboratory test consisting of a routine exfoliative cytology test (Papanicolaou test) provided to a woman for the early detection of cervical or vaginal cancer. The exam includes a clinical breast examination and a physician's interpretation of the results.

seeds. Small (1 mm or less) sources of radioactive material that are permanently placed directly into tumors.

Senning procedure. Flaps of intra-atrial septum and right atrial wall are used to create two interatrial channels to divert the systemic and pulmonary venous circulation.

sensitivity tests. Number of methods of applying selective suspected allergens to the skin or mucous.

sensorineural conduction. Transportation of sound from the cochlea to the acoustic nerve and central auditory pathway to the brain.

sentinel lymph node. First node to which lymph drainage and metastasis from a cancer can occur.

separate procedures. Services commonly carried out as a fundamental part of a total service and, as such, do not usually warrant separate identification. These services are identified in CPT with the parenthetical phrase (separate procedure) at the end of the description and are payable only when performed alone.

septectomy. 1) Surgical removal of all or part of the nasal septum. 2) Submucosal resection of the nasal septum.

serum. The clear liquid portion of the blood that remains after the clotting proteins and blood cells have been removed.

Shirodkar procedure. Treatment of an incompetent cervical os by placing nonabsorbent suture material in purse-string sutures as a cerclage to support the cervix.

short tandem repeat (STR). Short sequences of a DNA pattern that are repeated. Can be used as genetic markers for human identity testing.

sialodochoplasty. Surgical repair of a salivary gland duct.

single-lead device. Implantable cardiac device (pacemaker or implantable cardioverter-defibrillator [ICD]) in which pacing and sensing components are placed in only one chamber of the heart.

single-nucleotide polymorphism (SNP). Single nucleotide (A, T, C, or G that is different in a DNA sequence. This difference occurs at a significant frequency in the population.

sinus of Valsalva. Any of three sinuses corresponding to the individual cusps of the aortic valve, located in the most proximal part of the aorta just above the cusps. These structures are contained within the pericardium and appear as distinct but subtle outpouchings or dilations of the aortic wall between each of the semilunar cusps of the valve.

sleep apnea. Intermittent cessation of breathing during sleep that may cause hypoxemia and pulmonary arterial hypertension.

sleep latency. Time period between lying down in bed and the onset of sleep.

sleep staging. Determination of the separate levels of sleep according to physiological measurements.

somatic. 1) Pertaining to the body or trunk. 2) In genetics acquired or occurring after birth.

SPECT. Single photon emission computerized tomography. SPECT images are taken after the injection of a radionuclide using a special camera containing a detector crystal, usually sodium iodide. Images are captured as the gamma radiation from the radionuclide scintillates or gives off its energy in a flash of light when coming in contact with the crystal. This type of imaging is reported for the anatomical area and purpose such as detecting liver function or myocardial perfusion after an ischemic event.

speculoscopy. Viewing the cervix utilizing a magnifier and a special wavelength of light, allowing detection of abnormalities that may not be discovered on a routine Pap smear.

speech-language pathology services. Speech, language, and related function assessment and rehabilitation service furnished by a qualified speech-language pathologist. Audiology services include hearing and balance assessment services furnished by a qualified audiologist. A qualified speech pathologist and audiologist must have a master's or doctoral degree in their respective fields and be licensed to serve in the state. Speech pathologists and audiologists practicing in states without licensure must complete 350 hours of supervised clinical work and perform at least nine months of supervised full-time service after earning their degrees.

sphincteroplasty. Surgical repair done to correct, augment, or improve the muscular function of a sphincter, such as the anus or intestines.

spirometry. Measurement of the lungs' breathing capacity.

splint. Brace or support. 1) dynamic splint: brace that permits movement of an anatomical structure such as a hand, wrist, foot, or other part of the body after surgery or injury. 2) static splint: brace that prevents movement and maintains support and position for an anatomical structure after surgery or injury.

stent. Tube to provide support in a body cavity or lumen.

stereotactic radiosurgery. Delivery of externally-generated ionizing radiation to specific targets for destruction or inactivation. Most often utilized in the treatment of brain or spinal tumors, high-resolution stereotactic imaging is used to identify the target and then deliver the treatment. Computer-assisted planning may also be employed. Simple and complex cranial lesions and spinal lesions are typically treated in a single planning and treatment session, although a maximum of five sessions may be required. No incision is made for stereotactic radiosurgery procedures.

stereotaxis. Three-dimensional method for precisely locating structures.

Stoffel rhizotomy. Nerve roots are sectioned to relieve pain or spastic paralysis.

strabismus. Misalignment of the eyes due to an imbalance in extraocular muscles.

surgical package. Normal, uncomplicated performance of specific surgical services, with the assumption that, on average, all surgical procedures of a given type are similar with respect to skill level, duration, and length of normal follow-up care.

symblepharopterygium. Adhesion in which the eyelid is adhered to the eyeball by a band that resembles a pterygium.

sympathectomy. Surgical interruption or transection of a sympathetic nervous system pathway.

synchronous services. Those that entail real-time communication between the patient and/or family and a physician or other qualified health care professional (QHP) when both are located at different physical sites.

tarso-. 1) Relating to the foot. 2) Relating to the margin of the eyelid.

tarsocheiloplasty. Plastic operation upon the edge of the eyelid for the treatment of trichiasis.

tarsorrhaphy. Suture of a portion or all of the opposing eyelids together for the purpose of shortening the palpebral fissure or closing it entirely.

technical component. Portion of a health care service that identifies the provision of the equipment, supplies, technical personnel, and costs attendant to the performance of the procedure other than the professional services.

tendon. Fibrous tissue that connects muscle to bone, consisting primarily of collagen and containing little vasculature.

tendon allograft. Allografts are tissues obtained from another individual of the same species. Tendon allografts are usually obtained from cadavers and frozen or freeze dried for later use in soft tissue repairs where the physician elects not to obtain an autogenous graft (a graft obtained from the individual on whom the surgery is being performed).

tendon suture material. Tendons are composed of fibrous tissue consisting primarily of collagen and containing few cells or blood vessels. This tissue heals more slowly than tissues with more vascularization. Because of this, tendons are usually repaired with nonabsorbable suture material. Examples include surgical silk, surgical cotton, linen, stainless steel, surgical nylon, polyester fiber, polybutester (Novafil), polyethylene (Dermalene), and polypropylene (Prolene, Surilene).

tendon transplant. Replacement of a tendon with another tendon.

tenon's capsule. Connective tissue that forms the capsule enclosing the posterior eyeball, extending from the conjunctival fornix and continuous with the muscular fascia of the eye.

tenonectomy. Excision of a portion of a tendon to make it shorter.

tenotomy. Cutting into a tendon.

TENS. Transcutaneous electrical nerve stimulator. TENS is applied by placing electrode pads over the area to be stimulated and connecting the electrodes to a transmitter box, which sends a current through the skin to sensory nerve fibers to help decrease pain in that nerve distribution.

tensilon. Edrophonium chloride. Agent used for evaluation and treatment of myasthenia gravis.

terminally ill. Individual whose medical prognosis for life expectancy is six months or less.

tetralogy of Fallot. Specific combination of congenital cardiac defects: obstruction of the right ventricular outflow tract with pulmonary stenosis, interventricular septal defect, malposition of the aorta, overriding the interventricular septum and receiving blood from both the venous and arterial systems, and enlargement of the right ventricle.

therapeutic services. Services performed for treatment of a specific diagnosis. These services include performance of the procedure, various incidental elements, and normal, related follow-up care.

thoracentesis. Surgical puncture of the chest cavity with a specialized needle or hollow tubing to aspirate fluid from within the pleural space for diagnostic or therapeutic reasons.

thoracic lymphadenectomy. Procedure to cut out the lymph nodes near the lungs, around the heart, and behind the trachea.

thoracostomy. Creation of an opening in the chest wall for drainage.

thyroglossal duct. Embryonic duct at the front of the neck, which becomes the pyramidal lobe of the thyroid gland with obliteration of the remaining duct, but may form a cyst or sinus in adulthood if it persists.

total disc arthroplasty with artificial disc. Removal of an intravertebral disc and its replacement with an implant. The implant is an artificial disc consisting of two metal plates with a weight-bearing surface of polyethylene between the plates. The plates are anchored to the vertebral immediately above and below the affected disc.

total shoulder replacement. Prosthetic replacement of the entire shoulder joint, including the humeral head and the glenoid fossa.

trabeculae carneae cordis. Bands of muscular tissue that line the walls of the ventricles in the heart.

trabeculectomy. Surgical incision between the anterior portion of the eye and the canal of Schlemm to drain the aqueous humor.

tracheostomy. Formation of a tracheal opening on the neck surface with tube insertion to allow for respiration in cases of obstruction or decreased patency. A tracheostomy may be planned or performed on an emergency basis for temporary or long-term use.

tracheotomy. Formation of a tracheal opening on the neck surface with tube insertion to allow for respiration in cases of obstruction or decreased patency. A tracheotomy may be planned or performed on an emergency basis for temporary or long-term use.

traction. Drawing out or holding tension on an area by applying a direct therapeutic pulling force.

transcranial magnetic stimulation. Application of electromagnetic energy to the brain through a coil placed on the scalp. The procedure stimulates cortical neurons and is intended to activate and normalize their processes.

transcription. Process by which messenger RNA is synthesized from a DNA template resulting in the transfer of genetic information from the DNA molecule to the messenger RNA.

translocation. Disconnection of all or part of a chromosome that reattaches to another position in the DNA sequence of the same or another chromosome. Often results in a reciprocal exchange of DNA sequences between two differently numbered chromosomes. May or may not result in a clinically significant loss of DNA.

trephine. 1) Specialized round saw for cutting circular holes in bone, especially the skull. 2) Instrument that removes small disc-shaped buttons of corneal tissue for transplanting.

tricuspid atresia. Congenital absence of the valve that may occur with other defects, such as atrial septal defect, pulmonary atresia, and transposition of great vessels.

turbinates. Scroll or shell-shaped elevations from the wall of the nasal cavity, the inferior turbinate being a separate bone, while the superior and middle turbinates are of the ethmoid bone.

tympanic membrane. Thin, sensitive membrane across the entrance to the middle ear that vibrates in response to sound waves, allowing the waves to be transmitted via the ossicular chain to the internal ear.

tympanoplasty. Surgical repair of the structures of the middle ear, including the eardrum and the three small bones, or ossicles.

unlisted procedure. Procedural descriptions used when the overall procedure and outcome of the procedure are not adequately described by an existing procedure code. Such codes are used as a last resort and only when there is not a more appropriate procedure code.

ureterorrhaphy. Surgical repair using sutures to close an open wound or injury of the ureter.

vagotomy. Division of the vagus nerves, interrupting impulses resulting in lower gastric acid production and hastening gastric emptying. Used in the treatment of chronic gastric, pyloric, and duodenal ulcers that can cause severe pain and difficulties in eating and sleeping.

variant. Nucleotide deviation from the normal sequence of a region. Variations are usually either substitutions or deletions. Substitution variations are the result of one nucleotide taking the place of another. A deletion occurs when one or more nucleotides are left out. In some cases, several in a reasonably close proximity on the same chromosome in a DNA strand. These variations result in amino acid changes in the protein made by the gene. However, the term variant does not itself imply a functional change. Intron variations are usually described in one of two ways: 1) the changed nucleotide is defined by a plus or a minus sign indicating the position relative to the first or last nucleotide to the intron, or 2) the second variant description is indicated relative to the last nucleotide of the preceding exon or first nucleotide of the following exon.

vascular family. Group of vessels (family) that branch from the aorta or vena cava. At each branching, the vascular order increases by one. The first order vessel is the primary branch off the aorta or vena cava. The second order vessel branches from the first order, the third order branches from the second order, and any further branching is beyond the third order. For example, for the inferior vena cava, the common iliac artery is a first order vessel. The internal and external iliac arteries are second order vessels, as they each originate from the first order common iliac artery. The external iliac artery extends directly from the common iliac artery and the internal iliac artery bifurcates from the common iliac artery. A third order vessel from the external iliac artery is the inferior epigastric artery and a third order vessel from the internal iliac artery is the obturator artery. Note orders are not always identical bilaterally (e.g., the left common carotid artery is a first order and the right common carotid is a second order). Synonym(s): vascular origins and distributions.

vasectomy. Surgical procedure involving the removal of all or part of the vas deferens, usually performed for sterilization or in conjunction with a prostatectomy.

vena cava interruption. Procedure that places a filter device, called an umbrella or sieve, within the large vein returning deoxygenated blood to the heart to prevent pulmonary embolism caused by clots.

ventricular assist device. Temporary measure used to support the heart by substituting for left and/or right heart function. The device replaces the work of the left and/or right ventricle when a patient has a damaged or weakened heart. A left ventricular assist device (VAD) helps the heart pump blood through the rest of the body. A right VAD helps the heart pump blood to the lungs to become oxygenated again. Catheters are inserted to circulate the blood through external tubing to a pump machine located outside of the body and back to the correct artery.

ventricular septal defect. Congenital cardiac anomaly resulting in a continual opening in the septum between the ventricles that, in severe cases, causes oxygenated blood to flow back into the lungs, resulting in pulmonary hypertension.

vertebral interspace. Non-bony space between two adjacent vertebral bodies that contains the cushioning intervertebral disk.

volar. Palm of the hand (palmar) or sole of the foot (plantar).

Waterston procedure. Type of aortopulmonary shunting done to increase pulmonary blood flow. The ascending aorta is anastomosed to the right pulmonary artery.

Wharton's ducts. Salivary ducts below the mandible.

wick catheter. Device used to monitor interstitial fluid pressure, and sometimes used intraoperatively during fasciotomy procedures to evaluate the effectiveness of the decompression.

wound closure. Closure or repair of a wound created surgically or due to trauma (e.g., laceration). The closure technique depends on the type, site, and depth of the defect. Consideration is also given to cosmetic and functional outcome. A single layer closure involves approximation of the edges of the wound. The second type of closure involves closing the one or more deeper layers of tissue prior to skin closure. The most complex type of closure may include techniques such as debridement or undermining, which involves manipulation of tissue around the wound to allow the skin to cover the wound. The AMA CPT® book defines these as Simple, Intermediate and Complex repair.

xenograft. Tissue that is nonhuman and harvested from one species and grafted to another. Pigskin is the most common xenograft for human skin and is applied to a wound as a temporary closure until a permanent option is performed.

z-plasty. Plastic surgery technique used primarily to release tension or elongate contractured scar tissue in which a Z-shaped incision is made with the middle line of the Z crossing the area of greatest tension. The triangular flaps are then rotated so that they cross the incision line in the opposite direction, creating a reversed Z.

ZPIC. Zone Program Integrity Contractor. CMS contractor that replaced the existing Program Safeguard Contractors (PSC). Contractors are responsible for ensuring the integrity of all Medicare-related claims under Parts A and B (hospital, skilled nursing, home health, provider, and durable medical equipment claims), Part C (Medicare Advantage health plans), Part D (prescription drug plans), and coordination of Medicare-Medicaid data matches (Medi-Medi).

Appendix N — Listing of Sensory, Motor, and Mixed Nerves

This list contains the sensory, motor, and mixed nerves assigned to each nerve conduction study to improve coding accuracy. Each nerve makes up one single unit of service.

Motor Nerves Assigned to Codes 95907-95913

I. Upper extremity, cervical plexus, and brachial plexus motor nerves
   A. Axillary motor nerve to the deltoid
   B. Long thoracic motor nerve to the serratus anterior
   C. Median nerve
      1. Median motor nerve to the abductor pollicis brevis
      2. Median motor nerve, anterior interosseous branch, to the flexor pollicis longus
      3. Median motor nerve, anterior interosseous branch, to the pronator quadratus
      4. Median motor nerve to the first lumbrical
      5. Median motor nerve to the second lumbrical
   D. Musculocutaneous motor nerve to the biceps brachii
   E. Radial nerve
      1. Radial motor nerve to the extensor carpi ulnaris
      2. Radial motor nerve to the extensor digitorum communis
      3. Radial motor nerve to the extensor indicis proprius
      4. Radial motor nerve to the brachioradialis
   F. Suprascapular nerve
      1. Suprascapular motor nerve to the supraspinatus
      2. Suprascapular motor nerve to the infraspinatus
   G. Thoracodorsal motor nerve to the latissimus dorsi
   H. Ulnar nerve
      1. Ulnar motor nerve to the abductor digiti minimi
      2. Ulnar motor nerve to the palmar interosseous
      3. Ulnar motor nerve to the first dorsal interosseous
      4. Ulnar motor nerve to the flexor carpi ulnaris
   I. Other
II. Lower extremity motor nerves
   A. Femoral motor nerve to the quadriceps
      1. Femoral motor nerve to vastus medialis
      2. Femoral motor nerve to vastus lateralis
      3. Femoral motor nerve to vastus intermedius
      4. Femoral motor nerve to rectus femoris
   B. Ilioinguinal motor nerve
   C. Peroneal (fibular) nerve
      1. Peroneal motor nerve to the extensor digitorum brevis
      2. Peroneal motor nerve to the peroneus brevis
      3. Peroneal motor nerve to the peroneus longus
      4. Peroneal motor nerve to the tibialis anterior
   D. Plantar motor nerve
   E. Sciatic nerve
   F. Tibial nerve
      1. Tibial motor nerve, inferior calcaneal branch, to the abductor digiti minimi
      2. Tibial motor nerve, medial plantar branch, to the abductor hallucis
      3. Tibial motor nerve, lateral plantar branch, to the flexor digiti minimi brevis
   G. Other
III. Cranial nerves and trunk
   A. Cranial nerve VII (facial motor nerve)
      1. Facial nerve to the frontalis
      2. Facial nerve to the nasalis
      3. Facial nerve to the orbicularis oculi
      4. Facial nerve to the orbicularis oris
   B. Cranial nerve XI (spinal accessory motor nerve)
   C. Cranial nerve XII (hypoglossal motor nerve)
   D. Intercostal motor nerve
   E. Phrenic motor nerve to the diaphragm
   F. Recurrent laryngeal nerve
   G. Other
IV. Nerve Roots
   A. Cervical nerve root stimulation
      1. Cervical level 5 (C5)
      2. Cervical level 6 (C6)
      3. Cervical level 7 (C7)
      4. Cervical level 8 (C8)
   B. Thoracic nerve root stimulation
      1. Thoracic level 1 (T1)
      2. Thoracic level 2 (T2)
      3. Thoracic level 3 (T3)
      4. Thoracic level 4 (T4)
      5. Thoracic level 5 (T5)
      6. Thoracic level 6 (T6)
      7. Thoracic level 7 (T7)
      8. Thoracic level 8 (T8)
      9. Thoracic level 9 (T9)
      10. Thoracic level 10 (T10)
      11. Thoracic level 11 (T11)
      12. Thoracic level 12 (T12)
   C. Lumbar nerve root stimulation
      1. Lumbar level 1 (L1)
      2. Lumbar level 2 (L2)
      3. Lumbar level 3 (L3)
      4. Lumbar level 4 (L4)
      5. Lumbar level 5 (L5)
   D. Sacral nerve root stimulation
      1. Sacral level 1 (S1)
      2. Sacral level 2 (S2)
      3. Sacral level 3 (S3)
      4. Sacral level 4 (S4)

Sensory and Mixed Nerves Assigned to Codes 95907–95913

I. Upper extremity sensory and mixed nerves

  A. Lateral antebrachial cutaneous sensory nerve

  B. Medial antebrachial cutaneous sensory nerve

  C. Medial brachial cutaneous sensory nerve

  D. Median nerve

    1. Median sensory nerve to the first digit

    2. Median sensory nerve to the second digit

    3. Median sensory nerve to the third digit

    4. Median sensory nerve to the fourth digit

    5. Median palmar cutaneous sensory nerve

    6. Median palmar mixed nerve

  E. Posterior antebrachial cutaneous sensory nerve

  F. Radial sensory nerve

    1. Radial sensory nerve to the base of the thumb

    2. Radial sensory nerve to digit 1

  G. Ulnar nerve

    1. Ulnar dorsal cutaneous sensory nerve

    2. Ulnar sensory nerve to the fourth digit

    3. Ulnar sensory nerve to the fifth digit

    4. Ulnar palmar mixed nerve

  H. Intercostal sensory nerve

  I. Other

II. Lower extremity sensory and mixed nerves

  A. Lateral femoral cutaneous sensory nerve

  B. Medical calcaneal sensory nerve

  C. Medial femoral cutaneous sensory nerve

  D. Peroneal nerve

    1. Deep peroneal sensory nerve

    2. Superficial peroneal sensory nerve, medial dorsal cutaneous branch

    3. Superficial peroneal sensory nerve, intermediate dorsal cutaneous branch

  E. Posterior femoral cutaneous sensory nerve

  F. Saphenous nerve

    1. Saphenous sensory nerve (distal technique)

    2. Saphenous sensory nerve (proximal technique)

  G. Sural nerve

    1. Sural sensory nerve, lateral dorsal cutaneous branch

    2. Sural sensory nerve

  H. Tibial sensory nerve (digital nerve to toe 1)

  I. Tibial sensory nerve (medial plantar nerve)

  J. Tibial sensory nerve (lateral plantar nerve)

  K. Other

III. Head and trunk sensory nerves

  A. Dorsal nerve of the penis

  B. Greater auricular nerve

  C. Ophthalmic branch of the trigeminal nerve

  D. Pudendal sensory nerve

  E. Suprascapular sensory nerves

  F. Other

In the following table, the reasonable maximum number of studies per diagnostic category is listed that allows for a physician or other qualified health care professional to obtain a diagnosis for 90 percent of patients with that same final diagnosis. The numbers denote the suggested number of studies, although the decision is up to the provider.

Type of Study/Maximum Number of Studies

Indication	Limbs Studied by Needle EMG (95860–95864, 95867–95870, 95885–95887)	Nerve Conduction Studies (Total nerves studied, 95907-95913)	Neuromuscular Junction Testing (Repetitive Stimulation 95937)
Carpal Tunnel (Unilateral)	1	7	—
Carpal Tunnel (Bilateral)	2	10	—
Radiculopathy	2	7	—
Mononeuropathy	1	8	—
Polyneuropathy/Mononeuropathy Multiplex	3	10	—
Myopathy	2	4	2
Motor Neuronopathy (e.g., ALS)	4	6	2
Plexopathy	2	12	—
Neuromuscular Junction	2	4	3
Tarsal Tunnel Syndrome (Unilateral)	1	8	—
Tarsal Tunnel Syndrome (Bilateral)	2	11	—
Weakness, Fatigue, Cramps, or Twitching (Focal)	2	7	2
Weakness, Fatigue, Cramps, or Twitching (General)	4	8	2
Pain, Numbness, or Tingling (Unilateral)	1	9	—
Pain, Numbness, or Tingling (Bilateral)	2	12	—